❖

SIXTH EDITION

DISEASES

OF

POULTRY

❖

EDITED BY

M. S. Hofstad

WITH

B. W. Calnek
C. F. Helmboldt
W. M. Reid
H. W. Yoder, Jr.

**EDITORIAL BOARD FOR THE
AMERICAN ASSOCIATION OF
AVIAN PATHOLOGISTS**

❖

The Iowa State University Press, Ames

❖

© 1943, 1948, 1952, 1959, 1965, 1972. The Iowa State University Press
Ames, Iowa 50010. All rights reserved

Composed and printed by
The Iowa State University Press

First edition, 1943
Second edition, 1948
Third edition, 1952
Fourth edition, 1959
Fifth edition, 1965
Sixth edition, 1972

International Standard Book Number: 0–8138–0430–2
Library of Congress Catalog Card Number: 74–103841

❖

SIXTH EDITION

DISEASES OF POULTRY

❖

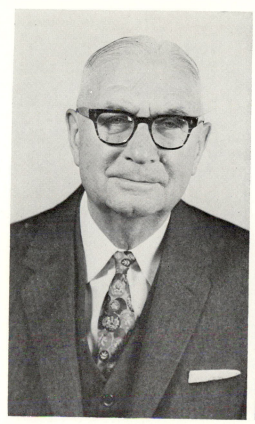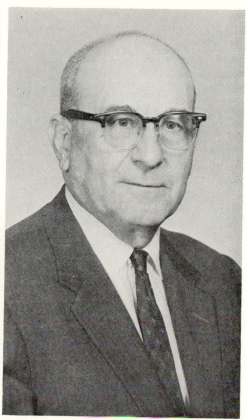

TO *H. E. Biester* AND *L. H. Schwarte*

❖

CONTRIBUTING AUTHORS

❖

B. R. BURMESTER
USDA Regional Poultry Research Laboratory, 3606 East Mt. Hope Road, East Lansing, Michigan 48823

E. E. BYRD
Department of Zoology, University of Georgia, Athens, Georgia 30601

B. W. CALNEK
Department of Avian Diseases, New York State Veterinary College, Cornell University, Ithaca, New York 14850

H. L. CHUTE
Department of Animal Pathology, University of Maine, Orono, Maine 04473

PHILIP H. COLEMAN
Department of Microbiology, Medical College of Virginia, Richmond, Virginia 23219

R. E. CORSTVET
Department of Veterinary Parasitology and Public Health, Oklahoma State University, Stillwater, Oklahoma 74074

C. H. CUNNINGHAM
Department of Microbiology & Public Health, Michigan State University, East Lansing, Michigan 48823

R. T. DuBOSE
Department of Veterinary Science, Virginia Polytechnic Institute, Blacksburg, Virginia 24061

B. C. EASTERDAY
Department of Veterinary Science, University of Wisconsin, Madison, Wisconsin 53706

T. N. FREDRICKSON
Department of Animal Diseases, University of Connecticut, Storrs, Connecticut 06268

W. B. GROSS
Department of Veterinary Science, Virginia Polytechnic Institute, Blacksburg, Virginia 24061

L. E. HANSON
Department of Veterinary Pathology and Hygiene, College of Veterinary Medicine, University of Illinois, Urbana, Illinois 61801

R. P. HANSON
Department of Veterinary Science, University of Wisconsin, Madison, Wisconsin 53706

K. L. HEDDLESTON
National Animal Disease Laboratory, Agricultural Research Service, USDA, Ames, Iowa 50010

C. F. HELMBOLDT
Department of Animal Diseases, University of Connecticut, Storrs, Connecticut 06268

S. B. HITCHNER
Department of Avian Diseases, New York State Veterinary College, Cornell University, Ithaca, New York 14850

M. S. HOFSTAD
Veterinary Medical Research Institute, College of Veterinary Medicine, Iowa State University, Ames, Iowa 50010

A. G. KARLSON
Microbiology Section, Mayo Clinic, Rochester, Minnesota 55901

L. KROOK
Department of Veterinary Pathology, New York State Veterinary College, Cornell University, Ithaca, New York 14850

LOUIS LEIBOVITZ
Long Island Duck Research Laboratory, Cornell University, Eastport, Long Island, New York 11941

P. P. LEVINE
Department of Avian Diseases, New York State Veterinary College, Cornell University, Ithaca, New York 14850

R. E. LUGINBUHL
Department of Animal Diseases, University of Connecticut, Storrs, Connecticut 06268

EVERETT E. LUND
Animal Disease and Parasitic Research Division, Beltsville Parasitological Laboratory, Agricultural Research Service, USDA, Beltsville, Maryland 20705

vii

J. G. MATTHYSSE
Department of Entomology and Limnology, New York State College of Agriculture, Cornell University, Ithaca, New York 14850

N. O. OLSON
Division of Animal and Veterinary Sciences, West Virginia University, Morgantown, West Virginia 26505

L. A. PAGE
National Animal Disease Laboratory, Agricultural Research Service, USDA, Ames, Iowa 50010

M. C. PECKHAM
Department of Avian Diseases, New York State Veterinary College, Cornell University, Ithaca, New York 14850

B. S. POMEROY
Department of Veterinary Microbiology and Public Health, Veterinary College, University of Minnesota, St. Paul, Minnesota 55108

H. GRAHAM PURCHASE
USDA Regional Poultry Research Laboratory, 3606 East Mt. Hope Road, East Lansing, Michigan, 48823

W. MALCOLM REID
Poultry Department, University of Georgia, Athens, Georgia 30601

A. S. ROSENWALD
Department of Epidemiology and Preventive Medicine, School of Veterinary Medicine, University of California, Davis, California 95616

M. L. SCOTT
Department of Poultry Science, Cornell University, Ithaca, New York 14850

G. H. SNOEYENBOS
Department of Veterinary Science, University of Massachusetts, Amherst, Massachusetts 01002

BELA TUMOVA
Institute for Epidemiology and Microbiology, Prague, Czechoslovakia, (Visiting Professor Department of Veterinary Science, University of Wisconsin, 1968–69)

EVERETT E. WEHR
Animal Disease and Parasite Research Division, Beltsville Parasitological Laboratory, Agricultural Research Service, USDA, Beltsville, Maryland 20705

J. E. WILLIAMS
USDA Southeast Poultry Research Laboratory, 934 College Station Road, Athens, Georgia 30601

R. L. WITTER
USDA Regional Poultry Research Laboratory, 3606 East Mt. Hope Road, East Lansing, Michigan 48823

R. YAMAMOTO
Department of Epidemiology and Preventive medicine, School of Veterinary Medicine, University of California, Davis, California 95616

H. W. YODER, JR.
USDA Southeast Poultry Research Laboratory, 934 College Station Road, Athens, Georgia 30601

DONALD V. ZANDER
Research Laboratory, Heisdorf & Nelson Farms, 14270 Redmond Wookinville Road, Redmond, Washington 98052

TABLE OF CONTENTS

❖

FOREWORD

❖

The fifth edition of *Diseases of Poultry*, edited by H. E. Biester and L. H. Schwarte, further solidified the position of this book as the standard in the field of avian diseases all over the world. The retirement of these editors has occasioned the launching of this completely revised sixth edition under the sponsorship of the American Association of Avian Pathologists with a five-member board serving as editors. This was a logical time to take stock, to attempt a reorientation, and to keep pace with the rapid changes in the avian disease picture.

Within a period of less than 50 years, poultry keeping has developed from a "pin money" farm activity or a hobby to a highly sophisticated industry, marketing products worth over $6 billion per year in the United States alone. The rapid evolvement of mass production and distribution methods has imposed increased and unique demands on those scientists working in the field of avian medicine. No longer are the effects of disease control practices or lack of them limited to farms or areas in any one country. Because of speedy international traffic and the dissemination of breeding stocks, the same disease problems have become worldwide in incredibly short periods of time. The avian pathologist and his decisions now have significant importance in places far distant from his laboratory.

Avian pathologists have responded to these disease challenges and have devised control methods which have stemmed losses quickly and effectively. But the fact remains that in the long run, disease eradication and not temporary control must be the ultimate goal. An outstanding example is the virtual disappearance of pullorum disease from breeding flocks in the United States, a disease which 30 years ago was one of the greatest causes of chick mortality. Most of the younger avian pathologists trained within recent years have never seen pullorum infection in young chicks. What makes this accomplishment even more noteworthy is that the eradication program was carried out under a voluntary, cooperative scheme.

To attempt disease eradication without complete knowledge of the natural history of the disease will be futile. Patient, intensive study of the epizootiology of the diseases and modification of flock management techniques are necessary to achieve the ultimate goal. This book is the most recent effort to present this basic information.

The rush of progress in dealing with immediate disease problems of the poultry industry has caused many to forget the significant role various avian species have played as research animals. In the field of nutrition the fowl has been of key importance. The word vitamin was coined by Eijkman when he demonstrated in 1897 the existence of what we now call thiamin deficiency. Vitamin K, folic acid, and B12 were other vitamins first discovered in work with poultry nutrition.

The practical application of genetic selection for control of plant diseases is well known. The breeding of fowl resistant to Marek's disease has been demonstrated as a practical possibility, and future editions of this book may well include significant sections on genetic resistance to various other diseases.

Not until the life cycle of avian malaria was worked out by Ross in 1898 did the missing parts of the human malaria transmission story fall into place.

Can one evaluate properly the stimulus that was given to virology when Goodpasture and Woodruff in 1931 cultivated the fowl pox virus for the first time in chicken embryos?

Little did we know that the first transmission of a solid tumor (sarcoma) to chickens with cell-free inocula by Peyton Rous in 1911 was to have such importance in resolving our leukosis problems 50 years later. The significance of this work to medical science was belatedly recognized by the awarding of a Nobel Prize to Rous in 1966.

More recently the cultivation of the RIF virus by Rubin in 1965 removed much of the expense and frustration that formerly accompanied research with avian leukosis. These findings stimulated tremendous activity in many laboratories where leukosis research had been abandoned. For the first time the groundwork was laid which eventually permitted clarification along strictly objective lines of the differences between Marek's disease and lymphoid leukosis. As this is being written, experimental vaccines for the protection of poultry against Marek's disease are being tested in the field. Favorable results obtained thus far bid fair to result in commercial vaccines for the protection of poultry against tumors and nerve lesions caused by Marek's disease. This will be the first time that prevention of tumors in food-producing animals on a large scale will have been accomplished.

If there is anything that avian pathologists have learned during the last 30 years, it is that poultry disease control in the face of fundamentally wrong husbandry practices will fail. Avian tuberculosis did not come under control until aged birds were shown to be unprofitable.

Chronic cholera and infectious coryza were constant scourges in the 30s and 40s when housing of multiple age groups was the usual practice. Again the economic superiority of pullet flocks initiated the "all in, all out" system and those diseases virtually disappeared. But now the large, expensive environment-controlled houses have caused poultrymen to keep more than one age group in a unit with the resultant reappearance of coryza and cholera. On the other hand, newer developments in poultry house ventilation and positive pressure, filtered air systems are showing promise in preventing exposure of birds to airborne infections.

Tremendous changes are taking place in poultry rearing practices. Not only will the approach to disease control have to be adapted to the new conditions but the diseases themselves will change in character. Infectious diseases will decline in importance; toxicologic, nutritional, genetic, and husbandry problems will demand increasing attention. Change is the order of life, and avian diseases are no exception.

This sixth edition of *Diseases of Poultry* is a worthy successor to the previous ones and presents the considerable achievements in the field without apologies.

P. P. LEVINE

❖

PREFACE

❖

THE PASSING of time has brought on the retirement of the previous editors of *Diseases of Poultry,* H. E. Biester and L. H. Schwarte. It was their wish that future editions of the book become the responsibility of the American Association of Avian Pathologists (AAAP), an organization concerned with all areas of avian medicine, including the publication of the *Journal of Avian Diseases.* This Association acknowledges the great contribution which Dr. Biester and Dr. Schwarte have made in editing previous editions; it is for this reason that the sixth edition is dedicated to these two men. Our hope is that future editions can maintain the high quality of the previous editions.

The AAAP selected an editorial board of five members to undertake the revision of the book for the sixth edition. Each member was assigned responsibility for a group of specific chapters.

To avoid going to a two-volume book, the board decided to eliminate several chapters not directly concerned with disease. The justification for eliminating anatomy, nutrition, genetics, and hematology was that these subjects were covered better in other publications and that the authors could not do justice to these areas in the allotted space.

Other changes in the book were made to avoid duplication. The material in the chapter on turkeys was incorporated into other appropriate chapters. A new chapter on neoplastic diseases was introduced to consolidate in one chapter the information on tumors of poultry.

An attempt was made to reduce the number of listed references at the end of each chapter by instituting a policy of selective reference citation. Many authors were able to reduce the number of references; others maintained approximately the same number by eliminating some and adding more recent references.

The editorial board expresses appreciation to the many previous authors who have made *Diseases of Poultry* the valuable reference and textbook that it has become. We welcome the new contributing authors whose efforts have made possible the sixth edition.

EDITORIAL BOARD
M. S. HOFSTAD, *Chairman*
B. W. CALNEK
C. F. HELMBOLDT
W. M. REID
H. W. YODER, JR.

❖

SIXTH EDITION

DISEASES OF POULTRY

❖

CHAPTER 1

PRINCIPLES OF DISEASE PREVENTION: DIAGNOSIS AND CONTROL

❖

D. V. ZANDER

Heisdorf & Nelson Farms, Inc.
Redmond, Washington

❖

DETAILED INFORMATION on the diseases of poultry, including diagnostic procedures and techniques and specific prevention and control measures for each disease, is contained in this book. This particular chapter acquaints the reader with basic principles of poultry sanitation and disease prevention and control. It also introduces the student to basic necropsy procedures and provides specific information on the usual insecticides and disinfectants, with special emphasis on formaldehyde fumigation. For information on the specific diagnostic techniques and control measures, the reader is referred to the chapters covering each disease.

This chapter will not cover all the detailed disease control methods adapted to modern trends or to all types of poultry, but will attempt only to outline and illustrate some fundamental concepts. Each ranch is different; therefore, the basic concepts must be applied according to conditions and facilities existing on individual ranches. To keep abreast of the flow of research and information, a constant review of current literature and recommendations applicable to specific diseases, special enterprises, and various geographic areas is necessary to supplement what is given here.

Standard textbooks on poultry and turkey production, husbandry, and nutrition are other sources of information (Taylor, 1949; Marsden and Martin, 1955; Card, 1961; Titus, 1961; Ewing, 1963).

HOST-PARASITE RELATIONSHIP

Disease results when normal body functions are impaired, and the degree of impairment determines the severity of the disease. Disease may occur due to deficiency of a vital nutrient or ingestion of a toxic substance. It may result from injury or physical stress with which the bird cannot cope, or it may be the consequence of the harmful action of infectious and parasitic agents.

Some nutrient deficiencies are temporary and reversible when the nutrient is supplied in adequate amounts; others are irreversible. Disease resulting from stress is related to the severity and duration of the stress. Injuries, such as extreme debeaking, tend to persist for a long time and may be permanent. Diseases caused by infectious and parasitic agents are frequently complex and depend upon characteristics of both host and parasite.

Whether or not disease results from an encounter of host and parasite depends on the number, type, and virulence of the parasite, the route of entry to the body, and the defense status and defense capabilities of the host. The latter is dependent partly on the nutritional status, partly on the environmental stresses, partly on the genetic ability of the host to organize resistance mechanisms, and partly on the kind and timing of the countermeasures (drugs, changed environment) employed by man.

Some virulent organisms overcome very rapidly the resistance of even the healthiest hosts. Less virulent strains or types cause moderate to severe illness, but most birds respond and return to a state of health. Still other strains or types cause no marked reaction, and the host shows little or no obvious symptoms of ill health. Some microorganisms are not considered pathogenic because they are usually found in and around those individuals considered "normal," but it must be recognized that the so-called "nonpathogenic" and low pathogenic organisms can also cause serious losses when the right circumstances exist. Severe physical stresses such as chilling, overheating, water deprivation, starvation, and concurrent infection by other disease agents can reduce the host's ability to resist and thus precipitate a disease condition which can be detected (e.g., clinical mycoplasmosis following infectious bronchitis, or clinical salmonellosis in chicks that have been chilled).

Coccidiosis provides a good example of the relationship of the number of invading organisms to the severity of the resulting infection, since the morbidity and mortality of the host species is usually proportional to the number of coccidial oocysts ingested. A similar situation exists for many other infectious diseases. A mild roundworm infection may not be serious, whereas a severe infection can be very detrimental to the health of the bird. The number of infective virus particles in a live virus vaccine (its titer) may be so low that a good immunizing infection does not occur following administration of the vaccine. A good reason for removing moribund and dead birds from a flock is to reduce the number of infectious organisms available to pen mates. Thorough washing and disinfecting of a building may not render it sterile but can reduce the number of infectious organisms to such a low level that there are too few to initiate a flock infection of sufficient magnitude to be recognizable as disease.

It is important to remember that man has the ability to alter the probability of a bird or flock becoming infected as well as the severity and outcome of an infection.

INFLUENCE OF MODERN POULTRY FARMING PRACTICES ON HOST AND PARASITE

Avian disease specialists must continually seek new knowledge about the nature and control of specific diseases. Meanwhile, those persons responsible for production of poultry meat, table eggs, hatching eggs, baby chicks and poults, feed ingredients, and mixed feeds should put into practice those basic techniques and management principles which will prevent the occurrence of disease. They should also provide the physical facilities necessary for control and elimination of those diseases which occasionally gain entrance so they do not become a perpetual burden. The economic losses due to disease can mean the difference between success or failure in the poultry business. Those who disregard the basic principles of disease prevention may succeed in times of a favorable market but do not remain competitive when the margin of profit is very small.

The poultryman who puts into practice the fundamental management practices which prevent disease outbreaks has very little need for detailed knowledge of the many infectious diseases which affect poultry. One does not need to be an expert on symptoms, lesions, and cures for diseases which are kept out of the flock through proper management.

When new farms and buildings are designed and constructed and the production programmed with the objective of excluding diseases or eradicating them when they gain entry, poultry can be maintained free of most common diseases in a practical manner with a minimum of effort. Facilities need not be new to be adequate. Frequently old farms can be enlarged and the production reprogrammed to exclude or eradicate diseases. Many old poultry buildings, hatcheries, and feed mills can be redesigned to greatly favor exclusion, eradication, or control of disease. Strict application of disease preventive management techniques has enabled poultrymen to maintain specific pathogen-free chickens on farms of usual design and construction (Chute et al., 1964).

The trend in all agricultural industries continues toward larger units, fewer farmers, and corporate enterprise. The chicken and turkey industries have been leaders in this trend which has placed emphasis on efficiency of operation and lower costs of production. In fact, survival in the industry has depended upon continual adoption of newer and more efficient practices. It is sometimes forgotten that efficiency of disease prevention is as important as efficiency of cleaning, feeding, bird handling, and egg processing. The resulting evolution of management systems has altered the emphasis in disease control practices and will continue to do so in the future. For example, the shift in housing of egg-laying flocks from floor pens to cages has altered the approaches to the control of intestinal diseases and parasites and increased the emphasis on control of cannibalism. New problems in feed formulation have arisen because certain vitamins and minerals normally found in the litter were not available to birds in cages.

Corporation farming accented the tendency toward integrated control and operation of two or more segments of the industry such as feed manufacturing, breeder flock management, hatchery operation, pullet rearing, broiler and turkey grow-out phases, laying farm production, egg processing, turkey and broiler slaughter and processing, and even retail distribution. Integration has concentrated under one decision-making body the disease control practices for millions of birds as well as several phases in the chain of production of eggs and meat. Thus sound health practices and emergency quarantine measures decided upon by one or a few individuals can be quickly and effectively applied to large numbers of birds. Through integration it has become economically practical to employ veterinarians full time and place responsibility for disease control directly in the hands of specialized avian pathologists. Disease considerations are sometimes reduced to simple cost accounting, whereby the economic loss from a disease and the costs of treating it (or of deliberately exposing the flocks to the infectious agent) are weighed against the cost of eradication and maintaining the clean status before determining the course of action.

Where established management and industry practices allow or contribute to the spread and propagation of some disease agent, attempts are frequently made to deliberately expose flocks to the disease at an opportune time. This practice is successful for some virus diseases and has led to the widespread use of specially prepared vaccines. The practice is much less successful for bacterial infections and is more likely to perpetuate the disease. Except for prevalent and highly contagious diseases for which effective vaccines are available, it is usually more economical to keep poultry free of disease than to burden them with it deliberately or by accident, provided the costs of eradication and maintaining a free status do not exceed the costs resulting from outbreaks of the disease.

Widespread and daily shipments of hatching eggs, poults, chicks, started pullets, and adult fowl across state and national boundaries have necessitated reevaluation of old concepts of health regulations. Specialized avian pathologists have evolved to guide the course of health control measures, and diagnostic facilities—both private and governmental—are available in major poultry producing areas of the world. Except where importation and usage are restricted by government regulation, high-quality vaccines and drugs are available wherever poultry is raised commercially. Breeding of poultry on a scientific basis has created strains of uniform quality with a high degree of resistance against those diseases for which satisfactory drugs and vaccines are not available. Good quality feed is the rule, not the exception.

Yet disease still takes a heavy toll from all types of poultry enterprise. The man who exercises the farm management decisions—whether it be the caretaker, owner, flock supervisor, corporate manager, or money lender—has the power to reduce these losses through management for disease control. He must be made aware of his responsibility and continually encouraged to develop a philosophy of disease prevention through management.

The cardinal principles of disease prevention and control are the same for the chicken hobbyist, fancy bird breeder, and game bird farmer as for the corporation with several million turkeys, broilers, or laying hens. The backyard flock maintained without regard for disease control can perpetuate a disease which constitutes a threat to a large productive industry. On the other hand, since most backyard flocks are not vaccinated, they may be susceptible to those diseases against which the large commercial flocks are vaccinated. The greatest hazard to commercial poultrymen created by fancy breeds and backyard flocks is the possible perpetuation of diseases which have been eradicated from the commercial poultry industry. For this reason, it is a sound principle that no employee of a commercial poultry unit have any poultry at home.

SOURCES OF INFECTION AND COUNTERMEASURES

Infections may gain entrance to a flock of birds from various sources some of which may more conveniently enter because of errors in management and industry practices. In order to understand why various preventive practices are recommended, it is important to review briefly the sources and route of infection.

MAN

Because of his mobility, duties, curiosity, ignorance, indifference, and carelessness, man constitutes one of the greatest potential causes of the introduction of disease. Rarely is this because he becomes infected and sheds the disease agent, but rather because he either tracks infectious diseases, uses contaminated equipment, or manages his flocks in such a way that spread of disease is inevitable.

Most frequently footwear is suspected as the means of transport of disease, but the hands can become contaminated with exudates when lesions and discharges are examined. Clothing can also become contaminated with dust, feathers, and excrement.

Neighbors

A frequent source of infection is the disease outbreak at the neighbor's ranch. Too frequently a poultryman will ask a neighbor over to look at his sick birds. Disease inspection visits among poultrymen is a common way of spreading disease. If a neighbor's flock is afflicted with a very interesting new disease, the best way to discuss it is by telephone. It is much better to warn a neighbor *not* to visit when a disease is in progress than to invite him over to see the flock.

Contract Work Crews

Much of the poultry farm work requires sporadic use of a crew of several workmen. Examples are blood testing, debeaking, vaccinating, inseminating, sexing, and moving birds from one location to another. The poultryman or farm manager frequently has difficulty in assembling a crew of people who are available and knowledgeable about handling poultry. He therefore contracts for crews of workmen who do such service work for many poultry enterprises. Such crews travel about the poultry community handling many flocks of birds and must be regarded as a potential source of infection. Thus they should take stringent precautions to safeguard the health of every flock they handle.

Visitors

Disease outbreaks in a community have been known to follow the path of a careless visitor. If visitors do not enter premises or buildings, they cannot track in diseases.

The source of a new or dreaded disease often is puzzling. World trade and world travel are becoming more commonplace. With high-speed travel by jet airliner it is not uncommon for a person to leave his farm or place of work in the morning and be visiting another farm or place of business in the opposite corner of the country or even on another continent the same day. Some disease agents can easily survive that long. All who travel should be ever cognizant of this fact and guard against introduction of disease onto the premises of client, competitor, friend, fellow poultryman, or into his own flocks when returning from a trip.

RECOVERED CARRIERS

Carrier birds are those which have apparently recovered from a clinical infection but still retain the infectious organism in some part of the body. While they appear healthy, the infectious agent continues to multiply in the body and to be eliminated into the environment. Like actively infected flocks they can perpetuate a disease on a farm and constitute a disease threat to other birds. Among the diseases known to be transmitted by carriers are histomoniasis, hexamitiasis, Leucocytozoon infection, coccidiosis, pullorum, fowl typhoid and other Salmonella infections, Arizona (paracolon) infection, tuberculosis, pasteurellosis, infectious coryza, laryngotracheitis, Mycoplasma (PPLO) infections, transmissible enteritis (bluecomb) of turkeys, lymphoid leukosis, and Marek's disease. Carrier birds can constitute a potential source of disease through the various industry practices noted below.

Multiple Ages

Multiple ages on a ranch constitute a serious disease potential from both actively infected fowl and recovered carriers, particularly if the various ages are closely associated. The disease agents which result in chronic infections or recovered carriers are passed by various means, including direct contact to each new susceptible flock brought onto the premises.

Started Pullets

Pullets are frequently reared to or near point-of-lay by a specialized pullet rearer or on a separate ranch unit belonging to the laying farm owner. This practice for many sound reasons has become established in the industry. Pullets can, however, constitute a potential source for introduction of a disease onto a lay ranch if they have been exposed on the pullet farm and as a result have become recovered carriers of some disease which does not exist on the lay ranch.

Force-Molted Hens

Force-molting of laying hens or breeders is frequently practiced, particularly during times of economic stress, to supply a special market, to meet an emergency hatching egg demand, or because it is deemed economical at the time. One advantage of keeping force-molted hens rather than rearing new replacement pullets is that the old hens are not apt to suffer a disease which normally occurs during the rearing age. If such flocks are force-molted and held in the same house, there is little danger of disease problems developing. On the other hand, a poultryman who collects "spent" hens for molting from many poultry farms and mixes them together on one ranch at one time is running a serious risk of disease, since any one of the force-molted groups may be carriers of a disease to which the other groups are susceptible.

Poultry Show Stock

Show birds may be exposed to actively infected or symptomless carrier birds from which they may contract disease. The contact-infected stock may not develop active symptoms until returned to the owner's farm where they may then be a source of new infection for all stock on the premises. Breeders of fancy birds and game birds and youths with poultry projects (4-H, Future Farmers of America) must recognize the extreme hazards of returning stock exhibited in community shows and fairs, and of introducing partly grown or adult birds onto their farms for special breeding purposes. A cardinal rule for show stock is that it should never be returned to the owner's farm. If birds must be shown, individuals should be selected which can be sold for market purposes after the exhibition is over.

Breeding Stock

Adult stock considered especially desirable for breeding purposes may be symptomless carriers and serve as a source of infection for the breeding farm. It is best to purchase such stock as hatching eggs or day-old chicks and to rear them in an isolated off-farm quarantine area until there is reasonable assurance that they are free of infection.

Mixing Species of Poultry

One species which is naturally very resistant to a disease may act as a carrier of that disease for another species which is very susceptible. Some death losses and debilitation from enterohepatitis occur in chickens, but in turkeys the losses can be disastrous. Therefore, even with the routine use of drugs to prevent blackhead, the two species should never be run together, and turkeys should not be run on a dirt yard or floor which has recently had chickens on it.

Also, a silent (inapparent) Mycoplasma infection in chickens may spread to turkeys and erupt into a full-blown case of sinusitis and air sac infection. Other diseases may be rather inocuous in one species of fowl but very serious in another. It is also advisable to keep meat and laying type chickens separated, because the same disease may have different economic importance in the two types.

Other Sources

HOSPITAL PEN. Sick birds from several pens congregated in one hospital pen or house and later taken back to their respective quarters may carry back not only the condition for which they were removed but one or more diseases contracted while in the hospital area. Hospital pens are, therefore, not recommended for routine segregation of sick birds, but if and when used for a special purpose (e.g., birds with transient paralysis), they should be temporary arrangements within the house and should hold birds from only one pen or house.

CULL PEN. The cull pen still exists on many poultry farms. Nonlaying hens are frequently culled from a flock and marketed for meat. Usually these present no health hazard for man or poultry. Cull birds in obvious poor health may or may not be afflicted with an infectious disease. The poultryman should suspect the worst and destroy such birds rather than hold them for slaughter.

BACKYARD AND PET FOWL. Poultry kept as pets or to supply household eggs or meat are just as capable of carrying and transmitting disease as the commercial flock. Pet barnyard fowl of a rare or interesting nature may also carry some disease to the commercial poultry. The risk to the invested enterprise is too great to permit such a part-time hobby.

EGG-BORNE DISEASES

Egg-borne diseases are those which are transmitted from the infected dam to the newly hatched offspring by means of the fertile egg. Some disease agents are carried inside the shell as a result of shedding into the egg prior to the addition of the shell and shell membranes. Others are carried on the shell or penetrate from the shell surface through the natural pores after the egg is laid and the surface contaminated.

The agent may gain entrance to the egg as a result of infection of the ovary and ovarian follicles (transovarian transmission), as a result of contamination of the free ovum in the peritoneal cavity, or by contact in the oviduct. Once the shell and membranes are added, the organism enjoys a protected location where it is not easily destroyed. From there it can later invade the developing embryo, and lesions are frequently observed in the tissues and organs of offspring at hatching. Transovarian transmission seems to be limited to only a few of the many diseases which affect poultry.

When the freshly laid egg cools from body temperature to nest, room, or cool-room temperature, a pressure differential occurs between the inside of the egg and the atmosphere. Any fluid on the shell surface is forced inward. Motile bacteria are aided by, but do not need, this pressure differential to penetrate the shell. The primary contamination of this nature is from enteric organisms, particularly salmonellae and coliforms, though other types of bacteria and also fungi may be drawn into the egg. (For preventive measures see Breeder Flock Management and Hatchery Sanitation.)

EQUIPMENT

Diseases and parasites can be carried on equipment. Poultry house cleaning equipment and vehicles usually have accumulations of litter and feces which can be a threat to other farms and houses where they may be taken on succeeding cleaning assignments. They should be washed free of litter and droppings before use on another farm or farm area.

Mites can be transported from farm to farm in the corrugations of egg cases which are taken into chicken houses. Mites are frequently found on eggs, so they can easily crawl off into spaces in the box and then crawl out in the next house. Wire crates and baskets do not offer these hiding places. Residues of Salmonella-contaminated eggs on egg flats may be a potential method of introducing disease.

Roundworm eggs, dried pox virus, coccidia, and other infectious material can be carried on crates, footwear, and vehicles, particularly on the floor and foot control pedals of the cab.

Inseminating equipment, particularly re-used inseminating tubes, offer an excellent method of transmitting disease if the crew does not exercise sanitary techniques.

Poultry hauling equipment likewise can disseminate infectious material through feathers, feces, blood, exudates, and skin encrustations left in the crates, or pick up infectious material at the slaughter plant. Hauling equipment should be washed and disinfected after use before being taken to another farm.

MISCELLANEOUS SOURCES OF DISEASE

Laboratory Exposure

Frequently a poultryman, particularly a small flock owner, hobbyist, or game bird owner, will want to return a bird home after the veterinarian has examined it at the laboratory. The diagnostic laboratory receives poultry which may be affected with any one of a whole host of infectious diseases. While in the receiving area or diagnostic facilities even for a short time, live poultry specimens have a good opportunity to pick up some disease agent. No birds should be returned from the laboratory to the farm, because exposed poultry could come down later with disease and be the source of a new infection.

A disease may be tracked from the laboratory surroundings to a farm by a careless laboratory worker, serviceman, or poultryman. Clean and frequently washed and disinfected laboratory areas are the responsibility of the veterinarian. Precautions against tracking disease from the laboratory to the farm are the responsibility of the poultryman and serviceman.

Rodents

Rodents contaminate feed and litter with their excrement. They are particularly hazardous to Salmonella control since they are frequently infected with these organisms and can perpetuate the disease on a farm.

Household Pets

Dogs and cats, like rodents, are capable of harboring enteric organisms which are infectious for poultry. When these pets are not confined to the household area but roam continually among the poultry in the pens and yards they constitute a serious health hazard. Dogs are just as capable of tracking contaminated material on their feet as man.

Wild Birds

Wild birds are capable of carrying a variety of diseases and parasites. Some cause illness in the wild birds; for others, the birds act as mechanical carriers. Every effort should be made to prevent their nesting in the poultry area. Imported zoological specimens are not a serious threat because of the location of the zoo, but they should be considered as a potential source of introduction of an unusual disease or parasite.

Insects

Many insects act as transmitters of disease. Some are intermediate hosts for blood or intestinal parasites; others are mechanical carriers of disease through their biting habits. Still others because of their feeding habits and hiding places appear to be mere reservoirs of disease where the infectious agent lives over from one flock to the next.

Feed

Certain feed ingredients may contain infectious agents, particularly Salmonella organisms, due to contamination at their source or anywhere along the production line or storage areas. Methods are available for sterilizing the feed, but they increase the cost of the final product.

FUNDAMENTAL MANAGEMENT FACTORS IN DISEASE PREVENTION

The more important physical principles of disease prevention include favorable geo-graphic location of farm unit in respect to other poultry units, proper location of the buildings in relation to each other and to prevailing wind currents, proper design of the building inside and out, and design and positioning of equipment. Long-range planning and programming of the operation, whether large or small, is very important and should take into account movement patterns of various vehicles and equipment, work traffic of regular and holiday caretakers and special work crews, the system of feed delivery and storage, and the system for moving eggs and flocks from the farm. An avian pathologist can be helpful in avoiding some of the common pitfalls, *but the most profitable time to consult with him is when the farm is being designed and the production programmed to avoid high disease risk situations, rather than after a disease hotbed has developed and serious trouble is already evident.* Most farms that have developed into disease hotbeds were designed, constructed, enlarged, or programmed without advance consultation with an avian pathologist.

It must be remembered that good disease prevention practices are perhaps best illustrated as a chain which is only as strong as the weakest link. Many sound principles can be discredited by failure to carry out one or two which are either overlooked or are not considered essential. While it may not always be possible to follow all of the practices, the more that are followed the greater are the chances of avoiding disease outbreaks.

ISOLATION

Not all poultrymen are going to follow the same disease control practices. A close neighbor may disregard sound principles and be burdened with diseases until economic pressures force him out of business. In the meantime, disease agents present on his ranch may be blown or carried by various vectors and fomites to closely adjacent ranches; thus a disease may occasionally gain entrance even on well-managed ranches. Until a disease has been eradicated from the ranch it may serve as a reservoir of disease for both future flocks and those on adjacent ranches. The closer the houses of one ranch are to those of another, the more likely is the spread from the infected to the healthy ranch.

Some highly concentrated poultry areas have developed because of some favorable condition such as a close market, an available slaughter or processing plant, a favorable location in respect to feed supply, cheap land, or favorable land zoning. Usually these areas progress into hotbeds of disease of one type or another. Such areas resemble huge "megafarms" with many managers each vaccinating, treating, or exposing birds as he sees fit without regard to the programs of other managers. Since such areas are in competition with all other areas for markets, several things may happen. Either the various advantages offset the disease losses or the additional cost of production due to disease prices the product (meat or eggs) out of the market. Poultrymen who do not reduce the disease loss go out of business, and many ranches are abandoned, purchased, or leased by other poultrymen. Some poultrymen move their operations to a less concentrated area where they usually escape disease, unless of course they take their problems with them knowingly or inadvertently through carelessness. Those who remain usually upgrade disease prevention practices by redesigning the houses and reprogramming the production cycle. Frequently the reprogramming proceeds all the way to a system of a single age of fowl on the ranch, permitting complete depopulation each year. This finally solves the major disease problem in most cases.

Another solution to area disease problems where ranches are too close even for systematic depopulation to succeed is to develop a coordinated *area* depopulation and restocking program. All flocks in a reasonably defined geographic area may be marketed at the same time and the houses refilled at the same time.

Most of the serious disease problems could be avoided if a philosophy of ranch isolation prevailed from the beginning of an enterprise. No exact minimum distance from other poultry farms can be stated because the desirable distance is influenced by prevailing winds, climate, type of houses, and other factors. The farther from other poultry farms, the less likelihood of contracting disease from neighbors' chickens. The degree of isolation of a farm is influenced as much by management philosophy as by economic considerations. This is illustrated by the cluster of farms shown in Figure 1.1 and the isolated farm shown in Figure 1.2 less than two miles away.

All of these farms were established in the same era of commercial poultry production.

One Age of Fowl per Farm

Removing carriers from a flock and premises is an effective way of preventing a recurrence of some diseases, but it is impossible or impractical for others. The best way to prevent infection from carrier birds is to remove the entire flock from the farm before any new replacements are added, and to rear young stock in complete isolation from older recovered birds, preferably on another farm and in an isolated area.

Where multiple ages of birds exist on a large farm, depopulation seems quite drastic, but when one considers the mortality, poor performance, and endless drug expense, it may be the most economical solution in the long run. Farm units of several hundred thousand laying hens, broilers, or turkeys of one age prove that size is no deterrent to the application of the sound principle of one age of bird on a farm with complete depopulation at the end of the production cycle.

Where only one age of bird is maintained on the ranch, depopulation occurs each time the pullets or poults are moved to the lay or breeder ranch, each time the broilers or turkeys are moved to slaughter, and each time the old layers or breeders are sent to market. Should a disease occur, the flock can be treated and handled in the best way possible until its disposal. The depopulated premises are then cleaned, disinfected, and left idle for a while before new healthy stock is brought in.

Ranch depopulation is most effective in controlling those disease agents which do not survive for long outside the bird. This applies to most respiratory infections (e.g., Mycoplasma infections, infectious coryza, laryngotracheitis). It is least effective in control of those disease agents having a resistant stage which survives for long periods in nature (e.g., coccidiosis, blackhead, intestinal parasites).

Started pullets and pullet rearing ranches are now an established specialized enterprise in the poultry industry. This system has made lay ranch and breeder ranch depopulation more practical and more successful. As on multiple-age lay ranches, serious disease problems may develop and persist on multiple-age rearing farms until these farms are reprogrammed for a single

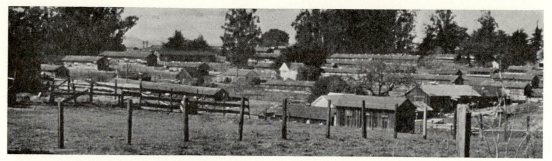

FIG. 1.1—Farms in this cluster are too close to each other to provide any reasonable degree of isolation. Diseases tend to remain endemic within such a group unless all are depopulated and restocked simultaneously.

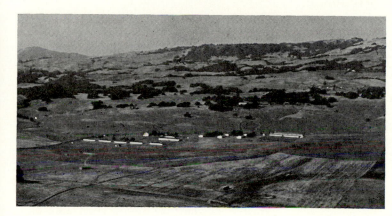

FIG. 1.2—Initial selection of a location for a poultry enterprise sufficiently isolated so that disease is not likely to spread from sick poultry on neighboring farms is a basic disease-prevention principle.

age or are divided into isolated units.

Started pullets should not be confused with "started chicks" and "started poults," the products of an old-time practice of rearing chicks or poults in batteries of cages for 1–6 weeks by the hatcheryman, usually at the hatchery, prior to sale to customers. In most cases the practice proved to be uneconomical, and one reason was that some diseases became established due to the multiple ages involved.

The same disease problems beset the broiler industry in the early stages of development when a continual weekly input of chicks into battery units and removal of finished broilers was attempted in order to supply a constant market. This practice also has largely been abandoned. With improved feeds, breeds, vaccines, cages, and housing, such a practice might someday be successfully reestablished but with much stricter precautions against entry of disease and with proper provision for depopulation if necessary.

In addition to sanitary practices, environment (temperature, humidity) plays an important part in the time interval necessary to prevent carry-over of disease. Disease germs begin to die out slowly after elimination from the body. Some (e.g., coryza) die out very quickly; others (e.g., parasites and coccidia) survive for months or years, depending on whether they develop a resistant stage and other factors discussed under individual diseases. It can be said, however, that the longer the premises remain vacant, the fewer are the disease agents that survive.

Dividing the Farm into Functional Units

For certain economic reasons (e.g., a breeding farm or a small specialized market trade) it is not always possible to limit the entire farm to a single age. In such instances the farm should be divided into separate quarantinable units or areas for different groups of birds, such as the rearing area, pedigree unit, production groups, and experimental birds. With a suitable ranch arrangement each area is periodically depopulated, cleared, and sanitized. Much stricter security procedures for personnel, bird, and equipment movements are necessary for this type of operation.

There is no reliable formula for minimum distances between houses or between units. Closed light-, temperature-, and ventilation-controlled houses appear to prevent building-to-building and ranch-to-ranch spread better than open houses. Greater distance can make up for some inadequacy in building design and equipment usage. Since each ranch and enterprise is different from all others, a good rule is for the poultryman to seek advice for his particular farm from specialists whose business it is to study diseases and how to control them.

The most important factor in dividing the farm into segregated units is not so much to facilitate daily separation of farm personnel, equipment, and poultry but to provide quarantinable units to prevent spread and to facilitate elimination of a disease should it occur. The affected unit can be immediately quarantined to contain the disease and prevent spread until that particular flock is removed and the unit cleaned and sterilized.

BUILDING CONSTRUCTION

Bird-Proofing

The first rule in poultry house construction is to exclude free-flying wild birds,

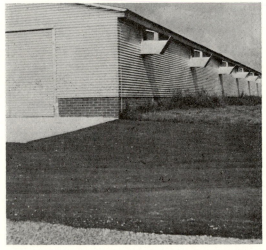

FIG. 1.3—This light-, temperature-, and ventilation-controlled house excludes wild birds and most flying insects. Concrete apron and paved roadway help prevent tracking of soil-borne diseases into the poultry house. (Schmidt-Ankum, Germany)

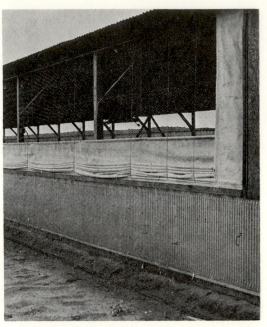

FIG. 1.4—Wild birds are effectively excluded from this open-type poultry house.

since many wild birds carry mites and harbor them in their nests. In addition, many species of wild birds have been found susceptible to some common viral and bacterial diseases of poultry and thus could act as carriers. Turkeys on range are especially vulnerable to infections carried by wild birds. For this reason and for generally improved sanitary practices, the present trend is to house turkeys, especially breeder turkeys and young growing turkeys, in closed or partially closed bird-proof houses. Ducks and other domestic waterfowl are also vulnerable to water-borne diseases and to diseases carried by wild birds, especially wild waterfowl.

Light- and temperature-controlled houses are usually bird-proof by reason of their construction (Fig. 1.3), but both ventilation and bird-proofing are also achievable in open-type houses in hot climates (Fig. 1.4). Bird-proofing is also an important feature of crate drying and storage sheds.

Building Entrances

An apron of concrete at the entrances to poultry houses helps prevent tracking of disease into the houses (Fig. 1.3). Rain and sunshine help keep the apron cleaned and sterilized. A water faucet, boot brush, and covered pan of disinfectant available on the apron for disinfecting footwear are further aids in keeping litter and soil-borne diseases out of the house. The disinfectant is useless, however, unless renewed frequently enough to insure a potent solution at all times.

Ventilation

Poultry buildings should be constructed to provide protection against the elements, yet not create artificial stress conditions such as excess dust, insufficient ventilation with ammonia buildup, excessive draft, damp litter, and situations which lead to injuries by mechanical equipment or sharp objects.

There are many advantages of closed light- and temperature-controlled houses over open houses, but one serious drawback has been the development in some instances of excessively dry and dusty litter. While Anderson et al. (1966) could not demonstrate significant deleterious effects of short-term inhalation of dust by test chickens, it has been observed in practice that colibacillosis outbreaks are frequently associated with inhalation of excessive dust. Dust, if created, must be carried from the building with ventilating air. This may require increased air movement, and precautions must be taken to prevent a stream of cold outside air from blowing directly onto chickens that are prevented by cage or pen arrangement from seeking a more comfortable area.

Coccidial oocysts require moisture to develop into the infective stage. Excessively dry litter inhibits their development and may so limit the number of infective oocysts that infection is too light for a good immune reaction. Conversely, improper ventilation can lead to excessively wet litter which favors the survival and development of coccidia and parasites.

Ammonia fumes tend to accumulate as a result of damp litter and improper ventilation, and if they reach a high enough concentration, they may cause a keratoconjunctivitis (Bullis et al., 1950; Wright and Frank, 1957). Exposure to as little as 20 ppm (parts per million) of ammonia for 72 hours or 50 ppm for 48 hours increased the infection rate and histopathological changes of the respiratory epithelium of chickens when subsequently exposed to Newcastle disease virus (Anderson et al., 1964). A concentration of 100 ppm of ammonia in the atmosphere was found to be deleterious to performance of broilers, replacement pullets, and laying hens (Charles and Payne, 1966a,b). The adverse effects of the high ammonia concentration appeared to be related to reduced feed intake, and the term "environmentally induced nutritional stress" was suggested by the authors to describe and explain the debilitating consequences.

Litter will dry better if it is stirred frequently with a rake or garden tiller, but in spite of all efforts, it may remain wet in the wintertime or in humid climates. If wetness and excess ammonia concentration persist in a house, the litter should be replaced and the ventilation improved.

Proper ventilation is an engineering science; a good policy is to seek the advice of someone knowledgeable in this field before installing any system. The influence of such environmental conditions as temperature, humidity, radiation, and atmospheric pollutants on virus diseases of poultry has been reviewed by Anderson and Hanson (1965).

Floors and Cages

All surfaces inside the building should be of impervious material to permit thorough washing. It is not possible to sterilize a dirt floor efficiently and adequately. Good concrete floors permit thorough washing and disinfection. However, concrete floors have the disadvantage in poultry houses of sometimes causing wet litter due to moisture condensation on the cool concrete surface. Proper preparation of the bed on which concrete is to be poured and proper curing after it is poured are essential to prevent the cracking which provides protected havens for infectious material.

Raised slatted floors have been used successfully for years for laying chickens, both for adults and for rearing birds. Such floors have alternating wooden pieces and spaces, each about ¾ in. wide (Fig. 1.5). This permits the droppings to fall through out of reach of the birds and prevents recycling infection of intestinal parasites and diseases. Since coccidial infection is thus avoided or greatly reduced, poor or no immunity to the parasite develops. This creates no problem for pullets destined for cages or slat-floored laying houses, because immunity to coccidiosis during the laying period in such houses would not be an im-

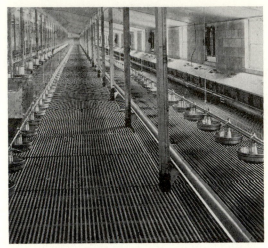

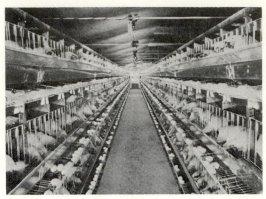

FIG. 1.5—Slat floors aid in control of intestinal diseases and parasites. Droppings fall through open spaces and out of reach of the poultry flock. (Creighton Bros., Warsaw, Ind.)

FIG. 1.6—Poultry are kept in cages in well-built, ventilated, light- and temperature-controlled houses in many countries throughout the world. Good housing reduces the stresses associated with variations in weather, and cages reduce intestinal diseases and parasitism. (Schmidt-Ankum, Germany)

portant consideration. However, if such pullets were transferred to litter-floored laying houses, they very likely would become seriously infected with coccidiosis. Commercial meat birds are inclined to develop leg problems and breast blisters if raised on complete slatted or wire floors. A modification of this system with part of the floor or yard raised slightly and covered with slats has been used for broiler breeders. The value of this system is increased further by placing the feed and water over the slatted area which encourages the collection of more droppings out of reach of the birds.

Keeping laying hens in some type of cage has become an accepted practice, both in closed houses (Fig. 1.6) and in open-type housing found in hot climates (Fig. 1.7). Cages and wire floors are widely used also to rear pullets destined for cages as adults. The system is so successful in preventing intestinal diseases that birds have no opportunity to develop immunity to them. Coccidiosis is almost certain to occur if chickens or other poultry reared in cages are transferred to litter floors. Of course drugs can be used successfully to control coccidiosis in birds transferred from cages to floors, but legal restrictions on their use in meat and egg-producing fowl seriously curtail the number of choices for this purpose in laying hens. There has been renewed interest in developing suitable cages

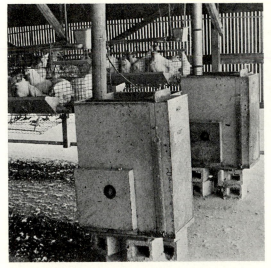

FIG. 1.7—In hot climates poultry are kept in cages in open-type houses. This practice prevents intestinal diseases and parasitism but subjects birds to temperature extremes. If the house is not bird-proof, external parasites are apt to be carried in by wild birds. Medicated feed can be placed in small feed tanks by hand for emergency flock treatment.

for breeder turkeys and commercial broilers. Such a development would be a distinct aid in eliminating many disease problems of soil and litter origin.

Feed and Water Medication Facilities

In spite of all precautions, poultry may become sick. This fact should be recognized from the start, and facilities for quick treatment by medication in the water or feed should be provided long before any trouble occurs. When birds are penned together by tens of thousands in one big pen, segregation and treatment of individual birds is impractical, so mass medication and vaccination are essential if any treatment is to be given at all.

Feed medication is not the best method of treatment because of the inappetence of sick birds and their inability to compete for feed. Water medication is somewhat better because the sick will frequently drink when they will not eat, but the medicaments that can be administered in the water are limited. Mass medication, while not completely successful in curing the sick, may hold the disease in check long enough for the host to make its own successful fight. Provision should also be made for mass vaccination through the drinking water as this has become an accepted and successful labor-saving practice. If the drinking water is chlorinated or otherwise treated, the sanitizing agent may destroy the vaccine, so provision must be made to permit use of untreated or distilled water for mixing and administering water vaccines.

If a building is constructed with a bulk water tank for gravity flow watering devices, the tank should be of plastic or lined with some nonreactive protective substance and be readily accessible for cleaning and for mixing medicaments. If the watering devices are operated on high pressure, the pipe leading into the pen should have a bypass system with proper valve arrangement so that a medicament proportioner can be installed quickly when needed. A metering device to measure the feed and water consumption is useful to keep track of the health of the flock (Fig. 1.8). Float regulated or continuous flow water troughs can spread disease within a house. Infectious coryza has been observed to spread down cage rows of chickens in the direction of water flow. The use of a watering system with small drinking cups (Fig. 1.9)

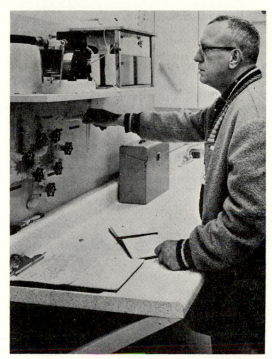

FIG. 1.8—*This poultry house is equipped with a proportioner which can be used to meter water consumption or to medicate merely by adjusting the proper water line valves located nearby.*

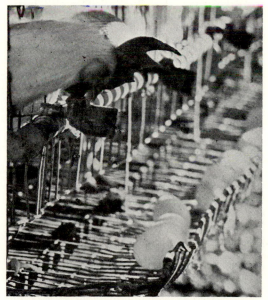

FIG. 1.9—*Separate small automatic drinking cups for each cage prevent spread of disease from pen to pen through the water supply.*

for individual small cage units will hinder the spread of disease through the drinking water.

Bulk feed delivery, metal bulk storage tanks, and automatic feeders are common in modern poultry keeping. These eliminate the possibility of rodent contamination since the feed is always in closed tanks rather than in bags or open bins, but the system leads to difficulties when short-term emergency medication in the feed is desirable and the bulk tank is full of feed. Two alternative systems are useful to avoid this stalemate. Either an additional smaller bulk tank may be installed just for emergency medicated feed, or a small dispensing tank may be interposed between the bulk tank and feed troughs (Figs. 1.7, 1.10) so emergency medicated feed can be put in the smaller tank by hand. Disposable paper bags have been developed which eliminate the danger of used feed bags as a source of mechanical carrier of disease from farm to farm.

Feeders and Waterers

Rats, mice, and other rodents should be kept out of feed because they may introduce Salmonella, paracolon, or other disease agents which can be the source of an outbreak in the poultry flock.

Litter scratched into the feed and water troughs and feed spilled in the litter in-

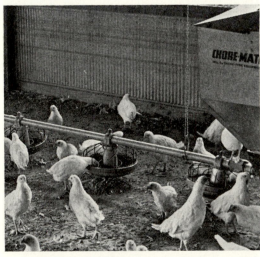

FIG. 1.10—Small feed tanks such as this one in a litter floor pen between the large bulk tank and the feed trough allow hand dumping of emergency medicated feed. Wire guards keep chickens out of the feeders.

crease the intake of litter and litter-borne disease agents. As an example, more coccidial oocysts and less coccidiostat are ingested, and a clinical infection may result. If poultry are permitted to consume litter, considerable mortality and depression can occur from impaction of the gizzard, and litter fragments may cause enteritis by mechanical irritation.

Feed troughs should have some type of guard to keep poultry out of them (Figs. 1.5, 1.10) and should not be overfilled so that feed is spilled into the litter. Feeders without guards permit defecation into the feed and encourage spread of diseases that are shed in the feces. Wet feed in the litter or in yards attracts wild birds and rodents and provides a good medium for growth of molds (fungi). Fungus toxins, if consumed, can make poultry sick. Feeders used in turkey yards should be in a covered area or designed to protect the feed from rainwater and sunlight to prevent mold growth and loss of vitamins.

Roost areas over screened dropping pits are common in floor laying and breeder hen houses to keep chickens away from their feces. Screened roost areas are also desirable in rearing houses to prevent piling by the birds and excessive fouling of the litter with feces, which in turn leads to packing and caking of the litter. Feeders and waterers over the roosting pits keep the birds on the roost area much of the daytime as well as at night, so that most of the droppings collect out of reach. Spilled water also falls under the roosts rather than into the litter, so the litter area stays drier.

Feeders and waterers are frequently set or hung over the litter area. In this case the waterer should be of a type which does not lend itself to spillage, or a raised wire frame should be placed under it (Fig. 1.11) with a drain area provided in the floor. Gravel may be added under the frame or it may be left empty. Here again, the aim is to prevent wetting of the litter which encourages coccidia and worm development and fungus growth. There are many good automatic, semiautomatic, and hand feeding devices available commercially.

PERSONNEL CONTROL

Company and Farm Personnel

Managers, supervisors, and owners are sometimes the worst offenders at breaking the sanitation rules. These people frequent-

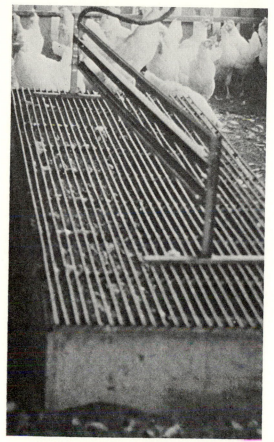

FIG. 1.11—*Raised concrete platform covered with a removable grill on which the waterer is placed. Spilled water collects in the pit and does not wet the litter. (HNJ Co., Japan)*

ly visit many different types of poultry enterprises, farms, and farm units, and disease agents do not respect authority or ownership. Such personnel, like veterinarians, should set a good example for the workmen. One of the most important aspects of disease control is an awareness on the part of everyone—owner; work force; feed and supply delivery men; egg, bird, and litter haulers; and all who visit or work on poultry farms—that each of them has an important role in the disease prevention program on a farm. Occasional educational conferences with the assembled work force on health goals and reasons for procedures used will foster this awareness. This is as important as the disease preventive measures established. An informed worker will be more effective in preventing the introduction and tracking of disease.

In designing buildings and farm layout and in programming production and management, it is important to make every disease preventive practice as easy and efficient as possible. Any procedures that are difficult will probably be done incorrectly.

Visitors and Customers

For some types of poultry enterprise it is deemed necessary to show either the birds or the premises to visitors rather frequently. In such cases an observation booth, platform, or fenced area should be provided for the purpose. Such an area should be sealed off from the poultry pens or hatchery. For maximum security the entry, access road, and observation area should be completely separated from the work area used by farm personnel. Such a facility for a hatchery is shown in Figure 1.12.

Visitors can be a minimum hazard if proper provisions are made to accommodate them and they cooperate fully with strict sanitary rules. When they must enter the poultry quarters, they should wear protective clothing such as clean or sterilized coveralls and hat in addition to disinfected rubber overshoes or other footwear. Most important is the disinfected footwear. Plastic footwear has limited use because it is

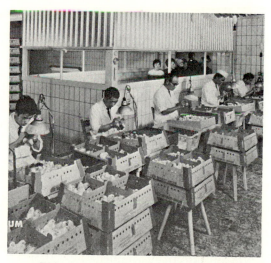

FIG. 1.12—*Sealed observation cubicle in this hatchery permits visitors to observe hatchery operations without tracking disease into the building. This observation booth is reached by a special walkway from a parking lot, and the entrance is located far from entrances used by hatchery personnel. (Schmidt-Ankum, Germany)*

easily punctured by gravel or other sharp objects. The sanitary precautions are most important when entering floor brooding and rearing houses but will help keep disease out of any house or pen.

SANITARY ENVIRONMENT

Grounds around Buildings

RODENT CONTROL. Piles of trash and unused equipment are good hiding and breeding places for rats, mice, and ground squirrels which may serve as reservoirs of disease and contaminate the troughs with their excrement. Feed spilled or left in troughs stacked carelessly aside is a good food supply for these rodents, and when this supply is exhausted, they will find any available route into the building where they have intimate contact with the poultry. Even if the buildings are rodent-proof, their excrement can be tracked in on footwear. It is more difficult to get rid of rodents once the premises are infested than to keep them out initially.

INSECT CONTROL. Many types of insects congregate in and under piles of trash and dead unmowed grass and weeds along fences and buildings. Many parasites and disease agents are either harbored from one generation to another in resident insects (e.g., Marek's disease), require an insect for an intermediate stage of development (e.g., tapeworms), or are simply carried from bird to bird mechanically or by biting (e.g., fowl pox virus). Countermeasures against insects are part of the sanitary environment and sanitary cleanup.

Some methods used to keep insects away from buildings are an apron of treated soil to prevent growth of all vegetation, an apron of hard surface material, or a border of well-mowed green grass. Spraying the area around buildings with an insecticide also prevents insect buildup, but the other methods have the additional advantage of reducing fire hazards to the buildings.

A good practice during cleanup is to spray the grounds, litter, and buildings with an insecticide immediately after removing the fowl; then allow a few days for effective insect kill before removing the litter preparatory to cleaning and disinfection. This is especially important when there is a history of an insect-borne disease in the previous brood. The building should be sprayed again after cleaning with an insecticide having a residual effect to prevent reinfestation.

Carcass Disposal Methods

When birds die because they have been overcome by disease agents, the carcasses remain as a source of infection for penmates and other poultry on the same or other farms. Likewise, hopelessly sick birds discharge infectious material into the environment and should be removed from the flock and killed in a manner which will not permit the spewing of blood or exudates (see Diagnostic Procedures). Whether due to a serious clinical infection or just the usual expected mortality, all carcasses should be disposed of by one of the following methods to prevent dissemination of any disease that may be plaguing the flock.

PIT OR TANK DISPOSAL. For small losses and "normal" attrition, a decomposition pit can be used. A suitable one is illustrated in Figure 1.13. Bigger and less elaborate ones can be built, but precautions should be taken that it is not located where it will contaminate drinking water supplies, that the roof or walls will not cave in, that animals will not dig into it, that flies and other insects cannot get into it, and above all that children cannot possibly fall into it. A suitable foolproof "manhole" is a five- or ten-gallon milk can with the bottom removed. It should be firmly fastened to the pit cover and fitted with a padlocking device. The pit cover should be sealed over with tar paper or plastic and should be strong enough to hold at least a foot of soil overlay.

An electrically heated septic tank for disposal of dead birds and waste products from large poultry farms and processing plants has been developed by the Agricultural Research Service, United States Department of Agriculture, in cooperation with the Maine and Connecticut Agricultural Experiment Stations (Anon. 1957). The method consists of digesting the carcasses and/or waste products in a heated septic tank. Heat is applied at 100° F and requires 2–3 kilowatt hours of electricity per day to maintain this temperature for the two weeks needed for destruction of all but the bones of carcasses. The system depends on mesophilic bacteria which multiply best at 90–100° F to accelerate decomposition. Neutralizing the mass at inter-

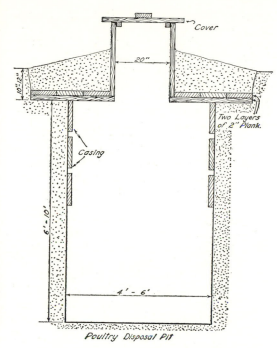

FIG. 1.13—Poultry disposal pit. Such a pit can be made any size that is convenient and is valuable for disposal of hatchery wastes as well as carcasses. (Hinshaw, Univ. Calif.)

vals with lime and adding hot water further accelerates the action and speed of decomposition.

BURNING. This is the surest way of destroying infectious material. Many smokeless, odorless incinerators for disposal of animal carcasses are available commercially. These devices are expensive but are handy and suitable for some purposes. Homemade incinerators of various types have been used successfully also, but they may create undesirable air pollution.

BURYING. For severe losses creating a serious disposal problem, a deep hole may be dug and the carcasses buried so animals cannot get at them. The best and easiest way is to use a backhoe and dig a deep narrow trench. Each day's collection of dead birds can be deposited and covered until the trench is filled.

COOKING OR RENDERING. Freshly dead poultry, like livestock, can be rendered into fertilizer or other products. The rendering temperature should be sufficient to sterilize the carcass. Cans used to haul the carcasses should be steam-cleaned and sterilized. Again, as in so many instances, it should be kept in mind that commercial or contract haulers of dead carcasses may introduce another disease from some other ranch outbreak unless precautionary measures are taken.

Cleaning the Buildings

A clean sanitized environment is good insurance against disease outbreaks from any cause. Stringent sanitary practices are frequently discredited because disease is tracked in after the buildings and equipment are cleaned and disinfected, or because some step in the total sanitary program was omitted and a focus of infection was preserved.

LITTER REMOVAL. When a house is depopulated the litter should be removed preparatory to cleaning. With the advent of easily applied commercial fertilizer, the decline of the diversified family farm, and development of huge specialized poultry farms, proper and economical disposal of litter and poultry manure has become a serious problem in the industry. There is no clearcut answer. A general recommendation is to remove it far enough from the buildings so that insects will not crawl or fly back into the houses, and to dry it, compost it, or spread it onto fields and work it into the soil. If cleaning is done while chickens are still present (e.g., cages), it should be remembered that contracted personnel, trucks, and equipment may recently have been on another farm where a disease outbreak occurred. A suitable concrete collection point with a separate access road for outside vehicles is recommended.

In some cases the nature of a disease that has occurred (e.g., pullorum) may dictate that extra precautions be taken with the litter. It may be advisable to remove and burn the litter or to thoroughly soak it with a disinfectant before removal from the house—both expensive procedures. *Any treatment of manure or litter must take into account the residual effects of the compounds used on plant life when the treated manure is spread on the land.* For most disease agents composting of the litter or droppings is sufficient. Composting can be done by piling above ground and covering with soil or a plastic sheet, or by digging a wide trench and burying below the ground level. Whatever is done with the litter, one must be ever cognizant of the fact that wherever the litter is spilled or piled, it remains as a disease reservoir for varying lengths of time. Equipment used to move it can carry the infection to another building or another farm, and this should especially be considered in relation to contracted cleaning and/or hauling services (and also haulers of new litter materials for a cleaned and disinfected house).

OUTSIDE RUNS. In the case of outside runs such as turkey and game bird ranges, the top soil should be scraped off and hauled some distance from the poultry. Sunlight and soil activity combine over a long period to destroy the pathogens. Anything that can be done to aid the destruction process is helpful. Removal of organic residues such as leaf beds and manure accumulations helps to reduce the danger for future broods. It is best to rotate the ranges or dirt yards so they stand idle for one complete flock cycle.

WASHING AND DISINFECTING. Once the litter or cage droppings have been removed the cleaning equipment, feeders, waterers, egg collecting equipment, walls, floors, roosts or cages, outside concrete or suspended runs, and entries to the buildings should be washed thoroughly and disinfected. If the supply of water is limited and washing is not possible, dry cleaning may suffice, provided it is thorough and includes scraping and sweeping or vacuuming the surfaces, corners, ledges, nests, and feeders. The amount of disinfectant used on dry-cleaned surfaces must be increased over that required for washed surfaces.

If possible to do so efficiently, it is preferable to clean the house without removing the equipment from the building. If not, all portable equipment should be removed from the house, soaked with water, then thoroughly washed and dried. A high-pressure water hose cleans equipment effectively. Equipment which cannot be removed should be washed in place and then the entire inside building surface completely washed clean. If the building has been constructed to facilitate good cleaning, a satisfactory job may be accomplished easily. If not, it may not be accomplished

at all, or only with great effort and expense. A large concrete apron equipped with racks and high-pressure hose is a good place to clean and stack equipment.

After washing, disinfection is in order (see section on disinfectants in this chapter). There are many good disinfectants sold under trade names. The one chosen should be used as recommended by the manufacturer. *The important thing is that the surfaces be clean before the disinfectant is applied. Disinfectants applied to dirt-encrusted surfaces are ineffective and wasted.* Not only are they inactivated by organic material in the dirt, but they never reach the infectious agents beneath the dirt. Thorough washing removes most of the infectious agents from the house and equipment, along with the dirt, and leaves a clean surface so the disinfectant can reach those that remain. Disinfectants are not cure-alls but only added sanitary insurance to a clean surrounding.

Two to four weeks of idleness or "down time" before a new flock is moved in is additional insurance against carry-over of disease.

Built-up Litter and Uncleaned Buildings

In some areas litter is reused for several broods before removal, resulting in built-up litter. It does not compost unless special effort is made to promote composting such as wetting and warming or by adding a composting starter. Sometimes a little new litter is added on top of the old under the brooders.

There are many differences of opinion on the advantages of providing a clean, sanitized environment over the practice of brooding and rearing on old built-up or composted litter. Certainly there are convincing arguments for monetary savings through reuse of litter, especially for broilers which have a relatively short grow-out time and in areas where litter material is scarce and costly. Some poultrymen have experimented and found this practice to be economically sound for their particular ranch conditions. Others have found it to be unsound or even disastrous.

One advantage claimed for "dirty" brooding is that the offspring become exposed early while they have parental antibodies to whatever disease may be present on the farm or in the area and carried over in the litter. Some have even suggested deliberate contamination of brooding quarters with litter from hen houses to expose chicks to certain viral agents carried by the hens. This is a risky theoretical approach to disease control with an uncertain outcome. It may result in success or disaster, depending upon unknown conditions or circumstances. Satisfactory results with old built-up litter may prevail as long as a serious litter-borne disease has not occurred in a previous brood, but there is always danger that a disease or parasite buildup may occur unknown to the poultryman until disaster overtakes the new flocks. In any event, the buildup of dust, enteric bacteria, and parasites increases the chance of parasitism and secondary and nonspecific infections in succeeding broods during stress periods.

Brooding and rearing young poultry on old or contaminated litter is counter to good sanitary practices and cannot be recommended by the writer as a sound disease prevention practice consistent with the ever greater demand for day-old chicks and poults free of all disease agents. *It does not make sense for poultrymen to demand disease-free chicks or poults and then brood them in dirty, non-disinfected quarters or on filth deliberately introduced into the brooding environment.*

HATCHERY MANAGEMENT

The building and equipment in which the fertile egg is converted to a day-old chick, poult, or other young fowl and the equipment used to deliver it to the farm must be clean and sanitary. An individual hatched from a pathogen-free egg will remain pathogen-free only if it hatches in a clean hatcher, is put in a clean box and held in a clean room where it can breathe clean air, and then is hauled to the farm in a clean delivery van. (No one appears to have studied the possible infection hazard of air circulated through chick delivery vans while driving past poultry houses in which actively infected chickens exist.)

DESIGN OF HATCHERY

A good hatchery design has a one-way flow of traffic from the egg entry room through egg traying, incubation, hatching, and holding rooms to van loading area. The clean-up area and hatch waste discharge should be off the hatch room with a separate load-out area. Each hatchery room should be designed for thorough washing and disinfecting. The ventilation system is equally important and must be designed to prevent recirculation of contaminated and dust-laden air. Gentry et al. (1962) found that hatcheries with poor floor designs and faulty traffic patterns were highly contaminated compared to those with one-way traffic flow.

IMPORTANCE OF GOOD SANITATION

Techniques have been devised for evaluating the sanitary status of commercial hatcheries by culturing fluff samples (Wright et al., 1959), by detecting microbial populations in hatchery air samples (Chute and Gershman, 1961; Gentry et al., 1962; Magwood, 1964), and by culturing various surfaces in the hatchery (Magwood and Marr, 1964). By relating the results of these techniques to hatchery management, it has been observed by Magwood (1964) that in clean air the bacterial counts of eggshells dropped quickly and low counts persisted on all surfaces to the completion of hatching. Chute and Barden (1964) found the fungal flora of hatcheries to be related to the management and sanitation programs of the hatchery.

In order to minimize bacterial contamination of eggs and hatching chicks, the hatchery premises must be kept free of reservoirs of contamination which readily becomes air borne (Magwood, 1964). Trays used for hatching should be thoroughly cleaned with water and then disinfected before eggs are placed in them. This can be done either by dipping in a tank of suitable disinfectant (see section on Disinfectants) or by fumigating with formaldehyde in the hatcher. Trays and eggs are frequently fumigated together when the eggs are transferred to the hatcher. Some fumigation is done during the hatch (at about 10% hatch), but concentrations which are low enough to avoid harming the hatching chick probably serve only to color the down a pleasing yellow color. Formaldehyde fumigation in one case increased the severity of mold infection rather than overcoming it (Wright et al., 1961). Wright (1958) emphasized the practical meaning of hatchery sanitation and how to attain it. He concluded: "No fumigation programme should be used to replace cleanliness but rather to supplement it."

As the chicks hatch, the exposed embryo

fluids collect bacteria from contaminated shells, trays, and ventilating air. The combination of nutritious embryo fluids and warm temperature forms an excellent environment for bacteria and they multiply very rapidly (Gentry et al., 1962). The cleaner the air and environment to begin with, the more delayed is the bacterial buildup, and as the hatch progresses, the less likely is the navel to become infected (oomphalitis).

The likelihood that newly hatched poultry will go into the brooder house pathogen-free increases with the distance between the hatchery and poultry farms and other potential dust and microbial aerosol sources. Other factors which aid in obtaining pathogen-free chicks and poults are hatchery cleanliness and sanitation, well-arranged traffic flow, and well-controlled ventilation.

BREEDER CODES

The breeder "code" is a designation used to denote the source of hatching eggs. It may denote breeders the same age on different farms, breeders on a particular farm, or any other breeder grouping. There have been frequent recommendations that all deliveries of chicks or poults to a particular brooder house or farm be from the same breeder code. If breeders are kept free of disease and fed a good breeder ration, if hatching eggs are produced clean and properly disinfected, and if chicks are hatched and handled in clean surroundings, keeping chicks of different breeder codes separated probably has little practical meaning. However, there is a tendency to keep breeders in larger flocks and to avoid as much as is practical the mixing of hatching eggs from breeder flocks of many different microbial, nutritional, and genetic backgrounds.

CHICK SEXERS

Unless the output of one hatchery is so great as to demand their full time, chick sexers must go from one hatchery to another. This introduces the possibility of carrying disease from infected to healthy chicks. Most sexers are aware of this hazard and are anxious to follow proper procedures. Facilities should be provided for them to store all their necessary equipment so that it can remain at the hatchery. They should have a clean area to change clothes and wash themselves and their equipment, and clean protective garments to wear (see Fig. 1.12). Their habits should be at least as clean as those of the hatchery crew.

FLOCK MANAGEMENT

HANDLING THE YOUNG

Chicks and poults hatch with a reserve food supply in unabsorbed yolk sufficient to sustain them for about 72 hours. Some offspring actually hatch one or two days before they are removed from the machine; therefore, they should receive feed and water as soon as possible, preferably within 24 hours of the time they are taken from the hatcher.

Brooder Temperature

Chilling, overheating, starvation, and dehydration are serious stress producers and can precipitate active infections from latent infections which might otherwise be overcome by the young without detectable symptoms. In a randomly split hatch of chicks from the same group of dams, those delivered to one farm can suffer much greater mortality than those delivered to other farms. This difference is associated with differences in environmental stresses. Young chicks and poults should be kept at a comfortable temperature at all times. The brooder temperature is usually started at 95° F and gradually reduced as the offspring mature. While thermometers are helpful, strict adherence to thermometer temperatures without regard to obvious discomfort of the chicks or poults is poor husbandry practice and courts disaster. An uncomfortable chick or poult lets the caretaker know about it. Its peeping should be heeded and the cause of discomfort corrected regardless of any thermometer reading.

Coccidiostats and Other Drugs

Floor-reared poultry receive coccidiostatic drugs in the feed from the first day either to prevent coccidiosis (broilers, turkeys, replacement pullets destined for cage adult housing) or to keep the disease under control until the bird develops active immunity (breeder flocks, replacement pullets destined for floor adult housing).

However the immunity developed by the

birds depends on a number of factors. The amount of feed and coccidiostat may vary among birds, and the number of viable sporulated oocysts will vary with differing humidity, temperature, and litter conditions. Depending on the relationship of these variable factors, the coccidial infection may be too mild to elicit good immunity, or it may be so severe that a frank outbreak occurs. There is no special management formula to overcome this dilemma other than a keen awareness of the variable factors and trying to maintain the proper physical environment which will favor the degree of infection desired.

Feed and Water Consumption and Medication

Scientific feed formulation is the business of highly trained nutrition experts, and quality feeds are the rule, not the exception. However, poultry eat the feed, not the formula, and occasionally problems do arise which are traceable to the feed (e.g., accidental omission of an ingredient, low potency vitamin supplement, moldy or toxic contamination of an ingredient).

More important in everyday disease control are the variations in feed consumption associated with hot or cold weather, housing changes, strain and age of bird, body weight, rate of lay, and the energy and fiber content of the feed. With a 10–20% lower feed consumption associated with one of these factors, there is also a lower intake of coccidiostat or other medicament in the feed by the same amount. Conversely, an increase in total feed consumption due to one of these factors increases the total intake of all feed ingredients, including drugs.

Increased water intake during hot weather can spell disaster through overconsumption of water medication. Sulfa toxicity has frequently occurred through failure to take into consideration the probable water intake. A given concentration of a drug in the water may fail to control a disease under circumstances where water consumption is very low, as in very cold weather. Also, if natural sources of water are available, particularly for range turkeys, the intake by some birds from the water trough may be light. Many are the tragedies from overdosing due to carelessness, miscalculation, or failure to consider feed and water

intake, weather, and other variables. When drugs are used in the feed, great care should be exercised in adding the same or other drugs to the water.

Immunization

Some diseases are so ubiquitous and so easily and rapidly spread that it is possible to avoid them only with extreme precautions, and little can be done to alter the course of an outbreak should it occur. Yet their prevention through vaccination is relatively harmless and inexpensive. This is particularly true of Newcastle disease, infectious bronchitis, and (for breeder flocks) avian encephalomyelitis. For these diseases, vaccination at the appropriate time (see individual diseases for recommendations) is just good common sense and is, in fact, a means of preventing spread of virulent forms of the disease in the industry.

Encounters with virulent and devastating disease agents have become less frequent and reliance on emergency drug treatments has declined as a result of increased knowledge of diseases, widespread saturation of the poultry population with mild and attenuated immunizing agents, elimination of egg-borne diseases, improved genetic resistance to disease, and improved health-protecting management practices. As a consequence, minor health improvements have become more important.

Surgical Procedures

Debeaking (surgical removal of the beak tips to prevent cannibalism) is commonly practiced on growing flocks, particularly those destined for cages as adults. When this is done properly there is no serious adverse effect on the chicken. However, proper debeaking is more an art than a science, and many birds are permanently handicapped by improper severe debeaking. Likewise, other surgical procedures such as removing certain toes, wattles, or combs must be done properly by one trained in the procedure if harm to the bird is to be avoided. Figure 1.14 shows a bird which was debeaked satisfactorily.

ADULT FLOCKS

The modern laying strains are bred for high egg production and can no longer be treated like jungle fowl. The most important management factor is maintaining the feed, water, and environmental conditions at the optimum condition for maximum efficient production. The same is required of meat bird, turkey, and other types of breeder hens. The egg production will be a good indicator of the success of the management. Many conditions arise which hamper performance, and it is important not only to keep disease out but also to prevent conditions which cause discomfort.

MANAGING THE BREEDER FLOCK AND HATCHING EGG SUPPLY

The breeder flock must be kept healthy and provided with a diet adequate to supply the fertile egg with all nutrients necessary, not only for normal embryonic development but also to maintain the offspring in a healthy condition until it consumes adequate feed. The flock should be managed so that egg-borne diseases are prevented by whatever techniques are available.

DIET, HEALTH, AND PARENTAL IMMUNITY

It bears emphasis here that a breeder ration is more than a laying ration. Laying rations which are adequate to sustain egg production are not always adequate to sustain good hatchability and good health of the young offspring. Many times production is satisfactory in breeder hens, but their embryos or chicks show symptoms and lesions of vitamin deficiency. The breeder ration must be adequate not only for performance of the breeder hen but also for the embryo and the chick.

Breeder hens that are in poor health for any reason frequently either fail to supply the embryo with some vital nutritional factor or perhaps pass some toxic material to the egg; thus the hatch is poor or the chicks are of poor quality and must be culled. While this occasionally happens with apparently healthy flocks also, a healthy breeder flock is the best insurance of good quality offspring.

Baby chicks and poults are delivered into many types of environment. In some poultry areas husbandry methods are such that chicks are exposed to some diseases from the first day of age. This type of management is not apt to survive, but for chicks exposed to disease at this early age, parental immunity may be an aid to disease prevention. How much parental immunity is necessary and against which diseases are debatable subjects and vary with the location where chicks are reared. Parental immunity is dissipated gradually after the chick hatches and usually does not last more than 2–4 weeks. In modern, well-run rearing facilities chicks and poults are well protected, not only against the elements but also against the introduction of disease from outside sources, for several weeks or beyond the time that a high initial parental immunity would be protective. Parental immunity in the chicks is of little concern in such cases. The cost of repeated vaccinations, in addition to possible adverse effects on health and egg production of breeders during the laying period, is hardly justified simply to attempt to insure high parental immunity in all the offspring. A high level of parental antibodies may adversely affect the response of the offspring to early vaccinations. A high level of passive parental antibodies may have real beneficial significance in controlling some diseases (e.g., duck virus hepatitis).

PREVENTING INTERIOR EGG-BORNE DISEASES

Various techniques are used for preventing disease agents from being carried to the offspring. The ideal situation is to have breeders free of all pathogens. For some diseases there is still no practical way of obtaining this utopian situation. For others (e.g., avian encephalomyelitis) the probability of the infection occurring during the egg-laying period with resultant egg transmission may be too great to permit the clean but susceptible status.

Immunization

In addition to routine immunization of breeders against several common diseases to prevent the adverse effects on egg production from inopportune infections, they should especially be immunized against avian encephalomyelitis during the growing period to insure that they do not become naturally infected during the period they are producing hatching eggs. While this may not be an absolute guarantee against egg transmission of the virus, it has been a practical means of preventing serious dissemination of the virus through infected offspring. Reluctance to use or permit usage of the vaccine in breeder flocks only encourages this type of dissemination.

Immunization at an early age to prevent infection and egg transmission during the laying period has been used with variable degrees of success with *Mycoplasma gallisepticum* also.

Test and Removal of Carriers

Carriers of some transovarially transmitted diseases can be detected by serologic means, and this procedure has been used to eliminate possible egg shedders from the breeding flocks. This has proven most successful for pullorum disease and fowl typhoid. The method has been so effective that its application in infected breeder flocks, along with management techniques, has been largely responsible for the eradication of these diseases from most commercial poultry enterprises.

Test and Slaughter of Infected Flocks

Where infected breeders are detected, the entire breeder flock may be discarded. This method is indicated where testing is not likely to detect all infected birds in the flock. It is a costly procedure and not warranted unless there is a definite advantage for the offspring and reasonable assurance that they will not become infected from other sources after delivery to the farm. It has been used successfully for eliminating Mycoplasma-infected turkey breeder flocks and some chicken breeder flocks. A modification of this procedure wherein the infected breeder flocks are quarantined from uninfected flocks rather than slaughtered has also been successful in eliminating Mycoplasma from many chicken breeding enterprises.

Destroying the Agent inside the Egg

A pressure differential between the atmosphere and the inside of the egg has been used to force antibiotics through the shell of incubating eggs to prevent transmission of Mycoplasma species from dam to offspring. This is done by dipping warm eggs into cold antibiotic solutions or by using special vacuum machines (Alls et al., 1963). Antibiotics have also been injected directly into eggs for this purpose.

Elevated egg temperature has also been used to destroy Mycoplasma inside the egg (Yoder, 1970).

PREVENTING EGGSHELL-BORNE DISEASES

Several procedures are used to overcome shell contamination which arises from intestinal contents and other environmental sources. Control involves preventing shell contamination or destroying the organisms before they penetrate the shell.

Producing Clean Hatching Eggs

Very dirty eggs should not be used for hatching. If they must be used, they should be dry-cleaned when gathered. The cleaner the egg surface, the less bacterial contamination there is on the shell.

The most important consideration in hatching egg sanitation is to manage the flock so that eggs are clean when gathered. Many factors enter into accomplishing this goal. Wire roll-out nests with or without automatic collecting devices generally result in clean eggs and a minimum of bacterial contamination. Egg breakage can be reduced by providing sufficient nests for the peak lay period.

The number of floor and yard eggs can be reduced by proper design and location of the nests which should be available when the maturing pullets need them. The location and design will vary with the type of house. Nests should be darkened and ventilated, and the hens must be prevented from roosting in them at night because they contaminate the area with fecal deposits. Conventional nests must be kept clean by continually replacing soiled nesting material.

Keeping the litter dry is an aid to preventing soiled nests and nest material. Here again, proper design and construction of the breeder house to create conditions conducive to keeping litter dry aids disease control at the hatching egg level.

Measures should be taken to prevent Salmonella infections through elimination of these pathogens from the feed (e.g., pelleting), keeping the feed clean by good feeding practices and storage facilities, and keeping natural carriers (rodents, wild birds, pets) out of the pens and houses. Preventing salmonellosis and other types of enteric infections also helps prevent wet droppings with resulting wet litter.

Above all, eggs should be gathered frequently, especially in the early part of the day when the hens are visiting the nests most frequently. They should be gathered in clean, dry equipment and held in a dry, dust-free area.

FUMIGATING THE EGGS. The shell surface of hatching eggs should be disinfected immediately after gathering (on-farm fumigation). If fumigation cannot be done on the farm, it should be done as soon as possible thereafter, preferably before the eggs enter the hatchery building or at the entrance to the egg processing area of the hatchery. The later the fumigation is done, the less effective it is because the longer the bacteria have had to penetrate the shell. Unfumigated eggs raise the possibility of carrying some serious infection into the hatchery when susceptible newly hatched chicks are present. (See section on fumigation under Disinfectants.)

WASHING AND LIQUID STERILIZATION. Washing of hatching eggs with warm detergent solution at a temperature always higher than that of the eggs entering the washing machine (at least 30° higher but not to exceed 130° F—suggested wash water temperature, 110–125° F), followed by sanitizing of the shells with a chlorine compound, quaternary ammonia product, or other sanitizing agent is a routine procedure for commercial eggs. The procedure has been employed successfully with hatching eggs, but some real disasters have occurred where thousands of eggs were contaminated rather than sanitized by using dirty water, especially in washing machines which recirculate wash water. Even if eggs are washed properly, very dirty eggs should be drycleaned first by sanding to prevent excessive pollution of the washing solution and equipment. If the iron content of the wash water exceeds 5 ppm, it favors certain types of bacteria and creates a serious egg spoilage problem.

If egg washing is done, it should be only with a type of machine (e.g., brush conveyor type using flow-through wash water principle) which will insure against contamination of the eggs with dirty wash or rinse water. Very careful supervision is also necessary to insure that all equipment is working properly at all times and that it is cleaned daily. In some types of machines if the washing system fails, a few contaminated eggs can contaminate the water and in turn contaminate thousands of other eggs before the problem is detected and corrected. Contaminated eggs in the incubator set off a chain reaction of exploding eggs which contaminate surrounding eggs, causing more exploders and more contamination. While washing and liquid sterilization of hatching eggs can be done satisfac-

torily, the procedure is subject to operational difficulties and should not be attempted on a routine basis without full knowledge of the hazards involved.

STORAGE FACILITIES. After fumigation or other shell sterilization, hatching eggs are frequently stored in a cool room (ca. 50° F) at the hatchery until set. Cool rooms should be clean and free of mold and bacteria and periodically disinfected to prevent recontamination of the shells. Clinical histories indicate that infection in young chicks may sometimes be traceable to fungus-contaminated hatching eggs, and infections have been produced experimentally by contaminating the shells with fungus spores (Wright et al., 1961).

HANDLING AN OUTBREAK OF DISEASE

OBSERVE THE NORMAL

A good poultryman watches feed and water consumption and egg production at all times, but more important, he observes normal sounds and actions of the flock. He senses immediately when any of these conditions are abnormal and interprets them as signs of abnormal health. When this happens it should be assumed that an infectious disease has gained entry and that it may be tracked elsewhere during the investigation period. In a modern factory-like poultry operation any disease creates serious disruption in the economic operation of both the farm and the plants processing the products from the farm. Serious infectious diseases can even create havoc. The following steps should be followed when disease is suspected.

LOOK FOR NONINFECTIOUS CONDITIONS

Take precautions against tracking, but investigate management errors immediately and first. A high percentage of the so-called disease problems referred to laboratories for diagnosis are noninfectious conditions related to management (e.g., debeaking errors; consumption of litter and trash; water deprivation; starvation; chilling of chicks; injury from rough handling, automatic equipment, or drug injection; electrical failures; cannibalism; smothering; and rodent and predator attacks). Bell (1966) observed marked reduction in lay due to water deprivation related to a debeaking system which resulted in long lower beaks making it difficult to obtain water when the water level was low in the troughs. These are conditions which do not require the services of a diagnostic laboratory. External parasites (mites, lice, ticks, etc.) can be determined by the poultryman if he will just examine some affected birds himself.

QUARANTINE THE FLOCK

In the event that no management factors can be found, the next step is to set up a quarantine of the pen, the building, the farm unit area, or the entire farm, depending upon the design and programming of the farm. If this emergency was anticipated when the farm was laid out and programmed originally, the quarantine will be a minor problem. Either establish separate caretakers for affected birds and apparently healthy ones or at least make sure the sick ones are visited last.

Submit Specimens or Call a Veterinarian

The owner or serviceman should submit typical specimens to a diagnostic laboratory or call a veterinarian to visit the farm and establish the diagnosis. Poultrymen should seek professional diagnoses rather than trying to hide some disease because of possible public recrimination. Veterinarians and servicemen can and should help dispel this apprehension by maintaining high ethical standards. Servicemen are frequently requested to examine the flock, select specimens for the laboratory, and initiate first aid procedures until the veterinarian can be called or visited. If so, he should wear protective footwear and clothing when he enters the house. *No other farm should be visited en route to the laboratory.*

Get a Diagnosis

It is important to get a diagnosis as soon as possible. The course of action taken will be determined by nature of the disease. A poultryman should not procrastinate for any reason when a disease threatens. If he does, the disease may get completely out of hand before he even finds out what it is. It is not always possible to treat a disease or check its deleterious effects, but it is important to identify any and all diseases that occur to plan effectively for the future. Veterinarians should also be cognizant of the poultryman's economic plight at such times and render advice and assistance as quickly as he is able to obtain information or make a judgment.

Special Precautions

In addition to causing serious losses in poultry, some diseases (e.g., ornithosis, erysipelas, and fungus infections) are especially hazardous for humans. When these conditions are diagnosed, extra precautions must be taken to insure against human infection. The proper government health authorities should be notified of ornithosis outbreaks, and all handling and processing personnel should be apprised of the disease, the hazards, and the necessary precautions.

Some diseases (e.g., Salmonella infections, ornithosis, laryngotracheitis, etc.) are "reportable" in some states, and when diagnosed must be reported immediately to the state animal disease control authorities in order that proper investigation and action can be taken to protect the general poultry industry.

NURSING CARE

Drugs

No drugs should be given until a diagnosis is obtained or a veterinarian consulted. If the wrong drug is given, it can be a useless waste of money, or it may be harmful or even disastrous. If an infectious disease is found and corrective drugs are applicable, they should be used very carefully according to directions.

Strict regulations govern the use of drugs in mixed feeds for food producing animals. For information write to the Food and Drug Administration, 200 C Street S.W., Washington, D.C. 20204. Feed manufacturers must have FDA clearance to include most drugs in mixed feeds. When treated flocks are to be marketed, a specified period of time, depending upon the drug used, must follow cessation of treatment to allow dissipation of drug residues from the tissues before slaughter. If the flock is producing table eggs when treated, the drug used must be one permitted for use in laying flocks or the eggs must be discarded during and for varying lengths of time after treatment—a costly alternative.

If the flock is producing hatching eggs when it becomes infected and there is danger that egg transmission of the infectious agent from dams to offspring may occur (e.g., salmonellosis, mycoplasmosis, epidemic tremor), the eggs should not be used for hatching until the danger has passed. It should be kept in mind also that in fertile eggs residues of drugs used to treat breeders may occasionally cause abnormalities in some of the embryos.

Tender Loving Care

Whether the flock consists of a few hundred individuals or tens of thousands, nursing care plays an important role in the outcome of a disease. Additional heat should be supplied to young chicks that begin huddling due to sickness. Clean and fresh (or medicated) water should be available at close range. Temporary waterers located more accessibly are sometimes necessary during sickness. If water founts are normally located where chickens must jump onto some raised device or turkeys must cross through hot sunlight to reach them, the sick will not have the energy or initiative to seek water. They will soon become dehydrated, an early step on the road to death. Birds on range or in yards tend to drink from the closest puddles, which may be thoroughly polluted.

The same principles are true for feed. Sick birds can be encouraged to eat if the caretaker will proceed through the house stirring feed and rattling feed hoppers or adding small quantities of fresh feed. Sometimes a little molasses in the feed or water (1 pt/gal) will encourage consumption. Some antibiotics appear to stimulate feed consumption when they are included in the diet. Anything that is added which proves distasteful to the bird should be removed immediately, however.

Sometimes birds become so depressed and moribund that the caretaker must walk among them frequently to rouse them so they will eat or drink.

Destroy Those That Will Not Recover

Kill hopelessly sick and crippled birds in a manner which will not permit the spewing of blood or exudates. (See Diagnostic Procedures.) Dead and destroyed birds should be disposed of immediately. (See Carcass Disposal.)

Disposition of the Flock

Do not move or handle the flock until it has recovered, unless the move is to a more favorable environment as part of the therapy. After the treatments, if any, have been completed and the flock appears to be completely healthy, it may be marketed or moved to permanent quarters, if such a move is part of the management program. *Some healthy carriers may remain.* If the flock is moved to another depopulated farm, this will present no problem except that occasionally a disease may flare up due to the stress of handling and moving. *If the recovered flock is moved to a multiple-age farm, carriers can introduce the disease into susceptible flocks already there. If the recovered flock is already in permanent quarters having multiple ages, newly introduced flocks may be exposed and come down with the disease—a common occurrence with many diseases.*

DIAGNOSTIC PROCEDURES

There are many satisfactory diagnostic and postmortem techniques. The technique and instruments used by one pathologist may vary considerably from those used by another. Some suggestions are offered here to guide the student and beginner. It is not *the* way to perform a postmortem examination; it is *a* way. The goal is to determine the cause of impaired performance, symptoms, or mortality by examining the tissues and organs, and to obtain the best specimens possible from the carcass to carry out microbiological, serological, histopathological, or animal inoculation tests. It is important that in the process infectious materials do not endanger the health of humans, livestock, or other poultry. By proceeding in an orderly fashion, some possible clue is less apt to be overlooked, and tissues will not be grossly contaminated prior to examination. It is well to remember at the outset that a blood sample or tissue specimen which is determined later to be superfluous can always be discarded, but it is very difficult to retrieve a sterile or suitable sample from the garbage can.

The techniques and procedures necessary to make an accurate diagnosis and to identify the specific disease agents are found in the technical information contained in the following chapters of this book. Additional aids in studying the infectious agents used for immunizing fowl can be found in *Methods for the Examination of Poultry Biologics* (Natl. Acad. Sci., 1963). Lucas and Jamroz (1961) should be consulted for detailed information on avian blood elements and methods for preparation and study. New information is continually being presented in *Avian Diseases,* a journal published by the American Association of Avian Pathologists.

ANAMNESIS

The pathologist who has not seen the ranch or the flock before attempting to diagnose the problem and recommend corrective measures is at a disadvantage at the outset. This disadvantage can be partially overcome by getting a *complete* history of the disease and all pertinent events leading up to the outbreak. The more information a pathologist has about the history and environment, the more directly he can proceed to solution of the problem. Unfortunately the history includes only those situations, events, and symptoms which the caretaker, owner, serviceman, or neighbor observed and remembered. Knowledge of management factors such as ventilation, feeding and watering systems, lighting program, debeaking practices, brooding and rearing procedures, routine medication and vaccination used, age, previous history of disease, location of farm, and unusual weather or farm events may make the difference between a diagnosis of the flock problem and the finding of a few miscellaneous conditions in a sample which may or may not be representative. The duration of the symptoms, the number sick and the number that have died, and when and where they were found dead are all important clues.

Poultrymen have developed a high degree of knowledge about poultry diseases and usually recognize those which result in dramatic or clear-cut symptoms and lesions. The veterinarian, therefore, is often confronted with obscure, undramatic, and complicated disease cases requiring extensive investigation to establish a diagnosis. Even if all indications are that the interruption in performance is most likely due to a management factor, the veterinarian must check all reasonable disease possibilities. This requires a systematic approach to be sure nothing is overlooked.

EXTERNAL EXAMINATION

Look for external parasites. Lice and northern fowl mites (*Ornithonyssus silviarum*) can be found on the affected chicken. If red mites (*Dermanyssus gallinae*) or blue bugs (*Argas persicus*) are suspected, an examination of roosting areas and cracks and crevices in the houses and around the yards must be made, because these species do not stay on the birds.

The general attitude of the live birds and all abnormal conditions should be carefully noted. It is very important to observe evidence of incoordination, tremors, paralytic conditions, abnormal gait and leg weakness, depression, blindness, and respiratory symptoms before the specimens are killed. It is very helpful to place the birds in a cage where they can be observed after they have become accustomed to the surroundings and perform at their best. It is sometimes advisable to save some of the affected birds to observe possible recovery from a transitory condition (transient paralysis), respiratory infection, chemical toxicity, or feed or water deprivation on the farm.

Examination should be made for tumors, abscesses, skin changes, beak condition, evidence of cannibalism, injuries, diarrhea, nasal and respiratory discharges, conjunctival exudates, feather and comb conditions, and the body fleshing condition. These are all useful clues.

OBTAINING BLOOD SAMPLES

Blood specimens may be taken at this time (or immediately after the bird is killed). Frequently it is desirable to have two (paired) blood samples several days apart to determine a rising or falling titer of immune bodies to some disease (e.g. Newcastle disease) in the serum. In this case a blood specimen may be taken from the main (brachial) wing vein, jugular vein, or by heart puncture and the bird saved for a second sample.

Venipuncture of the brachial vein is usually the simplest and best method under field conditions, especially when the bird is to be returned to the flock. Expose the vein to view by plucking a few feathers from the ventral surface of the humeral region of the wing. The vein will be seen lying in the depression between the biceps brachialis and triceps humeralis muscles. It is more easily seen if the skin is first dampened with 70% alcohol or other colorless disinfectant. The writer has found it convenient to extend both wings dorsally, grip them firmly together in the area of the wing web with the left hand, and insert the

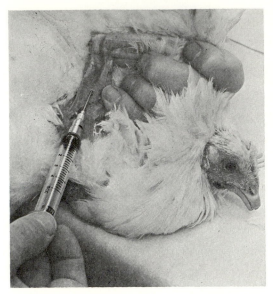

FIG. 1.14—Obtaining blood sample from the wing vein.

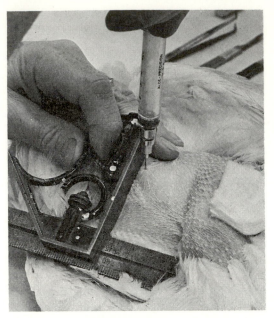

FIG. 1.15—This photo illustrates approximate location for insertion of needle for a lateral heart puncture.

needle into the vein of the right wing, holding the syringe with the right hand (Fig. 1.14). The needle should be inserted opposite to the direction of flow of the blood.

Heart puncture can be made anteromedially between the sternum and metasternum (Hofstad, 1950), laterally through the rib cage, or anteroposteriorly through the thoracic inlet. Only through experience can one learn exactly where and at what angle to insert the needle. It is best to practice these techniques on freshly killed specimens before attempting to bleed live birds. A general rule for the lateral puncture is to form an imaginary vertical line at the anterior end and at a right angle with the keel, and then palpate along the imaginary line. The heart beat can be felt and the needle inserted accordingly and to the proper depth (Fig. 1.15).

For heart puncture through the thoracic inlet, the bird should be held on its back with the keel up. The crop and contents are then pressed out of the way with a finger while the needle is guided along the ventral angle of the inlet. After penetrating the inlet, the needle is then directed horizontally and posteriorly along the midline until the heart is pierced (Fig. 1.16).

The site for heart puncture between the sternum and metasternum is (in a mature chicken) about an inch above and posterior to the point of the keel. The needle is di-

rected at approximately a 45-degree angle in an anteromedial direction toward the opposite shoulder joint. The needle should pass through the angle formed by the sternum and metasternum and directly into the heart (Fig. 1.17). For further details and illustrations see Hofstad (1950).

The size and length of needle required

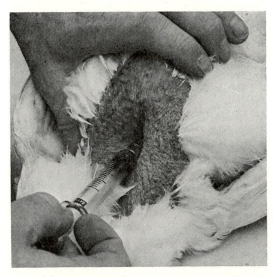

FIG. 1.16—Heart puncture through the thoracic inlet.

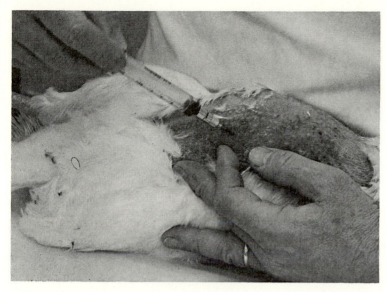

FIG. 1.17—Heart puncture can be made by inserting needle between the sternum and metasternum and directing it toward the opposite shoulder joint.

for heart and venipuncture will depend on the size of the bird. For young chicks and poults a ¾-in 20-gauge needle, and for mature chicks a 2-in 20-gauge needle, is satisfactory. Mature turkeys may require larger needles. *For quick and accurate bleeding it is essential that the needle be sharp.* Very slight vacuum should be developed in the syringe after insertion into the blood vessel or heart, because if there is too great a vacuum, the vessel wall may be drawn into and plug the beveled opening of the needle. It is sometimes necessary to rotate the needle and syringe to be sure the beveled opening is free in the lumen of the vessel.

For most serological studies the serum from 2 ml of blood is adequate. The blood should be removed aseptically and placed in a clean vial which is then laid horizontally, or nearly so, until the blood clots. An occasional sample may require a long time to clot. After the clot is firm, the vial may be returned to the vertical position to permit the serum to collect in a pool at the bottom. Frequently the serum from fat hens will appear milky due to the contained lipids. Placing the vials in an incubator will hasten syneresis. Never place a fresh sample in the refrigerator immediately after collection.

If an unclotted blood sample is required, it should be drawn into sodium citrate solution at the rate of 1.5 ml of 2% sodium citrate solution for each 10 ml of fresh blood, or deposited in a vial containing sodium citrate powder at the rate of 3 mg of sodium citrate to 1 ml of whole blood and the mixture quickly shaken. One way to prepare tubes for collecting sterile citrated blood is to add the proper amount of 2% sodium citrate solution to the collecting tubes ahead of time, then sterilize the solution and evaporate the moisture in an oven.

If a blood parasite or blood dyscrasia is suspected, smears of whole blood should be made on clean glass slides previously heated to promote rapid drying. For staining techniques see Lucas and Jamroz (1961).

A drop of blood for a wet mount or smear may be obtained from very small chicks by pricking the vein on the posteromedial side of the leg, or by pricking or cutting the immature comb.

METHODS OF KILLING BIRDS FOR POSTMORTEM

Breaking the Neck

Several methods can be used to kill fowl and each one has certain advantages. The quickest way to kill a small bird is to hold both wings over the back with one hand and the head with the other in such a way as to bend the head sharply vertically at the same time it is pulled firmly and quickly forward in a stretching manner (Fig. 1.18). This breaks the neck and spinal cord instantly. Holding both wings firmly prevents flapping and stirring of dust. If the neck is held firmly in the final position until struggling ceases, this prevents regurgi-

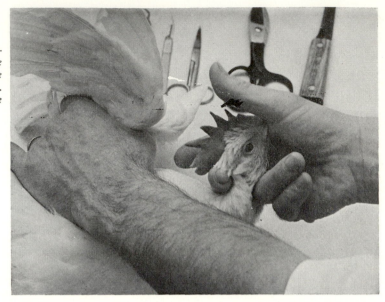

FIG. 1.18—To kill a small turkey or chicken, grasp the wings with one hand and the head with the other as shown. Then break the neck with one quick pull on the head.

tation and aspiration of crop contents into the respiratory passages.

Using a Burdizzo Forceps

Burdizzo forceps can be used for killing large chickens and turkeys (Fig. 1.19). It is difficult for one person to perform this operation and hold the bird at the same time, but it is quite easily done with the aid of an assistant. One advantage of this technique is that it also prevents regurgitation and aspiration of crop contents into the respiratory passages if the forceps are left clamped until struggling ceases.

Electrocution

Electrocution is a satisfactory method also. Clamps fixed to the end of electrical wires are fastened at opposite ends of the body of the bird, making sure the surfaces of attachment are damp to assure good electrical contact. The wires are then attached by means of a standard plug directly to 110-volt alternating house current. A switch is thrown to feed the electric current through the wires. This system has the advantage that the bird rarely struggles and thus does not stir up dust or regurgitate crop contents. With electrocution there is also less danger of agonal hemorrhages occurring or of blood spilling when tissue specimens are desired. *Obvious hazards to personnel and of short circuits on metal table tops should be kept in mind.*

Decapitation

Sudden decapitation with sharp scissors is satisfactory for very young specimens, especially when brain tissue is desired for bird passage or embryo inoculation. The

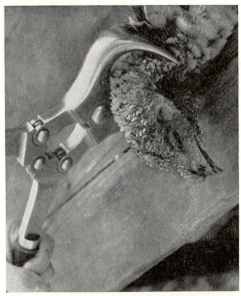

FIG. 1.19—Use of Burdizzo forceps in killing a turkey. When brought into a closed position carefully the jaws separate the vertebrae and sever the spinal cord and jugular vein without breaking the skin. (Hinshaw, Univ. Calif.)

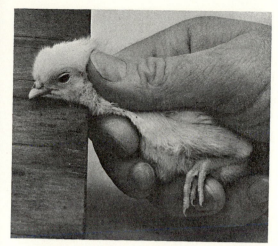

FIG. 1.20—*The neck of a small chick can be broken by pressing it against a sharp table edge.*

neck of young chicks can be broken easily by pressing firmly against a sharp table edge (Fig. 1.20) or by pinching between thumb and index finger.

Other

Magnesium sulfate solution or other euthanizing substances can be injected directly into the heart and cause sudden death. Death can be caused quickly also by injecting a large volume of air directly into the heart causing air embolism. Any injection method has the disadvantage of possible bacterial contamination of the blood stream and tissues.

POSTMORTEM PRECAUTIONS

If there is reason to suspect that the birds to be posted are infected with a disease which may be contagious for humans (e.g. ornithosis, erysipelas, equine encephalomyelitis), extra precautions are advisable. The carcass should be wet thoroughly with a disinfectant and the postmortem table surface should be wet with a disinfectant also. Good rubber gloves should be worn and care should be taken that neither the pathologist nor his assistants puncture the skin of their hands or inhale dust or aerosols from the tissues or feces during posting. All laboratory personnel who may come in contact with carcasses, tissues, or cultures should be apprised of the possible infectious nature and the precautions to be taken.

With some notable exceptions (see specific diseases) most commonly encountered poultry disease agents are not considered pathogenic for humans. Nevertheless, it would be wise to wear rubber gloves at all times while performing postmortem examinations until sufficient experience has been gained to anticipate and recognize possible human health hazards (ornithosis, erysipelas, mycosis, salmonellosis, equine encephalomyelitis, etc.). For a review of poultry diseases in public health, see Galton and Arnstein (1960). Posting specimens on metal trays which will fit into an autoclave facilitates quick sterilization of carcasses after the postmortem examination.

For routine postmortem examinations the writer has found a pair of postmortem shears to cut bones, a pair of enterotome scissors to incise the gut, a postmortem knife to cut skin and muscle, a scalpel for fine examination of tissues, and a pair of forceps to be adequate. These should be supplemented with sterile syringes, needles, vials, and petri dishes for collecting blood samples and tissue specimens as the situation dictates (Fig. 1.21).

POSTMORTEM TECHNIQUE

Exposing Internal Organs

The bird is laid on its back and each leg, in turn, drawn outward away from the body while the skin is incised between the leg and abdomen on each side (Fig. 1.22A). Both legs are then grasped firmly in the

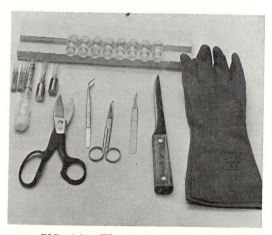

FIG. 1.21—*These instruments and equipment are adequate for most postmortem examinations of poultry.*

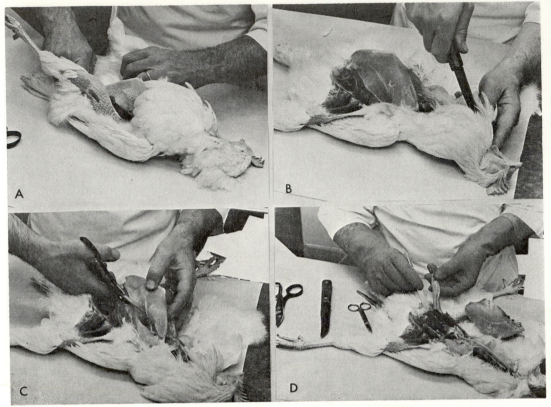

FIG. 1.22—Each pathologist develops his own technique for postmortem examination. This technique will aid the beginner. (A) Sever the skin and fascia between the legs and abdomen and break the legs out of the acetabular articulation. (B) Incise and reflect the skin from the vent to the beak. (C) Remove the breast, taking care not to sever large blood vessels. (D) Expose the viscera for examination.

area of the femur and bent forward, downward, and outward, until the heads of both femurs are broken free of the acetabular attachment so both legs will lie flat on the table.

The skin is cut between the two previous incisions at a point midway between keel and vent. The cut edge is then forcibly reflected forward, cutting as necessary, until the entire ventral aspect of the body, including the neck, is exposed (Fig. 1.22B). Hemorrhages of the musculature, if present, can be detected at this stage.

Either of two procedures is now used to expose the viscera. A postmortem knife is used to cut through the abdominal wall transversely midway between the keel and vent and then through the breast muscles on each side. Posting shears are used to cut first the rib cage and then the coracoid and clavicle on both sides (Fig. 1.22C).

With some care this can be done without severing the large blood vessels. The process may also be done equally well in reverse order, cutting first through the clavicle and coracoid and then through the rib cage and abdominal wall on each side. The sternum and attached structures can now be removed from the body and laid aside. The organs are now in full view and may be removed as they are examined (Fig. 1.22D).

If a blood sample has not previously been taken and the bird was killed just prior to postmortem examination, a sample can be removed by heart puncture at any stage that the heart is exposed to view.

Initiating Laboratory Procedures

IMPRESSION SMEARS. If the foregoing procedures have all been done aseptically, the internal organs will not be contaminated;

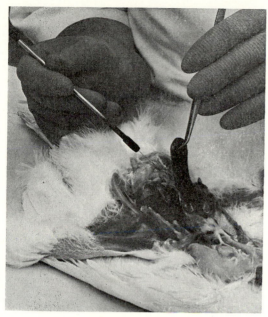

FIG. 1.23—If the abdominal cavity has been carefully opened, bacterial cultures can be taken from unexposed surfaces of the viscera without fear of extraneous contamination.

if exudates suggest the need, impression smears with sterile slides can now be taken.

BACTERIAL CULTURES. If gross lesions indicate bacterial cultures are needed, they can be made from the unexposed surfaces of the viscera without searing the surface (Fig. 1.23). If contamination has occurred, the surface of the organs should be seared with a hot iron designed for the purpose before inserting a sterile culture loop. Care must be taken not to sear the tissue excessively. It is often desirable to transfer large tissue samples aseptically to a sterile petri dish and take them to the bacteriological laboratory for initial culture in cleaner surroundings.

BILE SAMPLES. If infection with a vibrio species is suspected, a bile sample for wet mount examination or bacterial culture can be made at this point.

RESPIRATORY VIRUS ISOLATIONS. If a respiratory disease is suspected and virus culture or bird passage is desirable, an intact section of lower trachea, the bronchi, and upper portions of the lungs is removed aseptically with sterile scissors and forceps and

transferred to a sterile mortar and pestle for grinding, or to a sterile petri dish for temporary storage and later grinding. Other tissues (e.g. air sac tissue) can be added aseptically to the sample or transferred to other sterile containers for separate study. The trachea can now be incised, and if exudate is present, it can be added to the above collection or saved in separate vials.

Grinding of such specimens is facilitated by adding a portion of sterile sand or, preferably, alundum (mesh #60) to the mortar contents. The ground tissues are then transferred to sterile covered centrifuge tubes and spun at low speeds to prepare a supernate free of particulate matter for embryo, nutrient media, or cell culture inoculation or for inoculation of experimental birds.

Similar procedures can be followed for initial virus isolation from other visceral organs.

SALMONELLA CULTURES. All other visceral organs should be examined for lesions and, where indicated, cultures made and tissue specimens saved before the intestinal tract is cut. Once it is opened, gross contamination of other organs with gut contents is almost certain to occur. If Salmonella infection is suspected, selected sections of the gut are removed with sterile forceps and scissors and placed either directly into a sterile mortar and pestle or into a sterile petri dish for later culture. For routine examination the writer has used a single section comprising the lower ileum, proximal portions of the ceca and the cecal "tonsils," and proximal portion of the large intestine, all of which are minced and ground aseptically for the inoculum. Tissues of other visceral organs may be added to the gut collection or cultured separately. Alternatively, sterile swabs may be used to obtain samples from the exposed gut lining for Salmonella cultures. (See Chapter 3 for detailed culture technique.)

MISCELLANEOUS. After necessary cultures have been made the intestine may be laid out on newspaper or tabletop for examination for inflammation, exudates, parasites, foreign bodies, malfunctions, tumors, and abscesses. The various nerves, bone structure, marrow condition, and joints can now be examined. The sciatic nerve can be examined by dissecting away the musculature on the medial side of the thigh. Inside the body cavity the sciatic plexus is obscured by kidney tissue. These nerves can best be exposed by scraping away the kidney tissue with the blunt end of a scalpel. The nerves of the brachial plexuses are easily found on either side near the thoracic inlet and should be examined for enlargement. Examination of the vagus nerves in their entirety should be made. Otherwise, short enlargements are frequently overlooked.

The ease or difficulty with which the bones can be cut with the posting shears is an indication of their condition. The costochrondal junctions should be palpated and examined for enlargement ("beading") and the long bones cut longitudinally through the epiphysis to examine for abnormal calcification. The rigidity of the tibiotarsus or metatarsus should be tested by bending and breaking to check for nutritional deficiency. A healthy bone will make an audible snap when it breaks. Bones from a chicken deficient in vitamin D or minerals may be so lacking in mineral elements that they can be bent at any angle without breaking.

Joint exudate, if present, can be removed after first plucking the feathers and searing the overlying skin with a hot iron. After searing, the skin may be incised with a sterile scalpel and then the joint exudate removed with a sterile inoculating loop for culture seeding.

Paranasal sinus exudates can be removed in a manner similar to that used for the joint exudate.

EXPOSING AND REMOVING THE BRAIN. Removing the intact brain is not easy since the meningeal layers are attached firmly to the bony structures in some places. The following technique can be performed quickly and is satisfactory for examination and removal of the brain in most instances.

Remove the head at the atlanto-occipital junction and remove the lower mandible. Sear the cut surface with a hot searing iron and trim away excess loose tissue. Reflect the skin forward over the skull and upper mandible and hold it firmly in that position with one hand. Sterile instruments should be used for the succeeding steps if a portion of the brain is needed for animal passage, virus isolation, or fungus or bacterial culture.

With the sterilized tips of a pair of heavy-jawed posting shears nip just through the bone to the cranial cavity on both sides of the head, beginning at the occipital foramen and proceeding forward laterally to the midpoint at the anterior edge of the cranial cavity (Fig. 1.24A). Lift off the cut portion of bone and expose the entire brain (Fig. 1.24B).

If a portion is needed for culture or animal passage (e.g. avian encephalomyelitis virus suspect) and a portion also for histopathological examination (e.g. vitamin E deficiency), cut the brain medially from anterior to posterior along the midline with a sharp sterile scalpel blade. With sterile sharp curved scissors, cut the nerves and attachments carefully from one of the brain halves while the head is tipped upside down so the loosened portion will fall out into the jar of formalin as it is freed. The second half can now be removed aseptically, but without concern for preservation of tissue structure, to a sterile petri dish or sterile mortar and pestle. The separate halves may also be removed in reverse order (Figs. 1.24C, D). If all of the brain is required for either purpose, proceed with the proper precautions for the purpose intended. If the brain is destined only for sectioning, it may alternatively be fixed in situ and removed after fixing. Large brain portions should be incised longitudinally to permit good penetration of the fixative.

TISSUES FOR HISTOPATHOLOGICAL EXAMINATION. Frequently it is necessary to have stained tissue slices prepared. These are very often prepared by another department or sent to a special laboratory. The quality of the slide is no better than the quality of the specimen saved and the care taken to preserve it. For good preservation the tissue pieces should be saved immediately after death from killed birds, especially brain tissue which decomposes rapidly. The tissue specimens should be small to allow quick penetration of fixative, be gently incised with a sharp scalpel or razor blade to preserve the tissue structure, and be preserved in ten times their own volume of 10% formalin or other fixative. Zenker's fixative may be used for all tissues except brain and spinal cord. Bone pieces should be sawed with a sharp bone saw unless thin or soft enough to cut with scissors or scalpel. After proper labeling and dating

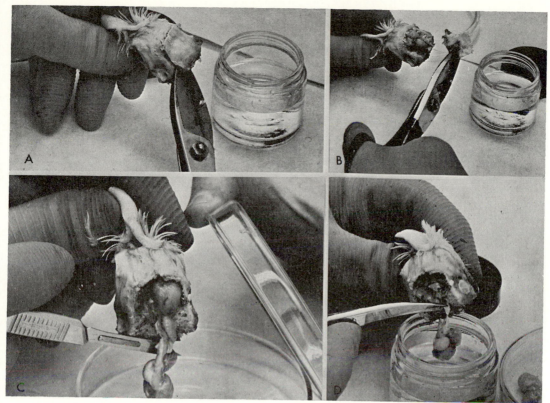

FIG. 1.24—*With a little practice the brain can be removed with a minimum of trauma.* **(A)** *Incise bone all the way around periphery of the cranial cavity with heavy posting shears.* **(B)** *Remove loosened portion of the bony skull.* **(C)** *Incise brain longitudinally with sterile, sharp scalpel and remove one-half for sterile culture technique.* **(D)** *Remove second half by dropping it into 10% formalin for histological techniques.*

they should be sent immediately to the processing laboratory.

Lung tissue usually floats on the surface of the fixing solution because air is trapped in the tissue. Satisfactory fixation can be accomplished by placing absorbent cotton over the tissue which serves to keep it immersed in the fixative. Methods to exhaust the air from the air spaces in the lung tissue by pulling a vacuum over the fixative during fixation can be used but are less satisfactory and may result in artifacts.

After fixing, bone tissue must be decalcified in order to cut it with a microtome. Nitric acid solution (10 parts nitric acid: 90 parts 70% alcohol) may be used for this purpose, and decalcification requires a week or more.

If eye tissue is to be saved for sectioning, a window should be cut through the scleral wall to allow fixative to quickly penetrate the vitreous body and thus reach the internal eye structures.

Any tissue held too long in formalin fixative becomes excessively hard. If processing is to be delayed, tissues should be transferred to 70% alcohol after 48 hours in fixative. Textbooks on histological techniques such as Luna (1968), Thompson (1966), and Preece (1965) should be consulted for detailed procedures.

Progressive Examination Hints

The following procedures during the course of postmortem examination may be helpful to the beginner in checking for some commonly encountered diseases. They are not intended as definitive diagnostic procedures. To arrive at a diagnosis, the student and beginning diagnostician must refer to the characteristic symptoms and lesions, diagnostic procedures, and characteristics of the infectious agent discussed under the specific diseases.

COCCIDIA. Observe and note the subserosa

before incising the intestine. Make wet mount smears of mucosal scrapings from various segments of the intestine and of cecal contents and examine directly under the microscope for suspended oocysts and merozoites and for stages undergoing development in the epithelial cells (tissue stages).

OTHER PROTOZOA. Make wet mounts of affected areas, adding a little warm physiological saline solution if necessary to provide fluid, and examine under microscope for Hexamita, histamonads, and trichomonads.

CAPILLARIA WORMS AND ASCARID LARVAE. Collect mucous exudate and deep mucosal scrapings and press into a thin layer between two thick pieces of plate glass. Examine before a strong light or under low-power magnification for the presence of the parasites. Under magnification look for double-poled, lemon-shaped eggs in the female capillaria.

FUNGUS. Make wet mount smears of scrapings of affected areas and add 20% sodium or potassium hydroxide. Digest with frequent warming for 15 minutes or more and examine under high-power magnification for mold hyphae.

VIBRIO. Examine fresh bile wet mounts under dark-field or phase illumination. Only positive findings have significance.

BACTEREMIA AND BLOOD PARASITES. Make fresh mounts, preferably with citrated blood, and examine under light- and dark-field illumination for viable organisms. Make fresh blood smears and air dry for staining by Giemsa, Gram, Wright's, or other methods.

EXUDATES. If infectious coryza is suspected, make thin smears of clear nasal or sinus exudate for staining by Giemsa, Gram, methylene blue, or other method. Inoculate appropriate media for culture of the organism.

ABSCESSES. Select appropriate culture media suitable for growth of a variety of infectious organisms which may be suspected of causing the abscess. Sear and incise the surface of the abscess and inoculate the culture media with material taken from the abscess with a sterile inoculating loop. Make smears from the abscess on clean glass slides, diluting with a drop of water if the material is too thick. Air dry and flame the slides and make Gram, acid-fast, or other stains as desired.

EMBRYO INOCULATION FOR VIRUS ISOLATIONS. For routine virus isolation attempts, centrifuged and/or filtered fine-ground suspensions of suspect tissues (trachea, bronchi, lung, liver, spleen, kidney, brain, bone marrow) or body fluids and exudates may be inoculated into the chorioallantoic cavity and yolk sac, and onto the chorioallantoic membrane of embryos at various stages of incubation. (See specific diseases for virus culture techniques. Also, see Cunningham [1966] for selection of the proper age of embryo and route of inoculation for various disease agents, as well as detailed inoculation procedures.) Figure 1.25 illustrates the various routes of inoculation of embryonating eggs. Since the purpose of virus isolation is to determine what viruses may be present, it is advisable to inoculate various ages of embryo by the various routes of inoculation. Several blind passages may be necessary before the culture attempt can reasonably be considered negative. A simple technique which does not require dropping the chorioallantoic membrane has been described by Gorham (1957).

The chorioallantoic membrane may be drawn away from the shell (dropped) to facilitate inoculation. First drill or punch a small hole in the shell over the air cell, then slowly drill another hole through the shell at a point on the side of the egg over the embryo while simultaneously applying mild suction through a rubber tube over the hole into the air cell. Due to the reduced pressure in the egg, air will force the chorioallantoic membrane slowly away from the inner shell membrane when the drill penetrates the latter. A strong (candling) light should be used while suction is applied to determine when the chorioallantoic membrane has dropped.

For yolk sac inoculation, the inoculating needle can be directed through the air cell and directly to the center of the egg. Some yolk can be withdrawn into the syringe to be sure of the location of the needle. There is less danger of injury to the embryo during this procedure if the eggs are first held several hours in a horizontal position and

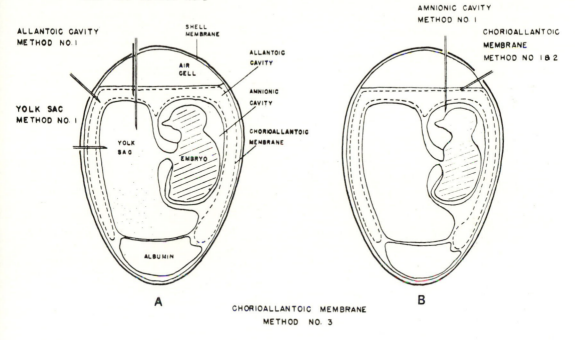

ALLANTOIC CAVITY METHOD NO. 2

YOLK SAC METHOD NO. 2

ALLANTOIC CAVITY
METHOD NO. 1

YOLK SAC
METHOD NO. 1

SHELL
MEMBRANE

AIR
CELL

ALLANTOIC
CAVITY

AMNIONIC
CAVITY

CHORIOALLANTOIC
MEMBRANE

YOLK
SAC

EMBRYO

ALBUMIN

A

AMNIONIC CAVITY
METHOD NO. 1

CHORIOALLANTOIC
MEMBRANE
METHOD NO 1 & 2

B

CHORIOALLANTOIC MEMBRANE
METHOD NO. 3

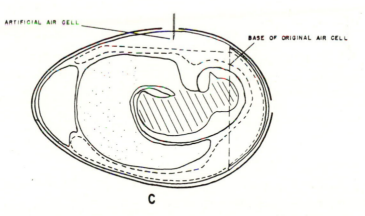

ARTIFICIAL AIR CELL

BASE OF ORIGINAL AIR CELL

C

FIG. 1.25—Routes of inoculation of embryonating chicken eggs. (Cunningham, 1966)

then placed upright, small end down, for the inoculation.

For chorioallantoic cavity inoculation, a hole is drilled over the edge of the air cell at a spot previously marked with the aid of a candling light. The cavity lies adjacent to the shell and can be easily penetrated from that point.

All holes should be sealed with hot paraffin or other suitable sterile material before reincubating.

Disposing of the Specimen

If a disease infectious for humans is suspected, the carcass should be autoclaved, incinerated, or otherwise rendered incapable of causing infection to laboratory or other personnel. Similar precautions should be followed during disposal of carcasses infected with a virulent poultry pathogen which presents a health hazard to the poultry industry. The posting area, instruments, and gloves should then be washed with a disinfectant solution.

DISINFECTANTS

To disinfect is "to free from pathogenic substances or organisms or to render them inert"; a disinfectant is an "agent that disinfects chiefly by destroying infective agents (pathogenic microorganisms) or rendering ferments inactive"; disinfection is "the act or process of destroying pathogenic germs or agents" (Dorland, 1951).

PROPERTIES

Among the properties of an ideal disinfectant are (1) low cost per unit of disinfecting value, (2) ready solubility in hard water, (3) relative safety for man and animals, (4) ready availability, (5) nondestructibility to utensils and fabrics, (6) stability when exposed to air, (7) absence of objectionable or lingering odor, (8) no residual toxicity, (9) effectiveness for a large variety of infectious agents, and (10) no deleterious accumulation of any portion of the disinfectant in meat or eggs. *For any disinfectant to be effective in economical quantities it must be applied to surfaces which have first been freed of debris and organic material by thorough washing or severe dry cleaning. When this basic condition is fulfilled, many disinfectants are highly efficient.*

TYPES

Many disinfectants of similar composition are sold under different trade names.

Before buying a product with an unfamiliar name, one should compare types and values with a well-known product. The directions for dilutions given by the manufacturer should be closely followed in making up a disinfectant for use. For a complete discussion of various disinfectants and sterilization methods in common use, consult Reddish (1957) and Lawrence and Block (1968). Additional references on disinfectants and their use are Phillips and Warshowsky (1958), Glick et al. (1961), and textbooks on pharmacology and therapeutics.

Phenol (Carbolic Acid)

Phenol is a chemical substance obtained from coal tar. In its pure form it occurs as colorless needles having a characteristic and familiar odor (e.g. lysol soap). It is usually sold in water solutions and is too expensive for general poultry house use. It is, however, the chemical used as a basis for determining the phenol coefficients of disinfectants (relative ability to kill specific test organisms when compared to that of phenol). See Prindle and Wright (1968) for a complete discussion of the phenolic compounds. In recent years commercial disinfectants containing phenolic compounds have been developed and marketed at cost values which permit wider use in poultry operations. Some have residual activity persisting after they have dried which has the advantage of continued suppression of bacterial and viral populations on sprayed surfaces.

Cresols

Cresols are compounds closely related chemically to phenol and having similar bactericidal properties. They are thick yellow or brown liquids, miscible with water but only slightly soluble. They form the bases for a large number of commercial brands of disinfectants made by combining cresol with soap.

A list of cresylic disinfectants permitted for use for official disinfection is published periodically by the United States Department of Agriculture, Agricultural Research Service, Animal Health Division. This list (Saulmon, 1968) will serve as a guide for the use of specific products.

Bis-phenols

Bis-phenols are compounds composed of two phenol molecules modified and joined together by various chemical linkages. Halogens, particularly chlorine, have been combined with the bis-phenols to increase their effectiveness, and some of the chlorophenols have high antifungal activity. Bisphenols are frequently combined with other phenolic compounds in disinfectants. See Gump and Walter (1968) for additional information.

Pine Oil

Pine oil has proved satisfactory as a disinfectant and has the advantage of being less injurious to the skin than the cresol compounds. The odor is also less objectionable and in fact is rather pleasant, which enhances its desirability for use in offices and lavatory areas. Since it is insoluble in water, it is used in the emulsion form with soap or other emulsifying agent.

Hypochlorites and Chlorinated Lime

Chlorine is the basis of the disinfectants known as hypochlorites, which contain about 70% available chlorine. Hypochlorites, according to Dychdala (1968), are available as powders containing calcium hypochlorite and sodium hypochlorite combined with hydrated trisodium phosphate and as liquids containing sodium hypochlorite. Chlorinated lime (bleaching powder), prepared by saturating slaked lime with chlorine gas, was one of the earliest recognized disinfectants. It has been largely supplanted by the more readily available hypochlorites.

The products containing sodium hypochlorite are essentially liquids ranging in concentrations from 1 to 15%. The 15% solutions are used to prepare 5% solutions with water for bleaches and sanitizing agents. Germicidal potency of hypochlorites is dependent upon both the concentration of available chlorine and the pH (acidity) of the solution, or upon the amount of hypochlorous acid formed, which is, in turn, dependent upon both factors. The influence of pH, especially in dilute solutions, is even greater than the percentage of available chlorine. Increasing the pH decreases the biocidal activity of chlorine, and decreasing the pH increases the activity. Germicidal activity is speeded up by raising the temperature.

If used according to directions, hypochlorites are highly efficient. These products are used for chlorination of water supplies, swimming pools, sewage effluents, and for preparation of bleaching and sanitizing solutions. Their principal use in the poultry industry is for egg washing and sanitizing and for disinfecting limited areas such as incubators, incubator and hatcher trays and other areas around the hatchery, egg breaking areas, small brooders, and water and feed containers, though they can also be used on cement surfaces. All surfaces to be disinfected with hypochlorite solutions must first be thoroughly cleaned in order to insure the greatest efficiency. Stock supplies should be kept in dark cool places, and the containers should be tightly sealed when not in use. Fresh solutions must be prepared daily.

All products containing chlorine must be handled with care because free chlorine is destructive to fabrics, leather, and metal.

Occasionally there is need to reduce, remove, or neutralize the chlorine from chlorinated water sources, particularly when administering water vaccines. The following methods have been suggested to the writer by public water department officials and others: aerate (this is the most commonly recommended method), boil, expose the water to sunlight in clear jugs (this converts the chlorine compounds to hydrochloric acid), pass through charcoal filters, add 4 ml of 10% solution of sodium thiosulphate to a gallon of chlorinated water, or add protein to the water. Gentry (1968) has suggested the addition of 1 lb dried milk per 50 gal water when mixing water vaccines. The efficacy of any of these methods is dependent upon the original concentration of chlorine in the water, and advice on a suitable method of dechlorination should be sought locally from the public water department officials. It may be cheaper and more practical to obtain distilled or potable nonchlorinated water for mixing and administering water vaccines.

Organic Iodine Combinations

Iodine has long been recognized as an effective germ killer. Many of the disadvantages of earlier products have been overcome by combining iodine in organic complexes, sometimes called "tamed iodine." The term "iodophor" refers to a combination of iodine with a solubilizing agent which slowly liberates free iodine when diluted with water. The term most frequently refers to formulas that consist of iodine complexed with certain types of surface-active agents that have detergent properties. These complexes are said to enhance the bactericidal activity of iodine and render the iodine nontoxic, nonirritating, and nonstaining if used as directed. The detergent also makes the products water soluble and stable under usual conditions of storage. There is no offensive odor and the detergent properties impart cleansing activity. See Gershenfeld (1968) for additional information on iodine compounds.

A group of commercial iodophors have been developed and marketed for a wide variety of disinfectant uses. Some of these products have a built-in indicator of germicidal activity because as the solution is used up, the normal amber color fades. When the solution is no longer effective it is colorless. The products can be mixed in cold and in hard water. The organic iodine products have a wide variety of uses in the industry. They can be applied without hazard to nearly all surfaces and are useful for disinfecting hatchery and incubator surfaces, incubator and hatcher trays, egg breaking areas, feeders and fountains, footwear, and poultry buildings. Like other disinfectants, these compounds are most effective on clean surfaces.

Quicklime
(Unslaked Lime, Calcium Oxide)

The action of quicklime depends on the liberation of heat and oxygen when the chemical comes in contact with water. On the poultry farm its use is limited to small yard areas that are damp and cannot be exposed to the sun, to the disinfection of drains and fecal matter, and to whitewashes. Adding chlorinated lime to quicklime at the rate of 1 lb/40 gal of wash increases its disinfecting value in whitewashes. As quicklime has a caustic action, birds should be kept away from it until it has become thoroughly dry.

Hydrated lime, according to Yushok and Bear (1944), when used as a preservative and deodorizing agent for poultry manure also has value as a partial disinfectant. Mixed with fresh manure at the rate of 200 lb/ton of manure, it was found to have a bactericidal effect in a 15-minute period. Similarly it prevented the sporulation of coccidial oocysts and the segmentation and embryonation of *Ascaridia galli* eggs. Another advantage of this use is that treated manure is unattractive to flies and rodents. Fly maggots are not produced in the treated dropping pits, and both mice and rats avoid them.

Lye

Lye is an excellent cleansing agent, valuable in any disinfecting program. A 2% solution of sodium hydroxide (soda lye) is a good disinfectant for many of the pathogenic microorganisms. It is frequently used along with broom action to simultaneously clean and disinfect floors that have first been swept free of debris.

Formaldehyde

Formaldehyde is a gas. It is sold commercially in a 40% solution (37% by weight) with water under the name of formalin. For spraying it is used in a 10% solution of formalin (that is, a 4% solution of formaldehyde). It may also be purchased as a powder known as paraformaldehyde (paraform, triformal). When heated this powder liberates formaldehyde gas, and if used in proper portions it may be substituted for formalin as a source of the gas. Manufacturer's directions on amounts to use for each type of equipment and the means of liberating the gas must be carefully observed. Figure 1.26 illustrates one method of heating paraformaldehyde powder to liberate formaldehyde gas. This electric pan should be equipped with a thermostat and a timer which can be controlled from outside the incubator or fumigation chamber.

Formaldehyde gas is often generated by mixing formalin and potassium permanganate ($KMnO_4$) in an earthenware crock or metal container. Because of the heat generated by the chemical reaction, glass containers should not be used. The container should be deep and have a volume several times that of the combined chemicals because considerable bubbling and splattering takes place.

The ratio in liquid measure of formalin is approximately twice the dry measure of potassium permanganate (e.g., 1 g $KMnO_4$ to 2 cc formalin, or 1 oz $KMnO_4$ to 2 oz formalin). If too much formalin is used, the excess will remain in the vessel. If too much potassium permanganate is used, the excess remains unchanged and is wasted. Potassium permanganate is poisonous. Both of these compounds must be kept in accident-proof containers in a safe place away from children.

A suitable fumigation cabinet consists of a source of heat, a fan to circulate the warm humid air and fumigant, a source of

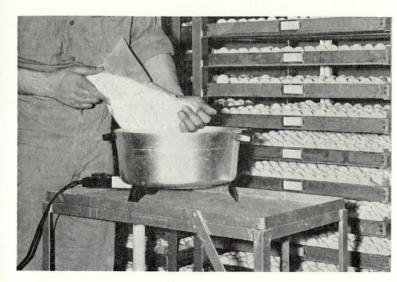

FIG. 1.26—An electrically heated pan for use in liberating formaldehyde gas from paraformaldehyde. (Vineland Poultry Laboratories)

humidifying moisture, and a method of generating formaldehyde gas. The box should be reasonably airtight, and an exhausting device from the fumigation box to the outside of the building is desirable.

Though a powerful disinfectant, formaldehyde has many disadvantages, especially its volatility, penetrating odor, caustic action, and tendency to harden the skin—properties which make it disagreeable to apply. It is extremely irritating to the conjunctiva and mucous membranes, and some people are very sensitive to it. Because of this, precautions must be taken to exhaust the gas to the exterior and prevent its escape into areas where people must work. Its chief advantages are as follows: (1) It can be used as a gas or vapor for fumigation of eggs and incubators or small rooms. (2) It is relatively nontoxic to animals and fowl. (3) It is an efficient disinfectant in the presence of organic matter. (4) It does not injure utensils and spraying equipment with which it comes in contact.

Formaldehyde gas is widely used in poultry enterprises for the fumigation of hatching eggs to destroy shell contaminants. Other uses are fumigation of incubators, hatchers, trays, egg containers, and equipment that might be ruined or inadequately penetrated by other disinfectants. It can be used for fumigating clothing and bulky utensils if necessary. Fumigation of poultry houses is, as a rule, impractical because of the difficulty in making them airtight, the large volumes required, and difficulties of establishing proper conditions for effective fumigation.

Fumigation of incubators and eggs has become an established practice in the industry and has varied little over the years. Various recommendations have been made for quantities, humidity, temperature, and time for adequate sterilization of the shells of hatching eggs. Stover (1964) and more recently Williams and Siegel (1969) have recommended a temperature of 70–75° F and 70% humidity. Approximately 60 g potassium permanganate and 120 cc formalin are used per 100 cu ft of cabinet space. Fumigation is for at least 20 minutes. When fumigation is completed, the exhaust ducts are opened and the gas exhausted. The writer considers these as minimum requirements for effective shell sterilization of eggs stacked in plastic flats in large commercial-type fumigation cabinets filled to capacity and, based on unreported work of associates, recommends greater quantities of chemicals (75 g $KNnO_4$:150 cc formalin per 100 cu ft of space), higher humidity (up to 90%), higher temperature (90° F), longer time (up to 30 minutes), and vigorous agitation of the gas during fumigation so it will penetrate the spaces and effectively sanitize the surfaces of eggs in the centers of large stacks. Pressed paper egg flats trap formaldehyde gas and may be disagreeable to handle for some time after fumigation; therefore, plastic flats or wire baskets are preferable for holding eggs for this purpose. Proper fumigation and subsequent aeration of the fumigated eggs creates somewhat of a dilemma, because excess ventilation of the egg surface may result in excess removal of carbon dioxide and perhaps other gases and thus reduce hatchability of fertile eggs (Becker et al., 1964). Determination of optimum sanitizing and storage methods of hatching eggs is a field of active research, and the reader should consult current issues of *Poultry Science* and other poultry publications for more information.

Similar procedures are used for fumigating the inside and the contents, including the eggs, of incubators and hatchers, but the quantity of formaldehyde is sometimes reduced. Most incubator manufacturers have recommendations for their type of machine.

Certain precautions are necessary after fumigation of hatching eggs. The incoming air for exhaustion must be clean, otherwise the humid surface of the egg can become recontaminated. During extremely cold weather, outside air must be warmed before entering the fumigation chamber to avoid overchilling the eggs. While humidity is essential for disinfective activity of the formaldehyde, the surface of the eggs should not become visibly wet during fumigation and should be dry when the eggs leave the fumigator. Fumigation in the incubators should not be done between the 12th and 84th hours of incubation because of the danger of injuring embryos at that stage of development (Stover, 1964). Also it should not be done at such high concentration after the hatch begins because of the danger of injuring the chick or poult.

Formaldehyde gas may be generated in incubators and hatchers by using approximately 20 cc formalin solution per 100 cu ft of space. The formalin is soaked onto enough cheesecloth so it does not drip and hung in the circulating currents in the incubator. The effectiveness of this method is limited because of the low concentration.

Chicks that have been overfumigated may develop a high-pitched, whistling-type chirp, and chick mortality in the hatchery or brooder house is an aftermath of excessive late fumigation.

A method of fumigation referred to by Glick et al. (1961) which is used for decontamination of large enclosed areas and which might be adapted for use in ventilating systems of large light- and temperature-controlled houses consists of liberation of formaldehyde gas by steam. In this system commercial grade formaldehyde solution (37%) with 12% methanol (5 parts 37% formaldehyde and 3 parts methyl alcohol adjusted to pH 5.0) is liberated into the space by a steam ejector at the rate of 1 ml formaldehyde for each cubic foot of air flow for 30 minutes. The methanol reduces deposits of polymers on interior surfaces of the treated spaces. The temperature of the space to be decontaminated must be maintained at above 70° F and the relative humidity above 70%.

For smaller spaces such as cabinets, small rooms, and incubators, a portable vaporizer such as the Hydro-mist Vaporizer Model H may be used to disperse the formaldehyde gas. This and other types commonly used for decontamination of air filtration systems are described by Decker et al. (1962).

Formaldehyde may be neutralized with ammonium hydroxide by using a quantity of 25–28% solution not to exceed one-half the quantity of formalin used in the fumigation. The ammonia may be released by sprinkling about in the fumigated area but not until the fumigated surfaces have dried completely.

Ethylene Oxide

Ethylene oxide is a colorless gas at ordinary temperatures, liquefying readily at 10.8° C and freezing at —111.3° C. The liquid is miscible with water and all organic solvents in all proportions. It is highly flammable and for this reason is dangerous to use by itself. It is now extensively used in the form of a low-pressure mixture with nonflammable chlorofluorohydrocarbons (Freons) in a disposable 16-oz can (Haenni et al., 1959). Chambers for utilization of such mixtures are described by Schley et al. (1960) and Glick et al. (1961). See also Phillips (1968) for more information on this disinfectant.

It probably has limited use in the poultry industry because of its flammability (somewhat comparable to diethylether) and need for dispensing under slight pressure. It does, however, have many advantages over formaldehyde gas and has been shown to be effective against many poultry pathogens, including viruses (Mathews and Hofstad, 1953).

Copper Sulfate (Bluestone)

Although copper sulfate and other salts of copper have a marked toxic effect upon some of the lower forms of life, they are not considered good general disinfectants. Copper sulfate is toxic to algae and fungi and has been used in attempts to check or prevent outbreaks of fungus diseases. It has been used in the feed at ½ lb per ton and sometimes 1 lb per ton for short periods without noticeable toxicity to chickens. Poultry will usually drink water containing copper sulfate at no greater concentration than 1:2,000 of water, but a greater concentration than 1:500 may be toxic when given as the only source of drinking water. Turkeys do not like water containing copper sulfate and will seek other water supplies if available. A 0.5% solution may be of value for disinfecting feed hoppers, water fountains, and areas around these in fungus-disease outbreaks.

Mercuric Chloride (Bichloride of Mercury, Corrosive Sublimate)

Although a powerful disinfectant, mercuric chloride is limited in usefulness by its cost, toxicity, and marked corrosive action on metals. It is commonly used in a 1:1,000 dilution with water. Because its value is markedly lowered by the presence of organic matter and because it has certain other undesirable properties, it cannot be recommended for disinfection of poultry equipment, houses, or litter.

Quaternary Ammonium Surface-Active Disinfectants (Quats)

There are several of these products now on the market, and they are considered to be good disinfectants if used according to directions. They are water clear, odorless, nonirritating to the skin, good deodorants, and have a marked detergent action. They contain no phenols, halogens, or heavy metals and are highly stable and relatively nontoxic. It is important to remember that quaternary ammonium compounds cannot be used in soapy solutions. It is also important that all surfaces to be disinfected be thoroughly rinsed with water to remove any residue of soap or anionic detergent before using a Quat for sterilizing purposes. Some hard-water minerals may interfere with the action of Quats. See Lawrence (1968) for more information on these compounds.

Quaternary ammonia compounds are used for washing eggs and disinfecting hatchery surfaces, incubator and hatcher trays, egg breaking equipment and areas, feeders and waterers, and footwear among other uses.

Sunlight and Ultraviolet Radiation

The sun's direct rays are the best disinfectant known. However, since the material to be treated must be in thin layers and exposed to the direct rays, this method is limited to yards and utensils that can be thoroughly cleaned before being exposed. The construction of most poultry houses prevents efficient disinfection by the sun. A cement platform fully exposed to the sun makes a convenient place for treating movable equipment. If properly constructed with a drain, such a platform can be used as a washing and disinfection rack. A concrete apron before the poultry house entry will be washed by rains or can be washed by hose in order to take advantage of the disinfecting power of the sun's rays (Fig. 1.3).

There are many types of germicidal (ultraviolet) lamps, but there is not enough scientific evidence available to warrant a recommendation for their general use in hatcheries or on poultry farms. For a complete review on the use of UV radiation in microbiological laboratories, the reader is referred to Phillips and Hanel (1960).

Hot Water

Hot water adds to the efficiency of most disinfectants and, if applied in the form of boiling water or live steam, is effective without the addition of any chemical. Detergents added to systems for generating and disseminating hot water and steam will increase cleaning and decontaminating efficiency. Live steam must be applied directly and at close range to the part to be disinfected.

Dry Heat

Dry heat in the form of a flame is effective provided the flame comes in contact with the bacteria to be killed. All methods involving direct flame are dangerous fire hazards and are not recommended except possibly on cement surfaces.

Many additional commercial disinfectants, mostly organic compounds, are available under trade names. Many of these are combinations of several individual disinfectants with complementary disinfecting properties. Some also have long residual activity. In order to choose disinfectants wisely, one must continually keep abreast of new product development through current valid scientific and lay publications.

Residues of disinfectants used to sanitize drinking fountains should be rinsed off with fresh water before water vaccines are given as they can be destructive to the vaccine virus.

DISINFESTANTS

PROPERTIES

Disinfestants (sometimes called parasiticides, insecticides, or pesticides) destroy animal parasites such as lice, mites, ticks, and fleas. They also destroy other undesirable insects (e.g. flies, beetles, ants, sow bugs). Some pesticides are highly toxic to man and livestock. Their use is recommended only as an adjunct to a properly conducted sanitary control program. Many disinfectants are also destructive to lice, mites, and other similar parasites, provided they come in contact with the parasite. Many, however, are useless as disinfestants.

Suitable insecticides are those which can be used on or around poultry without causing toxic effects from contact or ingestion and do not accumulate in the tissues or eggs as a result of ingestion or absorption.

The list of available and permissable commercial insecticides changes frequently. Chlorinated hydrocarbons such as DDT, so widely used in the past, have virtually been eliminated from use around food animals because of the ready storage of the insecticide in fatty tissue and in eggs (Bearse, 1966). Recently another old standby, sodium fluoride powder, has been banned from usage. Several other insecticides have found wide usage in the past, but populations of insects resistant to them have developed and rendered them ineffective. It is necessary to keep informed, through government and university advisers and industry representatives, on effective insecticides and the methods and areas where they may be used. Some of those permitted and effective at this writing are discussed below.

HANDLING PRECAUTIONS

The possible hazards to man and other animals from use of many of the modern pesticides must always be remembered when considering their use. Review references on this subject are Rogoff (1961) and Bearse (1966). A useful source of information on control of poultry mites is USDA leaflet No. 383, 1964.

A basic rule in handling insecticides is to keep them properly labeled and stored in a locked building reserved for that purpose only. Disposal of empty insecticide containers and discarded leftover insecticides is becoming more of a hazard and responsibility. Large drums should be returned to the supplier or heated to red heat for 5–10 minutes. Paper cartons should be burned. Small glass and metal containers should be broken or punctured so no one will use them for any purpose. In addition to the human hazard, discarded insecticides must not pollute lakes or streams nor become a hazard for honey bees.

TYPES

Crude Oil, Distillates, and Similar Cheap Oils

Petroleum oils applied to buildings and equipment are excellent and cheap agents for the destruction of lice, mites, and ticks but have been largely replaced by the more recently developed insecticides (e.g. malathion, Sevin) which are efficient and more easily applied.

Bullis and Van Roekel (1944) have reported that exposure of chicks to the fumes of coal-tar creosote oil, anthracene oil, and certain mite paints too soon after use in a brooder house may cause anasarca (ascites, watery belly).

Nicotine Sulfate

A 40% solution of nicotine sulfate (such as is sold under the trade name of Black Leaf 40), once in general use for controlling lice, has been largely replaced by newer pesticides. Its action depends on a volatile substance that penetrates the feathers of the birds when it is painted on the perches just before they go to roost. The method is not well adapted to control of lice on turkeys under rearing conditions where the perches are usually placed out of doors. It remains, however, a very effective insecticide for controlling lice and mites.

Malathion (O,O-dimethyl dithiophosphate of diethyl mercaptosuccinate)

This drug is effective against lice, mites, and flies and may be used as a spray in a 0.5% emulsion or as dust when applicable. The U.S. Food and Drug Administration (Agricultural Handbook No. 331, 1968) has accepted it for direct application as dust and has set a residue tolerance of 4 ppm as the amount which can be safely found in meat. They require a zero tolerance in eggs. Furman and Coates (1957) found it effective against the northern fowl mite *(Ornithonyssus sylviarum)* and nontoxic to chickens in the amounts used. Populations of insects and parasites resistant to this product will develop with long continued usage, and its effectiveness may decline (Reid and Botero, 1966).

Sevin (carbaryl)

Sevin is one of the newest chemicals to be developed for insect control. It is effective against the northern fowl mite and other insects and is relatively nontoxic to fowl. A residue tolerance of 5 ppm in meat and zero tolerance in eggs has been permitted (Agricultural Handbook, 1968).

Sulfaquinoxaline

This drug, used so widely for coccidiosis control and treatment of other internal infections, was found rather by accident to exert some control influence on mite infestations on birds receiving low levels in the feed. In an investigation of this phenomenon, Furman and Stratton (1963) found that continuous feeding of 0.033% sulfaquinoxaline in mash feed brought about a marked reduction in mites in two weeks and nearly complete elimination from infested hens in four weeks.

WARNING. This drug has recently been banned from feeds for hens laying eggs for human consumption.

Carbolineum

Carbolineum, a wood preservative, also repels mites and other insects for long periods of time after it is applied to the wood.

Sodium Fluoride

WARNING. This old-time remedy has recently been banned for use on poultry.

DDT (Dichloro-diphenyl-trichloroethane)

WARNING. While DDT, its derivatives, and other chlorinated hydrocarbon insecticides are highly effective, they accumulate in the fatty tissues and eggs in large quantities even from remote contact and thus have been banned from use around poultry destined for meat or egg production. The residues remain in tissues for long periods of time, and traces found in spot samples of poultry meat or eggs may lead to condemnation of entire lots. *The safest policy is not to use them anywhere around poultry houses, equipment, feed, or water supply.*

For additional information on insecticides for control of poultry pests see United States Department of Agriculture, Agricultural Handbook No. 331, 1968.

New organic insecticide products will undoubtedly continue to appear on the market, and one must continually be alert to announcements concerning their introduction and information on their use.

New synthetic materials are constantly finding usage in poultry house construction. If a new type of building material is used in house construction or a new disinfectant or disinfestant is to be introduced, the chemical should be tested on a piece of the building material before application to determine whether or not a deleterious chemical reaction may take place between some ingredient in the product and the building material.

REFERENCES

Agricultural Handbook 331. 1968. Suggested guide for the use of insecticides to control insects, p. 178. USDA, ARS and Forest Service.

Alls, A. A., W. J. Benton, W. C. Krauss, and M. S. Cover. 1963. The mechanics of treating hatching eggs for disease prevention. *Avian Diseases* 7:89–97.

Anderson, D. P., and R. P. Hanson. 1965. Influence of environment on virus diseases of poultry. *Avian Diseases* 9:171–82.

Anderson, D. P., C. W. Beard, and R. P. Hanson. 1964. The adverse effects of ammonia on chickens including resistance to infection with Newcastle disease virus. *Avian Diseases* 8:369–79.

———. 1966. Influence of poultry house dust, ammonia, and carbon dioxide on resistance of chickens to Newcastle disease virus. *Avian Diseases* 10:117–88.

Anonymous. 1957. Disposal of dead birds. *Agr. Res.* 5 (9): 14.

Bearse, G. E. 1966. Pesticide residues and poultry products: U.S.A. legislation and pertinent research. *World's Poultry Sci. J.* 22: 194–206.

Becker, W. A., J. V. Spencer, and J. L. Swartwood. 1964. The pre-incubation storage of turkey eggs in closed environments. *Poultry Sci.* 63:1526–34.

Bell, D. 1966. Water shortages can cut egg production. *Poultry Tribune* 72 (6): 30.

Bullis, K. L., and H. Van Roekel. 1944. Uncommon pathological conditions in chickens and turkeys. *Cornell Vet.* 34:313–20.

Bullis, K. L., G. H. Snoeyenbos, and H. Van Roekel. 1950. A keratoconjunctivitis in chickens. *Poultry Sci.* 29:386–89.

Card, L. E. 1961. *Poultry Production*, 9th ed. Lea & Febiger, Philadelphia.

Charles, D. R., and C. G. Payne. 1966a. The influence of graded levels of atmospheric ammonia on chickens. I. Effect on respiration and on the performance of broilers and replacement growing stock. *Brit. Poultry Sci.* 7:177–87.

———. 1966b. The influence of graded levels of atmospheric ammonia on chickens. II. Effects on the performance of laying hens. *Brit. Poultry Sci.* 7:189–98.

Chute, H. L., and Elizabeth Barden. 1964. The fungous flora of chick hatcheries. *Avian Diseases* 8:13–19.

Chute, H. L., and M. Gershman. 1961. A new approach to hatchery sanitation. *Poultry Sci.* 60:568–71.

Chute, H. L., D. R. Stauffer, and D. C. O'Meara. 1964. The production of specific pathogen-free (SPF) broilers in Maine. *Maine Agr. Expt. Sta. Bull.* 633.

Cunningham, C. H. 1966. *A Laboratory Guide in Virology*, 6th ed. Burgess Publ. Co., Minneapolis.

Decker, H. M., L. M. Buchanan, L. B. Hall, and K. R. Goddard. 1962. Air filtration of microbial particles. *U.S. Public Health Serv. Publ.* 953.

Dorland, W.A.N. 1951. *Medical Dictionary*, 22nd ed. W. B. Saunders Co., Philadelphia and London.

Dychdala, G. R. 1968. Chlorine and chlorine compounds, pp. 278–304. In Lawrence, C. A., and S. S. Block (eds.), *Disinfection, Sterilization, and Preservation*. Lea & Febiger, Philadelphia.

Ewing, W. R. 1963. *Poultry Nutrition*, 5th ed. Ray Ewing Co., Pasadena, Calif.

Furman, D. P., and W. S. Coates. 1957. Northern fowl mite control with malathion. *Poultry Sci.* 36:252–55.

Furman, D. P., and V. S. Stratton. 1963. Control of northern fowl mites, *Ornithonyssus sylviarum*, with sulphaquinoxaline. *J. Econ. Entomol.* 56:904–5.

Galton, Mildred M., and P. Arnstein. 1960. Poultry diseases in public health. *U.S. Public Health Serv. Publ.* 767.

Gentry, R. F. 1968. A.E. vaccination problems, p. 16. In *Summary of Proc. of Poultry Health Conf.* Coop. Ext. Serv., Univ. New Hampshire.

Gentry, R. F., M. Mitrovic, and G. R. Bubash. 162. Application of Andersen sampler in hatchery sanitation. *Poultry Sci.* 61:794–804.

Gershenfeld, L. 1968. Iodine, pp. 329–47. In Lawrence, C. A., and S. S. Block (eds.), *Disinfection, Sterilization, and Preservation*. Lea & Febiger, Philadelphia.

Glick, C. A., G. G. Gremillion, and G. A. Bodmer. 1961. Practical methods and problems of steam and chemical sterilization. *Proc. Animal Care Panel* 11:37.

Gorham, J. R. 1957. A simple technique for the inoculation of the chorioallantoic membrane of chicken embryos. *Am. J. Vet. Res.* 18:691–92.

Gump, W. S., and G. R. Walter. 1968. The bis-phenols, pp. 257–77. In Lawrence, C. A., and S. S. Block (eds.), *Disinfection, Sterilization, and Preservation*. Lea & Febiger, Philadelphia.

Haenni, E. O., W. A. Affens, H. G. Lento, A. H. Yeomans, and R. A. Fulton. 1959. New nonflammable formulations for sterilizing sensitive materials. *Ind. & Eng. Chem.* 51:685.

Hofstad, M. S. 1950. A method of bleeding chickens from the heart. *J. Am. Vet. Med. Ass.* 116:353–54.

Lawrence, C. A. 1968. Quaternary ammonium surface-active disinfectants, pp. 430–52. In Lawrence, C. A., and S. S. Block (eds.), *Disinfection, Sterilization, and Preservation*. Lea & Febiger, Philadelphia.

Lawrence, C. A., and S. S. Block (eds.). 1968. *Disinfection, Sterilization, and Preservation*. Lea & Febiger, Philadelphia.

Lucas, A. M., and C. Jamroz. 1961. *Atlas of Avian Hematology*. USDA, Agr. Monograph 25.

Luna, L. G. 1968. *Manual of Histological Staining Methods of the Armed Forces Institute of Pathology*, 3rd ed. Blakiston Div., McGraw-Hill, New York.

Magwood, S. E. 1964. Studies in hatchery sanitation. 1. Fluctuations in microbial counts of air in poultry hatcheries. *Poultry Sci.* 63:441–49.

Magwood, S. E., and H. Marr. 1964. Studies in hatchery sanitation. 2. A simplified method for assessing bacterial populations on surfaces within hatcheries. *Poultry Sci.* 63:1558–66.

Marsden, S. J., and J. H. Martin. 1955. *Turkey Management*, 6th ed. Interstate Co., Danville, Ill.

Mathews, J., and M. S. Hofstad. 1953. The inactivation of certain animal viruses by ethylene oxide (Carboxide). *Cornell Vet.* 43: 452–61.

Nat. Acad. Sci., Nat. Res. Council. 1963. *Methods for the Examination of Poultry Biologics*, 2nd ed. Publ. 1038.

Phillips, C. R. 1968. Gaseous sterilization, pp.

669–85. In Lawrence, C. A., and S. S. Block (eds.), *Disinfection, Sterilization, and Preservation*. Lea & Febiger, Philadelphia.

Phillips, C. R., and B. Warshowsky. 1958. Chemical disinfectants. *Ann. Rev. Microbiol.* 12:525.

Phillips, G. B., and E. Hanel. 1960. Use of ultraviolet radiation in microbiological laboratories. *U.S. Govt. Res. Rept.* 34 (2): 122. (Abstr.)

Preece, Ann. 1965. *A Manual for Histological Techniques*, 2nd ed. Little, Brown & Co., Boston.

Prindle, R. F., and E. S. Wright. 1968. Phenolic compounds, pp. 401–29. In Lawrence, C. A., and S. S. Block (eds.), *Disinfection, Sterilization, and Preservation*. Lea & Febiger, Philadelphia.

Reddish, G. F. (ed.). 1957. *Antiseptics, Disinfectants, Fungicides and Sterilization*, 2nd ed. Lea & Febiger, Philadelphia.

Reid, W. M., and H. Botero. 1966. How to control lice and mites. *Poultry Tribune* 72 (3): 22, 62, 66.

Rogoff, W. M. 1961. Chemical control of insect pests of domestic animals, pp. 153–81. In Metcalf, R. L. (ed.), *Advances in Pest Control Research*, Vol. 4. Interscience Publ. Inc., New York.

Saulmon, E. E. 1968. Cresylic disinfectants permitted for use in official disinfection. Rev. Sept. 1968. USDA, ARS, Animal Health Div. Memo 586.

Schley, D. G., R. K. Hoffman, and C. R. Phillips. 1960. Simple improvised chambers for gas sterilization with ethylene oxide. *Appl. Microbiol.* 8:15.

Stover, D. E. 1964. Hatching egg sanitation and fumigation for disease control. *The Bulletin*. Dept. of Agr., State of Calif. 53:147–50.

Taylor, L. W. (ed.). 1949. *Fertility and Hatchability of Chicken and Turkey Eggs*. John Wiley and Sons, Inc., New York.

Thompson, S. W. 1966. *Selected Histochemical and Histopathological Methods*, 1st ed. Charles C Thomas, Springfield, Ill.

Titus, Harry W. 1961. *The Scientific Feeding of Chickens*, 4th ed. Interstate Co., Danville, Ill.

USDA Leaflet 383. 1964. Poultry mites, How to control them. USDA, ARS, Entomology Res. Div.

Williams, J. E., and H. S. Siegel. 1969. Formaldehyde levels on and in chicken eggs following preincubation fumigation. *Poultry Sci.* 48:552–58.

Wright, G. W., and J. F. Frank. 1957. Ocular lesions in chickens caused by ammonia fumes. *Can. J. Comp. Med. Vet. Sci.* 21:225.

Wright, M. L. 1958. Hatchery sanitation. *Can. J. Comp. Med. Vet. Sci.* 22:62–66.

Wright, M. L., G. W. Anderson, and N. A. Epps. 1959. Hatchery sanitation. *Can. J. Comp. Med. Vet. Sci.* 23:288–90.

Wright, M. L., G. W. Anderson, and J. D. McConachie. 1961. Transmission of aspergillosis during incubation. *Poultry Sci.* 60: 727–31.

Yoder, H. W., Jr. 1970. Preincubation heat treatment of chicken hatching eggs to inactivate Mycoplasma. *Avian Diseases* 14:75–86.

Yushok, W., and F. E. Bear. 1944. Poultry manure, its preservation, deodorization and disinfection. *New Jersey Agr. Expt. Sta. Bull.* 707.

CHAPTER 2

NUTRITIONAL DEFICIENCY DISEASES

❖

M. L. SCOTT
Department of Poultry Science
Cornell University
Ithaca, New York

AND

L. KROOK
Department of Veterinary Pathology
N.Y.S. Veterinary College
Cornell University
Ithaca, New York

❖

ADEQUATE NUTRITION together with proper management and disease control is essential for maintenance of normal growth, egg production, hatchability, and long productive life in chickens and turkeys. Whenever a serious deficiency of one of the essential nutrients occurs, signs develop which in some instances are characteristic. These are frequently preceded and accompanied by nonspecific signs such as retarded uneven growth, rough feather development, decreased egg production, and lowered hatchability. When a deficiency is partial, these may be the only signs observed. This makes it difficult to recognize a partial nutritional deficiency, since nonspecific signs may be brought about by a number of causes including infectious diseases. It is important, therefore, that the veterinarian have up-to-date knowledge of nutritional deficiency diseases.

The food substances of importance in the nutrition of poultry are (1) proteins and amino acids, (2) carbohydrates, (3) fats, (4) vitamins, (5) essential inorganic elements, and (6) water. The recommended nutrient levels in diets for chickens and turkeys are given in Table 2.1.

PROTEINS AND AMINO ACIDS

The protein requirements of chickens and turkeys represent a requirement for the essential amino acids plus sufficient available nitrogen for use in the synthesis of nonessential amino acids.

A deficiency in "protein," therefore, is usually a deficiency of one or two of the most limiting essential amino acids. Poultry diets composed largely of corn and soybean meal, when formulated to contain enough protein to meet the nitrogen requirements, also will contain adequate amounts of most of the essential amino acids. In such diets methionine usually is the only amino acid which may be deficient. In some areas of the country where cottonseed meal, sunflower seed meal, or other plant protein sources may be used instead of soybean meal, a deficiency of lysine also may occur unless high-lysine supplements are added to the diets.

A marginal deficiency of protein, methionine, and/or lysine usually results in slower growth, decreased egg production, and decreased egg size in both chickens and turkeys.

In addition to their main function as building stones for the proteins required for growth of tissues and for the proteins deposited in eggs, many of the amino acids fulfill other functions. Characteristic deficiency diseases may occur when diets for chickens or turkeys are grossly deficient in certain amino acids. Creatine, which is physiologically essential for functioning of muscular tissue, is synthesized in the body from arginine, methionine, and glycine. Diets deficient in both vitamin E and sulfur-containing amino acids will cause the development of nutritional muscular dystrophy in young chicks. The amino acid tyrosine is used in the formation of the hormone thyroxine and certain pigments in the feathers of colored fowl. Lysine is needed in some indirect way for feather pigment formation in colored turkeys. Feather achroma in bronze turkeys fed a corn gluten meal diet was shown by Fritz et al. (1946) to be corrected by the addition

TABLE 2.1. Recommended Nutrient Levels for Chickens and Turkeys

Nutrient	Starting Chicks (0–8 wks)	Growing Chickens (8–22 wks)	Laying Hens (White Leghorn) (22–40 wks)	Laying Hens (White Leghorn) (after 40 wks)	Breeding Hens (White Leghorn) (22–40 wks)	Breeding Hens (White Leghorn) (after 40 wks)	Starting Poults (0–8 wks)	Growing Turkeys (8–16 wks)	Finishing Turkeys (16–24 wks)	Breeding Turkeys
Protein, minimum, %	21.5	16	18	16	18	16	28	22	16	18
Metabolizable energy, kcal/lb	1,350	1,350	1,350	1,350	1,350	1,350	1,250	1,350	1,400	1,300
Calcium, %	1.0	0.8	3.2	3.7	3.0	3.3	1.4	1.0	0.6	2.0
Phosphorus, available, %	0.5	0.4	0.5	0.55	0.5	0.55	0.7	0.6	0.5	0.6
Sodium, %	0.15	0.15	0.15	0.15	0.15	0.15	0.15	0.15	0.15	0.15
Chloride, %	0.15	0.15	0.15	0.15	0.15	0.15	0.15	0.15	0.15	0.15
Potassium, %	0.4	0.4	0.4	0.4	0.4	0.4	0.6	0.6	0.6	0.6
Magnesium, %	0.05	0.05	0.05	0.05	0.05	0.05	0.06	0.06	0.06	0.06
Iodide, ppm	0.35	0.35	0.30	0.30	0.30	0.30	0.35	0.30	0.30	0.30
Manganese, ppm	60	35	35	35	50	50	60	35	35	50
Iron, ppm	80	40	40	40	40	40	80	60	60	60
Copper, ppm	5	2	2	2	5	5	6	4	4	6
Zinc, ppm	50	35	35	35	50	50	70	60	50	70
Selenium, ppm	0.1	0.1	0.1	0.1	0.1	0.1	0.2	0.15	0.1	0.2
Methionine, %	0.45	0.32	0.36	0.32	0.36	0.32	0.56	0.44	0.32	0.36
Cystine, %	0.33	0.24	0.29	0.26	0.29	0.26	0.45	0.35	0.26	0.29
Lysine, %	1.1	0.8	0.72	0.64	0.72	0.64	1.4	1.1	0.8	0.9
Arginine, %	1.1	0.8	0.9	0.8	0.9	0.8	1.4	1.1	0.8	0.9
Tryptophan, %	0.22	0.16	0.18	0.16	0.18	0.16	0.28	0.22	0.16	0.18
Vitamin A, IU/lb	5,000	3,000	4,000	4,000	5,000	5,000	5,000	3,000	2,500	5,000
Vitamin D$_3$, IU/lb	500	300	500	500	500	500	600	600	600	600
Vitamin E, IU/lb	5	4	3	3	7.5	7.5	7	6	3	15
Vitamin K, mg/lb	1	1	1	1	1	1	1	1	1	1
Riboflavin, mg/lb	2	2	2	2	2.5	2.5	2.5	2	2	2.5
Nicotinic acid, mg/lb	15	12	12	12	15	15	35	30	30	20
Pantothenate, mg/lb	6.5	6	2.5	2.5	7.5	7	7	5	5	9
Folic acid, mg/lb	0.6	0.18	0.18	0.18	0.4	0.4	0.6	0.4	0.4	0.5
Choline, mg/lb	600	450	500	500	500	500	900	800	800	600
Vitamin B$_{12}$, mg/lb	0.005	0.003	0.003	0.003	0.005	0.005	0.005	0.003	0.003	0.005
Thiamin, mg/lb	1	1	1	1	1	1	1	1	1	1
Pyridoxine, mg/lb	2	1.5	1.5	1.5	2	2	1.8	1.5	1.5	2
Biotin, mg/lb	0.06	0.05	0.05	0.05	0.08	0.08	0.12	0.10	0.10	0.12

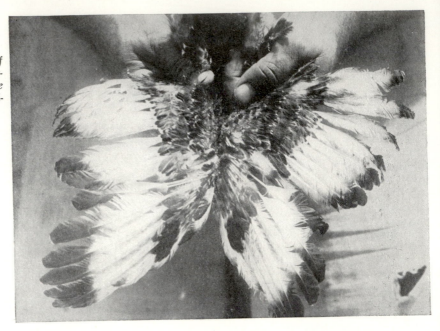

FIG. 2.1—Lack of normal feather pigmentation in Bronze poult caused by deficiency of lysine.

of lysine to the diet. The abnormal wing feather depigmentation of bronze poults caused by lysine deficiency is shown in Figure 2.1. Lysine deficiency may occur in commercial flocks of turkeys if the diet contains overheated soybean meal.

Methionine is a source of methyl groups for methylation processes in the body; it either exerts a sparing effect on choline or takes part in its synthesis when other necessary precursors are present in the diet. In this capacity it may help in the prevention of perosis.

Tryptophan is converted into nicotinic acid in the body of the chicken and the turkey; therefore, high levels of tryptophan may spare the requirements for nicotinic acid and thus help prevent enlarged hocks.

PROTEIN LEVEL AND FEATHERING

Feathers are composed chiefly of protein. Thus poor feathering will result from a lack of adequate protein in the diet. A relationship exists between protein deficiency and feather pulling, tail picking, and cannibalism.

UREMIC POISONING

Patterson (1928) suggested that nutritional gout or uremic poisoning in chickens, except that caused by vitamin A deficiency, may be due to the feeding of excess nitrogenous concentrates. This condition is char-

acterized by deposits of urates, particularly in the kidneys. Schlotthauer and Bollman (1934) were able to induce gout in turkeys by increasing the protein level of the diet to 40% by the addition of horse meat and also by the addition of 5% urea. Many interrelationships between amino acids, protein, minerals, and vitamins may be involved in kidney damage. Several diseases also may damage the kidneys and cause an increase in blood urates to a point of uremic poisoning. This effect undoubtedly is enhanced by excess protein in the diet but is not primarily caused by a high dietary level of protein.

CARBOHYDRATES

There is no specific deficiency disease attributed to a lack of dietary carbohydrates. Normal blood sugar levels can be maintained and growth is optimal in chickens fed diets containing energy in the form of fats (triglycerides), as long as the required metabolizable energy to protein ratios are maintained. Studies by Brambila and Hill (1965, 1966), Renner (1964), and Renner and Elcombe (1964) have shown, however, that when fats are hydrolyzed and glycerol removed, diets containing only proteins and free fatty acids fail to produce normal growth and cause paralytic signs. It is the current belief that chickens under these conditions may be unable to produce sufficient glucose to maintain their blood sugar levels, and that the glycerol moiety of fat is needed as a source of glucose in carbohydrate-free diets composed of proteins and triglycerides. These studies are of academic interest only, since carbohydrate-free diets are unlikely to be encountered in practical poultry production.

MILK AND MILK BY-PRODUCTS

Starch is the most important carbohydrate in feedstuffs and is readily digested and converted to glucose by poultry. In milk and milk by-products, however, carbohydrate is present as the disaccharide lactose. Although the digestive system of the chicken contains a limited amount of the enzyme lactase, hydrolysis of lactose appears to be very slow in chickens and turkeys. Therefore, while small amounts of dried milk by-products have beneficial effects in chickens and turkeys, high dietary levels of lactose retard growth. This effect is quite probably the result of two phenomena: (1) The slow rate of hydrolysis of lactose reduces uptake of sugar by the blood stream and thereby reduces the supply of available energy for growth. (2) Large amounts of unhydrolyzed lactose in the lower intestines and ceca stimulate the growth of acid-producing microorganisms. The tremendous multiplication of these microorganisms upsets digestion in the lower intestine and produces a severe diarrhea which flushes out many of the nutrients that might otherwise be absorbed.

FATS

Fats are important in the diet of poultry as concentrated sources of energy. In addition, they provide the unsaturated fatty acids linoleic and arachidonic. Growing chicks require approximately 1.5% linoleic acid for normal growth and development; approximately the same level is needed for maximum egg production and egg size. A lack of linoleic or arachidonic acid in the diet of young chicks results in suboptimal growth, enlarged fatty livers, and reduced resistance to respiratory infections (Ross and Adamson, 1961; Marion and Edwards, 1962; Hopkins et al., 1963; Hopkins and Nesheim, 1967).

IMPORTANCE OF ANTIOXIDANTS

When unprotected by natural or synthetic antioxidants, unsaturated fatty acids first lose hydrogen, forming fatty acid-free radicals. Through uptake of oxygen they are then converted into organic peroxides which eventually break down into ketones and aldehydes, giving rancid fat its characteristic odor. These peroxides destroy the essential fatty acids, markedly reduce the energy value of the diet, and may destroy the vitamin E and vitamin A activity of the feed. Vitamin E (which is present in many feedstuffs or is frequently added to poultry rations) is an effective antioxidant, but synthetic antioxidants also are used to prevent initiation of free radical formation and fatty acid oxidation.

VITAMINS

The term "vitamin" represents a heterogeneous group of fat-soluble and water-soluble chemical compounds essential in nutrition which bear no structural or necessary functional relationship to each other. All recognized vitamins with the exception of vitamin C are dietary essentials for poultry. Although the amounts of the various vitamins needed in poultry diets range from parts per million to parts per billion, each of them is required in exact amounts for normal metabolism and health. Many function as integral parts of vital enzymes. All appear to play various catalytic roles in the many chemical reactions concerned in digestion, intermediary metabolism, anabolism, and catabolism within the animal body.

A marked deficiency of a single vitamin in the diet of a chick or turkey poult results in breakdown of the metabolic process in which that particular vitamin is concerned. This causes a vitamin deficiency disease which in some instances exhibits characteristic macro- or microscopic changes. In several instances a single disease may result from a deficiency of any one of several vitamins. Perosis, for example, occurs in young chicks or poults when the diet is deficient in manganese or in any one of the following vitamins: choline, nicotinic acid, pyridoxine, biotin, or folic acid. Furthermore, the signs and pathologic changes of several different vitamin deficiencies are similar in appearance. As an example, the gross changes of either pantothenic acid or biotin deficiencies appear as severe dermatoses of the feet and of the areas around the mandibles and the eyes. Examination of the diet may be necessary to determine the cause of the deficiency.

After diagnosis of a specific vitamin deficiency, confirmatory evidence usually can be obtained upon determining by calculation or analysis the vitamin content of the diet that was fed to the chicken or turkey and comparing this with the known requirement for the particular vitamin.

Vitamin A, vitamin D, and riboflavin are the vitamins most apt to be deficient if special attention is not given to provide them when the feed is formulated. Recently, however, due to continued extraction and purification of many common ingredients and to the tendency to omit animal proteins and high-fiber ingredients such as alfalfa meal and wheat mill by-products from diets, the amounts of several other vitamins have decreased to levels that are sometimes deficient. These are vitamins E and K, pantothenic acid, vitamin B_{12}, nicotinic acid, and choline.

Present-day poultry rations are usually formulated to contain more than adequate amounts of all of the vitamins, providing margins of safety to compensate for possible losses during feed processing, transportation, storage, and variations in feed composition and environmental conditions. If a deficiency should occur it is usually due either to the inadvertent omission of a critical ingredient during mixing of the feed or to the destruction of one or more of the vitamins during processing of that ingredient. The fat-soluble vitamins A, D, and E are most prone to destruction. Under very severe conditions of processing or storage, thiamine and/or pantothenic acid may be destroyed. Special considerations in regard to each vitamin will follow.

VITAMIN A

Vitamin A is essential in poultry diets, not only for growth but also for optimal vision and to maintain the integrity of the mucous membrane. Since this membrane composes the epithelium lining all of those canals and cavities of the body which communicate with the external air (the alimentary canal and its branches, the respiratory tract and its connections, and the genitourinary tract), these are the areas in which lesions of vitamin A deficiency may be detected, either grossly or histologically, depending on the degree of deficiency.

Modern producers of vitamin A supplements have greatly enhanced the stability of vitamin A in two ways: (1) by mechanical means, wherein minute droplets of vitamin A are enveloped in a stable fat, gelatin, or wax, forming a small bead which prevents most of the vitamin from coming into contact with oxygen until it is digested in the intestinal tract of the animal; (2) through the use of effective antioxidants which markedly prolong the induction period preceding active oxidation of vitamin A, thereby allowing the vitamin to be consumed by the animals before this oxidation takes place. The chief antioxidant in current use is 6-ethoxy-1,2-dihydro-2,2,4-trimethylquinoline (ethoxyquin).

Signs of Deficiency

When adult chickens or turkeys are fed a diet severely deficient in vitamin A, signs and lesions develop usually within 2–5 months, depending upon the amount of vitamin A stored in the liver and other tissues of the body. As the deficiency progresses, chickens become emaciated and weak and their feathers are ruffled. Egg production decreases sharply; the length of time between clutches increases. Hatchability is decreased and there is an increase in embryonic malpositions and mortality in eggs from vitamin A deficient hens. A watery discharge from the nostrils and eyes is noted, and the eyelids are often stuck together. As the deficiency continues, an accumulation of milky white, caseous material forms in the eyes. At this stage of the disease the eyes fill with this white exudate to such an extent that it is impossible for the chicken to see unless the mass is removed; in many cases the eye is destroyed.

In adult turkeys receiving inadequate amounts of vitamin A most signs are similar to those in chickens. In addition to those described by Hinshaw and Lloyd (1934), Asmundson and Kratzer (1952) reported hatchability of eggs from vitamin A deficient turkey breeding stock to be greatly reduced and poults that did hatch suffered heavy mortality. After the flock was given high-potency vitamin A oil, the hens recovered except for blindness; hatchability of eggs increased and poult mortality decreased.

In many instances signs that cannot be differentiated from colds and infectious sinusitis are observed (Fig. 2.2). Moore (1953) described an ophthalmitis caused by

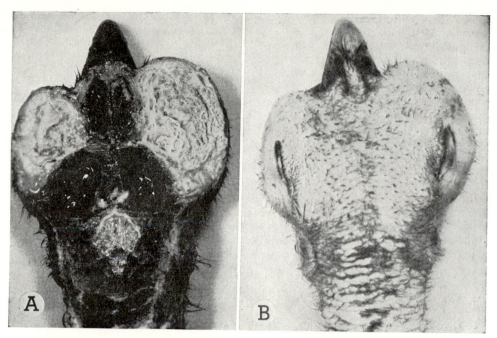

FIG. 2.2—*Extreme case of sinusitis in turkey hen suffering from vitamin A deficiency after being fed for 8 months on ration containing low level of vitamin A.* (**A**) *Sagittal section.* (**B**) *Note massive accumulation of whitish yellow caseous exudate typical of sinusitis associated with vitamin A deficiency in turkeys.* (*Hinshaw, Univ. Calif.*)

Aspergillus fumigatus, and Bierer (1956) described a keratoconjunctivitis, both of which could be mistaken for vitamin A deficiency. Therefore, it is desirable in all outbreaks of diseases in turkeys involving the head and/or respiratory tract to eliminate the possibility of vitamin A deficiency when making a diagnosis.

When young chicks or poults are given a vitamin A deficient diet, signs may appear at the end of the first week if the birds are progeny of hens fed a diet low in vitamin A. On the other hand, if they are progeny of hens receiving adequate amounts of vitamin A, signs and lesions of vitamin A deficiency may not appear until the 6th or 7th week of age, even though the chicks or poults are receiving a diet completely devoid of vitamin A. Breeding hens receiving adequate amounts of vitamin A store large quantities in their eggs which consequently provide the day-old chicks and poults with sufficient reserves to last for an extended period.

Vitamin A deficiency signs in chicks and poults are characterized by a cessation of growth, drowsiness, weakness, incoordination, emaciation, and ruffled plumage (Fig. 2.3). If the deficiency is severe they may show an ataxia not unlike that of vitamin

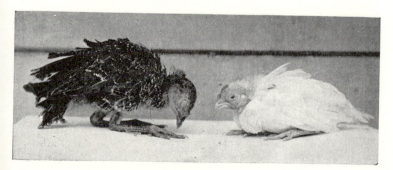

FIG. 2.3—*Five-week-old poult and 6-week-old chick, both showing typical signs of vitamin A deficiency.* (*Hinshaw, Univ. Calif.*)

E deficiency (encephalomalacia or crazy chick disease, Hill et al., 1961). The cause of ataxia in vitamin A deficient chicks may be better understood from the discovery by Woollam and Millen (1955) that one of the earliest signs of deficiency is increased cerebrospinal fluid pressure. The yellow pigment in the shanks and beaks in breeds of chickens that usually contain this pigment is lost, and the combs and wattles of the chicks are usually pale. In acute vitamin A deficiency lacrimation usually occurs, and a caseous material may be seen under the eyelids. Xerophthalmia is a definite lesion of vitamin A deficiency; not all chicks and poults exhibit this because in acute deficiency they often die of other causes before the eyes become affected.

Bone Development

According to Wolbach and Hegsted (1952, 1953), vitamin A deficiency in young ducks causes marked retardation and suppression of endochondral bone growth, and excess vitamin A accelerates this bone development. This may be due to alterations in the alkaline phosphatase content of the epiphyseal junction of the bone in ducks similar to that shown by Ludwig (1953) for vitamin A deficiency and hypervitaminosis A in rats. Studies reviewed by Wolf and Johnson (1960), however, indicate that effects of vitamin A upon bone development may be secondary to effects upon mucopolysaccharide biosynthesis in cartilage and connective tissues.

Internal Egg Quality

Bearse et al. (1953) reported that the incidence and severity of blood spots in eggs of two different strains of White Leghorn chickens was progressively increased as the level of vitamin A in the diet of the hens was decreased. Experiments conducted at Cornell University (Hill et al., 1961) confirm the finding that blood spots are increased in number and severity when hens are fed vitamin A deficient diets. These studies showed, however, that the amount of vitamin A required to minimize blood spot incidence is no higher than the vitamin A requirement for good production and health of the laying hens. Certain strains of chickens show a fairly high incidence of blood spots in their eggs which cannot be improved by increasing the vitamin A level in the diet above that needed for satisfactory egg production and health.

Intestinal Coccidiosis and Other Intestinal Parasites

Davies (1952) found that in chickens receiving adequate vitamin A in the form of natural sources of β-carotene and cryptoxanthin, infection with intestinal coccidiosis caused a reduction in liver stores of vitamin A to less than 10% of the uninfected controls. Erasmus et al. (1960) showed that although the severity of experimentally induced coccidiosis was similar in chicks receiving minimal requirements of vitamin A as compared to those receiving higher levels of the vitamin, recovery of surviving chicks as measured by improved appetites and growth rates was enhanced with increasing levels of vitamin A up to 10 times the minimal requirement under normal, nonstress conditions.

Ackert and associates (1931) reported that vitamin A deficient chicks were infected with significantly larger numbers and longer intestinal roundworms (Ascaridia lineata) than were found in comparable chicks receiving adequate vitamin A. This work was criticized because it is difficult to determine total numbers of roundworms in the intestinal tracts of chickens and because the number may vary considerably from day to day.

Pathology

Vitamin A deficiency lesions first appear in the pharynx and are largely confined to the mucous glands and their ducts. The original epithelium is replaced by a keratinizing epithelium which blocks the ducts of the mucous glands, causing them to become distended with secretions and necrotic materials. Small white pustules are found in the nasal passages, mouth, esophagus, and pharynx and may extend into the crop. The pustules range in size from microscopic lesions to 2 mm in diameter (Fig. 2.4). As the vitamin A deficiency progresses the lesions enlarge, are raised above the surface of the mucous membrane, and have a depression in the center. Small ulcers surrounded by inflammatory products may appear at the site of these lesions. This condition resembles certain stages of fowl pox, and the two conditions can be differentiated only by microscopic examina-

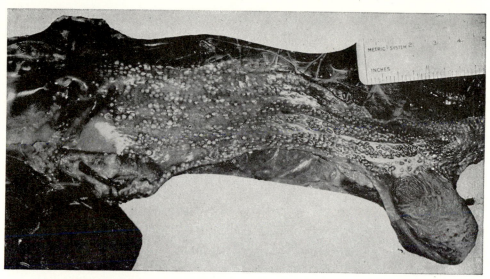

FIG. 2.4—Pustulelike lesions in pharynx and esophagus—vitamin A deficiency.
(Biester and Schwarte, North Am. Vet.)

tion. Due to the breakdown of the original mucous membrane, bacteria, viruses, and other pathogenic microorganisms may invade these tissues and enter the body, producing infections which are secondary to the original vitamin A deficiency signs.

Young chicks suffering from chronic vitamin A deficiency show lesions in the mucous membranes of the mouth, esophagus, crop, and respiratory tract and marked accumulation of urates in the renal tubules. In extreme cases even the ureters are filled with urates. According to Elvehjem and Neu (1932), the blood level of uric acid increases from a normal of about 5 mg to as high as 44 mg per 100 ml of whole blood during severe vitamin A deficiency. Deposits of urates have been found on the heart, pericardium, liver, and spleen of affected birds. Elvehjem and Neu (1932) found that vitamin A deficiency does not disturb uric acid metabolism but injures the kidney in such a way as to prevent normal excretion of uric acid.

The clinical signs and lesions of vitamin A deficiency of the respiratory tract are variable; it is difficult to differentiate this condition from infectious coryza, fowl pox, and infectious bronchitis. In vitamin A deficiency thin membranes and nasal plugs are usually limited to the cleft palate and its adjacent epithelium. They may be removed easily without bleeding. According

to Seifried (1930a,b) this is not true in fowl pox. Atrophy and degeneration of the respiratory mucous membrane and its glands occur. Later the original epithelium is replaced by a stratified squamous keratinizing epithelium. In the early stages of vitamin A deficiency in chickens the turbinates are filled with seromucoid water-clear masses which may be forced out of the nodules and cleft palate by the application of slight pressure. The vestibule becomes plugged and overflows into the paranasal sinuses. The exudate may also fill the sinuses and other nasal cavities, causing a swelling of one or both sides of the face. After the sinuses have filled, the tear ducts may become occluded. Upon removal of the inflammatory products the mucous membranes of the nasal passages, sinuses, mouth, and throat appear thin, rough, and dry.

Similar lesions may frequently be found in the trachea and bronchi. In the early stages these may be difficult to see, but as the condition progresses the mucous membrane is covered with a dry, dull, fine film which is slightly uneven, whereas the normal membrane is even and moist. In some cases small nodulelike particles may be found in or beneath the mucous membrane in the upper part of the trachea. These lesions are much more striking in the late stages of the deficiency and may be seen with the naked eye. The formation of a thin membranous covering over the mucosa of the trachea and bronchi is a lesion of vitamin A deficiency but is sometimes mistaken for infectious tracheitis. Smaller bronchi often are completely occluded by these membranes.

Histopathology

The first histologic lesion of vitamin A deficiency is an atrophy of the cytoplasm and loss of cilia in columnar ciliated epithelium of the respiratory tract (Seifried, 1930a). The nuclei often present marked karyorrhexis. A pseudomembrane formed by the atrophying and degenerating ciliated cells may hang as tufts on the basement membrane; later these are sloughed. During this process new cylindrical or polygonal cells may be formed either singly or in pairs and appear as islands beneath the epithelium. These new cells proliferate and their nuclei enlarge, containing less chromatin as they develop. Cell boundaries are less clearly defined; finally the columnar ciliated epithelial lining of the nasal cavities and communicating sinuses, the trachea, bronchi, and submucous glands are transformed into a stratified squamous keratinizing epithelium. Seifried (1930a) concluded that this process is not related to bacterial infection.

Histopathologic examination of tissues from the nasal passages of chicks serves as a sensitive indicator of borderline deficiencies of vitamin A (Jungherr, 1943). Chicks receiving suboptimal levels of vitamin A show lesions which resemble in basic character but not in severity those described by Seifried (1930a) for complete deficiency of vitamin A.

Further evidence that vitamin A is directly concerned with the differentiation of the mucous membrane was obtained by Fell and Mellanby (1953), who showed that explants of chick ectoderm, when grown in a tissue culture supplemented with a high level of vitamin A, failed to develop into typical keratinized epithelium. Instead the cells differentiated into mucus-secreting, often ciliated columnar epithelial cells resembling those of the nasal mucosa. Kahn (1954) showed that added vitamin A prevents keratinization that otherwise occurs in explants of rat vaginal epithelium.

Lesions in the glands of the tongue, palate, and esophagus are similar to those of the respiratory tract. As the disease progresses the collecting spaces fill with masses of mucus, degenerated cells, and inflammatory products. The epithelium of the ducts undergoes metaplasia and fills with keratinized stratified squamous epithelium. More or less complete occlusion results (Fig. 2.5). Desquamated cells from the metaplastic epithelium become more and more numerous. The glands become smooth and distended, although originally they were sacs with invaginations. These distended sacs finally completely fill with stratified keratinized epithelial cells. Seifried (1930b) believes that these lesions are responsible for the greater prevalence of bacterial in-

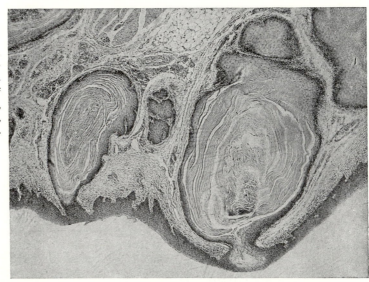

FIG. 2.5—Cross section through base of tongue showing final stage of process with dilatation of glands filled with stratified, more or less keratinized, homogeneous masses. ×50. (Seifried, J. Exp. Med.)

fections in the mouth cavity than in the crop and esophagus during avitaminosis A.

Adamstone (1947) conducted investigations to differentiate by histologic means between the ataxia of vitamin A deficiency and the encephalomalacia of vitamin E deficiency. Both vitamin A and vitamin E deficiencies in the chick are characterized by definite incoordination and imbalance of central nervous system origin. In vitamin A deficiency no gross lesions are noticed in the brain. Upon microscopic examination the vitamin A deficient cells are noted to lose their chromaticity but do not shrink. Nissl substance appears to break into fine granules and filaments before undergoing complete dissolution.

Embryos which are absolutely deficient in vitamin A show a characteristic syndrome. All of the embryos die—always in the same stage of development. The complete trunk and head are formed, and the head is rotated slightly to one side. No differentiation of major blood vessels occurs. An expanded area of vasculosa is seen forming a "blood ring" at the sinus terminalis. It appears that vitamin A is required for the cellular differentiation necessary for development of the vascular system of the embryo. Injection into the eggs of graded levels of vitamin A brings about progressively longer life of the embryo until an amount is reached which will produce a normal chick. Embryos which do not receive sufficient vitamin A cease to develop at the particular stage reached when the vitamin A supply is exhausted (Thompson et al., 1965).

Treatment of Deficiency

A chicken, turkey, or other poultry flock found to be severely deficient in vitamin A should be given a stabilized vitamin A preparation at a level of approximately 5,000 IU vitamin A per pound of ration.

Absorption of vitamin A is rapid; therefore, chickens or turkeys that are not in advanced stages of the deficiency should respond promptly. Hens in advanced stages of deficiency may return to production in less than one month after the diet is corrected, while others may die regardless of the level of vitamin A administered.

VITAMIN D

Vitamin D is required by poultry for the proper metabolism of calcium and phosphorus in the formation of normal bony skeleton, hard beaks and claws, and strong eggshells. A deficiency of vitamin D in young birds results in rickets. One of the primary actions of vitamin D is concerned with increasing the absorption of calcium (Wasserman and Taylor, 1966; Taylor and Wasserman, 1967).

Recently Trummel et al. (1969) discovered that a derivative of vitamin D_3, 25-hydroxycholecalciferol, is markedly more effective than cholecalciferol in bringing about resorption of calcium from bone in tissue culture. The results indicated a synergistic effect of 25-hydroxycholecalciferol and parathyroid hormone which indicated that the 25-hydroxy derivative may be the metabolically active form of vitamin D_3.

Whether vitamin D is also concerned in controlling serum phosphatase is not fully understood. A marked increase in serum phosphatase is perhaps the first indicator of a borderline rachitic condition. With the administration of vitamin D, provided the diet contains adequate phosphorus and calcium, the serum phosphatase decreases slowly toward normal. It may remain somewhat above normal for several months after all other signs of rickets have vanished. Vitamin D probably is concerned also in citric acid metabolism.

Although vitamin D_3 is produced on the skin of animals through the action of sunlight on precursors synthesized within the animal body, it is unlikely that this source of vitamin D is adequate for chickens and especially for turkeys reared in confinement. Further research is needed to determine the reason for the very high vitamin D requirements of turkeys as compared to chickens.

Signs of Deficiency

In laying hens in confinement, signs of vitamin D deficiency begin to occur about 2–3 months after they are deprived of vitamin D. The first sign is a marked increase in the number of thin-shelled and soft-shelled eggs, followed soon afterward by a marked decrease in egg production. Hatchability also is markedly reduced.

Individual hens may show temporary loss of use of the legs, with recovery after laying an egg which is usually shell-less. During the periods of extreme leg weakness the hens show a characteristic posture which has been described as a "penguin-type squat." Later the beak, claws, and keel become very soft and pliable. The sternum usually is bent and the ribs lose their normal rigidity and turn inward at the junction of the sternal and vertebral portions, producing a characteristic inward curve of the ribs along the sides of the thorax.

In addition to retarded growth, the first sign of vitamin D deficiency in chicks or poults is rickets, which is characterized by a severe weakness of the bones. Between 2 and 3 weeks of age the beaks and claws become soft and pliable and the birds walk with obvious effort and take a few unsteady steps before squatting on their hocks, whereupon they rest but at the same time sway slightly from side to side. Feathering is poor.

Pathology

In laying and breeding chicken and turkey hens receiving a deficient amount of vitamin D, the characteristic changes observed on necropsy are confined to the bones and parathyroid glands. The bones are soft and break easily. Well-defined knobs are present on the inner surface of the ribs at the costochondral junction (rachitic rosary). Many of the ribs show evi-

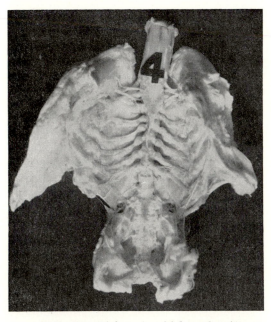

FIG. 2.6—Rickets in chicken showing severe beading and curvature of ribs and spinal column.

dence of pathologic fracture in this region. In chronic vitamin D deficiency marked skeletal distortions become apparent. The spinal column may bend downward in the sacral and coccygeal region, the sternum usually shows both a lateral bend and an acute dent near the middle of the breast. These changes reduce the size of the thorax with consequent crowding of vital organs. Histologic sections of the leg bones show a deficiency of calcium and an excess of osteoid tissue.

The most characteristic internal signs of vitamin D deficiency in chicks and poults are a beading of the ribs at their juncture with the spinal column and a bending of the ribs downward and posteriorly (Fig. 2.6).

Poor calcification can be observed at the epiphysis of the tibia or femur. By dipping the split bone in silver nitrate solution and allowing it to stand under an incandescent light for a few minutes, calcified areas are easily distinguished from areas of uncalcified cartilage (Fig. 2.7).

Hypervitaminosis D

Very high levels of vitamin D_3—2,000,000 IU or more per pound of diet—cause renal damage. This is due to dystrophic calcification of the kidney tubules also seen less often in the aorta and other arteries. Irradiated ergosterol (vitamin D_2), a very poor source of vitamin D for chickens and turkeys, is, however, quite toxic at high levels.

Treatment of Deficiency

Hooper et al. (1942) found that the feeding of a single massive dose of 15,000 IU vitamin D_3 cured rachitic chicks more promptly than when generous levels of the vitamin were added to the feed. This single oral dose protected cockerels against rickets for 8 weeks and pullet chicks for 5 weeks. In giving massive doses to rachitic chicks it should be remembered that excess vitamin D can be harmful. The dose should be scaled to the degree of deficiency, and excessive amounts of vitamin D should not be added to the feed.

VITAMIN E

Vitamin E deficiency produces encephalomalacia, exudative diathesis, and muscular dystrophy in chicks; enlarged hocks and dystrophy of the gizzard musculature in

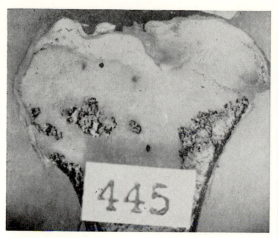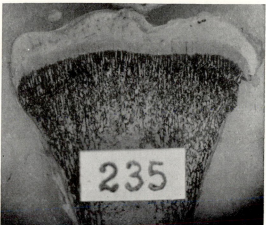

FIG. 2.7—*Tibia of severely vitamin D-deficient, rachitic chick (445) and normal chick (235), after staining with silver nitrate and exposure to light.*

turkeys; and muscular dystrophy in ducks. Vitamin E also is required for normal embryonic development in chickens, turkeys, and probably ducks.

In its alcoholic form vitamin E is a very effective antioxidant. It is an important protector in feeds of the essential fatty acids and other highly unsaturated fatty acids as well as vitamins A and D_3, the carotenes, and xanthophylls. Recently 0.04–0.1 ppm of selenium has been shown to prevent or cure exudative diathesis in vitamin E deficient chicks (Scott, 1962a,b), and 0.1–0.2 ppm effectively prevents myopathies of gizzard and heart in young poults (Scott et al., 1967).

Vitamin E plays a multiple role in the nutrition of poultry. It is required not only for normal reproduction but also (1) as nature's most effective antioxidant for prevention of encephalomalacia, (2) in a specific role interrelated with the action of selenium for prevention of exudative diathesis and turkey myopathies, and (3) in another role interrelated with both selenium and cystine for prevention of nutritional muscular dystrophy.

Signs and Pathology of Deficiency

No outward signs occur in mature chickens or turkeys receiving very low levels of vitamin E over prolonged periods. Hatchability of eggs from vitamin E deficient chickens or turkeys, however, is reduced markedly (Jensen et al., 1956). Embryos from hens fed rations low in vitamin E may die as early as the 4th day of incubation.

Testicular degeneration occurs in males deprived of vitamin E over prolonged periods of time (Adamstone and Card, 1934).

ENCEPHALOMALACIA IN CHICKS. Encephalomalacia is a nervous derangement characterized by ataxia, backward or downward retractions of the head (sometimes with lateral twisting), forced movements, increasing incoordination, a rapid contraction and relaxation of the legs, and finally complete prostration and death. Even under these conditions, complete paralysis of the wings or legs is not observed. The deficiency usually manifests itself between the 15th and 30th day of the chick's life, although it has been known to occur as early as the 7th and as late as the 56th day.

The cerebellum, the striatal hemispheres, the medulla oblongata, and the mesencephalon are affected most commonly in the order named. In chicks which are killed soon after the appearance of the signs of encephalomalacia, the cerebellum is softened and swollen and the meninges are edematous. Minute hemorrhages are often visible on the surface of the cerebellum. The convolutions are flattened. As much as four-fifths of the cerebellum may be affected, or lesions may be so small that they cannot be recognized grossly. A day or two after signs of encephalomalacia appear, necrotic areas present a greenish yellow opaque appearance.

In the corpus striatum necrotic tissue is frequently pale, swollen, and wet and in the early stages becomes sharply delineated from the remaining normal tissue. The greater portion of both hemispheres may be destroyed. In other cases the lesions are apparent only on microscopic examination. Medullary lesions are not so readily noted in a macroscopic examination. Flattening and general swelling of the ventral surface indicates the presence of internal lesions. After one is familiar with the disease a macroscopic diagnosis can be made correctly in approximately 90% of the cases (Pappenheimer et al., 1939).

Histologically the lesions include circulatory disturbances (ischemic necrosis) demyelination, and neuronal degeneration.

Meningeal, cerebellar, and cerebral vessels are markedly hyperemic and a severe edema usually develops. Capillary thrombosis often results in necrosis of varying extent.

In the normal chick cerebellum, the myelineated tracts exhibit a strongly positive reaction with Luxol Fast Blue (Fig. 2.8). In encephalomalacia the staining reaction

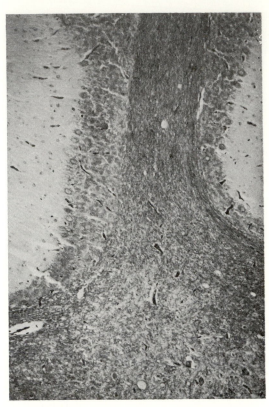

FIG. 2.9—Cerebellum, chick with encephalomalacia. Poor staining reaction of myelinated tract. Luxol Fast Blue, ×120.

is markedly diminished, diffusely or locally accentuated (Fig. 2.9).

Degenerative neuronal changes occur everywhere but are most prominent in the Purkinje cells and in the large motor nuclei. The ischemic cell change is most frequently encountered. The cells are shrunken and intensely hyperchromatic, and the nucleus is typically triangular. Peripheral chromatolysis with the Nissl substance packed along the periphery of the cell nucleus is also common (Fig. 2.10).

EXUDATIVE DIATHESIS IN CHICKS. Exudative diathesis is an edema of subcutaneous tissues (Fig. 2.11) associated with abnormal permeability of capillary walls (Dam and Glavind, 1939). In severe cases chicks stand with their legs far apart as a result of the accumulation of fluid under the ventral skin. This greenish blue, viscous fluid is easily seen through the skin since it usually contains some blood components from slight hemorrhages which appear through-

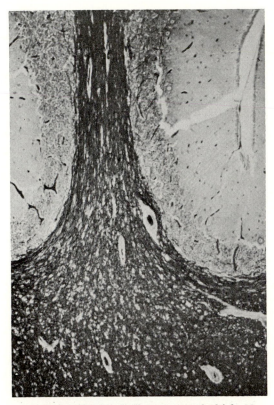

FIG. 2.8—Cerebellum, normal chick. Normal staining reaction of myelinated tract. Luxol Fast Blue, ×120.

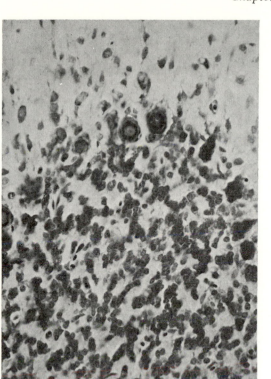

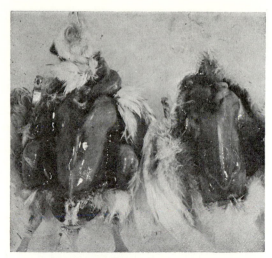

FIG. 2.11—*Exudative diathesis in chicks.*

The initial histologic change is hyaline degeneration. Mitochondria undergo swelling, coalesce, and form intracytoplasmic globules. Later the muscle fibers are disrupted transversely (Fig. 2.13, lower part). Extravasation separates groups of muscle

FIG. 2.10—*Cerebellum, Purkinje cell layer. Ischemic cell change in cells to the right; peripheral chromatolysis in cells on top and to the left. Cresyl Echt Violet, ×400.*

out the breast and leg musculature and in the intestinal walls. Distension of the pericardium and sudden deaths have been noted. The onset of the condition coincides with the appearance of peroxides in the tissues.

Chicks suffering from exudative diathesis show a low ratio of albumin to globulins (Goldstein and Scott, 1956).

MUSCULAR DYSTROPHY IN CHICKENS, DUCKLINGS, AND TURKEYS. When vitamin E deficiency is accompanied by a sulfur amino acid deficiency, chicks show signs of muscular dystrophy, particularly of the breast muscle, at about 4 weeks of age. The condition is characterized by light-colored streaks of easily distinguished affected bundles of muscle fibers in the breast (Fig. 2.12). A similar dystrophy occurs throughout all skeletal muscles of the body in vitamin E deficient ducks.

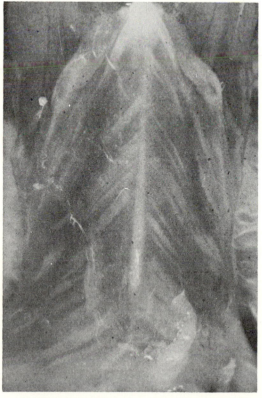

FIG. 2.12—*Muscular dystrophy in chicks.*

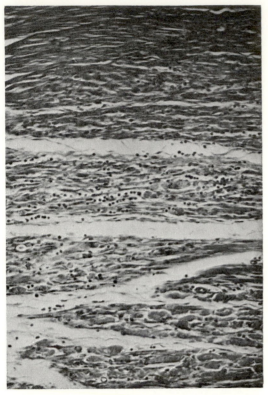

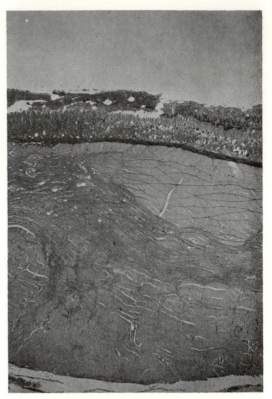

FIG. 2.13—*Pectoral muscle. Upper part shows proliferation of muscle nuclei and fibroblasts; lower part shows disruption of muscle fibers, separation of fibers, and bundle of fibers by edema. Dark spots in edema are heterophilic leukocytes. H & E, ×180.*

FIG. 2.14—*Gizzard, turkey. Chronic vitamin E deficiency. Extensive scar formation. Van Gieson, ×10.*

fibers and individual fibers. The transuded plasma usually contains erythrocytes and heterophilic leukocytes. In more chronic conditions, reparative processes dominate the picture. There is a pronounced proliferation of cell nuclei and also fibroplasia (Fig. 2.13, upper part), leaving a scar in the degenerate muscle.

Vitamin E and selenium deficiency in chickens and especially in turkeys may result in an extreme myopathy of the gizzard and heart muscles (Fig. 2.14) (Scott et al., 1967).

ENLARGED HOCK DISORDER IN TURKEYS. Turkeys receiving diets low in vitamin E and also containing readily oxidizable fats or oils may develop characteristic hock enlargements and bowed legs at approximately 2–3 weeks of age (Scott, 1953). If

poults are allowed to continue on these diets, hock enlargements usually disappear by the time the poults are 6 weeks of age, only to reappear in more severe form when they reach 14–16 weeks, especially in toms raised on wire or slat floors. Creatine excretion is increased and muscle creatine levels are reduced.

The development of enlarged hocks appears to be a peculiarity of turkeys and may result from a number of deficiencies and stresses. In addition to the need for adequate vitamin E, phosphorus, choline, glycine, nicotinic acid, zinc, and biotin are needed in adequate amounts for the prevention of enlarged hock disorders. The beneficial effect of vitamin E may be due to a protection of biotin which otherwise may be destroyed in the presence of rancidifying fats or oils (Scott, 1968). Two infectious diseases, synovitis and staphylococcic arthritis, also may show somewhat similar signs.

Treatment of Deficiency

If not too far advanced exudative diathesis and muscular dystrophy in chicks are readily reversed by administration of proper levels of vitamin E and selenium by injection, by oral dosing, or in the feed. Encephalomalacia may or may not respond to treatment with vitamin E, depending upon the extent of damage to the cerebellum. Gizzard myopathy in turkeys is prevented by supplementing deficient diets with either vitamin E or selenium. It is not affected by the dietary level of sulfur amino acids.

VITAMIN K

Vitamin K is required for the synthesis of prothrombin within the body. Since prothrombin is an important part of the blood-clotting mechanism, a deficiency of vitamin K results in a markedly prolonged blood-clotting time; an affected chick or poult may bleed to death from a slight bruise or other injury.

Signs and Pathology of Deficiency

Signs of vitamin K deficiency occur most frequently 2–3 weeks after chicks are placed on a vitamin K deficient diet. The presence of sulfaquinoxaline in the feed or drinking water may increase the incidence and severity of the condition. Large hemorrhages appear on the breast, legs, wings, and/or in the abdominal cavity. Chicks show an anemia which may be due partly to loss of blood but also to development of a hypoplastic bone marrow. Although blood-clotting time is a fairly good measure of vitamin K deficiency, a more accurate one is obtained by determining prothrombin time.

Treatment of Deficiency

Within 4–6 hours after vitamin K is administered to deficient chicks the blood clots normally, but recovery from the anemia or disappearance of the hemorrhages cannot be expected to take place promptly. This may account for the apparent failure to recover from some cases of "field hemorrhagic syndrome" upon treatment with menadione sodium bisulfite.

THIAMINE (VITAMIN B₁)

Thiamine is required by poultry for the metabolism of carbohydrates. In the body it becomes an important part of the enzyme carboxylase which is concerned in a number of reactions involving pyruvate, one of the end products of carbohydrate catabolism. Deficiency of thiamine in poultry leads to extreme anorexia, polyneuritis, and death.

Signs and Pathology of Deficiency

Polyneuritis is observed in mature chickens approximately 3 weeks after they are placed on a thiamine deficient diet. In young chicks it may appear before 2 weeks of age. The onset is sudden in young chicks, more gradual in mature birds. Anorexia is followed by loss of weight, ruffled feathers, leg weakness, and an unsteady gait. Adult chickens often show a blue comb. As the deficiency progresses apparent paralysis of the muscles occurs, beginning with the flexors of the toes and progressing upward, affecting the extensor muscles of the legs, wings, and neck. The chicken characteristically sits on its flexed legs and draws back the head in a "stargazing" position (Fig. 2.15). Retraction of the head is due to paralysis of the anterior muscles of the neck. The chicken soon loses the ability to stand or sit upright and topples to the floor where it may lie with the head still retracted.

The body temperature may drop to as low as 96° F. A progressive decrease in the respiratory rate occurs. Adrenal glands hypertrophy more markedly in females than males. The cortex is affected to a greater extent than the medulla. Apparently the degree of hypertrophy determines the degree of edema which occurs chiefly

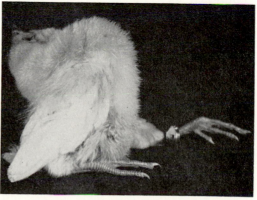

FIG. 2.15—*Typical "stargazing" pose displayed by chick suffering from thiamine deficiency.*

in the skin. The epinephrine content of the adrenal increases as the organ hypertrophies. Atrophy of the genital organs is more pronounced in the testes than in the ovaries. The heart shows a slight degree of atrophy; the right side may be dilated, the auricle being more frequently affected than the ventricle. Atrophy in the stomach and intestinal walls may be sufficiently severe to be easily noted.

Treatment of Deficiency

Chickens suffering from thiamine deficiency respond in a matter of a few hours to oral administration of the vitamin. Since thiamine deficiency causes extreme anorexia, supplementing the feed with the vitamin is not a reliable treatment until after the chickens have recovered from the acute deficiency via oral administration of thiamine.

RIBOFLAVIN (VITAMIN B₂)

Riboflavin forms the active part of over a dozen enzyme systems in the body. Important riboflavin-containing enzymes are: cytochrome reductase, diaphorase, xanthine oxidase, L- and D-amino acid oxidases, and histaminase, all of which are vitally associated with the oxidation-reduction reactions involved in cell respiration.

Signs and Pathology of Deficiency

When chicks are fed a diet deficient in riboflavin, they grow very slowly, become weak and emaciated; their appetite is fairly good; diarrhea develops between the 1st and 2nd week. The chicks do not walk except when forced to do so, and then frequently walk upon their hocks with the aid of their wings. The toes are curled inward when both walking and resting (Fig. 2.16). The chicks are usually found in a resting position. The wings often droop as though it were impossible for the chicks to hold them in the normal position. Leg muscles are atrophied and flabby, and the skin is

dry and harsh. Young chicks in advanced stages of deficiency do not move around but lie with their legs sprawled out.

Postmortem examination shows no marked abnormalities of internal organs, and bacteriologic examination reveals no specific infection of the blood or internal organs. In some cases the thymus shows congestion and premature atrophy.

A deficiency of riboflavin in the diet of hens results in decreased egg production, increased embryonic mortality, and an increase in size and fat content of the liver. Hatchability of eggs decreases within 2 weeks after hens are fed a riboflavin deficient diet, but improves to near normal levels within 7 days after adequate amounts of riboflavin are added to the diet. Embryos which fail to hatch from eggs of hens fed diets low in this vitamin are dwarfed and show a high incidence of edema, degeneration of Wolffian bodies, and defective down. The down is referred to as "clubbed," and results from a failure of the down feathers to rupture the sheaths, causing feathers to coil in a characteristic way.

Riboflavin deficiency in young turkeys is characterized by poor growth and incrustations in the corners of the mouth and on the eyelids. Severe dermatitis of the feet and shanks, marked by edematous swelling, desquamation, and deep fissures, appears in some deficient poults (McGinnis and Carver, 1947). It is noted that these signs of riboflavin deficiency in turkeys are similar to those of pantothenic acid deficiency in chickens.

In severe cases of riboflavin deficiency, chicks show a marked swelling and softening of sciatic and brachial nerves. The sciatic nerves usually show the most pronounced effects, sometimes reaching a diameter 4–5 times normal size.

Histologic examinations of affected nerves show degenerative changes in the myelin sheaths of the main peripheral nerve trunks. This may be accompanied by

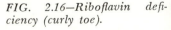

FIG. 2.16—Riboflavin deficiency (curly toe).

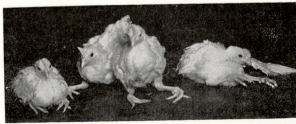

axis cylinder swelling and fragmentation. Schwann cell proliferation, myelin changes, gliosis, and chromatolysis occur in the spinal cord. In cases of curled-toe paralysis, degeneration of the neuromuscular end plate and muscle tissues is often found. This indicates that riboflavin is necessary for the normal functioning of the nervous system of the growing chick. Riboflavin is probably also essential for myelin metabolism of the main peripheral nerve trunks. No gross dystrophy develops although muscle fibers are in some cases completely degenerated. The sciatic nerve exhibits myelin degeneration in one or more of its branches. Similar changes are apparent in the brachial nerve trunks.

The nervous system of embryos which fail to hatch from eggs laid by hens fed riboflavin deficient diets shows degenerative changes very much like those described in riboflavin deficient chicks (Engel et al., 1940).

Treatment of Deficiency

Chicks receiving rations only partially deficient in riboflavin may recover spontaneously, indicating that the requirement rapidly decreases with age. Figure 2.17 shows a poult 35 days old, prostrate from riboflavin deficiency and with curled-toe paralysis. Figure 2.18 shows this same poult 5 days later after having been given two 100 μg-doses of riboflavin. This amount should be sufficient for treatment of riboflavin deficient chicks or poults, followed by incorporation of an adequate level in the ration. However, when the curled-toe deformity is of long standing, irreparable damage has occurred and administration of riboflavin no longer cures the condition.

PANTOTHENIC ACID

Pantothenic acid is the vitamin component of coenzyme A which is concerned in numerous reactions in carbohydrate, protein, and fat metabolism. This enzyme is involved in acetylation of choline in formation of acetylcholine, in formation of citrate, in fatty acid oxidation, in oxidation of keto acids resulting from deamination of amino acids, and in many other functions.

Signs and Pathology of Deficiency

Pantothenic acid is required for normal hatchability. Subcutaneous hemorrhage and severe edema are signs of pantothenic acid deficiency in the developing chicken embryo (Beer et al., 1963).

The signs of pantothenic acid deficiency

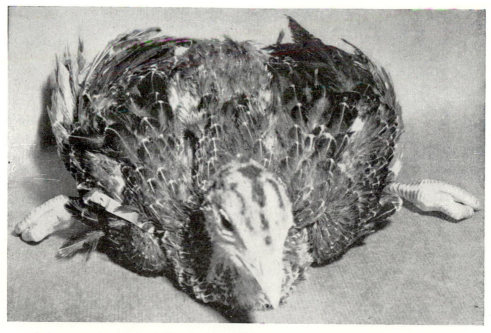

FIG. 2.17—A 35-day-old poult showing riboflavin deficiency with curled-toe paralysis. (Richardson, Tex. Agr. Expt. Sta.)

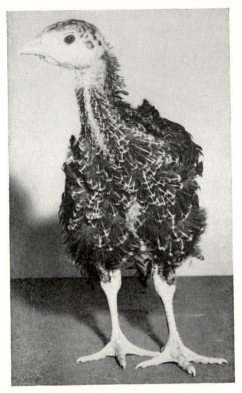

FIG. 2.18—Same poult (Fig. 2.17) 5 days later after having received two 100-μg doses of riboflavin. (Richardson, Tex. Agr. Expt. Sta.)

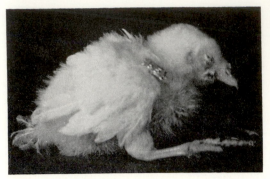

FIG. 2.19—Dermatosis of pantothenic acid deficiency in chick.

in chicks are difficult to differentiate from those of biotin deficiency. Deficiencies of either pantothenic acid or biotin result in dermatitis, broken feathers, perosis, poor growth, and mortality. Pantothenic acid deficient chicks are characterized by retarded and rough feather growth. Chicks are emaciated, and definite crusty scablike lesions appear in the corners of the mouth. The margins of the eyelids are granular, and small scabs develop on them. The eyelids frequently are stuck together by a viscous exudate; they are contracted, and vision is restricted (Fig. 2.19). There is slow sloughing of the keratinizing epithelium of the skin. The outer layers of skin between the toes and on the bottoms of the feet sometimes peel off, and small cracks and fissures appear at these points. These cracks and fissures enlarge and deepen so that the chicks move about very little. In some cases the skin layers of the feet of deficient chicks cornify, and wartlike protuberances develop on the balls of the feet.

Postmortem examination shows the presence of a puslike substance in the mouth and an opaque grayish white exudate in the proventriculus (Ringrose et al., 1931). The liver is hypertrophied and may vary in color from a faint to a dirty yellow. The spleen is slightly atrophied. The kidneys are somewhat enlarged. The nerves and myelinated fibers of the spinal cord show myelin degeneration (Phillips and Engel, 1939). These degenerating fibers occur in all segments of the cord down to the lumbar region.

Gillis et al. (1948) showed that the amount of pantothenic acid in the diet of breeding hens has a definite effect on the hatchability of eggs produced. Embryonic mortality was high when the hens were fed a diet low in pantothenic acid. Most mortality occurred during the last 2–3 days of the incubation period.

Treatment of Deficiency

Pantothenic acid deficiency appears to be completely reversible, if not too far advanced, by oral treatment or injection with the vitamin, followed by restoration of an adequate level of pantothenic acid in the diet.

Pantothenic acid deficiency in sufficient severity to cause characteristic symptoms has not been demonstrated to occur under field conditions. Robertson et al. (1949) noted that the disease known as "stunted chick disease" exhibits many of the signs characteristic of pantothenic acid deficiency. However, substitution of 5% liver meal for 5% meat scrap in the ration or injection of the chicks with 100 μg of pantothenic acid failed to provide any protection in the course of the disease.

Another field disease has been observed which may indicate a deficiency of pantothenic acid in chicken breeder rations under certain conditions. In this disease, first noted by Hill (1954, unpublished data), egg production and hatchability of fertile eggs are normal, but chicks are underweight and weak and may suffer up to 50% mortality during the first 24 hours after hatching. Hill (1954, unpublished data) and Fisher and Hudson (1956) found that injection of chicks with a mixture of B vitamins or with pantothenic acid alone repeatedly has reduced early mortality to normal levels. Beer et al. (1963) produced a very similar condition experimentally; they found that the peak day of embryonic mortality depends upon the degree of pantothenic acid deficiency, and that borderline deficiencies produce extremely weak chicks that fail to survive unless injected immediately with pantothenic acid (200 μg i.p.). Under field conditions it is possible that a pantothenic acid-vitamin B_{12} interrelationship or an interrelationship between pantothenic acid and some other nutrient is involved in this disease.

NICOTINIC ACID (NIACIN)

Nicotinic acid is the vitamin component in two important enzymes, nicotinamide adenine dinucleotide (NAD) and nicotinamide adenine dinucleotide phosphate (NADP). These coenzymes are involved in carbohydrate, fat, and protein metabolism. They are especially important in the metabolic reactions which furnish energy to the animal. Both NAD and NADP take part in the anaerobic and aerobic oxidation of glucose. In fat metabolism, NAD is required for glycerol synthesis and catabolism, for fatty acid synthesis, and for oxidation of the 2-carbon breakdown products of fats by way of the Krebs cycle. Both NAD and NADP are concerned in the degradation and synthesis of amino acids and the oxidation of amino acid residues.

Nicotinic Acid-Tryptophan-Pyridoxine Interrelationships

Briggs et al. (1946) showed that the nicotinic acid requirement of chicks and hens depends on the level of tryptophan in the diet. Later it was found that tryptophan is converted to nicotinic acid by the tissues of chickens, turkeys, and their developing embryos, and that pyridoxine (vitamin B_6) is required for this conversion.

Signs and Pathology of Deficiency

The main sign of nicotinic acid deficiency in young chicks, turkeys, and ducks is an enlargement of the hock joint and bowing of the legs similar to perosis (Scott and Heuser, 1954). The main difference between this condition and the perosis of manganese or choline deficiency is that in nicotinic acid deficiency the tendon of Achilles rarely slips from its condyles. Scott (1953) showed that both nicotinic acid and vitamin E are required for prevention of the disorder in turkeys. Briggs (1946) described further signs of nicotinic acid deficiency as inflammation of the mouth, diarrhea, and poor feathering. Poor feathering and "flightiness" are generally recognized signs of nicotinic acid deficiency.

No evidence has been obtained of any need to supplement practical diets of mature poultry with nicotinic acid, and no deficiency signs have been described.

Treatment of Deficiency

Supplementing a deficient ration with the required amounts of nicotinic acid usually brings about rapid recovery from all signs of deficiency, including hock enlargements and bowed legs in young chicks, ducklings, or poults. Nicotinic acid supplementation has little or no effect upon cases which have progressed to the extent that the tendon has slipped from its condyles (perosis) or upon advanced cases of "enlarged hock disorder" in adult tom turkeys.

PYRIDOXINE (VITAMIN B_6)

Pyridoxine is required in several enzymes, particularly those concerned with transamination and decarboxylation of amino acids. The coenzymes are pyridoxal phosphate and pyridoxamine phosphate.

Signs of Deficiency

Pyridoxine deficient chicks show depressed appetite, poor growth, perosis, and characteristic nervous signs. The chicks show jerky, nervous movements of the legs when walking and often undergo extreme spasmodic convulsions which usually terminate in death. During these convulsions chicks may run aimlessly about, flapping their wings and falling to their sides or rolling completely over on their backs, where they perform rapid jerking motions with their feet and heads. These signs may be distinguished from those of encephalomalacia (vitamin E deficiency) by the relatively greater intensity of activity of the chicks during a seizure caused by pyridoxine deficiency, which results in complete exhaustion and often in death.

In adult birds pyridoxine deficiency causes marked reduction of egg production and hatchability as well as decreased feed consumption, loss of weight, and death.

BIOTIN

Biotin takes part in carboxylation and decarboxylation reactions involving fixation of carbon dioxide.

Signs and Pathology of Deficiency

In biotin deficiency the dermatitis of the feet and skin around the beak and eyes is similar to that described for pantothenic acid (Fig. 2.20). Thus in making a differential diagnosis between biotin and pantothenic acid deficiencies, it is usually necessary to examine the composition of the diet and decide which vitamin is more likely to be deficient. This can be checked by feeding the diet to two groups of chicks, supplementing the feed for one group with biotin and the other with pantothenic acid.

Couch et al. (1948) reported that congenital perosis, ataxia, and characteristic skeletal deformities developed when hens were fed a low biotin diet which did not favor intestinal synthesis of the vitamin but these were prevented by adding biotin to the diet. These embryonic deformities consisted of a shortened tibiotarsus which was bent posteriorly, a much shortened tarsometatarsus, shortening of the bones of the wing and skull, and shortening and bending of the anterior end of the scapula.

According to Cravens et al. (1944), embryos from hens fed biotin deficient diets developed syndactylia, an extensive webbing between the third and fourth toes. These workers also observed that a large number of embryos which failed to hatch were chondrodystrophic, characterized by reduced size, a parrot beak, severely crooked tibia, and/or a much shortened or twisted tarsometatarsus. One peak of embryonic mortality occurred during the first week of incubation, a second during the last 3 days.

Perosis is also a characteristic deficiency sign of biotin avitaminosis. The young turkey requires about 2.5 times as much biotin as the young chick. Enlarged hocks and perosis due to biotin deficiency have been reported in commercial flocks of turkeys. This probably results from lack of availability of biotin from many feedstuffs plus possible loss of biotin in some feeds.

Treatment of Deficiency

If biotin deficiency is observed in chickens, one should investigate the possibility of the presence of uncooked egg white in the diet, since biotin deficiency in chickens is very difficult to produce even with highly purified feed ingredients unless raw egg white (avidin) is added to the diet. Biotin supplementation of a diet containing raw egg white may not correct the deficiency unless the level of biotin used is in excess of the biotin-combining capacity of the avidin present in the egg white. Under these conditions, removal of egg white from the diet and injection of a few micrograms of biotin should produce a quick recovery.

The available biotin content of a practical diet may in some instances provide only half of the biotin requirement of the young poult. Under severe stress conditions it might be necessary to add to poult starting diets as much as 0.125 mg biotin per kg of diet. This amounts to approximately 0.06 mg per lb of diet, or 120 mg per ton of turkey starting ration. Under

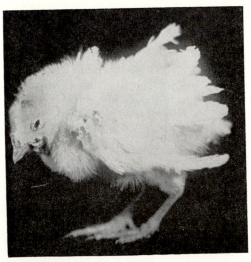

FIG. 2.20—A biotin-deficient chick.

most practical conditions, however, 80–100 mg per ton should be adequate. Since biotin carry-over from the breeder diet may be important in early nutrition of the young poult, it may be desirable also to add approximately this same level (80–100 mg biotin per ton) to turkey breeder diets.

FOLIC ACID (FOLACIN)

Folic acid is a part of the enzyme system concerned in "single carbon" metabolism. It is involved in the synthesis of purines and the methyl groups of such important metabolites as choline, methionine, and thymine. Folic acid, therefore, is required for normal nucleic acid metabolism and for the formation of the nucleoproteins required for cell multiplication.

Signs and Pathology of Deficiency

Folic acid deficiency in chicks is characterized by poor growth, very poor feathering, anemia, and perosis. It is required for pigmentation in the feathers of Rhode Island Red and Black Leghorn chicks. Thus folic acid, lysine, and iron appear to be required for prevention of achroma of feathers in colored poultry.

A deficiency in the breeding diet of chickens or turkeys causes a marked increase in embryonic mortality. The embryos die soon after pipping the air cell. According to Sunde et al. (1950a,b), a deformed upper mandible and bending of the tibiotarsus are lesions of embryonic deficiency. Poults show a characteristic "cervical paralysis" (Fig. 2.21) and die within 2 days after the onset of these signs unless folic acid is administered immediately. Poults show only a slight anemia.

Folic acid deficiency in chicks causes megaloblastic arrest of erythrocyte formation in the bone marrow, which results in a severe macrocytic anemia as one of the first signs in chicks. White cell formation also is reduced, causing a marked agranulocytosis. Further evidence that folic acid is necessary for cell mitosis is supplied by these discoveries: (1) Oviduct growth is not increased in estrogen-treated chicks unless the diet is supplemented with folic acid or, preferably, with the citrovorum factor (Kline and Dorfman, 1951). (2) Growth of the chicken embryo is inhibited by very small amounts of the folic acid antagonist 4-amino-folic acid, the inhibition being reversed by adding citrovorum factor (Cravens and Snell, 1950). (3) Rous sarcoma is inhibited completely either by folic acid deficiency or by feeding 4-amino-folic acid (Little et al., 1948).

Folic Acid-Choline Interrelationship

In the presence of adequate folic acid in the diet, only approximately 260 mg of choline are required to prevent perosis in chicks. When the diet is deficient in folic acid, an increase in the level of choline reduces the incidence and severity of perosis, but levels up to 900 mg of choline per lb of diet fail to prevent this disorder completely (Young et al., 1955).

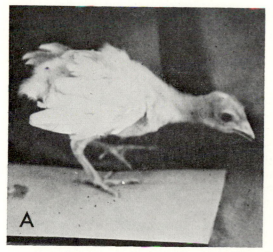 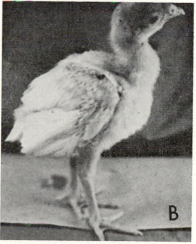

FIG. 2.21—(A) Cervical paralysis in poult suffering from folic acid deficiency. (B) Poult receiving same diet plus folic acid.

Treatment of Deficiency

A single intramuscular injection of 50 or 100 μg of pure pteroylglutamic (folic) acid causes a peak reticulocyte response—70% within 4 days in severely anemic folic acid deficient chicks (Robertson et al., 1947). The hemoglobin values and growth rates return to normal within one week. Oral administration of 50 μg of folic acid was much less effective, whereas the addition of 500 μg of folic acid per 100 g of feed caused recovery comparable to that obtained with injection of the vitamin.

VITAMIN B$_{12}$ (COBALAMIN)

Vitamin B$_{12}$ is concerned in nucleic acid synthesis, methyl synthesis, and carbohydrate and fat metabolism. One of its main enzyme functions involves the isomerization of methylmalonyl coenzyme A to form succinyl CoA.

Signs and Pathology of Deficiency

Signs of vitamin B$_{12}$ deficiency are slow growth, decreased efficiency of feed utilization, mortality, and reduced hatchability. Specific signs for vitamin B$_{12}$ deficiency have not been demonstrated in growing or mature poultry. Perosis may occur in vitamin B$_{12}$ deficient chicks or poults when the diet lacks choline, methionine, or betaine as sources of methyl groups. Addition of vitamin B$_{12}$ may prevent perosis under these conditions because of its effect upon the synthesis of methyl groups. Kline (1955) demonstrated that in vitamin B$_{12}$ deficient pullets maintained on a diet low in choline and methionine, oviduct response to treatment with diethylstilbestrol was significantly lower than in pullets receiving vitamin B$_{12}$. McGinnis et al. (1948) reported that a deficiency of vitamin B$_{12}$ increased the nonprotein nitrogen level in the blood of chicks, which was reduced to normal by feeding a liver concentrate rich in vitamin B$_{12}$. Olcese et al. (1950) reported a peak in embryonic mortality at the 17th day of incubation of eggs from vitamin B$_{12}$ deficient hens, and a myoatrophy of the legs in the vitamin B$_{12}$ deficient embryos. Other anomalies associated with vitamin B$_{12}$ deficiency in the embryos were hemorrhages and perosis.

Treatment of Deficiency

Peeler et al. (1951) showed that intramuscular injection of 2 μg of vitamin B$_{12}$ per

hen increased hatchability of eggs from the vitamin B$_{12}$ deficient hens from approximately 15 to 80% within one week. The addition of 4 mg of vitamin B$_{12}$ per ton of a breeding ration is sufficient to maintain maximum hatchability and to produce chicks having sufficient stores of the vitamin to prevent any deficiency during the first few weeks of life. Similar injections of young chicks followed by a similar supplementation of the chick ration also will correct a vitamin B$_{12}$ deficiency. Lillie et al. (1949) showed that when eggs laid by hens deficient in vitamin B$_{12}$ were injected with the crystalline vitamin, hatchability and subsequent growth of the chicks were improved.

CHOLINE

Choline is present in acetylcholine in the body phospholipids and acts as a methyl source in synthesis within the body of methyl-containing compounds such as methionine, creatine, and N-methylnicotinamide. Choline per se does not act as a methyl donor but first must be oxidized to the compound betaine, which can then donate one of its 3 methyl groups to a methyl acceptor such as homocysteine or glycocyamine for the formation of methionine or creatine respectively.

Signs and Pathology of Deficiency

In addition to poor growth, the outstanding sign of choline deficiency in chicks and poults is perosis (see section under manganese). Young turkeys have a high requirement for choline and therefore will show a high incidence of severe perosis unless special care is taken to supplement poult diets with choline. Perosis is first characterized by pinpoint hemorrhages and a slight puffiness about the hock joint, followed by an apparent flattening of the tibiometatarsal joint caused by a rotation of the metatarsus. The metatarsus continues to twist and may become bent or bowed so that it is out of alignment with the tibia. When this condition exists, the leg cannot adequately support the weight of the bird. The articular cartilage is deformed and the tendon of Achilles slips from its condyles.

When laying pullets which have received high-choline rearing diets are fed diets severely deficient in choline, the percentage of fat in the liver increases. In livers of choline deficient chickens the fat content is higher in females than in males. However, choline deficiency is rare in adult chickens and turkeys fed practical rations. Nesheim et al. (1967) have shown that pullets fed high choline levels during the 8–20-week growing period are more prone to show fatty livers when placed on purified low-choline laying diets than are pullets which have been fed minimum levels during the same growth period. These results indicate that maturing chickens can synthesize choline but will not fully develop this ability if given diets containing ample amounts of the vitamin.

Treatment of Deficiency

If a diagnosis of choline deficiency is noted in chicks or poults before severe signs of perosis have developed, the deficiency can be cured by supplementing the ration with sufficient choline to meet the requirements. Once the tendon has slipped in chicks or poults suffering from choline deficiency, the damage is irreparable.

VITAMIN C, INOSITOL, P-AMINOBENZOIC ACID, AND LIPOIC ACID

Under normal conditions vitamin C (ascorbic acid) is synthesized in adequate amounts by all species of poultry. A controversy has developed as to whether ascorbic acid supplementation of growing and laying diets produces beneficial results in growth, egg production, and eggshell quality, especially under conditions of prolonged heat stress (Perek and Kendler, 1963).

Inositol has been known for years to be an essential nutrient for certain yeasts and other microorganisms. Evidence from a number of studies indicates that inositol is not required in the diet of poultry.

A part of the folic acid molecule is p-aminobenzoic acid. Thus the presence of this compound in the diet aids the intestinal microorganisms in their synthesis of folic acid, which could benefit the chicken or turkey if the diet happened to be deficient in folic acid.

Lipoic acid (also referred to as protogen or thioctic acid) is a metabolite concerned in oxidative decarboxylation in carbohydrate (pyruvate) metabolism. Lipoic acid is synthesized in adequate amounts by chickens and turkeys.

ESSENTIAL INORGANIC ELEMENTS

The essential mineral elements are as important as amino acids and vitamins in the maintenance of life, well-being, and production in poultry. They enter into the composition of bones and give the skeleton the rigidity and strength needed to support the soft tissues. Minerals combine with protein, lipids, and other substances which make up the soft tissues of the body. They take part in maintenance of osmotic pressure and acid-base balance and exert specific effects on the ability of muscles and nerves to respond to stimuli. Minerals also are necessary for the activation of many of the enzymes of the animal body.

The inorganic elements which have been found essential for the maintenance of animal well-being are calcium, phosphorus, magnesium, potassium, sodium, chlorine, and the trace elements manganese, iron, copper, zinc, iodine, molybdenum, and selenium. Fluorine in small amounts is a constant constituent of several tissues, particularly bones. Traces of this element may be essential or at least beneficial for some species, but no direct evidence has been obtained with poultry. Analyses of the individual mineral constituents in the body of chickens show that the major portion of the calcium, phosphorus, magnesium, and zinc of the body is present in the bones. The other essential elements are distributed largely in muscles, other soft tissues, and body fluids.

CALCIUM AND PHOSPHORUS

Calcium and phosphorus are closely associated in metabolism, particularly in bone formation. The major portion of the calcium in the diet of the growing chick or poult is used for bone formation and in the mature hen for eggshell formation. Calcium also is essential for clotting of blood, is required along with sodium and potassium for normal beating of the heart, and is concerned in maintenance of the acid-base equilibrium.

In addition to its role in bone formation, phosphorus exercises important functions in metabolism of carbohydrates and fats; it enters into composition of important constituents of all living cells; and salts formed from it play an important part in maintenance of the acid-base balance. It apparently also is concerned in calcium transport in egg formation.

The utilization of calcium and phosphorus is dependent upon the presence of an adequate amount of vitamin D in the diet. In vitamin D deficiency, calcium and phosphorus deposition in the bones of growing chicks and poults is reduced, and the quantity of calcium in eggshells is decreased.

A deficiency of calcium, phosphorus, or vitamin D in the diet of growing chicks results in rickets (see section of this chapter dealing with vitamin D). In laying hens calcium deficiency results in reduced egg production, thin-shelled eggs, and a tendency to deplete the calcium content of the bones first by complete removal of the medullary bone, followed by a gradual removal of the cortical bone, finally causing the bones to become so thin that spontaneous fractures may occur, especially in the vertebrae, tibia, and femur. This condition may be associated with a syndrome commonly termed "cage layer fatigue" (Riddell et al., 1968). While a marginal calcium deficiency often has been found to be a triggering agent in cage layer fatigue, the syndrome apparently is not due to a simple deficiency of calcium but also is involved with other etiologic factors, one of which may be disease.

MAGNESIUM

Magnesium is closely associated with calcium and phosphorus in the body. It is essential for bone formation, about two-thirds of the magnesium in the body being present in the bone chiefly as a carbonate. It also is necessary for carbohydrate metabolism and for the activation of many enzymes. Eggshells contain about 0.4% magnesium.

Almquist (1942) found that the magnesium requirement of the chick is approximately 0.04% of the ration during the first few weeks of life. He observed that chicks fed a magnesium deficient diet grew slowly for approximately one week and then ceased growing and became lethargic. When disturbed these chicks frequently passed into a brief convulsion accompanied by gasping and finally into a comatose state sometimes ending in death.

The magnesium requirement of turkey poults fed a purified diet was reported by Sullivan (1962) to be about 0.0475%. The magnesium deficiency signs of poults were similar to those of chicks. Poults showed no evidence of toxicity when the diet contained 0.18% magnesium.

Excess Magnesium

Ordinary feedstuffs supply enough magnesium in practical poultry diets to meet requirements. It is possible, however, that under certain conditions rations may contain excess magnesium, producing detrimental effects. Alder (1927) found that feeding dolomite limestone with a high percentage of magnesium for 4 months caused egg production to decrease and eggshells to become progressively thinner; diarrhea, extreme irritability, and fright also were noted. All conditions cleared up shortly after substituting a high-grade limestone for the dolomite. Work with several species of animals, however, indicates that magnesium is less harmful when the diet contains liberal rather than marginal amounts of calcium and phosphorus.

SODIUM AND CHLORINE (SALT)

Sodium as chloride, carbonate, and phosphate is found chiefly in the blood and body fluids. Sodium is connected intimately with regulation of the hydrogen ion concentration of blood. Along with potassium and calcium in proper balance, it is essential for heart activity.

Signs of Deficiency

Animals receiving diets deficient in sodium not only fail to grow but also develop softening of the bones, corneal keratinization, gonadal inactivity, adrenal hypertrophy, changes in cellular function, impairment of food utilization, and decrease in both plasma and special fluid volumes. Cardiac output drops, mean arterial pressure falls, the hematocrit increases, elasticity of subcutaneous tissue decreases, adrenal function is impaired leading to a rise in blood urea, and a state of shock results which, if uncorrected, terminates in death. Deficiency of sodium markedly reduces the utilization of protein and energy and interferes with reproductive performance. Chicks fed a diet containing no added salt show retarded growth with decreased efficiency of food utilization. A lack of salt in the diet of laying hens results in decreased egg production and egg size, loss of weight, and cannibalism. Leach and Nesheim (1963) observed that chicks fed a purified diet containing 0.24% sodium and 0.4% potassium required 0.12% chlorine. They produced chloride deficiency by feeding young chicks a purified diet containing 190 mg chloride/kg diet. Chicks exhibited extremely poor growth rate, high mortality, hemoconcentration, dehydration, and a reduced blood chloride. In addition, deficient chicks showed nervous signs characteristic of chloride deficiency. When startled they fell forward with their feet outstretched behind them and lay paralyzed for several minutes, then appeared quite normal until they were frightened again (Fig. 2.22).

The addition of 1,200 mg chloride/kg basal diet resulted in optimal growth rate and prevented the deficiency. Although excess sodium and potassium did not affect the growth rate of deficient chicks, increasing the levels of these cations in the basal diet increased the incidence of mortality and nervous signs. Bromide (676–1,352 mg/kg) added to the basal diet partially counteracted most of the signs of chloride deficiency except the nervous signs. Higher levels of bromide were of no additional value. Iodide (537–1,074 mg/kg) depressed growth rate and produced mortality and nervous signs which suggested an antagonism between iodide and chloride. Fluoride (268 mg/kg) had no effect on the course of chloride deficiency.

Excessive amounts of salt in the ration are toxic to chickens. The lethal dose is approximately 4 gm/kg of body weight. Young chicks appear to be more susceptible to toxic effects of salt than older chickens; water consumption increases with increased salt content of the diet. Matterson et al. (1946) fed day-old turkey poults graded quantities of salt for 23 days and observed 25% edema and 25% mortality at 4.0% salt but none at 2.0%. Torrey and Graham

(1935) reported that ducks are more susceptible to salt poisoning than chickens.

The signs of salt intoxication are inability to stand, intense thirst, pronounced muscular weakness, and convulsive movements preceding death. Necropsy has revealed lesions in many organs, particularly hemorrhages and severe congestion in the gastrointestinal tract, muscles, liver, and lungs.

POTASSIUM

Potassium is widely distributed in feedstuffs of both plant and animal origin. The requirements of poultry, especially turkeys, for this element are rather high.

Potassium, in contrast to sodium, is found primarily in the cells of the body rather than in the body fluids; the soft tissues of the chicken contain more than three times as much potassium as sodium. The sodium and potassium contents of bones are approximately the same. Potassium is necessary for normal heart activity, reducing contractility of the heart muscle, and favoring relaxation. Potassium ions also appear to increase membrane permeability.

Signs of Deficiency

The main effect of potassium deficiency is an overall muscle weakness characterized by weak extremities, poor intestinal tone with distension, cardiac weakness, and weakness of the respiratory muscles and their ultimate failure. A low potassium level in the vital organs of animals may occur during severe stresses. Plasma potassium is elevated, causing the kidney (acting under the influence of the adrenocortical hormone) to discharge potassium into the

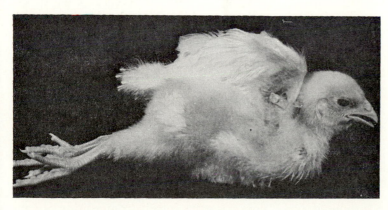

FIG. 2.22—*Characteristic sign of chloride deficiency.*

urine. During adaptation to the stress, the muscle will begin to retrieve its lost potassium. As liver glycogen is restored, potassium will return to the liver. This may result in a temporary prolongation of the general potassium deficiency throughout the body. Effects of administration of potassium salts to animals during and following severe stress periods have not been adequately investigated.

MANGANESE

Manganese is required by poultry for growth, reproduction, and prevention of perosis. Perosis is an anatomical deformity of the leg bones of young chickens, turkeys, pheasants, and other birds. It is characterized by gross enlargement of the tibiometatarsal joint, twisting, or bending of the distal end of the tibia and the proximal end of the metatarsus, and finally slipping of the gastrocnemius tendon from its condyles. This last lesion causes complete crippling in the affected leg; if both legs are affected, death usually results since the chick or poult cannot secure food and water. Early observers of perosis noted that it was most likely to occur under the crowded conditions of confinement rearing; that diets having a high mineral content tended to aggravate the condition; and that heavy breeds of chickens were more susceptible than light breeds.

In addition to its perosis-preventing properties, manganese is necessary for the formation of normal bones. Wilgus et al. (1937a,b) observed that frequently the leg bones of chicks fed perosis-producing diets were thickened and shortened. Manganese also has been reported to be necessary for maximum eggshell quality.

Lyons and Insko (1937) found that manganese deficiency resulted in very low hatchability of fertile eggs and chondrodystrophy in embryos. The peak of mortality for such embryos occurred on the 20th and 21st days of incubation. The chondrodystrophic embryos were characterized by very short thickened legs, short wings, "parrot beak," globular contour of head, protruding abdomen, and retarded down and body growth. Very marked edema was noted in about 75% of these embryos. The manganese content of the eggs producing chondrodystrophic embryos was less than that of normal eggs.

Chicks hatched from eggs produced by hens fed a diet deficient in manganese sometimes exhibit ataxia, particularly when excited (Caskey et al., 1944). The head may be drawn forward and bent underneath the body or retracted over the back. Ataxic chicks grow normally and reach maturity but fail to recover completely. They also retain the short bones characteristic of embryos and newly hatched chicks from manganese deficient dams (Caskey and Norris, 1940).

IODINE

Traces of iodine are required for normal functioning of the thyroid gland in poultry as in other animals. Thyroxine contains approximately 65% iodine and acts as an important regulating agent in body metabolism. When the intake of iodine is suboptimal, the thyroid tissue enlarges and so-called goiter results.

Iodine deficiency is found in areas in which the soil and consequently the feeds and drinking water contain insufficient amounts of this essential nutrient. In the United States these areas are primarily in the Northwest and in the Great Lakes region, but many other sections are either marginal or actually deficient. Iodine deficiency in poultry has been largely offset by the widespread use of fish meal and oyster shells, which contain significant amounts of iodine, and by addition to diets of stabilized iodine either in iodized salt or as part of the trace mineral premix.

Wilgus et al. (1941) reported that iodine deficiency results in enlarged thyroids and in some cases lower body weight in growing chicks. They observed congenital goiter in baby chicks hatched from hens receiving 0.025 ppm of iodine in the ration. The use of 0.25% iodized salt in chicken and turkey rations should prevent the development of iodine deficiency. This would supply 0.175 ppm in addition to that contained in the diet.

IRON AND COPPER

Both iron and copper are necessary for hemoglobin formation. Iron is present in heme, the iron porphyrin nucleus of hemoglobin. This nucleus is also one of the components of the cytochromes and the enzymes peroxidase and catalase. Copper also takes part in the activity of several enzymes but, while essential for hemoglobin formation, does not enter into its composition. In the

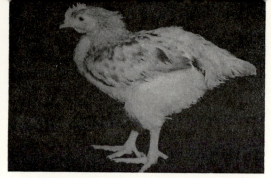

FIG. 2.23—*Deficient pigment formation in feathers of New Hampshire chick resulting from shortage of dietary iron. The chick was also anemic.*

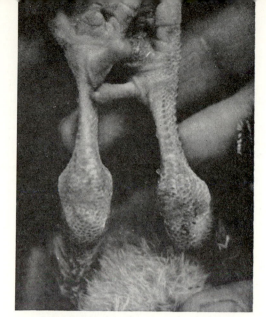

FIG. 2.24—*Enlarged hocks in turkey poult caused by zinc deficiency.*

absence of copper, dietary iron is absorbed and deposited in the liver and elsewhere, but hemoglobin formation does not occur and anemia results. Hill and Matrone (1961) concluded that the chick needs approximately 40 ppm of iron and 4 ppm of copper for maximum hemoglobin formation. Davis et al. (1962) presented evidence that the chick required approximately 65 ppm of iron when the diet contained 10 ppm of copper (Fig. 2.23).

The hemoglobin level of the blood of hens falls with the beginning of egg production, but this apparently is not related to the iron and copper content of the diet. Since hemoglobin level rises rapidly with the onset of broodiness, it is more probable that the low hemoglobin levels prevailing in egg production are due to changes in hormone mechanisms of the body rather than to iron and copper deficiencies.

ZINC

Traces of zinc appear to be necessary for life in all animals. It is a constituent of the enzyme carbonic anhydrase, and is necessary for activation of several other enzymes. Deficiency signs are retarded growth, poor feathering, enlarged hocks, and scaling of the skin, particularly on the feet (Fig. 2.24). Increasing the calcium content of the chick or poult diet from about 1.0 to 2.0% enhances the severity of zinc deficiency. The zinc requirement of poults is higher than that of chicks. Thus poults are more apt to show enlarged hocks and poor feathering of zinc deficiency unless special zinc supplements are added to the diet. The most dramatic embryonic abnormalities resulting from a nutritional deficiency appear when the breeding diet contains excess calcium and phosphorus, is high in phytic acid, and is deficient in zinc. Zinc deficient embryos may have only a head and complete viscera but no spinal column beyond a few vertebrae, no wings, no body wall, and no legs (Kienholz et al., 1961).

SELENIUM

Selenium has been shown to be an essential mineral element for both the chick and the turkey. Selenium prevents the development of "exudative diathesis" in young chickens and myopathy of the gizzard and heart in young turkeys (Scott, 1962a,b; Scott et al., 1967). See vitamin E.

WATER

The simple chemical compound water is of unequaled importance in the metabolism of all animals. Water holds this unique position in nutrition mainly because of its physical properties. Due to its solvent and polar properties it acts as a transport medium for other nutrients and products of metabolism and enhances cell reactions. Because of its high specific heat it can absorb the heat of reactions produced in the oxidation of carbohydrates and fats with little rise in temperature. Water evaporates readily, removing many calories of heat from the body as latent heat of vaporization. These and many other functions of water make it evident why the animal body is able to exist much longer without food than without water.

IMPORTANCE OF CONTINUOUS SUPPLY

Unlike larger farm animals, chickens and turkeys must have access to a continuous water supply since they drink only small amounts at a time. An insufficient amount of water results in decreased growth and egg production. During severely cold weather it is also necessary to keep the water warm. According to Beresford (1930), failure to warm drinking water for hens during cold weather lowers water consumption and reduces egg production. Lack of water causes development of loose, slimy gizzard linings which accompany early non-specific mortality in turkey poults (Hammond, 1944).

The quantity of water needed by chickens is related to the amount of some of the nutrients in the diet. The quantity drunk by chicks is correlated directly with the salt content of the diet (Heuser, 1952). This increases water elimination by increasing the water content of the feces.

REFERENCES

Ackert, J. E., M. F. McIlvaine, and N. Z. Crawford. 1931. Resistance of chickens to parasitism affected by vitamin A. *Am. J. Hyg.* 13:320–36.

Adamstone, F. B. 1947. Histologic comparison of the brains of vitamin A-deficient and vitamin E-deficient chicks. *Arch. Pathol.* 32:301–12.

Adamstone, F. B., and L. E. Card. 1934. The effects of vitamin E deficiency on the testis of the male fowl *(Gallus domesticus). J. Morphol.* 56:339–60.

Alder, B. 1927. The use of calcite and other natural deposits of calcium carbonate in the ration of laying hens. *Proc. Third World's Poultry Congr.,* pp. 231–34.

Almquist, H. J. 1942. Magnesium requirement of the chick. *Proc. Soc. Exp. Biol. Med.* 49:544–45.

Asmundson, V. S., and F. H. Kratzer. 1952. Observations on vitamin A deficiency in turkey breeding stock. *Poultry Sci.* 31:71–73.

Bearse, G. E., C. F. McClary, and H. C. Saxena. 1953. Blood spot incidence and the vitamin A level of the diet. *Poultry Sci.* 32:888. (Abstr.)

Beer, A. E., M. L. Scott, and M. C. Nesheim. 1963. The effect of a deficiency of pantothenic acid on the breeding performance of White Leghorn chickens. *Brit. Poultry Sci.* 4:243–53.

Beresford, H. 1930. Stock tank and poultry water heaters. *Agr. Eng.* 11:279–80.

Bierer, B. W. 1956. Keratoconjunctivitis in turkeys: A preliminary report. *Vet. Med.* 51:363–66.

Brambila, S., and F. W. Hill. 1965. Paralysis induced by feeding synthetic glycerides to chicks. *Proc. Soc. Exp. Biol. Med.* 118:845–47.

———. 1966. Comparison of neutral fat and free fatty acids in high lipid-low carbohydrate diets for the growing chicken. *J. Nutr.* 88:84–92.

Briggs, G. M., Jr. 1946. Nicotinic acid deficiency in turkey poults and the occurrence of perosis. *J. Nutr.* 31:79–84.

Briggs, G. M., Jr., A. C. Groschke, and R. J. Lillie. 1946. Effects of proteins low in tryptophane on growth of chickens and on laying hens receiving nicotinic acid-low rations. *J. Nutr.* 32:659–75.

Caskey, C. D., and L. C. Norris. 1940. Micromelia in adult fowl caused by manganese deficiency during embryonic development. *Proc. Soc. Exp. Biol. Med.* 44:332–35.

Caskey, C. D., L. C. Norris, and G. F. Heuser. 1944. A chronic congenital ataxia in chicks due to manganese deficiency in the maternal diet. *Poultry Sci.* 23:516–20.

Couch, J. R., W. W. Cravens, C. A. Elvehjem, and J. G. Halpin. 1948. Relation of biotin to congenital deformities in the chick. *Anat. Record* 100:29–48.

Cravens, W. W., and E. E. Snell. 1950. Reversal of aminopterin inhibition in the chick embryo with the *Leuconostoc citrovorum* factor. *Proc. Soc. Exp. Biol. Med.* 75:43–45.

Cravens, W. W., W. H. McGibbon, and E. E. Sebesta. 1944. Effect of biotin deficiency on embryonic development in the domestic fowl. *Anat. Record* 90:55–64.

Dam, H., and J. Glavind. 1939. Alimentary exudative diathesis and its relation to vitamin E. *Skand. Arch. Physiol.* 82:299–316.

Davies, A. W. 1952. Lowered liver vitamin A reserves in avian coccidiosis. *Nature* 170:849.

Davis, P. N., L. C. Norris, and F. H. Kratzer. 1962. Iron deficiency studies in chicks using treated isolated soybean protein diets. *J. Nutr.* 78:445–53.

Elvehjem, C. A., and V. F. Neu. 1932. Studies in vitamin A avitaminosis in the chick. *J. Biol. Chem.* 97:71–82.

Engel, R. W., P. H. Phillips, and J. G. Halpin. 1940. The effect of a riboflavin deficiency in the hen upon embryonic development of the chick. *Poultry Sci.* 19:135–42.

Erasmus, J., M. L. Scott, and P. P. Levine. 1960. A relationship between coccidiosis and vitamin A nutrition in chickens. *Poultry Sci.* 39:565–72.

Fell, Honor B., and E. Mellanby. 1953. Metaplasia produced in cultures of chick ectoderm by high vitamin A. *J. Physiol.* 119:470–88.

Fisher, H., and C. B. Hudson. 1956. Chick viability and pantothenic acid deficiency in the breeding diet—Case report. *Poultry Sci.* 35:487–88 (Research note.)

Fritz, J. C., J. H. Hooper, J. L. Halpin, and H. P. Moore. 1946. Failure of feather pigmentation in Bronze poults due to lysine deficiency. *J. Nutr.* 31:387–96.

Gillis, M. B., G. F. Heuser, and L. C. Norris. 1948. Pantothenic acid in the nutrition of the hen. *J. Nutr.* 35:351–63.

Goldstein, J., and M. L. Scott. 1956. An electrophoretic study of exudative diathesis in chicks. *J. Nutr.* 60:349–59.

Hammond, J. C. 1944. Lack of water a cause of loose, slimy gizzard linings accompanying early mortality in poults. *Poultry Sci.* 23: 477–80.

Heuser, G. F. 1952. Salt additions to chick rations. *Poultry Sci.* 31:85–88.

Hill, C. H., and G. Matrone. 1961. Studies on iron and copper deficiencies in growing chickens. *J. Nutr.* 73:425–31.

Hill, F. W., M. L. Scott, L. C. Norris, and G. F. Heuser. 1961. Reinvestigation of the vitamin A requirements of laying and breeding hens and their progeny. *Poultry Sci.* 40: 1245–54.

Hinshaw, W. R., and W. E. Lloyd. 1934. Vitamin A deficiency in turkeys. *Hilgardia* 8: 281–304.

Hooper, J. H., J. L. Halpin, and J. C. Fritz. 1942. The feeding of single massive doses of vitamin D to birds. *Poultry Sci.* 21:472. (Abstr.)

Hopkins, D. T., and M. C. Nesheim. 1967. The linoleic acid requirement of chicks. *Poultry Sci.* 46:872–81.

Hopkins, D. T., R. L. Witter, and M. C. Nesheim. 1963. A respiratory disease syndrome in chickens fed essential fatty acid deficient diets. *Proc. Soc. Exp. Biol. Med.* 114:82–86.

Jensen, L. S., M. L. Scott, G. F. Heuser, L. C. Norris, and T. S. Nelson. 1956. Studies on the nutrition of breeding turkeys. 1. Evidence indicating a need to supplement practical turkey rations with vitamin E. *Poultry Sci.* 35:810–16.

Jungherr, E. 1943. Nasal histopathology and liver storage in subtotal vitamin A deficiency of chickens. *Conn. Agr. Expt. Sta. Bull.* 250.

Kahn, R. H. 1954. Effect of estrogen and of vitamin A on vaginal cornification in tissue culture. *Nature* 174:317.

Kienholz, E. W., D. E. Turk, M. L. Sunde, and W. G. Hoekstra. 1961. Effects of zinc deficiency in the diets of hens. *J. Nutr.* 75:211–21.

Kline, Irene T. 1955. Relationship of vitamin B_{12} to stilbestrol stimulation of the chick oviduct. *Endocrinology* 57:120–28.

Kline, Irene T., and R. I. Dorfman. 1951. Citrovorum factor and oviduct response to stilbestrol in aminopterin-treated chicks. *Proc. Soc. Exp. Biol. Med.* 76:203–5.

Leach, R. M., Jr., and M. C. Nesheim. 1963. Studies on chloride deficiency in chicks. *J. Nutr.* 81:193–99.

Lillie, R. J., M. W. Olsen, and H. R. Bird. 1949. Role of vitamin B_{12} in reproduction in poultry. *Proc. Soc. Exp. Biol. Med.* 72: 598–602.

Little, P. A., A. Sampath, V. Paganelli, E. Locke, and Y. Subbarow. 1948. The effect of folic acid and its antagonists on Rous chicken sarcoma. *Trans. N.Y. Acad. Sci.* 10:91–98.

Ludwig, K. S. 1953. Vitamin A-mangel und uberdosierung und ihre Beziehungen zum Gehalt an alkalischer phosphatase der epiphysenfuge. *Int. Z. Vitaminforsch.* 25:98–103.

Lyons, M., and W. M. Insko, Jr. 1937. Chondrodystrophy in the chick embryo produced by manganese deficiency in the diet of the hen. *Ky. Agr. Expt. Sta. Bull.* 371.

McGinnis, J., and J. S. Carver. 1947. The effect of riboflavin and biotin in the prevention of dermatitis and perosis in turkey poults. *Poultry Sci.* 26:364–71.

McGinnis, J., P. T. Hsu, and W. D. Graham. 1948. Studies on an unidentified factor required by chicks for growth and protein utilization. *Poultry Sci.* 27:674–75. (Abstr.)

Marion, J. E., and H. M. Edwards, Jr. 1962. Observations on the influence of diet and age upon liver lipid changes in the chick. *J. Nutr.* 77:23–27.

Matterson, L. D., H. M. Scott, and E. Jungherr. 1946. Salt tolerance of turkeys. *Poultry Sci.* 26:539–41. (Research note.)

Moore, E. 1953. *Aspergillus fumigatus* as a cause of ophthalmitis in turkeys. *Poultry Sci.* 32:796–99.

Nesheim, M. C., R. M. Leach, Jr., and M. J. Norvell. 1967. The effect of rearing diet on choline deficiency in hens. *Proc. 1967 Cornell Nutr. Conf.*, pp. 57–60.

Olcese, O., J. R. Couch, J. H. Quisenberry, and P. B. Pearson. 1950. Congenital anomalies in the chick due to vitamin B_{12} deficiency. *J. Nutr.* 41:423–31.

Pappenheimer, A. M., M. Goettsch, and E. Jungherr. 1939. Nutritional encephalomalacia in chicks and certain related disorders of domestic birds. *Conn. Agr. Expt. Sta. Bull.* 229.

Patterson, F. D. 1928. Gout in poultry. *Vet. Med.* 23:73–74.

Peeler, H. T., R. F. Miller, C. W. Carlson, L. C. Norris, and G. F. Heuser. 1951. Studies of the effect of vitamin B_{12} on hatchability. *Poultry Sci.* 30:11–17.

Perek, M., and J. Kendler. 1963. Ascorbic acid as a dietary supplement for White Leghorn hens under conditions of climatic stress. *Brit. Poultry Sci.* 4:191–200.

Phillips, P. H., and R. W. Engel. 1939. Some histopathologic observations on chicks deficient in the chick antidermatitis factor or pantothenic acid. *J. Nutr.* 18:227–32.

Renner, Ruth O. A. 1964. Factors affecting the utilization of "carbohydrate-free" diets by the chick. I. Level of protein. *J. Nutr.* 84: 322–26.

Renner, Ruth O. A., and A. M. Elcombe. 1964. Factors affecting the utilization of "carbohydrate-free" diets by the chick. II. Level of glycerol. *J. Nutr.* 84:327–330.

Riddell, C., C. F. Helmboldt, E. P. Singsen, and L. D. Matterson. 1968. Bone pathology of birds affected with cage layer fatigue. *Avian Diseases* 12:285–97.

Ringrose, A. T., L. C. Norris, and G. F. Heuser. 1931. The occurrence of a pellagra-like syndrome in chicks. *Poultry Sci.* 10:166–77.

Robertson, E. I., Grace F. Fiala, M. L. Scott, L. C. Norris, and G. F. Heuser. 1947. Response of anemic chicks to pteroylglutamic acid. *Proc. Soc. Exp. Biol. Med.* 64:441–43.

Robertson, E. I., C. I. Angstrom, H. C. Clark, and M. Shimm. 1949. Field research on "stunted chick" disease. *Poultry Sci.* 28: 14–18.

Ross, E., and L. Adamson. 1961. Observations on the requirements of young chicks for dietary fat. *J. Nutr.* 74:329–34.

Schlotthauer, C. F., and J. L. Bollman. 1934. Experimental gout in turkeys. *Proc. Staff Meet. Mayo Clinic* 9:560–61.

Scott, M. L. 1953. Prevention of the enlarged hock disorder in turkeys with niacin and vitamin E. *Poultry Sci.* 32:670–77.

———. 1962a. Anti-oxidants, selenium and sulphur amino acids in the vitamin E nutrition of chicks. *Nutr. Abstr. Rev.* 32:1–8.

———. 1962b. Vitamin E in health and disease of poultry. *Vitamins Hormones* 20:621–32.

———. 1968. Rediscovery of biotin as a factor for prevention of leg weakness in turkeys. *Feedstuffs* 40 (11): 24.

Scott, M. L. and G. F. Heuser. 1954. Studies on leg weakness in turkeys, ducks and geese. *Proc. Tenth World's Poultry Congr.*, Sect. 11:255–58.

Scott, M. L., G. Olson, L. Krook, and W. R. Brown. 1967. Selenium-responsive myopathies of myocardium and of smooth muscle in the young poult. *J. Nutr.* 91:573–83.

Seifried, O. 1930a. Studies on A-vitaminosis in chickens. I. Lesions of the respiratory tract and their relation to some infectious diseases. *J. Exp. Med.* 52:519–31.

———. 1930b. Studies on A-vitaminosis in chickens. II. Lesions of the upper alimentary tract and their relation to some infectious diseases. *J. Exp. Med.* 52:533–38.

Sullivan, T. W. 1962. The magnesium requirement of turkeys, 0–4 weeks of age. *Poultry Sci.* 41:1686–87. (Abstr.)

Sunde, M. L., W. W. Cravens, H. W. Bruins, C. A. Elvehjem, and J. G. Halpin. 1950a. The pteroylglutamic acid requirement of laying and breeding hens. *Poultry Sci.* 29: 220–26.

Sunde, M. L., W. W. Cravens, C. A. Elvehjem, and J. G. Halpin. 1950b. The effect of folic acid on embryonic development of the domestic fowl. *Poultry Sci.* 29:696–702.

Taylor, A. N., and R. H. Wasserman. 1967. Vitamin D_3-induced calcium-binding protein: Partial purification, electrophoretic visualization, and tissue distribution. *Arch. Biochem. Biophys.* 119:536–40.

Thompson, J. N., J. M. Howell, G. A. J. Pitt, and Catherine I. Houghton. 1965. Biological activity of retinoic acid ester in the domestic fowl: Production of vitamin A deficiency in the early chick embryo. *Nature* 205:1006–7.

Torrey, J. P., and R. Graham. 1935. A note on experimental salt poisoning in ducks. *Cornell Vet.* 25:50–53.

Trummel, C. L., L. G. Raisz, J. W. Blunt, and H. F. DeLuca. 1969. 25-Hydroxycholecalciferol: Stimulation of bone resorption in tissue culture. *Science* 163:1450–51.

Wasserman, R. H., and A. N. Taylor. 1966. Vitamin D_3-induced calcium-binding protein in chick intestinal mucosa. *Science* 152: 791–93.

Wilgus, H. S., Jr., L. C. Norris, and G. F. Heuser. 1937a. The role of manganese and certain other trace elements in the prevention of perosis. *J. Nutr.* 14:155–67.

———. 1937b. The effect of various calcium and phosphorus salts on the severity of perosis. *Poultry Sci.* 16:232–37.

Wilgus, H. S., Jr., G. S. Harshfield, A. R. Patton, L. P. Ferris, and F. X. Gassner. 1941. The iodine requirements of growing chickens. *Poultry Sci.* 20:477. (Abstr.)

Wolbach, S. B., and D. M. Hegsted. 1952. Vitamin A deficiency in the duck. Skeletal growth and the central nervous system. *Arch. Pathol.* 54:548–63.

———. 1953. Hypervitaminosis A in young ducks. The epiphyseal cartilages. *Arch. Pathol.* 55:47–54.

Wolf, G., and B. C. Johnson. 1960. Vitamin A and mucopolysaccharide biosynthesis. *Vitamins Hormones* 18:439–55.

Woollam, D. H. M., and J. W. Millen. 1955. Effect of vitamin A deficiency on the cerebrospinal fluid pressure of the chick. *Nature* 175:41–42.

Young, R. J., L. C. Norris, and G. F. Heuser. 1955. The chick's requirement for folic acid in the utilization of choline and its precursors betaine and methylaminoethanol. *J. Nutr.* 55:353–62.

CHAPTER 3

AVIAN SALMONELLOSIS

❖

INTRODUCTION

❖

J. E. WILLIAMS

Southeast Poultry Research Laboratory
Agricultural Research Service
United States Department of Agriculture
Athens, Georgia

❖

AVIAN SALMONELLOSIS is an inclusive term designating a large group of acute or chronic diseases of fowl caused by any one or more members of the bacterial genus *Salmonella,* which is included in the large family Enterobacteriaceae.

The genus *Salmonella,* named for the late eminent USDA veterinarian Daniel E. Salmon, is composed of approximately 1,500 serological types, each with a specific serotype name. Serotype designations are presently derived from the place where the organisms are first isolated which has resulted in names representative of centers of population all over the world. The rapidity with which new types have been added to the ever-expanding list of salmonellae is illustrated by the fact that only about 60 types were recognized in the 1943 edition of this book.

Several new classification and nomenclature systems for the genus *Salmonella* have been recently suggested. Ewing (1963, 1967) proposed the "three species concept" of speciation that has been used by some writers and has appeared in the literature. Under this system the three species of *Salmonella* recognized are *S. cholerae-suis* (the type species of the genus), *S. typhi,* and *S. enteritidis.* All salmonellae other than *S.*

cholerae-suis and *S. typhi* are considered to be serotypes of *S. enteritidis* (e.g. *S. enteritidis,* serotype Pullorum; *S. enteritidis,* serotype Typhi-murium).

Kauffmann (1966) has proposed that the genus *Salmonella* be divided into 4 subgenera, the individual serotypes of which are considered bacterial species. A species is defined as "a group of serofermentative phage types." Edwards and Galton (1967) have reviewed developments leading up to this proposed system of classification and, along with most workers in the United States, did not subscribe to the species concept of Kauffmann but rather regarded the salmonella serotypes as subspecific or infrasubspecific entities.

In this chapter, the various serotypes will be designated in the traditional manner and the genus *Salmonella* discussed as a single group of organisms without division into subgenera or subspecies serotypes. Those working in the identification of salmonella cultures from poultry should be familiar with the "three species concept" of Ewing (1963) and the proposed salmonella subgenera as discussed by Kauffmann (1966), Ewing and Ball (1966), and Edwards and Galton (1967) in order to better appreciate the variations existent among members of the genus and to aid in the interpretation of unusual reactions in diagnostic media as occur with organisms in Kauffmann's proposed subgenus II.

A few salmonella serotypes are host specific. *S. typhi* infects only man, *S. dublin* is almost restricted to bovine animals, *S. abortus-equi* to the horse, *S. pullorum* to the chicken, and *S. cholerae-suis* to swine. Rarely do these types infect animals other than the host species, and if they do the infection dies out within the flock or herd in a comparatively short time. The great majority of salmonellae are ubiquitous, infecting and causing disease in a variety of animal species and man. Among such types are *S. typhi-murium, S. heidelberg, S. montevideo, S. infantis,* and *S. derby,* to name but a few (Taylor, 1967).

Domestic poultry constitutes the largest single reservoir of salmonella organisms existing in nature. Among all animal species, the salmonellae are most frequently reported from poultry and poultry products, due in part to the large population at risk and to active programs existing nationwide for their isolation and identification. Moran

---

et al. (1965) reported that almost 80% of the salmonellae from animals serotyped in the United States were from chickens and turkeys.

The two relatively host-specific, naturally nonmotile members of the genus, *S. pullorum* and *S. gallinarum*, causative organisms of pullorum disease and fowl typhoid respectively, are generally grouped separately from the motile salmonellae for purposes of discussion. The motile salmonellae, as they infect poultry, are designated *paratyphoid organisms* and the diseases they cause, *paratyphoid infections*. In Great Britain and some other parts of the world the general term avian salmonellosis, rather than paratyphoid, is used to define infection in poultry with any salmonellae other than *S. pullorum* and *S. gallinarum*.

Chronic intestinal carriers of motile salmonellae are common; however, paratyphoid infections, like pullorum disease, seldom occur in the acute, septicemic form except in young fowl or in mature birds under stress conditions such as virus diseases, inadequate diet, or unsanitary environment. Pullorum disease and fowl typhoid frequently infect the reproductive organs of adult chickens, establishing a chronic infection with direct passage of the organisms into the egg as formation takes place. Without the effective control of these two diseases through organized national regulatory programs, the profitable production of poultry would be impossible. Effective serological tests are available for the detection of carriers of pullorum disease and fowl typhoid among poultry breeding flocks, but these are presently lacking for paratyphoid organisms.

In addition to poultry, the motile salmonellae frequently infect all other warm- and cold-blooded animal species, including man. In the general human population, salmonella infection may be derived directly, or most often indirectly, from poultry and domestic animals. For any specific salmonella serotype to become important in human epidemiology it seems necessary for a buildup in population of that type to occur.

With the great expansion of the poultry industry, the widespread occurrence of avian salmonellosis has ranked it as one of the most important egg-borne bacterial diseases of poultry. As these infections recognize no international boundaries and few host barriers, nationwide programs to control them have been beset with numerous obstacles (Anon., 1969). Economically, avian salmonellosis is a problem of concern to all phases of the poultry industry from production to marketing. Pet store owners, zoological park administrators, pigeon and fancy bird raisers, and those interested in wild game are also concerned with these diseases. As they occur in poultry and poultry products, the normally motile salmonellae are also of very significant interest to those engaged in work in the field of public health.

Avian salmonellosis will be discussed in this chapter in three sections—pullorum disease, fowl typhoid, and paratyphoid infections.

REFERENCES

Anonymous. 1969. *An Evaluation of the Salmonella Problem.* Nat. Academy of Sciences, Bull. 1683, Nat. Res. Council, Washington, D.C.

Edwards, P. R., and Mildred M. Galton. 1967. Salmonellosis, pp. 1–63. In Brandly, C. A., and C. Cornelius, *Advances in Veterinary Science.* Academic Press, New York.

Ewing, W. H. 1963. An outline of nomenclature for the family Enterobacteriaceae. *Int. Bull. Bacteriol. Nomencl. Taxon.* 13:95–110.

———. 1967. *Revised Definitions of the Family Enterobacteriaceae, Its Tribes and Genera.* U.S. Dept. of HEW, Public Health Serv., NCDC, Atlanta, Ga.

Ewing, W. H., and M. M. Ball. 1966. *The Biochemical Reactions of Members of the genus Salmonella.* U.S. Dept. of HEW, Public Health Serv., NCDC, Atlanta, Ga.

Kauffmann, F. 1966. *The Bacteriology of Enterobacteriaceae.* Williams & Wilkins Co., Baltimore, Md.

Moran, Alice B., C. D. Van Houweling, and E. M. Ellis. 1965. The results of typing salmonella from animal sources in the United States. *Proc. Natl. Conf. on Salmonellosis,* U.S. Dept. of HEW, Public Health Serv., NCDC, Atlanta, Ga., pp. 33–37.

Taylor, Joan. 1967. Salmonellosis: The present position in man and animals. II. Public health aspects. *Vet. Record* 80:147–54.

PULLORUM DISEASE

G. H. SNOEYENBOS

*Department of Veterinary and
Animal Sciences
University of Massachusetts
Amherst, Massachusetts*

THE TERM pullorum disease is used to designate infections of avian species by *Salmonella pullorum*. The disease is most commonly spread by true egg transmission. It usually occurs in an acute systemic form in chicks and poults but in adults is most often localized and chronic.

"Bacillary white diarrhea" was used to designate the disease until the term pullorum disease was proposed in 1929; the latter term has since gained almost universal acceptance. In some areas of the world, including parts of Europe, *S. pullorum* and *S. gallinarum* are considered to be the same species. Reports of pullorum disease from these areas sometimes indicate either pullorum disease or fowl typhoid. The disease was once enzootic in many areas of the world but has been reduced in incidence to the point where it is rare in most advanced poultry producing areas. Virtual if not total eradication of the disease has been secured in some areas.

The major economic loss from pullorum disease in the United States at this time is indirect and due to the necessity of testing substantially all breeding flocks of chickens and turkeys to assure freedom from infection. Annual testing costs for chickens and turkeys in the United States have been estimated to exceed $5 million per year (B. S. Pomeroy, 1966, unpublished). Infections in man have occasionally been reported. Such infections have been produced by massive exposure following ingestion of contaminated foods and are characterized by rapid onset of severe symptoms of acute enteric infection followed by prompt recovery without treatment.

HISTORY

The etiological agent of pullorum disease was discovered by Rettger in 1899 and was described by him as a "fatal septicemia of young chicks" (1900). In a later report he designated it as "white diarrhea" (1909) and shortly thereafter expanded the term to "bacillary white diarrhea" to distinguish it from other diseases of chicks which might be classified under a common term of "white diarrhea," as was reported by Jones (1911). Reports in the lay press at the turn of the century cited by Rettger and Plastridge (1932) indicated that the disease was widespread in the United States and many foreign countries and caused mortality in chick flocks ranging upward to 100%. Losses were so high that intensive husbandry of chickens was seriously threatened. During the first decade of the twentieth century, investigators definitely proved that pullorum disease was an egg-borne infection. The cycle of infection involved an infected hen laying infected eggs, hatching infected chicks, which could remain infected throughout their life.

During the second decade Jones (1913b) announced the practical application of a macroscopic tube agglutination test for the detection of "carriers" of the organism. Extensive evaluation and development of this test for control and eradication of the disease were carried out in several of the eastern states which allowed inauguration of official state testing programs toward the close of the second decade.

The disease was first recognized in turkeys by Hewitt (1928) and within several years was identified in this species in several states and foreign countries. According to Hinshaw and McNeil (1940), the disease was introduced into turkeys from chickens principally by contact with infected chickens in commercial hatcheries or by brooding chicks and poults together. By 1940 the disease was widespread in turkeys and was responsible for severe economic losses.

Early epidemiological investigations demonstrated the possibility of transmission of infection in incubators and hatchers. The progressive development, starting near the turn of the century, of large hatcheries which used eggs from many flocks contrib-

Grateful acknowledgement is made to Dr. H. Van Roekel for providing the groundwork for this section.

uted a major means of disseminating the disease.

The major economic loss from pullorum disease and the promise of securing control of the disease through use of the agglutination test stimulated the organization of the Conference of Investigators and Workers in Bacillary White Diarrhea Control (Hinshaw, 1928), composed first of representatives from the New England states and later (Anon., 1930) enlarged to include other eastern states and provinces in Canada. This conference made a major contribution through concerted efforts to bring about standardization and uniformity of methods and to stimulate an interest in the practical eradication of the disease from breeding flocks.

The Conference of Research Workers in Animal Diseases of North America (Anon., 1933) formulated "Standard Methods of Diagnosis of Pullorum Disease in Barnyard Fowl" which were adopted by that organization and also by the United States Livestock Association in 1932. These methods of diagnosis have served as valuable guides in combating pullorum disease.

Schaffer et al. (1931) announced the development of a modified whole-blood test method in which stained antigen is employed. In view of its apparent simplicity it has been widely used, with the result that many infected birds have been detected and thus their removal from breeding flocks was made possible.

A voluntary National Poultry Improvement Plan administered by state agencies cooperating with the USDA, designed in part to secure control of pullorum disease in chickens, became operative in 1935. A National Turkey Improvement Plan organized along the same general lines became operative in 1943. Although these plans were recognized as being inadequate in many respects when formulated, they did represent highly significant steps toward reducing the incidence of the disease. The scientifically glaring shortcomings of the initial plans, which tolerated a low level of infection in officially tested flocks, reflected the interests of the industry which had helped formulate them. Industry cooperation was clearly essential for success of a disease control program of this scope. The plans allowed states to exceed minimum national requirements, with the result that state industries with the most stringent requirements generally made the most rapid progress in gaining control of the disease. A series of modifications of these plans in succeeding years have removed a number of the initial inadequacies. Total eradication on a national basis now appears technically feasible but awaits commitment of the industry to this ultimate goal.

INCIDENCE AND DISTRIBUTION

CHICKENS

Pullorum disease is worldwide in distribution and has been found in substantially all poultry producing areas of the world. Prior to the date the organism was discovered by Rettger (1900), the disease had apparently been observed in several areas in both the United States and Canada. As the poultry industry developed and became more intensified, the incidence of the disease became greater and the infection became widely disseminated throughout the United States and Canada. The monograph of Rettger and Plastridge (1932) indicates that the disease had become widespread in Europe, Japan, New Zealand, and perhaps other foreign countries by the end of the first World War. It is not clear whether the disease originated in America or in some other country. Currently the disease is rather common in many areas of the world. The geographic distribution is closely related to organized control efforts; such efforts have yielded variable results, but in some areas have resulted in virtual if not complete eradication (Wilson, 1967). Additional information on the flock and geographic incidence and distribution of the disease in North America is given in the section under Prevention and Control.

TURKEYS

The disease was first reported in turkey poults in Minnesota by Hewitt (1928). Reports by Tittsler (1932), Johnson and Anderson (1936), Hinshaw and McNeil (1940), and Carpenter et al. (1949) document the increasing geographic distribution and economic importance of the disease in turkeys during that period including work done between 1930 and 1937 which established that an egg-borne cycle of infection existed in turkeys as had been recognized earlier in chickens. Essentially all characteristics of the disease were found to be similar in the two species. The incidence and distribution of pullorum disease in turkeys has largely been a delayed reflection of the disease in chickens. Hinshaw and McNeil (1940) concluded that the disease had not become widely established in turkey breeding flocks until about 1935, and that infections recognized earlier were a result of contact with infected chickens in mixed hatching or growing operations. By 1939 the disease had become sufficiently established in California breeding stock to stimulate the development of a state control program. Many other turkey producing areas were encountering similar problems.

ETIOLOGY

CLASSIFICATION

Salmonella pullorum is a member of the family Enterobacteriaceae, is highly host adapted, and is one of the few members of the genus *Salmonella* which is nonmotile. In the first edition of *Bergey's Manual of Determinative Bacteriology* (1923) the organism was designated *Salmonella pullora*. In later editions the species name was changed to *pullorum*. In the seventh and most recent edition the designation *S. gallinarum* was used for both *S. pullorum* and *S. gallinarum,* a most unfortunate combination of two distinct pathogens.

MORPHOLOGY AND STAINING

The organism is a long slender rod (0.3–0.5 x 1–2.5μ) with slightly rounded ends. It readily stains with ordinary basic aniline dyes and is gram-negative. The cells occur singly, with chains of more than two bacilli rarely found. An occasional filament and large cell may be found in smear preparations. It is nonmotile, nonliquefying, nonchromogenic, nonsporogenic, and facultatively anaerobic.

GROWTH REQUIREMENTS

Salmonella pullorum grows readily on beef extract agar or broth and on other media of comparable nutritive value. The organism can be cultivated on special media such as dextrose-lactose agar (Mallmann and Snyder, 1929), brilliant green agar (Mallmann, 1929), Endo's agar and cysteine gelatin (Hinshaw, 1941), and sodium tartrate and mucate media (Mallmann, 1931), which may be of value in the differentiation from other organisms. Bushnell and Porter (1945) tested several types of media

for the cultivation and isolation of *S. pullorum.* They concluded that no single medium used was entirely satisfactory. In the selection of the medium for the isolation of *S. pullorum,* consideration must be given to the source of material to be examined. In isolating *S. pullorum* from the intestine, desoxycholate citrate, bismuth sulfite, and SS agar were found to be the most satisfactory. Tetrathionate broth was superior to either selenite M or selenite F as an enrichment medium.

Growth studies of *S. pullorum* strains in different media revealed that the rate of growth was in a declining order for nutrient broth, 1% tryptose-water, and a synthetic medium (Schoenhard and Stafseth, 1953). Other workers have demonstrated that the organism is capable of synthesizing glutamic acid and alanine when propagated in synthetic media containing threonine (Jones and Holtman, 1953). Also the virulence of the organism was maintained as readily in a synthetic medium as by animal passage (Gilfillan et al., 1955).

Stokes and Bayne (1957) showed that *S. gallinarum* was of intermediate growth rate between the slow growth of *S. pullorum* and the rapid growth rate of most salmonellae. The authors found that addition of yeast extract to trypticase soy agar improved the growth rate of *S. pullorum* and suggested that addition of yeast extract to selective media might be useful for the isolation of *S. pullorum* and other slow-growing salmonellae. Stokes and Bayne (1961) later demonstrated that *S. pullorum* is apparently unique among microorganisms in lacking ability to oxidatively assimilate a variety of amino acids and that this characteristic may explain the slow growth rate of the organism.

COLONIAL MORPHOLOGY

On meat extract agar (pH 7.0–7.2) heavily seeded with inoculum, the colonies appear discrete, smooth, glistening, homogeneous, entire, dome-shaped, transparent, and varying in form from round to angular. On chicken infusion agar the growth is slightly more luxuriant, with colonies possessing a lesser degree of transparency. On liver infusion agar the growth is even more luxuriant and markedly translucent. Crowded colonies remain small (1 mm or less), but isolated colonies may attain a diameter of 3–4 mm or more. Surface markings may appear as the colony increases in size and age, but as a rule the young colony on a heavily seeded plate changes little with age. Occasionally abnormal morphological strains are encountered (Van Roekel, 1935).

RESISTANCE TO CHEMICAL AND PHYSICAL AGENTS

Van Roekel et al. (1941) found *S. pullorum* to remain viable for at least 7 years and 8 months on a dry cloth maintained at room temperature. Allen and Jacob (1930) found that virulence was maintained for at least 14 months in a sample of contaminated soil and deduced that the infection could exist on premises from one year to the next. Kerr (1930) observed that *S. pullorum* remained viable in fecal emulsions for more than 3 months. Khasimov (1964) found that the organism survived for between 10 and 105 days on dirty woodwork inside poultry houses at temperatures ranging from −2° to +33° C and humidities of 31–75%. On similar wood placed out-of-doors the temperature range was −30° to +11° C and survival was 2–32 days. Survival in soil was 20–35 days in summer and 128–184 days in winter. Gubkin (1964) demonstrated survival of *S. pullorum* for 62 days on dirty wooden feeding troughs at temperatures ranging from −5° to +8° C at relative humidities of 65–75%.

Botts et al. (1952) reported that *S. pullorum* disappeared more rapidly from old built-up litter than from new cob litter. Tucker (1967) found substantially the same relationship between survival of the pathogen and period of litter use. He observed that survival was longer in dry than in wet litter and recognized that a number of factors may influence survival time in litter.

Tittsler (1930) found that boiling for 5 minutes was necessary to destroy *S. pullorum* in artificially contaminated chicken eggs. Winter et al. (1946) found *S. pullorum* to be less heat-resistant than the 15 paratyphoid serotypes studied.

Ayres and Taylor (1956) found that *S. pullorum* rapidly multiplied in the yolk of eggs stored at 20° C; at 10° C multiplication occurred after a 2-week storage period, and at 2° C the population slowly declined. The organism multiplied much more slowly in albumen than in yolk.

Miura et al. (1964) found that *S. pullorum* in naturally contaminated hatchery fluff held at room temperature was viable for less than a year in contrast to some paratyphoid species which persisted during a 5-year test period.

BIOCHEMICAL PROPERTIES

The following substances are fermented with acid, with or without gas production: arabinose, dextrose, galactose, levulose, mannitol, mannose, rhamnose, and zylose. Substances not attacked include adonite, dextrin, dulcitol, erythrol, glycerol, inositol, inulin, lactose, raffinose, sucrose, salicin, sorbite, and starch. Maltose is attacked very infrequently, as has been reported by Hendrickson (1927), Edwards (1928), Pacheco and Rodrigues (1936), and Hinshaw (1941). However, the results in some instances were attributed to the materials and methods employed for the cultivation of the organism. Edwards (1928) concluded that acid production in maltose by *S. pullorum* was made possible through hydrolization of the sugar by the alkali that slowly developed upon prolonged incubation. Hendrickson (1927) observed that when serum water was used for the sugar base, maltose was fermented by *S. pullorum*. Pacheco and Rodrigues (1936) encountered similar findings and claimed the acid production by the organism was the result of serum-enzyme hydrolysis of the sugar. Van-Roekel (1935) reported a laboratory strain which had been considered as a maltose nonfermenting organism, but after a lapse of several years since its original isolation it acquired and retained the ability to attack maltose. No plausible explanation could be given for the sudden change in the maltose-fermenting characteristic. Subsequent investigations (Van Roekel et al., 1937) revealed that strains which possessed a potential tendency to ferment maltose could be identified by cultivating them in a maltose-peptone solution for a period of time. Strains undergoing a change in behavior toward maltose would exhibit red and white colonies when plated on a modified Endo's medium (maltose substituted for lactose). Strains that produced both maltose-fermenting and nonmaltose-fermenting colonies exhibited only non-maltose-fermenting colonies after being subjected to animal passage. An apparently pure maltose-fermenting strain did not lose this property when subjected to animal passage. It is apparent that *S. pullorum* may vary in ability to ferment maltose, and for that reason this sugar is not always of value in the identification of the organism. Variation in the behavior of some strains may be observed occasionally, especially in regard to gas production. Litmus milk remains practically unchanged. Indole and acetylmethylcarbinol are not formed. Ornithine is rapidly decarboxylated. Hydrogen sulfide is produced more slowly than by most salmonellae, and nitrates are reduced.

American workers have regarded *S. pullorum* and *S. gallinarum* as distinct species since their initial isolation. Trabulsi and Edwards (1962) reviewed the evidence, based primarily on occasional fermentation of maltose by *S. pullorum* isolates and occasional isolates of *S. gallinarum* which fermented dulcitol upon prolonged incubation, which led some workers to conclude that the organisms belonged to a single species. Detailed biochemical studies of approximately 100 cultures of both *S. pullorum* and *S. gallinarum* demonstrated that only the ornithine decarboxylase test gave an absolute separation of the two. All of the *S. pullorum* cultures produced rapid decarboxylation of ornithine, whereas none of the *S. gallinarum* cultures gave positive reactions within a 7-day observation period. They concluded that *S. pullorum* and *S. gallinarum* constitute two distinct biochemical types. Costin et al. (1964) secured the same ornithine decarboxylation differentiation.

ANTIGENIC STRUCTURE AND TOXINS

The first evidence of antigenic form variation of *S. pullorum* was provided by Younie (1941) who found infection in the progeny of a flock negative to a standard agglutination test. Serum from infected chicks agglutinated homologous strain antigens but not standard antigens. Byrne (1943) and other investigators soon confirmed the presence of strains with differing antigenic composition. Edwards and Bruner (1946) explored the nature of the antigenic characteristics of *S. pullorum* and later extended these observations (Edwards et al., 1948). The antigenic composition was shown to be 9, 12_1, 12_2, 12_3; the presence of an O-1 antigen has been recognized in recent publications of the Kauffman-White schema. Form variation involves antigens 12_2 and 12_3, with standard strains containing a large amount of 12_3 and a very small amount of 12_2, whereas in variant strains the content of the two antigens is reversed. Edwards and Bruner (1946) recognized that standard strains of *S. pullorum* contained a small percentage of cells with strong 12_2 antigen and considered this to be the normal form of the organism. Later reports by Gwatkin and Bond (1947), Williams et al. (1949), and Snoeyenbos et al. (1950), among others, showed that initial field isolates are usually rather unstable unless they are in the variant form. Extensive examination of individual colonies, sometimes through succession transfers, is necessary to accurately determine the antigenic form of a culture. Most isolates tend to stabilize during passage on artificial media. Standard form cultures usually contain a small percentage of 12_2 predominant colonies even after long artificial cultivation. Variant form cultures are often pure or nearly pure for 12_2 predominant colonies upon initial isolation. The term intermediate has been used to designate cultures which contain appreciable amounts of both 12_2 and 12_3 factors. Colonies of intermediate strains are usually mixtures of both 12_2 and 12_3 predominant colonies or rarely are uniform and contain appreciable amounts of both factors in individual colonies. Strains may also vary in content of the O-1 antigen (Bassiouni et al., 1966; Kosters and Geissler, 1966).

Williams (1953a,b) reported that standard, intermediate, and variant types could be differentiated with an ammonium sulfate sedimentation test. An ammonium sulfate concentration of 310 g per liter completely cleared the supernatant fluid of standard type suspensions but had little or no effect on suspensions of the variant type and only partially cleared suspensions of intermediate types. A concentration of 470 g per liter was required to clear suspensions of variant and intermediate types.

Early reports of the incidence of the variant antigenic type of *S. pullorum* in the United States (Bivins, 1948; Heemstra, 1948; Willliams et al., 1949; Rhoades and Alberts, 1950; Snoeyenbos et al., 1952) indicated that as high as one-third of the isolates from some sections of the country were of the variant type. By 1950 only 13% of total isolates were of the variant type (Williams and McDonald, 1955), a reduction believed to be a result of extensive use of polyvalent testing antigens.

Tsubokura (1965, 1966) reported a series of experiments to elucidate the relationship between *S. pullorum* and the bacteriophages which had been found to be associated with them. The reports indicated that phage typing could be of value for type identification, epidemiological investigations, and genetic studies of *S. pullorum*.

The report of Williams and Harris (1956) on ammonium sulfate sedimentation of *S. gallinarum,* together with other work cited in the report, indicated lack of antigenic variation of *S. gallinarum*. Blaxland et al. (1956) reviewed publications to that date bearing on the relationship between *S. pullorum* and *S. gallinarum* and reported studies on 1,007 cultures of *S. pullorum* and 608 cultures of *S. gallinarum*. They concluded that antigenic differences between the two organisms, represented by the absence of antigenic variation in cultures of *S. gallinarum,* together with established biochemical and epidemiological differences, provided conclusive evidence that the two are separate and distinct species.

The toxicogenic properties of *S. pullorum* were investigated by Hanks and Rettger (1932), who observed that *S. pullorum* cells contained an extractable heat-resistant poison which is highly toxic for rabbits and is capable of killing guinea pigs and mice. Chicks revealed no noticeable symptoms of illness regardless of the route by which the toxin was introduced. They concluded that pullorum disease appears to be a septicemia rather than a toxemia.

PATHOGENESIS AND EPIZOOTIOLOGY

NATURAL HOSTS

Although the chicken appears to be the natural host of *S. pullorum,* the turkey has also proven to be an important host. The disease was initially introduced in turkeys by direct or indirect contact with infected chickens and soon became widespread and self-perpetuated in this species (Hinshaw and McNeil, 1940). The high degree of adaption of *S. pullorum* for the chicken, and to a lesser degree for the turkey, appears to have severely restricted pathogenicity for other hosts. Infections in other species have usually been minor and of little long-term significance.

Significant differences in susceptibility have been found among breeds of chickens. The lighter breeds, particularly Leghorns, have revealed fewer reactors among infected flocks than heavy breeds. Roberts and Card (1926) demonstrated differences in resistance among flocks and among chicks from different hens which could be ascribed to hereditary resistance. A series of trials was summarized by Roberts and Card (1935) which indicated that resistance to pullorum disease is dominant to susceptibility and that probably more than one gene is involved. Strains of chickens were developed which were relatively resistant to mortality following challenge as chicks through three generations. Later Roberts et al. (1939) reported that resistance and susceptibility of the domestic fowl to pullorum disease are related to the number of lymphocytes. Resistant chicks revealed a higher lymphocytic count than did the susceptibles. Increasing age of the chick also increased the degree of resistance as well as the number of lymphocytes. Scholes and Hutt (1942) claimed that high body temperatures and resistance to *S. pullorum* are closely associated. Later Scholes (1942) concluded that resistance to *S. pullorum* more likely depends upon body temperature differences than upon differences in the number of lymphocytes in the blood. While the observations reported by Roberts and Card (1935), Hutt and Scholes (1941), Scholes (1942), and Scholes and Hutt (1942) command academic interest, from a practical standpoint control of the disease through genetic selection of resistant stock does not appear to be an effective method of eliminating the disease from breeding flocks. This appraisal was supported by DeVolt et al. (1941) who stated that the development of pullorum-resistant strains is not now a satisfactory substitute for control and eradication programs by the agglutination test.

Test results over a period of years show a greater percentage of reactors among females than among males. The reason for this difference has not been determined but probably is related to the sequestered nature of local infections of ovarian follicles.

Age of Host Commonly Infected

Mortality from pullorum disease is usually confined to the first 2–3 weeks of age. Severens et al. (1944) concluded that resistance increases rapidly during the first 5–10 days of age in chicks coincident with increases in blood lymphocytes and body temperature. Jones (1913a) reported a natural outbreak among adult fowl. Plastridge and Rettger (1930) reported an acute outbreak in adult chickens which was caused by a highly pleomorphic strain of *S. pullorum.* Acute infections in adult chickens, particularly among brown-egg producing strains, have been reported from a variety of areas. Mortality in semimature and mature turkeys has also been observed.

A substantial percentage of chickens and turkeys which survive infection retain the infection with or without the presence of lesions.

UNUSUAL HOSTS

The disease has been reported in a variety of avian species other than the chicken and turkey but usually has not shown evidence of perpetuation between generations. Naturally occurring pullorum disease has been reported in ducks (Hinshaw and Hoffman, 1937; Beaudette, 1938; Chute and Gershman, 1963), guinea fowl (Bunyea, 1939), pheasants (Hendrickson and Hilbert, 1931; Van Roekel et al., 1947; Williams et al., 1949; Belding, 1955), quail (Emmel, 1936), sparrows (Dalling et al., 1928), canaries (Edwards, 1945), and the European bullfinch (Hudson and Beaudette, 1929). Goff (1932–34) reported serological evidence of *S. pullorum* infection in a pigeon loft. Nóbrega and Bueno (1944) found two wild uru (*Odontophorus capueira*), a gallinaceous bird, to be infected with *S. pullorum.* Canaries, goslings, turtledoves, goldfinches, greenfinches, and bitterns may be infected with *S. pullorum,* according to Villani (1937). Most of the infections reported in the above references were associated with infected chickens. Nevertheless, these findings caused many people to suspect that pullorum disease was so prevalent in wild birds that efforts to control the disease in chickens and other domestic fowl would be of little value. The striking progress achieved in eradicating pullorum disease from domestic birds in contact with wild birds has demonstrated that wild birds play no more than a minor role in the epizootiology of the disease.

A number of mammals are susceptible to *S. pullorum.* Rettger et al. (1916) produced infection in young rabbits, guinea pigs, and kittens by feeding eggs from infected chickens. Infections have been found in rabbits

(Olney, 1928), foxes (Benedict et al., 1941), and swine (Edwards and Bruner, 1943). Bruner and Moran (1949) reported the isolation of *S. pullorum* from a heifer, dog, fox, mink, and swine. Moran (1961) reported the isolation of the organism from two bovine and three mink sources. Sato (1967) infected wild rats (*Rattus norvegicus*) by massive oral exposure. No clinical signs were observed, but infected animals developed agglutinins and shed the organism in feces intermittently for a brief period. The organism persisted in lymph nodes for a longer period of time.

Human salmonellosis caused by *S. pullorum* has occasionally been reported. Mitchell et al. (1946) reviewed earlier reports and recorded what appeared to be the first extensive food-borne outbreak. Mc-Cullough and Eisele (1951) produced salmonellosis with four strains of *S. pullorum* by feeding 1.3–4 billion organisms. The pathogen was recovered from stools on the 1st or 2nd day of illness only, and was not recovered when fed at levels lower than those producing illness. Explosive onset of illness, high fever, prostration, and prompt recovery were noteworthy.

TRANSMISSION, CARRIERS, VECTORS

The primary role played by infected hatching eggs in transmitting pullorum disease was suspected very early in the course of investigations. The monograph by Rettger and Plastridge (1932) reviews work completed in 1910 by Rettger and colleagues which demonstrated that infected chicks excrete the pathogen in their droppings. Ingestion of such excreta by pen mates serves as an important means of transmission. By 1910 the same group of investigators had clearly demonstrated that infected chicks often become permanent carriers, capable of laying fertile infected eggs. Gage (1911) and others confirmed that infected chickens laid infected eggs. Refinement of culturing methods by Runnels and Van Roekel (1927) allowed them to demonstrate 33.7% of eggs laid by reacting hens to be carrying *S. pullorum.* The major cycle of infection of pullorum disease had been established but was extended by Hinshaw et al. (1926) who demonstrated transmission of infection within egg incubators and hatchers.

The infected egg was found by Rettger et al. (1916) to harbor sufficient numbers of the organism to produce infection when fed to young chicks and adult fowl. Van Roekel et al. (1932) made similar observations and concluded that the habit of egg eating or egg picking in an infected flock should be regarded as a hazard to an eradication program for such a flock.

The excreta of infected birds must be considered a means by which infection may spread to noninfected birds in a flock and from one farm to another. Kerr (1930) and Van Roekel et al. (1935) reported recovery of the organism from the feces of infected hens. Van Roekel et al. (1932, 1935) observed that fecal transmission of the disease among semimature and adult chickens apparently occurs very infrequently. Transmission was observed only after force-feeding repeated doses of feces from infected hens. The infection, as a rule, is spread among chicks and poults in cohabitation during the brooding stage, especially during the first days of age. According to Weldin and Weaver (1930), the chief source of the organism at this stage is the droppings. Litter, feed, and water soiled with infective droppings aid in the rapid spread of infection in chick flocks. Botts et al. (1952) reported that S. pullorum disappeared more rapidly from built-up litter than from new corncob litter. Tucker (1967) made similar observations and found that the survival time varied in built-up litter from 11 weeks in new litter to 3 weeks in old litter. A correlation was found between survival time and moisture level of the litter which favored survival in dry litter. The dissemination of the disease in an adult flock by means of feces or litter contaminated with S. pullorum may also be influenced by the numbers of organisms eliminated and the persistence of such elimination. Environmental contamination may constitute a major problem in the eradication of the disease in a short interval retesting or multiple testing program of an infected flock. Contamination of the exterior of the egg with feces and litter containing S. pullorum and penetration of the organism through the shell appear plausible (Stokes et al., 1956; Williams et al., 1968).

Furthermore, cannibalism in an infected flock may spread the disease. The abdominal viscera of infected birds in many instances are heavily contaminated with S. pullorum, and when such birds are eviscer-ated through cannibalistic habits of a flock, they may serve as a source of infection for other birds in the flock.

The important discovery of the organism in the egg established one phase in the cycle of infection. The most frequent spread of the disease occurs from the breeding female to its progeny by way of the egg. At the present time this is the most common mode of transmission. It is recognized that the greater the number of infected birds in a breeding flock, the greater will be the number of infected progeny. It has also been observed that one or two infected breeding birds may be responsible for serious infection in the progeny.

Gwatkin and Mitchell (1944) found that pullorum disease could be produced in chicks which had access to feed contaminated by infected flies and to the flies themselves, some of which were probably eaten by the chicks. S. pullorum was recovered from the feet and wings of flies at least 6 hours after exposure. The gastrointestinal tract of the flies was found to harbor the infection for at least 5 days.

Mortality is often increased by environmental factors such as extremes in temperature, unsanitary conditions, lack of or inadequate feed, and other diseases appearing concurrently. It is frequently observed that infected chicks which are subjected to unfavorable conditions in transit will manifest greater evidence of the disease than will chicks from the same source which are subjected to more favorable conditions.

Pullorum infection is likely to occur regardless of the portal of entry. Van Roekel et al. (1932) reported that pullorum disease can be reproduced in chickens by dropping suspensions of the organism on the conjunctiva, into an incision in the skin of the plantar surface of the foot, into the cloaca, and by oral administration. However, the oral route did not yield to the establishment of infection as readily as others that were investigated. Some investigators (Hinshaw et al., 1926; Doyle and Mathews, 1928; Bunyea and Hall, 1929) reported that infection may result from entrance of the organism into the respiratory and alimentary tracts. Jacobs et al. (1960) demonstrated transmission of infection to chicks from a contaminated debeaking machine. Gordon et al. (1953) showed that the infection could be spread by chick sexing instru-

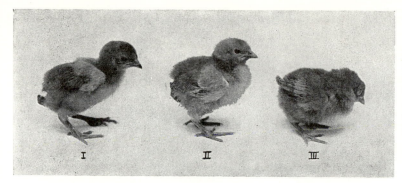

FIG. 3.1—Nine-day-old naturally infected pullorum disease chicks. S. pullorum was isolated from chicks II and III. Chick III died 2 days after it was photographed.

ments. Gorrie (1944) demonstrated that pullorum disease could be spread by contaminated infectious laryngotracheitis vaccine. Later experience in the United States convincingly demonstrated that contaminated vaccines could disseminate the disease widely. As few as 10 organisms per ml of vaccine infected chickens (Anon., 1954).

Dunlap (1931) reported infection in chicks which had been fed mash from an artificially contaminated feed bag. *S. pullorum* has seldom been found in animal feedstuffs but was isolated from two samples by Barkate (1968).

Hence it appears that *S. pullorum* may be eliminated and excreted from the host in various ways and in turn may enter the body through a variety of avenues. Apparently the portal of entry for posthatching infection is more often the digestive tract than other avenues.

SIGNS

Pullorum disease was first recognized among young chicks, and the malady may be considered as principally a chick or poult disease. Characteristics of the disease in both the chick and poult are so nearly identical that they may be considered as one. The signs exhibited by infected birds are not specific for pullorum disease, although in many cases a tentative diagnosis based on clinical evidence has been substantiated by the isolation of the etiologic agent. The disease occasionally is subclinical even when originating from egg transmission.

Chicks and Poults

If birds are hatched from infected eggs, moribund and dead birds may be observed in the incubator or within a short time after hatching. They manifest somnolence, weakness, and loss of appetite, and death may follow suddenly. In some instances evidence of the disease is not observed until several days (5–10) after hatching. The disease gains momentum during the following 7–10 days. The peak of mortality usually occurs during the 2nd or 3rd week of life. In some instances the birds exhibit lassitude, an inclination to huddle together under the hover, loss of appetite, drooping of wings, somnolence, and a distorted body appearance (Fig. 3.1). Affected birds frequently exhibit a shrill cry when voiding excreta and commonly develop an accumulation of chalk-white excreta, sometimes stained greenish brown, in and around the vent.

Jungherr (1935) reported that infected chicks manifest a febrile reaction as indicated by increased temperature of the legs. He also mentioned that affected chicks may appear as having been "dipped in water," which he explained as probably brought on by a water-logged condition of the body muscles which permits excess fluid to ooze through the skin. Hutyra et al. (1938) claimed that a febrile condition is responsible for the increased renal activity and elimination of the whitish material adhering to the vent and adjacent parts.

Labored breathing or gasping may be observed as a result of extensive pathology of the lungs. Anderson et al. (1948) found that lesions in the lungs of chicks which died from pullorum disease occurred as frequently in those infected per os as in those infected by an aerosol. Survivors may be greatly retarded in their growth and appear underdeveloped and poorly feathered (Fig 3.2). Van Roekel (1931) reported that among 29 6-week-old chicks exposed

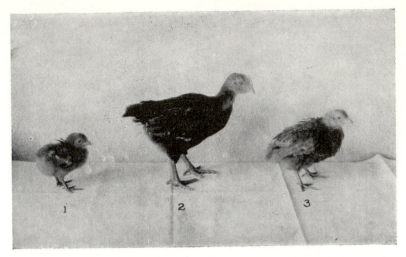

FIG. 3.2—Six-week-old chicks exposed to pullorum infection when 72 hours old. Weights: **No. 1, 115 g; No. 2, 488 g; No. 3, 193 g.**

to infection when 72 hours old, the range in weight varied from 90 to 558 g. In most instances it is advisable to destroy the survivors, clean and disinfect the quarters, and replace with clean stock. Chicks retarded in their growth do not mature into vigorous well-developed laying or breeding birds. However, some survivors may not reveal any great setback in growth but develop to maturity even though harboring the infection. Flocks which have passed through a serious outbreak usually reveal a high percentage of carriers at maturity.

Evans et al. (1955) reported blindness in chicks associated with salmonellosis. In one case *S. pullorum* was isolated from the anterior chamber of the eye and from the tibiotarsal joint. Fluctuating swellings of the tibiotarsal and the humeroradial and ulnar articulations have been ascribed to *S. pullorum* infection in chicks. Ferguson et al. (1961), Cosgrove and Lindenmaier (1961), and Davis et al. (1961) observed a relatively high incidence of localization of infection in joints and adjacent synovial sheaths of chicks which produced lameness and obvious swelling. Similar lesions in turkey poults were reported by Prier and Rhodes (1948). These observations suggest that some strains of the organism may have a predilection for these tissues.

Adults

Pullorum disease in a maturing or adult flock does not manifest the characteristics of an acute infection as a rule. Infection may spread within a flock for a long period of time without producing distinct signs. In contracting the infection the bird may exhibit little or no symptomatology. Infected individuals cannot, as a rule, be detected by their physical appearance.

Experimentally infected birds have exhibited limited and transient clinical manifestations. General depression and listlessness, accompanied by a partial or complete inappetence, may be the first signs following infection. Paleness of the comb and visible mucous membranes may be observed. Diarrhea may be noted. A febrile reaction accompanied by increased thirst has been observed. Occasionally adults may succumb to artificial or natural infection depending upon the dosage and virulence of the organism.

Natural epornitics in adult flocks have been observed. Jones (1913a) reported a natural outbreak among adult fowl which was attributed to feeding eggs discarded from an incubator. Evidence of disease was observed 16 days after feeding the infective eggs, and during a period of 6 weeks a loss of 50 birds among a flock of 700 hens was sustained. The symptoms noted were paleness of comb and mucous membranes, scaly shrunken and grayish appearance of the comb, listlessness, progressive depression, droopy wings, retraction of head and neck, inappetence, and usually diarrhea. The duration of the incubation period was from 16 days to 3 weeks. The course of the disease sometimes terminated fatally in 24 hours but usually continued 4–5 days or longer. A definite leukocytosis was observed. Plastridge and Rettger (1930) observed acute outbreaks of the disease caused by a highly pleomorphic strain of *S. pullorum* among adult flocks.

Pullorum disease definitely causes a reduction in fertility and hatchability. Bushnell et al. (1926), Dearstyne et al. (1929), and Runnells (1929) reported that more infertile eggs are laid by infected than by noninfected birds. However, some infected birds may lay a normal number of fertile eggs which hatch well. Beaudette et al. (1923a,b), Bushnell et al. (1926), Dearstyne et al. (1929), and Runnells (1929) observed that hatchability might be very seriously affected in eggs laid by infected birds. In one instance a difference of 18.2% in hatchability of fertile eggs laid by reacting and nonreacting birds was reported in favor of the latter.

Acute outbreaks have resulted in some flocks in which the infection was regarded as dormant among the carriers in the flock. Chronic carriers of the infection appear to be less able to withstand changes in environmental conditions and concurrent flock diseases, with the result that mortality occurs among carriers of the disease.

Losses also result from a decrease in egg production from infected adults, according to Runnells (1929), Dearstyne et al. (1929), and Asmundson and Biely (1930). The last-named authors report that average first-year egg production for nonreacting and reacting birds was 221 and 160 eggs respectively. A greater variation in production was noted among reactors than among the nonreactors. The egg production for the reactors was significantly lower than that of the nonreactors. On the contrary, Dearstyne et al. (1929) found that the reactor in its first-year egg production may be profitable and that variations in production may be expected, depending upon the localization and degree of infection.

MORBIDITY AND MORTALITY

Both morbidity and mortality are highly variable in chickens and turkeys and are influenced by age, strain susceptibility, nutrition, flock management, and characteristics of exposure. Mortality may vary from no losses to approximately 100% in serious outbreaks. The greatest losses usually occur during the 2nd week after hatching, with a rapid decline during the 3rd and 4th weeks of age. Morbidity is often much higher than mortality with some of the affected birds recovering spontaneously. Birds hatched from an infected flock and raised on the same premises will usually exhibit less mortality than those subjected to the stress of shipping.

GROSS LESIONS

Chicks and Poults

In birds that die suddenly in the early stages of brooding, the lesions are limited. The liver is enlarged and congested, and the normal yellow color may be streaked with hemorrhages. In the septicemic form, an active hyperemia may be found in other organs. The yolk sac and its contents reveal slight or no alteration. In more protracted cases, an interference with yolk absorption may occur, and the yolk sac contents may be yellowish in color and of creamy and cheesy consistency. Necrotic foci or nodules may be present in the cardiac muscle (Fig. 3.3), liver, lungs (Fig. 3.4), ceca, large intestine, and the muscle of the gizzard. Pericarditis may be observed in some instances. The liver may reveal punctiform hemorrhages and focal necrosis. The spleen may be enlarged (Fig. 3.5) and the kidneys congested or anemic with ureters prominently distended with urates. The ceca may contain a cheesy core, sometimes tinted with blood. The wall of the intestine may be thickened. Frequently peritonitis is manifested. Doyle and Mathews

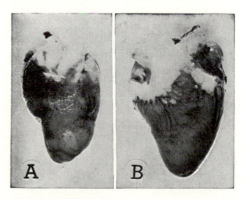

FIG. 3.3—*(A) Pullorum-diseased heart exhibiting nodular abscesses in myocardium (16-day-old chick). (B) Normal heart (17-day-old chick).*

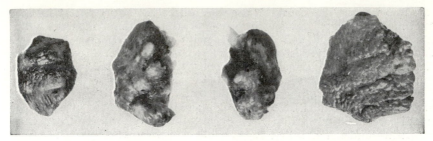

FIG. 3.4—(No. 1 from left) Normal lung (17-day-old chick). (Nos. 2, 3, 4) Pullorum-infected lungs exhibiting pneumonia and multiple abscesses (16-day-old chick).

(1928) report that the liver is the most consistent seat of gross lesions and is followed in order of frequency by the lungs, heart, gizzard, and ceca. Among chicks only a few days old, the lung lesions may consist only of a hemorrhagic pneumonia, whereas in older chicks yellowish gray nodules and areas of gray hepatization may be found. The nodules in the myocardium may attain sufficient size to cause a marked distortion in the shape of the heart.

Adults

The lesions found most frequently in the chronic carrier hen are misshapen, discolored, cystic ova (Fig. 3.6), peritonitis, and frequently an acute or chronic pericarditis. The diseased ova usually contain oily and cheesy material enclosed in a thickened capsule. These degenerated ovarian follicles may be closely attached to the ovary, but frequently they are pedunculated and may become detached from the ovarian mass. In such cases they may become embedded in the adipose tissue of the abdominal cavity. Ovarian and oviduct dysfunction may lead to abdominal ovulation or oviduct impaction, which in turn may bring about extensive peritonitis and adhesions of the abdominal viscera (Fig. 3.7). Ascites may also develop, particularly in the turkey. Advanced lesions of this type seldom, if ever, fail to yield S. pullorum on culture.

Lesions less extensive in nature may involve the heart (Fig. 3.8). Quite frequently pericarditis is observed in both females and males. The changes that have occurred in the pericardium, epicardium, and pericardial fluid appear to be dependent on the age of the disease process. In some cases the pericardium exhibits only a slight translucency, and the pericardial fluid may

be increased and turbid. In the more advanced stages the pericardial sac is thickened and opaque and the pericardial fluid is greatly increased in amount, containing considerable exudative material. This may be followed by permanent thickening of the pericardium and epicardium and partial obliteration of the pericardial cavity by adhesions. Occasionally small cysts containing amber-colored, cheesy material may be found embedded in the abdominal fat or attached to the gizzard or intestines. The organism can usually be recovered from such processes.

In the male the infection is frequently found in the reproductive organs (Fig. 3.9). Edwards and Hull (1929) reported the localization of the organism in the testicle and vas deferens.

Among birds dying from acute infection, Jones (1913a) observed marked emaciation, enlarged and distorted heart due to grayish white nodules, enlarged yellowish green and granular liver coated with fibrinous exudate, friable spleen of normal size with focal necrosis, minute necrotic foci of the pancreas, enlarged kidneys with parenchymatous degeneration, injection of mesenteric vessels, and a fibrinous exudate coating

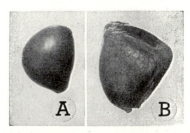

FIG. 3.5—(A) Normal spleen (17-day-old chick). (B) Pullorum-infected spleen exhibiting marked enlargement (16-day-old chick).

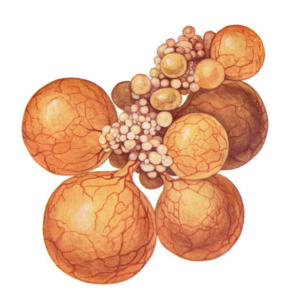

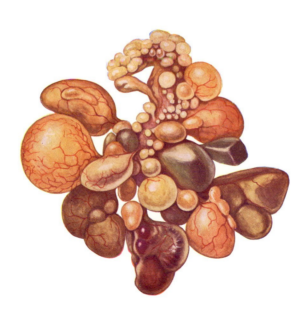

FIG. 3.6—**Top**, *normal ovary.* **Below**, *infected ovary* (S. pullorum). *(Storrs Agr. Expt. Sta.)*

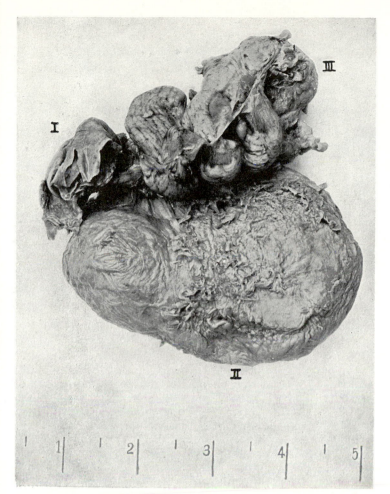

FIG. 3.7—*Impacted oviduct removed from infected hen. Parts I and II are funnel and albumen-secreting portions respectively. Part III is shell gland portion. Adhesions of the serosa.*

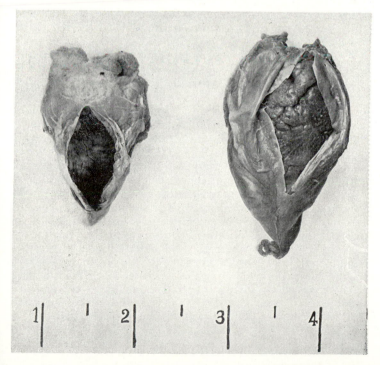

FIG. 3.8—**(Left)** *Normal heart.* **(Right)** *Infected heart exhibiting pericarditis and epicarditis.*

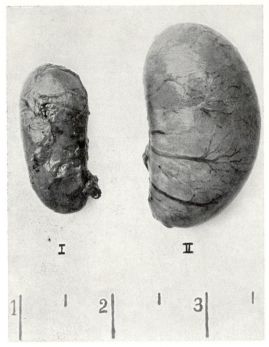

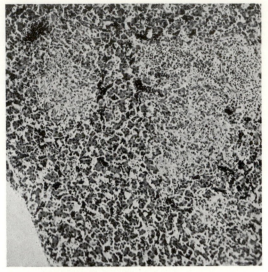

FIG. 3.10—Liver revealing focal degeneration and necrosis. ×100.

FIG. 3.9—Testicles removed from reacting adult male. Testis I—atrophic and very firm; S. pullorum isolated. Testis II—normal in size and texture; S. pullorum not isolated.

the abdominal viscera. Acute infections in adults may also occur which produce lesions indistinguishable from acute S. gallinarum infections.

HISTOPATHOLOGY

Gage and Martin (1916) in a study of the intestines of infected chickens found marked injury to the mucosa with hyperemia, hemorrhagic exudation, leukocytic infiltration, and in many instances marked thickening of the intestinal walls. The lesions observed were not specific as they corresponded to acute or chronic enteritis.

Doyle and Mathews (1928) state that in young chicks the livers show hyperemia, hemorrhages, focal degeneration, and necrosis (Fig. 3.10). They claim that the accumulation of endothelial leukocytes which replace the degenerated or necrotic liver cells is a characteristic cell reaction of the liver to S. pullorum infection. The histopathologic pulmonary lesions may consist of diffuse, acute congestion and hemorrhage in the early stages. Later, well-de-fined focal lesions appear which consist chiefly of a mononuclear infiltrating type of cell, serofibrinous exudate, and cellular debris. The larger lesions may involve several lobules, bronchioles, and bronchi terminating in necrosis. The nodules in the myocardium and in the muscle of the gizzard represent largely an infiltration with mononuclear cells and degenerative changes of the muscle fibers.

Suganuma (1960) studied 459 field cases of pullorum disease which included chicks and adult hens and roosters. The main pathological changes observed were: endothelial cell proliferative foci of the liver, focal necrosis of the myocardium, catarrhal bronchitis, catarrhal enteritis in chicks, and interstitial inflammation of the liver, lungs, and kidneys. No lesions were found in chicks under 10 days of age. Serositis, particularly in the pericardium, pleuroperitoneum, and serosa of the intestinal tract and mesentery, was found in a high percentage of cases and was regarded as the most characteristic lesion of the disease. This inflammatory change consisted of infiltration of lymphocytes, lymphocytic cells, plasma cells, and heterophils, and proliferation of fibrocytes, fibroblastic cells, histiocytes and histiocytic cells without accompanying exudative changes. Pericarditis was rarely observed. Edwards and Hull (1929) examined the infected gonad of a rooster and found a thickening of the tunica albuginea and complete obliteration of the seminiferous tubules. Multiple small abscesses and areas of round cell infiltration were found in the testes without evidence of spermatogenesis. The lumen of the vas deferens was enlarged and filled with a dense structureless homogenous exudate.

Histopathological lesions in turkeys apparently have not been studied and reported. They could be expected to be substantially identical to those found in the chicken.

IMMUNITY

The infected bird usually produces agglutinating antibodies within 3–10 days following infection which persist at varying levels for the duration of infection. Although such antibody production is an expression of immunity, the possible role of agglutinating antibodies in modifying the course of infection in the host is little understood. The general success in eradication of infection by elimination of carriers has not encouraged comprehensive investigation of the immune mechanism. High-titred serum from infected birds supports multiplication of *S. pullorum* in vitro; agglutinating antibodies in vivo probably serve a function in localizing infection.

DIAGNOSIS

A definitive diagnosis of pullorum disease requires isolation and identification of *S. pullorum*. Flock history and signs are of limited value in arriving at a diagnosis because of the similarity to a number of other diseases. Lesions, particularly in severely affected chicks and poults, may be highly suggestive and be used as a basis for a tentative diagnosis. Positive serological findings are of major value in detecting infection in a control program but should not be considered adequate for a definitive diagnosis. The delay in appearance of agglutinating antibodies following infection often results in mortality before antibody development. Van Roekel et al. (1932) detected agglutinating antibodies 6 days after exposure by cloacal inoculation, 7 days after ocular inoculation, and 10 days each after exposure by the oral and skin incision routes. Corpron et al. (1947) detected agglutinins in the serum of adult turkeys 3 days after intravenous exposure. Aggluti-

nins were detected in the feces of a small percentage of chickens after circulating antibodies had reached a relatively high level (E. R. Hitchner, 1952, unpublished).

ISOLATION OF *S. pullorum*

Acute Infections

Acute pullorum disease is characterized by a systemic infection which allows ready isolation from most body tissues. In such infections the liver is usually prominently involved and is a preferred organ to culture. Lesions which may occur in the spleen, myocardium or pericardium, lungs, gizzard, or yolk sac are also dependable for isolation. A bacteriological inoculating loop is satisfactory for transferring adherent tissues to culture media from chicks and poults; a cotton swab is preferable for making cultures from older birds as a larger amount of tissue is transferred.

Beef infusion agar in petri dishes is satisfactory for isolation by direct inoculation. Any other media of comparable nutritive value may also be used. Media containing inhibitory substances, such as brilliant green, are occasionally also inhibitory for salmonellae and should be used only if required because of decomposition of the specimens (Read and Reyes, 1968).

Chronic Infections

Cultural examination to identify localized chronic infections, represented by the carrier detected by serologic tests, must be detailed if reasonable accuracy is to be secured. An adequate outline for examination of such specimens is given in the *National Poultry and Turkey Improvement Plans* (Anon., 1969) as follows:

(a) The pericardial sac, peritoneum, oviduct, and any visible pathological tissues should be cultured on beef extract agar or tryptose agar by means of sterile swabs. Sterile technique should be followed. (Primary culture of these organs in a suitable nutrient broth and transfer to a suitable nutrient agar is optional.)

(b) The following organs should be aseptically collected for culture:

  (1) Heart (apex, pericardial sac, and contents if present);
  (2) Liver (portions exhibiting lesions or in grossly normal organs the drained gall bladder and adjacent liver tissues);

(3) Ovary-Testes (entire inactive ovary or testes, but if ovary is active use own judgment and include any atypical ova);

(4) Oviduct (if active include any debris and dehydrated ova);

(5) Pancreas; and

(6) Spleen.

(c) A composite sample of the organs listed should be ground in a sterile mortar or suitable blender. Individual organs may be used if desired. Nutrient broth should be added as a diluent. Ten ml of this suspension should be inoculated into 100 ml of either Selenite F broth or tetrathionate broth and into 100 ml of a suitable noninhibitory nutrient broth.

(d) After 24 hours incubation at 37° C a loopful of the broth cultures from each flask should be streaked on a suitable noninhibitory solid medium such as tryptose agar and one of the following media: SS, MacConkey, brilliant green, bismuth sulfite, or desoxycholate citrate lactose sucrose agar. If no suspicious colonies are observed after 24 hours incubation the enrichment broths should be restreaked on solid media.

(e) A portion of the crop wall and intestine to include the cecal tonsils are put into either Selenite F or tetrathionate broth and incubated for 24 hours at 37° C. Transfers should be made from the broth onto agar plates as indicated above.

Use of nonselective media demands careful aseptic techniques but has the advantage of securing more dependable isolation of *S. pullorum*. Also other bacteria capable of producing cross reactions with pullorum antigen may be more dependably demonstrated.

IDENTIFICATION OF CULTURES

Most isolates of *S. pullorum* produce typical reactions and can be identified promptly without resorting to a large bank of differential media. Familiarity with the characteristic small, smooth, translucent colony on nutrient media after 24-hr incubation often allows tentative identification. Careful initial culture of tissues on nonselective media should usually result in pure cultures. If pure cultures are not secured or if an enrichment medium has been used, it is often advantageous to transfer individual colonies to triple sugar iron agar slants for preliminary differentiation. *S. pullorum* on such slants produces a red slant with a yellow butt which shows delayed blackening from H₂S production.

The following reactions, which can be determined within 24 hours and provide identification of a number of other common pathogens, allow identification of most isolates:

DEXTROSE	Fermented with gas
LACTOSE	Not fermented
SUCROSE	Not fermented
MANNITOL	Fermented with gas
MALTOSE	Usually not fermented
DULCITOL	Not fermented
INDOLE	Not produced
UREA	Not hydrolyzed
MOTILITY	Nonmotile
AGGLUTINATION	Positive with Group D antiserum

Additional differential tests described under Etiology are necessary to identify isolates which produce nontypical reactions (chiefly fermentation of maltose or no gas production). Decarboxylation of ornithine by *S. pullorum* appears to be the single most dependable test for differentiating maltose-fermenting *S. pullorum* strains from *S. gallinarum*.

DIFFERENTIAL DIAGNOSIS

The signs and lesions produced by pullorum disease are not pathognomonic. Even the broadest spectrum of lesions which may develop in the chick, poult, or adult bird may be duplicated by infections with *S. gallinarum*. Other salmonella infections produce lesions of the liver, spleen, and intestines which cannot be distinguished grossly or microscopically from those produced by pullorum disease. Aspergillus or other molds may produce similar lesions in the lungs. Occasionally *S. pullorum* localizes in the major joints and tendon sheaths of considerable numbers of chicks and produces signs and lesions like those of *Mycoplasma synoviae* or other infectious agents which localize at these sites.

Local infections of *S. pullorum* in the adult carrier, particularly of the pericardium and ovary, may appear identical to those produced by other bacterial infections such as coliforms, staphylococci, micrococci, and other salmonellae. Birds of any age may be infected with *S. pullorum* and fail to show grossly discernible lesions.

A definitive diagnosis of pullorum disease can be made only following isolation and identification of *S. pullorum*.

TREATMENT

Reasonably effective prophylactic and therapeutic drugs were first discovered among the sulfonamides. Since that time other compounds including nitrofurans and several antibiotics have been found to be effective in reducing mortality from pullorum disease. No drug or combination of drugs has been found which is capable of eliminating infection from a treated flock. Sulfonamides in particular frequently suppress growth and may interfere with feed and water intake and egg production. Therapy, therefore, may have short-range economic merit but is no substitute for a sound eradication program.

SULFONAMIDES

Severens et al. (1945) appear to have been the first to report on the efficacy of sulfonamide medication for the control of mortality from pullorum disease. They found that sulfadiazine and sulfamerazine were the most effective in reducing chick mortality among seven sulfonamides tested. Sulfathiazole and sulfaguanadine were intermediate in effectiveness; sulfasuxidine, phthalylsulfathiazole, and sulfanilamide were least effective. Mullen (1946), in an extensive field trial in turkey poults, found that a 0.5% level of sulfamerazine in the mash for the first 5 days apparently reduced mortality in progeny of infected breeders from approximately 17% to 4%. A litter eating problem developed if the medication period was extended beyond 5 days. Bottorff and Kiser (1947) found sulfadiazine, sulfamethazine and sulfamerazine to be equally effective in preventing chick mortality which was reduced in the medicated groups from a minimum of 30% to a maximum of 56% compared to untreated controls. A maximum drug level of 0.75% in the starter mash was used for either 5 or 10 days starting at one day of age. Mortality recurred in all groups beginning 5 days after drug withdrawal. They made the significant observation, not found by Severens et al. (1945), that 90% of all survivors reacted to the whole-blood test for pullorum disease when tested at 12 weeks of age.

Pomeroy et al. (1948) tested the efficacy of nine sulfonamides against pullorum disease in chicks. Sulfadiazine, sulfamerazine,

sulfapyrazine, sulfaquinoxaline, and sulfamethazine were the most effective of the drugs tested. Neither sulfadiazine, sulfapyrazine, or sulfamethazine were found to be effective in reducing mortality in poults experimentally infected with *S. pullorum*. The authors concluded that results obtained from chicks treated with sulfonamides should not be considered applicable to turkeys without testing the drug for toxicity and effectiveness in turkeys. They found, as did Bottorff and Kiser (1947), that appreciable numbers of infected birds remained among medicated survivors. Later work by Anderson et al. (1948), Cole (1948), Dickinson and Stoddard (1949), Grumbles (1950), and Cooper et al. (1951) confirmed and extended the earlier work on the effect of sulfonamides on *S. pullorum* infection in chickens.

NITROFURANS

Smith (1954) appears to have been the first to report tests of nitrofurazone for the treatment of pullorum disease. In the trials reported, a concentration of 0.04% furazolidone in the feed for a 10–14-day period beginning shortly after exposure was highly effective in preventing mortality and carriers among chicks. Under the conditions of the trial, furazolidone was superior to either chloramphenicol or sulfamerazine. Gordon and Tucker (1955) and Wilson (1955, 1956) used furazolidone in mash at a 0.04% concentration and in some instances appeared to have eliminated *S. pullorum* from carrier birds. Henderson et al. (1960) fed chickens 0.011% furazolidone in the feed for 5 weeks starting at time of artificial exposure at 9–14 weeks of age. Infection developed in some birds during treatment without concurrent antibody development. They concluded that furazolidone interferes with antibody production and should not be used for at least 6 weeks before testing for pullorum disease. Richey and Morgan (1960) found infection in survivors of chickens treated at levels as high as 0.066% furazolidone from the 8th to the 20th day postexposure. Francis (1960) found that 0.011% furazolidone in the feed significantly reduced mortality from pullorum disease but that *S. pullorum* was still being excreted after the 4-week treatment period.

Bierer (1961) found furaltadone water

medication effective in reducing mortality in chicks infected with S. *pullorum*.

ANTIBIOTICS

Limited trials with chloramphenicol were reported by Smith (1954). A 0.5% concentration in the feed for 10 days following experimentally induced infection sharply reduced mortality but left many infected chicks. Chlortetracycline at a 200 mg/kg level in the ration was fed by Grausgruber and Kissling (1964) to suppress mortality in orally infected day-old chicks. The authors did not find interference with isolation of S. *pullorum* from infected chicks or adverse effect on agglutinin development even if the drug was administered for prolonged periods.

Colistin was found by Bionde and Schiavo (1966) and Schiavo and Bionde (1966) to increase survival of infected chick embryos and to markedly increase survival of infected chicks. S. *pullorum* was isolated from treated survivors.

Peresadin (1965) found S. *pullorum* more sensitive by in vitro tests to polymyxin than to chlortetracycline, oxytetracycline, or colistin. Limited trials in chickens allowed the suggestion that a 30–45-day treatment period with increasing dosage with advancing age be used for treatment.

DRUG RESISTANCE

Karyagin (1964) found that the minimum inhibitory concentration of chlortetracycline for 24 isolates of S. *pullorum* varied between 1.25 and 12.5 μg/ml. Resistance was increased as much as 32 times after 10 passages in increasing amounts of antibiotics. These strains lost pathogenicity for chicks and their biochemical properties changed. Relatively resistant strains with unchanged biochemical properties were obtained from infected birds treated with chlortetracycline. Similar changes in the 24 isolates in susceptibility, biochemical properties, and virulence occurred following passage in media containing increasing amounts of nitrofurazone. Increased resistance without decrease in virulence was found in isolates from birds treated with nitrofurazone. Sarkisov and Trishkina (1966) were unable to demonstrate increased resistance to chlortetracycline following a 30-day medication period.

PREVENTION AND CONTROL

It has long been established that chicken and turkey flocks can be developed and maintained free of pullorum disease by adhering to well-defined procedures. In the simplest sense, it may be stated that the only requirement is to establish breeding flocks free of S. *pullorum* and to hatch and rear their progeny under circumstances which preclude direct or indirect contact with infected chickens or turkeys.

MANAGEMENT PROCEDURES

Commonly accepted methods of management to prevent introduction of infectious agents are generally applicable to prevent introduction of S. *pullorum*. The fact that egg transmission plays a predominant role in the spread of infection makes it mandatory that only eggs from flocks known to be free of pullorum disease be introduced into hatcheries. Hinshaw et al. (1926) demonstrated that S. *pullorum* could be spread through the air of forced draft incubators. Fumigation of incubators and hatchers with formaldehyde was originally developed to decrease the spread of pullorum disease and to destroy residual infection during cleaning between hatches. Fumigation may have been of some benefit in the past when the disease was rampant but no longer has more than historical significance as an aid in control of pullorum disease. The reader interested in fumigation methods is referred to the discussion of this subject in the section on paratyphoid infections.

There should be no mixing of pullorum free stock at any time with other poultry or confined birds not known to be free of the disease. This principle applies on a farm basis; infected stock on a farm, even if in separate pens or buildings, compromises the status of all other birds on the farm.

ELIMINATION OF CARRIERS

The investigations already reviewed which established that pullorum disease was transmitted through the egg suggested a method of attack to secure control. The foundation of the control program was established by Jones (1913b) who reported the use of a macroscopic tube agglutination test for detecting infected chickens. Gage et al. (1914) and Rettger et al. (1915)

promptly substantiated this work and employed the test in statewide campaigns with the objective of detecting flocks free from the disease as well as eliminating the disease from flocks by detection and removal of reactors.

Early field testing results indicated that removal of reactors following a single test was not sufficient, as a rule, for the complete elimination of infected birds from a flock. Such results may be expected because of three possible intercurrent characteristics: (1) Serum agglutinin titers of infected birds tend to fluctuate and may for brief periods fail to produce significant agglutination at the usual finding dilution of 1:25 or 1:50 (Edgington, 1937). (2) There is a delay of at least several days between infection and development of agglutinins. (3) Environmental contamination may exist following removal of reactors which may serve as a source of infection at a later date.

As the obvious value of a serologic testing program as a tool to gain control of pullorum disease became apparent, a great deal of work by many investigators was accomplished to evaluate, refine, and modify the system. In addition to the macroscopic tube agglutination test, a rapid serum test was introduced by Runnells et al. (1927), and a stained antigen whole-blood test was developed by Schaffer et al. (1931). Biely et al. (1931) confirmed the accuracy of the rapid serum test for detecting infection in chickens. Gwatkin et al. (1941) reviewed the extensive literature which had then accumulated comparing the whole-blood test and the macroscopic tube agglutination test and reported extensive comparisons between the two tests for detecting infection in chickens. He concluded that the whole-blood test in competent hands could be used with results equally as satisfactory as those attained by the tube method under the conditions prevailing in Alberta.

The *National Poultry and Turkey Improvement Plans* (Anon., 1969) endorse three methods for testing chickens: (1) the standard tube agglutination test, (2) the stained antigen rapid whole-blood test, and (3) the rapid serum test. The choice of method is determined by many factors and objectives peculiar to a state or region. In some states the macroscopic tube agglutination method is considered the only official method for testing flocks. In other states the rapid serum method and the tube test are regarded as official. In many states all three methods may be employed, but the whole-blood test is the one most generally used.

Only two testing methods are endorsed by the *National Poultry and Turkey Improvement Plans* for testing turkeys: (1) the standard tube agglutination test and (2) the rapid serum test. A combination of *S. pullorum* and *S. typhi-murium* antigen is also approved. Winter et al. (1952) compared the efficacy of the whole-blood test and the tube agglutination test and found, as had most earlier workers to whom they refer, that the whole-blood test was less dependable to detect infected turkeys. Dickinson et al. (1944) found the rapid serum test to be acceptable for practical control use and only slightly less dependable than the tube agglutination test for detecting infection in turkeys.

The techniques and procedures for the official methods are described in detail by the Animal Husbandry Research Division, Agricultural Research Service, USDA, Beltsville, Md. (Anon., 1969). A brief review of each method follows.

Standard Tube Agglutination Test

The blood samples shall be collected by a properly qualified and authorized person. Suitable blood tubes, shipping containers, and bleeding and leg-banding equipment should be furnished by the agency in charge of the testing program. Blood tubes should be thoroughly cleaned and heated in a hot-air sterilizing oven. Cork stoppers should be boiled or washed and dried in a hot-air drying oven. Shipping containers for the blood samples should be constructed to permit washing and disinfection.

All birds tested should be officially legbanded. The blood tube is identified with the leg-band number inscribed on the etched portion of the tube or on a gummed label. A small amount of blood (0.5–2 ml) is collected from the median vein of the wing (Vena cutanea ulnaris) by incising the latter with a sharp-pointed lancet or knife (Figs. 3.11, 3.12) or by a 2-ml syringe and 20–22-gage needle washed with physiological saline. The latter method is particularly appropriate for bleeding turkeys. The tube is laid on its side permitting the blood to clot in a long slant. After the blood has

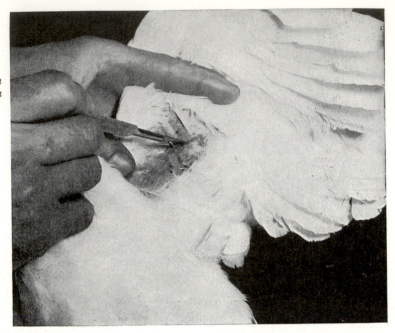

FIG. 3.11—Incising median vein of the wing (Vena cutanea ulnaris).

coagulated, the samples are packed in containers designed for shipment to the laboratory. In extremes of temperature, precautions should be taken against freezing or overheating; the blood samples should arrive at the laboratory in a fresh state and unhemolyzed condition for a satisfactory test. All hemolyzed or spoiled samples should be rejected. The laboratory should be equipped with adequate refrigeration facilities where blood samples should be retained until the sera have been tested and the results of the tests known. Occasionally a retest on the same serum may be necessary to determine the pullorum status of a bird.

The antigen for the tube test should be prepared from representative strains of S. pullorum which are known to contain the different antigenic components normally found in S. pullorum (Edwards and Bruner, 1946). Furthermore, the strains should possess high agglutinability with positive serum but should not agglutinate with negative or nonspecific sera. The following pullorum strains are widely used for the official tube test antigen with satisfactory results: strain 17 isolated in 1916, strain 19 isolated in 1911, strain 20 isolated in 1917. All of these strains are of the "standard" type and were originally isolated by Leo F. Rettger (Williams and MacDonald, 1955). Stock cultures of the antigen strains should be grown and maintained on nutrient agar medium composed of dry granular agar (Difco) 2.0%, Bacto peptone (Difco) 1.0%, beef extract (Difco) 0.4%, and water. The final pH should range from 7.0 to 7.2. The cultures should be transferred not more than once a month. Seed cultures should

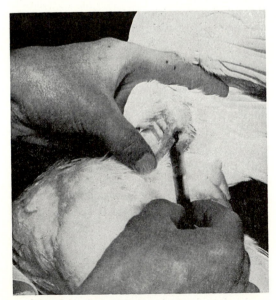

FIG. 3.12—Collecting blood into numbered etched tube.

be taken from the stock strains rather than from rapid serial transfers in order to avoid contaminants or possible variation in the characteristics of the organism. Large test tubes, Kolle flasks, or Blake bottles containing nutrient agar medium may be used for producing the antigen. After 48–72 hours incubation, the growth is washed off with sufficient phenolized (0.5%) saline (0.85%) solution to produce a very concentrated suspension. This suspension is filtered through sterile absorbent cotton or glass wool into sterile glass-stoppered bottles. The washings from each of the three strains are combined in equal volume-density, and the stock antigen is stored at 8–10° C. Anhydrous preparations of antigen have been demonstrated to be stable and comparable in sensitivity after reconstitution to undried antigen (Gershman et al., 1962).

An alternate medium, designated thiosulfate glycerin and frequently referred to as **TG** medium, may be used to prepare antigen. It is claimed that this medium provides an antigen of excellent specificity and greatly increases the yield of the antigen from a given volume of medium (Williams and MacDonald, 1955).

For routine testing, a dilute antigen is prepared from the stock antigen by diluting the latter with physiological saline solution containing 0.25–0.3% phenol. The turbidity of the antigen corresponds to 0.75–1.00 on the McFarland nephelometer scale, and the pH is adjusted to 8.2–8.5 by addition of dilute sodium hydroxide. The dilute antigen is prepared each day in order to reduce dissolution and plasmolysis to a minimum at the specified pH level.

The amount of diluted antigen employed in individual tests may vary from 1 to 2 ml; however, the amounts should be constant and placed in clean, clear test tubes. The sera are added to the test tubes containing the antigen with a serologic pipette or a serum delivery device which is accurately calibrated to deliver definite amounts. The maximum dilution employed for chickens must not exceed 1:50, and, according to available data, the 1:25 dilution appears to be the most efficient. The dilution for turkeys should not exceed 1:25. After the serum and antigen are well agitated, the mixture should be incubated for at least 20 hours at 37° C.

The results of the tests are interpreted as follows: *Negative test*—the fluid remains

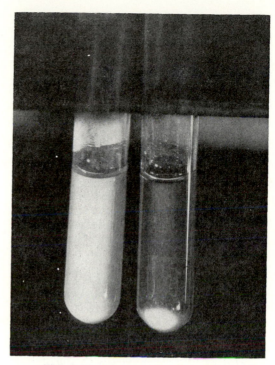

FIG. 3.13—*Macroscopic tube agglutination test.* **(Left)** *Negative reaction.* **(Right)** *Positive reaction.*

uniformly turbid. *Positive test*—the antigen reveals a distinct clumping, and clumps of cells have settled to the base of the tube with the supernatant fluid being clear (Fig. 3.13). Gradation of clumping or agglutination may occur between negative and positive tests. These may be designated as slightly or strongly *Suspicious.*

Stained Antigen, Rapid Whole-Blood Test

The stained antigen, rapid whole-blood test was first developed by Schaffer et al. (1931) and Coburn and Stafseth (1931). At the present time the antigen for this method is produced under a federal license from the Secretary of Agriculture, in accordance with specific directions. MacDonald (1947, unpublished) developed a colloidal-sulfur medium (K) for production of the whole-blood antigen. This medium produces an antigen which is superior to other stained antigens provided previously. Since July 1, 1953, all whole-blood crystal violet-stained antigen has been produced according to the K formula and is known as K antigen (Williams and MacDonald, 1955). Since July 1, 1957, all stained whole-blood antigens have been of the polyvalent type which contains both "standard" and "variant" type strains (Anon., 1969). In addition to K polyvalent antigen, there is a second whole-blood antigen product commercially available in the United States. This antigen, known as Redigen, is produced under the manufacturer's patented process (Patent No. 2,301,717). Its reading time is gauged in seconds since it reacts more rapidly than K antigen.

For a detailed description of the official procedure, reference should be made to the revised report on the *National Poultry and Turkey Improvement Plans* (Anon., 1969). Briefly the method may be described as follows: A wire loop, 3/16 inch in diameter made on the end of a 2½-inch length of noncorrosive wire (Brown and Sharpe gauge No. 24), is used to measure the blood. One end of the wire is inserted into a cork stopper which serves as a handle. A loopful of blood is taken from the punctured wing vein and contains approximately 0.02 ml when the blood appears to bulge out. The loopful of blood is mixed with the stained antigen which has been placed on a glass plate marked off in inch squares. The antigen is measured with a dropper whose tip is constructed to deliver 0.05 ml when held in a vertical position. An antigen-blood dilution of 2:1 or 3:1 has been reported to give the most satisfactory results. The loopful of blood is mixed with the antigen, and the mixture is spread out about an inch in diameter. The loop is washed in clean water and dried with cheesecloth or blotting paper. The glass plate is tilted several times to aid in the mixing of the blood and antigen; apparently the tilting has some influence on the speed of the agglutination. Reactions may occur within a few seconds or up to 2 minutes. Delayed reactions should be regarded as nonspecific. A positive reaction consists of the clumping of the stained cells floating in clear fluid (Fig. 3.14). The rapidity of the reaction and the size of the clumps are influenced by the agglutinin titer of the blood. Partial reactions should be regarded as suspicious and treated in the same manner as those observed in the other testing methods. Sometimes a very fine granulation appears which should be considered negative. Very infrequently agglutination of the red blood cells occurs and should not be confused with the clumping of the stained bacterial cells. The fine marginal flocculation, which may be observed before drying of the mixture, is to be considered negative. A negative reaction is one in which the mixture remains homogeneous for at least 2 minutes. Only those reactions which appear within 1 minute after the mixing of the blood and antigen should be considered definitely positive, while reactions delayed for 2 minutes should be considered suspicious.

In order to approach uniformity of results, the testing plate should be well lighted at all times, and the temperature should remain at a constant level. A temperature

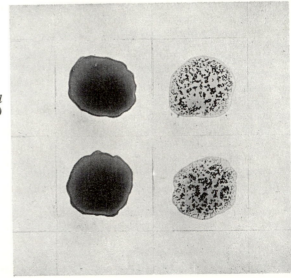

FIG. 3.14—Stained-antigen, whole-blood test. **(Left)** *Negative reaction.* **(Right)** *Positive reaction.*

of 75–85° F is considered satisfactory. The test plate should be free of dust and so constructed that it can be tilted with ease. The tested birds can be retained in either special holding equipment or crates and released as rapidly as the results of the test become known. All birds in the tested flock should be officially leg-banded. The accuracy of the results is greatly influenced by the competency of the testing agent and his thoroughness and care in conducting the test.

Rapid Serum Test

The rapid serum test for the detection of pullorum disease carriers was developed by Runnells et al. (1927). The blood samples may be collected in a manner similar to that described for the tube test. The antigen employed should consist of representative strains of *S. pullorum* which are of known antigenic composition and high agglutinability, but which are not sensitive to negative and nonspecific sera. The strains are suspended in 12% sodium chloride solution containing 0.5% phenol. The turbidity is adjusted to 50 times greater than tube 0.75 of McFarland's nephelometer.

A box with a glass top ruled off in inch squares and improvised with lighting and heating facilities is used for testing. The serum and antigen should be mixed thoroughly. Positive reactions may occur quickly, but delayed reactions may require several minutes (Fig. 3.15). Gradations of re-

actions occur in this method as in other methods.

Interpretation of Results

All suspicious and positive reacting tests should be reported to the agency responsible for disposition of infected birds. Also all broken, missing, and spoiled samples should be reported. A serologic diagnosis should be confirmed by bacteriologic examination of one or more reactors. If only suspicious reactions are observed in a flock, the strongest reacting birds should be submitted to the laboratory for retesting and a careful bacteriologic examination. In routine testing, flocks should not be condemned as infected on the basis of doubtful or atypical reactions, because such reactions may be due to infections other than *S. pullorum*. Nonpullorum reactions occasionally cause problems of interpretation. A variety of bacteria which possess antigens in common with or closely related to those of *S. pullorum* may infect birds and produce an agglutinin response. Garrard et al. (1948) reported that nonpullorum reactions occurred more frequently with variant than with standard form antigens. Infections with coliforms, micrococci, and streptococci, particularly those belonging to the Lancefield group D, were found to be responsible for a large percentage of nonpullorum reactions in chickens. Absorption tests indicated that the 12_2 factor was most frequently responsible for the cross-reactions. Other salmonellae with antigens common to *S. pullorum* may also produce cross-reactions. The serum of birds infected with bacteria antigenically related to *S. pullorum* often produces a low titer with an atypical type of agglutination; at times both the titer and character of agglutination are indistinguishable from those produced by pullorum disease. If no conclusive evidence of pullorum infection can be found, the flock should be regarded as negative. Occasionally it is advisable to retest groups of birds to clarify their status.

Miscellaneous Tests

A number of additional tests have been employed as a means of detecting infected birds. An intradermal test applied to the wattle was described by Ward and Gallagher (1917). Rettger and Plastridge (1932) summarized the work of several investigators with intradermal tests and concluded

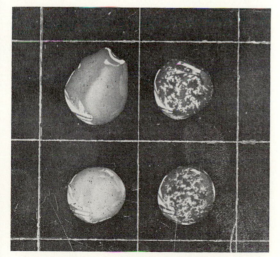

FIG. 3.15—Rapid serum agglutination test. (Left) Negative reaction. (Right) Positive reaction.

that the agglutination tests were more dependable.

Williams (1951) described a "spot test" for the detection of infected chickens. This test may serve as a useful adjunct to the agglutination test, especially in flocks in which suspicious reactors are detected.

A flocculation test was described by Roznowski and Foltz (1958). The antigen, which produced promising results from the limited work reported, was prepared by coating cholesterol crystals with an ecto-antigen extract of *S. pullorum*.

Rice and Gwatkin (1949) compared an indirect complement fixation test to the agglutination test. The test was too involved and expensive for routine work but offered promise for differentiating nonpullorum reactors from true reactors. Aoki et al. (1963) used an agar gel precipitin test to detect infected birds. The test was consistently negative with sera which produced nonspecific reactions with an agglutination test.

A rapid hemagglutination test with chloroform or ethyl alcohol washed antigens was reported by Ungureanu and Grecianu (1963) to be specific and to produce a higher titer than produced by the tube agglutination test. Sapre and Mehta (1967) described an indirect hemagglutination test for *S. pullorum* which detected antibodies earlier and in dilutions four times greater than by a bacterial agglutination test.

Andrews (1963) saturated serodiscs with serum and with whole blood of infected pheasants. Tube agglutination tests of whole-blood eluates for pullorum disease were unreadable, and the plate agglutination test of eluates was only about one-half as accurate as the serum tube agglutination test. Heutgens (1964) found that juices of either fresh or frozen muscle of affected chickens produced positive reactions with the whole-blood test, provided that tube agglutination titers of the donor bird had been 640 or higher.

National Control Program

The *National Poultry and Turkey Improvement Plans* (Anon., 1969) detail the specific criteria for establishing and maintaining official U.S. pullorum-typhoid clean flocks and hatcheries. These criteria are based on annual testing of breeding stock to assure freedom from infection, and routine management procedures on the farm and in the hatchery to prevent direct or indirect contact with infected or questionable stock. Chickens may be tested for accreditation after they reach 5 months of age, turkeys after 4 months of age.

If an attempt is to be made to free a flock of infection, retesting of the infected

TABLE 3.1 ❧ Retesting Data of Ten Infected Flocks

Flock Number		First Test	Second Test	Third Test	Fourth Test	Fifth Test	Results of Subsequent Season
1	No. of birds tested	189	152	48	. . .	. . .	467
	Percentage reactors	1.59	0.00	0.00	. . .	. . .	0.00
2	No. of birds tested	369	256	218	. . .	. . .	232
	Percentage reactors	0.54	0.39	0.00	. . .	. . .	0.00
3	No. of birds tested	125	98	91	. . .	. . .	201
	Percentage reactors	20.00	4.08	0.00	. . .	. . .	0.00
4	No. of birds tested	243	262	223	179	. . .	199
	Percentage reactors	11.11	1.15	0.00	0.00	. . .	0.00
5	No. of birds tested	464	444	433	397	. . .	1,087
	Percentage reactors	2.37	0.45	0.00	0.00	. . .	0.00
6	No. of birds tested	1,765	1,559	1,508	1,108	767	1,796
	Percentage reactors	3.17	0.13	0.00	0.00	0.00	0.00
7	No. of birds tested	2,079	1,929	1,811	1,648	1,337	2,132
	Percentage reactors	3.17	1.09	0.00	0.00	0.00	0.00
8	No. of birds tested	704	691	610	422	. . .	693
	Percentage reactors	8.24	8.83	0.16	0.00	. . .	0.00
9	No. of birds tested	2,722	2,413	2,284	1,929	. . .	3,707
	Percentage reactors	1.80	0.54	0.48	0.00	. . .	0.00
10	No. of birds tested	640	440	399	352	339	747
	Percentage reactors	27.34	4.32	1.00	0.00	0.00	0.00

flock should be done at 2–4-week intervals until two consecutive negative tests of the entire flock are secured at not less than 21-day intervals. In the majority of cases, infection can be eliminated from the flock through short interval testing. Two or three retests are often sufficient to detect all infected birds (Table 3.1). Occasionally infection continues to spread within a flock and the disease cannot be eliminated by repeated testing. The *National Poultry and Turkey Improvement Plans* have recently been revised to allow official accreditation based on annual testing of 25% (in some cases less) of the birds in hatchery supply flocks in a state, provided the state meets a number of specific regulatory provisions designed to detect and quarantine infected flocks.

Area Eradication

Early efforts to control pullorum disease were of necessity based on the objective of eliminating the disease from individual flocks and from the flocks of individual hatchery and breeding organizations. Striking progress has been made to date. Van Roekel (1964) reviewed progress in reducing the incidence of pullorum disease in the United States and suggested that the time had arrived to develop and implement area eradication programs. Table 3.2 compares the percentages of reactors among chickens tested in the member states and Canadian provinces of the Northeastern Conference on Avian Diseases during the initial years of official testing and 1966. The percentage of infected birds has been greatly reduced and in some states has been at a zero level for a number of years. A marked decline in the number of cases of pullorum disease in tested flocks and in all specimens submitted for diagnosis has also been observed (Table 3.3). A similar though more recent decline in percentage of positive reactors has been achieved throughout the United States in both chickens and turkeys (Tables 3.4, 3.5).

The very low rate of infection in commercial breeding stock, indicated by official reports of the control agencies, does not necessarily reflect the true incidence of infection. In many areas there are substantial numbers of small flocks of noncommercial chickens which have not been reached by pullorum control programs. Small breeding groups of "fancy" breeds of chickens

TABLE 3.2 ❧ Pullorum Testing Data Submitted By States and Canadian Provinces in Northeastern Conference on Avian Diseases

State	Year	Birds Tested	Percent Positive
Connecticut	1925	20,743	2.4
	1966	311,036	0.0
Delaware	1925	4,300	5.7
	1966	475,770	0.0
Maine	1921	2,730	22.3
	1966	722,283	0.005
Maryland	1927	3,725	21.0
	1966	518,997	0.0
Massachusetts	1921	24,718	12.5
	1966	478,860	0.005
New Hampshire	1926	35,237	2.5
	1966	348,150	0.0
New Jersey	1926	52,611	7.86
	1966	265,365	0.0
New York	1926	59,576	6.2
	1966	419,036	0.0
North Carolina	1932	64,702	4.02
	1966	5,739,629	0.0
Nova Scotia	1929	2,041	7.0
	1966	71,394	0.0
Ontario	1928	15,000	8.0
	1966	1,342,539	0.0001
Pennsylvania	1924	2,077	15.0
	1966	896,347	0.00044
Rhode Island	1925	8,175	6.97
	1966	48,078	0.0
Vermont	1928	8,555	7.4
	1966	42,464	0.01
Virginia	1925	13,000	20.0
	1966	821,039	0.012
West Virginia	1928	9,005	6.0
	1966	59,561	0.0

are commonly maintained for exhibition purposes. Owners of such stock frequently transfer birds between flocks without regard to fundamental disease control principles. During the years 1958–68 substantial numbers of such flocks, in addition to commercial breeding stock, have been tested in Massachusetts. In this period 6,278,328 chickens, turkeys, and pheasants in 2,159 flocks were tested, and 30 flocks were found to be infected. Of these, 2 were in commercial breeding chickens purchased from a questionable source, 5 were in egg producing flocks originating from questionable sources, and the remaining 23 infected flocks consisted of exhibition breeds of chickens. None of the flocks in the last group had a history suggesting they should

TABLE 3.3 ❧ Incidence of Pullorum Infection in Chickens and Turkeys in 14 Northeastern States as Detected Among Tested Flocks and Consignments Submitted for Diagnosis

State	1958		1962		1967	
	F*	D†	F*	D†	F*	D†
Connecticut	3	6	0	0	0	0
Delaware	3	6	0	0	0	1
Maine	0	1	0	0	0	0
Maryland	2	5	0	2	0	0
Massachusetts	3	7	0	2	3	3
New Hampshire	0	2	0	1	0	2
New Jersey	16	7	0	8	0	2
New York	3	13	0	12	0	5
North Carolina	5	37	16	29	0	0
Pennsylvania	12	37	1	13	1	4
Rhode Island	0	0	0	0	0	0
Vermont	0	4	0	4	1	2
Virginia	10	21	1	9	0	4
West Virginia	11	29	0	0	0	0
Total	68	175	18	80	5	23

* Infected tested flocks.
† Diagnosis among consignments submitted (data may sometimes include some infections detected by flock testing).

TABLE 3.4 ❧ Pullorum Disease Testing Summary of U.S. Chickens During 32-Year Period

Item	1935–36	1949–50	1962–63	1966–67
Number of flocks	9,191	111,422	21,272	12,377
Number of birds	4,329,364	37,237,674	35,236,200	38,327,497
Percentage of positive tests	3.66	0.72	0.005	0.001
Birds in pullorum-clean flocks	257,577	13,302,642	33,517,824	38,316,937

Source: Anon., 1969.

TABLE 3.5 ❧ Pullorum Disease Testing Summary of U.S. Turkeys During 23-Year Period

Item	1943–44	1949–50	1962–63	1966–67
Number of flocks	2,489	4,717	2,297	1,743
Number of birds	982,904	2,340,574	3,879,861	4,397,263
Percentage of positive tests	2.00	0.39	0.003	0.00005
Birds in pullorum-clean flocks	...	...	...	4,388,571

Source: Anon., 1969.

be free of pullorum disease. If only commercial breeding stock had been tested, as in many states, the record would have failed to show any infection, rather than the 23 flocks that were found during the last 7 years of the period. These results suggest that rather numerous unknown foci of infection may exist in many areas but that such infections might not greatly endanger well separated pullorum-negative commercial breeding stock. Nevertheless, such infected stock must pose a degree of danger which cannot be ignored in an eradication program.

The American Association of Avian Pathologists in 1965 voted to go on record as endorsing an effort to eradicate pullorum disease as a philosophy. It was significant that this body, composed of people with broad experience with the disease from all standpoints, considered eradication both possible and practical. It appears that a program to eradicate pullorum disease should be based on regulatory action which includes as a minimum: (1) mandatory reporting of all diagnoses, (2) epidemiological investigations and quarantine of all infected and suspicious flocks, and (3) limiting public exhibition and interstate movement of all chickens, turkeys, and hatching eggs unless accompanied by a history indicating freedom from pullorum disease.

REFERENCES

Allen, P. W., and M. Jacob. 1930. Sodium acid sulphate as a disinfectant against *Salmonella pullorum* in poultry-yard soils. *Tenn. Agr. Exp. Sta., Bull.* 143.

Anderson, G. W., J. B. Cooper, J. C. Jones, and C. L. Morgan. 1948. Sulfonamides in the control of pullorum disease. *Poultry Sci.* 27:172–75.

Andrews, R. D. 1963. Evaluation of tests for pullorum and Newcastle disease with whole-blood samples collected on serodiscs. *Avian Diseases* 7:193–96.

Anonymous. 1930. Eastern states conference of laboratory workers in pullorum disease control. *J. Am. Vet. Med. Ass.* 77:259–63.

Anonymous. 1933. Report of the conference of official research workers in animal diseases of North America on standard methods of pullorum disease in barnyard fowl. *J. Am. Med. Ass.* 82:487–91.

Anonymous. 1954. Report of the committee on transmissible diseases of poultry. *Proc. 58th Ann. Meet. U.S. Livestock Sanit. Ass.*, pp. 330–41.

Anonymous. 1969. *National Poultry and Turkey Improvement Plans and Auxiliary Provisions.* USDA, ARS, AHR Div., Beltsville, Md.

Aoki, S., M. Kashiwazaki, S. Sato, H. Watase, and C. Sakamato. 1963. Application of agar-jell precipitin test to the diagnosis of pullorum disease. *Nat. Inst. Animal Health Quart.* 3:175–84.

Asmundson, V. S., and J. Biely. 1930. Effect of pullorum disease on distribution of first year egg production. *Sci. Agr.* 10:497–507.

Ayres, J. C., and Betty Taylor. 1956. Effect of temperature on microbial proliferation in shell eggs. *Appl. Microbiol.* 4:355–59.

Barkate, J. A. 1968. Screening of feed components for salmonella with polyvalent H agglutination. *Appl. Microbiol.* 16:1272–74.

Bassiouni, A., M. Rifai, and K. Abbasi. 1966. The influence of the somatic factor O-1 on the agglutination reactions for detecting *S. gallinarum-pullorum* infections. *Vet. Med. J. Giza* 12:369–76.

Beaudette, F. R. 1938. Localized pullorum infection in the ovary of a duck. *J. Am. Vet. Med. Ass.* 92:100–101.

Beaudette, F. R., L. D. Bushnell, and L. F. Payne. 1923a. Study of an organism resembling *Bacterium pullorum* from unabsorbed yolk of chicks "dead in shell." *J. Infect. Diseases* 32:124–32.

———. 1923b. Relation of *Bacterium pullorum* to hatchability of eggs. *J. Infect. Diseases* 33:331–37.

Belding, R. C. 1955. The incidence of *Salmonella pullorum* in wild pheasants in southern Michigan. *Poultry Sci.* 34:1441–44.

Benedict, R. G., E. McCoy, and W. Wisnicky. 1941. Salmonella types in silver foxes. *J. Infect. Diseases* 69:167–72.

Biely, J., C. E. Sawyer, C. M. Hamilton, W. T. Johnson, and E. M. Dickinson. 1931. Accuracy of three cooperating laboratories in detecting pullorum disease by the agglutination test. *J. Am. Vet. Med. Ass.* 79:19–36.

Bierer, B. W. 1961. Furaltadone water medication against naturally induced *Salmonella pullorum* infection in stressed floor broilers. *Avian Diseases* 5:333–36.

Biondi, E., and A. Schiavo. 1966. Action of colimycin (colistin) on *Salmonella pullorum.* III. Studies on chicks. *Zooprofilassi* 21:637–58.

Bivins, J. A. 1948. A survey of the incidence of serological variants of *Salmonella pullorum* in Michigan. *Poultry Sci.* 27:629–34.

Blaxland, J. D., W. J. Sojka, and A. M. Smither. 1956. A study of *Salmonella pullorum* and *Salmonella gallinarum* strains isolated from field outbreaks of disease. *J. Comp. Pathol. Therap.* 66:270–77.

Bottorff, C. A., and J. S. Kiser. 1947. The use of sulfonamides in the control of pullorum disease. *Poultry Sci.* 26:335–39.

Botts, C. W., L. C. Ferguson, J. M. Birkeland, and A. R. Winter. 1952. The influence of litter on the control of salmonella infections in chicks. *Am. J. Vet. Res.* 13:562–65.

Bruner, D. W., and A. B. Moran. 1949. Salmonella infections of domestic animals. *Cornell Vet.* 39:53–63.

Bunyea, H. 1939. An outbreak of pullorum disease in young guinea fowl. *J. Am. Vet. Med. Ass.* 94:233–34.

Bunyea, H., and W. J. Hall. 1929. Some observations on the pathology of bacillary white diarrhea in baby chicks. *J. Am. Vet. Med. Ass.* 75:581–91.

Bushnell, L. D., and J. J. Porter. 1945. A study of methods for the isolation of *Salmonella pullorum.* *Poultry Sci.* 24:212–15.

Bushnell, L. D., W. R. Hinshaw, and L. F. Payne. 1926. Bacillary white diarrhea in fowl. *Kansas Agr. Exp. Sta. Tech. Bull.* 21.

Byrne, J. L. 1943. Variant or atypical strains of *Salmonella pullorum.* *Can. J. Comp. Med. Vet. Sci.* 7:227–38.

Carpenter, J. A., G. W. Anderson, R. A. Johnston, and E. H. Garrard. 1949. Pullorum disease in turkeys. *Poultry Sci.* 28:270–75.

Chute, H. L., and M. Gershman. 1963. Case report—*Salmonella pullorum* in a Muscovy (*Cairina muschata*) duck. *Avian Diseases* 7:168–69.

Coburn, D. R., and H. J. Stafseth. 1931. A field test for pullorum disease. *J. Am. Vet. Med. Ass.* 79:241–43.

Cole, R. K. 1948. Sulfonamides versus *Salmo-*

nella pullorum in adult chickens. *Poultry Sci.* 27:427–29.

Cooper, J. B., D. L. Morgan, G. W. Anderson, and J. C. Jones. 1951. Effect of sulfamerazine on pullorum reactors. *Poultry Sci.* 30:249–54.

Corpron, R., J. A. Bivins, and H. S. Stafseth. 1947. Pullorum disease studies in turkeys. *Poultry Sci.* 26:340–51.

Cosgrove, A. S., and P. R. Lindenmaier. 1961. Case report: Hock swellings as a primary lesion of *Salmonella pullorum* infection in broiler chickens. *Avian Diseases* 5:144–46.

Costin, I. D., L. Patricia, M. Garoiu, P. Onica, A. Pelle, and N. Dinu. 1964. Correlation between origin and biochemical behaviour of *Salmonella gallinarum* and *Salmonella pullorum* cultures. *Zentr. Bakteriol. Parasitenk. Abt. I. Orig.* 194:342–50.

Dalling, T., J. H. Mason, and W. S. Gordon. 1928. Bacillary white diarrhea (B.W.D.): *B. pullorum* isolated from sparrows. *Vet. Record* 8:329.

Davis, D. E., H. M. Sims, and N. Buchanan. 1961. A blister-like lesion associated with pullorum disease in broiler chicks. *Southeastern Vet.* 12:53–56.

Dearstyne, R. S., B. F. Kaupp, and H. S. Wilfong. 1929. Study of bacillary white diarrhea (pullorum disease). *N. Carolina State Coll. Agr. Expt. Sta. Bull.* 36.

DeVolt, H. M., G. D. Quigley, and T. C. Byerly. 1941. Studies of resistance to pullorum disease in chickens. *Poultry Sci.* 20:339–41.

Dickinson, E. M., and E. D. Stoddard. 1949. Sulfamerazine against *Salmonella pullorum* in adult chickens. *Poultry Sci.* 28:153–55.

Dickinson, E. M., A. S. Rosenwald, and D. R. Morrill. 1944. Comparison of the tube and rapid serum agglutination tests for the detection of pullorum disease in turkeys. *Oregon State Agr. Exp. Sta. Tech. Bull.* 6.

Doyle, L. P., and F. P. Mathews. 1928. The pathology of bacillary white diarrhea in chicks. *Purdue Univ. Agr. Expt. Sta. Res. Bull.* 323.

Dunlap, G. L. 1931. *Mass. Agr. Expt. Sta. Ann. Rept. Bull.* 271:281.

Edgington, B. H. 1937. Titre fluctuation in agglutination tests for pullorum disease in hens. *Poultry Sci.* 16:15–18.

Edwards, P. R. 1928. The fermentation of maltose by *Bacterium pullorum*. *J. Bacteriol.* 15:235–43.

———. 1945. An outbreak of *Salmonella pullorum* infection in canaries. *J. Am. Vet. Med. Ass.* 107:245.

Edwards, P. R., and D. W. Bruner. 1943. The occurrence and distribution of salmonella types in the United States. *J. Infect. Diseases* 72:58–67.

———. 1946. Form variation in *Salmonella pul-*

lorum and its relation to X strains. *Cornell Vet.* 36:318–24.

Edwards, P. R., and F. E. Hull. 1929. Bacillary white diarrhea and related diseases of chickens. *Kentucky Agr. Exp. Sta. Bull.* 296.

Edwards, P. R., D. W. Bruner, E. R. Doll, and G. S. Hermann. 1948. Further notes on variation in *Salmonella pullorum*. *Cornell Vet.* 38:257–62.

Emmel, M. W. 1936. Pullorum disease in captive quail. *J. Am. Vet. Med. Ass.* 89:716–17.

Evans, W. M., D. W. Bruner, and M. C. Peckham. 1955. Blindness in chicks associated with salmonellosis. *Cornell Vet.* 45:239–47.

Ferguson, A. E., M. C. Connell, and R. B. Truscott. 1961. Isolation of *Salmonella pullorum* from the joints of broiler chicks. *Can. Vet. J.* 2:143–45.

Francis, D. W. 1960. Treatment of natural infection of *Salmonella pullorum* in day-old chicks with furazolidone. *Avian Diseases* 4:63–73.

Gage, G. E. 1911. Notes on ovarian infection with *Bacterium pullorum* (Rettger) in the domestic fowl. *J. Med. Res.* 19:491–96.

Gage, G. E., and J. F. Martin. 1916. Notes on the histopathology of the intestines in young chicks infected with *Bacterium pullorum*. *J. Med. Res.* 29:149–55.

Gage, G. E., B. H. Paige, and H. W. Hyland. 1914. On the diagnosis of infection with *Bacterium pullorum* in the domestic fowl. *Mass. Agr. Exp. Sta. Bull.* 148:1–20.

Garrard, E. H., W. H. Burton, and J. A. Carpenter. 1948. Non-pullorum agglutination reactions. *Proc. Eighth World's Poultry Congr.*, pp. 626–31.

Gershman, M., H. L. Chute, and R. F. Cuozzo. 1962. The laboratory application of anhydrous *Salmonella pullorum* antigen. *Avian Diseases* 6:107–11.

Gilfillan, R. F., D. F. Holtman, and R. T. Ross. 1955. A synthetic medium for propagation and maintenance of virulent strains of *Salmonella pullorum*. *Poultry Sci.* 34:1283–88.

Goff, Ollia E. 1932–34. Pigeons react to pullorum test. *Rept. Okla. Agr. Exp. Sta.*, p. 140.

Gordon, R. F., and J. Tucker. 1955. The treatment of chronic carriers of *Salmonella pullorum* with furazolidone. *Vet. Record* 67:116–18.

Gordon, R. F., J. E. Lancaster, and J. Tucker. 1953. Chick sexing instruments as a means of spreading *S. pullorum* and the efficiency of formaldehyde in the sanitation of the optical tubes. *Vet. Record* 65:481–82.

Gorrie, C. J. R. 1944. Infectious laryngotracheitis vaccine in relation to transmission of pullorum disease. *Australian Vet. J.* 20:343–44.

Grausgruber, W., and R. Kissling. 1964. Influence of antibiotic food supplements on bacteriological and serological diagnosis of pullorum disease. *Wien. Tieraerztl. Monatsschr.* 51:814–22.

Grumbles, L. C., Helen E. Levy, and W. T. Oglesby. 1950. Sulfonamides in the control of pullorum disease in young chicks. *Poultry Sci.* 29:236–39.

Gubkin, S. M. 1964. Survival of paratyphoid bacteria in animal buildings. *Sb. Nauchni. Tr. Semipalatinsk. Zootekhn. Vet. Inst.* 12:157–65.

Gwatkin, R., and E. W. Bond. 1947. Studies in pullorum disease. XIX. Examination of colonies from regular and variant form cultures of *Salmonella pullorum*. *Can. J. Comp. Med. Vet. Sci.* 11:282–89.

Gwatkin, R., and C. A. Mitchell. 1944. Transmission of *Salmonella pullorum* by flies. *Can. J. Public Health* 35:281–85.

Gwatkin, R., I. W. Moynihan, C. W. Traves, and W. Roach. 1941. Comparison of the whole blood and tube agglutination test for pullorum disease. *Sci. Agr.* 21:335–49.

Hanks, J. H., and L. F. Rettger. 1932. Bacterial endotoxin. Search for a specific intracellular toxin in *S. pullorum*. *J. Immunol.* 22:283–314.

Heemstra, L. C. 1948. The importance of the variant problem in pullorum disease control. *Proc. 52nd Ann. Meet. U.S. Livestock Sanit. Ass.*, p. 274.

Henderson, W., G. L. Morehouse, and R. F. Cross. 1960. The effect of furazolidone on *Salmonella pullorum* and agglutination titers in chickens. *Avian Diseases* 4:223–30.

Hendrickson, J. M. 1927. The differentiation of *Bacterium pullorum* (Rettger) and *Bacterium sanguinarium* (Moore). *J. Am. Vet. Med. Ass.* 70:629–44.

Hendrickson, J. M., and K. F. Hilbert. 1931. Report of the Poultry Disease Laboratory at Farmingdale, Long Island. *N.Y. State Vet. Coll., Ann. Rept.* (1929–30), pp. 51–53.

Heutgens, H. W. 1964. A rapid method for determination of *S. gallinarum-pullorum* antibodies in poultry meat by the muscle juice press method and antibody reaction. Inaug. Diss. Tieraerztl. Hochschule, Hannover.

Hewitt, E. A. 1928. Bacillary white diarrhea in baby turkeys. *Cornell Vet.* 18:272–76.

Hinshaw, W. R. 1928. New England Conference of Laboratory Workers in Bacillary White Diarrhea Control. *J. Am. Vet. Med. Ass.* 73:263–64.

———. 1941. Cysteine and related compounds for differentiating members of the genus salmonella. *Hilgardia* 13:583–621.

Hinshaw, W. R., and H. A. Hoffman. 1937. Pullorum disease in ducklings. *Poultry Sci.* 16:189–93.

Hinshaw, W. R., and E. McNeil. 1940. Eradication of pullorum disease from turkey flocks. *Proc. 44th Ann. Meet. U.S. Livestock Sanit. Ass.*, pp. 178–94.

Hinshaw, W. R., C. W. Upp, and J. M. Moore. 1926. Studies in transmission of bacillary white diarrhea in incubators. *J. Am. Vet. Med. Ass.* 68:631–41.

Hudson, C. B., and F. R. Beaudette. 1929. The isolation of *Bacterium pullorum* from a European bullfinch (*Pyrrhula europa*). *J. Am. Vet. Med. Ass.* 74:929–32.

Hutt, F. B., and J. C. Scholes. 1941. Genetics of the fowl. XIII. Breed differences in susceptibility to *Salmonella pullorum*. *Poultry Sci.* 20:342–52.

Hutyra, F., J. Marek, and R. Manninger. 1938. *Special Pathology and Therapeutics of the Diseases of Domestic Animals*, Vol. I, 4th English ed. Alexander Eger, Chicago.

Jacobs, R. E., M. N. Frazier, and M. E. Tourtellotte. 1960. Hatchery spread of pullorum disease through debeaking. *Avian Diseases* 4:109–15.

Johnson, E. P., and G. W. Anderson. 1936. Pullorum disease in turkeys. *J. Infect. Diseases* 58:337–41.

Jones, A. W., and D. F. Holtman. 1953. Synthesis of glutamic acid and alanine by *Salmonella pullorum*. *J. Bacteriol.* 66:147–49.

Jones, F. S. 1911. Fatal septicemia or bacillary white diarrhea in young chickens. *N.Y. State Vet. Coll., Ann. Rept.* (1909–10), pp. 111–29.

———. 1913a. An outbreak of an acute disease in adult fowls due to *Bacterium pullorum*. *J. Med. Res.* 27:471–79.

———. 1913b. The value of the macroscopic agglutination test in detecting fowls that are harboring *Bacterium pullorum*. *J. Med. Res.* 27:481–95.

Jungherr, E. 1935. Diseases of brooder chicks. *Storrs Agr. Exp. Sta. Bull.* 202:20–24.

Karyagin, V. I. 1964. Development of resistance of *Salmonella pullorum*. I. To biomycin. II. To furazolidone. *Sb. Nauchni. Tr. Belorussk. Vet. Inst.*, pp. 31–49.

Kerr, W. R. 1930. Selective media for the cultivation of *Bacillus pullorum* and *Bacillus sanguinarium*. *J. Comp. Pathol. Therap.* 43:77–85.

Khashimov, A. U. 1964. Survival of *Salmonella pullorum* in the external environment. *Veterinariya* 41:21–24.

Kosters, J., and H. Geissler. 1966. The selection of *S. gallinarum-pullorum* strains for production of a standardized agglutination antigen. *Berlin. Muench. Tieraerztl. Wochschr.* 79:276–78.

McCullough, N. B., and C. W. Eisele. 1951. Experimental human salmonellosis. IV. Pathogenicity of strains of *Salmonella pullorum* obtained from spray-dried whole egg. *J. Infect. Diseases* 89:259–65.

Mallmann, W. L. 1929. *Salmonella pullorum* in the intestinal contents of baby chicks. *J. Infect. Diseases* 44:16–20.

———. 1931. Use of organic acids for the differentiation of *Salmonella pullorum* and *Salmonella gallinarum*. *Proc. Soc. Exp. Biol. Med.* 28:501–2.

Mallmann, W. L., and D. Snyder. 1929. Differential medium for *Salmonella pullorum, Salmonella gallinarum, Pasteurella avicida,* and *Escherichia coli*. *J. Infect. Diseases* 44:13–15.

Mitchell, R. B., F. C. Garlock, and R. H. Broh-Kahn. 1946. An outbreak of gastro-enteritis presumably caused by *Salmonella pullorum*. *J. Infect. Diseases* 79:57–62.

Miura, S., G. Sato, and T. Miyamae. 1964. Occurrence and survival of salmonella organisms in hatcher chick fluff from commercial hatcheries. *Avian Diseases* 8:546–54.

Moran, A. B. 1961. Occurrence and distribution of salmonella in animals in the United States. *Proc. 65th Ann. Meet. U.S. Livestock Sanit. Ass.,* pp. 441–48.

Mullen, F. E. 1946. Sulfamerazine as a prophylactic in pullorum disease in poults. *J. Am. Vet. Med. Ass.* 108:163–64.

Nóbrega, P., and R. C. Bueno. 1944. Pullorum Disease in the Uru (*Odontophorus capueira*). *Arquiv. Inst. Biol.* (Sao Paulo) 15:37–38.

Olney, J. F. 1928. *Salmonella pullorum* infection in rabbits. *J. Am. Vet. Med. Ass.* 73:631–33.

Pacheco, G., and C. Rodrigues. 1936. O grupo pullorum-gallinarum em provas bacteriologicas comparativas. *Mem. Inst. Oswaldo Cruz* 31:591–705.

Peresadin, A. V. 1965. Efficacy of polymyxin M in pullorum disease. *Veterinariya* 42:40–43.

Plastridge, W. N., and L. F. Rettger. 1930. An epidemic disease of domestic fowl caused by a hitherto undescribed organism of the *Salmonella pullorum* type. *J. Infect. Diseases* 47:334–39.

Pomeroy, B. S., R. Fenstermacher, and M. H. Roepke. 1948. Sulfonamides in the control of salmonellosis of chicks and poults. *J. Am. Vet. Med. Ass.* 112:296–303.

Prier, J. E., and H. E. Rhoades. 1948. Arthritis in turkeys associated with *Salmonella pullorum*. *Vet. Med.* 43:541.

Read, R. B., Jr., and A. L. Reyes. 1968. Variation in plating efficiency of salmonellae on eight lots of brilliant green agar. *Appl. Microbiol.* 16:746–48.

Rettger, L. F. 1900. Septicemia among young chickens. *N.Y. Med. J.* 71:803–5.

———. 1909. Further studies on fatal septicemia in young chickens, or "white diarrhea." *J. Med. Res.* 21:115–23.

Rettger, L. F., and W. N. Plastridge. 1932. Pullorum disease of domestic fowl. *Monograph Storrs Agr. Exp. Sta. Bull.* 178.

Rettger, L. F., W. F. Kirkpatrick, and R. E. Jones. 1915. Bacillary diarrhea of young chicks: Its eradication by the elimination of infected breeding stock (Fifth report). *Storrs Agr. Exp. Sta. Bull.* 85:151–67.

Rettger, L. F., T. G. Hull, and W. S. Sturges. 1916. Feeding experiments with *Bacterium pullorum*. The toxicity of infected eggs. *J. Exp. Med.* 23:475–89.

Rhoades, H. E., and J. O. Alberts. 1950. The incidence of serological variants of *Salmonella pullorum* in Illinois. *Poultry Sci.* 29:579–81.

Rice, C. E., and R. Gwatkin. 1949. Studies in pullorum disease. XXVI. A comparison of the titers obtained by indirect complement-fixation and agglutination methods for turkey sera. *Cornell Vet.* 39:183–94.

Richey, D. J., and C. L. Morgan. 1960. The effects of furazolidone on chicken *Salmonella pullorum* carriers. *Avian Diseases* 4:48–63.

Roberts, E., and L. E. Card. 1926. The inheritance of resistance to bacillary white diarrhea. *Poultry Sci.* 6:18–23.

———. 1935. Inheritance of resistance to bacterial infection in animals. A genetic study of pullorum disease. *Ill. Agr. Exp. Sta. Bull.* 419:467–96.

Roberts, E., J. M. Severens, and L. E. Card. 1939. Nature of the hereditary factors for resistance and susceptibility to pullorum disease in the domestic fowl. *Proc. Seventh World's Poultry Congr.,* pp. 52–54.

Roznowski, E. P. and V. D. Foltz. 1958. Flocculation tests for pullorum disease. *Am. J. Vet. Res.* 19:478–82.

Runnells, R. A. 1929. Bacillary white diarrhea. Pullorum infection of the domestic fowl. *Virginia Agr. Exp. Sta. Bull.* 265.

Runnells, R. A., and H. Van Roekel. 1927. Further observations on the occurrence of white diarrhea infection in eggs laid by hens reacting to the agglutination test. *Poultry Sci.* 6:229–32.

Runnells, R. A., C. J. Coon, H. Farley, and F. Thorp. 1927. An application of the rapid-method agglutination test to the diagnosis of bacillary white diarrhea infection. *J. Am. Vet. Med. Ass.* 70:660–62.

Sapre, V. A., and M. L. Mehta. 1967. Indirect hemagglutination test for the diagnosis of salmonellosis in poultry. *Indian Vet. J.* 44:647–52.

Sarkisov, A. Kh., and E. T. Trishkina. 1966. Antibiotic sensitivity of *Salmonella pullorum* isolated from chicks on farms where antibiotics have been used over a long period. *Tr. Vses. Inst. Eksperim. Vet.* 32:224–30.

Sato, G. 1967. Response of wild rats (*Rattus norvegicus*) bred in captivity to oral inoculation with *Salmonella pullorum, Sal-*

monella newington, and *Salmonella enteritidis. J. Infect. Diseases* 117:71–81.

Schaffer, J. M., A. D. MacDonald, W. J. Hall, and H. Bunyea. 1931. A stained antigen for the rapid whole blood test for pullorum disease. *J. Am. Vet. Med. Ass.* 79:236–40.

Schiavo, A., and E. Biondi. 1966. Action of colimycin (colistin) on *Salmonella pullorum.* II. Studies on chick embryos. *Zooprofilassi* 21:69–79.

Schoenhard, D. E., and H. J. Stafseth. 1953. Growth curves of *Salmonella pullorum* in different media. *J. Bacteriol.* 65:69–74.

Scholes, J. C. 1942. Experiments with X-rays on the roles of lymphocytes and body temperatures in the resistance of chicks to *Salmonella pullorum. Poultry Sci.* 21:561–65.

Scholes, J. C., and F. B. Hutt. 1942. The relationship between body temperature and genetic resistance to *Salmonella pullorum* in the fowl. *Cornell Univ. Agr. Exp. Sta. Mem.* 244.

Severens, J. M., E. Roberts, and L. E. Card. 1944. A study of the defense mechanism involved in hereditary resistance to pullorum disease of the domestic fowl. *J. Infect. Diseases* 75:33–46.

———. 1945. The effect of sulfonamides in reducing mortality from pullorum disease in the domestic fowl. *Poultry Sci.* 24:155–58.

Smith, H. W. 1954. The treatment of *Salmonella pullorum* infection in chicks with furazolidone, sulphamerazine, and chloramphenicol. *Vet. Record* 66:493–96.

Snoeyenbos, G. H., A. M. Crotty, and H. Van Roekel. 1950. Some antigenic characteristics of *Salmonella pullorum. Am. J. Vet. Res.* 11:221–25.

Snoeyenbos, G. H., B. A. Bachman, and H. Van Roekel. 1952. A survey of the incidence of antigenic forms of *Salmonella pullorum* in the United States. *Poultry Sci.* 31:1009–16.

Stokes, J. L., and H. G. Bayne. 1957. Growth rates of Salmonella colonies. *J. Bacteriol.* 74:200–206.

———. 1961. Oxidative assimilation of amino acids by salmonellae in relation to growth rates. *J. Bacteriol.* 81:118–25.

Stokes, J. L., W. W. Osborne, and H. G. Bayne. 1956. Penetration and growth of salmonella in shell eggs. *Food Res.* 21:510–18.

Suganuma, Y. 1960. Histopathological studies on serositis of pullorum disease. *Japan. J. Vet. Sci.* 22:175–82.

Tittsler, R. P. 1930. The sterilization of eggs infected with *Salmonella pullorum. Poultry Sci.* 9:107–10.

———. 1932. Pullorum disease in poults. *Poultry Sci.* 11:78–80.

Trabulsi, L. R., and P. R. Edwards. 1962. The differentiation of *Salmonella pullorum* and *Salmonella gallinarum* by biochemical methods. *Cornell Vet.* 52:563–69.

Tsubokura, M. 1965. Studies of *Salmonella pullorum* phage. I. Isolation of phages and their properties. *Japan. J. Vet. Sci.* 27:179–88.

———. 1966. Studies on *Salmonella pullorum* phage. V. Conversion of subtypes of *S. pullorum* by phage. *Japan. J. Vet. Sci.* 28:35–40.

Tucker, J. F. 1967. Survival of salmonellae in built-up litter for housing of rearing and laying fowls. *Brit. Vet. J.* 123:92–103.

Ungureanu, C., and A. Grecianu. 1963. Improvement of antigen for the rapid haemagglutination test for pullorum disease. *Lucrarile Inst. Patol. Igiena Anim.,* Bucuresti 12:315–22.

Van Roekel, H. 1931. Eleventh annual report on eradication of pullorum disease in Massachusetts. *Mass. Agr. Exp. Sta. Control Ser. Bull.* 58.

———. 1935. A study of variation of *Salmonella pullorum. Mass. Agr. Exp. Sta. Bull.* 319.

———. 1964. Is eradication of pullorum disease realistic? *J. Am. Vet. Med. Ass.* 144:19–23.

Van Roekel, H., K. L. Bullis, O. S. Flint, and M. K. Clarke. 1932. Twelfth annual report on eradication of pullorum disease in Massachusetts. *Mass. Agr. Exp. Sta. Control Ser. Bull.* 63.

———. 1935. Fifteenth annual report on eradication of pullorum disease in Massachusetts. *Mass. Agr. Exp. Sta. Control Ser. Bull.* 78.

———. 1937. Maltose-fermenting *S. pullorum* strains. *Mass. Agr. Exp. Sta., Ann. Rept. Bull.* 339.

———. 1941. Poultry disease control service. *Mass. Agr. Exp. Sta. Ann. Rept. Bull.* 378:103–7.

Van Roekel, H., K. L. Bullis, and G. H. Snoeyenbos. 1947. Twenty-seventh annual report of pullorum disease eradication in Massachusetts. *Mass. Agr. Exp. Sta. Control Ser. Bull.* 134.

Villani, S. 1937. Sulla recettivita di alcune specie di volatili all'infezione sperimentale da *B. pullorum. Profilassi* 10:148–50.

Ward, A. R., and B. A. Gallagher. 1917. An intradermal test for *Bacterium pullorum* infection in fowls. *USDA Bull.* 517.

Weldin, J. C., and H. J. Weaver. 1930. Transmission of pullorum disease from chick to chick. *Poultry Sci.* 9:176–83.

Williams, J. E. 1951. Use of the spot test in the diagnosis of pullorum disease. *Poultry Sci.* 30:125–31.

———. 1953a. Antigenic studies using ammonium sulfate. I. The relative sedimentation effect of ammonium sulfate on the various antigenic types of *Salmonella pullorum. Am. J. Vet. Res.* 14:458–64.

———. 1953b. Antigenic studies using ammonium sulfate. II. The macroscopic ammonium sulfate sedimentation test for distinguishing the antigenic forms of *Salmonella pullorum. Am. J. Vet. Res.* 14:465–70.

Williams, J. E., and M. E. Harris. 1956. Antigenic studies using ammonium sulfate. IV. The sedimentation effect of ammonium sulfate on *Salmonella gallinarum. Am. J. Vet. Res.* 17:535–37.

Williams, J. E., and A. D. MacDonald. 1955. The past, present and future of salmonella antigens for poultry. *Proc. Book, Am. Vet. Med. Ass.,* pp. 333–39.

Williams, J. E., B. S. Pomeroy, R. Fenstermacher, and A. Holland. 1949. The incidence of variant pullorum in Minnesota. *Cornell Vet.* 39:129–35.

Williams, J. E., L. H. Dillard, and Gaye O. Hall. 1968. The penetration patterns of *Salmonella typhimurium* through the outer structures of chicken eggs. *Avian Diseases* 12:445–66.

Wilson, J. E. 1955. The use of furazolidone in the treatment of infections of day-old chicks with *S. pullorum, S. gallinarum, S. typhimurium* and *S. thompson. Vet. Record* 67:849–53.

———. 1956. The treatment of carriers of *Salmonella pullorum* and *Salmonella gallinarum* with furizolidone. *Vet. Record* 68:748–51.

———. 1967. Pullorum disease in Scotland 1926–1966. *Brit. Vet. J.* 123:139–44.

Winter, A. R., G. F. Stewart, V. H. McFarlane, and M. Solowey. 1946. Pasteurization of liquid egg products. III. Destruction of salmonella in liquid whole eggs. *Am. J. Public Health* 36:451–59.

Winter, A. R., Blanche Burkhart, and H. Widley. 1952. Further studies on the whole blood and tube methods of testing turkeys for *Salmonella pullorum* infection. *Poultry Sci.* 31:399–404.

Younie, A. R. 1941. Fowl infection like pullorum disease. *Can. J. Comp. Med. Vet. Sci.* 5:164–67.

❖

FOWL TYPHOID

❖

B. S. POMEROY

Department of Veterinary Bacteriology and Public Health College of Veterinary Medicine St. Paul, Minnesota

❖

FOWL TYPHOID is a septicemic disease of domesticated birds. The course may be acute or chronic. The mortality may be moderate or very high, depending largely on the virulence of the inciting organism *Salmonella gallinarum*. It appears to be primarily a disease of chickens and turkeys, but in exceptional cases ducks, pheasants, peacocks, guineas, and a few other birds are attacked.

Grateful acknowledgement is made to Dr. W. J. Hall for providing the groundwork for this section.

Synonyms are infectious leukemia (Moore, 1895) and fowl typhoid (Curtice, 1902).

In 1966–67 the number of reported outbreaks of fowl typhoid in the United States was approximately 23 in chickens and 3 in turkeys, scattered over 12 states. At the present time (1969) fowl typhoid is not a reportable disease in 12 states. However, in 1967–68 there were 15 reported outbreaks in chickens and 3 in turkeys. The dramatic drop in outbreaks of fowl typhoid is related to the pullorum-typhoid control program. When the control of fowl typhoid was included in the National Plans programs in 1954 it resulted in the treatment of fowl typhoid in the same category as pullorum disease. It is estimated that the cost of the present pullorum-typhoid testing program exceeds $5 million annually in addition to administrative costs of state and federal supervision of these programs. Today fowl typhoid shares the economic cost of the pullorum-typhoid control program (B. S. Pomeroy, 1969, unpublished).

Salmonella gallinarum is rarely isolated from man and has little public health significance (Lerche, 1939; Cloud, 1943; Popp, 1947). The 1967 and 1968 annual reports of the National Communicable Disease Center reported no isolations of *S. gallina-*

rum from man (*Salmonella Surveillance,* 1967, 1968).

HISTORY

In 1888 a chicken breeder in England lost 400 chickens as a result of an infectious disease which was at first considered to be fowl cholera. Two hundred of these birds died in the first 2 months of the outbreak. Specimens were sent to Klein (1889) for necropsy and diagnosis. He reported it chiefly as an infectious enteritis. The intestinal mucosa and serosa were inflamed, and the feces appeared thin and greenish yellow. The spleen was enlarged 2–3 times; the liver was also somewhat enlarged, soft, flabby, and moist. The cause was an organism which he named *Bacillus gallinarum*. The same year he reported the disease among grouse, and in 1893 a similar disease among pheasants. The disease was investigated by Smith in Rhode Island in 1894 and more fully by Moore in Virginia and Maryland in 1895. Moore (1895) described the disease as "infectious leukemia" and named the organism *Bacillus sanguinarium*.

Klein observed small numbers of bacilli in the blood. They were nonmotile, gram-negative, and easily cultivated. Chickens inoculated subcutaneously became sick in 5–6 days and died 2–3 days later. A similar disease was described by Lucet (1891) in France. Lignières and Zabala (1905) described a disease which was probably identical with Klein's disease. The catarrhal enteritis and the swollen spleen attracted attention; gram-negative bacilli were observed in the blood. They were different from those described by Klein in that they first coagulated and later peptonized milk with an alkaline reaction.

Curtice (1902) studied the disease in Rhode Island and named it "fowl typhoid." The disease has been found in Germany, Hungary, Austria, France, Holland, and North and South America, as well as in Algiers. In Germany it was observed by Pfeiler and Rehse (1913). Van Straaten and Te Hennepe (1919) in Holland described the disease very fully.

On the basis of the postmortem observation, Klein believed that it was not cholera but a special disease. His suspicion was soon confirmed, because he ascertained that the newly discovered organism was different morphologically and biologically from that of fowl cholera.

INCIDENCE AND DISTRIBUTION

Fowl typhoid is worldwide in distribution. Some countries report complete absence to low sporadic incidence while others indicate the disease is widespread (Bigland, 1954; Coles, 1946; Glover and Henderson, 1946; Anon., 1967).

In a nationwide survey, Moore (1946b) found fowl typhoid to be widely distributed in the United States. During the period of 1939–46 there was a dramatic increase in the number of outbreaks of fowl typhoid in chickens and turkeys in 19 states, resulting in a disease of considerable economic importance; Delaware reported over 250 outbreaks in 1946 as compared to fewer than 25 outbreaks reported yearly prior to 1939. It was considered one of the greatest disease hazards to the poultry industry along the eastern seaboard.

ETIOLOGY

CLASSIFICATION

The causative agent of fowl typhoid belongs to the genus *Salmonella* within the family Enterobacteriaceae. It has received the following names: *B. gallinarum, B. sanguinarium, B. typhi gallinarum alacalifaciens, B. paradysenteriae gallinarum, Eberthella sanguinaria, Shigella gallinarum, Salmonella gallinarum,* and *S. enteritidis* serotype Gallinarum.

MORPHOLOGY AND STAINING

The organism is a relatively short, plump rod about $1.0–2.0\mu$ long and 1.5μ in diameter. The bacilli mostly occur singly but are occasionally united in pairs. They have a tendency to stain a little heavier at the poles than in the center. They are gram-negative, form no spores, have no capsules, and are nonmotile.

GROWTH REQUIREMENTS

Salmonella gallinarum grows readily on beef extract or infusion agar or in tryptose broth and other nutrient media adjusted to pH 7.2. It is aerobic, facultatively anaerobic, and grows best at 37° C. The organism will grow in selective enrichment media such as Selenite F and tetrathionate broths and on differential plating media such as MacConkey, bismuth sulfite, Salmonella-

Shigella, desoxycholate, desoxycholate citrate lactose sucrose, and brilliant green agars.

COLONIAL MORPHOLOGY

On meat extract or infusion agar (pH 7.0–7.2) the colony of the organism is small, blue-gray, moist, circular, and entire. Gelatin colonies are small, grayish white, entire. Gelatin stab growth has a slight, grayish white surface with filiform growth in the stab and no liquefaction. Growth in broth is turbid with heavy flocculent sediment.

BIOCHEMICAL PROPERTIES

Over the years there have been numerous studies comparing fermentation reactions of isolates of *S. pullorum* and *S. gallinarum*. (See Pullorum Disease). The following substances are usually metabolized with acid and without gas production: arabinose, dextrose, galactose, mannitol, mannose, rhamnose, xylose, fructose, maltose, dulcitol, and isodulcitol. Substances not fermented are lactose, sucrose, glycerol, salicin, and sorbitol. Ornithine is not decarboxylated and D-tartrate is utilized. Cysteine hydrochloride gelatin supports the growth of *S. gallinarum*. These media are helpful in differentiating *S. pullorum* and *S. gallinarum*. Indole is not formed and nitrates are reduced to nitrites.

RESISTANCE TO CHEMICAL AND PHYSICAL AGENTS

In general the resistance of this organism is about the same as that of the other members of the typhoid and paratyphoid groups.

The fowl typhoid organism is killed within 10 minutes at 60° C. It remains viable in the dark for 20 days in ordinary and in distilled water but dies in 24 hours when exposed to sunlight. When dried on glass plates and kept in the dark, the organism retains its viability for 89 hours; under the action of direct sunlight it is killed in a few minutes. The organism is killed by phenol in a 1:1,000 dilution, by bichloride of mercury in a 1:20,000 dilution, by 1% potassium permanganate in 3 minutes, and 2% formalin in 1 minute. Agar cultures rapidly lose their pathogenic character, although they retain their antigenic properties for some time. According to Altara, *S. gallinarum* in the virulent state can be demonstrated in the bone marrow of carcasses three months after chickens have died of fowl typhoid. No doubt under certain conditions it lives for much longer periods. Kaupp and Dearstyne (1924a) reported that although direct sunlight destroyed the organism in a short time, it remained viable for 20 days when stored in water in the dark.

In Moore's (1946b) national survey of fowl typhoid, 75% of the states reporting were uncertain as to the persistence of the organism in the soil, and 25% claimed that it persisted from year to year.

In the experiments of Hall et al. (1949a) there was little danger of starting an outbreak in susceptible birds when such birds were put into a fowl typhoid-contaminated pen one week or more after removal of all sick birds. It was evident that the causative organism did not survive long after leaving the bird's body.

The resistance of this organism to the action of bacteriophage is of some interest. D'Herelle (1919, 1922) examined the excreta of fowls and tested the bacteriophage for virulence against eight strains of bacteria. Bacteriophage activity was demonstrated from all excreta studied; some samples showed marked activity for all cultures used. This investigator claimed that his experiments with bacteriophage confirmed his conclusion that the immunity to an infection is assured at a time when the body contains a bacteriophage virulent for that organism. Mallmann (1931) criticizes these observations because of lack of controls. It was found that the bacteriophage from one organism was easily adapted to another by use of mixed cultures. Bacteriophage was of no value in treating chicks either naturally or artificially infected. Munné (1937) obtained several cultures of *S. gallinarum* and *S. pullorum,* all of which were equally susceptible to the action of bacteriophage.

In two experimental and one natural outbreaks of fowl typhoid, Hall et al. (1949b) saw no benefit from the administration of bacteriophage either in the drinking water in the experimental outbreak or by subcutaneous injection in the natural outbreak.

Orr and Moore (1953) tested *S. gallinarum* for longevity under various conditions. In cloth in the dark at room temperature the organisms remained alive for 228 days. On plastic cover slips some *S. gallinarum* organisms were viable up to 93 days. Organisms in distilled water in diffused light at room temperature were viable up to the time the water evaporated—88 days. *S. gallinarum* retained viability up to 43 days when subjected to daily freezing and thawing. A liver naturally infected with *S. gallinarum* was divided, one-half being kept at 7° C and the other half at −20° C. The organisms in the liver kept at 7° C survived two weeks, while those in the portion of liver kept at −20° C were still alive at 148 days, even though they were twice accidentally thawed.

Smith (1955a) found that the average survival time of *S. gallinarum* in feces from infected chickens was 10.9 days when kept in a range house and 2 days less in the open. Survival time was longer in naturally dried specimens than in those kept moist.

Tucker (1967) found that *S. gallinarum* persisted in built-up litter from 3 weeks in old litter to 11 weeks in new litter. When the infected pens were left unoccupied, the survival time in both types of litter was increased to more than 30 weeks.

ANTIGENIC STRUCTURE AND TOXINS

Salmonella gallinarum possesses the O antigens 1, 9, 12. There does not appear to be form variation involving 12 antigen as in *S. pullorum* (Edwards et al., 1948; Williams and Harris, 1956; Blaxland et al., 1956; Bassiouni et al., 1966; Kosters and Geissler, 1966; see Pullorum Disease).

Smith and Ten Broeck (1915) found a toxin in the filtrates of broth cultures of *S. gallinarum*. It appeared in the culture at the end of 2 days at 37° C and caused prompt death of a rabbit by the intravenous route. Death resulted within 2 hours and in many respects was like an anaphylactic shock. It was probably an endotoxin which was stable at 60° C for one hour. Boiling for 15 minutes reduced its activity.

PATHOGENICITY

The pathogenicity of fowl typhoid cultures has proved decidedly variable in the hands of different investigators, probably because they used cultures varying widely in virulence. Like most pathogenic microorganisms, *S. gallinarum* loses virulence rapidly on artificial media. Hence cultures of *S. gallinarum* should be passaged serially in their natural host, the chicken, before testing the pathogenicity of the organism. The pathogenicity of such cultures is best

maintained in the lyophilized or frozen state. With a uniformly pathogenic culture, most commonly used routes of exposure of chickens prove fatal. Kaupp and Dearstyne (1925) reported 16 deaths of 40 chickens artificially infected; 15 became visibly sick and 9 showed no symptoms. Similar results were reported at the Kansas station, whereas others report 20–90% loss.

Palmer and Baker (1928) studied six natural outbreaks of fowl typhoid on Delaware farms. Virulent strains from these outbreaks killed not over 33.3% of the test fowls, and the investigators concluded that 60–70% of fowls are naturally immune. Hall et al. (1948) found that feeding mash moistened with a broth culture of a stable virulent strain of *S. gallinarum* was an effective way of testing susceptibility to fowl typhoid. Of 20 groups of birds, aggregating 382, which were challenged by adding a broth culture of virulent strains of *S. gallinarum* to their mash, 367 (96%) died of fowl typhoid.

PATHOGENESIS AND EPIZOOTIOLOGY

NATURAL AND EXPERIMENTAL HOSTS

The disease was originally encountered in chickens and reported among grouse and pheasants (Klein, 1889). Natural outbreaks occur in chickens, turkeys, guinea fowl, peafowl, ducklings and game birds, quail, grouse, and pheasants. Lucet (1891) described what was probably an outbreak of the disease in turkeys but claimed that ducks, geese, and pigeons were not susceptible. Donatien et al. (1923) consider palmipeds to be refractory but found the turkey, guinea fowl, and peafowl among the susceptible species; ducks and geese were resistant. Pfeiler and Roepke (1917) mention the pheasant, turkey, and guinea fowl as susceptible in natural outbreaks, but that ducks, geese, and pigeons are not, although a duck which had been inoculated with a culture died a few days later. Kaupp and Dearstyne (1924b), Te Hennepe (1924), and Beck and Eber (1929) have observed the disease in ducks. Kaupp and Dearstyne (1925) state that turkeys are less susceptible than chickens, and that guineas, though slightly susceptible, yield to artificial inoculation. Fox (1923) isolated *B. sanguinarium* from an outbreak of disease among parrots in the Philadelphia Zoological Garden. Beck and Eber (1929) reported on the loss in ducklings 1–14 days old due to *B. gallinarum* infection. Truche (1923) found that pheasants, swans, grouse, sparrows, ring doves, and ostriches commonly became infected, but that the duck, goose, and turkey were more resistant. Johnson and Anderson (1933) reported outbreaks of the disease in ducklings, turkeys, and guinea fowl. The infection has been observed in wild birds, in quail, grouse, and pheasants. These birds are susceptible by feeding or injection of cultures. Te Hennepe (1939) stated that fowl typhoid had decreased in the Netherlands between 1929 and 1939 from a point at which it caused some 8% of the total deaths in adult birds to 0.7%. This was considered to be due to greater interest in poultry diseases and improved care of poultry. The disease was at one time one of the most important in Kansas. About 1935 it practically disappeared and is still quite uncommon. The reason for this is not known. El-Dine (1939) in Egypt stated that fowl typhoid was often mistaken for fowl cholera. He reported the disease mainly in chickens and turkeys, and stated that it had been reported in peacocks but had never been seen in pigeons, geese, or ducks. A vaccine was used to confer immunity.

The reports on the susceptibility of pigeons have been variable. Klein reported no success following subcutaneous injection of cultures. Lucet (1891) was unable to infect pigeons with 1.0-cc doses subcutaneously, while Moore (1895) killed pigeons within 8 days with 2.0 cc of a broth culture. Pfeiler and Roepke (1917) killed pigeons by injecting 1.0 cc of a 24-hour broth culture, but the heart blood of these birds would not cause infection in a second pigeon. Kaupp and Dearstyne (1924b) caused the pigeon to become sick on the 3rd or 4th day with recovery on the 15th day. Kraus (1918) produced death in a pigeon within 4 days by use of 1.0 ml of a 24-hour broth culture of the fowl typhoid organism. Te Hennepe and van Straaten (1921) claim that pigeons are not always susceptible to inoculation with these organisms. At the Animal Disease Station in 1946, four pigeons were killed in an average period of 4.5 days by intraperitoneal or intramuscular inoculation with 1.0 ml of a 5-hour broth culture of *S. gallinarum*.

Age of Host Commonly Infected

Although fowl typhoid frequently has been spoken of as a disease of adult birds, Beaudette (1925), Beach and Davis (1927), Martinaglia (1929), and Komarov (1932) reported the disease in young chicks. Moore (1946b), in a nationwide survey of fowl typhoid, reported that 11 states found the disease to be more common in birds under 6 months, 16 believed the disease to be more prevalent in older fowl, while 10 states reported that there was little difference in age susceptibility. Hall et al. (1949a) reported that in 25 hatches from typhoid reactors in their second year of lay, about every 4th hatch experienced a fowl typhoid outbreak, and losses up to 6 months of age amounted to 33.4% of the chicks hatched. Monthly distribution of mortality was as follows:

Month	Percent
1	25.6
2	13.5
3	24.9
4	19.2
5	13.8
6	2.7

As in pullorum disease, fowl typhoid losses often begin at hatching time; contrary to experience with pullorum disease, fowl typhoid losses continue through to laying age. In one experiment in which two lots of chicks were hatched from fowl typhoid reactors, 92.8% of the chicks hatched in one lot died within 16 days and in another lot 93.5% died within 11 days after hatching.

Epizootiologically there are a few peculiarities in regard to the disease. Van Heelsbergen (1929) states that according to his experience it is very difficult, in some cases at least, to infect chickens which come from a region to which fowl typhoid is indigenous. If chickens are imported from a part of the country where the disease is not known, infection is rather easy. It is suggested that the bacteriophage or acquired immunity is probably partly responsible.

St. John-Brooks and Rhodes (1923) found that strains of *S. gallinarum* produced lesions in young chicks indistinguishable from those associated with pullorum disease.

A relatively small number of avian species appear to be susceptible.

TRANSMISSION, CARRIERS, VECTORS

Like most other bacterial diseases, fowl typhoid is spread in several ways. Research on the transmission of fowl typhoid indicates that the infected bird, the reactor and carrier, is by far the most important means of perpetuating and spreading the disease. Such birds may infect not only their own generation but succeeding generations through egg transmission.

Evidence of egg transmission of *S. gallinarum* was reported by Beaudette (1925, 1930) and Beach and Davis (1927).

Nóbrega and Bueno (1942) cultured 1,465 fresh infertile eggs from 52 hens shown to be chronic carriers of fowl typhoid. These were reactors from three different flocks where severe outbreaks of fowl typhoid among chicks had been experienced. The incidence of *S. gallinarum* in the eggs from the three lots of fowls was 2.8, 0, and 1.73% respectively.

Moore (1946a) recovered *S. gallinarum* from 8.9% of 395 eggs cultured from a pen of 21 fowl typhoid reactors, some naturally and some artificially infected. He also conducted fowl typhoid transmission experiments with flies, turkey buzzards, and rats and also by mating and by air currents. No evidence was produced to indicate transmission of the disease by flies, by mating, or by air currents. Rats and turkey buzzards were found capable of transmitting fowl typhoid. Boney (1947) isolated *S. gallinarum* from one turkey egg of 374 cultured from a flock of pullorum reactors.

Gordeuk et al. (1949) found that fowl typhoid is transmitted from artificially infected birds to normal fowls by cohabitation. The mortality among normal birds was 60.9% in one group and 45.8% in another. In other exposure trials by contamination of feed or drinking water with a broth culture of *S. gallinarum* or with feces from fowl typhoid infected hens, mortality among normal pullets varied from 31.8% to 69.6% in four experiments with duplicate groups.

After culturing over 10,000 eggs from two flocks, one naturally infected and one artificially infected, Hall et al. (1949a) found that 50% of typhoid reactors laid infected eggs, and an average of 6% of all unhatched eggs were infected with *S. gallinarum*. That these infected eggs laid by typhoid carriers are highly virulent and may be the means of starting new outbreaks of fowl typhoid in laying flocks is indicated by six feeding trials in which 27 birds ranging in age from 8 weeks to 1 year were fed one or more infected eggs mixed in their mash, with death resulting in 21 in an average period of 10 days. These investigators also report that of 906 chicks hatched from these reactors 296, or 32.6%, died of the disease during the first 6 months with the heaviest loss in the first month.

Rao et al. (1952) recovered *S. gallinarum* from 13 of 36 (36%) eggs from a reactor flock.

Jordan (1956a) recovered, by a single swab, *S. gallinarum* from the fresh feces of 4 of 13 birds acutely ill of fowl typhoid. Single cloacal swabs were positive in 15 of 47 (93.6%). A total of 377 cloacal swabs were taken at intervals from 36 reactors which had recovered from fowl typhoid 3–18 months previously, but only one bird was positive for *S. gallinarum*.

Jordan (1956b) reported isolation of *S. gallinarum* from eggs laid by reactors to the rapid blood test:

From 3 of 23 eggs (13%) from 4 recovered birds.

From 13 of 274 eggs (4.75%) from 10 naturally recovered birds.

From none of 217 eggs from 4 birds, treated with Chloromycetin, that had recovered from fowl typhoid.

From 25 of 226 eggs (11%) from 2 recovered birds that received nitrofurazone.

Both *S. pullorum* and *S. gallinarum* were isolated from different eggs from one bird.

Attendants, feed dealers, chicken buyers, and visitors who travel from house to house and from farm to farm may carry the infection unless precautions are taken to disinfect footwear, hands, and clothing. Trucks, crates, and feed sacks are also important. Wild birds, animals, and flies may be important mechanical spreaders, especially if they have been feeding on carcasses of dead birds or on offal from packing plants or hatcheries.

INCUBATION PERIOD

Rao et al. (1952) reported *S. gallinarum* to be equally pathogenic to susceptible baby chicks and adults under natural conditions. The incubation period is 4–5 days, although this varies with the virulence of the organism, and the course of the disease is about 5 days. In a flock the losses from the disease may extend over a 2–3-week period with a tendency for recurrence.

SIGNS

Although the disease is encountered more frequently in growing and adult chickens and turkeys, it may be encountered in young chicks and poults resulting from egg transmission. The signs noted in young chicks and poults are quite similar to pullorum disease but are not specific for either disease.

Chicks and Poults

If birds are hatched from infected eggs, moribund and dead chicks may be seen on the hatching trays at the time the hatch is pulled. They show somnolence, poor growth, weakness, loss of appetite, and adherence of whitish material to the vent. Labored breathing or gasping may be noted as a result of involvement of the lungs.

Growing and Mature Fowl

CHICKENS. An acute outbreak in chickens may begin by a sudden drop in feed consumption with birds being droopy, ruffled, and having pale heads and shrunken combs. The bird's temperature may increase 2–5° within 2–3 days after exposure and remain high until a few hours before death. Death may occur within 4 days after exposure but usually in 5–10 days. In natural outbreaks the mortality in chicks as well as adults may vary from 10 to 50% or more. There may be intermittent recurrence of the disease (Hall et al., 1949a).

TURKEYS. In turkeys there may be increased thirst, loss of appetite, listlessness, tendency to separate from well birds, and green to greenish yellow diarrhea. The body temperature increases several degrees to as high as 112° F; before death it may drop to below normal. Losses may occur with no apparent previous clinical signs. The initial outbreak usually causes the heaviest mortality, followed by intermittent recurrence with the loss not as severe (Hinshaw, 1930).

MORBIDITY AND MORTALITY

Both morbidity and mortality may vary in chicken and turkey flocks. Hall et al. (1949a) reported, on extensive investigations of fowl typhoid in chickens, that the mortality varied from 10 to 50% or more, with the loss in two lots of chicks which

were hatched from fowl typhoid reactors of 92.8% within 16 days and 93.5% within 11 days. The seasonal incidence of fowl typhoid is coincidental with the period of most active egg production.

In turkeys losses may be as severe as in chickens. Hinshaw (1930) reported the average mortality in four outbreaks studied was 26.5%.

GROSS LESIONS

Chickens

In peracute cases little or no gross tissue changes are observed. In the more prolonged cases, however, marked changes begin to appear, the most common of which are swelling and redness of the liver, spleen, and kidneys. These lesions are frequently seen in young birds. In the subacute and chronic stages of the disease the greenish

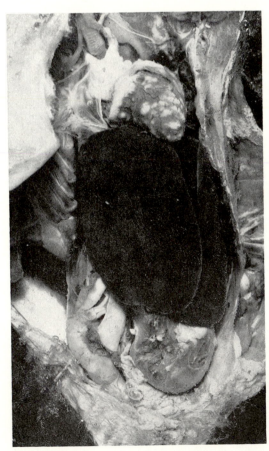

FIG. 3.16—Subacute fowl typhoid. Grayish white foci in myocardium and swollen "bronze" liver.

TABLE 3.6 ❧ Changes of the Blood with Fowl Typhoid

Date	Temperature (°C)	Number of Red Blood Corpuscles per cm	Number of White Blood Corpuscles per cm	Condition
Mar. 26	41.5	3,535,000	18,940	Healthy
Mar. 28	43.5	2,430,000	70,000	Chicken eats very little
Apr. 2	43.8	1,684,210	80,000	Blood very pale; chicken weak, refuses food
Apr. 3	41.3	1,745,000	245,000	Very weak, very many red blood corpuscles attacked by leukocytes
Apr. 4	...	...	...	Found dead

Source: Ward and Gallagher, 1920

brown or bronze and swollen livers are commonly seen. Other changes include grayish white foci of the miliary type in the liver and myocardium; pericarditis; peritonitis due to ruptured ova; hemorrhagic, misshapen, and discolored ova; and catarrhal inflammation of the intestines. In young chicks grayish white foci may sometimes be observed in the lungs, heart, and gizzard as in pullorum disease (Fig. 3.16).

In acute cases the blood picture is changed very little. If the disease lasts a few days, however, the changes mentioned in Table 3.6 are observed.

Gauger (1934) obtained the organism of fowl typhoid from focal lesions in the testicles of a rooster. The culture was pathogenic for other roosters by inoculation and feeding. Although various foci had been described, this was the first case described for focalization in the testicles.

Rao et al. (1952) reported the presence of a band of hemorrhage in the submucosa of the proventriculus, and cyanotic instead of anemic comb and wattles in the adult.

Smith (1955b) produced fowl typhoid in chickens by oral administration of *S. gallinarum*. Infection took place in the intestinal tract with localization in the intestinal wall, liver, and spleen. This was followed by a bacteremia and death or chronic disease with proliferative lesions in the intestinal and heart walls. Of 300 9-week-old cockerels, 45% died of the acute disease and 15% died in the chronic stage. *S. gallinarum* was shed in the feces up to 2–3 months after infection. This was associated with focal infection in the intestinal wall.

Turkeys

The lesions resemble those observed in chickens. Because of the short duration of this disease, the birds nearly always die while in good flesh. The muscles of the breast have a tendency to be congested and often appear as if partially cooked. The heart is usually swollen and contains small grayish necrotic areas or petechiae; in a few cases both have been observed. The liver is friable and is consistently enlarged two or three times its normal size; it is bronze- to mahogany-colored or covered with a mixture of bronze- and mahogany-colored streaks. Pinpoint areas of necrosis have been noted. On cutting the organ the blood flows readily. The spleen is always enlarged two or three times its normal size, is friable, and appears mottled. In most birds the lungs present a parboiled appearance and often are more firm than normal because of minute caseated abscesses. The kidneys are usually enlarged and may show some petechiae.

The crop usually contains food, which suggests paralysis of the digestive tract, since birds seldom eat after clinical signs appear. The mucous membrane of the proventriculus sloughs readily. The gizzard contains food, and the lining is easily removed. With a few exceptions the intestine appears anemic when viewed from the exterior, and ulcerations of the mucous membrane may be visible through the serosa. Ulceration is most severe in the duodenum; a few ulcers 1.0–4.0 mm in diameter have been observed throughout the intestine, extending to the ceca.

The enlarged mahogany- or bronze-streaked liver, the enlarged spleen, the area of necrosis in the heart, and the grayish lungs are pathognomonic. Hemorrhagic enteritis, especially of the duodenum, and marked ulceration of the intestine, although uncommon in chickens, are more or less consistent lesions in turkeys. *S. gallinarum* can readily be isolated from all organs. In birds that have been dead for some time, pure cultures are more easily isolated from the bone marrow than from the liver, spleen, and heart blood.

In young poults Johnson and Pollard (1940) described the following necropsy findings: (1) an increased percentage of large retained yolks, (2) slightly enlarged somewhat friable liver of a white creamy color, with the surface mottled with slight hemorrhagic areas, and (3) slight congestion in the anterior duodenum. The crops, gizzards, and intestines were always devoid of food, indicating lack of appetite for several hours before death. In adult carriers there is, as in the case of pullorum disease, a predilection for the reproductive organs.

Ducks

Beck and Eber (1929) recognized great loss from *S. gallinarum* infection among ducklings 1–14 days old. Maltose, dulcite, and dextrin were fermented with acid formation by the organism isolated. The disease picture was similar to the one observed in pullorum infection in chicks. The ducklings were sick only a short time. The anatomical changes were the following: hemorrhage in the pericardium, slight swelling of the spleen, catarrhal inflammation of the lungs and intestines. Small necrotic foci in the lungs, as frequently observed in chicks with pullorum disease, did not occur. In adult ducks the changes of the ovary and the yolk were frequently the same as those found in adult hens. Fowl typhoid organisms were isolated from the misshapen yolks.

Guinea Fowl

Beaudette (1938) states that the disease in the guinea is interesting because the affected birds show respiratory symptoms characterized by a severe congestion with collection of mucus in the nasal cleft and trachea. The lungs were congested, and the organism could be isolated from the nasal exudate.

HISTOPATHOLOGY

Dyakov (1966) reported finding in acute fowl typhoid a diffuse parenchymatous hepatitis and severe fatty dystrophy with occasional small necrotic foci in the parenchyma that was sometimes infiltrated with lymphocytes. The myocardium showed infarcts and large areas of fibrinoid necrosis

and sclerosis. Changes in the kidney, pancreas, intestine, and brain were similar to those in fowl cholera. There was severe hyperplasia of the reticuloendothelial system, particularly in the sinuses.

Garren and Barber (1955) studied the effect of fowl typhoid on the weight and histological changes in the pituitary, thyroid, adrenal, and bursae of Fabricius in New Hampshire (NH), Rhode Island Red (RIR), and White Leghorn (WL) young chickens. There were no statistically significant differences between the thyroid weights of the control and experimental groups. However, in the thyroid gland of the chicken dying of fowl typhoid the flat epithelium lining of the follicles showed decreased activity compared to cuboidal epithelium possessing the rounded nuclei characteristic of an active gland. Similar thyroid appearance was induced in the control group of chickens by restricting the feed and water intake to that of chickens infected with typhoid. In the infected chickens there was marked hypertrophy of interrenal tissue, the individual cells of interrenal tissue were larger, and the cytoplasm was less dense; only a small amount of medullary tissue remained. There was hypertrophy of the pituitary without consistent histological changes. The lymphatic follicles of the bursae were found in various stages of involution, suggesting a loss of cells from the follicles accompanied by a metaplasia of the cuboidal cells separating the medulla and cortex. Areas of cystlike formation were more numerous in infected birds than in the controls. The WL chickens used in the experiment survived the test period, whereas the mortality of NH chickens was 85% and RIR chickens 100%. The only pronounced changes in the tissues of the WL chickens were a decrease in the bursae weight and decrease in size of the follicles but no alterations.

IMMUNITY

Buxton and Allan (1963) conducted a series of experiments indicating that during early stages of fowl typhoid, circulating leukocytes develop a marked susceptibility to cytophilic antibodies in serum and later to bacterial polysaccharide. It was also shown that humoral antibodies, demonstrable by the antiglobulin hemagglutination test, have cytophilic properties. The results suggest that during acute infection, cellular antigen-antibody reactions occur which may result in development of a hypersensitive reaction.

Buxton and Davies (1963) used bacterial agglutination, hemagglutination, and antiglobulin hemagglutination tests to detect antibody production during the development of S. gallinarum infection in chickens. The antiglobulin hemagglutination test detected serum antibodies as early as 1 day after oral infection, and antibodies were detected in all birds at the time of death. The accumulation of bacterial polysaccharide in the tissues of infected birds was detected by a hemagglutination test. High but variable concentrations occurred in different organs of chickens which died from the disease. In birds that had recovered from an acute infection the concentration was low or undetectable. The authors postulated that an antigen-antibody reaction, developing as an anaphylactic type of hypersensitivity, may be closely associated with the production of symptoms and death of chickens infected with S. gallinarum.

Allan et al. (1968) found that following oral infection with live S. gallinarum organisms, serum collected on the 9th day and tested for the presence of hemagglutinating antibody (using erythrocytes modified with a Westphal lipopolysaccharide extract of S. gallinarum) had a high titer and on Sephadex fractionation and ultracentrifugal preparation showed a marked IgM response.

In some countries extensive efforts have been made to use immunizing agents to control fowl typhoid. In the United States efforts have been directed to control and eradicate fowl typhoid by the use of a testing program and elimination of infected carrier birds and use of clean flocks for breeding purposes.

Two areas have been extensively investigated to evaluate active immunity to fowl typhoid: (1) immunizing agents and (2) increasing resistance of the host.

Immunizing Agents

Various investigators have evaluated killed and modified live vaccines. McNutt (1926) experimented with various commercial vaccines and concluded that they had no value for the control of fowl typhoid. Wilson (1946) found that killed culture vaccines were ineffective in protecting against artificial exposure to S. gallinarum.

This was true of both autogenous and stock vaccines. However, when a dose of autogenous vaccine was followed by a dose of live culture, a solid and lasting immunity was produced.

Hall et al. (1949b) reported experiments on the use of various types of bacterial vaccines which were killed by different chemicals and with the exception of the crystal violet vaccines, were suspended in beeswax and peanut oil. The vaccines were administered by different routes and vaccinated birds were exposed 2–4 weeks later. No significant protection was observed.

Smith (1956) reported that a good protection was produced in chickens against oral infection by use of a smooth (9S) or rough (9R) attenuated vaccine. Killed vaccines had no effect. The immunity by the rough strain was limited to about 12 weeks, while that produced by the smooth strain was complete to at least 34 weeks. The 9R strain vaccine did not produce agglutinins, was nonlethal to day-old chicks, and did not cause a drop in egg production in laying hens. The 9S strain produced agglutinins, killed day-old chicks and caused marked drop in egg production.

Gordon et al. (1959) confirmed the efficiency of attenuated live vaccines in four breeds of chickens. Vaccination at 8 weeks of age produced better immunity than at 4 weeks of age. The 9S vaccine provided better immunity but interfered with the pullorum test.

Gordon and Luke (1959) confirmed the value of the 9R vaccine in the control of fowl typhoid in Northern Ireland. The vaccine strain was isolated 11 months after vaccination, and there was presumptive evidence that vaccination of adult birds may induce pathological changes in the ovary in some birds.

Harbourne (1957) conducted extensive field trials on 43 farms to assess the value of the two live attenuated vaccines. In 18 flocks where losses from fowl typhoid were slight, 0.9% of the deaths occurred in birds vaccinated with 9R, 0.4% in birds vaccinated with 9S, and 2.4% in unvaccinated controls. At 7 farms where losses from fowl typhoid were appreciable, 1% of the birds vaccinated with 9R, 1.7% vaccinated with 9S, and 11% of the unvaccinated birds died from fowl typhoid 14 days after start of the trial. At 2 farms the survivors were killed after blood testing. A smooth strain of S.

gallinarum was recovered from a high proportion of the birds in each of the three groups. In 5 flocks where fowl typhoid had previously been diagnosed, two-thirds of the birds of each flock received 9R vaccine and the remaining third was left unvaccinated. Significant losses from fowl typhoid occurred at 2 farms. At one of these farms vaccination apparently precipitated death. At the other, 5% of the vaccinated birds and 39% of the unvaccinated birds died from fowl typhoid.

Stoychev et al. (1963) found that both a killed vaccine prepared from a virulent *S. gallinarum* strain killed with 95% alcohol and a live vaccine from strain 9R produced good immunity under laboratory and field tests. The use of these vaccines in infected flocks in two injections at a 10-day interval markedly reduced the mortality in 15–20 days compared with unvaccinated controls.

Harbourne et al. (1963) reported that a freeze-dried 9R fowl typhoid vaccine was satisfactory under field conditions in reducing losses in infected flocks.

Increasing Resistance of the Host

Breeding and selection for resistant strains of birds may have value in control of the disease, but in the United States this approach has been secondary to a control and eradication program by testing and selection of clean breeding flocks. Lambert (1933) showed that selection for resistance to fowl typhoid in chickens resulted in a decided decrease in the mortality of selected stocks. Since *S. gallinarum* and *S. pullorum* are closely related organisms, it was decided to test fowl typhoid resistant stock for susceptibility to *S. pullorum* infection, and an *S. pullorum* stock for susceptibility to *S. gallinarum*. Results indicated that selection for resistance to one pathogen affords some protection to infection with one closely related. It was suggested that the resistance was to some extent due to nonspecific factors.

Garren and Hill (1959) made agglutinating antibody determinations for White Leghorns, Rhode Island Reds, and White Leghorn-Rhode Island Red crosses after inoculation with live and killed *S. gallinarum* cultures. White Leghorns consistently developed lower antibody titers than Rhode Island Reds whether induced by infection or by bacterin. Leghorn-Red crosses were intermediate between the two breeds in antibody titers but possessed almost the same marked resistance to fowl typhoid as observed for the Leghorn.

Prince and Garren (1966) found that resistance to *S. gallinarum* did not develop in some strains of WL chicks until they were 5–6 weeks of age. Extracts of pancreatic tissue plus a portion of the small intestine from WL chicks and extracts from RIR chicks were compared as to their activity against *S. gallinarum* and were found to have different levels of activity. A lysozyme was obtained from WL pancreatic-intestinal extracts which possessed the ability to inhibit *S. gallinarum*.

Prince (1967) reported there was depletion of the intestinal lysozyme after 4–5 days exposure to fowl typhoid in the RIR as compared to little depletion of lysozyme in the WL under similar conditions.

Freeman and Chubb (1964) found in fowl typhoid infected chickens the citric acid content of the blood rose but that of the liver fell significantly. The former may be due solely to anorexia; the latter, it was suggested, may be a result of the inhibition of the reaction between pyruvic and oxaloacetic acids. Pyruvic acid in the blood remained at its normal level, suggesting that other pathways for its metabolism were being utilized. A rise in the blood alpha-ketoglutaric acid concentration was also found.

Influence of Diet on Resistance

Various reports have suggested that diet may influence the resistance of chicks to fowl typhoid. Smith (1954) found that different infection rates were observed when different foods containing similar numbers of *S. gallinarum* were fed to chickens. The main reason for this was that certain properties of some of the foods had a profound influence on the bactericidal action of the gastric juice in the gizzard. One of these properties was physical consistency; another was the ability to maintain a relatively high pH in the gizzard. A diet of whole wheat only was especially effective in lowering the pH of the gastric juice with consequent destruction of *S. gallinarum* and a decrease in the infection rate. It is suggested that when a natural outbreak is diagnosed in a flock it would be worthwhile to alter the diet to whole wheat only until other methods of control can be instituted.

Hill and Garren (1955) demonstrated that high levels of all known required vitamins increase the resistance of chicks to fowl typhoid. The enhanced resistance observed when high levels of vitamins are fed is apparently not due to a uniform increase in requirements for all vitamins. Some vitamins must be increased over the requirement for growth many times more than others in order to bring about increased resistance to typhoid. In addition to the essential vitamins at high levels, an antioxidant is required in the diet in order to increase resistance of the chick to fowl typhoid. It was also found that it is possible to oversupplement the diet with vitamins insofar as obtaining maximum resistance to oral inoculation of the Salmonella organism. The exact mechanism of all the phenomena observed in these studies is not known.

Hill and Garren (1958) showed that the plasma ascorbic acid levels of chicks with fowl typhoid were reduced. Supplementation of the diet with 0.1% ascorbic acid resulted in an increased plasma ascorbic acid level at all times throughout the experimental period.

From the 6th to the 9th day, the period of heaviest mortality, the plasma ascorbic acid level of the basal-fed group was unchanged, while that of the supplemented group increased significantly. During this time, 20% of the basal-fed group died, while only 11.2% of the supplemented group died. This difference was statistically significant ($X^2 = 4.620$, P .05).

Chubb et al. (1958), testing the effect of feeding high levels of vitamins on the susceptibility of three breeds of chickens to experimental *S. gallinarum* infection, found that the administration of high levels of all the required vitamins in the diet for 4 weeks prior to infection or at infection had no effect on the average survival time or total mortality in 8-week-old Rhode Island Red or Brown Leghorn chickens. Neither did separation of these vitamins into the fat-soluble or water-soluble groups and their administration in the diet of high levels for 4 weeks prior to infection have any effect on the average survival time or total mortality in these two breeds.

With White Leghorn chickens infected with *S. gallinarum* a great variation in response to the high-level feeding of vitamins was encountered. Some results would suggest that the feeding of high levels of vitamins for 4 weeks prior to infection may increase the susceptibility of this breed to *S. gallinarum,* and this may possibly be associated with the fat-soluble group (A, D, E, and K).

Smith and Chubb (1957) found that the protein level of the diet affected the mortality rate of chickens infected with *S. gallinarum.* A simple diet of ground wheat plus 2.5% fish meal gave the highest resistance to *S. gallinarum* infection. A much higher or lower level of fish meal had an adverse effect on resistance to infection.

Starvation for 48 hours increased the severity of the disease.

Hill and Garren (1961) found that increasing the protein level of diets from 10% to 20–30% resulted in a progressively increased rate of mortality of chicks from *S. gallinarum* infection. The rate of mortality was not affected by the energy content of the diet. The acceleration of mortality was evident whether the protein was supplied by soybean meal or casein. Since the acceleration was noted when the organism was given either orally or intramuscularly, it was concluded that the effect of the increased protein level did not depend on a meeting of pathogen and diet in the intestinal tract. While total mortality was generally increased with increasing protein levels, the differences were not statistically significant in most of the comparisons.

Hill (1965) reported that chicks fed a copper-deficient diet were less susceptible to fowl typhoid. Hill (1966) found that varying levels of arginine and methionine ranging from deficiency to adequacy did not significantly affect the mortality of *S. gallinarum* infection.

DIAGNOSIS

A definitive diagnosis of fowl typhoid requires isolation and identification of *S. gallinarum.* The flock history, signs, and lesions may be highly suggestive of fowl typhoid. In growing and mature birds serological findings may be helpful in making a tentative diagnosis.

ISOLATION OF *S. gallinarum*

Acute Infection

Acute fowl typhoid is characterized by a systemic infection. *S. gallinarum* may be isolated from most of the visceral organs. The liver and spleen are usually involved and are preferred organs to culture. Lesions may occur in the lungs, heart, and gizzard, and these organs are dependable sites to culture. In the young chick and poult the yolk sac may be cultured. A bacteriological inoculating loop or cotton swab is satisfactory to transfer to culture media.

Beef extract or infusion or tryptose agar in tubes or petri dishes is satisfactory for primary isolation. Enrichment broths or selective media may also be used if the tissues are decomposed.

Chronic Infections

Chronic fowl typhoid is characterized by localized infection, and the infected organs may not show gross lesions. If a bird is submitted to the laboratory as a carrier as detected by serologic tests, detailed culturing of the internal organs is necessary. An outline for this examination is given in the section on Pullorum Disease.

IDENTIFICATION OF CULTURE

Salmonella gallinarum may be identified by bacteriological and serological methods. If pure cultures are obtained on primary isolation from tissues, special media may be inoculated. If the cultures are mixed, then single colony isolations may be made on triple sugar iron agar slants. *S. gallinarum* produces a red slant with a yellow butt with gas production and delayed blackening from H_2S production.

The following reactions occurring within 24 hours allow identification:

DEXTROSE	Fermented with no gas
LACTOSE	Not fermented
SUCROSE	Not fermented
MANNITOL	Fermented with no gas
MALTOSE	Fermented with no gas
DULCITOL	Fermented with no gas
ORNITHINE	Not fermented
INDOLE	Not produced
UREA	Not hydrolyzed
MOTILITY	Nonmotile
AGGLUTINATION ..	Positive with Group D antiserum

Additional differential tests are described under Etiology.

DIFFERENTIAL DIAGNOSIS

In young chicks and poults the signs and lesions produced by pullorum disease and fowl typhoid are quite similar but are different from other salmonella and the arizona infections. Aspergillus or other molds produce abscesses in the lungs but the lesions are more descrete than in fowl typhoid. Rarely *S. gallinarum* may localize in the joints and tendon sheaths which may be confused with other infections associated with synovitis.

In growing and mature chickens and turkeys other septicemic diseases may be confused with fowl typhoid such as fowl cholera, erysipelas, acute staphylococcosis, and acute colibacillosis. Blood or tissue smears stained with Gram's stain may be helpful in making a tentative differential diagnosis. Also the agglutination test may be helpful in chronic cases.

A final diagnosis of fowl typhoid can be made only by isolation and identification of *S. gallinarum*.

SEROLOGY

Several serological tests for fowl typhoid have been used under experimental and laboratory conditions. They are the bacterial agglutination, hemagglutination, and antiglobulin hemagglutination tests. The standard procedure in the United States for the detection of breeding flocks chronically infected with *S. gallinarum* is to use the standard strains of *S. pullorum* (1, 9, 12_3) for tube and serum plate antigens and both standard (1, 9, 12_3) and variant (1, 9, 12_2) strains of *S. pullorum* for the polyvalent rapid whole-blood plate antigens. These antigens will detect both *S. pullorum* and *S. gallinarum* infected flocks.

Numerous investigators in the development of control programs for fowl typhoid compared antigens prepared from various isolates of *S. gallinarum* with *S. pullorum* antigens with variable results (Moore, 1947; Hall et al., 1949b; Gwatkin and Dzenis, 1951; Lerche and Roots, 1958; Geissler, 1958; Molnar and Nagy, 1959; Kosters, 1965a,b,c; Kosters and Geissler, 1966).

The techniques and procedures for the official testing of chicken and turkey breeding flocks and interpretations of the tests are described in detail in the 1969 revision of Miscellaneous Publication No. 739 by USDA (Anon., 1969). (See pullorum section of this chapter for details of the testing procedures and preparations of antigens.)

TREATMENT

Effective prophylactic and therapeutic drugs have been developed against fowl typhoid, and these drugs have a role in salvaging flocks infected with the disease. Every effort should be made to eradicate the disease in areas that are amenable to this approach.

SULFONAMIDES

Sulfonamide drugs have been tried by numerous investigators with conflicting results. Hammond (1945) reported effective control by use of sulfathiazole. Holtman and Fisher (1946) studied an outbreak in battery-raised chickens which had caused 20% loss in 3 days. The flock was then divided into two parts. Group 1 received the usual care—removal of sick birds and cleaning and disinfection of batteries with a cresol solution. Group 2 was given sodium sulfathiazole in the drinking water for one week. At the end of the week 80% of the birds in group 1 had died. Losses in group 2 had been reduced to 4% with no losses during the last 3 days. However, losses in this group reappeared within 5 days but were controlled by the use of the drug.

The next year Holtman and Fisher (1947) were successful in controlling natural outbreaks of fowl typhoid in broilers by the use of sodium sulfamerazine (0.2%) in the drinking water. There was a loss of 62% in the controls compared to 4% in the treated birds when the drug was administered for 5 consecutive days each month for 2 months.

Simms (1946) reported on the use of sulfamerazine, sulfadiazine, and sodium sulfathiazole in broiler plants. The drugs were fed in 0.5–1.0% in wet mash. None of these drugs was satisfactory for controlling a virulent outbreak of the disease. Mortality was greatly reduced while the drugs were being fed, particularly in the case of sulfamerazine, but on discontinuance of its use, mortality rose again to nearly its former level. The same results were obtained from the use of these drugs in breeding flocks.

Moore (1946c) reported that sulfamerazine was effective in reducing death losses from fowl typhoid, while sulfathalidine and sulfasuxidine were not effective. The mortality varied from 33.3 to 83.3% for these two drugs. However, the former was given 5 days after exposure while the latter was started at the time of exposure.

Alberts (1950) used 0.4% sulfamerazine-mash mixture or 0.2% sodium sulfamerazine in the drinking water during a 7-day course of treatment. This prevented losses during the 7-day period of treatment and for 2 days after. The intermittent use of sulfamerazine or sodium sulfamerazine over a 21-day period was more effective in minimizing losses than was continuous feeding of the drug for 7 days.

NITROFURANS

After completing two large experiments on the effect of treating turkeys suffering from fowl typhoid with furazolidone (NF-180), Boney (1954) reported this drug to be effective in reducing mortality due to fowl typhoid when fed at the rate of 2 pounds per ton of feed for 7–10 days, or until mortality stops. He also recommended the use of sanitary procedures after an outbreak.

Grumbles et al. (1954) found furazolidone added to the feed at levels of 0.0055–0.011 to be effective in preventing mortality associated with fowl typhoid (*S. gallinarum*) infection in turkeys. The higher level at 0.011% was found to be more effective in severely infected birds. No evidence of toxicity or unpalatability was encountered. Exposed and treated birds have been shown susceptible to reinfection and to be carriers of *S. gallinarum*.

Richey (1954) reported that mortality was controlled promptly in field outbreaks of fowl typhoid in one chicken and two turkey flocks after feeding furazolidone (NF-180). Smith (1955c) found furazolidone to be greatly superior to the sulfonamides in treatment of experimental fowl typhoid in day-old and 9-week-old chickens. This was thought to be due to the fact that furazolidone is bactericidal while the sulfonamides are bacteriostatic in low concentration. Penicillin was of no value in treatment.

Fecal excretion of *S. gallinarum* could be stopped by feeding furazolidone in the mash at a concentration of 0.04% for 10 days. Chickens treated with furazolidone early but not late in the course of the experimental disease developed little immunity. Furazolidone was of value in treatment of chronic carriers of infection. Furazolidone, when fed continuously to young chicks in a low concentration (0.02–0.04%), slightly depressed the growth rate but was not toxic.

Wilson (1955) found that furazolidone in a concentration of 0.02% in the mash controlled mortality from *S. gallinarum* infection but that mortality recurred after treatment ceased. At the 0.04% level complete protection was obtained. When treatment was delayed until losses developed from the disease, results were less satisfactory but mortality was greatly reduced. Treatment begun at the earliest possible moment with 0.04% of furazolidone and continued for 7–10 days, together with the practice of sanitary measures, is recommended.

Wilson (1956) concludes that the administration of furazolidone in the mash in the treatment of carriers will result in a proportion of birds being sterilized of Salmonella and ultimately becoming negative to the agglutination test. A larger percentage continue to harbor the organism, especially in distorted ova, and remain reactors. Treated birds usually cease laying Salmonella-containing eggs. Wilson further predicts that furazolidone may prove even more valuable in the prevention of salmonellosis in turkeys and ducks as direct egg transmission is common in these species.

Titkemeyer and Schmittle (1957) used various levels of six different drugs to determine their effects on the recovery of *S. gallinarum* from inoculated White Leghorn chicks. Representing the sulfa drugs, sulfaquinoxaline at levels of 0.05% and 0.0175% in the feed or at 0.025% in the water and sulfamethazine at the level of 0.1% in the water resulted in an incidence of recovery of 82.5% as compared to 100% in the inoculated controls. At "growth-promoting" levels, chlortetracycline at levels of 18 g and 108 g per ton and penicillin at 4 g per ton of feed did not result in a significantly lower rate of recovery of the organism. At therapeutic levels, chlortetracycline at 200 g per ton of feed resulted in 80% recovery of the organism. With chlortetracycline in water, with neomycin alone or in combination with chlortetracycline in feed, the organism was recovered

from 90% of the chicks as compared to 100% of the infected control. Furazolidone at the rate of 100 g per ton of feed reduced the incidence of recovery of the organism to only 10%. With oral inoculation of the organism, the results were less conclusive in that often the organism could not be recovered regardless of whether the chick was medicated. Furazolidone seemingly prevented recovery of the organism in all 30 orally inoculated chicks. Time of administration of the medicaments, whether 48 hours before, at time of, or 48 hours after, did not alter significantly the recoverability picture.

Dijkstra (1959) states that treatment of fowl typhoid with chemotherapeutics and antibiotics nearly always gives unsatisfactory results because clinically healthy animals may remain carriers for a long time. Furazolidone, which has a bactericidal effect and apparently distinguishes itself favorably from the other drugs, cannot as a rule cure an infected flock.

Richey and Morgan (1959) artificially infected turkeys 10 days old with approximately 10^6 *S. gallinarum* cells. While mortality in the untreated control group was 100%, death losses were prevented by feeding chloramphenicol at 0.22% or furazolidone at 0.011 or 0.022% in feed starting 5 days before inoculation and continuing for 17 days.

When treatment was begun at the time of infection and continued for 12 days, deaths occurred in all groups. When medication was started 4 days after inoculation and continued for 8 days, more birds treated with furazolidone than chloramphenicol survived. Chloramphenicol given at the rate of one 50-mg capsule daily for 3 days was of little value in preventing deaths when given either at the time of inoculation or at the appearance of illness 4 days later.

Agglutination tests were negative in only one of the survivors medicated with chloramphenicol, but were negative in many of the survivors medicated with furazolidone.

Bierer et al. (1961) in four experiments found that prophylactic furaltadone water medication at 0.25 g/gal resulted in a marked reduction in mortality in pullorum disease in chicks, fowl typhoid in chicks and poults, and *S. typhi-murium* infection in poults.

Therapeutic medication at 0.25 g/gal resulted in a reduction in mortality in all four trials. However, mortality reduction was marked on the 0.5 g/gal level in three of four trials, but erratic results were obtained in poults with *S. typhi-murium* therapeutic medication.

In general, average body weights of all medicated groups at 10 days compared favorably with uninfected unmedicated controls but were lower in the infected unmedicated groups.

Further evaluation of furaltadone water medication in more extensive floor pen trials under field conditions is indicated.

Hall and Cartrite (1961) investigated the resistance of some strains of *S. gallinarum* to furazolidone and concluded that fowl typhoid is still a problem of major importance in Texas turkeys and chickens. Three of the four Texas Poultry Disease Investigation Laboratories reported one or more outbreaks of fowl typhoid that failed to respond to furazolidone therapy. Four isolates of *S. gallinarum* from such outbreaks were studied in the laboratory. All were sensitive in vitro to furazolidone; however, one strain developed resistance when serial passages were made in the presence of the drug. The same strain displayed resistance to the activity of furazolidone in experimentally infected turkeys when the drug was supplied in the feed at a level of 0.011% (2 lb NF-180 per ton).

Richey (1962) inoculated day-old chicks with *S. pullorum* or *S. gallinarum*. Medication with either of two soluble nitrofurans (nitrofurazone and furaltadone) in drinking water, alone and supplemented with furazolidone-medicated feed, prevented and reduced early (10-day) and total (4-week) mortality in all but one group (infected with *S. pullorum* and treated with furaltadone).

S. gallinarum-infected chicks succumbed rapidly. However, medication with furaltadone decreased both the early and total mortalities considerably. Appropriate time of medication rather than drug used accounted for the lowest number of infected survivors yielding a positive agglutination test.

In most cases average weight of surviving *S. pullorum*-infected birds was higher than that of the birds infected with *S. gallinarum*.

Stuart et al. (1962) isolated a strain of *S. gallinarum* from young breeder chickens that was resistant to 0.022% furazolidone, 0.011% nihydrazone, and 0.15% 3,5-dinitrobenzamide.

Tucker (1963) evaluated 28 drugs against experimental *S. gallinarum* infections and found only furaltadone as effective as furazolidone. At 0.04% in the drinking water it controlled mortality and did not give rise to a higher carrier rate in survivors.

Freedman et al. (1965) found that nihydrazone as well as furazolidone was highly effective prophylactically and therapeutically in experimental *S. gallinarum* infections in day-old chicks.

Stuart et al. (1967) studied two strains of *S. gallinarum* which were isolated from the same chicken breeder flock 39 days apart. The first isolate was sensitive to 0.011% furazolidone while the second was resistant to at least 0.022% of the drug. The premises on which the flock was located had a history of fowl typhoid and use of furazolidone for its control going back nearly 4 years.

Nagy and Fabian (1968) studied the effect of preventive and therapeutic levels of furazolidone on the agglutination titers of 57 chickens experimentally infected with *S. gallinarum*. The decrease in the percentage of high titers as demonstrable by the tube agglutination test was somewhat more pronounced in the treated groups than in the control group, but agglutinins remained demonstrable in each of the groups.

ANTIBIOTICS

Jones et al. (1944) reported on the use of streptomycin to protect chicken embryos from the action of the fowl typhoid organism.

Glantz and Gordeuk (1955) report that in vitro and in vivo tests of sensitivity of *S. gallinarum* to antibiotics were similar. Chloromycetin, when administered per os at the rate of 200 mg per bird per day or 1–2 g per pound of mash, gave excellent protection when started on the day of infection. A relapse occurred when the chloromycetin mash was discontinued. Aureomycin mixed with mash at the rate of 1 g per pound reduced losses to 25% and no relapse occurred when treatment was discontinued. Polymixin B and Terracon 180 had little therapeutic value.

Gale et al. (1963) found in in vivo studies that *S. gallinarum* developed no increased resistance to chlortetracycline at any of three dose levels tested in 6-day-old cockerels in 7–11 experiments covering 21–33 weeks. Resistance to sulfaethoxypyridazine and to sulfaquinoxaline emerged at one dose level in each of three passage series when these drugs were given separately. When four different combinations of chlortetracycline and sulfaethoxypyridazine were fed over 21–33 weeks, no significantly observable resistance to either of the drugs in combination was evidenced in the birds.

PREVENTION AND CONTROL

Fowl typhoid is a good example of a disease that has decreased in incidence in the United States by the application of basic procedures involving control programs aimed at breeding flocks, judicious use of effective drugs in the control and treatment of outbreaks, and recognition of the importance of the environment as a source of reinfection.

Flocks can be developed and maintained free of fowl typhoid by following well-defined management programs. The inclusion of fowl typhoid in the National Plans programs in 1954 recognized the importance of egg transmission in the cycle of this infection. Under the National Plans (Anon., 1969) chicken and turkey breeding flocks and their progeny are recognized as free of pullorum disease and fowl typhoid. As in the case of pullorum disease, chickens and turkeys are the primary hosts of *S. gallinarum*, and free-flying birds and other fowl are not major reservoirs of the infection. Thus eradication of the disease from chicken and turkey breeding flocks will go a long way in total elimination of these diseases from commercial poultry flocks. In some areas contaminated poultry ranges and pond water provide excellent means of perpetuation of fowl typhoid.

MANAGEMENT PROCEDURES

Management practices should be broadly applied that will prevent the introduction of fowl typhoid as well as other infectious diseases into a poultry population.

1. Chicks and poults should be obtained from sources free of pullorum and typhoid.
2. Chicks and poults should be placed in an environment that can be cleaned and sanitized to eliminate any residual salmo-

nella organisms from previous flocks. (See section on Resistance to Chemical and Physical Agents.)

3. Introduction of salmonellae from outside sources must be minimized.
   a. Although *S. gallinarum* does not commonly contaminate animal, poultry, and marine by-products, other salmonellae are commonly encountered. Poultry feeds free of salmonellae are highly desirable.
   b. Free-flying birds are commonly found carriers of salmonellae but *S. gallinarum* is rarely encountered. Poultry houses should be bird proof.
   c. Rats, mice, rabbits, and other pests may be carriers of salmonellae but are rarely found infected with *S. gallinarum*. Nevertheless, poultry houses should be rodent proof.
   d. Insect control is important, particularly against flies, poultry mites, lesser mealworm. These pests may provide a means of survival of salmonellae and other avian pathogens in the environment.
   e. Other animals such as dogs and cats may be carriers of salmonellae but rarely *S. gallinarum*. These animals should be kept from the poultry house.
   f. Potable water must be used as a source of drinking water or chlorinated water should be provided. In some sections of the country surface water is collected in open ponds for use as drinking water for livestock and poultry.
   g. Man may be a mechanical carrier of the organism on his footwear and clothing as well as poultry equipment, processing trucks, and poultry crates. Every precaution should be made to prevent introduction of *S. gallinarum* by fomites.
   h. Proper dead bird disposal is essential. *S. gallinarum* will survive in poultry carcasses for weeks depending on the ambient temperatures (Van Es and Olney, 1940; Hall et al., 1949a; Botts et al., 1952; Tucker, 1967).

ERADICATION PROGRAM

Elimination of Carriers

The principles established for the identification and elimination of pullorum disease infected flocks under the National Poultry and Turkey Improvement Plans are applicable to fowl typhoid.

Essentials of an Eradication Program for an Area

1. Pullorum disease and fowl typhoid must be mandatory reportable diseases.
2. Outbreaks are placed under quarantine and infected flocks are marketed under supervision.
3. All reports of pullorum disease and fowl typhoid are investigated by an authorized state or federal official.
4. Importation regulation shall require shipments of poultry and hatching eggs to be from sources considered free of pullorum disease and fowl typhoid.
5. Regulation shall require poultry going to public exhibition to be from flocks free from pullorum disease and fowl typhoid.
6. Total participation of the poultry breeding flocks and hatcheries shall be required in a pullorum-typhoid control program such as National Plans programs or their equivalent.

IMMUNIZATION

In the United States *S. gallinarum* killed bacterins are no longer produced by biological manufacturers operating under federal license. Live modified vaccines as currently used in England and other countries are not permitted in the United States. An autogenous bacterin may be prepared for use on an infected farm by a federally licensed manufacturer. With less than 50 reported outbreaks (1968) of fowl typhoid in chickens and turkeys and other fowl in the entire United States, there is no justification for the use of live or killed *S. gallinarum* vaccines. Field outbreaks may be adequately controlled by use of a medication program with quarantine measures established to prevent further spread. Supervision of marketing of the infected flock in a federal or state poultry processing plant and cleaning and disinfecting of the premises and equipment are essential aspects of handling an infected flock in areas under an eradication program.

REFERENCES

Alberts, J. O. 1950. The prophylactic and therapeutic properties of sulfamerazine in fowl typhoid. *Am. J. Vet. Res.* 11:421–25.
Allan, D., W. P. H. Duffus, and D. A. Higgins. 1968. Measurement of antigen-antibody complexes in *Salmonella gallinarum* infection. *Immunology* 14:575–81.
Anonymous. 1967. *Animal Health Yearbook.* FAO, WHO, OIE. Columbia Univ. Press, Irvington on Hudson, N.Y.
Anonymous. 1969. *National Poultry and Turkey Improvement Plans and Auxiliary Provisions.* USDA, ARS, AHR Div., Beltsville, Md.
Bassiouni, A., M. Rifai, and K. Abbasi. 1966. The influence of the somatic factor O-1 on the agglutination reactions for detecting *Salmonella gallinarum-pullorum* infections. *Vet. Med. J.* Giza 12:369–76.
Beach, J. R., and D. E. Davis. 1927. Acute infection of chicks and chronic infection of the ovaries of hens caused by the fowl-typhoid organism. *Hilgardia* 2:411–24.
Beaudette, F. R. 1925. The possible transmission of fowl typhoid through the egg. *J. Am. Vet. Med. Ass.* 67:741–45.
———. 1930. Fowl typhoid and bacillary white diarrhea. *Proc. 11th Int. Vet. Congr.*, London 3:705–23.
———. 1938. An outbreak of fowl typhoid in guineas. *J. Am. Vet. Med. Ass.* 92:695–98.
Beck, A., and R. Eber. 1929. Die wichtigsten bakteriellen Kuckenerkrankungen. Ihre Diagnose, Differentialdiagnose und Bekampfung. *Z. Infektkr. Haustiere* 35:76–95.
Bierer, B. W., H. D. Valentine, and C. L. Vickers. 1961. Furaltadone water medication: Its use in avian salmonellosis. *Avian Diseases* 5:214–18.
Bigland, C. H. 1954. Fowl typhoid controls in Alberta. *Proc. Am. Vet. Med. Ass. 91st Ann. Meet.* pp. 340–45.
Blaxland, J. D., W. J. Sojka, and A. M. Smither. 1956. A study of *S. pullorum* and *S. gallinarum* strains isolated from field outbreaks of disease. *J. Comp. Pathol. Therap.* 66:270–77.
Boney, W. A., Jr. 1947. Isolation of *Shigella gallinarum* from turkey eggs. *Am. J. Vet. Res.* 8:133–35.
———. 1954. Fowl typhoid yields to new drug. *Turkey World* 29:40.
Botts, C. W., L. C. Ferguson, J. M. Birkeland, and A. R. Winter. 1952. The influence of

litter on the control of Salmonella infections in chicks. *Am. J. Vet. Res.* 13:562–65.

Buxton, A., and D. Allan. 1963. Studies on immunity and pathogenesis of salmonellosis. I. Antigen-antibody reactions on circulating leucocytes of chickens infected with *Salmonella gallinarum. Immunology* 6:520–29.

Buxton, A., and J. M. Davies. 1963. Studies on immunity and pathogenesis of salmonellosis. I. Antibody production and accumulation of bacterial polysaccharide in the tissues of chickens infected with *Salmonella gallinarum. Immunology* 6:530–38.

Chubb, L. G., R. F. Gordon, and J. F. Tucker. 1958. The effect of high levels of vitamins on the susceptibility of chickens to *Salmonella gallinarium* infection. *Brit. Vet. J.* 114:55–68.

Cloud, O. E. 1943. Perforation with peritonitis from *Shigella gallinarum* (var. Duisburg). *Med. Bull. Veterans' Administration* 19:335–36.

Coles, J. D. W. A. 1946. Fowl typhoid. *South African Poultry, Pigeon, and Bird Magazine* 52:199.

Curtice, C. 1902. Fowl typhoid. *Rhode Island Agr. Expt. Sta. Bull.* 87.

D'Herelle, F. 1919. Sur le role du microbe bacteriophage dans la typhose aviaire. *Compt. Rend. Acad. Sci.* 169:932–34.

———. 1922. *The Bacteriophage: Its Role in Immunity.* Williams & Wilkins Co., Baltimore.

Dijkstra, R. G. 1959. Fowl typhoid: A review. *Tijdschr. Diergeneesk.* 84:375–82.

Donatien, A., E. Plantureaux, and F. Lestoquard. 1923. La typhose aviaire en Algerie. *Ann. Inst. Pasteur d'Algerie* 1:585.

Dyakov, L. 1966. Pathology of acute fowl typhoid with reference to differential diagnosis. *Nauchni Tr. Visshiya Vet. Med. Inst.* 16:13–22.

Edwards, P. R., D. W. Bruner, E. R. Doll, and G. S. Hermann. 1948. Further notes on variation in *Salmonella pullorum. Cornell Vet.* 38:257–62.

El-Dine, H. S. 1939. Important diseases of poultry in Egypt and their control. *Proc. Seventh World's Poultry Congr.*, pp. 229–31.

Fox, H. 1923. *Diseases of Captive Wild Animals and Birds,* 1st ed. Lippincott Co., Philadelphia.

Freedman, R., C. Johnson, and J. O'Connor. 1965. Comparative activity of nihydrazone and furazolidone against *Salmonella gallinarum* and *Escherichia coli* in chickens. *Poultry Sci.* 44:561–64.

Freeman, B. M., and L. G. Chubb. 1964. Effect of *Salmonella gallinarum* on certain Krebs cycle intermediates of domestic fowl. *J. Bacteriol.* 88:93–95.

Gale, G. A., J. S. Kiser, and T. F. McNamera. 1963. Bacterial resistance to chemotherapy. I. Effect of continuous feeding of chlortetracycline, sulfaethoxypyridazine, sulfaquinoxaline, and chlortetracycline-sulfaquinoxaline, and chlortetracycline-sulfaethoxypyridazine combinations on the development of resistance by *Salmonella gallinarum* in chickens. *Avian Diseases* 7:457–66.

Garren, H. W., and C. W. Barber. 1955. Endocrine and lymphatic gland changes occurring in young chickens with fowl typhoid. *Poultry Sci.* 34:1250–58.

Garren, H. W., and C. H. Hill. 1959. Agglutinating antibody titers of young White Leghorns and Rhode Island Reds following inoculation with live and inactivated *Salmonella gallinarum* cultures. *Poultry Sci.* 38:918–22.

Gauger, H. C. 1934. A chronic carrier of fowl typhoid with testicular focalization. *J. Am. Vet. Med. Ass.* 84:248–51.

Geissler, Von H. 1958. Vergleiche der Agglutinations Ergebnisse verschieden hergestellter Antigene bei der Infektion mit *Sal. gallinarum-pullorum. Berlin. Muench. Tieraerztl. Wochschr.* 71:328–30.

Glantz, P. J., and S. Gordeuk, Jr. 1955. *In vitro* and *in vivo* sensitivity of the fowl typhoid organism, *S. gallinarum* to antibiotics. *Poultry Sci.* 34:880–90.

Glover, J. A., and W. Henderson. 1946. Fowl typhoid. Report on a recent outbreak in Ontario. *Can. J. Comp. Med. Vet. Sci.* 10:241–49.

Gordeuk, S., Jr., P. J. Glantz, E. W. Callenbach, and W. T. S. Thorp. 1949. Transmission of fowl typhoid. *Poultry Sci.* 28:385–91.

Gordon, R. F., J. S. Garside, and J. F. Tucker. 1959. The use of living attenuated vaccines in the control of fowl typhoid. *Vet. Record* 71:300–305.

Gordon, W. A. M., and D. Luke. 1959. A note on the use of 9R fowl typhoid vaccine in poultry breeding flocks. *Vet. Record* 71:926–27.

Grumbles, L. C., F. K. Wills, and W. A. Boney, Jr. 1954. Furazolidone in the treatment of fowl typhoid in turkeys. *J. Am. Vet. Med. Ass.* 124:217–19.

Gwatkin, R., and L. Dzenis. 1951. Fowl typhoid. I. Comparison of antigenicity of sixteen gallinarum antigens. *Can. J. Comp. Med. Vet. Sci.* 15:15–20.

Hall, C. J., and H. T. Cartrite. 1961. Observations on strains of *Salmonella gallinarum* apparently resistant to furazolidone. *Avian Diseases* 5:382–92.

Hall, W. J. 1946. *Fowl Typhoid.* USDA Circ. 755, pp. 1–9.

Hall, W. J., D. H. Legenhausen, and A. D. MacDonald. 1948. A summary of results of fowl typhoid investigations. *Proc. 20th Ann. Meet. Northeast Conf. Lab. Workers in Pullorum Disease Control.*

————. 1949a. Studies on fowl typhoid. I. Nature and dissemination. *Poultry Sci.* 28:344–62.

Hall, W. J., A. D. MacDonald, and D. H. Legenhausen. 1949b. Studies on fowl typhoid. II. Control of the disease. *Poultry Sci.* 28:789–801.

Hammond, J. C. 1945. Sulfonamides in the control of fowl typhoid. *Poultry Sci.* 24:382–84.

Harbourne, J. F. 1957. The control of fowl typhoid in the field by use of live vaccines. *Vet. Record* 69:1102–7.

Harbourne, J. F., B. M. Williams, and I. H. Fincham. 1963. The prevention of fowl typhoid in the field using a freeze-dried 9R vaccine. *Vet. Record* 75:858–61.

Hill, C. H. 1965. Effect of copper deficiency on mortality from fowl typhoid and RPL 12 tumor. *Federation Proc.* 24:442.

————. 1966. Amino acid deficiencies and reaction of chicks to *Salmonella gallinarum.* *Avian Diseases* 10:383–89.

Hill, C. H., and H. W. Garren. 1955. The effect of high levels of vitamins on the resistance of chicks to fowl typhoid. *Ann. N.Y. Acad. Sci.* 63:186–94.

————. 1958. Plasma ascorbic acid levels of chicks with fowl typhoid. *Poultry Sci.* 37:236–37.

————. 1961. Protein levels and survival time of chicks infected with *Salmonella gallinarum.* *J. Nutr.* 73:28–32.

Hinshaw, W. R. 1930. Fowl typhoid of turkeys. *Vet. Med.* 25:514–17.

Hinshaw, W. R., and T. J. Taylor. 1933. A chronic carrier of fowl typhoid of turkeys. *J. Am. Vet. Med. Ass.* 82:922–26.

Holtman, D. F., and G. Fisher. 1946. Some observations on the control of fowl typhoid infection with sulfa drugs. *J. Bacteriol.* 51:401.

————. 1947. The application of sulfonamides to the control of typhoid in poultry. *Poultry Sci.* 26:478–88.

Johnson, E. P., and G. W. Anderson. 1933. An outbreak of fowl typhoid in guinea fowls (*Numida meleagis*). *J. Am. Vet. Med. Ass.* 82:258–59.

Johnson, E. P., and M. Pollard. 1940. Fowl typhoid in turkey poults. *J. Am. Vet. Med. Ass.* 96:243–44.

Jones, D., H. J. Metzger, A. Schatz, and S. A. Waksman. 1944. Control of gram-negative bacteria in experimental animals by streptomycin. *Science* 100:103–5.

Jordan, F. T. W. 1956a. The occurrence of *S. gallinarum* in the feces in fowl typhoid. *Poultry Sci.* 35:1026–29.

————. 1956b. The transmission of *S. gallinarum* through the egg. *Poultry Sci.* 35:1019–25.

Kaupp, B. F., and R. S. Dearstyne. 1924a. Chronic carriers of fowl typhoid. *J. Am. Vet. Med. Ass.* 64:329–33.

————. 1924b. Fowl typhoid. A comparison of various European strains with those of North America. *Poultry Sci.* 3:119–27.

————. 1925. The differential diagnosis of fowl cholera and fowl typhoid. *J. Am. Vet. Med. Ass.* 67:249–59.

Klein, E. 1889. Ueber eine epidemische Krankheit der Huehner, verursacht durch einen Bacillus—*Bacillus gallinarum.* *Zentr. Bakteriol. Parasitenk. Abt. I. Orig.* 5:689–93.

Komarov, A. 1932. Fowl typhoid in baby chicks. *Vet. Record* 12:1455–57.

Kosters, J. 1965a. Antigenic structure and serological behaviour of *Salmonella gallinarum.* I. Distribution of individual antigens in various strains. *Berlin. Muench. Tieraerztl. Wochschr.* 78:211–13.

————. 1965b. Antigenic structure and serological behaviour of *Salmonella gallinarum.* II. Antibody formation against various *S. gallinarum* strains. *Berlin. Muench. Tieraerztl. Wochschr.* 78:290–91.

————. 1965c. Antigenic structure and serological behaviour of *Salmonella gallinarum.* III. Differentiation of non-specific agglutination reactions. *Berlin. Muench. Tieraerztl. Wochschr.* 78:314–15.

Kosters, J., and H. Geissler. 1966. The selection of *Salmonella gallinarum-pullorum* strains for production of a standardized agglutination antigen. *Berlin. Muench. Tieraerztl. Wochschr.* 79:276–78.

Kraus, E. J. 1918. Zur Kenntnis des Huehnertyphus. *Zentr. Bakteriol. Parasitenk. Abt. I. Orig.* 82:282–303.

Lambert, W. V. 1933. A preliminary study of the reaction of two disease resistant stocks of chickens after infection with their reciprocal pathogens. *Proc. Iowa Acad. Sci.* 40:231–34.

Lerche, Von M. 1939. Salmonellainfektionen beim Gefluegel und ihre Bedeutung fur die Epidemiologie der Salmonellabakterien. *Proc. Seventh World's Poultry Congr.,* pp. 274–78.

Lerche, Von M., and E. Roots. 1958. Herstellung des *Salmonella gallinarum*-Trockenantigens fur die Agglutinationsreaktion. *Berlin. Muench. Tieraerztl. Wochschr.* 71:431–32.

Lignières, J., and Zabala. 1905. Sur une nouvelle maladie des poules. *Bull. Soc. Cent. Med. Vet.* 59:453–56.

Lucet, A. 1891. Dysenterie epizootique des poules et des dindes. *Ann. Inst. Pasteur* 5:312–31.

McNutt, S. H. 1926. Vaccination of poultry.

J. Am. Vet. Med. Ass. 69:472–77.

Mallmann, W. L. 1931. Studies on bacteriophage in relation to Salmonella and pullorum disease. *Mich. Agr. Expt. Sta. Bull.* 109.

Martinaglia, G. 1929. A note on *Salmonella gallinarum* infection of ten-day old chicks and adult turkeys. *J. S. African Vet. Med. Ass.* 1:35–36.

Molnar, I., and G. Nagy. 1959. Production of fowl typhoid antigen by fermentation. *Magy. Allatorv. Lapja* 14:386–87.

Moore, E. N. 1946a. Fowl typhoid transmission. *Delaware Agr. Expt. Sta. Bull.* 262:21.

———. 1946b. The occurrence of fowl typhoid. *Delaware Agr. Expt. Sta. Bull.* 19:20.

———. 1946c. The efficacy of recently developed sulfonamides against fowl typhoid. *Poultry Sci.* 25:309–11.

———. 1947. The agglutination test as a means of detecting fowl typhoid infection. *Cornell Vet.* 37:21–28.

Moore, V. A. 1895. Infectious leukemia in fowls—A bacterial disease frequently mistaken for fowl cholera. *USDA BAI 12th and 13th Ann. Rept.*, pp. 185–205.

Munne, J. V. 1937. Au sujet de la differentiation de *Salmonella pullorum* et *S. sanguinarium* au moyen d'un bacteriophage specifique. *Compt. Rend. Soc. Biol.* 126:1228–30.

Nagy, G., and L. Fabian. 1968. Serological response of chickens infected artificially with *Salmonella gallinarum* and treated with Tikofuran. *Acta Vet. Acad. Sci. Hung.* 18:53–55.

Nóbrega, P., and R. C. Bueno. 1942. Sobre a presenca da *Salmonella gallinarum* nos ovos de galinhas portadoras de tifo avairo. *Arquiv. Inst. Biol.* (Sao Paulo) 13:17–20.

Orr, Betty B., and E. N. Moore. 1953. Longevity of *S. gallinarum*. *Poultry Sci.* 32:800–805.

Palmer, C. C., and H. R. Baker. 1928. Fowl typhoid. *Delaware Agr. Expt. Sta. Bull.* 153.

Pfeiler, W. 1920. Identitatsnachweis fuer den Erreger der Kleinschen Huehnerseuche und den Pfeiler-Rehseschen Huehnertyphusbazillus. *Zentr. Bakteriol. Parasitenk. Abt. I. Orig.* 85:193–98.

Pfeiler, W., and A. Rehse. 1913. *Bacillus typhi gallinarum alcalifaciens* und die durch ihn verursachte Huehnerseuche. *Mitt. Kaiser Wilhelm Inst. Landwirtsch. Bromberg.* 5:306.

Pfeiler, W., and E. Roepke. 1917. Zweite Mitteilung ueber das Auftreten des Huehnertyphus und die Eigenschaften seines Erregers. *Zentr. Bakteriol. Parasitenk. Abt. I. Orig.* 79:125–39.

Popp, L. 1947. Fowl typhoid organism as cause of gastroenteritis in man. *J. Am. Vet. Med. Ass.* 111:314. (Abstr.)

Prince, W. R. 1967. Evidence for lysozyme depletion in Rhode Island Red chickens exposed to fowl typhoid. *Poultry Sci.* 46:1308.

Prince, W. R., and H. W. Garren. 1966. An investigation of the resistance of White Leghorn chicks to *Salmonella gallinarum*. *Poultry Sci.* 45:1149–53.

Rao, S. B. V., S. Narayanan, D. R. Ramnani, and J. Das. 1952. Avian salmonellosis: Studies on *Salmonella gallinarum*. *Indian J. Vet. Sci.* 22:199–208.

Richey, D. J. 1954. Furazolidone shows promise for control of fowl typhoid and pullorum diseases. *S. C. Agr. Res.* 1 (2):1–2.

———. 1962. Water-soluble nitrofuran therapy in pullorum and fowl typhoid in chicks. *Am. J. Vet. Res.* 23:102–5.

Richey, D. J., and C. L. Morgan. 1959. Treatment of *Salmonella gallinarum* infection in turkey poults with chloramphenicol and furazolidone. *Am. J. Vet. Res.* 20:659–61.

St. John-Brooks, R., and M. Rhodes. 1923. The organism of the fowl typhoid group. *J. Pathol. Bacteriol.* 26:433–39.

Salmonella Surveillance. 1967. Annual Summary, National Communicable Disease Center, Atlanta, Ga.

Salmonella Surveillance. 1968. Annual Summary, National Communicable Disease Center, Atlanta, Ga.

Simms, B. T. 1946. Tests of drugs and vaccine to control fowl typhoid. *Rept. Chief BAI*, USDA.

Smith, H. W. 1954. Food as a vehicle of infection: The effect of variations in the diet on the induction of *Salmonella gallinarum* infection. *Brit. J. Exp. Pathol.* 35:447–58.

———. 1955a. The longevity of *S. gallinarum* in the feces of infected chickens. *J. Comp. Pathol. Therap.* 65:267–70.

———. 1955b. Observations on experimental fowl typhoid. *J. Comp. Pathol. Therap.* 65:37–54.

———. 1955c. The chemotherapy of experimental fowl typhoid in fowls (*Gallus domesticus*). *J. Comp. Pathol. Therap.* 65:55–70.

———. 1956. The use of live vaccines in experimental *S. gallinarum* infection in chickens with observations on their interference effect. *J. Hyg.* 54:419–32.

Smith, H. W., and L. G. Chubb. 1957. The effect of feeding different levels of protein concentrates on the susceptibility of chickens to *S. gallinarum* infection. *J. Comp. Pathol. Therap.* 67:10–20.

Smith, H. W., and C. Ten Broeck. 1915. Agglutination affinities of a pathogenic bacillus from fowls (fowl typhoid) (*Bact. sanguinarium,* Moore) with the typhoid bacillus of man. *J. Med. Res.* 31:503–21.

Stoychev, S., M. Krustev, I. Slavkov, and I. Sumrov. 1963. Preparations of vaccines against fowl typhoid. *Izv. Vet. Inst. Zarazni. Parazitni* 8:177–82.

Stuart, E. E., R. D. Keenum, and H. W. Bruins. 1962. Experimental studies on an isolate of *Salmonella gallinarum* apparently resistant to furazolidone. *Avian Diseases* 7:294–303.

———. 1967. The emergence of a furazolidone-resistant strain of *Salmonella gallinarum*. *Avian Diseases* 11:139–45.

Te Hennepe, B. J. C. 1924. Combating poultry diseases by the state serum institute at Rotterdam. *Proc. Second World's Poultry Congr.*, pp. 219–28.

———. 1939. Combating poultry diseases in the Netherlands. *Proc. Seventh World's Poultry Congr.*, pp. 224–27.

Te Hennepe, B. J. C., and Van Straaten, H. 1921. Fowl septicemia. *Trans. First World's Poultry Congr.* 1:259.

Titkemeyer, C. W., and S. C. Schmittle. 1957. The effect of drugs on the isolation of *Salmonella gallinarum* from inoculated chicks. *Poultry Sci.* 36:1198–1206.

Truche, C. 1923. De la typhose aviaire. *Ann. Inst. Pasteur* 37:478–97.

Tucker, J. F. 1963. The chemotherapy of avian salmonellosis with particular reference to furaltadone. *Brit. Vet. J.* 119:544–48.

———. 1967. Survival of salmonellae in built-up litter for housing of rearing and laying fowls. *Brit. Vet. J.* 123:92–103.

Van Es, L., and J. F. Olney. 1940. An inquiry into the influence of environment on the incidence of poultry diseases: Fowl typhus. *Neb. Agr. Expt. Sta. Res. Bull.* 118.

Van Heelsbergen, T. 1929. *Handbuch der Gefluegelkrankheiten und Gefluegelzucht.* Ferdinand Enke, Stuttgart.

Van Straaten, H., and B. J. C. Te Hennepe. 1919. Die Kleinsche Huehnerseuche. *Folia Microbiol.* 5:103–25.

Ward, A. R., and B. A. Gallagher. 1920. *Diseases of Domesticated Birds.* Macmillan Co., New York.

Williams, J. E., and M. R. Harris. 1956. Antigenic studies using ammonium sulfate. IV. The sedimentation effect of ammonium sulfate on *Salmonella gallinarum*. *Am. J. Vet. Res.* 17:535–37.

Wilson, J. E. 1946. Fowl typhoid: Certain aspects of the experimentally produced disease. *Vet. Record* 58:269–71.

———. 1955. The use of furazolidone in the treatment of infections of day-old chicks with *S. pullorum, S. gallinarum, S. typhimurium*, and *S. thompson*. *Vet. Record* 67:849–53.

———. 1956. The treatment of carriers of *S. pullorum* and *S. gallinarum* with furazolidone. *Vet. Record* 68:748–51.

———. 1958. Fowl typhoid in Great Britain. *Agr. Rev.*, London 3:23.

❖

PARATYPHOID INFECTIONS

❖

J. E. WILLIAMS
*Southeast Poultry Research Laboratory
Agricultural Research Service
United States Department of Agriculture
Athens, Georgia*

❖

MOORE (1895) recorded the first authentic case of paratyphoid infection in domestic poultry in describing an outbreak of infectious enteritis in pigeons. With improvement of culture procedures for the isolation of salmonellae and a better definition of the characteristics of members of the genus, the frequent association of paratyphoid organisms with disease outbreaks in all types of poultry, as well as other animal species and man, was rapidly established.

Spray and Doyle (1921) described an early outbreak of paratyphoid infection in chickens, and Rettger et al. (1933) first reported the disease in turkey poults in the United States. Reference to the incidence and importance of paratyphoid infections in poultry has frequently been made in both the scientific and industry literature since the turn of the century. For a more complete review of earlier historical reports on paratyphoid infections in all avian species, reference can be made to the fifth edition of this book or to Henning (1939).

With growing interest in the problems of animal and human salmonellosis, numerous workshops, seminars, and conferences have been held on the subject in recent years. Notable among these have been the Animal Disease Eradication Salmonella Seminar (Anon., 1964a), Conference on the Destruction of Salmonellae (Anon., 1966), and the California Poultry Disease Control Programs Workshop (Anon., 1968c). The proceedings of each of these meetings is composed of reports of interest on the subject. The first national conference on salmonellosis was held at the National Communicable Disease Center of the U.S. Public Health Service in Atlanta, Georgia, in 1964. Specialists from all over the world thoroughly reviewed the status of salmonellosis in man, animals, and poultry up to that year. A comprehensive 217-page proceedings was issued following the meeting (Anon., 1965c). Reports such as those of the Scientific Advisory Committee of the Pacific Dairy and Poultry Association (Anon., 1964b), the World Association of Veterinary Food-Hygienists (Anon., 1967a), and the Committee on Salmonella of the National Research Council (Anon., 1969b) contain valuable information relative to salmonellae in poultry, poultry feeds, and poultry products. Various national and international committees have in recent years been established by professional organizations, public health agencies, and industry groups to study and make reports and recommendations on the many facets of salmonellosis in poultry, other animals, and man. These, as they concern poultry, have been reviewed by Huston (Anon., 1966).

There has never existed any official national program with the aim of eliminating paratyphoid infections from poultry flocks such as that in operation for the eradication of pullorum disease and fowl typhoid under the National Poultry (NPIP) and Turkey (NTIP) Improvement Plans (Anon., 1971a). Control of paratyphoid infections is directed toward blood testing programs for detection of carriers of S. typhi-murium and occasionally other serotypes, early on-the-farm fumigation of hatching eggs, and strict sanitation. These measures are discussed in more detail in the Prevention and Control section which follows. The National Plans also provide that the official state agency may at its own discretion take paratyphoid infections under consideration in determining the pul-

lorum-typhoid status of any chicken or turkey flock operating under the Plans.

The National Plans maintain a Committee on Salmonellosis and Related Enteric Diseases which advises on technical matters relating to these infections. The Animal Health Division of USDA in cooperation with the National Plans has instituted a salmonella reporting and epidemiologic service dealing with these infections as they occur in poultry flocks in the various states (Anon., 1967b). Independently this Division also maintains regional laboratories for serotyping salmonella and arizona cultures of animal origin, monitors poultry feeds for salmonella contaminants, and inspects plants that process raw feed ingredients.

INCIDENCE, DISTRIBUTION, AND ECONOMIC IMPORTANCE

Paratyphoid infections of poultry exist in all parts of the world; however, it has often been found that particular serotypes which were previously rare may progressively become very common in one region or country. The majority of new serotypes that are being added constantly to the genus *Salmonella* are usually not commonly found in nature, and approximately 70% of salmonella disease outbreaks at any one time in both animals and man are due to no more than 10 or 12 serotypes. Wilson (1948) called attention to the occurrence of 24 new salmonella types encountered in human cases of food poisoning in Great Britain. Six of these types were commonly found in poultry in the United States; however, they had not been found in Great Britain prior to the large-scale importation of egg powder during World War II.

Certain salmonella types have become widespread in a country or an area for a given period of time and then decreased in incidence to a point of little importance. Gordon and Buxton (1946) noted that S. thompson was first encountered in poultry in Great Britain in 1943 and subsequently ceased to be a problem. Buxton (1957a) stated that S. oranienburg, S. bareilly, and S. montevideo are more frequently isolated from poultry in the United States than in European countries, while S. enteritidis occurs more frequently among poultry in European countries than it does in North and South America.

SEROLOGICAL SURVEYS OF CULTURES OF AVIAN ORIGIN

More than two-thirds of approximately 25,000 salmonella cultures isolated from animals in the United States during the past 30 years were recovered from domestic poultry, primarily chickens and turkeys (Edwards and Galton, 1967). Martin and Ewing (1969) found that 33 salmonella serotypes account for almost 80% of the isolates from animal sources including poultry. Sanders et al. (1965) reported that in 1963 about 61% of all nonhuman isolates were obtained from chickens, turkeys, other wild and domestic fowl, and eggs and egg products.

Edwards et al. (1948c) reported on the serological analysis of 6,387 salmonella cultures isolated from fowl. Practically all of the cultures were derived from acute, fatal infections of young birds. A few were isolated from adult birds with acute infections, and many others from the intestines of adult birds that were apparently normal carriers. Fifty-eight different salmonella types, exclusive of *S. pullorum* and *S. gallinarum,* were recovered from fowl. *S. typhi-murium* was encountered most frequently, producing 30.8% of the outbreaks and composing 37.7% of the cultures. It was concluded that any salmonella type other than those types showing strict host adaptation, such as *S. typhi* and *S. abortus-equi,* may under proper circumstances cause highly destructive diseases in poultry. No correlation was found between the type of salmonella isolated and the severity of the disease; however, it was felt that such types as *S. typhi-murium, S. oranienburg, S. montevideo, S. bareilly,* and *S. newport* usually produced the highest percentages of mortality.

Moran (1959) cited typing data which indicated that *S. typhi-murium* was encountered 4 times as frequently in turkeys as in chickens in the United States in 1957. *S. heidelberg* and *S. infantis,* which had not been reported in fowl in the United States in the earlier report of Edwards et al. (1948c), comprised 8% and 6.7% respectively of the cultures from chickens.

The 5 most common salmonella serotypes isolated from chickens in the United States in 1967 were as follows in order of prevalence: (1) *S. heidelberg* (19.4%), (2) *S. typhi-murium* (15.5%), (3) *S. infantis*

(14.2%), (4) *S. thompson* (8.5%), and (5) *S. enteritidis* (4.5%) (Anon., 1968c). Three of these same serotypes in 1966 were among the top 5 salmonella types isolated from chickens (Anon., 1967c). In 1967 the 5 most common salmonella serotypes isolated from turkeys were: (1) *S. heidelberg* (23.8%), (2) *S. saint-paul* (12.2%), (3) *S. typhi-murium* (9.0%), (4) *S. schwarzengrund* (5.8%), and (5) *S. reading* (5.5%) (Anon., 1968a). In 1966, 4 of these same serotypes were among the top 5 salmonella types isolated from turkeys (Anon., 1967c), and *S. heidelberg* was most frequently encountered in turkeys that year also.

PROCESSING PLANTS AND MARKETED POULTRY

Woodburn and Stadelman (1968) have reported studies of the prevalence of salmonellae in poultry at the production and processing levels. Edwards and Galton (1967) have discussed the incidence of salmonella contamination in poultry processing plants and marketed poultry, and Sanders et al. (1965) have reviewed the results of a nationwide surveillance of animal, poultry, and human salmonellosis.

SEROTYPES FROM CHICKENS AND TURKEYS IN THE UNITED STATES

A total of 127 paratyphoid types that have been isolated from chickens and/or turkeys in the United States are listed in Table 3.7. Eleven new types not previously reported from poultry in the United States have been added to the list since the fifth edition of this book. The information included in the table has been developed from published reports and from data supplied by diagnostic laboratories, typing centers, and research workers in various parts of the country. While the listings may be incomplete, it is considered that most types that have been reported prior to 1970 from chickens and turkeys are represented. As additional laboratories are encouraged to submit cultures for typing, the listings will undoubtedly be considerably increased. Some of the types listed in Table 3.7 have not been associated with disease outbreaks but were recovered from the intestines of birds that were apparently normal carriers, and in some cases only on a single occasion. However, most of the cultures were derived from acute, fatal infections in young chicks or poults and were isolated from the internal organs or intestinal contents. Isola-

S. aberdeen (F)*	*S. litchfield* (C_2)
S. alabama (D_1)	*S. livingstone* (C_1)
S. alachua (O)	*S. lomita* (C_1)
S. albany (C_3)	*S. london* (E_1)
S. amager (E_1)	*S. madelia* (H)
S. amersfoort (C_1)	*S. manchester* (C_2)
S. amherstiana (C_3)	*S. manhattan* (C_2)
S. anatum (E_1)	*S. manila* (E_2)
S. arkansas (E_3)	*S. meleagridis* (E_1)
S. babelsberg (M)	*S. menston* (C_1)
S. bareilly (C_1)	*S. mgulani* (P)
S. berkeley (U)	*S. miami* (D_1)
S. berta (D_1)	*S. mikawasima* (C_1)
S. binza (E_2)	*S. minneapolis* (E_3)
S. blockley (C_2)	*S. minnesota* (L)
S. bovis-morbificans (C_2)	*S. mission* (C_1)
S. braenderup (C_1)	*S. montevideo* (C_1)
S. bredeney (B)	*S. muenchen (oregon)* (C_2)
S. budapest (B)	*S. muenster* (E_1)
S. california (B)	*S. new-brunswick* (E_2)
S. cambridge (E_2)	*S. new-haw* (E_2)
S. canoga (E_3)	*S. newington* (E_2)
S. cerro (K)	*S. newport (pueris)* (C_2)
S. champaign (Q)	*S. norwich* (C_1)
S. chester (B)	*S. onderstepoort* (H)
S. cholerae-suis (C_1)	*S. oranienburg* (C_1)
S. concord (C_1)	*S. orion* (E_1)
S. corvallis (C_3)	*S. panama (italiana)* (D_1)
S. cubana (G_2)	*S. paratyphi B (schottmuelleri)* (B)
S. denver (C_1)	*S. pensacola* (D_1)
S. derby (B)	*S. pomona* (M)
S. dublin (D_1)	*S. poona* (G_1)
S. duesseldorf (C_2)	*S. reading* (B)
S. eastbourne (D_1)	*S. rubislaw* (F)
S. edinburg (C_1)	*S. rutgers* (E_1)
S. eimsbuettel (C_1)	*S. saint-paul* (B)
S. enteritidis (D_1)	*S. san-diego* (B)
S. essen (B)	*S. san-juan* (C_1)
S. florida (H)	*S. schwarzengrund* (B)
S. fresno (D_2)	*S. senftenberg* (E_4)
S. gaminara (I)	*S. siegburg* (K)
S. give (E_1)	*S. simsbury* (E_4)
S. grumpensis (G_2)	*S. stanley* (B)
S. habana (G_2)	*S. takoradi* (C_2)
S. halmstad (E_2)	*S. taksony* (E_4)
S. hamilton (goerlitz) (E_2)	*S. tallahassee* (C_2)
S. harrisonburg (E_3)	*S. tel-aviv* (M)
S. hartford (C_1)	*S. tennessee* (C_1)
S. heidelberg (B)	*S. thomasville* (E_3)
S. hidalgo (C_2)	*S. thompson* (C_1)
S. hvittingfoss (I)	*S. typhi* (D_1)
S. illinois (E_2)	*S. typhi-murium* (B)
S. indiana (B)	*S. typhi-murium*
S. infantis (C_1)	(var. *copenhagen*) (B)
S. irumu (C_1)	*S. uganda* (E_1)
S. israel (D_1)	*S. uno* (C_2)
S. java (B)	*S. urbana* (N)
S. javiana (D_1)	*S. vejle* (E_1)
S. johannesburg (R)	*S. westerstede* (E_4)
S. kaapstad (B)	*S. westhampton* (E_1)
S. kentucky (C_3)	*S. wichita* (G_1)
S. kingston (B)	*S. worcester* (G_1)
S. kottbus (C_2)	*S. worthington* (G_1)
S. lexington (E_1)	*S. zanzibar* (E_1)

* Indicates antigenic group in the K-W Schema to which each serotype belongs.

tions from unabsorbed yolks, ovarian cysts, and oviducts represent only a small percentage of the culture types listed. Original references to the description of most of the salmonella types included in Table 3.7 are listed by Kauffmann (1966).

WORLDWIDE AVIAN SALMONELLOSIS

Buxton (1957a), in a comprehensive review of salmonellosis in animals, presented a worldwide survey of salmonella types occurring in poultry. A total of 90 types of paratyphoid organisms was reported from 12 species of fowl. Many of these serotypes were reported to have caused only a few minor epizootics and some to have been isolated only from apparently healthy birds. The reader seeking reference material on the host species, origin, and distribution of salmonella types occurring in poultry in various parts of the world is referred to this excellent review.

MULTIPLE SEROTYPES IN INDIVIDUAL FLOCKS AND BIRDS

The epizootiology of salmonella infections among individual flocks is often complex due to the wide distribution of the organisms in fowl and the practice of bringing eggs from different flocks together in one hatchery. Edwards and Bruner (1940) described an extensive study of multiple types of paratyphoids in individual flocks. Pomeroy and Fenstermacher (1941) reported that from one farm where poults had been accumulated from several sources over a period of 3 years, *S. typhi-murium*, *S. derby*, *S. give*, *S. oranienburg*, *S. senftenberg*, and *S. anatum* were isolated. From the same farm in previous years other salmonella types had been isolated. Hinshaw et al. (1944) also reported multiple types of salmonellosis on the same ranch.

Edwards et al. (1948a) found more than one salmonella type existing in the same flock in 165 instances. Akiyama et al. (1959) isolated 4 salmonella types from a group of 7-day-old chicks that were also found to be infected with *S. pullorum*. It was assumed that the organisms infected the eggs during incubation. Ballantyne (1953) reported the isolation from one turkey farm of 4 different serological types of salmonella. Boyer et al. (1962) reported multiple salmonella types in several individual cases of salmonellosis in both chicks

and poults. It was noted that simultaneous infections are not unusual.

The isolation of 2 or more salmonella types from a single bird was reported by Edwards et al. (1948a,b) in 51 cases of avian paratyphoid infections. Four salmonella types were recovered from the liver of one poult and 3 from the liver of a second.

ECONOMIC IMPORTANCE

From an economic viewpoint paratyphoid infections are among the most important bacterial diseases of the hatching industry and result in high death losses among all types of young poultry. The occurrence of this disease in valuable breeding stock is extremely costly. Because of its chronic nature and difficulty of eradication it is capable of terminating breeding operations in which large amounts of money may have been invested. Fertility, hatchability, and egg production may be seriously impaired (Graham and Michael, 1936; Pomeroy and Fenstermacher, 1941). The disease has a definite stunting effect on surviving birds and a debilitating influence on poultry of all ages, increasing their susceptibility to many other diseases.

ETIOLOGY

MORPHOLOGY AND STAINING

Organisms of the paratyphoid group are defined as serologically related, gram-negative, and nonsporogenic bacilli; 0.4–0.6 by 1–3μ in usual dimensions but occasionally forming short filaments (Fig. 3.17). They are normally motile by means of peritrichous flagella, but nonmotile variants with or without flagella may be encountered under natural conditions.

GROWTH REQUIREMENTS

Paratyphoids are facultative anaerobes and can be readily cultivated on initial isolation, from sources other than feces, on simple beef extract and beef infusion agars and broths. Optimum growth temperature is 37° C. When it is desired to obtain large yields of the organisms, media enhanced with serum, dextrose-starch, brain-heart infusion, beef heart infusion (McNeil and Hinshaw, 1951), colloidal sulfur and glycerin (MacDonald, 1947), or cysteine hydrochloride and glycerin (Harris and Williams, 1957) can be used. Gordon and Tucker

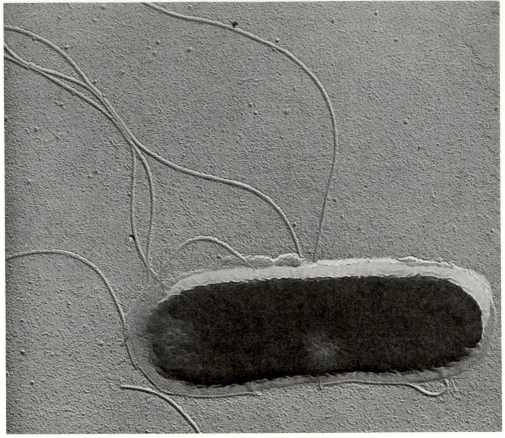

FIG. 3.17—Electron micrograph of single flagellated cell of Salmonella typhi-
murium. *Chromium shadowed, ×14,000.*

(1965) maintained stock laboratory cultures of *S. menston* on Dorset egg medium
stored at 4° C. (For further information
on growth requirements refer to Diagnosis
section.)

COLONIAL MORPHOLOGY AND GROWTH IN BROTH

Typical colonies of paratyphoids on agar
culture are round, slightly raised, and glistening with smooth edges. Colonies are
generally 1–2 mm in diameter depending
on the degree of dispersion on the plates.
Rough (R) colonies may be encountered
among both recently isolated strains and
those maintained in the laboratory on artificial media. These R forms are dull and
granular with irregular edges. From a practical standpoint, it is usually assumed that
morphologically rough strains of salmonella do not contain smooth antigens, and
such cultures cannot be typed serologically
or used in the preparation of antigens for
the agglutination test.

Smooth broth cultures after incubation
for 24 hours show a thick homogeneous
turbidity with no pellicle and very little
sediment. Rough cultures in broth have a
heavy, granular sediment and an almost
clear supernatant fluid. In order to avoid
the development of rough cultures, Kauffmann (1950) recommended that media employed for the storage of cultures should
contain no carbohydrates, and subculturing
should be done as infrequently as possible.
Lyophilization is the best method to prevent roughness of cultures.

BIOCHEMICAL PROPERTIES

The following biochemical reactions, as
described by Edwards and Ewing (1962),
are typical of practically all members of
the paratyphoid group:

DEXTROSE	Fermented with gas
LACTOSE	Not fermented
SUCROSE	Not fermented
MANNITOL	Fermented with gas
MALTOSE	Fermented with gas
DULCITOL	Usually fermented with gas
SALICIN	Not fermented
SORBITOL	Fermented with gas
ADONITOL	Not fermented
INOSITOL	Fermented or not fermented
INDOLE	Not produced
METHYL RED	Positive
VOGES-PROSKAUER ..	Negative
SIMMONS' CITRATE ..	Usually utilized
H₂S	Usually positive
UREA	Not hydrolyzed
GELATIN	Rarely liquefied
KCN	Negative
NITRATES	Reduced
MOTILITY	Positive
DECARBOXYLASES ...	
LYSINE	Positive
ARGININE	Positive, usually delayed
ORNITHINE	Positive
MALONATE	Negative
PHENYLALANINE DEAMINASE	Negative

Cultures that do not possess the above characteristics may be excluded from the paratyphoid group unless it can be established that they possess antigens of known salmonella types. *S. typhi-murium* var. *copenhagen,* a frequent cause of paratyphoid infection of pigeons, occasionally forms no acid and, more frequently, no gas in maltose broth when isolated from this species. Consequently this organism is sometimes confused with *S. pullorum* on initial examination. For a very comprehensive review of the biochemical reactions of paratyphoid organisms, reference can be made to Ewing and Ball (1966) and Kauffmann (1966).

Because of the delayed fermentative properties characteristic of some strains of the genus *Arizona,* prolonged incubation of fermentation broths is often advantageous. Sealing of the tubes with cork stoppers dipped in hot paraffin will hasten the reactions. Basal carbohydrate broths with Andrade's indicator have been very widely used for many years in the identification and study of salmonella cultures. Kauff-

mann (1966) recommended a basal 1% peptone broth with bromthymol blue as an indicator. Bromcresol purple has also been used by many laboratories as an indicator in the study of salmonella cultures.

Motility of paratyphoid cultures can be readily demonstrated through use of a semisolid medium as described by Edwards and Ewing (1962). This medium is also useful in the separation of flagellar phases for the preparation of antigens or typing sera.

RESISTANCE TO CHEMICAL AND PHYSICAL AGENTS

Heat, Cold, and Disinfectants

Paratyphoid organisms are quite susceptible to heat and the majority of the common disinfectants. Some salmonella strains such as *S. senftenberg,* strain 775W, may be 30 times or more heat resistant than usual strains (Ng et al., 1969). Bayne et al. (1965) found that it took only 5 minutes exposure to heat at 60° C to destroy 3×10^8 cells of *S. typhi-murium* per g sample of ground chicken meat; however, it took 10–15 minutes exposure at 65° C to destroy *S. senftenberg* 775W in similar samples. Winter et al. (1946) and Lancaster et al. (1952) reported paratyphoid organisms to be much more resistant to heat than *S. pullorum.* Salmonella organisms can survive for as long as 10 months at −25° C. Cresylic acid, lye, and phenolic compounds are frequently employed in the disinfection of poultry premises. Formaldehyde is also widely used as a disinfectant, particularly as a fumigant for eggs, incubators, and hatchery rooms.

Litter, Feedstuffs, and Dust

Adler et al. (1953) were able to isolate *S. typhi-murium* from litter 44 days after experimental infection of poults which were allowed to run on the litter. Smyser et al. (1963) found that *S. typhi-murium* had a short survival period in feedstuffs held at room temperature and contaminated with fewer than 10 organisms per gram. The organism was recovered for a longer period from feedstuffs stored at 4° C than from those stored at room temperature. It was suggested that feed samples for bacteriological examination should be refrigerated to prevent a possible decrease in the bacterial population.

Smyser et al. (1966) recovered *S. heidel-*

berg from contaminated litter, grit, feed, and dust held for extended periods at room temperature. Litter was positive at 18 months, when last tested. Tucker (1967) found that *S. thompson* survived 4–5 weeks in old litter and 8–20 weeks in new litter. When infected pens were left empty, the survival time in both types of litter increased to more than 30 weeks. Increased moisture reduced the viable salmonella count in the litter. Snoeyenbos et al. (1967b) reported *S. typhi-murium* to also survive better in new litter than in old litter, due apparently to the lower pH of the new litter.

Feces and Hatchery Fluff

Price et al. (1962) cited information to indicate that salmonella organisms may remain viable in duck feces for 28 weeks. Malathion in fly sprays was not found to kill the organisms in feces. Salmonellae were isolated by Baker et al. (1966) from dried feces collected from a turkey house that had been left unoccupied and uncleaned for 9 months after removal of the birds. Following a thorough steam cleaning, *S. chester* was still isolated from boards, cracks, and crevices in the house. This same serotype was known to have infected the flock occupying the house earlier. Miura et al. (1964) found that salmonella organisms would survive in hatchery fluff samples stored at room temperature for as long as 5 years.

Soil, Water, and Vegetation

Mair and Ross (1960) reported that *S. typhi-murium* was found to survive in urban garden soil in England for at least 280 days. Sato (1967b) isolated salmonella organisms from soil taken from turkey ranges that had not been in use for 7 months. It was suggested that salmonellae can survive for a long time in the soil, depending on sunlight, the nature of the soil, pH, humidity, and contamination of the soil with other species of bacteria.

Watts and Wall (1952) found that *S. typhi-murium* could survive for at least 119 days in ponds in Australia. Kraus and Weber (1958) demonstrated that salmonella organisms could survive from several weeks to 3 months in drinking water and natural surface water, being affected independently by the nutritional conditions and temperature of the water. Felsenfeld and Young (1945) demonstrated that salmonella could survive for several weeks on vegetables kept at room temperature. Steiniger (1961), in the examination of 100,000 samples of birds' feces found in nature, reported that salmonellae were more frequently isolated from feces found on vegetation than on stones and soil. Salmonella survived for 28 months on plant material allowed to dry slowly.

Egg Fluids, Albumen, and Whole Eggs

Hashimoto (1961) found *S. senftenberg*, in contrast to *S. pullorum*, to be resistant to the bactericidal properties of egg albumen, yolk, and various embryonic fluids. Watanabe et al. (1959b) demonstrated that embryonic fluid and serum had no bactericidal effect on *S. senftenberg*.

Anellis et al. (1954) reported that in egg albumen salmonella organisms were more rapidly destroyed by heat at a high pH, and Banwart and Ayres (1957) found that raising the pH of egg albumen to 9 or 10 caused a reduction in the number of surviving salmonella organisms during processing of the product. Lerche (1957) noted that the addition of 0.25–0.5% ammonia was necessary to destroy salmonellae in egg white. Cotterill (1968) found that pasteurization of egg albumen at high pH levels permitted the use of lower temperatures for salmonella destruction. It also reduced the chance of survival if the product should become recontaminated. The time required for the destruction of salmonellae in whole egg mixtures at 140° F has been found to vary from 7–9 minutes at pH 5.5 to 2–3.5 minutes at pH 8.0.

Simskaya (1955) demonstrated that inactivation of amylase in eggs can be used as an index to confirm the destruction of salmonella organisms in such eggs following heat treatment. Baldwin et al. (1968) studied the growth and destruction of *S. typhi-murium* in egg white foam products cooked electronically by microwaves. Products were rendered safer by this process, but the salmonellae were not always destroyed.

Eggshells, Filler Flats, and Egg Contents and Membranes

Buxton and Gordon (1947) found that *S. thompson* could survive on the surface of chicken eggs for at least 21 days under ordinary conditions of storage at room temperature. Gregory (1948), using an incubator at a temperature of 100° F and a wet bulb reading of 82–86° F, found that the shell surface of 2 of 26 turkey eggs contaminated with *S. typhi-murium* remained infected after 28 days. Pomeroy and Fenstermacher (1941) demonstrated that *S. typhi-murium* could survive in the contents of turkey eggs at incubator temperature for a period of at least 13 months. Lancaster and Crabb (1953a) reported that *S. typhi-murium* and *S. thompson* rapidly lose their viability on the shell of whole chicken eggs maintained under normal incubator temperature. At room temperature the organisms were found to survive for approximately 21 days on clean eggs and for a longer period on artificially dirty eggs. Increased humidity prolonged the viability of the organisms. Watanabe et al. (1959a) found that *S. senftenberg* survived for 10 days on the surface of the eggshell at room temperature.

Gordon and Tucker (1965) found *S. menston* to survive on the shell, in the membranes, and in the contents of chicken eggs from an infected flock stored for varying periods up to 8 weeks at room temperature. Rizk et al. (1966b) demonstrated that salmonellae survived better on the shell of experimentally infected eggs stored at 2° C than at 22–25° C; however, the number of organisms recovered from the interior of the shell and the membranes decreased in eggs stored at 2° C. Banwart (1964) found that autoclaving egg filler flats for 10 minutes at 255° F following contamination with salmonellae killed all the organisms; however, viable salmonellae were still present on contaminated filler flats stored at room temperature as long as 9 days without autoclaving.

Antibiotics and Infective Drug Resistance

Huey and Edwards (1958) found that 9% of *S. typhi-murium* strains isolated from poultry after 1956 were resistant to tetracyclines when compared with other cultures isolated prior to 1948. They attributed this to the use of antibiotics in poultry feeds. In further studies Ramsey and Edwards (1961) found that 29 of 100 *S. typhi-murium* cultures isolated from fowls in 1959 and 1960 were resistant to the tetracyclines. Garside et al. (1960) demonstrated a tenfold increase in resistance to chlortetracycline in the case of a single colony inoculum of *S. typhi-murium* administered to chicks receiving the antibiotic in their diet. The organisms were capable of resisting 210 ppm of chlortetracycline after 4 passages. Subsequent passage of the resistant cultures through chicks receiving no drug in their feed revealed that resistance declined gradually, but at the end of 14 weeks some strains were still four times as tolerant to the antibiotic as the normal strains. Hobbs et al. (1960) found that a strain of *S. typhi-murium* resistant to chlortetracycline grew more rapidly than spoilage organisms at 22° C on the skin of dressed poultry that had been immersed in slush ice containing 10 ppm chlortetracycline. Smith (1967), Schroeder et al. (1968), and Anon. (1969b) have reviewed infective drug resistance in salmonella cultures.

ANTIGENIC STRUCTURE AND TOXINS

The approximately 1,500 serotypes of the genus *Salmonella* presently recognized are listed in the Kauffmann-White diagnostic schema (Kauffmann, 1966). Most salmonella organisms possess both somatic (O) and flagellar (H) antigens. The O antigen is associated with the bacterial cell proper and is resistant to both alcohol and heat treatment. The H antigen is a part of the flagella and is both alcohol- and heat-labile. The various O antigenic factors are designated with arabic numerals while the H antigenic factors are divided into phases 1 and 2, which are usually designated with small letters and arabic numerals respectively. Thus the complete antigenic formula of *S. typhi-murium* is 1, 4, 5, 12 (O): i, 1, 2 (H).

Procedures for Serological Analysis

Highly specialized serological procedures have been developed for the antigenic analysis and classification of salmonella cultures. In conducting the antigenic analyses, sera containing agglutinins for specific antigenic factors are used in macroscopic plate and tube agglutination tests to determine first the O and subsequently the H antigenic structure of each culture. After the O and H antigenic factors of a culture have been determined, its identification merely requires reference to the Kauffmann-White schema. The schema includes 36 main serological groups, with groups C, D, E, and G possessing additional subgroups.

Most poultry diagnostic laboratories do

not find it practical to engage in the serological analysis of salmonella cultures, but rather rely upon one of USDA's several regional typing laboratories or the State Health Department laboratory for this service. Typing summaries listing all cultures isolated from poultry, other animals, and man are reported monthly and summarized annually in the National Communicable Disease Center's *Salmonella Surveillance Report* which was instituted nationally in 1963. This report, sponsored by the Public Health Service of the U.S. Department of Health, Education and Welfare, has contributed greatly to our understanding of salmonellosis in both animals and man.

It is strongly recommended that *all* salmonella cultures isolated from poultry be submitted for complete typing. This will permit cultures of avian origin to be examined at one central laboratory for better correlation, review, and distribution of results as accumulated. Thus accurate current information on the incidence and distribution of salmonella types among poultry will be available to guide the formulation of control programs for those types found to be of most importance. Knowledge of the serotypes, their incidence, and distribution is absolutely essential for determining reservoirs, vehicles, and routes of infection (Taylor, 1967).

Polyvalent Screening

Polyvalent sera for examination of salmonella cultures are very useful in preliminary culture screening. Methods for their preparation have been outlined by Edwards and Ewing (1962). These sera are generally employed in rapid slide tests and agglutination is easily read. They are available commercially. Kauffmann and Edwards (1947, 1957) described simplified methods for the serological identification of the most important salmonella types. Edwards et al. (1948c) found that 99.5% of all salmonella types from fowls they examined belonged to groups B, C, D, and E or were *S. worthington* or *S. minnesota*. This prompted them to suggest that a polyvalent serum covering the somatic and frequently occurring flagellar antigens of the above four groups and *S. worthington* and *S. minnesota* would be very helpful in the diagnosis and study of avian salmonellosis.

Spicer Screening Techniques

For the recognition of H antigens to establish a tentative salmonella diagnosis, the polyvalent antisera of Spicer (1956), which are commercially available in a slightly modified form, can be employed. This method can eliminate the need for sending a large number of duplicate cultures to the laboratory for typing. For a definitive identification of serotypes, most laboratories will do well to forward representative pure cultures to a reference laboratory that specializes in salmonella typing procedures (Edwards and Galton, 1967).

Antigenic Formulas and Type Distribution in Poultry

There is marked variation in the somatic and flagellar antigenic structure of salmonella types infecting poultry. The antigenic formula of each of 127 types of paratyphoids isolated from turkeys and chickens in the United States is listed in Table 3.8. Organisms representative of most of the major antigenic groups in the Kauffmann-White schema, with the exception of serological group A, have been isolated from chickens and turkeys.

Approximately 80% of all salmonella types isolated from turkeys and chickens in the United States are members of antigenic groups B, C, D, and E. The greatest number of paratyphoid types belong to group C followed by groups E, B, and D in sequence. Because of the very frequent occurrence of *S. heidelberg* and *S. typhimurium* in paratyphoid outbreaks in poultry in the United States, the greatest number of cultures isolated is representative of serological group B.

Serological Cross-Reactions in Avian Salmonellosis

As illustrated in Table 3.8, organisms within a given serological group share common somatic antigens. Flagellar antigens are also shared within and between groups. An example of the existence of common somatic antigenic factors in two separate groups of the Kauffmann-White schema is illustrated by organisms in groups B and D, which may possess both antigens 1 and 12. These common somatic antigens account for the fact that chickens and turkeys infected with *S. typhi-murium* (1, 4, 5, 12) or some other member of group B

TABLE 3.8 ❧ Antigenic Grouping of Paratyphoids Isolated from Chickens and/or Turkeys in United States

Group	Type	O-Antigen	H-Antigen Phase 1	H-Antigen Phase 2
A	....			
B	S. bredeney	1,4,12,27	l,v	1,7
	S. budapest	1,4,12	g,t	......
	S. california	4,5,12	m,t	......
	S. chester	4,5,12	e,h	e,n,x
	S. derby	1,4,5,12	f,g	......
	S. essen	4,12	g,m	
	S. heidelberg	1,4,5,12	r	1,2
	S. indiana	1,4,12	z	1,7
	S. java	1,4,5,12	b	(1,2)*
	S. kaapstad	4,12	e,h	1,7
	S. kingston	1,4,12,27	g,s,t	
	S. paratyphi B	1,4,5,12	b	1,2
	S. reading	4,5,12	e,h	1,5
	S. saint-paul	1,4,5,12	e,h	1,2
	S. san-diego	4,5,12	e,h	e,n,z_{15}
	S. schwarzengrund	1,4,12,27	d	1,7
	S. stanley	4,5,12	d	1,2
	S. typhi-murium	1,4,5,12	i	1,2
	S. typhi-murium (var. copenhagen)	1,4,12	i	1,2
C_1	S. amersfoort	6,7	d	e,n,x
	S. bareilly	6,7	y	1,5
	S. braenderup	6,7	e,h	e,n,z_{15}
	S. cholerae-suis	6,7	c	1,5
	S. concord	6,7	l,v	1,2
	S. denver	6,7	a	e,n,z_{15}
	S. edinburg	6,7	b	1,5
	S. eimsbeuttel	6,(7),(14)	d	1,w
	S. hartford	6,7	y	e,n,x
	S. infantis	6,7	r	1,5
	S. irumu	6,7	l,v	1,5
	S. livingstone	6,7	d	l,w
	S. lomita	6,7	e,h	1,5
	S. menston	6,7	g,s,t	......
	S. mikawasima	6,7	y	c,n,z_{15}
	S. mission	6,7	d	1,5
	S. montevideo	6,7	g,m,s	......
	S. norwich	6,7	e,h	1,6
	S. oranienburg	6,7	m,t	......
	S. san-juan	6,7	a	1,5
	S. tennessee	6,7	z_{29}	......
	S. thompson	6,7	k	1,5
C_2	S. blockley	6,8	k	1,5
	S. bovis-morbificans	6,8	r	1,5
	S. duesseldorf	6,8	z_4,z_{24}	......
	S. hidalgo	6,8	r	e,n,z_{15}
	S. kottbus	6,8	e,h	1,5
	S. litchfield	6,8	l,v	1,2
	S. manchester	6,8	l,v	1,7
	S. manhattan	6,8	d	1,5
	S. muenchen (oregon)	6,8	d	1,2
	S. newport	6,8	e,h	1,2
	S. takoradi	6,8	i	1,5
	S. tallahassee	6,8	z_4,z_{32}	......
	S. uno	6,8	z_{29}	......
C_3	S. albany	(8),20	z_4,z_{24}	......
	S. amherstiana	(8)	l,v	1,6
	S. corvallis	(8),20	z_4,z_{23}	......
	S. kentucky	(8),20	i	z_6
D_1	S. alabama	9,12	c	e,n,z_{15}
	S. berta	9,12	f,g,t	......
	S. dublin	1,9,12	g,p	......
	S. eastbourne	1,9,12	e,h	1,5
	S. enteritidis	1,9,12	g,m	......
	S. israel	9,12	e,h	e,n,z_{15}
	S. javiana	1,9,12	l,z_{28}	1,5

Group	Type	O-Antigen	H-Antigen Phase 1	H-Antigen Phase 2
D_1	S. miami	1,9,12	a	1,5
	S. panama (italiana)	1,9,12	l,v	1,5
	S. pensacola	9,12	m,t	......
	S. typhi	9,12,Vi	d	......
D_2	S. fresno	(9),46	z_{38}	......
E_1	S. amager	3,10	y	1,2
	S. anatum	3,10	e,h	1,6
	S. give	3,10	l,v	1,7
	S. lexington	3,10	z_{10}	1,5
	S. london	3,10	l,v	1,6
	S. meleagridis	3,10	e,h	l,w
	S. muenster	3,10	e,h	1,5
	S. orion	3,10	y	1,5
	S. rutgers	3,10	l,z_{40}	1,7
	S. uganda	3,10	l,z_{13}	1,5
	S. vejle	3,10	e,h	1,2
	S. westhampton	3,10	g,s,t	......
	S. zanzibar	3,10	k	1,5
E_2	S. binza	3,15	y	1,5
	S. cambridge	3,15	e,h	l,w
	S. halmstad	3,15	g,s,t	......
	S. hamilton (goerlitz)	3,15	z_{27}	......
	S. manila	3,15	z_{10}	1,5
	S. new-brunswick	3,15	l,v	1,7
	S. new-haw	3,15	e,h	1,5
	S. newington	3,15	e,h	1,6
E_3	S. arkansas	(3),(15),34	e,h	1,5
	S. canoga	(3),(15),34	g,s,t	......
	S. harrisonburg	(3),(15),34	z_{10}	1,6
	S. illinois	(3),(15),34	z_{10}	1,5
	S. minneapolis	(3),(15),34	e,h	1,6
	S. thomasville	(3),(15),34	y	1,5
E_4	S. senftenberg	1,3,19	g,s,t	......
	S. simsbury	1,3,19	z_{27}	......
	S. taksony	1,3,19	i	z_6
	S. westerstede	1,3,19	$1,z_{13}$	......
F	S. aberdeen	11	i	1,2
	S. rubislaw	11	r	e,n,x
G_1	S. poona	13,22	z	1,6
	S. wichita	1,13,23	d	......
	S. worcester	1,13,23	m,t	e,n,x
	S. worthington	1,13,23	z	l,w
G_2	S. cubana	1,13,23	z_{29}	......
	S. grumpensis	13,23	d	1,7
	S. habana	1,13,23	f,g	......
H	S. florida	1,6,14,25	d	1,7
	S. madelia	1,6,14,25	y	1,7
	S. onderstepoort	1,6,14,25	e,h	1,5
I	S. gaminara	16	d	1,7
	S. hvittingfoss	16	b	e,n,x
Further groups	S. alachua	35	z_4,z_{23}	......
	S. babelsberg	28	z_4,z_{23}	e,n,z_{15}
	S. berkeley	43	a	1,5
	S. cerro	18	z_4,z_{23}	......
	S. champaign	39	k	1,5
	S. johannesburg	1,40	b	e,n,x
	S. mgulani	38	i	1,2
	S. minnesota	21	b	e,n,x
	S. pomona	28	y	1,7
	S. siegburg	6,14,18	z_4,z_{23}	
	S. tel-aviv	28	y	e,n,z_{15}
	S. urbana	30	b	e,n,x

*( ) Indicates that this antigen may be absent.

may be detected when tested with *S. pullorum* (1, 9, 12) antigen. As would be expected, the serum titer of birds infected with *S. typhi-murium* is usually lower when tested with pullorum antigen than with an homologous antigen.

Hinshaw and McNeil (1943a) found that the 1:25 dilution tube agglutination test for pullorum disease in turkeys will detect about 25% of the *S. typhi- murium* reactors because of the cross agglutination in antigen 12. Burr et al. (1957) found that approximately 50% of a group of 13 chickens artificially infected with *S. heidelberg* (4, 5, 12) revealed no titer to *S. pullorum* tube agglutination antigen at a 1:25 dilution but gave at least a 2+ reaction at the same dilution with *S. heidelberg* antigen. Chang et al. (1957) reported that removal of the bursa of Fabricius in young chickens reduced antibody production following inoculation of *S. typhi-murium* antigen.

Bahr and Christensen (1933), Van Roekel and Bullis (1937), Sanders et al. (1943), Pomeroy and Fenstermacher (1944), Hinshaw and McNeil (1944), and Becker (1957) have discussed the difficulties encountered in testing chickens and turkeys for the control of pullorum disease when certain types of paratyphoid infections are present in flocks. Wilson (1947) reported the isolation of *S. typhi-murium* from 2 chickens that reacted with pullorum antigen.

Toxins

The pathogenic properties of salmonellae are due to endotoxins which are closely associated with the somatic portion of the organism. Vestal and Stephens (1966) suggested that differences in pathogenicity of salmonella serotypes for chicks may be due to the fact that the cells of some types are rapidly lysed following injection with the release of a large quantity of endotoxin and early mortality. Other serotypes, it was believed, must build up to a large number of cells over several days before sufficient endotoxin is released to cause mortality.

PATHOGENICITY

Mortality from paratyphoid infections of poultry is encountered most frequently during the first 2 weeks after hatching, with the highest losses occurring between the 6th and 10th days. The infection seldom causes mortality in birds more than 1 month old. Pigeons, parakeets, and canaries may be cited as exceptions, for the disease does occur more often in the acute form in adults of these species.

Young Birds

Mortality rates among broods of young birds under natural conditions usually vary from negligible to 10 or 20%; however, mortality rates of 80% or higher are encountered in severe outbreaks. Buxton (1958) called attention to the fact that nutrition may have a significant effect on the susceptibility of animals to salmonella infections and may be associated with factors concerning the development of immunity in the host and alterations in the virulence of the infecting organism.

POULTS. Bierer (1960) found turkey poults extremely susceptible to *S. typhi-murium* infection during the first 48 hours after hatching. Mitrovic (1956) reported that day-old turkey poults were very susceptible to experimental infection with *S. reading* with a mortality of 40%, while 2-week-old poults possessed extremely high resistance to the infection. Yamamoto et al. (1961a) studied the shedding of salmonella organisms in the feces of orally infected adult turkeys. They found that there was a marked decrease in the number of organisms shed by 14–21 days after infection.

CHICKS. The increased interest in salmonellosis as a disease of domestic chicken flocks is well illustrated by the growing number of reports appearing in the scientific literature on the subject. The frequent citing of chickens and eggs as a source of salmonellosis in man has no doubt contributed to the interest and pursuit of research in this field. In contrast to poults, chicks usually do not exhibit high mortalities when infected experimentally. Vestal and Stephens (1966) found that none of 9 salmonella serotypes studied for pathogenicity in chicks could be considered nonpathogenic. The strains studied were classified on the basis of being "highly pathogenic," "pathogenic," or "mildly pathogenic," depending on the mortality produced by experimental inoculation of chicks. *S. heidelberg, S. schwarzengrund,* and *S. saint-paul* were almost as pathogenic as *S. gallinarum* when injected into the yolk sacs of chicks. In contrast, *S. meleagridis* and *S. infantis* appeared to possess relatively low degrees of pathogenicity for baby chicks.

Milner and Shaffer (1952) infected day-old chicks with *S. typhi-murium* and obtained positive cloacal swabs 1–3 days later in 5% of those given 1–5 organisms, 51% for 10, 88% for 10^2, 95% for 10^3, 97% for 10^4, and 100% for 10^5. Infection by the oral route decreased rapidly with advancing age. Fatality rates in the chicks experimentally infected were not high, although bacteremia was easily demonstrated early through blood culture. Clemmer et al. (1960) found a wide variation in the response of chicks exposed to aerosol infection with various salmonella types. *S. typhi-murium* was found to be very invasive for lung tissue in contrast to the other types studied. Buxton and Gordon (1947) were able to produce a 44% mortality in chicks infected orally with *S. thompson*. Approximately 70% of the survivors remained intestinal carriers at 21 days of age. Gordon and Tucker (1965) reported that the cycle of infection of *S. menston* in poultry has been shown to be similar to that of *S. thompson* in that *S. menston* was shown to be present in adult chickens, the eggs laid by these birds, chicks hatched from these eggs, and the eggs laid by these progeny at maturity.

Sieburth and Johnson (1957) reported that orally administered *S. typhi-murium* organisms are very infective for the day-old chick with 100% infection arising from 10^2 and 50% mortality from $10^{3.5}$ viable organisms per chick. Sieburth (1957a) was able to produce a cumulative mortality of 27% in chicks 12 days postinoculation by administering approximately 160 viable *S. typhi-murium* cells orally to each bird at 1 day of age. *S. typhi-murium* recovery from the intestine and organs was 100%. Bierer (1961) found that *S. typhi-murium* infection could be induced experimentally in chicks by spraying broth cultures of the organism into incubators 1 day before hatching. Mortality was almost tripled in infected groups maintained in unheated brooders for a 10-day period. Hamada et al. (1958) found that chicks infected in the incubators usually acquire the infection through the respiratory and digestive organs and carry the greatest concentration of the organisms during the first week of

life. They may appear healthy and usually eliminate the infection in 4–6 weeks without therapy.

Shaffer et al. (1957) found marked variation in the response of day-old chicks to either peroral or parenteral inoculation with various antigenic types of salmonellae. The course of infection produced by *S. typhi-murium* included marked shedding of the organisms in the feces; frequent invasion and localization in tissues such as the spleen, liver, and lungs; and deaths from bacteremia. *S. paratyphi A*, a type that has not yet been isolated naturally from poultry in the United States, exhibited less evidence of invasiveness and caused no mortality. Henderson et al. (1960) administered 7 different salmonella serotypes orally in graduated doses to inbred White Leghorn day-old chicks. All 7 serotypes produced mortality varying from about 2% (*S. anatum*) to 80% (*S. typhi-murium*). Exposure to their own feces of chicks infected with *S. anatum* significantly increased but did not extend the period of mortality. Akiyama (1961) found that there was a low mortality rate in chicks artificially infected with *S. senftenberg* and the infection was rapidly shed by adult chickens.

Brownell and Sadler (1967) reported that in chicks experimentally infected with *S. typhi-murium*, shedders of the organisms were established much more commonly in birds infected at 2 days than at 4–8 weeks. Only a very small percentage of the latter birds infected with 10^4 organisms were found to be shedding them at any time. Stephens and Anderson (1967) inoculated newly hatched chicks in the yolk sacs with standardized suspensions of *S. anatum, S. heidelberg*, or *S. infantis* to determine if the growth patterns of the individual salmonella serotypes were associated with their relative degrees of pathogenicity. Growth patterns of the 3 serotypes were almost identical when each chick was inoculated with about 3.5×10^6 cells, but *S. heidelberg* was recovered more frequently from the liver and caused a much higher percentage of mortality than did either *S. anatum* or *S. infantis*. Results indicated that factors other than rate of multiplication in the yolk sac are responsible for observed differences between salmonella serotypes in degree of pathogenicity for chicks.

Snoeyenbos et al. (1969b) demonstrated

that 10 salmonella serotypes, a number of those most commonly found in poultry, were shown to spread rapidly from infected day-old chicks to pen mates reared on litter. Infection was almost always demonstrated in a majority or all contact chicks by the 3rd week of age. Mortality was confined chiefly to the infected principals and was low. Clinical signs of the infection were minimal or undetected.

Bierer and Eleazer (1965) were able to induce S. montevideo infection in week-old broiler chicks by feed and water deprivation. Brownell and Sadler (1967) also found that stressing chickens by water starvation before and after experimental infection with S. typhi-murium changed the pattern of fecal shedding of the organisms, which may make it more difficult to eliminate salmonellae from a flock.

Experimental efforts to produce chronic paratyphoid infections in both chicks and poults by oral administration of the organisms often result in the production of a disease of a transitory nature. During and a few weeks following the acute phase of infection, both tissues and intestinal cultures may readily yield positive isolations of the organisms administered. However, 1 or 2 months following oral infection most birds will be culturally negative. In actual field cases the course of the disease may be longer than would be expected under controlled experimental conditions.

Mortality from paratyphoid infection under natural conditions varies depending upon the environment, strain of infecting organism, and presence of concurrent infections. Schalm (1937) in studies of S. typhi-murium infection in chicks found a great contrast between the low mortality among chicks kept on the farm where hatched and the high mortality among chicks sold to others and transported to new quarters. Sieburth and Johnson (1957) found that the bluecomb agent, when administered to susceptible chicks in conjunction with S. typhi-murium, increased the mortality rate from 29 to 67%. Biddle and Cover (1957) reported the isolation of salmonella organisms from the respiratory tracts of chickens, some of which were infected with chronic respiratory disease.

Stephens et al. (1964) found that S. typhi-murium was recovered from the livers and spleens of chicks having concurrent coccidiosis infection more frequently than those inoculated with S. typhi-murium alone. It was felt that the coccidia may render the intestine more permeable to the salmonellae as occurs during certain vitamin deficiencies. Stephens and Vestal (1966) in further studies demonstrated that coccidiosis interferes with the rapid elimination of S. typhi-murium from the intestine and internal organs of chicks concurrently infected with these microorganisms.

Adult Birds

Adult birds infected with paratyphoid organisms generally show no outward symptoms; however, they may serve as intestinal carriers of the infection over long periods of time, as reported by Olesiuk et al. (1969). Paratyphoid infections exhibit no selectivity in their pathogenicity for specific strains or breeds of birds.

PATHOGENESIS AND EPIZOOTIOLOGY

NATURAL AND EXPERIMENTAL HOSTS

Paratyphoid infections occur in most species of warm- and cold-blooded animals. Many of the salmonella serotypes, particularly members of Kauffmann's subgenus II, have appeared only in cold-blooded animals. Buxton (1958), in discussing host specificity of salmonella strains, called attention to the need for fundamental information on the chemical pathology of the reactions between the bacteria and host tissues. It was felt that such information would provide a means of explaining the carrier state in salmonella infections. Edwards et al. (1948a) reported 111 serological types of salmonella which were encountered in a total of 47 warm- and cold-blooded animal species. Among domestic poultry, paratyphoid infections are most frequently encountered in turkeys and chickens.

Turkeys

Pfaff (1921) was the first to report on the occurrence of paratyphoid infection in turkeys. Rettger et al. (1933) described the disease in young poults in the United States. Lee et al. (1936) encountered an acute disease that caused 90% mortality among poults less than 5 weeks of age. In other flocks the losses were less, ranging from 40 to 70%. The organism recovered from the poults was found to be pathogenic for chicks, poults, guinea pigs, and rabbits.

Cherrington et al. (1937) found *S. typhi-murium* to be responsible for the loss of many poults on several turkey ranches in Idaho. The mortality was as high as 80% during the first week of brooding. Pomeroy and Fenstermacher (1939) first observed this infection in turkeys in Minnesota in 1932 when 4 poults were found infected with the disease. From 1932 to 1937 *S. typhi-murium* was recovered from poults which originated from 31 widely separated flocks. Hinshaw and McNeil (1943a) found that *S. typhi-murium* accounted for approximately 50% of the paratyphoid outbreaks in turkeys investigated by them. Hinshaw and McNeil (1943b) reported *S. newington* infection on 9 turkey ranches. The disease was apparently self-limiting and did not recur the following season. Gordon and Tucker (1957) isolated *S. infantis* from a turkey poult and cited this report as the first recorded isolation of this type from the turkey.

Chickens

There is little doubt that paratyphoid infections among chickens have existed for many years. Mazza (1899) was one of the first to describe a paratyphoid epizootic among chickens in various parts of northern Italy. He isolated an organism that was pathogenic for chickens and pigeons and possessed the biochemical characteristics of a salmonella. Pfeiler and Rehse (1913), Lütje (1921), and Spray and Doyle (1921) issued early reports of the recovery of paratyphoid organisms from chickens.

Doyle (1927) investigated an outbreak of *S. typhi-murium* infection in chicks and concluded that contaminated material might have been the means of introduction. Schalm (1937) reported a disease among chicks caused by an organism resembling *S. typhi-murium*.

Wilson (1944) reported several paratyphoid outbreaks in chicks due to *S. thompson* and one in which both *S. thompson* and *S. typhi-murium* were involved. Gordon and Buxton (1946) described the occurrence of *S. anatum*, *S. bareilly*, *S. california*, *S. london*, and *S. montevideo* for the first time in chicks in Great Britain, and the same authors (1945) isolated *S. thompson* on 44 occasions from 31 outbreaks of paratyphoid infection among chicks. The mortality varied from 20 to 80% and in one hatch a 100% loss occurred.

The incidence of paratyphoid in chickens has revealed an increase during recent years, as evidenced by the reports of Burr et al. (1957), Angstrom (1957), and Sieburth (1957a). Williams (1956 unpublished) investigated an outbreak of paratyphoid infection in chicks due to *S. typhi-murium*. The infection was confined to one large hatchery, and mortality varied from 10% among some hatches to as high as 90% among others. The virulence of the disease was apparently increased by repeated passage of the organism through succeeding generations of chicks. Van Roekel (1965) presented a comprehensive review of salmonellae in poultry and eggs.

Huygelen et al. (1958) described outbreaks of paratyphoid infection in chickens caused by 6 types of salmonellae. Mortality ranged from 12 to 75%, and attention was drawn to the role of these organisms in human food poisoning. Rao (1956) reported that *S. litchfield* infection in baby chicks caused a mortality of 50% on a large military poultry farm in India.

Geese and Ducks

Young geese and ducks are quite susceptible to paratyphoid infection, and outbreaks often become epizootic. Manninger (1918) reported the disease in 1–2-week-old ducks and geese and succeeded in isolating *S. paratyphi B* as the causative organism. Pfeiler (1920) and Weisgerber and Müller (1922) described outbreaks of paratyphoid infection in geese. Perek and Rabinovitz (1957) noted a mortality of 30% due to salmonellosis among young goslings during the first 3 weeks after hatching. Barckhausen (1961) isolated *S. typhi-murium* from the intestinal tract of a wild pale goose that he shot.

Rettger and Scoville (1920) described *S. anatum* as the cause of a disease in ducks known as "keel." This term has come to be accepted as a synonym for paratyphoid infection as it occurs in ducks. However, Price et al. (1962) have suggested that this is a misnomer as affected ducklings have clinical symptoms over a period of time and do not die suddenly ("keel over"), which was the origin of this terminology. Truscott (1956) reported a severe outbreak of *S. moscow* infection in ducklings. This salmonella type had not previously been identified from fowl in North America. In England and western Europe *S. enteritidis* in ducks has been reported by Warrack and Dalling (1933), Hohn and Herrmann (1935), Jansen (1936), and Clarenburg (1939).

Levine and Graham (1942) described an outbreak of paratyphoid in wood ducklings in which 400 of 500 birds died. S. typhi-murium was isolated from the heart blood and livers of a number of the ducklings. Garside and Gordon (1940) investigated an extensive outbreak of salmonellosis in ducklings. S. typhi-murium and S. enteritidis were recovered from the liver and pericardial fluid of a representative number of the birds examined. The losses among the 57,000 ducklings on one location were approximately 30% during the first month.

Edwards et al. (1948c) recorded 56 outbreaks of paratyphoid infection among ducks from which 90 cultures were examined. Of the 90 cultures, 62 were S. typhi-murium, and this type occurred in 32 of the 56 outbreaks. S. anatum was the second most frequent type and was involved in 8 outbreaks.

Dougherty (1953) reported that 38 of the 39 isolations of paratyphoids from ducks at the Long Island Duck Disease Research Laboratory during a 3-year period were S. typhi-murium. The other was S. give. Dougherty (1954) studied paratyphoid infection in the White Pekin duck. Mortality was found to start the first day after the ducks were out of the incubator. Losses varied from less than 1% to as high as 60%. Lucas (1956) described the loss of over 2,000 mallard ducklings on a private farm as the result of S. typhi-murium and S. anatum infections. Buxton (1957a) listed 31 types of paratyphoid organisms that have been isolated from ducks and 7 types from geese.

Brest Nielsen (1960) found S. typhi-murium to be the cause of high mortality among newly hatched mallard ducklings in Denmark. It was probable that the infection had been introduced with eggs from wild mallards. Dougherty (1961) has noted that paratyphoid infection is enzootic in the ducks on Long Island. Price et al. (1962) reported the isolation of 491 salmonella cultures from 7,029 accessions of ducks in New York during a 10-year period from 1950 to 1960; 93% of the cultures were S. typhi-murium and only 1% was S. anatum. Marthedal (1962) found that S. typhi-murium infection of ducklings and goslings in Denmark was 20 times as frequent as in

chicks during the period 1946–60. He suggested strict isolation of web-footed birds from chicks to prevent spread between species. Müller (1957b) indicated that ducks and other domesticated swimming birds appeared to be the primary source of S. typhi-murium infection in poultry in Denmark.

Pigeons

The first authentic report of pigeon paratyphoid was made by Moore (1895). He investigated a disease that affected squabs (and occasionally older pigeons) and was able to isolate an organism that was thought to be a variant of S. cholerae-suis. The pigeon fancier usually refers to paratyphoid infection as "megrims." Mohler (1904) reported an outbreak of paratyphoid in pigeons. Beaudette (1926b) described this disease in squabs, and Emmel (1929) associated salmonellosis in pigeons with arthritis.

Hoffmann and Edwards (1937) isolated paratyphoid organisms from pigeons which were believed to have transmitted the infection to rabbits on the same premises. Shirlaw and Iyer (1937) encountered an unusual loss among pigeons that were being used in the production of fowl pox vaccine. The organism isolated was S. enteritidis. Niemeyer (1939) recovered an organism from pigeons that was identified as S. typhi-murium. The organism was recovered from 3 of 14 pigeons examined.

Gauger et al. (1940) published a comprehensive study of pigeon paratyphoid. The etiological type was S. typhi-murium var. copenhagen. These authors listed 26 references to paratyphoid epizootics in pigeons. Edwards et al. (1948c) found that 97.5% of all cultures of S. typhi-murium isolated from pigeons were S. typhi-murium var. copenhagen. Moran (1961) reported a similar high incidence of this variety in pigeons. This organism, unlike typical S. typhi-murium strains, lacks the somatic antigen 5. It is a unique example of a paratyphoid type exhibiting host specificity, and has resulted in most investigators suspecting direct or indirect association with pigeons as the source of infection when this type is encountered in other species of animals. Van Dorssen (1955) reported a serological and cultural study of 223 S. typhi-murium strains isolated from pigeons in the Netherlands. He concluded that there does not exist any specific pigeon type of this organism as has been reported by some workers. Pigeons surviving paratyphoid outbreaks often become chronic carriers, excreting the organisms intermittently in their feces. Epizootics may occur among adult flocks, especially if their resistance is lowered by other conditions.

Faddoul and Fellows (1965) presented a review of paratyphoid infection in pigeons and reported that the greatest number of outbreaks in their 10-year study occurred in birds under 1 year of age.

Other Birds

Edwards et al. (1948c) reported 10 serological types of salmonella isolated from pheasants. *S. bredeney* was recovered from 7 outbreaks.

Graham (1936) studied an outbreak of paratyphoid among quail in which *S. oranienburg* was found to be the causative organism. Cunningham (1941) encountered an acute paratyphoid infection among quail chicks in which the heaviest mortality occurred in chicks 3–9 days old. *S. bredeney* was isolated as the causative organism.

Hinshaw et al. (1942) isolated *S. bredeney* and *S. typhi-murium* from a group of chukar chicks. This report clearly indicated the isolation of multiple salmonella types from a single outbreak wherein a 48.2% mortality occurred among a group of 1,061 chicks. Francis et al. (1960) reported the isolation of *S. derby* and *S. anatum* from chukar partridges.

Beaudette and Edwards (1926) investigated paratyphoid in canaries and parrots. In one bird store 200 birds of all ages became infected and mortality was 35%. *S. typhi-murium* was found to be the causative organism. Emmel and Stafseth (1929) reported several outbreaks of an epizootic of paratyphoid that occurred in canary bird stores throughout the state of Michigan. The disease was highly infectious, and the mortality was high. The incubation period was 4–5 days and the course of the disease varied from 2 to 4 days. *S. typhi-murium* was isolated from the internal organs.

Beaudette (1926a) reported that *S. typhi-murium* readily infected parrots as well as canaries. No differentiation could be made between the strains of *S. typhi-murium* isolated from the parrots and those previously isolated from canaries. Altman (1940) studied an outbreak of paratyphoid among a group of 170 canaries of all ages. The incidence of infection and mortality was greater in the young birds. Approximately 60% of the infected birds died. *S. cholerae-suis* was isolated as the etiological agent. Keymer (1959) reported that heavy losses occur in canaries and other passerine birds from *S. typhi-murium* infection. Meyer and Eddie (1934, 1939) reported the isolation of salmonella organisms from tropical psittacine birds including parrots, parrotlets, paroquets, and conures.

Meyer (1942), Buxton (1957a), and Kaye et al. (1961) have reported on the isolation of salmonella organisms from budgerigars (parakeets). Meyer (1942) demonstrated that 37% of parakeets from a single dealer were infected with *S. typhi-murium*. Burkhart et al. (1962) experimentally infected parakeets and canaries with *S. typhi-murium* and *S. heidelberg*. Stone (1960) cited salmonella as an infectious cause of gastroenteritis in parakeets as encountered in veterinary practice.

Buxton (1957a) reported the isolation of *S. panama, S. paratyphi B,* and *S. typhi* from sea birds. Brest Nielsen (1969) isolated *S. typhi-murium* from seagulls in Denmark, and Williams and Dodson (1960) reported the isolation of 3 salmonella types from gulls. Salisbury (1958) reported that from 1948 to 1957 *S. typhi-murium* was isolated from a seagull, mallard duck, pigeon, parakeet, goose, and pheasant as well as other species of poultry in New Zealand. Strauss et al. (1957) isolated *S. typhi-murium* from the black-headed gull. Muller (1965) reported gulls to be commonly infected with salmonellae.

Sieburth (1958a) was unable to isolate any salmonella organisms from the livers or intestines of 17 penguins cultured during a survey in the Antarctic region. A history of salmonellosis was suggested in the ringed penguin, skua gull, and 2 sheath bills by serological tests.

Hudson (1942) encountered an outbreak of paratyphoid infection among a flock of guinea fowl with a reported loss of 60 birds during a period of 6 weeks. *S. bredeney* was isolated from the infraorbital sinuses.

Manninger (1913) examined the intestinal flora of various birds. From 3 birds belonging to the family of finches he recovered *S. paratyphi B.* Keymer (1959) reported that he has observed *S. typhi-murium* infection in the gouldian finch, the black-crested finch, the cordon bleu, the cut-throat, and the domestic variety of the Bengalese finch. Gordon and Buxton (1946) reported the isolation of paratyphoid organisms from a sparrow. Deom (1960) isolated a strain of *S. california* from a sparrow for the first time in the Congo. Dózsa (1961) reported the isolation of *S. typhi-murium* from the intestinal tract of 52 of 266 captured sparrows in Budapest. Edwards et al. (1948c) reported the isolation of paratyphoids from the following avian species not mentioned above: a peafowl, partridges, Japanese robins, a secretary bird, a diamond dove, a yellow-winged sugar bird, and callistes. Moran (1961) reported the isolation of *S. typhi-murium* from the following types of "other birds": cockatoo, hoatzin, hornbill, and parrot.

Cope et al. (1955) in a study of salmonella in zoo birds, animals, and reptiles isolated 8 types of paratyphoid from a total of 20 species of fowl maintained in the Detroit Zoological Park. Csiszár et al. (1961) studied salmonellosis among birds of a zoological garden and found that approximately 27% of the infected birds exhibited gastroenteritis. Such infections were not deemed to constitute a hazard to zoo visitors, but the danger for attendant personnel was stressed. Bigland et al. (1962), following a typing survey in Alberta, Canada, extending for 12 years, expressed the opinion that salmonella organisms are seldom found in free-living wild birds and animals. Wilson and Macdonald (1967) reported 4 outbreaks of *S. typhi-murium* infection in wild birds involving greenfinches and sparrows. These authors concluded that while salmonellosis in wild birds is a potential hazard to man and domestic animals, the low incidence of the disease in the general population of wild birds suggests that they are not an important reservoir of the pathogens.

Hudson and Tudor (1957) isolated *S. typhi-murium* from several varieties of free-flying birds including starlings, sparrows, rusty blackbirds, and a cowbird originating from 4 outbreaks in 3 areas of north central New Jersey during a period of 2 years. They called attention to the possibility that these birds may spread the infection to man and domestic animals. Vallée et al. (1959) reported the isolation of *S. johannesburg* from Bengali birds during an enzootic in a commercial bird shop. No treatment was found effective. Petzelt and Steininger (1961) isolated 18 types of salmonella from chaffinches, house sparrows, black-headed gulls, starlings, and blackbirds captured in the area of a sewage purification plant of a big city.

Wilson and Macdonald (1967) reviewed literature on reports of salmonella infections in wild birds. Faddoul et al. (1966) in a 5-year survey reported the isolation of salmonellae from a chukar, pigeon, pheasant, canary, gull, duck, hornbill, parakeet, sparrow, and cowbird among other avian species. Wilson and Macdonald (1967) reported *S. typhi-murium* infection from house sparrows, a feral pigeon, a herring gull, a wood pigeon, 2 gannets, and a number of greenfinches. Snoeyenbos et al. (1967a) isolated salmonellae from wild grackles, cowbirds, starlings, and gulls in Massachusetts with sufficient frequency to suggest that these avian species may play a role in the epidemiology of salmonellosis in domestic poultry. Macdonald et al. (1968) described a severe outbreak of salmonellosis due to *S. hessarek* in blackbirds, starlings, and house sparrows in Scotland. Wilson and Macdonald (1967) found *S. typhi-murium* in feral pigeons, greenfinches, a tawny owl, a hooded crow, a rook, a red-throated diver, a mallard, and a mute swan. The organism was also isolated from the viscera of two mice in the gizzard of the tawny owl.

The reader seeking additional historical information on paratyphoid outbreaks in various species of fowl is referred to the comprehensive review of Henning (1939).

Other Animals

Unlike the causative organisms of pullorum disease and fowl typhoid, the paratyphoids are common pathogens of most species of domestic and wild mammals. Cattle, swine, sheep, goats, dogs, cats, horses, mink, and foxes are among the many animal species that may be chronically infected and shed the organisms in large numbers in their feces. In these animals paratyphoid usually occurs as an acute disease only in the very young or in old, debilitated animals under extreme conditions of stress. A voluminous amount of literature has been accumulated on salmonella infections of animals other than poultry, and for a review of this subject the reader is referred to Buxton (1957a). Schnurrenberger et al. (1968) reported that in 26 instances salmonellae were isolated from 976 domestic animals, 325 wild birds, 253 wild mammals, and 217 feed samples during a survey of 7 farms in 6 Illinois counties. The organisms were recovered from opossums, rats, a beef steer, cats, a pig, a starling, and pelleted feed samples. There was little evidence of interspecific transmission of salmonellosis.

Craige (1944), Wolff et al. (1948), Adler et al. (1951), Galton et al. (1952), Stucker et al. (1952), McElrath et al. (1952), and Mackel et al. (1952) have reported studies of paratyphoid isolations from the feces of dogs. Dogs and cats often carry salmonella organisms in their digestive tract without showing any clinical symptoms. Bruner and Moran (1949) reported 26 salmonella types recovered from dogs. Approximately 40% of the cultures were *S. typhi-murium*. Thirty-four cultures isolated from cats included 17 salmonella serotypes. Jungerman and Grumbles (1960) isolated salmonella organisms from 9 of 100 mature healthy dogs studied. Two of the dogs were infected with more than 1 type. The infection was of a transient nature and cultures were negative 6 weeks later. Baker et al. (1966) reported the isolation of *S. chester* from a red fox at the entrance of a turkey house where this type had been a problem.

Rats and mice are frequently intestinal carriers of paratyphoid organisms, particularly *S. typhi-murium* and *S. enteritidis*. When *S. enteritidis* is encountered in poultry it is logical to suspect these rodents as a possible source of the infection. Sato (1967a) demonstrated that wild rats could be readily infected experimentally with *S. newington* and *S. enteritidis* with fecal excretion and final localization of the infecting organisms in the submaxillary nodes.

Insects

Salmonellae have also been isolated from various insects including flies, fleas, and cockroaches. It is known that *S. enteritidis* can be transmitted through the complete life cycle of flies and that the infection may continue as long as 4 weeks within flies (Ostrolenk and Welch, 1942; Greenberg, 1959). Greenberg et al. (1963), Greenberg (1964), and Greenberg and Bornstein (1964) noted that salmonellae persisted in flies from the maggot to the adult stage, and found that the organisms could be recovered from tagged flies up to 3 miles from their point of origin. Twelve salmonella serotypes were recovered from domestic flies in a Mexican slaughterhouse, and it was demonstrated that *S. typhi-murium* could be transmitted from dog feces to man by flies.

Kaye et al. (1961) noted paratyphoid isolations from the housefly, tick, louse, flea, and cockroach. Buxton (1957a) cited references indicating that ticks may remain carriers for more than 30 days after oral infection. Casas et al. (1968) demonstrated that the lesser mealworm *Alphitobius diaperinus* (Panzer), alive or dead, can be a carrier of *S. typhi-murium* with a potential for contaminating feed for poultry flocks and food for humans. Julseth et al. (1969) reported that the hide beetle *Dermestes maculatus* can be a carrier of salmonellae and might be infected and potentially harbor the organisms for long periods in environments which all types of poultry inhabit.

Reptiles

McNeil and Hinshaw (1946) isolated *S. san-diego* and *S. newport* from Galapagos turtles, *S. montevideo* from a Gila monster, and *S. manhattan* from an iguana. Hinshaw and McNeil (1945) examined 41 snakes caught on ranches in 7 localities in California; 11 of the snakes yielded salmonellae on culture. Bövre and Sandbu (1959) isolated 19 types of salmonella from 27 tortoises in Oslo. Feeley and Treger (1969) demonstrated that *S. braenderup* could penetrate through the shell of turtle eggs and infect the egg contents.

Man

Most of the salmonella types recovered from poultry have also been found to infect man, causing gastroenteritis or occasionally a more serious septicemic type infection. Turkey, chicken, eggs and egg products, which together were responsible for 48% of the food-borne outbreaks of human salmonellosis reported in 1967, accounted for 33.8% of all nonhuman isolations (Anon., 1968b). Edwards (1958) and Quist (1962) reported a 7-fold increase of salmonella infections other than typhoid fever in humans in the United States from 1949 to 1960 and noted that these infections in poultry constitute the major source of human disease. Quist (1963) indicated that the sources most often incriminated in food-borne outbreaks of salmonellosis in the United States are poultry and poultry products.

Salmonellosis has been cited as one of the most frequent and important causes of food poisoning in humans and has been estimated to cause financial losses of $10–100 million a year (Eickhoff, 1966). A later report (Anon., 1969b) has set the economic loss from the disease in man at $300 million due to about 2 million human salmonellosis cases annually. Botes (1965) suggested that the domestic fowl is one of the important, if not the most important, avenues of salmonellosis in humans and cited 15 references in support of this. The role of poultry products and eggs in the transmission of salmonella infections to man has been reviewed by McCullough (1958), Galton et al. (1964), Botes (1965), Taylor (1967), and Edwards and Galton (1967).

Direct transmission of salmonella infections from fowl to humans has occasionally been reported. Hinshaw et al. (1944) recorded the transmission of 2 types of paratyphoids (*S. panama* and *S. montevideo*) to man, believed to have occurred as a result of handling infected poults. Kaye et al. (1961) described a case of *S. typhi-murium* infection in an infant who was allowed to crawl in the droppings of a pet parakeet that was infected. Hinshaw and McNeil (1948, 1951) recorded 7 cases of gastroenteritis among poultry caretakers resulting from contact with acute outbreaks of paratyphoid in fowl. Darby and Stafseth (1942) reviewed the literature with reference to 35 types of the genus *Salmonella* found in poultry in the United States. Most of these types have also been incriminated in pathological conditions in man. Anderson et al. (1955) reported several cases of *S. typhimurium* infection in children, with a likely source of the infection being Easter chicks. *S. typhi-murium* was recovered from the stools of the children and also the chicks. Gordon and Tucker (1965) demonstrated that with the increased occurrence of *S. menston* in poultry the incidence in man also increased in Great Britain.

PROCESSING PLANTS AND MARKETED POULTRY. Gunderson et al. (1954) and Galton et al. (1955) have discussed the occurrence and distribution of paratyphoid organisms in poultry processing plants. Florin and Nilsson (1959) cited the very important influence of techniques in slaughter on the contamination of carcasses in the case of intestinal salmonellosis of poultry. Recognizing this fact, many poultry processing plants in the United States have established laboratory control testing services to monitor the presence of salmonella organisms in their operations.

Brobst et al. (1958) were successful in isolating salmonellae from chickens and ducks being prepared for market as well as from vats in poultry processing plants in western Pennsylvania. They concluded that potentially these salmonellae are a serious menace to those who handle the birds and to the families that may receive them. Van Keulen (1959) described the role played by animal-borne salmonellosis in human infections. Attention was drawn to the significance of infection through the medium of foodstuffs of poultry and animal origin, whether primarily or secondarily infected. Better hygiene in the production and handling of foodstuffs of animal origin was stressed. McCroan et al. (1963) noted that measures to avoid the contamination of animal feeds and improved sanitary and decontamination practices in abattoirs and poultry processing plants would materially reduce the number of grossly infected animal carcasses now being marketed.

Morris and Ayres (1960) found that 0–9% of the samples obtained from turkey processing plants and 7–14% of the samples from chicken processing plants were positive on culture for salmonellae. Specimens were taken from 10 sampling stations including the scald tanks, carcass surfaces, and final rinse water. Twenty-eight salmonella cultures were isolated from chickens and 12 from turkeys. Dixon and Pooley (1961) isolated salmonella organisms from 13.8% of 544 specimens taken at a poultry plant in Great Britain.

No salmonella or arizona organisms were isolated from the livers of fresh market poultry (turkeys and chickens) being processed in 1 of 8 processing plants on 67 days over a period of 4 years (Sadler et al., 1965). The same findings were reported by Salzer et al. (1964) following the culturing of 200 turkey giblet samples. In a continuation of an earlier survey of market poultry for salmonellae and arizonae, Sadler and Corstvet (1965) isolated these organisms from fecal specimens of 5.25% of turkeys, 0.54% of chicken hens, and 1.05% of chicken fryers in 8 large federally inspected processing plants.

Glezen et al. (1966) surveyed for salmonella contamination in 2 poultry processing plants following a febrile gastroenteritis outbreak in humans thought to be due to salmonellae originating from chicken served at a supper. Only 4 of 1,017 samples from various areas in a large well-equipped plant yielded salmonellae, but from a smaller plant, 208 (21%) of 1,000 specimens were infected with the organisms. In the smaller plant, methods of processing permitted a few infected birds to contaminate many others during the washing and chilling procedures. Wilder and MacCready (1966) found poultry and frozen whole egg to be frequent reservoirs of salmonellae in Massachusetts. Bacteriologic examinations of 2,057 samples from within poultry processing plants yielded 230 (11.2%) cultures positive for salmonellae. Glezen et al. (1966) reported that salmonellae do not persist or multiply in poultry processing plants if the daily clean-up procedures are adequate. Even in plants that from time to time show a high degree of salmonella contamination, the organisms are prevalent only periodically. Better practices and equipment in poultry processing plants would decrease gross contamination of dressed birds. Magwood et al. (1967) found that 6 of 345 market chicken carcasses received from processing plants across Canada yielded salmonellae. Examinations of surfaces and samples from the plants gave positive salmonella isolations from 25 (14%). The evidence indicated that salmonella-infected flocks were frequently slaughtered and that salmonella contamination could become widespread in a plant during processing. Most of the organisms were eliminated during processing, but opportunity exists for recontamination during subsequent handling.

Thomson et al. (1967) studied the effects of 6 decontaminating chemicals and distilled water on a suspension of S. *typhimurium* inoculated on the breast skin surface of broilers. A significant reduction in salmonella counts was effected by spraying all treatment solutions, including distilled water. Carcasses sprayed with 100 and 200 ppm chlorine showed significantly reduced salmonella counts compared with unsprayed controls and with carcasses sprayed with distilled water. Nilsson and Regner (1963) and Wabeck et al. (1968) have also reported on the use of chlorine to destroy salmonellae on dressed chicken and turkey carcasses. Woodburn and Stadelman (1968) reported the isolation of salmonellae from both the production and processing facilities for broilers and ducklings in 4 plants. Retail birds were also found to be infected. The patterns of recovery indicated that good sanitation and equipment lowered the incidence of salmonellae on the retail product but did not eliminate in-plant contamination. In the poultry houses it was suggested that thorough cleaning and sanitizing are needed between broods, since salmonellae can frequently be recovered from dry house dust as well as litter, waterers, and feeders.

Bryan et al. (1968) investigated farms supplying turkeys to a processing plant where salmonellae were frequently detected. Salmonella cultures of the same serotype were found in the feed and water on the farm, in feces taken from delivery trucks, processed turkey products, and plant processing equipment. Subsequent spray washing did not remove all the salmonella organisms.

Galbraith (1961) noted that salmonella infections of humans are usually conveyed by the contamination of food with intestinal contents of animals. Yet the cycle of infection from animals to man is often long and devious and despite full investigation may remain obscure. Felsenfeld et al. (1950), in a survey of salmonella organisms in market meat, eggs, and milk, called attention to the need for proper inspection of certain foods intended for human consumption. Brandly (1951) and Dolman (1954) have also emphasized the public health significance of salmonella infections of poultry. Abelseth and Robertson (1953) implicated S. *typhi-murium* infection of turkeys as a definite public health hazard.

Cherry et al. (1946) isolated a nonmotile salmonella from frozen turkeys. Browne (1949) was able to isolate salmonellae from the skin of turkeys that had been frozen for 13 months. Schneider and Gunderson (1949) recovered 4 salmonella types from the skin of 4.4% of 1,014 eviscerated chickens. Felsenfeld (1949) reported a case of human infection with *S. cubana* from eating a New York dressed chicken infected with this organism.

Savage (1956) noted that the incidence of salmonella food poisoning in Great Britain was increasing. Meat and egg products were cited as the chief sources of the infection in man. Canale-Parola and Ordal (1957) found 5 of 40 poultry pies sampled to contain salmonella organisms. They recommended that manufacturers improve technology and sanitary procedures used in preparing the pies and give longer baking periods. Similar studies have been reported by Litsky et al. (1957). Beloian and Schlosser (1963) reported that baked foods that reach a temperature of 71° C (160° F) or higher in the slowest heating region can be considered safe from any salmonella organisms that may be present in the ingredients. Woodburn et al. (1962) found that 10 minutes in boling water destroyed salmonellae in boned chicken packaged in polyester polyethylene laminated bags.

Mackel et al. (1959) studied an outbreak of human gastroenteritis due to *S. typhi-murium* among 300 inmates of a penal institution. The patients had eaten roasted turkey which had been sliced on the same chopping block on which the uncooked fowl had been prepared. Those persons eating only reheated meat did not become ill. *S. typhi-murium* was recovered from more than 100 persons who had eaten the meat as well as from turkey necks that had been frozen. Spink (1960) traced an outbreak of *S. thompson* infection involving 35 people in Great Britain to a broiler shop. The organism was isolated from cooked chicken, the manager of the shop, his assistant, and from living broilers at a packing station supplying the shop.

Tailyour and Avery (1960) cultured the viscera and intestinal contents of 523 market-weight turkeys in Vancouver, British Columbia, for salmonella. Four birds (0.76%) were found to be harboring *S. derby*. Wilson et al. (1961) found approximately 17% of 525 raw poultry specimens in the Cincinnati area contaminated with salmonellae. Eighteen serotypes were encountered during the study, and isolations showed an increasing trend from supermarket through general store, meat market, and poultry market. Eight percent of

household turkey specimens were positive for salmonella. Sadler et al. (1961) random-sampled market meat birds for salmonella organisms. Infected or carrier birds were found being processed on 43% of the sampling days for turkeys, 26% for chicken fryers, and 12% for hens.

Morris and Ayres (1960) and Wilson et al. (1961) have reviewed the incidence of salmonellae in commercially processed poultry and poultry products. Woodburn (1964) isolated salmonellae from 72 (27%) of 264 broiler-fryer type chickens that were purchased in retail stores in Indiana in 1963; 13 different serotypes were identified, the more common being *S. infantis, S. reading,* and *S. blockley.* Baker et al. (1966) found a high percentage of culled turkeys to be infected with salmonellae. Saulmon (1966b) pointed out the public health danger of human food contamination resulting from poultry without clinical signs or pathologic evidence of disease that might otherwise be detected during inspection.

Walker (1960) called attention to the increased incidence of salmonellosis in humans in Great Britain, and cautioned that the use of antibiotics in broiler rations is resulting in the emergence of resistant salmonella strains. Such strains may cause an increase in the carrier rate and may multiply more rapidly in contaminated carcasses. It has been suggested (Anon., 1961) that the carcasses of poultry for the market may be immersed in slush ice containing 10 ppm of chlortetracycline for 2 hours to inhibit the growth of salmonellae. Attention is called to the development of chlortetracycline-resistant salmonella strains when this drug is given to birds as a feed additive. Garside et al. (1960) reported that birds receiving antibiotics for the prevention or treatment of salmonella infections may be a public health hazard because of the large number of infected carrier birds remaining in such flocks.

EGGS AND EGG PRODUCTS. Raw, frozen, and dried eggs are rather frequently implicated in salmonella infections in man. Cockburn (1965) has presented an early historical tracing of human salmonella infections due to contaminated eggs and egg products. An outbreak due to raw eggs containing *S. tennessee* was reported by Watt (1945). Blaxland and Blowers (1951) implicated *S. typhi-murium* in duck eggs as a cause of human food infection. Such occurrences have been frequently reported in Europe. Salmonellosis in man has also been reported following the consumption of pudding containing infected pigeon eggs (Clarenburg and Dornickx, 1932).

The occurrence of salmonellae in egg powder has been extensively studied by Schneider (1946) and Solowey et al. (1946, 1947). McCullough and Eisele (1951a,b,c,d), in detailed clinical studies of experimental salmonellosis in human volunteers, were able to establish the pathogenicity of 6 salmonella types which had been isolated from spray-dried whole egg powder. Cultures were administered in graduated doses in eggnogs, and the following salmonella types were used in these studies: *S. meleagridis, S. anatum, S. newport, S. derby, S. bareilly,* and *S. pullorum.*

Alves de Oliveira and Gomes (1954) described a hospital epidemic of *S. typhimurium* infection involving 200 persons and resulting in 3 deaths. The outbreak was traced to eggs consumed in the diet. Newell et al. (1955) traced 2 outbreaks of paratyphoid fever *(S. paratyphi B)* in humans to the consumption of cream-filled cakes. The same phage type of *S. paratyphi B* was found in unopened cans of Chinese frozen whole egg used by the bakeries, in some members of the staff, and in the patients. Buxton (1957b) called attention to the fact that human foods composed of eggs and egg products are a common source of salmonella food infection in man. It was emphasized that the rate of infection is much higher among eggs with cracked and fecal-contaminated shells than among those laid under clean, hygienic conditions.

McCullough (1958) discussed the importance of poultry and poultry products, especially eggs, in the epidemiology of salmonellosis in humans in the United States. In one epidemiological investigation, *S. infantis* was isolated from poultry feedstuffs, eggs, and patients that had eaten lightly cooked and uncooked egg products (Newell et al., 1959). Taylor (1960) called attention to the importance of eggs and egg products in the transmission of salmonella infections to man. It was noted that the infection is more often traced to frozen eggs, dried eggs, and other egg products.

Philbrook et al. (1960) reported an outbreak of *S. typhi-murium* food poisoning traced to infected chicken eggs consumed in

eggnogs by patients at an institution in Massachusetts. Eggnogs consumed in the institution are now pasteurized. Fey and Wiesmann (1960) described a family outbreak of salmonellosis in Switzerland caused by imported egg powder which contained 5 different salmonella types. Attention has been called (Anon., 1961) to the public health significance of salmonellae in poultry and the fact that eggs that may be contaminated with the organisms should be cooked well. Hobbs (1961) referred to the importance of poultry products in transmitting salmonellosis to humans, and listed pasteurization of egg products and the pelleting of animal feeds as factors that would help to reduce this transmission. Galbraith (1961) cited bulk egg products as an important source of salmonella organisms for humans in Great Britain. Thatcher and Montford (1962) reported that 14 different salmonella types were isolated from 119 egg-containing cake mixes of which 65 contained salmonellae. The importance of breaking the animal-to-animal chain of infection in the control of salmonellosis was emphasized.

Taylor (1963) has reviewed the salmonella serotypes isolated from egg products and found in human infections in the United Kingdom. During a hospital-associated epidemic of *S. derby* infection (Anon., 1963a) in the United States it was recommended that cracked and unclean eggs should not be used. It was further suggested that commercial products containing eggs or egg products should be cooked well. McCroan et al. (1963) described 5 poultry-related outbreaks of salmonellosis in humans directly traceable to egg powder, fresh eggs, baby chicks, and mature chickens. Gandon (1963) outlined measures that should be taken to improve the freedom of eggs and egg products from salmonella organisms.

Galton et al. (1964) have reviewed the public health aspects of salmonellosis in man as related to poultry and eggs. Rizk et al. (1966b) have noted that the incidence of salmonellae on or in market eggs depends on the environmental condition of the eggs, handling and storage, and physical structure of the shell. Ayres et al. (1967) traced 2 large salmonellosis outbreaks to contaminated frozen egg products used to prepare baked meringue pies. Contaminated poultry rations fed to supply flocks and the bulk handling of cracked and dirty eggs without pasteurization were blamed for the outbreaks cited. Salmonella isolations were reported from liquid egg products and an egg breaking machine.

CONTROL OF INFECTIONS IN POULTRY PRODUCTS. Procedures involved in the destruction of salmonellae in all types of egg products and various poultry meats were thoroughly reviewed during the Conference on Destruction of Salmonellae held in 1966 at Albany, California (Anon., 1966). Cunningham et al. (1965) have discussed the pasteurization of liquid egg white for the destruction of salmonella contaminants. Regulations regarding pasteurization of egg products for destruction of salmonellae have been reviewed by Edwards and Galton (1967). McCroan et al. (1963) have pointed out that currently the protection of man against salmonella infections depends on proper cooking and handling of poultry, eggs, and meat by housewives, on adequate disinfection of uncanned meat by commercial processors, and on use of properly processed egg or animal products in uncooked foods.

Bowmer (1964) presented a comprehensive review of the challenge of salmonellosis as a disease of poultry and other animals and as a major public health problem. He listed 50 recommendations for the control and ultimate eradication of salmonella infections with specific responsibilities for the 10 official groups involved in implementing the recommendations made. Glezen et al. (1966) and Malhotra et al. (1968) have suggested that the elimination of salmonellae from animal by-products and poultry feeds would decrease the likelihood of infection of poultry before processing and at the same time lessen the public health hazard presently existent in poultry products.

Saulmon (1966b) thoroughly reviewed control programs for salmonellosis in poultry and other animals and animal products as these relate to the elimination of salmonellosis as one of the foremost public health problems of animal origin. In a related report Saulmon (1966a) discussed the activities of the USDA salmonella work group in developing recommendations on elimination of salmonellae from animal feeds and environments as a contribution to the better control of the disease in man. It has

been suggested (Anon., 1967a) that until the attainment of virtually salmonella-free animals is possible, a high standard of sanitation should be maintained on rearing and production farms, during transport, in holding pens, during slaughter, in meat processing plants, butcher shops, supermarkets, restaurants, and homes.

A 330-page report (Anon., 1969b) from the National Academy of Sciences points toward major new government efforts to reduce salmonella contamination in eggs, poultry meat, and other foods and also as an environmental pollutant. Taylor (1967) noted that the greatest reduction in human infection is expected to follow the application of simple hygienic principles at all stages from the birth of the food animal to the appearance of the cooked meal on the plate of the consumer.

TRANSMISSION, CARRIERS, VECTORS

The wide distribution of paratyphoid organisms under natural conditions contributes materially to their rapid spread. Bowmer (1964) has noted that most poultry flocks are exposed to salmonella organisms at some stage of their lives. Preventive efforts to be successful must give first consideration to the means by which the disease is transmitted. A significant symposium (Anon., 1963b) on the epidemiology of salmonellosis in poultry, other animals, and man was held during the American Public Health Association meeting in 1962.

The frequent isolation of paratyphoid organisms from eggs has resulted in reference to the disease as an egg-borne infection. However, in consideration of the spread of paratyphoid infections through the medium of the egg, it is important that a distinction be drawn between direct ovarian transmission and transmission through shell penetration.

Direct Ovarian Transmission

DUCKS. Numerous investigators (Dalling and Warrack, 1932; McGaughey, 1932; Warrack and Dalling, 1933) have recovered paratyphoid organisms from the yolk of duck eggs, providing ample evidence that direct ovarian transmission is quite common in this species. Hole (1932) and Clarenburg (1939) have also shown that duck eggs may be infected as a result of localization of the organism in the ovary.

TURKEYS. Paratyphoid infections of turkeys may occasionally be directly transmitted through the ovaries. However, experimental evidence does not indicate that infected turkeys produce a high percentage of infected eggs. Cherrington et al. (1937) reported the isolation of *S. typhi-murium* from the ovaries of two turkeys. The results of these investigations indicated that the infection was transmitted from the ovaries of the breeding hens to fertile eggs. Lee et al. (1936) investigated the direct ovarian transmission of *S. typhi-murium* infection of turkeys and were able to recover the organism from the ovarian tissues of infected hens. Pomeroy and Fenstermacher (1939) reported the isolation of *S. typhi-murium* from the ovaries and oviducts of 3 of 10 naturally infected turkeys. Hinshaw and McNeil (1943a) were able to isolate *S. typhi-murium* from the ovaries and oviducts of turkeys. Gauger and Greaves (1946a) isolated *S. typhi-murium* from the ovary of a turkey hen. Yamamoto et al. (1961a) reported the isolation of *S. typhi-murium* from the ovaries of an adult turkey that was experimentally infected.

CHICKENS. There is little evidence in the literature to suggest that direct ovarian transmission is a common occurrence in chickens. Wilson (1950) reported the isolation of *S. typhi-murium* from chicken eggs and suggested the possibility of direct ovarian transmission. Taylor (1967) has also suggested that salmonella serotypes may become established in a chicken flock causing an infection of the ovary which results in direct transmission of such organisms as *S. typhi-murium, S. thompson,* and *S. menston* through the egg. Clarenburg and Romijn (1954) were successful on one occasion in isolating *S. bareilly* from the ovary of an infected chicken. Others have made similar reports; however, isolations of paratyphoid organisms from ovarian tissues of chickens are not common. This is in direct contrast to the cycle of pullorum disease in chickens.

Mundt and Tugwell (1958) were unable to recover salmonellae from the contents of eggs laid by White Leghorn pullets experimentally infected orally and intravenously with various types of paratyphoid organisms. However, the organisms were recovered from shells of eggs laid by the most severely infected group 24 days after infection and from feces 35 days after infection. Smyser and Van Roekel (1959) cultured eggs of reacting chickens from a flock known to be infected with *S. typhi-murium*. The organism was isolated from egg contents on one occasion.

Forsythe et al. (1967) were unable to establish a localized infection of the reproductive tracts of hens by direct ovarian inoculation of *S. anatum*. None of the eggs produced by such hens was contaminated with *S. anatum*. Ovarian inoculation with *S. pullorum* resulted in an ovarian infection and the production of eggs containing these organisms.

Snoeyenbos et al. (1969a) isolated motile salmonellae from the ovary, peritoneal cavity, or both sites from a total of 63 semimature or mature chickens of 1,050 submitted for bacteriological examination as reactors to the pullorum-typhoid tube agglutination test. In a few cases pathological ovarian follicles were found and the pathogen was isolated on direct plate cultures. It was suggested that at least some nonhost-adapted salmonellae produce local infections of the ovary and peritoneum of laying chickens which allows contamination of the egg contents prior to shell formation. Although the incidence of such infection is probably low, these studies suggest that true egg transmission may sometimes contribute to the transmission of avian salmonellosis.

Eggshell Contamination and Penetration

FECAL CARRIER. Fecal contamination of eggshells with paratyphoid organisms during the process of laying or from contaminated nests, floors, or incubators after laying is of foremost importance in the spread of the disease. Intestinal carriers of the organisms are common (Gauger and Greaves, 1946c, 1947; Gibbons and Moore, 1946; Chase, 1947). Buxton and Gordon (1947) reported an instance in which *S. thompson* infected the gallbladder of a chicken and the organisms were excreted in the feces for at least 18 months. Yamamoto et al. (1961a) inoculated *S. typhi-murium* into the crop of adult turkeys and found that the organisms were generally shed in higher numbers in the cecal than in the other intestinal feces. Cloacal swabs were positive (83.4%) at 14 days and also (27.8%) at autopsy 35–

44 days postinoculation. Total positive isolations were increased to 67% when all methods of culture (swab, direct fecal, and visceral organs) were considered.

Perek and Rabinovitz (1957) were able to obtain positive fecal cultures of *S. enteritidis* for a period of 3 months from a naturally infected adult flock of geese. After 7 months fecal cultures were negative. Bacteriological examination of all internal organs was also negative at that time. Pulst (1960) found that geese infected orally with *S. typhi-murium* excreted the organism for 18–26 days after infection, and one goose became a chronic carrier. All of the birds developed agglutinin titers which disappeared in about 4 weeks. Yamamoto et al. (1961a) found that *S. typhi-murium* could be recovered from the surface of eggs laid by experimentally infected adult turkeys; however, subsequent culture of the contents of incubated eggs yielded negative results.

Forsythe et al. (1967) were unable to isolate *S. lexington* and *S. anatum* from the reproductive organs of chickens infected orally with the organisms. However, salmonellae were recovered from the feces of these birds, indicating that indirect contamination of egg contents is possible by shell contamination. Wilson (1945) isolated *S. typhi-murium* and *S. thompson* from the outside of eggshells and suggested that the mixing of such eggs with clean eggs is a means of spreading the infection in the incubator.

Mellor and Banwart (1965) were unable to recover *S. derby* from the shells of eggs or egg meats from hens that received the organisms by feeding and by inoculation. Neither was *S. derby* recovered from any of the hens upon sacrifice or from any of the chicks from these hens. *S. derby* was found in the feces of 2 birds receiving contaminated feed and 4 birds given a weekly inoculation of the organism. Olesiuk et al. (1969) reported only a very few fresh or incubated eggs, out of thousands cultured, to carry *S. typhi-murium* organisms in flocks experimentally infected and containing fecal carriers. Board et al. (1964) reported the isolation of only one salmonella strain, *S. senftenberg*, from the shell of a lightly soiled egg during an extensive survey of microbial contamination of eggshells and egg packing materials.

Forsythe et al. (1967) suggested from their work that the main source of salmonella contamination of the contents of chicken eggs is shell contamination resulting from fecal contact. Mellor and Banwart (1965) concluded that most of the salmonellae infecting eggs are not interior but shell surface contamination. Smyser et al. (1966) isolated *S. heidelberg* from the contents of only a small percentage of eggs laid by hens known to be intestinal carriers of the organisms. Most of the isolations from the shell surfaces resulted from the eggs being contaminated in the nests. Gordon and Tucker (1965) found 200 (5.6%) of 3,584 stored eggs laid by poultry which had received food contaminated with *S. menston* to be infected with the organism. The majority of the isolations were made from the shells of the eggs.

SHELL PENETRATION. Schalm (1937) was able to demonstrate that *S. typhi-murium* in fecal material smeared on the surface of chicken eggs was capable of penetrating the shell and multiplying within the egg. These findings suggested a means by which paratyphoid organisms might be introduced into the incubator by contaminated eggs with subsequent spread to the hatched chicks or poults. Board (1964) described two phases involving multiplication of invading bacteria in the course of shell membrane penetration and infection of the egg contents by salmonellae and other bacterial types. The second phase began when the yolk made contact with the shell membranes. An historical review dating to 1895 of experimental studies of salmonella penetration of chicken eggshells has been presented by Williams et al. (1968).

Rizk et al. (1966a) used brightened salmonella cells to infect the surface of eggs, and the fluorescent spots of bacterial growth were subsequently detected using ultraviolet light. Williams and Whittemore (1967) described procedures for experimental study of the penetration of salmonella organisms through the outer egg structures. These methods, designed to closely simulate natural conditions, were based on the use of chicken feces containing salmonella organisms which were used to infect the egg surface. Penetration into three areas of the outer egg structures was subsequently determined after varying periods and conditions of incubation.

Maclaury and Moran (1959) found that freshly laid eggs, cooling in contact with contaminating organisms, will draw the organisms through the shell openings. The bacteria may be recovered on the day of contamination from the inside of the shells of 84–95% of the eggs. Beach (1936) also called attention to the role of contamination on the eggshell in the transmission of the infection. Buxton and Gordon (1947) noted that the average diameter of the pores of chicken eggs varied from 6 to 13μ, which would readily permit paratyphoid organisms to penetrate the shell when conditions are favorable. Shell imperfections of larger dimensions exist on most eggs, affording areas which can be easily penetrated by salmonellae.

Wilson (1948) reported the examination of 1,023 chicken eggs, from 60 of which *S. thompson* was isolated; 45 yielded the organism from the outside of the shell and 17 from the contents. It was felt that penetration of the shell readily occurred as the eggs were stored for a period of 14 days and no effort was made to keep the various eggs apart. Cantor and McFarlane (1948) isolated strains of *S. montevideo* and *S. anatum* from 13 (0.6%) of 2,132 samples of eggshell scrapings. Bigland and Papas (1953) found shell penetration in 8% of eggs contaminated with *S. typhi-murium,* 3% contaminated with *S. oranienburg,* and 16% with *S. kentucky.* No penetration was found when *S. bareilly* was used.

Wright and Frank (1956) demonstrated that a few eggs are penetrated by *S. typhi-murium* on the 1st day and the great majority by the end of the 7th day. Watanabe et al. (1958) were unable to isolate *S. senftenberg* from the eggs of adult hens that were artificially infected with the organism and reacted positively to both somatic and flagellar antigens of *S. senftenberg*. These workers were able, however, to isolate *S. senftenberg* from the shell membranes of dead embryonated eggs, suggesting that these organisms may invade the shell during incubation. Gordon and Tucker (1965) found *S. menston* on the shell and in the membranes, albumen, and yolks of eggs from chickens fed the organisms. Birds receiving high doses of the bacteria in their feed yielded the organisms from the outer egg structures as well as their contents within 24 hours of being laid.

Williams et al. (1968) found that the penetration of *S. typhi-murium* through all the outer structures of chicken eggs could oc-

cur as early as 6 minutes using eggs incubated at 99° F. Defects in shell structure rather than shell thickness determined the degree to which salmonella bacteria could penetrate into eggs. The markedly increased permeability of cracked eggs was also established. Moisture aided the penetration process. Williams and Dillard (1968) found chicken eggs to be more resistant to shell penetration by *S. typhi-murium* as embryonic development took place in the eggs during incubation.

Temperature and moisture play an important part in the rate of penetration of the eggshell by paratyphoids. Buxton and Gordon (1947) demonstrated that *S. thompson* could readily penetrate the shell of chicken eggs stored at 37° C, but penetration was less common in eggs stored at room temperature. Gregory (1948) reported the penetration of *S. typhi-murium* and *S. bredeney* through the shell of chicken and turkey eggs under different conditions of humidity. Stokes et al. (1956) found that salmonellae were able to penetrate the eggshell membrane and contaminate the yolk if a temperature favorable to the growth of the bacteria was maintained.

Ellemann (1959) reported that *S. typhi-murium* did not penetrate the shells of eggs stored for more than 2 months at 4° C. However, penetration was demonstrated as early as 4 days when eggs were stored at 30° C. It was further noted that storage of eggs is most favorable in a cold room with a low relative humidity. Clise and Swecker (1965) demonstrated that the shells of eggs from hens given a feed naturally contaminated with *S. worthington* and housed together and using a common nest were found to contain the organism on culture. After such eggs were stored unrefrigerated for 1 week *S. worthington* was isolated from the shells and yolks. Wilson (1948) demonstrated that the virulence of the organism is important in the rate of eggshell penetration. He found that after repeated passage, penetration of the shell could occur more readily.

Pomeroy and Fenstermacher (1941) found that *S. typhi-murium* organisms, when mixed with sterile turkey feces and smeared on one third of the surface of turkey eggs, were able to penetrate the eggshell during incubation and invade the egg contents. In one group 17.6% and in a second group 16% of the eggshells were penetrated. Gauger and Greaves (1946a) recovered *S. typhi-murium* from the shells of 27 eggs and the shells and contents of 6 of 117 eggs laid by a group of turkeys experimentally infected with this organism. Stover (1964) indicated that penetration of turkey eggshells may occur within a few hours and continue for many days. Williams and Dillard (1969) demonstrated that turkey eggs without pigmentation were much more likely to be penetrated by *S. typhi-murium* than normal pigmented eggs. There were more gross openings in the shells of such eggs, which were also thinner than speckled eggs.

Schaaf (1936) found that in the case of duck eggs penetration occurred in 5 days, while Lerche (1936) reported that at room temperature penetration required 15 days.

Organisms that have gained entrance into the egg are able to multiply rapidly in the yolk and subsequently infect the developing embryo, which may die or hatch to serve as a source of infection for other young birds. Egg albumen has very little inhibitory effect on salmonellae that penetrate the shell (Buxton and Gordon, 1947; Gregory, 1948; Lancaster and Crabb, 1953a).

Spread in Incubator, Hatchery, Brooder, and Environment

Contaminated eggshells and other debris of the hatch may also serve as a source of the infection in the incubator. From the incubator the organisms may be distributed by air currents throughout the hatchery and a high level of salmonella aerosol infection established. Samples of air taken within the hatchery may remain positive for several weeks or months, and the infection may spread to subsequent hatches through this means. Contaminated down and dust may carry the organisms and be inhaled by susceptible young birds. Adler et al. (1953) demonstrated that poults could be infected with *S. typhi-murium* by the intranasal route.

Paratyphoid infection, when established in the brooder, is rapidly transmitted by inhalation, fecal contamination of feed and water, or direct consumption of fecal matter by young birds. Repeated passage of the organisms results in an infection of increased severity.

The disease may be transmitted directly to young birds from older fowl that are chronic intestinal carriers of the infection but exhibit no visible symptoms. The unusual method by which pigeons feed their young may contribute to the spread from the older birds to the young of this species. Gauger and Greaves (1946b) demonstrated that contaminated drinking water could serve as a source of the disease in an infected environment. Adler et al. (1953) were able to recover *S. typhi-murium* from the dust, litter, and feathers for 71, 44, and 37 days respectively following experimental infection of poults by the oral route. In an infected environment the disease may also be readily transmitted through mechanical means such as litter and feces adhering to footwear, feed bags, shipping crates, or brooding equipment.

Poultry Feedstuffs

Evidence has been presented that poultry feeds may be a common and very important source of paratyphoid organisms. Galton et al. (1964), Pomeroy et al. (1965), and Edwards and Galton (1967) have reviewed the role of poultry feeds and feed ingredients in the epidemiology of salmonellosis in poultry and man. Edwards et al. (1948a) isolated *S. typhi-murium* and *S. bareilly* from chicken feed in the middle 1940s. Wilson (1948) suggested that the incorporation into poultry feed of dried egg powder unfit for human consumption may have been a source of some of the new salmonella types introduced into Great Britain. Erwin (1955) reported the recovery of 3 strains of *S. oranienburg* during the bacteriological culture of 206 poultry feed samples. Butler and Mickel (1955) studied samples of wheat from different sources and found that 17.2% were contaminated with rodent pellets and 3.9% were contaminated with bird pellets. Becker (1957) emphasized the necessity of bacteriological examination of feed products of animal origin to insure that these products do not serve to carry salmonella infections to poultry. Müller (1957b) cited the relationship between salmonella outbreaks in Denmark and the importation of salmonella-contaminated meat, bone, and fish meals used in animal feed manufacture.

Boyer et al. (1958) conducted bacteriological examinations of samples taken from 51 unopened sacks of poultry feed and 4 fish meal and 21 meat scrap samples. From 5 of the turkey starter mash samples, 6 salmonella serotypes were isolated. No salmonellae were recovered from the chicken and duck feeds or the fish meal. Several salmonella types were isolated from meat scrap samples. An outbreak of *S. thomasville* infection in poults was associated with the consumption of contaminated feed.

Pomeroy (1958) has emphasized that feed ingredients may become contaminated with salmonellae on the farm, in storage bins, boxcars, terminal elevators, and feed mills. Bergsma (1959) has drawn special attention to salmonella-contaminated products of animal origin which have been substituted in the production of poultry feeds. He felt that this is one of the principal reasons that poultry are the chief reservoir of salmonellae.

Watkins et al. (1959) did not find salmonellae in freshly cooked poultry feed materials from 7 processing plants. Salmonella organisms were apparently introduced into the by-products as a result of recontamination of the cooked product in the processing plant. It was found that one-half of the salmonellae isolated from chickens and turkeys in the state of Texas were also present in animal by-products used as poultry feed ingredients.

Gordon (1959) reported that of 71 samples of complete poultry feeds examined, 8% yielded salmonellae. It appeared probable that the organisms were present in relatively small numbers in contaminated material, although it was stressed that multiplication may occur in mashes under suitable conditions of moisture and temperature. Moran (1960) called attention to the fact that in 1957 only 60 salmonella cultures from feed products of animal origin were serotyped; however, in 1958, 555 cultures of the same origin were received for typing. This sharp increase was interpreted to reflect the interest in the occurrence of salmonellae in feed products. She indicated that control of salmonellosis can begin only after strict standards of sanitation, rigidly enforced, are applied to production of animal feed ingredients.

Taylor (1960) noted that it is both possible and practical to treat animal feed and feed constituents with heat to destroy salmonellae which they contain. Such a practice was cited as having a potentially profound effect on the general incidence of salmonella infections. Pelleting of poultry feeds has been suggested as an effective measure to destroy salmonella organisms

that may be present (Hobbs, 1961). Rasmussen et al. (1964) found that the severity of heat treatment required to destroy salmonellae in naturally contaminated feed meals will vary considerably with different products.

Quesada et al. (1960) found that fish meal imported into Italy from Angola was contaminated with *S. binza,* which was found to be pathogenic for chickens. Bischoff (1961) reported on the salmonella types isolated from egg products and feeds of animal origin. A total of 113 salmonella types was recovered, and the strict bacteriological control of imported products was emphasized.

Morehouse and Wedman (1961) reported a survey of salmonella and other disease-producing organisms in animal by-products. Egg products, poultry by-products, and meat scraps were among the feed constituents found to contain salmonellae. It was concluded that salmonella organisms present in animal by-products and finished rations are a potential disease threat to poultry as well as other animal species. Wedman (1961) called attention to the potential disease problem resulting from the "cycling" of a number of salmonella serotypes from farms to processing plants and back to farms by animal by-products incorporated into feeds. It was felt that realistic, workable measures to minimize the chance for exposure of poultry to salmonellae occurring in animal by-products and rations are desirable and essential. Niven (1961) pointed out some of the problems that industry encounters in efforts to eliminate salmonellae from rendered animal by-products used in the manufacture of animal feeds. The need for further information concerning the real significance of this problem to animal health was emphasized.

Pomeroy and Grady (1961) conducted bacteriological examinations of 980 samples of animal by-products used in manufacturing poultry feeds in 22 states and Canada. Salmonellae were isolated from 175 of the samples and 43 serotypes were identified. Many of the same types have been isolated from poultry submitted to diagnostic laboratories. The authors pointed out that if continued progress is to be made in reducing the incidence of paratyphoid infections in poultry, every effort must be made to eliminate the contamination of feed ingredients with salmonellae. Thomas (1961) discussed the beneficial effects of legal measures that have been taken to restrict the use of salmonella-contaminated ingredients in the production of animal feeds in Belgium. Imported tankage, meat scrap meal, fish meal, and related products are presently being sampled and examined by the U.S. Food and Drug Administration. Those lots found contaminated with salmonellae are refused entry unless they are sufficiently heated to destroy the organism.

Grumbles and Flowers (1961) cultured for salmonellae 136 samples of cottonseed and/or soybean oil meal used in the preparation of poultry feeds. Six salmonella types were isolated from 5.14% of the samples. This study is especially significant since it demonstrates that salmonellae may also be present in feed constituents of vegetable origin. These authors stated that "a method of processing and handling poultry feed and feed ingredients to assure freedom from salmonella contamination must be developed before a satisfactory control program for paratyphoid infections in turkeys can be carried out." Galbraith (1961) traced outbreaks of *S. saint-paul* in Great Britain to chicks and in turn to meat meal imported from the United States and used in preparing feed for the flock of chickens involved. Quist (1962) reported the isolation of 13 serotypes of salmonellae from 60 samples of protein supplement used in poultry feed manufacture. He also pointed out that two significant factors that have influenced the high rates of paratyphoid infection in poultry are infection through egg transmission and exposure of birds to feeds heavily contaminated with salmonellae.

Boyer et al. (1962) described in detail 2 cases of salmonellosis in turkey poults and 1 case in chicks in which it was possible to correlate salmonella serotypes causing the infections with those isolated from samples of feed that the birds were receiving. In 2 other cases the types of salmonellae isolated from the birds were not identified with the types recovered from the feed. It was emphasized that no control program for salmonellosis in poultry will be of much value until a way can be found to keep these organisms out of the feed. Burr and Helmboldt (1962) during a one-year period cultured 131 fish meal, 161 meat scrap, and 145 poultry by-products before incorporation into finished poultry feeds. Fifty-six salmonella isolations were made from an average of 12.8% of the samples, and 10 salmonella types were represented. These workers called attention to serological cross-reactions that can occur as a result of such infections during pullorum-typhoid testing. Galbraith et al. (1962), in a survey of salmonella organisms in pet foods and garden fertilizers in Great Britain, found 27% of raw horse meat samples, 16% of other raw meat, 12% of prepared pet food, and 13% of garden fertilizers to contain salmonellae.

Gordon and Tucker (1965) were able to create a salmonella carrier status in young chicks by contaminating chicken feed with *S. menston*. Older birds so infected were found to lay eggs containing the organisms. Clise and Swecker (1965) isolated 94 salmonella cultures involving 27 serotypes from 71 by-product samples used in preparing poultry feeds. Faddoul and Fellows (1966) cultured 285 bags of poultry mash and found only 3 bags to yield salmonella organisms. Forsythe et al. (1967) reported that the role of feed contamination and its relation to the salmonella problem in poultry and man has been overemphasized. *S. typhi-murium* and *S. heidelberg*, two of the most comon salmonella serotypes in animals and man, are seldom isolated from animal and poultry feedstuffs.

Snoeyenbos et al. (1967b) noted that the population of salmonellae in dry poultry feed reached a relatively stable number in a short time and persisted for a long time. The organisms were present very frequently in the mash rations on the farm as they found 19% of the farm samples salmonella-positive. Indirect evidence suggested that the level of contamination was usually low. Feed was demonstrated to be the direct sources of both *S. california* and *S. oranienburg* infections in chickens. Dawkins and Robertson (1967) in a survey of animal feeds found that the most heavily contaminated materials were imported bone meal and both home-produced and imported meat and bone meals. Vegetable protein derivatives were comparatively free of salmonellae.

Kaufmann and Feeley (1968) conducted 3 salmonella culture surveys of a vertically integrated broiler operation at intervals over a 2-year period. Salmonellae were isolated from 18.2% of 1,400 fecal samples and from 29.3% of 324 samples of feed and feed ingredients. A self-perpetuating cycle of infection was suggested by the isolation of the same serotype from the live birds, their feed, and poultry meal which was derived from rendered offal from the company's own processing plant. One type involved frequently *(S. eimsbeuttel)* was not commonly isolated from poultry in the United States at the time. The hatcheries appeared to be unimportant in the perpetuation of infection in this operation. The data supported the concept that feed contamination is a very important link in the cycling of salmonellae in domestic poultry.

Rendering Plants and Rendered By-Products

The interests of the Animal Health Division of USDA in salmonella contamination of poultry feeds have stimulated a number of reported surveys of the incidence of salmonella contaminants in rendering plants.

Clise and Swecker (1965) found 8 of 11 offal reduction plants in Maryland to be producing supplements containing salmonellae. Moyle (1966) reported 10.8% of the samples he studied in a rendering plant to be contaminated with a total of 12 different serotypes of salmonella. No correlation was found in this study between the incidence of salmonellae and plant sanitation. Allred et al. (1967) reported results of a survey to determine the salmonella contamination rate in 4 categories of feed ingredients and in 3 finished feed categories in 26 states; 12,770 samples were collected at 724 feed mills. Of all feed ingredients, animal by-products revealed the highest degree of salmonella contamination (31.07%) and grain the lowest (0.66%). In the finished poultry feed category, 5.23% of 1,606 samples cultured were positive for salmonellae. *S. montevideo* was the most common serotype encountered during this survey.

Orthoefer et al. (1968) found 180 (34.5%) of 527 environmental swabs, aerosol samples, and bulk samples from an animal protein rendering plant to yield salmonellae on culturing. Included were 7 of the most prevalent nonhuman isolates and 6 of the most common isolates from humans. The main factors responsible for the widespread contamination appeared to be inadequate sanitation, airborne dispersion, and insufficient cooking. Timoney (1968) conducted a survey in 5 rendering plants to determine the routes of contamination of animal by-products by salmonellae. Of 224 samples 59 were positive for salmonellae and 15 different serotypes were found.

Loken et al. (1968) sampled protein feed supplements produced by rendering plants for salmonellae and other enteric organisms. Isolations of salmonellae were more frequent from products with high counts; however, 6% of the samples with total counts of less than 1,000 per g and 14% of the samples with coliform counts of less than 1 per g contained salmonellae. Flies were found to be a potential source of contamination in the plants. Wilson (1969) reported that of 14,512 rendered animal and marine products intended for use in the preparation of animal and poultry feeds, 2,278 (15.7%) were positive for salmonellae. At the initial inspection, at least 1 positive sample was obtained from 295 of 718 plants (41.1%). The most common serotype isolated from these products in 1968 was *S. montevideo. S. typhi-murium,* the salmonella serotype most frequently isolated from both human and nonhuman sources, accounted for only 1.8% of total isolates.

The USDA cooperative state/federal program for salmonella control in animal feeds and feed ingredients has been intensified. In 1968 it provided for approximately 2,500 rendering plant inspections with testing of finished products. At least one epidemiological study was made of each plant showing a salmonella-positive sample. Recommended sanitation guidelines for salmonella control in the processing of poultry and animal by-products (Anon., 1964c) and industrial fishery products (Anon., 1965a) are available from the Agricultural Research Service of USDA. A survey indicated that 43% of the renderers who received the guidelines had made an evaluation of their rendering operation for salmonellae. It is expected that with state or federal officials working with renderers, nearly all can be stimulated to initiate and maintain a salmonella control program.

Methods for Salmonella Isolation from Feeds and By-Products

Recommended laboratory procedures for the isolation of salmonellae from animal feeds and meat by-products were revised in 1967 by the National Conference of Veterinary Laboratory Diagnosticians and published in ARS 91-68 (Anon., 1968b). Malhotra et al. (1968) described a modified membrane filter technique for the quantitative determination of *S. typhi-murium* in artificially contaminated poultry feed and feed ingredients. A contamination level as low as 3–8 organisms per g of feed sample was detectable. Overall recovery rate averaged 61–68%. The membrane filter technique was found to offer a better potential for salmonella detection in feedstuffs than standard procedures in general use at the present time.

Barkate (1968) described methods for the detection and identification of salmonellae in feed components using a polyvalent H antiserum prepared by mixing together Spicer-Edwards H antisera (Difco) to screen suspicious colonies. Salmonellae were detected by this method within 60 hours whereas conventional methods require at least 4 days. Fluorescent antibody techniques are also being studied and applied for the rapid detection of salmonellae in fresh feed samples and animal by-products.

As Edwards (1958) has noted, it is obvious that in any effort to eradicate salmonellosis from domestic animals it is necessary to take into consideration the continuous seeding of the population through infected feedstuffs.

Spread from Other Animal Sources and Man

Rats and mice are frequent carriers of the organisms, and their droppings may readily contaminate feed supplies. Pigeons, sparrows, and various other species of wild birds may also serve as a source of the infection for domestic poultry flocks. Brest Nielsen (1960) has suggested that wild birds are a source of salmonella infections in Danish poultry flocks.

Attention has already been drawn to dogs, cats, swine, cattle, sheep, and goats as sources of paratyphoid infections for poultry. Gwatkin and Mitchell (1944) and McNeil and Hinshaw (1944) have discussed the part that snakes, flies (*Musca domestica*), and cats may play in the transmission of the infections to poultry. Man must also be recognized as a possible source of the disease (Gordon and Buxton, 1946). This source may involve not only the caretakers but also waste products of human

source. Hinshaw et al. (1944) record instances of humans transmitting the infection to poults. Poultry may serve as a source of salmonellosis for other animal species on the farm. Ladehoff (1959) cited evidence that *S. typhi-murium* infection in calves was introduced by apparently healthy geese and ducks.

Mortelmans et al. (1958) isolated 5 serotypes of salmonella from chicks shipped into the Belgian Congo from other parts of Africa and Europe by air. They called attention to the importance of air shipments as a means of rapid spread of salmonellosis among poultry. Rao and Gupta (1961) also reported on the isolation of salmonellae from imported chickens in India.

Direct Spread among Adult and Young Chickens

In transmission among adult poultry the feces of infected carriers are probably the most common source of the organisms. The bacterial population and the nature of the environment are among the many factors that determine the extent of such transmission. Smyser et al. (1966) concluded that paratyphoid infections do not spread readily between adjacent groups of chickens. Snoeyenbos et al. (1967b) did not find direct transmission of established salmonella flock infections between houses even though there was ample opportunity for transfer of large numbers of salmonellae from pen to pen. Litter from pens containing chicks known to be infected with *S. montevideo* was found to yield a high percentage of positive samples (87.5%) during the first 16 weeks and then sharply decline to very low levels. Brownell and Sadler (1967) were able to isolate salmonellae from an infected environment (litter, water, feed, dust) beginning on the 2nd day and continuing until the 57th day after transfer.

SIGNS

The signs of paratyphoid infections in both young birds and adults closely resemble those observed in pullorum disease, fowl typhoid, avian arizonosis, and several other diseases. A differential diagnosis based on signs and necropsy findings is not possible.

Young Birds

Basically paratyphoid infection is a disease of young fowl with environmental conditions, degree of exposure, and the presence of concurrent infections having an important influence on the severity of an outbreak. In acute outbreaks with deaths occurring in the incubator or during the first few days after hatching no signs may be noted. In such instances the infection is acquired by egg transmission or early incubator exposure. A high proportion of pipped and unpipped eggs containing dead embryos may be observed.

Signs of paratyphoid infections in all species of young fowl are very similar and include the following: a progressive state of somnolence evidenced by a tendency to stand in one position with head lowered, eyes closed, wings drooping, and feathers ruffled; a marked anorexia and increased water consumption; a profuse, watery diarrhea with pasting of the vent; and a tendency of the birds to huddle together near the source of heat. Respiratory signs are not commonly observed. Clemmer et al. (1960) found that experimentally produced pulmonary infections in chicks were usually self-limited although 2–3 weeks may be required for autosterilization.

In experimental exposure studies of turkey poults orally administered broth cultures of *S. typhi-murium,* Pomeroy (1944) observed that losses started 2–3 days after exposure and discontinued by the time the poults were 2 weeks old. When signs are observed in young birds 1 week of age or older, contact exposure or an outside source of the disease should be considered.

Emmel (1936) described a paralytic condition in chicks which he was able to produce by parenteral inoculation of the endotoxin of *S. typhi-murium.* Rasmussen (1962) described the frequency with which *S. typhi-murium* is associated with arthritis in ducks. Lee et al. (1936) reported that chicks orally infected with *S. typhi-murium* died between the 5th and 12th days, most losses occurring between the 5th and 8th days. Evans et al. (1955) have described blindness in chicks associated with salmonellosis. Lannek et al. (1962) reported conjunctivitis in natural *S. typhi-murium* infection in chicks. Salisbury (1958) found navel infection in young chicks from which *S. typhi-murium* was isolated. Bierer (1961) demonstrated that a navel route of infection was established by the incubator-spray inoculation of baby chicks with *S. typhi-murium.* The organism was also recovered from livers, unabsorbed yolks, and ceca of chicks so infected.

Dougherty (1953) and Price et al. (1962) found that ducklings infected with paratyphoid usually die slowly, tremble and gasp for air and very often have pasted vents. The eyelids of ducklings frequently become swollen and edematous. Truscott (1956) reported that infected ducklings appeared drowsy and weak. Perek and Rabinovitz (1957) found that goslings with salmonella infection were sluggish and refused feed or ate very little but consumed large quantities of water. Diarrhea was observed in some birds.

Das et al. (1959) reported that pigeons infected with salmonellosis demonstrated anorexia, greenish diarrhea, droopiness, and death within 2–3 days. Infected squabs are often retarded in growth, underweight, and exhibit a general depression and listlessness, accompanied by a partial or complete inappetence (Faddoul and Fellows, 1965).

Altman (1940) observed that infected canaries seemed to "puff up," developed convulsions, and died within 2–3 days. Constipation was observed in some cases; later, diarrhea developed. The droppings were greenish in color and in some instances bloody. Keymer (1959), in discussing paratyphoid infection in canaries and other passerine birds, noted that incubation takes 4–5 days, and the infection is usually acute. The birds will die 2–4 days after the plumage becomes ruffled and greenish diarrhea is observed. Vent feathers usually become matted with droppings and convulsions often precede death. Surviving birds are apparently carriers and can infect susceptible birds.

Adult Birds

Mature fowl generally exhibit no outward signs of the infection. Acute outbreaks in semimature and adult birds under natural conditions are rare. However, adults in infected flocks are often chronic carriers of paratyphoid organisms in their internal organs and intestinal tracts. Wilson (1948) found that adult chickens may remain intestinal carriers of *S. typhi-murium* and *S. thompson* for periods up to 9–16 months.

Experimental paratyphoid infection of adult chickens and turkeys by either the parenteral or oral route of administration will result in an acute disease of short duration. Signs during the acute stage will include loss of appetite, increased water consumption, diarrhea, dehydration, and general listlessness. Recovery is rapid in most cases, and death losses do not usually exceed 10%. Kashiwazaki et al. (1966) described the signs and pathological findings during a field outbreak of *S. typhi-murium* infection in adult chickens. Watery diarrhea, general depression and listlessness, droopy wings and ruffled feathers were listed.

GROSS LESIONS AND HISTOPATHOLOGY

Young Birds

Lesions may be entirely absent in extremely severe outbreaks. In outbreaks which permit the development of advanced cases, the following lesions are most commonly observed: emaciation; dehydration; coagulated yolks; congested liver and spleen with hemorrhagic streaks or pinpoint, necrotic foci; congested kidneys; and pericarditis with adhesions. However, both heart and lung lesions are not as frequently observed as in pullorum disease. Hemorrhagic enteritis involving the duodenum is a common occurrence in poults. Cecal cores are occasionally observed. Ballantyne (1953) reported that in cases which he studied, caseous ceca were found in 33% of poults infected with *S. oranienburg*, in 46% of poults infected with *S. typhi-murium,* and in 20% of poults with *S. newport.* The same condition occurred in 33% of chicks with *S. typhi-murium* infection.

Lukas and Bradford (1954), in an effort to classify necropsy findings of paratyphoid outbreaks encountered among poults during a survey in California, found: (1) systemic involvement with lesions such as pericarditis, necrotic foci in the liver and heart, air sac involvement, central nervous system disturbance, and severe catarrhal enteritis with cecal cores (20.8% of specimens); (2) uncomplicated catarrhal enteritis (33.2% of specimens); (3) enteritis complicated with Coccidium, Hexamita, or sinusitis-air sac infection (28.4% of specimens); (4) other findings such as water starvation, ascites, mycosis (15% of specimens); (5) no gross lesions (2.5% of specimens). *S. typhi-murium* was most frequently involved in systemic cases, while other common types such as *S. anatum* and *S. manhattan* were more common in cases with uncomplicated diarrhea.

Truscott (1956), on necropsy of ducklings infected with *S. moscow,* found the livers of the birds bronze in color and covered with small gray areas of focal necrosis. The air sacs were somewhat opaque with yellow fibrinous plaques. Dougherty (1961) described in detail the pathology of *S. typhi-murium* and *S. enteritidis* infection in the White Pekin duckling. Gross enlargement of the liver with or without focal necrosis, formation of caseous plugs in the ceca, and enlargement and mottling of the rectum were the predominant lesions. Pericarditis, epicarditis, and myocarditis were found. Central nervous lesions consisted of thickened meninges in about one-third of the typical salmonellosis cases confirmed by bacteriological studies. Price et al. (1962), in necropsy studies of ducklings infected with salmonellae, found necrotic foci in the liver, cheesy plugs in the ceca, impaction of the rectum, and blanching of the kidneys. Rasmussen (1962) described the pathology of arthritis in slaughter ducks due predominantly to *S. typhi-murium.* Among 827 arthritic ducks, *S. typhi-murium* was isolated from 12% of the inflamed hock joints, 75% of the knee joints, and 52% of the hip joints. Perek and Rabinovitz (1957) found that at autopsy, goslings revealed pale flesh with some necrotic foci on the livers.

Arthritis is commonly observed in paratyphoid infection of pigeons (Emmel, 1929). It most frequently involves the wing joints and is evident as soft subcutaneous swellings. Swelling of the eyelids is also a common symptom in pigeons. Faddoul and Fellows (1965) found that the formation of a salmonella abscess of the brain was often observed in pigeon paratyphoid. Das et al. (1959) described yellowish green fibrinous deposits in the oral cavity, at the base of the tongue, and on the upper palate of pigeons infected with *S. typhi-murium.* Paratyphoid infection in pigeons must be differentiated from other diseases, notably trichomoniasis, ornithosis, tuberculosis, colibacillosis, erysipelas, ulcerative enteritis, and staphylococcal arthritis.

Adult Birds

Acutely infected adult fowl may reveal congested and swollen liver, spleen, and kidneys and hemorrhagic or necrotic enteritis, pericarditis, and peritonitis. Khera et al. (1965) described an outbreak of avian salmonellosis in maturing pullets and hens caused by *S. stanley.* In these adult laying birds the disease was characterized by necrotic and hyperplastic lesions in the oviduct and suppurative and necrotic lesions in the ovaries. The lesions often progressed to generalized peritonitis. Kashiwazaki et al. (1966) noted marked gross and microscopic pathology in the ovarian tissues of adult birds infected with *S. typhi-murium.*

Leg weakness in mature birds is not uncommon. Higgins et al. (1944) encountered a flock of 24-week-old turkeys infected with paratyphoid in which 10% of the birds were so severely affected with an arthritic condition that they were unsuitable for marketing. Chaplin and Hamilton (1957) reported a synovitis in turkeys, similar to that ascribed to intravenous staphylococcal inoculation, following intravenous inoculation of broth cultures of *S. thompson.*

In an infected environment under natural conditions the disease is constantly transmitted among adults through consumption of the organisms; however, the period that the birds are infected may be transient. The degree to which adult chickens and turkeys become chronic carriers is dependent upon the number of organisms to which they are exposed, the virulence of the strains, and the general condition of the infected individuals.

Chronic adult carriers of paratyphoid infections are often submitted for necropsy as reactors to serological tests for pullorum disease or *S. typhi-murium* infection. Emaciation; necrotic ulcers in the intestines; enlarged liver, spleen, or kidneys; nodules on the heart; and distorted ovules may occasionally be noted. Pathological changes in ovarian tissues as a result of paratyphoid infection are not so distinctive or common as those observed in the case of chronic carriers of pullorum disease. Chronically infected adults frequently exhibit no lesions. This is particularly true of intestinal carriers.

DIAGNOSIS

Clinical observations and necropsy findings may be suggestive of paratyphoid infection when a supportive history is available, and may permit one to reach a tentative diagnosis as a basis for early treatment or control recommendations. However, the final diagnosis of paratyphoid infections is dependent on the isolation and identification of the causative organisms. Procedures for this purpose require approximately 48–72 hours.

Faddoul et al. (1966), in summarizing a 5-year survey involving 245 salmonella isolations from avian species, reported a total of 24 serotypes recovered from diagnostic materials. *S. typhi-murium* was the most common and was identified from the greatest variety of avian species. In 78% of the positive consignments from chickens and 70% of those from turkeys, salmonella organisms were isolated only from the intestinal tract.

Snoeyenbos et al. (1967b) have suggested that detection on a practical basis of paratyphoid-infected flocks remains one of the most serious unsolved problems in controlling salmonellosis of poultry. It was demonstrated that chicks subclinically infected with salmonellae may contaminate litter on which they are reared sufficiently to allow rather dependable isolation of the pathogen from this material. These investigators suggested that litter samples can be used as a practical method of detecting salmonella-infected chicken flocks.

The culture of cloacal swabs taken from living birds has been studied as a diagnostic procedure for paratyphoid infection; however, its reliability seems to be limited since fecal excretion of the organisms may be intermittent (Wilson, 1948). These procedures have often been employed, however, as a general measure in the detection of supply flocks that may contain salmonella carriers. Magwood and Bigland (1962) found that carrier turkeys yielded salmonellae from cloacal swabs only intermittently which emphasized that failure to isolate the organisms did not prove absence of infection in flocks. Recovery of salmonellae from swabs or from dead-in-the-shell embryos indicated the likelihood of clinical disease in the progeny.

Olesiuk et al. (1969) found that the culture of the floor litter was more effective than serologic tests or cloacal swab culture for detecting experimental *S. typhi-murium* infection. Snoeyenbos et al. (1967b) reported nest litter to give the highest frequency of salmonella isolations during the study of various environmental samplings to detect the organisms.

Miura et al. (1964) sampled 300 hatchery fluff samples from commercial hatcheries in Japan and found 52.7% of them infected with salmonellae. They suggested that the examination of fluff samples from a series of hatches may be used for the measurement of salmonella contamination in commercial hatcheries instead of the bacteriological culture of dead-in-the-shell embryos. The bacteriological examination of yolk material from embryos dying between days 19 and 21 proved a practical method of detecting carrier flocks in Great Britain.

ISOLATION AND IDENTIFICATION OF CAUSATIVE AGENT

Tissues, Feces, Eggs and Egg Products, Feedstuffs, Litter, and Vaccines

Cultures taken directly from fresh organs of diseased birds are made on beef infusion agar slants or plates, which are incubated for 24 hours at 37° C. Intestinal cultures are subjected to selective enrichment in liquid broths, after which they are streaked on selective agar plates. This technique is also useful in the bacteriological examination of specimens that are in a state of decomposition or are likely to be contaminated with other organisms. Essentially the same procedures are used for the isolation of salmonellae from all the sources listed above, and therefore these will be discussed together in this section and differences noted where applicable.

There are many liquid enrichment broths and selective agars that have been recommended for the isolation of salmonellae from fecal specimens. These have been reviewed by Edwards and Ewing (1962), Kauffmann (1966), and Edwards and Galton (1967). Several media have been established, through practice, as most universally useful in the diagnosis of paratyphoid infections of poultry. For initial enrichment of fecal cultures most laboratories employ either tetrathionate broth with 1:100,000 brilliant green and 5% bile, or selenite broth. Some laboratories use both of these media (available commercially in dehydrated form) in the examination of each fecal specimen. About 1 g of fecal material is used to inoculate each 10–15 ml of selective broth.

Stokes and Osborne (1955) and Osborne and Stokes (1955) developed a modified selenite-brilliant green medium for the isolation of salmonellae. This medium, through the addition of 0.05% sodium sulfapyridine, was found to be sufficiently selective and sensitive to permit isolation of salmonellae, even when only one viable cell was present in 100 g of commercial, naturally contaminated dried egg. Galton et al. (1952) reported that the addition of 0.125 mg of sodium sulfathiazole to each 100 ml of tetrathionate broth suppressed the multiplication of proteus organisms. Galton (1961) recommended the addition of 6 ml of a 10% solution of Tergitol No. 7 to each 100 ml of tetrathionate-brilliant green broth for the isolation of salmonellae from animal feed products.

North (1961) reported that preenrichment of dried egg products in lactose broth, followed by enrichment in selenite-cystine or tetrathionate, was more sensitive than direct enrichment in selective media for detecting salmonellae when present in small numbers. Smyser et al. (1963) found selenite-brilliant green-sulfapyridine (SBG sulfa), selenite-cystine, and tetrathionate broths to be more effective than selenite broth and selenite-brilliant green enrichment for the recovery of S. typhi-murium from artificially contaminated feedstuffs. Little difference was noted between the preenrichment method and direct inoculation method in the ability to recover salmonellae from feedstuffs stored at 4° C. Gordon and Tucker (1965) cultured shells, shell membranes, dead-in-the-shell embryos, albumen, and yolk enriched in Selenite F broth in the isolation of S. menston from chicken eggs. Carlson et al. (1967) did not find the addition of Tergitol to modified selenite enrichment broth to significantly increase the number of positive salmonella isolates from meat and bone meal. Snoeyenbos et al. (1967b) used selenite-brilliant green-sulfapyridine broth (Difco) for sample enrichment during the isolation of salmonellae from animal by-products used in poultry feeds, floor and nest litter, water samples, rubber egg transfer cups, and fresh tissues of infected birds. Forsythe et al. (1967) in isolating salmonellae from experimentally infected chickens employed lactose preenrichment of cultures followed by transfer to selenite-cystine broth and plating on brilliant green agar.

Although temperatures of incubation of broths used by most investigators are 35° C and 37° C, Harvey and Thomson (1953) and Dixon (1961) recommended a selective temperature of 43° C for incubation of selenite broth. Carlson et al. (1967) found a distinct advantage in incubating selenite-brilliant green-sulfapyridine enrichment broth at 43° C and plating after 48 hours for isolating salmonellae from meat and bone meal and from poultry litter. Woodburn (1964) also reported that the incubation of poultry meat samples in Selenite F cystine broth at 43° C rather than 37° C gave more salmonella isolations. McCoy (1962) found that incubating tetrathionate broth at 43° C was lethal to salmonellae. Smyser and Snoeyenbos (1969) found SBG sulfa broth incubated for 48 hours at 43° C to be the preferred enrichment medium for the isolation of salmonellae from poultry litter and animal feedstuffs.

In the isolation of paratyphoid organisms, it is usually advantageous to make two platings from enrichment broths, the first after 24 hours and the second after 48 or 72 hours.

The most widely used solid plating media for isolation of salmonellae are brilliant green agar, SS agar, desoxycholate citrate agar, and bismuth sulfite agar. There is some variation in preferences for these plating media among various diagnostic laboratories. Edwards et al. (1948c) stated that the most satisfactory method for examination of intestinal material from fowl for paratyphoid organisms is the use of tetrathionate-brilliant green broth plated after 24 hours incubation on the brilliant green agar of Kauffmann (1950). Galton et al. (1954) recommended the addition of 8–16 mg of sodium sulfadiazine per 100 ml of brilliant green agar to inhibit growth of pseudomonads and coliforms on plates. Smyser et al. (1963) reported that brilliant green agar yielded best results in the isolation of salmonellae from poultry feeds.

Bloom et al. (1958), in culture studies of sewage, found a selenite-brilliant green enrichment medium to be superior to tetrathionate broth in the isolation of salmonellae. Yamamoto et al. (1961b) did not find the number of salmonellae in turkey feces to change appreciably when samples were held 24–48 hours at 4° C. Ringer's solution and Hajna's preservative were effective as suspending media to maintain the organisms. Selenite-cystine broth enrichment with subsequent plating on brilliant green agar gave the most favorable results in the isolation of *S. typhi-murium* from infected tissues and other material.

Methods for bacteriological examination of reactors to serological tests for paratyphoid infections are identical to those used in the cultural examination to identify localized chronic pullorum infection. These are outlined in the pullorum section of this chapter and in the auxiliary provisions of the *National Poultry and Turkey Improvement Plans* (Anon., 1971a). Yamamoto et al. (1962) proposed cultural procedures for the examination of turkeys reacting to serological tests for *S. typhi-murium*.

All selective plating media are examined after 24 hours incubation at 37° C for colonies typical of salmonellae. Suspected colonies are picked by touching the tip of a platinum needle to the center of the colony and transferred by stab and streak to triple sugar iron (TSI) agar slants. The inoculated tubes are incubated for 24 hours at 37° C. Slants which have a typical acid butt (yellow), with or without gas, and an alkaline slant (red) are selected for further study as possible salmonella cultures. Hydrogen sulfide production is indicated by blackening of the agar due to iron sulfide precipitation. Ewing et al. (1960) described the decarboxylase reactions of salmonella and arizona strains and pointed out their value in taxonomy of the groups.

In order to eliminate *Proteus* spp., it is advantageous to test the suspected salmonella cultures for urease production. The urea agar of Christensen (1946), which permits a reading at 6–8 hours, or the rapid urease test of Stuart et al. (1945) may be used.

Those cultures that are negative to the urease test should be transferred to the following media for final identification: dextrose, lactose, sucrose, mannitol, maltose, dulcitol, malonate, and salicin; peptone medium for indol production; semisolid medium for motility; and gelatin. A Gram's stain of each culture should also be prepared. Checking each culture with a polyvalent salmonella typing serum is helpful in identification. Marthedal (1962) used a biochemical and serological scheme for classifying *S. typhi-murium* strains of avian origin in Denmark.

Typical reactions of paratyphoids, ari-

TABLE 3.9 ❧ Typical Reactions of Paratyphoid, Arizona and Citrobacter Cultures on Diagnostic Media

Media	Paratyphoid	Arizona	Citrobacter
Dextrose	+	+	+
Lactose	—	d	(+) or +
Sucrose	—	—	d
Mannitol	+	+	+
Maltose	+	+	+
Dulcitol	+	—	d
Malonate	—	+	d
Urease	—	—	d
KCN	—	—	+
Gelatin	—	(+)	—
Lysine decarboxylase	+	+	—
Beta galactosidase	—	+	+ or —
Jordan's tartrate	+	—	+
Motility	+	+	+

Abbreviations: $+$ = positive within 1–2 days incubation; (+) = positive reaction after 3 or more days; — = no reaction; + or — = majority of strains positive, occasional cultures negative; (+) or + = majority of reactions delayed, some occur within 1–2 days; d = different reactions: +, (+), or —.

zonae, and citrobacters on diagnostic media are listed in Table 3.9.

Johnson et al. (1966) described methods for identifying members of the family Enterobacteriaceae based on primary differentiation of the various groups using Kligler iron agar and lysine-iron agar. For identification of salmonella and arizona group organisms from stools, triple sugar iron agar and lysine-iron agar were employed. Wenger and McMurray (1967) reported the application of PathoTec urease and lysine decarboxylase test paper strips for the presumptive identification of salmonellae. The PathoTec procedures used as a part of an isolation and identification scheme proved practical and reliable for screening poultry, poultry products, and feed ingredients for salmonella contamination and gave presumptive identification of salmonellae 1 day earlier.

Banwart et al. (1968) described a screening method for detecting salmonellae in pasteurized dried whole egg in which hydrogen sulfide production and mannitol fermentation were determined while the egg sample was being incubated in lactose broth. Samples showing a positive reaction can be tested further by enrichment in selenite or tetrathionate broth followed by selective plating. In further studies Banwart and Kreitzer (1969) successfully used inverted tubes of media to test mannitol fermentation and H_2S production in detecting presumptively salmonella-positive samples of dried egg. Lactose broth as an enrichment was better than either nutrient broth or mannitol broth when the inverted tube test was used. Belliveau et al. (1968) have proposed a simple, rapid method of identifying the Enterobacteriaceae including the genera *Salmonella* and *Arizona*. The method involves the use of five common, readily available media: triple sugar iron agar, lysine-iron agar, SIM media, ortho-nitro-phenol-Beta-D-galactoside (ONPG), and urea broth.

Haglund et al. (1964) combined selective cultural methods with fluorescent antibody techniques to detect salmonellae in eggs and egg products within 24 hours in the presence of Pseudomonadaceae and other Enterobacteriaceae. The techniques were specific when flagellar antibodies were used. The somatic antibodies would not give specific reactions without absorption techniques. Absorption and interference techniques indicated the test was specific for salmonellae. Forsythe et al. (1967) utilized the fluorescent antibody method to detect salmonellae in the feces of infected chickens. Thomason et al. (1959) have discussed the application of fluorescent antibody to identify salmonellae in fecal specimens and described the problems of cross serological reactivity encountered with these methods.

Because of the interest in salmonella organisms occurring in poultry feedstuffs, recommended procedures for the isolation of salmonellae from animal feeds and meat by-products have been developed and published (Anon., 1968b). Snoeyenbos et al. (1967b) found it advantageous to bacteriologically examine animal by-products at the plant rather than the finished feed at the farm for effective salmonella isolation. Dilution of constituents in the feed hindered recovery of the contaminants. They found a large number of salmonella serotypes in 51.8% of the samples of by-products cultured. The methods outlined by Lewis and Angelotti (1964) and Edwards and Galton (1967) can also be referred to in culturing poultry feeds for enteric organisms. Smyser et al. (1963) found that the use of multiple samples in the examination of poultry feeds for salmonellae increased the chances of recovering the organisms.

Hobbs (1963), Silliker et al. (1964), and Anon. (1965b) discussed in detail techniques for the isolation of salmonellae from eggs and egg products. Standard procedures for detection of salmonella organisms in live poultry vaccines of egg-embryo origin have also been described (Anon., 1971b).

Bacteriophage Typing

The application of phage typing in studying the epidemiology of various salmonella serotypes in man and animals has been reviewed by Edwards and Galton (1967). Garside et al. (1960) used phage-typing of *S. typhi-murium* in distinguishing a single strain of this organism in experimental studies of antibiotic resistance. Anderson and Williams (1956) have described a bacteriophage-typing scheme for salmonella strains of animal origin. They suggested that more extensive veterinary use of this procedure will aid in tracing the distribution of particular types of salmonellosis in animals. Taylor (1967) referred to the great contribution of phage typing of *S. typhi-murium* to the study of the disease as it occurs in man and in animals.

SEROLOGY

All salmonellae isolated in pure culture and identified biochemically should be submitted for serological typing. This subject has been discussed in the Antigenic Structure portion of this section to which reference may be made. Serological testing procedures and antigens for the detection of salmonella carriers in poultry flocks are described in the Prevention and Control section which follows.

TREATMENT

Medicinal therapeutic measures may be employed to reduce mortality in acute outbreaks of paratyphoid infections and to aid in preventing the development and spread of the disease. All such measures have the disadvantage of being incapable of eliminating the infection from treated birds. The demonstration by Yurchenco et al. (1953) that certain of the furan ring type of chemicals (nitrofurans) have marked activity against gram-negative bacteria opened a new field in the therapy of salmonellosis of poultry. Wolfgang (1958) reviewed recent progress in nitrofuran research.

The use of chemical therapeutic measures for paratyphoid infections in domestic poultry flocks should be restricted to flocks intended for market use. Young birds that have undergone an acute outbreak of paratyphoid infection, even when drug therapy is used, are not a safe source of future breeding stock. Birds that have received treatment may remain carriers of the organisms as therapeutic measures are not capable of completely eliminating the infection. While advances have been made in the prevention of paratyphoid and reduction of losses through treatment, therapeutic measures are of little value in any long-range program to eliminate paratyphoid infections from poultry flocks.

Individual or flock therapy may be indicated in acute outbreaks of paratyphoid infections among birds maintained in zoological parks, for treating household pets such as parakeets or canaries (Burkhart et al., 1962), and for flocks of wild birds maintained on refuges (Lucas, 1956; Jones, 1959).

SULFONAMIDES

The sulfonamide drugs have been demonstrated to have some effect in reducing the mortality from paratyphoid infections. Sulfamethazine and sulfamerazine have been most widely used and are usually administered as feed additives. Feeding of the sulfonamides at the therapeutic level should be intermittent to prevent the development of toxicity from the treatment. Turkey poults are particularly susceptible to the toxic effects of the drugs. Soluble forms of some of the sulfonamide drugs are available for addition to the drinking water. This method of administration is advantageous when the birds do not consume feed in quantity. Sulfonamide-resistant bacterial forms may develop from continued treatment.

Clark (1946) reported that sulfamerazine in the mash at a level of 0.3% or higher was effective as a prophylactic measure against paratyphoid infection of chicks and poults. Peterson (1947) encountered a serious outbreak of *S. typhi-murium* infection in which sulfamerazine at a 0.5% concentration in the mash was ineffective. Eveleth et al. (1947) reported that 0.4% sodium sulfamerazine in the drinking water or 0.5% sulfamerazine in the mash was found useful in reducing death losses from paratyphoid infections in poults and chicks.

Pomeroy et al. (1948) reported that sulpha-methazine, sulfadiazine, and sulfamerazine reduced death losses from *S. typhi-murium* infection in chicks 50%; however, the drugs proved to be only half as effective when fed to poults. Price et al. (1962) used soluble sulfamethazine in the drinking water at the rate of 1 oz per gallon of water for 2 days in the treatment of salmonellosis of ducklings.

ANTIBIOTICS

The antibiotics have not been extensively used in the treatment of paratyphoid infections of poultry. In general, they have proved less effective than other medicinal treatments available. Recommendations have been made (Anon., 1969a,b) that the use of higher levels of antibiotics for prophylactic purposes in poultry flocks should not be permitted from the standpoint of human health.

Lukas and Bradford (1954) reported that Terramycin and chlortetracycline (Aureomycin) were the drugs of choice in controlling paratyphoid outbreaks in poults. The effective concentrations were 100 ppm of soluble Terramycin in the water and 250 g of Terramycin or chlortetracycline per ton of feed. The duration of treatment was determined by flock response. Other flocks that received sulfonamide therapy had a higher percentage of losses and stunted birds than the antibiotic-treated group. Garside et al. (1960) found that chlortetracycline gave a measure of protection against experimental infection with *S. typhi-murium* in chicks, the mortality rate in antibiotic-fed chicks being approximately one-half that in chicks not receiving the antibiotic.

Ravaioli and Orfei (1952) found Chloromycetin and Terramycin to change the fermentative properties of salmonellae isolated from treated birds. McCarty (1953) reported neomycin to be beneficial in the treatment of *S. derby* infection in geese, and Schoop and Moser (1954) found that streptomycin was used with some success in the therapy of pigeons infected with *S. typhi-murium*.

Field applications are being made of antibiotics administered by vaccination as a routine preventive for paratyphoid infections in poults; however, experimental data to support this practice have not been published.

NITROFURANS

Furazolidone (N-(5-nitro-2-furfurylidene)-3-amino-2-oxazolidone), one of the nitrofuran derivatives of furfural, has been found to be effective in reducing mortality in acute outbreaks of several types of paratyphoid infections. Subtherapeutic levels of the drug are recommended to decrease the development and spread of paratyphoid infections. Furazolidone is marketed under the trade name nf-180.

In recommended concentrations, furazolidone has a low toxicity for host tissues and acts by interrupting the enzymatic metabolic processes of the microbial cell, preventing cell multiplication (Paul, 1956). The drug has a low solubility which permits the extended maintenance of a rather high concentration in the intestinal tract of treated birds. Smith (1955) demonstrated, however, that furazolidone is usually totally absorbed near the middle of the avian intestinal tract. The drug is generally administered at a concentration of 0.0055% (50 g per ton) fed in the mash on a continuous basis as a preventive of paratyphoid infections in birds over 2 weeks of age, or at the level of 0.011% (100 g per ton) as a preventive in birds during the first 2 weeks after hatching. A dosage schedule of 0.011–0.022% (200 g per ton) in the mash fed for 2 weeks is recommended for treatment of acute outbreaks of paratyphoid infections. The drug is usually added at the required level by the feed manufacturer.

Paratyphoid organisms are apparently more resistant than *S. pullorum* and *S. gallinarum* to the inhibitory action of furazolidone both in laboratory tests and in field therapy trials. Smith (1955) during in vitro sensitivity studies found that the 9 strains of *S. typhi-murium* included in his tests were 2–4 times as resistant to furazolidone as was *S. pullorum*. Harwood (1956) indicated that furazolidone only rarely eliminated paratyphoids from infected birds although clinical response in reducing mortality from the disease was excellent.

Smith (1955) reported that furazolidone fed at a level of 0.04% in the mash continually for 10 days was very effective in reducing the mortality associated with experimental *S. typhi-murium* infection in poults and chicks. It was found that a high proportion of treated birds become carriers of *S. typhi-murium* even when treatment was started 3 days before infection. The organisms were more frequently recovered from the feces than from the organs of experimentally infected birds. Repeating the treatment or increasing the concentration of furazolidone was not found to decrease the carrier rate.

Wilson (1955) conducted experiments to test the efficacy of furazolidone in treating *S. typhi-murium* and *S. thompson* infections in chicks. Both 0.02% and 0.05% levels of the drug were used in these experiments. Results were inconclusive as the disease did not develop to any degree in control groups that received no treatment. Harwood (1956) suggested that a combination treatment of furazolidone and sulfonamide may prove useful in reducing losses in extremely severe paratyphoid epizootics of poultry.

Sieburth (1957a) studied the effect of 0.011% furazolidone on the mortality rate of chicks experimentally infected with *S. typhi-murium* at 1 day of age. Uninfected controls and furazolidone-treated groups both experienced 7% mortality, while the infected groups that received no treatment experienced a mortality of 27%. However, 100% of the intestinal cultures and a majority of the organ pools from the surviving chicks contained detectable numbers of *S. typhi-murium*. The drug also had an inhibitory effect on the development of *S. typhi-murium* agglutinins detectable by a conventional agglutination test. Agglutinins were demonstrable, however, through the use of an indirect hemagglutination test.

Beattie (1960) used furazolidone with excellent results in the treatment of experimental *S. thompson* infection in chicks; however, Khera et al. (1965) employed the drug to no avail during an outbreak of *S. stanley* infection in maturing pullets and hens. Botes (1965) reported that furazolidone medication caused almost immediate cessation of losses due to avian salmonellosis.

Lannek et al. (1962) reported studies of the nitrofurazone compound Tiafur in the treatment of experimental and spontaneous salmonella infections in chicks. Mortality was considerably reduced and clinical symptoms were markedly suppressed by a level of 0.1% Tiafur in the feed. A long-time treatment with low doses (0.01 and 0.04%) gave more chicks the chance to survive without eliminating infection and consequently left more carriers. Bierer and Barnett (1962a) studied the use of the nitrofuran feed additive nihydrazone (Nidrafur) at the 0.011 and 0.022% levels in the therapy of incubator-induced *S. typhi-murium* infection in chicks. The drug was found to be effective in lowering death losses from the infection and also in increasing the body weights of birds being treated.

Belding and Mayer (1958) reported that furazolidone added to the mash of poults at a level of 0.011% for 2 weeks followed by a 0.0055% level for 3 weeks reduced the mortality due to *S. san-diego* infection by 50%. Treatment was started at the time the poults were experimentally infected. Aureomycin and sulfamethazine were found to have no appreciable effect in reducing mortality from the infection. Treatment with either Aureomycin and sulfamethazine or furazolidone reduced the number of infected carriers.

Bierer and Vickers (1960b) found that furazolidone in the feed or soluble nitrofurans in the drinking water drastically reduced mortality from experimentally induced *S. typhi-murium* and *S. heidelberg* infection in poults. The soluble nitrofurans used were NF-248 and solubilized furaltadone at levels of 0.0066 and 0.0264% respectively in the drinking water. These drugs did not depress water consumption. Solubilized furaltadone would have been the nitrofuran of choice if it was not feasible or desirable to medicate through the feed. Bierer et al. (1961b), in further studies of water-soluble furaltadone medication, found that the drug administered at the rate of 0.25 g/gal of water resulted in a marked reduction in mortality from *S. typhi-murium* infection in poults. Using furaltadone prophylactically in the drinking water at the levels of 0.25, 0.5, and 1 g/gal, Bierer and Barnett (1962b) found the drug to reduce mortality from *S. typhi-murium* infection in turkey poults from 70–80% to 20–30%. Bierer (1963) reported that both 0.011% and 0.0165% nihydrazone (Nidrafur) reduced mortality due to *S. typhi-murium* infection in turkey poults. However, this drug seemed to retard growth at effective therapeutic levels in turkeys.

Lucas (1956) reported that furazolidone at the level of 0.011% in the feed was used successfully to control outbreaks of *S. typhi-murium* and *S. anatum* infections in wild mallard ducks. Tablets of the drug were also found to be effective in individual treatment at a dosage of 50 mg daily. Agglutination tests using *S. anatum* and *S. typhi-murium* antigens revealed the presence of reactors after treatment. Truscott (1956) found that a level of 0.011% furazolidone in the feed did not alleviate an outbreak of salmonellosis among ducklings. However, when the concentration was increased to 0.0165% and strict sanitation measures instituted in the brooding pens, the infection was brought under control. Price et al. (1962) indicated that treatment of paratyphoid-infected ducklings was usually limited to rigid culling. Sulfamethazine in the drinking water was recommended as medication in more serious outbreaks.

Jones (1959) recommended furazolidone as the drug of choice in the treatment of salmonella and arizona infections of game birds. Francis et al. (1960) reported that pheasants and quails may effectively be treated for salmonellosis with 0.011–0.022% furazolidone for 7–10 days followed by 0.0055% for another 7–10 days.

Keymer (1959) recommended a compound consisting of nitrofurazone and furazolidone added to the drinking water in the treatment of salmonellosis of canaries and other passerine birds. Treated birds may remain carriers of the organisms. Burkhart et al. (1962) reported treatment of parakeets and canaries with several water-soluble nitrofurans following experimental paratyphoid infections. Furaltadone (NF-260) and a second nitrofuran (NF-248) in a 6% propylene carbonate solution, administered in the drinking water, controlled *S. typhi-murium* infection in parakeets when used for 2 weeks at the level of 300 mg total nitrofuran per liter of water. This combination at 150- and 200-mg levels gave 100% protection against *S. typhi-murium* infection in canaries. It was emphasized that increased water consumption during paratyphoid infections makes the use of water-soluble nitrofurans preferable. Also pet birds like parakeets and canaries consume seeds which makes it impossible to administer the drugs in the feed.

Taylor (1967) noted that with the more frequent use of drugs such as ampicillin, tetracycline, and furazolidone there has been an increase in the number of drug resistant strains of *S. typhi-murium* in both animals and man, the increase corresponding in time with the use of these drugs in animal feedstuffs and prophylaxis.

PREVENTION AND CONTROL

MANAGEMENT PROCEDURES

Adult intestinal carriers serve as the chief source of paratyphoid infections in most species of poultry. Fecal contamination of hatching eggs by the chronic carrier or from an infected environment is the means by which infections are generally introduced into the incubator and subsequently into the brooder. Because of the wide natural distribution of salmonella organisms, the numerous antigenic types, and the lack of adequate methods to detect carriers among adult flocks, *hatchery and flock sanitation is the most important factor in the prevention and control of paratyphoid infections of poultry.*

Flocks that experience acute outbreaks of paratyphoid with high losses at a young age or those that are known to carry the infection at any age should not be used as a source of eggs for hatching purposes. Early disposal of such flocks is usually the most desirable program to follow. Agglutination tests have been employed to detect infected flocks; however, procedures for this purpose have not been developed to the degree of accuracy of serological tests for the detection of pullorum disease and fowl typhoid. For prevention of the infections, replacement stock and hatching eggs should be obtained from a source that is known to be paratyphoid-free. The birds should be maintained at all times in an environment where exposure to the organisms is kept at a minimum. Goetz (1962) discussed the California program used for the control of *S. typhi-murium* and arizonosis in turkeys. The program is based on the following principles: (1) stocking the breeding flock from a known clean source; (2) bacteriological sampling of all poult mortality up to 21 days of age; (3) tube agglutination testing of all potential breeding stock with *S. pullorum*, *S. typhi-murium*, and arizona antigens; and (4) routine bacteriological examination of samples of 10-day dead embryos from the hatchery.

Paratyphoid infections when encountered in valuable breeding stock constitute a particular problem. Special measures are necessary in such cases, and eradication efforts often extend over a period of several

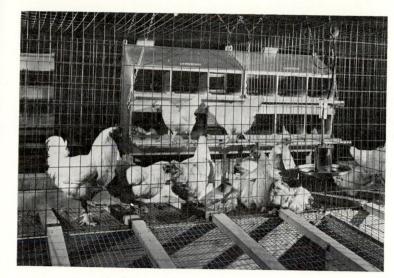

FIG. 3.18—Wire-floored houses with rollaway nests for production of hatching eggs with a minimum of fecal contamination (Courtesy Indian River Poultry Farms, Lancaster, Pa.)

years involving considerable financial loss. The most practical way to control the disease among birds in the pet or bird store is by means of depopulation and thorough cleaning and disinfection of the premises. A critical examination should be made of the source of supply for replacements in order to prevent recurrent infection.

An effective program for prevention and control of paratyphoid infections of poultry should give consideration to the following measures.

Hatchery and Egg Sanitation

EGG PRODUCTION, COLLECTION, HANDLING, AND STORING. The use of only clean eggs for hatching purposes will lessen the chances of introducing the infection into the incubator through fecal contamination. Adequate numbers of nests and clean laying houses should be provided. There is a growing interest in the use of wire floors and rollaway nests for hatching egg flocks (Fig. 3.18). Fertility levels of 95–97% have been obtained with White Leghorn breeders housed at 2/3 sq ft space per bird on sloping wire floors with a ratio of males to females of 1:12. Quarles et al. (1970) demonstrated that much less degree of bacterial shell contamination occurred when eggs were collected from wire-floored houses than from houses with conventional nests and litter floors.

Eggs should be collected at frequent intervals, fumigated, and stored in a cool place for as short a period as possible before setting. Cleaned and disinfected containers should be used in collecting the eggs, and the person making the collections should be certain that he does not serve as a source of contamination from organisms that may be present on his clothing or hands. Dirty eggs should not be used for hatching purposes and should be collected in a separate container from hatching eggs. The cleaning of eggs with cold water or wiping with a damp cloth hastens bacterial penetration and facilitates the transfer of infection from egg to egg (Gordon et al., 1956). It is best to remove dirt and dried feces from eggs by dry sanding (Fig. 3.19).

Racks or crates used for storing eggs should be new or properly cleaned and disinfected. Contact of the eggs should be kept at a minimum during storage since one egg may serve as a source of contamina-

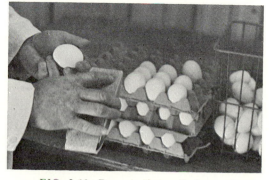

FIG. 3.19—Dry sanding soiled eggs immediately after collection. Abrasive must be changed frequently to prevent spread of contamination.

tion for many others. Maclaury and Moran (1959) stressed the fact that if warm, freshly laid eggs do not come in contact with contaminated soil or fecal material while they are cooling, the chances of their being infected with salmonella organisms are greatly decreased. If it is necessary to transport eggs before setting, new crates are most desirable for this purpose. Dirty crates should never be used. Pomeroy (1958) has pointed out that contaminated eggshells may serve as an important means of introducing salmonella and arizona organisms into a hatchery. Attention to sanitation on the farm at the supply flock level to obtain salmonella-free hatching eggs is an essential part of a paratyphoid control program.

EGG DIPPING, SPRAYING, AND WASHING. Egg dipping and spraying procedures have been proposed and are presently in use for the destruction of salmonellae on the surface of both hatching and market eggs prior to penetration of the organisms through the shell and shell membranes. To be effective such procedures must be properly applied and utilized immediately after egg collection. Wash solutions can become excessively contaminated with organic matter and bacteria to the extent that dipping practices can do more harm than good. For this reason they are not universally recommended or applied for prevention of egg-borne salmonellosis.

Gordon et al. (1956) reviewed the literature on germicidal dipping of hatching eggs and noted that "the dipping of hatching eggs in germicidal solution on the same day on which they are collected from the nests has been regarded for some years as a fruitful method for the control of avian salmonellosis and other egg-borne diseases." They presented detailed instructions on the field application of disinfectant dips for the destruction of salmonellae on the shells of freshly laid hatching eggs.

Quaternary ammonium compounds, formalin, sodium hydroxide, and sodium orthophenylphenate have been studied for dipping and washing hatching eggs (Wilson, 1948). According to Lancaster et al. (1952), solutions of sodium hypochlorite, sodium P-toluene-sulphonchloramide, cetyltrimethyl ammonium bromide, and chloro-m-xylenol were each successful in removing S. *pullorum* from the shells of artificially infected eggs but not S. *typhi-murium* or

S. *thompson*. It was their opinion that the practice was of no value in controlling egg rot during storage. Gordon et al. (1956) studied the germicidal effects of nine chemical dipping solutions for the destruction of S. *typhi-murium* and S. *thompson* organisms experimentally deposited on shells of chicken eggs. Most of the compounds effectively sanitized the shell surfaces and did not affect flavor of the egg contents nor hatchability of dipped eggs. Dipping solutions were maintained at a temperature higher than the eggs. These authors felt that there is a place for an early egg dipping program to disinfect the shell and prevent salmonellae and other types of organisms from penetrating into the egg.

Frank and Wright (1956) reported that 0.5% sodium hydroxide was effective within 5 minutes in disinfecting pieces of eggshell infected with S. *typhi-murium*. However, dipping whole eggs in sodium hydroxide at concentrations up to 2% for 5 minutes failed to prevent penetration of the eggshell by the organism at both incubator and room temperature. It was felt that penetration of the shells may have occurred before the disinfectant had a chance to act or that the organism was protected by some physical property related to the pores of the shell.

Mundt and Tugwell (1958) and Beattie (1960) have suggested dipping eggs in germicides as a reliable method of salmonellosis control. Bierer et al. (1961a) found that none of 24 chemical egg-washing compounds was effective in killing S. *typhi-murium* when used at 2.5–4 times manufacturers' recommendations. Quaternary ammonium compounds were found to be entirely unsatisfactory. One percent zinc sulfate was found to be superior to the other chemicals used from the standpoint of causticity, toxicity, odor, and staining. Bierer et al. (1961c) used 8 commercial compounds advertised as detergents or detergent-sanitizers in egg-washing experiments. The compounds were 52–92% effective in removing or destroying artificially induced S. *typhi-murium* eggshell contamination. Bierer and Barnett (1961) demonstrated that egg-wash germicides should be tested at 38° C or lower to avoid the germicidal effect of the water itself in experimental studies.

Rizk et al. (1966a) studied the application of several disinfectants to destroy salmonellae on the surface of market shell eggs subsequent to dipping in liquid cultures of the organisms. None of the disinfectants applied could eliminate salmonellae from the shell membrane system after the organisms had penetrated the shell. Quaternary ammonium compounds were considered the most effective compounds used for destruction of organisms on the shell surface and exhibited a residual germicidal effect when eggs were infected with salmonellae after dipping. March (1969) found a higher proportion of shell eggs were heavily contaminated (5 x 10⁶ organisms per egg) after washing than when received at grading stations in British Columbia. No salmonellae were detected in the 3,995 eggs examined. It was concluded that salmonella contamination of intact shell eggs does not constitute a serious public health hazard in the area studied. For a recent review of egg-washing procedures to reduce the microbial counts on the shell, the reader may refer to the report of Ayres et al. (1967).

PREINCUBATION FUMIGATION. Early on-the-farm fumigation of hatching eggs with formaldehyde gas has been found to be very effective in the prevention of egg-borne paratyphoid infections. Wilson (1949) stated that fumigation of eggs with formaldehyde gas is probably the most important factor in paratyphoid prevention. Early fumigation is essential since there exists no means of destroying salmonella organisms once they have penetrated the eggshell. Carlson and Snoeyenbos (1968) studied the bactericidal effect on *S. typhimurium* of injecting tetracycline HCl, neomycin, kanomycin sulfate, ampicillin anhydrous, naladixic acid, chloramphenicol, and dihydrostreptomycin in several chicken embryo test systems. Even at embryo-toxic dose levels, none was sufficiently salmonellacidal to indicate that they have practical value for destroying paratyphoid organisms that may be present in hatching eggs.

The fumigation of eggs undergoing incubation and embryonic development with any level of formaldehyde gas is risky and not generally recommended. In the event paratyphoid organisms are on the shells of the eggs prior to setting time, penetration is likely to have already occurred in the incubator and fumigation will be of no benefit. Furthermore, the developing embryo may be killed by the gas if variations occur from recommended procedures, especially excessive extension of the period of fumigation or the development of extremely high levels of the fumigant resulting from repeated fumigations.

Marcellus et al. (1930) have demonstrated that chicken embryos are most susceptible to injury from formaldehyde gas between the 24th and 96th hours. Fumigation during this period must be avoided. Lancaster (1962) reviewed information relating to formaldehyde fumigation of eggs with high levels of the gas. It was pointed out that earlier studies on the period of maximum susceptibility of embryos are not necessarily applicable when higher levels of the fumigant are used. With these larger amounts the period of embryonic susceptibility appeared to be prolonged from the 2nd to the 6th or even 8th day of incubation. Since Harry and Binstead (1961) were able to demonstrate that hatchability may be adversely affected when embryos are exposed to high levels of formaldehyde gas between the 3rd and 9th days of incubation, preincubation on-the-farm fumigation as a standard procedure was highly recommended. The degree to which hatchability was affected was influenced by the particular flock involved and the preincubational storage period.

Fumigation of hatching eggs as soon after being laid as possible, preferably within 2 hours, is highly recommended. The fumigation of fresh hatching eggs with levels of the gas several times that recommended here does not adversely affect hatchability during the short period they are exposed to the gas. If the period of exposure at these high levels is extended to several hours, hatchability is significantly lowered. A room or cabinet sized proportionally to the number of eggs should be provided (Fig. 3.20). Such cabinets are available commercially (Wolfe and Fulenwider, 1967). Fans can be used to circulate and exhaust the gas from enclosed areas. Eggs for fumigation should be placed on racks which will permit good air circulation. Stover (1964) provided detailed information on preparing and handling turkey eggs during all stages of preincubation formaldehyde fumigation procedures.

Formaldehyde gas is provided by mixing 0.6 g potassium permanganate with 1.2 ml formalin (40%) for each cubic foot of space

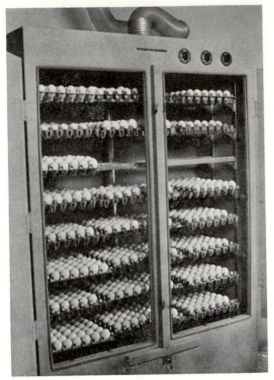

FIG. 3.20–Front view of on-the-farm fumigation cabinet with automatic controls for cycling the fumigant and exhausting the gas prior to removal of eggs. Metal bars for suspending eggs on plastic racks permit complete exposure of entire egg surface to the gas.

in the cabinet or room. The chemicals should be mixed in an earthenware or enamelware container having a capacity of at least 10 times the volume of the total ingredients. The gas should be circulated within the enclosure for 20 minutes, then expelled.

Humidity for this type of fumigation is not too critical, but the temperature should be around 70° F. Both heat and water are generated during the release of the gas in this procedure. In areas of the country where extremely low humidities are not common, a relative humidity of 70% or higher is generally generated during the reaction in the compact cabinet. When humidity is extremely low, moisture can be released from a small steam bath in the cabinet.

Formaldehyde as a fumigant gas can also be generated by heating paraformaldehyde (Formaldegen), a white powder with a very pungent odor. No moisture is generated in this process, and therefore it is important that water be added to the hot plate at the time the gas is released. Manufacturers' instructions should be closely followed in using this product for the fumigation of eggs and poultry buildings. Very little residue remains in this process which facilitates cleaning operations.

Harry (1954a) did not find that there was any residual protective effect from salmonella contamination on the shell surface of fresh eggs afforded by high-level formaldehyde fumigation. Williams and Siegel (1969) found that adsorbed formaldehyde on the surface of fresh hatching eggs fumigated with high levels of the gas rapidly disappeared on storage of eggs at room temperature. The fumigant could be easily washed from the surface and did not penetrate the shell and membranes into the egg substance to any degree.

Two illustrated bulletins in which the importance of preincubation fumigation of turkey hatching eggs is discussed have been published by the California Department of Agriculture (Stover, 1960, 1964).

Buxton and Gordon (1947), Wilson (1948, 1949, 1951), Clarenburg and Roepke (1952), Lancaster and Crabb (1953a,b), Lancaster et al. (1954), Harry (1954a), Clarenburg and Romijn (1954), and Frank and Wright (1955) have studied the use of formaldehyde gas in the fumigation of eggs and incubators contaminated with paratyphoid organisms. Buxton and Gordon (1947) and Wilson (1949) have recommended that fumigation for the destruction of paratyphoid organisms on the shell surface should be done before incubation. Penetration of the shell was found to proceed far more rapidly in the warm humid atmosphere of the incubator, and usually to occur during the 1st week of incubation.

Wilson (1951) recommended the fumigation of eggs for a period of 30 minutes with formaldehyde gas produced by the addition of 1.5 ml formalin to 1.0 g potassium permanganate per cu ft of incubator space. This concentration of the gas was invariably lethal for *S. typhi-murium* on eggshells and on down but normally had no adverse effect on hatchability. Humidity was not a factor as this treatment was found to be effective even under ordinary atmospheric conditions. The high concentration of the gas was recommended particularly following an actual outbreak of paratyphoid infection.

Frank and Wright (1955) studied the susceptibility of 19 salmonella serotypes to formaldehyde fumigation. Test organisms were placed on pieces of egg shell and string. Fumigation with 1.5 ml formalin and 0.75 g potassium permanganate per cu ft of incubator space killed all organisms in 20 minutes, while a number survived 10 minutes fumigation. When 1.0 ml formalin and 0.5 g potassium permanganate per cu ft were used, 30 minutes were required to kill all organisms. *S. pullorum* was found to be more susceptible than the paratyphoids to the lethal effects of formaldehyde gas.

Harry (1954b) found that removal of residual formaldehyde remaining after fumigation could be accomplished by adding 33% ammonia solution to the incubator in a volume equal to one-half that of the formalin used. This limited the escape of irritant concentrations of formaldehyde from the incubators.

When an airborne infection of salmonella organisms has become established in a hatchery, it may be necessary to fumigate the entire hatchery with high levels of formaldehyde gas to destroy the organisms. Close attention should also be given to contaminated egg sources which are usually responsible for introduction of the infection into the hatchery. Blood testing and the culture of eggs from supply flocks are often useful adjuncts in locating the source of the infection.

Price et al. (1962) recommended that duck eggs be fumigated on the 2nd day of incubation for a period of 15 minutes using 1 oz formalin and 0.5 oz potassium permanganate to every 80 cu ft of incubator space. Rasmussen (1962) also discussed hygienic measures to control the spread of duck salmonellosis.

CLEANING INCUBATORS AND HATCHING ROOMS. After each hatch incubators should be thoroughly cleaned of the debris of the hatch, washed with detergent and hot water, disinfected, and fumigated with a high level of formaldehyde gas. At least 1.2 ml formalin (40%) and 0.6 g potassium permanganate per cu ft of incubator space should be used with an exposure period of 1 hour. Higher levels of the gas may be used if desired. Wright et al. (1959) discussed the use of formalin fumigation for destruction of general bacterial and fungal flora in hatcheries. General disinfection procedures for incubators and hatching rooms and additional recommendations on formaldehyde fumigation of eggs and incubators are discussed in Chapter 1.

HATCHERY SANITATION. Restrictions should be placed on hatchery personnel to insure that they do not introduce infections into the hatchery from older fowl or from other animals with which they come in contact in their daily operations. It should be determined that no human carriers exist among the personnel. Visitors to the hatching area should be restricted. Boxes used to ship birds should be new, and trucks employed for transporting operations should be kept clean and be frequently disinfected. There should be a constant campaign to eliminate rats, mice, and flies in the vicinity of the hatchery.

Sanitation during Brooding Period

For prevention of paratyphoid infections during brooding it is important that the young birds be constantly isolated from sources of infection. Personnel that are in contact with older birds and other animals should take precautions not to introduce the infection through droppings that may adhere to the shoes, clothing, or hands. It is a good practice under these conditions to wear overshoes that can be disinfected and coveralls that can be frequently changed. Bierer (1960) emphasized the importance of starting poults on cleaned and disinfected premises and possibly administering preventive medication in the initial feed and water in preventing paratyphoid infections. All types of animals should be restricted from the brooding area.

Gordon and Tucker (1965) found that when salmonella-contaminated feed is given to poultry, water containers may become infected either by fecal contamination or by the birds carrying infected food on their beaks. Multiplication of the organisms under these conditions is rapid, and they can survive for as long as 6 months in feed samples. Feed and water containers should be situated where they cannot be contaminated by droppings and should be frequently cleaned and disinfected. Live steam is very effective for this purpose. A detailed sanitation program for the poultry industry has been outlined (Anon., 1947) in which cresylic disinfectants are recommended. The standard dilution of cresylic disinfectant used is 4 fl oz to each gallon of water (about 3%). Commercial lye, 2% in water, is also a very effective disinfectant when used as a hot solution. Odorless disinfection is available through the use of sodium orthophenylphenate in an aqueous or detergent solution.

Young birds that die or are sick should be promptly submitted to the diagnostic laboratory for examination. It is the responsibility of the laboratory to conduct complete bacteriological examinations to detect any salmonellae that may be present. All salmonella cultures isolated should be typed serologically, with up-to-date and complete records maintained relative to the salmonella types recovered from each flock within an area. This information is essential in guiding the use of specific antigens in serological tests for the disease in breeding flocks. Information derived from typing the organisms also aids in tracing the origin of disease outbreaks. Periodic summarizing of this information within each state would be most helpful to those engaged in paratyphoid control activities.

Flock Sanitation

Magwood and Bigland (1962) found environmental sanitation in the flock and hatchery to have a major influence on the frequency of clinical outbreaks of salmonellosis in poultry flocks. Rodents and other pests around poultry yards serve as an important source of salmonella organisms for semimature and adult flocks. Mice and rats may pass large numbers of the organisms in their excreta and are able to contaminate feed supplies and water as well as litter and poultry yards.

A more satisfactory sanitation code must be developed and adopted to insure that salmonella organisms are not present in the feed which the flock consumes. Edwards and Galton (1967) noted that every effort should be made to provide salmonella-free poultry feeds to reduce the incidence of salmonellosis in poultry, eggs, and poultry products. Kaufmann and Feeley (1968) suggested that if salmonellosis can be eradicated in single broiler operations by using salmonella-free feed, it can be eradicated from the industry as a whole if all feeds can be made salmonella-free.

Even the strictest measures are not always successful in keeping salmonella infections out of poultry flocks. Morello et al. (1965) reported on colonies of laboratory mice wherein, even with the most rigid control over food, bedding, sanitation, and overall animal maintenance, salmonellae persisted and were recovered on cultural tests.

Perhaps one of the most promising future methods for the prevention of salmonellosis in poultry flocks will be the production of hatching eggs on wire floors equipped with rapid mechanized means of removal followed by immediate egg fumigation. Smyser et al. (1966) found that 11 chickens which were fecal shedders of salmonellae became negative within several days after being placed in individual wire-floored cages in a clean environment. The studies of Brownell and Sadler (1967) indicated that if chickens are maintained on wire and are unable to cycle salmonella infections through contaminated litter, feed, water, and other means, the majority of the infected individuals will eventually eliminate the infection from the intestinal tract even after massive doses of the organisms have been administered. Similar favorable results from the use of wire floors are suggested by the work of Quarles et al. (1970).

An active rodent eradication campaign is an essential part of the general salmonella control program. Dogs, cats, sheep, cattle, horses, and swine should never have access to poultry operations.

Birds that have received therapy for paratyphoid infections should not be kept for breeding purposes. Neither should breeding flocks be treated for these infections and then maintained as a source of hatching eggs. Garside et al. (1960) found that a large number of carriers remained among groups of chicks receiving therapeutic levels of chlortetracycline. They emphasized that such a practice increases the problem of control of salmonellosis in poultry. Goetz (1962) reported an incident in which it was necessary to abandon turkey raising operations because *S. typhi-murium* was indigenous in the wildlife of the area. The organism was isolated from gopher snakes, ground squirrels, and owls shot on the premises.

Saulmon (1966b) has suggested that the problem of providing salmonella-free shell eggs will involve elimination of infected birds following identification by available or improved blood testing techniques, maintenance of flocks in a manner which will minimize the carrier problem, and development of carefully controlled sanitary routines in the collection, packaging, and distribution system.

Serological Testing

PROCEDURES. Procedures for serological detection of adult carriers of paratyphoid infections have not been accepted or applied on the scale of those employed for detection of pullorum disease and fowl typhoid. The tube agglutination test for *S. typhi-murium* has been most frequently used as a supplementary measure to other means of control or as a method for locating infected flocks. This procedure has been most widely applied in testing turkey breeding flocks. Moran et al. (1965) noted that since the development of a typhi-murium agglutination test antigen, *S. typhi-murium* infection has been reduced in turkeys.

Intestinal carriers may reveal no serological response to the agglutination test, and titers of birds that do react may fluctuate widely, as reported by Pomeroy and Fenstermacher (1943), Buxton and Gordon (1947), Lee (1957), and Smyser et al. (1966). Testing programs for paratyphoids are further complicated by the large number of antigenic types of the organism infecting poultry and the need for refinements in methods of producing antigens for the test.

Buxton (1958) noted that the agglutination test is of value in controlling salmonellosis in turkeys provided it is used in conjunction with hygienic measures to prevent reinfection. The agglutination test was found to give some idea of the rate of multiplication of the organism in the host, and the carrier animal usually revealed a low titer. Bierer and Vickers (1960a) reported that in nitrofuran-medicated poults there was a definite suppression of agglutinin production to the extent that *S. typhimurium* experimentally infected birds treated with nitrofurans did not react to any serological tests. McCapes et al. (1967) applied the tube agglutination test for *S. typhi-murium* in selecting turkeys free of the infection for experimental use. However, the antibody response of adult turkey hens to vaccination with *S. typhi-murium* bacterin as measured by the tube agglutination test for this serotype was quite erratic.

There also appeared to be no connection between the number of dams showing titers of 1:25 or higher and the apparent resistance of their offspring to challenge.

Specific antigens for the salmonella type involved must be prepared in the laboratory. Laboratory personnel conducting the tests and interpreting the results must be thoroughly familiar with salmonella serology and the variations that may arise during testing procedures. The history of each flock tested must be carefully considered. Representative reactors to the agglutination test should be submitted for complete bacteriological examination and laboratory confirmation of the presence of the infection.

The agglutination test has been applied in testing most species of fowl for paratyphoid. The use of the test has been sporadic in most areas, being applied as conditions warranted. In 1970 approximately 8 states in the United States were using the macroscopic tube agglutination test on a large scale to detect *S. typhi-murium* in turkey breeding flocks. At least 3 states (Minnesota, California, and Texas) have official rules and regulations including blood testing programs that have been adopted for the control of *S. typhi murium* infection of turkeys.

Turkey flocks in the United States can be blood tested under the *National Turkey Improvement Plans* (Anon., 1971a) and classified as U.S. Typhimurium Controlled if no reactors are found on the last test with *S. typhi-murium* somatic tube agglutination antigen. Also under the Plan a single combination antigen made up of equal quantities of pullorum and typhi-murium antigen can be officially used as a screening test for turkeys. All sera revealing suspicious and positive reactions to the combination antigen are reset with individual antigens. Saulmon (1966b) suggested that attention should be directed to the development of polyvalent antigens for poultry blood testing that will provide a more critical screening of birds that may be infected with more than one salmonella serotype.

Müller (1957b) reported that in Denmark the selling of ducklings, goslings, and turkey poults hatched in incubators is allowed only when the hatching eggs originate from flocks in which no reactors to the *S. typhi-murium* and *S. enteritidis* tube agglutination tests have been found 1 month before the beginning of the hatching season. Williams (1969) has described a device for the restraint of large fowl such as turkeys during the collection of blood samples for agglutination tests for avian salmonellosis or other diseases.

DeLay et al. (1954) reported that 7,578 of 593,341 turkeys tested with S. typhi-murium antigens by the tube agglutination method reacted in the diagnostic dilution of 1:25. Of this number 4,486 were from flocks subsequently found to have S. typhi-murium carriers. The O antigen was found to be most useful in detecting carriers, and birds revealing positive tests to both O and H antigens were found most likely to yield S. typhi-murium on culture. They emphasized that a testing program for S. typhi-murium is most effective when it is possible to practice complete replacement of all flocks shown to harbor carriers of the organisms. Pomeroy et al. (1957a) also recommended that in a control program based on the use of the agglutination test, reacting flocks should be disposed of, equipment and housing cleaned and disinfected, and replacement birds secured from a known clean source.

Belding and Mayer (1958) studied the use of the tube agglutination test to detect turkeys experimentally infected with S. san-diego. Only about one-third of the infected birds were detected by the test under the conditions of their experiment. Bierer and Vickers (1960a) found the rapid serum plate test using stained antigen for S. typhi-murium to be superior to the tube agglutination test or the rapid whole-blood test in detecting turkeys demonstrated bacteriologically to be carriers of the organism. However, serological tests were not entirely effective in detecting the infection. Stover (1961) pointed out that serological testing for S. typhi-murium in turkeys has helped to detect the infection in flocks that were subsequently disposed of or in which rigid sanitation including early high-level fumigation of eggs was applied.

Yamamoto et al. (1961a) reported a positive correlation of 33.6% between serological findings and isolation at 14 days after crop-induced S. typhi-murium infection in adult turkeys. The percentage correlation had increased to 38.8% at necropsy 35–44 days postinoculation. Yamamoto et al. (1962) found in Oregon that turkeys reacting as 3+ and 4+ to the agglutination test

for S. typhi-murium had a higher isolation rate of the organism on culture. It was apparent, however, that a flock could not be considered infected on the basis of serology alone. Isolation rate on a flock or per-bird basis was optimal when 3 or 4 suspected birds per flock were examined. Serological testing was recommended merely as a part of the entire control program. Goetz (1962) described the role of the tube agglutination test for S. typhi-murium in the paratyphoid control program in California.

Schalm (1937), Buxton and Gordon (1947), Wilson (1948), Clarenburg and Romijn (1954), Gwatkin and Dzenis (1954), Gwatkin and Grinewitsch (1955a,b), and Sieburth (1957a,b) have reported the use of the agglutination test to detect carriers of paratyphoid infections in chicken flocks. Buxton and Gordon (1947) reported that in known infected flocks, the use of blood testing was believed to have merit as an adjunct to hygienic measures in the hatchery. Müller (1957a) used the agglutination test in examining 30,596 blood samples from ducks, geese, turkeys, and chickens from 1,356 flocks in the Danish islands. It was found that 26.4% of the flocks contained reactors to S. typhi-murium and S. enteritidis antigens. Infection was confirmed by bacteriological culture in 41 of 361 reactors from 197 flocks. S. typhi-murium infected birds were found on one farm where the farmer and his family had experienced S. typhi-murium gastroenteritis.

Smyser and Van Roekel (1959), in the study of a supply flock to an institution where an outbreak of salmonella food poisoning had occurred, serologically tested 5,050 chickens with the tube agglutination test for S. typhi-murium. Ninety-four reacting birds were detected, and 9 of the higher-titered reactors were cultured. S. typhi-murium was isolated from 2 birds. Müller (1961), reporting on the progress of the elimination of salmonellosis in poultry of the Danish islands, noted that more extensive serological testing programs should be conducted for S. typhi-murium infection.

Ruedy et al. (1966) did not detect antibodies to typhi-murium somatic antigen in a survey of chicken flocks in Wisconsin. Smyser et al. (1966) studied S. heidelberg infection in 3 breeding flocks of chickens which manifested no visible signs of the disease. Cloacal swab culture methods for detection of carriers were more reliable than were serum agglutination tests for somatic antibodies. Salmonellae were recovered from the environment of one farm during a 5-month period. At necropsy there was no correlation between a bird's serological response and the recovery of *S. heidelberg*.

Brownell and Sadler (1967) did not find the tube agglutination test for *S. typhi-murium* infection to be of much, if any, value in detecting carriers in chickens. No correlation could be demonstrated between serological response and the ability to isolate salmonellae from rectal swabs or from tissues at necropsy. Following experimental infection of chickens with *S. typhi-murium*, Olesiuk et al. (1969) found the agglutination test using somatic typhi-murium antigen to be of very low efficiency in detecting birds that were fecal carriers of the organisms.

Levine and Graham (1942) and Gordon and Garside (1944) have reported on the use of paratyphoid antigens to test ducks. Lucas (1956) used furazolidone treatment and blood testing in the elimination of paratyphoid infection from mallard ducks. Perek and Rabinovitz (1957) concluded that agglutination tests of sera of geese for the detection of salmonella carriers is of negligible value since agglutinins may be present for several types of salmonella. Jungherr and Wilcox (1934) and Gauger et al. (1940) tested pigeons for paratyphoid, and Cunningham (1941) used serological procedures in an attempt to control paratyphoid infection in quail.

PARATYPHOID ANTIGENS. Various procedures have been recommended for the preparation of antigens for use in conducting serological tests for paratyphoid of poultry, as reviewed by Williams and MacDonald (1955). The techniques usually employed in the United States for the preparation of tube agglutination antigen closely follow those recommended by McNeil and Hinshaw (1951), the Committee on Salmonellosis of the North Central Regional Poultry Disease Conference (Pomeroy et al., 1957b), or the *National Poultry and Turkey Improvement Plans* (Anon., 1971a). Yamamoto et al. (1962) also described methods for the preparation and standardization of *S. typhi-murium* antigen for testing turkeys. Salmonella antigens and serological testing

procedures for avian species have been discussed in a recent comprehensive review (Anon., 1971b).

Presently all testing being conducted nationally for *S. typhi-murium* infection in turkeys under the NTIP is conducted using an antigen of the somatic (O) type in the macroscopic tube agglutination test. No official tests are being carried out for the detection of flagellar (H) agglutinins. With only a few exceptions the recommendations given in the Pullorum Disease section of this chapter for preparing, standardizing, using, and reading test results with the pullorum-typhoid tube agglutination test can be applied equally to the tube agglutination antigen for *S. typhi-murium*.

A single strain of *S. typhi-murium*, designated P-10, is used for the preparation of typhi-murium tube agglutination antigen in the United States (Williams, 1968). This strain possesses only somatic (O) antigens as it is naturally nonmotile, unlike most Group B organisms in the Kauffmann-White Schema. Strain P-10, which has antigens 4, 5, and 12, grows very well on common laboratory media. It yields an antigen of high stability and excellent sensitivity. The culture is best maintained by transferring every 3 months to new nutrient agar stabs which are maintained in the dark at room temperature.

Before the culture is used for antigen preparation it should be carefully checked for smoothness. The culture may be grown in veal infusion broth (Difco) for 18–24 hours at 37° C, then plated on veal infusion agar for single colony selection. After 18–24 hours incubation at 37° C, single colonies are picked and transferred to veal infusion agar slants. After incubation, growth from the slants is inoculated into veal infusion broth, which is incubated for 18–24 hours at 37° C before use in seeding the production agar bottles.

Veal infusion agar (Difco) prepared according to the manufacturer's directions from the dehydrated state is used as the antigen production medium. It is dispensed into Kolle flasks, Blake or Roux bottles, or other suitable containers and sterilized in the autoclave. The medium is allowed to harden with the bottles in a flat position to provide as much agar surface as possible.

The seeded production bottles are incubated for 24–48 hours at 37° C after which the growth is harvested in 0.5% phenolized saline solution. The antigen suspensions are standardized and used in the same manner as standard pullorum tube agglutination antigen discussed in the Pullorum Disease section of this chapter. A diagnostic dilution of 1:25 is recommended for routine use.

Tube agglutination antigens can be prepared for most other salmonella serotypes using the procedures outlined here for *S. typhi-murium* antigen. These antigens are also standardized and used in the same manner. Several antigen strains may need to be examined before a satisfactory one is found. Hypersensitivity is the main problem that will be encountered in the preparation and use of such antigens. A great deal of selection and experimentation may be needed to develop a satisfactory antigen, and judgment will need to be used in the interpretation of test results.

The reader interested in the preparation and use of flagellar type antigens for avian paratyphoid testing should refer to the report of McNeil and Hinshaw (1951).

Bassiouni (1965) described a method for preparing desiccated *S. typhi-murium* somatic and flagellar antigens. The dry somatic antigen when reconstituted was very similar to a liquid antigen in sensitivity; however, the flagellar antigen gave less comparative results.

Gauger et al. (1940) and Gwatkin and Grinewitsch (1955b) experimented with whole-blood antigens for the detection of *S. typhi-murium* infection in naturally and artificially infected fowl. Infected birds were not always detected by the antigens used. Clarenburg and Romijn (1954), using *S. bareilly* stained whole-blood antigen, were able to detect several infected birds; however, a large number of nonspecific reactions occurred with the antigen.

Blaxland et al. (1958) described the preparation and use of a stained whole-blood *S. typhi-murium* antigen for testing chickens, turkeys, and ducks by the rapid macroscopic plate method. The test with this antigen was found to be in close agreement with the tube agglutination test when dealing with birds revealing typically positive reactions. More nonspecific reactions were encountered with the *S. typhi-murium* stained antigen than with conventional *S. pullorum* plate antigens.

Khera et al. (1965) found an outbreak of *S. stanley* infection in adult laying hens to be controlled by whole-blood testing of the flock with subsequent segregation and destruction of serological reactors. Kashiwazaki et al. (1966) described a malachite green stained rapid whole-blood antigen that was used with some success for detection of *S. typhi-murium* infection in chickens.

Harris and Williams (1957) demonstrated a bacterial hemagglutinin in 17 of 22 strains of *S. typhi-murium* examined. The hemagglutinin was heat labile and disappeared upon prolonged storage of cultures. The results of this study indicated the necessity of carefully selecting strains free of hemagglutinating activity for the production of diagnostic antigens that are to be used with avian whole blood. Williams and Whittemore (1966) confirmed the frequent natural occurrence of hemagglutinating properties in strains of *S. typhi-murium* following studies involving 565 cultures of avian origin.

Sieburth and Johnson (1957) and Sieburth (1957a,b, 1958b) have described an indirect hemagglutination test that may be of value in screening for the detection of salmonella infections of poultry. Chicken erythrocytes sensitized with material liberated from boiled bacterial cells are used as the antigen in the test. A single polyvalent antigen was found to be capable of detecting several antigenic types of the infection. Hemagglutinins occurred in the blood of infected birds at a higher titer and appeared earlier than conventional agglutinins. It was stated that the indirect hemagglutination test, unlike the agglutination test, detected antibodies in chickens receiving furazolidone treatment. Sieburth (1960) further refined the antigen for the indirect hemagglutination test by developing methods for the production of more stable and standard antigen preparations.

Magwood and Bigland (1962) found the overall performance of the bacterial agglutination and hemagglutination tests to demonstrate an equal but unsatisfactory degree of efficacy in detecting turkeys infected with salmonellosis. Both tests failed to identify half of the infected birds and also one infected flock. Many nonspecific reactions were detected with the hemagglutination test.

Rice et al. (1960) applied the modified direct complement-fixation test for detection of salmonella antibodies in heat-inactivated turkey serum. Reactions recorded with partially purified somatic antigens were group specific. Magwood and Annau (1961) adsorbed crude and partially purified extracts containing salmonella somatic antigens on polystyrene latex particles. The latex particles were used in agglutination tests to detect salmonella agglutinins in turkey sera. The antigen revealed serological specificity and was agglutinated by antibodies for the homologous salmonella groups. Results with this testing procedure appeared encouraging, but the practical value of the test in naturally infected birds has not been determined.

In 1970 there was no official testing program for the control of paratyphoid infections in all avian species on a nationwide basis. Heemstra (1952) pointed out the responsibility of the veterinary profession in helping the poultry industry seek a solution to this problem. The application of serological procedures for the diagnosis of paratyphoid infections is dependent to a large degree on facilities available in state laboratories for conducting the tests. Furthermore, the importance of the paratyphoid problem in a particular area will indicate the desirability of using testing procedures as an ancillary measure to the general control program for the disease.

Immunization

Bacterins and attenuated live cultures for use as vaccines in the prevention of avian paratyphoid infections have been studied experimentally but have never had wide application under field conditions in the United States. Khera et al. (1965) reported that they used a formolized broth culture vaccine prepared from a strain of *S. stanley* during an outbreak due to this serotype in a chicken flock. After vaccination, mortality due to this infection ceased to occur. Botes (1965) experimentally studied attenuated live cultures of *S. typhimurium* for preventive vaccination of chickens. The vaccine could not be properly evaluated because control birds resisted fatal infection when challenged.

McCapes et al. (1967) reported the use of 4 isolates of *S. typhi-murium* in the preparation of an experimental whole-broth aluminum hydroxide adsorbed bacterin for vaccination of turkey hens. Poults from dams receiving the bacterin exhibited measurable resistance to yolk sac challenge with both *S. typhi-murium* and *S. schwarzengrund* but not with *S. anatum*. Challenge of poults from *S. typhi-murium*-vaccinated dams produced 39.7% mortality in 10 days, whereas challenge of poults from unvaccinated dams produced 85.6% mortality in the same period. It was felt that further challenge trials needed to be conducted to fully ascertain the range of poult protection obtained through the use of single-serotype vaccination of dams. While trials such as these indicate that some resistance can be stimulated to paratyphoid infection in the young by vaccination of dams, it is unlikely that such practices will ever have a place in programs aimed at complete elimination of salmonella infections from poultry flocks.

REFERENCES

Abelseth, M. K., and H. E. Robertson. 1953. *Salmonella typhimurium* infection in 1952 turkey flocks—A public health hazard. *Can. J. Public Health* 44:263–65.

Adler. H. E., E. H. Willers, and M. Levine. 1951. Incidence of salmonella in apparently healthy dogs. *J. Am. Vet. Med. Ass.* 118:300–304.

Adler, H. E., M. A. Nilson, and W. J. Stadelman. 1953. A study of turkeys artificially infected with *Salmonella typhimurium*. *Am. J. Vet. Res.* 14:246–48.

Akiyama. Y. 1961. Studies on salmonella infections in chicks. II. Observations on chicks hatched from eggs artificially infected with *S. pullorum* and *S. senftenberg*. *Japan. J. Bacteriol.* 16:460–67.

Akiyama, Y., S. Watanabe, and R. Sakazaki.

1959. A survey on salmonella infection among chicks and embryonating eggs in Aomori Prefecture. *J. Japan. Vet. Med. Ass.* 12:210–12.

Allred, J. N., J. W. Walker, V. C. Beal, Jr., and F. W. Germaine. 1967. A survey to determine the salmonella contamination rate in livestock and poultry feeds. *J. Am. Vet. Med. Ass.* 151:1857–60.

Altman, I. E. 1940. *Salmonella suipestifer* infection in canaries. *J. Am. Vet. Med. Ass.* 97:601.

Alves de Oliveira, J. J., and J. F. Gomes. 1954. Isolamento e caracterizacao de *S. typhimurium* em ovos de galinha, por ocasiao de um surto occorrido no hospital da C.U.F. *Rev. Cienc. Vet.* 49:389–99.

Anderson, A. S., H. Bauer, and C. B. Nelson.

1955. Salmonellosis due to *Salmonella typhimurium* with Easter chicks as likely source. *J. Am. Med. Ass.* 158:1153–55.

Anderson, E. S., and R. E. O. Williams. 1956. Bacteriophage typing of enteric pathogens and staphylococci and its use in epidemiology. *J. Clin. Pathol.* 9:94–127.

Anellis, A., J. Lubas, and M. M. Rayman. 1954. Heat resistance in liquid eggs of some strains of the genus *Salmonella*. *Food Res.* 19:377–95.

Angstrom, C. I. 1957. Case report—A paratyphoid outbreak in a poultry breeding flock. *Avian Diseases* 1:52–53.

Anonymous. 1947. *Outline of a Sanitation Program for the Poultry Industry*. USDA, ARS, Animal Health Div., Hyattsville, Md.

Anonymous. 1961. Infection from poultry. *Lancet* 1:38.

Anonymous. 1963a. *Salmonella derby* epidemic—Follow-up report. *Morbidity and Mortality Weekly Report*, U.S. Dept. of HEW 12:230.

Anonymous. 1963b. Symposium—epidemiology of salmonellosis. *Public Health Rept.* 78:1065–88.

Anonymous. 1964a. *Proceedings of the Salmonella Seminar*. USDA, ARS, Animal Health Div., Hyattsville, Md.

Anonymous. 1964b. *Salmonella Facts Summarized for the Poultry and Egg Industry*. Scient. Advis. Committee, Pacific Dairy and Poultry Ass., Los Angeles, Cal.

Anonymous. 1964c. *For Salmonella Control—Recommended Sanitation Guidelines for Processors of Poultry and Animal By-products*. USDA, ARS 91–47.

Anonymous. 1965a. *Sanitation Guidelines for Salmonella Control in Processing Industrial Fishery Products*. USDA, ARS 91–51.

Anonymous. 1965b. *Method of Salmonella Detection of Grading Branch*, Poultry Division, Consumer and Marketing Serv., USDA, pp. 39–42.

Anonymous. 1965c. *Proceedings National Conference on Salmonellosis*. U.S. Dept. of HEW, Public Health Serv., NCDC, Atlanta, Ga.

Anonymous. 1966. *The Destruction of Salmonellae*. West. Reg. Res. Lab., USDA, ARS, Albany, Cal.

Anonymous. 1967a. *Destination of Salmonella Contaminated Foods and Feeds*. World Ass. of Vet. Food-Hygienists.

Anonymous. 1967b. *Salmonella in Livestock and Poultry*. ARS 91–48–5, USDA, ARS, Animal Health Div., Hyattsville, Md.

Anonymous. 1967c. *Salmonella Surveillance—Annual Summary 1966*. U.S. Dept. of HEW, Public Health Serv., NCDC, Atlanta, Ga.

Anonymous. 1968a. *Salmonella Surveillance—Annual Summary 1967*. U.S. Dept. of HEW, Public Health Serv., NCDC, Atlanta, Ga.

Anonymous. 1968b. *Recommended Procedure For the Isolation of Salmonella Organisms from Animal Feeds and Feed Ingredients*. ARS 91–68, USDA, ARS, Animal Health Div., Hyattsville, Md.

Anonymous. 1968c. *Poultry Disease Control Programs—A Workshop Report*. Univ. Calif., Davis.

Anonymous. 1969a. *The Use of Drugs in Animal Feeds*. Proceedings of a symposium. Nat. Acad. Sci. Publ. 1679, Nat. Res. Council, Washington, D.C.

Anonymous. 1969b. *An Evaluation of the Salmonella Problem*. Nat. Acad. Sci. Publ. 1683, Nat. Res. Council, Washington, D.C.

Anonymous. 1971a. *National Poultry and Turkey Improvement Plans and Auxiliary Provisions*. USDA, ARS, ASR Div., Beltsville, Md.

Anonymous. 1971b. *Methods for the Examination of Poultry Vaccines. Methods for the Identification and Quantitation of Avian Pathogens*. Nat. Acad. Sci. Publ. Nat. Res. Council, Washington, D.C. (In press).

Ayres, J. C., A. A. Kraft, R. G. Board, G. S. Torrey, and S. S. Rizk. 1967. Sanitation practices in egg handling and breaking plants and the application of several disinfectants for sanitizing eggs. *J. Appl. Bacteriol.* 30:106–16.

Bahr, L., and N. P. C. Christensen. 1933. Investigations concerning the *B. pullorum* and bacteria pertaining to the salmonella group. *Brit. Vet. J.* 89:561–69.

Baker, E. D., F. A. Van Natta, and A. R. McLaughlin. 1966. *Salmonella* isolations on a turkey farm—A field study. *Avian Diseases* 10:131–34.

Baldwin, Ruth E., Marion Cloninger, and M. L. Fields. 1968. Growth and destruction of *Salmonella typhimurium* in egg white foam products cooked by microwaves. *Appl. Microbiol.* 16:1929–34.

Ballantyne, E. E. 1953. Salmonella infections of poultry in Alberta. *Proc. Book, Am. Vet. Med. Ass. 90th Ann. Meet.*, pp. 355–58.

Banwart, G. J. 1964. Elimination of salmonellae from inoculated filler flats. *Poultry Sci.* 43:939–41.

Banwart, G. J., and J. C. Ayres. 1957. The effect of pH on the growth of *Salmonella* and functional properties of liquid egg white. *Food Technol.* 11:244–46.

Banwart, G. J., and Madeleine J. Kreitzer. 1969. Further studies on the screening technique for determining *Salmonella*-negative samples of pasteurized dried egg. *Poultry Sci.* 48:235–40.

Banwart, G. J., A. J. Mercuri, and T. Ryan. 1968. Screening method for determining *Salmonella*-negative samples of dried egg. *Poultry Sci.* 47:598–603.

Barckhausen, J. 1961. Aufenthalt und Verhalten einer Jungen Blaessgans mit Maeuse-typhus *(Salmonella typhi-murium). Deut. Tieraerztl. Wochschr.* 68:660.

Barkate, J. A. 1968. Screening of feed components for salmonella with polyvalent H agglutination. *Appl. Microbiol.* 16:1872–74.

Bassiouni, A. 1965. A dry antigen for the detection of *Salmonella typhimurium* infection in poultry. *Egyptian Vet. Med. J.* 11:121–29.

Bayne, H. G., J. A. Garibaldi, and H. Lineweaver. 1965. Heat resistance of *Salmonella typhimurium* and *Salmonella senftenberg* 775W in chicken meat. *Poultry Sci.* 44:1281–84.

Beach, J. R. 1936. Remarks made during discussion of paratyphoid infections of poultry. *Proc. 6th World's Poultry Congr.* 3:410.

Beattie, W. E. 1960. Avian infection with *Salmonella thompson*—Observations. *Poultry Sci.* 39:1233.

Beaudette, F. R. 1926a. B. *aertrycke* infection in canary birds and parrots. *J. Am. Vet. Med. Ass.* 68:642–43.

———. 1926b. B. *aertrycke* as the etiological agent in a disease affecting squabs. *J. Amer. Vet. Med. Ass.* 68:644–52.

Beaudette, F. R., and P. R. Edwards. 1926. The etiology of a canary bird epizootic. *J. Bacteriol.* 12:51–55.

Becker, W. 1957. Salmonellosen beim Hausgefluegel. *Berlin. Muench. Tieraerztl. Wochschr.* 70:168–70.

Belding, R. C., and M. L. Mayer. 1958. Furazolidone in the treatment of salmonella infections of turkeys. 2. Effect on acute paratyphoid infection in poults. *Poultry Sci.* 37:463–67.

Belliveau, R. R., J. W. Grayson, and T. J. Butler. 1968. A rapid, simple method of identifying Enterobacteriaceae. *Am. J. Clin. Pathol.* 50:126–28.

Beloian, A., and G. C. Schlosser. 1963. Adequacy of cooking procedures for the destruction of salmonellae. *Am. J. Public Health* 53:782–91.

Bergsma, C. 1959. Veterinaire Problemen bij de Epidemiologie der Salmonellosen. *Tijdschr. Diergeneesk.* 84:872–91.

Biddle, E. S., and M. S. Cover. 1957. The bacterial flora of the respiratory tract of chickens affected with chronic respiratory disease. *Am. J. Vet. Res.* 18:405–8.

Bierer, B. W. 1960. Effect of age factor on mortality in *Salmonella typhimurium* infection in turkey poults. *J. Am. Vet. Med. Ass.* 137:657–58.

———. 1961. A method of inducing *Salmonella typhimurium* infection in chicks. *J. Am. Vet. Med. Ass.* 139:790.

———. 1963. The use of nihydrazone against *Salmonella typhimurium* and *Salmonella gallinarum* infections in turkeys. *Poultry Sci.* 42:465–68.

Bierer, B. W., and B. D. Barnett. 1961. Effect of increasing wash water temperature on eggs contaminated with salmonella. *Poultry Sci.* 40:1379. (Abstr.)

———. 1962a. Nihydrazone and the salmonella infections. *Poultry Sci.* 41:1291–94.

———. 1962b. Furaltadone water medication and the salmonelloses. *Proc. 12th World's Poultry Congr.*, pp. 283–85.

Bierer, B. W., and T. H. Eleazer. 1965. Clinical salmonellosis accidentally induced by feed and water deprivation of one-week-old broiler chicks. *Poultry Sci.* 44:1606–7.

Bierer, B. W., and C. L. Vickers. 1960a. Nitrofuran medication for experimental *Salmonella typhimurium* infection in poults. *Avian Diseases* 4:22–37.

———. 1960b. Evaluation of water soluble nitrofurans in experimental salmonella infection in turkey poults. *Vet. Med.* 55:78–82.

Bierer, B. W., B. D. Barnett, and H. D. Valentine. 1961a. Experimentally killing *Salmonella typhimurium* on egg shells by washing. *Poultry Sci.* 40:1009–14.

Bierer, B. W., H. D. Valentine, and C. L. Vickers. 1961b. Furaltadone water medication: Its use in avian salmonellosis. *Avian Diseases* 5:214–18.

Bierer, B. W., H. D. Valentine, B. D. Barnett, and W. H. Rhodes. 1961c. Germicidal efficiency of egg washing compounds on eggs artificially contaminated with *Salmonella typhimurium. Poultry Sci.* 40:148–52.

Bigland, C. H., and G. Papas. 1953. Experiment in egg penetration by salmonella. *Can. J. Comp. Med. Vet. Sci.* 17:105–9.

Bigland, C. H., G. S. Wilton, H. N. Vance, and H. C. Carlson. 1962. Salmonellosis of animals in Alberta, 1949–1960. *J. Am. Vet. Med. Ass.* 140:251–53.

Bischoff, J. 1961. Vorschlaege zur Aenderung der Verordnung zum Schutze gegen Infektion durch Erreger der Salmonellagruppe in Eiprodukten vom 17. Dezember 1956. *Berlin. Muench. Tieraerztl. Wochschr.* 74:70–71.

Blaxland, J. D., and A. J. Blowers. 1951. *Salmonella typhimurium* infection in duck eggs as a cause of human food poisoning. *Vet. Record* 63:56–59.

Blaxland, J. D., W. J. Sojka, and A. M. Smither. 1958. Avian salmonellosis in England and Wales 1948–56, with comment on its prevention and control. *Vet. Record* 70:374–82.

Bloom, H. H., W. N. Mack, and W. L. Mallmann. 1958. Enteric viruses and salmonellae isolation. II. Media comparison for salmonellae. *Sewage Ind. Wastes* 30:1455–60.

Board, R. G. 1964. The growth of gram-negative bacteria in the hen's egg. *J. Appl. Bacteriol.* 27:350–64.

Board, R. G., J. C. Ayres, A. A. Kraft, and R. H. Forsythe. 1964. The microbiological contamination of egg shells and egg packing materials. *Poultry Sci.* 43:584–95.

Botes, H. J. W. 1965. Live vaccines in the control of salmonellosis. *J. S. African Vet. Med. Ass.* 36:461–74.

Bövre, K., and P. Sandbu. 1959. Salmonella excreting tortoises in Oslo. *Acta Pathol. Microbiol. Scand.* 46:339–42.

Bowmer, E. J. 1964. The challenge of salmonellosis. Major public health problem. *Am. J. Med. Sci.* 247:467–501.

Boyer, C. I., D. W. Bruner, and J. A. Brown. 1958. Salmonella organisms isolated from poultry feed. *Proc. 30th N.E. Conf. on Avian Diseases.*

Boyer, C. I., S. Narotsky, D. W. Bruner, and J. A. Brown. 1962. Salmonellosis in turkeys and chickens associated with contaminated feed. *Avian Diseases* 6:43–50.

Brandly, C. A. 1951. Poultry diseases as public health problems. *Public Health Rept.* 66:668–72.

Brest Nielsen, B. 1960. *Salmonella typhimurium* carriers in seagulls and mallards as a possible source of infection to domestic animals. *Nord. Veterinaermed.* 12:417–24.

Brobst, D., J. Greenberg, and H. M. Gezon. 1958. Salmonellosis in poultry and poultry processing plants in Western Pennsylvania. *J. Am. Vet. Med. Ass.* 133:435–37.

Browne, A. S. 1949. The public health significance of salmonella on poultry and poultry products. Ph.D. thesis, Univ. Calif. Berkeley.

Brownell, J. R., and W. W. Sadler. 1967. Salmonella carriers. *Proc. Western Poultry Disease Conf.*, Univ. Calif., Davis, pp. 14–16.

Bruner, D. W., and Alice B. Moran. 1949. Salmonella infections of domestic animals. *Cornell Vet.* 39:53–63.

Bryan, F. L., J. C. Ayres, and A. A. Kraft. 1968. Contributory sources of salmonellae on turkey products. *Am. J. Epidemiol.* 87:578–91.

Burkhart, D. M., R. W. Wolfgang, and P. D. Harwood. 1962. Salmonellosis in parakeets and canaries treated with nitrofurans in the drinking water. *Avian Diseases* 6:275–83.

Burr, W. E., and C. F. Helmboldt. 1962. Salmonella species contaminants in three animal by-products. *Avian Diseases* 6:441–43.

Burr, W. E., M. Tourtellotte, R. E. Luginbuhl, and E. L. Jungherr. 1957. *Salmonella heidelberg* infection as a problem in pullorum disease control. *Avian Diseases* 1:298–304.

Butler, R. L., and C. E. Mickel. 1955. Insect and rodent contamination of grain. *Univ. Minn. Agr. Exp. Sta. Tech. Bull.* 431, p. 20.

Buxton, A. 1957a. *Salmonellosis in Animals.*

A review. Commonwealth Agricultural Bureaux, Farnham Royal, Bucks, England.

———. 1957b. Public health aspects of salmonellosis in animals. *Vet. Record* 69:105–9.

———. 1958. Salmonellosis in animals. *Vet. Record* 70:1044–52.

Buxton, A., and R. F. Gordon. 1947. The epidemiology and control of *Salmonella thompson* infection of fowls. *J. Hyg.* 45:265–81.

Canale-Parola, E., and Z. J. Ordal. 1957. A survey of the bacteriological quality of frozen poultry pies. *Food Technol.* 11:578–82.

Cantor, A., and V. H. McFarlane. 1948. Salmonella organisms on and in chicken eggs. *Poultry Sci.* 27:350–55.

Carlson, Virginia L., and G. H. Snoeyenbos. 1968. The effect of antibacterials on *Salmonella typhimurium* within hatching eggs. *Avian Diseases* 12:606–14.

Carlson, Virginia L., G. H. Snoeyenbos, B. A. McKie, and C. F. Smyser. 1967. A comparison of incubation time and temperature for the isolation of salmonella. *Avian Diseases* 11:217–25.

Casas, E. de las, B. S. Pomeroy, and P. K. Harein. 1968. Infection and quantitative recovery of *Salmonella typhimurium* and *Escherichia coli* from within the lesser mealworm, *Alphitobius diaperinus* (Panzer). *Poultry Sci.* 47:1871–75.

Chang, T. S., M. S. Rheins, and A. R. Winter. 1957. The significance of the bursa of Fabricius in antibody production in chickens. 1. Age of chickens. *Poultry Sci.* 36:735–38.

Chaplin, W. C., and C. M. Hamilton. 1957. A synovitis in turkeys produced by *Salmonella thompson*. *Poultry Sci.* 36:1380–81.

Chase, F. E. 1947. The occurrence and distribution of salmonella types in fowl. II. Studies of artificial *S. bareilly* and *S. oranienburg* infections in hens. *Can. J. Res.* 25:316–25.

Cherrington, V. A., E. M. Gildow, and P. Moore. 1937. Paratyphoid in turkeys. *Poultry Sci.* 16:226–31.

Cherry, W. B., L. A. Barnes, and P. R. Edwards. 1946. Observations on a monophasic salmonella variant. *J. Bacteriol.* 51:235–43.

Christensen, W. B. 1946. Urea decomposition as a means of differentiating proteus and paracolon cultures from each other and from salmonella and shigella types. *J. Bacteriol.* 52:461–66.

Clarenburg, A. 1939. Paratyphoid in ducks in relation to public health. *Proc. 7th World's Poultry Congr.*, pp. 233–36.

Clarenburg, A., and C. G. J. Dornickx. 1932. Voe dselvergiftiging bij Mensch in Verband met Duiven—Paratyphose. *Tijdschr. Diergeneesk.* 59:670–76.

Clarenburg, A., and W. J. Roepke. 1952. *S. bareilly*—Infectie bij kuikens. *Tijdschr. Diergeneesk.* 77:174–78.

Clarenburg, A., and C. Romijn. 1954. The effectiveness of fumigation with the formaldehyde-potassium permanganate and the influence on the hatchability. *Proc. 10th World's Poultry Congr.*, pp. 214–16.

Clark, C. H. 1946. Sulfamerazine in paratyphoid disease of poults and chicks. *J. Am. Vet. Med. Ass.* 109:279.

Clemmer, Dorothy I., J. L. S. Hickey, J. F. Bridges, D. J. Schliessmann, and M. F. Shaffer. 1960. Bacteriologic studies of experimental air-borne salmonellosis in chicks. *J. Infect. Diseases* 106:197–210.

Clise, J. D., and E. E. Swecker. 1965. Salmonellae from animal by-products. *Public Health Rept.* 80:899–905.

Cockburn, W. C. 1965. Salmonella, retrospect and prospect. *Proc. Nat. Conf. on Salmonellosis*, U.S. Dept. of HEW, Public Health Health Serv., NCDC, Atlanta, Ga., pp. 185–91.

Cope, E. J., W. K. Appelhof, and P. C. Martineau. 1955. Salmonella isolated from animals, birds, and reptiles in a metropolitan zoo. *Cornell Vet.* 45:3–9.

Cotterill, O. J. 1968. Equivalent pasteurization temperatures to kill salmonellae in liquid egg white at various pH levels. *Poultry Sci.* 47:354–65.

Craige, J. E. 1944. The isolation of *Salmonella anatum* from the feces of a dog. *J. Am. Vet. Med. Ass.* 105:33–34.

Csiszár, V., I. Dózsa, and J. Takács. 1961. A budapesti allatkerti allatok salmonellas fertozottsege. *Magy. Allatorv. Lapja* 16:373–76.

Cunningham, C. H. 1941. Paratyphoid infection in quail. *J. Am. Vet. Med. Ass.* 99:217.

Cunningham, F. E., J. A. Garibaldi, K. Ijichi, and H. Lineweaver. 1965. Pasteurization of liquid egg white. *World's Poultry Sci. J.* 21:365–69.

Dalling, T., and G. K. Warrack. 1932. Ducks and salmonella infection. *J. Pathol. Bacteriol.* 35:655.

Darby, C. W., and H. J. Stafseth. 1942. Salmonella infections common to man, animals, and birds. *Proc. 46th Ann. Meet. U.S. Livestock Sanit. Ass.*, pp. 189–202.

Das, M. S., M. B. Chakravorty, and G. K. Ghosh. 1959. Occurrence of avian salmonellosis in West Bengal. *Indian Vet. J.* 36: 403–8.

Dawkins, H. C., and L. Robertson. 1967. Salmonellas in animal feeding stuffs. *Monthly Bull. Ministry Health, Public Health Lab. Serv.* 26:215–21.

DeLay, P. D., T. W. Jackson, E. E. Jones, and D. E. Stover. 1954. A testing service for the control of *Salmonella typhimurium* infection in turkeys. *Am. J. Vet. Res.* 15:122–29.

Deom, J. 1960. Un type rare de Salmonella isole chez un passereau au Conge Belge. *Rev. Pathol. Gen. Comparee* 60:249–56.

Dixon, J. M. S. 1961. Rapid isolation of salmonellae from faeces. *J. Clin. Pathol.* 14:397–99.

Dixon, J. M. S., and F. E. Pooley. 1961. Salmonellae in a poultry processing plant. *Monthly Bull. Ministry Health, Public Health Lab. Serv.* 20:30–33.

Dolman, C. E. 1954. Some ways in which animal health affects human health. *Can. J. Comp. Med. Vet. Sci.* 18:35–50.

Dougherty, E. 1953. Disease problems confronting the duck industry. *Proc. Book, Am. Vet. Med. Ass. 90th Ann. Meet.*, pp. 359–65.

———. 1954. Paratyphoid infection in the White Pekin duck. *Proc. 26th Ann. Conf. Lab. Workers in Pullorum Disease Control.*

———. 1961. The pathology of paratyphoid infection in the White Pekin duck, particularly the lesions in the central nervous system. *Avian Diseases* 5:415–30.

Doyle, T. M. 1927. *B. aertrycke* infection of chicks. *J. Comp. Pathol. Therap.* 40:71–75.

Dózsa, I. 1961. A hazivereb (*Passer d. domesticus*), mint *Salmonella typhimurium*—Reservoir. *Magy. Allatorv. Lapja* 16:144–45.

Edwards, P. R. 1958. Salmonellosis: Observations on incidence and control. *Ann. N.Y. Acad. Sci.* 70:598–613.

Edwards, P. R., and D. W. Bruner. 1940. The occurrence of multiple types of paratyphoid bacilli in infections of fowls, with special reference to two new Salmonella species. *J. Infect. Diseases* 66:218–21.

Edwards, P. R., and W. H. Ewing. 1962. *Identification of Enterobacteriaceae.* Burgess Publ. Co., Minneapolis.

Edwards, P. R., and Mildred M. Galton. 1967. Salmonellosis, pp. 1–63. In Brandly, C. A., and C. Cornelius, *Advances in Veterinary Science.* Academic Press, New York.

Edwards, P. R., D. W. Bruner, and Alice B. Moran. 1948a. The genus *Salmonella*: Its occurrence and distribution in the United States. *Ky. Agr. Exp. Sta. Bull.* 525.

———. 1948b. Further studies on the occurrence and distribution of salmonella types in the United States. *J. Infect. Diseases* 83:220–31.

———. 1948c. Salmonella infections of fowls. *Cornell Vet.* 38:247–56.

Eickhoff, T. C. 1966. Economic losses due to salmonellosis in humans, p. 17. In *The Destruction of Salmonellae.* West. Reg. Res. Lab., USDA, ARS, Albany, Cal.

Ellemann, G. 1959. Temperaturens betydning

for indvaekst af *Salmonella typhi-murium* i hønseaeg. *Nord. Veterinarmed.* 11:341–49.

Emmel, M. W. 1929. Arthritis in pigeons caused by *Salmonella schottmulleri. J. Am. Vet. Med. Ass.* 28:367–70.

———. 1936. The importance of endotoxin of *Salmonella sertrycke* in the development of fowl paralysis. *Vet. Med.* 31:436.

Emmel, M. W., and H. J. Stafseth. 1929. *Salmonella aertrycke* infection in the canary bird. *J. Am. Vet. Med. Ass.* 75:230–31.

Erwin, L. E. 1955. Examination of prepared poultry feeds for the presence of salmonella and other enteric organisms. *Poultry Sci.* 34:215–16.

Evans, W. M., D. W. Bruner, and M. C. Peckham. 1955. Blindness in chicks associated with salmonellosis. *Cornell Vet.* 45:239–47.

Eveleth, D. F., A. I. Goldsby, and F. M. Bolin. 1947. The treatment of pullorum disease and paratyphoid infections with sulfamerazine. *N. Dakota Agr. Exp. Sta. Bull.* 9:163–65.

Ewing, W. H., and M. M. Ball. 1966. *The Biochemical Reactions of Members of the Genus Salmonella.* U.S. Dept. of HEW, Public Health Serv., NCDC, Atlanta, Ga.

Ewing, W. H., B. R. Davis, and P. R. Edwards. 1960. The decarboxylase reactions of Enterobacteriaceae and their value in taxonomy. *Public Health Rept.* 18:77–83.

Faddoul, G. P., and G. W. Fellows. 1965. Clinical manifestations of paratyphoid infection in pigeons. *Avian Diseases* 9:377–81.

———. 1966. A five-year survey of the incidence of salmonellae in avian species. *Avian Diseases* 10:296–304.

Faddoul, G. P., G. W. Fellows, and J. Baird. 1966. A survey of the incidence of salmonellae in wild birds. *Avian Diseases* 10:89–94.

Feeley, J. C., and M. D. Treger. 1969. Penetration of turtle eggs by *Salmonella braenderup. Public Health Rept.* 84:156–58.

Felsenfeld, O. 1949. Notes on *Salmonella cubana. Poultry Sci.* 28:142–43.

Felsenfeld, O., and V. M. Young. 1945. The viability of salmonella on artificially contaminated vegetables. *Poultry Sci.* 24:353–55.

Felsenfeld, O., V. M. Young, and T. Yoshimura. 1950. A survey of salmonella organisms in market meat, eggs, and milk. *J. Am. Vet. Med. Ass.* 116:17–21.

Fey, H., and E. Wiesmann. 1960. Die Gefahr des Salmonellenimportes mit Eiprodukten und Tierischen Futtermitteln. *Schweiz. Med. Wochschr.* 90:791–93.

Florin, S. O., and T. Nilsson. 1959. The influence of slaughter technique on contamination of the meat in cases of intestinal salmonellosis of poultry. *Proc. 8th Nordic Vet. Congr.*

Forsythe, R. H., W. J. Ross, and J. C. Ayres.

1967. Salmonellae recovery following gastrointestinal and ovarian inoculation in the domestic fowl. *Poultry Sci.* 46:849–55.

Francis, D. W., H. Campbell, and G. R. Newton. 1960. The use of furazolidone for chukar partridges. *Avian Diseases* 4:218–23.

Frank, J. F., and G. W. Wright. 1955. Susceptibility of salmonella organisms to formaldehyde fumigation. *Can. J. Comp. Med. Vet. Sci.* 19:71–75.

———. 1956. The disinfection of eggs contaminated with *Salmonella typhimurium. Can. J. Comp. Med. Vet. Sci.* 20:406–10.

Galbraith, N. S. 1961. Salmonellosis in man and animals. 2. Studies on human salmonellosis in relation to infection in animals. *Vet. Record* 73:1296–1303.

Galbraith, N. S., C. E. D. Taylor, P. Cavanagh, J. G. Hagan, and J. L. Patton. 1962. Pet foods and garden fertilizers as sources of human salmonellosis. *Lancet,* 1:372–74.

Galton, Mildred M. 1961. Laboratory procedures for the isolation of salmonella from human and animal food products. *Proc. 65th Ann. Meet. U.S. Livestock Sanit. Ass.,* pp. 434–40.

Galton, Mildred M., J. E. Scatterday, and A. V. Hardy. 1952. Salmonellosis in dogs. I. Bacteriological, epidemiological, and clinical considerations. *J. Infect. Diseases* 91:1–5.

Galton, Mildred M., W. D. Lowery, and A. V. Hardy. 1954. Salmonella in fresh and smoked pork sausage. *J. Infect. Diseases* 95:232–35.

Galton, Mildred M., D. C. Mackel, A. L. Lewis, W. C. Haire, and A. V. Hardy. 1955. Salmonellosis in poultry and poultry processing plants in Florida. *Am. J. Vet. Res.* 16:132–37.

Galton, Mildred M., J. H. Steele, and K. W. Newell. 1964. Epidemiology of salmonellosis in the United States, pp. 421–44. In Van Oye, E., *The World Problem of Salmonellosis.* Junk Publishers, The Hague, Netherlands.

Gandon, Y. 1963. Les salmonella des oeufs et ovoproduits francais et etrangers. *Ann. Inst. Pasteur* 104:584–97.

Garside, J. S., and R. F. Gordon. 1940. Salmonella infections of ducks and ducklings. *J. Comp. Pathol. Therap.* 53: 80–89.

Garside, J. S., R. F. Gordon, and J. F. Tucker. 1960. The emergence of resistant strains of *Salmonella typhimurium* in the tissues and alimentary tracts of chickens following the feeding of an antibiotic. *Res. Vet. Sci.* 1:184–99.

Gauger, H. C., and R. E. Greaves. 1946a. Bacterial examination of shells and contents of eggs laid by turkeys naturally and artificially infected with *Salmonella typhimurium. Poultry Sci.* 25:119–23.

———. 1946b. Isolation of *Salmonella typhimurium* from drinking water in an infected environment. *Poultry Sci.* 25:476–78.

———. 1946c. Isolation of *Salmonella typhimurium* from the feces of turkeys. *Poultry Sci.* 25:232–35.

———. 1947. Isolation of *Salmonella typhimurium* from the feces of artificially infected poults. *Poultry Sci.* 26:48–51.

Gauger, H. C., R. E. Greaves, and F. W. Cook. 1940. Paratyphoid of pigeons. Serological, bacteriological, and hematological studies of spontaneously infected birds. *N. Carolina State Coll. Agr. Exp. Sta. Bull.* 62.

Gibbons, N. E., and R. L. Moore. 1946. A note on artificially infected fowl as carriers of salmonella. *Poultry Sci.* 25:115–18.

Glezen, W. P., M. P. Hines, Mildred Kerbaugh, Minnie E. Green, and J. Koomen, Jr. 1966. Salmonella in two poultry processing plants. *J. Am. Vet. Med. Ass.* 148:550–52.

Goetz, M. E. 1962. The control of paracolon and paratyphoid infections in turkey poults. *Avian Diseases* 6:93–99.

Gordon, R. F. 1959. Broiler diseases. *Vet. Record* 71:994–1003.

Gordon, R. F., and A. Buxton. 1945. The isolation of *Salmonella thompson* from outbreaks of disease in chicks. *J. Hyg.,* 44:179–83.

———. 1946. A survey of avian salmonellosis in Great Britain. *Brit. Vet. J.* 102:187–206.

Gordon, R. F., and J. S. Garside. 1944. Salmonella infections in ducks. Observations on the value of the agglutination test in the eradication of infection and investigations on the cycle of infection via the egg. *J. Comp. Pathol. Therap.* 54:61–76.

Gordon, R. F., and J. F. Tucker. 1957. The isolation of *Salmonella infantis* from a turkey poult. *Monthly Bull. Ministry Health, Public Health Lab. Serv.* 16:71–72.

———. 1965. The epizootiology of *Salmonella menston* infection of fowls and the effect of feeding poultry food artificially infected with salmonella. *Brit. Poultry Sci.* 6:251–64.

Gordon, R. F., E. G. Harry, and J. F. Tucker. 1956. The use of germicidal dips in the control of bacterial contamination of the shells of hatching eggs. *Vet. Record* 68:33–38.

Graham, R. 1936. Salmonella isolated from baby quail. *J. Am. Vet. Med. Ass.* 88:763–64.

Graham, R., and Viola M. Michael. 1936. Studies on incubator hygiene. *Poultry Sci.* 15:83–87.

Greenberg, B. 1959. Persistence of bacteria in developmental stages of housefly. I. Survival of enteric pathogens in normal and aseptically reared host. *Am. J. Trop. Med. Hyg.* 8:405–11.

———. 1964. Experimental transmission of *Salmonella typhimurium* by houseflies to man. *Am. J. Hyg.* 80:149–56.

Greenberg, B., and A. Bornstein. 1964. Fly dispersion from a rural Mexican slaughterhouse. *Am. J. Trop. Med. Hyg.* 13:881–86.

Greenberg, B., G. Varela, A. Bornstein, and H. Hernandez. 1963. Salmonellae from flies in a Mexican slaughterhouse. *Am. J. Hyg.* 77:177–83.

Gregory, D. W. 1948. Salmonella infections of turkey eggs. *Poultry Sci.* 27:359–66.

Grumbles, L. C., and A. I. Flowers. 1961. Epidemiology of paratyphoid infections in turkeys—Species encountered and possible sources of infection. *J. Am. Vet. Med. Ass.* 138:261–62.

Gunderson, M. F., H. W. McFadden, and T. S. Kyle. 1954. *The Bacteriology of Commercial Poultry Processing.* Burgess Publ. Co., Minneapolis.

Gwatkin, R., and L. Dzenis. 1954. Salmonellosis. I. Agglutination tests in experimental infections in chickens. *Can. J. Comp. Med. Vet. Sci.* 18:155–67.

Gwatkin, R., and C. Grinewitsch. 1955a. Salmonellosis. II. Comparison of whole blood agglutination test and faecal cultures in chickens and turkeys infected by mouth with *Salmonella typhimurium. Can. J. Comp. Med. Vet. Sci.* 19:113–15.

———. 1955b. Salmonellosis. III. Blood cultures and agglutination tests on chickens infected by mouth with *Salmonella typhimurium. Can. J. Comp. Med. Vet. Sci.* 19:174–76.

Gwatkin, R., and C. A. Mitchell. 1944. Transmission of *Salmonella pullorum* by flies. *Can. J. Public Health* 35:281–85.

Haglund, J. R., J. C. Ayres, A. M. Paton, A. A. Kraft, and L. Y. Quinn. 1964. Detection of salmonella in eggs and egg products with fluorescent antibody. *Appl. Microbiol.* 12:447–50.

Hamada, S., H. Hashimoto, T. Tasaka, and Y. Tsuchiya. 1958. Studies on chick salmonellosis. II. *Salmonella senftenberg* infection in chicks. *Japan. J. Vet. Res.* 6:181–95.

Harris, M. E., and J. E. Williams. 1957. The hemagglutinating properties of *Salmonella typhimurium. Am. J. Vet. Res.* 18:432–36.

Harry, E. G. 1954a. The influence of certain chemico-physical characteristics of formaldehyde on its use as a disinfectant. *Proc. 10th World's Poultry Congr.,* pp. 217–21.

———. 1954b. Studies on disinfection of eggs and incubators. IV. The use of ammonia in formaldehyde fumigation practice. *Brit. Vet. J.* 110:380–87.

Harry, E. G., and J. A. Binstead. 1961. Studies on disinfection of eggs and incubators. V. The toxicity of formaldehyde to the developing embryo. *Brit. Vet. J.* 117:532–39.

Harvey, R. W. S., and S. Thomson. 1953. Optimum temperature of incubation for isolation of salmonellae. *Monthly Bull. Ministry Health, Public Health Lab. Serv.* 12:149–50.

Harwood, P. D. 1956. Clinical applications of nitrofurans—past and present. *Proc. 1st Nat. Symp. on Nitrofurans in Agr.* Hess and Clark, Ashland, Ohio, pp. 12–23.

Hashimoto, K. 1961. Studies on the bactericidal action of embryonating eggs against *S. pullorum* and *S. senftenberg*. II. The bactericidal action of various liquid materials of embryonating eggs. *Japan. J. Bacteriol.* 16(6):447–51.

Heemstra, L. C. 1952. Salmonella infections in chickens and turkeys. *Proc. Am. Vet. Med. Ass. 89th Ann. Meet.*, pp. 314–19.

Henderson, W., J. Ostendorf, and Georgia L. Morehouse. 1960. The relative pathogenicity of some salmonella serotypes for chicks. *Avian Diseases* 4:103–9.

Henning, M. W. 1939. The antigenic structure of salmonellas obtained from domestic animals and birds in South Africa. *Onderstepoort J. Vet. Sci. Animal Ind.* 13:79–189.

Higgins, W. A., J. B. Christiansen, and C. H. Schroeder. 1944. A *Salmonella enteritidis* infection associated with leg deformity in turkeys. *Poultry Sci.* 23:340–41.

Hinshaw, W. R., and Ethel McNeil. 1943a. The use of the agglutination test in detecting *Salmonella typhimurium* carriers in turkey flocks. *Proc. 47th Ann. Meet. U.S. Livestock Sanit. Ass.*, pp. 106–21.

————. 1943b. *Salmonella newington* infection in turkeys. *Poultry Sci.* 22:415–20.

————. 1944. The importance of group agglutinations in pullorum testing programs. *Proc. 48th Ann. Meet. U.S. Livestock Sanit. Ass.*, pp. 165–70.

————. 1945. Salmonella types isolated from snakes. *Am. J. Vet. Res.* 6:264–66.

————. 1948. Avian salmonellosis; its economic and public health significance. *Proc. 8th World's Poultry Congr.*, pp. 599–604.

————. 1951. Salmonella infection as a food industry problem. *Advan. Food Res.* 3:209–40.

Hinshaw, W. R., T. J. Taylor, and Ethel McNeil. 1942. *Salmonella bredeney* infection in birds. *Cornell Vet.* 32:337–39.

Hinshaw, W. R., Ethel McNeil, and T. J. Taylor. 1944. Avian salmonellosis. Types of salmonella isolated and their relation to public health. *Am. J. Hyg.* 40:264–78.

Hobbs, Betty C. 1961. Public health significance of salmonella carriers in livestock and birds. *J. Appl. Bacteriol.* 24:340–52.

————. 1963. Techniques for the isolation of salmonellae from egg and egg-products. *Ann. Inst. Pasteur* 104:621–37.

Hobbs, Betty C., J. C. Reeves, J. S. Garside, R. F. Gordon, E. M. Barnes, D. H. Shrimpton, and E. S. Anderson. 1960. Antibiotic treatment of poultry in relation to *Salmonella typhimurium*. *Monthly Bull. Ministry Health, Public Health Lab. Serv.* 19:178–93.

Hoffmann, H. A., and P. R. Edwards. 1937. The spontaneous transmission of IV—Variants of *Salmonella aertrycke* from pigeons to rabbits. *Am. J. Hyg.* 26:135–37.

Hohn, J., and W. Hermann. 1935. Die Typen der Gaertnerbakterien und die Quelle ihrer Infektion in der Tierwelt. *Zentr. Bakteriol. Parasitenk. Abt. I. Orig.* 133:183–96.

Hole, N. 1932. Salmonella infections in ducklings. *J. Comp. Pathol. Therap.* 45:161–71.

Hudson, C. B. 1942. An outbreak of paratyphoid in guineas. *J. Am. Vet. Med. Ass.* 100:438.

Hudson, C. B., and D. C. Tudor. 1957. *Salmonella typhimurium* infection in feral birds. *Cornell Vet.* 47:394–95.

Huey, Carolyn R., and P. R. Edwards. 1958. Resistance of *Salmonella typhimurium* to tetracyclines. *Proc. Soc. Exp. Biol. Med.* 97:550–51.

Huygelen, C., J. Mortelmans, and J. Vercruysse. 1958. Infekties door *Salmonella saint paul, Salmonella senegal, Salmonella vejle, Salmonella infantis, Salmonella braenderup* en *Salmonella thompson*, als oorzaak van kuikensterfte. *Vlaams Diergeneesk. Tijdschr.* 27:201–15.

Jansen, J. 1936. Endenkuikensterfte door *S. typhi-murium* en *S. enteritidis* var. Essen. *Tijdschr. Diergeneesk.* 63:140–42.

Johnson, J. G., L. J. Kunz, W. Barron, and W. H. Ewing. 1966. Biochemical differentiation of the Enterobacteriaceae with the aid of lysine-iron-agar. *Appl. Microbiol.* 14:212–17.

Jones, T. J. 1959. The control of game bird diseases. *Mod. Game Breeding and Hunting Club News* 29:12–14.

Julseth, R. M., J. K. Felix, W. E. Burkholder, and R. H. Deibel. 1969. Experimental transmission of Enterobacteriaceae by insects. I. Fate of salmonella fed to the hide beetle *Dermestes maculatus* and a novel method for mounting insects. *Appl. Microbiol.* 17:710–13.

Jungerman, P. F., and L. C. Grumbles. 1960. Salmonella organisms in mature, healthy dogs. *Southwestern Vet.* 13:208–10.

Jungherr, E., and K. S. Wilcox. 1934. *Salmonella aertrycke* as an etiologic agent of paratyphoid in pigeons. *J. Infect. Diseases* 55:390–401.

Kashiwazaki, M., S. Aoki, T. Horiuchi, S. Shoya, and S. Namioka. 1966. An outbreak of paratyphoid infection due to *Salmonella typhimurium* in adult chickens. *Nat. Inst. Animal Health Quart.* 6:144–51.

Kauffmann, F. 1950. *The Diagnosis of Salmonella Types.* Charles C Thomas, Springfield, Ill.

———. 1966. *The Bacteriology of Enterobacteriaceae.* Williams & Wilkins Co., Baltimore.

Kauffmann, F., and P. R. Edwards. 1947. A simplification of the serologic diagnosis of salmonella cultures. *J. Lab. Clin. Med.* 32:548–53.

———. 1957. A revised, simplified Kauffmann-White schema. *Acta Pathol. Microbiol. Scand.* 41:242–46.

Kaufmann, A. F., and J. C. Feeley. 1968. Culture survey of salmonella at a broiler-raising plant. *Public Health Rept.* 83:417–22.

Kaye, D., H. R. Shinefield, and E. W. Hook. 1961. The parakeet as a source of salmonellosis in man. Report of a case. *New Eng. J. Med.* 264:868–69.

Keymer, I. F. 1959. Specific diseases of the canary and other passerine birds. *Mod. Vet. Pract.* 40(17): 32–35.

Khera, S. S., S. B. V. Rao, and K. K. Agarwal. 1965. Avian salmonellosis—An outbreak of egg-peritonitis simulating *Salmonella pullorum* infection caused by *Salmonella stanley. Indian J. Vet. Sci.* 35:126–30.

Kraus, P., and G. Weber. 1958. Untersuchungen ueber die Haltbarkeit von Krankheitserregern in Trink- und Oberflaechenwasser. *Zentr. Bakteriol. Parasitenk. Abt. I. Orig.* 171:509–23.

Ladehoff, G. 1959. Beitrag zur Epidemiologie von *Salmonella typhi murium* in Schleswig-Holstein. Inaug. diss., Hanover.

Lancaster, J. E. 1962. A note on the toxicity of formaldehyde to the developing chicken embryo. *Can. J. Comp. Med. Vet. Sci.* 26:139–40.

Lancaster, J. E., and W. E. Crabb. 1953a. Studies on disinfection of eggs and incubators. I. The survival of *Salmonella pullorum, thompson,* and *typhi-murium* on the surface of hen's egg and on incubator debris. *Brit. Vet. J.* 109:139–48.

———. 1953b. Studies on disinfection of eggs and incubators. II. The value of formaldehyde gas with particular reference to the concentration resulting from the addition of formalin to potassium permanganate. *Brit. Vet. J.* 109:390–97.

Lancaster, J. E., R. F. Gordon, and J. Tucker. 1952. The disinfection, prior to incubation of hen eggs contaminated with *Salmonella pullorum. Brit. Vet. J.* 108:418–31.

Lancaster, J. E., R. F. Gordon, and E. G. Harry. 1954. Studies on disinfection of eggs and incubators. III. The use of formaldehyde at room temperature for the fumigation of eggs prior to incubation. *Brit. Vet. J.* 110: 238–46.

Lannek, N., N. O. Lindgren, and T. Nilsson.

1962. Therapeutical experiments with a new nitrofuran compound (Tiafur) in salmonellosis of chicks. *Avian Diseases* 6:228–38.

Lee, C. D. 1957. Evaluation of the paratyphoid (*Salmonella typhimurium*) program in Iowa 1956–57. *Proc. 8th Ann. North Central Reg. Poultry Disease Conf.*

Lee, C. D., G. Holm, and C. Murray. 1936. Paratyphoid infection in turkeys. *J. Am. Vet. Med. Ass.* 89:65–76.

Lerche, M. 1936. Zur Entstehung Bakterieller Lebensmittelschaedingungen durch Gefluegel und Gefluegelprodukte. *Deut. Tieraerztl. Wochschr.* 44:531–33.

Lerche, M. 1957. Ueber die Abtoetung von Salmonella-Bakterien im Weissei. *Berlin. Muench. Tieraerztl. Wochschr.* 70:436–38.

Levine, N. D., and R. Graham. 1942. Paratyphoid in baby wood ducks. *J. Am. Vet. Med. Ass.* 100:240–41.

Lewis, K. H., and R. Angelotti. 1964. *Examination of Foods for Enteropathogenic and Indicator Bacteria.* U.S. Dept. of HEW, Public Health Serv., Publ. 1142, pp. 100–113.

Litsky, W., I. S. Fagerson, and C. R. Fellers. 1957. A bacteriological survey of commercially frozen beef, poultry and tuna pies. *J. Milk Food Technol.* 20:216–19.

Loken, K. I., Kathleen H. Culbert, R. E. Solee, and B. S. Pomeroy. 1968. Microbiological quality of protein feed supplements produced by rendering plants. *Appl. Microbiol.* 16:1002–5.

Lucas, F. R. 1956. Use of furazolidone in a field outbreak of salmonellosis in mallard ducks. *J. Am. Vet. Med. Ass.* 129:529–31.

Lukas, G. N., and D. R. Bradford. 1954. Salmonellosis in turkey poults as observed in routine necropsy of 1,148 cases. *J. Am. Vet. Med. Ass.* 125:215–18.

Lütje, F. 1921. Abort und Sterilitaet der Stuten. *Deut. Tieraerztl. Wochschr.* 29: 448–55.

McCapes, R. H., R. T. Coffland, and L. E. Christie. 1967. Challenge of turkey poults originating from hens vaccinated with *Salmonella typhimurium* bacterin. *Avian Diseases* 11:15–24.

McCarty, R. T. 1953. Neomycin sulfate treatment of *Salmonella derby* infection in geese. *J. Am. Vet. Med. Ass.* 122:386–87.

McCoy, J. H. 1962. The isolation of salmonella. *J. Appl. Bacteriol.* 25:213–24.

McCroan, J. E., T. W. McKinley, A. Brim, and C. H. Ramsey. 1963. Five salmonellosis outbreaks related to poultry products. *Public Health Rept.* 78:1073–80.

McCullough, N. B. 1958. Food in the epidemiology of salmonellosis. *J. Am. Dietet. Ass.* 34:254–57.

McCullough, N. B., and C. W. Eisele. 1951a. Experimental human salmonellosis. I. Pathogenicity of strains of *Salmonella meleagridis* and *Salmonella anatum* obtained from spray-dried whole egg. *J. Infect. Diseases* 88:27–89.

———. 1951b. Experimental human salmonellosis. II. Immunity studies following experimental illness with *Salmonella meleagridis* and *Salmonella anatum*. *J. Immunol.* 66:595–608.

———. 1951c. Experimental human salmonellosis. III. Pathogenicity of strains of *Salmonella newport, Salmonella derby,* and *Salmonella bareilly* obtained from spray-dried whole egg. *J. Infect. Diseases* 89:209–13.

———. 1951d. Experimental human salmonellosis. IV. Pathogenicity of strains of *Salmonella pullorum* obtained from spray-dried whole egg. *J. Infect. Diseases* 89:259–65.

MacDonald, A. D. 1947. K antigen for the detection of pullorum disease in poultry. *Proc. 19th Ann. Conf. Lab. Workers in Pullorum Disease Control.*

Macdonald, J. W., M. J. Everett, and M. Maule. 1968. Blackbirds with salmonellosis. *Brit. Birds* 61:85–87.

McElrath, H. B., M. M. Galton, and A. V. Hardy. 1952. Salmonellosis in dogs. III. Prevalence in dogs in veterinary hospitals, pounds, and boarding kennels. *J. Infect. Diseases* 91:12–14.

McGaughey, C. A. 1932. Bacteria of the enteric group among poultry. *Brit. Vet. J.* 88:16–26.

Mackel, D. C., Mildred M. Galton, H. Gray, and A. V. Hardy. 1952. Salmonellosis in dogs. IV. Prevalence in normal dogs and their contacts. *J. Infect. Diseases* 91:15–18.

Mackel, D. C., F. J. Payne, and C. I. Pirkle. 1959. Outbreak of gastroenteritis caused by *S. typhimurium* acquired from turkeys. *Public Health Rept.* 74:746–48.

Maclaury, D. W., and Alice B. Moran. 1959. Bacterial contamination of hatching eggs. *Kentucky Agr. Exp. Sta. Bull.* 665.

McNeil, Ethel, and W. R. Hinshaw. 1944. Snakes, cats, and flies as carriers of *Salmonella typhimurium*. *Poultry Sci.* 23:456–57.

———. 1946. Salmonella from Galapagos turtles, a Gila monster and an iguana. *Am. J. Vet. Res.* 7:62–63.

———. 1951. Procedures for conducting the agglutination test for detection of salmonella carriers in turkey flocks. *Vet. Med.* 46:360–62.

Magwood, S. E., and E. Annau. 1961. The adsorption of somatic antigens of salmonella by polystyrene latex particles. *Can. J. Comp. Med. Vet. Sci.* 25:69–73.

Magwood, S. E., and C. H. Bigland. 1962. Salmonellosis in turkeys: Evaluation of bacteriological and serological evidence of infection. *Can. J. Comp. Med. Vet. Sci.* 26:151–59.

Magwood, S. E., Charlotte Rigby, and P. H. J. Fung. 1967. Salmonella contamination of the product and environment of selected Canadian chicken processing plants. *Can. J. Comp. Med. Vet. Sci.* 31:88–91.

Mair, N. S., and A. I. Ross. 1960. Survival of *Salmonella typhimurium* in the soil. *Monthly Bull. Ministry Health, Public Health Lab. Serv.* 19:39–41.

Malhotra, F. C., W. Henderson, and L. W. Tiffany. 1968. Quantitative determination of salmonella organisms from poultry feedstuffs. *Avian Diseases* 12:29–37.

Manninger, R. 1913. Ueber eine durch den *Bazillus paratyphi B* verursachte Infektions-Krankheit der Finken. *Zentr. Bakteriol. Parasitenk. Abt. I. Orig.* 70:12–14.

———. 1918. Ueber Paratyphus beim Wassergefluegel. *Allatorv. Lapok.* (Abstr. in *Jahresbr. Vet. Med.* 38:160.)

Marcellus, F. N., R. Gwatkin, and J. S. Glover. 1930. Incubator disinfection in the control of *Salmonella pullorum*. *Proc. 4th World's Poultry Congr.*, pp. 401–8.

March, B. E. 1969. Bacterial infection of washed and unwashed eggs with reference to salmonellae. *Appl. Microbiol.* 17:98–101.

Marthedal, H. E. 1962. Occurrence of *Salmonella typhi-murium* infections in poultry in Denmark 1934–1960. Epizootiological studies. *Proc. 12th World's Poultry Congr.*, pp. 278–82.

Martin, W. J., and W. H. Ewing. 1969. Prevalence of serotypes of salmonella. *Appl. Microbiol.* 17:111–17.

Mazza, C. 1899. Bakteriologische Untersuchungen ueber einer neuerdings aufgetretene Huehnerepizootie. *Zentr. Bakteriol. Parasitenk. Abt. I. Orig.* 26:181–85.

Mellor, D. B., and G. J. Banwart. 1965. *Salmonella derby* contamination of eggs from inoculated hens. *J. Food Sci.* 30:333–36.

Meyer, K. F. 1942. The ecology of psittacosis and ornithosis. *Medicine* 21:175–206.

Meyer, K. F., and Bernice Eddie. 1934. Latent psittacosis and *Salmonella psittacosis* infection in South American parrotlets and conures. *Science* 79:546–48.

———. 1939. Psittacosis in importations of psittacine birds from South American and Australian continent. *J. Infect. Diseases* 65:234–41.

Milner, K. C., and M. F. Shaffer. 1952. Bacteriologic studies of experimental salmonella infections in chicks. *J. Infect. Diseases* 90:81–96.

Mitrovic, M. 1956. First report of paratyphoid infection in turkey poults due to *Salmonella reading*. *Poultry Sci.* 35:171–74.

Miura, G., G. Sato, and T. Miyamae. 1964. Occurrence and survival of salmonella organisms in hatcher chick fluff from commercial hatcheries. *Avian Diseases* 8:546–54.

Mohler, J. R. 1904. Infectious enteritis of pigeons. *USDA BAI 21st Ann. Rept.*, p. 29.

Moore, V. A. 1895. On a pathogenic bacillus of the hog-cholera group associated with a fatal disease in pigeons. *USDA BAI Bull.* 8, pp. 71–76.

Moran, Alice B. 1959. Salmonella in animals: A report for 1957. *Avian Diseases* 3:85–88.

———. 1960. Salmonella and arizona cultures of animal origin: 1958. *Avian Diseases* 4:73–78.

———. 1961. Occurrence and distribution of salmonella in animals in the United States. *Proc. 65th Ann. Meet. U.S. Livestock Sanit. Ass.*, pp. 441–48.

Moran, Alice B., C. D. Van Houweling, and E. M. Ellis. 1965. The results of typing salmonella from animal sources in the United States. *Proc. Nat. Conf. on Salmonellosis*, U.S. Dept. of HEW, Public Health Serv., NCDC, Atlanta, Ga., pp. 33–37.

Morehouse, L. G., and E. E. Wedman. 1961. Salmonella and other disease-producing organisms in animal by-products—A survey. *J. Am. Vet. Med. Ass.* 139:989–95.

Morello, J. A., T. A. DiGenio, and E. E. Baker. 1965. Significance of salmonellae isolated from apparently healthy mice. *J. Bacteriol.* 89:1460–64.

Morris, T. G., and J. C. Ayres. 1960. Incidence of salmonellae on commercially processed poultry. *Poultry Sci.* 39:1131–35.

Mortelmans, J., C. Huygelen, and J. Vercruysse. 1958. Le transport de poussins par avion, moyen de dispersion des salmonellae. *Bull. Soc. Pathol. Exotique* 51:294–97.

Moyle, A. I. 1966. Salmonellae in rendering plant by-products. *J. Am. Vet. Med. Ass.* 149:1172–76.

Muller, Gertrude. 1965. Salmonella in bird feces. *Nature* 207:1315.

Müller, J. 1957a. Om salmonellainfektioner hos svømmefugle. *Medlemsbl. danske Dyrlaeg.* 40:631–35.

———. 1957b. Le probleme des Salmonelloses au Danemark. *Bull. Off. Int. Epizoot.* 48:323–33.

———. 1961. Om bekaempelsen af salmonellose hos fjerkrae. *Nord. Veterinarmed.* 13:617–28.

Mundt, J. O., and R. L. Tugwell. 1958. The relationship of the chicken egg to selected paratyphoids. *Poultry Sci.* 37:415–20.

Newell, K. W., B. C. Hobbs, and E. J. G. Wallace. 1955. Paratyphoid fever associated with Chinese frozen whole egg. *Brit. Med. J.* 2:1296–98.

Newell, K. W., R. McClarin, C. R. Murdock, W. N. Macdonald, and H. L. Hutchinson. 1959. Salmonellosis in Northern Ireland, with special reference to pigs and salmonella contaminated pig meal. *J. Hyg.* 57:92–105.

Ng, H., H. G. Bayne, and J. A. Garibaldi. 1969. Heat resistance of salmonella: The uniqueness of *Salmonella senftenberg* 775 W. *Appl. Microbiol.* 17:78–82.

Niemeyer, W. E. 1939. Paratyphoid and trichomonas infection in pigeons. *J. Am. Vet. Med. Ass.* 94:434–35.

Nilsson, T., and B. Regner. 1963. The effect of chlorine in the chilling water on salmonellae in dressed chicken. *Acta Vet. Scand.* 4:307–12.

Niven, C. F. 1961. Industry's role in reducing the incidence of salmonella in animal feeds. *Proc. 65th Ann. Meet. U.S. Livestock Sanit. Ass.*, pp. 453–57.

North, W. R., Jr. 1961. Lactose pre-enrichment method for isolation of salmonella from dried egg albumin. *Appl. Microbiol.* 9:188–95.

Olesiuk, Olga M., V. L. Carlson, G. H. Snoeyenbos, and C. F. Smyser. 1969. Experimental *Salmonella typhimurium* infection in two chicken flocks. *Avian Diseases* 13:500–508.

Orthoefer, J. G., Minnie Schrieber, J. B. Nichols, and N. Schneider. 1968. Salmonella contamination in a rendering plant. *Avian Diseases* 12:303–11.

Osborne, W. W., and J. L. Stokes. 1955. A modified selenite brilliant-green medium for the isolation of salmonella from egg products. *Appl. Microbiol.* 3:295–99.

Ostrolenk, M., and H. Welch. 1942. The house fly as a vector of food poisoning organisms in food producing establishments. *Am. J. Public Health* 32:487–94.

Paul, H. E. 1956. Research background on the nitrofurans. *Proc. 1st Nat. Symp. on Nitrofurans in Agr.* Hess and Clark, Ashland, Ohio, pp. 6–11.

Perek, M., and S. Rabinovitz. 1957. The value of faeces examinations in detection of carriers of salmonellosis in geese. *Brit. Vet. J.* 113:511–14.

Peterson, E. H. 1947. Field studies of sulfamerazine in the control of pullorum and some other diseases of domestic birds. *North Am. Vet.* 28:298–300.

Petzelt, J., and F. Steininger. 1961. Die Vogel der Klaeranlage von Hannover und die von ihnen Ausgeschiedenen Salmonellen. *Arch. Hyg. Bakteriol.* 145:605–19.

Pfaff, Fr. 1921. Eine Truthuehnerseuche mit Paratyphus-Befund. *Z. Infektkr. Haustiere* 22:285–98.

Pfeiler, W. 1920. Beitrag zur Kasuistik des Huehnertyphus. *Z. Fleisch Milch Hyg.* 30:267–69.

Pfeiler, W., and A. Rehse. 1913. Ueber das Vorkommen von Bakterien aus der Gruppe der Fleischvergifter bei Voegeln. Paratyphus B-Infektion beim Huhn. *Zentr. Bakteriol. Parasitenk. Abt. I. Orig.* 68:174–81.

Philbrook, F. R., R. A. MacCready, H. Van Roekel, E. S. Anderson, C. F. Smyser, F. J. Sanen, and W. M. Groton. 1960. Salmonellosis spread by a dietary supplement of avian source. *New Eng. J. Med.* 263:713–18.

Pomeroy, B. S. 1944. Salmonellosis of turkeys. Ph.D. thesis, Univ. Minn.

———. 1958. The control of paratyphoid infections and typhimurium testing programs. *Rept. Nat. Plans Conf.,* USDA, ARS, AHR Div., Beltsville, Md., pp. 15–22.

Pomeroy, B. S., and R. Fenstermacher. 1939. Paratyphoid infection of turkeys. *J. Am. Vet. Med. Ass.* 94:90–97.

———. 1941. Paratyphoid infection of turkeys. *Am. J. Vet. Res.* 2:285–91.

———. 1943. Salmonella infections of breeding turkeys. *Am. J. Vet. Res.* 4:199–208.

———. 1944. Salmonella infections in turkeys. *Am. J. Vet. Res.* 5:282–88.

Pomeroy, B. S., and Margaret K. Grady. 1961. Salmonella organisms isolated from feed ingredients. *Proc. 65th Ann. Meet. U.S. Livestock Sanit. Ass.,* pp. 449–52.

Pomeroy, B. S., R. Fenstermacher, and M. H. Roepke. 1948. Sulfonamides in the control of salmonellosis of chicks and poults. *J. Am. Vet. Med. Ass.* 112:296–303.

Pomeroy, B. S., R. Fenstermacher, Florence Jones, and L. E. Jenkins. 1957a. The control of paratyphoid and related enteric infections of turkeys. *Proc. 8th Ann. North Central Reg. Poultry Disease Conf.*

Pomeroy, B. S., R. C. Belding, J. E. Williams, L. E. Erwin, G. S. Vickers, and Alice Moran. 1957b. Report of the Committee on Salmonellosis (1957) for North Central Regional Poultry Disease Conference. *Proc. 8th Ann. North Central Reg. Poultry Disease Conf.*

Pomeroy, B. S., Y. Siddiqui, and Margaret K. Grady. 1965. Salmonella in animal feeds and feed ingredients. *Proc. Nat. Conf. on Salmonellosis,* U.S. Dept. of HEW, Public Health Serv., NCDC, Atlanta, Ga., pp. 74–77.

Price, J. I., E. Dougherty, and D. W. Bruner. 1962. Salmonella infections in White Pekin duck. A short summary of the years 1950–60. *Avian Diseases* 6:145–47.

Pulst, H. 1960. Ein Beitrag zur Salmonellose beim Wassergefluegel. *Mh. Vet. Med.* 15:226–30.

Quarles, C. L., R. F. Gentry, and G. O. Bressler. 1970. Bacterial contamination in poultry houses and its relationship to egg hatchability. *Poultry Sci.* 49:60–66.

Quesada, A., R. Izzi, and V. Maggio. 1960. Sulla presenza di germi del genere salmonella nelle farine di pesce impiegate per la confezione dei mangimi. *Soc. Ital. Sci. Vet. Atti.* 14:757–62.

Quist, K. D. 1962. Salmonella in poultry as related to human health. *Rept. Nat. Plans Conf.,* USDA, ARS, AHR Div., Beltsville, Md., pp. 24–30.

———. 1963. Salmonellosis in poultry. *Public Health Rept.* 78:1071–73.

Ramsey, C. H., and P. R. Edwards. 1961. Resistance of salmonellae isolated in 1959 and 1960 to tetracyclines and chloramphenicol. *Appl. Microbiol.* 9:389–91.

Rao, S. B. V. 1956. Isolation of *Salmonella litchfield* from an outbreak in chicks in the Indian Union. *Indian J. Vet. Sci.* 26:131–34.

Rao, S. B. V., and B. R. Gupta. 1961. The isolation of *Salmonella weltevreden* and *Salmonella dublin* in an outbreak of salmonellosis in imported chicks. *Indian J. Med. Res.* 49:6–8.

Rasmussen, O. G., R. Hansen, N. J. Jacobs, and O. H. M. Wilder. 1964. Dry heat resistance of salmonellae in rendered animal by-products. *Poultry Sci.* 43:1151–57.

Rasmussen, P. G. 1962. *Salmonella typhimurium*—ledbetaendelser hos slagteaender. Ledbetaendelsernes aetiologi og fjerkraekontrolmaessige bedømmelse. *Nord. Veterinarmed.* 14:39–52.

Ravaioli, L., and Z. Orfei. 1952. La cloromicetina e la terramicina nella terapia della salmonellosi aviare. *Soc. Ital. Sci. Vet. Atti.* 6:536–37.

Rettger, L. F., and M. Scoville. 1920. *Bacterium anatum* n.s. the etiologic factor in a widespread disease of young ducklings known in some places as "keel." *J. Infect. Diseases* 26:217–29.

Rettger, L. F., W. N. Plastridge, and R. Cameron. 1933. Endemic paratyphoid infection in turkeys. *J. Infect. Diseases* 53:272–79.

Rice, C. E., S. E. Magwood, and E. Annau. 1960. A modified direct complement-fixation test for the detection of antibodies for salmonella antigens in turkey sera. *Can. Vet. J.* 1:132–37.

Rizk, S. S., J. C. Ayres, and A. A. Kraft. 1966a. Disinfection of eggs artificially inoculated with salmonellae. *Poultry Sci.* 45:764–69.

———. 1966b. Effect of holding condition on the development of salmonellae in artificially inoculated hens' eggs. *Poultry Sci.* 45:825–29.

Ruedy, D. D., E. D. Baker, and M. E. Teal. 1966. The incidence of *Mycoplasma gallisepticum, Salmonella pullorum,* and *Salmonella typhimurium* and newcastle disease virus antibodies in certain Wisconsin chickens. *Avian Diseases* 10:407–9.

Sadler, W. W., and R. E. Corstvet. 1965. Second survey of market poultry for salmonella infection. *Appl. Microbiol.* 13:348–51.

Sadler, W. W., R. Yamamoto, H. E. Adler, and G. F. Stewart. 1961. Survey of market poultry for salmonella infection. *Appl. Microbiol.* 9:72–76.

Sadler, W. W., R. Yamamoto, and R. E. Corstvet. 1965. Bacteriological survey of market poultry livers. *Poultry Sci.* 44:993–98.

Salisbury, R. M. 1958. Salmonella infections in animals and birds in New Zealand. *New Zealand Vet. J.* 6:76–86.

Salzer, R. H., A. A. Kraft, and J. C. Ayres. 1964. Bacteria associated with giblets of commercially processed turkeys. *Poultry Sci.* 43:934–38.

Sanders, E., P. S. Brachman, E. A. Friedman, J. Goldsby, and C. E. McCall. 1965. Salmonellosis in the United States. Results of nationwide surveillance. *Am. J. Epidemiol.* 81:370–84.

Sanders, R. G., B. S. Pomeroy, and R. Fenstermacher. 1943. Cross-agglutination studies between *Salmonella pullorum* and other microorganisms isolated from turkeys positive to the pullorum test. *Am. J. Vet. Res.* 4:194–98.

Sato, G. 1967a. Response of wild rats *(Rattus norvegicus)* bred in captivity to oral inoculation with *Salmonella pullorum, Salmonella newington,* and *Salmonella enteritidis. J. Infect. Diseases* 117:71–81.

———. 1967b. Detection of salmonella and arizona organisms from soil of empty turkey yards. *Jap. J. Vet. Res.* 15:53–55.

Saulmon, E. E. 1966a. Activities of the USDA salmonella work group. *Rept. Nat. Plans Conf.,* USDA, ARS, AHR Div., Beltsville, Md., pp. 19–27.

———. 1966b. Control of salmonella contamination in eggs, feeds, and feed products. *J. Am. Vet. Med. Ass.* 149:1691–97.

Savage, W. 1956. Problems of salmonella food poisoning. *Brit. Med. J.* 2:317–23.

Schaaf, J. 1936. Remarks made during discussion of paratyphoid infections of poultry. *Proc. 6th World's Poultry Congr.* 3:409.

Schalm, O. W. 1937. Study of a paratyphoid infection in chicks. *J. Infect. Diseases* 61:208–16.

Schneider, M. D. 1946. Investigations of salmonella content of powdered whole egg with not more than 2% moisture content. II. General survey on the occurrence of species of salmonella in high quality egg powder. *Food Res.* 11:313–18.

Schneider, M. D., and M. F. Gunderson. 1949. Investigators shed more light on salmonella problem. *U.S. Egg and Poultry Magazine* 55:10.

Schnurrenberger, P. R., L. J. Held, R. J. Martin, K. D. Quist, and M. M. Galton. 1968. Prevalence of salmonella species in domestic animals and wildlife on selected Illinois farms. *J. Am. Vet. Med. Ass.* 153:442–45.

Schoop, G., and K. Moser. 1954. Zur Therapie der Salmonellen-Infektion (Fluegellachme) der Tauben. *Berlin. Muench. Tieraerztl. Wochschr.* 67:53–54.

Schroeder, S. A., Pamela M. Terry, and J. V.

Bennett. 1968. Antibiotic resistance and transfer factor in salmonella, United States 1967. *J. Am. Med. Ass.* 205:903–6.

Shaffer, M. F., K. C. Milner, Dorothy I. Clemmer, and J. F. Bridges. 1957. Bacteriologic studies of experimental salmonella infections in chicks. II. *J. Infect. Diseases* 100:17–31.

Shirlaw, J. F., and S. G. Iyer. 1937. A note on a variety of *S. enteritidis* isolated from pigeons. *Indian J. Vet. Sci.* 7:231–42.

Sieburth, J. M. 1957a. The effect of furazolidone on the cultural and serological response of *Salmonella typhi-murium* infected chickens. *Avian Diseases* 1:180–94.

———. 1957b. Indirect hemagglutination studies on salmonellosis of chickens. *J. Immunol.* 78:380–86.

———. 1958a. Respiratory flora and diseases of Antarctic birds. *Avian Diseases* 2:402–8.

———. 1958b. The indirect hemagglutination test in the avian salmonella problem. *Am. J. Vet. Res.* 19:729–35.

———. 1960. Stable, standardized, sensitized chicken erythrocytes for the polyvalent indirect hemagglutination test. *Am. J. Vet. Res.* 21:1084–89.

Sieburth, J. M., and E. P. Johnson. 1957. Observations on stress factors and serological response in *Salmonella typhi-murium* infection of chicks. *Avian Diseases* 1:122. (Abstr.)

Silliker, J. H., R. H. Deibel, and P. T. Fagan. 1964. Isolation of salmonellae from food samples. VI. Comparison of methods for the isolation of salmonella from egg products. *Appl. Microbiol.* 12:224–28.

Simskaya, A. M. 1955. Gigienicheskaya otsenka teplovoi obrabotki utinykh yaits. *Vop. Pitaniya* 14:34–39.

Smith, H. W. 1955. The treatment of experimental *Salmonella typhimurium* infection in turkey poults and chicks. *Vet. Record* 67:749–53.

———. 1967. Salmonellosis: The present position in man and animals. I. Laboratory aspects with particular reference to chemotherapy and contact. *Vet. Record* 80:142–47.

Smyser, C. F., and G. H. Snoeyenbos. 1969. Evaluation of several methods of isolating salmonellae from poultry litter and animal feedstuffs. *Avian Diseases* 13:134–41.

Smyser, C. F., and H. Van Roekel. 1959. Detection of *Salmonella typhimurium* infection in an egg producing chicken flock. *Avian Diseases* 3:485. (Abstr.)

Smyser, C. F., J. Bacharz, and H. Van Roekel. 1963. Detection of *Salmonella typhimurium* from artificially contaminated poultry feed and animal by-products. *Avian Diseases* 7:423–34.

Smyser, C. F., N. Adinarayanan, H. Van Roekel, and G. H. Snoeyenbos. 1966. Field and laboratory observations on *Salmonella heidelberg* infection in three chicken breeding flocks. *Avian Diseases* 10:314–29.

Snoeyenbos, G. H., E. W. Morin, and D. K. Wetherbee. 1967a. Naturally occurring salmonella in "blackbirds" and gulls. *Avian Diseases* 11:642–46.

Snoeyenbos, G. H., V. L. Carlson, B. A. McKie, and C. F. Smyser. 1967b. An epidemiological study of salmonellosis of chickens. *Avian Diseases* 11:653–67.

Snoeyenbos, G. H., C. F. Smyser, and H. Van Roekel. 1969a. Research note—Salmonellae infections of the ovary and peritoneum of chickens. *Avian Diseases* 13:668–70.

Snoeyenbos, G. H., V. L. Carlson, C. F. Smyser, and Olga M. Olesiuk. 1969b. Dynamics of salmonella infection in chicks reared on litter. *Avian Diseases* 13:72–83.

Solowey, M. E., E. H. Spaulding, and H. E. Goresline. 1946. An investigation of a source and mode of entry of salmonella organisms in spray-dried whole-egg-powder. *Food Res.* 11:380–90.

Solowey, M., E. H. Spaulding, and C. Chemerda. 1947. Microbiology of spray-dried whole egg. II. Incidence and types of salmonella. *Am. J. Public Health* 37:971–82.

Spicer, C. C. 1956. A quick method of identifying *Salmonella* H antigens. *J. Clin. Pathol.* 9:378–79.

Spink, M. S. 1960. Broilers. *Lancet,* September 24, pp. 707–8.

Spray, R. S., and L. P. Doyle. 1921. Paratyphoid bacilli from chicks. *J. Infect. Diseases* 28:43–47.

Steininger, F. 1961. Wie Lange Halten sich Salmonellen aus verregnetem Abwasser auf Pflanzen? *Berlin. Muench. Tieraerztl. Wochschr.* 74:389–92.

Stephens, J. F., and E. L. Anderson. 1967. Growth of salmonella in chickens' yolk sacs and its relationship to pathogenicity. *Appl. Microbiol.* 15:1468–72.

Stephens, J. F., and O. H. Vestal. 1966. Effects of intestinal coccidiosis upon the course of *Salmonella typhimurium* infection in chicks. *Poultry Sci.* 45:446–50.

Stephens, J. F., B. D. Barnett, and D. F. Holtman. 1964. Concurrent *Salmonella typhimurium* and *Eimeria necatrix* infections in chicks. *Poultry Sci.* 43:352–56.

Stokes, J. L., and W. W. Osborne. 1955. A selenite brilliant green medium for the isolation of salmonella. *Appl. Microbiol.* 3:217–20.

Stokes, J. L., W. W. Osborne, and H. G. Bayne. 1956. Penetration and growth of salmonella in shell eggs. *Food Res.* 21:510–18.

Stone, R. M. 1960. Pet bird practice. *J. Am. Vet. Med. Ass.* 137:364–72.

Stover, D. E. 1960. Fumigation of hatching eggs. *The Bulletin, Dept. of Agr., State of California,* Sacramento 48:30–33.

———. 1961. The salmonella infections (pullorum, typhoid, and paratyphoid). In *Disease, Environmental, and Management Factors Related to Poultry Health.* USDA, ARS 45-2, pp. 45–48.

———. 1964. Hatching egg sanitation and fumigation for disease control. *The Bulletin, Dept. of Agr., State of California,* Sacramento 53:147–50.

Strauss, J., B. Bednř, and V. Serý. 1957. The incidence of ornithosis and salmonellosis in the black-headed gull *(Larus* ridibundus L.). II. Isolation and identification of the virus of ornithosis from the black-headed gull with simultaneous isolation of S. *(Salmonella) typhi-murium. J. Hyg. Epidemiol. Microbiol. Immunol.* (Prague) 1:230.

Stuart, C. A., E. Van Stratum, and R. Rustigian. 1945. Further studies on urease production by proteus and related organisms. *J. Bacteriol.* 49:437–44.

Stucker, C. L., M. M. Galton, J. Cowdery, and A. V. Hardy. 1952. Salmonellosis in dogs. II. Prevalence and distribution in greyhounds in Florida. *J. Infect. Diseases* 91:6–18.

Tailyour, J. M., and R. J. Avery. 1960. A survey of turkey viscera for salmonellae, British Columbia. *Can. J. Public Health* 51:75–77.

Taylor, Joan. 1960. Food poisoning. (b) Salmonella and salmonellosis. *Roy. Soc. Health J.* 80:253–59.

———. 1963. The serotypes of salmonella isolated from foods. *Ann. Inst. Pasteur* 104:660–69.

———. 1967. Salmonellosis: The present position in man and animals. II. Public health aspects. *Vet. Record* 80:147–54.

Thatcher, F. S., and J. Montford. 1962. Egg products as a source of salmonellae in processed foods. *Can. J. Public Health* 53:61–69.

Thomas, J. 1961. Salmonelles isolees en Belgique chez les animaux et dans les denrees alimentaires d'origine animale. *Ann. Med. Vet.* 105:206–18.

Thomason, B. M., W. B. Cherry, and P. R. Edwards. 1959. Staining bacterial smears with fluorescent antibody. VI. Identification of salmonellae in fecal specimens. *J. Bacteriol.* 77:478–86.

Thomson, J. E., G. J. Banwart, D. H. Sanders, and A. J. Mercuri. 1967. Effect of chlorine, antibiotics, B-propiolactone, acids, and washing on *Salmonella typhimurium* on eviscerated fryer chickens. *Poultry Sci.* 46:146–51.

Timoney, J. 1968. The sources and extent of salmonella contamination in rendering plants. *Vet. Record* 83:541–43.

Truscott, R. B. 1956. *Salmonella moscow* isolated from ducks in Ontario. *Can. J. Comp.*

Med. Vet. Sci. 20:345–46.

Tucker, J. F. 1967. Survival of salmonellae in built-up litter for housing of rearing and laying fowls. *Brit. Vet. J.* 123:92–103.

Vallée, A., L. LeMinor, P. Collin, and R. Girardin. 1959. Enzootie de paratyphose a *Salmonella johannesburg* chez des bengalis. *Rec. Med. Vet. Ecole Alfort* 135:383–84.

Van Dorssen, C. A. 1955. *Salmonella typhimurium* Typen uit Duiven. *Tijdschr. Diergeneesk.* 80:1188–1201.

Van Keulen, A. 1959. Salmonellosis als Zoonose. *Tijdschr. Diergeneesk.* 84:1102–17.

Van Oye, E. 1964. *The World Problem of Salmonellosis.* Junk Publishers, The Hague, Netherlands.

Van Roekel, H. 1965. Salmonella in poultry and eggs. *Proc. Nat. Conf. on Salmonellosis,* U.S. Dept. of HEW, Public Health Serv., NCDC, Atlanta, Ga., pp. 78–83..

Van Roekel, H., and K. L. Bullis. 1937. Salmonella infections in chickens. *J. Am. Vet. Med. Ass.* 91:48–58.

Vestal, O. H., and J. F. Stephens. 1966. The relative pathogenicity of selected paratyphoids for chicks. *Avian Diseases* 10:502–7.

Wabeck, C. J., D. V. Schwall, G. M. Evancho, J. G. Heck, and A. B. Rogers. 1968. Salmonella and total count reduction in poultry treated with sodium hypochlorite solutions. *Poultry Sci.* 47:1090–94.

Walker, J. H. C. 1960. The broiler industry—Transmission of salmonella infection. *Roy. Soc. Health J.* 80:142–45.

Warrack, G. H., and T. Dalling. 1933. Salmonella infections in young ducklings and duck eggs. *Brit. Vet. J.* 89:483–91.

Watanabe, S., K. Hashimoto, and T. Kume. 1958. Studies on salmonella infection in hen's eggs during incubation with special reference to the mode of infection with *S. pullorum* and *S. senftenberg.* II. Transmission of salmonella from infected hens to laid eggs. *Bull. Nat. Inst. Animal Health* (Tokyo) 36:1–9.

Watanabe, S., K. Hashimoto, T. Kume, M. Murata, and R. Sakazaki. 1959a. Studies on salmonella infection in hen's eggs during incubation with special reference to the mode of infection with *S. pullorum* and *S. senftenberg.* III. Salmonella infection of embryonated eggs through the egg shell. *Bull. Nat. Inst. Animal Health* (Tokyo) 37:47–60.

Watanabe, S., T. Kume, K. Hashimoto, and R. Sakazaki. 1959b. Studies on salmonella infection in hen's eggs during incubation with special reference to the mode of infection with *S. pullorum* and *S. senftenberg.* IV. Natural resistance of chick embryos against *S. pullorum* and *S. senftenberg. Bull. Nat. Inst. Animal Health* (Tokyo) 37:61–69.

Watkins, J. R., A. I. Flowers, and L. C. Grumbles. 1959. Salmonella organisms in animal products used in poultry feeds. *Avian Diseases* 3:290–301.

Watt, J. 1945. An outbreak of salmonella infection in man from infected chicken eggs. *Public Health Rept.* 60:835–39.

Watts, P. S., and M. Wall. 1952. The 1951 *Salmonella typhi-murium* epidemic in sheep in South Australia. *Australian Vet. J.* 28:165–68.

Wedman, E. E. 1961. Findings and recommendations of the United States Department of Agriculture task force on salmonella in animal by-products and feeds. *Proc. 65th Ann. Meet. U.S. Livestock Sanit. Ass.,* pp. 458–63.

Weisgerber, and Ch. Müller. 1922. Untersuchungen ueber eine seuchenhafte Erkrankung der jungen Gaense in der Provinz Ostpreussen mit Paratyphus Befund. *Deut. Tieraerztl. Wochschr.* 30:663–65.

Wenger, D. M., and B. L. McMurray. 1967. Abbreviated salmonella screening procedures with Pathotec urease and lysine decarboxylase test papers. *Avian Diseases* 11:503–8.

Wilder, A. N., and R. A. MacCready. 1966. Isolation of salmonella from poultry, poultry products, and processing plants in Massachusetts. *New Eng. J. Med.* 274:1453–60.

Williams, J. E. 1968. History, morphology, and biochemical and antigenic properties of *Salmonella typhimurium,* strain P-10. *Avian Diseases* 12:512–17.

———. 1969. A restraining device for large fowl. *Avian Diseases* 13:234–38.

Williams, J. E., and L. H. Dillard. 1968. Salmonella penetration of fertile and infertile chicken eggs at progressive stages of incubation. *Avian Diseases* 12:629–35.

———. 1969. Salmonella penetration of the outer structures of white- and speckled-shell turkey eggs. *Avian Diseases* 13:203–10.

Williams, J. E., and A. D. MacDonald. 1955. The past, present, and future of salmonella antigens for poultry. *Proc. Am. Vet. Med. Ass. 92nd Ann. Meet.,* pp. 333–39.

Williams, J. E., and H. S. Siegel. 1969. Formaldehyde levels on and in chicken eggs following preincubation fumigation. *Poultry Sci.* 48:552–58.

Williams, J. E., and A. D. Whittemore. 1966. Hemagglutinating properties of 565 avian strains of *Salmonella typhi-murium* isolated in the U.S.A. *Proc. 13th World's Poultry Congr.,* pp. 389–94.

———. 1967. A method for studying microbial penetration through the outer structures of the avian egg. *Avian Diseases* 11:467–90.

Williams, J. E., L. H. Dillard, and Gaye O. Hall. 1968. The penetration patterns of *Salmonella typhimurium* through the outer structures of chicken eggs. *Avian Diseases* 12:445–66.

Williams, R. B., and M. W. Dodson. 1960.

Salmonella in Alaska. *Public Health Rept.* 75:913–16.

Wilson, E., R. S. Paffenbarger, M. J. Foter, and K. H. Lewis. 1961. Prevalence of salmonellae in meat and poultry products. *J. Infect. Diseases* 109:166–71.

Wilson, J. E. 1944. Observations on fowl paralysis and some current conditions in poultry problems. *Vet. Record* 56:521–24.

———. 1945. Infected egg shells as a means of spread of salmonellosis in chicks and ducklings. *Vet. Record* 57:411–13.

———. 1947. The isolation of *S. typhi-murium* from fowls which gave a positive agglutination test with *S. pullorum* antigen. *Brit. Vet. J.* 103:101–4.

———. 1948. Avian salmonellosis. *Vet. Record* 60:615–24.

———. 1949. The control and prevention of infectious disease in the hatchery. *Brit. Vet. J.* 105: 463–66.

———. 1950. The occurrence of *S. typhimurium* in hen eggs and its implications. *Vet. Record* 62:449–50.

———. 1951. The control of salmonellosis in poultry with special reference to fumigation of incubators. *Vet. Record* 63:501–3.

———. 1955. The use of furazolidone in the treatment of infections of day-old chicks with *S. pullorum, S. gallinarum, S. typhimurium,* and *S. thompson. Vet. Record* 67:849–53.

Wilson, J. E., and J. W. Macdonald. 1967. Salmonella infection in wild birds. *Brit. Vet. J.* 123:212–19.

Wilson, S. T. 1969. Cooperative state-federal salmonella program in rendering plants—fiscal year 1968. *Salmonella Surveillance.* U.S. Dept. of HEW, NCDC, Rept. 81, p. 5.

Winter, A. R., G. F. Stewart, V. H. McFarlane, and M. Solowey. 1946. Pasteurization of liquid egg products. III. Destruction of salmonella in liquid whole eggs. *Am. J. Public Health* 36:451–59.

Wolfe, L. W., and J. L. Fulenwider. 1967. *Automatic egg fumigator.* U.S. Patent 3,326,114.

Wolff, A. H., N. D Henderson, and G. L. McCallum. 1948. Salmonella from dogs and the possible relationship to salmonellosis in man. *Am. J. Public Health* 38:403–8.

Wolfgang, R. W. 1958. Recent progress in nitrofuran research. *Proc. 2nd Nat. Symp. on Nitrofurans in Agr.* Hess and Clark, Ashland, Ohio, pp. 14–22.

Woodburn, Margy. 1964. Incidence of salmonellae in dressed broiler-fryer chickens. *Appl. Microbiol.* 12:492–95.

Woodburn, Margy, and W. J. Stadelman. 1968. Salmonellae contamination of production and processing facilities for broilers and ducklings. *Poultry Sci.* 47:777–82.

Woodburn, Margy, M. Bennion, and G. Vail. 1962. Destruction of salmonellae and staphylococci in precooked poultry products by heat treatment before freezing. *Food Technol.* 16 (6): 98–100.

Wright, G. W., and J. F. Frank. 1956. Penetration of eggs by *Salmonella typhi-murium. Can. J. Comp. Med. Vet. Sci.* 20:453–57.

Wright, M. L., G. W. Anderson, and N. A. Epps. 1959. Hatchery sanitation. *Can. J. Comp. Med. Vet. Sci.* 23:288–90.

Yamamoto, R., H. E. Adler, W. W. Sadler, and G. F. Stewart. 1961a. A study of *Salmonella typhimurium* infection in market-age turkeys. *Am. J. Vet. Res.* 22:382–87.

Yamamoto, R., W. W. Sadler, H. E. Adler, and G. F. Stewart. 1961b. Comparison of media and methods for recovering *Salmonella typhimurium* from turkeys. *Appl. Microbiol.* 9:76–80.

Yamamoto, R., J. G. Kilian, W. E. Babcock, and E. M. Dickinson. 1962. Some observations on serological testing for *Salmonella typhi-murium* in breeder turkeys. *Avian Diseases* 6:444–54.

Yurchenco, J. A., M. C. Yurchenco, and C. R. Piepoli. 1953. Antimicrobial properties of furoxone (N-5-Nitro-2-furfurylidene-3-amino-2-oxazolidone). *Antibiot. Chemotherapy* 3:1035–39.

CHAPTER 4

AVIAN ARIZONOSIS

❖

J. E. WILLIAMS

Southeast Poultry Research Laboratory
Agricultural Research Service
United States Department of Agriculture
Athens, Georgia

❖

THE GENUS *Arizona* consists of motile bacteria that conform to the definitions of the family Enterobacteriaceae and the tribe Salmonelleae. These organisms, formerly referred to as "paracolon" bacteria, are related to members of the genera *Salmonella* and *Citrobacter* but can be readily distinguished from them by biochemical tests and serological typing. The lack of fermentation of lactose by salmonellae and its fermentation by most of the arizonae is one of the most obvious differences between these two groups. Other biochemical differences are presented in Table 3.9 in Chapter 3.

Reference to members of the genus *Arizona* as "paracolons" will be found in the following pages of this chapter only in the interest of accuracy of prior literature citations. As used here it is not intended to denote a specific group of bacteria, since the recent systematic classification of microorganisms in the family Enterobacteriaceae has rendered obsolete the imprecise term "paracolon" (Fields et al., 1967).

The disease caused by arizona serotypes in poultry is indistinguishable clinically from salmonellosis and is referred to as *arizona infection* or *avian arizonosis*. The avian and mammalian host range for the arizonae, like the salmonelleae, is unlimited. A few arizona serotypes are host-adapted.

Hinshaw and McNeil (1946a), Edwards et al. (1956, 1959), Goetz (1962), Kowalski and Stephens (1968), and Snoeyenbos and Smyser (1969) point out that avian arizonosis poses a problem of considerable economic importance to the turkey industry. Sato and Adler (1966d) reported that hatchability is adversely affected by these infections and production is reduced. As both an avian and human disease, arizonosis is likely to occupy a position of increasing importance with additional attention being given to its detection and control.

HISTORY

The first-described culture now recognized as a member of the genus *Arizona* was isolated from fatal infections of certain reptiles by Caldwell and Ryerson (1939). These investigators classified the organism as a *Salmonella* sp. (Dar-es-salaam, var. from Arizona). Kauffmann (1941) after a careful study of the flagellar antigens of one of the original cultures, designated the organism *S. arizona*. It was recognized that the arizona culture fermented lactose and liquefied gelatin, and Kauffmann (1945, personal communication) agreed that this organism should be classified separately from the salmonellae. Prior to the Caldwell and Ryerson isolation, Lewis and Hitchner (1936) reported the recovery of slow lactose-fermenting bacteria from a disease of chicks resembling salmonellosis. This infection was probably due to a member of the genus *Arizona* and may represent the first report of avian arizonosis.

INCIDENCE AND DISTRIBUTION

Arizonosis occurs worldwide and has been found in all areas where poultry is raised. The exact incidence of the disease in the United States has not been determined as all outbreaks are not regularly reported; however, the growing literature indicates that these infections are being encountered more frequently, particularly among young turkeys.

In 1939 when arizonosis was first recognized in turkeys, poults from individual hatcheries were found to harbor a single serotype of the infection, and it was possible to trace the source to certain hatcheries. Through the interchange of eggs and supply flocks this situation changed and infection with multiple types of arizona organisms became the rule. Many of the cultures have come from normal carriers.

ETIOLOGY

CLASSIFICATION

Since 1939 repeated attempts have been made to find a generally acceptable taxonomic position for this group of bacteria intermediate between the salmonellae and other Enterobacteriaceae. Several classification systems have come and gone during the past 30 years, and a wide variety of names and designations has been applied to the organisms. Their exact taxonomic position and nomenclature are yet to be resolved but are presently on a sounder basis than at any time previously.

Stuart et al. (1943) and Borman et al. (1944) classified the "paracolon" organisms in a specific genus *Paracolobactrum,* an appendix to the tribe Eschericheae, and recognized three species: *Paracolobactrum aerogenoides, Paracolobactrum intermedium,* and *Paracolobactrum coliforme.* This general classification was adopted by the seventh edition of *Bergey's Manual of Determinative Bacteriology* (Breed et al., 1957) with the addition of the species *Paracolobactrum arizonae.* Neither this scheme nor another one in which the "paracolon" bacteria were classified in the Arizona, Bethesda-Ballerup, and Providence groups has had universal application and is mainly of historical interest.

The work of the late P. R. Edwards and associates, as cited by Martin et al. (1967), established the biochemical and antigenic similarity of the arizonae and salmonellae. Enough differences were found between the two groups, however, to justify classification of the arizona bacteria in a separate genus. Kauffmann and Edwards (1952) first employed the generic term *Arizona* and the species name *Arizona arizonae,* which was also used by Ewing (1963) for members of the genus *Arizona* (genus II of the tribe Salmonelleae). Kauffmann (1966) subsequently included the arizonae in his subgenus III of the genus *Salmonella,* designating them *Salmonella arizonae* and listing their antigenic formulas only in the simplified Kauffmann-White schema.

More recently Ewing and his colleagues (Ewing et al., 1965; Ewing and Fife, 1966; Ewing and Ball, 1966; Ewing, 1967; and Martin et al., 1967) have further clarified the definition by which the biochemical and antigenic characteristics of members of the genus *Arizona* may be readily differentiated from salmonellae and other Enterobacteriaceae. A new type species name *Arizona hinshawii* has been proposed by Ewing (1969) to replace the unacceptably redundant *A. arizonae* and to pay due honor to the pioneering work of W. R. Hinshaw on arizona infections in turkeys, reptiles, and other animals as cited in the following pages. The type species designation *A. hinshawii* will be used in this chapter.

MORPHOLOGY AND STAINING

The arizonae resemble other enteric organisms. They are gram-negative, nonsporogenic bacilli which are motile by peritrichous flagella. Most arizona strains grow best at 37° C and are facultative anaerobes with optimum growth under normal atmospheric conditions.

GROWTH REQUIREMENTS

Members of the genus *Arizona* can be readily cultivated on ordinary liquid and solid laboratory media, revealing an abundant growth similar to that of the salmonellae. Many strains produce a putrid odor, although this characteristic is not consistent.

Most arizona cultures grow very well on SS and brilliant green agars as well as other solid media recommended for isolation of salmonellae. On initial isolation on these media the colonies sometimes resemble those of salmonellae, but may develop an indicator change typical of lactose fermenters after incubation for several days or weeks. Rapid lactose-fermenting strains cannot be distinguished from normal coliforms, which are usually inhibited by these media. The use of bismuth sulfite plating medium was recommended by Martin et al. (1967) to aid in preliminary recognition of arizona strains before they are possibly discarded as coliforms. Mushin (1949) found desoxycholate agar more effective than SS agar in isolation of arizona cultures from humans. Bruner and Peckham (1952) reported the use of Selenite F as a liquid enrichment for the isolation of arizonae from poults.

COLONIAL MORPHOLOGY

On veal infusion agar smooth colonies have unbroken borders, are raised, dome-shaped, and translucent with a glistening appearance identical to salmonellae. With extended incubation colonies may develop dark brown centers. Rough (R) colonies have irregular edges and a corrugated appearance. When transferred with a loop such colonies are very dry and brittle.

BIOCHEMICAL PROPERTIES

Investigations of Edwards et al. (1959), Edwards and Ewing (1962), Ewing and Fife (1966), and Martin et al. (1967) have indicated the biochemical and antigenic homogeneity of the arizonae. Cultures possessing the following biochemical characteristics are almost invariably classifiable serologically as members of the genus *Arizona* (Edwards and Ewing, 1962; Ewing and Fife, 1966):

DEXTROSE	Fermented with gas
LACTOSE	Fermented, usually promptly
SUCROSE	Not fermented as a rule
MANNITOL	Fermented with gas
MALTOSE	Fermented with gas
DULCITOL	Not fermented
INOSITOL	Not fermented
INDOLE	Not produced as a rule
METHYL RED	Positive
VOGES-PROSKAUER	Negative
JORDAN'S TARTRATE ..	No reaction
H₂S	Positive
UREA	Not hydrolyzed
GELATIN	Liquified slowly
KCN	Negative as a rule
NITRATES	Reduced
MOTILITY	Positive
BETA-GALACTOSIDASE .	Positive
DECARBOXYLASES	
LYSINE	Positive
ARGININE	Positive, usually delayed
ORNITHINE	Positive
MALONATE	Positive
PHENYLALANINE	
DEAMINASE	Negative

The majority of arizona cultures, unlike salmonellae, ferment lactose within 1–2 days, but some produce acid from lactose only after 7–10 days or longer incubation. Edwards et al. (1956) reported that cultures of one serotype characteristically failed to ferment lactose. Occasional strains have been encountered which ferment sucrose rapidly, but these are the exception.

Arizona cultures on preliminary screening are occasionally mistaken for salmonellae; however, such errors are not of great importance since the organisms of both groups produce clinically identical diseases in poultry, and prevention and control measures are the same for both. The failure of arizona cultures to ferment dulcitol and inositol or to utilize D-tartrate, their slow liquefaction of gelatin, and their positive reactions in sodium malonate (Schaub, 1948) and beta galoctosidase (LeMinor and Ben Hamida, 1962) are most useful in distinguishing them from members of the salmonella group.

A summary tabulation of biochemical and other differential tests for identification of paratyphoid, arizona, and citrobacter strains is presented in Table 3.9 in Chapter 3. Sieburth (1957), Ewing et al. (1965), Ewing and Fife (1966), and Ewing and Ball (1966) have reviewed media for the differentiation of salmonella and arizona cultures.

Ellis et al. (1957) tested a total of 1,136 salmonella and 621 arizona cultures for their ability to utilize the organic acids D-tartrate, citrate, mucate, and malonate during an incubation period of 20 hours. Reaction patterns on these media were divisible into two groups, one of which was composed almost exclusively of salmonella and the other essentially of arizona strains. Edwards et al. (1959) utilized these organic acids in further differential tests for salmonella and arizona strains. Especially useful for the purpose is the organic acid sodium malonate which is utilized with most arizona strains and not utilized with salmonella cultures. Tests should be read after 24 and 48 hours (Edwards and Ewing, 1962). Ewing et al. (1965) have presented a comprehensive review of the biochemical reactions of arizonae and discussed procedures for differentiating them from members of the genera *Salmonella* and *Citrobacter*.

Citrobacter

For purposes of classification and identification, the arizona group of bacteria must be differentiated not only from the salmonellae but also from the closely related genus *Citrobacter* of the tribe Salmonelleae. Members of this genus are not known to be pathogenic for poultry, but from a diagnostic standpoint they may be confused with arizona and salmonella cultures on initial isolation from fecal specimens. The former Bethesda-Ballerup "paracolons" *(P. intermedium)* are included in the genus *Citrobacter* along with cultures previously classified as *Escherichia freundii.* While members of the genus *Citrobacter* are antigenically related to the salmonella and arizona groups, they must be differentiated from them biochemically.

Members of the genus *Citrobacter* are motile and usually ferment lactose; however, some cultures attack lactose slowly or not at all. Sucrose and salicin may or may not be fermented; indole is usually negative; gelatin is usually not liquefied; and dulcitol is usually fermented. The potassium cyanide (KCN) and lysine decarboxylase tests are most valuable in distinguishing *Citrobacter* strains from those of the arizona and salmonella groups. *Citrobacter* cultures grow in KCN medium while arizona and salmonella strains as a rule do not. *Citrobacter* strains are lysine-negative while arizona and salmonella strains are positive. Procedures for determining these reactions are described by Edwards and Ewing (1962). These authors as well as Ewing et al. (1965) have defined and characterized the genus. For further information on the biochemical differentiation of the genus *Citrobacter* from the paratyphoids and arizonae, the reader may refer to Table 3.9 in Chapter 3.

RESISTANCE TO CHEMICAL AND PHYSICAL AGENTS

Arizona bacteria have environmental survival properties very similar to the salmonellae. They are readily destroyed by heat and the common disinfectants. Jamison (1956) found arizona bacteria more resistant than *S. pullorum* to formaldehyde gas as a fumigant.

Kowalski and Stephens (1967) were able to recover arizona organisms from 2 of 4 water samples 5 months (but not 6 months) after the water was contaminated, and from feed samples 17 months after they were infected. Sato (1967) recovered arizona organisms from soil samples from turkey ranges which had stood vacant for 6–7 months.

Rosenwald (1965) and Kowalski and Stephens (1968) cited information to indicate that arizona organisms will survive in shady poultry yards for at least 6 months. Gerlach et al. (1968) found the albumen of eggs from birds vaccinated with arizona serotype 7:1,7,8 bacterin to show bactericidal activity toward *A. hinshawii* 7:1,7,8 in contrast to bacteriostatic activity only exhibited by the albumen of eggs from unvaccinated birds.

ANTIGENIC STRUCTURE

Arizona strains are related serologically to the salmonellae and other Enterobacteriaceae, and the procedures for study and identification of their antigenic structure are identical to those discussed with reference to the paratyphoid organisms in the previous chapter. Both somatic (O) and flagellar (H) components are demonstrable, and their antigenic formulas are designated with Arabic numerals only. Monophasic, diphasic, and triphasic strains are recognized, and all phases must be identified before the serological type can be established. Arizona serotypes delineated by serological methods are epidemiologically significant.

Although the simplified salmonella serotyping methods of Edwards and Kauffmann were earlier applied to the genus *Arizona,* the establishment of a separate and distinct antigenic schema for the genus has been necessary (Anon., 1965) to distinguish epidemiologically significant antigenic differences.

The arizona bacteria have many somatic and flagellar antigenic components which are related to antigens of the salmonellae (Anon., 1965). Schiff et al. (1941) reported 1 indole-negative "paracolon" with the complete somatic antigens of *S. onderstepoort* and 4 others with all or a part of the somatic antigens of other salmonellae. Edwards et al. (1943) isolated 1 "paracolon" culture with all the somatic and all but a minor flagellar antigen of a salmonella type.

The serotype nomenclature system used in designating members of the genus *Salmonella* has not been applied to the arizonae. In writing arizona antigenic formulas commas are used to separate O antigen factors, a colon to distinguish the O and H antigens, commas to separate H antigenic factors within a single phase, and a hyphen or dash to separate the first phase from the second and the second from the third, etc. Thus the monophasic type species of the genus would be designated *A.*

hinshawii 1,2:1,2,5. *A. hinshawii* 7:27–31–38 is an example of a triphasic member of the genus. When a monophasic variety of a normally diphasic form is encountered, it is noted in writing the formula, e.g. 1,4:26 monophasic or simply 1,4:26 mono.

Arabic numerals used to designate arizona antigenic components do not refer to the same antigenic factors as exist in salmonella strains. For example, arizona H antigen 1 which is related to salmonella H antigen Z_4 is not identical to salmonella H antigen 1. The reader seeking synonyms and antigenic formulas for earlier arizona serotypes designated by the "PC" system can refer to the bulletin of Edwards et al. (1947).

By examining the somatic and flagellar antigens of 373 arizona cultures, Edwards et al. (1947) were able to demonstrate 19 O groups and 55 distinct serological types. Martin et al. (1967) described a revised antigenic schema for the genus *Arizona* including 34 O groups, 43 H antigens and 322 serological types. Antigenic schema for the genus *Arizona* are presently issued periodically by the Public Health Service's National Communicable Disease Center and kept current through the publication of supplements.

Sanders et al. (1943) and Burton and Garrard (1948) reported that atypical reactions in routine testing with *S. pullorum* antigen may be due to certain "paracolon" strains. The organisms may occasionally be recovered from tissues of adult chickens and turkeys submitted for routine bacteriological examination as reactors to the blood test for pullorum disease (Gauger, 1946).

Edwards et al. (1956, 1959) found *A. hinshawii* 7:1,7,8 to be more frequently isolated than any other type in the United States and reported that it comprised almost one-fourth of the total cultures studied and was isolated from 408 outbreaks of infection. This has continued to be the predominant arizona serotype in both animals and man in this country. In 1947 most of the outbreaks of serotype 7:1,7,8 infection in poults were from eggs produced by a single cooperative turkey breeder association in a western state. This type is now found in turkeys in all parts of the United States.

Moran (1959a) serologically typed 155 members of the arizona group isolated from animals; 138 of the cultures were isolated from turkeys and were confined to 2 serological types, namely 7:1,2,6 and 7:1,7,8. The number of each of these arizona serotypes was approximately the same as the number of cultures of *S. typhi-murium* typed in 1957 from turkeys. *A. hinshawii* 7:1,7,8 and 7:1,2,6 are also the serotypes most commonly isolated from man (Martin et al., 1967). Moran (1960) reported the serological typing in 1958 of 119 arizona strains, 74.7% of which were isolated from turkeys and only 4.2% from chickens. In 1959 the same author (Moran, 1961) typed 91 arizona cultures from chickens and turkeys, of which 93% were isolated from turkeys and 7% from chickens.

PATHOGENICITY

Like the salmonellae, arizona bacteria can invade the bloodstream especially of young fowl, and high mortality has been reported (Edwards et al., 1956). Worcester (1965) noted that arizona bacteria can penetrate the wall of the intestinal tract and stay there indefinitely. Young chicks and poults are most frequently infected during the first 3 weeks after hatching. Kowalski and Stephens (1967) cite persistence without a host as one of the prominent characteristics of the arizonae.

Lewis and Hitchner (1936) recorded a mortality of 32–50% in chicks from the infection. These investigators were able to reproduce the disease under laboratory conditions in day-old chicks by subcutaneous and oral inoculations. Guinea pigs were also found susceptible to the infection by parenteral inoculation.

Edwards et al. (1947) administered arizona organisms orally to a group of White Leghorn chicks. Deaths continued for 1 week with a mortality of 16.6%. Of a group of Rhode Island Red chicks placed in the same pen as contacts, 26.6% died. Arizona bacilli serologically identical with the organisms administered were recovered from the livers and intestines of every chick that died.

Kowalski and Stephens (1968) found the first death in poults orally inoculated at 1 day of age with arizona organisms to occur after 4 days. The peak of mortality in the inoculated birds occurred on the 10th day. A mortality of 15% occurred in poults inoculated with arizona organisms at 1 day of age while 2% of contact poults died. Goetz and Quortrup (1953) recorded the mortality rates among poults infected with *A. hinshawii* 7:1,7,8 varied from 0.5 to 50% and occurred from the 4th or 5th day through the 3rd week. Adler and Rosenwald (1968) indicated that about 10% of infected poults die during arizona outbreaks. Snoeyenbos and Smyser (1969) reported a mortality of approximately 50% from an *A. hinshawii* 7:1,7,8 outbreak in turkey poults.

Adler and Rosenwald (1968) found that storage of hatching eggs at room temperature markedly increased susceptibility of embryos to arizona organisms, and Gerlach et al. (1968) demonstrated high embryo mortality in stored turkey eggs inoculated in the air cell with 7–20 colony-forming units of arizona serotype 7:1,7,8.

PATHOGENESIS AND EPIZOOTIOLOGY

NATURAL AND EXPERIMENTAL HOSTS

Like salmonellae, arizona organisms recognize no host barriers, are widely distributed in nature, and have been found in a large segment of man's environment. The frequent isolation of arizona bacteria particularly from reptiles and fowl is notable. All ages of fowl may be infected with arizonosis, but mortality usually occurs only in young birds up to 3 weeks of age. Adult birds generally show no signs of the infection.

Edwards et al. (1947, 1956, 1959) reported the identification of arizona strains from humans, turkeys, chickens, canaries, ducks, parrots, a pheasant, a macaw, reptiles, sheep, swine, dogs, a mink, a cat, a Gila monster, a capybara, monkeys, guinea pigs, and opossums. Arizona cultures isolated from fowls and reptiles over a 20-year period composed almost 75% of the cultures studied. Excluding chickens, turkeys, reptiles, and man, Martin et al. (1967) isolated arizonae from about 20 other animals which included dogs, swine, sheep, cats, rabbits, hedgehogs, baboons, and rats. Host adaptation does occasionally occur in arizona infections. Serotype 26:23–30 is very common in monkeys; serotype 26:29–30 occurs often in sheep.

Poultry

Among poultry, arizonosis is most frequently encountered in turkeys. Peluffo et al. (1942) and Edwards et al. (1943) reported a group of arizonae which were isolated from poults as well as adult turkeys under natural conditions. Mortality varied from 15 to 60%. The average mortality was 35%. Cultures isolated from the same group of birds were of the same serological type and the birds had a common hatchery source.

Hinshaw and McNeil (1944) reported the occurrence of a single serotype of arizona as a cause of mortality in poults. They also reported the presence of this same serotype in snakes found on the premises and believed to be carriers of the infection. In further investigations Hinshaw and McNeil (1946a,b) isolated a number of cultures of *A. hinshawii* 7:1,7,8 from poults and snakes. On one turkey ranch where a 70% mortality occurred, the greatest losses were observed during the first 3 weeks, but losses continued for 5 weeks. Gauger (1946) isolated *A. hinshawii* 7:1,7,8 from an adult turkey.

Bruner and Peckham (1952) reported the isolation of *A. hinshawii* 7:1,7,8 from poults which experienced a mortality of 5%. Pomeroy et al. (1957) studied 120 outbreaks of arizona infections in young turkeys. Four arizona serotypes were isolated. Serotype 7:1,7,8 was encountered most frequently.

Perek (1957) encountered a severe outbreak of arizona infection in chicks in Israel. The organisms isolated proved to be highly infectious for chicks up to 4 weeks but not for adult birds. Bigland and Quon (1958) described 8 outbreaks of *A. hinshawii* 7:1,2,6 infection in poults, chicks, and an adult hen in Alberta. This was the first report of arizona infections among poultry in Alberta. Mortality occurred up to 4 weeks of age and varied from 10% in chicks to 50% in poults. Galton (1953) recovered 13 cultures of *A. hinshawii* 10:1,2,5 in a poultry processing plant.

Martin et al. (1967) reported following an 18½-year survey that only 4.2% of 4,438 arizona cultures studied were isolated from chickens, 45% from turkeys, 21.1% from reptiles, 12.2% from man, and 6.2% from other animals. By far the lowest percentage of outbreaks of arizonosis was reported in chickens, since only 5.7% of 2,423 outbreaks studied occurred in this species contrasted to 54.3% in turkeys. Other avian species found to be infected with arizona organisms included cockatoo, parakeet, duck, canary, and hawk. In contrasting the period 1948–59 with that of 1959–66, an unexplained drop of approximately 50%

in the number of outbreaks and arizona cultures isolated from turkeys and chickens during the later period was found.

Dougherty (1953) cited 2 occasions on which he isolated arizona organisms from duck livers revealing lesions very similar to those produced by paratyphoid infections. Edwards et al. (1947, 1956) indicated that arizona bacteria may cause heavy losses among canaries in which the bacteria may be isolated from ocular tissues in cases of iritis. Edwards et al. (1959) reported that *A. hinshawii* 13:13,14 was the only causative agent recognized in 2 highly fatal outbreaks of disease in canaries.

Reptiles and Other Animals

Fey et al. (1957) discussed pathological changes encountered in 6 cases of arizona infections of reptiles and described the biochemical and serological properties of the causative organisms isolated. Edwards et al. (1961) reported the isolation of 7, and Fife and Ewing (1967) the isolation of 8 previously undescribed cultures of arizona bacteria from reptiles. Goetz and Quortrup (1953) were able to recover arizona strains from gophers, and Hinshaw and McNeil (1947) cited fence lizards as carriers of the organisms. LeMinor et al. (1958) described the high percentage of reptiles that are infected with arizonae in nature. Sato et al. (1966) reported the isolation of arizonae from a normal snake and cited work to indicate that salmonella and arizona organisms could be recovered from about 5% of frogs and earthworms in Japan.

Johnson et al. (1951) reported infection of the bovine udder with arizona bacteria. Ryff and Browne (1952) isolated a diphasic arizona type (26:29–30) from aborted fetuses in ewes.

Man

Arizona infection as a disease in humans is very similar to salmonellosis in its epidemiology, pathogenesis, symptomology, and control. The recovery of arizona cultures from man has increased markedly with improved procedures for their recognition and identification. Martin et al. (1967) reported a twofold rise in total outbreaks in man for the period 1959–66 compared to an earlier period. Galton (1956), Edwards et al. (1956, 1959), and Martin et al. (1967) have reviewed the occurrence of arizonosis in man.

Gastroenteritis with symptoms of vomiting, diarrhea, and fever is the most common form of the disease in man (Stuart et al., 1943). However, certain serotypes (e.g. 7:1,2,6 and 7:1,7,8) have a predilection for producing infections outside the intestinal tract (Martin et al., 1967) which have been encountered with increasing frequency in man. Certain arizona serotypes seem to have a greater invasive potential in humans, as evidenced by frequent septic foci in various organs (Edwards et al., 1956). Arizona bacteria have been reported to cause gastroenteritis in man (Murphy and Morris, 1950) as well as febrile illnesses with bacteremia (Edwards and Fife, 1962).

Arizona infections of man have been associated with chronic enterocolitis (Luippold, 1947), endocarditis (Friedman and Goldin, 1949), pneumonia (Kraft, 1951), otitis media and sickle cell disease (Butt and Morris, 1952), osteomyelitis (Fisher, 1953), meningoencephalitis (Edwards et al., 1959), and arthritis (Guckian et al., 1967). Two fatal cases of arizona infection in humans attributed to *A. hinshawii* 7:1,2,6 were described by Krag and Shean (1959). One case involved a liver abscess and the other was a chronic osteomyelitis compounded by a septic arthritis of the knee. Lystad (1962) studied 51 "paracolon" strains responsible for a nosocomial outbreak of urinary tract infection in man.

From the above brief review it is clear that extraintestinal isolations of arizona bacteria from pathological conditions in humans are perhaps more common than salmonellae. This disease may with time pose a major public health threat. Fields et al. (1967) presented a bacteriological and clinical reappraisal of the so-called "paracolon" group of bacteria. This is a timely review and an excellent source of information on the clinical phases of arizonosis in man.

Evidence indicates that a cycle similar to that which exists in salmonella infections between man and animals, including all types of poultry, exists with the arizonae. The importance of animals and animal products such as meat and eggs in spreading the infection to humans must be considered in the epidemiology of the disease in man. Buttiaux and Kesteloot (1948) drew attention to the likelihood that certain arizona infections in humans were contracted from contaminated eggs or egg powder. Ueda et al. were cited by Sato et al. (1966) as isolating arizona organisms from chickens and eggs which caused food poisoning.

TRANSMISSION, CARRIERS, VECTORS

The transmission cycle of arizona infections in poultry is identical with that established for motile salmonellae discussed in the previous chapter. Infected adult birds are frequently intestinal carriers and spreaders of arizona organisms for long periods (Edwards et al., 1943). Wild birds (McClure et al., 1957), rats and mice (Goetz, 1962), and reptiles (Hinshaw and McNeil, 1944, 1947) have been cited as common sources of the organisms for poultry flocks. Arizonae have also been isolated from commercial poultry feed (Erwin, 1955).

Transmission of arizona infections through eggs has been reported by Edwards et al. (1943, 1947, 1956, 1959), Hinshaw and McNeil (1946a), Bruner and Peckham (1952), and Jamison (1956). Goetz et al. (1954) were able to isolate arizona 7:1,7,8 from the eggs and embryos of turkey hens reacting to the agglutination test for this serotype. Hinshaw and McNeil (1946a), Gauger (1946), and Sato and Adler (1966d) reported the recovery of arizona organisms from the ovaries of adult turkeys, suggesting that transovarian transmission can occur in this species. Sato and Adler (1966d) demonstrated that ingestion of arizona organisms by adult turkeys may cause a systemic involvement which may be followed by ovule localization and provide a potential source of egg-borne arizona infection.

The frequent presence of arizona organisms within both chicken and turkey eggs (Edwards et al., 1943; Goetz et al., 1954) is accepted as resulting primarily from contamination of the shell surface by feces that contain arizona organisms, with eventual penetration of the shell (Sato and Adler, 1966d). Williams and Dillard (1968) found arizona organisms to have a penetration pattern through the outer structures of chicken eggs very similar to that of S. typhimurium and demonstrated that A. hinshawii 7:1,7,8 could readily penetrate the shell and shell membranes of chicken eggs incubated at 99° F.

The frequent isolation of members of the genus Arizona from egg powder by Edwards et al. (1947) suggested wide distribution of the organisms on the surface of chicken eggs in the United States. Kowalski and Stephens (1968) reported the isolation of A. hinshawii 7:1,7,8 from the shell of soiled turkey eggs. Sato and Adler (1966d) were able to isolate arizona organisms from the shell surface of eggs laid by experimentally infected adult turkeys. All of the egg contents were negative for arizonae on culture after incubation for 14 days.

Edwards et al. (1943) pointed out that arizona infections may be carried for long periods by adult fowl which were infected as poults. Hinshaw and McNeil (1946a) reported that 5 of 7 infected turkeys yielded the organisms from the intestines, and Sadler et al. (1961) also made intestinal isolations of Arizona organisms. Sato and Adler (1966c) reported that 50% of a group of poults naturally infected with arizona organisms continued to have arizona-positive cloacal swabs for as long as 11 weeks. Four of 16 birds yielded the organisms from the rectum, cecum, and ileum on necropsy. The same investigators (1966d) demonstrated that adult turkeys experimentally infected with arizona serotypes 7:1,7,8 and 7:1,2,6 became fecal shedders of the organisms. Adler and Rosenwald (1968) reported that arizona infections in adult turkeys are confined primarily to the intestinal tract.

Arizonosis of a particular type may become established in a hatchery and then spread to a distant establishment through eggs purchased from the original infected hatchery. Edwards et al. (1947) cited instances in which arizona infection with organisms of a certain serological type was traced from egg sources in a far western state to points as far away as Minnesota, North Carolina, and Pennsylvania. Bigland and Quon (1958) suspected that arizona infections were introduced with eggs shipped into Canada from certain western states of the United States.

Edwards et al. (1959), in an epizootiological study of arizona 10:1,2,5 infection in chickens, traced the spread of the disease from a southern state to the Midwest and then back to the broiler producing areas of the Southeast. This same type of the organism has appeared in man, dogs, and cats. Jamison (1956) noted that since arizona infections usually started in poults in California in late April or May, it was suspected that the breeding flocks were infected from some outside source.

Fecal contamination may spread the infection from other animal species to poultry. Goetz (1962) found an arizona infection rate of 90% in rats and 50% in mice on the premises of a turkey ranch where the infection was a problem in poults. Various types of wild birds, reptiles, and many common animal species can also infect poultry flocks and establish fecal carriers.

Arizona infections are transmitted in the incubator and brooder by direct contact and through contaminated feed and water. The role of direct contact in spreading the infection among chicks and poults was illustrated by the reports of Edwards et al. (1947) and Kowalski and Stephens (1968). Goetz et al. (1954) did not feel that arizona infections are frequently transmitted to healthy poults during the brooding period. Erwin (1955) reported the isolation of 73 "paracolon" cultures during the bacteriological examination of 206 prepared poultry feed samples.

SIGNS

While symptoms of arizonosis in poultry are not specific, infected poults and chicks may appear listless and develop diarrhea, leg paralysis, twisted necks, and pasting of the down around the vent (Hinshaw and McNeil, 1946a). Infected birds tend to sit on their hocks and huddle together. Bruner and Peckham (1952) reported that infected poults revealed signs of weakness, ataxia, and trembling.

Jamison (1956) observed nervous symptoms in arizona-infected poults as a result of the organisms localizing in the brain. Perek (1957) observed that death from arizonosis in chicks was accompanied by convulsions. Bigland and Quon (1958) noted that arizona infections in chicks and poults revealed sudden death preceded for 1–2 hours by shivering, huddling, and anorexia. In birds 2–3 weeks old, diarrhea, droopiness, twisted heads, and evidence of blindness in one or both eyes were seen up to 2 days prior to death. The blindness was caused by caseous material covering the retina.

Kowalski and Stephens (1968) found blindness to occur in 13% of poults inoculated with arizona serotype 7:1,7,8 and in 6% of the contacts. Blindness was more frequent in females than in males, and more often seen in the left eye than the right eye. Nervous symptoms along with recovery of the organisms from infected brains were observed earlier in inoculated birds than contact birds. Adler and Rosenwald (1968) did not believe that infected eyes during arizona infections were a likely source of the organisms for other fowl that come in contact with birds so infected. Sato and Adler (1966d) noted that rarely can clinical signs of arizonosis be noted in adult turkeys and they seldom die from this infection.

GROSS LESIONS AND HISTOPATHOLOGY

The lesions described by Lewis and Hitchner (1936) in chicks artificially infected with "paracolon" bacteria were typical of a generalized septicemia and included peritonitis; retained yolk sacs; enlarged yellowish, mottled, or inflamed liver; and discolored heart. Similar lesions were noted in chicks by Edwards et al. (1947) and in poults by Bruner and Peckham (1952). Goetz and Quortrup (1953) found caseous plugs similar to those seen in pullorum disease in arizona-infected poults. Hinshaw and McNeil (1946a) noted marked congestion of the duodenum and ocher or mottled livers to be common in arizona infection. Arizona organisms were recovered from adult turkeys, 2 of which had small, caseous mesenteric lesions and 3 had cystic ovules. Cheesy exudates in the abdominal cavities readily yielded cultures of *A. hinshawii* 7:1,7,8 in the experimental studies of Kowalski and Stephens (1968).

Eye lesions resulting in opacity and partial or complete blindness are frequently seen in arizonosis of poults. Sato and Adler (1966c) selected poults naturally infected with arizonae from a flock known to be carriers by observing the birds for ocular lesions. Jamison (1956) called attention to the cloudiness of the eyes in infected poults which is also observed in Newcastle disease. The organisms can be readily recovered from the infected eye tissues.

Bigland and Quon (1958) described eye lesions as a common occurrence in arizona infections. They found a heavy, yellowish white, cheesy exudate covering the retinae. Affected eyes became quite dry and failed to grow normally. Other lesions included caseation of the ceca and tiny lung abscesses.

Sato and Adler (1966c) in studying natural arizona infection in turkeys found eyeballs from affected eyes shriveled and various amounts of yellowish cheesy exudate covering the retinae. Pure cultures of *A. hinshawii* 7:1,7,8 were obtained from the contents of the affected eyeballs. These same authors found yellowish caseous exudate in the air sacs, abdominal or thoracic cavity, and retained yolks in arizona-infected turkeys.

Histological changes due to arizona infection of chicks were observed by Perek (1957) as fatty degeneration of the liver and distinct capillary congestion of the kidneys.

DIAGNOSIS

Symptoms and lesions are of little value in differentiating avian arizonosis from salmonellosis. Findings on necropsy must be substantiated by recovery and identification of the causative bacteria. In arizona infections the organisms can usually be recovered from the liver, spleen, heart blood, lungs, kidneys, unabsorbed yolk, and intestines. Bigland and Quon (1958) were able to readily isolate arizona strains from the caseous material covering the retinae of affected eyes. They called attention to the need to differentiate this infection from that due to *Aspergillus fumigatus* when eye involvement occurs.

ISOLATION AND IDENTIFICATION
OF CAUSATIVE AGENT

Cultural procedures outlined and discussed in the previous chapter for pullorum disease and paratyphoid infections are employed. Moran (1959b) reported procedures and media for isolation and identification of arizona strains from fresh specimens. The history of the outbreak as well as the degree of infection indicated by culture results must be considered. Recovery of the organisms from the intestinal tract alone of poults and chicks may be of little significance. Goetz and Quortrup (1953) used the cloacal swab and culture technique in an effort to detect carriers of arizona organisms in adult turkey flocks which had suffered a severe outbreak as poults. Results were negative. Sato and Adler (1966c) re-

ported the recovery of arizona serotype 7:1,7,8 from the heart, lungs, gallbladder, spleen, testes, kidneys, bursa, peritoneum, retained yolk, and intestinal contents of naturally infected turkeys.

Snoeyenbos and Smyser (1969) were able to isolate arizona organisms from infected litter in turkey houses for as long as 6 weeks after a clinical outbreak of arizonosis in poults. It was felt that litter culturing may have some value in epidemiological studies and as an aid in identifying arizona-infected flocks of turkeys as part of a program to control this group of pathogens. Worcester (1965) and Sato and Adler (1966c) reported that cloacal swabs are not a very sensitive method for detecting intestinal carriers over 12 weeks of age. The methods outlined by Lewis and Angelotti (1964) and those cited in the paratyphoid section of Chapter 3 can be applied in culturing poultry feeds for arizonae.

Arizona organisms may be discarded as coliforms, and in the past many probably have been. When extended incubation is not practiced some may be classified as salmonella strains on initial isolation. The increasing evidence of the pathogenicity for fowl of members of the genus *Arizona* indicates the necessity for studying this group of organisms more closely.

Sato and Adler (1966c,d) and Kowalski and Stephens (1968) used selenite cystine broth (Difco) in the enrichment of fecal and organ tissue cultures for the isolation of arizonae from poults and adult turkeys. Platings were made on brilliant green agar. Edwards and Galton (1967) have reported that bismuth sulfite agar is especially effective for isolation of arizona organisms. Edwards and Fife (1961) described lysine-iron agar slants for preliminary detection of arizona strains that rapidly ferment lactose. Salmonella and arizona strains produce a distinctive reaction as they regularly form lysine decarboxylase and produce large amounts of hydrogen sulfide. Kowalski and Stephens (1967) discussed the tendency of certain arizona strains to lose ability to produce hydrogen sulfide in diagnostic media. Williams and Dillard (1968) did not find the addition of neo-tetrazolium chloride to a standard tetrathionate broth to interfere with the growth of *A. hinshawii* 7:1,7,8.

For further information on the biochemical characteristics of the arizonae useful in differential laboratory diagnosis, see the Etiology section of this chapter or Table 3.9 in Chapter 3.

SEROLOGY

Serological analysis of cultures is essential in epizootiological studies of arizona infections of fowl. If facilities for complete identification of the organisms are not readily available, cultures should be submitted to one of USDA's regional salmonella-arizona typing laboratories or to the National Animal Disease Laboratory, Box 70, Ames, Iowa 50010, where the cultures may be studied more closely biochemically and typed antigenically. Goetz and Quortrup (1953) reported the use of a polyvalent antiserum in screening cultures that were suspected to be arizona strains.

Edwards and Galton (1967) noted that it is essential to use a polyvalent arizona antiserum in the preliminary examination of cultures since arizona types may not be agglutinated by salmonella polyvalent antiserum. Kowalski and Stephens (1968) reported employing formalized broth cultures and arizona polymonophasic antiserum in the serological identification of arizona cultures. Snoeyenbos and Smyser (1969) used arizona flagellar polyvalent, salmonella flagellar Z_{32}, and salmonella somatic 18 antisera in screening cultures suspected to be arizonae.

Serological testing procedures and antigens for the diagnosis of avian arizonosis are discussed in the Prevention and Control section of this chapter.

TREATMENT

The use of chemical therapeutic measures may reduce losses in acute outbreaks of arizonosis and may be recommended to prevent the spread of the disease in market flocks. Hinshaw and McNeil (1946a), in their study of *A. hinshawii* 7:1,7,8 infection of turkeys, reported the administration of sulfamerazine to a group of 8-day-old poults that had shown a 12% mortality previous to this treatment. The drug was used at a dosage of 0.25% in the mash for 3 days. Marked improvement was noted in the treated group compared to untreated controls. Cessation of treatment resulted in increased losses. A favorable response was noted when the same treatment was administered to both groups of birds for 3 more days. When the survivors were tested with the agglutination test 6 months later, no reactors were found. Goetz et al. (1954) reported that the use of various combinations of sulfonamides and antibiotics had little effect upon mortality from arizona infections of poults.

Although supportive data are lacking, parenteral inoculation of very young poults with antibiotics has recently been extensively applied in the field for prevention of arizonosis.

Harwood (1956), Jamison (1956), and Pomeroy et al. (1958) have reported on the use of furazolidone (nf-180) in the treatment of arizona infections. Jamison (1956) described the experimental use of furazolidone in the feed of adult turkey flocks in California as a preventive against arizonosis. It was recommended that 100 g of the drug be added to each ton of feed for 1 week each month. The same level of the drug for 5–7 days was recommended in treating acute outbreaks of the disease in poults. This level of treatment was also suggested for the first 2 weeks of brooding as a preventive in poults from breeding flocks suspected of having arizonosis. Higher levels of furazolidone may be recommended and prove more effective in treating particularly severe outbreaks. It is possible that treated birds may remain intestinal carriers of the causative organism. Harwood (1956) has suggested the use of a combination treatment consisting of a sulfonamide in the drinking water and furazolidone in the feed for treatment of severe outbreaks of the disease.

Pomeroy et al. (1958) found that furazolidone fed to poults at a level of 100 g or higher per ton reduced the mortality from arizona infection 50% when administered at the time the poults were experimentally exposed to the organisms. The 200 g per ton level of the drug was more effective in reducing poult mortality and in eliminating arizona isolations from surviving birds. When treatment was started before exposure, the 100 g per ton level of the drug was found to have a preventive effect on development of the disease. Goetz (1962) reported that intensive furazolidone treatment of laying turkeys infected with arizonae did not eliminate the presence of the organisms in the eggs of such turkeys.

PREVENTION AND CONTROL

MANAGEMENT PROCEDURES

Since arizona infections of fowl are transmitted in the same manner as paratyphoid infections, the control program for this disease is identical to that for paratyphoid infection as outlined in the previous chapter.

Adler and Rosenwald (1968) recommended the following measures involving egg handling for prevention of arizona infections in turkeys: gather eggs frequently, do not use floor eggs, clean nesting boxes frequently, clean slightly dirty eggs with an abrasive, keep egg-receiving rooms separate from other buildings, fumigate all hatching eggs as soon as possible after gathering, after fumigation use a separate egg handler in another room to take eggs from racks, store eggs in clean boxes at 55–60° F, and always prevent eggs from sweating. Sanitation was cited as of prime importance in controlling arizonae during egg handling, artificial insemination, and hatching operations.

On-the-farm preincubation formaldehyde fumigation of hatching eggs as soon as possible after they are laid, preferably within 2 hours, is highly recommended for breaking the transmission cycle of this disease. Shell contamination by fecal carriers is the usual means of spread of the organisms to young birds. The penetration pattern of arizona organisms through the shell of avian eggs is apparently identical to that established for *S. typhi-murium* (Williams and Dillard, 1968) and can be very rapid.

The level of fumigant used for on-the-farm fumigation of eggs should be 1.2 ml formalin mixed with 0.6 g potassium permanganate per cu ft of cabinet space for a 20-minute period. Refer to the Prevention and Control section of Chapter 3 (Paratyphoid Infections) for further information on preincubation fumigation procedures.

Jamison (1956) recommended that high levels of formaldehyde fumigant be used for destruction of arizonae on eggshells and fumigation carried out as soon as the eggs are set and the temperature and humidity are up to regular operating levels. It was recommended that the eggs be fumigated again with the high level of fumigant just before they are transferred to the hatching trays.

SEROLOGICAL TESTING

Because of the large number of antigenic types of arizona strains, any control program involving use of the agglutination test to detect infected adults must be based on the location and disposal of infected breeding flocks. Rosenwald (1965) and Worcester (1965) reported that serological tests were not entirely effective to detect or to help control arizona infections in turkeys. Their use in California for this purpose has not been highly successful (Adler and Rosenwald, 1968).

Specific types of antigen must be prepared and used in each case. From the small percentage of reactors to the agglutination test found by Hinshaw and McNeil (1946a), it appeared that the infection may be more easily shed than is pullorum disease. Goetz et al. (1954) used an experimental plate agglutination antigen to test serum samples from turkey flocks infected with *A. hinshawii* 7:1,7,8. In one flock containing 1,414 birds, 6 reactors were found, 5 of which yielded arizona organisms on culture. A retest of the flock 1 month later revealed no reactors. Other flocks tested contained many reactors and were disposed of.

Goetz (1962) described the use of a flagellar tube agglutination test for arizona infection in turkeys. Reference may be made to the section on Prevention and Control of paratyphoid infections in Chapter 3 for a discussion of the California control program for arizona infections in turkeys.

Sato and Adler (1966c) found naturally infected turkeys to have positive O agglutination reactions at some time during the period they were observed; however, some of the same birds were negative when tested with H antigen. The H agglutinins disappeared earlier than did O agglutinins. All infected birds did not reveal positive O agglutination tests at the time of necropsy. There was little correlation between serological results and persistence of infection. The same investigators (1966d) used a formalin-treated broth culture of actively motile arizona strains in preparing flagellar antigen for serologically testing adult turkeys for arizona serotypes 7:1,2,6 and 7:1,7,8. The somatic antigen of the same strains was prepared by growing the cultures on beef heart infusion agar and treating the heavy cell suspension harvested with ethanol.

Sato and Adler (1966d) used serum dilutions as low as 1:6.25 in serological tests for arizona infections in experimentally infected turkeys. Flagellar agglutination was read after incubation for 2 hours in the water bath at 51–52° C. Somatic agglutination was read after the reactants were left overnight in the refrigerator or at room temperature following 2 hours at 37° C. Both somatic and flagellar agglutinins were found in rather high titers in turkeys artificially infected with 2 arizona serotypes. Sato and Adler (1966b) found that because of the nonspecific hemagglutinating qualities of turkey sera, the indirect hemagglutination test was unsuitable as a diagnostic serological procedure. The antiglobulin test provided the most specific enhancing effect for O agglutination.

Methods for preparing and using arizona antigens for serological testing of chickens and turkeys have been reviewed in a recent publication (Anon., 1971).

IMMUNIZATION

Efforts have been made to apply several types of bacterins for production of immunity to arizona infections in turkey breeding stock and in the progeny of vaccinated breeder stock. Holte (1965) found that there is a reduction in the shedding of arizona serotype 7:1,7,8 when vaccinated breeders are exposed to the organisms, and bacterin vaccination protected the hens from systemic infection, thus preventing transmission of arizonae through the egg. Parental immunity was found to be transmitted to the poults of vaccinated hens. This author concluded that vaccination of turkeys against arizona infections appeared to be beneficial; however, it was not considered as a substitute for other disease control procedures but rather as ancillary to sanitary measures.

Sato and Adler (1966a) found varying degrees of protection afforded by arizona bacterins in both mice and turkeys. A formalin-treated whole culture in aluminum hydroxide gel provided the best protection. In attempting to estimate the efficacy of arizona bacterins, these investigators took as a gauge of immunity the migration of various numbers of organisms to the spleen following intramuscular challenge. Miyamae and Adler (1967) found a high degree of protection offered by arizona bacterin with an aluminum hydroxide adjuvant in intraperitoneally challenged mice; however, no significant protection against oral exposure was afforded by the bacterin. In turkeys a chrome-alum-treated arizona bacterin provided the best protection to both oral and intraperitoneal challenge. Aluminum hydroxide bacterin and endotoxin appeared to render birds more susceptible to oral challenge. Trypticase soy broth (BBL) produced the least amount of smooth to rough dissociation in arizona cultures during the preparation of experimental bacterins.

Gerlach et al. (1968) found serum from unimmunized turkey hens had both bacteriostatic and bactericidal effects on cultures of *A. hinshawii* 7:1,7,8. There was no inhibitory activity in the serum of birds vaccinated with arizona bacterin or in naturally infected breeders. Inhibition of growth was not associated with the presence of agglutinating antibodies; in fact, the opposite appeared to be true.

Adler and Rosenwald (1968) in experimental studies of arizona bacterins to immunize turkeys found one bacterin that almost completely prevented infection of the internal organs even when the challenge dose was extremely high. None of the bacterins studied reduced the fecal shedding rate during the first 21 days after challenge; however, vaccinated turkey hens were found to have a bactericidal substance in the albumen of their eggs. It was concluded that additional research is needed if a satisfactory bacterin to produce immunity to arizona infections in turkeys is to become a reality.

The establishment of the arizonae as a group of considerable pathogenic importance for fowl suggests that all efforts with an objective toward the prevention and control of avian salmonellosis must take into consideration these closely related organisms.

REFERENCES

Adler, H. E., and A. S. Rosenwald. 1968. Paracolon control: What we know and need to know. *Turkey World* 43:18.

Anonymous. 1965. *Antigenic schema for the genus Arizona.* U.S. Dept. of HEW, Public Health Serv., NCDC, Atlanta, Ga.

Anonymous. 1971. *Methods for the examination of poultry vaccines. Methods for the identification and quantitation of avian pathogens.* Nat. Acad. Sci., Nat. Res. Council, Washington, D.C. (In press).

Bigland, C. H., and A. B. Quon. 1958. Infections of poultry with arizona paracolon in Alberta. *Can. J. Comp. Med. Vet. Sci.* 22:308–12.

Borman, E. K., C. A. Stuart, and K. M. Wheeler. 1944. Taxonomy of the family Enterobacteriaceae. *J. Bacteriol.* 48:351–67.

Breed, R. S., E. G. D. Murray, and N. R. Smith. 1957. *Bergey's Manual of Determinative Bacteriology,* 7th ed. Williams & Wilkins Co., Baltimore.

Bruner, D. W., and M. C. Peckham. 1952. An outbreak of paracolon infection in turkey poults. *Cornell Vet.* 42:22–24.

Burton, W. H., and E. H. Garrard. 1948. Non-pullorum agglutination reactions. IV. Reactions with pullorum antigen from fowl inoculated with coliform types. *Can. J. Comp. Med. Vet. Sci.* 12:20–25.

Butt, E., and J. F. Morris. 1952. Arizona paracolon recovered from middle ear discharge. *J. Infect. Diseases* 91:283–84.

Buttiaux, R., and A. Kestleloot. 1948. Les "B paracoli" du group Arizona, leur pouvoir pathogene chez l'homme. *Ann. Inst. Pasteur* 75:379–81.

Caldwell, M. E., and D. L. Ryerson. 1939. Salmonellosis in certain reptiles. *J. Infect. Diseases* 65:242–45.

Dougherty, E. 1953. Disease problems confronting the duck industry. *Proc. 90th Ann. Meet. Am. Vet. Med. Ass.,* pp. 359–65.

Edwards, P. R., and W. H. Ewing. 1962. *Identification of Enterobacteriaceae.* Burgess Publ. Co., Minneapolis.

Edwards, P. R., and Mary A. Fife. 1961. Lysine-iron agar in the detection of arizona cultures. *Appl. Microbiol.* 9:478–80.

———. 1962. Eleven undescribed arizona serotypes isolated from man. *Antonie van Leeuwenhoek, J. Microbiol. Serol.* 28:402–4.

Edwards, P. R., and Mildred M. Galton. 1967. Salmonellosis, pp. 1–63. In Brandly, C. A., and C. Cornelius (eds). *Advances in Veterinary Science.* Academic Press, New York.

Edwards, P. R., W. B. Cherry, and D. W. Bruner. 1943. Further studies on coliform bacteria serologically related to the genus *Salmonella. J. Infect. Diseases* 73:229–38.

Edwards, P. R., M. G. West, and D. W. Bruner.

1947. Arizona group of paracolon bacteria. *Kentucky Agr. Exp. Sta. Bull.* 499.

Edwards, P. R., Alma C. McWhorter, and Mary A. Fife. 1956. The arizona group of Enterobacteriaceae in animals and man. Occurrence and distribution. *Bull. World Health Organ.* 14:511–28.

Edwards, P. R., Mary A. Fife, and Carolyn H. Ramsey. 1959. Studies on the arizona group of Enterobacteriaceae. *Bacteriol. Rev.* 23:155–74.

Edwards, P. R., E. H. Kampelmacher, Mary A. Fife, and P. A. Guinee. 1961. Seven new arizona serotypes isolated from reptiles. *Antonie van Leeuwenhoek, J. Microbiol. Serol.* 27:110–12.

Ellis, R. J., P. R. Edwards, and Mary A. Fife. 1957. The differentiation of the salmonella and arizona groups by utilization of organic acids. *Public Health Rept.* 15:89–93.

Erwin, L. E. 1955. Examination of prepared poultry feeds for the presence of salmonella and other enteric organisms. *Poultry Sci.* 34:215–16.

Ewing, W. H. 1963. An outline of nomenclature for the family Enterobacteriaceae. *Int. Bull. Bacteriol. Nomencl. Taxon.* 13:95–110.

———. 1967. *Revised definitions for the family Enterobacteriaceae, its tribes and genera.* U.S. Dept. of HEW, NCDC, Atlanta, Ga.

———. 1969. *Arizona hinshawii comb. nov. Int. J. Syst. Bacteriol.* 19:1.

Ewing, W. H., and M. M. Ball. 1966. *The biochemical reactions of members of the genus Salmonella.* U.S. Dept. of HEW, NCDC, Atlanta, Ga.

Ewing, W. H., and Mary A. Fife. 1966. A summary of the biochemical reactions of *Arizona arizonae. Int. J. Syst. Bacteriol.* 16:427–33.

Ewing, W. H., Mary A. Fife, and B. R. Davis. 1965. *The Biochemical Reactions of Arizona arizonae.* U.S. Dept. of HEW, Public Health Serv., NCDC, Atlanta, Ga.

Fey, H., P. R. Edwards, and H. Stünzi. 1957. Arizona-Infektionen bei Reptilien mit Isolierung von 4 Neuen Arizonatypen. *Schweiz. Z. Allgem. Pathol. Bakteriol.* 20:27–40.

Fields, B. N., M. M. Uwaydah, L. J. Kunz, and M. N. Swartz. 1967. The so-called "paracolon" bacteria. A bacteriologic and clinical reappraisal. *Am. J. Med.* 42:89–106.

Fife, Mary A., and W. H. Ewing. 1967. *Eight Previously Undescribed Serotypes of the Genus Arizona.* U.S. Dept. of HEW, Public Health Serv., NCDC, Atlanta, Ga.

Fisher, R. H. 1953. Multiple lesions of bone in Letterer-Siwe disease. *J. Bone Joint Surg.* 35A:445–64.

Friedman, I. A., and Goldin, M. 1949. Paracolon endocarditis. *Am. J. Clin. Pathol.* 19:840–45.

Galton, Mildred M. 1953. Sanitation problems in poultry processing plants. *Proc. Public Health Vet. Meet.* NCDC, Atlanta, Ga.

———. 1956. Poultry diseases transmissible to man including summary report of outbreaks. *Congressional Record,* June 18, pp. 10531–38.

Gauger, H. C. 1946. Isolation of a type 10 paracolon bacillus from an adult turkey. *Poultry Sci.* 25:299–300.

Gerlach, Helga, H. E. Adler, and A. S. Rosenwald. 1968. Observations on immune factors associated with arizona group infections in turkeys. *Avian Diseases* 12:681–86.

Goetz, M. E. 1962. The control of paracolon and paratyphoid infections in turkey poults. *Avian Diseases* 6:93–99.

Goetz, M. E., and E. R. Quortrup. 1953. Some observations on the problems of arizona paracolon infections of poults. *Vet. Med.* 48:58–60.

Goetz, M. E., E. R. Quortrup, and J. E. Dunsing. 1954. Investigations of arizona infections in poults. *J. Am. Vet. Med. Ass.* 124:120–21.

Guckian, J. E., E. H. Byers, and J. E. Perry. 1967. Arizona infection of man. *Arch. Internal Med.* 119:170–75.

Harwood, P. D. 1956. Clinical applications of nitrofurans—Past and present. *Proc. 1st Nat. Symp. on Nitrofurans in Agr.* Hess and Clark, Ashland, Ohio, pp. 12–23.

Hinshaw, W. R., and Ethel McNeil. 1944. Gopher snakes as carriers of salmonellosis and paracolon infections. *Cornell Vet.* 34:248–54.

———. 1946a. The occurrence of type 10 paracolon in turkeys. *J. Bacteriol.* 51:281–86.

———. 1946b. Paracolon type 10 from captive rattlesnakes. *J. Bacteriol.* 51:397–98.

———. 1947. Lizards as carriers of salmonella and paracolon bacteria. *J. Bacteriol.* 53:715–18.

Holte, R. J. A. 1965. Paracolon arizona immunization trials in turkeys. *Proc. 69th Ann. Meet. U.S. Livestock Sanit. Ass.,* pp. 539–42.

Jamison, S. L. 1956. Paracolon infection. *Pacific Poultryman,* March, 62:40–42.

Johnson, S. D., D. W. Bruner, and J. M. Murphy. 1951. Infection of the bovine udder with paracolon bacteria. *Cornell Vet.* 41:283–88.

Kauffmann, F. 1941. Ueber mehrere neue Salmonella-Typen. *Acta Pathol. Microbiol. Scand.* 18:351–66.

———. 1966. *The Bacteriology of Enterobacteriaceae.* Williams & Wilkins Co., Baltimore.

Kauffmann, F., and P. R. Edwards. 1952. Classification and nomenclature of Enterobacteriaceae. *Int. Bull. Bacteriol. Nomencl. Taxon.* 2:2–8.

Kowalski, L. M., and J. F. Stephens. 1967. Persistence of *Arizona paracolon* 7:1,7,8 in feed and water. *Poultry Sci.* 45:1586–87.

———. 1968. Arizona 7:1,7,8 infection in young turkeys. *Avian Diseases* 12:317–26.

Kraft, J. R. 1951. Paracolon pneumonia. *Am. J. Clin. Pathol.* 21:666–71.

Krag, D., and D. B. Shean. 1959. Serious human infections due to bacilli of the arizona group. *Calif. Med.* 90:230–33.

LeMinor, L., and F. Ben Hamida. 1962. Advantages de la recherche de la β-galactosidase sur celle de la fermentation du lactose en milieu complexe dans le diagnostic bacteriologique, en particulier des Enterobacteriaceae. *Ann. Inst. Pasteur* 102:267–77.

LeMinor, L., Mary A. Fife, and P. R. Edwards. 1958. Sur le *Salmonella* et *Arizona* hebergees par les viperes de France. *Ann. Inst. Pasteur* 95:326–33.

Lewis, K. H., and R. Angelotti. 1964. *Examination of Foods for Enteropathogenic and Indicator Bacteria.* U.S. Dept. of HEW, Public Health Serv., Publ. 1142, pp. 100–113.

Lewis, K. H., and E. R. Hitchner. 1936. Slow lactose-fermenting bacteria pathogenic for young chicks. *J. Infect. Diseases* 59:225–35.

Luippold, G. F. 1947. A paracolon organism antigenically related to the Sachs Q-1030 bacillus and associated with chronic enterocolitis. *Gastroenterology* 8:358–66.

Lystad, A. 1962. An unusual *Paracolobactrum aerogenoides* as the cause of nosocomial urinary tract infection. *Acta Pathol. Microbiol. Scand.* 54:400–411.

McClure, H. E., W. C. Eveland, and A. Kase. 1957. The occurrence of certain Enterobacteriaceae in birds. *Am. J. Vet. Res.* 18:207–9.

Martin, W. J., Mary A. Fife, and W. H. Ewing. 1967. *The Occurrence and Distribution of the Serotypes of* Arizona. U.S. Dept. of HEW, Public Health Serv., NCDC, Atlanta, Ga.

Miyamae, T., and H. E. Adler. 1967. Comparative studies on immunogenicity of arizona (7:1,7,8) adjuvant bacterins in mice and turkeys. *Avian Diseases* 11:380–92.

Moran, Alice B. 1959a. Salmonella in animals. A report for 1957. *Avian Diseases* 3:85–88.

———. 1959b. Serotypes of salmonella and arizona organisms in animals: 1958. *Avian Diseases* 3:440–42.

———. 1960. Salmonella and arizona cultures of animal origin: 1958. *Avian Diseases* 4:73–78.

———. 1961. Salmonella and arizona cultures from agricultural sources: 1959. *Avian Diseases* 5:147–49.

Murphy, W. J., and J. F. Morris. 1950. Two outbreaks of gastroenteritis apparently caused by a paracolon of the arizona group. *J. Infect. Diseases* 86:255–59.

Mushin, R.: 1949. Studies on paracolon bacilli. *Australian J. Exp. Biol. Med. Sci.* 27:543–56.

Peluffo, C. A., P. R. Edwards, and D. W. Bruner. 1942. A group of coliform bacilli serologically related to the genus *Salmonella*. *J. Infect. Diseases* 70:185–92.

Perek, M. 1957. Isolation of a paracolobactrum organism pathogenic to chicks. *J. Infect. Diseases* 101:8–10.

Pomeroy, B. S., R. Fenstermacher, Florence Jones, and L. E. Jenkins. 1957. The control of paratyphoid and related enteric infections of turkeys. *Proc. 8th Ann. North Central Reg. Poultry Dis. Conf.*

Pomeroy, B. S., J. R. Juhl, and J. T. Tumlin. 1958. Arizona-type paracolon infection of turkeys. *Proc. 2nd Nat. Symp. on Nitrofurans in Agr.* Hess and Clark, Ashland, Ohio, pp. 138–44.

Rosenwald, A. S. 1965. New facts on paracolon control. *Poultry Meat* 2:T–25.

Ryff, J. F., and J. Browne. 1952. Paracolon abortion in ewes. *J. Am. Vet. Med. Ass.* 121:266.

Sadler, W. W., R. Yamamoto, H. E. Adler, and G. F. Stewart. 1961. Survey of market poultry for salmonella infection. *Appl. Microbiol.* 9:72–76.

Sanders, R. G., B. S. Pomeroy, and R. Fenstermacher. 1943. Cross-agglutination studies between *Salmonella pullorum* and other microorganisms isolated from turkeys positive to the pullorum test. *Am. J. Vet. Res.* 4:194–98.

Sato, G. 1967. Detection of salmonella and arizona organisms from soil of empty turkey yards. *Japan. J. Vet. Res.* 15:53–55.

Sato, G., and H. E. Adler. 1966a. A study on the efficacy of arizona bacterin in turkeys. *Avian Diseases* 10:239–46.

———. 1966b. Serologic tests for arizona group infections. *Avian Diseases* 10:247–54.

———. 1966c. Bacteriological and serological observations on turkeys naturally infected with arizona 7:1,7,8. *Avian Diseases* 10:291–95.

———. 1966d. Experimental infection of adult turkeys with arizona group organisms. *Avian Diseases* 10:329–36.

Sato, G., A. Sato, and S. Miura. 1966. Isolation of arizona from a snake (*Elaphe climacophora*) in Hokkaido. *Japan. J. Vet. Res.* 14:63–64.

Schaub, I. G. 1948. The cultural differentiation of paracolon bacilli. *Bull. Johns Hopkins Hosp.* 83:367–82.

Schiff, F., S. Bornstein, and I. Saphra. 1941. The occurrence of salmonella O-antigens in coliform organisms. *J. Immunol.* 40:365–72.

Sieburth, J. M. 1957. A procedure for the differentiation of salmonella and arizona groups from other enteric organisms. *Avian Diseases* 1:348. (Abstr.)

Snoeyenbos, G. H., and C. F. Smyser. 1969. Isolation of arizona 7:1,7,8 from litter of pens housing infected turkeys. *Avian Diseases* 13:223–24.

Stuart, C. A., K. M. Wheeler, R. Rustigian, and A. Zimmerman. 1943. Biochemical and antigenic relationships of the paracolon bacteria. *J. Bacteriol.* 45:101–19.

Williams, J. E., and L. H. Dillard. 1968. Penetration of chicken egg shells by members of the arizona group. *Avian Diseases* 12:645–49.

Worcester, W. W. 1965. Californians report results of tests on paracolon control. *Feedstuffs* 37:6.

CHAPTER 5

AVIAN PASTEURELLOSIS

❖

K. L. HEDDLESTON

National Animal Disease Laboratory
United States Department of Agriculture
Ames, Iowa

❖

PASTEURELLOSIS is a general term used to designate any disease caused by the *Pasteurellae,* a group of loosely related, widely distributed bacteria.

In poultry these diseases are fowl cholera, pseudotuberculosis, infectious serositis, and goose influenza. Goose influenza is very similar to infectious serositis, and there is reason to believe that the causative agent *Pasteurella septicaemiae* is identical with *P. anatipestifer,* the causative agent of infectious serositis. Therefore, goose influenza will not be included as a separate disease but will be discussed under infectious serositis. The avian influenza viruses are discussed in Chapter 20. *P. haemolytica* and *P. gallinarum* are discussed under differential diagnosis of fowl cholera.

❖

FOWL CHOLERA

❖

FOWL CHOLERA (avian cholera, avian pasteurellosis, avian hemorrhagic septicemia) is an infectious disease affect-

ing domestic and feral birds. It usually appears as a septicemic disease associated with high morbidity and mortality, but chronic or benign conditions occur often. This disease is of historical importance because of its role in the early development of bacteriology, and because in 1879 it was one of four diseases which the Veterinary Division of the USDA was created to investigate.

HISTORY

Several epornitics among fowls occurred in Europe during the latter half of the eighteenth century. The disease was studied in France by Chabert in 1782 and Maillet in 1836 who first used the term fowl cholera. Huppe in 1886 used the term hemorrhagic septicemia, and Lignieres in 1900 used the term avian pasteurellosis. Benjamin in 1851 gave a good description of the disease and demonstrated that it could be spread by cohabitation. With this knowledge of the disease he formulated procedures for its prevention. About the same time Renault, Reynal, and Delafond demonstrated its transmissibility to various species by inoculation. In 1877 and 1878, Perroncito of Italy and Semmer of Russia found in the tissues of affected birds a bacterium which had a rounded form and occurred singly or in pairs. Shortly thereafter, Toussant in 1879 confirmed these observations and proved that this bacterium was the sole cause of the disease (history according to Gray, 1913).

Pasteur (1880a) isolated the organism and grew pure cultures in chicken broth. In further studies Pasteur (1880b, 1881) used the fowl cholera organism to perform his classic experiments in the attenuation of bacteria for use in producing immunity. Salmon (1880) appears to have been the first to study the disease in the United States. A good description of the signs of the disease, however, was reported as early as 1867 in Iowa where losses of chickens, turkeys, and geese had occurred (*USDA Monthly Report,* 1867).

INCIDENCE

Fowl cholera occurs sporadically or enzootically in most countries of the world. At times it causes high mortality; at others

Grateful acknowledgment is made of the assistance of K. R. Rhoades in preparing this chapter, R. M. Glazier in preparing photographs, A. E. Ritchie in preparing electron micrographs, and previous works of G. S. Harshfield, W. R. Hinshaw, G. H. Snoeyenbos, and N. D. Levine.

Year	Chickens	Turkeys	Others	Total
Northeastern				
1962	307*	56	169	532
1963	282	97	39	418
1964	216	81	99	396
1965	163	117	34	314
1966	131	103	61	295
North central				
1962	118	109	14	241
1963	123	102	13	238
1964	118	101	12	231
1965	103	103	4	210
1966	83	137	15	235
Southeastern				
1962	490	159	7	656
1963	485	184	6	675
1964	462	252	8	722
1965†	305	145	13	463
1966	491	232	22	745

Source: *Avian Diseases.* 1967, 11:703, 708, 727.
* Each unit approximates an outbreak of fowl cholera.
† June through December.

the losses are nominal. Alberts and Graham (1948a) reported a loss of 68% within 6 days in a flock of 5½-month-old turkeys. Vaught et al. (1967) reported that over 1,000 wild geese died of fowl cholera in one night. In studying the chronic respiratory form of fowl cholera in chickens, Hall et al. (1955) observed that the mortality was low but infection persisted for at least 4 years.

Fowl cholera is more prevalent in late summer, fall, and winter. This seasonal occurrence is one of circumstance rather than lowered resistance, except that chickens become more susceptible to fowl cholera as they reach maturity. The incidence of fowl cholera in turkeys has increased in certain areas during the past few years (Table 5.1).

ETIOLOGY

CLASSIFICATION

The bacterium *Pasteurella multocida* (*mul to ci′ da*) is the causative agent of fowl cholera. In the past it has been given many names, some of which are as follows: *Micrococcus gallicidus,* 1883; *M. cholerae gallinarum,* 1885; *Octopsis cholerae gallinarum,* 1885; *Bacterium cholerae gallinarum,* 1886; *Bacillus cholerae gallinarum,* 1886; *Pasteurella cholerae-gallinarum,* 1887; *Coccobacillus avicidus,* 1888; *P. avi-*
cida, 1889; *Bacterium multicidum,* 1899; *P. avium,* 1903; *Bacillus avisepticus,* 1903; *Bacterium avisepticum,* 1903; *Bacterium avisepticus,* 1912; *P. aviseptica,* 1920 (Breed et al., 1957; Buchanan et al., 1966).

For a while each isolant of *P. multocida* was given a name corresponding to the animal from which it was isolated, such as *P. avicida* or *P. aviseptica,* *P. muricida* or *P. muriseptica.* In 1929 it was suggested that all isolants be referred to as *P. septica* which is used to a limited extent in current literature (Wilson and Miles, 1964). However, *P. multocida,* which was proposed by Rosenbusch and Merchant (1939), has been accepted as the official name in *Bergey's Manual* and is now used almost exclusively in the United States.

MORPHOLOGY

Pasteurella multocida is a gram-negative, nonmotile, nonsporeforming rod occurring singly, in pairs, and occasionally as chains or filaments. It measures 0.2–0.4×0.6–2.5μ but tends toward pleomorphicity after repeated subculture. A capsule can be demonstrated in recently isolated cultures, using indirect methods of staining (Fig. 5.1). In tissues, blood, and recently isolated cultures the organism stains bipolar (Fig. 5.2).

GROWTH REQUIREMENTS

Pasteurella multocida grows aerobically or anaerobically. The optimal growth temperature is 37° C. The optimal pH range is 7.2–7.8, but it will grow in the range of 6.2 through 9.0, depending on the composition of the medium. In liquid media, maximum growth is obtained in 16–24 hours. The broth becomes cloudy, and in a few days a sticky sediment collects at the bottom. With some isolants a flocculent precipitate occurs.

The bacterium will grow on meat infusion media, but growth is enhanced when the medium is enriched with enzymatic digest of peptone, casein hydrolysate, or avian serum. Blood or serum from some animals inhibits growth of *P. multocida.* Inhibition is greatest from blood of horses, cattle, sheep, and goats; blood of chickens, ducks, swine, and water buffalo has little or no inhibitory action (Ryu, 1961). Two selective media (Das, 1958; Morris, 1958) and a chemically defined medium (Watko, 1966) have been described for growth and isolation of the organism. The medium of

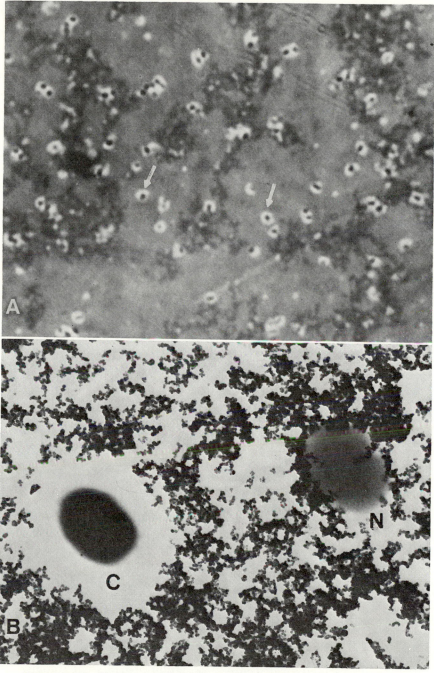

FIG. 5.1—*Virulent* Pasteurella multocida *from iridescent colonies grown 20 hours on surface of dextrose starch agar.* (**A**) *Encapsulated cells (arrows). Jasmin, ×2,000.* (**B**) *Electron photomicrograph of encapsulated cell (C) and nonencapsulated cell (N) suspended in India ink, ×19,000.*

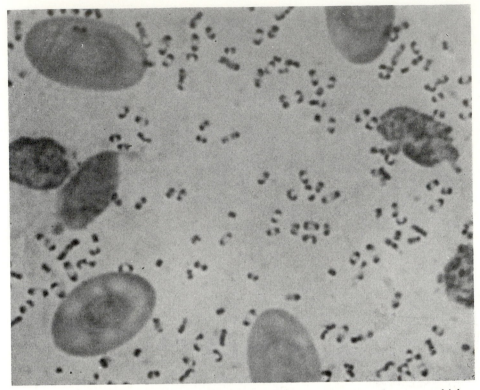

FIG. 5.2—*Acute fowl cholera.* Pasteurella multocida *in liver imprint from chicken (note bipolarity). Wright,* ×2500.

Morris is of value in differentiating some of the *Pasteurellae.* Banerji and Mukherjee (1954) found that pantothenic acid and nicotinamide are essential for growth. Dextrose starch agar with 5% avian serum is an excellent medium for isolating and growing *P. multocida.*

COLONIAL MORPHOLOGY AND RELATED PROPERTIES

Colonial morphology is one of the most useful characteristics in the study of *P. multocida.* On primary isolation from birds with fowl cholera, colonies of *P. multocida* may be strongly or weakly iridescent, sectored with variable iridescence, or blue with little or no iridescence (Fig. 5.3). Small rough colonies with variable iridescence may occasionally be observed. Iridescence, which varies from reddish to bluish and is related to the capsule, is used synonymously with fluorescence which has often been used to describe colonies of *P. multocida.* The composition of the medium determines to a certain extent the degree and type of iridescence. Occasionally an isolant

produces blue colonies, but when serum is added to the medium, sectored or iridescent colonies are produced. Examination of 18–24-hour colonies with a stereomicroscope using obliquely transmitted light (Fig. 5.4) is helpful when observing colonial morphology (Henry, 1933). Iridescent colonies on primary isolation from acute cases of fowl cholera are circular (2–3 mm), smooth, convex, translucent, glistening, and butyrous with a tendency to coalesce. As the colony ages it usually loses these distinguishing properties, becomes larger and viscous, and may adhere to the medium when picked with an inoculating loop. Blue colonies often isolated from the chronic type of cholera or derived by dissociation of iridescent colonies are circular (1–2 mm), smooth, slightly convex or flat, translucent, butyrous, and discrete.

Anderson et al. (1929) observed that a highly virulent isolant which produced smooth (iridescent) colonies later dissociated on subculture and produced rough (blue) colonies. Organisms from the smooth colonies were approximately 3–4 million

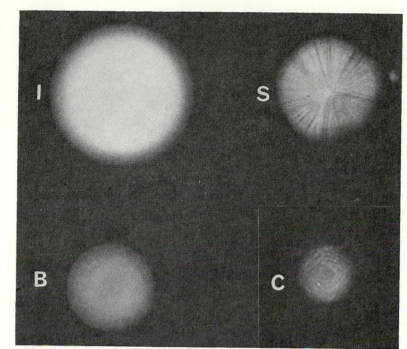

FIG. 5.3—Pasteurella multocida 20-hour colonies from birds with fowl cholera. (I) Iridescent, (S) sectored, (B) blue, (C) rough on surface of dextrose starch agar illuminated by oblique transmitted light. ×20.

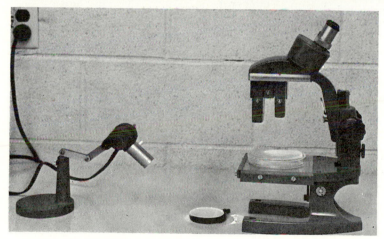

FIG. 5.4—Arrangement of stereomicroscope with obliquely transmitted light for inspection of colonial morphology.

times more virulent for pigeons than those from rough colonies. Hughes (1930) studied the colonial morphology of 210 cultures from cases of fowl cholera and distinguished 3 types. One type, fluorescent, was associated with outbreaks of acute fowl cholera and was highly virulent. The second type, blue, was of low virulence and occurred in flocks in which cholera was enzootic. A third type, intermediate, was intermediate in its properties of fluorescence and virulence.

In a study of 28 cultures, 15 of which originated from cases of fowl cholera, Car-

ter and Bigland (1953) described three principal colonial variants as follows: (1) mucoid, with moderate mouse virulence, (2) smooth, which included fluorescent and intermediate colonies and was highly virulent for mice, and (3) rough, which is equivalent to blue colonies and was of low virulence for mice. Carter and Annau (1953) extracted polysaccharides from fluorescent, intermediate, and mucoid colonies. The extract from the mucoid colonies contained hyaluronic acid and was nonimmunogenic and nontoxic for mice. The extract from fluorescent and intermediate colonies was immunogenic and nontoxic for mice. In a later report Carter (1957) described colonial variation and three principal colonial types: (1) mucoid—largest, with flowing margins, moist, and reddish fluorescence, (2) smooth—smaller, discrete, and greenish iridescence, (3) smooth—smaller than other two colonial types, noniridescent with a gray or grayish blue appearance.

Webster and Burn (1926) described, in cultures from rabbits, a "watery mucoid" type of colony having different properties than those of the iridescent colonies described by Hughes. This type of colony is also frequently observed in cultures from the respiratory tracts of cattle and swine but not from poultry. The "watery mucoid" colony may be autolytic and contain both individual cells and filamentous forms. Dwarf satellite colonies are infrequently observed close to the "watery mucoid" colony. Cells from this type of colony are avirulent for poultry and less virulent for mice than those from iridescent colonies.

Heddleston et al. (1964) reported that a virulent isolant of *P. multocida* of avian origin produced iridescent colonies that dissociated in vitro and produced blue colonies which were similar to the rough colonies described by Anderson et al. (1929). Organisms from blue colonies also mutated and produced gray colonies that have not been reported in primary cultures from birds. Organisms from iridescent colonies occurred singly or in pairs; did not agglutinate in immune serum; and were encapsulated and virulent for chickens, turkeys, rabbits, and mice when administered on the mucous membranes of the upper air passages. Organisms from blue colonies occurred singly or in pairs, agglutinated in immune sera, were nonencapsulated and avirulent when applied to the mucous membranes of chickens and mice, but were virulent for rabbits and slightly virulent for turkeys. Cells from gray colonies occurred only as chains (Fig. 5.5) and were nonencapsulated and avirulent. Killed organisms from all three colonial forms induced immunity in chickens. Antigens extracted with hot saline from highly virulent encapsulated cells of fluorescent colonies by Yaw and Kakavas (1957) actively immunized chickens and mice, whereas the less virulent nonencapsulated cells from blue colonies immunized chickens more effectively than mice.

BIOCHEMICAL PROPERTIES

The following properties were determined from over 300 isolants of *P. multocida* associated with fowl cholera:

GALACTOSE	Fermented without gas
GLUCOSE	Fermented without gas
LEVULOSE	Fermented without gas
MANNITOL	Fermented without gas
MANNOSE	Fermented without gas
SORBITOL	Fermented without gas
SUCROSE	Fermented without gas
XYLOSE	Usually fermented without gas
GLYCEROL	Usually fermented after 5 days
DULCITOL	Usually not fermented
ARABINOSE	Usually not fermented
LACTOSE	Usually not fermented
MALTOSE	Usually not fermented
RAFFINOSE	Usually not fermented
TREHALOSE	Usually not fermented
DEXTRIN	Not fermented
INOSITOL	Not fermented
INULIN	Not fermented
RHAMNOSE	Not fermented
SALICIN	Not fermented
INDOLE	Almost always produced
CATALASE	Produced
AMMONIA	Produced
HYDROGEN SULFIDE	Usually produced in 1–14 days
UREASE	Not produced
ACETYL METHYL CARBINOL	Not produced
METHYL RED	Negative
NITRATES	Reduced
GELATIN	Not liquified
LITMUS MILK	Not changed
BLOOD	Not hemolyzed
MACCONKEY'S AGAR	No growth

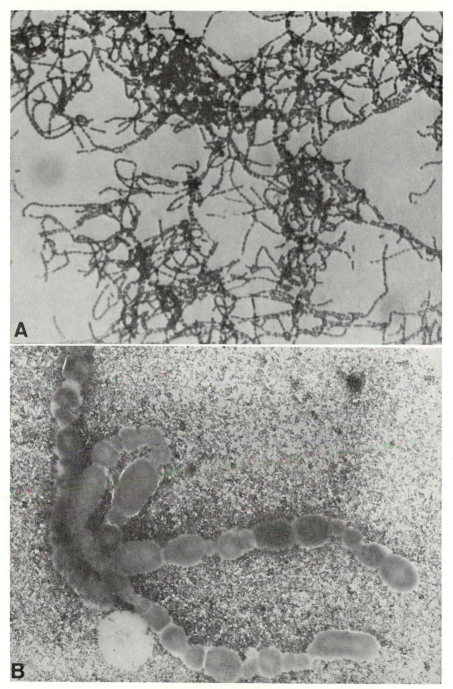

FIG. 5.5—Chain formation of P. multocida *from gray colony (laboratory mutant).* (A) *Gram's stain,* ×1,200. (B) *Electron photomicrograph of cells suspended in India ink,* ×9,000.

Significant differential characteristics are listed in Table 5.2.

RESISTANCE TO CHEMICAL AND PHYSICAL AGENTS

Pasteurella multocida is easily destroyed by ordinary disinfectants, sunlight, drying, or heat, being killed within 15 minutes at 56° C and 10 minutes at 60° C. A 1% solution of formaldehyde, phenol, sodium hydroxide, beta-propiolactone, or glutaraldehyde and a 0.1% solution of benzalkonium chloride killed within 5 minutes 4.4×10^8 organisms of *P. multocida* per ml suspended in 0.85% sodium chloride at 24° C.

Das (1958) observed that cotton swabs saturated with blood from infected mice contained viable organisms after 118 hours but not after 166 hours (at which time the swabs were completely dry), and that films of blood on glass contained viable organisms after 24 but not 30 hours. Das also reported that infected blood sealed in glass tubes and held in a cold room contained viable organisms after 221 days. Skidmore (1932) observed that the organism survived in dried turkey blood on glass for 8 but not 30 days at room temperature. In studies of the influence of environment on the incidence of fowl cholera, Van Es and Olney (1940) found that the infection hazard had apparently disappeared from a poultry yard 2 weeks after the occurrence of the last death and the removal of birds.

The influence of temperature on the viability and virulence of *P. multocida* was studied by Nobrega and Bueno (1950), who observed that broth cultures stored in sealed tubes at an average room temperature of 17.6° C were still virulent after 2 years; at 2–4° C they were nonviable after 1 year. With controlled experiments Dimov (1964) observed that *P. multocida* died rapidly in soils with moisture content of less than 40% At a moisture content of 50% and temperature of 20° C, it survived for 5–6 days at pH 5.0, 15–100 days at pH 7.0, and 24–85 days at pH 8.0. A culture survived without loss of virulence for 113 days in soil with 50% moisture at 3° C and pH 7.15.

Cultures may be maintained without dissociation or loss of virulence in the lyophilized state or sealed in glass tubes and stored at —23° C or colder (Watko and Heddleston, 1966). Lyophilized cultures tested after 26 years by the writer were still virulent for chickens, and a culture sealed in a rubber-stoppered bottle containing beef infusion broth with 50% horse serum and held at room temperature was virulent after 20 years.

ANTIGENIC STRUCTURE AND STRAIN CLASSIFICATION

A variety of criteria has been used to group isolants of *P. multocida* including colonial morphology, immunology, zoology, enzyme production, lysogeny, and serology. Each method has some value but no one method has been proved sufficiently meaningful for epizootiologic studies.

Carter (1955) studied numerous isolants from various animals (using an indirect hemagglutination test) and found four serotypes, two (A and D) of which were isolated from fowl and various other animals. The indirect hemagglutination test in conjunction with the serum agglutination test was used by Namioka and Bruner (1963) who found four serotypes (5:A, 8:A, 9:A and 2:D) associated with fowl cholera. Serotypes 5:A, 8:A and 9:A contained a common hemagglutinating antigen as well as specific agglutinating antigens.

Serologic grouping of *P. multocida* is often difficult or impossible because of the inability of encapsulated cells to agglutinate or the absence of hemagglutinating antigens which have been reported to be related to the capsule. Cross-reactions often occur between different serotypes because of common antigens shared by all isolants. Sixteen common antigens were demonstrated by Prince and Smith (1966) using immunoelectrophoresis. Serologic methods that have been used for typing *P. multocida* were recently reviewed by Carter (1967).

Rosenbusch and Merchant (1939) placed isolants of *P. multocida* into three groups on the basis of fermentation of xylose, arabinose, and dulcitol. Group I fermented arabinose and dulcitol but not xylose; Group II fermented xylose but not arabinose or dulcitol; Group III was variable but more nearly like Group I. Dorsey (1963a) studied the fermentation reactions of 409 isolants of fowl origin and found that 81.42% were of Group I, 16.87% were of Group II, and 1.71% were of Group III; 23 isolants could not be grouped on the basis of these reactions. Usually there was correlation in the agglutinating and immunizing properties of the isolants within a biochemical group, but exceptions were encountered (Dorsey, 1963b).

The ability to immunize poultry with killed organisms has been used to group isolants of *P. multocida* associated with fowl cholera. The vaccinated birds are resistant to infection to the homologous strain and others of the same immunogenic type but become ill or die when exposed to organisms of a different immunogenic type. Two immunogenic types (prototypic strains X-73 [ATCC 11039] and P-1059 [ATCC 15742]) have been reported (Heddleston, 1962). In addition, these two strains differed in their serologic, pathogenic, and biochemical properties. The two strains were type A by the indirect hemagglutination test, but strain X-73 was type 1 and P-1059 was type 3 by the agglutination test of Little and Lyon (1943). A third immunogenic type has been recognized and will be described later.

Phage sensitivity as a basis for grouping *P. multocida* has been investigated. Rifkind and Pickett (1954) found 84 of 118 isolants from various hosts were sensitive to one or more of 16 bacteriophages. Kirchner and Eisenstark (1956) examined 25 cultures of avian origin and found that 11 were lysogenic. They divided the 11 bacteriophages into 5 groups as to their host range and 3 groups on plaque morphology. Saxena and Hoerlein (1959) demonstrated lysogeny in 63 of 112 cultures from various hosts. One phage caused lysis of 8 different cultures, while several were lysogenic for only 1 or 2 cultures. Results of these investigations demonstrated the possibility of a phage grouping system for *P. multocida*, but further studies are necessary before a valid interpretation can be made.

PATHOGENICITY

Pathogenicity or virulence of *P. multocida* in relation to fowl cholera is complex and quite variable, depending on the strain of *P. multocida*, the host species, variations within the strain or host, and the conditions of contact between the two. The ability of *P. multocida* to invade and reproduce in the host is related to a capsule (Fig. 5.1) which surrounds the organism (Manninger, 1919). Loss of ability of a virulent strain to produce the capsule results in loss of virulence (Heddleston et al., 1964). Many

isolants from cases of fowl cholera have large capsules but are of low virulence. Therefore, the ability to invade and grow in the host is apparently related to some chemical substance associated with the capsule rather than with its physical presence.

P. multocida usually enters the tissues of birds through mucous membranes of the pharynx or upper air passages, but it may also enter through the conjunctiva or cutaneous wounds. Hughes and Pritchett (1930) were unable to infect chickens by placing a culture in a gelatin capsule and inserting it into the esophagus, but chickens were infected when culture was dropped on the roof of the nasal cleft. Arsov (1965) infected birds by mouth using P-35 labeled culture and observed that the portal of infection was the mucous membrane of the mouth and pharynx but not the esophagus, crop, or proventriculus. The eustachian tube was suggested by Olson and McCune (1968) as the most likely route of infection which localizes in the air spaces of the cranial bone, middle ear, and meninges.

Turkeys are much more susceptible to infection with *P. multocida* than chickens, and mature chickens are more susceptible than young chickens (Heddleston, 1962). Hungerford (1968) observed heavy losses in mature chickens but no losses in birds up to 16 weeks of age in a case involving 90,000 birds. When testing the infectivity of an isolant or the susceptibility of a host, cohabitation is the most natural method of exposure. However, unless the host is highly susceptible and the isolant highly invasive, results may be slow. Therefore, it is often advantageous to swab the nasal cleft with a cotton swab saturated with the culture, or, if a more severe exposure is required, the culture can be injected parenterally.

TOXINS

Toxins are produced by *P. multocida* which give rise to pathologic processes. A dried culture filtrate of *P. multocida* was first demonstrated to produce signs of toxicity in chickens by Pasteur (1880a). Salmon (1880) repeated this work and described signs resulting from toxicity which were similar to those observed in cases of acute fowl cholera. Pirosky (1938) obtained a toxic and protective antigen from capsulated and noncapsulated *P. multocida* of avian origin by the trichloracetic acid extraction procedure of Boivin. Kyaw (1944), using the developing chick embryo in the study of pathogenesis, suggested that a toxin was produced in vivo by *P. multocida*. Rhoades (1964) observed severe acute general passive hyperemia in chickens that died from acute fowl cholera. This lesion was considered to be indicative of shock and was attributed to the action of endotoxin. Heddleston et al. (1966) demonstrated that a loosely bound endotoxin could be washed from *P. multocida* with cold formalized saline solution. This endotoxin was a nitrogen-containing phosphorylated lipopolysaccharide, readily inactivated under mild acid conditions. Signs of acute fowl cholera were induced in chickens by injection of fractional amounts of the endotoxin.

PATHOGENESIS AND EPIZOOTIOLOGY

NATURAL AND EXPERIMENTAL HOSTS

Domestic fowl, game birds raised in captivity, and small feral birds (sparrows, starlings, robins, etc.) that visit poultry yards are susceptible to fowl cholera. Most reported outbreaks and disease studies have involved chickens, turkeys, geese, and ducks.

Fowl cholera is a very serious problem for the individual turkey grower whose entire flock may die in a few days. The disease may spread so rapidly that control measures are often limited. The disease usually occurs in young mature turkeys, but all ages are highly susceptible. Under experimental conditions 90–100% of mature turkeys may die within 48 hours when exposed to a highly virulent strain of *P. multocida* by swabbing the palatine cleft or by contact with infected birds.

The disease in turkeys was first reported in detail by DeVolt and Davis (1932) who described an outbreak in a flock of 175 turkeys in Maryland where the mortality was 17%. Alberts and Graham (1948a) described outbreaks in 4 flocks of turkeys in which mortality was 17–68%. They emphasized that environmental stressors such as changes in climate, nutrition, injury, and excitement may have influenced the incidence and course of the disease.

In chickens death losses from fowl cholera usually occur in laying flocks because chickens under 16 weeks of age are quite resistant. When an epornitic does occur in young chickens, it is usually caused by serotype 1 in conjunction with some other malady. Mortality varies from 0 to 20%, but greater losses have been reported. In addition to death losses, there is a drop in egg production and often a persistent localized infection in many of the birds. Chickens are more susceptible to fowl cholera after withdrawal of feed and water or after an abrupt change of diet (Bolin and Eveleth, 1951). Heat or rough treatment on a shaking machine increased the incidence in chickens exposed experimentally (Juszkiewicz, 1966a,b).

Under experimental conditions 90–100% of mature chickens exposed by swabbing the palatine cleft may die within 24–48 hours, depending on the strain of *P. multocida* used, but only 10–20% usually die within a 2-week period when exposed by contact with the infected birds. Pritchett et al. (1930a) observed a mortality of 35–45% in three houses of pullets. In one house 45% of the birds died within 4 weeks. In a flock of 45 birds which had survived an acute outbreak the previous year, no losses were observed, but the number of birds with localized lesions increased during the winter. In South Carolina and adjoining areas, fowl cholera exists mainly as a persistent subacute and chronic disease that clinically resembles avian monocytosis (Bierer, 1962).

Domestic geese and ducks are also highly susceptible to fowl cholera. Curtice (1902) reported the disease in geese in Rhode Island where about 3,200 of a flock of 4,000 died in a short period of time. Van Es and Olney (1940) recognized the marked susceptibility of geese to fowl cholera in using them to test for persistence of viable organisms in lots after removal of infected chickens. Fowl cholera in ducks is a serious problem on Long Island where it was diagnosed on 32 of 68 commercial duck farms. Losses usually occur in ducks over 4 weeks of age, and mortality may reach 50% (Dougherty, 1953a).

Birds of prey, waterfowl, and other birds kept in zoological gardens occasionally succumb to infection. *P. multocida* has been isolated from over 35 species of feral birds. During a 2½-year survey Faddoul et al. (1967) isolated *P. multocida* from 13 (7 species) of 248 feral birds submitted to the diagnostic laboratory. Jakšić et al. (1964) described an acute epornitic among pheasants in which 1,700 died. An outbreak in the San Francisco Bay area was reported to have been responsible for an estimated loss of 40,000 waterfowl (Rosen and Bischoff, 1949). Gershman et al. (1964) observed a serious outbreak among eider ducks *(Somateria mollissima)* in their nesting area 6 miles off the coast of Maine where over 200 birds died and more than 100 nests were lost. Over 60,000 waterfowl died of fowl cholera during the winter of 1956–57 at the Muleshoe National Wildlife Refuge in Texas (Jensen and Williams, 1964).

P. multocida from birds with fowl cholera will usually kill rabbits and mice, but other animals are resistant to infection. According to Heddleston and Watko (1963), rabbits, mice, pigeons, and sparrows died of acute septicemia when exposed intranasally to an isolant of *P. multocida* from an acute case of fowl cholera; but rats, ferrets, guinea pigs, a sheep, a pig, and a calf did not show any clinical response to the same organism. One of 5 rats, 1 of 2 mink, and 11 of 19 mice fed viscera of infected chickens developed nasal infection, pneumonia, and fatal septicemia respectively. A calf died of acute septicemia in less than 18 hours after injection of the organism intramuscularly. Guinea pigs given intramuscular injections developed necrosis at the site of injection while those given intraperitoneal injection usually died.

Horses, cattle, sheep, pigs, dogs, and cats are refractory to infection per os, and subcutaneous inoculation results in localized abscesses. All of these animals may succumb, however, to intravenous inoculation.

TRANSMISSION, CARRIERS, AND VECTORS

How fowl cholera is introduced into a flock is often difficult or impossible to determine. It may occur after adding newly purchased stock to the breeding flock or adding pullets to an older population. There is no limit to the duration of the chronic carrier state in fowl cholera other than the life of the bird. Free-flying birds having contact with poultry may be a source of fowl cholera organisms. Transmission of the organism through the egg seldom if ever occurs. A study of more than 2,000 fresh and embryonated eggs from chickens infected with chronic fowl cholera yielded no evidence that *P. multocida* was transmitted through the egg (Report of the Chief of BAI, USDA, 1951).

Pritchett et al. (1930a,b) and Pritchett and Hughes (1932) examined three infected commercial flocks of White Leghorns for *P. multocida* and found that many birds harbored the organisms in the nasal clefts. The presence of the bacterium was related to the severity of the upper respiratory infection in the flocks. They concluded that the enzootic focus of infection was "healthy" nasal carriers or "roup cold" cases. These studies as well as those of Van Es and Olney (1940) and Hall et al. (1955) proved that survivors of an epornitic of fowl cholera may be reservoirs of infection. Dorsey and Harshfield (1959) reported a higher incidence of fowl cholera during late summer and fall months in South Dakota. Carrier birds among the older flock, held over for a second year, provided a reservoir of infection for young susceptible pullets housed with them.

Most species of farm animals may be carriers of *P. multocida*. Generally these organisms, except for those from swine and possibly those from cats, are avirulent for fowls. Iliev et al. (1963a) isolated *P. multocida* from the tonsils of 34 of 75 slaughtered cattle, 14 of 27 sheep, and 102 of 162 pigs. Isolants from cattle and sheep were not pathogenic for fowls, but all 18 isolants from pigs in areas where fowl cholera was common were highly pathogenic for fowls. Only 2 of 47 isolants from pigs in areas having a low incidence of fowl cholera were pathogenic. They also (Iliev et al., 1963b) reported that healthy pigs which were carriers of *P. multocida* transmitted infection to fowls in the same enclosure. Two isolants, serotypes 1:A and 5:A, from lungs of pigs with pneumonia were studied by Murata et al. (1964). Serotype 5:A was highly virulent for chickens and serotype 1:A was avirulent. They found no cross-immunity in chickens between the 2 serotypes.

Contaminated crates, feed bags, or any equipment used previously for poultry may serve in introducing fowl cholera into a flock. The carcasses of birds that die of acute fowl cholera are thoroughly permeated with organisms and may serve as an infection source, especially as fowls tend to consume such materials. Mice and other rodents may also serve as sources of infection. Hendrickson and Hilbert (1932) were able to isolate *P. multocida* from the blood of a naturally infected chicken for 49 days preceding death. They noticed a rapid increase in number of organisms immediately preceding and following death, and the organisms remained viable in a cadaver for 11 days at room temperature and for 2 months at ice box temperature.

The possibility that insects may serve as vectors of fowl cholera has been investigated. Skidmore (1932) experimentally transmitted fowl cholera to turkeys by feeding them flies that had previously fed on infected blood. He pointed out that under natural conditions, ingestion of flies might be a means of introducing the disease into a flock. Transmission by flies, however, is probably not common, as indicated by the studies of Van Es and Olney (1940). Although fowl cholera was maintained in two lots of chickens during the height of the fly season, there was no spread of the disease to adjoining lots separated only by poultry netting. Iovčev (1967) observed that larvae, nymphs, and adult ticks *(Argas persicus)* contained *P. multocida* after feeding on infected hens.

In review of the literature, Henderson (1963) reported that *P. multocida* had been isolated from most regions of the body of man, with the respiratory tract frequently involved. One may assume, therefore, that man may also be a source of infection for poultry.

Dissemination of *P. multocida* within a flock is primarily by excretions from the mouth (Fig. 5.6), nose, and conjunctiva of diseased birds that contaminate their environment, particularly the feed and water. Feces very seldom contain viable *P. multocida.* Reis (1941) found *P. multocida* in the feces from 1 of 9 birds just before death. In the remaining 8 birds the organisms were isolated only in feces collected in the cloaca of dead birds. Iliev et al. (1965) demonstrated that *P. multocida* labeled with P-32 was inactivated in the proventriculus, and the feces contained no viable *P. multocida.*

SIGNS OF INFECTION

Acute

The signs of infection which occur in acute fowl cholera are often present for only a few hours before death. Unless in-

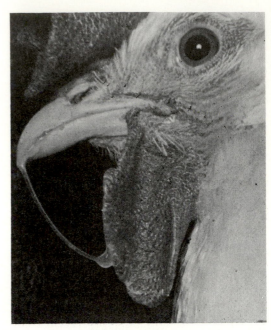

FIG. 5.6—*Acute fowl cholera. Excretion (more evident than usual) from mouth contaminates feed and water with* P. multocida.

fected birds are observed during this period, death may be the first indication of disease. Signs which often occur are fever, anorexia, ruffled feathers, mucous discharge from the mouth, diarrhea, and increased respiratory rate. Cyanosis often occurs immediately prior to death and is most evident in the unfeathered areas of the head, such as the comb and wattles. Fecal material associated with the diarrhea is initially watery and whitish in color but later becomes greenish and contains mucus. Birds which survive the initial acute septicemic stage may later succumb to the debilitating effects of emaciation and dehydration, may become chronically infected, or may recover.

Chronic

Chronic fowl cholera may follow an acute stage of the disease or result from infection with organisms of low virulence. The signs are generally related to localized infections. Wattles (Fig. 5.7), sinuses, leg or wing joints, foot pads, and sternal bursae often become swollen. Exudative conjunctival (Fig. 5.8) and pharyngeal lesions may be observed, and torticollis (Fig. 5.9) sometimes occurs. Tracheal rales and dysp-

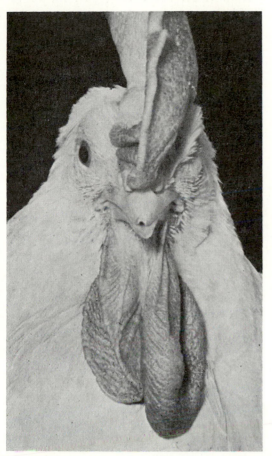

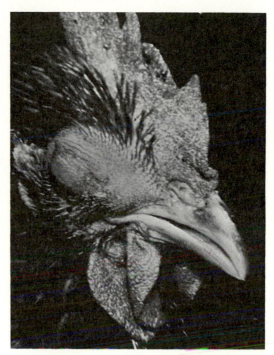

FIG. 5.8—Chronic fowl cholera. Serous inflammation of conjunctiva and adjacent tissue.

FIG. 5.7—Chronic fowl cholera. Swollen wattle resulting from localized infection.

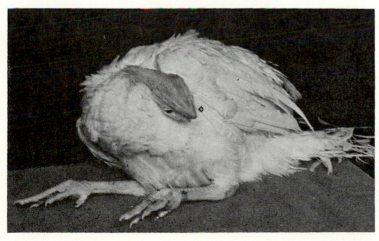

FIG. 5.9—Chronic fowl cholera. Torticollis resulting from meningeal infection.

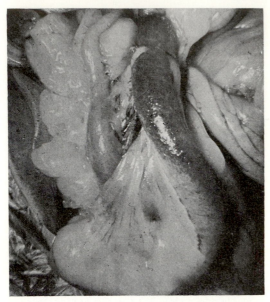

FIG. 5.10—Acute fowl cholera. Hyperemia in chicken duodenum.

nea may result from respiratory tract infections. In the past the term "roup" was used to indicate a condition in which signs were associated with chronic infections of cephalic mucous membranes. The term was not limited to fowl cholera but includ-

ed other diseases as well (Moore, 1895). Chronically infected birds may succumb, remain infected for long periods, or recover.

GROSS AND MICROSCOPIC LESIONS

The lesions of fowl cholera are not constant but vary both in type and severity. The greatest variation is related to the course of the disease, whether acute or chronic. Although it is convenient for descriptive purposes to refer to either acute or chronic fowl cholera, it is sometimes difficult to categorize the disease in this manner. The signs of infection and lesions which occur may be intermediate to those described for acute and chronic forms of the disease.

Acute

When the course of the disease is acute most of the postmortem lesions are associated with vascular disturbances. General hyperemia usually occurs, is most evident in the veins of the abdominal viscera, and may be quite pronounced in the small vessels of the duodenal mucosa (Figs. 5.10, 5.11). Large numbers of bacteria can usually be observed microscopically in the hyperemic vessels. Petechial and ecchymotic hemorrhages are frequently found

FIG. 5.11—Acute fowl cholera. Marked hyperemia of chicken duodenum. H & E, ×150.

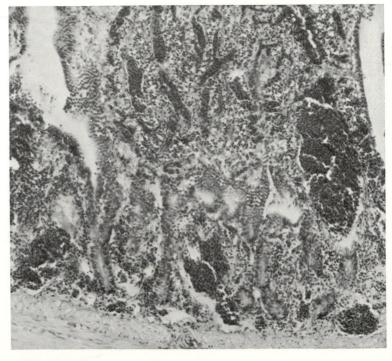

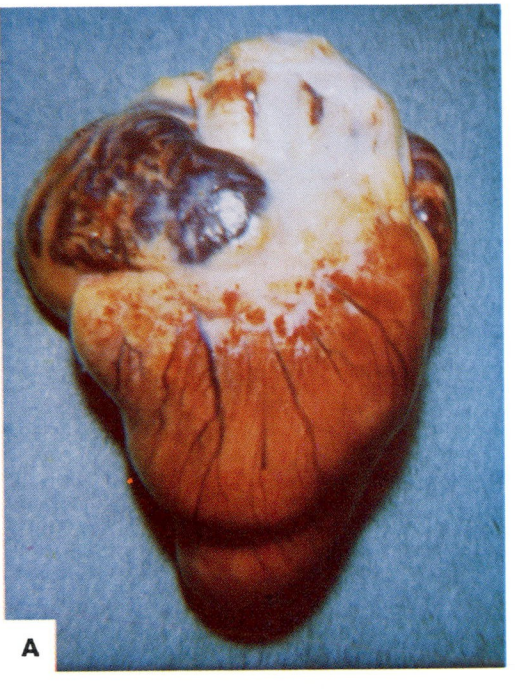

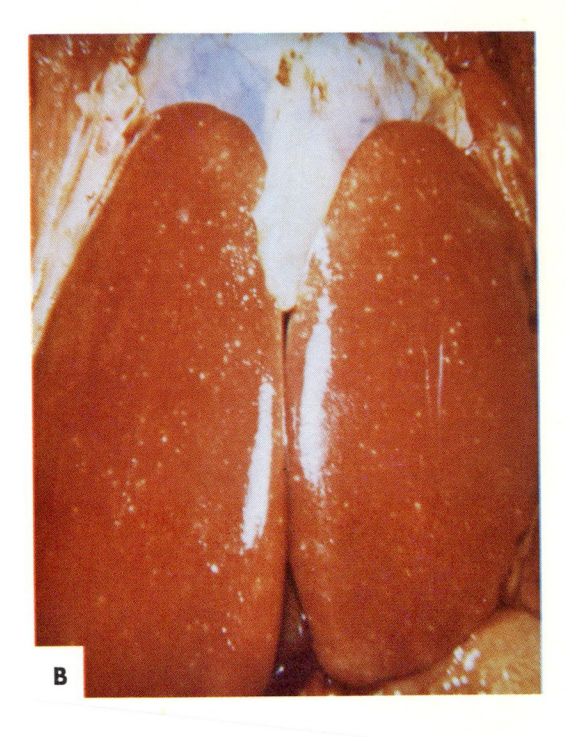

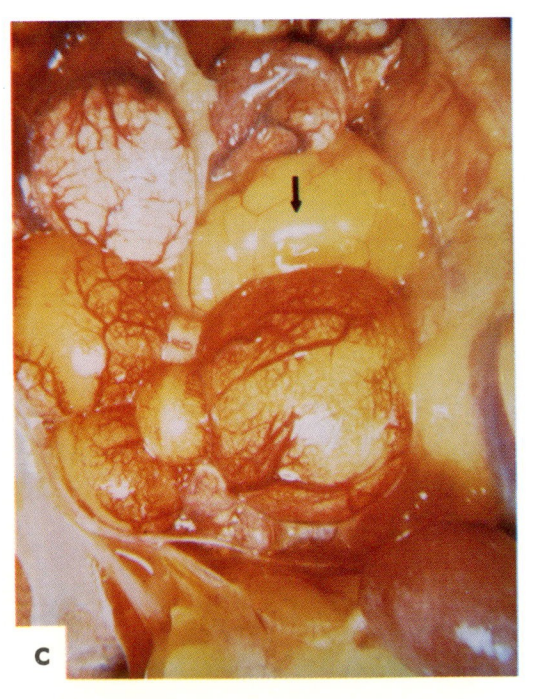

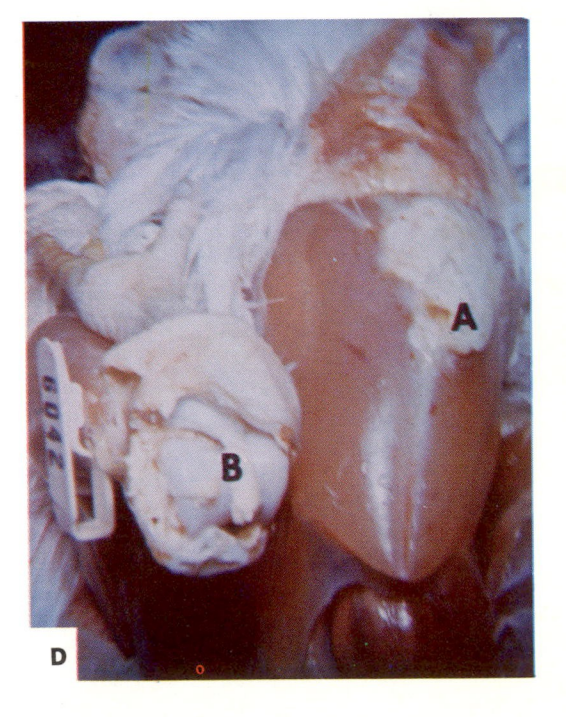

FIG. 5.12—(A) Acute fowl cholera. Subepicardial hemorrhages in a chicken. (B) Acute fowl cholera. Multiple necrotic foci in chicken liver. (C) Acute fowl cholera. Flaccid ovarian follicle (arrow) with thecal blood vessels less evident than normal. (D) Chronic fowl cholera. Caseous exudate in sternal bursa (A) and hock joint (B) of turkey.

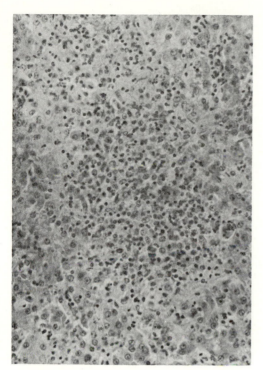

FIG. 5.13—Acute fowl cholera. Coagulative necrosis and heterophilic infiltration in turkey liver. H & E, ×375.

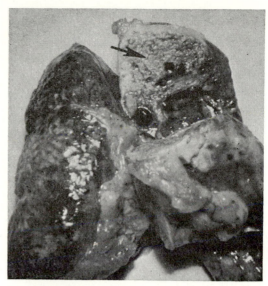

FIG. 5.15—Chronic fowl cholera. Pneumonic area (arrow) in cut surface of turkey lung.

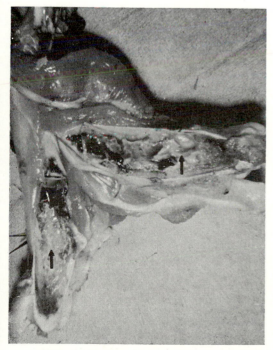

FIG. 5.14—Chronic fowl cholera. Caseous exudate (arrows) in turkey humerus.

and may be widely distributed. Subepicardial (Fig. 5.12-A) and subserosal hemorrhages are common, as are hemorrhages in the lung, abominal fat, and intestinal mucosa. Increased amounts of pericardial and peritoneal fluid frequently occur.

The livers of acutely affected birds may be swollen and usually contain multiple small focal areas (Fig. 5.12-B) of coagulative necrosis and heterophilic infiltration (Fig. 5.13). Some of the less virulent *P. multocida* do not produce necrotic foci in the liver. Heterophilic infiltration also occurs in the lungs and certain other parenchymatous organs (Rhoades, 1964). The lungs of turkeys are affected more severely than those of chickens, with pneumonia being a common sequela. Large amounts of viscid mucus may be observed in the digestive tract, particularly in the pharynx, crop, and intestine.

Ovaries of laying hens are commonly affected. Mature follicles often appear flaccid, and thecal blood vessels which are normally easily observed are less evident (Fig. 5.12-C). Yolk material from ruptured follicles may be found in the peritoneal cavity. Immature follicles and ovarian stroma are often hyperemic.

Chronic

Chronic fowl cholera is usually characterized by localized infections, in contrast

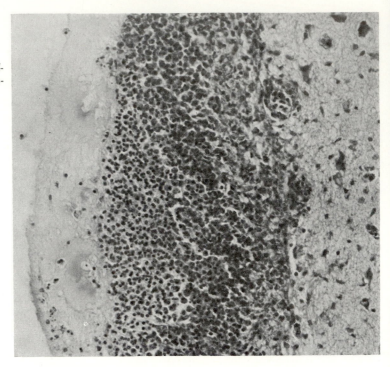

FIG. 5.16—Chronic fowl cholera. Fibrino-suppurative meningitis in turkey.

to the septicemic nature of the acute disease. These localized infections generally become suppurative and may be widely distributed anatomically. They often occur in the respiratory tract and may involve any part, including sinuses and pneumatic bones (Fig. 5.14). Pneumonia (Fig. 5.15) is an especially common lesion in turkeys. Infections of the conjunctiva and adjacent tissues occur (Fig. 5.8), and facial edema may be observed. Localized infections may also involve the hock joints (Fig. 5.12-D), sternal bursa (Fig. 5.12-D), foot pads, peritoneal cavity, and oviduct.

Chronic localized infections can involve the middle ear and cranial bones and have been reported to result in torticollis. In turkeys torticollis and eventual death can be associated with infections of the cranial bones, middle ear, and meninges. In a study of naturally infected turkeys exhibiting torticollis, Olson (1966) described lesions which occurred at these sites. The outstanding gross lesion was yellowish caseous exudate in the air spaces of the calvarial bones. Heterophilic infiltration and fibrin were consistently observed in the air spaces, middle ear, and meninges. Multinuclear giant cells were often associated with necrotic masses of heterophils in the air spaces. Similar lesions were found in

experimentally exposed turkeys (Olson and McCune, 1968). Localized meningeal infections (Fig. 5.16) without involvement of cranial bones or the middle ear have been observed in turkeys exhibiting torticollis (Rhoades, unpublished), as have cerebellar infections (Fenstermacher and Pomeroy, 1941).

IMMUNITY

Pasteur (1881) used an avirulent culture, attenuated by prolonged growth on artificial medium, and produced immunity that protected fowls against subsequent exposure. In field use his method did not prove practical, because uniform attenuation could not be obtained and heavy losses sometimes occurred in vaccinated flocks. This method is used occasionally in Europe.

Since Pasteur's classical work there have been numerous attempts to produce efficient vaccines against fowl cholera, but results have not been consistent. However, there can be little doubt that a substantial but not absolute immunity can be induced in fowl using killed *P. multocida* vaccines under controlled conditions (Dougherty, 1953b; Heddleston and Hall, 1958; Heddleston and Reisinger, 1959, 1960; Chute et al., 1962; Bierer, 1962; Boyer and Brown,

1963; Dorsey, 1963b; Bhasin and Biberstein, 1968). Killed *P. multocida* vaccines are usually prepared by growing selected immunogenic strains on a suitable medium and suspending in formalized saline solution. The killed organisms are usually incorporated with an adjuvant and injected subcutaneously.

Under field conditions losses due to fowl cholera sometimes occur in vaccinated flocks. This failure may be due to a concomitant disease, environmental stressors, or an improperly prepared or administered vaccine. Heddleston and Reisinger (1960) demonstrated that stress caused by changing the social or peck order of vaccinated males as well as fowl pox infection in chickens at time of vaccination and exposure significantly reduced the efficacy of vaccination. It was also observed that an isolant of *P. multocida* recovered from a fowl cholera outbreak in previously vaccinated turkeys differed immunologically from the culture used in preparing the vaccine (Heddleston, 1962). Apparently more critical studies under various field conditions are needed to determine the reasons for vaccine failure.

In a recent study Heddleston and Rebers (1968) reported that oral administration of killed *P. multocida* induced immunity in young chickens and turkeys. The quantity of vaccine required to induce immunity by this method was considerably larger than that required for parenteral administration.

Passive immunity for the prevention of fowl cholera was studied by Kitt in 1892, who used immune horse sera. This method was used frequently, but because of the short duration of passive immunity it is used little if any at the present time. Bolin and Eveleth (1951) reported that *P. multocida* antiserum prepared in chickens gave maximum protection 16–24 hours after injection. Protection began to decline after 48 hours and had disappeared 192 hours after injection.

DIAGNOSIS

A presumptive diagnosis of fowl cholera may be made from clinical observations, necropsy findings, or isolation of *P. multocida,* but a conclusive diagnosis should be based on all three findings. Signs and lesions of the disease were described previously.

ISOLATION AND IDENTIFICATION

Pasteurella multocida can be isolated readily from viscera of birds that die of acute cholera and usually from lesions of chronic cases, but it is less likely to be isolated from dehydrated, emaciated survivors of an acute outbreak. A tentative diagnosis of acute cholera can be made by demonstrating bipolar organisms in liver imprints (Fig. 5.2) using Wright's staining method (Report of Poultry Disease Subcommittee, 1969). Immunofluorescent technique can be used to identify *P. multocida* in tissue or exudate (Marshall, 1963).

Bone marrow, heart blood, liver, meninges, or localized lesions are preferred for culturing. To isolate *P. multocida,* sear the tissue or exudate with a spatula and obtain a specimen by inserting a sterile cotton swab or wire loop through the seared surface. If birds are living, squeeze mucus from the nostril or insert a cotton swab into the nasal cleft. Transfer the specimen to peptone broth and streak on dextrose starch agar containing 5% chicken serum or other suitable media. Specimens may also be streaked on MacConkey and blood agar media to aid in identification.

Colonies characteristic of *P. multocida,* as described under the section on etiology, are transferred to dextrose starch agar slants which are incubated 18–24 hours. Tubes of phenol red broth base containing 1% glucose, lactose, sucrose, mannitol, and maltose are then inoculated with the growth from the slant. The fermentation of glucose, sucrose, and mannitol without gas is characteristic of *P. multocida.* Lactose is usually not fermented, but some avian isolants will ferment lactose. Inoculate 2% tryptose in 0.85% NaCl solution, incubate 24 hours at 37° C, and test for indole (Kovac's test). Indole is almost always produced by *P. multocida.* There should be no hemolysis of blood and no growth on MacConkey agar (Table 5.2).

Inoculation of animals may be used as an aid for isolating *P. multocida.* Rabbits, hamsters, or mice are inoculated subcutaneously or intraperitoneally with 0.2 ml of exudate or minced tissue from an infected bird. If *P. multocida* is present, the animal usually dies within 24–48 hours, and the organism can be isolated in pure culture from the heart, blood or liver.

Serologic diagnosis of fowl cholera by the

TABLE 5.2 ❧ Differential Test for
*Pasteurella multocida (multo.), P. anatipestifer
(anati.), P. pseudotuberculosis (pseudo.),
P. haemolytica (haemo.), and P. gallinarum (gall.)*

Test	Pasteurella				
	multo.	anati.	pseudo.	haemo.	gall.
Hemolysis	−	−	−	+	−
MacConkey	−	−	+u	+u	−
Indol	+	−u	−	−	−
Motility	−	−	+	−	−
Urease	−	−u	+	−	−
Gelatin	−	+u	−	−	−
Glucose	+	−	+	+	+
Lactose	−u	−	−	+u	−
Sucrose	+	−	+u	+	+
Maltose	−u	−	+	+	+

Note: u = usually.

rapid whole-blood agglutination, serum-plate agglutination, or agar diffusion tests has limited value in chronic cholera and no value with the acute form of the disease.

DIFFERENTIAL DIAGNOSIS

Pasteurella gallinarum and *Pasteurella haemolytica* are two closely related bacteria which may be isolated from diseased poultry and incorrectly identified as *P. multocida*. *P. gallinarum* was first described by Hall et al. (1955), who isolated it along with *P. multocida* from chickens with other maladies characterized by inflammation of the upper respiratory tract. Clark and Godfrey (1960) found *P. gallinarum* associated with a respiratory disease complex of chickens in southern California. Gilchrist (1963), in a survey of avian respiratory diseases in New South Wales, reported finding *P. gallinarum, P. haemolytica,* and *P. multocida.* Harbourne (1962) isolated *P. haemolytica* on four occasions from the livers of young chickens and turkeys. *P. haemolytica* was isolated from young chickens with salpingitis which was often accompanied by nasal catarrh, helminth infection, or leukosis; the organism was also isolated from the lungs of fowl with chronic respiratory disease and infectious bronchitis (Nicolet and Fey, 1965).

Differential characteristics of the various species of *Pasteurella* that may be isolated from poultry are listed in Table 5.2.

TREATMENT

Antibacterial chemotherapy has been used extensively in the treatment of fowl cholera with varying success, depending to a large extent on the promptness of treatment.

SULFONAMIDES

Several of the sulfonamides have been employed both experimentally and in natural outbreaks. The main disadvantages of the sulfonamides are their bacteristatic instead of bactericidal action, their inability to cure localized abscesses, and their toxic effect on the birds. Kiser et al. (1948) reported 63–85% reduction in mortality due to experimentally produced fowl cholera compared to untreated controls, using sulfamethazine and sodium sulfamethazine. In natural outbreaks the mortality was reduced 45–75%. Favorable results were obtained with 0.5–1% of the drug in the food or 0.1% in the drinking water.

Alberts and Graham (1948b) employed 0.5% sulfamerazine in mash feed for 5 days in a field outbreak of fowl cholera in turkeys. The mortality was 1.9% in the treated group as compared with 50% in untreated birds. Fowl cholera recurred four times after cessation of treatment, and each time losses were arrested after the turkeys were again given the sulfamerazine-mash mixture. In experimental infection in turkeys, sodium sulfamerazine at oral dosage rates of 143 and 107.25 mg/kg body weight effectively reduced mortality. In chickens 0.2% sodium sulfamerazine in the drinking water or 0.4% sulfamerazine in the mash checked the mortality in an established outbreak 2 days after treatment was started (Alberts, 1950). Sulfaquinoxaline in amounts of 0.05–0.01% in drinking water was completely prophylactic in experimental fowl cholera when treatment was started 24 hours before the birds were inoculated. Peterson (1948) treated two natural outbreaks in turkey flocks successfully with 1:2,000–1:4,000 dilution of the drug in drinking water. He found sulfamethazine and sodium sulfamerazine also were markedly effective in reducing experimental cholera, but sulfadiazine, sulfathiazole, and sulfanilamide were much less effective. Sulfaquinoxaline was used by Delaplane (1945) at the rate of 0.1 and 0.05% in the mash in the prophylaxis of fowl cholera in chickens. Nelson (1955) reported favorable results in controlling mortality in turkeys with a concentration of 0.025% sulfaquinoxaline in drinking water for 5–7 days. He stated further that administration of sulfaquinoxaline one day out of four usually controls later mortality and permits the grower to finish the birds for market. Dorsey and Harshfield (1959) confirmed the usefulness of several sulfonamide drugs in checking losses from fowl cholera if treatment is carried out in early stages of an outbreak. They also noted frequent recurrence of mortality after treatment was discontinued and unsatisfactory results of treatment after the disease had become chronic.

Sulfadimethoxine in drinking water was observed by Mitrovic (1967) to be highly effective in arresting experimentally induced fowl cholera; it was effective, palatable, and safe at the level of 0.05% for chickens and 0.025% for turkeys. Sulfaethoxypyridazine was reported by Stuart et al. (1966) to be effective in controlling fowl cholera in chickens and turkeys. The effectiveness of the drug was dependent in part on the size of dose and duration and promptness of treatment.

ANTIBIOTICS

Streptomycin given intramuscularly in dosage of 150,000 μg prevented deaths when administered before or at the time of inoculation of *P. multocida* in adult turkeys. When treatment was delayed for 6–24 hours or when dosage was reduced, chronic infection resulted (McNeil and Hinshaw, 1948). Chlortetracycline reduced losses in chicks about 80% when given at the rate of 40 mg/kg body weight intramuscularly a half-hour after parenteral inoculation of the organism (Little, 1948). Chicks that received mash containing 1 mg/g had 50% fewer losses than untreated controls. In an outbreak of fowl cholera in pheasants, however, Alberts and Graham (1951) did not observe any beneficial results when 1 mg/g mash was fed. When chlortetracycline was given intramuscularly, a slight reduction in mortality was recorded.

Chloramphenicol (20 mg/kg body weight) in a single intramuscular injection was effective in treating fowl cholera, but in flocks where fowl cholera and fowl typhoid or fowl pox were concurrently present, chloramphenicol treatment was not successful (Horváth et al., 1962). Water-soluble erythromycin at the rate of 1 lb/50 gal drinking water halted mortality in two flocks of Muscovy ducklings infected with *P. multocida* (Hart, 1963).

Antibiotics used in rations at very low levels for promotion of growth, according to the experiments of Dorsey and Harshfield (1959), did not significantly influence the course of fowl cholera infection in inoculated birds. At therapeutic levels, birds that received penicillin and streptomycin in the feed died at about the same rate as the controls. No deaths occurred in groups which received sulfaquinoxaline or sulfamerazine. These workers found oxytetracycline and chlortetracycline also effective in preventing mortality in experimental fowl cholera, although a comparatively high level in the mash was necessary. In these trials, treatment was initiated 24–48 hours before subcutaneous inoculation of the birds with virulent organisms. In an induced outbreak of fowl cholera in a small flock of laying birds, the mortality was 80% in an untreated group compared to 12% in a group which received mash containing oxytetracycline at the level of 500 g/ton. In six natural outbreaks, oxytetracycline at this level in the feed checked mortality, but losses returned in three flocks after withdrawal of the antibiotic.

PREVENTION AND CONTROL

MANAGEMENT PROCEDURES

Prevention of fowl cholera can be effected by eliminating the reservoirs of *P. multocida* or by preventing their access to poultry flocks. Good management practices, therefore, with emphasis on sanitation as prescribed by Zander (Chapter 1), are the best means of preventing fowl cholera. Unlike many bacterial diseases, fowl cholera is not a disease of the hatchery. Infection therefore occurs after the birds are in the hands of the producer, and consideration must be given to the many ways that infection might be introduced into a flock.

The primary source of infection is usually sick birds or those that have recovered and still carry the causative organism. Only young birds should be introduced as new stock, and these birds raised in a clean environment completely isolated from other birds. The isolation should be extended to the housing. Unless separate houses can be provided for first- and second-year laying flocks, the older flock should be marketed in its entirety. Different species of birds should not be raised on the same premises. The danger of mixing birds from different flocks cannot be overemphasized. Farm animals (particularly pigs, dogs, and cats) should not have access to the poultry area. Water fountains should be self-cleaning and feeders covered to prevent contamination as much as possible.

The fact that *P. multocida* has been recovered from many species of free-flying birds warrants consideration of this source of infection to poultry with measures to prevent their association with the flock. The raising of turkeys in areas where fowl cholera is a serious problem may warrant their confinement in houses where free-flying birds, rodents, and other animals can be excluded. If an outbreak of fowl cholera occurs, the flock should be quarantined and disposed of as soon as economically feasible. All housing and equipment should be cleaned and disinfected before repopulation.

IMMUNIZATION

Vaccination should be considered in areas where fowl cholera is prevalent, but it should not be substituted for good sanitary practices. Birds should be vaccinated at 6–8 weeks of age and revaccinated 8–10 weeks later if they are being held as breeders.

REFERENCES

Alberts, J. O. 1950. The prophylactic and therapeutic properties of sulfamerazine in fowl cholera. *Am. J. Vet. Res.* 11:414–20.

Alberts, J. O. and R. Graham. 1948a. Fowl cholera in turkeys. *North Am. Vet.* 29:24–26.

———. 1948b. Sulfamerazine in the treatment of fowl cholera in turkeys. *Am. J. Vet. Res.* 9:310–13.

———. 1951. An observation on Aureomycin therapy of fowl cholera in pheasants. *Vet. Med.* 46:505–6.

Anderson, L. A. P., M. G. Coombes, and S. M. K. Mallick. 1929. On the dissociation of *Bacillus avisepticus.* Part I. *Indian J. Med. Res.* 29:611–22.

Arsov, R. 1965. The portal of infection in fowl cholera. *Nauchni Tr. Visshiya Vet. Med. Inst., Prof. G. Pavlov* 14:13–17. (*Vet. Bull.* 36:710.)

Banerji, T. P. and R. Mukherjee. 1954. Nutritional requirements of *Pasteurella septica. Current Sci. India* 22:177–78. (*Vet. Bull.* 25:4.)

Bhasin, J. L., and E. L. Biberstein. 1968. Fowl cholera in turkeys—The efficacy of adjuvant bacterins. *Avian Diseases* 12:159–68.

Bierer, B. W. 1962. Treatment of avian pasteurellosis with injectable antibiotics. *J. Am. Vet. Med. Ass.* 141:1344–46.

Bolin, F. M., and D. F. Eveleth. 1951. The use of biological products in experimental fowl cholera. *Proc. Am. Vet. Med. Ass. 88th Ann. Meet.,* pp. 110–12.

Boyer, C. I., Jr., and J. A. Brown. 1963. Protection of turkeys vaccinated with fowl cholera bacterins. *Avian Diseases* 7:165–67.

Breed, R. S., E. G. D. Murray, and N. R. Smith. 1957. *Bergey's Manual of Determinative Bacteriology.* Williams & Wilkins Co., Baltimore.

Buchanan, R. E., J. G. Holt, and E. F. Lessel. 1966. *Index Bergeyana.* Williams & Wilkins Co., Baltimore.

Carter, G. R. 1955. Studies on *Pasteurella multocida.* I. A hemagglutination test for the identification of serological types. *Am. J. Vet. Res.* 16:481–84.

———. 1957. Studies on *Pasteurella multocida.* II. Identification of antigenic characteristics and colonial variants. *Am. J. Vet. Res.* 18:210–13.

———. 1967. Pasteurellosis: *Pasteurella multocida* and *Pasteurella hemolytica,* pp. 321–79. In Brandly, C. A., and C. Cornelius, *Advances in Veterinary Science,* Vol. II. Academic Press, New York and London.

Carter, G. R., and E. Annau. 1953. Isolation of capsular polysaccharides from colonial variants of *Pasteurella multocida. Am. J. Vet. Res.* 14:475–78.

Carter, G. R., and C. H. Bigland. 1953. Dissociation and virulence in strains of *Pasteurella multocida* isolated from a variety of lesions. *Can. J. Comp. Med.* 17:473–79.

Chute, H. L., D. C. O'Meara, and M. Gershman. 1962. Bacterins and drugs for the control of experimental fowl cholera. *Avian Diseases* 6:7–13.

Clark, D. S., and J. F. Godfrey. 1960. Atypical *Pasteurella* infections in chickens. *Avian Diseases* 4:280–90.

Curtice, C. 1902. Goose septicemia. *Univ. Rhode Island Agr. Exp. Sta. Bull.* 86:191–203.

Das, M. S. 1958. Studies on *Pasteurella septica* (*Pasteurella multocida*). Observations on some biophysical characteristics. *J. Comp. Pathol. Therap.* 68:288–94.

Delaplane, J. P. 1945. Sulfaquinoxaline in preventing upper respiratory infection of chickens inoculated with infective field material containing *Pasteurella avicida. Am. J. Vet. Res.* 6:207–8.

DeVolt, H. M., and C. R. Davis. 1932. A cholera-like disease in turkeys. *Cornell Vet.* 22:78–80.

Dimov, I. 1964. Survival of avian *Pasteurella*

multocida in soils at different acidity, humidity and temperature. *Nauchni Tr. Visshiya Vet. Med. Inst., Sofia* 12:339–45. (*Vet. Bull.* 35:349.)

Dorsey, T. A. 1963a. Studies on fowl cholera. I. A biochemic study of avian *Pasteurella multocida* strains. *Avian Diseases* 7:386–92.

———. 1963b. Studies on fowl cholera. II. The correlation between biochemic classification and the serologic and immunologic nature of avian *Pasteurella multocida* strains. *Avian Diseases* 7:393–402.

Dorsey, T. A., and G. S. Harshfield. 1959. Studies on fowl cholera. *S. Dakota State Univ. Agr. Exp. Sta. Bull.* 23:1–16.

Dougherty, E. 1953a. Disease problems confronting the duck industry. *Proc. Am. Vet. Med. Ass. 90th Ann. Meet.*, pp. 359–65.

———. 1953b. The efficacy of several immunizing agents for the control of fowl cholera in the White Pekin duck. *Cornell Vet.* 43:421–27.

Faddoul, G. P., G. W. Fellows, and J. Baird. 1967. Pasteurellosis in wild birds in Massachusetts. *Avian Diseases* 11:413–18.

Fenstermacher, R., and B. S. Pomeroy. 1941. Encephalitis-like symptoms in turkeys associated with a *Pasteurella sp. Cornell Vet.* 31:295–301.

Gershman, M., J. F. Witter, H. E. Spencer, and A. Kalvaitis. 1964. Case report: Epizootic of fowl cholera in the common eider duck. *J. Wildlife Management* 28:587–89.

Gilchrist, P. 1963. A survey of avian respiratory disease. *Australian Vet. J.* 39:140–44.

Gray, H. 1913. Some diseases of birds, pp. 420–32. In Hoare, E. W., *A System of Veterinary Medicine*, Vol. I. Alexander Eger, Chicago.

Hall, W. J., K. L. Heddleston, D. H. Legenhausen, and R. W. Hughes. 1955. Studies on pasteurellosis. I. A new species of *Pasteurella* encountered in chronic fowl cholera. *Am. J. Vet. Res.* 16:598–604.

Harbourne, J. F. 1962. A hemolytic coccobacillus recovered from poultry. *Vet. Record* 74:566–67.

Hart, L. 1963. Treatment of duck cholera with erythromycin. *Australian Vet. J.* 39:92–93.

Heddleston, K. L. 1962. Studies on pasteurellosis. V. Two immunogenic types of *Pasteurella multocida* associated with fowl cholera. *Avian Diseases* 6:315–21.

Heddleston, K. L., and W. J. Hall. 1958. Studies on pasteurellosis. II. Comparative efficiency of killed vaccines against fowl cholera in chickens. *Avian Diseases* 2:322–35.

Heddleston, K. L., and P. A. Rebers. 1968. Fowl cholera: Active immunity induced in chickens and turkeys by oral administration of killed *Pasteurella multocida*. *Avian Diseases* 12:129–34.

Heddleston, K. L., and R. C. Reisinger. 1959. Studies on pasteurellosis. III. Control of experimental fowl cholera in chickens and turkeys with an emulsified vaccine. *Avian Diseases* 3:397–404.

———. 1960. Studies on pasteurellosis. IV. Killed fowl cholera vaccine adsorbed on aluminum hydroxide. *Avian Diseases* 4:429–35.

Heddleston, K. L., and L. P. Watko. 1963. Fowl cholera: Susceptibility of various animals and their potential as disseminators of the disease. *Proc. 67th Ann. Meet. U.S. Livestock Sanit. Ass.*, pp. 247–51.

Heddleston, K. L., L. P. Watko, and P. A. Rebers. 1964. Dissociation of a fowl cholera strain of *Pasteurella multocida*. *Avian Diseases* 8:649–57.

Heddleston, K. L., P. A. Rebers, and A. E. Ritchie. 1966. Immunizing and toxic properties of particulate antigens from two immunogenic types of *Pasteurella multocida* of avian origin. *J. Immunol.* 96:124–33.

Henderson, A. 1963. *Pasteurella multocida* infection in man; a review of the literature. *Antonie Van Leeuwenhoek, J. Microbiol. Serol.* 29:359–67.

Hendrickson, J. M., and K. F. Hilbert. 1932. The persistence of *P. avicida* in the blood and organs of fowls with spontaneous fowl cholera. *J. Infect. Diseases* 50:89–97.

Henry, B. S. 1933. Dissociation in the genus *Brucella*. *J. Infect. Diseases* 52:374–402.

Horváth, Z., M. Padányi, and Z. Palatka. 1962. Chloramphenicol in the treatment of fowl cholera. *Magy. Allatorv. Lapja* 17:332–36. (*Vet. Bull.* 33:290.)

Hughes, T. P. 1930. The epidemiology of fowl cholera. II. Biological properties of *P. avicida*. *J. Exp. Med.* 51:225–38.

Hughes, T. P., and I. W. Pritchett. 1930. The epidemiology of fowl cholera. III. Portal of entry of *P. avicida*; reaction of the host. *J. Exp. Med.* 51:239–48.

Hungerford, T. G. 1968. A clinical note on avian cholera. The effect of age on the susceptibility of fowls. *Australian Vet. J.* 44:31–32.

Iliev, T., A. Arsov, I. Dimov, G. Girginov, and E. Iovchev. 1963a. Swine, cattle, and sheep as carriers and latent sources of pasteurella infection for fowl. *Nauchni Tr. Visshiya Vet. Med. Inst. Sofia* 11:281–88. (*Vet. Bull.* 34:129.)

Iliev, T., R. Arsov, E. Iovchev, and G. Girginov. 1963b. Role of swine in the epidemiology of fowl cholera. *Nauchni Tr. Visshiya Vet. Med. Inst., Sofia* 11:289–93. (*Vet. Bull.* 34:129.)

Iliev, T., R. Arsov, and V. Lazarov. 1965. Can fowls, carriers of *Pasteurella*, excrete the organism in faeces? *Nauchni Tr. Visshiya*

Vet. Med. Inst., Prof. G. Pavlov 14:7–12. (*Vet. Bull.* 26:710.)

Iovčev, E. 1967. The role of *Argas persicus* in the epidemiology of fowl cholera. *Angew. Parasitol.* 8:114–17. (*Vet. Bull.* 38:71.)

Jakšić, B. L., M. Dordević and B. Marković. 1964. Fowl cholera in wild birds. *Vet. Glasn.* 18:725–30. (*Vet. Bull.* 35:544.)

Jensen, W. I., and C. S. Williams. 1964. Botulism and fowl cholera, pp. 333–41. In Linduska, J. P., *Waterfowl Tomorrow.* U.S. Government Printing Office, Washington, D.C.

Juszkiewicz, T. 1966a. Hyperthermia and prednisolone acetate as provocative factors of *Pasteurella multocida* infection in chickens. *Polskie Arch. Weterynar.* 10:141–51.

———. 1966b. Effects of shaking and premedication with methylprednisolone on some biochemical indices associated with *Pasteurella multocida* infection of cockerels. *Polskie Arch. Weterynar.* 10:129–40.

Kirchner, C., and A. Eisenstark. 1956. Lysogeny in *Pasteurella multocida. Am. J. Vet. Res.* 17:547–48.

Kiser, J. S., J. Prier, C. A. Bottorff, and L. M. Greene. 1948. Treatment of experimental and naturally occurring fowl cholera with sulfamethazine. *Poultry Sci.* 27:257–62.

Kyaw, M. H. 1944. Pathogenesis of *Pasteurella septica* infection in developing chick embryo. *J. Comp. Pathol.* 54:200–206.

Little, P. A. 1948. Use of Aureomycin in some experimental infections in animals. *Ann. N.Y. Acad. Sci.* 51:246–53.

Little, P. A., and B. M. Lyon. 1943. Demonstration of serological types within the nonhemolytic *Pasteurellae. Am. J. Vet. Res.* 4:110–12.

McNeil, E., and W. R. Hinshaw. 1948. The effect of streptomycin on *Pasteurella multocida* in vitro, and on fowl cholera in turkeys. *Cornell Vet.* 38:239–46.

Manninger, R. 1919. Concerning a mutation of the fowl cholera bacillus (translated title). *Zentr. Bakteriol. Abt. I. Orig.* 83:520–28.

Marshall, J. D. 1963. The use of immunofluorescence for the identification of members of the genus *Pasteurella* in chemically fixed tissues. Ph.D. thesis, Univ. Maryland.

Mitrovic, M. 1967. Chemotherapeutic efficacy of sulfadimethoxine against fowl cholera and infectious coryza. *Poultry Sci.* 46:1153–58.

Moore, V. A. 1895. A preliminary investigation of diphtheria in fowls. *USDA BAI Bull.* 8, pp. 39–62.

Morris, E. J. 1958. Selective media for some *Pasteurella* species. *J. Gen. Microbiol.* 19:305–11.

Murata, M., T. Horiuchi, and S. Namioka. 1964. Studies on the pathogenicity of *Pasteurella multocida* for mice and chickens on the basis of O-groups. *Cornell Vet.* 54:293–307.

Namioka, S., and D. W. Bruner. 1963. Serological studies on *Pasteurella multocida.* IV. Type distribution of the organisms on the basis of their capsule and O groups. *Cornell Vet.* 53:41–53.

Nelson, C. L. 1955. The veterinarian in poultry practice. *Proc. 92nd Ann. Meet. Am. Vet. Med. Ass.*, pp. 306–10.

Nicolet, J., and H. Fey. 1965. Role of *Pasteurella haemolytica* in salpingitis of fowls. *Schweiz. Arch. Tierheilk.* 107:329–34. (*Vet. Bull.* 36:133.)

Nobrega, R., and R. C. Bueno. 1950. The influence of the temperature on the viability and virulence of *Pasteurella avicida. Bol. Soc. Paulista Med. Vet.* 8:189–94.

Olson, L. D. 1966. Gross and histopathological description of the cranial form of chronic fowl cholera in turkeys. *Avian Diseases* 10:518–29.

Olson, L. D., and E. L. McCune. 1968. Experimental production of the cranial form of fowl cholera in turkeys. *Am. J. Vet. Res.* 29:1665–73.

Pasteur, L. 1880a. Sur les maladies virulents et en particulier sur la maladie appelee vulgairement cholera des poules. *Compt. Rend. Acad. Sci.* 90:239–48, 1030–33.

Pasteur, L. 1880b. De l'attenuation du virus du cholera des poules. *Compt. Rend. Acad. Sci.* 91:673–680.

Pasteur, L. 1881. Sur les virus-vaccins du cholera des poules et du charbon. *Comptes Rendus des Travaux du Congres International des Directeurs des Stations Agronomiques, Session de Versailles,* pp. 151–62.

Peterson, E. H. 1948. Sulfonamides in the prophylaxis of experimental fowl cholera. *J. Am. Vet. Med. Ass.* 113:263–66.

Pirosky, I. 1938. Sur l'antigen glucidolipidique des *Pasteurella. Compt. Rend. Soc. Biol.* 127:98–100.

Prince, G. H., and J. E. Smith. 1966. Antigenic studies on *Pasteurella multocida* using immunodiffusion techniques. III. Relationship between strains of *Pasteurella multocida. J. Comp. Pathol. Therap.* 76:321–32.

Pritchett, I. W., and T. P. Hughes. 1932. The epidemiology of fowl cholera. VI. The spread of epidemic and endemic strains of *Pasteurella avicida* in laboratory populations of normal fowl. *J. Exp. Med.* 55:71–78.

Pritchett, I. W., F. R. Beaudette, and T. P. Hughes. 1930a. The epidemiology of fowl cholera. IV. Field observations of the "spontaneous" disease. *J. Exp. Med.* 51:249–58.

———. 1930b. The epidemiology of fowl cholera. V. Further field observations of the spontaneous disease. *J. Exp. Med.* 51:259–74.

Reis, J. 1941. On the presence of *Pasteurella avicida* in feces of infected birds. *Arquiv. Inst. Biol.* (Sao Paulo) 12:307–9. Report of the Chief of the Bureau of Animal Industry, USDA. 1951. Fowl cholera, p. 44.

Report of Poultry Disease Subcommittee on Animal Health, Agr. Bd., Div. of Biol. and Agr. Nat. Acad. Sci. 1969. *Methods for the Examination of Poultry Biologics,* 3rd ed. (In press.)

Rhoades, K. R. 1964. The microscopic lesions of acute fowl cholera in mature chickens. *Avian Diseases* 8:658–65.

Rifkind, D., and M. J. Pickett. 1954. Bacteriophage studies on the hemorrhagic septicemia *Pasteurellae. J. Bacteriol.* 67:243–46.

Rosen, M. N., and A. I. Bischoff. 1949. The 1948–49 outbreak of fowl cholera in birds in the San Francisco Bay area and surrounding counties. *Calif. Fish Game* 35:185–92.

Rosenbusch, C., and I. A. Merchant. 1939. A study of the hemorrhagic septicemia *Pasteurellae. J. Bacteriol.* 37:69–89.

Ryu, E. 1961. Studies on *Pasteurella multocida.* VI. The relationship between inhibitory action of blood and susceptibility of animals to *Past. multocida. Japan. J. Vet. Sci.* 23:357–61.

Salmon, D. E. 1880. Investigations of fowl cholera. *Rept. U.S. Comm. Agr.,* pp. 401–45.

Saxena, S. P., and A. B. Hoerlein. 1959. Lysogeny in Pasteurella. I. Isolation of bacteriophages from *Pasteurella* strains isolated from shipping fever and those from other infectious processes. *J. Vet. Animal Husbandry* 3:53–66.

Skidmore, L. V. 1932. The transmission of fowl cholera to turkeys by the common house fly (*Musca domestica* Linn) with brief notes on the viability of fowl cholera microörganisms. *Cornell Vet.* 22:281–85.

Stuart, E. E., R. D. Keenum, and H. W. Bruins. 1966. Efficacy of sulfaethoxypyridazine against fowl cholera in artificially infected chickens and turkeys, and its safety in laying chickens and broilers. *Avian Diseases* 10:135–45.

USDA Monthly Report. 1867. Poultry Diseases. pp. 216–17.

Van Es, L., and J. F. Olney. 1940. An inquiry into the influence of environment on the incidence of poultry diseases. *Univ. Nebraska Agr. Exp. Sta. Res. Bull.* 118, pp. 17–21.

Vaught, R. W., H. C. McDougle, and H. H. Burgess. 1967. Fowl cholera in waterfowl at Squaw Creek National Wildlife Refuge, Missouri. *J. Wildlife Management* 31:248–53.

Watko, L. P. 1966. A chemically defined medium for growth of *Pasteurella multocida. Can. J. Microbiol.* 12:933–37.

Watko, L. P., and K. L. Heddleston. 1966. Survival of shell-frozen, freeze-dried, and agar slant cultures of *Pasteurella multocida. Cryobiology* 3:53–55.

Webster, L. T., and C. G. Burn. 1926. Biology of *Bacterium lepisepticum.* III. Physical, cultural, and growth characteristics of diffuse and mucoid types and their variants. *J. Exp. Med.* 44:343–56.

Wilson, G. S., and A. A. Miles. 1964. *Topley and Wilson's Principles of Bacteriology and Immunity.* Williams & Wilkins Co., Baltimore.

Yaw, K. E., and J. C. Kakavas. 1957. A comparison of the protection-inducing factors in chickens and mice of a type 1 strain of *Pasteurella multocida. Am. J. Vet. Res.* 18:661–64.

❖

AVIAN PSEUDOTUBERCULOSIS

❖

AVIAN PSEUDOTUBERCULOSIS is a contagious disease of domestic, feral, and caged birds. It is characterized by an acute septicemia of short duration, followed by a chronic focal infection which gives rise to caseous swellings and nodules resembling lesions of avian tuberculosis in many of the visceral organs. Research on this disease has been limited, and most reported observations have dealt with case reports.

HISTORY AND DISTRIBUTION

The causative agent *Pasteurella pseudotuberculosis* was first isolated from a guinea pig inoculated with material from a subcutaneous tubercular lesion on the forearm of a child (Malassez and Vignal, 1883). Since then the organism has been isolated from many species of mammals and birds. In describing a case of pseudotuberculosis in a blackbird, Beaudette (1940) gave an extensive review of the disease in birds. He credited Riech in 1889 and Kinyoun in 1906 with making the first isolation from birds in Europe and the United States respectively.

Avian pseudotuberculosis has been reported in many countries and probably occurs throughout the world. However, because of its minor economic importance, it is seldom investigated or reported. It occurs sporadically in domestic poultry but occasionally causes severe losses in turkeys.

ETIOLOGY

CLASSIFICATION

The causative agent *P. pseudotuberculosis* has been given many names in the past (Buchanan et al., 1966): *Streptobacillus pseudotuberculosis-rodentium*, 1894; *Bacterium pseudotuberculosis-rodentium*, 1896; *Bacillus pseudotuberkulosis*, 1889; *Bacterium pseudotuberculosis*, 1900; *Corynebacterium rodentium*, 1932; *C. pseudotuberculosis*, 1925; *P. pseudotuberculosis*, 1929; *C. pseudotuberculosis-rodentium*, 1933; *Malleomyces pseudotuberculosis-rodentium*, 1933; *Shigella pseudotuberculosis*, 1935; *Yersinia rodentium*, 1944; *Pasteurella rodentium*, 1944; *P. pseudotuberculosis rodentium*, 1947; *Cillopasteurella pseudotuberculosis-rodentium*, 1953.

The inclusion of this organism in the genus *Pasteurella* has been questioned (Hutyra et al., 1938; Meyer, 1965). A new genus *Yersinia* was proposed by Smith and Thal (1965) for *P. pseudotuberculosis, P. pestis,* and a closely related bacterium *Yersinia enterocolitica* or *Pasteurella "X"* (Knapp and Thal, 1963).

CELLULAR MORPHOLOGY AND STAINING

The organism is a gram-negative rod 0.5 $\times$ 0.8–5.0μ. Coccoid and long filamentous forms also occur. The coccoid forms usually show some bipolar staining. According to Cook (1952) it is slightly acid-fast, which can be demonstrated in pus or imprint smears using a modified Ziehl-Neelsen staining method. Neither spores nor visible capsules are formed, although at 22° C an envelope may be seen in India ink preparations. Single rods occasionally show peri-trichous flagella which develop at a temperature between 20 and 30° C.

GROWTH REQUIREMENTS AND COLONIAL MORPHOLOGY

Pasteurella pseudotuberculosis grows in the presence or absence of oxygen. The optimal temperature is 30° C. Burrows and Gillett (1966) studied 7 strains of various serotypes and observed that some strains when grown at 28° C required thiamine or pantothenate. At 37° C most strains could grow with the addition of any 3 of 4 factors—glutamic acid, thiamine, cystine, and pantothenate; other strains required all 4 factors and nicotinamide.

Good growth occurs in ordinary peptone broth. Growth at 22° C is diffuse, with some clumped masses and occasionally ring and pellicle formation. Cultivation at 37° C, especially in acid media, accelerates dissociation. On plain agar it forms colonies smooth to slimy, granular, translucent, grayish yellow, butyrous, 0.5–1 mm in diameter. On agar containing blood the colonies grow to 2–3 mm in diameter by the 2nd day. At 37° C the colonies are thin, dry, and irregular with rough edges. Growth occurs on MacConkey's agar. *P. pseudotuberculosis* is motile at 25° C but not at 37° C. Motility is best demonstrated in semi-solid medium.

BIOCHEMICAL PROPERTIES

The following properties are characteristic of *P. pseudotuberculosis:*

ARABINOSE	Fermented without gas
DEXTRIN	Fermented without gas
FRUCTOSE	Fermented without gas
GLUCOSE	Fermented without gas
GLYCEROL	Fermented without gas
MALTOSE	Fermented without gas
MANNITOL	Fermented without gas
MANNOSE	Fermented without gas
MELIBIOSE	Fermented without gas
RHAMNOSE	Fermented without gas

TREHALOSE	Fermented without gas
XYLOSE	Usually fermented without gas
SALICIN	Usually fermented without gas
SUCROSE	Usually fermented without gas
DULCITOL	Not fermented
INOSITOL	Not fermented
LACTOSE	Not fermented
RAFFINOSE	Not fermented
SORBITOL	Not fermented
UREASE	Produced
CATALASE	Produced
AMMONIA	Produced
HYDROGEN SULFIDE	Usually not produced
NITRATES	Reduced
METHYLENE BLUE	Reduced
BLOOD	Not hemolyzed
INDOLE	Not produced
GELATIN	Not liquified
MACCONKEY'S AGAR	Usually growth

Differential characteristics are listed in Tables 5.2 and 5.4.

RESISTANCE TO CHEMICAL AND PHYSICAL AGENTS

Pasteurella pseudotuberculosis is easily destroyed by sunlight, drying, heat, or ordinary disinfectants. It remains viable for years on sealed agar slants or when lyophilized.

ANTIGENIC STRUCTURE

There are 5 serotypes on the basis of thermostable O antigens, 2 of which are subdivided by absorption agglutination. In addition to the O antigens there are 5 thermolabile H antigens (Table 5.3) (Thal, 1966).

TABLE 5.3 ✿ Serotypes and Antigens of *Pasteurella pseudotuberculosis*

Serotype	Subtype	O Antigen	H Antigen
I	IA	1,2,3	a,c
	IB	1,2,4	a,c
II	IIA	1,5,6	a,d
	IIB	5,7	a,d
III		1,8	a
IV	A	1,9,11	b
		1,9,11	a,b
	B	1,9,12	a,b,d
V		1,10	a,e,b

Thal (1954) studied 186 strains of *P. pseudotuberculosis;* of these, 33 were isolated from eight species of birds. All were biochemically identical; there were 5 serologically distinct groups. Most strains in group III produced thermolabile exotoxins which were convertible to toxoids. Experimentally, anti-infection immunity was produced with live avirulent strains, thus protecting against infection with atoxic strains and subtoxic culture doses of toxic strains. Antitoxic immunity protected against toxin and, to a degree, against infection with toxic strains but not against infection with atoxic strains.

Mair (1965) studied the type distribution of *P. pseudotuberculosis* in Great Britain during the years 1961–64; 177 strains were isolated from 39 different species of mammals and birds. Sixty-five isolates were from 26 species of birds; 39 of these 65 isolates were type IA, 16 type IB, 6 type IIA, 2 type IIB, and 2 type IV. Of 17 isolates from turkeys, 9 were type IA and 8 were type IB.

EPIZOOTIOLOGY

NATURAL AND EXPERIMENTAL HOSTS

Pseudotuberculosis has been reported in turkeys, ducks, geese, chickens, guinea fowl, and caged and free-flying birds. It has also been reported in many species of mammals. Of the laboratory animals, guinea pigs, rabbits, mice, monkeys, and baboons are quite susceptible; white rats and hamsters are refractory.

Pseudotuberculosis occurs quite frequently in turkeys, with losses as high as 80% (Rosenwald and Dickinson, 1944; Karlsson, 1945; Mathey and Siddle, 1954; Adamec and Matoušek, 1965). Kiliam et al. (1962) isolated *P. pseudotuberculosis* from 9-month-old turkey hens. The organism was considered unusual in that it resembled *Salmonella pullorum* on brilliant green agar, was agglutinated by *S. pullorum* antiserum, and after 24 hours incubation at 37° C resembled *S. pullorum* by producing acid and no gas from dextrose and mannitol and failing to change lactose, sucrose, maltose, dulcitol, or salicin. Serum from sensitized guinea pigs, chickens, and turkeys which agglutinated homologous antigen failed to agglutinate either *S. pullorum* or *S. typhi-murium*.

Pseudotuberculosis among stock doves in

Hampshire, England, was observed by Clapham (1953). In a search for the source of infection, *P. pseudotuberculosis* was isolated from a lark, a wood pigeon, a jackdaw, a rook, and a hare. The organism was also isolated from a rabbit in Hertfordshire and from two pigeons from Norfolk. The authors had isolated the organism previously from gray partridge, pheasant, and bobwhite quail. Seven outbreaks among pigeons in Denmark were reported by Marthedal and Velling (1954). They also had observed the infection in a turkey and 7 outbreaks in ornamental birds (canaries, snow-buntings, and waxwings). An epornitic of pseudotuberculosis in common grackles (*Quiscalus quiscula*) occurred at a major winter roost of Icteridae in Maryland (Clark and Locke, 1962). Mortality and morbidity were extensive and continued for several weeks until spring roost breakup. The occurrence of extensive infection in a large migratory bird population has major epizootiological significance.

Pseudotuberculosis in humans, once thought to be a rare and fatal septicemic disease, is now recognized as occurring quite often in Europe as an enteric form causing symptoms of appendicitis (Surgalla, 1965).

TRANSMISSION, PATHOGENESIS, AND INCUBATION PERIOD

Body excretions of diseased birds or mammals that contaminate soil, food, or water are important factors in dissemination of the disease. Predisposing causes are apparently important; as a rule, the only birds affected are those whose resistance has been lowered by inadequate feeding, exposure to cold, or worm infestation. Very young birds are particularly susceptible. During cold and wet weather in the fall, considerable losses may occur among young turkeys.

In susceptible birds the organism gains entrance to the bloodstream through breaks in the skin or through the mucous membranes, perhaps mostly (but not necessarily exclusively) in the digestive tract. Thus a bacteremia is established. Usually the bacteremic condition is of short duration, but the bacteria are not all destroyed. Some of them establish foci of infection in one or more organs such as the liver, spleen, lungs, or intestines, giving rise to tubercularlike lesions. Such lesions have also been found in the mesentery and breast muscles.

The incubation period of artificial infection varies considerably and is dependent on the virulence of the organism, the amount of inoculum, the avenue of introduction, and the host species. Sparrows and canaries are very susceptible and may die in 1–3 days from small doses of organisms injected subcutaneously, intramuscularly, or intraperitoneally. Feeding of cultures is usually ineffective unless some intestinal inflammation is present to act as a predisposing influence. Canaries fed mustard seed for the purpose of causing intestinal irritation have sickened 5 days after being given cultures by mouth, death resulting 2 days later. Judging from the various reports available, the incubation period may vary from 3 to 6 days in acute attacks and 2 or more weeks in chronic cases.

SIGNS

The signs vary considerably. In very acute cases the birds may die suddenly without warning, or they may live a few hours or a few days after showing the first signs. Such cases are usually marked by sudden appearance of diarrhea and the usual manifestations of acute septicemia. Usually, however, the course of this disease extends over 2 or more weeks, in which case the signs appear 2–4 days before death. In such cases the birds will show weakness, dull and ruffled feathers, and difficult breathing. Diarrhea is also a common sign in such cases. Occasionally the disease will run a more protracted course, when emaciation and extreme weakness or paralysis may be evident. Such manifestations as stiffness, difficulty in walking, droopiness, somnolence, constipation, and discoloration of the skin have also been observed. In early stages of the chronic form of the disease the birds may eat normally, but the appetite is usually completely lost 1 or 2 days before death.

LESIONS

In highly acute cases, the only changes observed are swelling of the spleen and enteritis. Subacute or chronic cases result in enlargement of the liver, spleen, and lungs. Yellowish white foci the size of millet seed may be found in the liver, spleen, lungs, and breast muscles. There is usually

severe enteritis which is sometimes hemorrhagic. The serous cavities may sometimes
contain an increased amount of fluid.

DIAGNOSIS

A definite diagnosis can be established
only by isolation and identification of the
organism, since the symptoms and lesions
are very similar to those of several other
diseases such as fowl cholera, fowl typhoid,
paratyphoid, spirochetosis, tuberculosis,
and certain forms of the leukosis complex.
In making a bacteriological examination,
one must remember that in acute cases the
organism can be found in blood but in
chronic cases it must be sought in tissues.

ISOLATION AND IDENTIFICATION

Primary isolation is made by streaking
specimens from liver or spleen on blood or
trypticase soy agar, or inoculating trypticase soy broth followed by streaking onto
agar after 3–5 hours incubation at 37° C.
The inoculated agar is incubated for 24
hours at 30–37° C and observed for colonies
as previously described. The medium of
Paterson and Cook (1963) is recommended
for the isolation of *P. pseudotuberculosis*
from feces. The surface of the agar is inoculated by streaking a suspension of 10%
feces in phosphate buffer (pH 7.6) and incubating at 37° C for 24–48 hours.

DIFFERENTIAL DIAGNOSIS

The bacterium *P. pseudotuberculosis* is
quite similar in many respects to *P. pestis*
and *Bordetella bronchiseptica*. Although

TABLE 5.4 ❧ Differential Characteristics of
Pasteurella pseudotuberculosis, P. pestis,
and *Bordetella bronchiseptica*

Test	*Pasteurella pseudotuberculosis*	*pestis*	*Bordetella bronchiseptica*
Urease	+	−	+
Oxidase	−	−	+
Lysine decarboxylase	−	−	+
Indol	−	−	−
Citrate	−	−	+
Rhamnose	+	−	−
Esculin	+	...	−
Hemolysis	−	−	+
Motility at 25° C	+	−	+

these two organisms are not likely to be
encountered in poultry, they may be carried by rodents having access to the poultry
area.

Farkas-Himsley (1963) observed that *P.
pseudotuberculosis* could be differentiated
from *B. bronchiseptica* by the utilization of
citrate as a sole source of carbon, presence
of lysine decarboxylase and oxidase, hydrol-
yzation of esculin, and fermentation of
rhamnose (Table 5.3). A summary of differential tests of *P. pseudotuberculosis, P.
pestis,* and *B. bronchiseptica* is listed in
Table 5.4.

TREATMENT AND PREVENTION

No medical treatment or vaccine is available. Therefore, one must depend on sanitary and hygienic procedures (Chapter 1)
for combatting this disease.

REFERENCES

Adamec, Z., and K. Matoušek. 1965. Pseudotuberculosis in turkeys. *Veterinarstvi* 15:158–
60. (*Vet. Bull.* 1966:65.)

Beaudette, F. R. 1940. A case of pseudotuberculosis in a blackbird. *J. Am. Vet. Med. Ass.*
97:151–57.

Buchanan, R. E., J. G. Holt, E. F. Lessel. 1966.
Index Bergeyana. Williams & Wilkins Co.,
Baltimore.

Burrows, T. W., and W. A. Gillett. 1966. The
nutritional requirements of some *Pasteurella*
species. *J. Gen. Microbiol.* 45:333–45.

Clapham, P. A. 1953. Pseudotuberculosis
among stock-doves in Hampshire. *Nature*
172:353.

Clark, M. C., and L. N. Locke. 1962. Case report: Observations on pseudotuberculosis in
common grackles. *Avian Diseases* 6:506–10.

Cook, R. 1952. A method of demonstrating
Pasteurella pseudotuberculosis in smears
from animal lesions. *J. Pathol. Bacteriol.*
64:228–29.

Farkas-Himsley, H. 1963. Differentiation of
Pasteurella pseudotuberculosis and *Bordetel-
la bronchiseptica* by simple biochemical test.
Am. J. Vet. Res. 24:871–73.

Hutyra, F., J. Marek, and R. Manninger. 1938.
*Special Pathology and Therapeutics of the
Diseases of Domestic Animals,* Vol. I. Alex-
ander Eger, Chicago.

Karlsson, Karl-Fredrik. 1945. Pseudotuber-
kulos hos honsfaglar. *Scand. Vet. Tidskr.*
35:673–87.

Kiliam, J. G., R. Yamamoto, W. E. Babcock,
and E. M. Dickinson. 1962. An unusual aspect of *Pasteurella pseudotuberculosis* in

turkeys. *Avian Diseases* 6:403–5.

Knapp, W., and E. Thal. 1963. Biochemical, serological, pathogenic, and immunological properties of bacteria provisionally designated *"Pasteurella X"* from chinchillas (Translated title). *Zentr. Bakteriol. Parasitenk. Abt. I. Orig.* 190:472–84.

Mair, N. S. 1965. Sources and serological classification of 177 strains of *Pasteurella pseudotuberculosis* isolated in Great Britain. *J. Pathol. Bacteriol.* 90:275–78.

Malassez, L., and W. Vignal. 1883. Tuberculose zoologique (forme on espice de tuberculose sans bacillis). *Arch. Physiol. Norm. Pathol.* Ser. 3, 2:369–412.

Marthedal, H. E., and G. Velling. 1954. Pasteurellosis and pseudotuberculosis among fowls in Denmark. *Nord. Veterinarmed.* 6:651–65.

Mathey, W. J., Jr., and P. J. Siddle. 1954. Isolation of *Pasteurella pseudotuberculosis* from a California turkey. *J. Am. Vet. Med. Ass.* 125:482–83.

Meyer, K. F. 1965. *Pasteurella* and *Francisella*, pp. 659–97. In Dubos, R. J., and J. G. Hirsch, *Bacterial and Mycotic Infections of Man*, 4th ed. Lippincott, Co., Philadelphia and Montreal.

Paterson, J. S., and R. Cook. 1963. A method for the recovery of *Pasteurella pseudotuberculosis* from faeces. *J. Pathol. Bacteriol.* 85:241–42.

Rosenwald, A. S., and E. M. Dickinson. 1944. A report on *Pasteurella pseudotuberculosis* infection in turkeys. *Am. J. Vet. Res.* 5:246–49.

Smith, J. E., and E. Thal. 1965. A taxonomic study of the genus *Pasteurella* using a numerical technique. *Acta Pathol. Microbiol. Scand.* 64:213–23.

Surgalla, M. J. 1965. *Pasteurella pseudotuberculosis* information as background for understanding plague. *Public Health Rept.* 80:825–28.

Thal, E. 1954. Untersuchungen ueber *Pasteurella pseudotuberculosis* unter besonder Beruecksichtigun ihres immunologisches Verhaltens. Thesis, Berlingska Boktryckeriet, Lund, Sweden.

———. 1966. Weitere Untersuchungen ueber die thermolabilen Antigene der *Yersina pseudotuberculosis* (Syn. *Pasteurella pseudotuberculosis*). *Zentr. Bakteriol. Parasitenk. Abt. I. Orig.* 200:56–65.

❖

INFECTIOUS SEROSITIS

❖

INFECTIOUS SEROSITIS (new duck disease, duck septicemia, anatipestifer infection) is a relatively new but serious disease affecting domestic ducks. It is a septicemic disease characterized by fibrinous peritonitis, pericarditis, and airsacculitis. Very little research has been reported on this disease.

Signs and lesions of infectious serositis in ducks and those reported in geese affected with goose influenza are similar, and the causative agents *Pasteurella anatipestifer* and *P. septicaemiae* cannot be differentiated on the basis of reported characteristics. Goose influenza, therefore, will not be described as a separate disease but will be discussed in the section on differential diagnosis.

HISTORY AND DISTRIBUTION

Infectious serositis was first described in 1932 in ducks from 3 duck ranches on Long Island, New York, where several thousand ducks had died (Hendrickson and Hilbert, 1932). The report referred to a new disease, and the disease became known in that area as "new duck disease." Six years later the disease was observed in ducks from a commercial duck farm in Illinois and reported as duck septicemia (Graham et al., 1938). The designation infectious serositis was applied by Dougherty et al. (1955) after a comprehensive pathological study.

Infectious serositis in ducks has also been recognized in England (Asplin, 1955), Canada (Taylor, 1955), the Netherlands (Donker-Voet, 1962), and the Soviet Union (Avrorov et al., 1964).

ETIOLOGY

CLASSIFICATION

The causative bacterium was isolated and characterized by Hendrickson and Hilbert (1932) who gave it the name *Pfeifferella anatipestifer*. The bacterium was later studied by Bruner and Fabricant (1954) who compared its characteristics with those of the *Brucellae, Pasteurellae, Moraxellae, Actinobacilli,* and *Hemophili.* They concluded that the organism had more in common with the *Moraxellae* and proposed the name *Moraxella anatipestifer.* However, it was listed in *Bergey's Manual* as *Pasteurella anatipestifer* (Breed et al., 1957).

Whether or not this organism belongs in the genus *Pasteurella* is dubious since it differs from other *Pasteurellae* by liquifying gelatin and not fermenting carbohydrates. Little is known of the antigenic structure of *P. anatipestifer* or of its resistance to chemical and physical agents.

MORPHOLOGY AND STAINING

It is a gram-negative, nonmotile, nonsporeforming rod occurring singly, in pairs, and occasionally as filaments. The cells vary in size from 0.2–0.4 x 1–5μ. Many cells stain bipolar with Wright's stain, and a capsule can be demonstrated in preparations with India ink.

GROWTH REQUIREMENTS AND COLONIAL MORPHOLOGY

The organism grows well on chocolate agar or trypticase soy agar. Maximum growth usually occurs in 48–72 hours at 37° C. Growth is more abundant with increased carbon dioxide (Graham et al., 1938).

The organism was typed as a strict aerobe by Hendrickson and Hilbert (1932) on the basis of results obtained with the pyrogallic acid and sodium hydroxide procedure for removing oxygen. However, since carbon dioxide would also be depleted by reacting with the sodium hydroxide, neither oxygen nor carbon dioxide was available to the organism.

Colonies on chocolate agar, when grown 24 hours at 37° C in a candle jar, are 1–1.5 mm in diameter, convex, transparent, glistening, and butyrous. Older colonies are larger and viscous. Colonies on clear media are iridescent when observed with obliquely transmitted light.

BIOCHEMICAL PROPERTIES

Gelatin is usually liquefied. Litmus milk may slowly become alkaline. Carbohydrates are not fermented, although Asplin (1955) reported 2 of 5 strains produced a slight amount of acid in glucose and maltose after 7 days. Indole (usually) and hydrogen sulfide are not produced. Nitrates are not reduced and starch is not hydrolyzed. There is no growth on MacConkey's agar and no hemolysis of blood agar. Urease is occasionally produced. (Differential characteristics are listed in Table 5.2.)

PATHOGENESIS AND EPIZOOTIOLOGY

NATURAL AND EXPERIMENTAL HOSTS

Infectious serositis is primarily a disease of young ducklings. Ducks under 2 weeks of age usually die 1–2 days after signs appear; older birds may survive a week or more.

Adverse environmental conditions or concomitant disease often predispose the birds to outbreaks of infectious serositis. Mortality may vary from 5 to 75%

The disease can be induced in healthy ducks by exposure to a culture of *P. anatipestifer.* There is wide variation, however, in the virulence of the organism in ducks, depending on the strain of organism and route of exposure. Mortality can be produced most consistently by injection of the organism intravenously or into the foot pad. The disease can also be produced by subcutaneous, intraperitoneal, or intratracheal routes of exposure. Feeding of the organism to birds has not been successful in producing the disease.

Chickens, geese, pigeons, rabbits, and mice have been reported to be refractory to infection with *P. anatipestifer,* but guinea pigs may succumb to inoculation of large doses intraperitoneally. The writer observed that 8×10^6 organisms inoculated into the foot pad killed 5 of 7 day-old chicks, and 4×10^6 organisms produced the same signs and lesions in 2-week-old White Chinese goslings as were produced in White Pekin ducklings.

Infection normally takes place through wounds, scratches, or punctures of the skin, particularly of the feet (Asplin, 1956). The results of an experiment by Asplin shown below emphasize this point.

EXPOSURE	No. DUCKLINGS	No. DIED	SIGNS
Intranasal	10	0	None
Intraocular	10	0	None
Oral	10	0	None
Cohabitation	10	0	None
Foot web stab	7	7	...

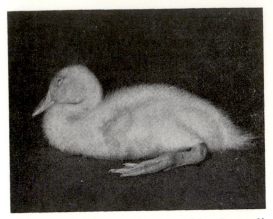

FIG. 5.17—Infectious serositis. Incoordinated and droopy duckling.

Ducklings which recover from the disease are resistant to subsequent infection (Hendrickson and Hilbert, 1932; Graham et al., 1938; Asplin, 1955).

SIGNS

Signs most often observed in infectious serositis are diarrhea, ocular discharge, and ataxia (Fig. 5.17). Mild coughing may occur (Dougherty et al., 1955), and affected ducks often rapidly become emaciated (Graham et al., 1938). Ducks which survive may be stunted (Pickrell, 1966).

LESIONS

The most obvious gross lesion in infectious serositis is fibrinous exudate which involves serosal surfaces in general but is most evident in the pericardial cavity and over the surface of the liver (Figs. 5.18, 5.19, 5.20). In addition to fibrin the exudate contains a few inflammatory cells, primarily mononuclear cells and heterophils.

Fibrinous airsacculitis is common. Mononuclear cells are the predominant cell type in the exudate. Multinuclear giant cells and fibroblasts may be observed in chronic cases (Dougherty et al., 1955), and the exudate may be partially calcified (Pickrell, 1966). The lungs of infected ducks may be unaffected (Dougherty et al., 1955), there may be interstitial cellular infiltration and proliferation of lymphoid nodules adjacent to parabronchi (Pickrell, 1966), or there may be an acute fibrino-purulent pneumonia (Graham et al., 1938).

Liver lesions which have been observed in the acute stage of the disease are mild periportal mononuclear leukocytic infiltration, cloudy swelling, and hydropic degeneration of parenchymal cells. In less acute cases moderate periportal lymphocytic infiltration may be observed (Pickrell, 1966).

Infections of the central nervous system can produce a fibrinous meningitis. Spleens may be enlarged and mottled. Mucopurulent exudate in nasal sinuses and caseous exudate in oviducts have been associated with this infection (Dougherty et al., 1955). Jortner et al. (1969) studied the central nervous system of naturally infected ducklings and described diffuse fibrinous men-

FIG. 5.18—Infectious serositis produced by foot pad inoculation. Fibrinous epicarditis (A), pericarditis, and perihepatitis (B). Forceps hold exudate from surface of liver.

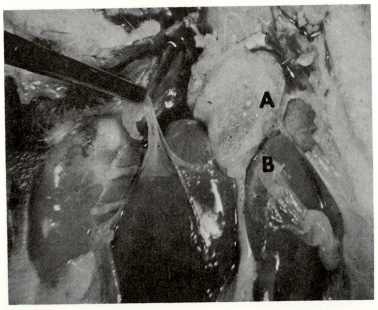

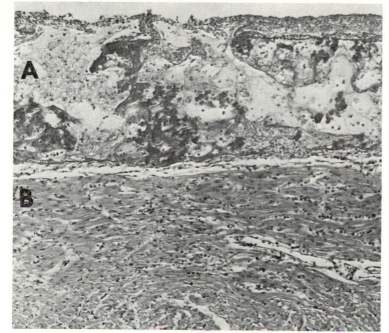

FIG. 5.19—Infectious serositis. Fibrinous exudate (A) over surface of heart (B). H & E, ×150.

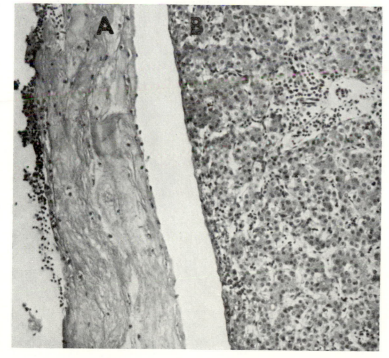

FIG. 5.20—Infectious serositis. Fibrinous exudate (A) over surface of liver (B). H & E, ×300.

ingitis with leukocytic infiltration in and around the walls of meningeal blood vessels. Extensive exudate was observed in the ventricular system. Slight to moderate leukocytic and microglial infiltrates were observed in subpial and periventricular brain tissue.

DIAGNOSIS

Like fowl cholera, a presumptive diagnosis may be made from clinical observations, necropsy findings, or isolation of *P. anatipestifer*, but a conclusive diagnosis should be based on the results of all three.

ISOLATION AND IDENTIFICATION

The bacterium can be isolated most readily when the birds are in the acute stage of the disease. Suitable tissues for culturing the organism are bone marrow, heart blood, liver, spleen, lung, brain, and exudates from the eye, trachea, or peritoneal cavity. Specimens should be taken aseptically, streaked over chocolate agar medium, and incubated 24–72 hours at 37° C under increased carbon dioxide. The candle jar is satisfactory. Colonies should be selected for inoculation of the differentiating media listed in Table 5.2. *P. anatipestifer* usually liquifies gelatin but does not ferment carbohydrates. Other characteristics are listed in Table 5.2.

Immunofluorescent procedure can be used to identify *P. anatipestifer* in tissue or exudate from infected birds (Marshall et al., 1961).

DIFFERENTIAL DIAGNOSIS

Goose influenza (Levine, 1965) and infectious serositis are probably the same disease with the exception that one has been described as a disease of geese and the other a disease of ducks. Information in the literature about the causative agents leads one to believe that they are the same organism. To resolve the question as to whether there are 2 distinct bacteria, *P. anati-*

pestifer and *P. septicaemiae* (Breed et al., 1957), both organisms should be studied simultaneously. The writer has not been successful in obtaining a culture of *P. septicaemiae* for comparative studies.

Riemer (1904), who was one of the first to study the disease in geese, used the term "septicaemia anserum exsudativa." He found that the causative bacterium was more pathogenic for geese than for ducks, but the lesions were the same in both species of birds when exposed artificially.

Loeffler (1910) studied a disease of geese, which he named goose influenza, and concluded that it was the same disease as reported by Riemer and other investigators. He found that the causative organism was pathogenic for both geese and ducks, and the lesions were similar in both species.

Miklovichné Kis Csatári (1965), on the other hand, studied an epornitic of goose influenza and reported that the causative organism was pathogenic for geese but not for ducks.

Asplin (1955) studied an epornitic of infectious serositis in ducks and reported that the causative organism was pathogenic for ducks but not for geese. He noted the close morphological and biochemical resemblance of the organism that he isolated to the one described by Riemer.

TREATMENT AND CONTROL

Two percent sulphamezathine (which was toxic) in the drinking water or 2,000 units of penicillin inoculated twice a day intramuscularly for 5 days prevented symptoms in ducks exposed experimentally to *P. anatipestifer* (Asplin, 1955). A combination of penicillin and dihydrostreptomycin was superior to oxytetracycline in reducing mortality and increasing weight gains in 20–25-day-old ducks that had signs of infection (Ash, 1966).

To prevent infectious serositis one must use the usual sanitary and hygienic procedures described in Chapter 1.

REFERENCES

Ash, W. J. 1967. Antibiotics and infectious serositis in White Pekin ducklings. *Avian Diseases* 11:38–41.

Asplin, F. D. 1955. A septicaemic disease of ducklings. *Vet. Record* 67:854–58.

———. 1956. Experiments on the transmission of a septicaemic disease of ducklings. *Vet. Record* 68:588–90.

Avrorov, A. A., E. M. Kozhevnikov, and B. A. Gladkov. 1964. Pathology of duck influenza. *Tr. II Vses. Konf. Patol. Anat. Zhivotn. Mosk. Vet. Akad.* 1963, pp. 171–76. (*Vet. Bull.* 36:405.)

Breed, R. S., E. F. Lessel, Jr., and E. Heist Clise. 1957. Genus I. Pasteurella *Trevisan*, 1887, pp. 395–402. In Breed, R. S., E. G. D.

Murray, and N. R. Smith (eds.). *Bergey's Manual of Determinative Bacteriology*, 7th ed. Williams & Wilkins, Baltimore.

Bruner, D. W., and J. Fabricant. 1954. A strain of *Moraxella anatipestifer (Pfeifferella anatipestifer)* isolated from ducks. *Cornell Vet.* 44:461–64.

Donker-Voet, J. 1962. A disease in ducklings caused by *Moraxella anatipestifer. Tijdschr. Diergeneesk.* 87:741–46.

Dougherty, E., L. Z. Saunders, and E. H. Parsons. 1955. The pathology of infectious serositis of ducks. *Am. J. Pathol.* 31:475–80.

Graham, R., C. A. Brandly, and G. L. Dunlap. 1938. Studies on duck septicemia. *Cornell Vet.* 28:1–8.

Hendrickson, J. M., and K. F. Hilbert. 1932. A new and serious septicemic disease of young ducks with a description of the causative organism, *Pfeifferella anatipestifer*, N.S. *Cornell Vet.* 22:239–52.

Jortner, B. S., R. Porro, and L. Leibovitz. 1969. Central-nervous system lesions of spontaneous *Pasteurella anatipestifer* infection in ducklings. *Avian Diseases* 8:27–35.

Levine, N. D. 1965. Goose influenza *(septicaemia anserum exsudativa)*, pp. 469–71. In

Biester, H. E., and L. H. Schwarte (eds.). *Diseases of Poultry*, 5th ed. Iowa State Univ. Press, Ames.

Loeffler, F. 1910. Ueber eine im Jahre 1904 in Klein-Kiesow bei Greifswald beobachtete Gaenseseuche. *Arch. Wiss. Prakt. Tierheilk* 36:289–98.

Marshall, J. D., Jr., P. A. Hansen, and W. C. Eveland. 1961. Histobacteriology of the genus *Pasteurella*. I. *Pasteurella anatipestifer. Cornell Vet.* 51:24–34.

Miklovichné Kis Csatári, M. 1965. A libainfluenza jarvanyos eloforfulasa hazankban. *Magy. Allatorv. Lapja* 20:148–51.

Pickrell, J. A. 1966. Pathologic changes associated with experimental *Pasteurella anatipestifer* infection in ducklings. *Avian Diseases* 10:281–83.

Riemer, Von Stabsarzt. 1904. Kurze Mitteilung ueber eine bei Gaensen beobachtete exsudative Septikaemie und deren Erreger. *Zentr. Bakteriol. Parasitenk. Abt. I. Orig.* 37:641–48.

Taylor, J. R. E. 1955. Studies on infectious serositis of ducks in Canada. *Proc. 27th Ann. Meet. Northeast Conf. Lab. Workers in Pullorum Disease Control.*

CHAPTER 6

TUBERCULOSIS

❖

ALFRED G. KARLSON, D.V.M., PH.D.
Consultant in Microbiology, Mayo Clinic
Professor of Comparative Pathology
Mayo Graduate School of Medicine
(University of Minnesota)
Rochester, Minnesota

❖

TUBERCULOSIS of poultry is a contagious disease caused by *Mycobacterium avium*. The disease is characterized by its chronicity, its persistence in a flock when once established, and its tendency to induce unthriftiness, decrease of egg production, and finally death.

Tuberculosis of chickens was first recognized as a related but separate entity by Cornil and Mégnin (1884). Koch (1890) maintained for many years that tubercle bacilli were always the same regardless of the species in which they might occur. However, Rivolta, and later Maffucci (1890), showed that the microorganism of tuberculosis of chickens is dissimilar to that of bovine tuberculosis. Koch (1902) finally abandoned his previous position and declared that tuberculosis of poultry is unlike tuberculosis of human beings and that the disease in man is dissimilar to that of cattle.

Although tuberculosis of chickens has long been recognized as a contagious disease, it has continued to spread throughout most of the world. With the available information on the nature of avian tuberculosis, its eradication is entirely feasible. The more important reasons for elimination of tuberculosis of poultry are as follows:

(1) affected birds are unthrifty; (2) tuberculous chickens are undesirable for human food; (3) diseased birds produce fewer eggs; (4) tuberculous chickens are the source of tuberculosis of sheep and especially of swine; (5) avian tubercle bacilli are capable of sensitizing cattle to mammalian tuberculin; (6) avian tubercle bacilli in a few instances have been isolated from lesions in man. Unfortunately, in the United States the presence of tuberculosis of chickens continues to be accepted with a certain complacency, and we have failed thus far to formulate a program that can be expected to eradicate the disease. The noteworthy results obtained in eradication of bovine tuberculosis should stimulate the attack on the disease in chickens.

INCIDENCE AND DISTRIBUTION

Tuberculosis of chickens is worldwide in distribution but occurs most frequently in the North Temperate Zone. The highest incidence of infection in the United States occurs in flocks of the north central states (Fig. 6.1), which include North Dakota, South Dakota, Kansas, Nebraska, Minnesota, Iowa, Missouri, Wisconsin, Illinois, Michigan, Indiana, and Ohio. Available data indicate that in some areas more than 50% of the flocks may be infected (USDA, 1969). The incidence of the disease in western and southern states is low. The explanation for this is not entirely obvious, although there are several possible contributing factors such as climate, flock management, and duration of the infection. The necessity to keep the birds closely confined during winter months provides favorable conditions for spread of the disease.

The difficulty of tuberculin-testing all chickens in the United States, or even a majority of the flocks, makes it impossible to obtain exact data on the incidence of tuberculous infection of chickens. Figures from meat inspection reports may be of interest. In 1968 tuberculosis was the cause for condemning 0.13% of 160.6 million mature hens slaughtered under federal inspection (USDA, 1969). However, this figure may be deceiving because the hens may not be representative of the average farm flock. Furthermore, visual inspection may not disclose all infected birds. Of particular interest is the finding by Schack-Steffenhagen and Seeger (1967) that *M. avium* was found in livers of 3.38% of ma-

Revision of a chapter prepared for previous editions by William H. Feldman, Emeritus Staff, Mayo Clinic, Rochester, Minn. The photographs are from previous editions.

MATURE CHICKENS INSPECTED

And Number Condemned for Tuberculosis

Fiscal Year 1968

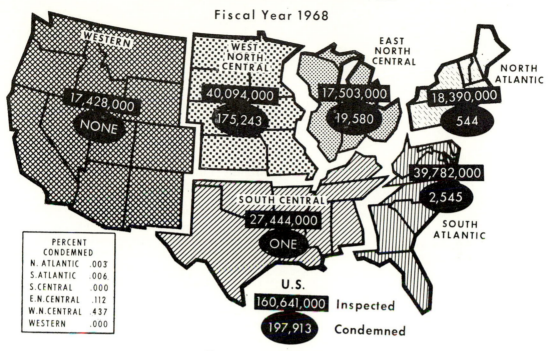

SOURCE: CROP REPORTING BOARD.

FIG. 6.1—Relative incidence of tuberculosis of poultry in United States based on data compiled by Agricultural Research Service, USDA. Note that highest percentage of condemnations for tuberculosis for the year 1968 was among chickens in 7 states comprising western north central area. (Courtesy A. F. Ranney, USDA)

ture chickens imported into Germany from the United States and Holland, including livers with no gross lesions.

In fiscal year 1968, tuberculin tests were done by the USDA in 15 states on 73 small flocks; 23 flocks or 31.5% had reactors (USDA, 1969). These figures may be misleading unless it is remembered that the incidence of infection varies greatly in different sections of the country. In fact there has been a significant reduction in the prevalence of the disease, due in considerable part to the changing concept of poultry husbandry. During the past several years increasing emphasis has been placed on the desirability of maintaining all-pullet flocks rather than adult birds.

In Canada the incidence of tuberculosis of chickens varies greatly in different areas—from 1 to 26%. Avian tuberculosis occurs in some Latin American countries but the incidence is variable—low in Bra-

zil, common in Uruguay, widespread in Venezuela as of 1946, and has been reported in Argentina. Isolated cases of avian tubercle bacillus infections in man have been found in various Latin American countries (Myers and Steele, 1969).

Considerable recent information exists on the occurrence of avian tuberculosis in certain European countries. It is said to be rare in Finland (Vasenius, 1965; Stenberg and Turunen, 1968) but is not uncommon in Norway (Fodstad, 1967) and Denmark (Andersen, 1965). Avian tuberculosis occurs in Germany (Hiller et al., 1967), Switzerland (Schneider and Riggenbach, 1963), Great Britain (Lesslie and Birn, 1967), Yugoslavia (Simeonov, 1967), and Poland (Bekajo, 1963). In Australia avian tuberculosis is unknown in Queensland and West Australia, but it does occur in other states (Kovacs, 1962). In South Africa the incidence of tuberculosis in poultry is low (Worthington, 1967). It is rare also in Kenya and Rhodesia (Myers and Steele, 1969). It is likely that in other countries infections occur in domestic and wild fowl, but the incidence and distribution cannot be determined because bacteriologic studies are not universally done. Tuberculosis in swine due to *M. avium* has been reported in countries other than the foregoing (Karlson, 1970) and in man (Kubin et al., 1966). Further discussion on the prevalence of tuberculosis in animals may be found in the report by Myers and Steele (1969).

AGE IN RELATION TO INCIDENCE

The incidence of infection depends on the age of the chickens. This is well illustrated by data obtained from reports on poultry slaughtered under federal inspection. From April through September 1968, a period of 6 months, 1,231 million young chickens were slaughtered; only 17 of these were recorded as having tuberculous lesions. In contrast, 67.7 million mature chickens were inspected and 47,382 had tuberculous lesions. It is of interest that the 17 tuberculous young chickens were reported from the western north central states and that 89% of the tuberculous mature hens were reported from this region (USDA, 1968). Schack-Steffenhagen and Seeger (1967) found *M. avium* in livers of 3.38% of mature chickens imported into Germany from Holland and from the United States but could not demonstrate the microorganisms in broilers. These authors concluded that tuberculosis is commoner in older birds.

Tuberculosis appears to be less prevalent in young fowl not because the younger birds are more resistant to infection but because in older birds the disease has had a greater opportunity to become established due to a longer period of exposure. Although tuberculous lesions are usually less severe in young chickens than in adult birds, extensive or generalized tuberculosis in young chickens has been observed. Such a bird is an important source of dissemination of virulent tubercle bacilli and must be considered a menace to other fowl and to susceptible mammals.

ETIOLOGY

The most characteristic feature of *M. avium* is its acid-fastness. The organisms are bacillary in character, but clublike, curved, and crooked forms are also seen in some preparations. Cords are not formed. Branching infrequently occurs. Most of the bacteria have rounded ends and vary in length from 1 to 3μ. Spores are not produced, and the organism is nonmotile. Reproduction of the avian tubercle bacillus is by simple fission. Spherical or conical granules occur in the endoplasm anywhere along the length of the bacterium.

CULTURAL DISTINCTIONS

The avian tubercle bacillus is not as exacting in its temperature requirements as are the human and bovine forms of the organism. The avian form will grow at temperatures ranging from 25 to 45° C, although the most favorable temperature is between 39 and 40° C. *M. avium* is aerobic. On original isolation, growth is enhanced by an atmosphere of 5–10% carbon dioxide (Stafseth et al., 1934).

For original isolation of the organisms from naturally infected material, one of the special media designed for culturing tubercle bacilli is desirable. Both glycerinated and nonglycerinated media are satisfactory, but the colonies are larger if the medium contains glycerin (Fig. 6.2). On media containing whole egg or egg yolk and incubated at 37.5–40° C, the bacteria usually will become evident in 10 days to 3 weeks as small, slightly raised, discrete, grayish white colonies. If the inoculum is rich in bacteria, the colonies will be numerous and may tend to coalesce into granulated masses, but there is slight if any tendency for the individual colonies to spread. The colonies are hemispherical and do not penetrate the medium. If the medium contains glycerin, the colonies gradually change from grayish white to light ocher. They become darker as the age of the culture increases. Karlson et al. (1962) described a culture of *M. avium* which was bright yellow but typical in all other respects.

Subcultures on solid media show evidence of growth within a few days and reach a maximal development in 3–4 weeks. Such cultures usually appear moist and unctuous, the surface eventually becoming roughened. The growth is creamy or sticky and is readily removable from the underlying medium. In liquid media growth occurs at the bottom as well as at

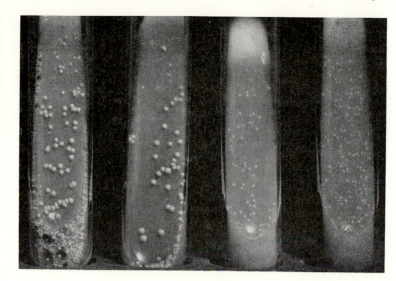

FIG. 6.2—Mycobacterium avium. Primary isolation on egg yolk agar showing enhancement of growth in the presence of glycerin (two slants at left) compared with growth on nonglycerinated medium (two slants at right).

the surface. Growth in liquid media usually may be dispersed readily by shaking to form a turbid suspension, which is in contrast to the flocculent or granular growth of mammalian tubercle bacilli.

A definite relationship appears to exist between type of colony and virulence. Moehring and Solotorovsky (1965) compared cultures isolated from tuberculous chickens and certain similar nonchromogenic mycobacteria from man and found that pure cultures with smooth, transparent colonies were virulent for chickens; in contrast, variants with smooth-domed or rough colonies were avirulent for chickens regardless of source. These results suggest that some nonchromogens or so-called Battey bacilli may be avirulent variants of *M. avium.*

Although most strains of *M. avium* are smooth and moist when first isolated, cultures of avian tubercle bacilli have been noted that were rough, dry, and crumbly. The occurrence of such strains is sufficient reason for caution in designating the type of any tubercle bacillus without tests for identification.

BIOCHEMICAL PROPERTIES

Cultures of *M. avium* and certain nonchromogenic strains from man and swine have been studied with an attempt to delineate differences. There appear to be no significant biochemical distinctions between avian tubercle bacilli known to be virulent for chickens and the nonchromogenic strains commonly called "Battey ba-

cilli" or "Group III mycobacteria" and having little or no virulence for chickens. However, this group (including *M. avium*), also called "*M. avium* complex," has features which separate it from other species or groups of mycobacteria.

M. avium does not produce niacin, does not hydrolyze Tween 80, is peroxidase-negative, produces catalase, does not have urease or arylsulfatase, and does not reduce nitrate; there are variations in these features, particularly in the results of tests for arylsulfatase. Mycobacteria possess amidases that appear to be specific for certain species or for closely related groups. For example, avian tubercle bacilli are singularly lacking in certain amidases except for pyrazinamidase and nicotinamidase (Bönicke, 1962).

Detailed discussions of the biochemical features of *M. avium* and related microorganisms may be found in Bönicke (1962), Kubín et al. (1966), Engbaek et al. (1968), and in Internationales Symposium über atypische Mykobakterien, *Z. Tuberk.* 127: 1–148, 1967.

SENSITIVITY IN VITRO TO ANTITUBERCULOSIS DRUGS

Generally speaking, *M. avium* is resistant to the commonly used antituberculosis drugs compared to *M. tuberculosis* and *M. bovis.* On approximately 50 strains of *M. avium* from chickens and swine and 11 from human patients, the author found that in egg yolk agar most strains will grow in 10 μg but not in 50 μg of streptomycin, in more than 10 μg of para-aminosalicylic acid, and in more than 40 μg of isoniazid/ml of medium. On the same kind of medium, a relative resistance was shown to ethambutol, ethionamide, viomycin, and pyrazinamide. The inhibitory concentration is variable, however, depending on the medium and procedure. Other reports are in agreement that *M. avium* has a high degree of resistance to antituberculosis agents (Kubín et al., 1966; Engbaek et al., 1968).

SEROLOGIC TYPES

The notable contributions of Schaefer (1965) have demonstrated a number of serotypes of *M. avium* which appear to be stable even during years of artificial culture. These studies indicate that strains of *M. avium* can be identified by serologic procedures, including those that have lost their virulence for fowl. Certain serotypes occur mainly in animals and others are found mainly among the Battey strains from human patients and from swine. Some serotypes of *M. avium* found in animals have also been isolated from man. The ability to identify stable serotypes of avian tubercle bacilli provides a means of studying origin and distribution of specific strains.

PATHOGENICITY

Fowl

All species of birds are capable of being infected with avian tubercle bacilli. Generally speaking, domesticated fowl are affected more frequently than those living in a wild state. Tuberculosis may occur in ducks, geese, swans, peacocks, pigeons, and turkeys. Parrots and canaries may be infected with avian tubercle bacilli. Reports of tuberculosis in domestic fowl other than chickens have been made by Scrivner and Elder (1931), Hinshaw et al. (1932), Hinshaw (1933a,b), Feldman (1938), Francis (1958), Huitema and Van Vloten (1959), Bekajlo (1963), and Vallette et al. (1967). Among wildfowl, tuberculosis is uncommon. However, in wild birds that frequent farm premises where tuberculosis is prevalent in chickens, the disease may be expected to develop. Pheasants seem to be unusually susceptible to infection by the avian tubercle bacillus; the disease has also been observed in sparrows, crows, barn owls, cowbirds, blackbirds, eastern sparrow hawks, starlings, and wood pigeons.

Accounts of tuberculosis in wild birds and reviews of the literature may be found in reports by Feldman (1938), McDiarmid (1948), Mitchell and Duthie (1950), Francis (1958), Høybråten (1959), Wilson and Macdonald (1965), Bickford et al. (1966), Švrček et al. (1966), Matějka and Kubín (1967), and Karlson et al. (1970).

Tuberculosis is common among birds in many zoological gardens. In the unnatural environment of captivity, the incidence of the disease frequently equals or even exceeds that for domestic species of fowl. The infectious agent in nearly all instances is the avian tubercle bacillus. Tuberculosis in the parrot is usually due to either the human or the bovine type of bacillus.

Ratcliffe (1946) presented evidence that the incidence of tuberculosis in captive wild birds was related to dietary factors that can be remedied. After a change of diet to provide adequate protein, vitamin B complex elements, vitamins A and D, and iodized salt, the frequency of the disease in the bird collection of the Philadelphia Zoological Garden was reduced significantly.

TURKEYS. Turkeys are not commonly affected with tuberculosis. The disease in most instances is contracted from infected chickens and is chronic in character. Information regarding tuberculosis in turkeys has been contributed by Hinshaw et al. (1932) who examined at necropsy a total of 88 birds; tuberculosis was found in 45, or 51.15%. The disease was found in only 1 of 11 birds less than 1 year of age, whereas 28 (65.12%) of 43 over 2 years of age were tuberculous. Additional information of the disease in turkeys may be found in Feldman (1938) and Francis (1958).

Mammals

The avian tubercle bacillus has a definite pathogenicity for some important species of domesticated mammals and at least a slight pathogenicity for others (Feldman, 1938; Francis, 1958). This fact should be recognized if the problem of eliminating tuberculosis is to be attacked and eventually solved.

Under conditions of natural exposure it is very exceptional for extensive tuberculosis due to avian tubercle bacilli to de-

TABLE 6.1 ❧ Comparative Pathogenicity of *Mycobacterium avium* for Certain Mammals

Animal	Susceptibility
Cat	Highly resistant
Cattle	Infection occurs; usually localized
Deer	Infection reported
Dog	Highly resistant
Goat	Assumed to be relatively resistant
Guinea pig	Relatively resistant
Hamster	Susceptible (intratesticularly)
Horse	Assumed to be highly resistant
Man	Highly resistant
Marsupials	Infection reported
Mink	Readily infected
Monkey	Highly resistant
Mouse	Relatively resistant
Rabbit	Readily infected
Rat	Relatively resistant
Sheep	Moderately susceptible
Swine	Readily infected

velop in mammals other than rabbits and swine. Infection may occur, but the disease in most mammals remains localized. However, the microorganisms may multiply in the tissues for a considerable period and induce sensitivity to tuberculin. Although spontaneous infection of mammals may not be of comparable severity to that which develops in fowl, it is possible to produce extensive changes in many species of mammals by introducing the infective agent artificially. The relative pathogenicity of *M. avium* for many of the domesticated mammals is summarized in Table 6.1.

CATTLE. Avian tubercle bacilli have a limited pathogenicity for cattle. The lesions usually remain localized, but a few cases of generalized tuberculosis due to *M. avium* have been described. Of particular importance is the sensitivity to mammalian tuberculin which may be induced in cattle by infection with *M. avium* (Karlson, 1962; Lesslie and Birn, 1967; Cassidy et al., 1968). The interpretation of the tuberculin test in cattle is difficult if tuberculous poultry or swine exist on the same premises.

In the United States the importance of avian tuberculosis is made clear by a recent report that avian tubercle bacilli were isolated from lesions in 10–20% of reactor cattle and from 50% of lesions in other slaughter cattle. Also avian tubercle bacilli were isolated from cattle that had reacted to the Johnin test but had no evidence of Johne's disease (Ranney, 1966). In Great Britain 11.2% of tubercle bacilli isolated from reactor cattle during 1953–65 were identified as *M. avium* (Lesslie and Birn, 1967). Concern about avian tuberculosis in cattle and the effect on eradication programs has been expressed in Norway (Fodstad, 1967), Denmark (Andersen, 1965), Germany (Schliesser, 1967), and Czeckoslovakia (Matějka and Kubín, 1967). Additional accounts of *M. avium* infection in cattle may be found by referring to the reports cited herein.

SWINE. In an infected environment swine readily become infected with avian tubercle bacilli. Since the beginning of federal supervision of abattoirs in the United States, it has been noted that the incidence of tuberculosis in swine exceeds that in cattle. Among approximately 72.3 million swine slaughtered during fiscal year 1968, there were 981,947 or 1.35% retained as suspect for tuberculous lesions. In the same year 28.1 million cattle were examined and only 1,509 or 0.005% were retained for tuberculosis (USDA, 1969).

The explanation for the great difference in the incidence of tuberculous lesions in swine compared to that in cattle became apparent many years ago when it was established that most of the disease in swine was due to the avian tubercle bacillus (Van Es and Martin, 1925; Graham and Tunnicliff, 1926). Tuberculosis will remain an unnecessary economic burden on the swine industry until the disease is eliminated from chickens and other barnyard fowl. Data presented in Table 6.2 reveal a grad-

TABLE 6.2 ❧ Incidence of Tuberculosis in Swine as Determined in Federally Inspected Abattoirs (USDA, 1969)

Fiscal Year	Number Slaughtered	Percent Retained*	Condemned on Final Inspection Number	Condemned on Final Inspection Percent
1932	45,852,422	11.4	37,509	0.08
1937	36,226,309	9.5	15,854	0.04
1942	50,133,871	8.0	13,357	0.03
1947	45,073,370	8.5	10,756	0.02
1952	63,965,522	4.4	10,368	0.016
1957	62,238,519	2.9	7,146	0.011
1962	67,109,539	2.2	5,503	0.008
1967	68,675,841	1.5	4,080	0.006
1968	72,325,507	1.3	3,951	0.005

* Carcasses suspected of tuberculosis and retained for additional inspection.

ual but definite decrease of tuberculosis in swine in the United States. A similar decrease has been noted in Canada (J. F. Frank, 1968, personal communication), Denmark (Andersen, 1965), and Germany (Schliesser, 1967). One reason for a decrease in prevalence of tuberculosis in swine may be the lowering of the incidence in poultry as a result of the increasing practice of maintaining all-pullet flocks (Karlson, 1970).

MAN. The literature contains a number of instances in which it was claimed that avian tubercle bacilli were responsible for a tuberculous infection in human beings. However, very few of the published reports of such cases contain unequivocal proof necessary to substantiate the diagnosis. Although tuberculosis in chickens is rather common in the United States, the first case in human beings in this country with adequate proof was not published until 1947 (Feldman) followed by a second case in 1949 (Feldman et al.).

With the decline in incidence of tuberculosis in man, an increasing interest is being given to mycobacteria other than *M. tuberculosis*. The result is that an increasing number of infections with *M. avium* are being recognized.

Most of the infections in man have involved the pulmonary system and have in some cases been associated with pulmonary silicosis (Karlson and Feldman, 1953; Karlson et al., 1955). Involvement of the skin and lymph nodes has been seen. The relatively uncommon occurrence of avian tubercle bacillus infection in man, even where the disease is common in poultry, indicates that human beings are extremely resistant to this infection. Details of the reported cases may be found in reviews of the literature by Forschbach et al. (1965), Kubín et al. (1966), Tacquet et al. (1966), and Schack-Steffenhagen et al. (1966), each of which has many references.

PATHOGENESIS AND EPIZOOTIOLOGY

TRANSMISSION

Of primary importance in the establishment of an infected environment are certain factors characteristic of the disease in the natural host. The tremendous number of tubercle bacilli exuded from ulcerated tuberculous lesions of the intestine creates a constant source of virulent bacteria. Although other sources of infection exist, there is none that equals infective fecal material in the dissemination of avian tuberculosis. Fecal discharges may contain tubercle bacilli from lesions of the liver and of the mucosa of the gallbladder expelled through the common duct. The respiratory tract is also a potential source of infection, especially if lesions occur in the tracheal mucosa.

The infective environment, comprising as it does the bacilli-laden soil and litter, is the factor of greatest importance in transmission of the disease to noninfected animals. The longer the premises have been occupied by infected birds and the more concentrated the poultry population, the more prevalent the infection is likely to be.

Avian tubercle bacilli may persist in soil for a long time. Schalk et al. (1935) found an infected barnyard to have viable and virulent *M. avium* in the litter and soil after 4 years. These workers could also demonstrate that the bacteria remained viable in carcasses buried 3 feet deep for 27 months. This ability of avian tubercle bacilli to survive outside the host presents a serious hazard to poultry and swine.

Role of Eggs

The possibility that avian tuberculosis might be transmitted through the eggs from tuberculous hens has long been a pertinent point. The problem has been approached in two ways: (1) by inoculating eggs with tubercle bacilli and noting whether or not tuberculosis develops in the birds hatched from the infected eggs, and (2) by observing whether or not tuberculosis develops in chickens hatched from eggs from naturally infected hens. It has been demonstrated many times that some of the artificially inoculated eggs will hatch and that the chicks hatched from such eggs will be infected with tubercle bacilli. From a practical point of view, such observations are of doubtful importance to the fundamental question: Are eggs from naturally infected chickens likely to produce tuberculous chicks? The most convincing evidence to the contrary is that furnished by the investigations of Fitch and Lubbehusen (1928) and Schalk et al. (1935), who raised many hundreds of chicks hatched from eggs of naturally infected hens without tuberculosis having been observed in a single instance. Similar conclusions have been made by others (Feldman, 1938; Francis, 1958). However, *M. avium* has been isolated by culture of eggs from naturally infected chickens. In Germany Fritzsche and Allam (1965) found that avian tubercle bacilli were demonstrable in 3.55% of 899 eggs from 58 flocks in which avian tuberculosis existed. In contrast, of 650 eggs from 7 commercial poultry farms only 0.31% had *M. avium;* these came from a single large farm where a few tuberculin-positive chickens were found. Also, these workers found that avian tubercle bacilli would not survive in eggs after 6 minutes of boiling; in the preparation of scrambled eggs 2 minutes of frying was sufficient to kill the bacteria. Studies in Poland by Bojarski (1968) revealed that *M. avium* could be cultured from 8% of 175 eggs from naturally infected hens. However, avian tubercle bacilli were recovered by culture from 8 (33.3%) of 24 eggs from artificially infected hens.

Other Sources

Other sources of dissemination of avian tubercle bacilli are carcasses of tuberculous fowl that die of the disease and offal from chickens that are dressed for food. It is also conceivable that cannibalism might play a part in the transmission of tuberculosis from one chicken to another.

Avian tubercle bacilli may be transmitted from one place to another by persons whose shoes have become soiled with fecal matter of the poultry yard. The equipment used in care and maintenance of infected poultry flocks (crates and feed sacks) also might be responsible for transfer of infective bacteria from diseased to healthy flocks.

As previously mentioned, wild birds and pigeons may be infected with avian tubercle bacilli and are therefore capable of spreading *M. avium* to poultry flocks. Swine may have ulcerative intestinal lesions due to avian tubercle bacilli and thus constitute a source of infection for other animals and birds. Birds such as sparrows, starlings, and pigeons that feed in farm yards are potential sources of avian tuberculosis.

SIGNS

Few symptoms of the disease in chickens are pathognomonic. However, if the disease is prevalent in a flock, several or most of the signs may be evident in different birds.

Ordinarily if the infection has progressed sufficiently to affect the physical condition, the bird will be less lively than its mates.

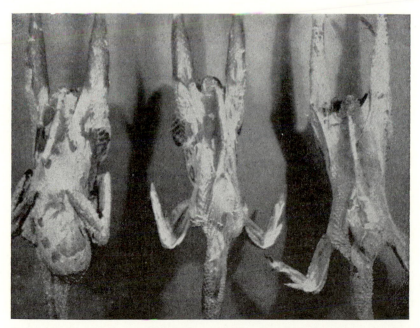

FIG. 6.3—Carcasses of tuberculous chickens from flock in which disease was rampant. Note extreme atrophy of pectoral muscles.

The affected fowl fatigues easily and appears depressed. Although the appetite usually remains good, a progressive and striking loss of weight commonly occurs. The thinness of the tuberculous bird is especially noticeable in the breast muscles (Fig. 6.3). The pectoral muscles are often atrophied, and the breastbone becomes strikingly prominent and may be deformed. In extreme instances most of the body fat eventually disappears, and the face of the affected bird appears smaller than it would normally.

The feathers assume a dull and ruffled appearance. The comb, wattles, and earlobes often become anemic and thinner than normal, and the uncovered epidermis has a peculiar dryness. Occasionally, however, the comb and wattles have a bluish discoloration. Icterus, indicative of hepatic changes, may be noted.

Even though the disease is severe, the temperature of the affected bird remains within the normal range. In many instances the bird reveals a unilateral lameness and walks with a peculiar jerky, hopping gait, probably due to tuberculous involvement of the bone marrow of the leg. Infrequently a wing may droop, owing to tuberculous involvement of the humeral scapulocoracoid articulation which may rupture and discharge thin or caseous material. Paralysis due to tuberculous arthritis sometimes occurs.

If the affected chicken is greatly emaciated, one may detect nodular masses along the intestine by palpation of the abdomen. The great hypertrophy of the liver of many tuberculous birds, however, may make this procedure difficult or impossible. Most tuberculous chickens have lesions along the intestinal tract, and if these are ulcerative, severe diarrhea results. The enteric disturbance induces extreme weakness, and the affected bird assumes a sitting position as a result of exhaustion.

Affected birds may die within a few months or live for many months, depending on the severity or extent of the disease. An affected bird may die suddenly as a consequence of hemorrhage from rupture of the affected liver or spleen.

In summary, the presence of tuberculosis in a poultry flock is suggested by (1) unthriftiness, (2) gradual loss of weight, (3) wasting of the breast muscles, and (4) loss of color in the comb and wattles.

However, such signs lead only to a presumptive diagnosis. The most expedient way to diagnose the disease is by postmortem examination. The lesions are rather characteristic, but some other conditions must be differentiated from tuberculosis. These include neoplasia, enterohepatitis, and possibly fowl cholera and fowl typhoid. The presence of numerous acid-fast bacilli in the lesions is especially significant because they do not occur in any other known disease of chickens.

GROSS LESIONS

Lesions of the disease are seen most frequently in the liver, spleen, intestines, and bone marrow. The bacillemia, which probably occurs intermittently and perhaps early in most instances, provides for a generalized distribution of lesions. None of the tissues, with the possible exception of the central nervous system, appears to be immune from infection. Some of the organs such as the heart, ovaries, testes, and skin are affected infrequently and cannot be considered organs of predilection. Wojaczek-Steffke (1964) reviewed some of the reports on the distribution of lesions in tuberculous chickens and presented his own findings. Of 306 tuberculin-positive chickens, 260 had tuberculous lesions distributed as follows: liver 77%, lungs 44%, spleen 43.5%, intestine 11.5%, and ceca 4.0%. In addition, lesions were found in the air sacs five times, kidneys twice, myocardium twice, and bursa of Fabricius once. Francis (1958) reviewed the available literature and found that for turkeys, ducks, and pigeons the lesions predominate in liver and spleen but occur also in many other organs.

The distribution of lesions in the turkey as found by Hinshaw et al. (1932) was as follows: liver 95.6%, spleen 67.3%, intestine 45.6%, lungs 32.6%, ovaries 32.2%, thymus 29%, testes 25%, mesentery 21.7%, pancreas 12.9%, muscle 11.7%, bones 7.4%, skin 6.2%, gizzard 5.7%, esophagus 4.7%, pericardium 4.5%, proventriculus 3.7%, kidneys 3.5%, oviduct 3%, and myocardium 2.2%.

Tuberculosis in fowl is characterized by the occurrence of irregular grayish yellow or grayish white nodules of varying sizes in the organs of predilection such as liver, spleen, and intestine (Figs. 6.4, 6.5, 6.6). Involvement of the liver and spleen results in hypertrophy which is often significant.

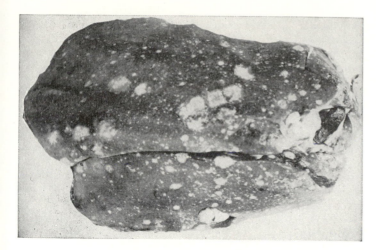

FIG. 6.4—*Tuberculous lesions in liver of naturally infected chicken.*

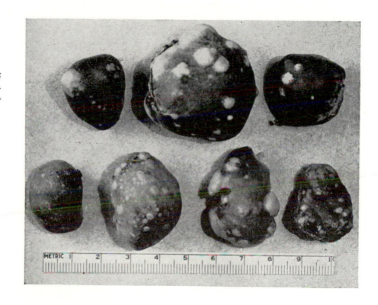

FIG. 6.5—*Spleens from chickens naturally infected with tuberculosis. Note variation in number and size of lesions.*

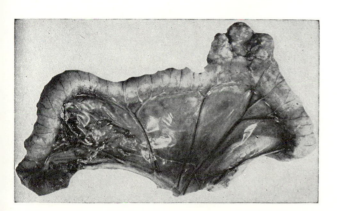

FIG. 6.6—*Large nodulated lesions of tuberculosis in wall of small intestine of chicken.*

Fatal hemorrhage may result from rupture of the enlarged liver or spleen. The tuberculous nodule varies in size from a structure that is barely discernible to a huge mass that may measure serveral centimeters in diameter. Large nodules frequently have an irregular knobby contour, with smaller granulations or nodules often present over the surface. Lesions near the surface in such organs as the liver and spleen are enucleated easily from the adjacent tissues. The nodules are firm but can be incised easily since mineral salts are not present. On cross section a fibrous nodule containing a variable number of small yellowish foci or a single soft, yellowish central region, which is frequently caseous, may be observed. The latter is surrounded by a fibrous capsule, the continuity of which often is interrupted by small circumscribed necrotic foci. The fibrous capsule varies in thickness and consistency depending on the size and duration of the lesions. It is barely discernible or apparently absent in the smaller lesions and measures 0.1–0.2 cm in thickness in the larger nodules.

The number of lesions is also variable, ranging from a few to innumerable. It is rather common to observe a few nodular lesions in organs such as the liver and spleen associated with an enormous number of lesions of minute to moderate size. The variation in size of such lesions is a consequence of successive episodes of reinfection from previously established lesions, usually of the same organ. Involvement of the lungs is usually less severe than that of the liver or spleen (Fig. 6.7).

The marked tendency of the disease to disseminate to several organs indicates that tuberculous bacillemia is common. This tendency of the bacilli to circulate with the bloodstream provides the explanation for frequent involvement of the bone marrow (Figs. 6.8, 6.9). Infection of the bone marrow probably occurs very early in the course of the disease and is characterized by hypertrophy of the myeloid tissues, by disappearance of most of the bony spicules, and finally by the formation of tuberculous nodules which may be numerous and visible to the unaided eye or few and microscopic.

HEMATOLOGY

Reliable data on the effects of a natural tuberculous infection on the circulating blood of chickens are somewhat meager. Some workers have reported anemia associated with a reduction in total number of erythrocytes. Other observations have indicated that a marked increase occurs in the number of large lymphocytes and a decrease in the small lymphocytes. The work of Olson and Feldman (1936) on a relatively small number of naturally infected chickens indicated that the erythrocyte and thrombocyte counts and the values for hemoglobin were within the limits of normal. Although in this material the disease was presumably of long duration, anemia was not observed. Leukocytosis was the most striking and consistent finding, the

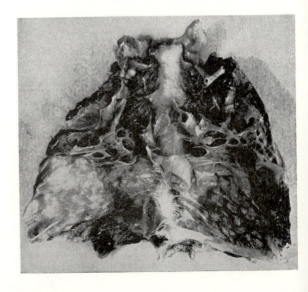

FIG. 6.7—Massive tuberculous involvement of lung of naturally infected chicken.

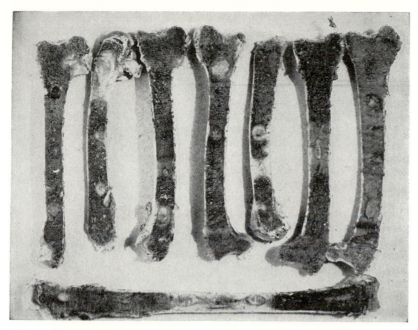

FIG. 6.8—Several femurs and one tibia from chickens naturally infected with tuberculosis showing lesions in myeloid tissue and some well-marked osteoplastic changes due to the infection.

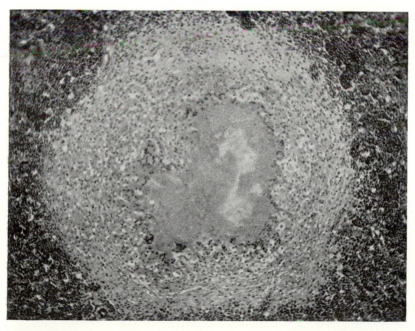

FIG. 6.9—Small tuberculous nodule in bone marrow of naturally infected chicken. Central necrotic region is surrounded by zone of dense connective tissue. ×100.

number of monocytes and heterophils being increased. The degree of leukocytosis was, for the most part, in direct ratio to the extent and severity of the disease.

HISTOPATHOLOGY

In chickens the tubercle may be observed experimentally 10–14 days after infection occurs as a closely packed collection of pale-staining cells with vesiculated nuclei. These epithelioid cells are derived from fixed tissue elements known as histiocytes (Fig. 6.10). The latter cells phagocytose tubercle bacilli early in the reactive process.

The cellular mass, or primary tubercle, gradually expands as histiocytes proliferate at the periphery, and within 3–4 weeks signs of retrogression can be detected in the epithelioid cells of the central zone. This retrogression is due partly to the avascularity of the structure and partly to the toxic substances of the tubercle bacilli. As the cellular mass becomes larger, the epithelioid cells have a tendency to fuse and form syncytia. The outlines of the individual cells become less distinct or disappear. Vacuoles appear, and the staining reaction is more acidophilic. This is followed within a week or so by a necrobiotic change resembling coagulation necrosis. The nuclei of the epithelioid cells become pyknotic and may disappear, while the cellular mass, excepting the peripheral portion, becomes fused and stains deeply with eosin. The tubercle bacilli have multiplied and appear singly or in clumps throughout the necrotic tissue.

While the epithelioid cells in the central zone undergo necrobiotic changes, there persists an outer zone of epithelioid syncytia which appears as a mantle around the entire periphery. From these, giant cells are developed. The nuclei of the giant cells are situated distally to the central zone of necrosis, and the cells are arranged rather frequently in palisade formation. Large vacuoles often occur in the cytoplasm of the giant cells. Immediately peripheral to the zone of giant cells there occurs a more or less diffuse collection of epithelioid cells and their progenitors, histiocytes (Fig. 6.11). Fibrocytes and minute blood vascular channels also occur near the outer portion of the peripheral area. Although tubercle bacilli are more numerous in the central or necrotic zone of the tubercle, they also occur in large numbers in the epithelioid zone, adjacent and distal to the giant cells.

The final phase in the formation of a tubercle is the development of a zone of encapsulation consisting of fibrous con-

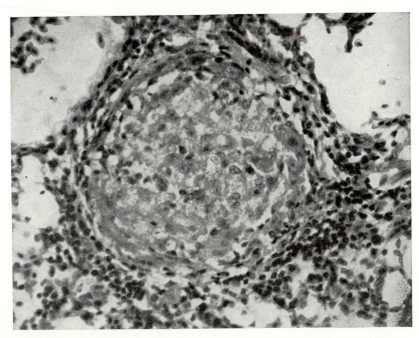

FIG. 6.10—Young epithelioid tubercle in lung of chicken. ×440.

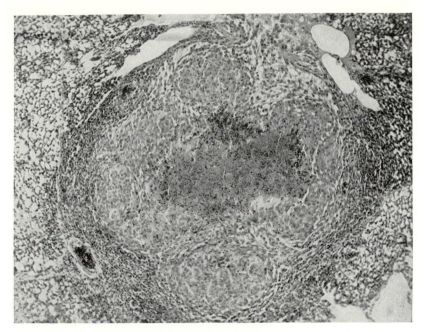

FIG. 6.11—Developing tubercle in lung of chicken showing activity of third or tuberculogenic zone. ×100.

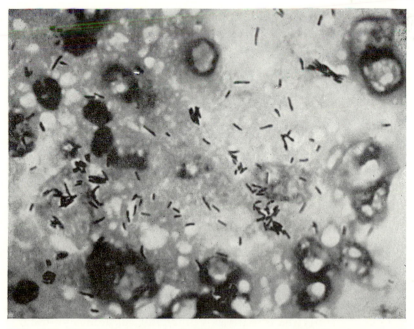

FIG. 6.12—Numerous tubercle bacilli in smear preparation from small lesion of lung of naturally infected chicken. Ziehl-Neelsen, ×1,600.

nective tissue, histiocytes, some lymphocytes, and an occasional eosinophilic granulocyte. New tubercles develop in the epithelioid zone immediately peripheral to the giant cells. As a consequence, a tubercle as recognized grossly consists of the original or parent tubercle and several smaller or adjacent ones.

The nature of the degenerative process which occurs in the central zone of the tubercle is somewhat unusual in that the integrity of the cells is maintained for a considerable period before disintegration. Caseation necrosis eventually occurs and may affect all or part of the central zone.

Calcification of the tubercle occurs rarely in fowl. Amyloidlike degeneration of portions of the surrounding parenchymal elements sometimes is observed in the liver, spleen, and kidney.

Acid-fast bacilli occur in great numbers in smears of lesions and in appropriately stained sections (Fig. 6.12).

Microscopically, lesions of tuberculosis in the turkey vary considerably. In some, tubercles like those seen in tuberculosis of chickens are present. In other instances the lesions are diffuse with extensive destruction of the surrounding parenchyma. Cytoplasmic masses or large giant cells may be numerous, and large numbers of eosinophilic granulocytes are commonly present. Some of the lesions become circumscribed by a broad, dense zone of fibrous connective tissue. Conditions that may simulate tuberculosis and which must be excluded from the diagnosis are mycosis, enterohepatitis, and certain forms of neoplasia. Proof of diagnosis is dependent on laboratory studies to establish the microorganism as *M. avium*.

Detailed descriptions of gross and microscopic lesions of tuberculosis in the different organs of chickens will be found in Feldman (1938) and Francis (1958).

DIAGNOSIS

A presumptive diagnosis of tuberculosis in fowl can usually be made on the basis of gross lesions. However, finding acid-fast organisms in smears of infected liver, spleen, or other organs stained with a stain such as the Ziehl-Neelsen is very helpful in diagnosis. The inoculation of suitable media to isolate and identify the causative agent is necessary for a definite diagnosis of avian tuberculosis.

TUBERCULIN TEST

When administered properly, the tuberculin test provides a satisfactory procedure for determining whether or not tuberculosis is present in a flock.

Technique

The equipment consists of a sterile tuberculin syringe (1-ml capacity) and a supply of sterile hypodermic needles one-half inch (1.3 cm) in length and of 25–26 gauge. Absorbent cotton and 70% alcohol should also be available. The tuberculin should be that prepared for intradermic use from avian tubercle bacilli. Tuberculin prepared from mammalian strains of tubercle bacilli may elicit positive reactions in tuberculous chickens, but the results are generally unsatisfactory. The reactions to avian tuberculin are usually more pronounced.

The bird should be restrained so that the head is entirely immobile. The surface of the wattle should be cleaned with alcohol; other attempts to clean or disinfect the skin are unnecessary. The needle is inserted carefully into the lateral aspect of the dermis, and 0.03–0.05 ml of tuberculin is forced into the tissue. A small bleb or a small diffuse blanched area will appear where the tuberculin was deposited. Although fairly satisfactory results may follow if the tuberculin is injected into the subcutaneous tissue, it is a better practice to inject the tuberculin intradermally.

Reaction

After 48 hours the chickens are examined. The opposite uninjected wattle is used for comparison. A positive reaction is indicated by soft swelling in the tissues of the injected wattle (Fig. 6.13). Some reactions are small; others result in pronounced swelling which increases the thickness of the wattle 1–5 times. The swelling is due largely to edema which occurs in the zone of connective tissue that lies between the layers of the dermis. To a lesser extent the swelling is due to the increased width of the corium, which is filled with closely packed mononuclear histiocytic cells, a few eosinophilic granulocytes, and a variable number of lymphoid cells and lymphocytes. After 48 hours the swelling gradually subsides and usually disappears within 5 days.

Sometimes a negative reaction will ap-

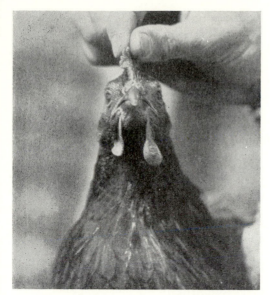

FIG. 6.13—*Positive reaction in left wattle of tuberculous chicken 48 hours after intradermal injection of avian tuberculin.*

pear in a bird that is definitely tuberculous, and conversely a positive result is sometimes obtained in chickens in which signs of tuberculosis cannot be demonstrated. In the latter instance, failure to find lesions of tuberculosis does not imply that tubercle bacilli are not present in the tissues of the chicken. If the disease is in an early stage, lesions are likely to be too small to be noted grossly or too few to be found by the ordinary methods of examination. A definitely positive tuberculin test indicates that the bird has been exposed to avian tubercle bacilli.

Tuberculin is a bacteria-free concentrated filtrate prepared from a liquid culture of tubercle bacilli and, as used for the diagnosis of tuberculosis in chickens, may be considered harmless to normal birds. If retests are done after an interval of one month, false positive reactions will not occur. In other words, in chickens the usual diagnostic dose of tuberculin does not sensitize the nontuberculous bird to subsequent injections of the same product.

The preparation of tuberculin for veterinary use in the United States is briefly described by Karlson (1967).

The tuberculin test has been utilized to a limited extent in diagnosing tuberculosis of turkeys. However, for the most part the results have been less satisfactory than for chickens. Certain difficulties are encountered also in tuberculin testing of pigeons and ducks. For pigeons Švrček et al. (1966) applied the test in the submandibular area. For Japanese quail the tuberculin may be injected intradermally in the area around the vent (Karlson et al., 1970). Generally speaking, the test is of limited value in diagnosing tuberculosis in these birds.

The usefulness of the tuberculin test in the diagnosis of tuberculosis in turkeys has not been adequately established. Hinshaw et al. (1932), using avian tuberculin, injected the snood, the mucosa of the anus, the wattle, the skin of the edge of the wing web, and the skin at the center of the wing web. The results of the tests indicated that (1) the reactions in the wattle agreed with the findings at postmortem examination in only 11.1% of the birds, and (2) there was agreement between the tuberculin reaction in the wing web and the findings at postmortem examination in 75.68% of the animals. From the meager information available, one must conclude that the intradermic tuberculin test has been less reliable for detecting tuberculosis in turkeys than in chickens. It would seem desirable to investigate the reliability of the rapid agglutination test as a means of detecting tuberculosis in live turkeys.

RAPID AGGLUTINATION TEST

A whole-blood agglutination test of possible diagnostic value for tuberculosis in fowl was described by Karlson et al. (1950). The antigen is a 10% suspension of avian tubercle bacilli in 0.85% sodium chloride solution containing 0.5% phenol. Blood is obtained by pricking the comb with a sharp instrument such as an 18-gauge needle. A drop of the fresh blood is mixed with a drop of the antigen on a warm plate. The appearance of agglutination in 1 minute is considered a positive test, as shown in Figure 6.14.

Observations indicate that in chickens the whole-blood agglutination test may have a reliability comparable to that of the tuberculin test. Recently Hiller et al. (1967) reported studies comparing the agglutination test and the tuberculin test in flocks where, on the same farm, so-called nonspecific tuberculin reactions were found in cattle. In 290 flocks, 38.3% of the birds reacted to the serologic test compared to 18.4% to the tuberculin test. Of 501 chick-

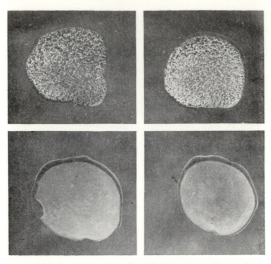

FIG. 6.14—*Results of four tests from four different chickens, two of which were tuberculous and two of which were not.*

Preparations illustrated in upper row show characteristic agglutination. Blood was obtained from chickens that had reacted positively to tuberculin, and lesions of tuberculosis were found at necropsy. Preparations shown in the lower row failed to agglutinate. Negative reactions agreed with results of tuberculin tests, and at necropsy lesions were not found. (From Karlson et al., 1950. Reproduction by permission of Am. J. Vet. Res.)

ens reacting only to the serologic test, 77.2% had postmortem or bacteriologic evidence of tuberculosis. It was concluded that the agglutination test was more useful than the tuberculin test for detecting infected birds in a diseased flock; however, the occurrence of false positive agglutination reactions in healthy birds is a drawback. The procedure offers certain practical advantages. The birds need to be handled only once, and samples of blood submitted for agglutination tests for pullorum disease may also be examined for the presence of specific mycobacterial agglutinins. The reliability of the rapid agglutination test as a diagnostic procedure for the detection of tuberculosis in other fowl should be explored.

PREVENTION AND CONTROL

The widespread distribution of the disease, its high incidence in some areas, and the importance of the poultry and the swine industries make it imperative that measures be devised for control and eradication of the disease.

The tuberculin test is of considerable practical value. The removal of chickens that react eliminates many foci of infection. The test enables one to detect many infected fowl before the disease reaches a severe or chronic state, and if repeated tests are made and reactors are removed, dissemination of the bacteria to the environment may be reduced. The whole-blood agglutination test also may serve to detect infected birds. Hiller et al (1967) concluded from their investigations that this rapid serologic test was more useful than the tuberculin test for detecting tuberculous chickens in a diseased flock.

If the residual flock is permitted to occupy the same infective premises, a continuing source of infection remains. This provides opportunity for new infections to occur indefinitely since in the soil avian tubercle bacilli may remain viable and virulent for years. Furthermore, neither the tuberculin test nor the agglutination test can be depended on with certainty for detection of every tuberculous fowl. As long as one infected bird remains in a flock, dissemination of the disease to healthy fowls is possible. Consequently, means other than the tuberculin test must be resorted to if a more satisfactory control of avian tuberculosis is to be expected.

It has been stated frequently that avian tuberculosis can be controlled if all birds in the flock are disposed of after the first laying season. This practice has much to commend it, especially since it is economically sound from the point of view of egg production. Older birds usually produce fewer eggs than the younger ones, and, furthermore, the mortality from nonbacterial diseases such as neoplasia is greater among older hens than among pullets. Another factor in favor of the disposal of the older stock is that tuberculosis is usually more severe in the older birds, which are as a consequence more likely to become depots of dissemination.

Procedures for establishing and maintaining tuberculosis-free flocks should include the following: (1) Abandon the old equipment and establish other facilities on new soil. Ordinarily it is impractical to render an infected environment satisfactorily safe by disinfection. (2) Provide proper fencing or other measures to prevent unrestricted movement of chickens, thus preventing exposure from previously infected premises. (3) Eliminate the old flock, burning the carcasses of birds that show lesions of tuberculosis. (4) Establish a new flock in the new environment from tuberculosis-free stock. (5) Eliminate from the swine herd all reactors to avian and mammalian tuberculin. If the chickens in a clean flock are prevented from having access to an infected environment and are protected against accidental exposure to tubercle bacilli, it is reasonable to believe they will remain free from tuberculosis.

The measures just mentioned for the elimination of avian tuberculosis are not complicated. The additional profits that will accrue from a tuberculosis-free flock maintained in a hygienic environment will compensate for the initial expense and work necessary to establish the new flock

and new facilities. Furthermore, the general health of the birds will be better, and diseases other than tuberculosis will be controlled more satisfactorily. The benefits will also be reflected in a decrease in tuberculosis in swine. The importance of avian tuberculosis in the infection of swine is such that if chickens were maintained entirely separate and apart from swine, the incidence of tuberculosis of swine due to *M. avium* would be reduced.

Recommendations for the control of tuberculosis in turkeys include the following: (1) Prevent contact with tuberculous chickens; premises and housing previously used by tuberculous chickens are to be avoided. (2) When tuberculosis is discovered in a flock of turkeys, the entire flock should be destroyed. (3) If a flock is to be reestablished, the new stock should be limited to day-old poults.

REFERENCES

Andersen, S. 1965. Fjerkraetuberkulosens udbredelse i Danmark. *Medlemsbl. danske. Dyrlaeg.* 2:54–59.

Bekajlo, R. 1963. Wytepowanie grulicy u g'si rzeznych. *Med. Weterynar. (Poland)* 19:254–55.

Bickford, A. A., G. H. Ellis, and H. E. Moses. 1966. Epizootiology of tuberculosis in starlings. *J. Am. Vet. Med. Ass.* 149:312–18.

Bojarski, J. 1968. Badania nad wystepowaniem *Mycobacterium* w jajach kur tuberkulinododatnech. *Med. Weterynar. (Poland)* 24:21–23.

Bönicke, R. 1962. Identification of mycobacteria by biochemical methods. *Bull. Int. Union Against Tuberc.* 32:13–68.

Cassidy, D. R., L. G. Morehouse, and H. A. McDaniel. 1968. *Mycobacterium avium* infection in cattle: A case series. *Am. J. Vet. Res.* 29:405–10.

Cornil, V., and P. Mégnin. 1884. Tuberculose et diphtherie des gallinaces. *Compt. Rend. Soc. Biol.* 36:617–21.

Engbaek, H. C., B. Vergmann, I. Baess, and M. W. Bentzon. 1968. *Mycobacterium avium:* A bacteriological and epidemiological study of *M. avium* isolated from animals and man in Denmark. Part 1. Strains isolated from animals. Part 2. Strains isolated from man. *Acta Pathol. Microbiol. Scand.* 72:277–312.

Feldman, W. H. 1938. Avian tuberculosis infections. Williams & Wilkins Co., Baltimore.

———. 1947. Animal tuberculosis and its relationship to the disease in man. *Ann. N.Y. Acad. Sci.* 48:469–505.

Feldman, W. H., D. W. Hutchinson, V. M.

Schwarting, and A. G. Karlson. 1949. Juvenile tuberculous infection, possibly of avian type. *Am. J. Pathol.* 25:1183–95.

Fitch, C. P., and R. E. Lubbehusen. 1928. Completed experiments to determine whether avian tuberculosis can be transmitted through the eggs of tuberculous fowls. *J. Am. Vet. Med. Ass.* 72:636–49.

Fodstad, F. H. 1967. En oversikt over mycobakterielle infeksjoner hos dyr påvist i Norge i 1966. *Medl. bl. Norske Veterinaerforen.* 19:314–27.

Forschbach, G., G. Kielwein, and K. Dedié. 1965. Kritische Stellungnahme zum Nachweis des *Mycobacterium avium* in vom Menschen stammenden Untersuchungsmaterial. *Prax. Pneumol.* 19:204–17.

Francis, J. 1958. *Tuberculosis in Animals and Man: A Study in Comparative Pathology.* Cassell and Co., London.

Fritzsche, K., and M. S. A. M. Allam. 1965. Ein Beitrag zur Frage der Kontamination der Huehnerei mit Mycobakterien. *Arch. Lebensmittelhyg.* 16:248–50.

Graham, R., and E. A. Tunnicliff. 1926. Fowl tuberculosis in swine. *Trans. Ill. State Acad. Sci.* 19:138–43.

Hiller, K., T. Schliesser, G. Fink, and P. Dorn. 1967. Zur serologischen Diagnose der Huehnertuberkulose. *Berlin. Muench. Tieraerztl. Wochschr.* 80:212–16.

Hinshaw, W. R. 1933a. Tuberculosis of avian origin in Muscovy ducks. *J. Am. Vet. Med. Ass.* 82:111–13.

———. 1933b. Tuberculosis of human origin in an Amazon parrot. *Am. Rev. Tuberc.* 28:273–78.

Hinshaw, W. R., K. W. Niemann, and W. H.

Busic. 1932. Studies of tuberculosis of turkeys. *J. Am. Vet. Med. Ass.* 80:765–77.

Høybråten, P. 1959. Tuberkulosetilfeller hos fugler. *Nord. Veterinarmed.* 11:780–86.

Huitema, H., and J. Van Vloten. 1959. Aviare tuberculose. *Tijdschr. Diergeneesk.* 84:6–30.

Karlson, A. G. 1962. Nonspecific or cross-sensitivity reactions to tuberculin in cattle, pp. 147–81. In Brandly, C. A., and E. L. Jungherr, *Advances in Veterinary Science*. Academic Press, New York.

———. 1967. The genus Mycobacterium, pp. 441–65. In Merchant, I. A., and R. A. Packer (eds.), *Veterinary Bacteriology and Virology*, Iowa State Univ. Press, Ames.

———. 1970. Tuberculosis in swine. In Dunne, H. W. (ed.), *Diseases of Swine*. Iowa State Univ. Press, Ames.

Karlson, A. G., and W. H. Feldman. 1953. Mycobacteria of human origin resembling *Mycobacterium avium*. *Proc. 15th Int. Vet. Congr.*, Part I, 1:159–63.

Karlson, A. G., M. R. Zinober, and W. H. Feldman. 1950. A whole blood, rapid agglutination test for avian tuberculosis—A preliminary report. *Am. J. Vet. Res.* 11:137–41.

Karlson, A. G., H. A. Andersen, and G. M. Needham. 1955. Isolation of avian tubercle bacilli in human silicosis. *Diseases Chest* 28:451–57.

Karlson, A. G., C. L. Davis, and M. L. Cohn. 1962. Skotochromogenic *Mycobacterium avium* from a trumpeter swan. *Am. J. Vet. Res.* 23:575–79.

Karlson, A. G., C. O. Thoen, and R. Harrington, 1970. Japanese quail: Susceptibility to avian tuberculosis. *Avian Diseases* 14:39–44.

Koch, R. 1890. Ueber bakteriologische Forschung. *Wien Med. Bl.* 13:531–35.

———. 1902. Address before the Second General Meeting, *Trans. Brit. Congr. Tuberc.* 1:23–35.

Kovacs, N. 1962. Nichtklassifizierte Mykobakterien. *Zentr. Bakteriol. Parasitenk. Abt. I. Orig.* 184:46–58.

Kubín, M., K. Dvorsky, R. Eisnerova, L. Mezensky, K. Franc, and M. Matějka. 1966. Pulmonary and nonpulmonary disease in humans due to avian mycobacteria. II. Microbiologic analysis of strains isolated. *Am. Rev. Respirat. Diseases* 94:31–39.

Lesslie, I. W., and K. J. Birn. 1967. Tuberculosis in cattle caused by the avian type tubercle bacillus. *Vet. Record* 80:559–64.

McDiarmid, A. 1948. Occurrence of tuberculosis in the wild wood-pigeon. *J. Comp. Pathol. Therap.* 58:128–33.

Maffucci, A. 1890. Beitrag zur Aetiologie der Tuberculose (Huehnertuberculose). *Zentr. Allgem. Pathol. Pathol. Anat.* 1:409–16.

Matějka, M., and M. Kubín. 1967. Vrabce (*Passer domesticus*) jako zdroj infekce aviar-

nimi mykobakteriemi pro skot. *Vet. Med. Praha* 12:491–97.

Mitchell, C. A., and R. C. Duthie. 1950. Tuberculosis of the common crow. *Can. J. Comp. Med. Vet. Sci.* 14:109–17.

Moehring, Joan M., and M. R. Solotorovsky. 1965. Relationship of colonial morphology to virulence for chickens of *Mycobacterium avium* and the nonphotochromogens. *Am. Rev. Respirat. Diseases* 92:704–13.

Myers, J. A., and J. H. Steele. 1969. *Bovine Tuberculosis: Control in Man and Animals*. Warren H. Green, St. Louis.

Olson, C., Jr., and W. H. Feldman. 1936. The cellular elements and hemoglobin in the blood of chickens with spontaneous tuberculosis. *J. Am. Vet. Med. Ass.* 89:26–34.

Ranney, A. F. 1966. The status of the state-federal tuberculosis eradication program. *Proc. 70th Ann. Meet. U.S. Livestock Sanit. Ass.*, pp. 194–207.

Ratcliffe, H. L. 1946. Tuberculosis in captive wild birds: Decrease of its incidence following a change in diets. *Am. Rev. Tuberc.* 54:389–400.

Schack-Steffenhagen, G., and J. Seeger. 1967. Untersuchungen ueber das Vorkommen von Gefluegeltuberkelbakterien bei auslaendischen Schlachthuehnern. *Zentr. Bakteriol. Parasitenk. Abt. I. Orig.* 202:204–11.

Schack-Steffenhagen, G., K. Petzoldt, and R. Larson. 1966. Gefluegeltuberkulose bei Schlachthuehnern und ihre Bedeutung als Infektionsquelle fuer den Menschen. *Zentr. Bakteriol. Parasitenk. Abt. I. Orig.* 201:363–72.

Schaefer, W. B. 1965. Serologic identification and classification of the atypical mycobacteria by their agglutination. *Am. Rev. Respirat. Diseases* 92 (part 2): 85–93.

Schalk, A. F., L. M. Roderick, H. L. Foust, and G. S. Harshfield. 1935. Avian tuberculosis: collected studies. *N. Dakota Agr. Exp. Sta. Tech. Bull.* 279.

Schliesser, T. 1967. Die epidemiologische Situation bei der Tuberkulose der Tier nach der Tilgung der Rindertuberkulose. *Zentr. Bakteriol. Parasitenk. Abt. I. Orig.* 205:300–308.

Schneider, P. A., and C. Riggenbach. 1963. Reactions a la tuberculose bovine et tuberculose aviare. *Schweiz. Arch. Tierheilk.* 105:417–22.

Scrivner, L. H., and C. Elder. 1931. Cutaneous and subcutaneous tuberculosis in a turkey. *J. Am. Vet. Med. Ass.* 79:244–47.

Simeonov, L. A. 1967. Results of testing with avian sensitin in Yugoslavia. *Z. Tuberk.* 127:89–92.

Stafseth, H. J., R. J. Biggar, W. W. Thompson, and Lisa Neu. 1934. The cultivation and egg-transmission of the avian tubercle bacillus. *J. Am. Vet. Med. Ass.* 85:342–59.

Stenberg, H., and A. Turunen. 1968. Differenzierung aus Haustieren isolierter Mykobakterien. *Zentr. Veterinaermed. B.* 15:494–503.

Svrček, S., O. J. Vrtiak, B. Kapitančik, T. Pauer, and Z. Koppel. 1966. Vol'ne zijuce vtactvo a domace holuby ako zdroje aviarnej tuberkulozy (Wild birds and domestic pigeons as sources of avian tuberculosis). *Rozhledy Tuberk.* 26:659–67.

Tacquet, A., B. Devulder, F. Tison, and B. Polspoel. 1966. Le role pathogene pour l'homme des mycobacteries du groupe avium. *Rev. Pathol. Gen. Comparee* 66:459–75.

USDA. 1968. *Poultry Slaughtered under Federal Inspection and Poultry Used in Canning and Other Processed Food.* Pou 2–1 June 1968 to Nov. 1968. Statistical Reporting Serv., Crop Reporting Board. Washington, D.C.

———. 1969. *Cooperative State-Federal Tuberculosis Eradication Program. Statistical Tables Fiscal Year 1968.* Washington, D.C.

Vallette, L.-R., G. de Saint Aubert, and J. Cherby. 1967. Un cas de tuberculose pulmonaire chez le canard, la pintade, et la poule. *Bull. Soc. Sci. Vet. Lyon* 69:241–46.

Van Es, L., and H. M. Martin. 1925. An inquiry into the cause of the increase of tuberculosis of swine. *Univ. Nebraska Agr. Exp. Sta. Res. Bull.* 30.

Vasenius, H. 1965. Tuberculosis-like lesions in slaughter swine in Finland. *Nord. Veterinaermed.* 17:17–21.

Wilson, J. E., and J. W. Macdonald. 1965. Tuberculosis in wild birds. (Letter to the editor.) *Vet. Record* 77:177.

Wojaczek-Steffke, E. 1964. Ueber das Vorkommen von Lungentuberkulose beim Haushuhn. *Monatsh. Veterinaermed.* 19:427–29.

Worthington, R. W. 1967. Mycobacterial PPD sensitins and the nonspecific reactor problem. *Onderstepoort J. Vet. Res.* 34:345–438.

CHAPTER 7

INFECTIOUS CORYZA

❖

R. YAMAMOTO

*Department of Epidemiology and
Preventive Medicine
School of Veterinary Medicine
University of California, Davis*

❖

INFECTIOUS CORYZA is an acute respiratory disease of chickens caused by *Hemophilus gallinarum*. The clinical syndrome has been variously described in the early literature as roup, contagious or infectious catarrh, cold, and uncomplicated coryza (Beach, 1920; De Blieck, 1931; Nelson, 1932; Beach and Schalm, 1936). Since the disease was proven to be infectious and affected primarily the nasal passages, the name "infectious coryza" was adopted (Beach and Schalm, 1936). Infectious coryza may occur in growing chickens and in layers, with the greatest economic losses resulting from increased number of culls and marked reduction (10–40%) in egg production. The disease is limited primarily to chickens and has no public health significance.

HISTORY

As early as 1920 Beach held the view that infectious coryza was a distinct clinical entity. The etiologic agent eluded detection for a number of years since the disease often was masked in mixed infections, and with fowl pox in particular. In 1931 De Blieck (1931, 1932) isolated a hemophilic bacterium from such a mixed infection and reproduced coryza in fowl pox-immune chickens. He called the organism *Bacillus hemoglobinophilus coryzae gallinarum*.

Within a short period of time other investigators reported isolation of a similar organism from cases of infectious coryza (Nelson, 1932, 1933; Delaplane et al., 1934; Schalm and Beach, 1934). Eliot and Lewis (1934) and Delaplane et al. (1934) independently proposed the binomial *Hemophilus gallinarum* for the organism which prevailed over the name proposed by DeBlieck. The currently suggested nomenclature is *Haemophilus gallinarum* (Breed et al., 1957).

INCIDENCE AND DISTRIBUTION

Hemophilus gallinarum infections were rather common during the 1930s and early 1940s and then almost disappeared. The decreased prevalence of the disease was attributed to better methods of isolation rearing, to the practice of disposing of the laying flock at the end of the laying season, and to the failure of the organism to survive outside the bird. However, the disease appears to have increased in prevalence somewhat in recent years. It is an important problem in California (Clark and Godfrey, 1961; Page, 1962a) and continues to be diagnosed sporadically in several other states (Angstrom et al., 1965; Henderson, 1967; Murphy et al., 1968). Based on reports in the literature and from communication with various workers, it would appear that *H. gallinarum* has a worldwide distribution, being found wherever chickens are raised (Chu, 1954; Yoder, 1965). Currently, infectious coryza is of major economic importance in Mexico (Garrido, 1968, personal communication) and in Japan (Watanabe, 1967) where the poultry industry is developing at an accelerated pace.

ETIOLOGY

CLASSIFICATION, MORPHOLOGY, AND STAINING

Hemophilus gallinarum is a gram-negative, polar-staining, nonmotile bacterium. In 24-hour cultures it appears as short rods or coccobacilli $1–3\mu$ in length and $0.4–0.8\mu$ in width, with a tendency for filament formation. The organism undergoes degeneration within 48–60 hours, showing fragments and indefinite forms. Subcultures to fresh medium at this stage will again yield the typical rod-shaped morphology. The bacilli may occur singly, in pairs, or as short chains (Delaplane et al., 1934; Schalm

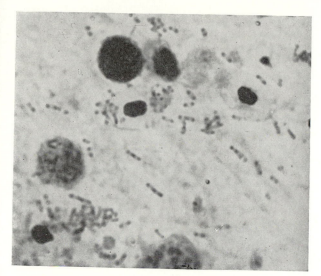

FIG. 7.1—Hemophilus gallinarum *in film of nasal exudate.* ×810.

and Beach, 1936a). The organism detected in the sinus exudate of the infected chicken has bipolar staining characteristics (Fig. 7.1).

GROWTH REQUIREMENTS

Schalm and Beach (1936a,b) found that their strains required two growth factors—an X-factor (hemin) and a V-factor (nicotinamide adenine dinucleotide; NAD). Serum from defibrinated horse blood contained both factors. More recently Page (1962a) and Biberstein et al. (1963) showed that the X-factor was not essential since media devoid of hemin readily supported growth of the organism. The reduced form of NAD (2.5 μg per ml of medium) (Page, 1962a) or its oxidized form (20–100 μg per ml) Sato and Shifrine, 1965; Cundy, 1965a) was essential for growth. Other sources of the V-factor used by various workers have been yolk from chicken eggs (Cunningham and Stuart, 1944), fresh yeast extract (Roberts et al., 1964), and chicken or sheep sera (Bornstein and Samberg, 1954; Page, 1962a). Rabbit or bovine sera were unsatisfactory Bornstein and Samberg, 1954). A number of bacterial species excrete the V-factor and consequently have been used as "feeder" cultures to support the growth of *H. gallinarum* (Schalm and Beach, 1936b; Page, 1962a).

H. gallinarum is a facultative anaerobe (Eliot and Lewis, 1934). However, most workers have considered that an atmosphere containing carbon dioxide or reduced oxygen tension was necessary for op-

timum growth (Schalm and Beach, 1936b). Page (1962a) demonstrated that *H. gallinarum* was not dependent on carbon dioxide as such but was microaerophilic. He obtained good growth with reduced oxygen tension as well as under complete anaerobic conditions.

COLONIAL MORPHOLOGY

Tiny dewdrop colonies up to 0.3 mm in diameter develop on suitable media. The characteristic satellitic growth particularly around staphylococcus colonies was observed by the earliest workers. Schalm and Beach (1936a) reported that the minimal and maximal temperatures of growth were 25 and 45° C respectively, with the optimal range being 34–42° C. The organism is commonly grown at 37–38° C.

BIOCHEMICAL PROPERTIES

Various broth media enriched with 5–10% chicken serum have been used to determine the biochemical properties of *H. gallinarum* (Bornstein and Samberg, 1954; Clark and Godfrey, 1961; Page, 1962a; Kato and Tsubahara, 1962a). The organism ferments a number of sugars without gas formation; at least nine different fermentation patterns have been recorded by various workers. Glucose is consistently fermented by all isolates; the carbohydrates which are frequently fermented are galactose, mannose, levulose, sucrose, maltose, dextrin, and starch; those infrequently fermented are mannitol and trehalose. The commonly used carbohydrates which are not fermented are lactose, inulin, xylose, and salicin. Whether the variations in the fermentation pattern of the various isolates reflect differences in serotypes or in strains within serotypes is yet to be elucidated. However, these differences apparently do not reflect differences in the pathogenicity of the organisms (Page, 1962a; Kato and Tsubahara, 1962a).

Hydrogen sulfide and indole are not produced, gelatin is not liquified, and litmus and methylene blue milk are not changed (Bornstein and Samberg, 1954). Nitrates are reduced (Clark and Godfrey, 1961; Page, 1962a), and catalase activity is absent (Page, 1962a).

RESISTANCE TO PHYSICAL AND CHEMICAL AGENTS

Eliot and Lewis (1934) found that the organism suspended in water did not survive at a temperature of 45° C for 6 minutes and not more than 2 minutes at 50° C. When suspended in hemolyzed blood broth, the organism was killed at 55° C in 4–6 minutes but survived at 50° C for 10 minutes. Page (1962b) reported that the organism in infectious exudate suspended in tap water was viable at 3 but not at 4 hours. Organisms which were cultivated on agar medium and then suspended in tap water were nonviable within 4–12 minutes. Formalin added at a concentration of 0.25% to infected chicken embryo fluids killed the organism within 24 hours at 6° C (Page et al., 1963).

De Blieck (1934) found that a saline suspension of nasal exudate held at 37° C for 24 hours had lost its infectivity for chickens. Such suspensions held at 22° C were infectious at 24 but not at 96 hours. Eliot and Lewis (1934) found that infectious exudate or tissue which was held at 37° C for 24 hours (and on occasion up to 48 hours) was still infectious; at 4° C the exudate remained infectious for several days. Thus it appears that the survival time of *H. gallinarum* is governed to some extent by the menstrum and by the temperature.

The organism may be maintained on blood agar plates by weekly passages. Young cultures maintained in a candle jar will remain viable for 2 weeks at 4° C. Chicken embryos 6–7 days old may be inoculated with single colonies or with broth cultures via the yolk sac; the yolk from

embryos dead in 24–48 hours will contain a large number of organisms which may be frozen at —20 to —70° C or lyophilized. Titers in frozen yolk material may drop a hundredfold; consequently, serial embryo passages should be made at monthly intervals to maintain cultures by this method. The organism has survived for at least 10 years in the lyophilized state (Yoder, 1965).

ANTIGENIC TYPES

At least three antigenic types of *H. gallinarum* have been described (Page, 1962a; Kato and Tsubahara, 1962a; Page et al., 1963). Page classified his organisms with the plate agglutination test into serotypes A, B, and C. Type A, represented by strain 0083, was the one most commonly encountered in California. Bacterins prepared from each of the serotypes showed some degree of protection against the heterologous types (Page et al., 1963), indicating that they shared common antigens. Kato and Tsubahara (1962a) also described three pathogenic serotypes of *H. gallinarum;* however, it is not known whether these are identical with Page's isolates.

Nonpathogenic hemophili have also been described which are strongly catalase-positive, grow aerobically, require the V-factor for growth, and some strains produce pigment in the presence of glucose (Page, 1962a; Roberts et al., 1964). These organisms should be designated only as *Hemophilus* species at this time and should not be confused with *H. gallinarum*.

PATHOGENICITY

The characteristic feature of the disease is a coryza of short incubation which develops within 24–48 hours after intranasal or intrasinus inoculation with either culture or exudate. The duration of the disease seems to vary, however, with the inoculum. Various studies have shown that the coryza produced by culture was of much shorter duration (6–14 days) than that produced by infectious sinus exudate (50 days or more) (Nelson, 1933; Schalm and Beach, 1936a). These early workers felt that the organism rapidly lost virulence on artificial cultivation which accounted for the shorter duration of the culture-induced disease; 30–40 transfers on artificial media in most cases rendered the organism completely avirulent (Nelson, 1933; De Blieck, 1934). However, since these studies were conducted at a time when *M. gallisepticum* was still an unknown entity, the prolonged course of the exudate-induced disease could very well have been due to an infection complicated with this and possibly other agents. A coryza of short incubation and long duration has since been convincingly demonstrated in mixed infections of *H. gallinarum* and *M. gallisepticum* (Nelson, 1938; Adler and Yamamoto, 1956). On the other hand, Schalm and Beach (1936a) showed that the virulence of attenuated laboratory cultures could be increased to simulate the exudate-induced disease by rapid serial passages through chickens. A study of this nature has not been repeated in recent years in chickens known to be free of common poultry pathogens to clearly demonstrate that *H. gallinarum* is capable of producing a disease of long duration.

The variation of the severity and duration of the disease in different outbreaks is influenced also by the virulence of the organism. While infectious coryza is considered to cause minimal mortality, Delaplane et al. (1933) described outbreaks in which mortality was extremely high. The organism isolated by these workers was highly toxigenic. Subcutaneous inoculation of chickens with the organism resulted in severe local swelling and generalized toxic reactions; chickens inoculated via the nasal cavity showed extensive edema extending into the head and neck region.

Page (1962a) also described a highly virulent isolate (strain 0083) which produced airsacculitis in 60% of the chickens inoculated by the intranasal route; air sac lesions have been described by early workers as an incidental feature to the main involvement of the upper respiratory tract (Beach and Schalm, 1936). The observations that the disease in natural outbreaks may vary in its severity and course may thus be due to pure or mixed infections and to variation in virulence of the organism. Individual differences in resistance of birds may also be a factor (Beach and Schalm, 1936).

Cundy (1965a) characterized the endotoxin of *H. gallinarum* (strain 0083) to be a lipopolysaccharide similar to that of other gram-negative bacteria. The endotoxin killed chicken embryos in 24 hours when inoculated onto the chorioallantoic membrane and produced petechial hemorrhages in the skin and perivascular hemorrhage and edema in the brain. In a small group of chickens studied, the endotoxin was antigenic but not protective. Toxic reactions were not observed in chickens inoculated intravenously or intramuscularly.

PATHOGENESIS AND EPIZOOTIOLOGY

NATURAL AND EXPERIMENTAL HOSTS

The chicken is the natural host for *H. gallinarum*. While all ages are susceptible, older birds appear to react more severely to the disease. Chickens 3–5 days of age are somewhat resistant (Eliot and Lewis, 1934; Kato and Tsubahara, 1962b); however, Eliot and Lewis (1934) routinely produced coryza in 7-day-old chickens by intranasal inoculation. Beach and Schalm (1936) found that chickens 4 weeks to 3 years of age were susceptible but observed considerable individual variation in resistance to the disease. Kato and Tsubahara (1962b) reproduced typical signs of coryza in 90% of chickens 4–8 weeks of age and in 100% of chickens 13 weeks of age and older. The incubation period was shortened and the course of the disease tended to be longer in older birds.

The disease has been diagnosed infrequently in pheasants (Delaplane et al., 1934; Angstrom et al., 1965; Henderson, 1967), and one case has been reported in guinea fowls (Angstrom et al., 1965). Cundy (1965b) described an experimental *H. gallinarum* infection in the Japanese quail (*Coturnix coturnix*) which was suggestive of a toxic reaction rather than a true coryza. The following species have been found to be refractory to experimental infection: pigeon, sparrow, duck, crow, rabbit, guinea pig, and mouse (Delaplane et al., 1934; De Blieck, 1934; Beach and Schalm, 1936; Page, 1962a; Yamamoto and Clark, 1966). Delaplane et al. (1934) indicated that turkeys were refractory to infection with *H. gallinarum;* De Blieck (1934) and Beach and Schalm (1936) reported that this species was susceptible. The description of the disease by the latter workers, however, suggested that *M. gallisepticum* may have been a complicating factor. Recent studies in this laboratory indicated that turkeys were quite resistant to intrasinus inoculation with *H. gallinarum,* but the organism multiplied profusely and persisted for at least 4 weeks when inoculated into turkeys previously infected with *M. gallisepticum* (Yamamoto and Matsumoto, 1968, unpublished).

Natural infections of *H. gallinarum* have not been observed in turkeys.

TRANSMISSION AND INCUBATION PERIOD

The chronic or healthy carrier birds in flocks which have experienced the disease serve as the main reservoir of infection. The disease seems to occur most frequently in the fall and winter months, although such seasonal patterns may be coincidental to management practices (such as introduction of susceptible replacement pullets onto farms where the disease is present). On farms where multiple age groups are brooded and raised the spread of the disease to successive age groups can almost be predicted, with infection occurring in a matter of 1–6 weeks after such birds are moved from the brooder house to growing cages near older groups of infected birds (Clark and Godfrey, 1961).

In recent years, however, hemophilus epizootics have been observed in California on isolated ranches in which only one age group of birds was being raised at any one time (Yamamoto and Clark, 1966). Free-flying birds such as sparrows were suspected as possible vectors; however, these workers were unable to transmit the disease to chickens using sparrows as the intermediary host. While airborne transmission was postulated as one possible means by which such isolated outbreaks may occur, it is evident that the source of such outbreaks remains obscure and needs further clarification.

The incubation period after experimental inoculation is 18–36 hours. Susceptible birds exposed by contact to infected cases usually have signs of the disease in 1–3 days.

SIGNS

The most prominent features are involvement of the nasal passages and sinuses with a serous to mucoid nasal discharge, edema of the face, and conjunctivitis. Figure 7.2 illustrates the typical facial swelling. Swollen wattles may be evident, particularly in males. Infections of the lower respiratory tract may also occur, causing rales and difficult breathing (Beach and Schalm, 1936).

The birds may have diarrhea, and feed and water consumption usually is decreased; in growing birds this means an increased number of culls and in laying flocks

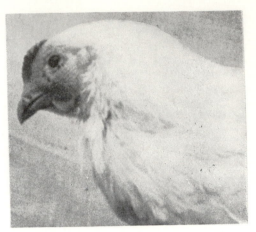

FIG. 7.2–*Artificial infection with infectious coryza showing facial edema.*

a reduction in egg production. A foul odor may be detected in flocks where the disease has become chronic and complicated with other bacteria.

MORBIDITY AND MORTALITY

The virulence of the organism may alter the course of the disease. While highly toxigenic strains such as that described by Delaplane et al. (1934) may cause high mortality, the disease if uncomplicated is usually one of low mortality and high morbidity. Complicating factors such as poor housing, parasitism, and inadequate nutrition may add to the severity and duration of the disease.

The disease is usually more severe and prolonged with resulting increased mortality when complicated with other agents such as fowl pox (Beach and Schalm, 1936), *M. gallisepticum* (Nelson, 1938; Adler and Yamamoto, 1956; Kato, 1965b), infectious bronchitis (Yoshimura et al., 1966; Raggi et al., 1967), pasteurella (Clark and Godfrey, 1961), and infectious laryngotracheitis (Mohamed et al., 1969). (See section on Pathogenicity.)

GROSS LESIONS

Hemophilus gallinarum produces an acute catarrhal inflammation of the mucous membranes of the nasal passages and sinuses. There is frequently a catarrhal conjunctivitis and subcutaneous edema of the face and wattles. Pneumonia and airsacculitis may also be present (Page, 1962a,b).

HISTOPATHOLOGY

Histopathologic studies are limited (Adler and Page, 1962; Fujiwara and Konno, 1965; Raggi et al., 1967). Fujiwara and Konno (1965) studied the response of chickens from 12 hours to 3 months after intranasal inoculation. The essential changes in the nasal cavity, infraorbital sinuses, and trachea consisted of sloughing, disintegration, and hyperplasia of the mucosal and glandular epithelia, and edema and hyperemia with heterophil infiltration in the tunica propria of the mucous membranes. The pathological changes first observed at 20 hours reached maximum severity by 7–10 days with subsequent repair occurring within 14–21 days. In birds with involvement of the lower respiratory tract, an acute catarrhal bronchopneumonia was observed with heterophils and cell debris filling the lumen of the secondary and tertiary bronchi; the epithelial cells of the air capillaries were swollen and showed hyperplasia. The catarrhal inflammation of the air sacs was characterized by swelling and hyperplasia of the cells with abundant heterophil infiltration.

IMMUNITY

Virtually all of the early investigators have indicated that chickens which have recovered from active infection possessed varying degrees of immunity to reexposure (Nelson, 1932; De Blieck, 1934; Schalm and Beach, 1936a; Page et al., 1963). Recovered birds are immune for at least 1 year. Resistance to reexposure among individual birds may develop as early as 2 weeks after initial exposure by the intrasinus route (Sato and Shifrine, 1964). Information is not available on passive immunity to *H. gallinarum* infection.

DIAGNOSIS

ISOLATION AND IDENTIFICATION OF CAUSATIVE AGENT

Many different media have been developed to support the growth of *H. gallinarum*. The interested reader is referred to the papers of Bornstein and Samberg (1954) and Kato (1965a) for excellent reviews of the early literature concerning these media.

While *H. gallinarum* is considered to be a fastidious organism, it is not difficult to isolate, requiring simple media and procedures. Specimens should be taken from two or three chickens in the acute stage of the disease (1–7 days incubation). The skin under the eyes is seared with a hot iron spatula and an incision made into the sinus cavity with sterile scissors. A sterile cotton swab is inserted deep into the sinus cavity where the organism is found most often in pure form. Tracheal and air sac exudates also may be taken on sterile swabs. The swab is streaked on a blood agar (horse, bovine, sheep, avian, or rabbit) plate. The plate is then cross-streaked with a staphylococcus and incubated at 37° C in a large screw-cap jar in which a candle is allowed to burn out. Growth of small translucent colonies adjacent to the feeder culture in 24–48 hours indicates *H. gallinarum*. These should be tested for catalase activity by placing a loopful of the culture into a drop of 3% hydrogen peroxide. A diagnosis of infectious coryza may be based on a history of a rapidly spreading disease in which coryza is the main manifestation, together with the isolation of a catalase-negative, gram-negative bacterium showing satellitic growth. The organism may be characterized further by biochemical and serologic tests (see sections on Biochemical Properties and Serology).

Another efficient and useful diagnostic procedure is to inoculate the sinus exudate or culture into 2 or 3 normal chickens by the intrasinus route. The production of a coryza in 24–48 hours is diagnostic; however, the incubation period may be delayed up to a week if only a small number of organisms is present in the inoculum, such as in cases of long standing.

SEROLOGY

Agglutination tests have been developed by several investigators (Kato et al., 1962; Sato and Shifrine, 1964; Yamamoto and Somersett, 1964). Brain heart infusion broth (Difco) supplemented with 100 μg per ml of NAD (Sato and Shifrine, 1965) or with reduced NAD (2.5 μg per ml) and 1% horse serum (Yamamoto and Somersett, 1964) have been used to propagate the organism in large quantities. Kato (1965a) compared several infusion broths and found that cultures grown in chicken meat infusion broth of Hofstad and Doerr (1956) supplemented with 5% chicken serum yielded the most sensitive antigens. The optimal pH was found to be in the range of 6.6–6.8.

Since agglutinins to infection with *H. gallinarum* are not detected until 7–14 days after infection by either the plate or tube tests, the procedure has limited diagnostic value. Probably the serologic tests will find greatest application for studies on antigenic analyses of serotypes, to follow the immune response in bacterin studies, and for epidemiological investigations. In the last case, the test may be used to check flocks for evidence of past infections prior to their movement from one farm to another if one is concerned about introducing infection through carrier birds. The presence of more than one serotype in an area may complicate the serologic interpretation, although available data indicate that common antigens are shared by the different serotypes. Agglutinins to *H. gallinarum* may be detected up to one year or longer after infection.

Other serologic tests which have been developed are the direct complement fixation (Kato et al., 1962), agar-gel diffusion (Sato and Shifrine, 1965), and indirect hemagglutination (Cundy, 1965a). The direct fluorescent antibody technique has been applied to identify *H. gallinarum* in cultures and from infected tissues (Corstvet and Sadler, 1964; Peters et al., 1968).

DIFFERENTIAL DIAGNOSIS

A field diagnosis of *H. gallinarum* infection is difficult to make since other diseases such as chronic respiratory disease, chronic fowl cholera, fowl pox, and A-avitaminosis may produce similar clinical signs. Since *H. gallinarum* infections often occur in mixed infections, one should consider the possibility of other bacteria or viruses as complicating the disease, particularly if the mortality is high and the disease takes on a prolonged course (see sections on Pathogenicity and Morbidity and Mortality).

TREATMENT

Various sulfonamides and antibiotics are useful in alleviating the severity and course of the disease; however, none of the therapeutic agents in current use have been found to be bactericidal. Relapse often occurs after the treatment is discontinued, and the carrier state is not eliminated. Various drugs have been added to the feed or water or administered parenterally.

Sulfathiazole was one of the earliest sulfonamides to be extensively used in the treatment of infectious coryza (Page, 1962b). This drug has been used at the rate of ½ lb/100 lb of mash (Heiman, 1943; Wernicoff and Goldhaft, 1944). Improvement in the flock is observed usually within a week after treatment if other complicating agents or factors are not involved. Streptomycin at a dose of 200 mg per bird, intramuscularly, also has been found to be effective in treating infectious coryza (Bornstein and Samberg, 1955). However, Page (1962b) found his test isolate to be relatively resistant to dihydrostreptomycin and sulfathiazole, and sensitive to erythromycin and oxytetracycline. Erythromycin given for 4 days in the drinking water reduced the spread of infection among susceptible chickens, but following its removal a relapse in the flock was apparent. Good and Hanley (1967) reported favorable results with erythromycin in the treatment of infectious coryza; however, birds with mixed infections responded poorly. Spectinomycin (500 mg/gal of water) administered for 7 days reduced the spread and significantly modified the course of the disease without completely eliminating the organisms (Hanley et al., 1968; Yamamoto and Matsumoto, 1968, unpublished data). Mitrovic (1967) reported that sulfadimethoxine given in the drinking water at the rate of 0.05% for 6 days was effective, palatable, and safe in the treatment of infectious coryza. While tylosin tartrate has been used most extensively for the treatment of mycoplasma infections, a report from Egypt indicated that this antibiotic was effective in the treatment of a bacteriologically confirmed field outbreak of infectious coryza when administered subcutaneously at a dose of 37.5 mg per bird (Farid et al., 1966). A new nitrofuran Furmizole appears to have some promise, according to a report from Japan (Ota et al., 1967), but as is the case with other therapeutic agents, apparently it is not completely bactericidal.

PREVENTION AND CONTROL
MANAGEMENT PROCEDURES

Since recovered carrier birds are the main source of infection, such practices as buying breeding males or started chicks should be discouraged. Only day-old chicks should be secured for replacement purposes unless the source is known to be free of the disease. Isolation rearing and housing away from old stock are desirable practices for prevention of this disease.

IMMUNIZATION

A more recent approach to the prevention of infectious coryza has consisted of various vaccination procedures (Clark and Godfrey, 1961; Tennison and Siddle, 1961; Page et al., 1963). Several commercial formalin-killed products prepared from chicken embryos are available which may be autogenous or may contain 2–3 strains or serotypes. These products may contain adjuvants, stabilizers, or saline diluents. The bacterins which are generally injected in birds 10–20 weeks of age yield optimal results when injected 2–3 weeks prior to the expected natural outbreak. Two injections given approximately 3 weeks apart before 20 weeks of age seem to result in better performance of layers than a single injection (Price et al., 1967; Bell, 1968). Clark and Godfrey (1961) showed that the bacterin significantly reduced losses due to complicating respiratory diseases in growing birds in hemophilus endemic areas. Page et al. (1963) showed that the bacterin afforded minimal protection of the upper respiratory tract but did significantly protect against the occurrence of airsacculitis and a drop in egg production. Extensive field studies by Price et al. (1967) indicated that the various commercial bacterins generally mimimize losses due to mortality and reduction in egg production. Bell (1968) reported that the bacterin significantly reduced the severity of clinical signs following exposure to *H. gallinarum* and prevented the loss of up to 13 eggs per hen housed. His study also showed that birds vaccinated at 16 weeks of age maintained a significant degree of immunity to challenge up to 27 weeks of age.

Another approach to prevention of infectious coryza in endemic areas has been the practice of controlled exposure. The practice has been based on the observation that pullets which have experienced the disease during their growing period are generally protected against a later drop in egg production. The usual procedure has been to vaccinate the birds between 15 and 18 weeks of age and expose them to the live organism (culture or carrier birds from the same ranch) at 20 weeks of age. Individual birds showing severe signs may be injected with antibiotics. Controlled exposure has its danger, particularly if the disease is complicated with other agents, and should be performed under careful veterinary supervision (Allen, 1967).

While still in the experimental stages, a broth-propagated bacterin has been developed which seems to give a better index of protection against clinical coryza than egg-propagated products (Matsumoto and Yamamoto, 1967).

Page et al. (1963) indicated that chickens exposed to bacterins prepared from different serotypes showed some degree of cross protection, but more recent studies indicate that such protection may be minimal (Matsumoto and Yamamoto, 1968, unpublished data).

ERADICATION

It is necessary to depopulate flocks which have experienced the disease, because recovered birds remain reservoirs of infection. The method of eradication depends upon circumstances on the farm—size of the flock, facilities, and purpose of the flock. The infected birds may be marketed at once and the premises cleaned before new chicks are brought on the place. Another more popular method is to treat the affected flock and keep it isolated until new stock has been raised in isolation as replacements. After the infected or recovered birds are marketed, the house should be cleaned and disinfected before housing clean stock. Since the organism may survive in exudate for several days at colder temperatures, it would be advisable to allow the cleaned house to remain vacant for about one week, particularly during the cooler part of the year.

REFERENCES

Adler, H. E., and L. A. Page. 1962. *Haemophilus* infections in chickens. II. The pathology of the respiratory tract. *Avian Diseases* 6:1–6.

Adler, H. E., and R. Yamamoto. 1956. Studies on chronic coryza (Nelson) in the domestic fowl. *Cornell Vet.* 46:337–43.

Allen, J. A. 1967. Comments on coryza. *Proc. First Ann. Poultry Health Symp.*, Univ. Calif., Davis.

Angstrom, C. I., H. L. Chute, and M. S. Cover. 1965. Report of the committee on nomenclature and reporting of disease. N.E. Conf. on Avian Diseases, June, 1965. *Avian Diseases* 9:611–16.

Beach, J. R. 1920. The diagnosis, therapeutics, and prophylaxis of chicken-pox (contagious epithelioma) of fowls. *J. Am. Vet. Med. Ass.* 58:301–12.

Beach, J. R., and O. W. Schalm. 1936. Studies of the clinical manifestations and transmissibility of infectious coryza of chickens. *Poultry Sci.* 15:466–72.

Bell, D. 1968. A field evaluation of an infectious coryza bacterin. *Proc. Second Ann. Poultry Health Symp.*, Univ. Calif., Davis.

Biberstein, E. L., P. D. Mini, and M. G. Gills. 1963. Action of *Haemophilus* cultures on δ-aminolevulinic acid. *J. Bacteriol.* 86:814–19.

Bornstein, S., and Y. Samberg. 1954. The therapeutic effect of streptomycin on infectious coryza of chickens caused by *Hemophilus gallinarum*. II. Isolation and culture of *Hemophilus gallinarum*, and some of its biochemical reactions. *Am. J. Vet. Res.* 15:612–16.

———. 1955. The therapeutic effect of streptomycin on infectious coryza of chickens caused by *Hemophilus gallinarum*. V. The effect of parenteral streptomycin in high dosage on egg production and growth in birds affected with infectious coryza. *Poultry Sci.* 34:896–904.

Breed, R. S., E. G. D. Murray, and N. R. Smith. 1957. *Bergey's Manual of Determinative Bacteriology*, 7th ed. William & Wilkins Co., Baltimore.

Chu, H. P. 1954. The identification of infectious coryza associated with Nelson's coccobacilliform bodies in fowls in England and its similarity to the chronic respiratory disease of chickens. *Proc. 10th World's Poultry Congr.*, Edinburgh, pp. 246–51.

Clark, D. S., and J. F. Godfrey. 1961. Studies of an inactivated *Hemophilus gallinarum* vaccine for immunization of chickens against infectious coryza. *Avian Diseases* 5:37–47.

Corstvet, R. E., and W. W. Sadler. 1964. The diagnosis of certain avian diseases with the fluorescent antibody technique. *Poultry Sci.* 43:1280–88.

Cundy, K. R. 1965a. Isolation and characterization of an endotoxin from *Haemophilus gallinarum*. Ph.D. thesis, Univ. Calif., Davis.

———. 1965b. Susceptibility of Japanese quail (*Coturnix coturnix japonica*) to experimental infection with *Haemophilus galli-*

narum. *Avian Diseases* 9:272:84.

Cunningham, C. H., and H. O. Stuart. 1944. Egg-yolk medium for the cultivation of *Hemophilus gallinarum*. *Am. J. Vet. Res.* 5:142–46.

De Blieck, L. 1931. Een haemoglobinophile bacterie als oorzaak van coryza infectiosa gallinarum. *Tijdschr. Diergeneesk.* 58:310–14. (English summary.)

———. 1932. A haemoglobinophilic bacterium as the cause of contagious catarrh of the fowl (coryza infectiosa gallinarum). *Vet. J.* 88:9–13.

———. 1934. Coryza infectiosa gallinarum. *Proc. 12th Int. Vet. Congr.* 3:161–82.

Delaplane, J. P., H. O. Stuart, and H. Bunyea. 1933. A preliminary report on an apparently new respiratory disease of chickens. *J. Am. Vet. Med. Ass.* 82:772–74.

Delaplane, J. P., L. E. Erwin, and H. O. Stuart. 1934. A hemophilic bacillus as the cause of an infectious rhinitis (coryza) of fowls. *Rhode Island Agr. Expt. Sta. Bull.* 244.

Eliot, C. P., and M. R. Lewis. 1934. A hemophilic bacterium as a cause of infectious coryza in the fowl. *J. Am. Vet. Med. Ass.* 84:878–88.

Farid, A., M. Y. Khalil, and K. H. Abbassi. 1966. A note on fowl coryza in U.A.R. *Arab. Vet. Med. Ass. J.* 26:81–86.

Fujiwara, H., and S. Konno. 1965. Histopathological studies on infectious coryza of chickens. II. Findings in experimentally infected cases. *Nat. Inst. Animal Health Quart.* 5:86–96.

Good, R. E., and J. E. Hanley. 1967. A chronic sinus infection in Florida chickens. *Southwestern Vet.* 20:297–99.

Hanley, J. E., R. B. Davis, and E. M. Sunka. 1968. An evaluation and comparison of spectinomycin and spectinomycin-erythromycin combinations for infectious coryza. *Avian Diseases* 12:1–3.

Heiman, V. 1943. Sulfathiazole for colds in chickens. *Vet. Med.* 38:26–28.

Henderson, W. 1967. Summary principal poultry diseases diagnosed North Central poultry disease conference area 1966. *Avian Diseases* 11:703–8.

Hofstad, M. S., and Laverne Doerr. 1956. A chicken meat infusion medium enriched with avian serum for cultivation of an avian pleuropneumonia-like organism, *Mycoplasma gallinarum*. *Cornell Vet.* 46:439–46.

Kato, K. 1965a. Infectious coryza of chickens. IV. Studies on the nutrition of *Haemophilus gallinarum*. *Bull. Nat. Inst. Animal Health* 50:10–14.

———. 1965b. Infectious coryza of chickens. V. Influence of *Mycoplasma gallisepticum* infection on chickens infected with *Haemophilus gallinarum*. *Nat. Inst. Animal Health Quart.* 5:183–89.

Kato, K., and H. Tsubahara. 1962a. Infectious coryza of chickens. II. Identification of isolates. *Bull. Nat. Inst. Animal Health* 45: 21–26. (English summary in *Nat. Inst. Animal Health Quart.*, 1962, 2:239.)

———. 1962b. Infectious coryza of chickens. III. Susceptibility of chickens of different ages. *Bull. Nat. Inst. Animal Health* 45:27–32. (English summary in *Nat. Inst. Animal Health Quart.*, 1962, 2:239–40.)

Kato, K., T. Sato, and H. Tsubahara. 1962. Infectious coryza of chickens. I. Clinical and etiological observations. *Bull. Nat. Inst. Animal Health* 45:15–20. (English summary in *Nat. Inst. Animal Health Quart.*, 1962, 2:238–39.)

Matsumoto, M., and R. Yamamoto. 1967. Immunogenicity of preparations of *Haemophilus gallinarum* bacterin. *Poultry Sci.* 46: 1290. (Abstr.)

Mitrovic, M. 1967. Chemotherapeutic effcacy of sulfadimethoxine against fowl cholera and infectious coryza. *Poultry Sci.* 46:1153–58.

Mohamed, Y. S., P. D. Moorhead, and E. H. Bohl. 1969. Preliminary observations on possible synergism between infectious laryngotracheitis virus and *Hemophilus gallinarum.* *Avian Diseases* 13:158–62.

Murphy, C. D., C. F. Hall, and H. W. Yoder, Jr. 1968. Disease reports of the Southern Conference on Avian Diseases (SCAD) 1967. *Avian Diseases* 12:737–54.

Nelson, J. B. 1932. Etiology of an uncomplicated coryza in the domestic fowl. *Proc. Soc. Exp. Biol. Med.* 30:306–7.

———. 1933. Studies on an uncomplicated coryza of the domestic fowl. I. The isolation of a bacillus which produces a nasal discharge. *J. Exp. Med.* 58:289–95.

———. 1938. Studies on an uncomplicated coryza of the domestic fowl. IX. The cooperative action of *Hemophilus gallinarum* and the coccobacilliform bodies in the coryza of rapid onset and long duration. *J. Exp. Med.* 67:847–55.

Ota, S., S. Watanabe, and C. Kuniyasu. 1967. Efficacy of a new nitrofuran compound, Furamizole (NF161) against experimentally induced infection of *Mycoplasma gallisepticum* and *Haemophilus gallinarum* in chickens. *Japan. World Vet. Poultry Ass.*, p. 15. (English summary.)

Page, L. A. 1962a. *Haemophilus* infections in chickens. I. Characteristics of 12 *Haemophilus* isolates recovered from diseased chickens. *Am. J. Vet. Res.* 23:85–95.

———. 1962b. *Haemophilus* infections in chickens. III. Factors in intraflock transmission of infectious coryza and its chemical and antibiotic therapeusis. *Avian Diseases* 6: 211–25.

Page, L. A., A. S. Rosenwald, and F. C. Price. 1963. *Haemophilus* infections in chickens.

IV. Results of laboratory and field trials of formalinized bacterins for the prevention of disease caused by *Haemophilus gallinarum.* *Avian Diseases* 7:239–56.

Peters, R. L., J. E. Faber, and H. M. DeVolt. 1968. Identification of *Haemophilus gallinarum* in artificially infected chickens. *Poultry Sci.* 47:123–29.

Price, F. C., R. Yamamoto, and A. S. Rosenwald. 1967. Where are we on coryza research? *Pacific Poultryman* 73:42–54.

Raggi, L. G., D. C. Young, and J. M. Sharma. 1967. Synergism between avian infectious bronchitis virus and *Haemophilus gallinarum.* *Avian Diseases* 11:308–21.

Roberts, D. H., B. S. Hanson, and L. Timms. 1964. Observations on the incidence and significance of *Haemophilus gallinarum* in outbreaks of respiratory disease among poultry in Great Britain. *Vet. Record* 76:1512–16.

Sato, S., and M. Shifrine. 1964. Serologic response of chickens to experimental infection with *Hemophilus gallinarum,* and their immunity to challenge. *Poultry Sci.* 43:1199–1204.

———. 1965. Application of the agar gel precipitation test to serological studies of chickens inoculated with *Haemophilus gallinarum.* *Avian Diseases* 9:591–98.

Schalm, O. W., and J. R. Beach. 1934. The etiology of a respiratory disease of chickens. *Science* 79:416–17.

———. 1936a. Studies of infectious coryza of chickens with special reference to its etiology. *Poultry Sci.* 15:473–82.

———. 1936b. Cultural requirements of the fowl coryza bacillus. *J. Bacteriol.* 31:161–69.

Tennison, L. B., and P. J. Siddle. 1961. Limited study with *Haemophilus* cultures. *Avian Diseases* 5:352–54.

Watanabe, M. 1967. Poultry disease in Japan. *Japan. World Vet. Poultry Ass.* pp. 1–8.

Wernicoff, N. E., and T. M. Goldhaft. 1944. The field use of sulfathiazole in some diseases of poultry. *Cornell Vet.* 34:199–213.

Yamamoto, R., and G. T. Clark. 1966. Intra- and interflock transmission of *Haemophilus gallinarum.* *Am. J. Vet. Res.* 27:1419–25.

Yamamoto, R., and D. T. Somersett. 1964. Antibody response in chickens to infection with *Haemophilus gallinarum.* *Avian Diseases* 8:441–53.

Yoder, H. W., Jr. 1965. Infectious coryza and avian mycoplasmosis, pp. 405–11. In Biester, H. E., and L. H. Schwarte (eds.), *Diseases of Poultry,* 5th ed. Iowa State Univ. Press, Ames.

Yoshimura, S., Y. Odagiri, and Y. Tomo. 1966. Aetiological studies on the respiratory disease complex of chickens in Osaka prefecture and its neighborhood. *J. Japan. Vet. Med. Ass.* 19:111–15. (English summary.)

CHAPTER 8

AVIAN MYCOPLASMOSIS

❖

INTRODUCTION

❖

HARRY W. YODER, Jr.

*USDA Southeast Poultry
Research Laboratory
Athens, Georgia*

❖

DURING recent years approximately 20 serotypes of mycoplasma have been characterized from avian sources. Those serotypes representing significant pathogens have been given genus and species designations, as have a few of lesser importance. Thus it has become necessary to discuss the entire group under the broad designation of avian mycoplasmosis, with more complete treatises presented for only the three most significant members: *Mycoplasma gallisepticum*, *M. meleagridis*, and *M. synoviae*.

HISTORY

Mycoplasma were probably first encountered in chickens by Nelson (1933, 1935, 1936, 1939), and the condition designated as "chronic respiratory disease" was described by Delaplane and Stuart (1943). The infection in turkeys was described by Dodd (1905) and named "infectious sinusitis" by Dickinson and Hinshaw (1938). Markham and Wong (1952) and Van Roekel and Olesiuk (1953) reported on the successful cultivation of the organisms from chickens and turkeys and noted their similarity. Grumbles et al. (1953) and Van Roekel and Olesiuk (1953) described some of the cultural and biochemical characteristics of mycoplasma (probably *M. gallisepticum*) from chickens and turkeys. Comparative studies by Jacobs et al. (1953), White et al. (1954), and Gianforte et al. (1955) indicated that their isolates were all antigenically similar.

SEROTYPING

Mycoplasma representing different serotypes became apparent during studies by Adler et al. (1957, 1958) and Chu (1958). Yamamoto and Adler (1958a,b) characterized 5 serotypes. Kleckner (1960) described 8 serotypes, designated A through H, including the previous 5. Yoder and Hofstad (1962) characterized the Iowa 695 serotype. All of these serotypes were included in the 12 serotypes (A through L) which were characterized by Yoder and Hofstad (1964) and in the 19 serotypes (A through S) characterized by Dierks et al. (1967). Isolates found to represent serotypes O and P confirmed the differences noted earlier by Moore et al. (1960). Roberts (1964b) added at least one new serotype, represented by isolate WRI.

Some of these serotypes, especially E and G, were not distinguishable by the colony inhibition technique employed by Fabricant (1960, 1962, personal communication) and Kelton and Van Roekel (1963). Dierks et al. (1967) and Fabricant (1968, personal communication) noted the similarity of serotypes B and M, as well as that of E and G. Frey (personal communication), using complement fixation tests with one representative strain of each of the 19 previously reported "serotypes," placed them in 8 antigenic groups (Table 8.1). Newer techniques may alter future groupings, and additional serotypes will undoubtedly be added.

CLASSIFICATION

Edward and Freundt (1956) suggested a revised classification for the entire pleuropneumonia group, and Freundt (1957) published the major aspects of it in the 7th edition of *Bergey's Manual of Determinative Bacteriology*. A single genus, *Mycoplasma*, was placed in the family Mycoplasmataceae under the Mycoplasmatales order. Edward and Freundt (1967) proposed Mollicutes as the name of the separate new class recently created. The only avian member originally listed was *Mycoplasma gallinarum*, a nonpathogenic spe-

TABLE 8.1 ❧ Avian Mycoplasma Relationships as Demonstrated by Complement Fixation
(Expressed as reciprocal of highest reacting dilution of antiserum)

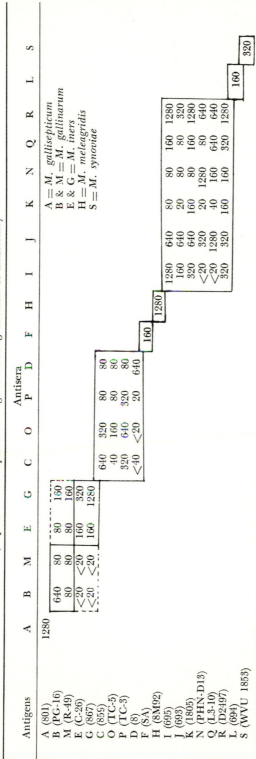

Antigens	A	B	M	E	G	C	O	P	D	F	H	I	J	K	N	Q	R	L	S
A (801)	1280																		
B (PG-16)	640	80	80	80	160														
M (R-49)	80	80	80	80	160														
E (C-26)		<20	<20	160	320														
G (867)		<20	<20	160	1280														
C (855)						640	320	80	80										
O (TC-5)						40	160	80	80										
P (TC-3)						320	640	320	80										
D (8)						<40	<20	20	640										
F (SA)										160									
H (8M92)											1280								
I (695)												1280	640	80	80	160	1280		
J (693)												160	640	20	80	80	320		
K (1805)												320	640	160	80	160	1280		
N (PHN-D13)												<20	320	20	1280	80	640		
Q (L3-10)												<20	1280	40	160	640	640		
R (D2497)												320	320	160	160	320	1280		
L (694)																		160	
S (WVU 1853)																			320

A = *M. gallisepticum*
B & M = *M. gallinarum*
E & G = *M. iners*
H = *M. meleagridis*
S = *M. synoviae*

Antisera

Source: Unpublished data prepared by M. L. Frey, Veterinary Medical Research Institute, Iowa State University.
Solid lines enclose reaction between serotypes which were considered to be closely enough related to include in one species. Broken lines enclose reactions between serotypes which have a one-way relationship only.
All reactions not indicated were negative at 1/20.

cies found to represent the B serotype of Kleckner (1960) by Fabricant (1960). Edward and Kanarek (1960) proposed the name *Mycoplasma gallisepticum* for the typical pathogen which causes chronic respiratory disease of chickens and infectious sinusitis of turkeys, and *M. iners* for a relatively nonpathogenic species representing serotype G. Yamamoto et al. (1965) designated *M. meleagridis* for the H serotype, and Olson et al. (1964) named the infectious synovitis serotype *M. synoviae*. Adler and Shifrine (1964) described *M. laidlawii* var. *inocuum* as a saprophytic member from a chicken sinus. Roberts (1964a) described *M. anatis,* an isolate from ducks.

CHARACTERIZATION

A summary concerning the major aspects of mycoplasma associated with poultry is presented in Table 8.2.

Space will not permit a detailed description of each serotype so far described, but an effort will be made to mention some of the most pertinent characteristics as summarized by Dierks et al. (1967).

Mycoplasma from avian sources generally require a complete medium containing 10–15% added serum from animal blood and further supplemented with some yeast-derived component. *M. synoviae* requires the addition of reduced nicotinamide adenine dinucleotide (NAD).

They tend to grow rather slowly, usually prefer 37–38° C, and are rather resistant to thallium acetate and penicillin which are frequently employed in media to retard the growth of contaminant bacteria. Colonies form on agar media incubated in an especially moist area for 3–10 days at 37° C. Variations in colony morphology have been described but cannot be relied upon to differentiate the various serotypes. Typical colonies are very small (0.1–1.0 mm), smooth, circular, and somewhat flat with a more dense central elevation (Fig. 8.4). Individual cells vary from 0.2 to 0.5μ and are basically coccoid to coccobacilliform, but slender rods, filaments, and ring forms have been described employing Giemsa-stained films.

Fermentation of carbohydrates is variable, but all serotypes may be divided into those which ferment glucose with the production of acid (serotypes A, C, D, F, I, J, K, N, O, P, Q, R, and S) and those which do not. At least certain isolates of sero-

types A, H, I, J, K, N, P, and S hemagglutinate chicken or turkey erythrocytes. Other characteristics which aid in the differentiation of serotypes are the reduction of tetrazolium and the presence of arginine decarboxylase, as described by Fabricant (1968, personal communication).

M. gallisepticum, M. meleagridis, and *M. synoviae* are considered to be pathogenic for certain avian hosts under various conditions, but the status of the pathogenicity of other serotypes is less clear. Certain isolates of serotypes C, E, I, J, M, and Q seem to elicit at least a lymphofollicular response when injected directly into the air sacs of experimental birds. Egg transmission of the pathogens *M. gallisepticum, M. meleagridis,* and *M. synoviae* is well documented and has been strongly suggested for serotypes I, Q, and R in turkeys.

It is necessary to employ various serological procedures to definitely identify a given isolate of avian mycoplasma. Agglutination procedures have been the most common, but the hemagglutination-inhibition procedure has been employed for serotypes A, H, I, and S. Other procedures have also been employed: complement fixation (Frey and Hanson, 1969), growth inhibition (Fabricant, 1960; Dierks et al., 1967), fluorescent antibody (Corstvet and Sadler, 1964), polyacrylamide-gel electrophoresis (Razin, 1968), and agar gel diffusion (Too, 1967).

L-PHASE ORGANISMS AND MYCOPLASMA

The possible relationship of avian mycoplasma to so-called L-phase organisms of various bacteria was postulated by McKay and Taylor (1954) and Kelton and Gentry (1957). McKay and Truscott (1960) reported the apparent reversion of mycoplasma to organisms resembling *Haemophilus gallinarum.* However, further study by Rogul et al. (1965) showed that *H. gallinarum, M. gallinarum,* and *M. gallisepticum* were genetically dissimilar, based on DNA base-ratio and homology studies, and consequently were of different phylogenetic origin.

Kelton et al. (1960) and Gentry (1960) reported on the apparent reversion of numerous cultures of avian mycoplasma (apparently *M. gallisepticum* and *M. gallinarum*) to various bacteria, especially micrococci. Gentry (1960) did classify the pathogenic strains as mycoplasma but con-

TABLE 8.2 ❧ Characteristics of Avian Mycoplasma

Serotype	Species	Isolate	Origin	Original Source	Ferments Glucose	Hemagglutination	Pathogenicity*
A	M. gallisepticum	X95	Chicken trachea	Markham	+	++++	+
A	M. gallisepticum	S6	Turkey brain	Zander	++	++++	++++
A	M. gallisepticum	A5969	Chicken trachea	Van Roekel	++	+	+++
A	M. gallisepticum	801	Turkey air sac	Hofstad	++	+	−
B	M. gallinarum	Fowl	Chicken trachea	Edward	−	−	−
B	M. gallinarum	54-537	Chicken trachea	Kleckner	−	−	±
C		C	Chicken trachea	Adler	++	−	±
C		DIVA	Chicken trachea	Kleckner	++	−	E
D		NY	Chicken trachea	Markham	++	−	E
D		R39A	Chicken trachea	Fabricant	++	−	E
E		DPR-2	Chicken trachea	Kleckner	−	−	E
E		640	Chicken trachea	Hofstad	−	−	−
E		C26	Chicken trachea	Fabricant	−	−	−
F		SA	Turkey trachea	Adler	+	−	E
G	M. iners	M	Chicken trachea	Edward	−	−	−
G	M. iners	O	Chicken pericardium	Adler	−	−	E
H	M. meleagridis	N	Turkey air sac	Adler	−	+	+++
H	M. meleagridis	1300	Turkey air sac	Yoder	−	++	+++
H	M. meleagridis	E-2	Turkey yolk sac	Rhoades	−	+++	±
I		695	Turkey air sac	Hofstad	+++	+	±
J		693	Turkey hock joint	Hofstad	++	+++	−
K		1805	Chicken oviduct	Yoder	++	+	−
L		694	Pigeon turbinate	Hofstad	−	−	−
M		R49	Chicken trachea	Fabricant	−	−	±
N		PHND13	Turkey air sac	Fabricant	++++	+	−
O		TC5	Chicken trachea	Moore	++++	±	−
P		TC3	Chicken trachea	Moore	++++	+	−
Q		L3-10	Turkey yolk sac	Fabricant	+	−	±
R		D2497	Turkey air sac	Fabricant	+	−	±
S	M. synoviae	1853	Turkey hock joint	Olson	+++	++	S
S	M. synoviae	1331	Turkey sinus	Yoder	+++	−	S
:	M. anatis		Duck sinus	Roberts	+++	+	−
:			Turkey air sac	Roberts	++	+	−
:	M. laidlawii var. inocuum	WRI	Chicken sinus	Adler	+	−	−

* Pathogenicity symbols: + = extensive airsacculitis in inoculated turkeys; ± = slight to moderate airsacculitis in inoculated turkeys; − = nonpathogenic for chickens or turkeys; E = periarticular abscesses in chicken embryos; S = synovitis in chickens and turkeys.

sidered others as L-phase organisms of bacteria. The issue is still controversial, with some feeling that apparent reversions are mainly due to the removal of inhibitors

from media supporting the growth of true mycoplasma in addition to suppressed bacteria which then revert to their vegetative form.

REFERENCES

Adler, H. E., and M. Shifrine. 1964. *Mycoplasma laidlawii* var. *inocuum* comb. nov. *J. Bacteriol.* 87:1245.

Adler, H. E., R. Yamamoto, and J. Berg. 1957. Strain differences of pleuropneumonia-like organisms of avian origin. *Avian Diseases* 1:19–26.

Adler, H. E., J. Fabricant, R. Yamamoto, and J. Berg. 1958. Symposium on chronic respiratory disease of poultry. I. Isolation and identification of pleuropneumonia-like organisms of avian origin. *Am. J. Vet. Res.* 19: 440–47.

Chu, H. P. 1958. Differential diagnosis and control of respiratory diseases of poultry. *Vet. Record* 70:1064–78.

Corstvet, R. E., and W. W. Sadler. 1964. The diagnosis of certain avian diseases with the fluorescent antibody technique. *Poultry Sci.* 43:1280–88.

Delaplane, J. P., and H. O. Stuart. 1943. The propagation of a virus in embryonated chicken eggs causing a chronic respiratory disease of chickens. *Am. J. Vet. Res.* 4: 325–32.

Dickinson, E. M., and W. R. Hinshaw. 1938. Treatment of infectious sinusitis of turkeys with argyrol and silver nitrate. *J. Am. Vet. Med. Ass.* 93:151–56.

Dierks, R. E., J. A. Newman, and B. S. Pomeroy. 1967. Characterization of avian mycoplasma. *Ann. N.Y. Acad. Sci.* 143:170–89.

Dodd, S. 1905. Epizootic pneumoenteritis of the turkey. *J. Comp. Pathol. Therap.* 18: 239–45.

Edward, D. G., and E. A. Freundt. 1956. The classification and nomenclature of organisms of the pleuropneumonia group. *J. Gen. Microbiol.* 14: 197–207.

———. 1967. Proposal for Mollicutes as name of the class established for the order Mycoplasmatales. *Int. J. Syst. Bacteriol.* 17:267–68.

Edward, D. G., and A. D. Kanarek. 1960. Organisms of the pleuropneumonia group of avian origin: Their classification into species. *Ann. N.Y. Acad. Sci.* 79:696–702.

Fabricant, J. 1960. Serological studies of avian pleuropneumonia-like organisms (PPLO) with Edward's technique. *Avian Diseases* 4:505–14.

Freundt, E. A. 1957. Order X. Mycoplasmatales, Freundt, 1955, pp. 914–26. In Breed, R. S., E. G. D. Murray, and N. R. Smith (eds.), *Bergey's Manual of Determinative Bacteriology*, 7th ed. Williams & Wilkins Co., Baltimore.

Frey, M. L., and R. P. Hanson. 1969. A complement fixation test for the study of avian mycoplasmas. *Avian Diseases* 13:185–97.

Gentry, R. F. 1960. Differentiation of avian PPLO and bacterial L forms. *Ann. N.Y. Acad. Sci.* 79:403–9.

Gianforte, E. M., E. L. Jungherr, and R. E. Jacobs. 1955. A serologic analysis of seven strains of pleuropneumonia-like organisms from air sac infection in poultry. *Poultry Sci.* 34:662–69.

Grumbles, L. C., E. Phillips, W. A. Boney, Jr., and J. P. Delaplane. 1953. Cultural and biochemical characteristics of the agent causing infectious sinusitis of turkeys and chronic respiratory disease of chickens. *Southwestern Vet.* 6:166–68.

Jacobs, R. E., E. L. Jungherr, R. E. Luginbuhl, and E. Gianforte. 1953. Serological studies on air sac infection. *Proc. 25th Ann. Meet. Northeast Conf. Lab. Workers in Pullorum Disease Control.* Univ. Mass., Amherst.

Kelton, W. H., and R. F. Gentry. 1957. Studies on chronic respiratory disease. II. The reversion of so-called "PPLO" to bacterial L-forms. *Avian Diseases* 1:347. (Abstr.)

Kelton, W. H., and H. Van Roekel. 1963. Serological studies of mycoplasma (PPLO) of avian origin. *Avian Diseases* 7:272–86.

Kelton, W. H., R. F. Gentry, and E. H. Ludwig. 1960. Derivation of Gram-positive cocci from pleuropneumonia-like organisms. *Ann. N.Y. Acad. Sci.* 79:410–21.

Kleckner, A. L. 1960. Serotypes of avian pleuropneumonia-like organisms. *Am. J. Vet. Res.* 21:274–80.

McKay, K. A., and J. R. E. Taylor. 1954. The reversion of L type cultures previously described as pleuropneumonia-like and associated with chronic respiratory disease to an organism resembling *Hemophilus gallinarum*. *Can. J. Comp. Med. Vet. Sci.* 18: 7–12.

McKay, K. A., and R. B. Truscott. 1960. Reversion of avian pleuropneumonia-like organisms to bacteria. *Ann. N.Y. Acad. Sci.* 79:465–80.

Markham, F. S., and S. C. Wong. 1952. Pleuropneumonia-like organisms in the etiology of turkey sinusitis and chronic respiratory disease of chickens. *Poultry Sci.* 31:902–4.

Moore, R. W., L. C. Grumbles, and J. N. Beasley. 1960. Pathological, serological and cultural characteristics of ten avian strains of pleuropneumonia-like organisms. *Ann. N.Y. Acad. Sci.* 79:556–61.

Nelson, J. B. 1933. Studies on an uncomplicated coryza of the domestic fowl. II. The relation of the "bacillary" coryza to that produced by exudate. *J. Exp. Med.* 58: 297–304.

———. 1935. Coccobacilliform bodies associated with an infectious fowl coryza. *Science* 82:43–44.

———. 1936. Studies on an uncomplicated coryza of the domestic fowl. VI. Coccobacilliform bodies in birds infected with the coryza of slow onset. *J. Exp. Med.* 63: 515–22.

———. 1939. Growth of fowl coryza bodies in tissue culture and in blood agar. *J. Exp. Med.* 69:199–209.

Olson, N. O., K. M. Kerr, and A. Campbell. 1964. Control of infectious synovitis. 13. The antigen study of three strains. *Avian Diseases* 8:209–14.

Razin, S. 1968. Mycoplasma taxonomy studied by electrophoresis of cell proteins. *J. Bacteriol.* 96:687–94.

Roberts, D. H. 1964a. The isolation of an influenza A virus and a mycoplasma associated with duck sinusitis. *Vet. Record* 76:470–73.

———. 1964b. Serotypes of avian mycoplasma. *J. Comp. Pathol. Therap.* 74:447–56.

Rogul, M., Z. A. McGee, R. G. Wittler, and S. Falkow. 1965. Nucleic acid homologies of selected bacteria, L-forms and mycoplasma species. *J. Bacteriol.* 90:1200–1204.

Too, K. 1967. Immunological study of *Mycoplasma gallisepticum*, especially by the agar gel diffusion test: Preliminary report. *Japan. J. Vet. Res.* 15:110.

Van Roekel, H., and O. M. Olesiuk. 1953. The etiology of chronic respiratory disease. *Proc. 90th Ann. Meet., Am. Vet. Med. Ass.,* pp. 289–303.

White, F. H., G. I. Wallace, and J. O. Alberts. 1954. Serological and electron microscope studies of chronic respiratory disease agent of chickens and of turkey sinusitis agent. *Poultry Sci.* 33:500–507.

Yamamoto, R., and H. E. Adler. 1958a. Characterization of pleuropneumonia-like organisms of avian origin. I. Antigenic analysis of seven strains and their comparative pathogenicity for birds. *J. Infect. Diseases* 102:143–52.

———. 1958b. Characterization of pleuropneumonia-like organisms of avian origin. II. Cultural, biochemical, morphological and further serological studies. *J. Infect. Diseases* 102:243–50.

Yamamoto, R., C. H. Bigland, and H. B. Ortmayer. 1965. Characteristics of *Mycoplasma meleagridis* sp. n., isolated from turkeys. *J. Bacteriol.* 90:47–49.

Yoder, H. W., Jr., and M. S. Hofstad. 1962. A previously unreported serotype of avian mycoplasma. *Avian Diseases* 6:147–60.

———. 1964. Characterization of avian mycoplasma. *Avian Diseases* 8:481–512.

❖

MYCOPLASMA GALLISEPTICUM INFECTION

❖

HARRY W. YODER, Jr.
USDA Southeast Poultry Research Laboratory Athens, Georgia

❖

Mycoplasma gallisepticum infection is commonly designated as chronic respiratory disease (CRD) of chickens and infectious sinusitis of turkeys. It is characterized by respiratory rales, coughing, nasal discharge, and frequently in turkeys a sinusitis. The clinical manifestations are usually slow to develop and the disease has a long course. Air sac disease designates a severe airsacculitis which is the result of *M. gallisepticum* infection complicated by some respiratory virus infection and also usually *Escherichia coli*.

Airsacculitis in chickens and airsacculitis and sinusitis in turkeys continue to be significant causes of condemnations at the time of slaughter. Most of this loss is related directly or indirectly to *M. gallisepticum* infection, with or without complicating factors. The economic losses due to downgrading of carcasses, reduced feed and egg production efficiency, and increased medication costs are additional factors which make this one of the costliest disease problems confronting the poultry industry. Conducting adequate prevention and control programs is also expensive. Fortunately the disease is of little or no public health significance beyond the condemnations for unwholesomeness.

HISTORY

The first accurate description of the disease in turkeys was probably made by Dodd (1905) in England under the name of "epizootic pneumoenteritis." Graham-Smith (1907) described it as "swollen head" in turkeys in England also. Tyzzer (1926) apparently was the first to describe turkey sinusitis in the United States. Dickinson and Hinshaw (1938) named the disease "infectious sinusitis" of turkeys.

Nelson (1935) described coccobacilliform bodies associated with an infectious coryza in chickens. He found them to be associated with the coryza of slow onset and long duration (Nelson, 1936a,b, 1938) and eventually was able to grow the coccobacilliform bodies in embryonating eggs, tissue culture, and cell-free medium (Nelson, 1936c, 1939). Smith et al. (1948) studied Nelson's agent and found it grew well in ascitic peptic digest plates and in infusion broth enriched with 30% horse serum. From cultural and morphological characteristics they concluded that Nelson's coccobacilliform bodies could be included in the pleuropneumonia group of organisms.

Beach and Schalm (1936) produced sinusitis in turkeys following intranasal inoculation with nasal exudate from chickens with coryza. They, like Nelson, apparently were studying *Mycoplasma gallisepticum* infection, sometimes in addition to *Hemophilus gallinarum* infection. This is further supported by the finding of Adler and Yamamoto (1956b) that a combination of *H. gallinarum* and avian pleuropneumonialike organisms *(M. gallisepticum)* resulted in a disease of rapid onset and long duration which Nelson (1938) produced with a combination of *H. gallinarum* and coccobacilliform bodies.

Delaplane and Stuart (1943) cultivated an agent in embryos isolated from chickens with a chronic respiratory disease, and later from turkeys with sinusitis (Delaplane, 1949). Markham and Wong (1952) and Van Roekel and Olesiuk (1953) reported on successful cultivation of the organisms from chickens and turkeys and noted their similarity, and Markham and Wong (1952) suggested that they were members of the pleuropneumonia group (mycoplasma).

INCIDENCE AND DISTRIBUTION

The disease has become an important flock problem in chickens and turkeys in all areas of the United States. It is also present in chickens in Canada (Fahey et al., 1953), Holland (De Blieck, 1950), Brazil (Garust and Nóbrega, 1956), the Philippines (Quizon, 1958), India (Pathak and Singh, 1961), Japan (Tajima et al., 1958), England (Chu, 1958), Germany (Hartwigk, 1958), Switzerland (Keller, 1958), Egypt (Eissa, 1956), France (Brion et al., 1958), Australia (Cottew, 1956), South Africa (Coles and Cumming, 1959), Czechoslovakia (Stricker and Fišera, 1955), and Finland (Estola, 1967). Similar reports concerning the infection in turkeys have been made from England (Graham-Smith, 1907), Australia (Hart, 1940), Italy (Valcarenghi, 1960), France (Brion et al., 1958), and South Africa (Coles and Cumming, 1959). Thus *M. gallisepticum* infection appears to be worldwide in distribution.

ETIOLOGY

CLASSIFICATION

Mycoplasma gallisepticum (Edward and Kanarek, 1960) is a pathogenic species within the genus *Mycoplasma* of the family Mycoplasmataceae under the order Mycoplasmatales (Freundt, 1957). Mollicutes was proposed as the name of the separate

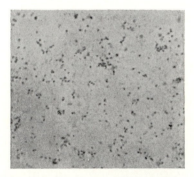

FIG. 8.1—*Smear of sedimented broth culture of* Mycoplasma gallisepticum. *Giemsa,* ×885. *(Hofstad, Iowa State Univ.)*

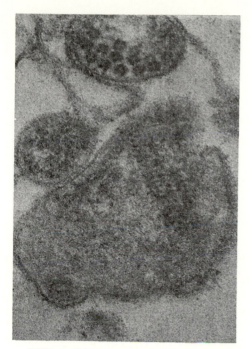

FIG. 8.2—Mycoplasma gallisepticum strain JA, 96-hour culture. Cells with ribosomes arranged in corncoblike pattern on longitudinal section; others seen on cross section. Electron micrograph of thin section. ×94,000. (Domermuth et al., 1964b)

new class recently created (Edward and Freundt, 1967).

MORPHOLOGY AND STAINING

The organism stains well with Giemsa's stain but is weakly gram-negative. It is generally coccoid, approximately 0.25–0.5μ in size (Fig. 8.1). It has been studied by electron microscopy, and some variation in morphology has been found. Shifrine et al. (1962) studied the edge of growing colonies and concluded that the elementary cells were hexagonal and originated from within larger cells or by fragmentation of peripheral filaments.

The use of thin section techniques with negative staining has made it possible to study their ultrastructure and modes of multiplication. Domermuth et al. (1964a,b) noted internal cellular dense bodies which appeared to be developing elementary bodies. Similar dense bodies were observed in protrusions extending from the surface of the cells (Fig. 8.2). Ribosomes were present in some of their preparations (Fig. 8.3).

Dutto et al. (1965) noted similar internal dense areas within the mother cells, in cell protrusions, and in daughter cells. Part of the growth cycle resembled budding, as also noted by Domermuth et al. (1964a). Morowitz and Maniloff (1966) described

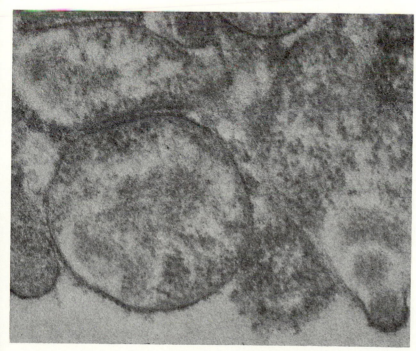

FIG. 8.3—Mycoplasma gallisepticum strain W, 96-hour culture. Small elementary body (lower left) contains cytoplasm of marked electron density. One semilunar and two spherical condensations are located within a protrusion of the cell membrane (lower right). Electron micrograph of thin section. ×94,000. (Domermuth et al., 1964b)

mainly a binary fission scheme. They observed ribosomes, dense polar bodies, and obvious cell divisions into similar daughter cells. It is probable that more than one mode of cell replication is possible, depending upon various cell and environmental conditions.

GROWTH REQUIREMENTS

Mycoplasma gallisepticum requires a rather complex medium enriched with 10–15% heat-inactivated swine, avian, or horse serum. Concentrated serum fraction (Difco) may also serve as an enrichment. Several media have been developed for the isolation and growth of *M. gallisepticum* (Markham and Wong, 1952; Grumbles et al., 1953; Adler and Yamamoto, 1956c; Hofstad and Doerr, 1956; Fabricant, 1959). Comparisons of different media have been made (Adler et al., 1954; Lecce and Sperling, 1954; Taylor et al., 1957; Taylor and Fabricant, 1957; Fabricant, 1958, 1959; Adler and Berg, 1960; Frey et al., 1968). It is apparent that several types of liquid or agar media will support the growth of mycoplasma of avian origin, with certain purposes altering the final choice. A liquid medium is desirable for antigen production, but the use of a broth overlay on an agar slant apparently is of some added value for making original isolations and maintaining cultures (Adler et al., 1954; Fabricant et al., 1962; Yamamoto and Bigland, 1964; Yoder and Hofstad, 1964). Media and techniques for antigen production have been described by Adler and Yamamoto (1956a), Hall (1962), and Vardaman (1967). Growth generally is optimal in medium at approximately pH 7.8 incubated at 37–38° C. Colonies form on agar medium containing the usual mycoplasma ingredients but require prolonged incubation (2–5 days) in a very moist atmosphere (Fabricant et al., 1962).

Frey et al. (1968) developed a medium which incorporated all of the essential ingredients including yeast autolysate and dextrose. (The formula for Frey's medium is listed in the section on *M. synoviae* infection.) The basic ingredients are available as a commercial formulation (Albimi). When prepared with 10–15% swine serum it is a convenient and very efficient medium for the cultivation of most mycoplasma. The inclusion of phenol red and dextrose makes it possible to detect growth in tubes employed in mass culturings, as does the addition of 0.0025% 2,3,5 triphenyl tetrazolium chloride as an indicator (Yoder and Hofstad, 1964).

M. gallisepticum may also be propagated in embryonated chicken eggs. See sections on Pathogenicity and Isolation and Identification.

COLONIAL MORPHOLOGY

Mycoplasma gallisepticum can be grown on serum-enriched agar medium inoculated with broth or agar culture material. It is very difficult to obtain colony growth direct from original exudates. Inoculated agar plates must be incubated at 37° C in a very moist atmosphere for 3–5 days. The technique of incubating plates in a sealed candle jar is not essential, although it is effective (Fabricant et al., 1962). Evidence of colony growth is best studied with the aid of a dissecting microscope with indirect lighting. The characteristic colonies appear as tiny, smooth, circular, translucent masses with a dense, raised central area (Fig. 8.4). They rarely are more than 0.2–0.3 mm in diameter and frequently occur in ridges along the streak line since closely adjacent colonies readily coalesce.

Yoder and Hofstad (1964) and Dierks et al. (1967) noted certain variations in the colonies of isolates representing the numerous serotypes of avian mycoplasma but could not definitely determine the serotype of an organism by its colony characteristics.

BIOCHEMICAL PROPERTIES

Biochemical and related biological properties of *M. gallisepticum* have been reported by numerous workers including Yamamoto and Adler (1958b), Kleckner (1960), Yoder and Hofstad (1964), and Dierks et al. (1967). *M. gallisepticum* ferments glucose and maltose with the production of acid but not gas. It does not ferment lactose, dulcitol, or salicin. Sucrose is rarely fermented; the results with galactose, fructose, trehalose, and mannitol are variable.

Yoder and Hofstad (1964) reported that *M. gallisepticum* reduced 2,3,5 triphenyl tetrazolium chloride incorporated into medium as a growth indicator. Yamamoto and Adler (1958b) reported on its reduction of tetrazolium-blue.

Yamamoto and Adler (1958b) observed a browning type of partial hemolysis of avian

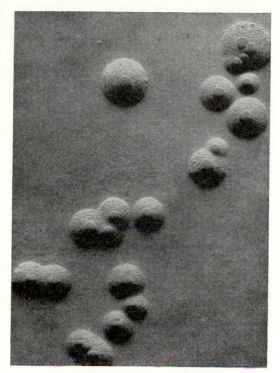

FIG. 8.4—*Colonies of* Mycoplasma galli-septicum *on 20% chicken serum agar plate.* ×40. *(Hofstad, Iowa State Univ.)*

erythrocytes in a tube test procedure. Yoder and Hofstad (1964) reported that *M. galli-septicum* caused complete hemolysis of horse erythrocytes incorporated into agar medium. *M. gallisepticum* agglutinates erythrocytes of turkeys and chickens (Ya-mamoto and Adler, 1958b). See further discussion under hemagglutination-inhibition test in section on Serology.

RESISTANCE TO CHEMICAL AND PHYSICAL AGENTS

It is assumed that most of the commonly employed chemical disinfectants are effective against *M. gallisepticum*, but reports appear to be lacking on this subject. Its resistance to penicillin and low concentration (1:4,000) of thallous acetate makes these valuable additives to mycoplasma culture media as inhibitors of bacterial contamination. The inactivation of mycoplasma by beta-propiolactone was described by Roberts (1964).

M. gallisepticum remained viable in chicken feces for 1–3 days at 20° C, on muslin cloth for 3 days at 20° C or 1 day at 37° C, and in egg yolk for 18 weeks at 37° C

or 6 weeks at 20° C (Chandiramani et al., 1966). Broth suspensions of infective chorioallantoic membranes lost their infectivity after 1 hour of exposure at 45° C, after 20 minutes at 50° C, or by the third week at 5° C (Hofstad, 1959). However, Olesiuk and Van Roekel (1952) found infective allantoic fluid remained infective for 4 days in the incubator, for 6 days at room temperature, and for 32–60 days in the refrigerator. Yoder (1970) found that *M. gallisepticum* was inactivated in infected chicken hatching eggs which just reached 114° F during a 12–14-hour heating procedure. Fabricant (1953) recovered the organism from 60%, 35%, and 13% of infective materials stored at −25° C for 1, 2, and 3 years respectively. Yoder and Hofstad (1964) found broth cultures remained viable for 2–4 years when stored at −30° C. They also recovered viable *M. gallisepticum* from lyophilized broth culture stored at 4° C for at least 7 years, and from lyophilized infective chicken turbinates stored at 4° C for 13–14 years.

The sensitivity of *M. gallisepticum* to various antibiotics is discussed in the section on Treatment.

STRAIN CLASSIFICATION

Various strains within the species *M. gallisepticum* should not be confused with the numerous serotypes which have been characterized from avian sources within the entire genus *Mycoplasma*. Certain isolates of *M. gallisepticum* have come to be known more commonly by their isolate designations which sometimes are called strains. The S6 strain of Zander (1961) is probably the best example. Other commonly designated strains are listed in the introductory part of this chapter. Reports have not been published showing any major antigenic differences among the numerous isolates of *M. gallisepticum*. However, certain ones are preferred for antigen production and others for bird inoculation, due to differences in their adaptations to certain media and experimental hosts or due to their relative pathogenicity.

PATHOGENICITY

Inoculum

Isolates of *M. gallisepticum* vary widely in their relative pathogenicity, depending upon the nature of the isolate, its method of propagation, and the number of passages through which it has been maintained. The route of infection and type of host are also factors influencing the observed degree of pathogenicity. Hofstad and Doerr (1956) found that one isolate produced turkey sinusitis after 33 serial broth passages, another was similarly infective after 50 broth passages, but 2 others were not infective after 75 and 95 broth passages. Infective yolk from inoculated embryonated chicken eggs is generally considered to be more capable of producing infection than broth-passaged mycoplasma (Fabricant and Levine, 1963; Yoder and Hofstad, 1964).

Chicken and Turkey

The pathogenicity for chickens and turkeys of various serotypes of mycoplasma including *M. gallisepticum* was determined in studies by Yamamoto and Adler (1958a), Kleckner (1960), Yoder and Hofstad (1964), Rhoades et al. (1965), Dierks et al. (1961), Kerr and Olson (1967), and Madden et al. (1967b).

In general, turkeys appeared to be more susceptible than chickens; inoculated turkeys developed more severe sinusitis, airsacculitis, and tendovaginitis. Yoder and Hofstad (1964) found that inoculation of the tendovaginal cavity in the region of the hock and foot pad of chickens resulted in the production of antibodies and usually severe to moderate tendovaginitis, while inoculated air sacs in the same chickens showed little or no gross response.

EMBRYONATED CHICKEN EGGS

Inoculation of broth cultures or exudates containing *M. gallisepticum* in 7-day-old embryonated chicken eggs via the yolk sac route usually results in embryo deaths within 5–7 days. One or more yolk passages may be necessary before typical deaths and lesions are produced. Dwarfing, generalized edema, liver necrosis, and enlarged spleens are most typical (Van Roekel et al., 1952; Chute and Cole, 1954). The organism reaches its highest concentration in the yolk sac, yolk, and chorioallantoic membrane just prior to death of the embryo (Hofstad, 1952; Luginbuhl and Jungherr, 1953; Gentry et al., 1967).

The joint abscesses noted in some infected embryos by Moulton and Adler (1957), Calnek and Levine (1957) and Von Roekel et al. (1957) were described by Chute (1960)

as being primarily subcutaneous periarticular granulomas with necrotic centers and a border of epithelioid cells, some of which had coalesced to form giant cells. However, Yoder and Hofstad (1964) concluded that such lesions were produced by mycoplasma representing other serotypes than that of *M. gallisepticum*.

PATHOGENESIS AND EPIZOOTIOLOGY

NATURAL AND EXPERIMENTAL HOSTS

Mycoplasma gallisepticum infection occurs naturally in chickens and turkeys. It has also been isolated from natural infections in pheasants (Osborn and Pomeroy, 1958a), chukar partridges (*Alectoris graeca*) by Wichmann (1957) and Yoder and Hofstad (1964), in a peacock (*Pavo cristatus*) by Wills (1955), and from bobwhite quail (*Colinus virginianus*) by Madden et al. (1967a). Reports by Winterfield (1953) and Gianforte et al. (1955) suggested that *M. gallisepticum* infection occurred in pigeons.

Pigeons and partridges were included as susceptible hosts by Jungherr et al. (1953). However, Yoder and Hofstad (1964) were not able to produce the infection in pigeons or quail by inoculation with infective yolk material. Van Roekel and Olesiuk (1953) reported that guinea fowl and pheasants were readily infected.

Embryonated chicken eggs have been employed as experimental hosts by numerous investigators since the early reports of Delaplane and Stuart (1943), and Van Roekel et al. (1952).

TRANSMISSION

Direct contact of susceptible birds with infected carrier chickens or turkeys causes outbreaks of the disease, and it is also spread by air-borne dust or droplets (Fahey and Crawley, 1955a; Anderson and Beard, 1967). Spread by contact with contaminated equipment is commonly assumed but has not been well documented (Olesiuk et al., 1967). Evidence that the infection may be transmitted through the egg in chickens was reported by Van Roekel et al. (1952), Cover and Waller (1954), and Fahey and Crawley (1954b). Egg transmission in turkeys has been reported by Jerstad et al. (1949), Hofstad (1957a), and Osborn and Pomeroy (1958b). *M. gallisepticum* was isolated from the oviduct of infected chickens and semen of infected roosters by Yoder and Hofstad (1964). Egg transmission has been successfully produced following experimental infection of susceptible chickens (Fabricant and Levine, 1963; Yoder and Hofstad, 1965; and Yoder, 1969). Benton et al. (1967) isolated *M. gallisepticum* from a commercial laryngotracheitis vaccine, but they did not determine if it could cause transmission of *M. gallisepticum* infection in vaccinated birds.

INCUBATION PERIOD

Delaplane and Stuart (1943) and Van Roekel et al. (1952) found the incubation period to vary from 4 to 21 days in experimental transmission. Hofstad (1952) found that 65% of 233 chicks had symptoms of nasal discharge between 11 and 18 days following inoculation of infective turbinate material. Sinusitis often develops in experimentally inoculated turkeys within 7–10 days. Under natural conditions it is very difficult to determine the exact date of exposure; so many variable factors seem to influence the onset and extent of clinical infection that meaningful incubation periods cannot be stated. In the author's experience it seems evident that numerous chicken and turkey flocks develop clinical infection near the onset of egg production, suggesting a low level of inherent infection (probably due to egg transmission) which precipitates due to a series of stressing events. This apparent long extension of the incubation period is especially common in the offspring from infected chickens or turkeys which have been hatched from eggs dipped in antibiotic solutions for the control of *M. gallisepticum* infection. The possible role of contamination from other sources of the infection is not always clear and can rarely be proved beyond reasonable doubt.

SIGNS

Chickens

The most characteristic signs of the natural disease in adult flocks are tracheal rales, nasal discharge, and coughing. Feed consumption is reduced and the birds lose weight. In laying flocks egg production declines but is usually maintained at a lowered level. However, flocks may have serological evidence of infection with no obvious clinical signs, especially if they encountered the infection at a younger age

and have partially recovered. Male birds frequently have the most pronounced signs, and the disease is often more severe during the winter months. In broiler flocks most outbreaks occur between 4 and 8 weeks of age. The signs are frequently more marked than observed in mature flocks. The severe outbreaks observed in broilers are frequently due to complications (see Morbidity and Mortality).

Turkeys

A nasal discharge with foaming of the eye secretions frequently precedes the more typical swelling of the paranasal sinuses due to sinusitis. Sometimes partial to complete closing of the eyes results from severe sinus swelling (Fig. 8.5). The appetite remains near normal as long as the bird can see to eat. As the disease progresses the affected birds become thin. Tracheal rales, coughing, and labored breathing may become evident if tracheitis or airsacculitis is present. In breeding flocks there may be a drop in egg production or at least a lowered egg production efficiency.

MORBIDITY AND MORTALITY

Chickens

The infection usually affects nearly all of the chickens in a flock but is variable in severity and duration. It tends to be more severe and of longer duration in the cold months of the year and affects younger birds more severely than mature birds, although there may be a considerable loss from lowered egg production.

While *M. gallisepticum* is considered the primary cause of chronic respiratory disease, other organisms frequently cause complications (Biddle and Cover, 1957). Severe air sac infection, frequently designated as complicated CRD or air sac disease, is undoubtedly the more commonly encountered condition in the field. Newcastle disease or infectious bronchitis may precipitate outbreaks of *M. gallisepticum* infection (Van Roekel et al., 1957). *Escherichia coli* (especially O-group 2) has been found to be a frequent complicating organism (Wasserman et al., 1954; Gross, 1956; Glantz et al., 1962). The affect of *M. gallisepticum*, *E. coli*, and infectious bronchitis virus in singly and in multiply infected chickens was studied by Gross (1961a) and Fabricant and Levine (1962). They reproduced

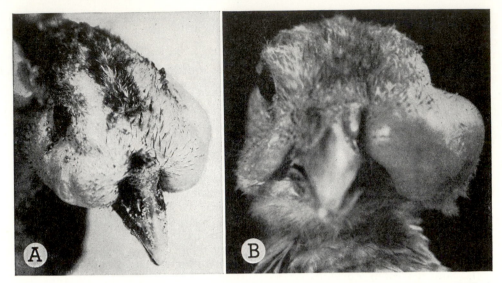

FIG. 8.5—(A) Advanced case of infectious sinusitis involving both sides of face. (B) Similar case after exudate in one sinus has been removed. (Hinshaw, Univ. of Calif.)

a severe air sac infection when all three agents were combined. They further noted that *E. coli* could not readily infect the air sacs unless they were previously invaded by *M. gallisepticum* alone or in combination with either infectious bronchitis virus (Gross, 1961b, 1962) or Newcastle disease virus. Adler et al. (1962) and Blake (1962) noted increased severity and duration of the disease when both *M. gallisepticum* and infectious bronchitis were present. The possible significance of the virus isolated by Fahey and Crawley (1954a) from outbreaks of chronic respiratory disease is still not clear. However, it was reported to be a reovirus by Petek et al. (1967).

Mortality is negligible in adult flocks, but in broilers it may be very low in the uncomplicated disease to as much as 30% in the complicated outbreaks. Retarded growth, downgrading of carcasses, and condemnations constitute still further losses.

Turkeys

The disease affects most of the turkeys in a flock, although some of them may not exhibit sinusitis and the lower respiratory form of the infection may be most prominent. The infection will last for weeks and months in untreated flocks. Condemnations are primarily due to airsacculitis and related systemic effects rather than to sinusitis as such.

GROSS LESIONS

The gross lesions consist primarily of catarrhal exudate in the nasal and paranasal passages, trachea, bronchi, and air sacs. Sinusitis is usually most prominent in turkeys but is also observed in chickens and other affected avian hosts. The air sacs frequently contain caseous exudate, although they may only present a "beaded" or lymphofollicular appearance. Some degree of pneumonia may be observed (Van Roekel et al., 1952). In severe cases of typical air sac disease in chickens there is

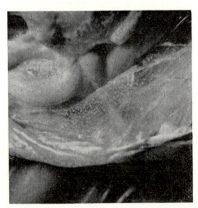

FIG. 8.6—Lymphofollicular or "beading" reaction in air sac of experimentally inoculated turkey. (Van Roekel et al., Univ. of Mass.)

fibrinous or fibrino-purulent perihepatitis and pericarditis along with massive airsacculitis (Gross, 1961a, 1962; Fabricant and Levine, 1962). *M. gallisepticum*-induced salpingitis of chickens and turkeys was reported by Domermuth et al. (1967).

HISTOPATHOLOGY

The microscopic pathology has been studied by Jungherr et al. (1953) and by Van Roekel et al. (1957). They found marked thickening of the mucous membrane of the affected tissues due to infiltration with mononuclear cells and hyper-

plasia of the mucous glands (Fig. 8.6). Focal areas of lyphoid hyperplasia (lymphofollicular reaction) were commonly found in the submucosa (Figs. 8.7, 8.8, 8.9). Johnson (1954) regarded these as specific for chronic respiratory disease. Hitchner (1949) found them characteristic in his study of the pathology of infectious sinusitis of turkeys. However, Barber (1962) observed similar lesions in apparently normal turkeys and suggested that the presence of lymphofollicular lesions may be of limited diagnostic value. In the lungs, in addition to pneumonic areas and lymphofollicular

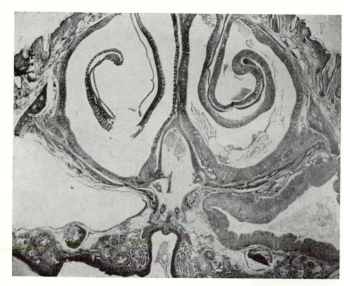

FIG. 8.7—*Section through nasal passages and sinuses of experimental chicken. Unilateral mucosal thickening of sinus and nasal passage.* ×6. (*Van Roekel et al., Univ. of Mass.*)

FIG. 8.8—*Section of sinus in chicken. Subepithelial infiltration of mononuclear cells and lymphofollicular reaction.* ×36. (*Van Roekel et al., Univ. of Mass.*)

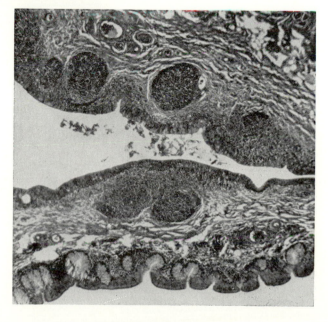

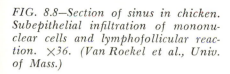

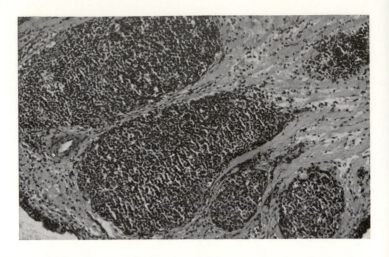

FIG. 8.9—Air sac of 7-week-old experimental chicken. Lymphofollicular reaction. ×100. (Van Roekel et al., Univ. of Mass.)

changes, granulomatous lesions were also found. Van Roekel et al. (1957) found granulomatous lesions in lungs of about 22% of field cases in chickens but in only 7% of experimentally inoculated chickens.

IMMUNITY

Birds which have recovered from clinical signs of the disease have some degree of immunity. Such flocks, however, carry the organism and can transmit the disease to susceptible stock by contact or by egg transmission to their progeny. A review of the literature concerning the immune response to *M. gallisepticum* is included in the report by Luginbuhl et al. (1967). For immunization procedures see the section on Prevention and Control.

DIAGNOSIS

ISOLATION AND IDENTIFICATION OF CAUSATIVE AGENT

Suspensions of tracheal or air sac exudates, turbinates, lungs, or fluid sinus exudate may be cultured directly in suitable broth or agar overlay medium. (See media formulations under Growth Requirements.) Extraneous bacterial contamination is usually controlled by the inclusion of thallous acetate (1:4,000) and penicillin (up to 2,000IU per ml) in the medium. Contaminants may also be eliminated by filtering the suspension through a series of Selas filters beginning with the 01 and continuing through the 015 and then the 02. Both the 015 and 02 filtrates should be cultured. Membrane filters of 0.45–0.60μ average pore diameter may also be used (Tourtellotte, 1963). Viable my-

coplasma can pass through still finer filters, but their number may be too drastically reduced.

Cultures should be incubated at least 5–7 days at 37° C. Growth may not be evident, but 2 or 3 serial passages of 0.5–1.0-ml transfers to new tubes of media at 3–5-day intervals may increase the number of isolations. The inclusion of triphenyl tetrazolium or phenol red with sufficient dextrose provides a growth indicator system. *M. gallisepticum* reduces the tetrazolium to produce a red color in the medium, or it ferments dextrose to change the phenol red to a yellow color as the medium becomes acid.

Cultures can be further identified by preparing Giemsa-stained films which should reveal small coccoid organisms, often in clumps, when examined through the oil immersion lens of a microscope (Fig. 8.1). Enriched agar medium may be inoculated from the broth cultures to study colonial morphology. The inoculated plates must be incubated at 37° C in a very moist atmosphere for 3–5 days before being examined for typical mycoplasma colonies. The hemagglutinating ability of cultures may also be determined. Inoculation of sinuses, air sacs, or tendon sheaths of young chickens or turkeys may be done to determine the pathogenicity of the culture. Sections prepared for histopathology might also be of aid in making a diagnosis.

The inoculation of 7-day embryonated chicken eggs via the yolk sac with original exudates may be employed as a further means of isolating *M. gallisepticum*, but the inoculum must be relatively free of bacterial contamination. Death of embryos should occur within 5–8 days, but one or more serial passages of harvested yolk material might be required before embryo deaths and typical lesions are noted.

However, proof that isolates truly are *M. gallisepticum* must be determined by serological procedures. Antigens can be prepared and then tested with known antiserum representing *M. gallisepticum*. Such testing of recently isolated cultures is rarely very satisfactory. One of the best methods is to test the serum from experimentally inoculated chickens or turkeys with known *M. gallisepticum* antigen.

SEROLOGY

Serological procedures are available to aid in the diagnosis of *M. gallisepticum* infection. A positive serological test, together with history and symptoms typical of the disease, would constitute a presumptive diagnosis pending isolation and identification of the organisms. Jungherr et al. (1953) first recognized the possibilities of certain serological procedures in *M. gallisepticum* infection. The rapid serum plate test was used by Adler (1954). Antigen is prepared according to the procedure of Adler and Yamamoto (1956a), Hofstad and Doerr (1956), or Hall (1962). The test is performed by placing a drop of serum on a white porcelain or glass plate and mixing with a drop of stained antigen. After the drops are mixed to make a spot about 2 cm in diameter, the plate is rotated gently and the test read within 2 minutes. Turkey serum reacts more slowly than chicken serum.

The tube agglutination test was found more reliable than the plate test by Jungherr et al. (1955). It was also found more reliable than the plate test in testing turkey serum (Hofstad, 1957b). The antigen prepared for the plate test can be used in the tube test when diluted 1:20 in phenolized (0.25%) buffered saline (pH 7). For routine flock testing, it is suggested that the 1:12.5 dilution (.08 ml serum plus 1 ml antigen) be used. The test is read after overnight incubation at 37° C. Clearing of the supernatant fluid, with clumps of antigen covering the entire bottom of the tube, is indicative of a positive test.

The hemagglutination-inhibition (HI) test has been used by Fahey (1954), Fahey and Crawley (1954b), Crawley and Fahey (1957), Hofstad (1957b), Hall et al. (1961), Yoder and Hofstad (1964), Newnham (1964), and Dierks et al. (1967).

The procedure of the HI test is essentially the same as the one used in Newcastle disease. The antigen used may be prepared by growing a suitable hemagglutinating strain of *M. gallisepticum* in broth. The antigen should be harvested at the peak of hemagglutinating (HA) activity. The organism is centrifuged out at 4,500 RPM for 1 hour in a refrigerated centrifuge. It is then suspended in 50% glycerin and stored in the freezer. The HA titer is determined by making twofold dilutions in 0.5-ml amounts of buffered saline (pH 7) containing a 1:1,000 dilution of normal serum. Washed 0.25% chicken or turkey red blood cells are added in 0.5-ml amounts to each dilution of the antigen. The test is read when the cell controls have sedimented, usually after 1 hour at room temperature. Agglutination is recognized by a uniform layer of cells covering the entire bottom of the tube, while in the negative tube a button of cells is found in the center of the bottom (Fig. 8.10). No elution occurs, so the test can be read at any time after 1 hour. If turkey cells are used, usually a twofold higher titer is obtained than with chicken cells.

The HI procedure can be used for both chicken and turkey serum. When testing chicken serum 4 HA units are used, while 2 HA units can be used for turkey serum. One HA unit is contained in the highest dilution of antigen which causes complete agglutination of 0.5 ml of 0.25% red blood cells. To set up the test, a series of 10 tubes is placed in a rack for each chicken serum sample to be tested. To tube 1 is added 0.8 ml of diluent, to tube 2 is added 0.5 ml of antigen containing 8 HA units, and to tubes 3 through 10 is added 0.5 ml of antigen containing 4 HA units. Using a 1-ml pipette, 0.2 ml of serum is removed from the serum sample and placed in tube 1 to make a 1:5 dilution of serum. Tube 1 becomes the serum control. The contents of tube 1 are mixed with the pipette, and a 0.5-ml amount is transferred to tube 2. Using the same pipette, twofold dilutions are continued through tube 10, discarding 0.5 ml from tube 10 after mixing has been done. Negative and positive sera should be included as controls. A 0.5-ml amount of 0.25% red cell suspension is then added to

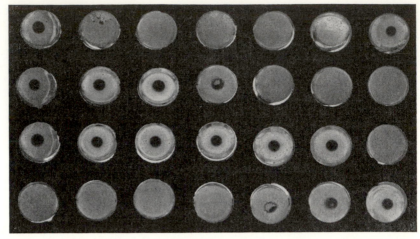

FIG. 8.10—*Hemagglutination-inhibition (HI) test.* **(Bottom row)** *Titration of antigen* (M. gallisepticum). *From left to right: 4 tubes show agglutination of red cells; tube 5 is intermediate; tubes 6 and 7 show normal settling of red cells.* **(Top row)** *Negative serum in HI test: tube 1 is serum control; tubes 2–5 show agglutination of cells; tube 6 is saline blank with no red cells; tube 7 is cell control.* **(Second row from top)** *Positive serum—low titer: tube 1 is serum control; tubes 2 and 3 show complete inhibition; tube 4 shows partial inhibition; tubes 5–7 show no inhibition.* **(Third row from top)** *Positive serum—higher titer: inhibition through tube 6.* (Hofstad, Iowa State Univ.)

each tube; the rack is shaken and set at room temperature for 1 hour, after which the test can be read. A positive serum will inhibit agglutination to a certain dilution of serum. The results may be recorded as HI units (highest dilution of serum in which there is complete inhibition × the HA units used). For example, if the end point of inhibition is the 1:320 dilution, the serum would contain 320×4, or 1,280 HI units.

Other serological procedures have been developed employing formalinized antigen for the HI test (Adler and DaMassa, 1967), an antiglobulin test for the detection of *M. gallisepticum* antibodies (Adler et al., 1964) and the use of the fluorescent antibody technique (Noel et al., 1964; Corstvet and Sadler, 1964). The use of saline diluted yolk from fresh eggs as a source of antibodies employed with rapid plate test antigen was described by Devos et al. (1968).

It is important to note that Olson et al. (1965) found definite cross-reactions when certain *M. synoviae* positive serum samples were tested with *M. gallisepticum* plate antigen. This was confirmed by Roberts and Olesiuk (1967) employing the rapid serum plate test but not with the tube

agglutination, agar gel diffusion, and *M. gallisepticum* HI test. Vardaman and Yoder (1969) noted the cross-reaction with the plate test also, but demonstrated little or no cross-reactions employing HI procedures for both *M. synoviae* and *M. gallisepticum*. The transient cross-reaction to *M. gallisepticum* plate antigen by serum from chickens and turkeys several days after injections with erysipelas bacterin noted by Boyer et al. (1960) was also confirmed by Roberts and Olesiuk (1967).

DIFFERENTIAL DIAGNOSIS

Chickens

Care must be taken to differentiate *M. gallisepticum* infection from the other common respiratory diseases of chickens. Newcastle disease and infectious bronchitis virus and/or antibodies may be present as separate entities or as part of the complicated CRD problem. Infectious coryza and fowl cholera usually can be identified by cultural studies. *M. synoviae* infection may be present alone or in addition to *M. gallisepticum*. The application of both of their serological test procedures may be necessary in some cases.

Turkeys

The presence of a respiratory disease including sinusitis in a turkey flock may at times be due to such things as fowl cholera, ornithosis, *M. synoviae* infection, or vitamin A deficiency as well as the more usual *M. gallisepticum*. Specific cultural and serological procedures are needed to differentiate them. Avian influenza A infection might also be considered. See the review by Bankowski et al. (1968).

TREATMENT

M. gallisepticum is susceptible to contact with certain antibiotics: streptomycin, oxytetracycline, chlortetracycline, erythromycin, magnamycin, spiramycin, and tylosin (Wong and James, 1953; Domermuth and Johnson, 1955; Yamamoto and Adler, 1956; Hamdy et al., 1957; Kiser et al., 1961; Yoder et al., 1961; Newnham and Chu, 1965). However, some strains of *M. gallisepticum* have been reported to be rather resistant to streptomycin, erythromycin, and spiramycin (Fahey, 1957; Yoder et al., 1961; Domermuth, 1958, 1960; Kiser et al., 1961).

Various antibiotics and chemicals have been injected or administered in the feed or water for the treatment of chronic respiratory disease (Peterson, 1953; Carson et al., 1954; White-Stevens and Zeibel, 1954; Cover, 1955; Fahey and Crawley, 1955b; Lecce and Sperling, 1955; Adler et al., 1956; Olesiuk and Van Roekel, 1959; Olesiuk et al., 1957, 1964, 1965; Olson et al., 1959, 1960; Barnes et al., 1960, 1961; Gross, 1961b; Heishman et al., 1960, 1962; Kiser et al., 1960; Gale et al., 1967).

The results of the various treatment studies have been variable, probably reflecting the varied complicating infections present in a wide spectrum of age groups under diverse conditions. In many cases it is doubtful if the small increase in weight gains or egg production and moderate reduction of carcass condemnations is sufficient to cover the cost of treatment. However, some of the more commonly employed treatments which tend to provide favorable results include the use of oxytetracycline or chlortetracycline at 200 g per ton of feed for at least several days. Such broad-spectrum antibiotics have been potentiated with approximately 0.5% terephthalic acid and sometimes a reduced cal-

cium ration. However, terephthalic acid is not cleared by the Food and Drug Administration for use in poultry rations. Tylosin has been injected subcutaneously at 3–5 mg per lb of body weight or administered at 2–3 g per gal of drinking water for 3–5 days. Antibiotic injections of infected breeding stock to control egg transmission have been used (see Control).

PREVENTION AND CONTROL

MANAGEMENT PROCEDURES

Strict isolation of the flock should be maintained to avoid introduction of the disease into a clean flock. A comprehensive list of sanitation and isolation procedures has been reported by Chute et al. (1964). The concept of raising poultry free of *M. gallisepticum* infection was based on the finding of some flocks naturally free of the disease in early studies by Jungherr et al. (1955) and Van Roekel et al. (1958). Dunlop and Strout (1956) obtained some negative groups by hatching and rearing small groups of a few hundred chicks in isolation and separating the clean groups from the infected by serological procedures. Current control programs are supported by the use of serological testing as a means of monitoring the status of flocks either found to be free of the disease or in which effort has been made to eliminate the infection. Most of the breeder turkeys in the United States are within some state-sponsored control program based on serological testing, with proved reactor flocks strictly eliminated for breeding purposes (Anon., 1965). Thus immunization and medication of breeding stock are mainly practiced with chickens.

IMMUNIZATION

Various inactivated vaccine preparations were reported to be of limited value in preventing *M. gallisepticum* infection by Prier and Dart (1951), Adler et al. (1960), and Warren et al. (1968). Attempts to immunize young birds with infective *M. gallisepticum* preparations inoculated intramuscularly have not been very satisfactory (Adler et al., 1960; Domermuth, 1962). Infective preparations inoculated via the respiratory route of young chickens gave somewhat better protection against subsequent challenge (McMartin and Adler, 1961), and the chickens apparently remained free of the clinical disease during their subsequent laying period (Luginbuhl et al., 1967). The use of live virulent cultures of *M. gallisepticum* for "controlled exposure" in young chickens as a possible means of eliminating egg transmission has been studied by several groups (Olson et al., 1962b, 1964; Fabricant and Levine, 1963; Vardaman, 1965; Heishman et al., 1966; and Luginbuhl et al., 1967). Although egg transmission was reduced to a low level in most of these studies, only the report by Fabricant and Levine (1963) demonstrated complete elimination of egg transmission following controlled exposure. The possible benefit of some reduction in egg transmission must be evaluated in the light of the hazard of perpetuation of the disease and the production of flocks which will be reactors when tested by the serological procedures employed with most other control efforts.

MEDICATION OF BREEDERS

Attempts to eliminate egg transmission of *M. gallisepticum* by the medication of breeder flocks or their progeny have been conducted by Crawley and Fahey (1955), Adler et al. (1956) and Van Roekel et al. (1958). They reported that monthly injections of 200 mg of streptomycin and dehydrostreptomycin in infected breeders were not consistently effective in eliminating egg transmission. Peterson (1966) reported on the successful elimination of the disease from breeder flocks by the repeated injection of chicks with tylosin in oil plus the use of chlortetracycline in the feed. Further reports on the value of such a procedure apparently have not been published.

EGG DIPPING

The preincubation immersion of warmed (100° F) hatching eggs in cold (35–40° F) solutions of antibiotics (especially tylosin or erythromycin at 400–1,000 ppm) for 15–20 minutes has also been explored as a means of eliminating egg transmission of the disease due to the effects of the absorbed antibiotic (Chalquest and Fabricant, 1959; Levine and Fabricant, 1962; Olson et al., 1962a; Stuart and Bruins, 1963; Hall et al., 1963; Yoder and Hofstad, 1965; Inglis and Jones, 1966). Alls et al. (1963, 1964) reported on various factors affecting the permeability of dipped eggs and on the mechanics of the dipping process. In general, the reports have indicated that the dipping process has reduced but not completely eliminated the possibility of egg transmission. The influence on hatchability has not been consistently favorable, and bacterial contamination of dipped eggs has sometimes been a problem. Smit and Hoekstra (1967) devised a procedure for injecting tylosin into the air cell of hatching eggs, but their preliminary results were inconclusive.

EGG HEATING

Still another approach to somehow break the egg transmission cycle has been reported by Yoder (1970). Room temperature (78° F) eggs were heated in a forced air incubator during a 12–14-hour period to just reach an internal temperature of 115.0° F. Hatchability was usually reduced 8–12%, but *M. gallisepticum* and *M. synoviae* appeared to be inactivated. Field studies are necessary before the procedure can be properly evaluated.

CONTROL PROGRAM

Turkeys

Turkey breeders have generally adopted the various state-supported infectious sinusitis control programs which specify that breeding stock be selected only from apparently normal flocks proved to be serologically negative for *M. gallisepticum* upon a series of 10% sample tests, sometimes augmented with at least one 100% test at pullorum testing time. See the details in the USDA ARS Report (Anon. 1965). Proved reactor flocks are eliminated as breeders.

Chickens

Although no consistently effective procedure has been developed for the control of *M. gallisepticum* infection in chickens, the application of one or more of the currently available procedures may lead to establishment of clean replacement breeders. Regardless of methods employed to eliminate the infection, serological testing is an important part of the procedure to determine and monitor the *M. gallisepticum* status of flocks and their progeny. Repeated sample testing is usual, with at least one 100% test at pullorum testing time, followed by further sample testing at 30–60-day intervals. These procedures are variable, but in general a clean status is not established until serologically negative progeny flocks are produced from serologically negative parent flocks. See the details in the USDA ARS Report (Anon., 1965). Also see the section on Serology for a discussion of possible cross-reactions with serum from *M. synoviae* infected birds and

M. gallisepticum plate test antigen.

Reports on the benefits of raising *M. gallisepticum* free broilers have been made by Moulthrop (1962) and Chute and Reese (1968).

REFERENCES

Adler, H. E. 1954. A rapid slide agglutination test for the diagnosis of chronic respiratory disease in the field and in laboratory-infected chickens and turkeys. *Proc. 90th Ann. Meet. Am. Vet. Med. Ass.*, pp. 346–49.

Adler, H. E., and J. Berg. 1960. Cultivation of Mycoplasma of avian origin. *Avian Diseases* 4:3–12.

Adler, H. E., and A. J. DaMassa. 1967. Use of formalinized *Mycoplasma gallisepticum* antigens and chicken erythrocytes in hemagglutination and hemagglutination-inhibition studies. *Appl. Microbiol.* 15:245–48.

Adler, H. E., and R. Yamamoto. 1956a. Preparation of a new pleuropneumonia-like organism antigen for the diagnosis of chronic respiratory disease by the agglutination test. *Am. J. Vet. Res.* 17:290–93.

———. 1956b. Studies on chronic coryza (Nelson) in the domestic fowl. *Cornell Vet.* 46:337–43.

———. 1956c. A minced chicken embryo medium for cultivating pleuropneumonia-like organisms. *Poultry Sci.* 35:1396–97.

Adler, H. E., R. Yamamoto, and R. A. Bankowski. 1954. A preliminary report of efficiency of various mediums for isolation of pleuropneumonia-like organisms from exudates of birds with chronic respiratory disease. *Am. J. Vet. Res.* 15:463–65.

Adler, H. E., R. Yamamoto, and S. F. Extrom. 1956. Control of egg transmitted pleuropneumonia-like organisms in two hatcheries through medication of the foundation stock. *J. Am. Vet. Med. Ass.* 128:313–15.

Adler, H. E., D. A. McMartin, and M. Shifrine. 1960. Immunization against Mycoplasma infections of poultry. *Am. J. Vet. Res.* 21:482–85.

Adler, H. E., D. A. McMartin, and H. Ortmayer. 1962. The effect of infectious bronchitis virus on chickens infected with *Mycoplasma gallisepticum*. *Avian Diseases* 6:267–74.

Adler, H. E., A. J. DaMassa, and W. W. Sadler. 1964. Application of the anti-globulin technique for the detection of *Mycoplasma gallisepticum* antibodies. *Avian Diseases* 8:576–79.

Alls, A. A., W. J. Benton, W. C. Krauss, and M. S. Cover. 1963. The mechanics of treating hatching eggs for disease prevention. *Avian Diseases* 7:89–97.

Alls, A. A., M. S. Cover, W. J. Benton, and W. C. Krauss. 1964. Treatment of hatching eggs for disease prevention—Factors affecting permeability and a visual detection of drug absorption. *Avian Diseases* 8:245–56.

Anderson, D. P., and C. W. Beard. 1967. Aerosol studies with avian Mycoplasma. II. Infectivity of *Mycoplasma gallisepticum* for chickens and turkeys. *Avian Diseases* 11:60–64.

Anonymous. 1965. *Report of the Second Study Group on* Mycoplasma gallisepticum *Infection in Chickens and Turkeys*. USDA, ARS 91–55, p. 16.

Bankowski, R. A., R. D. Conrad, and B. Reynolds. 1968. Avian influenza A and paramyxo viruses complicating respiratory disease diagnosis in poultry. *Avian Diseases* 12:259–78.

Barber, C. W. 1962. The lymphofollicular nodules in turkey tissues associated with *Mycoplasma gallisepticum* infection. *Avian Diseases* 6:289–96.

Barnes, L. E., E. E. Ose, and F. O. Gossett. 1960. Treatment of experimental PPLO infections in young chickens with tylosin, a new antibiotic. *Poultry Sci.* 39:1376–81.

Barnes, L. E., E. E. Ose, and L. F. Ellis. 1961. Tylosin treatment of experimental *Mycoplasma gallinarum* infections of chickens and turkeys. *Antimicrobial Agents Ann.* 1960:605–11.

Beach, J. R., and O. W. Schalm. 1936. Studies on the clinical manifestations and transmissibility of infectious coryza of chickens. *Poultry Sci.* 15:466–72.

Benton, W. J., M. S. Cover, and F. W. Melchior. 1967. *Mycoplasma gallisepticum* in a commercial laryngotracheitis vaccine. *Avian Diseases* 11:426–29.

Biddle, E. S., and M. S. Cover. 1957. The bacterial flora of the respiratory tract of chickens affected with chronic respiratory disease. *Am. J. Vet. Res.* 18:405–8.

Blake, J. T. 1962. Effects of experimental chronic respiratory disease and infectious bronchitis on pullets. *Am. J. Vet. Res.* 23:847–53.

Boyer, C. I., Jr., J. Fabricant, and J. A. Brown. 1960. Non-specific plate agglutination reactions with PPLO antigens. *Avian Diseases* 4:546–47. (Abstr.)

Brion, A., M. Fontaine, M. P. Fontaine, and C. Pilet. 1958. Sur l'existence en France de la maladie respiratoire chronique des volailles. *Acad. Vet. France Bul.* 31:105–10.

Calnek, B. W., and P. P. Levine. 1957. Studies on experimental egg transmission of pleuropneumonia-like organisms in chickens. *Avian Diseases* 1:208–22.

Carson, J. R., R. D. Eaton, and R. E. Luginbuhl. 1954. The effect of injections of an oil suspension of Terramycin on egg production and egg quality in hens affected with chronic respiratory disease. *Poultry Sci.* 33:589–96.

Chalquest, R. R., and J. Fabricant. 1959. Survival of PPLO injected into eggs previously dipped in antibiotic solutions. *Avian Diseases* 3:257–71.

Chandiramani, N. K., H. Van Roekel, and O. M. Olesiuk. 1966. Viability studies with *Mycoplasma gallisepticum* under different environmental conditions. *Poultry Sci.* 45:1029–44.

Chu, H. P. 1958. Differential diagnosis and control of respiratory diseases of poultry. *Vet. Record* 70:1064–78.

Chute, H. L. 1960. Pathology of PPLO and other agents in chicken embryos. *Ann. N.Y. Acad. Sci.* 79:741–49.

Chute, H. L., and C. R. Cole. 1954. Lesions in chicken embryos produced by pleuropneumonia-like organisms from chronic respiratory disease of chickens and infectious sinusitis of turkeys. *Am. J. Vet. Res.* 15:108–18.

Chute, H. L., and R. S. Reese. 1968. Mycoplasma problems in integrated poultry companies. *Maine Agr. Expt. Sta. Bull.* 657.

Chute, H. L., D. R. Stauffer, and D. C. O'Meara. 1964. The production of specific pathogen free broilers in Maine. *Maine Agr. Expt. Sta. Bull.* 633.

Coles, J. D. W. A., and R. B. Cumming. 1959. Chronic respiratory disease: Its nature and eradication. *J. S. African Vet. Med. Ass.* 30:5–14.

Corstvet, R. E., and W. W. Sadler. 1964. The diagnosis of certain avian diseases with the fluorescent antibody technique. *Poultry Sci.* 43:1280–88.

Cottew, G. S. 1956. A chronic respiratory disease of poultry in Queensland. *Australian Vet. J.* 32:249–51.

Cover, M. S. 1955. The therapeutic use of antibiotics for chronic respiratory disease in three laying flocks. *Poultry Sci.* 34:686–90.

Cover, M. S., and E. F. Waller. 1954. The presence of chronic respiratory disease in pipped eggs. *Am. J. Vet. Res.* 15:119–21.

Crawley, J. F., and J. E. Fahey. 1955. A proposed plan for the control of chronic respiratory disease of chickens. *Poultry Sci.* 34:707–16.

———. 1957. The use of the hemagglutination-inhibition test for the control of PPLO infection in poultry. *J. Am. Vet. Med. Ass.* 130:187–90.

De Blieck, L. 1950. The treatment of *Coryza infectiosa gallinarum* type II (Nelson) with streptomycin. *Vet. Record* 62:787.

Delaplane, J. P. 1948. Some recent observations of lesions in chick embryos induced by the virus of a chronic respiratory disease of chickens. *Cornell Vet.* 38:192–95.

———. 1949. Cultivation of the chronic respiratory disease virus in chick embryos. *Proc. 53rd Ann. Meet. U.S. Livestock Sanit. Ass.,* pp. 193–201.

Delaplane, J. P., and H. O. Stuart. 1943. The propagation of a virus in embryonated chicken eggs causing a chronic respiratory disease of chickens. *Am. J. Vet. Res.* 4:325–32.

Devos, A., N. Viaene, L. Spanoghe, and L. Devriese. 1968. An egg-yolk agglutination test to detect *Mycoplasma gallisepticum* infection. *Rec. Med. Vet.* 144:421–28.

Dickinson, E. M., and W. R. Hinshaw. 1938. Treatment of infectious sinusitis of turkeys with argyrol and silver nitrate. *J. Am. Vet. Med. Ass.* 93:151–56.

Dierks, R. E., J. A. Newman, and B. S. Pomeroy. 1967. Characterization of avian Mycoplasma. *Ann. N.Y. Acad. Sci.* 143:170–89.

Dodd, S. 1905. Epizootic pneumo-enteritis of the turkey. *J. Comp. Pathol. Therap.* 18:239–45.

Domermuth, C. H. 1958. *In vitro* resistance of avian PPLO to antibacterial agents. *Avian Diseases* 2:442–49.

———. 1960. Antibiotic resistance and mutation rates of Mycoplasma. *Avian Diseases* 4:456–66.

———. 1962. Vaccination of chickens with *Mycoplasma gallisepticum*. *Avian Diseases* 6:412–19.

Domermuth, C. H., and E. P. Johnson. 1955. An in vitro comparison of some antibacterial agents on a strain of avian pleuropneumonia-like organism. *Poultry Sci.* 34:1395–99.

Domermuth, C. H., M. Nielsen, E. A. Freundt, and A. Birch-Andersen. 1964a. Gross morphology and ultrastructure of *Mycoplasma gallisepticum*. *J. Bacteriol.* 88:1428–32.

———. 1964b. Ultrastructure of Mycoplasma species. *J. Bacteriol.* 88:727–44.

Domermuth, C. H., W. B. Gross, and R. T. Dubose. 1967. Mycoplasmal salpingitis of chickens and turkeys. *Avian Diseases* 11:393–98.

Dunlop, W. R., and R. G. Strout. 1956. State wide testing for PPLO infection of poultry. *Proc. 60th Ann. Meet. U.S. Livestock Sanit. Ass.,* pp. 197–202.

Dutta, S. K., R. E. Dierks, and B. S. Pomeroy. 1965. Electron microscopic studies of the morphology and the stages of development of *Mycoplasma gallisepticum. Avian Diseases* 9:241–51.

Edward, D. G., and E. A. Freundt. 1967. Proposal for Mollicutes as name of the class established for the order Mycoplasmatales. *Int. J. Syst. Bacteriol.* 17:267–68.

Edward, D. G., and A. D. Kanarek. 1960. Organisms of the pleuropneumonia group of avian origin: Their classification into species. *Ann. N.Y. Acad. Sci.* 79:696–702.

Eissa, Y. M. 1956. La maladie respiratoire chronique des volailles en Egypte. *Bull. Off. Int. Epizoot.* 46:170–83.

Estola, T. 1967. Studies on the occurrence of *Mycoplasma gallisepticum* in Finland. *Finsk. Vet. Tidskr.* 73:102–4.

Fabricant, Catherine G., P. J. Van Demark, and J. Fabricant. 1962. The effect of atmospheric environment upon the growth of *Mycoplasma gallisepticum. Avian Diseases* 6:328–32.

Fabricant, J. 1953. The viability of the agent of chronic respiratory disease at minus 25° C. *Proc. 25th Ann. Conf. Lab. Workers in Pullorum Disease Control.* (Abstr.)

———. 1958. A re-evaluation of the use of media for the isolation of pleuropneumonia-like organisms of avian origin. *Avian Diseases* 2:409–17.

———. 1959. Swine serum and CO_2 in the isolation of avian PPLO. *Avian Diseases* 3:428–39.

———. 1960. Serological studies of avian pleuropneumonia-like organisms (PPLO) with Edward's technique. *Avian Diseases* 4:505–14.

Fabricant, J., and P. P. Levine. 1962. Experimental production of complicated chronic respiratory disease infection ("air sac" disease). *Avian Diseases* 6:13–23.

———. 1963. Infection in young chickens for the prevention of egg transmission of *Mycoplasma gallisepticum* in breeders. *Proc. 17th World Vet. Congr.,* pp. 1469–74.

Fahey, J. E. 1954. A hemagglutination inhibition test for infectious sinusitis of turkeys. *Proc. Soc. Exp. Biol. Med.* 86:38–40.

———. 1957. Infectious sinusitis of turkeys caused by antibiotic-resistant pleuropneumonia-like organisms. *Vet. Med.* 52:305–7.

Fahey, J. E., and J. F. Crawley. 1954a. Studies on chronic respiratory disease of chickens. II. Isolation of a virus. *Can. J. Comp. Med. Vet. Sci.* 18:13–21.

———. 1954b. Studies on chronic respiratory disease of chickens. III. Egg transmission of a pleuropneumonia-like organism. *Can. J. Comp. Med. Vet. Sci.* 18:67–75.

———. 1954c. Studies on chronic respiratory disease of chickens. IV. A hemagglutination inhibition diagnostic test. *Can. J. Comp. Med. Vet. Sci.* 18:264–72.

———. 1955a. Studies on chronic respiratory disease of chickens. V. Air-borne spread of the CRD agents. *Can. J. Comp. Med. Vet. Sci.* 19:53–56.

———. 1955b. Studies on chronic respiratory disease of chickens. VI. The effects of antibiotics on the clinical and serological course of CRD. *Can. J. Comp. Med. Vet. Sci.* 19:281–86.

Fahey, J. E., J. F. Crawley, and W. R. Dunlop. 1953. Studies on chronic respiratory disease of chickens. Observations on outbreaks in Canada in a two-year period. *Can. J. Comp. Med. Vet. Sci.* 17:294–98.

Freundt, E. A. 1957. Mycoplasmatales, pp. 914–26. In Breed, R. S., E. G. D. Murray, and N. R. Smith (eds.), *Bergey's Manual of Determinative Bacteriology.* 7th ed. Williams & Wilkins Co., Baltimore.

Frey, M. L., R. P. Hanson, and D. P. Anderson. 1968. A medium for the isolation of avian Mycoplasmas. *Am. J. Vet. Res.* 29:2163–71.

Gale, G. O., H. W. Layton, A. L. Shor, and G. A. Kemp. 1967. Chemotherapy of experimental avian Mycoplasma infections. *Ann. N.Y. Acad. Sci.* 143:239–55.

Garust, A. T., and P. Nóbrega. 1956. Chronic respiratory disease in Brazil. *Arquiv. Inst. Biol.* (Sao Paulo) 23:35–38.

Gentry, R. F., C. T. Kantor, and D. Marthouse. 1967. Factors influencing the growth and storage of *M. gallisepticum* propagated in embryonated chicken eggs. *Ann. N.Y. Acad. Sci.* 143:256–67.

Gianforte, E. M., E. L. Jungherr, and R. E. Jacobs. 1955. A serologic analysis of seven strains of pleuropneumonia-like organisms from air sac infection in poultry. *Poultry Sci.* 34:662–69.

Glantz, P. J., S. Narotsky, and G. Bubash. 1962. *Escherichia coli* serotypes isolated from salpingitis and chronic respiratory disease of poultry. *Avian Diseases* 6:322–28.

Graham-Smith, G. S. 1907. Some observations on "swollen head" in turkeys. *J. Agr. Sci.* 2:227–43.

Gross, W. B. 1956. *Escherichia coli* as a complicating factor in chronic respiratory disease of chickens and infectious sinusitis of turkeys. *Poultry Sci.* 35:765–71.

———. 1961a. The development of "air sac disease." *Avian Diseases* 5:431–39.

———. 1961b. The effect of chlortetracycline, erythromycin and nitrofurans as treatments for experimental "air sac disease." *Poultry Sci.* 40:833–41.

———. 1962. Blood cultures, blood counts and temperature records in an experimentally produced "air sac disease" and uncomplicated *Escherichia coli* infection in chickens. *Poultry Sci.* 41:691–700.

Grumbles, L. C., E. Phillips, W. A. Boney, Jr., and J. P. Delaplane. 1953. Cultural and biochemical characteristics of the agent causing infectious sinusitis of turkeys and chronic respiratory disease of chickens. *Southwestern Vet.* 6:166–68.

Hall, C. F. 1962. *Mycoplasma gallisepticum* antigen production. *Avian Diseases* 6:359–62.

Hall, C. F., R. W. Moore, and L. C. Grumbles. 1961. Eradication of infectious sinusitis in a hatchery operation by serological testing. *Avian Diseases* 5:168–77.

Hall, C. F., A. I. Flowers, and L. C. Grumbles. 1963. Dipping of hatching eggs for control of *Mycoplasma gallisepticum*. *Avian Diseases* 7:178–83.

Hamdy, A. H., L. C. Ferguson, V. L. Sanger, and E. H. Bohl. 1957. Susceptibility of pleuropneumonia-like organisms to the action of the antibiotics erythromycin, chlortetracycline, hygromycin, magnamycin, oxytetracycline, and streptomycin. *Poultry Sci.* 36:748–54.

Hart, L. 1940. Sinusitis in turkeys. *Australian Vet. J.* 16:163–68.

Hartwigk, H. 1958. Nachweis von pleuropneumonia-aehnlichen Organismen (PPLO) beim Gefluegel. *Berlin. Muench. Tieraerztl. Wochschr.* 71:45–50.

Heishman, J. O., N. O. Olson, and D. C. Shelton. 1960. Control of chronic respiratory disease. II. The effect of low calcium diet, terephthalic acid and chlortetracycline. *Avian Diseases* 4:413–18.

Heishman, J. O., N. O. Olson, and C. J. Cunningham. 1962. Control of chronic respiratory disease. IV. The effect of a low calcium diet and high concentrations of chlortetracycline in the isolation of Mycoplasma from experimentally infected chicks. *Avian Diseases* 6:165–70.

———. 1966. Control of chronic respiratory disease. VII. The effect of controlled versus natural infection of chickens with *Mycoplasma gallisepticum* on egg transmission. *Avian Diseases* 10:189–93.

Hitchner, S. B. 1949. The pathology of infectious sinusitis of turkeys. *Poultry Sci.* 28:106–18.

Hofstad, M. S. 1952. Chronic respiratory disease. *Progr. Rept. Vet. Med. Res. Inst.*, Iowa State Coll., Ames.

———. 1957a. Egg transmission of infectious sinusitis of turkeys. *Avian Diseases* 1:165–70.

———. 1957b. A serological study of infectious sinusitis in turkeys. *Avian Diseases* 1:170–79.

———. 1959. Chronic respiratory disease, pp. 320–30. In Biester, H. E., and L. H. Schwarte (eds.), *Diseases of Poultry*, 4th ed. Iowa State Univ. Press, Ames.

Hofstad, M. S., and L. Doerr. 1956. A chicken meat infusion medium enriched with avian serum for cultivation of an avian pleuropneumonia-like organism, *Mycoplasma gallinarum*. *Cornell Vet.* 46:439–46.

Inglis, J. M., and R. C. Jones. 1966. Effect of dipping eggs in spiramycin to inactivate *Mycoplasma gallisepticum*. *J. Comp. Pathol. Therap.* 76:225–29.

Jerstad, A. C., C. M. Hamilton, and V. E. Smith. 1949. Preliminary report of probable egg transmission of infectious sinusitis of turkeys. *Vet. Med.* 44:272–73.

Johnson, E. P. 1954. The specificity of lymphofollicular lesions in the diagnosis of chronic respiratory disease. *Cornell Vet.* 44:230–39.

Jungherr, E. L., R. E. Luginbuhl, and R. E. Jacobs. 1953. Pathology and serology of air sac infection. *Proc. 90th Ann. Meet. Am. Vet. Med. Ass.*, pp. 303–12.

Jungherr, E. L., R. E. Luginbuhl, M. Tourtellotte, and W. E. Burr. 1955. Significance of serological testing for chronic respiratory disease. *Proc. 92nd Ann. Meet. Am. Vet. Med. Ass.*, pp. 315–21.

Keller, H. 1958. Ueber die Isolierung von Pleuropneumonie-aehnlichen Erregern bei Huehnern. *Schweiz. Arch. Tierheilk.* 100:45–51.

Kerr, K. M., and N. O. Olson. 1967. Pathology in chickens experimentally inoculated or contact-infected with *Mycoplasma gallisepticum*. *Avian Diseases* 11:559–78.

Kiser, J. S., F. Popken, and J. Clemente. 1960. Antibiotic control of an experimental *Mycoplasma gallinarum* (PPLO) infection in chickens. *Ann. N.Y. Acad. Sci.* 79:593–607.

———. 1961. The development of resistance to spiromycin, streptomycin and chlortetracycline by *Mycoplasma gallisepticum* in chick embryos. *Avian Diseases* 5:283–91.

Kleckner, A. L. 1960. Serotypes of avian pleuropneumonia-like organisms. *Am. J. Vet. Res.* 21:274–80.

Lecce, J. G., and F. G. Sperling. 1954. Chronic respiratory disease. I. The isolation of pleuropneumonia-like organisms as a diagnostic aid. *Cornell Vet.* 44:441–49.

———. 1955. Chronic respiratory disease. III. The effect of treatment on the pleuropneumonia-like organism flora of avian tracheas. *J. Am. Vet. Med. Ass.* 127:54–56.

Levine, P. P., and J. Fabricant. 1962. Effect of dipping eggs in antibiotic solutions on PPLO transmission in chickens. *Avian Diseases* 6:72–85.

Luginbuhl, R. E., and E. L. Jungherr. 1953. The growth curve of a chronic respiratory disease agent in embryonating eggs. *Poultry Sci.* 32:912. (Abstr.)

Luginbuhl, R. E., M. E. Tourtellotte, and M. N. Frazier. 1967. *Mycoplasma gallisepticum*—control by immunization. *Ann. N.Y. Acad. Sci.* 143:234–38.

McMartin, D. A., and H. E. Adler. 1961. An immunological phenomenon in chickens following infection with *Mycoplasma galli-*

septicum. J. Comp. Pathol. Therap. 71: 311–23.

Madden, D. L., W. H. Henderson, and H. E. Moses. 1967a. Case report: Isolation of *Mycoplasma gallisepticum* from bobwhite quail *(Colinus virginianus). Avian Diseases* 11:378–80.

Madden, D. L., R. E. Horton, and N. B. Mc-Cullough. 1967b. *Mycoplasma gallisepticum* infection in germfree and conventional chickens. Experimental studies with a culture of low virulence. *Am. J. Vet. Res.* 28: 517–26.

Markham, F. S., and S. C. Wong. 1952. Pleuropneumonia-like organisms in the etiology of turkey sinusitis and chronic respiratory disease of chickens. *Poultry Sci.* 31:902–4.

Morowitz, H. J., and J. Maniloff. 1966. Analysis of the life cycle of *Mycoplasma gallisepticum. J. Bacteriol.* 91:1638–44.

Moulthrop, I. M. 1962. A report on broilers from parents free of *Mycoplasma gallisepticum. Avian Diseases* 6:161–64.

Moulton, J. E., and H. E. Adler. 1957. Pathogenesis of arthritis in chicken embryos caused by a pleuropneumonia-like organism. *Am. J. Vet. Res.* 18:731–34.

Nelson, J. B. 1935. Cocco-bacilliform bodies associated with an infectious fowl coryza. *Science* 82:43–44.

———. 1936a. Studies on an uncomplicated coryza of the domestic fowl. V. A coryza of slow onset. *J. Exp. Med.* 63:509–13.

———. 1936b. Studies on an uncomplicated coryza of the domestic fowl. VI. Coccobacilliform bodies in birds infected with the coryza of slow onset. *J. Exp. Med.* 63:515–22.

———. 1936c. Studies on an uncomplicated coryza of the domestic fowl. VII. Cultivation of the coccobacilliform bodies in fertile eggs and in tissue cultures. *J. Exp. Med.* 64:749–58.

———. 1938. Studies on an uncomplicated coryza in the domestic fowl. IX. The co-operative action of *Hemophilus gallinarum* and the coccobacilliform bodies in the coryza of rapid onset and long duration. *J. Exp. Med.* 67:847–55.

———. 1939. Growth of the fowl coryza bodies in tissue culture and in blood agar. *J. Exp. Med.* 69:199–209.

Newnham, Audrey G. 1964. The hemagglutination-inhibition (HI) test and a study of its use in experimental avian respiratory mycoplasmosis. *Res. Vet. Sci.* 5:245–55.

Newnham, Audrey G., and H. P. Chu. 1965. An "in vitro" comparison of the effect of some antibacterial, antifungal and antiprotozoal agents on various strains of mycoplasma (pleuropneumonia-like organisms: PPLO). *J. Hyg.* 63:1–23.

Noel, J. K., H. M. Devolt, and J. E. Faber. 1964. Identification of *Mycoplasma galli-*

septicum in lesion tissue by immunofluorescence. *Poultry Sci.* 43:145–49.

Olesiuk, Olga M., and H. Van Roekel. 1952. Cultural attributes of the chronic respiratory disease agent. *Proc. 24th Ann. Conf. Northeast Lab. Workers in Pullorum Disease Control.* (Abstr.)

———. 1959. The effects of antibiotics on experimental chronic respiratory disease in chickens. *Avian Diseases* 3:457–70.

Olesiuk, Olga M., H. Van Roekel, and L. P. Beninato. 1957. Influence of chemotherapeutic agents on experimental chronic respiratory disease in chickens and turkeys. *Poultry Sci.* 36:383–95.

Olesiuk, Olga M., H. Van Roekel, and N. K. Chandiramani. 1964. Antibiotic medication of chickens experimentally infected with *Mycoplasma gallisepticum* and *Escherichia coli. Avian Diseases* 8:135–52.

———. 1965. Control of experimental *Mycoplasma gallisepticum* infection in young chickens with tylosin and other antibiotics. *Avian Diseases* 9:67–77.

Olesiuk, Olga M., H. Van Roekel, and D. H. Roberts. 1967. Transmission and eradication of *Mycoplasma gallisepticum* in chickens. *Poultry Sci.* 46:578–99.

Olson, N. O., D. C. Shelton, and J. O. Heishman. 1959. Control of chronic respiratory disease. I. The effects of chlortetracycline (CTC) and terephthalic acid (TPA). *Avian Diseases* 3:443–51.

Olson, N. O., J. O. Heishman, and D. C. Shelton. 1960. Control of chronic respiratory disease. III. Isolation of Mycoplasma as influenced by potentiated chlortetracycline and time interval after exposure. *Avian Diseases* 4:419–28.

Olson, N. O., T. R. Hash, J. O. Heishman, and Ann Campbell. 1962a. Dipping of hatching eggs in erythromycin for the control of Mycoplasma. *Avian Diseases* 6:191–94.

Olson, N. O., J. O. Heishman, and D. C. Shelton. 1962b. Control of chronic respiratory disease. V. Artificial exposure of young chicks to *Mycoplasma gallisepticum. Avian Diseases* 6:171–77.

Olson, N. O., J. O. Heishman, and C. J. Cunningham. 1964. Control of chronic respiratory disease. VI. The effect on egg transmission of early exposure of chicks to *Mycoplasma gallisepticum. Avian Diseases* 8:215–20.

Olson, N. O., R. Yamamoto, and H. Ortmayer. 1965. Antigenic relationship between *Mycoplasma synoviae* and *Mycoplasma gallisepticum. Am. J. Vet. Res.* 26:195–98.

Osborn, O. H., and B. S. Pomeroy. 1958a. Case report—Isolation of the agent of infectious sinusitis of turkeys from naturally infected pheasants. *Avian Diseases* 2:370–72.

Osborn, O. H., and B. S. Pomeroy. 1958b. The effect of antibiotics on the infectious sinusitis agent of turkeys. Part 1. Egg transmission. *Avian Diseases* 2:180–86.

Pathak, R. C., and C. M. Singh. 1961. Occurrence of pleuropneumonia-like organisms in poultry in India. *Agra Univ. J. Res. Sci.*, Pt. 2, 10:155–69.

Petek, M., B. Felluga, G. Borghi, and A. Baroni. 1967. The Crawley agent: An avian reovirus. *Arch. Ges. Virusforsch.* 21:413–24.

Peterson, E. H. 1953. Terramycin injections control chronic respiratory disease in two pullet flocks. *Vet. Med.* 48:311–14.

———. 1966. Eradication of chronic respiratory disease from breeder farm flocks. *J. Am. Vet. Med. Ass.* 149:160–64.

Prier, J. E., and G. Dart. 1951. Immunological and serological studies on infectious sinusitis of turkeys. *Cornell Vet.* 41:38–46.

Quizon, A. S. 1958. A survey of the occurrence of chronic respiratory disease (CRD) in the Philippines. *Philippine J. Animal Ind.* 19:69–71.

Rhoades, K. R., W. K. Kelton, and K. L. Heddleston. 1965. Serologic, pathologic, and symptomatic aspects of Mycoplasmosis of turkeys. *Can. J. Comp. Med. Vet. Sci.* 29:169–72.

Roberts, D. H. 1964. The inactivation of Mycoplasma by beta-propiolactone. *Brit. Vet. J.* 120:479–80.

Roberts, D. H., and Olga M. Olesiuk. 1967. Serological studies with *Mycoplasma synoviae*. *Avian Diseases* 11:104–19.

Shifrine, M., J. Pangborn, and H. E. Adler. 1962. Colonial growth of *Mycoplasma gallisepticum* observed with the electron microscope. *J. Bacteriol.* 83:187–92.

Smit, T., and J. Hoekstra. 1967. Treatment of hatching eggs against Mycoplasma infections by injecting tylosin tartrate into the air cell. *Tijdschr. Diergeneesk.* 92:1190–94.

Smith, W. E., J. Hillier, and S. Mudd. 1948. Electron micrograph studies of two strains of pleuropneumonialike (L) organisms of human derivation. *J. Bacteriol.* 56:589–601.

Stricker, F., and J. Fišera. 1955. Chronicka chroba dychodiel hydiny. *Vet. Casopis.* 6:199–207.

Stuart, E. E., and H. W. Bruins. 1963. Preincubation immersion of eggs in erythromycin to control chronic respiratory disease. *Avian Diseases* 7:287–93.

Tajima, M., T. Miyamoto, and H. Nagashima. 1958. An outbreak of chronic respiratory disease of chickens in Japan. *Nippon Inst. Biol. Sci. Bull. Biol. Res.* 3:43–52.

Taylor, J. R. E., and J. Fabricant. 1957. Studies on the isolation of the pleuropneumonia-like organism of chronic respiratory disease of fowls. *Cornell Vet.* 47:112–26.

Taylor, J. R. E., J. Fabricant, and P. P. Levine.

1957. A comparison of four *in vitro* methods for the isolation of the pleuropneumonia-like organism of chronic respiratory disease from tracheal exudate. *Avian Diseases* 1:101–4.

Tourtellotte, M. E. 1963. The isolation of Mycoplasma from grossly contaminated material by use of membrane filters. *Proc. 35th N. E. Conf. Avian Diseases, Univ. Mass.*

Tyzzer, E. E. 1926. The injection of argyrol for the treatment of sinusitis in turkeys. *Cornell Vet.* 16:221–24.

Valcarenghi, G. 1960. Un episodio di sinusite infettiva. *Veterinaria Ital.* 11:113–17.

Van Roekel, H., and Olga M. Oesiuk. 1953. The etiology of chronic respiratory disease. *Proc. 90th Ann. Meet. Am. Vet. Med. Ass.*, pp. 289–303.

Van Roekel, H., Olga M. Olesiuk, and H. A. Peck. 1952. Chronic respiratory disease of chickens. *Am. J. Vet. Res.* 13:252–59.

Van Roekel, H., J. E. Gray, N. L. Shipkowitz, M. K. Clarke, and R. M. Luchini. 1957. Etiology and pathology of the chronic respiratory disease complex in chickens. *Univ. Mass. Agr. Expt. Sta. Bull.* 486.

Van Roekel, H., Olga M. Olesiuk, and L. P. Beninato. 1958. Symposium on chronic respiratory diseases of poultry. III. Epizootiology of chronic respiratory diseases in chickens. *Am. J. Vet. Res.* 19:453–63.

Vardaman, T. H. 1965. The resistance and carrier status of chickens exposed to *Mycoplasma gallisepticum* under field conditions. *Proc. 69th Ann. Meet. U.S. Livestock Sanit. Ass.*, pp. 303–10.

———. 1967. A culture medium for the production of *Mycoplasma gallisepticum* antigen. *Avian Diseases* 11:123–29.

Vardaman, T. H., and H. W. Yoder, Jr. 1969. Preparation of *Mycoplasma synoviae* hemagglutinating antigen and its use in the hemagglutination-inhibition test. *Avian Diseases* 13:654–61.

Warren, J., L. B. Senterfit, and F. Sieiro. 1968. Inactivated culture vaccine against *Mycoplasma gallisepticum* infection in chickens. *Am. J. Vet. Res.* 29:1659–64.

Wasserman, B., V. J. Yates, and D. E. Fry. 1954. On so-called air sac infection. *Poultry Sci.* 33:622–23.

White-Stevens, B., and H. G. Zeibel. 1954. The effect of chlortetracycline (Aureomycin) on the growth efficiency of broilers in the presence of chronic respiratory disease. *Poultry Sci.* 33:1164–74.

Wichmann, R. W. 1957. Case report—PPLO infection in chukar partridges (*Alectoris graeca*). *Avian Diseases* 1:222–27.

Wills, F. K. 1955. Isolation of pleuropneumonia-like organisms from a peacock (*Pavo cristatus*). *Southwestern Vet.* 8:258–59.

Winterfield, R. W. 1953. Pigeons as a source

of the turkey sinusitis agent. *Vet. Med.* 48:124–25.

Wong, S. C., and C. G. James. 1953. The susceptibility of the agents of chronic respiratory disease of chickens and infectious sinusitis of turkeys to various antibiotics. *Poultry Sci.* 32:589–93.

Yamamoto, R., and H. E. Adler. 1956. The effect of certain antibiotics and chemical agents on pleuropneumonia-like organisms of avian origin. *Am. J. Vet. Res.* 17:538–42.

———. 1958a. Characterization of pleuropneumonia-like organisms of avian origin. I. Antigenic analysis of seven strains and their comparative pathogenicity for birds. *J. Infect. Diseases* 102:143–52.

———. 1958b. Characterization of pleuropneumonia-like organisms of avian origin. II. Cultural, biochemical, morphological and further serological studies. *J. Infect. Diseases* 102:243–50.

Yamamoto, R., and C. H. Bigland. 1964. Pathogenicity to chicks of Mycoplasma associated with turkey airsacculitis. *Avian Diseases* 8:523–31.

Yoder, H. W., Jr. 1970. Preincubation heat treatment of chicken hatching eggs to inactivate Mycoplasma. *Avian Diseases* 14:75–86.

Yoder, H. W., Jr., and M. S. Hofstad. 1964. Characterization of avian Mycoplasma. *Avian Diseases* 8:481–512.

———. 1965. Evaluation of tylosin in preventing egg transmission of *Mycoplasma gallisepticum* in chickens. *Avian Diseases* 9:291–301.

Yoder, H. W., Jr., C. L. Nelson, and M. S. Hofstad. 1961. Tylosin, an effective antibiotic for treatment of PPLO turkey sinusitis. *Vet. Med.* 56:178–80.

Zander, D. V. 1961. Origin of S6 strain Mycoplasma. *Avian Diseases* 5:154–56.

MYCOPLASMA MELEAGRIDIS INFECTION

R. YAMAMOTO

*Department of Epidemiology and Preventive Medicine
School of Veterinary Medicine
University of California, Davis*

Mycoplasma meleagridis (N strain PPLO, H serotype) is the cause of an egg transmitted disease of turkeys in which the primary lesion is an airsacculitis in the progeny. The organism is a specific pathogen of turkeys.

Following the original study of Adler et al. in 1958, research on this organism and its effect on turkey production was not extensively pursued. However, with the reduction in the prevalance of *M. gallisepticum* infection in the turkey population in recent years, more attention is now being focused on *M. meleagridis*. The observations that *M. meleagridis* is widely distributed and could be responsible for airsacculitis in as high as 50% of the progeny of *M. gallisepticum*-free turkeys have suggested that the disease may be more important economically than heretofore recognized.

HISTORY

Adler et al. (1958) were the first to show that airsacculitis in day-old poults could be associated with a mycoplasma other than *M. gallisepticum*. Airsacculitis was seen in samplings of poults from each of 10 breeding flocks from four states. Mycoplasma was recovered from 9 of 10 sources of which only one proved to be *M. gallisepticum*. The mycoplasma isolated from the remaining 8 sources was shown to be antigenically related and was named the N strain. In his consecutive alphabetical designation of serotypes of avian mycoplasma, Kleckner (1960) placed the N strain into the H serotype. The latter designation has been used widely (Yoder and Hofstad, 1964; Dierks et al., 1967). Recently Yamamoto et al. (1965a) proposed the species designation of *M. meleagridis* for this avian serotype. The clinical syndrome has been referred to as "day-old type" airsacculitis (Kumar et al., 1963).

INCIDENCE AND DISTRIBUTION

Mycoplasma meleagridis is distributed widely among turkey flocks in the United States (Adler et al., 1958; Kumar et al., 1963; Yoder and Hofstad, 1964; Mohamed et al., 1966; Dierks et al., 1967), Canada (Bigland, 1961; Cloutier and Filion, 1965; Bigland and Benson, 1968), and Great Britain (Fraser, 1966a). Adler et al. (1958) isolated the organism from air sac lesions of poults from 8 of 10 breeding flocks. Bigland (1961) reported observing airsacculitis in poults during 1954–61 in which no pathogenic agent could be consistently isolated. Kumar et al. (1963) observed airsacculitis in 24% of 1,197 first-run, cull, and pipped poults from breeders testing serologically negative to *M. gallisepticum*. The lesions were distributed among all of 21 consignments which made up their samples. In 13 consignments of 183 poults ranging in age from 1 to 13 weeks, air sac lesions were seen in each consignment and in 23% of the poults. Mycoplasma was the only agent consistently isolated from the lesions. Bigland et al. (1964) found that the air sac lesion rate in cull poults from 18 strains of turkeys free of *M. gallisepticum* increased from 13 to 60% through 9 consecutive hatches; mycoplasma showing cultural characteristics of *M. meleagridis* were isolated from representative samples. More recently Bigland and Benson (1968) found a mean lesion rate of 65% among 1,932 cull poults from a Saskatchewan turkey flock over a 20-week period of lay; *M. meleagridis* was recovered from a high percentage of the lesions. Yoder and Hofstad (1966) observed airsacculitis in approximately 50% of pipped embryos from 118 supply flocks from five states. Similar lesions were seen in 20% of poults examined from 1 day to 13 weeks of age from 62 flocks. *M. meleagridis* was isolated from the majority of lesions from embryos and poults examined; *M. gallisepticum* could not be incriminated in any of the cases studied.

Thus to date, no commercial turkey flock examined has been found free of *M. meleagridis*. Only 4 flocks associated with research stations in California (Yamamoto, 1967), Minnesota (Dierks et al., 1967), Ohio (Mohamed and Bohl, 1968a), and Iowa (Yoder and Hofstad, 1966) are known to be free of this agent. These small flocks were composed of selected individuals naturally free of the disease or were produced by experimental procedures.

ETIOLOGY

CLASSIFICATION

Mycoplasma meleagridis (Yamamoto et al., 1965a) was designated as the "N" strain by Adler et al. (1958) and was placed in the H serotype by Kleckner (1960), Yoder and Hofstad (1964), and Dierks et al. (1967).

MORPHOLOGY AND STAINING

Giemsa-stained smears of broth cultures of *M. meleagridis* show coccoid bodies approximately 0.4μ in diameter, similar to those of *M. gallisepticum* (Yamamoto and Adler, 1958; Yoder and Hofstad, 1964). The coccoid bodies may appear singly, in pairs, or in small clusters.

GROWTH REQUIREMENTS

Mycoplasma meleagridis is a facultative anaerobe. Growth is optimal at 37–38° C and slight at 40–42° C. While the organism will not grow at room temperature (22–24° C), freshly seeded cultures on agar held for 6 days at room temperature will develop upon subsequent incubation at 37° C (Yamamoto et al., 1965a).

Most isolates of *M. meleagridis* grow poorly or not at all in broth (Yoder and Hofstad, 1964; Yamamoto et al., 1965a; Mohamed et al., 1966); however, this characteristic may be governed by the type of basal medium used, as recently reported by Frey et al. (1968a).

A 10–20% addition of serum to the basal medium is required for growth of *M. meleagridis*. Swine serum (Mohamed and Bohl, 1967) or horse serum (Adler et al., 1958) are satisfactory; however, both turkey (Yoder and Hofstad, 1964) and chicken sera (Adler and Berg, 1960) generally are unsatisfactory. The suitability of certain sera may be influenced by the basal medium; for example, Yoder and Hofstad (1964) found that *M. meleagridis* grew poorly if at all in turkey meat infusion broth supplemented with yeast autolysate (5%) and turkey serum (20%), but grew satisfactorily on agar medium of the same constituents. Replacement of the turkey serum with horse serum (15%) resulted in better growth in broth. A yeast source appears to be essential for optimal growth. Frey et al. (1968a) compared several commercial preparations and found yeast autolysate (Albimi) to be the most satisfactory and as efficient as fresh yeast autolysate. On occasion fresh isolates appear to grow more favorably adjacent to staphylococcus colonies, suggesting that the particular lot of medium was inadequate in supplying certain growth factors; however, the organism does not require nicotinamide adenine dinucleotide (NAD) other than what may be provided in the complex ingredients added to the media. The fastidious and delicate nature of this organism is exemplified in the observation that from time to time certain batches of media do not support growth of the organism. In such cases the source of the problem often can be traced to one of the ingredients such as the serum, yeast supplement, basal medium, or agar.

Since Adler et al. (1958) first reported the isolation of *M. meleagridis* on Difco PPLO media, some modifications have been made through the years which have not been specifically reported in the literature. The media and procedures incorporating these modifications are as follows. Solid medium consists of PPLO broth (Difco) to which is added 1.55% Bacto agar, 1% yeast autolysate (Albimi), and 10–15% horse serum. The enrichment medium consists of a 10% horse blood agar slope (Tryptose blood agar base, Difco) overlaid with 2.5 ml of broth of the same constituents as the solid medium without the agar. The pH of the broth or agar medium is adjusted to 7.4–7.6 before sterilizing at 15 lbs for 15 minutes. The serum is filter-sterilized and inactivated at 56° C for 30 minutes before use. Thallium acetate and penicillin are added to the broth and agar media at final concentrations of 1:4,000 and 1,000 units per ml respectively. The pH of the final media is between 7.6 and 7.8.

Mohamed and Bohl (1967) obtained satisfactory results with PPLO agar (Difco) supplemented with 0.5% starch, 0.05% trypticase (BBL), 1% yeast hydrolysate, and 10% swine serum for primary isolation of *M. meleagridis*. In addition to penicillin and thallium acetate, 50 units Mycostatin per ml were added to their medium to obviate excessive contamination problems.

Others (Kumar et al., 1963; Frey et al., 1968a) have reported PPLO basal media (Difco) to be generally unsatisfactory for primary isolation of *M. meleagridis*, although in such cases one or more of the ingredients such as serum, yeast product, or thallium acetate may not have been of the same source or concentration as that used by Yamamoto et al. (1966b). The poor results obtained with the available dehydrated media have stimulated these workers to develop other media. Frey et al. (1968a) developed a new medium, designated FM, which was modified after Papageorgiou, a French formulation for growth of *M. gallisepticum*. When supplemented with 10–15% horse serum, the FM agar medium was more efficient than *viande foie* (VF) medium for primary isolation of *M. meleagridis*. The latter was equally as efficient as avian meat infusion medium. While new isolates grew well on VF broth on first passage, several passages were required before adaptation occurred in either FM or avian meat infusion broths. The FM medium is now available as a dehydrated product called Mycoplasma broth base (Albimi). Other studies have indicated that VF (Kumar et al., 1963; Dierks et al., 1967) and avian meat infusion (Yoder and Hofstad, 1964) media are highly efficient for primary isolation and maintenance of *M. meleagridis* although both must be prepared from fresh ingredients.

COLONIAL MORPHOLOGY

Colonies on agar medium after 2–3 days incubation appear small and flat (0.04–0.2 mm in diameter) with rough-appearing centers or ill-defined nipples. Nippling of the colonies is more prominent in laboratory-adapted strains than in fresh isolates (Yamamoto et al., 1965a).

BIOCHEMICAL PROPERTIES

The organism does not ferment dextrose or other carbohydrates nor reduce tetrazolium salts (Yoder and Hofstad, 1964; Yamamoto et al., 1965a). Yoder and Hofstad (1964) reported that the organism hemolyzes horse erythrocytes when incorporated at the 2% level into turkey meat infusion agar. Most isolates do not possess hemagglutinating activity against turkey (Yoder and Hofstad, 1964) or chicken erythrocytes (Yamamoto et al., 1965a). Of many isolates studied Yamamoto et al. (1965a) reported finding one which possessed this activity. More recently Rhoades (1969) reported the isolation of another hemagglutinating strain of *M. meleagridis*.

RESISTANCE TO CHEMICAL AND PHYSICAL AGENTS

Very little is known specifically about the resistance of *M. meleagridis* to certain chemical and physical agents. However, it is assumed that most chemical disinfectants would be effective against it. (See section on Treatment for information on antibiotic sensitivity).

The stationary phase of *M. meleagridis* (strain 529) grown in broth medium of pH ranges of 7.0–7.8 was less than 5 days; it was extended 25–30 days at a high titer (viable counts of $10^7/ml$) at pH ranges of 8.4–8.7 (DaMassa and Adler, 1969). Thus under proper environmental conditions *M. meleagridis* may survive at high titers for prolonged periods.

Isolates of *M. meleagridis* may be maintained for at least 2 months by mincing colonies on agar in 3% sucrose and freezing at —20 to —70° C. Yoder and Hofstad (1964) found broth overlaid agar slant cultures to be viable after at least 2 years storage at —30° C. Lyophilized cultures remain viable for at least 5 years (Yamamoto et al., 1965a).

ANTIGENIC STRUCTURE

Studies by several investigators have shown *M. meleagridis* to be a distinct serotype, unrelated to other avian mycoplasma. The agglutination (Adler et al., 1958; Yoder and Hofstad, 1964), fluorescent antibody (Corstvet and Sadler, 1964), antiglobulin (Adler and DaMassa, 1964), growth inhibition (Dierks et al., 1967), complement fixation (Newman, 1967; Frey and Hanson, 1969), and polyacrylamide gel electrophoresis (Razin, 1968) tests have been used to identify and differentiate *M. meleagridis* from other avian mycoplasma. Isolates recovered from various sites of the turkey (sinus, trachea, lung, air sac, bursa of Fabricius, vagina, and semen) were found to be antigenically related (Yamamoto et al., 1965b).

PATHOGENICITY

Only recently conclusive evidence has been presented to prove that *M. meleagridis* could cause air sac lesions in turkeys. This has been possible through the establishment of small groups of *M. meleagridis*-free turkeys at various research stations as indicated earlier. Dierks et al.

(1967) observed airsacculitis in a high percentage of poults inoculated via the air sacs and sinus with 8 isolates of *M. meleagridis*. Yamamoto and Bigland (1965) inoculated day-old poults with isolates of *M. meleagridis* recovered from the air sac, semen, and oviduct of turkeys. The air sac lesions seen at necropsy 3 weeks after inoculation were indistinguishable from those seen in natural infections. In another study when turkey embryos were inoculated via the yolk sac at 7 or 14 days of incubation with varying numbers of mycoplasma, the incidence of airsacculitis in the poults at hatching ranged from 30 to 100% with a mean of 72% (Yamamoto and Bigland, 1966). The organism evidently was highly infectious in that air sac lesions were detected in 37 and 50% of two groups of poults inoculated during embryonic development, with 3.5 and 0.6 colony-forming units (CFU) per embryo respectively. The high infectivity and low mortality caused by *M. meleagridis* in turkey embryos as indicated in this and other studies would suggest that this organism has attained an ideal host-parasite relationship. Studies to prove that the organism is responsible for various deleterious conditions in the turkey become extremely difficult under such conditions.

M. meleagridis will grow to high titers in the yolk sac of developing chicken embryos without causing excessive mortality (Yoder and Hofstad, 1964). Airsacculitis may be observed if inoculated embryos are allowed to hatch; however, the lesion rate is much lower in chicken than in turkey embryos (Yamamoto and Ortmayer, 1966).

PATHOGENESIS AND EPIZOOTIOLOGY

NATURAL AND EXPERIMENTAL HOSTS

Turkeys of all ages are susceptible to air sac infection with *M. meleagridis* when inoculated via the air sac, trachea, or by aerosol (Yamamoto and Bigland, 1965; Kumar, 1967; Mohamed and Bohl, 1968a). Chickens are refractory to infection with *M. meleagridis* when inoculated via the air sac (Adler, 1958; Yamamoto and Bigland, 1964a; Yoder and Hofstad, 1966). A mycoplasma believed to be *M. meleagridis* was isolated from the sinus exudate of a Japanese quail *(Coturnix coturnix)* in cohabitation with turkeys. Young chickens inoculated via the air sac with this isolate responded with agglutinins to *M. meleagridis* antigen without producing lesions (Yamamoto and Bigland, 1964a). However, since the organism was not subjected to critical antigenic analysis, definite proof of susceptibility of the quail must await further study.

TRANSMISSION

The primary mode by which the organism is perpetuated is through egg transmission. Studies by various workers indicate that the primary mechanism by which infection of the reproductive tract of the female occurs is through insemination with mycoplasma-contaminated semen (Yamamoto et al., 1966b; Mohamed et al., 1966; Kumar, 1967; Mohamed and Bohl, 1967; Yamamoto, 1967). Hens proven to be free of infection of the oviduct are rapidly converted to a positive status when inseminated even once with contaminated semen. By this route of infection, average airsacculitis rates of 10–25% in first-run poults over a season's lay have been reported under commercial and experimental conditions (Yamamoto et al., 1966b; Mohamed and Bohl, 1967; Kumar, 1967). The egg transmission rate among individual hens may vary from 10 to 60% (Yamamoto et al., 1966b). However, there is apparently no regular pattern as to the sequence of infected eggs laid (Mohamed and Bohl, 1967). The transmission starts out at a low rate during the first 2–3 weeks of lay, reaches a maximum at midseason, and gradually declines toward the end of the laying season (Bigland et al., 1964; Benson, 1967; Kumar, 1967). There seems to be some intracyclic fluctuation in the transmission pattern during the laying season (Yamamoto et al., 1966b; Kumar, 1967), but it has not been possible to relate such changes to the insemination schedule.

Egg transmission does not occur in hens in which the organism is found only in the upper respiratory tract such as the sinus (Yamamoto, 1967; Kumar, 1967; Mohamed and Bohl, 1967) and is minimal in hens infected via the air sacs and subsequently inseminated with clean semen (Kumar, 1967).

A comparative study of the persistence of *M. meleagridis*, *M. synoviae*, and *M. gallisepticum* in the genitalia of adult turkeys indicated that *M. meleagridis* favored this environment more than the other two species did (Yamamoto and Ortmayer, 1967c).

Although the exact site in the reproductive system where the organism penetrates the developing egg is not known, it appears not to be in the gonads; numerous isolation attempts from the ovules of hens known to be transmitting the organism have generally failed to yield the organism (Yamamoto et al., 1966b; Yamamoto, 1967; Mohamed and Bohl, 1967). Furthermore, egg transmission occurs at a high rate in the absence of active airsacculitis. However, the organism has been recovered frequently from various sites of the oviduct with greatest frequency in the vagina and uterus (Yamamoto et al., 1966b; Mohamed and Bohl, 1968a).

In hens which received contaminated semen, organisms were found as high as the magnum in some cases (Kumar, 1967). The report by Joshi and Yamamoto (1968, unpublished data), indicated that the number of organisms in the uterovaginal region may reach a relatively higher titer (10^4 CFU/swab) in hens inseminated with contaminated semen twice and thereafter with clean semen, with no evidence of egg transmission. Furthermore, high levels of infection in the uterovaginal region were not sustained in hens which were repeatedly inseminated with contaminated semen, although such hens did transmit the organism through their eggs. It thus appears that the conditions necessary for egg transmission are more complex than mere infection of the lower oviduct. The critical site of egg penetration probably occurs in the area of the fimbria or upper magnum soon after the yolk is released from the ovules. The isolation of the organism from yolk sac and yolk of fresh eggs (Kumar, 1967; Mohamed and Bohl, 1967) would also tend to support the above hypothesis.

While gross lesions (if any) in poults from infected dams are limited to the air sacs, the organism may be widely distributed in various tissues including the sinus, trachea, lungs, air sac, bursa of Fabricius, intestine, and cloaca. Cloacal infection detected at hatching can persist through maturity; semen taken from such males will contain mycoplasma (Yamamoto, 1967; Yamamoto and Ortmayer, 1968, unpublished data). The organism apparently remains localized in the region of the cloaca and phallus and does not ascend the vas deferens or testes (Yamamoto, 1967). Histologic study of the phallus and accessory organs suggests that one of the possible sites where the organism localizes is in the region of the submucosal glands (Gerlach et al., 1968). The mycoplasma isolation rates from the phallus or semen of turkeys from naturally infected flocks may range from 13 to 32%.

Recent studies have indicated that *M. meleagridis* may infect the oviduct of virgin hens by way of a descending infection early in life (Reis et al., 1971) or by an ascending infection from infection foci in the cloaca or bursa of Fabricius after the occluding plate is perforated at sexual maturity (Matzer and Yamamoto, 1970). Infection rates of 19–57% have been found in flocks in which cultures were taken from the vagina of virgin females. While such hens probably contribute to the overall egg transmission rate, particularly when the incidence is high, it is generally believed that venereal infection (due to artificial insemination) plays a major role in initiating and sustaining the egg transmission rate during the laying season.

LATERAL TRANSMISSION AND INCUBATION PERIOD

Kumar (1967) demonstrated that transmission in the hatcher by the respiratory route is a definite possibility. Noninfected poults hatched and held with infected poults in the incubator for 24 hours yielded the organism from their trachea and yolk sacs. However, Yamamoto and Ortmayer (1967b) were unable to demonstrate hatcher transmission when the hatcher contacts were separated immediately from the infected poults after hatching. These latter workers showed that lateral transmission occurred when noninfected poults were placed in cohabitation with infected poults at 1 day of age. Agglutinins were detected in the principals at 3 weeks and in the contacts at 4 weeks of age. When the poults were necropsied at 10 weeks of age, the organism was recovered from the sinuses of the majority of the contact poults, and to a lesser degree from the trachea, air sac, bursa of Fabricius, and cloaca. The isolation from the latter tissues suggests that lateral transmission may be another potential method which could lead to genital infection. Other studies

have indicated that the organism localizes primarily in the sinuses and trachea by lateral transmission (Mohamed and Bohl, 1967; Kumar, 1967; Frey et al., 1968b). Beard and Anderson (1967) showed that *M. meleagridis* can survive in the air for at least 6 hours, which strengthens the idea of airborne transmission. While further study is needed to show the relative importance of lateral transmission in growing birds in contributing to genital infection, apparently this mode is not important once a bird has reached sexual maturity. Infected adult females have been placed in cages adjacent to noninfected females with no evidence of egg transmission occuring in the latter. Similarly, clean males held in the same room with phallus-infected males were found to produce noninfected semen throughout the production period (Yamamoto, 1967; Yamamoto and Ortmayer, 1968, unpublished data).

SIGNS

Although some respiratory distress may be observed if the birds are carefully examined during the early morning or late evening hours, there generally is a lack of respiratory signs in affected flocks. Sternal bursitis was observed by Yamamoto and Bigland (1965) when poults were inoculated via the sinus and air sac. While sinusitis is not a regular feature of the disease, one or two birds with sinusitis may be observed in flocks of several thousand turkeys (Dierks et al., 1967).

MORBIDITY AND MORTALITY

It has been mentioned previously that nearly all flocks of turkeys are serologically positive for *M. meleagridis*. However, clinical manifestations are not always apparent. Moderate airsacculitis may be present with no great reduction in growth performance. A number of conditions such as reduced hatchability, poor liveability and growth performance, skeletal deformities, and condemnation at processing due to airsacculitis have been suggested as being directly or indirectly related to infection with *M. meleagridis*.

Growth Performance

Benson (1967) and Bigland and Benson (1968) could not relate poor feathering and other deficiency syndromes to *M. meleagridis* infection in growing poults. However, a significant difference in weight gains was observed between poults with and without air sac lesions studied during the first 3 weeks of life.

A marked increase in the incidence and prevalence of leg weakness problems (first observed in 1966) in turkey flocks throughout the country has caused some consternation among turkey growers. The clinical syndrome which includes bowing, twisting, and shortening of the tarsometatarsal bones with occasional hock joint swelling without exudation was seen in turkeys 3–12 weeks of age. Crooked necks caused by deformation of the cervical vertebrae also were seen in some flocks. The morbidity ranged from 5 to 10% and on occasion reached higher levels; severely affected birds had to be culled from the flock. The problem did not appear to be associated with a particular strain of bird or sex predilection, nor could it be traced to any particular feed or feeding regime. The incidence appeared to increase with the progression of the laying season (Peterson, 1966, personal communication; Nelson, 1968, personal communication). A similar clinical syndrome was first observed in England in 1965 and called the "turkey syndrome-65" (Report of a Working Party, 1965, 1966). The condition has also been seen in Canada as early as 1954 (Bigland, personal communication).

Peterson (1968) found a positive correlation among birds with the above-described skeletal deformities with the presence of airsacculitis and corresponding high agglutination titers to *M. meleagridis*. On the other hand, Frazer (1966b) reported observing turkey flocks with high prevalence of airsacculitis in the absence of leg deformities.

More detailed studies have been conducted on these problems relating to skeletal deformities in young turkeys by Grasso (1968) and Reis et al. (1970) but the etiology is not clearly elucidated.

Reproductive Performance

Cherms and Frey (1967) could not relate infertility in turkeys to infection of the reproductive tract with *M. meleagridis*. Yamamoto and Ortmayer (1967a) found that the infection had no adverse effect on egg production, fertility, or early incubation mortality. However, there was a significant increase in poult yield between eggs hatched from noninfected versus infected hens. The decreased poult yield in the infected group was attributed to late incubation mortality. In another study where a large number of organisms was inoculated directly into the yolk sac of developing embryos, hatchability was not affected (Yamamoto and Bigland, 1966).

Air Sac Lesions and Condemnations

Airsacculitis has been reported to be one of the major causes of condemnation of fryer-roaster turkeys, particularly in the central areas of the United States (Kumar et al., 1966; Anderson et al., 1968). *M. meleagridis* has been implicated as the underlying cause of such condemnations in view of its widespread distribution and high prevalence within individual turkey flocks. Since air sac lesions caused by uncomplicated *M. meleagridis* infection regress in a matter of 16 weeks, it would appear that other agents or factors may be involved in the overall picture. Kumar et al. (1963) found a high incidence of airsacculitis in fryer-roaster turkeys at processing in which mycoplasma and bacteria such as pasteurella, salmonella, and *E. coli* were isolated from the air sacs. However, the condemnations were no greater in such flocks than those in which only mycoplasma were isolated. Apparently in the flocks with the mixed infections the bacterial disease was controlled by medication prior to marketing. The condemnations of each of several flocks, which approximated 1%, were generally due to air sac infection. Frey et al. (1968b) conducted a thorough bacteriologic and virologic investigation of turkeys up to 16 weeks of age from 18 *M. gallisepticum*-free flocks in which airsacculitis was prevalent; *M. meleagridis* was the only agent of pathogenic significance which was consistently isolated from such lesions. Adler (1958) reported negligible condemnation in turkeys infected with *M. meleagridis* singly or in combination with *M. gallisepticum* when marketed at approximately 30 weeks of age. However, Kumar et al. (1966) reported significantly high condemnation rates (5%) due to air sac infections in turkey flocks marketed at 15–26 weeks of age. Anderson et al. (1968) observed a twofold or greater increase in the incidence of air sac lesions caused by *M. meleagridis* in turkeys raised to 12 weeks of age in a high dust environment

(0.6–1.0 mg per cu ft) as compared to turkeys raised in a low dust environment (0.1–0.4 mg per cu ft). The lesions were more severe in birds raised under such conditions. Environmental stress factors in aggravating *M. meleagridis* airsacculitis were also suggested by Brown (1967). Turkeys selected, following cold stress, for low plasma corticosterone were found to be more resistant to development of air sac lesions than birds selected for high levels of plasma corticosterone. Thus the available data suggest that the interaction of several factors governs the pathogenesis of severe airsacculitis in growing birds.

GROSS LESIONS

Air sac lesions seen in day-old poults are generally confined to the thoracic air sacs. These lesions are characterized by thickening of the walls with adherence of a yellow exudate to the tissue and occasionally the presence of various sized flecks of caseous material free in the lumen (Adler et al., 1958; Bigland and Yamamoto, 1964). Extension of such lesions to the abdominal air sacs is a common occurrence by 3–4 weeks of age. Lesions produced by *M. meleagridis* have been reported to be not as extensive or fulminating as those described for *M. gallisepticum* (Kumar et al., 1963; Dierks et al., 1967). Although some respiratory distress may be observed if the birds are carefully examined during the early morning or late evening hours, the striking feature is the general lack of respiratory signs in affected flocks.

Reports by various workers indicate that air sac lesions caused by *M. meleagridis* regress by about 16–30 weeks of age (Adler, 1958; Bigland, 1961). In more recent studies in which sequential samplings were taken from poults infected during embryonic development, it was found that lesions seen at hatching were still present in a high percentage (but in a stage of regression) by 10 weeks of age; by 16 weeks the lesions were nearly healed, and they were absent in the majority of poults at 20 weeks of age (Yamamoto and Ortmayer, 1968, unpublished data).

HISTOPATHOLOGY

Microscopically the air sacs of affected birds are thickened 8–20 times normal with heavy and diffuse lymphocytic infiltration and many large lymphofollicular areas;

some vascularization with an increase in connective tissue may be evident. The lesions are similar to those described for *M. gallisepticum* (Yamamoto and Bigland, 1965).

Cherms and Frey (1967) could not relate the lymphocytic infiltration in the uterus and vagina of naturally infected hens specifically to *M. meleagridis* infection. Gerlach et al. (1968) examined histologically the terminal papillae, ampule of the vas deferens, lymphfold and phallus, and vascular body of males experimentally infected with *M. meleagridis*. The only significant change was an extensive lymphofollicular formation in the region of the mucous type glands in the submucosa of the lymphfold.

IMMUNITY

The study of Mohamed and Bohl (1968a) indicates that turkeys are capable of developing active immunity when inoculated by the intravenous or various respiratory routes with *M. meleagridis*. Maximum agglutinin antibody response was obtained at 4 weeks, while the organism persisted in the trachea up to 7 weeks after infection. Upon reexposure by the same routes at 21 weeks after initial exposure, tracheal cultures remained negative and the secondary antibody response was of much lower magnitude than the initial response. At necropsy, 6 weeks after the second exposure, only caseated plaques were seen in the air sacs, and the organism could not be isolated from various respiratory or reproductive tissues. It was suggested that the immunity which developed in the respiratory tract was not related to agglutinating antibodies since the organism persisted in the trachea beyond the time of maximal antibody response following initial exposure; secondly, on reexposure an anamnestic response (agglutinating antibody) did not occur even though the birds were immune at that time.

Yamamoto et al. (1968) found that hens infected via the oviduct during one breeding season were free of such infections at the start of the second laying season; among five adult males infected via the phallus, the organism persisted for 55–344 days. Kumar (1967) reported that naturally infected males, selected at sexual maturity, shed the organism in their semen up to 13 but not beyond 14 weeks of production. Hens infected via the oviduct remained carriers up to 15 weeks but were negative at 19 weeks. These findings are consistent with the observation that egg transmission rate declines during the latter part of the laying season and may be related to an active immune mechanism.

Passive antibodies (agglutinins) may be detected in a high percentage of poults from infected dams which persist for approximately 2 weeks after hatching (Yamamoto and Bigland, 1964b; Bigland and Yamamoto, 1964; Mohamed and Bohl, 1968a). Such antibodies appear not to protect against development of air sac lesions in infected embryos (Yamamoto et al., 1966b; Mohamed and Bohl, 1968a).

DIAGNOSIS

ISOLATION AND IDENTIFICATION OF CAUSATIVE AGENT

Mycoplasma meleagridis may be readily isolated on several commercially available and laboratory prepared media. Suspected tissue suspensions or samplings of exudates on cotton swabs may be streaked directly on agar medium, but it is generally best to inoculate broth or overlay enrichment medium with 4–6 days incubation before plating on agar. The various media are described in detail under the section on Growth Requirements.

The broth overlay enrichment medium on agar slants, as a modification of the original medium described by Adler et al. (1958), is especially effective for the isolation of *M. meleagridis* from materials likely to contain a minimum of organisms. This is often the case in the late stages of infection. For large sampling studies in the field (e.g., swabbing of oviducts or phallus) culturing directly into overlay broth facilitates transport to the laboratory as well as serving as an initial enrichment. The addition of polymyxin B to the broth overlay (10 μg per ml) together with penicillin and thallium acetate facilitates isolation of *M. meleagridis* from highly contaminated sources such as the cloaca and phallus (Ortmayer and Yamamoto, 1968, unpublished data).

Media prepared from fresh meat infusions have proved to be highly efficient for primary isolation (Kumar et al., 1963; Yoder and Hofstad, 1964; Dierks et al., 1967), but the FM medium developed by

Frey et al. (1968a) is very adequate and now available commercially (mycoplasma broth base—Albimi).

Once growth is apparent in original isolation medium, usually after 4–6 days incubation, agar plates should be streaked and placed in a sealed container with added moisture. The plates should be incubated at 37° C for 5–7 days before being examined for colonies under the dissecting microscope. The plates should be incubated at least 10 days before being discarded as negative.

Isolates of *M. meleagridis* may be identified further by their inability to ferment glucose or maltose and by their inability to reduce certain tetrazolium salts, as described by Yamamoto and Adler (1958) and Yoder and Hofstad (1964). Isolates of *M. meleagridis* have been reported to be culturally distinct from certain other serotypes on primary agar isolation (Yamamoto and Bigland, 1964a), but definitive identification of *M. meleagridis* isolates may be made with a number of serologic tests as indicated earlier (see Antigenic Structure). Dierks et al. (1967) incorporated 5% rabbit hyperimmune anti-*M. meleagridis* serum in the agar medium. The criterion of specificity was based on complete inhibition of growth of undiluted cultures plated on such media. However, as many as 30 injections of antigen into rabbits were required before satisfactory growth-inhibiting antibodies could be obtained. The direct fluorescent antibody test is another rapid identification procedure (Corstvet and Sadler, 1964). Colony imprints on coverslips may be prepared and examined immediately or stored at −20 to −70° C for several months. By this procedure the specifically labeled antiserum will detect *M. meleagridis* colonies in the presence of mixed cultures.

In the absence of any of the more detailed tests, one may inoculate the unknown broth or agar culture intravenously into chickens and check for specific agglutinins 1–3 weeks after inoculation (Yamamoto et al., 1965b; Mohamed and Bohl, 1968a).

SEROLOGY

The plate and tube agglutination tests have been used by various workers (Adler, 1958; Bigland and Yamamoto, 1964; Newman, 1967; Mohamed and Bohl, 1968a).

Mohamed and Bohl (1968a) found an excellent correlation between the presence of antibodies and isolation of the organism in the sinus, air sac, or both in naturally infected poults necropsied at 14 weeks of age. In poults with air sac lesions the tube agglutination titer of 1:320, detected at 3 weeks of age, persisted at the same level up to the time of necropsy. Lower titers (0–80) were detected in poults in which the organism had localized only in the sinus; antibodies in such poults generally were first detected at 7 weeks of age, suggesting infection by contact. The tube test was more sensitive than the plate test. Observations generally similar to that described by Mohamed and Bohl were reported by others (Yamamoto et al., 1966b; Yamamoto and Ortmayer, 1967b).

The plate and tube agglutination antigens were prepared and standardized in essentially the same manner as described for *M. gallisepticum* (Mohamed and Bohl, 1968a).

A hemagglutination-inhibition test also has been developed and reported to be as effective as the agglutination test in detecting antibodies to *M. meleagridis* infection (Rhoades, 1969). As mentioned earlier, however, not all isolates of *M. meleagridis* possess hemagglutinating activity.

A modified direct complement fixation test and indirect hemagglutination test also have been developed (Newman, 1967).

DIFFERENTIAL DIAGNOSIS

Air sac lesions caused by *M. meleagridis* must be differentiated from those caused by *M. gallisepticum,* other mycoplasma serotypes, and possibly other agents. While lesions produced by *M. gallisepticum* are often more extensive and exudative than those produced by *M. meleagridis,* such a criterion is of little value for definitive diagnosis. However, based on a high lesion rate in poults from dams free of *M. gallisepticum,* one could make a tentative diagnosis of *M. meleagridis* infection since other agents produce such lesions only sporadically if at all. Definitive diagnosis must be based on cultural, serological, and other laboratory procedures.

TREATMENT

Using antibiotic sensitivity discs as their test procedure, Yamamoto et al. (1966a) reported that tylosin, chloromycetin, tetra-cycline, and oxytetracycline were active; novobiocin and neomycin were variable; and kanamycin, streptomycin, erythromycin, and oleandomycin were inactive against 23 isolates of *M. meleagridis.* Using the tube dilution method with 46 isolates, Newman (1967) found tylosin to be the most active followed closely by erythromycin. Oxytetracycline, magnamycin, magnamycin-oxytetracycline, spiramycin, and chloromycetin were intermediate in activity; chlortetracycline, dihydrostreptomycin, and novobiocin were the least active. Considering that different testing procedures were used by these investigators, the results in general are in agreement with the exception of the activity reported for erythromycin. The reason for this apparent discrepancy is not known. During in ovo (turkey embryos) trials with two isolates, it was found that tylosin was the most active; tetracycline, chlortetracycline, and streptomycin were variable; and erythromycin showed no activity. The test dose of antibiotic was 1 mg per embryo and the criteria of efficacy were based on prevention of air sac lesions and failure to isolate the organism (Yamamoto et al., 1966a). Common to both studies was the finding that the different isolates varied in their sensitivity to certain antibiotics, which points out the importance of prior sensitivity testing of several isolates before mass medication programs are contemplated (e.g. egg dipping) with a particular antibiotic.

The various treatment regimes used have been directed primarily at reducing the incidence of air sac infections. Parenteral injections or water medication of turkeys in production with tylosin have not been successful in reducing the egg-transmitted disease (Bigland et al., 1964; Kumar et al., 1966). Injections of day-old poults with erythromycin, streptomycin, or neomycin did not effectively prevent lateral spread of *M. meleagridis* infection (Yamamoto et al., 1966b). However, dipping of hatching eggs in antibiotic solutions has been shown to significantly reduce the incidence of air sac infection (Kumar et al., 1966; Bigland, 1968; Peterson, 1968; Mohamed and Bohl, 1968b; Nestor and Mohamed, 1968), concomitant with improved hatchability (Peterson, 1968, personal communication; Kumar et al., 1966), improved growth performance (Bigland, 1968; Nelson, 1968, personal

communication), reduced incidence of skeletal deformities (Peterson, 1968; Nelson,
1968, personal communication), and reduced condemnation at processing (Kumar
et al., 1966; Nelson, 1968, personal communication). Whether all or any of these
events are related to the reduction of incidence of *M. meleagridis* infection is presently not known or clearly elucidated.

The dipping procedure involves immersion of eggs, previously warmed at 37° C
for 2–4 hours, in a cold antibiotic solution
(4° C) for 15–20 minutes (Kumar et al.,
1966; Newman, 1967; Nestor and Mohamed, 1968). Tylosin has been used most extensively, and at concentrations from 1,000
to 3,000 ppm. Bigland et al. (1964) reported
that dipping of prewarmed (24° C) hatching eggs in erythromycin, 950 ppm at 4° C
for 10 minutes, did not significantly reduce
the incidence of air sac lesions. In another
study, Bigland (1968) reported that dipping
of eggs in spiramycin (1,000 ppm) reduced
the air sac lesion rate 72% and mycoplasma
isolation rate 84% over the controls. Disinfectants such as zephiran (1,000 ppm),
Wescodyne (0.45%) (Newman, 1967), and
Iosan (0.34%) (Nestor and Mohamed, 1968)
are added to the antibiotic solution to aid
in reducing bacterial contamination. The
vacuum procedure for incorporating antibiotics into the egg also is being used in
the field.

PREVENTION AND CONTROL

MANAGEMENT PROCEDURES

Since *M. meleagridis* is essentially a venereal infection, strict sanitary procedures
should be practiced during collection of
semen and insemination of hens to minimize cross-contamination. Such procedures
as determining the presence of an egg in
the uterus by vaginal palpation may lead
to increased incidence of vaginal carriers
(Mohamed and Bohl, 1967). Since the organism may be present in the cloaca of
day-old poults, strict sanitary procedures to
reduce cross-contamination during sexing
should be considered. Hatchery-borne infections and lateral transmission during the
growing period are possibilities; but until
such time that clean stocks become available, it would appear that strict isolation
procedures would be of little value. Furthermore, in a naturally infected flock, one
would expect the sanitary procedures insti-

tuted to minimize cross-contamination to
merely delay and possibly alter the egg
transmission rate without actually preventing it. However, all of the above-men-
tioned factors should be considered if attempts are being made to produce *M. meleagridis*-free turkeys.

CONTROL AND ERADICATION

The currently used procedure of dipping
hatching eggs in antibiotic (tylosin) solution
should be considered only as a control measure since all reports indicate approximately
5% of the poults originating from such eggs
may still remain infected. Such procedures
may have application for commercial meat
birds to improve general performance (see
Treatment).

While practical and proven procedures
for eradication of *M. meleagridis* from basic
breeders have not yet been developed, certain experimental approaches may be considered. Based on the premise that not all
turkeys in a flock would be infected, Yamamoto et al. (1966b) applied serologic and
cultural procedures to detect such individuals. Nonreactors detected by the serologic
test were in turn cultured (semen or phallus
of the males and oviduct of the females) at
least three times prior to insemination. Turkeys testing negative by these criteria were
selected for study. It was necessary to conduct such procedures through two generations before a *M. meleagridis*-free flock was
produced (Yamamoto, 1967).

Newman (1967) produced *M. meleagridis*-
free turkeys by double-dipping eggs in tylosin. The procedure consisted of immersing
prewarmed eggs (4 hours at 37° C) in tylosin (3,000 ppm) solution held at 5° C for 15
minutes; the eggs were reincubated at 37° C
for 4 hours and then dipped again for 15
minutes. It was essential that the eggs were
taken from the first week or two of the laying cycle at the time of lowest egg transmission; the procedure was not successful when
applied to eggs taken later in the season.

With the finding that the male is the
main contributor to infection of the female
oviduct and the belief that lateral transmission does not contribute significantly to
ultimate egg transmission, Kumar (1967)
considered dipping of hatching eggs in
tylosin with subsequent monitoring of the
males by culture during the growing season. Mohamed and Bohl (1968b) suggested
that dipping of eggs followed by serological

testing of the poults might be a method of producing M. meleagridis-free turkeys.

It would appear from these studies that dipping of eggs in antibiotic solution together with a monitoring system including serologic and cultural procedures, particularly during the early growing period, would be required to produce M. meleagridis-free turkeys. The efficacy of the dipping procedure may be immediately evaluated by examination of the hatch debris, pipped embryos, and cull poults for air sac

lesions and presence of the organism. The development of resistant strains of mycoplasma should be kept in mind, particularly at the basic breeder level where treated birds must necessarily be recycled in the operation (Newman, 1967).

Work is in progress at various stations to determine the effect of treating semen with antibiotic to eliminate the organism; it is still premature for definitive conclusions (Kumar et al., 1968; Mohamed and Bohl, 1968b).

REFERENCES

Adler, H. E. 1958. A PPLO agglutination test for the detection of infectious sinusitis of turkeys. *Poultry Sci.* 37:1116–23.

Adler, H. E., and J. Berg. 1960. Cultivation of Mycoplasma of avian origin. *Avian Diseases* 4:3–12.

Adler, H. E., and A. J. DaMassa. 1964. Enhancement of Mycoplasma agglutination titer by use of anti-globulin. *Proc. Soc. Exp. Biol. Med.* 116:608–10.

Adler, H. E., J. Fabricant, R. Yamamoto, and J. Berg. 1958. Isolation and identification of pleuropneumonia-like organisms of avian origin. *Am. J. Vet. Res.* 19:440–47.

Anderson, D. P., R. R. Wolfe, F. L. Cherms, and W. E. Roper. 1968. Influence of dust and ammonia on the development of air sac lesions in turkeys. *Am. J. Vet. Res.* 29:1049–58.

Beard, C. W., and D. P. Anderson. 1967. Aerosol studies with avian Mycoplasma. I. Survival in the air. *Avian Diseases* 11:54–59.

Benson, Margaret L. 1967. Cellular and other aspects of *Mycoplasma meleagridis* infection in cull and normal turkey poults. Master's thesis, Univ. Saskatchewan.

Bigland, C. H. 1961. Air sac infection in turkeys. *Can. Poultry Rev.* (Nov.), pp. 68, 70.

———. 1968. Experimental control of *Mycoplasma meleagridis* in turkeys by the temperature differential dipping of eggs in tylosin and spiramycin. *Poultry Sci.* 47:1656. (Abstr.)

Bigland, C. H., and M. L. Benson. 1968. *Mycoplasma meleagridis* ("N" strain Mycoplasma-PPLO): Relationship of air sac lesions and isolations in day old turkeys (*Meleagridis gallopavo*). *Can. Vet. J.* 9:138–41.

Bigland, C. H., and R. Yamamoto. 1964. Study of natural and experimental infection of Mycoplasma associated with turkey airsacculitis. *Avian Diseases* 8:531–38.

Bigland, C. H., W. Dungan, R. Yamamoto, and J. C. Voris. 1964. Airsacculitis in poults from different strains of turkeys. *Avian Diseases* 8:85–92.

Brown, K. I. 1967. Environmentally imposed stress, pp. 101–13. In Carter, T. C. (ed.),

Environmental Control in Poultry Production. Oliver and Boyd, Edinburgh.

Cherms, F. L., and M. L. Frey, 1967. *Mycoplasma meleagridis* and fertility in turkey breeder hens. *Avian Diseases* 11:268–74.

Cloutier, S., and R. Filion. 1965. Essais d'isolement de PPLO a partir de dindes negatives a l'antigene S6. *Can. Vet. J.* 6:137–42.

Corstvet, R. E., and W. W. Sadler. 1964. The diagnosis of certain avian diseases with the fluorescent antibody technique. *Poultry Sci.* 43:1280–88.

Da Massa, A. J., and H. E. Adler. 1969. Effect of pH on growth and survival of three avian and one saprophytic Mycoplasma. *Applied Microbiol.* 17:310–16.

Dierks, R. E., J. A. Newman, and B. S. Pomeroy. 1967. Characterization of avian Mycoplasma. *Ann. N.Y. Acad. Sci.* 143:170–89.

Fraser, D. McK. 1966a. The "N" strain of Mycoplasma in the turkey—a review. *Poultry Rev.* 6:3–5.

———. 1966b. *Mycoplasma meleagridis* and turkey bad leg syndrome. *Vet. Record* 78:323.

Frey, M. L., and R. P. Hanson. 1969. A complement fixation test for the study of avian Mycoplasmas. *Avian Diseases* 13:185–97.

Frey, M. L., R. P. Hanson, and D. P. Anderson. 1968a. A medium for the isolation of avian Mycoplasmas. *Am. J. Vet. Res.* 29:2163–71.

Frey, M. L., D. P. Anderson, and R. P. Hanson. 1968b. Airsacculitis relation to Mycoplasmas in turkeys free of *Mycoplasma gallisepticum*. *Avian Diseases* 12:693–99.

Gerlach, Helga, R. Yamamoto, and Herrad B. Ortmayer. 1968. Zur pathologie der phallus-infektion der puten mit *Mycoplasma meleagridis*. *Archiv. Gefluegelk.* 32:396–99.

Grasso, P. 1968. Pathological changes in tarsometatarsus from turkeys affected with turkey syndrome '65 (Turkey Y-disease). *Vet. Record* 82:758–61.

Kleckner, A. L. 1960. Serotypes of avian pleuropneumonia-like organisms. *Am. J. Vet. Res.* 21:274–80.

Kumar, M. C. 1967. Studies on the transmission of *Mycoplasma meleagridis* in turkeys. Ph.D. thesis, Univ. Minn.

Kumar, S., R. E. Dierks, J. A. Newman, C. I. Pfow, and B. S. Pomeroy. 1963. Airsacculitis in turkeys. I. A study of airsacculitis in day-old poults. *Avian Diseases* 7:376–85.

Kumar, M. C., S. Kumar, R. E. Dierks, J. A. Newman, and B. S. Pomeroy. 1966. Airsacculitis in turkeys. II. Use of tylosin in the control of the egg transmission of *Mycoplasma* spp. other than *Mycoplasma gallisepticum* in turkeys. *Avian Diseases* 10:194–98.

Kumar, M. C., J. A. Newman, S. H. Kleven, and B. S. Pomeroy. 1968. Control of *Mycoplasma meleagridis* in turkeys. *Poultry Sci.* 47:1688. (Abstr.)

Matzer, N., and R. Yamamoto. 1970. Genital pathogenesis of *Mycoplasma meleagridis* in virgin turkey hens. *Avian Diseases* 14:321–29.

Mohamed, Y. S., and E. H. Bohl. 1967. Studies on the transmission of *Mycoplasma meleagridis*. *Avian Diseases* 11:634–41.

———. 1968a. Serologic studies on *Mycoplasma meleagridis* in turkeys. *Avian Diseases* 12:554–66.

———. 1968b. The use of serologic methods for the control of *Mycoplasma meleagridis* in turkeys. *Poultry Sci.* 47:1697–98. (Abstr.)

Mohamed, Y. S., S. Chema, and E. H. Bohl. 1966. Studies on Mycoplasma of the "H" serotype *(Mycoplasma meleagridis)* in the reproductive and respiratory tracts of turkeys. *Avian Diseases* 10:347–52.

Nestor, K. E., and Y. S. Mohamed. 1968. Tylosin and PPLO in turkeys. *Drumstick* 12:11, 21.

Newman, J. A. 1967. The detection and control of *Mycoplasma meleagridis*. Ph.D. thesis. Univ. Minn.

Peterson, I. L. 1968. Field significance of *Mycoplasma meleagridis* infection. *Poultry Sci.* 47:1708–9. (Abstr.)

Razin, S. 1968. Mycoplasma taxonomy studied by electrophoresis of cell proteins. *J. Bacteriol.* 96:687–94.

Reis, R., J. M. L. DaSilva, and R. Yamamoto. 1970. Pathologic changes in the joint and other organs of turkey poults after intravenous inoculation of *Mycoplasma meleagridis*. *Avian Diseases* 14:117–25.

Reis, R., N. Matzer, and R. Yamamoto. 1971. Pathogenesis of *Mycoplasma meleagridis* in diethylstilboestrol treated turkey embryos and poults. *J. Comp. Pathol.* 81:235–43.

Report of Working Party. 1965. A new syndrome in turkey poults. *Vet. Record* 77:1292.

———. 1966. Turkey syndrome '65. *Vet. Record* 71:805–6.

Rhoades, K. R. 1969. A hemagglutination-inhibition test for *Mycoplasma meleagridis* antibodies. *Avian Diseases* 13:22–26.

Yamamoto, R. 1967. Localization and egg transmission of *Mycoplasma meleagridis* in turkeys exposed by various routes. *Ann. N.Y. Acad. Sci.* 143:225–33.

Yamamoto, R., and H. E. Adler. 1958. Characterization of pleuropneumonia-like organisms of avian origin. II. Cultural, biochemical, morphological and further serological studies. *J. Infect. Diseases* 102:243–50.

Yamamoto, R., and C. H. Bigland. 1964a. Pathogenicity to chicks of Mycoplasma associated with turkey airsacculitis. *Avian Diseases* 8:523–31.

———. 1964b. Serological evidence that "N" Mycoplasma causes an airsacculitis in turkeys. *Bacteriol. Proc.*, p. 47. (Abstr.)

———. 1965. Experimental production of airsacculitis in turkey poults by inoculation with "N"-type Mycoplasma. *Avian Diseases* 9:108–18.

———. 1966. Infectivity of *Mycoplasma meleagridis* for turkey embryos. *Am. J. Vet. Res.* 27:326–30.

Yamamoto, R., and Herrad B. Ortmayer. 1966. Pathogenicity of *Mycoplasma meleagridis* for turkey and chicken embryos. *Avian Diseases* 10:268–72.

———. 1967a. Effect of *Mycoplasma meleagridis* on reproductive performance. *Poultry Sci.* 46:1340. (Abstr.)

———. 1967b. Hatcher and intraflock transmission of *Mycoplasma meleagridis*. *Avian Diseases* 11:288–95.

———. 1967c. Localization and persistence of avian mycoplasma in the genital system of the mature turkey. *J. Am. Vet. Med. Ass.* 150:1371. (Abstr.)

Yamamoto, R., C. H. Bigland, and Herrad B. Ortmayer. 1965a. Characteristics of *Mycoplasma meleagridis* sp. n., isolated from turkeys. *J. Bacteriol.* 90:47–49.

Yamamoto, R., Herrad B. Ortmayer, C. H. Bigland, M. L. Seely, and R. E. Corstvet. 1965b. Isolation of "N" Mycoplasma from different sites of the turkey. *Poultry Sci.* 44:732–36.

Yamamoto, R., C. H. Bigland, and Herrad B. Ortmayer. 1966a. Sensitivity of *Mycoplasma meleagridis* to various antibiotics. *Poultry Sci.* 45:1139. (Abstr.)

Yamamoto, R., C. H. Bigland, and I. L. Peterson. 1966b. Egg transmission of *Mycoplasma meleagridis*. *Poultry Sci.* 45:1245–57.

Yamamoto, R., Herrad B. Ortmayer, and C. S. Joshi. 1968. Persistence of *Mycoplasma meleagridis* in the genitalia of experimentally infected turkeys. *Poultry Sci.* 47:1734. (Abstr.)

Yoder, H. W., Jr., and M. S. Hofstad. 1964. Characterization of avian Mycoplasma. *Avian Diseases* 8:481–512.

———. 1966. *Mycoplasma meleagridis* infection in turkeys. *J. Am. Vet. Med. Ass.* 148:1351. (Abstr.)

MYCOPLASMA SYNOVIAE INFECTION

❖

N. O. OLSON

*Division of Animal
and Veterinary Sciences
West Virginia University
Morgantown, West Virginia*

❖

Mycoplasma synoviae infection is commonly designated as infectious synovitis, an acute to chronic infectious disease of chickens and turkeys involving primarily the synovial membranes of joints and tendon sheaths producing an exudative synovitis, tenosynovitis, or bursitis.

HISTORY

Infectious synovitis was first described by Olson et al. (1954) and Wills (1954) in two separate areas of the United States. They published additional reports concerning the disease in chickens (Wills and Delaplane, 1955; Olson et al., 1956) as did Lecce et al. (1955) and Cover et al. (1956). Snoeyenbos and Olesiuk (1955) described a similar condition in turkeys.

INCIDENCE AND DISTRIBUTION

The disease is observed primarily in growing birds 4–12 weeks of age in the broiler growing regions of the United States. It has been seen in replacement flocks of laying chickens with increased frequency during recent years. On one occasion signs were not noted until the birds were in production. It usually appears in turkeys when they are 10–20 weeks old, but it seems to be a serious flock problem less frequently than in chickens.

Infectious synovitis has been reported from England (Carnaghan, 1959), Canada (Bigland and Brown, 1955), Norway (Badstue, 1961), Germany (Burtscher, 1961), France (Guillon et al., 1962), and South Africa (Cole, 1964, personal communication) and is probably worldwide in distribution.

ETIOLOGY

CLASSIFICATION

Infectious synovitis was thought to be caused by a large particle virus or rickettsia by early workers (Wills, 1954; Lecce et al., 1955; Cover et al., 1956; Olson et al., 1956). Lecce (1960) noted colonies typical of mycoplasma as satellites adjacent to micrococcus colonies on PPLO agar. This was confirmed by Chalquest and Fabricant (1960) who incorporated beta-diphosphopyridine nucleotide (DPN) in their medium. It was designated as serotype S by Dierks et al. (1967). Olson et al. (1964b) studied several isolates and proposed the name *Mycoplasma synoviae* (MS).

Identification is based on typical colony and cell morphology, biochemical characteristics, special requirements for growth, and serological reactions.

MORPHOLOGY AND STAINING

In stained preparations *M. synoviae* appear as pleomorphic coccoid bodies or rods approximately 0.2μ in diameter and 0.4μ in length. Staining is accomplished by spreading a thin film of broth on a clean slide and allowing it to dry at room temperature. The film is fixed by flooding the slide with Bouin's fixative for 5–10 minutes. The slide is washed in running water until the yellow color in the fixative disappears. Ten drops of Giemsa blood stain is placed in 10 ml of water. The slide is flooded with the diluted Giemsa and allowed to stain for 30 minutes. The stain is washed off with running water and allowed to air dry before observation at 1,000 magnification.

GROWTH REQUIREMENTS

Nicotinamide adenine dinucleotide (NAD) is required for growth (Chalquest and Fabricant, 1960). Reports that yeast may be used for NAD (previously sometimes called diphosphopyridine nucleotide [DPN]) does not apply to all *M. synoviae* (Lecce, 1960). Serum is essential for growth, and swine serum is preferred (Chalquest, 1962). Growth on agar is accomplished by incubation of plates in a jar (candle jar) in which part of the oxygen has been removed by burning a candle. Although growth will occur in broth, an agar over-laid with broth improves growth, especial-ly on primary isolation. Diaphasic cultur-ing also improves growth. The latter meth-od involves seeding agar, incubating for 3 days, spreading colonies with a bent glass rod, reincubating for 24 hours, and placing broth on the agar with a final incubation period of 3–4 days. On primary isolation tissue antigens, toxins, or both are present; therefore, transfer in 24 hours is essential. All transfers are made with a pipette using a 10% inoculum. Transfer of 0.1 ml from a broth overlay to a well in an agar plate and adding broth to the level of the agar followed by incubation in a candle jar for 7 days improves isolation percentage. The plates are observed in 7 days at 30 magni-fication using indirect lighting. Colonies are observed floating in the broth, on the glass surface at the bottom of the well or on the agar. The floating colonies are light brown and easily distinguished from floating debris which is usually in the cen-ter of the well and is nearly colorless. If only one or two floating colonies are seen it is necessary to transfer to broth overlay medium. After incubation for 3–7 days, 0.1 ml is transferred to an agar plate which is incubated in a candle jar for an addi-tional 7 days before observing for colonies.

The medium described below (Chal-quest, 1962) gives excellent growth and is composed of the following ingredients (C-Medium):

PPLO broth or agar (Difco)	90 ml
Swine serum	10 ml
NAD	1 ml of 1% solution
Cysteine*	1 ml of 1% solution
Trypticase (BBL†)	1 ml of 5% solution
Soluble starch	0.5 g
Thallium acetate	0.25 ml of 1% solution
Phenol red	0.25 ml of 1% solution
Penicillin	1,000 units/ml

* Not used in agar.
† Baltimore Biological Laboratory.

Excellent growth in broth is obtained in 24 hours using Frey's medium as outlined.

Formula:

Mycoplasma broth base (Albimi)	22.5 g
Eagle essential vitamins (100×)	25.0 ml
Dextrose	10 g
Swine serum	120 ml
Oxidized NAD (Coenzyme I)	0.1 g
Cysteine · HCl	0.1 g
Phenol red	25 mg
Distilled H₂O	1,000 ml

Procedure for preparation:[1]
Dissolve Frey medium base in 970 ml dis-tilled water. Add phenol red at a 0.25% concentration. Add Eagle basal medium vitamins, dextrose, and swine serum which has been previously inactivated at 56° C for 35 minutes. Dissolve NAD and cysteine • HCl in the remaining 30 ml of distilled H₂O. (NAD must be in a reduced form and this procedure insures reduction.) Af-ter 10 minutes add this solution to the medium. With 0.1 N NaOH, adjust the pH of the medium to 7.7. All glassware, filter pads, tubes, and pipettes employed for the cultivation of *M. synoviae* in this medium must be prerinsed with deminer-alized or distilled water to prevent inhibi-tion of growth by inorganic impurities. This medium must be sterilized by filtra-tion. Passage of the organism at daily in-tervals is performed by transferring 0.3–0.5 ml of culture to uninoculated tubes of me-dium.

For original isolation, the yolk sac route of inoculation of 5–7-day-old embryonat-ing chicken eggs is the preferred method. Passage of the agent in embryonating chick-en eggs, using 0.25 ml of a 1:10 dilution of inoculum, results in mean day of death of the embryos as follows: yolk 6.7 days, am-niotic 8.6 days, chorioallantoic membrane 12 days, allantoic sac 12.9 days (Lecce et al., 1955). Those embryos which die 4–10 days postinfection are edematous and hemor-rhagic (Fig. 8.11). The hemorrhages of the skin are not obvious in those that die later. The liver, spleen, and kidneys are enlarged, and the liver is frequently mottled or con-tains necrotic foci. Petechiae frequently appear on the chorioallantoic membrane

---

1. Source of materials:
   Mycoplasma broth base (Albimi)—Pfizer Diag-nostic Division, Chas Pfizer & Co., Inc., 300 W. 43rd St., New York, N.Y.
   Eagle essential vitamins—Microbiological Asso-ciates, Bethesda, Md.
   Coenzyme I—Nutritional Biochemical Corpora-tion, Cleveland, Ohio.

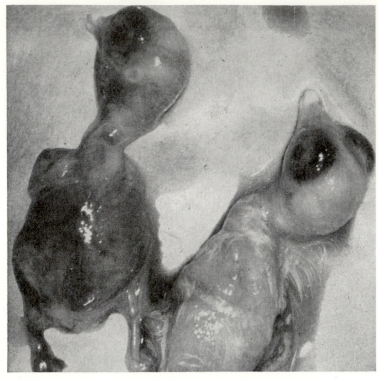

FIG. 8.11—Two 15-day-old embryos. Infectious synovitis-inoculated embryo on left is edematous and has numerous hemorrhages in the skin. Embryo on right is normal.

(CAM). Plaques were produced on the CAM by 2 of 9 isolates and by the isolate described by Thayer et al. (1958). The latter lesion is probably related to the viral arthritis agent (Olson et al., 1964b).

COLONIAL MORPHOLOGY

The colonies on solid media are best observed with a dissecting microscope at 30 magnification using indirect lighting and appear as raised, round, slightly latticed colonies with or without centers. Higher magnification ($\times 100$) is obtained by removing the condensor from a light microscope and using reflected light from a mirror. The colonies are from less than 1 to 3 mm in diameter, depending on the number of colonies present, suitability of medium, and age of culture. Growth is seen on solid medium in 3–7 days, and in 10–14 days a crystalline film develops on the surface of the agar or broth.

BIOCHEMICAL PROPERTIES

The biochemical characteristics of M. synoviae have been described by Chalquest and Fabricant (1960), Yamamoto et al. (1965), and Dierks et al. (1967). M. synoviae ferments glucose and maltose with the production of acid but not gas in suitably enriched media. It does not ferment lactose, dulcitol, salicin, or trehalose. Some isolates of M. synoviae are capable of hemagglutinating chicken and turkey erythrocytes. Its ability to reduce tetrazolium salts appears to be very limited.

RESISTANCE TO CHEMICAL AND PHYSICAL AGENTS

Resistance to disinfectants has not been determined but is probably similar to other mycoplasma. M. synoviae is not stable at pH 6.9 or lower. No critical studies have been made on resistance to heat, but it is believed to be sensitive to temperatures above 39° C. It will withstand freezing; however, the titer is reduced. End points have not been reached, but in yolk material M. synoviae is viable after 7 years at —63° C and after 2 years at —20° C. Broth cultures are viable after 2 years if treated in the following manner: 12 ml broth culture, 12 ml swine serum, and 1 ml 10% glucose solution are combined, dispensed in 1-ml vials, sealed, and frozen by reducing the temperature 2° per minute until —60° C is reached. Thawing is accomplished in an ice water bath.

ANTIGENIC STRUCTURE

Antigen may be prepared for testing against specific antiserum (Olson et al., 1963; Vardaman and Yoder, 1969). Fabricant (1960) employed the growth inhibition technique, and Corstvet and Sadler (1964) used colony imprints for the fluorescent antibody technique as a method for the antigenic identification of *M. synoviae*.

Information available to date indicates a single serotype of *M. synoviae* (Olson et al., 1964b; Dierks et al., 1967). Serum from chickens infected with *M. synoviae* occasionally agglutinates *M. gallisepticum* plate antigen (Olson et al., 1964b, 1965). The reverse occurs less frequently. Roberts and Olesiuk (1967) suggested that the cross-reactions were related to the presence of the rheumatoid factor and could be stimulated by tissue reactions. Cross-reactions are absent when the hemagglutination inhibition or the tube agglutination test is used. Other unknown factors are also involved in nonspecific agglutination reactions.

PATHOGENICITY

Most effort has been made in selecting pathogenic isolates. There appears to be as much variation within isolates as between isolates in their ability to produce typical disease. Passage in embryos, tissue culture, or broth reduces its ability to produce typical infection. Embryo passage appears to have less effect on pathogenicity than broth passage. Carnaghan (1961) reproduced the disease in chickens after 50 embryo passages. Three to four passages in broth reduces the number of organisms, pathogenicity, or both so that it is difficult to reproduce the typical disease.

PATHOGENESIS AND EPIZOOTIOLOGY

NATURAL AND EXPERIMENTAL HOSTS

Chickens and turkeys are the natural hosts of *M. synoviae*. Pheasants and geese are susceptible by artificial inoculation (Sevoian et al., 1958). Roberts and Olesiuk (1967) found *M. synoviae* agglutinins in cage-reared pheasants. Rabbits, rats, guinea pigs, mice, pigs, and lambs are not susceptible to experimental inoculation.

Natural infection in chickens has been observed as early as 1 week (Thayer et al., 1958), but generally the acute infection is seen when chickens are 4–16 and turkeys are 10–24 weeks old. Acute infection occasionally occurs in adult chickens. Chronic infection follows the acute phase and may persist for 5 years or longer. The chronic stage may be seen at any age and in some flocks may not be preceded by an acute infection.

TRANSMISSION

Lateral transmission readily occurs by direct contact. *M. synoviae* has been demonstrated in the respiratory tract of contact control chickens 1–4 weeks following infection of the principals (Olson et al., 1964a). Spread between batteries in the same room occurs. In many respects the spread appears to be similar to the spread of *M. gallisepticum* (Olson and Kerr, 1967). Transmission occurs via the respiratory tract, and usually 100% of the birds become infected though none or only a few develop joint lesions.

Carnaghan (1961) reviewed the literature on egg transmission of *M. synoviae*. He demonstrated vertical transmission in natural and artificially infected chickens. Hemsley (1965) further documented egg transmission. Using the agglutination test antigen, it is possible to demonstrate infection in dams and offspring even though no clinical signs have been seen in either. Chute et al. (1968) found approximately 50% of the flocks hatched from infected dams to be free of the infection. It is believed that vertical transmission plays the major role in the spread of *M. synoviae* in chickens and turkeys. For this reason all eggs used for live virus vaccine production should be obtained from *M. synoviae*-free flocks.

Arthropods apparently are not vectors of *M. synoviae*. However, Turner et al. (1963) demonstrated the infectious agent in the blood of mosquitoes and mites at 3, 6, and 24 but not 72 hours after feeding on infected chickens. Maceration of engorged infected northern fowl mites *Culex pipiem* and *Aedes sollicitans* resulted in infection when inoculated into susceptible chickens. Even though their feeding trials were negative, one cannot completely rule out arthropod transmission of *M. synoviae*.

INCUBATION PERIOD

Infectious synovitis has been seen in chicks 6 days old (Thayer et al., 1958), suggesting that the incubation period can be relatively short in birds apparently infected by egg transmission of *M. synoviae*. The incubation period following contact exposure is generally 11–21 days. Antibodies may be detected before clinical disease becomes evident. In birds experimentally infected by inoculation at 3–6 weeks of age with joint exudate from infected birds or yolk from infected embryos, the order of susceptibility and incubation period is as follows: foot pad 2–10 days, intravenously 7–10 days, intracranially 7–10 days, intraperitoneally 7–14 days, intrasinusly 14–20 days, conjunctival instillation 20 days. Birds are also susceptible to intramuscular inoculation. Intratracheal inoculation results in infection of the trachea and sinus as early as 4 days and readily spreads to contact birds. The incubation period varies with the amount and pathogenicity of the inoculum. Sevoian et al. (1958) reported an incubation period as short as 3 days in intravenously inoculated birds. The agent has been found in nearly all body tissues but not in bile or intestinal contents. In intravenously inoculated birds the blood was infective by the 8th hour but not by the 4th. In intramuscularly inoculated birds the blood was infective by the 48th hour but not by the 32nd. The agent was present in the blood until the 15th day. The duration of the septicemia is not known, but it was not present at 52 days after inoculation (Benton and Cover, 1959).

SIGNS

Chickens

The first observable signs in an affected flock are pale comb, lameness, and retarded growth. As the disease progresses, the feathers become ruffled and the comb shrinks. In some cases the comb is bluish red. Swellings usually occur around the joints, and breast blisters are common. The hock joints and foot pads are principally involved, but in some birds all joints become affected. However, birds are occasionally found with a generalized infection but not having apparent swelling of the joints. The birds become listless, dehydrated, and emaciated (Fig. 8.12). Although birds are severely affected, many of them continue to eat and drink if placed near feed and water. A greenish discoloration of the droppings, which contain large amounts of uric acid or urates, is frequently seen.

The acute signs described above are followed by slow recovery; however, synovitis may persist for as long as 5 years. In other instances the acute phase is absent or not noticed and only a few chronically infected birds are seen in a flock. Chickens infected via the respiratory tract may show slight rales in 4–6 weeks or may be asymptomatic.

Turkeys

Infectious synovitis generally causes the same type of signs in turkeys as in chickens (Snoeyenbos and Olesiuk, 1955). Lameness is the most prominent symptom. Warm fluctuating swellings of one or more joints of lame birds are usually found. Occasionally there is an enlargement of the sternal bursa. Severely affected birds lose weight, but many birds less severely affected make satisfactory weight gains when separated from the flock. In experimentally infected turkeys (Olson et al., 1956), the first noticeable sign is failure to grow (Fig. 8.13).

Respiratory signs are not usually observed in turkeys, but Sadler and Corstvet (1965) reported respiratory stress in turkey poults which had been inoculated via the foot pad at 2 weeks of age but not in those inoculated intratracheally at 6, 10, 14, and 18 weeks of age. Yoder (1964) isolated *M. synoviae* via chicken embryo inoculation from sinus exudate obtained from turkey flocks exhibiting a very low incidence of sinusitis in the absence of *M. gallisepticum* infection. Confirmation that turkey sinus exudate Iowa #1331 was *M. synoviae* was published by Vardaman and Yoder (1969).

MORBIDITY AND MORTALITY

Chickens

The morbidity varies from 2 to 75%, with 5–15% being most usual. Respiratory involvement is generally asymptomatic, but 90–100% of the birds may actually be infected. Mortality is usually low, ranging from less than 1 to 10%. In experimentally infected chickens mortality may vary from 0 to 100%, depending upon route of inoculation and dose of inoculum.

Turkeys

Morbidity in infected flocks is usually low (1–20%), but mortality from trampling

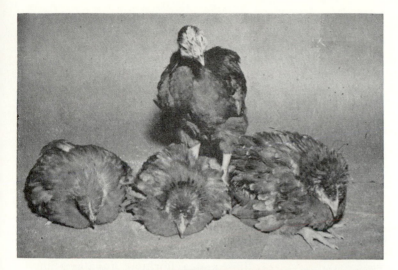

FIG. 8.12—*Experimental chickens with infectious synovitis. Contact control bird (standing) and three typically infected birds in advanced stage of the disease.*

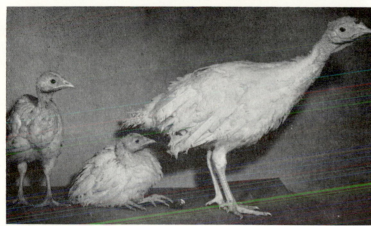

FIG. 8.13—*Two experimental turkeys with infectious synovitis* (left) *and isolated control turkey* (right).

and cannibalism may be significant (Snoeyenbos, 1956). The number of serologically positive birds in a flock may approach 100%, although outward signs may not be apparent.

GROSS LESIONS

Chickens

In early stages of the disease necropsy reveals a viscous, creamy-to-gray exudate involving the synovial membranes of the joints, keel bursae, and tendon sheaths (Fig. 8.14). As the disease progresses, this exudate becomes caseous. Caseous exudate is occasionally found over the skull, along the neck, and rarely extends into the muscles and air sacs. When birds become severely emaciated and dehydrated before caseous exudate develops, there is occasion-

ally no fluid about the joints. In chronic cases the surfaces of the affected joints are frequently yellow to orange.

In early stages of the disease, splenomegaly generally occurs. The liver is frequently enlarged, occasionally mottled, greenish or dark red. The kidneys are usually swollen, mottled, and/or pale. These changes occur in approximately 50% of the birds and become more pronounced and frequent as the severity of the disease increases. Even though some birds are severely affected, their internal organs appear normal. In birds experimentally inoculated via the foot pad, infection frequently localizes in the inoculated foot, and no gross internal lesions are noted.

Generally no gross lesions are seen in the respiratory tract. Occasionally considerable mucus is found in the trachea of a few

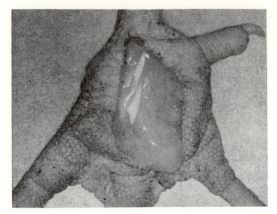

FIG. 8.14—Foot of 7-week-old turkey showing purulent exudate in foot pad 22 days after experimental inoculation. Similar exudates are seen in chickens.

chickens inoculated intranasally. The specificity of this lesion might be questioned. Attempts to isolate a virus from this mucus have not been successful. Recent studies on extensive air sac lesions observed in broiler flocks suffering moderate condemnations for airsacculitis suggest that *M. synoviae* was part of the complex cause of the lesions (Yoder, 1969, personal communication). However, further work is needed to clarify this situation.

Turkeys

Noticeable swellings in joints are not always present; however, when the hock joints are opened, a small amount of purulent exudate is present. The agent is recovered from this exudate after injection into embryonating eggs, and inoculation of the exudate into chickens produces signs and lesions of synovitis. Lesions in the respiratory tract are not common, but reference has been made to an occasional sinusitis (Yoder, 1964). Extensive air sac lesions were noted in 2 flocks of turkeys proved to be free of *M. gallisepticum,* although condemnations due to airsacculitis varied from 8 to 11% when the turkeys were marketed at 20–24 weeks of age. *M. synoviae* was isolated from several of the air sac lesions, and the flocks were proved to be consistently positive for *M. synoviae* agglutinins (Yoder, 1969, personal communication).

HISTOPATHOLOGY

The microscopic lesions (Sevoian et al., 1958) of the brain consist of vascular endo-thelial thickening and adventitial proliferation in the cerebrum, cerebellum, and optic lobe; degeneration of some of the Purkinje cells; and occasionally cerebellar lesions similar to those of encephalomalacia. The latter lesion was not observed by Moorhead et al. (1967).

In the liver, perivascular, periportal, and interparenchymal cellular hyperplasia of the reticular cells of the reticulo-endothelial system occurs. The sinusoids are dilated and the parenchymal cells are atrophied. There is proliferation of the bile duct epithelium. The connective tissue framework of the heart, gizzard, and interlobular septa of the lungs reveals a similar reticular cell hyperplasia. Occasionally focal mononuclear infiltration and necrosis of the myocardium and a fibrinous inflammation of the pericardium are seen. A reticular cell or lymphocytic hyperplasia or both decrease the sinusoidal areas of the spleen. A granulocytic hyperplasia of bone marrow occurs, and atrophy of the thymus and bursa of Fabricius results from lymphoid degeneration in the medulla and cortex.

Heterophil hyperplasia is common in the acute phase of the infection 7–20 days post-inoculation and to a lesser extent during an 8-month observation period associated with the vessels or connective tissue framework of the heart, gizzard, intestines, liver, and lungs (Kerr, 1965; Kerr and Olson, 1967). Casorso and Jungherr (1959) found the embryo response to infectious synovitis to be similar to that described in birds. Although they did not describe heterophil hyperplasia for infectious synovitis, they did for several strains of mycoplasma.

Giemsa-stained smears made from creamy synovial fluid reveal many large macrophage cells, lymphocytes, plasma cells, and heterophils. In many cases the heterophils predominate. No bacteria are found.

The changes in the blood components have been studied (Olson et al., 1957b; Shelton et al., 1957; Sevoian et al., 1957). Average determinations for 31 experimentally inoculated birds were as follows: erythrocytes 1,680,000 per mm³, leukocytes 80,810 per mm³, hemoglobin 6.5 g per 100 ml of blood. Differential count gave the following percentages: lymphocytes 41.9, heterophils 31.9, monocytes 19.3, eosinophils 0.23, basophils 1.1, immature leukocytes 6.1. The thrombocyte count increased and hematocrit decreased. The gamma globulin is increased and albumin is decreased (Shelton and Olson, 1960). The rheumatoid factor is present in serum of affected chickens associated with the euglobulin fraction (Porter and Gooderham, 1966). Blood abnormalities increased as the severity of infectious synovitis increased, generally reaching a maximum shortly before death. The changes were most severe between the 6th and 26th days following foot pad inoculation. In severely affected birds the erythrocytes showed anisocytosis, poikilocytosis, polychromatophilia, and achromia. Immature erythrocytes of varying degrees were present. When the birds showed signs of recovery, the blood changes showed evidence of returning to normal. Similar blood changes have been noted in experimentally infected turkeys.

IMMUNITY

Cassidy and Grumbles (1959) were not able to demonstrate immunity to the infectious synovitis agent; however, Wichmann et al. (1960) found that after 9 passages in tissue culture the pathogenicity was reduced but not its antigenicity. Carnaghan (1962) demonstrated a neutralizing antibody in chicken serum which persisted for 30 weeks. Birds exposed intranasally were resistant to subsequent foot pad challenge (Olson et al., 1964a). Parenteral inoculation of *M. synoviae* frequently overwhelms the bird before adequate resistance can develop.

Passive immunity was conferred on chicks by inoculation of immune serum (Carnaghan, 1962). Hyperimmune rabbit serum prepared against *M. synoviae* inhibits colony growth on agar (Fabricant, 1960; Chalquest and Halfhill, 1962).

DIAGNOSIS

ISOLATION AND IDENTIFICATION

A positive diagnosis may be made by isolation and identification of *M. synoviae*. Isolation from acutely infected birds is not difficult, but from chronically infected birds isolation is difficult or impossible. The use of 5–7-day-old embryonating chicken eggs is more efficient than artificial media for original isolation. A 1:5 to 1:10 dilution of joint exudate, liver, or spleen in nutrient broth is inoculated in 0.25-ml amounts into the yolk sac. Yolk or allantoic fluid or both are harvested from dead embryos. Embryos should show typical lesions as described previously. Allantoic fluid may be plated directly on agar plates for identification. The medium and isolation methods are described under growth characteristics.

Mycoplasma isolates should be plated on PPLO media containing 10% swine serum and 0.01% NAD and on similar media without NAD. Preliminary identification is possible if growth occurs only on the plate containing NAD. Identification of colony imprints by the direct fluorescent antibody technique (Corstvet and Sadler, 1964) is the preferred method if facilities are available. Chickens and turkeys may be inoculated via the foot pad with 0.25 ml of yolk from infected embryos or joint exudate, and typical lesions should develop in 4–10 days. Preinoculation and four-week postinoculation sera should be tested against *M. synoviae* and *M. gallisepticum* antigens. Both chicken and turkey serum should show agglutinins to *M. synoviae* plate test antigen within 30–60 seconds and no reaction to *M. gallisepticum*. However, *M. gallisepticum* antigen may be agglutinated on occasion, but the reaction is somewhat delayed and usually lower in titer (Olson et al., 1965).

SEROLOGY

Antigen is available commercially for the rapid serum plate test. Adequate directions for use are given with each package. Generally 0.02 ml of serum is mixed with an equal amount of antigen on a glass plate. The plate is gently rotated and observed against a black background with indirect lighting. Agglutination with most antigens occurs within 1 minute at room temperature. Heating and storage of the antigen at room temperature for any length of time results in autoagglutination; therefore, only the amount to be used in one day is removed from the bottle. Sterile pipettes should be used to remove antigen. The antigen and serum should be stored at refrigerator temperature but allowed to come to room temperature before conducting tests. Antigen should be tested with known positive and negative serum each day. Vardaman and Yoder (1969) described the use of a hemagglutination antigen for use in the hemagglutination-inhibition test for *M. synoviae* employing chicken and turkey serum samples. It should be remembered that it requires 2–4 weeks for antibodies to develop in infected birds (Olson et al., 1963).

DIFFERENTIAL DIAGNOSIS

A presumptive diagnosis may be made on the basis of pale comb, droopiness, emaciation, leg weakness, breast blisters, enlarged foot pads or hock joints, splenomegaly, and enlarged liver or kidneys. Bacteria as a cause of synovitis or arthritis must be eliminated by bacteriological procedures. Medium 110 (Difco) is suggested for the isolation of staphylococcus. *E. coli,* pasteurella, and salmonella may also be present as primary causes of synovitis. *M. gallisepticum* may also be a cause of breast blisters (Domermuth, 1962) and joint lesions (Olson et al., 1956; 1964b). Inoculation of one strain of fowl pox virus into the foot pad of chickens caused growth of the virus in the synovial membranes with enlargement; but Newcastle disease, infectious bronchitis, and laryngotracheitis virus did not.

Fibrosis of the metatarsal extensor digital flexor tendons and marked heterophil infiltration of the myocardium associated with the viral arthritis agent help to differentiate it from *M. synoviae* (Olson and Solomon, 1968). Serum from viral arthritis-infected chickens does not agglutinate *M. synoviae* antigen, but one must bear in mind that *M. synoviae* agglutinins may be present without obvious joint involvement. Antigen prepared from ground chorioallantoic membranes from embryos inoculated with the virus arthritis agent will react in a double gel diffusion test with serum from viral arthritis-inoculated birds tested at least 3 weeks postinoculation. Turkeys and chickens should be inoculated with yolk from infected embryos or joint exudates. *M. synoviae* should cause infection in turkeys and chickens, but the viral arthritis agent should infect only chickens (Olson, unpublished data).

TREATMENT

CHICKENS

A summary of data obtained from field and experimental studies indicates that chlortetracycline (50–100 g per ton of feed) given continuously will provide satisfactory control of infectious synovitis. Higher concentrations (approximately 200 g per ton of feed) are needed to control synovitis af-ter infection has occurred in a flock. Severely infected birds show improvement after treatment, but such a procedure is not considered practical. Effectiveness of the antibiotics appears to be related to pathogenicity of the agent, availability of the antibiotic, age of the bird, and the presence of intercurrent infections. The concentration of the antibiotic used in treating field outbreaks should be adjusted according to the severity of the infection.

The order of effectiveness of several antibacterial compounds was as follows: chlortetracycline, oxytetracycline, furazolidone, tetracycline, chloramphenicol, carbomycin, and NF-153 (Shelton et al., 1957). In another study (Shelton and Olson, 1957) the order of efficacy of three antibiotics given in the feed was chlortetracycline, oxytetracycline, and tetracycline, but equal results were obtained when daily injections of these drugs were given.

The antibiotics are bacteriostatic at the usual levels used. For this reason continuous medication is recommended; however, the cost may exceed the value of treatment. Potentiation of the tetracycline antibiotics approximately two times is possible by reducing the calcium content of the ration to 0.19% (Price and Zolli, 1959) or replacing calcium carbonate with calcium sulphate (Stokstad et al., 1959). The use of terephthalic acid for potentiation of tetracycline antibiotics is not approved for use in poultry feed.

Dihydrostreptomycin injections (25 mg/lb body weight) satisfactorily controlled infectious synovitis if given at the time of experimental inoculation. If given 4 or more days after inoculation, only slight benefit was noted. Increasing the dose to 200 mg/lb of body weight increased its effectiveness slightly (Shelton and Olson, 1957–58; Snoeyenbos et al., 1958). The literature concerning treatment is reviewed by Messersmith (1965).

TURKEYS

Protection is afforded by chlortetracycline at 200 g/ton of feed during prophylactic medication of turkeys. Partial protection is produced by levels as low as 50 g/ton. The comparative efficacy in turkeys of the tetracycline antibiotics has not been determined. Treatment of affected birds with streptomycin or chlortetracycline has given discouraging results. However, it is generally concluded that chlortetracycline or oxytetracycline at the rate of 200 g/ton of feed for 5–7 consecutive days may at least reduce the spread and severity of the infection in turkey flocks.

PREVENTION AND CONTROL

Mycoplasma synoviae is egg-transmitted, and the only effective method of control is to select chickens or turkeys from flocks free of the infection. Since *M. synoviae* antigen became available commercially in 1968, there has not been time to develop any official control program. However, some primary breeders have started surveillance programs for *M. synoviae* (Olson et al., 1968; Chute et al., 1968).

Hatchery managers have been able to trace outbreaks of *M. synoviae* infection in broilers to a specific breeder flock, but usually by the time the transmitting breeder

flock is found the transmission is low or no longer of clinical significance. Slaughter of infected breeder flocks cannot be a universal recommendation at this time.

Antibiotic treatment of the breeders does not appear to be effective in eliminating *M. synoviae*. Egg dipping for the control of *M. synoviae* has not been reported. However, in vitro studies employing cultures of *M. synoviae* held for 20 days indicated that it was inhibited by more than 0.15 μg of tylosin per ml (Olson, unpublished data). As with *M. gallisepticum*, such procedures are mainly practical for primary breeders only.

Yoder (1970) reported that the preincubation heat treatment of chicken hatching eggs might be employed to eliminate *M. synoviae*, but the procedure has not yet been evaluated extensively.

REFERENCES

Badstue, P. B. 1961. Infectious synovitis. *Nord. Veterinaermed.* 13:561–70.

Benton, W. J., and M. S. Cover. 1959. The infectivity of blood and tissues from chickens with infectious synovitis. *Avian Diseases* 3:361–70.

Bigland, C. H., and J. A. Brown. 1955. A suspected case of infectious synovitis in Alberta. *Can. J. Comp. Med. Vet. Sci.* 19:251–54.

Burtscher, H. 1961. Zum Vorkommen der infektiosen Synovitis in Oesterreich. *Wien Tieraerztl. Monatsschr.* 48:850–72.

Carnaghan, R. B. A. 1959. An outbreak of infectious synovitis in chickens. *Vet. Record* 71:81–85.

———. 1961. Egg transmission of infectious synovitis. *J. Comp. Pathol. Therap.* 71:279–85.

———. 1962. Immunity in infectious synovitis of chickens. *J. Comp. Pathol. Therap.* 72:433–38.

Casorso, R. D., and E. L. Jungherr. 1959. The response of the developing chicken embryo to certain avian pathogens. *Am. J. Vet. Res.* 20:547–57.

Cassidy, D. R., and L. C. Grumbles. 1959. Immunity studies on avian infectious synovitis. *Avian Diseases* 3:126–35.

Chalquest, R. R. 1962. Cultivation of the infectious-synovitis-type pleuropneumonia-like organisms. *Avian Diseases* 6:36–43.

Chalquest, R. R., and J. Fabricant. 1960. Pleuropneumonia-like organisms associated with synovitis in fowls. *Avian Diseases* 4:515–39.

Chalquest, R. R., and J. Halfhill. 1962. Preparation of antigen and antiserum for the infectious synovitis-type pleuropneumonia-

like organisms. *J. Bacteriol.* 84:591–92.

Chute, H. L., E. S. Bryant, R. Cuozzo, and N. O. Olson. 1968. A preliminary survey of the serological incidence of *Mycoplasma synoviae* in Maine chickens. *Proc. 40th N.E. Conf. on Avian Diseases.*

Chute, H. L., R. F. Cuozzo, and D. D. King. 1968–69. Experimental infectious synovitis testing in Maine chickens. *Res. Life Sci.,* Univ. Maine, pp. 46–47.

Corstvet, R. E., and W. W. Sadler. 1964. The diagnosis of certain avian diseases with the fluorescent antibody technique. *Poultry Sci.* 43:1280–88.

Cover, M. S., and W. J. Benton. 1957. The distribution of the infectious synovitis agent in the tissues of artificially infected chickens. *Avian Diseases* 1:312–19.

Cover, M. S., J. N. Geleta, and E. F. Waller. 1956. The etiology of an arthritic disease of chickens. *Am. J. Vet. Res.* 17:12–15.

Dierks, R. E., J. A. Newman, and B. S. Pomeroy. 1967. Characterization of avian Mycoplasma. *Ann. N.Y. Acad. Sci.* 143:170–89.

Domermuth, C. H. 1962. Experimental production of "breast blisters" by S-6 type Mycoplasma. *Avian Diseases* 6:135–40.

Fabricant, J. 1960. Serological studies of avian pleuropneumonia-like organisms (PPLO) with Edward's technique. *Avian Diseases* 4:505–14.

Guillon, J. C., L. Renault, and E. Petit. 1962. Quelques aspects de la synovite infectieuse aviaire en France. *Rec. Med. Vet. Ecole Alfort* 138:5–19.

Hemsley, L. A. 1965. Experiences of infectious synovitis in broiler breeding stock and broiler chickens, with particular reference to the natural spread of the disease. *Brit. Vet. J.* 121:76–82.

Kerr, K. M. 1965. Three synovitis producing agents in chickens. Thesis, West Virginia Univ.

Kerr, K. M., and N. O. Olson. 1964. Control of infectious synovitis. 14. The effect of age of chickens on the susceptibility of three agents. *Avian Diseases* 8:256–63.

———. 1967. Cardiac pathology associated with viral and mycoplasmal arthritis in chickens. *Ann. N.Y. Acad. Sci.* 143:204–17.

Lecce, J. G. 1960. Porcine polyserositis with arthritis. Isolation of a fastidious pleuropneumonia organism and *Hemophilus influenzae suis. Ann. N.Y. Acad. Sci.* 79:670–76.

Lecce, J. G., F. G. Sperling, L. Hayflick, and W. Stinebring. 1955. Tendovaginitis with arthritis, a new syndrome of chickens: Isolation and characterization of an infectious agent. *J. Exp. Med.* 102:489–98.

Messersmith, D. H. 1965. Avian infectious synovitis: A review of the literature. *World's Poultry Sci. J.* 21:358–64.

Moorehead, P. D., R. F. Cross, and W. Henderson. 1967. Pathological manifestations of experimental infectious synovitis and staphylococcosis in chickens. *Avian Diseases* 11:354–65.

Olson, N. O., and K. M. Kerr. 1967. The duration and distribution of synovitis producing agents in chickens. *Avian Diseases* 11:569–85.

Olson, N. O., and D. P. Solomon. 1968. A natural outbreak of synovitis caused by the viral arthritis agent. *Avian Diseases* 12:311–16.

Olson, N. O., J. K. Bletner, D. C. Shelton, D. A. Munro, and G. C. Anderson. 1954. Enlarged joint condition in poultry caused by an infectious agent. *Poultry Sci.* 33:1075. (Abstr.)

Olson, N. O., D. C. Shelton, J. K. Bletner, D. A. Munro, and G. C. Anderson. 1956. Studies of infectious synovitis in chickens. *Am. J. Vet. Res.* 17:747–54.

Olson, N. O., D. C. Shelton, and D. A. Munro. 1957a. Infectious synovitis control by medication. Effect of strain differences and pleuropneumonia-like organisms. *Am. J. Vet. Res.* 18:735–39.

Olson, N. O., D. C. Shelton, D. A. Munro, and R. Bletner. 1957b. Preliminary blood studies in chickens with a synovitis caused by the infectious synovitis agent, pleuropneumonia-like organisms and a combination of the two agents. *Avian Diseases* 1:82–91.

Olson, N. O., K. M. Kerr, and A. Campbell. 1963. Control of infectious synovitis. 12. Preparation of an agglutination test antigen. *Avian Diseases* 7:310–17.

Olson, N. O., H. E. Adler, A. J. DaMassa, and R. E. Corstvet. 1964a. The effect of intranasal exposure to *Mycoplasma synoviae* and infectious bronchitis on development of lesions and agglutinins. *Avian Diseases* 8:623–31.

Olson, N. O., K. M. Kerr, and A. Campbell. 1964b. Control of infectious synovitis. 13. The antigen study of three strains. *Avian Diseases* 8:209–14.

Olson, N. O., R. Yamamoto, and H. Ortmayer. 1965. Antigenic relationship between *Mycoplasma synoviae* and *M. gallisepticum. Am. J. Vet. Res.* 26:195–98.

Olson, N. O., H. L. Chute, R. F. Cuozzo, and E. S. Bryant. 1968. Experiences with *Mycoplasma synoviae* test program. *Poultry Sci.* 47:1704. (Abstr.)

Porter, P., and K. R. Gooderham. 1966. Changes in serum proteins and identification of a rheumatoid factor in a field outbreak of avian infectious synovitis. *Res. Vet. Sci.* 7:25–34.

Price, E. K., and Z. Zolli, Jr. 1959. The influence of dietary calcium, phosphorus and terephthalic acid on antibiotic control of of experimental infectious synovitis. *Avian Diseases* 3:135–36.

Roberts, D. H., and O. M. Olesiuk. 1967. Serological studies with *Mycoplasma synoviae. Avian Diseases* 11:104–19.

Sadler, W. W., and R. E. Corstvet. 1965. The effect of experimental *Mycoplasma synoviae* infection on the wholesomeness of young adult turkeys. *Am. J. Vet. Res.* 26:1421–28.

Sevoian, M., G. H. Snoeyenbos, H. Basch, and I. Reynolds. 1957. Studies of infectious synovitis. *Avian Diseases* 1:121–22. (Abstr.)

———. 1958. Infectious synovitis. I. Clinical and pathological manifestations. *Avian Diseases* 2:499–513.

Shelton, D. C., and N. O. Olson. 1957. Infectious synovitis control. 7. Comparison of tetracycline antibiotics. *Poultry Sci.* 38:1309–15.

———. 1957–58. Infectious synovitis control. 9. The efficacy of dihydrostreptomycin sulfate as related to time of experimental infection. *Antibiot. Ann.,* pp. 272–78.

———. 1960. Serum proteins of chicks with infectious and mycoplasma synovitis. *Poultry Sci.* 39:112–17.

Shelton, D. C., J. K. Bletner, N. O. Olson, G. C. Anderson, and C. E. Weakley, Jr. 1957. Control of infectious synovitis. 1. Continuous feeding of antibiotics and the influence of diethylstilbestrol and coccidiostats. *Poultry Sci.* 36:113–21.

Snoeyenbos, G. H. 1956. Infectious synovitis in turkeys. *Proc. Poultry Pathol. Conf.,* American Cyanamid Co. (Abstr.)

Snoeyenbos, G. H., and O. M. Olesiuk. 1955. Studies of an agent producing arthritis in turkeys. *Proc. Ann. Conf. Lab Workers in Pullorum Disease Control.*

Snoeyenbos, G. H., H. I. Basch, and M. Sevoian. 1958. Infectious synovitis. II. Drug prophylaxis and therapy. *Avian Diseases* 2:514–30.

Stokstad, E. L. R., C. N. Huhtanen, W. L. Williams, and T. H. Jukes. 1959. The effect of calcium levels on aureomycin absorption. *Poultry Sci.* 38:1251. (Abstr.)

Thayer, S. C., R. G. Strout, and W. R. Dunlop. 1958. Observations on infectious synovitis. *Poultry Sci.* 37:449–54.

Turner, E. C., N. L. Wehrheim, D. H. Messersmith, and J. W. Davis. 1963. Transmission studies of avian infectious synovitis by selected arthropod vectors. *Poultry Sci.* 42:1434–41.

Wichmann, R. W., R. A. Bankowski, and A. J. DaMassa. 1960. The cultivation and modification of the avian infectious synovitis agent in tissue culture. *Avian Diseases* 4: 152–64.

Wills, F. K. 1954. Preliminary report on transmission of an agent producing arthritis in chickens. *Texas Agr. Expt. Sta. Prog. Rept.* 1674:1–2.

———. 1955. Study of an unidentified agent producing arthritis in chickens. *Southwestern Vet.* 8:146–58.

Wills, F. K., and J. P. Delaplane. 1955. Transmission and therapy studies on an agent which produces arthritis in chickens. *Proc. Book, Am. Vet. Med. Ass.* 350–57.

Vardaman, T. H., and H. W. Yoder, Jr. 1969. Preparation of *Mycoplasma synoviae* hemagglutinating antigen and its use in the hemagglutination-inhibition test. *Avian Diseases* 13:654–61.

Yamamoto, R., C. H. Bigland, and H. B. Ortmayer. 1965. Characteristics of *Mycoplasma meleagridis* sp. n. isolated from turkeys. *J. Bacteriol.* 90:47–49.

Yoder, H. W., Jr. 1964. Studies on the etiology of turkey sinusitis and airsacculitis not associated with *Mycoplasma gallisepticum. Proc. 8th Poultry Pathol. Conf.*, American Cyanamid Co., pp. 25–26. (Abstr.)

———. 1970. Preincubation heat treatment of chicken hatching eggs to inactivate Mycoplasma. *Avian Diseases* 14:75–86.

CHAPTER 9

AVIAN
VIBRIO INFECTIONS

❖

M. C. PECKHAM

Department of Avian Diseases
New York State Veterinary College
Ithaca, New York

❖

VIBRIONIC HEPATITIS

❖

AVIAN VIBRIONIC HEPATITIS is a contagious bacterial disease of young and mature chickens characterized by low mortality, high morbidity, and chronic course. The disease was first described as a hepatitis by Delaplane et al. (1955). Sevoian et al. (1958) and Hofstad et al. (1958) called the disease avian infectious hepatitis. Peckham (1958) used the terminology avian vibrionic hepatitis to give the disease an etiologic-pathologic title that would aptly describe and distinguish it from other vibrio infections or diseases of the liver.

Accurate estimates giving the cost of avian vibrionic hepatitis to the poultry industry have not been published. Its overall adverse effect on weight gains and egg production is no doubt much greater than suspected because of the insidious nature of the disease.

The infection of humans with the organism has not been reported, and it would appear that it is not a public health hazard.

HISTORY

Probably the first successful transmission of this disease and description of the gross and microscopic pathology was given (albeit unknowingly) by Blakemore (1939). He was attempting to transmit neurolymphomatosis and regarded the liver lesions and granulocytes as an early inflammatory response caused by the leukosis agent. The inocula he used were liver suspensions which he injected intraperitoneally into young chicks. The chicks showed signs and liver lesions within 7 days. The heart was enlarged and pale and the pericardial sac contained coagulated serum. Focal necrosis, illustrated by excellent photographs, was present in the liver. The histopathological lesions described in the heart and liver are in accord with those found in avian vibrionic hepatitis.

Tudor (1954) reported a liver degeneration of unknown origin but with histopathological lesions similar to those later described for vibrionic hepatitis. Delaplane et al. (1955) were the first to isolate the causative organism and reproduce the disease. Lukas (1955) described an infectious hepatitis that had many similarities to the disease described by Tudor (1954) and Delaplane et al. (1955). Hofstad (1956) was the first to recognize this disease as being caused by a vibrio, and this was confirmed by subsequent reports (Hofstad et al., 1958; Peckham, 1958; Sevoian and Calnek, 1959). Moore (1958) reported the results of characterization studies with the agent and bird inoculation studies. Sevoian et al. (1958) described the clinical and pathological manifestations, and Winterfield et al. (1958) studied the characteristics of the etiologic agent and the effects of drugs on the course of the disease.

INCIDENCE AND DISTRIBUTION

Reports of the northeastern states diagnostic laboratories (Angstrom, 1966, 1967) indicated that the incidence varied from 0 to 5% between adjoining states. Most reports were in birds over 20 weeks of age but some were in birds younger than 4 weeks. The average number of cases from all the states included in these reports was approximately 1% of all accessions. This low percentage of avian vibrionic hepatitis cases is in sharp contrast to the 13.4% reported by Gerlach and Gylstorff (1967) in Germany.

The disease has been identified throughout the United States and Canada. Voüte and Grimbergen (1959) reported vibrionic hepatitis of chickens in the Netherlands. There are many reports of the disease in Germany (Bisping et al., 1963; Kölbl, 1964; Winkenwerder and Maciak, 1964; Vielitz et al., 1965; Gerlach and Gylstorff, 1967). In Italy Rinaldi et al. (1964) isolated vibrios from chickens with hepatitis. The disease was reported in Switzerland (Bertschinger, 1965).

ETIOLOGY

The disease is caused by a gram-negative, motile, microaerophilic bacterium of the genus *Vibrio.*

CLASSIFICATION

Mathey and Rissberger (1964) proposed to designate the avian hepatitis vibrio as *Vibrio hepaticus,* n. sp. However, in view of the marked variation in the biochemical and serological properties of the avian vibrios that have been studied, it would be difficult to propose criteria for the type species to distinguish it from variants (Whenham et al., 1961; Kölbl, 1964; Fletcher and Plastridge, 1964; Winkenwerder and Bisping, 1964; Speck, 1965; Gerlach and Gylstorff, 1967). More study of the biochemical and antigenic properties of the isolates is needed before any workable classification can be evolved.

MORPHOLOGY AND STAINING

The vibrio appears as short comma forms, S-shaped forms, and long spirals (Figs. 9.1, 9.2). On some occasions, partic-ularly in older cultures, the organism has a coccoid morphology. It can easily be stained with any aniline dye.

GROWTH REQUIREMENTS

Avian vibrio can be isolated and cultured by using an enriched medium and incubating under reduced oxygen tension. Hofstad et al. (1958) were the first investigators to successfully propagate the vibrio on artificial medium by using chicken infusion medium containing 20% chicken serum. Peckham (1958) grew the organism on 10% horse blood agar, in Bacto-thiol, in PPLO liquid media with added serum fraction without inhibitors, on chicken infusion agar incubated under 10% carbon dioxide, and in thioglycollate with 1% chicken or horse serum. Both Peckham and Bertschinger (1965) noted that some strains were difficult to subculture on artificial media, and Hagan (1964) confirmed their observation that when older cultures had reached a coccoid morphology, subculture was extremely difficult. However, Bertschinger (1965) reported that reversion of coccoid forms to comma and S-shaped forms was accomplished by subculture. Vielitz et al. (1965) reported that some strains that had been passed many times could no longer be subcultured and occasionally primary isolates exhibited this phenomenon.

Bisping et al. (1963) used thioglycollate to which were added 2% agar and 10% ox blood. Inhibitors added to this basic medium were either brilliant green or a com-

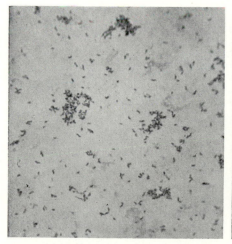
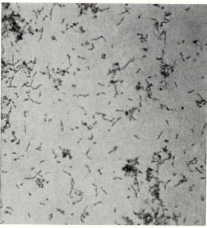

FIG. 9.1—*(Left) Smear of sedimented 96-hour broth culture of vibrio. (Right) Smear of 6th day culture illustrating spiral forms. Giemsa, ×885. (Hofstad, Iowa State Univ.)*

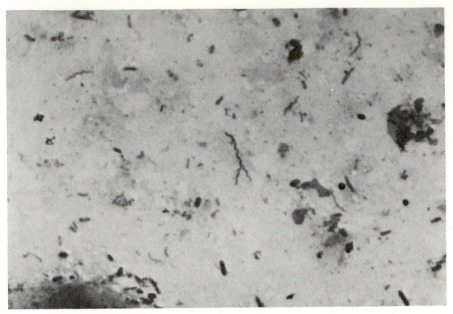

FIG. 9.2—Cecal smear illustrating spiral vibrio forms. ×1,500.

bination of bacitracin, polymyxin, and no-vobiocin. The inoculated plates were incubated under 20% vacuum with a gas mixture of which 10% was normal atmosphere and 70% was a mixture of a gas containing 95% nitrogen and 5% carbon dioxide. Results obtained with the antibiotic medium proved it was much superior to the brilliant green medium.

Fletcher and Plastridge (1964) maintained stock cultures in thiol medium (Difco). However, it should be emphasized that once cultures are adapted to artificial media their growth requirements may be less fastidious than those necessary for primary isolation. Hagan (1964) used Bacto brilliant green agar and Bacto blood agar base with 8% defibrinated chicken blood. Isolations were more frequent with the brilliant green medium. Truscott and Stockdale (1966) isolated vibrio on fresh 10% sheep's blood agar incubated under 10% carbon dioxide. Cultures were maintained in brucella broth (Albimi) containing 0.1% agar.

Vibrios can readily be propagated in embryonated chicken eggs by inoculation of either the yolk sac or chorioallantoic sac (Delaplane et al., 1955; Winterfield and Sevoian, 1957; Hofstad et al., 1958).

The organism grows more readily in the yolk sac, and this route of inoculation is preferred for primary isolation or to obtain yolk with a high titer of organisms. Hofstad et al. (1958) recorded a titer of 10 × 10⁵ ELD_{50} per ml of yolk following yolk sac inoculation. Embryo mortality occurred 4 days postinoculation with congestion of the yolk sac and embryo.

COLONIAL MORPHOLOGY

Thackrey and Johnstone (1964) described typical vibrio colonies as small, moist, round, smooth-edged, raised, almost transparent, and colorless.

BIOCHEMICAL PROPERTIES

The biochemical properties of avian vibrios have been extensively studied and compared with those of vibrios isolated from domestic animals and humans.

There is not unanimity among investigators at the present time in regard to the properties of the avian vibrio; this may be due to variations in technique, different media, or intrinsic differences in the strains.

Most investigators found the vibrio to be catalase-positive, microaerophilic, nonhemolytic, and motile (Peckham, 1958; Whenham et al., 1961; Kölbl, 1964).

Carbohydrates not consistently utilized were xylose and mannitol (Peckham, 1958; Gerlach and Gylstorff, 1967). Whenham et al. (1961) occasionally found acid formation in mannitol, maltose, and lactose.

Peckham (1958) and Gerlach and Gylstorff (1967) did not find acid production from dextrose, whereas Whenham et al. (1961) recorded positive results. Reduction of nitrate to nitrite was not found by Peckham (1958) and Kölbl (1964) but was evident in the strains examined by Voûte and Grimbergen (1959) and Bertschinger (1965). Gerlach and Gylstorff (1967) found 3 strains positive for nitrite production and some strains negative.

Whenham et al. (1961) and Gerlach and Gylstorff (1967) did not find H₂S production in Kliglers iron agar, and Fletcher and Plastridge (1964) reported all strains H₂S negative. Kölbl (1964) reported H₂S production. Avian vibrios vary in their tolerance to NaCl. Bisping et al. (1963) did not obtain growth in 3% NaCl, whereas Gerlach and Gylstorff (1967) found 2 strains that would tolerate 3% NaCl and all isolates would grow in 1% NaCl. Fletcher and Plastridge (1964) found their strains would tolerate 1.6% NaCl but not 2% NaCl. Some strains isolated by Truscott and Stockdale (1966) would tolerate 1% NaCl whereas others would not replicate. Avian vibrio will grow in 1% glycine (Fletcher and Plastridge, 1964; Bertschinger, 1965; Truscott and Stockdale, 1966). Indole is not produced (Peckham, 1958; Voûte and Grimbergen, 1959).

Deaminase and/or deamidase activity was detected when aspartic acid or asparagin was the substrate (Fletcher and Plastridge, 1964).

The avian organism will grow at 45° C, but vibrios isolated from humans and *Vibrio fetus* Types I and II do not (Fletcher and Plastridge, 1964; Bertschinger, 1965). There is little growth of chicken vibrios at 30° C but good growth of *Vibrio fetus* Types I and II (Bertschinger, 1965). Bryans and Smith (1960) found 3 avian isolates tolerant to 1% ox bile and 0.1% Selenite. Galactose, arabinose, and mannose are not utilized (Basden et al., 1968).

RESISTANCE TO CHEMICAL AND PHYSICAL AGENTS

Chemical

Among the antibiotics and chemicals tested, those that exhibited the most consistent inhibitory action against vibrios were streptomycin, dihydrostreptomycin, and derivatives of the nitrofurans (furazolidone, furoxon, furacin) (Delaplane et al., 1955; Hofstad et al., 1958; Winterfield et al., 1958; Gerlach and Gylstorff, 1967).

Varying degrees of susceptibility were shown by different isolates to the following antibiotics: oxtetracycline, chlortetracycline, tetracycline, neomycin, erythromycin, chloramphenicol, and magnamycin. Some strains showed slight susceptibility to penicillin by in vivo embryo tests. Delaplane et al. (1955) found their agent resistant to chlortetracycline and oxytetracycline; Winterfield et al. (1958) found all but one strain susceptible to chlortetracycline. Gerlach and Gylstorff (1967) tested the antibiotic sensitivity of 10 isolates and found 3 resistant to chlortetracycline and oxytetracycline. The same authors found most strains highly susceptible to erythromycin but one strain proved resistant. Whenham et al. (1961) found vibrio resistant to sulfamerazine but did not find any strains resistant to chloramphenicol or tetracycline. There is general agreement that the vibrio is resistant to bacitracin, polymyxin B sulfate, and novobiocin. Bisping et al. (1963) used bacitracin, novobiocin, and polymyxin B sulfate to control contaminants when isolating vibrio from tissues. Hofstad et al. (1958) found vibrio susceptible to thallous acetate. Winterfield et al. (1958) reported that sulfamethazine and sulfaquinoxaline had some prophylactic effect against experimental infection in birds.

Physical

Avian vibrios are able to withstand prolonged storage and wide variation in temperature. Yolk cultures of vibrio maintain viability for at least 2 years at —25° C (Hofstad et al., 1958). Lyophilized cultures are viable after 20 months. The organism remains viable in tissues and bile stored at 4° C for 6 days (Peckham, 1958). When cultures on blood agar were stored at 4° C under 10% carbon dioxide they remained viable for 14 days and could be easily subcultured, whereas cultures held at room temperature consisted only of coccoid forms and could not be subcultured (Hagan, 1964). Gerlach and Gylstorff (1967) found 6 weeks as the maximum survival time for fluid thioglycollate cultures kept at —25° C. Winterfield et al. (1958) found yolk cultures viable after 2 but not 3 weeks held at 37.5° C.

Filtration

The bacterium is filterable through a Selas 02 filter but is retained by the Selas 03 filter (Hofstad et al., 1958). Winterfield et al. (1958) passed the agent through a .45μ Millipore filter but not through the .30μ size. The agent passed through a 2μ Seitz pad but not a Seitz EK filter. They estimated the size of the agent to be between 280 and 470 mμ.

STRAIN CLASSIFICATION

It is becoming apparent that vibrios isolated from the digestive tract and parenchymatous organs of chickens vary in their biochemical, serological, and pathogenic properties (Speck, 1965; Truscott and Stockdale, 1966; Gerlach and Gylstorff, 1967).

Speck (1965) investigated the possibility of separating different strains of avian vibrios by the complement fixation test. Phenol-soluble antigens were prepared by heating vibrio suspensions 30 minutes at 80° C. Antiserum was obtained from hyperimmunized rabbits. By cross-reactions with 18 strains, two heterogeneous groups were recognized. Five antigens fitted into neither group and reacted only with homologous antiserum. Three strains did not give clear-cut complement fixation with the antiserum.

Truscott and Stockdale (1966) demonstrated that vibrios isolated from the bile and cecal contents were similar in somatic antigen structure and reacted alike in selected biochemical tests. Pathogenicity studies indicated that the strains varied in virulence. Gerlach and Gylstorff (1967) found their strains to have similar biochemical and virulence properties but a variable antigenic structure.

Basden et al. (1968) used nucleic acid homology studies and demonstrated that a relationship existed between vibrios isolated from the bile and cecal contents of the same bird.

PATHOGENESIS AND EPIZOOTIOLOGY

NATURAL HOST

Chickens are the primary species in which natural infection has been reported. The disease is usually seen in pullets coming into production or after they have been in production several months (Sevoian et al., 1958). Peckham (1958) isolated vibrios from chickens varying in age from 2 to 17 months. Vibrios were isolated from 8–14-day-old chickens by Bisping et al. (1963) and from 1–18-month-old chickens by Gerlach and Gylstorff (1967).

Grünberg and Otte (1963) isolated vibrio from 2-day and 8-day-old bustards (*Otis tarda* L.). This vibrio had the same biochemical properties and produced the same histopathologic lesions in domestic chicks as the etiologic agent of vibrionic hepatitis.

EXPERIMENTAL HOSTS

Turkey poults were infected by intramuscular or intraperitoneal inoculation with the production of hydropericardium, pale myocardium, enlarged spleen, and an enlarged and necrotic liver (Winterfield et al., 1958; Peckham, 1958; Rinaldi et al., 1964).

Swiss white mice were slightly susceptible to intracerebral inoculation and occasionally manifested nervous signs. Vibrios were recovered from the brains (Delaplane et al., 1955; Peckham, 1958).

Delaplane et al. (1955) and Rinaldi et al. (1964) produced necrosis in the livers of rabbits by intraperitoneal injection. Winterfield et al. (1958) confirmed these findings and produced mortality in young rabbits but found hamsters and mice refractory to intraperitoneal inoculation. Delaplane et al. (1955) and Rinaldi et al. (1964) reported no pathogenic effects following inoculation of guinea pigs. Rinaldi et al. (1964) found ducklings not susceptible to intraperitoneal inoculation.

TRANSMISSION

Delaplane et al. (1955) infected day-old chicks by intracerebral, oral, subcutaneous, and intraperitoneal inoculation. Sevoian et al. (1958) confirmed these observations and found lesions 48 hours postinoculation, with the maximum liver lesions occurring between 5 and 12 days. Lesions persisted for at least 9 weeks in older chickens, and vibrios were reisolated.

Egg

The natural transmission of vibrio in ovo to newly hatched chicks has not been conclusively established. That the possibility exists has been suggested by experimental and field observations. Hofstad et al. (1958) reported liver lesions in newly hatched chicks following chorioallantoic sac inoculation. Kölbl (1964) isolated vibrios from chicks that hatched following chorioallantoic sac inoculation. Narotsky and Taylor (1958) found gross and microscopic lesions of hepatitis in chicks hatched from infected flocks. They did not isolate vibrio from these chicks. Peckham (1958) recorded the isolation of vibrio from the ovary of a naturally infected bird. Sevoian and Calnek (1959) incubated 1,200 eggs collected for 8 weeks following experimental infection of laying birds. All embryos that died were cultured but vibrio could not be isolated. Abdallah and Winkenwerder (1966) were unsuccessful in isolating vibrio from 176 dead embryos and 242 infertile eggs collected from infected flocks.

Feces

Once vibrio has made its appearance in a flock, by whatever means, its dissemination throughout the group by fecal contamination seems inevitable. The presence of vibrio in the ceca, intestine, and feces of infected birds has been adequately demonstrated (Kölbl, 1964; Winkenwerder and Maciak, 1964; Levina, 1964; Truscott and Stockdale, 1966; Kölbl and Willinger, 1967).

Voûte and Grimbergen (1959) postulated that transmission probably occurred via the feces. Truscott and Stockdale (1966) established that vibrios isolated from the bile and ceca of the same bird had similar somatic antigens, biochemical properties, and virulence. They further stated that the presence of vibrio in feces is an indication that the disease is transmitted by fecal contamination. Kölbl and Willinger (1967) conclusively proved that the disease quickly and readily spreads by contact. They infected young chicks by oral inoculation and demonstrated vibrio in the ceca of contact controls 24 hours later. Controls not in contact with infected birds were negative. In another experiment, 4 chickens 3 months old were inoculated orally and 5 days later were placed in contact with 4 controls. Fecal cultures from the 8 chickens were positive for vibrio 48 hours after contact exposure. Vibrio could still be found in the ceca 49 days after oral inoculation.

INCUBATION PERIOD

Sevoian et al. (1958) found lesions in chicks 48 hours after inoculation, with maximum changes occurring between 5 and 12 days. Moore (1958), using a laparotomy technique, observed that some birds with signs and lesions spontaneously recovered. Therefore, if in experimental studies birds are necropsied too late after infection, lesions may not be present.

SIGNS

Characteristically the course of the disease is one of insidious onset and persistent duration. Occasionally in pullet flocks the onset is signaled by increased mortality. Pullet flocks may fail to peak at expected production levels and mature flocks may fail to maintain normal production. Sevoian et al. (1958) observed a 25–35% drop in production. Individual birds show loss of weight, listlessness, and a scaly shrunken comb. Diarrhea in individual birds or the entire flock has frequently been reported (Whenham et al., 1961; Bisping et al., 1963; Vielitz et al., 1965).

No adverse effect on shell quality or internal egg quality has been reported. Information is not available as to the effect of hepatitis on fertility or hatchability.

Vielitz et al. (1965) and Gerlach and Gylstorff (1967) reported that hepatitis in broilers caused liver lesions and poor weight gains.

MORBIDITY AND MORTALITY

Usually a small percentage of the flock shows signs at any one time, and the disease may persist in an untreated flock for many weeks (Sevoian et al., 1958). Birds severely affected are listless, stay on the roosts, or stand apart from the flock. Occasionally a bird may die in excellent flesh from an acute infection and show evidence of having laid within the past 48–72 hours. Mortality rates of 2% (Vielitz et al., 1965), 5% (Bisping et al., 1963), and 15% have been reported (Sevoian et al., 1958).

GROSS LESIONS

The most striking lesions occur in the liver and represent inflammatory and necrotic processes. Less than 10% of clinically infected birds have gross liver lesions. Therefore one cannot rely on gross lesions to establish a diagnosis. Liver lesions are variable in extent, size, and number. Enlargement and discoloration may be the only changes. Small stellate yellow necrotic foci may be disseminated throughout the liver parenchyma (Figs. 9.3-A, E, F). Large irregular focal hemorrhagic areas or circumscribed small hemorrhagic foci may be seen beneath the liver capsule. Hematocysts may occur beneath the liver capsule and occasionally rupture of the liver will be evident by a large blood clot adhering to the surface of the liver (Fig. 9.3-A). Severely affected livers may be friable and have large cauliflowerlike necrotic areas throughout (Figs. 9.3-E, F) (Sevoian et al., 1958). In chronic cases induration and atrophy of the liver may be accompanied by ascites and hydropericardium (Fig. 9.3-B). The kidneys may be pale and enlarged. Ovarian changes range from a collapsed balloon appearance of several follicles to complete regression with only a cluster of pea size follicles remaining. Enlargement of the heart with absence of muscle tone may be accompanied by hydropericardium (Delaplane et al., 1955). In some cases areas of necrosis are observed in the heart muscle (Fig. 9.3-C). In young chickens the heart is pale and encased with an amber-colored gelatinous exudate. Splenic enlargement may be accompanied by a large yellow friable infarct involving most of the parenchyma (Fig. 9.3-D).

Intestinal lesions consist of catarrhal enteritis with either petechiation or marked inflammation of the mucosal surface.

HISTOPATHOLOGY

An excellent description of the histopathological changes was given by Sevoian et al. (1958). Early infections were characterized by lymphocytic and granulocytic infiltration of the portal area. More advanced lesions were focal accumulations of lymphocytes and granulocytes accompanied by focal necrosis (Fig. 9.4). The necrotic areas varied in shape and size and had random distribution. There was bile duct proliferation. Fatty metamorphosis, congestion, and hemorrhage occurred in the liver. Connective tissue was increased around the portal and interlobular areas. The liver capsule was edematous and infiltrated by inflammatory cells. Occasionally

granulomas with fibrinoid necrosis were present.

The spleen had decreased lymphopoietic activity and occasionally had granulomas. The kidneys had infiltration of heterophils and lymphocytes in interstitial areas and in focal areas of necrotic parenchymal cells. The tubules were dilated and contained casts of heterophils. The bone marrow had an increase of large immature myelocytes. Mononuclear infiltration of the myocardium was more common in young chickens.

Casorso and Jungherr (1959) reported liver lesions in embryos as focal necrosis, accumulations of heterophils, bile duct proliferation and bile stasis, and regenerating liver cells around the hepatic vessels.

Hematology

Sevoian et al. (1958) noted that hematological abnormalities in chicks were most pronounced between the 2nd and 21st days postinoculation. The heterophil, thrombocyte, and total leukocyte counts increased. Hemoglobin and hematocrit values were lowered, and erythrocyte and lymphocyte counts decreased.

IMMUNITY

The development of agglutinating antibodies in infected birds is evidence that a protective mechanism is being stimulated. However, in most bacterial infections the immune status is of short duration, and the presence of circulating antibodies does not necessarily mean absence of infection. The success of the pullorum control program lies in the ability of the agglutination test to detect birds that are harboring the bacteria. Gerlach and Gylstorff (1967) demonstrated that vibrio agglutinins develop and reach their maximum titer within 2–3 weeks postinoculation. Nevertheless, Sevoian et al. (1958) were able to isolate vibrio from chickens 9 weeks postinfection. Kölbl and Willinger (1967) isolated vibrio from the ceca of chickens 49 days after infection. It is quite apparent that any immunity that does develop is not sufficient to eliminate the infecting organism from the host. Vielitz et al. (1965) stated that in the course of vibrionic hepatitis either no immunity or only a very incomplete immunity developed.

DIAGNOSIS

The diagnosis of avian vibrionic hepatitis is aided by the history, appearance of

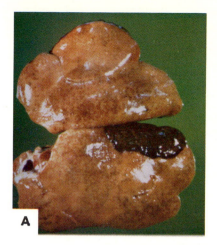

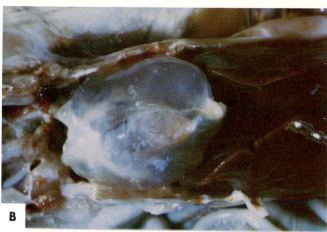

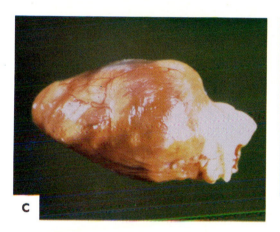

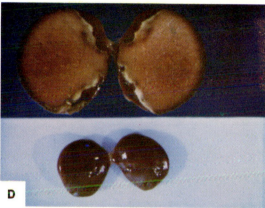

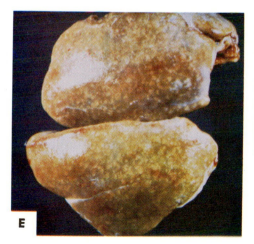

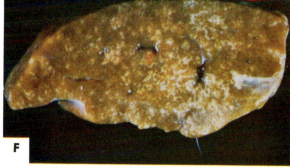

FIG. 9.3—(A) Liver with subcapsular hemorrhage and focal areas of necrosis. (B) Hydropericardium of bird affected with hepatitis. (C) Heart with necrosis in myocardium. (D) Enlarged spleen with infarct compared with normal spleen. (E) Liver with stellate foci from chicken affected with vibrionic hepatitis. (F) Cut surface of liver shown in (E).

the flock, gross and microscopic lesions, serology, and demonstration or isolation of the vibrio. Rarely will all the diagnostic criteria be present in an individual bird or in a single accession. The significance attributed to the demonstration or isolation of vibrio from a single bird must be evaluated by critical analysis of the history and performance of the flock.

Angstrom (1959, personal communication) and Bisping et al. (1963) noted that birds with marked liver lesions sometimes failed to yield vibrio on culture and birds without gross lesions were positive on culture. Vibrio was isolated from a bird that came from a flock laying 80% (Peckham, 1958). Thackrey and Johnstone (1964) stated that although vibrios have etiologic significance it does not necessarily follow that a bird or flock is ill at the time of isolation. They suggested that some form of stress occurs to precipitate the clinical disease. This is further substantiated by the work of Sevoian and Calnek (1959), who isolated vibrio from an uninoculated healthy appearing control and stated that the infection is widespread and its significance varies from flock to flock.

ISOLATION OF CAUSATIVE AGENT

Vibrios were isolated from the liver, spleen, kidneys, bile, heart, and pericardial fluid (Delaplane et al., 1955; Winterfield and Sevoian, 1957; Hofstad et al., 1958; Peckham, 1958). Early investigators used liver suspensions inoculated into the yolk sac of 5–8-day chicken embryos. This method was tedious and expensive and often not feasible for the average diagnostic laboratory. Peckham (1958) isolated vibrio from chickens by aspirating bile from the gallbladder and inoculating a few drops onto 10% blood agar plates which were incubated under 10% carbon dioxide for 24 hours. Colonies were not visible but the area inoculated with bile was mucoid and had sharp, raised edges. A small block of the inoculated area on the agar was cut out, inverted on a microscope slide, and pushed off. The resulting smear was stained and examined by oil immersion. Despite the fact that no colonies were visible, a confluent mass of vibrios was regularly seen by microscopic examination in positive cases. In comparative studies, if vibrio were not found in those plates examined at 24 hours, they were not found on agar plates incubated beyond 24 hours. Hagan (1964) in an extensive series of controlled studies reported optimum incubation time of 18–24 hours and found a heavy density of vibrios on agar smears. Voûte and Grimbergen (1959) found an abundance of vibrios after incubation of agar plates for 18 hours. From the standpoint of the diagnostician who is invariably pressed for a quick diagnosis, the fact that a positive diagnosis can

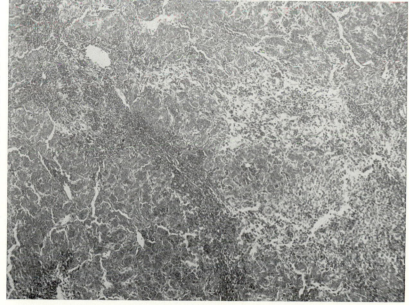

FIG. 9.4—*Liver section of field case of vibrionic hepatitis. Hemorrhage around central vein. Light area to right of center is devoid of liver cord cells and contains erythrocytes, heterophils, and some lymphocytes. ×96. (Hofstad, Iowa State Univ.)*

be made in 24 hours is of paramount importance.

Vibrios can be isolated from the liver by smearing the cut surface on appropriate agar and incubating the plate under reduced oxygen tension (Kölbl, 1964; Gerlach and Gylstorff, 1967). However, they are found more frequently and in greater concentration in the bile (Sevoian and Calnek, 1959).

Vibrios can be seen in stained bile smears or in bile suspensions with the phase-contrast microscope (Whenham et al., 1961; Eleazer et al., 1964; Vielitz et al., 1965). The correlation between positive microscopic observations and positive cultures is high, but in some instances vibrios are seen in bile but are not cultured and in other cases microscopic examination of the bile is negative but the cultures are positive. This method is not for the inexperienced as particulate matter in the bile may resemble vibrios.

Vibrios can be seen in cecal and intestinal contents with the phase-contrast microscope. Kölbl (1964) observed red foci 2–4 mm in diameter in the mucosa of the intestine where vibrios were found.

Vibrios can also be seen in stained smears of cecal and intestinal contents (Truscott and Stockdale, 1966). In experimentally infected chickens cecal smears were positive more often than vibrio isolations from bile. Vibrios isolated from the bile and ceca of the same bird had similar somatic antigenic components. Vibrios can be isolated from cecal contents using a series of Millipore filtrations, as described by Truscott and Morin (1964).

Vibrios can be cultured from the intestinal tract and ceca. Winkenwerder and Maciak (1964) used fluid thioglycollate media (Difco) with 2% agar and 10% ox blood and added to each ml of substrate 25 units of bacitracin, 20 units of polymyxin-B-sulfate and .025 mg of novobiocin. The inoculated plates were placed in an anaerobic jar which was evacuated to 10% of normal atmospheric pressure and refilled to 80% with a gas mixture of 95% nitrogen and 5% carbon dioxide. They compared the rate of vibrio isolations from flocks suspected of having hepatitis with isolations from clinically normal flocks. From 114 suspect birds 86% were positive on culture; 36% of the cultures were positive from normal appearing chickens. Of the 98 isolations from the suspicious birds, 62 were simultaneously recovered from the intestinal tracts of birds which also yielded vibrios from either heart blood, liver, or bile. Thirty-three birds yielded vibrios from only the intestinal tract, indicating that vibrios are more prevalent in the intestinal tract than in the bile or viscera.

Vibrios can be isolated from the bile, heart, liver, spleen, and kidney by inoculation of suspensions into the yolk sac of 5–8-day embryos. Mortality usually occurs 3–5 days postinoculation (Delaplane et al., 1955; Winterfield et al., 1958; Hofstad et al., 1958). Bacterial contamination is controlled by using 1,000 units of bacitracin and 10,000 units of polymyxin per ml of inoculum (Winterfield et al., 1958; Hagan, 1964). Vibrios can be demonstrated in the yolk or allantoic fluid by examination of stained smears (Peckham, 1958), by phase-contrast microscopic examination (Kölbl, 1964), and by culture of these fluids (Hofstad et al., 1958).

Hagan (1964) studied the comparative efficacy of artificial media and embryos for isolating vibrios from bile by inoculating aliquot samples on blood agar and in the yolk sac of chick embryos. Of the 110 samples, 33 were positive on agar and in embryos, 2 were positive only on agar, and 6 were positive in embryos only. The vibrio isolation rates were 31.8% by blood agar culture and 35.5% by embryo inoculation. The results indicated that blood agar is an adequate medium for routine culture of bile from field cases.

The recovery rate of vibrio from clinical cases is of importance to the diagnostician. Peckham (1958) was able to isolate vibrio from bile in 25% of the accessions suspected of having hepatitis on the basis of history and necropsy. Hagan (1964) was able to isolate vibrio from 46.7% of the accessions classified as presumptive hepatitis and from 20% of the birds. In accessions not classified as presumptive hepatitis, 2.3% were positive and only 0.8% of the birds were positive. The results in this trial would indicate that the diagnostician may expect to isolate vibrios on blood agar from 20% of the bile samples in slightly less than 50% of the cases.

Bisping et al. (1963) isolated vibrios from 25% of 395 hens; 58% of the isolations were from bile, 27% simultaneously from bile and liver, and 15% from only the liver.

Winkenwerder and Maciak (1964) obtained similar results and isolated vibrios from bile in 28% of the birds suspected of having hepatitis. However, they achieved 86% isolations from suspected flocks by the combined total of positive cultures from ceca, jejunum, heart blood, liver, and bile. Cecal cultures yielded 72% positive isolations, and 28% of the birds yielded vibrios from only the intestinal tract. This work and subsequent reports indicate that vibrios can be found more often in the intestinal tract than in the bile or liver (Kölbl and Willinger, 1967).

SEROLOGY

The use of serology for diagnosis of infected birds or flocks may play a role in the control of this disease in the future. However, standardization of antigens and development of uniform techniques have not been established.

Kölbl (1964) found that strains of vibrio that swarmed on agar were unsatisfactory as antigens as they autoagglutinated. A satisfactory antigen strain maintained a constant S form when passed on agar. Cultures were washed from agar with 1:5,000 merthiolate solution, washed twice, and used at 0.03% concentration for the tube agglutination test. Tenfold dilutions of serum and antigen were incubated 24 hours and then left at room temperature 18 hours before reading. The first 2 weeks postinfection titers reached 1:10 and at 2–4 weeks 1:80.

Truscott and Stockdale (1966) compared the antigenic structure of bile and cecal isolates. Antigen was heated 10 minutes at 100° C to remove the flagellar (H) antigen. Hyperimmune serum produced by multiple injections of antigen reached a maximum agglutination titer of 1,280 at 3 weeks. Somatic antigens prepared from cecal and bile isolates from the same bird were similar. Using cross-absorption tests they demonstrated different somatic antigen types. However, as there was some cross-absorption of the agglutinins by different antigens it indicated antigen similarities in different strains.

Gerlach and Gylstorff (1967) used the rapid slide agglutination test and compared the sera of 100 birds with 6 antigens. Sera from 42 birds were positive, and from 21 of these birds vibrios were isolated from the liver, bile, or heart and 21 were negative on culture. There were marked differences in the agglutination titers against the 6 antigens. Nine of the birds negative on culture had positive histological lesions, and 12 birds were without lesions. One bird had a negative titer but was positive on culture. The authors mentioned that this was probably a recent infection without sufficient time elapsing for agglutinating antibodies to form. The 57 birds negative to the agglutination test had neither history nor lesions of hepatitis, and cultural attempts were negative. In experimentally infected chicks, agglutinins appeared in 14 days and reached a maximum titer in 21 days.

DIFFERENTIAL DIAGNOSIS

Several other diseases have similar clinical signs and gross lesions and must be considered in making a diagnosis of vibrionic hepatitis. Pullorum disease, fowl typhoid, and leukosis produce enlargement of the liver with color changes and foci varying in size and number. The stained antigen rapid plate test is a valuable aid in detecting pullorum and fowl typhoid, and a positive test should be supplemented by the inoculation of appropriate media. Leukosis often produces tumors in organs other than the liver, and a thorough examination should aid in confirming a diagnosis. Histological examination of affected viscera will give supportive evidence.

A diagnosis of avian vibrionic hepatitis based on isolation or demonstration of the vibrio and characteristic gross and microscopic pathology is preferred. It should be kept in mind that isolation of the organism is not always successful and histological changes are not pathognomonic. The history of the flock is of prime consideration in establishing a flock diagnosis and interpreting laboratory findings. Recommendations should be made on the basis of flock history, performance of the flock, and future plans for the flock.

TREATMENT

Winterfield et al. (1958) conducted prophylactic and therapeutic trials in experimentally infected chicks. Prophylactic activity was demonstrated by chlortetracycline, oxytetracycline, and furazolidone administered in the feed; by sulfaquinoxaline and sulfamethazine in water; and by streptomycin injections. Oxytetracycline, furazolidone, and streptomycin gave the best results. As a therapeutic measure in chicks, furazolidone and streptomycin appeared more effective. The injection of 5 mg streptomycin per chick was less effective than 0.022% furazolidone in the feed. Sevoian and Calnek (1959) noted a high degree of efficacy by the prophylactic administration of 250–300 g furazolidone per ton of feed for 5–6 days, or a single injection of 250 mg dihydrostreptomycin in mature chickens. Despite the treatment, relapse or reinfection was noted.

Bisping et al. (1963) noted a beneficial effect following furazolidone medication and recommended not less than 400 g per ton of feed for 8 days. They also observed relapses in older birds. Vielitz et al. (1965) used 400 g furazolidone per ton of feed for 4 days followed by a level of 200 g for 10 days. Relapses were noted with this treatment. They also used 400 g furazolidone per ton of feed for 14 days without superior results. It was observed that a delay in treatment a few days after the onset of signs led to unsatisfactory results.

PREVENTION AND CONTROL

MANAGEMENT PROCEDURES

Those management security measures employed to prevent the introduction of most bacterial diseases to a poultry farm will be useful in preventing the introduction of vibrionic hepatitis. The chain of infection is best broken at the fomite link. Contaminated chick boxes, egg cases, and feed bags must be disinfected before reuse. Servicemen must take every precaution to prevent the spread of diseases. Animals and wild birds must be regarded as potential hazards. A steam cleaning and disinfecting of the building and all equipment should precede the introduction of new birds. Studies have not been made to determine how long the vibrio survives under natural conditions. When vibrio infection becomes established on a farm, only the most stringent security measures will prevent its spread to each new flock. Separate caretakers and equipment should be used for

the new flock. One can assume from reports already discussed that once a flock is infected, it remains so indefinitely and is continually discharging vibrios via the feces. If serological techniques become standardized and reach high confidence levels, they will be useful in detecting infected flocks and appropriate measures can be instituted.

The role played by stress factors and concomitant diseases in converting a latent infection to a clinical outbreak must be considered. Bisping et al. (1963) reported they rarely saw hepatitis without accompanying diseases such as ascarids, capillaria, Marek's disease, pox, and mycoplasma. Thackrey and Johnstone (1964) said their experience suggested some form of stress often occurred to precipitate the clinical disease. Winkenwerder and Maciak (1964) believed that vibrio may play the role of a facultative pathogenic saprophyte since they could isolate vibrio from the intestine of clinically normal hens. They found a high percentage of hepatitis cases with worm infestations. Voûte and Grimbergen (1959) also noted parasites in hepatitis cases.

Gerlach and Gylstorff (1967) noted their cases often had capillaria, intestinal coccidiosis, or *Escherichia coli* infection. The only controlled study on the influence of stress on the exacerbation of symptoms or lesions was done by Sevoian et al. (1958) who vaccinated birds with fowl pox after inoculation with vibrio. They found that this stress factor did not alter the course of experimental infection.

It may well be that management practices that are favorable for perpetuating worm populations are also conducive to the establishment of vibrionic hepatitis as a flock problem.

IMMUNIZATION

There are no reports of successful immunization against vibrionic hepatitis. By the nature of the disease which is characterized by a protracted course in a flock with the development of carriers, it appears that it would be most difficult to develop effective immunization techniques.

REFERENCES

Abdallah, I. S., and W. Winkenwerder. 1966. Haussperlinge (*Passer domesticus* L.) als Uebertrager von Vibronen. *Zentr. Veterinaermed.* 13:338–44.

Angstrom, C. I. 1966. Report of the committee on nomenclature and reporting of diseases. N.E. Conf. on Avian Diseases. *Avian Diseases* 10:535–41.

————. 1967. Report of the committee on nomenclature and reporting of diseases. N.E. Conf. on Avian Diseases. *Avian Diseases* 11:727–33.

Basden II, E. H., M. E. Tourtellotte, W. N. Plastridge, and J. S. Tucker. 1968. Genetic relationship among bacteria classified as vibrios. *J. Bacteriol.* 95:439–43.

Bertschinger, H. U. 1965. Nachweis von Vibrionen bei Huehnern mit Hepatitis. *Zentr. Veterinaermed.* 12:33–40.

Bisping, W., U. Freytag, and H. Krauss. 1963. Festellung der Vibrionenhepatitis der Huehner in Nordwestdeutschland. *Berlin. Muench. Tieraerztl. Wochschr.* 76:456–61.

Blakemore, F. 1939. The nature of fowl paralysis (neurolymphomatosis). *J. Comp. Pathol. Therap.* 52:144–59.

Bryans, J. T., and A. G. Smith. 1960. Physiological properties of pathogenic and nonpathogenic vibrio species isolated from cattle, sheep and chickens. *Cornell Vet.* 50:331–33.

Casorso, D. R., and E. L. Jungherr. 1959. The response of the developing chicken embryo to certain avian pathogens. *Am. J. Vet. Res.* 20:547–57.

Delaplane, J. P., H. A. Smith, and R. Moore. 1955. An unidentified agent causing a hepatitis in chickens. *Southwestern Vet.* 8:356–61.

Eleazer, T. H., H. S. Powell, D. E. Roebuck, and B. W. Bierer. 1964. Direct phase microscopic examination of bile as an aid in diagnosing avian vibrionic hepatitis. *J. Am. Vet. Med. Ass.* 144:380.

Fletcher, R. D., and W. N. Plastridge. 1964. Difference in physiology of vibrio spp. from chickens and man. *Avian Diseases* 8:72–75.

Gerlach, Helga, and Irene Gylstorff. 1967. Untersuchungen ueber biochemische Eigenschaften, Pathogenitaet und Resistenzspektrum gegen Antibiotika bei Vibrio Metschnikovii. *Berlin. Muench. Tieraerztl. Wochschr.* 8:153–55.

Grünberg, W., and E. Otte. 1963. Vibrionen-Hepatitis bei Trappenkuecken (*Otis tarda* L.). *Wien. Tieraerztl. Monatsschr.* 50:862–69.

Hagan, Jean. 1964. Diagnostic techniques in avian vibrionic hepatitis. *Avian Diseases* 8:428–37.

Hofstad, M. S. 1956. *Report of Progress in Veterinary Medical Research.* Iowa State Coll.

Hofstad, M. S., E. H. McGehee, and P. C. Bennett. 1958. Avian infectious hepatitis. *Avian Diseases* 2:358–64.

Kölbl, O. 1964. Nachweis der Vibrionenhepatitis bei Huehnern in Oesterreich. *Wien. Tieraerztl. Monatsschr.* 51:165–70.

Kölbl, O., and H. Willinger. 1967. Tierex-

perimentelle Untersuchungen zur Vibrionenhepatitis der Huehner. *Wien. Tieraerztl. Monatsschr.* 54:84–91.

Levina, I. G. 1964. Vibrionic enterohepatitis of chickens. *Veterinariia Moscow* 41:20–22.

Lukas, G. N. 1955. Avian infectious hepatitis —A preliminary report. *J. Am. Vet. Med. Ass.* 126:402–6.

Mathey, W. J., and A. C. Rissberger. 1964. A turkey sinus vibrio (*Vibrio meleagridis,* n. sp.) compared with the avian hepatitis vibrio (*Vibrio hepaticus,* n. sp.). *Poultry Sci.* 43:1339. (Abstr.)

Moore, R. W. 1958. Studies on an agent causing hepatitis in chickens. *Avian Diseases* 2:39–54.

Narotsky, S., and J. R. E. Taylor. 1958. Case Report. Clinical evidence suggesting the possibility of egg transmission of avian hepatitis. *Avian Diseases* 2:541–42.

Oehring, H. 1963. Ist die Blaettchenmethode als Schnelltest zur bakteriellen Sensibilitatsbestimmung geeignet? *Deut. Gesundheitsw.* 18:2200–2202.

Peckham, M. C. 1958. Avian vibrionic hepatitis. *Avian Diseases* 2:348–58.

Rinaldi, A., G. Mandelli, G. Cervio, and E. Ratti. 1964. Osservazioni sull'epatite vibrionica dei polli in Italia. *Clin. Vet.* 87:321–35.

Sevoian, M., and B. W. Calnek. 1959. Avian infectious hepatitis. III. Treatment of chickens in egg production. *Avian Diseases* 3:302–11.

Sevoian, M., R. W. Winterfield, and C. L. Goldman. 1958. Avian infectious hepatitis. I. Clinical and pathological manifestations. *Avian Diseases* 2:3–18.

Speck, J. 1965. Die serologische Differenzierung von Huehner-Vibrionen mittels Komplementbindungsreaktion. *Zentr. Veterinaermed.* 12:541–46.

Thackrey, D. J., and H. C. Johnstone. 1964. Diagnosis of avian vibrionic hepatitis in San Diego County, California. *Avian Diseases* 8:310–12.

Truscott, R. B., and E. W. Morin. 1964. A bacteriological agent causing bluecomb disease of turkeys. II. Transmission and studies of the etiological agent. *Avian Diseases* 8:27–35.

Truscott, R. B., and P. H. G. Stockdale. 1966. Correlation of the identity of bile and cecal vibrios from the same field cases of avian vibrionic hepatitis. *Avian Diseases* 10:67–73.

Tudor, D. C. 1954. A liver degeneration of unknown origin in chickens. *J. Am. Vet. Med. Ass.* 125:219–20.

Vielitz, E., H. Landgraf, and R. Kirsch. 1965. Zur Diagnostik and Therapie der Vibrionenhepatitis. *Tieraerztl. Umschau.* 20:216–21.

Voûte, E. J., and A. H. M. Grimbergen. 1959. Vibrio hepatitis bij kippen. *Tijdschr. Diergeneesk.* 23:1380–82.

Whenham, G. R., H. C. Carlson, and A. Aksel. 1961. Avian vibrionic hepatitis in Alberta. *Can. Vet. J.* 2:3–7.

Winkenwerder, W., and W. Bisping. 1964. Kulturelle, serologische und experimentelle Untersuchungen mit von Huehnern und Rinden isolierten Vibrionen. *Zentr. Veterinaermed.* 11:603–14.

Winkenwerder, W., and T. Maciak. 1964. Vibrionenfunde bei Huehnern aus erkrankten bestaenden und bei Schlachthuehnern. *Deut. Tieraerztl. Wochschr.* 71:625–27.

Winterfield, R. W., and M. Sevoian. 1957. Isolation of a causal agent of an avian hepatitis. *Vet. Med.* 52:273–74.

Winterfield, R. W., M. Sevoian, and C. L. Goldman. 1958. Avian infectious hepatitis. II. Some characteristics of the etiologic agent. Effect of various drugs on the course of the disease. *Avian Diseases* 2:19–39.

❖

VIBRIO METSCHNIKOVII INFECTION

❖

Vibrio metschnikovii infection is an acute disease of young chickens characterized by sudden onset, high mortality, diarrhea, and severe enteritis. Gamaléia (1888a) first reported the disease in Odessa, Russia. He isolated vibrio from dead chickens and conducted cultural and inoculation experiments with the organism. Krause and Windrath (1919) reported the disease in Germany in newly imported sunbirds (*Leiothrix luteus* L.). Csukás (1930) reported the disease in Hungary in geese that were being force-fed. Kujumgiev (1957) reported the disease from Bulgaria in turkeys and pheasants.

INCIDENCE AND DISTRIBUTION

The incidence of the disease is extremely low if one is to judge by less than half a dozen reports in almost a century since its first description. It was reported only in European countries, and all reports other than the original by Gamaléia (1888a,b) were in birds other than chickens.

ETIOLOGY

The organism was called *Vibrio metschnikovii* (Gamaléia, 1888a) and also referred to as the paracholera vibrio.

MORPHOLOGY AND STAINING

The bacteria are seen in the blood of inoculated pigeons as short, thick, curved rods with rounded ends. Occasionally they are in spiral form with 5–10 turns. They are motile and stain gram-negative.

CULTURAL CHARACTERISTICS

According to Gamaléia (1888a), the organism is easily cultivated on ordinary media and forms a pellicle in veal bouillon. Gelatin is liquified and milk is coagulated. The addition of sulfuric acid to peptone cultures gives an orange color indicative of indole production. The organism survives 2 minutes at 50° C but not 5 minutes.

Krause and Windrath (1919) isolated a vibrio from sunbirds (*Leiothrix luteus* L.) which had properties similar to those of *V. metschnikovii*. They observed the vibrio would grow on potato slices and at room or incubator temperature. On agar the colonies were round, sharply circumscribed, and transparent. Litmus milk became alkaline.

Kujumgiev (1957) reported reduction of nitrate to nitrite; hemolysis on blood agar; catalase production; and acid production in sucrose, galactose, maltose, glucose, levulose, mannitol, and sorbitol.

Kuzdas and Morse (1956) reported the following characteristics for a strain of *V. metschnikovii* obtained from the American type culture collection: slight catalase production, growth in 3.5% NaCl, no reduction of nitrate, urease negative, and acid production in litmus milk. Litmus milk plus 0.1% agar gave an alkaline zone at the surface, and there was growth in semisolid broth with 8% dextrose.

PATHOGENESIS AND EPIZOOTIOLOGY

NATURAL AND EXPERIMENTAL HOSTS

Gamaléia (1888a) reported pigeons were highly susceptible and died within 24–48 hours after intramuscular inoculation, but oral inoculation of pigeons had no effect. Oral infection of young chicks caused mortality. Rabbits and gophers were refractory. Guinea pigs died 48 hours after oral inoculation. Krause and Windrath (1919) killed rats, mice, and guinea pigs by parenteral inoculation. Pigeons and nightingales died within 18–48 hours after intramuscular injection. Hens and rabbits were refractory to injections. None of the animals or birds died after oral inoculation.

Gamaléia (1888b) found that species ordinarily refractory to oral inoculation or injection were highly susceptible when the organism was introduced into the respiratory tract. Pigeons, guinea pigs, mature chickens, and rabbits were susceptible to this mode of infection.

Kujumgiev (1957) easily killed pigeons by intramuscular injection, guinea pigs by subcutaneous inoculation, and only a few chicks by oral inoculation.

Csukás (1930) killed mice, pigeons, and guinea pigs but not rabbits by subcutaneous inoculation.

TRANSMISSION

The consistent finding of the organism in the intestinal tract of infected birds would indicate that feces play a role in dissemination of the disease. Birds and animals were experimentally infected by oral inoculation and suggested a means of transmission which could easily occur in nature. Gamaléia (1888b) found that instillation of the organism in the respiratory tract was a more successful method of infecting hosts and concluded that this was the natural method. He confined pigeons, chicks, and guinea pigs in the same cages with infected animals, and they did not contract the disease.

SIGNS AND LESIONS

The signs in chickens resemble those of fowl cholera but the course is less acute.

The body temperature is normal whereas in cholera the body temperature is elevated. Affected birds are listless, sleepy, and have diarrhea. Death ensues in 2–3 days. The disease in sunbirds was acute and killed several hundred in a few days.

At necropsy a consistent finding is hyperemia of the digestive tract. The intestines contain yellowish, green liquid and some blood. The spleen is always pale and small; other organs appear normal.

IMMUNITY

Gamaléia (1888a) reported that *V. metschnikovii* was similar to the vibrio of Asiatic cholera. When he vaccinated pigeons with *V. metschnikovii* they were immune to challenge with Asiatic cholera. Pigeons vaccinated against Asiatic cholera were refractory to *V. metschnikovii*.

DIAGNOSIS

ISOLATION AND IDENTIFICATION OF CAUSATIVE AGENT

The organism can be isolated from the viscera and intestinal tract and is not fastidious in its growth requirements; 5% blood agar will suffice for primary isolation. Kujumgiev (1957) reported isolation of the organism from the intestinal tract on nutrient agar. Studies have not been published on the antibiotic sensitivity of the organism, but certain bacterial inhibitors might prove of value in making isolations from the intestine. Identification of the organism would be aided by determination of its biochemical properties and its pathogenicity for pigeons.

DIFFERENTIAL DIAGNOSIS

The disease syndrome most likely to be confused with vibrio infection is fowl cholera. However, in fowl cholera the liver is brick red, friable, and studded with focal necrosis. Petechiation of the serous surfaces is characteristic of fowl cholera. In fowl cholera the characteristic bipolar rods can be seen in smears of heart blood. Isolation of the organism is necessary for a definitive diagnosis.

TREATMENT AND PREVENTION

Modern chemicals and antibiotics have not been evaluated for either prophylaxis or therapy of the disease. Drugs effective against vibrionic hepatitis should be considered in the treatment of *V. metschnikovii*. Prevention must depend on the usual

management and sanitation measures employed in the control of diseases of similar epidemiological nature.

❖

MISCELLANEOUS VIBRIOS

❖

TURKEY. Peterson et al. (1959) reported a 50% drop in the fertility of turkey eggs associated with vibriosis. Vibrios were isolated from 80% of the infertile eggs. They postulated that the low fertility was the result of infection of the oviduct, but they did not mention any attempts to isolate vibrio from this organ.

Biochemical determinations were done with the organism, but the authors did not indicate its relationship to previously described vibrio. It was found that the continuous administration of oxytetracycline at the rate of 50 g per ton of feed beginning at the onset of production was associated with improved fertility.

Mathey and Rissberger (1964) isolated a hemolytic vibrio (*V. meleagridis* n. sp.) from sinus exudate of turkeys with sinusitis. The organism was catalase-negative and H_2S positive. Intramuscular inoculation of Japanese quail, chicks, or poults caused severe reaction and death in day-old birds.

PIGEON. Spanedda (1941) isolated a vibrio from the viscera of pigeons during a severe disease outbreak. Necropsy revealed hemorrhages in the viscera and pectoral muscles. The organism did not hemolyze

blood, did not liquify gelatin, was indole-negative, H_2S-negative, did not reduce nitrate, and did not coagulate milk. Pigeons died within 20 hours following intramuscular injection, and mice were killed by intraperitoneal injection. Guinea pigs were not susceptible. In view of differences in biochemical properties and host pathogenicity compared to *V. metschnikovii*, the name *Vibrio columbae* was proposed by Spanedda (1941).

PENGUIN. Fraser (1961) isolated an anaerobic vibrio from the viscera of an adult King penguin. The organism required strict anaerobiosis and would not grow under 10% carbon dioxide or in embryonating eggs. Indole, H_2S, and catalase were not produced. Guinea pigs, mice, and pigeons were refractory to inoculation. It did not resemble either *V. metschnikovii* or the vibrio causing avian vibrionic hepatitis.

SPARROW. Abdallah and Winkenwerder (1966) isolated vibrio from 20 of 106 sparrows (*Passer domesticus* L.). Inoculation of the vibrio into young chicks produced slight inflammatory changes in the liver. The characteristics of the isolated vibrio were similar to *V. fetus* Types I and II.

CHICKEN. Peckham (1962) isolated a hemolytic vibrio from sinus exudate of chickens affected with a respiratory disease. The vibrio grew on blood agar inoculated under 10% carbon dioxide. Inoculation of the organism into the nasal sinus of 3-week-old chickens produced a sinusitis and nasal discharge. Hemolytic vibrios were reisolated from the nasal passages and palatine cleft of the inoculated birds.

REFERENCES

Abdallah, I. S., and W. Winkenwerder. 1966. Haussperlinge (*Passer domesticus* L.) als Uebertraeger von Vibrionen. *Zentr. Veterinaermed.* 13:338–44.

Csukás, Z. 1930. Paracholera vibrio okozta elhullasok libafalkakban. *Allatorv. Lapok* 53:173–76.

Fraser, G. 1961. Isolation of an anaerobic vibrio from a King penguin (*Aptenodytes longirostris*). *Avian Diseases* 5:243–50.

Gamaléia, M. N. 1888a. *Vibrio metschnikovii* (n. sp.) et ses rapports avec le microbe du cholera asiatique. *Ann. Inst. Pasteur* 2:482–88.

————. 1888b. *Vibrio metschnikovii* son mode naturel d'infection. *Ann. Inst. Pasteur* 2: 552–57.

Grünberg, W., and E. Otte. 1963. Vibrionen-Hepatitis bei Trappenkueken (*Otis tarda* L.). *Wien. Tieraerztl. Monatsschr.* 50:862–70.

Krause, W., and H. H. Windrath. 1919. Ueber eine durch einen Vibrio veranlasste Seuche der Sonnenvoegel (*Leiothrix luteus* L. chinesische Nachtigall). *Berlin. Muench. Tieraerztl. Wochschr.* 35:468–69.

Kujumgiev, I. 1957. Prima segnalazione dell'infezione da *Vibrio metschnikovii* (Paracholera aviario) nei tacchini e fagiani. *Vet. Ital.* 8:1094–1102.

Kuzdas, C. D., and E. V. Morse. 1956. Physiological characteristics differentiating vibrio fetus and other vibrios. *Am. J. Vet. Res.* 17:331–36.

Mathey, W. J., and Rissberger, A. C. 1964. A turkey sinus vibrio (*Vibrio meleagridis* n. sp.) compared with the avian hepatitis vibrio (*Vibrio hepaticus* n. sp.). *Poultry Sci.* 43:1339.

Peckham, M. C. 1962. Isolation of a hemolytic vibrio from respiratory cases. *Ann. Rept. N.Y. State Vet. Coll. for 1961–62,* p. 60.

Peterson, E. H., R. D. Hendrix, and C. E. Worden. 1959. Low fertility in turkeys associated with vibriosis. *J. Am. Vet. Med. Ass.* 135:219–22.

Spanedda, A. 1941. Su di un nuovo vibrione agente etiologico di una epidemia nei piccioni. *Giorn. Batteriol. Immunol.* 26:518–20.

CHAPTER 10

ERYSIPELAS

❖

A. S. ROSENWALD

Agricultural Extension Service
University of California
Davis, California

AND

R. E. CORSTVET

Department of Veterinary Parasitology
and Public Health
Oklahoma State University
Stillwater, Oklahoma

❖

ERYSIPELAS in birds is generally an acute, fulminating infection of individuals within a flock. The infection and disease have been reported from many different vertebrate species, either as a contaminant (fish) or an infection, but in birds its primary importance is as a disease of turkeys. It is caused by *Erysipelothrix insidiosa* (previously called *E. rhusiopathiae*), which also causes swine erysipelas in pigs and erysipeloid in man.

Outbreaks of economic significance are only occasional in bird species other than turkeys. Occasional losses of individual birds within a flock have been reported, and a few economically significant outbreaks in chickens and ducklings have occurred (Levine, 1965). *E. insidiosa* has been involved in natural outbreaks of erysipelas in pheasants and ducks (Graham et al., 1939; Hudson, 1949; Hudson et al., 1952).

The disease not only causes death but frequently affects the fertilizing capacity of male turkeys. Further marketing losses may result from condemnation losses higher than normal or from downgrading due either to lack of finish or, more particularly, to postmortem evidence of septicemias (Fig. 10.1). Affected chicken flocks have been reported to suffer depression of egg production, and ducklings were reported by Graham et al. (1939) to have death losses exceeding 10%.

The public health hazard of *E. insidiosa* as a local, septicemic, and occasionally fatal infection has been pointed out by many authors including Klauder (1926, 1944) and Klauder et al. (1943), who indicated that it was particularly a disease of fish handlers, butchers, and kitchen workers. To that list should be added veterinarians and turkey growers. Numerous presumptive diagnoses of the infection have been made in turkey flocks as a result of infection of a turkey handler or a member of an insemination crew. In most cases the disease is preceded by injury, such as a cut. Silberstein (1965) reported endocarditis and encephalitis in man, successfully treated with penicillin. Sadler and Corstvet (1965) showed that grossly normal birds may remain carriers of the organism in various organs, such as the cecal tonsil, cloaca, and liver. Even though only a few surviving infected birds carry this organism, they could remain a source of infection to man.

HISTORY

Sporadic cases of infection were reported from various avian species prior to 1936, when Beaudette and Hudson (1936) were the first to call attention to the economic significance of the disease in turkeys on the American continent. In fairly rapid succession outbreaks in turkeys were reported from all over the United States, and Graham et al. (1939) reported the previously mentioned duck outbreak. Detailed information is supplied by Beaudette and Hudson (1936), Levine (1965), and Hinshaw (1965) as well as by the extensive reference list cited by Woodbine (1950); but it is sufficient to say that the disease has become of major economic concern to turkey growers in many parts of the United States. The infection continues to be reported from time to time in individuals or small groups of other species of birds, but since the advent of widespread artificial insemination of turkeys, prevention of erysipelas has become a major problem facing producers of turkey hatching eggs and, in some areas, of market turkeys.

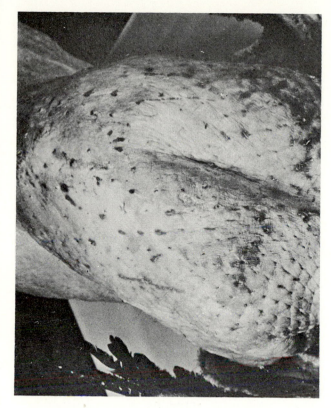

FIG. 10.1—Erysipelas. Bruised blue-black discoloration of skin on breast of New York dressed turkey. In good flesh when slaughtered, this bird was rejected when dressed and, on examination, was bacteriologically positive for E. insidiosa. (Rosenwald, 1941)

Following introduction of the use of a bacterin in the early 1950s, and the availability of penicillin as a treatment regime in outbreaks, various programs of preventive vaccination and/or treatment have been followed. Despite this, as recently as 1969 more than a hundred cases of postinsemination erysipelas in turkey hens were reported from fewer than 1,000 diagnostic cases (McDonald, personal communication).

Despite the concern of the industry, little has been published on the disease in birds in the last several years, and very little research work has been done on it. The antigenic components of the causative organism, however, have received considerable study.

INCIDENCE AND DISTRIBUTION

The adaptiveness of the organism is indicated by the isolation of this bacterium from a wide variety of animals. The disease has a worldwide distribution; in general it occurs sporadically in poultry populations.

Though the disease in turkeys was originally reported more frequently among the males, there is no evidence of a sex differential in susceptibility. Field observations indicate that the portal of entry for the organism is breached more frequently in the male than in the hen. With artificial insemination and the frequent handling of the females, however, the percentage of occurrence among hens has increased markedly in the last 10 years.

ETIOLOGY

CLASSIFICATION

The disease is caused by *Erysipelothrix insidiosa* (synonym *Erysipelothrix rhusiopathiae*) which belongs to the family Cornyebacteriaceae and is said by some workers to resemble *Listeria* sp. (Barber, 1939; Nelson and Shelton, 1963). Those same investigators, however, demonstrated marked cultural and antigenic differences between *E. insidiosa* and *Listeria* sp. This organism has a high lipid content in its cell wall (almost 30%), in this way resembling some of the *Mycobacterium* species. It resembles gram-negative bacteria in that it has a rather low hexosamine content, but it differs from gram-negative bacteria in having a limited complement of amino acids (Kalf and White, 1963).

MORPHOLOGY AND STAINING

The organisms are slender, highly pleomorphic, nonmotile rods. They stain as clumps of curved beaded or filamented gram-positive organisms which decolorize easily. Short rods, often arranged in short chains, are found in smooth colonies; the larger rough colonies have rods that are filamentous, with branching and beading.

GROWTH REQUIREMENTS

The organism grows slowly at 4° C and more rapidly at 35–37° C. Reduced oxygen or increased carbon dioxide favors isolation, as does serum, which also enhances growth, but none is essential. The organism grows moderately well in thioglycollate broth and in various other broths containing serum or serum extracts; it grows especially well in deep stabs of semisolid medium prepared by adding 0.5% agar to tryptose phosphate broth.

COLONIAL MORPHOLOGY

Erysipelothrix insidiosa grows readily though sparsely on ordinary culture media. Colony forms range from dewy, discrete, pinpoint (smooth) to opaque, flat, dry, pinhead type (rough); all adhere tenaciously to solid media. A test-tube brush type of growth (lateral radiating projections) occurs 48 hours postinoculation in gelatin stab culture incubated at 21° C.

BIOCHEMICAL PROPERTIES

Erysipelothrix insidiosa ferments galactose, dextrose, lactose, and levulose anaerogenically. Lead acetate agar or triple-sugar iron (TSI) agar is sometimes browned, indicating H_2S production, and l-oxylose is occasionally fermented. Litmus milk is occasionally acidified slightly without coagulation. Alpha hemolysis occurs in a medium containing 5–10% horse or bovine blood after 2–3 days incubation at 37° C in an atmosphere of 5–10% carbon dioxide. The organism is catalase-negative does not produce indole, does not reduce nitrates, is Voges-Proskauer-negative and methyl red-negative, does not hydrolyze esculin, and does not reduce 0.1% methylene blue. White and Shuman (1961) found that the fermentation pattern varied with

the medium, the indicator, and the method of measuring acid production and stated that the most dependable medium was Andrade's base plus serum. Of three methods used to measure acid production (chemical indicator, change in pH, production of titrable acidity) they found that the chemical indicator gave the most valid, reproducible results.

RESISTANCE TO CHEMICAL AND PHYSICAL AGENTS

Erysipelothrix insidiosa is fairly resistant to various environmental and chemical factors. It is very resistant to desiccation and may survive the smoking and pickling used for processing meat. Apart from tissues, it is killed at 70° C in 5–10 minutes. The organism can remain viable in the soil and is said to multiply in alkaline soils during the warmer months (Vallee, 1930). This indicates that it can compete effectively with normal soil flora and thus remain a soil-borne source of infection. The organism is destroyed in a short time by a 1:1,000 concentration of bichloride of mercury, 0.5% NaOH solution, 3.5% liquid cresol compound, or 5% solution of phenol; it is resistant to formalin. Its survival and possible multiplication in soil makes disinfection of premises extremely difficult. The various sulfanilamides are not effective in vivo against *E. insidiosa*. Penicillin, broad-spectrum antibiotics, and in some instances streptomycin are effective in vitro and in vivo.

ANTIGENIC STRUCTURE

Erysipelothrix insidiosa has been shown to contain antigens that are genus-specific, Flourescent antibody techniques showed no cross-reaction with *Listeria monocytogenes* or with certain other bacterial species (Marshall et al., 1959; Nelson and Shelton, 1963). *Erysipelothrix* and *Listeria* are two prominent genera of the same family but with different antigens.

Apparently all strains of *E. insidiosa* have at least one antigen in common. Precipitation tests demonstrated that there are 6 different serologic groups, designated A through E, and one group (N) which does not have antigen soluble in hydrochloric acid. Murase et al. (1959) surveyed 17 avian strains isolated in the United States and Canada. Of these, 9 were found to belong to Group A and 5 to Group B, whereas 3 had no classified antigenicity. Those workers stated that the majority of the avian strains belonged to Group A, and they found that a strain of *E. insidiosa* isolated in Japan from ducks cross-precipitated with a strain recovered from fish. That finding, they say, "supports the opinion of Iwaschina who attributed the cause of a duck epizootic which occurred in 1942 in Japan to the dried fish used as feed."

Truszczyński (1963) has shown that polysaccharide fractions of serotypes A and B contain two different antigenic components; one (composed of galactose) is the type-specific antigen, and the other (composed of xylose) is the species antigen. The additional 3 protein antigens isolated from serotypes A and N were identical. Those designated A, B, and N serotypes are not the same as the alphabetically designated antigens purified from a single unspecified serotype (Kalf and White, 1963; Kalf and Grece, 1964).

Kalf and White (1963) and Kalf and Grece (1964) have shown that the A antigen is a rather large heat-stable mucopeptide fragment of the cell wall. The B antigen differs from the A antigen in that it does not contain glucosamine and phenylalanine but does contain proline. C antigen appears to be the generic-type antigen, reacting with antiserum prepared against different serologic types of the organism. Unlike the heat-stable A and B antigens, it is heat-labile (destroyed at 100° C in 4 minutes) and is protein in nature.

The physiopathologic properties of the various isolated antigens have evidently not been ascertained.

STRAIN CLASSIFICATION

Strain classification is for the most part based on serologic activity, not biological or biochemical activity. According to White and Shuman (1961), the fermentation pattern of a particular strain did not vary to any great extent. There is no reported correlation between the serologic group or biochemical pattern of strains of *E. insidiosa* isolated from birds and the production of the septicemic, urticarial, or endocardial form of erysipelas or of the carrier state (Murase et al., 1959; White and Kalf, 1961).

PATHOGENICITY

Turkeys

Erysipelothrix insidiosa is pathogenic for turkeys at any age following exposure by a variety of parenteral routes. In natural outbreaks it appears that the organism is more pathogenic for (or causes more disease in) tom turkeys than female turkeys, whereas experimentally there is no difference. The only record of erysipelas in young poults (Rosenwald, 1940) was based on isolation of the organism from a single week-old poult and apparently did not represent a flock outbreak. In retrospect this was an infection of a single bird or may have been a laboratory contaminant.

Other Species

Virulent cultures of *E. insidiosa*, administered either subcutaneously, intramuscularly, or intraperitoneally, produced a septicemia in chickens less than 14 days old (Malik, 1962). In older birds septicemia could be produced only by intrapalpebral or subconjunctival instillation of the pathogen along with injury to that tissue. Hydrocortisone not only increased the susceptibility of the chicken to *E. insidiosa* but shortened the course of infection and increased mortality, thus appearing to increase pathogenicity. Parenteral injection of the organism regularly kills mice (*Mus musculus*), pigeons, and turkeys. Guinea pigs and chickens usually survive such injections.

PATHOGENESIS AND EPIZOOTIOLOGY

Van Es and McGrath (1936) cited Nocard and Leclainche as saying in 1903 that "at the present state of our knowledge it is impossible to explain the mysterious behavior of the contagion." Basically this is still true. Experiments have shown that the organism may be shed in the feces of a very few turkeys for up to 41 days postinoculation (Corstvet, 1967 and unpublished data). It has been shown that the organism can survive in soil (Woodbine, 1950; Blackmore and Gallagher, 1964) and that soil may serve as a source of the organism. Though soil is known to harbor the organism for long periods under certain conditions, and though swine and sheep as well as various species of wildlife can harbor the infection, no clear-cut relationship has been established even between the presence of the infection in prior years among the same species (for instance, turkeys) and subsequent outbreaks of the disease among flocks (Rosenwald and Dickinson, 1941).

NATURAL AND EXPERIMENTAL HOSTS

The organism has been isolated in nature not only from turkeys, chickens, and ducks but also from swine, sheep, cattle, marine and freshwater fish, mud hens, parrots, sparrows, canaries, finches, thrushes, blackbirds, doves, quail, wild mallards, white storks, herring gulls, golden eagles, pheasants, starlings, peacocks, parakeets, geese, various captive wild birds and mammals, chipmunks, a wide variety of rodents, meadow and house mice, dolphins, and crocodiles (Woodbine, 1950; Kilian et al., 1958; Blackmore and Gallagher, 1964; Levine, 1965; Geraci et al., 1966; Jasmin and Baucom, 1967; Faddoul et al., 1968). From the reports it appears that the susceptibilities of various avian populations differ. The age of the host evidently has no effect on whether it will be susceptible to *E. insidiosa;* no detailed research has been done in this area, however.

The experimental hosts are the pigeon, turkey, chicken, budgerigar, mouse, and rat (Blackmore and Gallagher, 1964; Geissinger, 1968a,b).

Erysipelas in chickens is relatively uncommon in the United States. It has occurred in chickens from 6 weeks to 13 months of age (Evans and Narotsky, 1954; Kilian et al., 1958; Hall, 1963). Natural outbreaks in turkeys usually occur at 20 weeks of age or older.

TRANSMISSION, CARRIERS, VECTORS

The actual portal of entry and pathogenesis of *E. insidiosa* infection in birds (and in fact in animals other than man) has not been definitively established. Contaminated material as the source of infection and entry through breaks in the mucous membranes or skin have been suggested. Experimentally Corstvet infected turkeys by per os inoculation of freshly isolated virulent organisms grown in chicken embryo yolk sac and obtained up to 50% mortality. Broth culture instilled per os, intranasally, or into the conjunctival sac (without damaging continuity of the membrane) was not infectious (Grenci, 1943). Corstvet

also found that parenteral inoculation of virulent cultures caused local multiplication followed by septicemia, resulting in 80–100% mortality in susceptible turkeys.

Sadler and Corstvet (1965) showed that some few turkeys infected subcutaneously remained carriers for variable periods. Asymptomatic carriers of *E. insidiosa* could not be detected at antemortem or postmortem inspection. The number of organisms used to challenge the turkeys, the route of inoculation (per os or parenteral), the administration of antibiotics, the time after vaccination and challenge, and the age of the turkey apparently did not influence this carrier state, which is produced in a very few turkeys. The reasons for the production of a carrier turkey are undetermined at present.

Cannibalism and fighting among birds apparently result in increased losses. Permitting carcasses of infected dead turkeys to remain on the premises to be picked at or eaten by surviving pen mates also speeds the spread and increases degree of loss, though at unpredictable rates. Erysipelas in turkeys usually results in a generalized infection. The organism can be isolated from the esophagus, proventriculus, duodenum, cecal tonsils, large intestine, cloaca, heart muscle, blood, liver, spleen, pancreas, wing and hock joints, and bone marrow. Isolations from carriers are most frequent from the cecal tonsils, cloaca, liver, and spleen (Corstvet and Holmberg, 1968; Corstvet, unpublished data).

The role of vectors in transmission is not known. Wellman (1950) found that this pathogen could be transmitted mechanically from sick mice to pigeons by the stable fly, horse fly, mosquito, and other biting flies. An outbreak of erysipelas in chickens in England reported by Hall (1963) was interesting in that the disease occured in pullets after they escaped from their pen and gained access to an area that 8 years previously had housed pigs affected with erysipelas. Hall speculated that the disease started with pullets that had gained access to the soil of a barn floor contaminated with many years of accumulated pig feces. Pullets confined nearby were not infected. Madsen (1937) suggested that rain washing contaminated feces from a sheep corral initiated an outbreak in turkeys on range.

Fish meal and fish in general have been

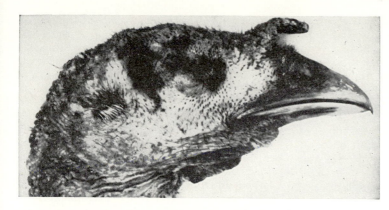

FIG. 10.2—*Erysipelas. Erysipeloid lesion on face of turkey involving major portion of eyelids and area posterior to them. (Oregon Agr. Expt. Sta.)*

cited as probable sources of infection for avian species (Murase et al., 1959; Grenci, 1943; Blackmore and Gallagher, 1964).

INCUBATION PERIOD

In natural outbreaks the incubation period cannot be readily ascertained. The disease is usually manifested in many birds at one time. Experimental subcutaneous exposure of turkeys to 10^4–10^6 organisms usually kills the majority of the turkeys in 44–70 hours; a few may die after 96–120 hours. With per os exposure, signs of infection generally occur 2–3 days later and the death rate is lower. Occasionally a turkey dies 2–3 weeks after per os exposure. A subcutaneous inoculum of 10^2 instead of 10^4 or 10^6 organisms delays clinical signs by about 24 hours. The incubation period does not seem to vary among turkeys 7, 12, 16, and 20 weeks of age, or between the sexes.

SIGNS

Turkeys

Outbreaks usually start suddenly, with losses of one to several birds, and owners may suspect that the deaths are due to poisoning, stampede injuries, or predators. A few droopy birds, especially toms, may be noticed, but these somnambulant individuals are usually easily aroused. Just prior to death there may be some very droopy birds with unsteady gait. Some birds have cutaneous lesions (Fig. 10.2), and affected males may have swollen, purplish turgid snoods (flashy tubular appendage on dorsal surface of the head) (Fig. 10.3). Gradual emaciation, weakness, and signs of anemia occur in some cases where endocarditis is the cause of death; other turkeys with vegetations (especially those in vaccinated flocks) may die suddenly without signs,

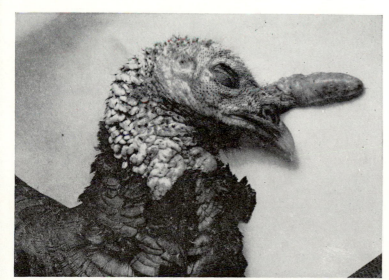

FIG. 10.3—*Erysipelas. Swollen snood with purplish discoloration which, according to Rosenwald and Dickinson, is pathognomonic for the disease. Swelling may also be seen in outbreaks of fowl cholera. (Rosenwald and Dickinson, 1941)*

probably as a result of emboli (Dickinson, unpublished data). Sudden losses of hens 4–5 days after artificial insemination, with peritonitis and perineal congestion and skin discoloration, have been reported by McDonald (unpublished data).

Other birds

The main clinical signs in chickens are general weakness, depression, diarrhea, and sudden death. In laying chickens egg production may be decreased. However, Kilian et al. (1958) reported no immediate drop in egg production in laying pullets, although signs were evident, and later there was about a 50–70% drop. Affected ducks, pheasants, and quail generally are depressed, have diarrhea, and die suddenly.

MORBIDITY AND MORTALITY

Turkeys

Morbidity and mortality are frequently about the same in turkeys unprotected by vaccination. In previously immunized flocks, however, some of the birds may be depressed and recover. Both morbidity and mortality vary, from sickness or death of occasional birds in good condition to a sudden loss of several birds within 24–48 hours. Mortality ranges from much less than 1% to as high as 25 or 50% of a given group, though adjacent groups of birds may not be affected. There have been reports of more than 12–15% mortality in unmedicated flocks, but losses reported are probably reduced by prior immunization, early treatment, or possible early sale of apparently normal birds from affected flocks. Unvaccinated turkeys inoculated parenterally with 4–10 million virulent organisms usually die at the rate of 80–100%.

Other birds

As in turkeys, morbidity and mortality rates approximate each other in other birds since most sick birds die. It is difficult to state exact figures for mortality in chickens, ducks, pheasant, quail, and turkeys, although in chickens it has been reported to be from 5% (Hall, 1963) to 25% (Evans and Narotsky, 1954).

GROSS LESIONS

The gross lesions in birds are septicemic with generalized congestion; degeneration of the fat on the anterior edge of the thigh; degeneration and hemorrhage in the pericardial fat; hemorrhage in the heart muscle; and a friable enlarged liver, spleen, and, usually, kidney. Other gross lesions may be a fibrinopurulent exudate in the joints and pericardial sac, fibrin plaques on the heart muscle, thickening of the proventriculus and gizzard wall with ulceration, small yellow nodules in the ceca, vegetative endocarditis, and dark crusty skin lesions. In ducks the lesions are similar to those observed in other avian species with the addition of dark congested areas in the webs of the foot.

In a study of field cases in turkeys, Rosenwald and Dickinson (1941) observed that most were characterized by congestion and intramuscular and subpleural hemorrhages. Of 54 necropsies of natural cases in which erysipelas was diagnosed culturally, 46 showed intramuscular or subpleural ecchymotic and suffusion hemorrhages which Beaudette and Hudson (1936) considered of great diagnostic significance. In 12 toms the tubular leader or snood was turgid with an irregular reddish-purple color (Fig. 10.3). When present, this lesion has appeared to be pathognomonic of this infection. Two birds showed cyanotic erysipeloid lesions of the skin (Fig. 10.2). One showed endocardial vegetations of the right atrioventricular muscle flap.

The liver was often swollen and mottled from congestion, with increased friability and areas of degeneration or anemic infarction. Although the liver was slightly swollen and presented a "cooked appearance" in peracute experimental cases, this condition was noted also in some of the field cases.

The spleen was consistently highly engorged with blood and was purplish black or showed diffuse congestion with petechiae and ecchymoses.

Abdominal fat was usually tinged red and petechiated. Ecchymotic and suffusion hemorrhages under the gizzard serosa were noted in many cases, especially in birds infected experimentally. All visceral blood vessels appeared highly injected. Intense enteritis, either catarrhal or sanguinocatarrhal, was seen.

Kidney and sex organs were congested and frequently showed petechiae or ecchymoses under the serous surface. Sharply outlined rose-colored spots or areas of congestion or hemorrhage were frequent on the pancreas.

Hydropericardium was common, as were petechial and ecchymotic hemorrhages on the pericardium and epicardium. Other lesions noted with varying frequency in field outbreaks were diffuse skin reddening and a dirty brick-red muscle color. An occasional bird that died had no lesions other than slight catarrhal enteritis and petechiae on the heart fat.

Postinsemination losses in turkey hens with peritonitis, subcutaneous perineal hemorrhage, or congestion have been seen (McDonald, personal communication).

Endocarditis and skin lesions are rare in experimentally infected turkeys but have been reported in some chronic cases, especially vaccinated birds (Dickinson, unpublished). In some field cases and intravenously challenged birds vaccinated twice or more with bacterin, congestive heart failure with vegetations of the atrioventricular valves (sometimes extending as much as 7 cm into the aorta) have been found. Sadler and Corstvet (1965) found carrier turkeys usually free of lesions.

IMMUNITY

Active

Published reports of the use of bacterins have dealt mainly with turkeys or swine. There is no reason, however, to suspect that bacterins would not also protect other avian species. Bacterins have been used successfully for immunizing turkeys (Adler and Nilson, 1952; Adler and Spencer, 1952; Dickinson et al., 1953; Cooper et al., 1954, 1957; Boyer and Brown, 1957; Mitrovic et al., 1961; Hinshaw, 1965; Levine, 1965). The immunity induced by proper use of a good bacterin prevents disease under field and experimental conditions. Bacterin in conjunction with penicillin at the beginning of an outbreak will usually control losses. The immunity produced in turkeys by one injection of bacterin does not last very long. Response is more effective from two or more doses at intervals of at least 2–4 weeks. Under experimental conditions, effective immunity lasted 4 weeks following subcutaneous administration of a commercial bacterin to turkeys 4 and 12 weeks old. Between 4 and 8 weeks after vaccination

the immunity, as measured by death of challenged turkeys, declined. Four weeks postvaccination, all turkeys are generally refractory to a subcutaneous challenge with 10^7 organisms; 8 weeks postvaccination, up to 39% of the vaccinates succumb from infection. Experiments with turkeys 4–7 weeks old have shown that effective immunity (one that protects against death) begins to decline between 4 and 5 weeks after vaccination.

Passive

Swine erysipelas antiserum (horse origin) has not proved uniformly successful in controlling erysipelas in various avian species. Treatment with antiserum alone is said to be of some value if administered very early, but it is not practical because of expense and lack of efficacy.

DIAGNOSIS

ISOLATION AND IDENTIFICATION OF CAUSATIVE AGENT

Since gross lesions at necropsy of birds dead from *E. insidiosa* infection are not pathognomonic and usually indicate a septicemia, diagnosis depends on demonstration and identification of the causative agent. Differentiation from fowl cholera by such isolation is especially necessary because of general similarity of outbreaks.

Rapid presumptive diagnosis is provided by the presence in liver, spleen, heart blood, or bone marrow smears of clumps and segregated gram-positive, beaded, slender, pleomorphic rods.

Isolation of the erysipelas organism from sick birds which are killed and then cultured is neither as easy nor as frequently positive as culturing from birds dead of the disease. Detecting the organism from a carrier requires multiple samples from various tissues. Finely grinding minced, affected tissue prior to inoculation into enrichment broth facilitates isolation and recovery of *E. insidiosa* from endocardial lesions which is otherwise difficult.

With birds dead from the infection, however, the liver, spleen, or bone marrow will suffice. Useful inhibitory media are the sodium azide-crystal violet medium described by Packer (1943) and the medium described by Wood (1965), which is tryptose phosphate broth with 5% horse serum plus kanomycin, neomycin, vancomycin, and novobiocin. These media are the most satisfactory ones described, though they do not completely prevent the growth of other organisms. For primary isolation, recovery is favored by inoculated solid media incubated in an atmosphere of 5–10% carbon dioxide or reduced oxygen. Ordinary atmosphere is suitable after a few passages on artificial media. Typical colonies composed of gram-positive rods are selected and placed in triple-sugar iron medium (Vickers and Bierer, 1958) or Kligler's lead acetate medium and incubated for 24 hours at 37° C. *E. insidiosa* will produce a blackening (due to H_2S production) along the line of the stab before there is a very noticeable change in the color of the medium. This is an excellent presumptive test for *E. insidiosa*.

The mouse, pigeon, or budgerigar may be used for a confirmatory protection test using erysipelas antiserum. One group of the experimental animals is inoculated parenterally with a 24-hour culture of the isolate; another group is inoculated with *E. insidiosa* antiserum and immediately thereafter with the isolate. The unprotected group should die within 4 days, whereas the animals receiving antiserum will live.

E. insidiosa may be detected in tissues using the fluorescent antibody technique (Marshall et al., 1959; Nelson and Shelton, 1963; Corstvet and Sadler, 1964). Therefore this technique may also be used as a confirmatory test in diagnosis.

Sudden losses of adolescent turkeys in good flesh but with septicemic lesions, intramuscular and subpleural ecchymotic and suffusion hemorrhages, and erysipeloid swelling of the snood point toward erysipelas. Also a significant finding is a marked hemorrhagic condition of the skin and fascial and muscular tissues of the breast. In many cases the predominant losses will be in the males; but in breeding flocks sudden losses in hens with peritonitis, subcutaneous and cutaneous discoloration, and a history of insemination just prior to this suggest *E. insidiosa* infection. The diagnosis is further validated by demonstration of the typical organisms in blood, tissues, and especially bone marrow smears or identification of the organism by culture. Particularly helpful with decomposed specimens are bone marrow culture and smear.

Since cases of hemorrhagic enteritis with subcutaneous blotch hemorrhages and other erysipelaslike lesions have been observed, and since some of the general lesions of fowl cholera in turkeys are similar, either demonstration or isolation of the organism is of critical diagnostic significance.

TREATMENT

The antibiotic of choice for an outbreak in market or breeder turkeys is a rapid-acting form of penicillin. In view of the present uncertain status of penicillin for use in food animals, label directions should be carefully followed. As soon as diagnosis is definitely established, potassium or sodium penicillin should be administered intramuscularly at the rate of about 10,000 units per pound of body weight (200,000–300,000 units), and a full dose of erysipelas bacterin administered simultaneously (see below). Control has usually been attained by giving penicillin (1,000,000 units/gal) in the drinking water as a "stopgap" measure. As the sole control measure, however, this almost invariably fails.

All birds in the affected flock should be treated. Some recommendations suggest the use of procaine penicillin or other longer-acting derivatives, and under certain circumstances these may be used successfully, but in outbreaks rapid-acting formulations are almost mandatory. Penicillin plus streptomycin can also be used. In meat-bird flocks, care should be taken to observe the required withdrawal periods for the antibiotic used.

Turkeys, and possibly other birds, with advanced signs of the disease at treatment often will not recover. Erythromycin and broad-spectrum antibiotics have been found effective in treating *E. insidiosa* (Levine, 1965; Hinshaw, 1965).

Comparative studies are lacking on the efficacy of various antibiotics for controlling *E. insidiosa* infection in avian populations, though in vitro studies have shown the organism to be resistant to neomycin (Fuzi, 1963). Sulfonamides have no value.

Oxytetracycline was not effective administered in water at the rate of 2 g/gal to turkeys infected subcutaneously with 10^7 organisms and showing signs at the time of administration of the antibiotic.

Beneficial management practices in handling an outbreak of erysipelas in a flock of turkeys include thorough decontamination of the equipment, prompt removal of dead birds and other carrion from the premises, encouraging adequate feed and water intake, and handling the birds as little and as gently as possible or practical. If unlimited range is available it might be desirable to move the flock to clean ground, but it must be realized that such a practice may contaminate the new range.

PREVENTION AND CONTROL

MANAGEMENT PROCEDURES

It has been suggested, though not established, that various stresses may make avian species more susceptible to *E. insidiosa* infection. When an outbreak has occurred in a particular pen or area on the premises, it is usually not advisable to move the infected flock to new areas, since some birds may seed the additional area by shedding the organism.

The presence of decaying material and the beginning of rainy, cold weather, which frequently coincide with sexual maturity of the birds, seem to be related to outbreaks. There seems to be an occasional relationship (Madsen, 1937) between contaminated range, previous outbreaks in the same or other species, and losses from erysipelas, though no consistent pattern has been determined.

Under the circumstances it is impossible to make clear-cut and specific recommendations for management procedures which would be successful in preventing or controlling outbreaks. A general suggestion is the use of clean disinfected equipment and the rotation of ranges for turkeys away from areas known to be previously contaminated. Certain disinfectants, notably 1–2% sodium hydroxide (lye) solution, are effective against *E. insidiosa;* phenols, *liquor cresolis compositus* and related disinfectants, iodine, and certain household soaps are moderately effective (Hinshaw, 1965). Formalin is ineffective.

Since contaminated fish meal may be a source of infection (Grenci, 1943), care in selecting feedstuffs is also recommended.

With no specific and effective recommendations for management control of this disease in turkeys, it is suggested that turkeys be properly immunized in areas where erysipelas is known to be a problem.

IMMUNIZATION

With the application of formalin-inactivated, aluminum hydroxide-adsorbed *E. insidiosa* bacterin for turkeys, a regimen of immunization can be suggested for meat turkeys as well as those kept for hatching egg production. Since the disease in other species is so sporadic, immunization for species other than turkeys is not generally recommended unless known danger from the infection occurs.

Only bacterins produced in media containing serum additives have been found effective. It is important that the strains of organisms used for bacterin preparation be immunogenic and only 1 or 2 passages removed from isolation or repassage through turkeys. There appears to be little relationship, however, between virulence and immunogenicity of a given isolate. It is also well to remember that effective immunization of mice or swine is not adequate demonstration of the ability of a bacterin to protect turkeys. Especially in the case of erysipelas, extrapolation of results from mice to turkeys is most misleading. Cultures avirulent for turkeys and without immunogenicity for them may both kill and provide protection in mice. The immunizing capacity of bacterins for turkeys can be properly assessed only with challenge of vaccinated turkeys.

Suggested for meat turkeys in areas of high risk is a single dose of the bacterin inoculated subcutaneously at the dorsal surface of the neck behind the atlas. The original investigation and demonstration of efficacy were based on intramuscular injection of the bacterin (Adler and Spencer, 1952; Dickinson et al., 1953); however, because of the possibility of sterile abscesses (with consequent downgrading at slaughter), subcutaneous inoculation is used currently. Whether the different route of inoculation accounts for the lack of immunizing efficacy reported in the last few years is not known. It might be due to a change in procedure of manufacture or a higher challenge risk.

For turkeys kept as breeders, at least two doses of the bacterin, given at intervals of no less than 4 weeks, should be administered prior to the onset of egg production.

The first dose may be given at 16–20 weeks of age (at selection time), and an additional dose (2 ml per hen and 4 ml per tom) given just prior to the beginning of lay.

Infected birds which recover without treatment are apparently solidly immune to reinfection, but so-called avirulent or modified live vaccines have not been successful in turkeys (Osebold et al., 1950). Infections aborted by treatment (Van Es et al., 1945) or with the use of antiserum apparently do not induce permanent resistance to reinfection and death. While sur-vivors of simultaneous antiserum-virulent culture inoculations were resistant, this has no practical application.

Improved bacterins properly used, adequate testing of the biologicals, planned immunization programs based on flock and premises history, and proper diagnosis of disease outbreaks as a basis for prompt treatment must be combined for most effective prevention of erysipelas.

Care should be taken in handling suspected turkeys because *E. insidiosa* is also a human pathogen.

REFERENCES

Adler, H. E., and M. A. Nilson. 1952. Immunization of turkeys against swine erysipelas with several types of bacterins. *Can. J. Comp. Med. Vet. Sci.* 16:390–93.

Adler, H. E., and G. R. Spencer. 1952. Immunization of turkeys and pigs with an erysipelas bacterin. *Cornell Vet.* 42:238–46.

Barber, Mary. 1939. A comparative study of *Listerella* and *Erysipelothrix*. *J. Pathol. Bacteriol.* 48:11–23.

Beaudette, F. R., and C. B. Hudson. 1936. An outbreak of acute swine erysipelas infection in turkeys. *J. Am. Vet. Med. Ass.* 88:475–83.

Blackmore, D. K., and G. L. Gallagher. 1964. An outbreak of erysipelas in captive wild birds and mammals. *Vet. Record* 76:1161–64.

Boyer, C. I., and J. A. Brown. 1957. Studies on erysipelas in turkeys. *Avian Diseases* 1:42–52.

Cooper, M. S., G. R. Personeus, and B. R. Choman. 1954. Laboratory studies on the vaccination of mice and turkeys with an *Erysipelothrix rhusiopathiae* vaccine. *Can. J. Comp. Med. Vet. Sci.* 18:83–92.

Cooper, M. S., G. R. Personeus, and R. C. Percival. 1957. Laboratory studies on erysipelas. 4. Duration of immunity in turkeys vaccinated with an adsorbed vaccine. *Poultry Sci.* 36:266–69.

Corstvet, R. E. 1967. Pathogenesis of *Erysipelothrix insidiosa* in the turkey. *Poultry Sci.* 46:1247. (Abstr.)

Corstvet, R. E., and C. H. Holmberg. 1968. The carrier state of *Erysipelothrix insidiosa* in turkeys. *Poultry Sci.* 47:1662. (Abstr.)

Corstvet, R. E., and W. W. Sadler. 1964. The diagnosis of certain avian diseases with fluorescent antibody technique. *Poultry Sci.* 43:1280–88.

Dickinson, E. M., A. C. Jerstad, H. E. Adler, M. Cooper, W. E. Babcock, E. E. Johns, and C. A. Bottorff. 1953. The use of an *Erysipelothrix rhusiopathiae* bacterin for the control of erysipelas in turkeys. *Proc. 90th Ann. Meet. Am. Vet. Med. Ass.,* pp. 370–75.

Evans, W. M., and S. Narotsky. 1954. Two field cases of *Erysipelothrix rhusiopathiae* infection in chickens. *Cornell Vet.* 44:32–35.

Faddoul, G. R., G. W. Fellows, and J. Baird. 1968. Erysipelothrix infection in starlings. *Avian Diseases* 12:61–66.

Fuzi, M. 1963. A neomycin sensitivity test for the rapid differentiation of *Listeria monocytogenes* and *Erysipelothrix rhusiopathiae*. *J. Pathol. Bacteriol.* 85:524–25.

Geissinger, H. D. 1968a. Acute and chronic *Erysipelothrix rhusiopathiae* infection in white mice. *J. Comp. Pathol. Therap.* 78:79–88.

———. 1968b. Acute and chronic *Erysipelothrix rhusiopathiae* infection in rats. *Zentr. Veterinaermed.* (B) 15:392–405.

Geraci, J. R., R. M. Sauer, and W. Medway. 1966. Erysipelas in dolphins. *Am. J. Vet. Res.* 27:597–606.

Graham, R., N. D. Levine, and H. R. Hester. 1939. *Erysipelothrix rhusiopathiae* associated with a fatal disease in ducks. *J. Am. Vet. Med. Ass.* 95:211–16.

Grenci, Catherine M. 1943. The isolation of *Erysipelothrix rhusiopathiae* and experimental infection of turkeys. *Cornell Vet.* 33:56–60.

Hall, S. A. 1963. A disease in pullets due to *Erysipelothrix rhusiopathiae*. *Vet. Record* 75:333–34.

Hinshaw, W. R. 1965. Erysipelas in turkeys, pp. 1271–76. In Biester, H. E., and L. H. Schwarte (eds.), *Diseases of Poultry,* 5th ed. Iowa State Univ. Press, Ames.

Hudson, C. B. 1949. *Erysipelothrix rhusiopathiae* infection in fowl. *J. Am. Vet. Med. Ass.* 115:36–39.

Hudson, C. B., J. J. Black, J. A. Bivins, and D. C. Tudor. 1952. Outbreaks of *Erysipelothrix rhusiopathiae* infection in fowl. *J. Am. Vet. Med. Ass.* 121:278–84.

Jasmin, A. M., and J. Baucom. 1967. *Erysipe-

lothrix insidiosa infections in the caiman *(Caiman crocodilus)* and the American crocodile *(Crocodilus acutus)*. *Am. J. Vet. Clin. Pathol.* 1:173–77.

Kalf, G. F., and Mary Ann Grece. 1964. The antigenic components of *Erysipelothrix rhusiopathiae*. III. Purification of B- and C-antigens. *Arch. Immunol. Therap. Exp.* 107:141–46.

Kalf, G. F., and T. G. White. 1963. The antigenic components of *Erysipelothrix rhusiopathiae*. II. Purification and chemical characterization of a type-specific antigen. *Arch. Immunol. Therap. Exp.* 102:39–47.

Kilian, J. G., W. E. Babcock, and E. M. Dickinson. 1958. Two cases of *Erysipelothrix rhusiopathiae* infection in chickens. *J. Am. Vet. Med. Ass.* 133:560–62.

Klauder, J. V. 1926. Erysipeloid and swine erysipelas in man. *J. Am. Med. Ass.* 86:536–41.

———. 1944. *Erysipelothrix rhusiopathiae* infection in swine and in human beings. Comparative study of cutaneous lesions. *Arch. Dermatol.* 50:151–59.

Klauder, J. V., D. W. Kramer, and Leslie Nicholas. 1943. *Erysipelothrix rhusiopathiae* septicemia: Diagnosis and treatment. Report of a fatal case of erysipeloid. *J. Am. Med. Ass.* 122:938–43.

Levine, N. D. 1965. Erysipelas, pp. 461–69. In Biester, H. E., and L. H. Schwarte (eds.), *Diseases of Poultry*. Iowa State Univ. Press, Ames.

Madsen, D. E. 1937. An erysipelas outbreak in turkeys. *J. Am. Vet. Med. Ass.* 91:206–8.

Malik, Z. 1962. Susceptibility of chicks to experimental rhusiopathiae infection. (Translated title. Synopsis in English; text in Russian.) *Vet. Casopis* 11:89–94.

Marshall, J. D., W. C. Eveland, and C. W. Smith. 1959. The identification of viable and nonviable *Erysipelothrix insidiosa* with fluorescent antibody. *Am. J. Vet. Res.* 20:1077–80.

Mitrovic, M., P. J. Matisheck, and L. C. Lynch. 1961. Studies on the antigenicity in turkeys of an erysipelas bacterin made from *Erysipelothrix rhusiopathiae* strains H_4 and H_7. *Avian Diseases* 5:328–33.

Murase, N., K. Suzuke, and T. Nakahara. 1959. Studies on the typing of *Erysipelothrix rhusiopathiae*. II. Serological behaviours of the strains isolated from fowls including those from cattle and humans. *Japan. J. Vet. Sci.* 21:177–81.

Nelson, J. D., and Sharon Shelton. 1963. Immunofluorescent studies of *Listeria monocytogenes* and *Erysipelothrix insidiosia*. *J. Lab. Clin. Med.* 62:935–42.

Osebold, J. W., E. M. Dickinson, and W. E. Babcock. 1950. Immunization of turkeys against *Erysipelothrix rhusiopathiae* with avirulent live culture. *Cornell Vet.* 40:387–91.

Packer, R. A. 1943. The use of sodium azide (NaN_3) and crystal violet in a selective medium for streptococci and *Erysipelothrix rhusiopathiae*. *J. Bacteriol.* 46:343–49.

Rosenwald, A. S. 1940. Swine erysipelas in a week-old turkey poult. *J. Am. Vet. Med. Ass.* 96:268–69.

Rosenwald, A. S., and E. M. Dickinson. 1941. A report of swine erysipelas in turkeys. *Am. J. Vet. Res.* 2:202–13.

Sadler, W. W., and R. E. Corstvet. 1965. The effect of *Erysipelothrix insidiosa* infection on wholesomeness of market turkeys. *Am. J. Vet. Res.* 26:1429–36.

Silberstein, E. P. 1965. *Erysipelothrix* endocarditis. Report of a case with cerebral manifestations. *J. Am. Med. Ass.* 191:862–64.

Truszczyński, M. 1963. Immunological characterization of antigenic extracts obtained from bacteria with different methods. II. Serotypes of *Erysipelothrix insidiosa*. *Arch. Immunol. Therap. Exp.* 11:259–79.

Vallee, M. 1930. Sur l'etiologie du rouget. *Rev. Pathol. Comparee* 30:857–58. (Abstr.)

Van Es, L., and C. B. McGrath. 1936. Swine erysipelas. *Nebraska Agr. Expt. Sta. Res. Bull.* 84:1–47.

Van Es, L., J. F. Olney, and I. C. Blore. 1945. The effect of penicillin on *E. rhusiopathiae* infected pigeons. *Nebraska Agr. Expt. Sta. Res. Bull.* 141:1–15.

Vickers, C. L., and B. W. Bierer. 1958. Triple sugar iron agar as an aid in the diagnosis of erysipelas. *J. Am. Vet. Med. Ass.* 133:543–44.

Wellmann, G. 1950. The transmission of swine erysipelas by a variety of blood-sucking insects to pigeons. *Zentr. Bakteriol. Parasitenk. Abt. I. Orig.* 155:109–15.

White, T. G., and G. F. Kalf. 1961. The antigenic components of *Erysipelothrix rhusiopathiae*. I. Isolation and serological classification. *Arch. Biochem. Biophys.* 95:458–63.

White, T. G., and R. D. Shuman. 1961. Fermentation reactions of *Erysipelothrix rhusiopathiae*. *J. Bacteriol.* 82:595–99.

Wood, R. F. 1965. A selective liquid medium utilizing antibiotics for isolation of *Erysipelothrix insidiosa*. *Am. J. Vet. Res.* 26:1303–8.

Woodbine, M. 1950. *Erysipelothrix rhusiopathiae*. Bacteriology and chemotherapy. *Bacteriol. Rev.* 14:161–78.

CHAPTER 11

ULCERATIVE ENTERITIS (QUAIL DISEASE)

M. C. PECKHAM

Department of Avian Diseases
New York State Veterinary College
Cornell University
Ithaca, New York

ULCERATIVE ENTERITIS is an acute bacterial infection in young chickens, turkey poults, and upland game birds characterized by sudden onset and rapidly increasing mortality. The disease was first seen in quail in enzootic proportions and was termed "quail disease." However, it has since been recognized that many avian species other than quail are susceptible, and the species designation has been superseded by the pathological term "ulcerative enteritis," pending precise identification of the etiological agent.

Increasing outbreaks of the disease have occurred in broiler and replacement flocks the past few years and represent a substantial loss to the poultry industry (Angstrom, 1968, personal communication). The constant threat of this disease to our game birds, either in confinement or in the wild, constitutes a menace to our wildlife conservation programs.

The infection of humans with this disease has not been reported.

HISTORY

One of the first reports of quail disease in the United States was by Morse (1907), who indicated that the disease was causing serious losses in quail and grouse in Great Britain and was becoming a menace to the game bird population of the United States.

The next two decades yielded several scattered reports of outbreaks in quail and grouse (Gallagher, 1924; Levine, 1932; Barger et al., 1934; LeDune, 1935). Infection in wild turkeys was reported by Shillinger and Morley (1934), and Bullis and Van Roekel (1944) first reported the disease in domestic turkey poults. Other domestic birds found susceptible were the pigeon (Glover, 1951; Peckham, 1963) and the chicken (Shillinger and Morley, 1934; Witter, 1952; Jungherr, 1955). The pheasant, blue grouse, and California quail were added to the list of susceptible game birds by Buss et al. (1958). Periodically reports were published as to the identity of the etiological agent, but complete agreement was lacking (Morley and Wetmore, 1936; Bass, 1939, 1941b; Peckham, 1959, 1960). Treatment of ulcerative enteritis with sulfonamides gave unfavorable results as reported by Churchill and Coburn (1945) and Rosen and Bischoff (1949). The first breakthrough in treatment was the discovery by Kirkpatrick et al. (1950) that streptomycin was highly effective.

INCIDENCE AND DISTRIBUTION

The incidence of the disease during the past decade is increasing, as indicated by reports of the diagnostic laboratories. Ulcerative enteritis represented 9% of all poultry diagnostic accessions between the ages of 4 and 20 weeks (N.Y.S. Vet. Coll. Ann. Rept. 1966–67). The disease is widespread throughout the poultry industry in the United States. Harris (1961) reported several outbreaks occurring in quail reared in England.

ETIOLOGY

The isolation and identification of the etiologic agent have been the subject of several investigations. Morley and Wetmore (1936) reported the isolation of an organism from the liver of diseased quail with which they produced ulcerative enteritis when inoculated into quail. The organism, which they named *Corynebacterium perdicum,* was described as a gram-positive, pleomorphic, aerobic, nonmotile rod. The organism could not be isolated on solid media and on primary culture grew poorly in fluid media. The organism retained its virulence for 7 subcultures but the majority of cultures soon lost their virulence.

Bass (1941a) described the isolation of a

gram-negative, anaerobic bacillus from the intestine and liver of infected quail. He used thioglycollate media modified by the addition of 0.1% agar and was able to reproduce the clinical syndrome by feeding quail cultures grown in artificial media.

Durant and Doll (1941) tested 70 bacterial cultures they had isolated from quail by aerobic and anaerobic culture. None of these cultures reproduced ulcerative enteritis when fed to quail. On the basis of histological studies and the character of the disease, they concluded the disease was probably of bacterial origin.

Peckham (1959, 1960) reported on the isolation of a gram-positive, spore-forming rod from the blood, liver, and intestine of infected quail. When this organism was fed or injected into quail they died in 48–96 hours with lesions of ulcerative enteritis. The same organism was isolated from the livers of chickens and turkeys affected with ulcerative enteritis and was capable of reproducing the clinical syndrome when fed to quail, thus establishing that the disease seen in chickens, turkeys, and quail was caused by the same organism.

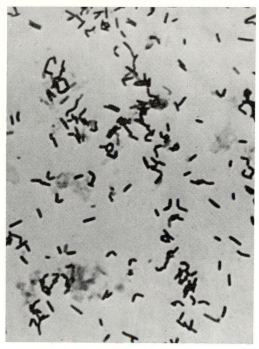

FIG. 11.1—*Smear of quail bacillus from 48-hour culture on yolk agar.* ×1,000.

CLASSIFICATION

The organisms isolated by Bass (1939) and Peckham (1959, 1960) have not been classified.

MORPHOLOGY AND STAINING

The bacillus described by Peckham (1959) is 3–4μ long and occurs singly as a straight rod or a slightly curved rod with rounded ends. Occasionally organisms undergoing binary fission are found joined at the ends by a fine strand. It was noted that variations in morphology occurred with continued passage in artificial media. Coccoid forms, pleomorphic forms, and chains were sometimes seen (Fig. 11.1). However, the organism still retained its rod-shaped morphology after 14 serial passages in embryos. In embryo cultures subterminal spores are readily formed. The spores occupy the terminal third of the cell and have a cylindrical form with rounded ends (Fig. 11.2) and stain readily with Wirtz spore stain. The bacillus is gram-positive in young cultures, in smears from liver with focal areas of necrosis, and in yolk smears from dead embryos. Organisms in old cultures lose the gram-positive stain more readily than those from fresh cultures.

GROWTH REQUIREMENTS

The organism is fastidious in its growth requirements when first isolated from birds. Enriched media and reduced oxygen tension facilitate growth. Peckham (1959, 1960) first isolated the organism in the yolk sac of embryonating chicken eggs. Yolk harvested from the dead embryos was inoculated into thioglycollate medium enriched with 3–10% horse serum or defibrinated horse blood. After adaptation to thioglycollate, growth occurred as a granular mass in the lower two-thirds of the tube. Following 8–10 serial passages in thioglycollate at 48–96-hour intervals, growth was established on yolk agar, PPLO agar (Difco) with 3% serum fraction, Dorset's egg slants without glycerol, Loeffler's serum agar slants, and 5% horse blood agar incubated in 10% CO_2, 63% methane, and 27% air. Macheak (1960, personal communication) inoculated yolk cultures into many types of broth media used in anaerobe propagation and differentiation, but multiplication was attained only in brain-liver and Thiogel (Difco) media. After 6 serial passages in brain-liver medium he obtained growth on freshly poured egg yolk agar plates in-

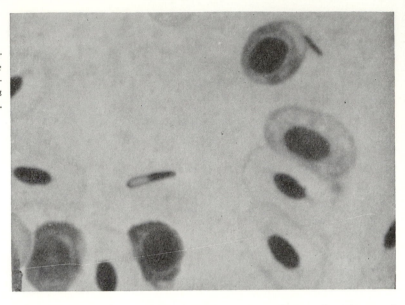

FIG. 11.2—Blood smear from quail with ulcerative enteritis. Note two bacteria, one of which has a subterminal spore. ×2700.

cubated either aerobically or anaerobically for 4–5 days. Growth was more rapid under aerobic conditions provided high humidity was maintained in the incubator.

COLONIAL MORPHOLOGY

On yolk agar light growth occurs in 48 hours as discrete, smooth, raised, white, circular colonies 1–2 mm in size. After adaptation, growth is not as moist and becomes confluent (Peckham, 1960). Macheak (1960, personal communication) reported three types of colonial growth were evident on yolk agar. One type of colony ranged in size from pinpoint to 1 mm, was round and transparent, and when viewed under the dissecting microscope was observed to grow on the surface of the agar as well as at various subsurface levels. The second type of colony occurred as a spreading mucoid growth with lobated margin and gray-white color. The third type of colony was discrete, round, white, with an entire margin, and somewhat raised with an umbonate center.

BIOCHEMICAL PROPERTIES

Because of the difficulty in cultivating this organism in artificial media its biochemical properties have not been determined.

RESISTANCE TO CHEMICAL AND PHYSICAL AGENTS

The effect of chemicals and disinfectants on the ulcerative enteritis organism has not been studied. The organism by virtue of its spore-forming capabilities is extremely resistant and will remain viable after storage at −20° C for 5 years. It will survive 70° C for 3 hours, 80° C for 1 hour, and 100° C for 3 minutes (Peckham, 1960). The resistance of the organism to heat facilitates isolation as it can be freed of bacterial and viral contaminants by heat treatment.

PATHOGENICITY

Yolk cultures are pathogenic for quail by intramuscular, intraperitoneal, and oral routes of administration. Cultures grown on artificial media were not pathogenic. Death occurred within 1–3 days following intramuscular and intraperitoneal inoculation and within 3–12 days following oral inoculation. A large white area of degeneration occurred at the site of intramuscular injection (Peckham, 1960).

PATHOGENESIS AND EPIZOOTIOLOGY

NATURAL AND EXPERIMENTAL HOSTS

Ulcerative enteritis is found in a wide range of avian hosts, but quail are undoubtedly among the most susceptible species. Natural infections were found in the following species: common bobwhite (*Colinus virginianus*), California quail (*Lophortyx californicus vallicola*), Gambel quail (*Lophortyx gambeli*), mountain quail (*Oreortyx pictus*), scaled quail (*Callipepla squamata*), and sharp-tailed grouse (*Pedioecetes phasianellus campestris*)

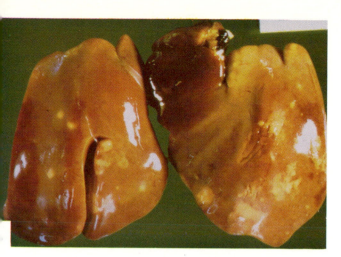

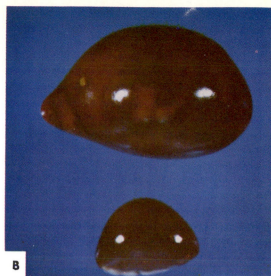

B

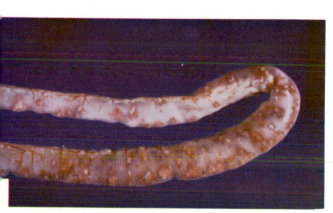

FIG. 11.5—Lesions of ulcerative enteritis. (A) Focal areas of necrosis in liver of chicken. (B) Enlarged hemorrhagic and necrotic spleen compared to normal spleen below. (C) Yellowish lenticular ulcers visible through serosal surface of intestine. (D) Ulceration of intestinal mucosa of affected bird.

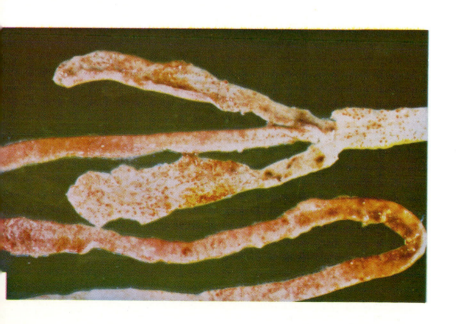

(Morse, 1907); ruffed grouse *(Bonasa umbellus)* (Levine, 1932); domestic turkey *(Meleagris gallopavo)* and chicken *(Gallus gallus domesticus)* (Shillinger and Morley, 1934; Durant and Doll, 1941); European partridge *(Perdix perdix)* and wild turkey *(Meleagris gallopavo)* (Durant and Doll, 1941); chukar partridge *(Alectoris graeca)* (Levine and Goble, 1947); pigeon *(Columba livia)* (Glover, 1951); pheasant *(Phasianus colchicus)* and blue grouse *(Dendragapus obscurus)* (Buss et al., 1958); and crested quail *(Lophortyx c. californicus)* (Harris, 1961).

Experimental infections have proved easiest in the quail, although chickens are frequently infected under natural conditions. The disease in chickens often accompanies or follows coccidiosis, hemorrhagic syndrome, and other diseases and stress conditions. Infectious material of known virulence for quail failed to reproduce the infection when repeatedly fed to pigeons, rabbits, guinea pigs, and white mice (Shillinger and Morley, 1934). Intraperitoneal injections of yolk cultures were nonpathogenic for 3-week-old mice (Peckham, 1959). The organism was nonpathogenic for guinea pigs when injected into the thigh muscles using the calcium chloride technique described by Smith (1954). Shillinger and Morley (1934) demonstrated that the disease in chickens was the same that occurred in quail by feeding intestinal contents from chickens to quail and producing ulcerative enteritis.

The disease is more frequently seen in young birds, with cases occurring in chickens 4–12 weeks of age (Peckham, 1960), in turkeys 3–8 weeks of age (Bullis and Van Roekel, 1944), and in quail 4–12 weeks of age. An outbreak was reported in adult quail by Kirkpatrick and Moses (1953).

TRANSMISSION

The disease can readily be transmitted to quail by feeding feces or intestinal suspensions from infected birds (Bass, 1941a). Peckham (1960) transmitted the disease from chickens and turkeys to quail by feeding intestinal suspensions or liver suspensions taken from infected birds. Levine (1932) was able to transmit the infection to grouse by giving them flies that had been allowed to feed on intestinal contents. The "carrier" status of recovered birds or survivors in a flock has not been critically studied. Morris (1948) stated that the chronic carrier has been established as one of the most important factors in perpetuation of the disease and described the use of the complement fixation test to detect carriers.

INCUBATION PERIOD

The acute form of the disease following experimental infection resulted in death within 1–3 days. The course of the disease in a flock following experimental infection is approximately 3 weeks, with the peak of mortality occurring 5–14 days postinoculation. Bass (1941b) stated that when wide distribution had occurred in quail stock, it took 6–10 months for all infected birds to die.

SIGNS

Birds dying acutely may exhibit no premonitory signs. These birds are usually well muscled and fat and have feed in the crops. Quail often exhibit watery white droppings (Fig. 11.3). As the disease progresses infected birds become listless, humped up, with eyes partly closed and feathers dull and ruffled. In birds affected a week or longer there is a marked atrophy of the pectoral muscles leading to extreme emaciation.

MORBIDITY AND MORTALITY

Losses in young quail may approach 100% in a matter of a few days. In chickens losses range from 2 to 10%. As chickens are more resistant to ulcerative enteritis than quail, recovery following infection is more likely to occur.

GROSS LESIONS

Gross lesions are variable in extent and number, depending upon the time elapsing between infection and death. Acute lesions in quail are characterized by a marked hemorrhagic enteritis in the duodenum. Small punctate hemorrhages may be visible in the intestinal wall. In chronic cases the lesions become more prominent and extensive. Ulcers may occur in any portion of the intestine and ceca (Fig. 11.4). Small yellow foci with hemorrhagic borders may be seen on the serosal and mucosal surfaces (Fig. 11.5-C, D). As the ulcers increase in size, the hemorrhagic border tends to disappear. The ulcers may be lenticular or roughly circular in outline and sometimes

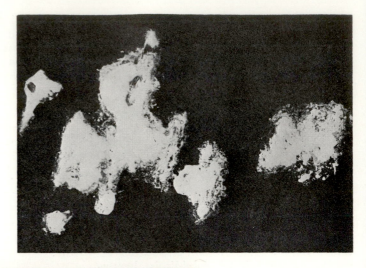

FIG. 11.3—Ulcerative enteritis. Characteristic watery white droppings from infected quail.

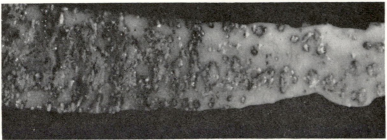

FIG. 11.4—Ulceration of intestinal mucosa of chicken.

coalesce to form large necrotic diphtheritic patches. The lenticular shape is more common in the upper portion of the intestine. The ulcers may be deep in the mucosa, or in older lesions they may be superficial and have raised edges (Fig. 11.6). Ulcers in the ceca may have a central depression filled with dark-staining material that cannot be rinsed off. Perforation of the ulcers commonly occurs resulting in peritonitis and intestinal adhesions.

Liver lesions vary from a light yellow mottling to large irregular yellow areas of necrosis along the edges (Fig. 11.5-A). Other liver lesions are disseminated gray foci or small yellow circumscribed foci which are sometimes surrounded by a light yellow halo effect. The spleen may be congested, enlarged, and hemorrhagic (Fig. 11.5-B). Gross lesions are absent in the other organs. Peckham (1960) described an unusual lesion of ulcerative enteritis in poults characterized by a necrotic, diphtheritic membrane occupying the middle third of the intestine. This combination of necrosis and sloughing of the intestinal mucosa ap-

peared similar to the lesion produced by *Eimeria brunetti* infection in chickens (Fig. 11.7).

HISTOPATHOLOGY

A detailed description of the histopathology of ulcerative enteritis in quail was given by Durant and Doll (1941). Intestinal sections from acute cases revealed desquamation of mucosal epithelium, edema of the intestinal wall, vascular engorgement, and lymphocytic infiltration. The lumen of the intestine contained desquamated epithelium, blood cells, and fragments of mucosa. Early ulcers were small hemorrhagic necrotizing areas involving the villi and penetrating into the submucosa. Cells adjacent to these areas exhibited coagulation necrosis with karyolysis and karyorrhexis. Lymphocytic and granulocytic infiltration occurred in the area adjacent to the necrosis. Small clumps of bacteria were present in the necrotic tissue. Older ulcers appeared as thick masses of granular acidophilic coagulated material mixed with cellular detritus and bacteria (Fig. 11.8). Gran-

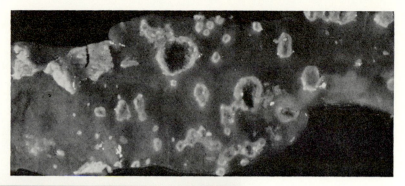

FIG. 11.6—Craterlike ulcerations in intestines from natural case of ulcerative enteritis in poult.

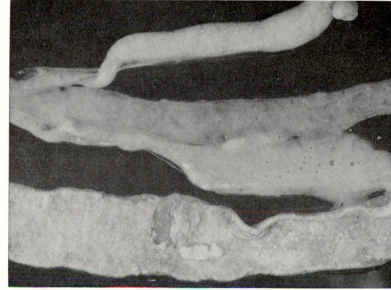

FIG. 11.7—Necrotic diphtheritic membrane in intestine of poult with "quail disease."

ulocytes and lymphocytes infiltrated the area surrounding the ulcer (Fig. 11.9). In the submucosa and muscularis small blood vessels near the ulcers were occasionally occluded by bacteria. Liver lesions comprised clearly demarcated foci of necrosis scattered through the parenchyma (Harris, 1961; Fig. 11.10).

IMMUNITY

In some cases it appears that active immunity is stimulated in the survivors of a natural outbreak. Kirkpatrick et al. (1950) challenged 22 survivors of a natural outbreak without any noticeable effect. The controls had 85% mortality. However, it has been observed by several investigators that survivors in groups treated with antibiotics may remain highly susceptible to infection (Kirkpatrick et al., 1952b; Peckham, 1962). This susceptibility was not influenced by variations in dosage of anti-

biotics, the time when treatment was administered in relation to onset of infection, or duration of treatment.

DIAGNOSIS

The diagnosis of ulcerative enteritis has depended primarily upon clinical and pathological findings. The presence of typical intestinal ulceration accompanied by necrosis of the liver is usually the basis for a clinical diagnosis. Syndromes that resemble ulcerative enteritis must be considered in making a differential diagnosis. As an aid in confirming the diagnosis, a stained smear of the liver will reveal the causative rod-shaped bacilli, subterminal spores, and free spores.

ISOLATION AND IDENTIFICATION
OF CAUSATIVE AGENT

Peckham (1959, 1960) reported in detail techniques for isolation and cultivation of

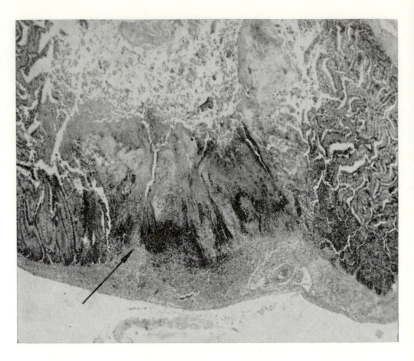

FIG. 11.8—Transverse section of quail intestine with large ulceration. ×80.

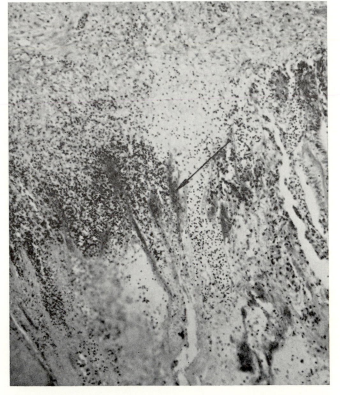

FIG. 11.9—Higher magnification of area indicated by arrow in Fig. 11.8. Note cellular infiltration and dark linear masses (arrow) of bacteria. ×160.

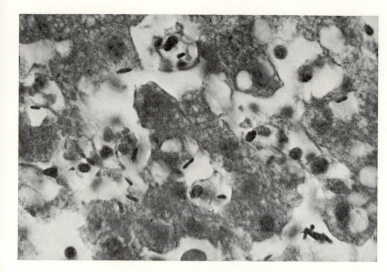

FIG. 11.10—*Histological section of quail liver revealing necrosis and presence of ulcerative enteritis organisms. Gram, ×2,700.*

the causative bacterium. Although the organism is found in the liver, intestine, and occasionally blood of infected birds, it is very fastidious in its growth requirements. The preferred technique for primary isolation is inoculation of liver suspensions into the yolk sac of 5–7-day-old embryonated chicken eggs which will die 48–72 hours postinoculation. Embryos inoculated via the chorioallantoic sac usually survive. The bacilli and spores can be readily seen in yolk smears of dead embryos. Growth of the organism in artificial media can be accomplished by inoculating yolk cultures into thioglycollate enriched with 10% horse serum. The fact that the bacillus is a spore former and resistant to heating facilitates isolation. Liver samples that might contain surface contamination can be prepared for embryo or media inoculation by triturating the tissue with a small amount of diluent followed by heating at 80° C for 20 minutes or 100° C for 3 minutes. As biochemical and serological properties of the organism have not been adequately studied to identify it, the only means of proving isolation of the causative agent is by oral inoculation of quail.

SEROLOGY

Morris (1948) described the use of the complement fixation test in the detection of ulcerative enteritis in quail. He stated that the chronic carrier was an important factor in the perpetuation of ulcerative enteritis and developed a complement fixation test to detect these carriers. Antigen was prepared from livers and hearts of birds dying with quail disease. Details for performing the test are described in the report. The specificity of the test was demonstrated in a field trial consisting of 403 birds; 46 birds reacted positively to the test and 9 of these died of quail disease. There was no mortality in the group reacting negatively.

DIFFERENTIAL DIAGNOSIS

The lesions caused by ulcerative enteritis could be mistaken for those of coccidiosis, hemorrhagic syndrome, and histomoniasis. Frequently coccidiosis precedes or accompanies ulcerative enteritis (Fig. 11.11). Both diseases may be present in the same or different specimens submitted for diagnosis (Witter, 1952; Peckham, 1959). Bullis and Van Roekel (1944) noted that coccidiosis and ulcerative enteritis were often associated in poults. Buss et al. (1958) found coccidia in pheasants affected with ulcerative enteritis. It is vital that the diagnostician make a distinction between the two diseases as treatment for one disease may be valueless or even harmful for the other. Jungherr (1955) indicated that ulcerative enteritis was increasing in turkey poults and chickens (Fig. 11.12). He stated that some cases of coccidiosis did not respond to the usual coccidiostats because of complications with ulcerative enteritis, and only when the treatment was changed to antibiotics or furazolidone did the flock improve.

Chickens with ulcerative enteritis manifest signs similar to those of coccidiosis; consequently many flock owners medicate

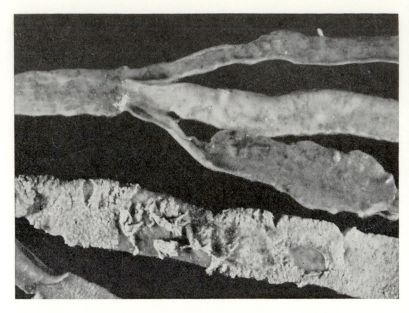

FIG. 11.11—Combined ulcerative enteritis and E. brunetti infection in intestine of chicken. Note small ulcers in ceca and rectum. Diphtheritic membrane is due to coccidial infection.

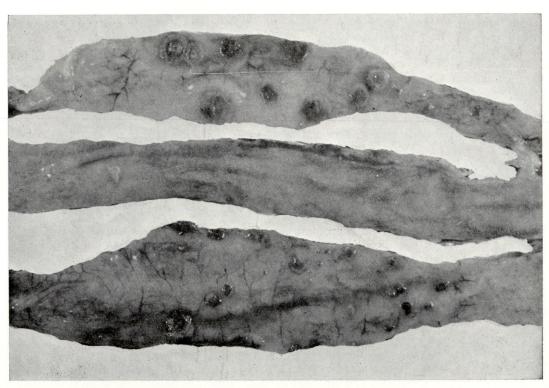

FIG. 11.12—Cecal ulcerations in poult affected with ulcerative enteritis.

with a coccidiostat before obtaining a diagnosis. Sulfonamides are widely used in the control of coccidiosis but have proved ineffective against ulcerative enteritis. Churchill and Coburn (1945) reported the failure of sulfaguanidine, sulfathalidine, and sulfasuxidine to prevent infection in artificially infected quail. Rosen and Bischoff (1949) reported that 1% sulfamethazine and 0.25% sulfaquinoxaline in mash feed for 3 days had no effect on the course of ulcerative enteritis in quail.

Coccidiosis does not cause focal necrosis in the liver and an enlarged hemorrhagic spleen. When these lesions are accompanied by ulcerations in the ceca and intestine, the diagnostician can make a presumptive diagnosis of ulcerative enteritis. Supportive evidence can readily be obtained by staining liver smears to demonstrate the bacilli and spores.

The hemorrhagic syndrome may produce punctate hemorrhages in the wall of the intestine and irregular light-colored areas on the edges of the liver similar to lesions of ulcerative enteritis. However, pale bone marrow and intramuscular hemorrhages are commonly found in hemorrhagic syndrome but rarely in ulcerative enteritis. It is not uncommon for flocks affected with hemorrhagic syndrome to have ulcerative enteritis as a complicating disease. Gray et al. (1954) noted intestinal and cecal ulcerations with large areas of necrosis in the liver of chickens with hemorrhagic disease. All of the flocks had been treated with coccidiostats to no avail. Although adequate therapy is lacking for hemorrhagic syndrome, prompt recognition of ulcerative enteritis affords early treatment of this condition.

Histomoniasis produces caseous cores in the ceca and necrotic areas of varying size in the liver. This combination of cecal and liver lesions seen in chickens, poults, and other birds makes it imperative that the cecal ulcerations and liver necrosis of ulcerative enteritis be distinguished from histomoniasis. An enlarged hemorrhagic spleen and intestinal ulcerations are characteristic of ulcerative enteritis. Histological examination of the liver or ceca will reveal the histomonads.

TREATMENT

Kirkpatrick et al. (1950, 1952a,b) and Kirkpatrick and Moses (1953) reported that streptomycin administered by injection or in water or feed had a prophylactic and therapeutic value against ulcerative enteritis in quail. Chloromycetin at a level of 500 g per ton of mash gave complete protection. Streptomycin at a level of 60 g per ton of mash gave complete protection when administered prophylactically. One gram of streptomycin per gallon of drinking water gave complete protection when administered prior to or concomitant with artificial infection. The majority of quail that survived following treatment with streptomycin or chloromycetin remained highly susceptible to reexposure. After reexposure of the survivors from groups treated with streptomycin in the water, Kirkpatrick concluded that development of immunity was not influenced by variations in dosage of antibiotic, time when treatment was started, or duration of treatment. Kirkpatrick and Moses (1953) treated a natural outbreak of ulcerative enteritis with 5 g streptomycin/gal drinking water for 1 day, followed by 1 g per gal for 19 days. The treated birds sustained 4% mortality and the controls 21%.

Peckham and Reynolds (1962) reported on the efficacy of furazolidone, bacitracin, streptomycin, and chlortetracycline in the control of experimental ulcerative enteritis in quail. Their results confirmed those of Kirkpatrick et al. (1952b); it was found that prophylactic administration of streptomycin at a level of 2 g per gal of drinking water for 25 days gave complete protection against artificial exposure. One hundred grams of bacitracin per ton of feed also gave complete protection. However, 40% mortality was experienced in the groups receiving 200 g of furazolidone or chlortetracycline per ton of mash. In one drug trial, quail receiving streptomycin in the water or bacitracin in the feed were completely refractory to challenge after medication was discontinued. However, in another trial two groups receiving bacitracin were 100% susceptible to challenge after discontinuing medication.

PREVENTION AND CONTROL

MANAGEMENT PROCEDURES

Ulcerative enteritis in chickens tends to follow in the wake of other diseases such as coccidiosis and hemorrhagic syndrome. Therefore, management procedures designed to control these diseases will also aid in reducing losses from ulcerative enteritis. It has been noted that ulcerative enteritis tends to recur on the same farm in each succeeding flock, and a meticulous and vigorous clean-up program should ensue between new lots of birds. As the infectious organism is in the droppings and remains viable indefinitely in the litter, every precaution should be used to prevent carrying the infection from one group to another.

Game farm managers should exercise caution with regard to overgrazing ranges or overcrowding birds. Placing birds on 0.5-in wire mesh is recommended on farms where the disease is a problem. Survivors of an outbreak may be carriers and should not be mixed with unexposed birds.

IMMUNIZATION

In preliminary studies Bass (1941b) reported that he was able to immunize quail by intramuscular injection of killed cultures. Peckham (1962) reported the results of 4 preliminary trials in which attempts were made to immunize quail by single and multiple intramuscular injections of heat-attenuated or untreated yolk cultures. Although some trials gave encouraging results, others indicated no protection was given by the vaccination procedures. At the present time vaccines or techniques for their production are not available for ulcerative enteritis.

REFERENCES

Barger, E. H., S. E. Park, and R. Graham. 1934. A note on so-called quail disease. *J. Am. Vet. Med. Ass.* 84:776–83.

Bass, C. C. 1939. Observations on the specific cause and nature of "quail disease" or ulcerative enteritis in quail. *Proc. Soc. Exp. Biol. Med.* 42:377–80.

———. 1941a. Quail disease—Some important facts about it. *Louisiana Conserv. Rev. Summer*, pp. 11–14.

———. 1941b. Specific cause and nature of ulcerative enteritis of quail. *Proc. Soc. Exp. Biol. Med.* 46:250–52.

Bullis, K. L., and H. Van Roekel. 1944. Uncommon pathological conditions in chickens and turkeys. *Cornell Vet.* 34:313–20.

Buss, I. O., R. D. Conrad, and J. R. Reilly. 1958. Ulcerative enteritis in the pheasant, blue grouse and California quail. *J. Wildlife Management* 22:446–49.

Churchill, Helen M., and D. R. Coburn. 1945. Sulfonamide drugs in the treatment of ulcerative enteritis of quail. *Vet. Med.* 40:309–11.

Durant, A. J., and E. R. Doll. 1941. Ulcerative enteritis in quail. *Missouri Agr. Expt. Sta. Res. Bull.* 325:3–27.

Faddoul, G. 1958. *Ann. Rept. Waltham Field Sta.*, Waltham, Mass.

Gallagher, B. A. 1924. *Am. Game Prod. Ass. Bull.* Apr., pp. 14–15.

Glover, J. S. 1951. Ulcerative enteritis in pigeons. *Can. J. Comp. Med. Vet. Sci.* 15:295–97.

Gray, J. E., G. H. Snoeyenbos, and I. M. Reynolds. 1954. The hemorrhagic syndrome of chickens. *J. Am. Vet. Med. Ass.* 125:144–51.

Green, R. G., and J. E. Shillinger. 1933. Minnesota wild-life disease investigation (monthly report). Oct. USDA, Bur. Biol. Surv. (Mimeo.)

Harris, A. H. 1961. An outbreak of ulcerative enteritis amongst bobwhite quail *(Colinus virginianus)*. *Vet. Record* 73:11–13.

Jungherr, E. 1955. The bloody trio of poultry diseases. *Eastern States Cooperator* 31:6–8.

Kirkpatrick, C. M., and H. E. Moses. 1953. The effects of streptomycin against spontaneous quail disease in bobwhites. *J. Wildlife Management* 17:24–28.

Kirkpatrick, C. M., H. E. Moses, and J. T. Baldini. 1950. Streptomycin studies in ulcerative enteritis in bobwhite quail. I. Results of oral administration of the drug to manually exposed birds in the fall. *Poultry Sci.* 29:561–69.

———. 1952a. The effects of several antibiotic products in feed on experimental ulcerative enteritis in quail. *Am. J. Vet. Res.* 13:99–100.

———. 1952b. Streptomycin studies in ulcerative enteritis in bobwhite quail. II. Concentrations of streptomycin in drinking water suppressing the experimental disease. *Am. J. Vet. Res.* 13:102–4.

LeDune, E. K. 1935. Ulcerative enteritis in ruffed grouse. *Vet. Med.* 30:394–95.

Levine, P. P. 1932. A report on an epidemic disease in ruffed grouse. *Trans. 19th Am. Game Conf.*, pp. 437–41.

Levine, P. P., and Frans C. Goble. 1947. Diseases of grouse, pp. 401–42. In Bump, G., et al. (eds.), *The Ruffed Grouse*. N.Y. State Conserv. Dept., Albany.

Morley, L. C., and P. W. Wetmore. 1936. Discovery of the organism of ulcerative enteritis. *Proc. N. Am. Wildlife Conf.*, Senate

Comm. Print, 74th Congr., 2nd session, Washington, D.C. 1936:471–73.

Morris, A. J. 1948. The use of the complement fixation test in the detection of ulcerative enteritis in quail. *Am. J. Vet. Res.* 9:102–3.

Morse, G. B. 1907. Quail disease in the United States. USDA, *BAI Circ.* 109.

New York State Veterinary College. 1966–67. *Ann. Rept. Poultry Diagnostic Lab.*, p. 184.

Peckham, M. C. 1959. An anaerobe, the cause of ulcerative enteritis, (Quail disease). *Avian Diseases* 3:471–77.

———. 1960. Further studies on the causative organism of ulcerative enteritis. *Avian Diseases* 4:449–56.

———. 1962. Immunization trials against ulcerative enteritis in quail. *Ann. Rept. N.Y. State Vet. Coll.*, 1961–62.

———. 1963. Poultry diagnostic accessions. *Ann. Rept. N.Y. State Vet. Coll.*, 1962–63.

Peckham, M. C., and R. Reynolds. 1962. The efficacy of chemotherapeutic drugs in the control of experimental ulcerative enteritis. *Avian Diseases* 6:111–18.

Pickens, E. N., H. M. DeVolt, and J. E. Shillinger. 1932. An outbreak of quail disease in bobwhite quail. *Maryland Conservationist* 9 (Spring): 18–19.

Rosen, M. H., and A. I. Bischoff. 1949. Field trials of sulfamethazine and sulfaquinoxaline in the treatment of quail ulcerative enteritis. *Cornell Vet.* 39:195–98.

Shillinger, J. E. 1940. Diseases of game birds. *Vet. Med.* 35:124–27.

Shillinger, J. E., and L. C. Morley. 1934. Studies on ulcerative enteritis in quail. *J. Am. Vet. Med. Ass.* 84:25–33.

Smith, L. DS. 1954. *Introduction to the Pathogenic Anaerobes.* Univ. Chicago Press, Chicago, Ill.

Stoddard, H. L. 1931. *The Bobwhite Quail— Its Habits, Preservation and Increase.* Charles Scribner's Sons, New York.

Witter, J. F. 1952. Observations on apparent complications of coccidiosis in broiler flocks. *Proc. 24th Ann. Conf. Lab. Workers in Pullorum Disease Control,* Univ. Maine.

CHAPTER 12

MISCELLANEOUS BACTERIAL DISEASES

❖

W. B. GROSS

Department of Veterinary Science
Virginia Polytechnical Institute
Blacksburg, Virginia

❖

ANTHRAX

❖

CHICKENS AND TURKEYS are very resistant to anthrax. However, ducks and pigeons may become infected (Hofherr, 1910). The disease occurs naturally in the ostrich (Theiler, 1912).

Snoeyenbos (1965) has reviewed much of the literature on anthrax in birds.

Anthrax is caused by *Bacillus anthracis*, an aerobic, sporeforming, gram-positive organism. The disease occurs naturally in cattle, sheep, goats, swine, camels, and other mammals as well as man.

A presumptive diagnosis of anthrax may be made if blood smears of freshly killed infected birds reveal many gram-positive, large, rod-shaped bacilli. However, a definite diagnosis should be based on isolating the organism and demonstrating its pathogenicity in mice, rabbits, cavies, or hamsters.

REFERENCES

Hofherr, O. 1910. Experimentelle Beitraege zur Milzbrandinfektion des Gefluegels durch Fuetterung. *Zentr. Bakteriol. Parasitenk. Abt. I. Orig.* 55:434–64.
Snoeyenbos, G. H. 1965. Anthrax, pp. 432–35. In Biester, H. E., and L. H. Schwarte (eds.), *Diseases of Poultry,* 5th ed. Iowa State Univ. Press, Ames.
Theiler, A. 1912. Anthrax in the ostrich. *Agr. J. Union S. Africa* 4:370–79.

❖

BOTULISM

❖

BOTULISM POISONING of birds is caused by ingesting the toxin of *Clostridium botulinum*. Synonyms are limber neck and western duck sickness.

HISTORY

The history of botulism in birds has been reviewed by Levine (1965). Paralysis of chickens following ingestion of fly larvae (*Lucillia caesar* and *L. sericata*) was reported by Bengston (1923) who identified the Type C strains of *Cl. botulinum* from the larvae. Wetmore (1918) studied losses in waterfowl in the western part of the United States and concluded that the losses were due to alkali poisoning. However, Kalmbach (1930) and Giltner and Couch (1930) later demonstrated that similar losses in waterfowl were due to botulism.

INCIDENCE AND DISTRIBUTION

Modern methods of raising chickens and turkeys have reduced the incidence of botulism. However, outbreaks occur commonly in ducks and other waterfowl, particularly in the western regions of North and South America. Outbreaks may occur on pheasant farms (Vadlamudi et al., 1959; Lee et al., 1962). The distribution of botulism is apparently worldwide, having been reported from many countries (Kalmbach and Gunderson, 1934; Levine, 1965).

ETIOLOGY

Botulism is caused by the toxin produced by *Clostridium botulinum* under anaerobic conditions. The organism itself does not produce disease. *Cl. botulinum* is a saprophyte found in soil and mud in most parts of the world. It can also be found in intestinal contents and feces, but this may not have any relationship to the disease.

MORPHOLOGY AND STAINING

Clostridium botulinum is a large bacillus with rounded ends. It may occur singly, in pairs, or in short chains. Spores are situated terminally causing a bulging of the cell. The spores are extremely resistant to heat, requiring 5 hours of boiling or 10 minutes autoclaving at 120° C for inactivation. Young cultures are gram-positive.

TOXINS AND STRAIN CLASSIFICATION

There are five types of *Cl. botulinum* based on specific toxins produced and on different biochemical and serologic reactions.

Botulism neurotoxin is one of the most toxic substances known. The minimum lethal dose (MLD) for cavies is 0.00012 mg/kg when administered subcutaneously (Bengston, 1924); under similar circumstances the MLD of cobra venom is 0.002 mg/kg. The intraperitoneal LD_{50} for mice of purified toxins is 10^8 per mg of nitrogen (Smith and Holdeman, 1968). The toxic oral dose is 50–100 times greater (Licciardello et al., 1967). The toxin is relatively heat-stable. Six minutes at 80° C are required for destruction. Losses in birds are most commonly due to Types A and C, depending on the geographic location of the outbreak. Types B and E have also been incriminated in bird botulism. Type A is found in the mountainous areas of western North and South America where it is very common. Type B has been found in eastern United States, England, Europe, and China. Type C is worldwide in distribution. Type E poisoning is associated with water and fish and is found in and around the North Sea and the Great Lakes, particularly on Green Bay of Lake Michigan. Since identification of *Cl. botulinum* types is difficult, a text such as that of Smith and Holdeman (1968) should be consulted before attempts at isolation and identification are made.

PATHOGENESIS AND EPIZOOTIOLOGY

The disease has occurred in many species of birds. Kalmbach (1939) has reported vultures to be extremely resistant to botulism toxin, withstanding as much as 300,000 lethal doses for guinea pigs.

When birds die, the *Cl. botulinum* in their digestive tracts is able to invade the muscle and in the anaerobic environment will grow and produce toxin. After the carcass becomes flyblown, toxin accumulates in and on the surface of fly larvae. Birds, particularly pheasants, are fond of fly larvae and can be poisoned following the ingestion of only a few larvae. Lee et al. (1962) found that one gram of fly larvae contained 180,000 mouse LD_{50} and that pheasants died after eating 8 or more larvae. *Cl. botulinum* from the intestines of birds dead from botulism poisoning or any other disease invade the decomposing tissues and so perpetuate the outbreak. The organism can produce toxin in other anaerobic organic matter such as feed.

SOURCE OF TOXIN IN WESTERN DUCK SICKNESS

Western duck sickness occurs primarily in shallow alkaline waters, particularly in western United States and Canada. Type C toxin is most commonly implicated. It occurs during the summer and fall months, and outbreaks cease with the advent of cold weather.

One hypothesis as to the pathogenesis is that following storms large amounts of aquatic plants accumulate and decompose on the windward shores of the lakes. In the alkaline anaerobic environment *Cl. botulinum* proliferates and produces toxin. Ducks and other waterfowl die as the result of ingesting this material. Anaerobiosis is aided by the growth of *Pseudomonas aeruginosa* in the decaying vegetation (Quortrup and Sudheimer, 1943).

A more probable hypothesis is that among the aquatic vegetation are insect larvae which die as the result of the anaerobic conditions caused by the decaying vegetation. Botulism organisms in their intestines invade the tissue and produce toxin (Bell et al., 1955). Ingestion of these dead toxin-containing organisms by ducks results in their becoming sick from the botulism toxin and the seeding of their intestinal tracts with *Cl. botulinum*. After the death of the ducks their bodies become toxic from the *Cl. botulinum* invading the decomposing tissue from their intestines. Fly larvae feeding on the floating carcasses become toxic and fall into the shallow water where they are ingested by the bottom-feeding ducks, thus perpetuating the outbreak. Due to the frequent presence of *Cl. botulinum* in the mud of such lakes, the intestines of many ducks are already seeded and an outbreak can begin if ducks are killed by any cause. Most losses may be due to dehydration rather than entirely to the toxin itself. Cooch (1964) reported that ducks can withstand 4 times as much toxin when provided with fresh water as when

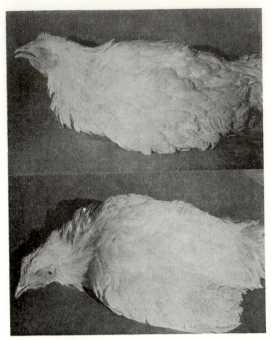

FIG. 12.1—Botulism in chicken showing partial paralysis of wing and lower eyelid, difficult breathing caused by partial paralysis of respiratory muscles, and ruffled hackle feathers.

provided with water of high mineral content, such as from the alkaline lakes. The salt gland of ducks is especially sensitive to botulism toxin. Moving birds to fresh water greatly increases survival.

SIGNS

Birds become sick within a few hours to 1 or 2 days after ingesting toxic material. The earliest signs are those of drowsiness, weakness, and some impairment of flying or walking. An early sign in roosters is the frequent raising of their hackle feathers. If birds have ingested large doses of toxin, the signs progress to complete paralysis of the wings, legs, and neck. The characteristic limp neck has led to the common name of "limberneck" for the disease (Fig. 12.1).

The feathers become ruffled; in severe cases the feathers may be easily removed. Frequently chickens die without neck paralysis or loose feathers. The birds die in a coma. If small doses of the botulinus toxin are ingested, recovery may take place after mild signs of incoordination.

PATHOLOGY

There are no gross lesions except that the anterior portion of the alimentary tract is usually empty. There is no microscopic pathology since the toxin apparently interferes with the output of acetylcholine from the peripheral cholinergic nerves at the neuromuscular junction (Van Heyningen and Arseculeratne, 1964).

DIAGNOSIS

Characteristic paralytic signs in the absence of gross lesions and the presence of carcasses suggest botulism. Demonstration of the toxin may be done directly in the sick birds by injecting appropriate antitoxin which should result in many recoveries. The botulinus toxin may also be demonstrated by injecting serum or extracts of intestinal contents intraperitoneally (0.3 ml) into mice. Paralysis occurs in 1 or 2 days if toxin is present. Mice which have been protected with the appropriate type of antitoxin will survive, giving additional proof of botulism. *Cl. botulinum* is a common inhabitant of intestinal contents, soil, and mud, and its presence has no diagnostic significance.

TREATMENT

Administration of Type C antitoxin, even to extremely sick birds, greatly reduces losses. However, the protective effect of the passive antibodies disappears within a short time and the birds again become susceptible. Affected birds should have access to clean fresh water.

PREVENTION AND CONTROL

Proper management procedures can aid greatly in preventing losses from botulism. Since dead and decomposing carcasses may be a source of the toxin, these should be collected frequently from the environment and incinerated or buried. In case of botulism in large flocks of wild waterfowl, it may be desirable to herd ducks away from shores of potentially dangerous lakes and provide suitable feeding areas.

IMMUNIZATION

Pheasants, quail, and ducks have been immunized with two injections of *Cl. botulinum* Type C toxoid (Boroff and Reilly, 1962). Kaufmann and Crecelius (1967) report that repeated small doses of Type E toxin immunize gulls against Type E botulism toxin.

REFERENCES

Bell, J. F., G. W. Sciple, and A. A. Hubert. 1955. A micro-environmental concept of the etiology of avian botulism. *J. Wildlife Management* 19:352–57.

Bengston, Ida A. 1923. A toxin-producing anaerobe isolated principally from fly larvae. *Public Health Rept.* 38:340–44.

———. 1924. Studies on organisms concerned as causative factors in botulism. *U.S. Public Health Serv., Hyg. Lab. Bull.* 136.

Boroff, D. A., and J. R. Reilly. 1962. Studies of the toxin of *Clostridium botulinum.* VI. Botulism among pheasants and quail, mode of transmission and degree of resistance offered by immunization. *Intern. Arch. Allergy Appl. Immunol.* 3:809–16.

Cooch, F. G. 1964. Preliminary study of the survival value of a salt gland in prairie antidae. *Auk* 81:380–93.

Giltner, L. T., and J. F. Couch. 1930. Western duck sickness and botulism. *Science* 72:660.

Kalmbach, E. R. 1930. Western duck sickness produced experimentally. *Science* 72:658.

———. 1939. American vultures and the toxin of *Clostridium botulinum. J. Am. Vet. Med. Ass.* 94:187–91.

Kalmbach, E. R., and M. F. Gunderson. 1934. Western duck sickness: A form of botulism. *USDA Tech. Bull.* 411, pp. 1–82.

Kaufmann, O. W., and E. M. Crecelius. 1967. Experimentally induced immunity in gulls to Type E botulism. *Am. J. Vet. Res.* 28: 1857–62.

Lee, V. H., S. Vadlamudi, and R. P. Hanson. 1962. Blow fly larvae as a source of botulinum toxin for game farm pheasants. *J. Wildlife Management* 26:411–13.

Levine, N. D. 1965. Botulism, pp. 456–61. In Biester, H. E., and L. H. Schwarte (eds.), *Diseases of Poultry,* 5th ed. Iowa State Univ. Press, Ames.

Licciardello, J. J., J. T. R. Nickerson, A. Ribici Crystal, and S. A. Coldblith. 1967. Thermal inactivation of Type E botulism toxin. *Appl. Microbiol.* 15:249–56.

Quortrup, E. R., and R. L. Sudheimer. 1943. Some ecological relations of *Pseudomonas aeruginosa* to *Clostridium botulinum* Type C. *J. Bacteriol.* 45:551–54.

Smith, L. DS., and Lillian Holdeman. 1968. *Cl. botulinum,* pp. 282–318. In *Pathogenic Anaerobic Bacteria.* Charles C Thomas, Springfield, Ill.

Vadlamudi, S., V. H. Lee, and R. P. Hanson. 1959. Botulism Type C outbreak on a pheasant game farm. *Avian Diseases* 3:344–50.

Van Heyningen, W. E., and S. M. Arseculeratne. 1964. Exotoxins. *Am. Rev. Microbiol.* 18:195–216.

Wetmore, A. 1918. The duck sickness in Utah. *USDA Bull.* 672.

❖

OTHER CLOSTRIDIAL
INFECTIONS
(Gangrenous Dermatitis,
Necrotic Enteritis)

❖

CLOSTRIDIA are part of the etiology of gangrenous dermatitis (gangrenous cellulitis) and necrotic enteritis of chickens and turkeys. Isolations have also been made from chicks, eggs, viscera, and joints.

Clostridial infections are not thought to be common in birds and the economic loss is small. Avian infections do not appear to be a significant source of infection for man or other animals.

HISTORY

Infection of the skin, subcutaneous tissue, and muscle was first described by Niemann (1930). Many subsequent reports were reviewed by Saunders and Bickford (1965). Necrotic enteritis of chickens was first described by Parish (1961). Peterson (1964, 1967) described infection of joints and chicks. The presence of clostridia in the yolk sacs of eggs was observed by Harry (1957).

INCIDENCE AND DISTRIBUTION

Clostridia are commonly found in soil, dust, and intestinal contents. They can frequently be isolated from apparently normal liver and other organs, probably as a result of bacteremia originating from the intestines. Normally they cannot grow in aerobic tissue, and they also resist destruction by the host. The incidence of infection is low and probably depends on an injury or other infection to destroy tissue. Losses in infected flocks range between 1 and 60%

ETIOLOGY

Clostridium perfringens Type A and *Cl. septicum* have been isolated from gangrenous dermatitis of chickens and turkeys. *Cl. perfringens* Type C has been isolated from cases of necrotic enteritis. *Cl. novyi* and *Cl. sporogenes* have been isolated from hock joint arthritis and surrounding tissue by Peterson (1964, 1967). He also isolated *Cl. sporogenes* from livers, spleens, and hearts of day-old chicks, most frequently (40%) from cull birds. *Cl. sporogenes* produced myohemorrhages and pale bone marrow when inoculated into chicks.

Clostridia are large anaerobic ($0.8 \times 2\mu$ or larger) gram-positive rods which usually have spores. They are obligate anaerobes. They grow readily on ordinary media incubated in Brewer jars containing hydrogen or a mixture of 3–10% hydrogen in carbon dioxide or nitrogen. The colony morphology is variable. When grown on blood, agar colonies of most pathogens are surrounded by a zone of beta hemolysis. Clostridia are catalase-negative, which separates them from the aerobic sporeformers which are catalase-positive.

Clostridia bacteria and spores are easily destroyed by oxidizing disinfectants such as chlorine and iodine. They are resistant to the phenols, cresolic disinfectants, and quaternary ammonia compounds. Autoclaving at 120° F for 20 minutes will destroy the spores. A wide variety of specific toxins is produced by the clostridia. Classification into species is made on the basis of a large number of biochemical properties. The presence of many nonpathogenic sporeformers (which may be in tissue) makes the separation difficult. A recent text such as the one by Smith and Holdeman (1968) should be consulted before attempting the separation of the clostridia into species.

PATHOGENESIS AND EPIZOOTIOLOGY

GANGRENOUS DERMATITIS
(WOUND INFECTIONS)

This disease occurs in 4–16-week-old chickens and in turkeys. In most cases staphylococci were also isolated from the lesions. Both organisms are common inhabitants of the skin. Infection usually follows wounds, injuries, or severe bruises which produce the initial necrosis or anaerobiosis necessary for the growth of the clostridia. The staphylococci help to create necrosis and anaerobiosis. The disease was reproduced following the intramuscular or subcutaneous injection of both clostridia and staphylococci (Frazier et al., 1964; Saunders and Bickford, 1965). Initial necrosis which will greatly favor the expression of pathogenicity can be produced by diluting the bacteria in 15% $CaCl_2$ just before intramuscular inoculation. A wound infection following caponization was described by Weymouth et al. (1963) from which *Cl. perfringens* could be isolated.

Signs and Lesions

The signs of infection are necrosis of the skin and deeper tissues of the thigh, lumbar area, breast, wing tips, wattles, and feet. There is a hemorrhagic necrotizing myositis which often contains gas. Livers are often swollen, greenish brown, and contain focal areas of necrosis. Kidneys are darkened and there are petechiae on the heart. Some birds have pale bone marrow. Microscopically there is a serosanguinous infiltration of the skin and subcutaneous tissue. There is myositis with fragmentation of the muscle bundles and loss of striation (Fig. 12.2). Edema is often severe. Many large gram-positive rods are present in the subcutaneous tissue and muscles. Similar bacteria are found in necrotic tissue of the liver and proventriculus (Saunders and Bickford, 1965).

NECROTIC ENTERITIS

Necrotic enteritis is an infrequently reported disease of 6–8-week-old chickens. The disease was well described by Parish (1961). Only Type C of *Cl. perfringens* has been isolated from cases of necrotic enteritis. The condition could be reproduced following the oral administration of *Cl. perfringens* Type C to birds which were dosed orally with a thick suspension of chalk, sodium bicarbonate, and opium (Parish, 1961).

A similar condition was described by Nairn and Bamford (1967) in Australia from birds receiving a specific lot of feed. They could reproduce the condition only by administering *Cl. perfringens* Type C

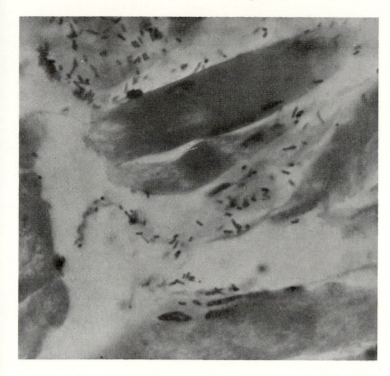

FIG. 12.2—Muscle infected with Clostridium perfringens *Type C. Section shows edema, fragmentation, and degeneration of the muscle; bacteria; and absence of inflammatory cells. H & E, ×1,200.*

orally to chickens receiving the same feed which was being fed during a natural outbreak.

Apparently under some circumstances *Cl. perfringens* Type C proliferates in the lower small intestine which results in toxin-induced necrotic enteritis. Enterotoxemia of sheep is a similar condition.

Signs and Lesions

The disease causes loss of appetite and dark feces which are occasionally blood-stained. Death losses range between 5 and 50%.

Lesions consist of thickened areas particularly of the distal third of the small intestine. The wall is congested and the lumen contains hemorrhagic material. A necrotic layer consisting of degenerate cells and large numbers of gram-positive rods adheres to the surface or is free in the lumen. The contiguous mesentery is edematous and congested. The liver is congested and contains variable numbers of 2–3-mm sharply defined necrotic areas. In chronic cases there are also emaciation and pale bone marrow. At times there is hemorrhagic necrosis of the feet.

Microscopically the villi are partly or completely denuded of epithelium. The tips are necrotic and fused by fibrin, cellular debris, and large numbers of gram-positive bacteria. Cellular infiltration is minimal. Liver lesions are sometimes extensive and consist of degeneration and necrosis without bacteria. Bone marrow is degenerate and has few areas of erythroid or myeloid activity.

DIAGNOSIS

Clostridium infection can be diagnosed if many large gram-positive rods can be seen in stained smears from infected tissue. The organisms can be easily grown anaerobically. Great care should be exercised to prevent contamination from the skin, soil, dust, or intestinal contents. There are no other large gram-positive anaerobic organisms which infect poultry.

TREATMENT AND PREVENTION

Most clostridia are susceptible to tetracyclines although a few avian isolates are resistant. Clostridia are very susceptible to penicillin and bacitracin. The prevention of bruises and injuries and wounds would reduce the incidence of gangrenous dermatitis.

REFERENCES

Frazier, M. N., W. J. Parizek, and E. Garner. 1964. Gangrenous dermatitis of chickens. *Avian Diseases* 8:269–73.

Harry, E. G. 1957. The effect on embryonic and chick mortality of yolk contamination with bacteria from the hen. *Vet. Record* 69: 1433–40.

Nairn, M. D., and V. W. Bamford. 1967. Necrotic enteritis of broiler farms in western Australia. *Australian Vet. J.* 43:49–54.

Niemann, K. W. 1930. *Clostridium welchii* infection in the domesticated fowl. *J. Am. Vet. Med. Ass.* 77:604–6.

Parish, W. E. 1961. Necrotic enteritis in fowl. *J. Comp. Pathol. Therap.* 71:377–413.

Peterson, E. H. 1964. *Clostridium novyi* isolated from chickens. *Poultry Sci.* 43:1062–63.

———. 1967. The isolation of *Clostridium sporogenes* from the viscera of day-old chicks. *Poultry Sci.* 46:527–28.

Saunders, J. R., and A. A. Bickford. 1965. Clostridial infections of growing chickens. *Avian Diseases* 9:317–26.

Smith, L. DS., and Lillian Holdeman. 1968. *Pathogenic Anaerobic Bacteria*. Charles C Thomas, Springfield, Ill.

Weymouth, D. K., M. Gershman, and H. L. Chute. 1963. Report of clostridium in capons. *Avian Diseases* 7:342–43.

❖

BRUCELLOSIS

❖

BRUCELLOSIS is an infection caused by *Brucella abortus, Br. suis,* or *Br. melitensis,* which are found throughout the world in cattle, swine, goats, and sheep as well as other mammals including man. Brucellae have not been recovered from naturally infected birds. Furthermore, experimental infections suggest that birds are not important reservoirs of infection and that they are probably not sources of human infection.

HISTORY

Several reports of spontaneous brucellosis of chickens based on mortality and positive agglutination tests have been reviewed by Snoeyenbos (1965). In none of these cases were brucellae isolated from the chickens. When chickens were fed massive doses of brucellae, serum agglutinins were present for up to 5 weeks and bacteria were shed in the feces for up to 4 weeks. Infection spread to uninoculated pen mates (Felsenfeld et al., 1951). Agglutination also occurred with pullorum antigen.

ETIOLOGY

Brucella abortus, Br. melitensis, and *Br. suis* are closely related small gram-negative, nonmotile coccobacilli. Growth is favored by the presence of serum in the agar such as Huddleson's medium, chocolate agar, or tryptose agar. The addition of 2.5% glucose or erythritol increases growth. An atmosphere of about 10% carbon dioxide is necessary for growth which occurs best at 37° C. Two days or more may be required for colonies to appear. Colonies are small, bluish, and translucent with regular margins and a smooth glistening surface. Brucellae are relatively susceptible to heat and chemical disinfectants. The three species can be separated by differences in their antigenic structure. All species are pathogenic in susceptible hosts when in the smooth form.

DIAGNOSIS

A diagnosis of brucellosis in poultry should be based on isolation of the causative organism. The isolation of small gram-negative, nonmotile bacilli which are aerobic or carboxyphilic, catalase-positive, urease-positive, and do not produce acids from sugars in peptone water is highly suggestive of members of the genus *Brucella*.

PREVENTION AND CONTROL

Since it has been demonstrated experimentally that chickens can become infected if given large doses of brucellae, chickens should be kept away from brucella-infected mammals, and aborted fetuses should not be fed to poultry.

REFERENCES

Felsenfeld, Oscar, Viola Mae Young, E. Ishihara Loeffler, Janet Sachiko, and W. F. Scholder. 1951. A study of the nature of brucellosis in chickens. *Am. J. Vet. Res.* 12:48–54.

Snoeyenbos, G. H. 1965. Brucellosis, pp. 427–32. In Biester, H. E., and L. H. Schwarte (eds.), *Diseases of Poultry,* 5th ed. Iowa State Univ. Press, Ames.

❖

LISTERIOSIS

❖

SPORADIC OUTBREAKS of a septicemic disease caused by *Listeria monocytogenes* have been reported from temperate zones throughout the world in many kinds of birds and mammals. Mortality in chickens varies greatly, usually being low but occasionally reaching 40%. Avian infections may be a source of a few human infections, since many women giving birth to infected infants have had recent contact with sick or dead birds (Gray and Killinger, 1966). Conjunctivitis was reported by Felsenfeld (1951) among poultry dressing plant workers who had processed apparently normal chickens from which *L. monocytogenes* could be isolated.

HISTORY

Listeria was first isolated by Murray et al. (1926) from a septicemic infection in rabbits and cavies. The first report of infections in chickens was made by Seastone (1935). An excellent review has been made by Gray and Killinger (1966).

INCIDENCE AND DISTRIBUTION

Most reports are from the temperate zones of both hemispheres where *L. monocytogenes* is commonly found in soil and feces. Thamm (1962) reports that listeriosis occurs mainly in regions with loamy soil, marl, or humus but rarely from regions with chalky or sandy soil. Kruger (1963) reports isolations from maize, rye, and grass silage.

ETIOLOGY

Listeria monocytogenes is a gram-positive coccoid to rod-shaped nonsporeforming bacterium (1–3 × 0.5μ) which has a tendency to form long filaments, particularly in older cultures. Motility by peritrichate flagella, which can be observed at 20–25° C, is characterized by tumbling.

Growth on the surface of agar is usually sparse. Smooth surface colonies on nutrient agar are convex, circular, transparent, 0.2–0.4 mm in diameter, have a smooth surface and entire edge, and appear bluish green particularly when viewed by oblique transmitted light. On glucose agar the colonies may reach 1–3 mm in a few days. There is a narrow zone of beta hemolysis on blood agar. The addition of 0.5–1% glucose greatly improves the growth rate in broth. Within 24 hours there is a fairly dense, even turbidity which tends to settle. Acid without gas is produced on glucose, maltose, lactose, sucrose, trehalose, rhamnose, and salicin. There is no fermentation of arabinose, dulcitol, inulin, raffinose, or xylose. It is methyl red-positive, catalase-positive, and aerobic, and acetylmethylcarbinol is produced. It does not liquify gelatin nor produce H₂S or urease. It grows between 4 and 42° C and is somewhat resistant to heat, being killed in 60 minutes at 55° C. In milk it can be killed by 75° C in 10 seconds. It can grow in 10% salt solution at pH 9.6 and can survive in 20% salt. It can survive for years at 4° C in broth and for long periods of time on silage, hay, or in soil.

By means of flagella antigens, Robbins and Griffin (1945) were able to identify 4 antigenic groups which have no geographic or host animal significance. There are no toxins.

Cavies, mice, rabbits, poults, cattle, and sheep are susceptible; rats and pigeons are somewhat resistant. Human infection occasionally occurs and results in septicemia, abortions, and infant meningitis. Canaries appear to be the most susceptible birds.

PATHOGENESIS AND EPIZOOTIOLOGY

The most common avian hosts are chicken, turkey, goose, duck, and canary. Other species such as parrot, snow owl, eagle, grouse, and partridge have also been found to be infected (Gray, 1958). Birds of all ages have been infected.

Artificially infected birds shed the organism in their nasal secretions and feces but not from their eggs. Listeria grow in artificially inoculated eggs and can be transformed from the rough to smooth form by egg passage. The organism can be recovered from infected tissue by inoculation of 10-day chick embryos via the allantoic route (Dedie, 1955). It has survived in soil 1–2 years and resisted repeated freezing and thawing (Lehnert, 1960). Listeria can at times be recovered in large numbers from silage (Gray and Killinger, 1966). According to Weidenmuller (1964) the organism spreads rapidly by contact with infected birds, being found temporarily in the feces and nasal mucosa.

Gray (1958) reviewed many reports which suggest that listeriosis is frequently associated with other diseases such as coccidiosis, infectious coryza, enteritis, avian leukosis complex, worm infections, and salmonellosis. Outbreaks tend to recur on the same premises.

It appears that listeriosis in birds frequently is an inapparent infection with shedding of the organism from the feces and nasal secretions. Brem and Eveland (1968) suggest that the carrier state may be maintained intracellularly as the L form. Under special incompletely understood circumstances, it becomes septicemic and can result in chronic or acute disease. The reservoir is probably soil, plant materials, and feces from carriers. The incubation period in turkeys ranges from 16–20 hours (Malewitz et al., 1957) to 14–52 days (Bolin and Eveleth, 1961), depending on the severity of infection and age of the birds.

SIGNS

The signs of infection are those of septicemic infection such as depression and at times death. In some birds there are signs attributable to central nervous system damage, the most common being torticollis. Diarrhea and emaciation are reported in experimental infection (Bolin and Eveleth, 1961).

GROSS AND MICROSCOPIC LESIONS

Gross lesions are variable and characteristic of septicemia. The most frequent lesions of the heart are multiple areas of degeneration or necrosis of the myocardium and frequently congestion and pericarditis. The liver may be swollen, have a greenish color, or have small necrotic areas. Spleens may be enlarged or mottled. No gross lesions are associated with brain pathology. There may be petechia on the heart and proventriculus.

Microscopically the periphery of areas of degeneration and necrosis frequently contains bacteria. Bacteria can also be seen in Kupffer cells and in circumscribed areas in the brain. Infiltration with lymphoid cells, macrophages, and plasma cells are characteristic. An increase in blood monocytes may be noted. Inoculated birds have increased H agglutination titers even though no signs or lesions are observed. Titers begin to rise 2 weeks after inoculation and reach 1:40 to 1:320 4–6 weeks after exposure.

DIAGNOSIS

The organism can frequently be isolated from the blood, liver, spleen, myocardium, and at times the brain. Growth is improved if ½–1% glucose is added to the medium. Samples which are negative on original culture may yield organisms if they are macerated and kept refrigerated for up to 2 months. This may be influenced by the ease with which *L. monocytogenes* transforms between the bacterial and L forms (Brem and Eveland, 1968). Isolation can also be made in the allantoic sac of 10-day-old embryos.

Diagnosis is made by isolating a gram-positive, nonacid-fast, nonsporeforming bacillus which is catalase-positive, motile, aerobic, and attacks sugars by fermentation.

TREATMENT

The sensitivity of *L. monocytogenes* to antibiotics and drugs has been reviewed by Levine (1965). Listeria are resistant to most antibiotics, particularly at the lower levels.

Tetracyclines at high levels are the antibiotics of choice.

PREVENTION

Avoiding keeping birds on infected premises and keeping them away from sheep and cattle which may be infected might be helpful. Artificial immunization has not been successful in preventing losses.

REFERENCES

Bolin, F. M., and D. F. Eveleth. 1961. Experimental listeriosis of turkeys. *Avian Diseases* 5:229–31.

Brem, A. M., and W. C. Eveland. 1968. L. forms of *Listeria monocytogenes*. *J. Infect. Diseases* 118:181–87.

Dedie, K. 1955. Beitrag zur Epizootiologie der Listeriose. *Arch. Exp. Vet. Med.* 9:251–64.

Felsenfeld, D. 1951. Diseases of birds transmissible to man. *Iowa State Coll. Vet.* 13: 89–92.

Gray, M. L. 1958. Listeriosis in fowls. *Avian Diseases* 2:296–314.

Gray, M. L., and A. H. Killinger. 1966. *Listeria monocytogenes* and listeria infections. *Bacteriol. Rev.* 30:309–82.

Kruger, W. 1963. Das Vorkommen von *Listeria Monocytogenes* in den verschiedenen Silagen und dessen aetiologische Bedeutung. *Arch. Exp. Veterinaermed.* 17:181–203.

Lehnert, C. 1960. Die Tanazitaet von *Listeria Monocytogenes* in der Aussenwelt. *Zentr. Bakteriol. Parasitenk. Abt. I. Orig.* 180:350–56.

Levine, N. D. 1965. Listeriosis, pp. 451–56. In Biester, H. E., and L. H. Schwarte (eds.), *Diseases of Poultry*, 5th ed. Iowa State Univ. Press, Ames.

Malewitz, T. D., M. L. Gray, and E. M. Smith. 1957. Experimentally induced listeriosis in turkey poults. *Poultry Sci.* 36:416–19.

Murray, E. G. D., R. A. Webb, and M. B. R. Swann. 1926. A disease of rabbits characterized by large mononuclear leucocytosis, caused by a hitherto undescribed bacillus, *Bacterium monocytogenes* (n. sp.). *J. Pathol. Bacteriol.* 29:407–39.

Robbins, M. L., and A. M. Griffin. 1945. Studies on *Listeria monocytogenes*. II. The effect of heat and alcohol on the stable (somatic) antigens. *J. Immunol.* 50:237–45.

Seastone, C. V. 1935. Pathogenic organisms of the genus *Listerella*. *J. Exp. Med.* 62:203–12.

Thamm, H. 1962. Zur Epizootiologie der Listeriose. *Monatsh. Veterinaermed.* 17:224–37.

Weidenmuller, H. 1964. Listeriosis in poultry. *Tieraerztl. Umschau* 19:388–89.

✦

STAPHYLOCOCCOSIS

✦

STAPHYLOCOCCAL INFECTIONS of poultry are worldwide and are occasionally responsible for chronic and acute infections. Most losses, occasionally up to 30% (Williams and Gaines, 1942), occur in turkeys. The chief disease conditions are pyogenic localization in tendon sheaths, joints, and bursas (synovitis, arthritis); wound infections; septicemia; spondylitis; omphalitis; emaciation; and bacterial endocarditis.

HISTORY

Lucet (1892) proved that a staphylococcus was the cause of an arthritis in geese. Isolation of staphylococci from joint infections of pheasants was reported by Hale and Purchase (1931). Since then there have been numerous reports of joint bursa and tendon sheath infections, particularly in turkeys. Staphylococci were isolated from the yolk sacs of chicks and poults with omphalitis by Volkman (1929). Staphylococci were isolated from bacterial endocarditis by Povar and Brownstein (1947) and from spondylitis by Carnaghan (1966). Infection of the air sacs has been reported by Salana et al. (1964).

ETIOLOGY

Staphylococcus aureus (*S. pyogenes*, *S. pyogenes aureus*, *S. citreus*) are gram-positive cocci occurring in pairs and irregular clusters. Old cultures may contain some gram-negative cells. It is nonmotile, nonsporeforming, facultatively anaerobic, catalase-positive, and ferments glucose (anaerobically) with the production of acid. It is also Voges-Proskauer-positive, coagulase-positive, and phosphatase-positive and reduces nitrate. S. aureus is separated from the nonpathogenic Staphylococcus epidermidis (S. albus) by its ability to produce coagulase. S. aureus grows readily on ordinary laboratory media. Colonies are circular, smooth, orange to white, glistening, butyrous, and entire. Broth cultures are usually turbid but may clear with a sediment. Staphylococci are among the more resistant nonsporeforming bacteria. They are usually killed by exposure to 60° C for 30 minutes. They are relatively resistant to mercuric chloride, phenol, and salt and are relatively susceptible to dyes such as crystal violet and malachite green.

Staphylococci can be separated into subgroups by serological analysis of their antigenic structure (Oeding, 1960). Bacteriophage typing of staphylococci from human and animal sources is widely practiced. Examination of isolates from avian sources has been conducted by Smith et al. (1961) and Carnaghan (1966), who found that some of the avian isolates belong to human phage types.

S. aureus may produce a wide variety of toxins and enzymes such as hemolysins, leucocidin, coagulase, enterotoxin, hyaluronidase, and lipase. The ability of bacteriophage to induce the formation of staphylococcal toxins and increase pathogenicity is reviewed by Zabriskie (1966). All isolates of S. aureus are considered to be pathogenic.

INCIDENCE AND DISTRIBUTION

Staphylococcus aureus is a common inhabitant of the skin and mucous membranes of all animals. Staphylococcus epidermidis, the nonpathogenic coagulase negative species, is also found in similar habitats. The manner by which S. aureus gets from the skin and mucous membranes to the lesions is unknown.

Staphylococci have been isolated from the yolk (and albumin) of about 7% of examined dead embryos by Harry (1957), Sato et al. (1961), and Itagaki and Tsubokura (1960). Most (about 2/3) were coagulase-negative. Sato et al. (1961) determined that the coagulase-positive, but not coagulase-negative, isolates were pathogenic for rabbits and chickens. Almost all of the isolates from down from incubators were coagulase-negative and nonhemolytic.

Salana et al. (1964) report the growing of 2,700 colonies per cu ft of air in the house of a flock with a respiratory disease caused by S. aureus.

PATHOGENESIS AND EPIZOOTIOLOGY

EGG AND YOLK SAC INFECTIONS

Staphylococci have been isolated from dead embryos and dead early-hatched chicks but much less frequently than Escherichia coli, salmonellae, and enterococci (Harry, 1957; Sato et al. 1961). Their importance in eggs is not clear since both coagulase-positive and coagulase-negative strains are isolated and because of the relatively low incidence of contamination. They are a possible means for the spread of pathogenic staphylococci between generations. Early infection of eggs with S. aureus tends to produce rapid death. If an avirulent staphylococcus is inoculated 48 hours before a virulent staphylococcus, mortality is greatly reduced (McCabe, 1965). Omphalitis in newly hatched poults has been described by Williams and Gaines (1942), who presented evidence that infected hatchery workers might be a source of infection.

ARTHRITIS-SYNOVITIS DISEASE

Poults 3 weeks of age and older frequently experience severe losses from a septicemic staphylococcal infection that localizes in the joints and tendon sheaths. It is most prevalent between 9 and 16 weeks of age and in poults hatched from January to March (Smart and Miner, 1961). Similar joint infections have been reported in 25–40-day-old chicks by Schiavo and Biondi (1963). The intravenous inoculation of S. aureus into chickens or turkeys usually results in a high incidence of joint and tendon infections. Some isolates cause a disease characterized by emaciation. Other isolates often cause bacterial endocarditis following intravenous inoculation.

Willemart and Verger (1965) report synovitis in 14–16-week-old pullets. Natural and experimental infection in young chicks characterized by depression and lameness was described by Smith (1954).

Experimental infection in turkeys has been described by Smart et al. (1968). They found that bacteria were rapidly cleared from the blood in about 6 hours, the bacteria being retained in the spleen, lungs, and liver. The retained bacteria multiplied in the internal organs and reappeared in the blood by 12 hours, reaching levels of about 10^5 in the blood, liver, and spleen. Signs of infection such as depression and joint infections occurred within 48–120 hours. Issar (1966) found that pretreatment with prednisolone resulted in a fulminating infection by *S. aureus*.

Experimental work by Miner et al. (1968) and others suggests that there is first a bacteremia of unknown origin followed by localization of the bacteria in the parenchymatous organs, especially the liver. Toxins then make the joints and synovial sheaths especially susceptible to the later localization of infection which then results in the production of pus. Frank Craig of the University of North Carolina (1968, personal communication) has observed that injuries to the tendons and ligaments predisposes them to infection. In addition to incubator spread, Hinshaw and McNeil (1952) suggest thorns and other foot injuries as well as mosquitoes.

Signs

The signs of infection are fever, bacteremia (particularly early in infection), swelling of the tibiotarsal joint and adjacent tendon sheaths. Less frequently there are femorotibial joint infection and abscesses of the feet and keel. Similar clinical signs can be produced following the intravenous inoculation of virulent culture. Birds are lame and show reluctance to move.

Lesions

The lesions consist of swollen joints which contain serous to caseous exudate (Fig. 12.3). The liver is swollen and congested. Synovial membranes are thickened and edematous. Microscopically there is degeneration of hepatic cells and an increase in perivascular foci of mononuclear cells and heterophils. Early in infection the synovial membranes of the joints and tendon sheaths have focal thickening consisting of rounded synovial cells followed by stratification. Later there is considerable infiltration of heterophils and foci of staphylococci can be seen (Fig. 12.4).

SPONDYLITIS

Carnaghan (1966) described the natural occurrence of an infection of the 5th, 6th, and 7th cervical vertebrae due to *S. aureus* (*S. pyogenes*) which results in spinal cord compression and lameness of chickens.

The disease could be reproduced following the intravenous inoculation of a coagulase-positive or coagulase-negative isolate. Vertebral lesions developed 33–50 days postinoculation although bacteria could be isolated from the vertebrae a week after inoculation. Many inoculated birds died of staphylococcal septicemia.

SKIN AND WOUND INFECTIONS

Staphylococci have been isolated from skin and wound infections, usually in combination with *Clostridium perfringens* Type

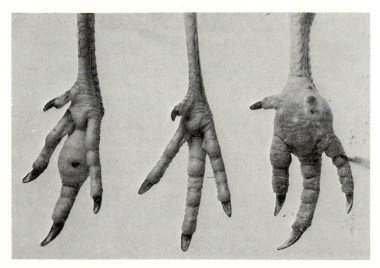

FIG. 12.3—Staphylococcal infection of feet (left and right) and normal foot (center) of Hungarian partridge. (M. C. Peckham, Cornell Univ.)

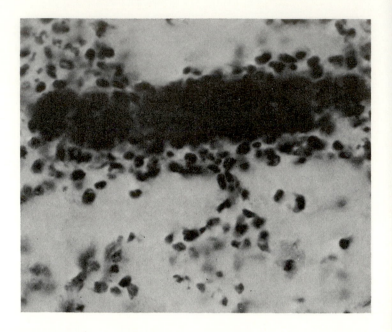

FIG. 12.4—Necrotic muscle showing mass of Staphylococcus aureus *surrounded by necrotic heterophils. H & E, ×1,500.*

A. The relationship of staphylococci to the infection is not clear since lesions can be reproduced by clostridia alone. Staphylococci may at times create the initial necrosis which is necessary for growth of the clostridia.

DIAGNOSIS

The isolation of gram-positive cocci from lesions characteristic of staphylococcal infections is diagnostic if the isolated organism ferments glucose anaerobically and produces catalase and coagulase. Since most coagulase-negative staphylococci are nonpathogenic, they should be inoculated intravenously into chickens or turkeys to determine their pathogenicity. Staphylococci are common inhabitants of the skin and mucous membrane, and great care should be made to avoid contamination from these sources.

TREATMENT

The treatment of staphylococcal synovitis has been reviewed by Smart and Miner (1961). Antibiotics such as streptomycin,

penicillin, oxytetracycline, chlortetracycline, and novobiocin are at times effective if they are given at high levels early in the disease. According to these authors, novobiocin is particularly effective.

Since many isolates are resistant to one or more antibiotics, drug sensitivity should be determined early in the course of the disease so that use of an ineffective drug can be avoided. Smith and Crabb (1960) found that feeding of low levels of penicillin and chlortetracycline to chickens greatly increased the incidence of resistant isolates from their skin and nasal cavities as well as from their caretakers.

PREVENTION AND CONTROL

Diets of birds should be compounded so that ligament, tendon, and joint abnormalities are minimal. Injuries to ligaments and tendons should be avoided. Persons with staphylococcal infection should not handle eggs or young birds. Vaccines have not proved beneficial in preventing infection (Smith, 1954).

REFERENCES

Carnaghan, R. B. A. 1966. Spinal cord compression of fowls due to spondylitis caused by *Staphylococcus pyogenes. J. Comp. Pathol. Therap.* 76:9–14.

Hale, N., and H. S. Purchase. 1931. Arthritis and periostitis in pheasants caused by *Staphylococcus pyogenes aureus. J. Comp. Pathol. Therap.* 44:252–57.

Harry, E. G. 1957. The effect on embryonic and chick mortality of yolk contamination with bacteria from the hen. *Vet. Record* 69:1433–40.

Hinshaw, W. R., and Ethyl McNeil. 1952. Staphylococcosis (synovitis) in turkeys. *Poultry Sci.* 31:320–27.

Issar, S. L. 1966. The influence of prednisolone on the morbid anatomy of induced *Staphylococcus aureus* and *Staphylococcus epidermis* infection in chickens. (Kansas State Univ.) *Dissertation Abstr.* 26:7265.

Itagaki, K., and M. Tsubokura. 1960. Bacteriological investigation on infection among embryonating hens' eggs and baby chicks. (In Japanese, English summary.) *J. Jap. Vet. Med. Ass.* 13:439–42.

Lucet, A. 1892. De l'osteo-arthrite aigue infectieuse des jeunes vies. *Ann. Inst. Pasteur* 6:841–50.

McCabe, W. R. 1965. Staphylococcal interference in infections in embryonated eggs. *Nature* 205:1023.

Miner, M. L., R. A. Smart, and A. E. Olson. 1968. Pathogenesis of staphylococcal synovitis in turkeys: Pathologic changes. *Avian Diseases* 12:46–60.

Oeding, P. 1960. Antigenic properties of *Staphylococcus aureus*. *Bacteriol. Rev.* 24:374–96.

Povar, M. L., and B. Brownstein. 1947. Valvular endocarditis in the fowl. *Cornell Vet.* 37:49–54.

Salana, P., D. P. Anderson, M. L. Frey, and R. P. Hanson. 1964. Epizootiological study of *Staphylococcus aureus* infection in turkeys. *Poultry Sci.* 43:1364.

Sato, G., S. Miura, T. Miyamae, M. Nakegawa, and I. Akiharu. 1961. Characteristics of staphylococci isolated from dead chick embryos and from pathological conditions in chickens. *Japan. J. Vet. Res.* 9:1–13.

Schiavo, A., and E. Biondi. 1963. Treatment of avian staphylococcosis. *Acta. Med. Vet.,* Napoli 9:199–205.

Smart, R. A., and M. L. Miner. 1961. Treatment of staphylococcal synovitis of turkeys. *Poultry Sci.* 40:676–83.

Smart, R. A., M. L. Miner, and R. V. Davis. 1968. Pathogenesis of staphylococcal synovitis in turkeys: Cultural retrieval in experimental infection. *Avian Diseases* 12:37–46.

Smith, H. W. 1954. Experimental staphylococcal infection in chickens. *J. Pathol. Bacteriol.* 67:81–87.

Smith, H. W., and W. E. Crabb. 1960. The effect of diets containing tetracycline and penicillin on the *Staphylococcus aureus* flora of the nose and skin of pigs and chickens and their attendants. *J. Pathol. Bacteriol.* 79:243–49.

Smith, W., J. Whitney, A. Garth, M. L. Miner, E. Blommer, and M. L. Jensen. 1961. A phage-typing system for staphylococci from turkeys with synovitis. *Am. J. Vet. Res.* 22:388–90.

Volkman, F. 1929. Omphalitis in baby chicks and turkeys. *J. Am. Vet. Med. Ass.* 75:647–49.

Willemart, V. P., and M. Verger. 1965. Enzootic staphylococcal synovitis of pullets. *Rec. Med. Vet. Ecole Alfort* 141:523–30.

William, R. B., and L. L. Gaines. 1942. The relationship of infectious omphalitis in poults and impetigo staphylogenes in man. *J. Am. Vet. Med. Ass.* 101:26–28.

Zabriskie, J. B. 1966. Viral-induced bacterial toxin. *Ann. Rev. Med.* 17:337–50.

STREPTOCOCCOSIS

❖

STREPTOCOCCAL INFECTIONS of poultry, although not common, are of worldwide distribution. They cause acute or chronic infections with losses up to 50%. Although *Streptococcus fecalis* is a pathogen in many animals and man, the bird does not appear to be a source.

HISTORY

Acute streptococcal septicemia of chickens was first described by Nörgaard and Mohler in 1902. *Str. fecalis* infection in chickens has been reported by Povar and Brownstein (1947), Agrimi (1956), and Gross and Domermuth (1962). Huhtanen and Pensack (1965) present evidence that *Str. fecalis* is responsible for some growth depression in chicks. A review of *Str. zooepidemicus* infections was made by Peckham (1966).

ETIOLOGY

The genus *Streptococcus* is composed of bacteria which are gram-positive spheres in pairs or chains, nonmotile, nonspore-forming, facultatively anaerobic, catalase-

TABLE 12.1 ❧ Differentiation of Streptococci of Avian Origin

Species	Pathogenicity	Hemolysis on Chicken Blood Agar	Biochemical Differentiation
Str. zooepidemicus	High	β	Does not grow at pH 9.6 nor in presence of 6.5% NaCl
Str. fecalis	High	Neg or B*	Ferments sorbitol, liquefies gelatin†
Str. faecium	Slight	α	Ferments arabinose
Str. durans	Slight	α	Ferments neither sorbitol nor arabinose

* Str. fecalis var. zymogenes.
† Str. fecalis var. liquefaciens.

negative, and attack sugars fermentatively. Str. zooepidemicus (occasionally referred to as Str. gallinarum) belongs to antigenic group C; Str. fecalis, Str. faecium, and Str. durans belong to group D (enterococci). The streptococci which might be encountered from avian sources can be differentiated according to the plan in Table 12.1. The enterococci can be differentiated from Str. zooepidemicus by their ability to grow at pH 9.6 and in the presence of 6.5% NaCl and by their strong reduction of litmus milk. The enterococci can usually be differentiated by the fermentation of arabinose and sorbitol. Str. faecium ferments arabinose, Str. fecalis ferments sorbitol, and Str. durans ferments neither. Some isolates of Str. fecalis can be placed into variety liquifacious if they liquify gelatin or into variety zymogenes if they are beta hemolytic. The relationship of pathogenicity to those characteristics is unknown.

PATHOGENESIS AND EPIZOOTIOLOGY

Streptococcus zooepidemicus infects primarily mature chickens. Experimentally, rabbits, mice, turkeys, pigeons, ducks, and geese are reported to be susceptible. In contrast Str. fecalis affects poultry of all ages and may be a serious problem in young chicks. The source and route of infection of Str. zooepidemicus is unknown although carriers exist for several months. Str. fecalis is a common intestinal inhabitant of most birds and mammals. Most intestinal isolates from healthy birds are pathogenic when administered intravenously. This and other enterococci can be readily recovered from the air of poultry houses. Aerosol transmission of Str. zooepidemicus and Str. fecalis was accomplished by Agrimi (1956) with resultant acute septicemia. He also re-

ported egg transmission of Str. fecalis from infected hens with misshapen ova. Harry (1957) reported isolating enterococci from 75 of 411 dead embryos. An isolate of Str. fecalis was reported (Moore and Gross, 1968) to alter the intestine so that intestinal bacteria such as bacteroides, catenabacteria, and streptococci produced liver granulomas in turkeys. Isolates of Str. faecium and Str. durans have also produced bacterial endocarditis following intravenous inoculation of chickens. Their pathogenicity is markedly less than Str. fecalis. The incubation period ranges from 1 day

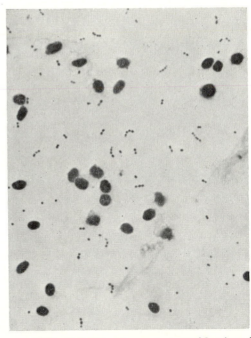

FIG. 12.5—Streptococcus zooepidemicus in blood of naturally infected chicken. Gram, ×800. (M. C. Peckham, Cornell Univ.)

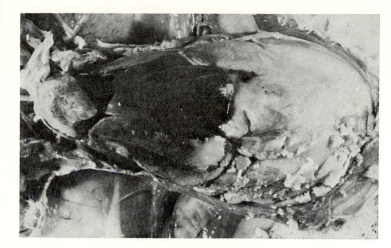

FIG. 12.6—Streptococcus zoo-epidemicus infection showing perihepatitis and peritonitis. (M. C. Peckham, Cornell Univ.)

to several weeks following experimental inoculation.

SIGNS

Among the signs of *Str. zooepidemicus* infection are lassitude, yellowish droppings, pale comb and wattles, emaciation, anorexia, and bloodstained tissue and feathers in the head region. *Str. zooepidemicus*-infected birds may have body temperatures of over 109° F and tend to have persistent bacteremia (Fig. 12.5). *Str. fecalis*-infected birds may have subnormal temperature or temperature of 107–108° F. Bacteremia tends to be persistent with great variation in number of bacteria present. Heterophil counts are greatly increased and may exceed 120,000 per mm³. Most visibly sick birds eventually die of the infection.

GROSS LESIONS

The gross lesions of acute *Str. zooepidemicus* infection (Fig. 12.6) are characterized by enlarged spleen, slightly enlarged liver (with or without small red or light-colored foci), sanguinous fluid in the pericardial sac and under the skin of the keel, and peritonitis. Joint infection, salpingitis, dehydration, bacterial endocarditis, misshapen ova, pericarditis, perihepatitis, and emaciation are found in less acute infections. Most isolates of *Str. fecalis* produce bacterial endocarditis. Acute infections of 10–

20-day-old chicks due to *Str. fecalis* as well as a high incidence of embryo infection and mortality were described by Agrimi (1956).

Streptococci can usually be demonstrated in sections stained with tissue gram stains. Necrotic areas in the liver, spleen, and myocardium are common. Frequently there is little cellular reaction, but in some sections there is massive infiltration with heterophils and macrophages. In chronic infection plasma cells are common.

DIAGNOSIS

Streptococci can be easily isolated on blood agar from the blood, liver, spleen, and other lesions. The differential medium of Domermuth and Gross (1969) is helpful in isolating and identifying enterococci. Identification of *Str. zooepidemicus* or *Str. fecalis* from infected tissue constitutes a diagnosis. *Str. zooepidemicus* is in Lancefield serotype C, while the enterococci are in type D. Sharpe and Shattock (1952) describe methods for detecting serogroups within group D.

TREATMENT

Drugs such as penicillin, erythromycin, novobiocin, oleodromycin, tetracyclines, and nitrofurans have proved of value, particularly in acute infections. Isolates should be tested for drug sensitivity.

REFERENCES

Agrimi, P. 1956. Studio sperimentale su alcuni focali di streptococcosi nel pollo. *Zooprofilassi* 11:491–501.
Domermuth, C. H., and W. B. Gross. 1969. A solid medium for isolation and tentative identification of fecal streptococci. *Avian Diseases* 13:394–99.
Gross, W. B., and C. H. Domermuth. 1962.

Bacterial endocarditis of poultry. *Am. J. Vet. Res.* 23:320–29.

Harry, E. G. 1957. The effect on embryonic and chick mortality of yolk contamination with bacteria from the hen. *Vet. Record* 69:1433–40.

Huhtanen, C. H., and J. M. Pensack. 1965. The role of *Streptococcus faecalis* in the antibiotic growth effect in chickens. *Poultry Sci.* 44 (3): 830–34.

Kernkamp, H. C. H. 1927. Idiopathic streptococcic peritonitis in poultry. *J. Am. Vet. Med. Ass.* 70:585–96.

Moore, W. E. C., and W. B. Gross. 1968. Liver granulomas of turkeys—Causative agents and

mechanism of infection. *Avian Diseases* 12: 417–22.

Nörgaard, V. A., and J. R. Mohler. 1902. Apoplectiform septicemia in chickens. *USDA BAI Bull.* 36.

Peckham, M. C. 1966. An outbreak of streptococcosis (apoplectiform septicemia) in White Rock chickens. *Avian Diseases* 10:413–21.

Povar, M. L., and Bernard Brownstein. 1947. Valvular endocarditis in the fowl. *Cornell Vet.* 37:49–54.

Sharpe, M. Elisabeth, and P. M. Frances Shattock, 1952. The serological typing of group D streptococci associated with outbreak of neonatal diarrhea. *J. Gen Microbiol.* 6: 150–65.

✤

BACTERIAL ENDOCARDITIS

✤

BACTERIAL ENDOCARDITIS was first reported to be associated with streptococcic peritonitis by Kernkamp (1927). Povar and Brownstein (1947) described 38 cases in mature chickens. Valvular lesions were found by Peckham (1966) in chickens inoculated with *Streptococcus zooepidemicus*. The experimental infection and pathology were described by Gross and Domermuth (1962).

Sporadic mortality which totals less than 0.5%, occurring over a period of many months, is the usual history for infected flocks.

ETIOLOGY

Isolates of *Staphylococcus aureus* or *Str. fecalis* (Povar and Brownstein, 1947; Gross and Domermuth, 1962) and less frequently *Str. zooepidemicus* (Kernkamp, 1927; Peckham, 1966), *Pasteurella multocida* (Gross and Domermuth, 1962) or *Erysipelothrix insidiosa* (Helmboldt, personal communication) have been found in natural cases and

have produced valvular lesions following intravenous inoculation.

Infected chickens or turkeys are depressed and have pale and shrunken combs and wattles. Body temperature may be normal or as high as 108° F. Blood pressure may be decreased. Heterophil blood counts may be greatly increased to as high as 120,000 or more. The etiological bacterium can be frequently isolated from the blood, but there may be fewer than 20 bacteria per ml. Almost all birds with lesions die 5–28 days after inoculation. Incidence of lesions is related to dose of exposure.

PATHOLOGY

Lesions consist of vegetations on the heart valves and secondary septic infarcts of the liver (Figs. 12.7, 12.8, 12.9) and spleen. The vegetations range from less than 1 mm in diameter to those which may fill the lumen of the valve. The mitral and aortic valves are most frequently involved (Fig. 12.10). Vegetations are rare on the pulmonary and right atrioventricular valves. Infarcts of the liver, heart, and spleen are cream to light brown and tend to be hard with sharp margins.

Valvular vegetations consist of varying proportions of fibrin and bacteria (Fig. 12.11). The infected valves are edematous and have little cellular infiltration. Anitschkow myocytes are common—in fact numerous in the fibrous portion of the valve. There may be a diffuse myocarditis. The lesion begins with slight edema of the valve which soon loosens the surface endo-

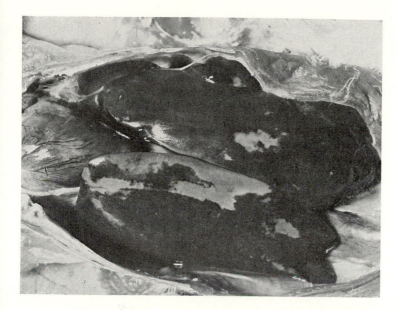

FIG. 12.7—Bacterial endocarditis. Specimen shows infarcts of liver and myocardium.

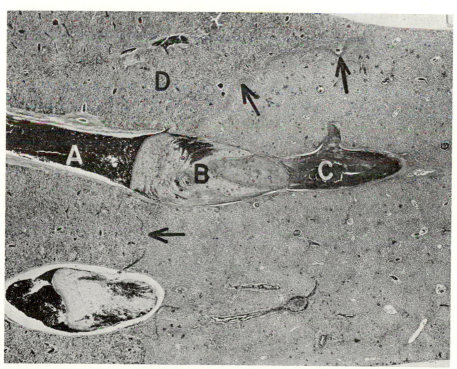

FIG. 12.8—Bacterial endocarditis caused by Streptococcus fecalis. Section of recent liver infarct shows septic thrombus (**B**), portion of vessel filled with necrotic erythrocytes (**C**), margin of infarcted area (**arrows**), portion of vessel adjacent to the thrombus (**A**), relatively normal liver tissue (**D**). H & E, ×10.

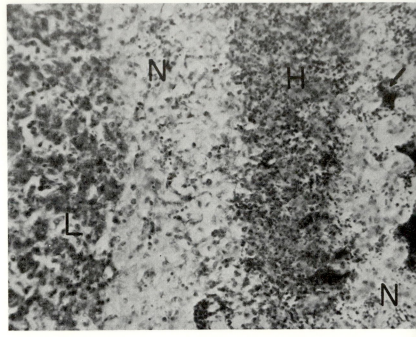

FIG. 12.9—Margin of liver infarct associated with bacterial endocarditis showing clumps of bacteria (arrows), necrotic area (N), zone of necrotic heterophils (H), and relatively normal liver tissue (L). H & E, ×400.

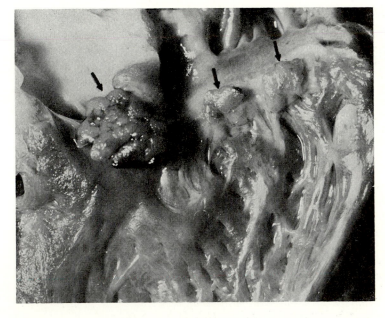

FIG. 12.10—Bacterial endocarditis showing vegetations of mitral valve (arrows).

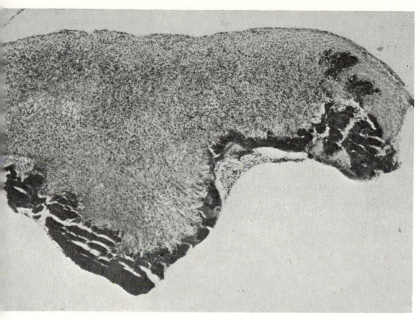

FIG. 12.11—Bacterial endocarditis. Section of leaf of mitral valve shows clumps of bacteria on surface and thickening caused by fibrosis and infiltration by heterophils and macrophages. H & E, ×30.

FIG. 12.12—Detail of valvular lesion in Fig. 12.11 showing clumps of bacteria with heterophilic debris. H & E, ×280.

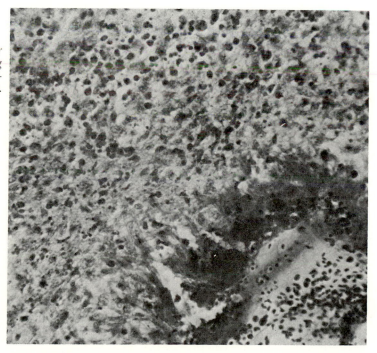

thelium. Fibrin is deposited to form a distinct pink band—a nonbacterial thrombocytic deposit. This apparently is so unusual that bacteria stick to it easily and colonies build up rapidly (Fig. 12.12). Infarcts of the liver are characterized by septic thrombi of branches of the portal vein followed by necrosis of the affected tissue. Clumps of bacteria are present throughout the necrotic area. A band of heterophils just within the border of the necrotic area is the characteristic lesion. Infarcts of the myocardium, liver, and spleen are characterized by septic thrombi and necrosis. Healing of myocardial infarcts is rapid by replacement of the necrotic muscle with fibrinous tissue. In the brain a vasculitis is common. Usually a few heterophils are scattered about. Some birds even have microscopic granulomas. Most of these lesions are in the neostriatum.

DIAGNOSIS AND CONTROL

Diagnosis is made by finding vegetations on the valves of the heart, usually with secondary infarcts of the myocardium, liver, or spleen. Many birds have edematous thickened margins of the valves which can be distinguished from vegetations by the absence of fibrin. The causative bacterium can be isolated from the blood, valves, and infarcts of the liver and spleen. No methods of control have been developed.

REFERENCES

Gross, W. B., and C. H. Domermuth. 1962. Bacterial endocarditis of poultry. *Am. J. Vet. Res.* 23:320–29.

Kernkamp, H. C. H. 1927. Odiopathic streptococcic peritonitis in poultry. *J. Am. Vet. Med. Ass.* 70:585–96.

Peckham, M. C. 1966. An outbreak of streptococcosis (apoplectiform septicemia) in White Rock chickens. *Avian Diseases* 10:413–21.

Povar, M. L., and Bernard Brownstein. 1947. Valvular endocarditis in the fowl. *Cornell Vet.* 37:49–54.

❖

COLIBACILLOSIS

❖

Escherichia coli infection includes colibacillosis, Hjärre's disease, coligranuloma, peritonitis, salpingitis, synovitis, omphalitis, air sac disease, and all other disease conditions caused entirely or partly by *E. coli*. Collectively the various diseases caused by *E. coli* infections are responsible for major economic losses to the poultry industry. Most of the serotypes isolated from poultry are pathogenic only for birds, but a few are also associated with disease conditions of other animals. Avian sources of *E. coli* do not seem to be important sources for infections in other animals. The various serotypes of *E. coli* are intestinal inhabitants of all animals, and therefore their distribution is widespread.

E. coli has been associated with many disease conditions of poultry since it was first described by Lignières (1894).

INCIDENCE AND DISTRIBUTION

Various strains of *E. coli* probably infect most mammals and birds. Most infections are reported in chickens, turkeys, and ducks.

E. coli is a common inhabitant of the intestinal tracts of animals at a concentration of 10^6 per g or less, and its presence in drinking water is considered indicative of fecal contamination. Harry and Hemsley (1965a) found that 10–15% of the intestinal coliforms belong to pathogenic serotypes. The intestinal strains were not necessarily of the same serotype as those from the pericardial sac of the same bird. Egg transmission of pathogenic *E. coli* is common and can be responsible for high mortality of chicks. Newly hatched chicks have a higher incidence of pathogenic coliforms in the gut than the eggs from which they hatch (Harry and Hemsley, 1965b), which suggests rapid spread after hatching. The most important source of egg infection seems to be from fecal contamination of the surface with subsequent penetration of the shell and membranes. Coliform bacteria can be found in litter and fecal matter. Dust in poultry houses may contain 10^5–10^6 of *E. coli* bacteria per g. These bacteria persist for long periods of time, particularly when dry (Harry, 1964a). There was a reduction of 84–97% in 7 days following wetting of the dust with water. Sawow and Pawlow (1967) could reproduce coliform septicemia by means of oral and aerosol exposure of 5–6-day-old chicks. Feed is often contaminated with pathogenic coliforms which can be destroyed by hot pelleting. Rodent droppings often contain pathogenic coliforms.

ETIOLOGY

Escherichia coli (Bacterium coli) is a gram-negative, nonacid-fast, uniform staining, nonsporeforming bacillus, usually 2–3 $\times$ 0.6μ. The organism may be variable in size and shape. Many strains are motile and have peritrichous flagella.

GROWTH REQUIREMENTS

Escherichia coli grows on ordinary nutrient media at temperatures of 18–44° C or lower. On agar plates incubated for 24 hours at 37° C the colonies are low, convex, smooth, and colorless. They are usually 1–3 mm in diameter with granular structure and an entire margin. *E. coli* grows well in broth, producing turbid growth.

BIOCHEMICAL PROPERTIES

Acid and gas are produced in glucose, maltose, mannitol, xylose, glycerol, rhamnose, sorbitol, and arabinose but not in dextrin, starch, or inisitol. A few strains require up to a week to ferment lactose. Fermentation of adonitol, sucrose, salicin, raffinose, and dulcitol are variable. *E. coli* produces positive methyl red and negative Voges-Proskauer reactions. No H_2S is produced on Kligler's medium. It does not grow in the presence of KCN, attack urea, liquify gelatin, or grow in citrate medium. Isolates of *E. coli* from poultry are simi-

lar to isolates from other sources. Pathogenic isolates cannot be differentiated from nonpathogens by means of biochemical tests.

ANTIGENIC STRUCTURES

The various serotypes of *E. coli* are classified according to the Ewing (1956) scheme. Current knowledge about the antigenic structure of *E. coli* and its antigenic relationship to other species has been reviewed by Sojka (1965). The current classification lists 141 O antigen, 89 K antigen, and 49 H antigen serotypes.

O Antigen Somatic

The O or somatic antigen is the endotoxin which is liberated on autolysis of smooth cells. It is composed of a polysaccharide-phospholipid complex with a protein fraction (Harvey and Carne, 1960) resistant to boiling. Ewing et al. (1956) and Sojka (1965) discuss the methods of preparing O antisera. Briefly, O antisera agglutinate antigen at high titers (usually over 1:2,560) when the antigen-antibody mixture is incubated at 50° C for 24 hours.

K Antigens

The K antigens are polymeric acid containing 2% reducing sugars (Webster et al., 1952). These antigens are associated with virulence, are on the surface of the cell, interfere with O agglutination, and can be removed by heating to 100° C for 1 hour; however, some strains require heating for 2½ hours at 121° C. On the basis of heat stability, the K antigens are subdivided into L, A, and B antigens. Antisera are prepared in rabbits by inoculating live organisms intravenously. Tube agglutination titers are determined by incubating antigen-antibody mixtures at 37° C for 2 hours and overnight at 4° C. Titers are low (1:100–1:400). Most can be identified by the slide agglutination test (serum diluted 1:2–1:10).

H Antigen (flagellar)

Flagellar (H) antigens are not often used in the antigenic identification of *E. coli* isolates and are not correlated with pathogenicity. They are destroyed by heating at 100° C and are proteins. Tube agglutination tests are read after incubation at 37° C for 2 hours. Siccardi (1966) found that 57% of 607 isolations were motile.

TABLE 12.2 ❧ Serotypes of *E. coli* Isolated from Poultry

O Serotype	Sojka, 1961, G.B.	Glantz, 1962, USA	Stepkovits, 1967, Bulgaria	Savov, 1965, Hungary	Siccardi, 1966, USA	Hensley, 1965, G.B.
			percent			
1	10	3		25	14	1
2	41	25	4	14	26	65
3			6			
6	1					1
8	3			4		3
15	2	2	6		2	
18	3	2			2	
35			15			
71	3			1		
74			9			
78	11	16	28	14	15	2
87			19			
88		5			2	
95			9			
109		11				
Other serotypes	13	24	2		33	4
Not typed	13	12	2	42	2	28
Total cultures examined	243	122	97	130	607	1,611

The reports of Ewing et al. (1956) and Sojka (1965) should be consulted before attempting antigenic differentiation of *E. coli*. Many workers have determined the O antigens of isolates from poultry diseases. Examples of the worldwide distribution of *E. coli* serotypes isolated from diseases of poultry are recorded in Table 12.2. Only serotypes reported by more than one investigator, or which accounted for over 5% of the cultures examined by any author, are recorded separately. Many other serotypes were isolated infrequently. By far the most common serotypes are 01:K1(L), 02:K1(L) and 078:K80(B). Edwards and Ewing (1954) isolated serotype 02:K1:H5 from 30 cases of acute coliform septicemia in chickens.

PATHOGENESIS AND EPIZOOTIOLOGY

Siccardi (1966) tested all known serotypes of *E. coli* for their ability to kill 13-day-old embryos following allantoic inoculation, and for their ability to cause pericarditis and mortality in 3-week-old chicks following air sac inoculation. His results indicate that 74 of 154 serotypes of *E. coli* proved to be pathogenic for either chicks or embryos or both. Other O serotypes might be considered to be pathogenic if other routes of inoculation were utilized. The reason that only 3 pathogenic serotypes are commonly isolated from poultry is unknown.

Neither the endotoxin nor the hemolysins are associated with the disease-producing ability of *E. coli* in birds.

Serotypes of *E. coli* frequently isolated from septicemia in poultry are not among those pathogenic for man. Serotype 078:K80 is commonly isolated from cattle and sheep.

EMBRYO AND EARLY CHICK MORTALITY

Between 0.5 and 6% of eggs from normal hens were found to contain *E. coli* by Savov (1966). His experimentally inoculated hens shed *E. coli* in up to 26.5% of their eggs. Pathogenic strains accounted for 43 of 245 isolates from dead embryos (Harry, 1964a). Normal yolk sac contents change from yellow-green viscid material to caseous material or to yellow-brown watery material when contaminated with *E. coli*. It can at times be isolated from chicks' normal-appearing yolk material. Harry (1957) found that *E. coli* was present in the yolk sacs of about 70% of the chicks with "mushy chick disease," which was characterized by edema and infected yolk. Other commonly isolated bacteria were proteus, bacilli, and enterococci.

Fecal contamination of eggs was considered to be the most important source of infection. Other sources may be ovarian infection or salpingitis (Ardrey et al., 1968). There was an increase of infection shortly after hatching, and the incidence of infection was reduced about 6 days after hatching.

The yolk sac of embryos is the focus of infection (Fig. 12.13). Many embryos die before hatching, particularly late in incubation. Some die at or shortly after the time of hatching, with losses continuing up to 3 weeks later. It was found by Siccardi (1966) that as few as 10 organisms of serotype 01a:K1:H7 would cause 100% mortality of day-old chicks when inoculated into the yolk sac. In many cases there is also omphalitis. Chicks or poults living more than 4 days often have pericarditis as well as infected yolks. There may be no em-

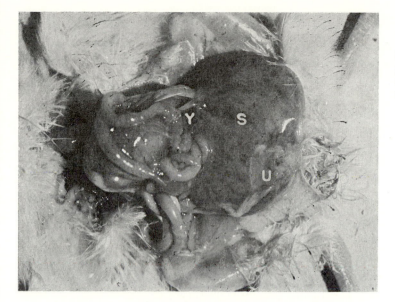

FIG. 12.13—Coliform-infected yolk sac of 6-day-old chick showing yolk stalk (Y), yolk sac (S), and umbilicus (U).

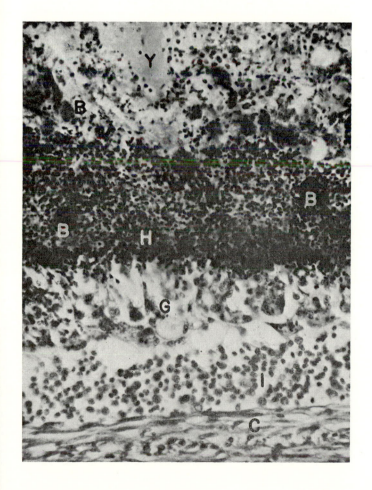

FIG. 12.14—Wall of coliform-infected yolk sac. Section shows outer connective tissue layer of yolk sac wall (C), layer of inflammatory cells containing heterophils and macrophages (I), layer of giant cells (G), zone of necrotic heterophils (H) containing masses of bacteria (B), and yolk (Y). H & E, ×220.

bryo or chick mortality, the only manifestation being retained infected yolk and reduced weight gain. The microscopic reaction in the wall of infected yolk sacs appears to be mild. The wall is edematous. There is an outer connective tissue layer followed by a layer of inflammatory cells containing heterophils and macrophages, a layer of giant cells, a zone of necrotic heterophils and masses of bacteria and then the inner infected yolk contents (Fig. 12.14). In some yolk sacs there are a few plasma cells.

Omphalitis and other yolk sac infections have been experimentally reproduced by exposing eggs to *E. coli* broth cultures by Reid et al. (1960), Gross (1964), and Siccardi (1966). Dipping at 18 days of incubation resulted in a higher incidence of infection than dipping at 1 day. Low brooding temperature or fasting increases the incidence of infection and mortality.

RESPIRATORY TRACT INFECTION (AIR SAC DISEASE)

Escherichia coli often infects the respiratory tracts of birds which are infected with various combinations of infectious bronchitis, Newcastle disease, and mycoplasmosis. This is commonly called "air sac disease." There are often secondary pericarditis and perihepatitis (Fig. 12.15). Occasionally panophthalmitis and salpingitis occur. "Air sac disease" occurs chiefly in 5–12-week-old broilers with a maximum incidence at 6–9 weeks. Important economic losses occur as the result of mortality and condemnation of birds at time of slaughter.

The lesions of uncomplicated coliform "air sac disease" can be easily reproduced by inoculating pathogenic serotypes of *E. coli* via the air sac. Airsacculitis occurs within an hour. Bacteremia and pericarditis may develop by 6 hours. Lesions are well developed 48 hours after inoculation. Most mortality occurs during the first 5 days. Recovery is usually rapid if birds survive the initial infection although a few birds with persistent anorexia become emaciated and die.

Respiratory tracts which are experimentally infected with various combinations of mycoplasma and respiratory viruses such as infectious bronchitis virus (IBV) and Newcastle disease virus (NDV) become extremely susceptible to invasion by *E. coli* via the respiratory route (Gross, 1961b; Fabricant and Levine, 1962). Vaccine strains of IBV and NDV may result in almost as much increase in coliform susceptibility as field strains. Mycoplasmal infection results in increased susceptibility to *E. coli* about 12–16 days after inoculation, and susceptibility persists for at least 30 days. Respiratory tracts infected with IBV or NDV in addition to mycoplasma become more susceptible to *E. coli,* and the susceptible period begins earlier and persists longer. Infection with IBV or NDV alone results in a lower level of susceptibility to *E. coli* aerosols than mixed infection. Although uninfected chicken respiratory tracts are relatively resistant to inhaled *E.*

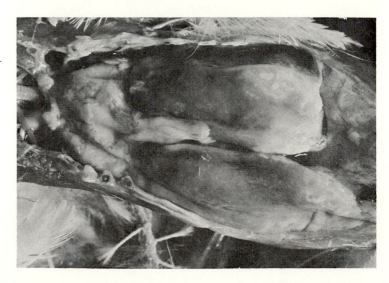

FIG. 12.15—Coliform pericarditis and perihepatitis.

coli, losses are reported with no signs of respiratory disease (Carlson and Whenham, 1968). Increased social interaction seems to increase the susceptibility of respiratory disease infected air sacs to *E. coli.* Inhaled coliform contaminated dust is probably one of the most important sources for infecting susceptible air sacs.

Pathology

Infected air sacs are thickened and often have a caseous exudate on the respiratory surface. Microscopically the earliest lesions consist of edema and infiltration by heterophils. Mononuclear phagocytes are frequently seen 12 hours after inoculation. Later the mononuclear phagocytes are most common, with giant cells lining the margins of necrotic areas. There is much fibroblastic proliferation and accumulation of vast numbers of necrotic heterophils in the caseous exudate. Lesions of the predisposing respiratory disease are usually present and consist of lymphoid follicles, epithelial hyperplasia, and epithelial lined air passages which may contain heterophils (Figs. 12.16, 12.17).

PANOPHTHALMITIS

Panophthalmitis is an uncommon manifestation of *E. coli* septicemia. There is hypopyon, usually of one eye, which is blind (Fig. 12.18). Most birds die shortly after the onset of lesions although some recover. Microscopically there are infiltrations of heterophils and mononuclear phagocytes throughout the eye, and giant cells form around necrotic areas (Fig. 12.19). The choroid becomes hyperemic and there is complete destruction of the retina.

PERICARDITIS

Most serotypes of *E. coli* cause pericarditis after they become septicemic. Borstein and Samberg (1953) reported a coliform infection in geese characterized by pericarditis and perihepatitis. Pericarditis is usually associated with myocarditis and results in marked changes in the electrocardiogram (Gross, 1966), often before macroscopic lesions appear. The pericardial sac becomes cloudy and the epicardium becomes edematous and is covered with a light-colored exudate. Often the pericardial sac fills with a light yellow fibrinous exudate. Microscopically at first there are many heterophils in the epicardium. In less than 24 hours the macrophages become most common. Within the myocardium, particularly close to the epicardium, there are accumulations of lymphoid cells, and by 7–10 days there are many plasma cells (Fig. 12.20). Pericarditis-myocarditis results in reduction of carotid artery blood pressure from a norm of about 150 to 40 mm of mercury just before death.

SALPINGITIS

When the left greater abdominal air sac is infected by *E. coli,* many females develop a chronic salpingitis which is characterized by a large caseous mass in a dilated thin-walled oviduct (Gross, 1958; Fabricant and Levine, 1962). The caseous mass contains many necrotic heterophils and bacteria which persist for many months. The size of the caseous mass may increase with time. Affected birds frequently die during the first 6 months after infection and most never lay. Salpingitis may also occur following entry of coliform bacteria from the vagina in laying hens.

The tissue reaction in the oviduct is surprisingly mild and consists largely of the accumulation of heterophils just under the epithelium (Fig. 12.21). High estrogenic activity seems to be associated with growth of coliforms in the oviduct. Infection can be reproduced by inoculating large (10^9) doses of bacteria into the uterus or oviduct. Stilbestrol implants increase susceptibility and result in increased numbers of coliforms in the oviduct.

ACUTE SEPTICEMIA

An acute infectious disease which resembled fowl typhoid and fowl cholera from which *E. coli* could be isolated was described by Twisselmann (1939). Affected birds were in good flesh and had full crops which suggests the acute nature of the infection. The most characteristic lesions were a green liver and congested pectoral muscles. In some cases there were small white focal areas in the liver. As in other coliform septicemias, there was a tendency toward pericarditis and peritonitis. Twisselmann was unable to reproduce the condition.

This disease continues to cause acute losses in mature and growing chickens and turkeys. There are no reports of experimental reproduction of the condition even

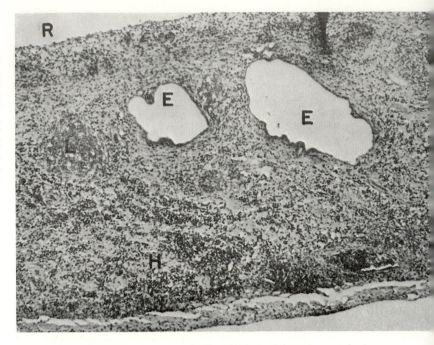

FIG. 12.16—Air sac infected with Mycoplasma gallisepticum *followed by* E. coli *aerosol exposure. Section shows respiratory surface (**R**), epithelium-lined air passages (**E**), lymphoid follicles (**L**), and area containing many heterophils (**H**). H & E, ×110.*

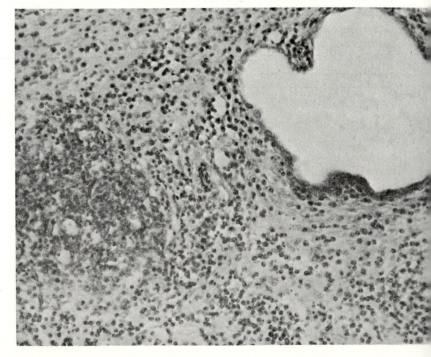

FIG. 12.17—Air sac infected with Mycoplasma gallisepticum *followed by* E. coli *aerosol exposure showing epithelium-lined air passage, lymphoid follicle, and heterophil infiltration. ×400.*

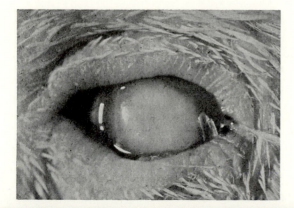

FIG. 12.18—Coliform panophthalmitis of left eye of chicken.

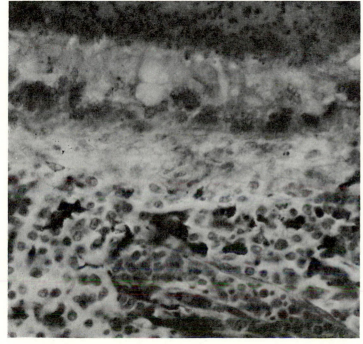

FIG. 12.19—Coliform panophthalmitis. Section shows (from top to bottom) necrotic mass in vitreous humor lined with giant cells, completely degenerate retina, and hyperemic choroid containing many mononuclear phagocytes. H & E, ×600.

though the same serotypes are also isolated from other diseases in poultry.

SYNOVITIS

Isolates of *E. coli* have been recovered from joint infections of chickens. Lesions could be reproduced following the intravenous inoculation of a broth culture of an isolate identified as 015 (Gross, 1961a). Synovitis is frequently a sequel to bacteremia. Many birds recover in about a week, while others remain chronically infected and may become emaciated.

COLIGRANULOMA

Coligranuloma of chickens and turkeys is characterized by typical granuloma of the liver, ceca, duodenum, and mesentery but not of the spleen (Figs. 12.22, 12.23, 12.24). It is relatively uncommon; however, individual flocks may have mortality of as much as 75% (Hamilton and Conrad, 1958).

The first report of granulomas was made by Hjärre and Wramby (1945) who isolated a mucoid coliform organism from the lesions. Well-developed coligranuloma is histologically similar to tubercular granuloma (Figs. 12.25, 12.26), but the acid-fast stain differentiates the two. The lesions could be reproduced following intramuscular inoculation of ground granulomas or intravenous inoculation of the isolated mucoid coliform bacteria. Granulomas could also be reproduced in the rabbit.

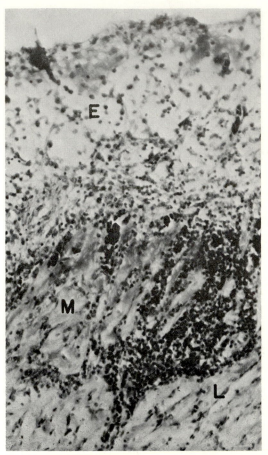

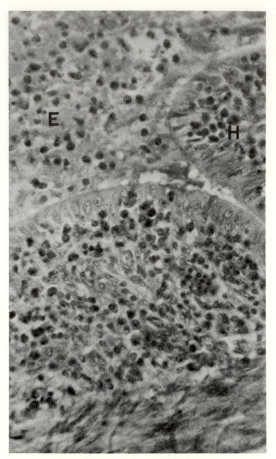

FIG. 12.20—Coliform-infected heart wall showing epicardium (E) which is edematous and contains mononuclear inflammatory cells and myocardium (M) which contains large infiltrations of lymphoid cells (L). H & E, ×100.

FIG. 12.21—Coliform salpingitis showing exudate containing heterophils (E) in lumen and heterophils (H) passing through epithelium. H & E, ×500.

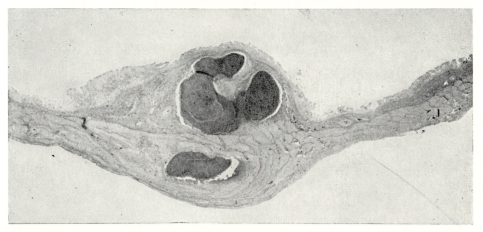

FIG. 12.22—Longitudinal section of cecum through a granuloma. Enlarged. (Hjärre, State Vet. Med. Inst., Stockholm, Sweden)

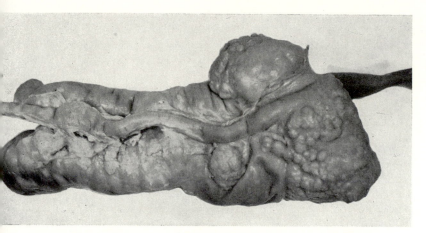

FIG. 12.23—Ceca containing granulomae (Hjärre, State Vet. Med. Inst., Stockholm, Sweden)

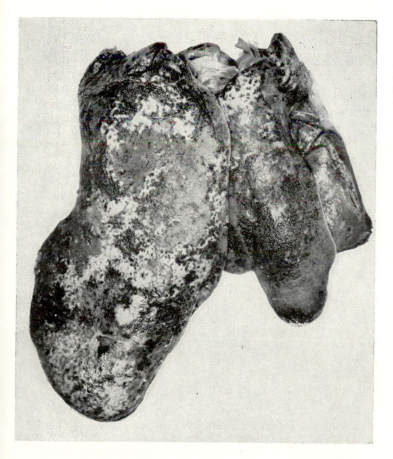

FIG. 12.24—Liver from chicken with coligranuloma. (Hjärre, State Vet. Med. Inst., Stockholm, Sweden)

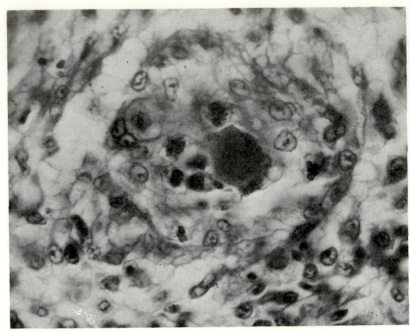

FIG. 12.25—Early coliform granuloma showing central mass of bacteria and surrounding heterophils, macrophages, and fibroblasts. H & E, ×1,200.

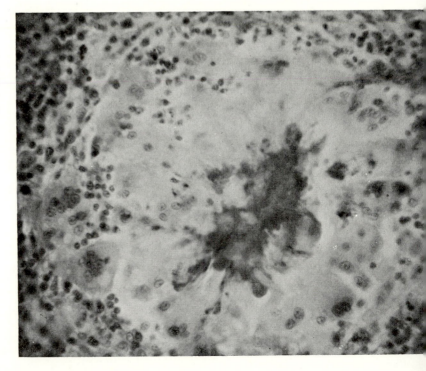

FIG. 12.26—Old coliform granuloma showing small necrotic area surrounded by large giant cells. H & E, ×1,200.

According to Helmboldt (personal communication), *E. coli* occasionally causes serosal lesions resembling leukosis. There is confluent coagulation necrosis involving as much as half of the liver. Only scattered heterophils are seen and at the edge of the necrotic areas a few histiocytes attempting to form giant cells. This lesion is possibly the precursor to Hjärre's disease.

COLIFORM SEPTICEMIA OF DUCKS
(NEW DUCK DISEASE, ANATIPESTIFER
SYNDROME, DUCK SEPTICEMIA)

The characteristics and etiologies of diseases that produce lesions of pericarditis, perihepatitis, and airsacculitis in ducklings have been described by Leibovitz (1968, personal communication). The most common causes of these infections are *E. coli* and *Pasteurella anatipestifer*, although other agents may produce similar necropsy findings. Coliform septicemia of ducks is characterized by a moist granular to curdlike exudate on the abdominal and thoracic viscera and on the surfaces of all the air sacs. The exudate varies in thickness. A characteristic odor is often noted when affected birds are necropsied. The liver is frequently swollen, dark, and bile-stained. The spleen is swollen and dark. The organism can usually be recovered from any of the internal organs.

Coliform septicemia occurs throughout the growing season but becomes more frequent in the late fall and winter months. All ages of ducklings are susceptible. Distribution of losses suggests that individual farms rather than hatcheries are the source of infection.

Differential diagnosis involves distinguishing this infection from *P. anatipestifer* infection. The latter is characterized by a more limited involvement of the respiratory tract and a dry, thin transparent covering over the visceral organs. When the exudate is thick, it is yellow and firm. Casts of such thick exudates may be found in the nasal sinuses, respiratory tract, and oviduct. *P. anatipestifer* is more difficult to recover by cultural means. It is most frequently isolated from the respiratory tract, heart blood, and brain of affected birds, less frequently from other internal organs. Dual infections of ducklings are seldom encountered.

ENTERITIS

Enteritis caused by *E. coli* is important in humans, calves, and swine. While there are a few reports of enteritis in poultry in which *E. coli* has been suggested as playing a part, there has not been enough conclusive research to indicate an *E. coli* etiology. During acute *E. coli* infections there are often very fluid yellowish droppings. This is associated not with enteritis but with increased water loss from the urine.

Pathogenic strains of *E. coli* apparently cause no growth depression or other adverse effects when confined to the digestive tract (Siccardi and Pomeroy, 1964). Stephens et al. (1965) were unable to increase the incidence of colisepticemia in normal and mycoplasma-infected 2-week-old chicks by means of *Eimeria necatrix* infection.

DIAGNOSIS

ISOLATION AND IDENTIFICATION
OF CAUSATIVE AGENT

Material should be streaked on either eosin methylene blue (EMB) agar, MacConkey agar, or tergitol 7 agar as well as noninhibitory media. Care should be made to avoid fecal contamination. A presumptive diagnosis of *E. coli* infection can be made if the majority of the colonies are characteristically dark with a metallic sheen on EMB agar, brick red on MacConkey agar, and yellow on tergitol 7 agar. A few strains of *E. coli* are slow lactose fermenters and appear as nonlactose-fermenting colonies. A definite diagnosis of *E. coli* can be made if the gram-negative bacillus does almost all of the following: produces indole; does not attack urea; fails to produce H_2S; does not liquify gelatin; does not grow on citrate medium; gives positive methyl red and negative Voges-Proskauer reaction; ferments glucose, mannite, and maltose with the production of acid and gas.

Antigenic identification of the isolate might be helpful, particularly when done as part of an epidemiological investigation.

DIFFERENTIAL DIAGNOSIS

Lesions similar to those described as being caused by *E. coli* can be caused by a wide variety of other organisms.

Synovitis-arthritis can also be caused by

mycoplasma, staphylococci, salmonellae, *Streptobacillus moniliformis* (Boyer et al., 1958), and other organisms. A great variety of organisms such as aerobacters, proteus, salmonellae, bacilli, staphylococci, enteric streptococci, and clostridia are frequently isolated (often as mixed cultures) from the yolk sacs of embryos and chicks (Harry, 1957). Pericarditis can also be caused by chlamydia. Peritonitis is sometimes caused by pasteurellae or streptococci. Acute septicemic diseases are caused by pasteurellae, salmonellae, streptococci, and other organisms. Granulomas of the liver have many causes, including highly anaerobic bacteria such as *Catenabacterium*.

TREATMENT

Escherichia coli is sensitive to streptomycin, chloramphenicol, chlortetracycline, nitrofurans, neomycin, oxytetracycline, and sulfa drugs. Isolates of *E. coli* from poultry may be resistant to drugs, but this is less frequently encountered with the nitrofurans, chloramphenicol, and neomycin. It is advisable to determine the drug sensitivity of the strains of *E. coli* involved in a disease condition so that an ineffective drug can be avoided. Even a highly effective drug may not result in improvement of the flock if too little drug is used. Smith (1967) was able to transmit infectious drug resistance to tetracycline in 37 of 38 attempts with *E. coli*.

PREVENTION AND CONTROL

Methods which reduce the introduction of pathogenic serotypes into poultry flocks are essential to the control of the colibacillosis.

E. coli infection of the respiratory tract of birds can be reduced by raising mycoplasma-free birds and by reducing the exposure of birds to viruses causing respiratory diseases. Reducing the level of *E. coli*-contaminated dust in the air of poultry houses by means of increased ventilation will reduce respiratory tract exposure. Methods for reducing the level of pathogenic *E. coli* in the intestinal tract and feces are unknown, although consideration that pelleted feed has fewer *E. coli* than mash and that rodent droppings are a source of pathogenic *E. coli* should not be overlooked. The most important source for the transmission of pathogenic *E. coli* between flocks is fecal contamination of hatching eggs. Transmission can be reduced by fumigating or disinfecting eggs 1½–2 hours after they are laid and by discarding cracked eggs or eggs with fecal contamination. If infected eggs are broken during incubation, their contents are a serious source of infection to other eggs, especially when personnel and egg handling equipment are soiled. Eggs are particularly susceptible just before hatching. Methods for preventing incubator dissemination are unknown. However, venting incubators to the outside and having as few breeder flocks as possible represented in each incubator will help reduce losses. More contaminated chicks survive if they are kept warm and are not starved.

REFERENCES

Ardrey, W. B., C. F. Peterson, and Margaret Haggart. 1968. Experimental colibacillosis and the development of carriers in laying hens. *Avian Diseases* 12:505–11.

Borstein, S., and Y. Samberg. 1953. Colibacillosis in geese caused by *Escherichia freundii*. (In Hebrew, English summary.) *Pefnat. Veterinarith* 10:95–103, 136–38.

Boyer, C. I., Jr., D. W. Bruner, and J. A. Brown. 1958. A streptobacillus, the cause of tendon sheath infection in turkeys. *Avian Diseases* 2:418–27.

Carlson, H. C., and G. R. Whenham. 1968. Coliform bacteria in chicken broiler house dust and their possible relationship to colisepticemia. *Avian Diseases* 12:297–302.

Edwards, P. R., and W. H. Ewing. 1954. Studies on a coliform type isolated from the organs of fowls. *Cornell Vet.* 44:50–56.

Ewing, W. H., H. W. Tatum, B. R. Davis, and R. W. Reavis. 1956. Studies on the serology of the *Escherichia coli* group. Communicable Disease Center, Atlanta, Georgia.

Fabricant, J., and P. P. Levine. 1962. Experimental production of complicated chronic respiratory disease infection (Air Sac Disease). *Avian Diseases* 6:13–23.

Glantz, P. J., S. Narotsky, and G. Bubash. 1962. *Escherichia coli* serotypes isolated from salpingitis and chronic respiratory disease of poultry. *Avian Diseases* 6:322–28.

Gross, W. B. 1958. Symposium on chronic respiratory diseases of poultry. II. The role of *Escherichia coli* in the cause of chronic respiratory disease and certain other respiratory diseases. *Am. J. Vet. Res.* 19:448–52.

———. 1961a. Case report: A synovitis caused by a strain of *Escherichia coli. Avian Diseases* 5:218–20.

———. 1961b. The development of "air sac disease." *Avian Diseases* 5:431–39.

———. 1964. Retained caseous yolk sacs caused by *Escherichia coli. Avian Diseases* 8:438–41.

———. 1966. Electrocardiographic changes of *Escherichia coli*-infected birds. *Am. J. Vet. Res.* 27:1427–36.

Gross, W. B., and P. B. Siegel. 1959. Coliform peritonitis of chickens. *Avian Diseases* 3: 370–73.

Hamilton, C. M., and R. D. Conrad. 1958. Extreme mortality in Hjärre's disease (coli-granuloma in chickens. *J. Am. Vet. Med. Ass.* 132:84–85.

Harry, E. G. 1957. The effect on embryonic and chick mortality of yolk contamination with bacteria from the hen. *Vet. Record* 69: 1433–40.

———. 1964a. The survival of *E. coli* in the dust of poultry houses. *Vet. Record* 76:466–70.

———. 1964b. A study of 119 outbreaks of *Coli septicaemia* in broiler flocks. *Vet. Record* 76:443–49.

Harry, E. G., and L. A. Hemsley. 1965a. The association between the presence of septicemia strains of *Escherichia coli* in the respiratory and intestinal tracts of chickens and the occurrence of *Coli septicaemia. Vet. Record* 77:35–40.

———. 1965b. The relationship between environmental contamination with septicemia strains of *Escherichia coli* and their incidence in chickens. *Vet. Record* 77:241–45.

Harvey, D. G., and P. J. Carne. 1960. Studies on some chemical aspects of the pathological activities of strains of *Escherichia coli* of bovine origin. *J. Comp. Pathol. Therap.* 70:84–108.

Hemsley, L. A., and E. G. Harry. 1965. Coliform pericarditis *(Coli septicaemia)* in broiler chickens: A three-year study on one farm. *Vet. Record* 77:103–7.

Hjärre, A., and G. Wramby. 1945. Undersokningar over en med specifika granulom forlopande honssjukdom orsakad av mukoida kolibacterier (Koli-granulom). *Skan. Veterinaertidskr.* 35:449–507.

Lignières, J. M. 1894. Septicemie a coli-bacille chez la poule. *Compt. Rend. Soc. Biol.* 46: 135–37.

Lindgren, Nils Olof. 1964. On the aetiology of salpingitis and salpingo-peritonitis of the domestic fowl, a statistical and experimental investigation. Thesis. (Akad. Avh. Veterinarhogsk) Ivar Haeggstroms Tryckeri AB, Stockholm.

Reid, Malcolm, T. A. Maag, F. M. Boyd, A. L. Kleckner, and S. C. Schmittle. 1960. Embryo and baby chick mortality and morbidity induced by a strain of *Escherichia coli. Poultry Sci.* 40:1497–1502.

Savov, D. 1965. Investigations into pathogenic strains of *Escherichia coli* isolated from fowls. (In Bulgarian, English summary.) *Vet. Med. Nauki* (Sofia) 2:825–32.

———. 1966. Pathogenic *Escherichia coli* carriage in fowl. (In Bulgarian, English summary.) *Vet. Med. Nauki* (Sofia) 3:519–25.

Sawow, von D., and N. Pawlow. 1967. Untersuchungen zur experimentellen Koliinfektion an Huhnerkuken. *Monatsh. Veterinaermed.* 22 (4): 151–55.

Siccardi, F. J. 1966. Identification and disease producing ability of *Escherichia coli* associated with *E. coli* infection of chickens and turkeys. M. S. thesis. Univ. Minnesota.

Siccardi, F. J., and B. S. Pomeroy. 1964. Effect of *E. coli* on the growth rate, morbidity and mortality in monocontaminated and conventional White Rock chickens. *Poultry Sci.* 43:1361. (Abstr.)

Smith, H. W. 1967. Incidence of infective drug resistance in strains of *Escherichia coli* isolated from diseased human beings and domestic animals. *Vet. Record* 80:464–69.

Sojka, W. J. 1965. Escherichia coli *in Domestic Animals and Poultry.* Commonwealth Agr. Bur., England.

Sojka, W. J., and R. B. A. Carnaghan. 1961. *Escherichia coli* infection in poultry. *Res. Vet. Sci.* 2:40–52.

Stephens, J. F., R. O. Taylor, and B. D. Barnett. 1965. Coccidiosis as a stress factor in the development of air sac disease. *Poultry Sci.* 44:165–69.

Stipkovits, L., and T. Bereznai. 1967. Relationship between gross lesions and *Escherichia coli* serotypes in chronic respiratory disease (CRD) of poultry. *Acta Vet. Acad. Sci. Hung.* 17:183–88.

Twisselmann, N. M. 1939. An acute infectious disease of pullets apparently caused by *E. coli communis. J. Am. Vet. Med. Ass.* 94: 235–36.

Webster, M. E., M. Landy, and M. E. J. Freeman. 1952. Studies on Vi antigen II purification of Vi antigen from *Escherichia coli* 5396/38. *J. Immunol.* 69:135–42.

❖

SPIROCHETOSIS

❖

SPIROCHETOSIS (*Borrelia anserina* infection) is usually an acute disease of many species of fowl characterized by fever, depression, cyanosis of the head, and diarrhea. While the disease has no major significance in the United States, it is of great economic importance in many areas of the world.

HISTORY

Spirochetosis was first described by Sakharoff (1891). He reported on an extensive outbreak among geese in the Caucasus. The disease was first recorded in India in 1908 by Pease (Rao et al., 1954). The first case of spirochetosis in the United States was among turkeys in California (Hoffman and Jackson, 1946). About one year later another outbreak occurred in California turkeys (McNeil et al., 1949). The disease was also reported in pheasants in California (Mathey and Siddle, 1955) and in chickens from other southwestern states (Francis, 1956; Rokey and Snell, 1961).

INCIDENCE AND DISTRIBUTION

Spirochetosis is prevalent in many countries where the tick vector *Argas persicus* Oben 1818 is present. Knowles et al. (1932) in their review of the disease list spirochetosis as a cause for mortality in 33 different regions or countries up to that time. The disease is prevalent and causes serious losses in Egypt (Morcos et al., 1946; Ahmed and Elsisi, 1966). Rao et al. (1954) reported that the disease is a serious hazard to poultry in most North Indian provinces but some parts of southern India are free of the disease.

Spirochetosis is not common in the United States even though the tick and other vectors are present in the southern states.

ETIOLOGY

The causative organism is *Borrelia anserina* (Breed et al., 1957). Synonyms are

Revised by M. S. Hofstad, Veterinary Medical Research Institute, Iowa State University, Ames.

Spirochaeta anserina (Sakharoff, 1891), *Spirochaeta gallinarum, Spirochaeta anatis,* and *Treponema anserina.* The organism belongs in the order Spirochaetales and family Treponemataceae. *Borrelia* differs from the other two genera of this family in that it stains readily with ordinary aniline dyes, whereas *Treponema* and *Leptospira* require Giemsa's stain or silver impregnation. For additional information on spirochetes the reader is referred to the review by Stavitsky (1948).

MORPHOLOGY AND STAINING

Borrelia anserina is loosely spiraled with 5–6 spirals (Fig. 12.27). The length varies from 7 to 21μ with an average of 14μ (McNeil et al., 1949). The organism is motile by a single, short, delicate flagellum at each end (Knowles et al., 1932). The spirochete has no terminal hook which differentiates it from leptospira. *B. anserina* stains readily with aniline dyes as well as with Giemsa's stain. In the late stages of the disease, stained blood smears show the spirochetes in clumps (Fig. 12.28).

GROWTH REQUIREMENTS

Cultures

Cultivation of the organism in artificial medium has not been very successful. Noguchi (1912) succeeded in growing the spirochete by using a piece of fresh tissue such as rabbit kidney or pectoral muscle of chicken, ascitic fluid, and paraffin oil. He was able to make 15 serial passages, and the culture was still virulent after 13 passages.

Kligler et al. (1938a) also succeeded in growing the organism for vaccine production. They used two different media; the simpler one was 2 parts Tyrode's solution and 1 part rabbit serum using 10 ml per tube. The tubes were inoculated with 0.5 ml infective blood during the early stage of the disease and incubated at 30° C. Maximum growth occurred by the 6th day. However, Morcos et al. (1946) using Kligler's procedure had poor success in propagating the organism beyond the 1st passage. Mathey and Siddle (1955) also failed to grow the organism in Schüffner's medium and in Tyrode's solution with 10% rabbit serum.

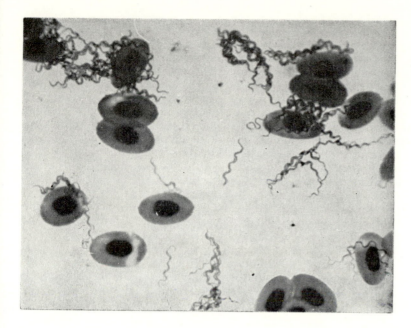

FIG. 12.27—Borrelia anserina *in turkey blood in early stages of disease.* ×1,200. *(McNeil et al., 1949)*

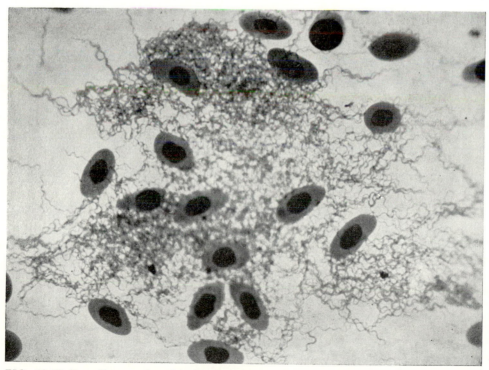

FIG. 12.28—Borrelia anserina *showing clumping in late stage of disease.* ×1,200. *(McNeil et al., 1949)*

Chickens

Borrelia anserina is propagated and kept viable in the laboratory by passaging it every 2 or 3 weeks in young chicks. Morcos et al. (1946) passaged every 3 weeks in chickens 2 months old. The infected chickens were bled on the 2nd day, the blood was allowed to clot, and the serum in which the spirochetes were abundant was stored in the refrigerator for 2–3 weeks.

McNeil et al. (1949) maintained two strains by serial passage in chicks every 5 days. At first mortality in the chicks was 35%, but after 2 years the mortality increased to 85%. Blood of the chicks contained spirochetes for an average of 7 days.

Embryonating Chicken Eggs

Knowles et al. (1932) succeeded in growing the organism in embryonating chicken eggs. Mathey and Siddle (1955) also used embryonating eggs to grow the spirochete which they isolated from pheasants. The organism grew equally well in the yolk sac, the allantoic sac, and on the chorioallantoic membrane. The spirochetes were most numerous in the embryo and membranes, with only a few in the extra-embryonic fluids.

RESISTANCE TO CHEMICAL AND PHYSICAL AGENTS

Borrelia anserina is not very resistant outside the host and must maintain itself in some vector between bird hosts. In the laboratory the spirochete can be maintained by bird passage where it may be stored for as long as 3–4 weeks in serum from clotted infected blood. McNeil et al. (1949) found liver and spleen from infected birds to remain infective for chicks for 31 days when stored at 32° F. They also reported the spirochetes to be soluble in 10% ox bile and 10% saponin.

STRAIN CLASSIFICATION

Little is known about strain differences of *Borrelia anserina*. Kligler et al. (1939b) reported on experiments using the agglutinating and spirocidal action of specific immune serum and cross-immunity challenge to study the antigenic relationship of different strains. Their studies demonstrated the existence of antigenically distinct types. However, no additional reports in the literature were found confirming the existence of serologically different strains.

PATHOGENICITY

Borrelia anserina is pathogenic primarily for fowl. Nonavian species are generally resistant except rabbits which may have a transient infection. Experimentally in chicks, the routes of inoculation giving the shortest incubation period and greatest mortality are intravenous, intramuscular, and subcutaneous in that order (McNeil et al., 1949). However, the organism may be given by other routes such as oral, nasal, and rectal to produce infection. Older birds tend to be more resistant with lower mortality. Morcos et al. (1946) report that the native Egyptian breeds are more resistant than imported breeds. McNeil et al. (1949) observed that adult turkeys are more resistant than chickens. Packchanian (1950) found chicks 2 weeks old or older to be more resistant than 3–4-day-old chicks.

PATHOGENESIS AND EPIZOOTIOLOGY

NATURAL AND EXPERIMENTAL HOSTS

Geese, turkeys, chickens, ducks, pheasants, grouse, and canaries have been reported to be natural hosts for *Borrelia anserina*. In the review by McNeil et al. (1949) the following birds have been experimentally infected: crows, myna, cominos, capuchins, turtledoves, pigeons, guinea fowl, partridges, magpies, larks, and sparrows. Knowles et al. (1932) report the turtledove and sparrow to be very susceptible. Pigeons and guinea fowl are rather resistant. Morcos et al. (1946) found only 1 of 8 pigeons susceptible. They report guinea fowl, doves, kites, crows, and hawks refractory. All ages are susceptible, but older birds tend to be more resistant and many recover spontaneously.

TRANSMISSION, CARRIERS, VECTORS

Spirochetosis can apparently be transmitted directly from bird to bird. McNeil et al. (1949) fed bile-stained droppings from infected birds to poults and they developed infection in 5 days. Dzhankov et al. (1968) found spirochetes in the mouth and cloaca during spirochetemia, but the organism disappeared from there and other organs 24–48 hours after disappearance of spirochetes from the blood. Marchoux and Salimbeni (1903) reported a natural outbreak of spirochetosis in Brazil and were the first to incriminate the tick *Argas persicus* as a vector. Zuelzer (1936) reported good evidence that Culex mosquitoes may also serve as vectors. Mites may serve as mechanical carriers of the organism but are not true vectors. Dickie and Barrera (1964) were unable to detect spirochetes in experimental chickens beyond the 13th day postinoculation. Dzhankov et al. (1968) likewise found no evidence of carriers.

Infection in Argas persicus

Ticks become infective via bite in 6–7 days and remain infective up to 430 days. In ticks that are fed, the spirochete develops regardless of the temperature, and transmission is possible at all times of the year. The ticks may infect the host by bite or the birds may become infected by eating infected ticks. Infected ticks lay infected ova and thus pass on the spirochetes to the next generation of ticks. Spirochetes are difficult to demonstrate in the tick, but it is believed that they occur as tiny, slender spirochetes and not in some different form (Knowles et al., 1932).

INCUBATION PERIOD

In chickens the incubation period is 3–8 days. In experimentally inoculated birds the temperature usually increases in 24–48 hours, and spirochetes may be in the blood as early as 24 hours depending on route of inoculation and dosage. Knowles et al. (1932) found the incubation period in young chicks to be 3–4 days after oral ingestion of infected blood and mortality was 77%; after percutaneous inoculation with infective blood it was 4 days; after intramuscular or intravenous inoculation it was 24 hours with 100% mortality; after bites by ticks it was 6–7 days with 33% mortal-

ity; after ingestion of ticks it was 6–7 days and 53% mortality; and after ingestion of tick ova it was 7–12 days and 57% mortality.

SIGNS

Infected birds are visibly sick with droopy, cyanotic heads and ruffled feathers (Fig. 12.29). They have elevated body temperatures which in turkeys may reach 110° F or higher (McNeil et al., 1949). The birds are depressed and stop eating. They have a greenish diarrhea, increased thirst, and finally may become paralyzed.

MORBIDITY AND MORTALITY

The morbidity varies from 10 to near 100%. McNeil et al. (1949) reported 20% and 11% morbidity in two flocks of turkeys. The morbidity varies with age and circumstances under which infection occurs. Mortality also varies from 1–2% as reported by McNeil et al. (1949) up to 100% in more susceptible birds and where vectors are numerous. Knowles et al. (1932) report chicks a few weeks old invariably die after experimental inoculation. They report old birds resistant, with few deaths, and that old birds die 1–2 days after disappearance of spirochetes from the blood, while young ones die at the height of infection with many spirochetes in the blood.

GROSS LESIONS

Hinshaw (1965) states that the most characteristic lesion at necropsy of dead birds is the marked enlargement and mottling of the spleen due to ecchymotic hemorrhages (Fig. 12.30). The liver may be enlarged, containing small hemorrhages and minute

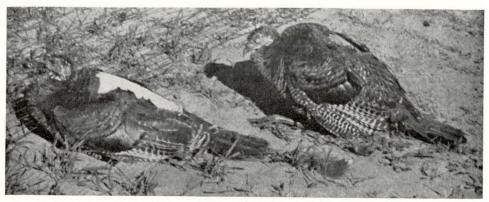

FIG. 12.29—Spirochetosis. Typical attitudes seen in acute outbreaks in turkey flocks. (Hinshaw, 1965)

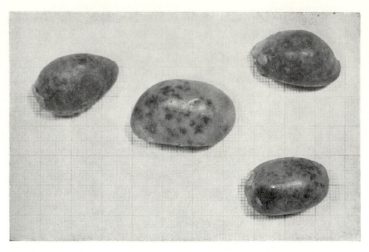

FIG. 12.30—Spleens of adult turkey hens infected with spirochetosis show typical mottling and ecchymosis. Approximately three-fourths normal size. (Hinshaw, 1965)

areas of necrosis. Occasionally liver infarcts may be observed. The kidneys are enlarged and pale. A greenish mucoid enteritis is usually present.

HISTOPATHOLOGY

The microscopic lesions of spirochetosis have been studied by Rokey and Snell (1961) and by McNeil et al. (1949). The latter workers described the changes as follows:

The characteristic structure of the spleen was not lost. The reticular cells were increased in number and size. They presented a foamy appearance due to the ingestion of lipoid material. The centers of the groups of reticular cells underwent hyalinization at times. Massive areas of hemorrhage were present (Fig. 12.31). This was the result of the rupture of the walls of veins and sinusoids. The endothelial cells lining these structures were swollen and presented the foamy appearance seen in the primitive reticular cells. The diffuse lymphatic tissue was undergoing rapid growth. The cells consisted of young large- and medium-sized lymphocytes and hemocytoblasts. Numerous mitotic figures were present. In poults spirochetes occurred in foci throughout the spleen but did not appear to have been phagocytized by the reticular cells.

The liver showed congestion and an increase in the periportal lymphoid deposits. The cells of these deposits consisted of lymphocytes in all stages, hemocytoblasts, and large phagocytic cells with vacuolated cytoplasm. Various stages of erythropoiesis were present. The endothelial cells lining the sinusoids were swollen and vacuolated. The perenchymal cells showed various degrees of fatty degeneration. Silver stains showed the majority of the spirochetes to be in the intercellular spaces and in the bile capil-

laries. Those within the hepatic cells underwent fragmentation or coiled upon themselves to form small rings.

The lungs showed generalized congestion and edema. The endothelial cells of the capillaries contained excess blood pigment. Some endothelial cells had hypertrophied so as to occlude the lumen of the vessel. Their cytoplasm was vacuolated, giving a foamy appearance. Small foci of hyaline necrosis were present throughout. The lymphoid nodules showed hemorrhage and hyperplasia.

The kidneys showed marked congestion and some hemorrhage. The glomeruli and convoluted tubules appeared normal. There was marked degeneration and desquamation with hyaline casts in the collecting tubules. The interstitial tissue showed lymphocytic infiltration. No spirochetes could be demonstrated in the kidney of the adults outside of the larger blood vessels. In poults spirochetes could be found in the intercellular spaces and in the lumens of the tubules.

The myocardial fibers presented a vacuolated appearance. In some areas this was so pronounced as to obliterate the cross striations. Spirochetes did not invade the heart tissue.

The seminiferous tubules appeared unaffected. The interstitial cells were large and filled with lipoid. The most striking feature was a prominent lymphocytic infiltration around the blood vessels. The ovary showed congestion and hemorrhage.

The intestines showed a marked degree of catarrhal enteritis. The lymphoid follicles in the submucosa were hypertrophied, and there was a generalized lymphocytic infiltration of the submucosa. The tips of some of the villi were necrotic. The most severe injury occurred in the jejunum. The pancreas appeared normal except for slight vacuolization of the secreting cells.

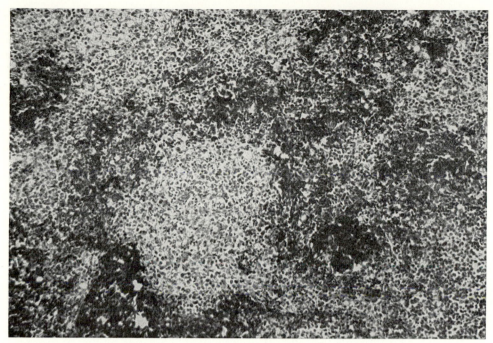

FIG. 12.31—Section of spleen showing massive areas of hemorrhage. ×150. *(McNeil et al., 1949)*

The cerebrum and medulla showed a perivascular gliosis. The meninges showed a lymphocytic infiltration.

IMMUNITY

Birds recovered from the natural disease or birds immunized with vaccines are immune to challenge for 6 months or longer. El Dardiry (1945) found recovered chickens immune for at least 13 months. Passive immunity conferred by injection of hyperimmune serum prepared in fowl or goats will serve to protect birds against challenge for 3 weeks (Morcos et al., 1946).

DIAGNOSIS

Finding spirochetes in stained blood smears from typically sick birds constitutes a diagnosis. The blood smears may be stained with Giemsa's stain. The spirochetes may also be seen by examining wet preparations by dark-field illumination. The spirochetes may not be observed in the blood during late stages of the disease. In such cases, a technique of demonstrating antibodies in the spleen from dead birds has been described by Nobrega and Reis (1947). A 30% suspension of the spleen is made to which is added 10% fresh rabbit serum. To each 1 ml of this is added 0.25 ml of a 1:10 dilution of known infected blood. After 1½ hours incubation at 37° C, the material is injected intramuscularly into 1–2-month-old cockerels. Other cockerels are inoculated with spleen suspensions only and others with infected blood. If the spleen protects the birds against infection (spirochetes in the blood on the 4th day) it indicates the dead bird possessed antibodies in its spleen and had died from the disease.

Isolation of the organism in 6-day-old embryonating chicken or turkey eggs can be done by inoculating infective blood into the yolk sac. Spirochetes may be demonstrated 2–3 days later by examining allantoic fluid which contains embryonic blood since spirochetes are found predominantly in the embryo and chorioallantoic membrane.

SEROLOGY

Kligler et al. (1938b) described a spirocidal test for antibodies. Serial dilutions of the serum are made in Tyrode's solution and 0.4 ml is added to small tubes. To these dilutions is added 1 drop of fresh rabbit serum and 1 or 2 drops of defibrinated infected blood. The tubes are shaken and incubated at 30° C. Drops from each tube are examined at ½, 1, and 2 hours under the dark-field microscope. The tubes are then kept at room temperature and examined again at 24 hours. The degree of agglutination and dissolution serves as a measure of serum antibodies.

Fluorescent Antibody Test

Gross and Ball (1964) used a direct fluorescent antibody technique to detect *Borrelia anserina* in the tissues and blood of infected chickens. They found, during the acute stages, organisms confined to the vascular system in the liver, spleen, lungs, kidney, and brain. Antigens could not be demonstrated in tissues of recovered and challenged immune birds.

TREATMENT

Borrelia anserina is sensitive to penicillin; McNeil et al. (1949) found 10,000 units of penicillin to be the minimum effective dose for turkeys. This dosage was found satisfactory in treating sick turkeys early in the course of a field outbreak of spirochetosis. These workers also found two arsenicals, neoarsphenamine and mepharsen, effective in treating experimental spirochetosis. The former was used in a dosage of 10 mg per kg intramuscularly while mepharsen was given at half that level.

Packchanian (1950) studied the effectiveness of drugs against spirochetosis using 3–4-day-old chicks. Thirteen were ineffective in 2-mg daily doses. Effective drugs were neoarsphenamine, mepharsen, tryparsamide, and penicillin G. Hsiang and Packchanian (1951) tested 11 antibiotics against experimental spirochetosis in 3–4-day-old chicks. Aureomycin in 1-mg daily doses for 2 days; bacitracin in 1-mg daily doses for 3 days, Chloromycetin in 10-mg daily doses for 4 days; and dihydrostreptomycin, penicillin G, streptomycin sulfate, and Terramycin in single 10-mg doses were all effective. Actidione, neomycin, polymyxin B, and antibiotic Q-19 failed to produce a cure when given in maximum tolerance doses. Hinshaw (1965) reported that sulfonamides and streptomycin were not effective in controlling the disease in turkeys.

PREVENTION AND CONTROL

Management procedures which serve to prevent the disease would be eliminating ticks from areas where birds are raised. Area control of mosquitoes might also serve to prevent the disease in an endemic region. Controlling the disease during an outbreak was effected by using penicillin in treating sick turkeys as soon as they were observed (McNeil et al., 1949).

IMMUNIZATION

In countries where the disease is endemic, prevention is best accomplished by immunization. Various vaccines have been used against avian spirochetosis, including simultaneous immune serum and infective blood, and infected tissues inactivated with formalin or phenol. Active immunization using these different vaccines have generally induced a satisfactory immunity for 6 months.

Types of Vaccine

Rao et al. (1954) have reviewed some of the earlier types of vaccines. Nobrega and Reis (1941) successfully used a formalin-inactivated vaccine prepared from 12-day-old chicken embryos inoculated with *B. anserina*. Morcos et al. (1946) used a vaccine composed of equal parts of infected citrated blood, liver, and spleen diluted 1:4 in saline and treated with 1% phenol for 10 days in the refrigerator. It was used in 2 doses of 0.5 ml each subcutaneously at a 5-day interval. The immunity of the birds withstood challenge 6 months later.

Rao et al. (1954) prepared experimental vaccines in embryos from 3 field strains without success. A laboratory strain which had been maintained for 2 years was passaged rapidly in birds to enhance its virulence. This strain in the form of citrated blood was then injected into 7-day-old embryos via yolk sac route. The inoculated eggs were incubated for 7 days. Only those embryos having high concentrations of spirochetes in their blood (40–50 per microscopic field) were used. Embryos and membranes were ground in a blender for 1 minute, diluted with saline, and inactivated with formalin. Challenge tests 12 months after vaccination found the birds immune.

Uppal and Rao (1966) prepared a lyophilized chicken embryo vaccine containing *B. anserina* and found that it induced an immunity in chickens. Gupta and Rao (1967) found the yield of this lyophilized vaccine 25% greater if prepared in 13-day-old chicken embryos and the embryos inoculated into the allantoic sac rather than on the chorioallantoic membrane.

Reshetnyak (1966) prepared a vaccine from citrated blood of artificially infected geese. The blood was held at 2–5° C for 2–3 days, then diluted with 0.5% phenolized saline and held at 30° C for 2–3 days, with occasional agitation, for lysis of the spirochetes to occur. After filtration a subcutaneous injection of 0.5 ml of the hemolysate vaccine was effective. Immunity persisted for at least 1 year. The vaccine was economical to produce and immunogenicity was retained after 8–9 months storage.

REFERENCES

Ahmed, A. A. S., and M. A. Elsisi. 1966. Observations of aegyptianellosis and spirochaetosis of poultry in Egypt. *Vet. Med. J.* (Giza) 11:139–46.

Breed, R. S., E. G. D. Murray, and N. R. Smith. 1957. *Bergey's Manual of Determinative Bacteriology,* 7th ed. Williams & Wilkins Co., Baltimore.

Dickie, C. W., and J. Barrera. 1964. A study of the carrier state of avian spirochetosis in the chicken. *Avian Diseases* 8:191–95.

Dzhankov, I., I. Sumrov, T. Lozeva, and P. Panev. 1968. Carriage and secretion of *Treponema anserinum* Sakharoff in chickens. *Vet. Med. Nauki* (Sofia) 5:33–37.

El Dardiry, A. H. 1945. Studies on avian spirochetosis in Egypt. Ministry of Egypt, *Tech. Sci. Serv. Bull.* 243:1–78.

Francis, D. W. 1956. A case of fowl spirochetosis in New Mexico. *Poultry Sci.* 35:1142–43. (Abstr.)

Gross, Wendy M., and Meridian R. Ball. 1964. Use of fluorescein-labeled antibody to study *Borrelia anserina* infection (avian spirochetosis) in the chicken. *Am. J. Vet. Res.* 25:1734–39.

Gupta, B. R., and S. B. V. Rao. 1967. Studies on the preparation of spirochaete vaccine. Part II. Research on its economic aspects. *Indian Vet. J.* 44:96–103.

Hinshaw, W. R. 1965. Spirochaetosis, pp. 1308–14. In Biester, H. E., and L. H. Schwarte (eds.), *Diseases of Poultry,* 5th ed. Iowa State Univ. Press, Ames.

Hoffman, H. A., and T. W. Jackson. 1946. Spirochetosis in turkeys. *J. Am. Vet. Med. Ass.* 109:481–86.

Hsiang, Chin-Min, and A. A. Packchanian. 1951. A comparison of eleven antibiotics in the treatment of *Borrelia anserina* infection (spirochetosis) in young chicks. *Texas Rept. Biol. Med.* 9:34–45.

Kligler, I. J., D. Hermoni, and M. Perek. 1938a. Immunization of chickens with *Spirochaeta gallinarum. J. Comp. Pathol. Therap.* 51: 197–205.

———. 1938b. Studies on fowl spirochaetosis. II. Presence of serologically differentiated types of spirochaetes. *J. Comp. Pathol. Therap.* 51:206–12.

Knowles, R., B. M. Das Gupta, and B. C. Basu. 1932. Studies in avian spirochaetosis. *Indian Med. Res. Mem.* 22:1–113.

McNeil, Ethyl, W. R. Hinshaw, and R. E. Kissling. 1949. A study of *Borrelia anserina* infection (spirochetosis) in turkeys. *J. Bacteriol.* 57:191–206.

Marchoux, E., and A. Selimbeni. 1903. La spirillose des poules. *Ann. Inst. Pasteur* 17: 569–80.

Mathey, W. J., and P. J. Siddle. 1955. Spirochetosis in pheasants. *J. Am. Vet. Med. Ass.* 126:123–26.

Morcos, Z., O. A. Zaki, and R. Zaki. 1946. A concise investigation of fowl spirochaetosis in Egypt. *J. Am. Vet. Med. Ass.* 109:112–16.

Nobrega, P., and A. S. Reis. 1947. O diagnostico da espiroquetose aviaria em animals mortos. *Arquiv. Inst. Biol.* (Sao Paulo) 18: 91–96.

Nobrega, P., and J. Reis. 1941. Producao da vacina contra a espiroquetose aviaria em ovos embrionados. *Arquiv. Inst. Biol.* (Sao Paulo) 12:87–92.

Noguchi, H. 1912. Cultivation of *Spirochaeta gallinarum. J. Exp. Med.* 16:620–28.

Packchanian, A. A. 1950. Chemotherapy of *Borrelia anserina* infections (spirochetosis) in young chicks. *Texas Rept. Biol. Med.* 8:78–85.

Rao, S. B. V., B. M. Thakral, and M. R. Dhanda. 1954. Studies on fowl spirochaetosis with special reference to penicillin therapy and the development of an eggadapted vaccine for its control. *Indian Vet. J.* 31:1–14.

Reshetnyak, V. Z. 1966. Specific preventive measures against avian spirochetosis. *Proc. 13th World's Poultry Congr.* (Kiev), pp. 420–23.

Rokey, N. W., and V. N. Snell. 1961. Avian spirochetosis *(Borrelia anserina)* epizootics in Arizona poultry. *J. Am. Vet. Med. Ass.* 138:648–52.

Sakharoff, M. N. 1891. *Spirochaeta anserina* et la septicemie des oies. *Ann. Inst. Pasteur* 5:564–66.

Stavitsky, A. B. 1948. Characteristics of pathogenic spirochetes and spirochetoses with special reference to the mechanisms of host resistance. *Bacteriol. Rev.* 12:203–55.

Uppal, D.R., and S. B. V. Rao. 1966. Studies on the preparation of a spirochaete vaccine (Part I). *Indian Vet. J.* 43:191–95.

Zuelzer, M. 1936. *Culex,* a new vector of *Spirochaeta gallinarum. J. Trop. Med. Hyg.* (London) 39:204.

CHAPTER 13

CHLAMYDIOSIS
(ORNITHOSIS)

LESLIE A. PAGE

National Animal Disease Laboratory
Animal Disease and Parasite
Research Division
Agricultural Research Service, U.S.D.A.
Ames, Iowa

ORNITHOSIS is a naturally occurring, systemic, contagious, occasionally fatal disease of nonpsittacine birds caused by organisms of the bacterial species *Chlamydia psittaci* (family Chlamydiaceae, order Chlamydiales.)

Chlamydiosis, a recent term meaning infection or disease caused by the presence of organisms of the genus *Chlamydia,* denotes infection of birds, mammals, arthropods, or any other member of the animal kingdom by any species of *Chlamydia.* Chlamydiosis as it originally occurred in man and psittacine birds was called psittacosis (Morange, 1895) and later, parrot fever. The term ornithosis was introduced in 1941 by Meyer to differentiate the disease in domestic and wild fowl from that in psittacine birds. This distinction proved to be artificial since it is now known that except for epizootiologic variations, psittacosis and ornithosis are essentially the same disease and that strains of *C. psittaci* originally isolated from either psittacine or nonpsittacine birds can be used interchangeably to reproduce an identical disease in birds of either group.

For the purposes of this book, this chapter is restricted to a discussion of ornithosis as it appears in birds raised commercially for meat or egg production—turkeys, ducks, pigeons, chickens, and pheasants.

Over the last three decades acute ornithosis in turkeys and ducks periodically has resulted in serious agricultural losses when sporadic epornitics have affected large concentrations of birds in commercial breeding establishments. Ornithosis in pigeons is a chronic disease in this reservoir host, affecting a large proportion of the total population of this species; it becomes an economic factor only when large numbers of birds in a poorly managed operation die as a result of the disease plus concurrent infection and environmental stress. Aside from the hazard to public health in such a situation, the economic loss is small compared to that caused by ornithosis in turkeys and ducks.

In the United States agricultural losses attributed to ornithosis reached a peak in the period from 1954 through 1956 when mortality and meat and egg condemnation losses in turkeys alone approached $0.5 million annually. In Europe epornitics in ducks, geese, chickens, and turkeys also caused periodic losses for more than a decade prior to 1963. During this period public health interest on both continents was deeply aroused by the fact that the disease appeared concurrently in humans whose occupations involved the production, handling, or processing of infected fowl. As the incidence of epornitics increased, the disease became an occupational hazard in segments of the poultry industry. In Czechoslovakia ornithosis became the most frequent zooanthroponosis as well as one of the most important infectious diseases of persons in the poultry industry. Between 1949 and 1960 there were 1,072 recorded cases in Czechoslovakia, 54% of which were associated with contact with ducks, 29% with geese, 10% with chickens, 4% with turkeys, and 3% with pigeons and pheasants (Strauss, 1967). A sharp rise in the incidence of psittacosis in U.S. citizens occurred in 1954 when there were 563 cases reported, 200 (35.5%) of which were associated with the processing of turkeys and 33 (5.9%) related to contact with chickens (Andrews, 1957). Meyer (1965) tabulated the worldwide incidence of human psittacosis for the years 1931–63 that resulted from contact with domestic fowl. He found that there were 5,390 cases: 756 (14%) associated with turkeys, 1,251 (23%) with ducks, 680 (12.5%) with pigeons, 285 (5.3%) with chickens, 192 (3.6%) with sea-

TABLE 13.1 ❧ Reports of Epornitics of Chlamydiosis (Ornithosis) in Poultry in United States, 1960–70

Year	State	Affected Species	Degree of Loss	Basis for Diagnosis	Investigator
1960	Oregon	Turkey	None reported	Agent isolation	E. M. Dickinson
1961	Texas	Turkey	Significant condemnation losses	Agent isolation	L. Passera
1964	Oregon	Chicken Pigeon Pheasant	No significant losses	Positive serology only	L. A. Page and K. Erickson
1965	Virginia	Turkey	20% mortality; severe losses	Agent isolation	W. S. Thompson and L. A. Page
1966	Virginia	Duck	10% mortality; severe losses	Agent isolation	E. C. Roukema and L. A. Page
	Texas	Turkey	"moderate"	Agent isolation	L. C. Grumbles
1967	California	Turkey	Moderate with 3% mortality	Agent isolation	J. A. Newman
1968	Minnesota	Turkey (4 flocks)	None	Positive serology	B. S. Pomeroy
	Georgia	Turkey	High condemnations	Positive tissue antigen (FA & CF)	H. W. Yoder and L. A. Page
1969	South Carolina	Turkey	Mild condemnations	Positive serology	T. H. Eleazer and L. A. Page
	California	Turkey	Low mortality; moderate condemnations	Agent isolation	D. L. Bristow and G. Lucas

All reports were personal communications to the author.

shore birds, and 2,226 (41.5%) with undifferentiated "poultry."

Agricultural losses due to ornithosis were markedly reduced in the 1960s. While over 500 epornitics were reported for the 1950s, only 11 reports were recorded for the 1960s (Table 13.1). Reasons for the reduction in incidence are not definitely established; it has been suggested that the reduced incidence is due in part to a decrease in the intermingling of chlamydia-carrying wild water fowl with domestic birds, improvements in the management of birds, increased awareness of the disease, more rapid diagnosis and treatment. Concurrent cases in humans have also been reduced. Thus as of 1969 the disease is not a widespread economic or public health factor, but its potential for damage remains high.

HISTORY

Detailed discussions of the history and epidemiology of ornithosis and psittacosis have appeared elsewhere (Meyer, 1959, 1965, 1967); however, the significant studies influencing the understanding of ornithosis in poultry bear brief mention.

Following a decade of worldwide investigations in the 1930s of the etiology and epidemiology of psittacosis in man and psittacine birds, a similar disease was observed in poultry. Transmissability of the disease in commercial squabs was demonstrated in South Africa by Coles (1940). Serologic surveys of domestic birds, stimulated by concurrent disease in humans, pointed to infections in pigeons in the United States (Meyer, et al., 1942a) and in turkeys and ducks in the United States and Europe (Eddie and Francis, 1942; Korns, 1955; Strauss, 1956). In the middle and late 1940s ornithosis epornitics in domestic ducks and turkeys caused numerous individual agricultural losses and human infections, but between 1951 and 1956 a widespread series of epornitics of unusual virulence caused such economic and public health damage that the disease became a matter of national concern. Subsequently support of research and study of turkey ornithosis by commercial, academic, and governmental agencies was promptly increased. The resultant investigations focused on ornithosis microbiology (Meyer and Eddie, 1953; Page, 1956), epizootiology (Mason and Irons, 1954; Irons et al., 1955; Meyer, 1959), serology (Gogolak and Ross, 1955; Volkert and Matthiesen, 1956; Benedict and McFarland, 1956; Benedict and O'Brien, 1958; Neal and Davis, 1958; Page and Bankowski, 1960; Brumfield et al., 1961; Rice, 1961), histopathology (Beasley et al., 1959, 1961), pathogenesis (Page, 1959a), chemotherapy and control (Meyer and Eddie, 1955; Meyer, 1955; Davis and Delaplane, 1958; Moore and Watkins, 1960). These studies formed the basis for recommendations and needed reforms in the management of birds in areas of high incidence of ornithosis (Texas, Minnesota-Wisconsin, California-Oregon) and for the treatment, handling, and processing of birds suspected of having ornithosis.

During the 1960s the incidence of severe epornitics in poultry in the United States and Europe declined, although serologic surveys continued to indicate that the infection of reservoir hosts—pigeons, wild birds, and mammals—is still prevalent. A significant role for arthropods in the transmission and perpetuation of ornithosis agents in nature was suggested by the intriguing observations of Eddie et al. (1962, 1969) and others. At this writing research is continuing on this important aspect of chlamydial epizootiology, but conclusive evidence that the etiologic agents of ornithosis are transmitted and maintained in nature by arthropods is lacking.

Scientific attention also returned to the microbiology of the disease agent and its classification and nomenclature. In a series of published lectures and a review, J. W. Moulder of the University of Chicago convincingly summarized the morphologic and biochemical evidence that revealed the bacterial nature of the etiologic agents of psittacosis, ornithosis, lymphogranuloma venereum, trachoma, and related diseases (Moulder, 1964, 1966). Further studies by Gordon and Quan (1965) resulted in the discovery of two distinct groups of chlamydiae, separated on the basis of their microbiologic characters alone and not upon their epidemiology or presumed tissue preferences as was done previously. This work permitted a simplified classification and

nomenclatural system to be established, thereby ending two decades of international disagreement (Page, 1966, 1968).

Research interest in the development of effective ornithosis vaccines for use in domestic birds declined during the 1960s. This was attributed in part to the facts that the urgency for such an immunization program had diminished, that past attempts to immunize domestic birds against ornithosis were largely inconclusive, and that antibiotic treatment of affected flocks was relatively efficacious. In fact, none of the attempts to protect man, domestic birds, or mammals by immunization procedures against the various forms of chlamydiosis have been decisive. This failure presents a continuing challenge to immunologists and to those in governmental agencies concerned with the control of animal disease.

ETIOLOGY

CLASSIFICATION

The etiologic agent of ornithosis is an obligately intracellular bacterium, *Chlamydia psittaci*, of the family Chlamydiaceae, order Chlamydiales, and class Schizomycetes. The names of the higher taxa to which this class belongs have not yet been agreed upon since it is now generally conceded that bacteria should be classified in a kingdom other than Plantae or Animalia.

For many years chlamydial organisms were often called "large viruses," because they were large enough to be seen with a light microscope and could be cultivated only in living cells. However, their nonviral nature has been satisfactorily demonstrated in numerous studies of their morphology, mode of reproduction, chemistry, and metabolism (see below). They are a unique group of organisms among a spectrum of widely varying bacteria which include such unusual microorganisms as the trichomes of the orders Hyphomicrobiales and Caryophanales, the slime molds of the order Myxobacteriales, the algaelike Beggiatoales, the spirally twisted Spirochaetales, and the common rod or spherically shaped microbes of the orders Eubacteriales and Pseudomondales.

The nomenclatural history of the chlamydiae has been marked by the publication of at least seven well-intentioned but contradictory classification proposals by French, American, and Russian taxonomists. Thus the world's literature of the last two decades contains references to these organisms as members of the genera *Chlamydozoon, Miyagawanella, Ehrlichia, Chlamydia, Rickettsiaformis, Bedsonia,* or *Rakeia.* This confusion of names led many investigators, until recently, to refer to the organisms as agents of the psittacosis-lymphogranuloma venereum-trachoma (PLT) group, or as PLT agents. The genus name *Chlamydia* has now been officially established and internationally accepted. Taxonomically all of the etiologic agents of the diseases listed below have been placed in this genus because of their common morphology, mode of reproduction, and group antigen. Only two species are recognized, and these are separated on the basis of stable differences in intracellular colonial morphology—production of glycogen, and growth inhibition by sodium sulfadiazine. A key to their differentiation, to be published in the 8th Edition of *Bergey's Manual of Determinative Bacteriology,* is as follows:

Key to the Species of *Chlamydia*

1. Forms compact microcolony in a vesicle 2–12μ in diameter in the cytoplasm of the host cell. The microcolony contains iodine-staining carbohydrate and lipid detectable by staining with iodine-potassium iodide solution following methanol fixation. Growth of the organisms in the yolk sac of the chicken embryo is inhibited by sodium sulfadiazine (1 mg per embryo):
   1. *Chlamydia trachomatis*
2. Forms microcolonies of organisms in vesicles in the cytoplasm of the host cell. The vesicle wall tends to rupture early in microcolony development, and the organisms become distributed throughout the cytoplasm. Iodine-staining compounds are not formed in microcolonies. Growth of the organisms in the yolk sac of the chicken embryo is not inhibited by sodium sulfadiazine (1 mg per embryo):
   2. *Chlamydia psittaci*

Specific diseases or conditions caused by organisms of the genus *Chlamydia* in man and animals are:

Chlamydia trachomatis
   Trachoma in man
   Inclusion conjunctivitis in man
   Lymphogranuloma venereum in man
   Urethritis in man
   Arthritis in man
   Murine pneumonitis

Chlamydia psittaci
   Psittacosis in man and psittacine birds
   Ornithosis in nonpsittacine birds
   Feline, ovine, bovine, caprine, equine, lapine, and porcine pneumonitis
   Ovine, bovine, and porcine polyarthritis
   Sporadic bovine encephalomyelitis
   Enzootic ovine abortion, epizootic bovine abortion
   Bovine enteritis
   Cavian conjunctivitis, ovine conjunctivitis
   Lapine septicemia
   Subclinical intestinal infection in domestic cattle and sheep.

MORPHOLOGY AND MODE OF REPRODUCTION

Chlamydiae are nonmotile spheroids ranging between 0.3 and 1.5μ in diameter, depending upon their stage of development in a unique, obligately intracellular growth cycle. Within hours after being phagocytized by the host cell, the elementary body or small, dense infectious form of the organism enlarges to a thin-walled, reticulated spheroid 0.6–1.5μ in diameter, called initial body (Figs. 13.1, 13.2). This large form, which contains nuclear fibrils and

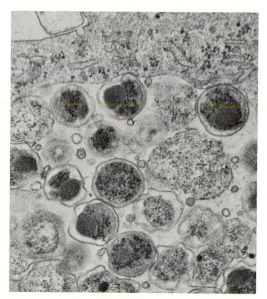

FIG. *13.1—Small (0.3μ diameter), dense, infectious forms of* C. psittaci *within cytoplasmic vesicle of host cell. Organisms have dense nuclei and clusters of ribosomes. Several large, amorphous initial bodies are also present. Electron micrograph of ultrathin section. ×40,000. (Anderson et al., 1965)*

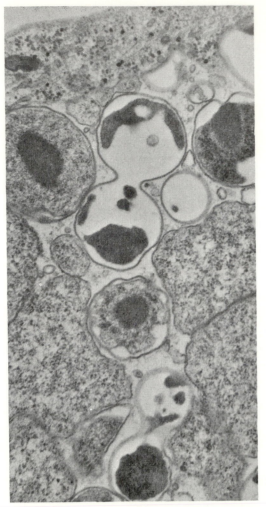

FIG. 13.2—Large vegetative forms of C. psittaci *in process of dividing within cytoplasmic vesicle. Electron micrograph of ultrathin section.* ×40,000. (Anderson et al., 1965)

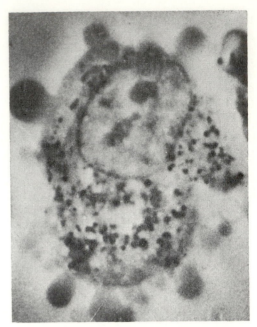

FIG. 13.3—Phase contrast micrograph of mononuclear cell from peritoneum of mouse infected with NJ-1 turkey strain of C. psittaci. Cytoplasm of cell is filled with chlamydiae in all stages of growth. ×4,500. (Page, 1967)

ribosomal elements, represents the vegetative phase of the organism and multiplies by fission. Daughter organisms gradually reduce in size and become dense spherules approximately 0.3μ in diameter containing nuclear material and ribosomes and bounded by a cytoplasmic membrane and rigid cell wall. Growth, multiplication, and maturation of the organisms occur over a period of 30 hours or less within a vesicle in the cytoplasm of the host cell. The wall of the vesicle apparently originates from the cytoplasmic membrane of the host cell which invaginates as it engulfs the organism. After the chlamydiae begin to mul-

tiply, the vesicle wall of C. psittaci microcolonies ruptures and the organisms become distributed throughout the cytoplasm (Fig. 13.3). This type of chlamydial microcolony is characteristic of C. psittaci and is distinguished from the rigid, compact microcolonies of C. trachomatis (Fig. 13.4).

TINCTORIAL CHARACTERISTICS

The microcolonies of each species can be distinguished further by staining sections of infected tissues or monolayers of infected cell cultures with an alcoholic solution of 5% iodine-potassium iodide for several hours after fixing them in cold methanol for several hours. Microcolonies in cells in conjunctival exudate from trachomatous humans may be stained in Lugol's iodine for 10 minutes without prior fixation with positive results, according to some investigators. Carbohydrate (glycogen) and lipid produced by microcolonies of C. trachomatis stain a dark tan (Fig. 13.5), whereas microcolonies of C. psittaci which produce no iodine-staining carbohydrate and lipid remain the same light tan color as the background.

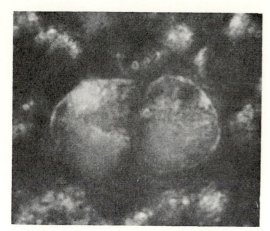

FIG. 13.4—*Dark-field micrograph of two murine tissue culture cells containing compact microcolonies of* C. trachomatis. *Rigid vesicle distorts cell and forces cell nucleus to one side.* ×4,000.

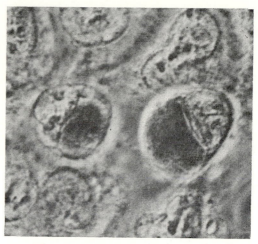

FIG. 13.5—*Phase contrast micrograph of two murine tissue culture cells infected with* C. trachomatis *and stained with iodine solution. Carbohydrate (glycogen) produced by chlamydial microcolony stains dark brown in contrast with tan background.* ×4,000.

In wet mounts of impression smears of infected tissues or exudates, intracellular chlamydiae are large enough to be seen at magnifications of ×800 or more in microscopes equipped with phase contrast optics (Fig. 13.6). They are readily visualized by dark-field illumination (Fig. 13.7). With either technique, however, they cannot be distinguished from contaminating intracellular *Mycoplasma* organisms. When bright-field optics only are available, chlamydiae may be visualized in impression smears of infected tissues by staining the smears with Giemsa's, Castenada's, Macchiavello's or Gimenez's methods after appropriate fixation. They appear dark purple with Giemsa, blue with Castenada, and red with Macchiavello's and Gimenez's stains against contrasting backgrounds. Gimenez's method is best for staining chlamydiae in impression smears of yolk sacs of infected chicken embryos (Gimenez, 1964). In infected cell cultures, chlamydiae stain especially well with Giemsa solution or with acridine orange but do not stain readily in tissue sections without proper fixation. Acridine orange is a nonspecific nucleic acid stain which causes microbial ribonucleic acid to appear green and deoxyribonucleic acid to appear red. Observing fresh infected tissue smears in wet mounts under phase contrast optics avoids the time loss and microscopic

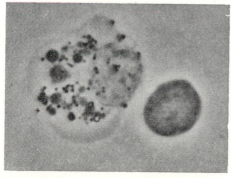

FIG. 13.6—*Phase contrast micrograph of chlamydia-laden mononuclear cell in air sac exudate of turkey infected with* C. psittaci. ×4,000.

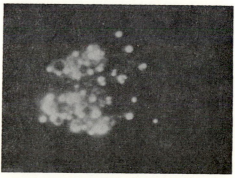

FIG. 13.7—*Dark-field micrograph of same cell at same magnification as Fig. 13.6.*

artifacts associated with staining methods. All chlamydiac are gram-negative.

METABOLISM AND BIOCHEMICAL PROPERTIES

Chlamydiae have limited enzymatic capabilities when compared with free-living, colonizing bacteria, but when separated from the host cell they are capable of producing carbon dioxide from glucose when provided with energy-rich phosphates (ATP) and certain organic and inorganic cofactors (Weiss, 1967). Other compounds known to be catabolized by chlamydiae are pyruvic acid and glutamic acid. The products of this catabolism are carbon dioxide and 2- and 4-carbon residues. Since chlamydiae apparently are unable to synthesize their own high-energy compounds and are dependent upon the host cell for the source of these compounds, they have been described as "energy parasites" (Moulder, 1964). While chlamydiae are dependent upon the host cell for metabolic energy, they are able to synthesize their own DNA, RNA, protein, and in the case of *C. trachomatis* the vitamin folic acid. RNA and DNA have been demonstrated in both initial bodies and elementary bodies of chlamydial organisms, but the ratio of RNA to DNA is greater in the initial bodies.

Tests for homology between DNAs of strains of *C. trachomatis* and *C. psittaci* have shown them to be distinct, thereby substantiating the separation of the two species.

The cell walls of chlamydiae are similar in chemical composition to those of gram-negative bacteria; that is, the distribution of amino acids in chlamydial cell walls is close to that of the cell walls of *Escherichia coli*, the wall content being largely protein (70%), lipid (5.1%), and the remainder presumably carbohydrate (Manire and Tamura, 1967). The cell walls of the elementary bodies have a greater variety of amino acids and larger proportion of lipid than those of the initial bodies. Elementary body walls are rigid envelopes with a layer of hexagonally packed macromolecular structures 100 Å across. In contrast, the walls of the initial bodies are fragile and nonrigid, are destroyed by brief low-frequency (10 kc) sonic treatment, lyse upon standing, and are trypsin-permeable (Tamura and Manire, 1967).

Intact organisms contain approximately 64% protein, 15% nucleic acid, 20% lipid, and small amounts of carbohydrate.

ANTIBIOTIC SENSITIVITIES

The multiplication of strains of both *C. psittaci* and *C. trachomatis* (except for experimental mutants) are strongly inhibited by appropriate concentrations of tetracyclines, chloramphenicol, and erythromycin and less strongly by penicillin. Some strains of both species are inhibited by D-cycloserine. All strains of *C. trachomatis* are inhibited by sodium sulfadiazine. By varied mechanisms, tetracyclines, chloramphenicol, and erythromycin inhibit synthesis of protein on chlamydial ribosomes. Penicillin inhibits chlamydial cell wall synthesis in the same manner as in ordinary bacteria and causes the development of spheroplasts. D-cycloserine acts similarly, but the drug's action can be reversed by alanine. The inhibition of multiplication by sodium sulfadiazine reflects the organism's ability to produce folic acid, and, as is well known, sulfadiazine inhibition can be reversed by p-aminobenzoic acid. Certain antibiotics have little or no effect on the growth of chlamydiae, and this fact can be useful in selecting for viable chlamydiae in suspensions containing contaminating bacteria. Concentrations of 1 mg each of streptomycin sulfate, vancomycin, and kanomycin sulfate, per ml of solution may be used for this purpose.

PROPAGATION OF THE ORGANISMS

At present *C. psittaci* can be cultivated only in susceptible animals or in cell cultures. The most commonly used hosts are chicken embryos, mice, and guinea pigs. Cell cultures of murine, avian, or human origin are satisfactory also for the isolation or propagation of chlamydiae. Cell cultures of bovine, ovine, or other vertebrate origin probably are susceptible but have not been thoroughly tested. Growth of chlamydiae in cultures of cells from ectothermic vertebrates has been successful.

Chicken Embryo

All strains of *C. psittaci* grow and multiply in the yolk sac of chicken embryos. This host is preferable to mice for propagation purposes since chlamydiae multiply to a much higher titer in the yolk sac membrane than they do in mouse tissues, thereby providing a more concentrated source of organisms for preparation of antigens or for metabolic studies.

The average number of days to death of embryos infected with chlamydiae is directly related to the number of organisms inoculated, the optimum temperature of incubation (37–39° C), and the strain of organism used. The relationship of inoculum number to average number of days to death is reproducible and useful for experimental purposes, but it must first be determined empirically for each strain under the prevailing laboratory conditions.

Mice and Guinea Pigs

Most strains of *C. psittaci* from avian hosts may be isolated and propagated in mice (3–4 weeks of age; intracerebral, intranasal, or intraperitoneal route of inoculation). On the other hand, many strains from birds fail to grow in guinea pigs. Some strains, such as those causing ovine polyarthritis or bovine encephalomyelitis, grow rapidly and produce severe lesions and death in guinea pigs but have no effect in mice. In the titration of such strains in chicken embryos, mice, and guinea pigs, the highest titer for the suspension of organisms is obtained in guinea pigs.

Cell Cultures

All strains of *C. psittaci* isolated from birds multiply satisfactorily in secondary cell cultures derived from chicken embryo tissues and in common mammalian cell lines such as HeLa, Chang human liver, murine L, or McCoy cells. All of the chlamydial strains isolated from birds will readily cause plaques in primary chicken embryo cell cultures overlaid with agar, and this procedure may be useful in cloning strains or characterizing them serologically by plaque-reduction tests (Piraino, 1969). Strains from mammals will not develop plaques in chicken embryo cell cultures but will in murine L cells (Banks et al., 1970).

Propagation of chlamydiae in cell cultures is particularly adapted to studies of the intracellular growth cycle, colonial and plaque morphology, and iodine reaction of chlamydial strains. Chlamydiae-infected cell cultures may also be used for preparation of antigens, but the infectivity titer and potency of these cultures is usually lower than that obtained in the yolk sac of chicken embryos.

RESISTANCE TO CHEMICAL AND PHYSICAL AGENTS

Chlamydiae are very susceptible to chemicals that affect their lipid content or the integrity of their cell walls. Even in a milieu of tissue debris, they are rapidly inactivated by surface-active compounds such as quaternary ammonium compounds and lipid solvents. They are somewhat less susceptible to dilute solutions of protein denaturants, acids, and alkalies (methanol, ethanol, ammonium or zinc sulfate, phenol, hydrochloric acid, and sodium hydroxide). Infectivity is destroyed within minutes, however, by exposure to common disinfectants such as benzalkonium chlorides (Roccal, Zephiran), alcoholic iodine solution, 70% ethanol, 3% hydrogen peroxide, and silver nitrate; but they are resistant to cresyl compounds and lime (Tarizzo and Nabli, 1967). Dilute suspensions (20%) of infectious tissue homogenates are inactivated by incubation for 5 minutes at 56° C, 48 hours at 37° C, 12 days at 22° C, and 50 days at 4° C (Page, 1959b).

The infectious dense forms of the organism in yolk sac membranes or mouse tissues may be preserved indefinitely at −20° C or below, although the initial freezing and subsequent thawing incurs a titer loss of 1–2 logs. Infectivity of the suspension is destroyed after 6 freeze-thaw cycles (Page, 1959b). The thin-walled, large forms of the organism are inactivated at −70° C.

Cell walls of the dense forms are disrupted by ultrasonication at frequencies above 100 kc or by treatment of the intact organisms with sodium desoxycholate.

ANTIGENIC STRUCTURE AND TOXINS

Chlamydiae have a thermostable (100° C, 30 min.), phenol-stable (0.5%), lipoglycoprotein antigen that is common to all strains of both chlamydial species. The antigen is soluble in ether or in aqueous solutions of sodium lauryl sulfate from which it can be precipitated with acid; is resistant to trypsin, chymotrypsin, and papain; but is inactivated by periodate. Antibodies to this genus-wide group antigen are produced in animals infected with any chlamydial agent, but these antibodies are not necessarily related to immunity to challenge with any strain.

The cell walls of the organisms contain strain-specific antigens which can be differentiated by complement fixation, cell culture plaque reduction, embryo infectivity neutralization, and toxin neutralization tests. The toxigenicity of each strain, as measured in mice, appears to be associated with cell wall components neutralizable by specific antiserum. The toxin-neutralization test formerly was used to separate "species" of psittacosis agents, but many cross-reactions were apparent. Antigenically distinct toxins were found in chlamydiae isolated from fowl, humans, cats, sheep, and cattle; but it was soon observed that the specificity of the toxin was not necessarily correlated with the species of host from which the organisms were isolated.

The cell wall antigens are primarily protein and are more heat-sensitive than the group antigen. Chemical diversity of cell wall components is responsible for the variations between strains in the specificity of neutralizing antibodies and immunity. The numerous serotypes and immunotypes distinguished by various methods do not as yet illustrate a clear-cut pattern that is practical for epizootiologic purposes. To account for all of the individual variants in the face of numerous cross-reactions, one must postulate that the organisms have a constantly changing mosaic of surface determinants which in turn modify in varying degree the specificity of base cell wall structures.

PATHOGENICITY

In terms of natural pathogenicity for domestic fowl, strains of *C. psittaci* isolated from these hosts fall into two general categories:

1. Highly virulent strains that cause acute epornitics in which 5–30% of the affected birds die. Strains of this type have been isolated most often from turkeys and occasionally from unaffected wild birds. These strains have been labeled "toxigenic," because in natural and experimental hosts they produce rapidly fatal disease with lesions characterized by extensive vascular congestion and inflammation of vital organs. The toxigenicity of a strain can be measured experimentally by inoculating large numbers of yolk sac-propagated chlamydiae intravenously into mice. The end point is lethal toxic shock within 48 hours after inoculation. Toxigenic strains have a broad spectrum of pathogenicity for laboratory animals. Most often such strains are the ones that cause serious human infections—some of them fatal—in poultry handlers and laboratory research workers. Examples of such strains are coded as NJ-1 (Page, 1956), TT (Meyer and Eddie, 1953), VT-1 (Page, 1966, unpublished observations) from turkeys, the Borg strain from egrets, the Oregon gull strain (Dickinson et al., 1957).

2. Strains of low virulence that cause slowly progressive epornitics with a mortality rate of less than 5% in the birds when uncomplicated by secondary bacterial or parasitic infection. Strains of this type have often been isolated from pigeons, ducks, turkeys (occasionally), sparrows, and other wild birds. Birds infected with these strains usually do not develop the severe vascular damage that is evident in birds infected with toxigenic strains, nor do they have such obvious clinical signs. The mouse toxigenicity titers of these strains are of much lower order than those of the highly virulent strains. Unless unusually high exposure does alter the balance between infection and resistance, humans are less susceptible to strains commonly found in pigeons and ducks.

Ornithosis in pigeons and ducks may often be accompanied by concurrent infection with salmonellae. In such cases mortality rates among the birds are high, chlamydiae are shed in very large numbers, and humans and animals in the immediate environment of the infected birds are exposed to doses that result in clinical disease.

Strains of both high and low virulence appear to have equal ability to spread rapidly among a flock, as determined by serologic tests. Such studies show that more than 90% of birds in any one enclosure have developed antibodies to the chlamydial group antigen by the time clinical signs of disease appear in the flock.

In terms of experimental pathogenicity for specific hosts where the age and breed of host and the route and number of organisms inoculated are defined, various strains of *C. psittaci* appear to have recognizable pathogenicity differences (Fig. 13.8). Titrations of toxigenic strains in laboratory

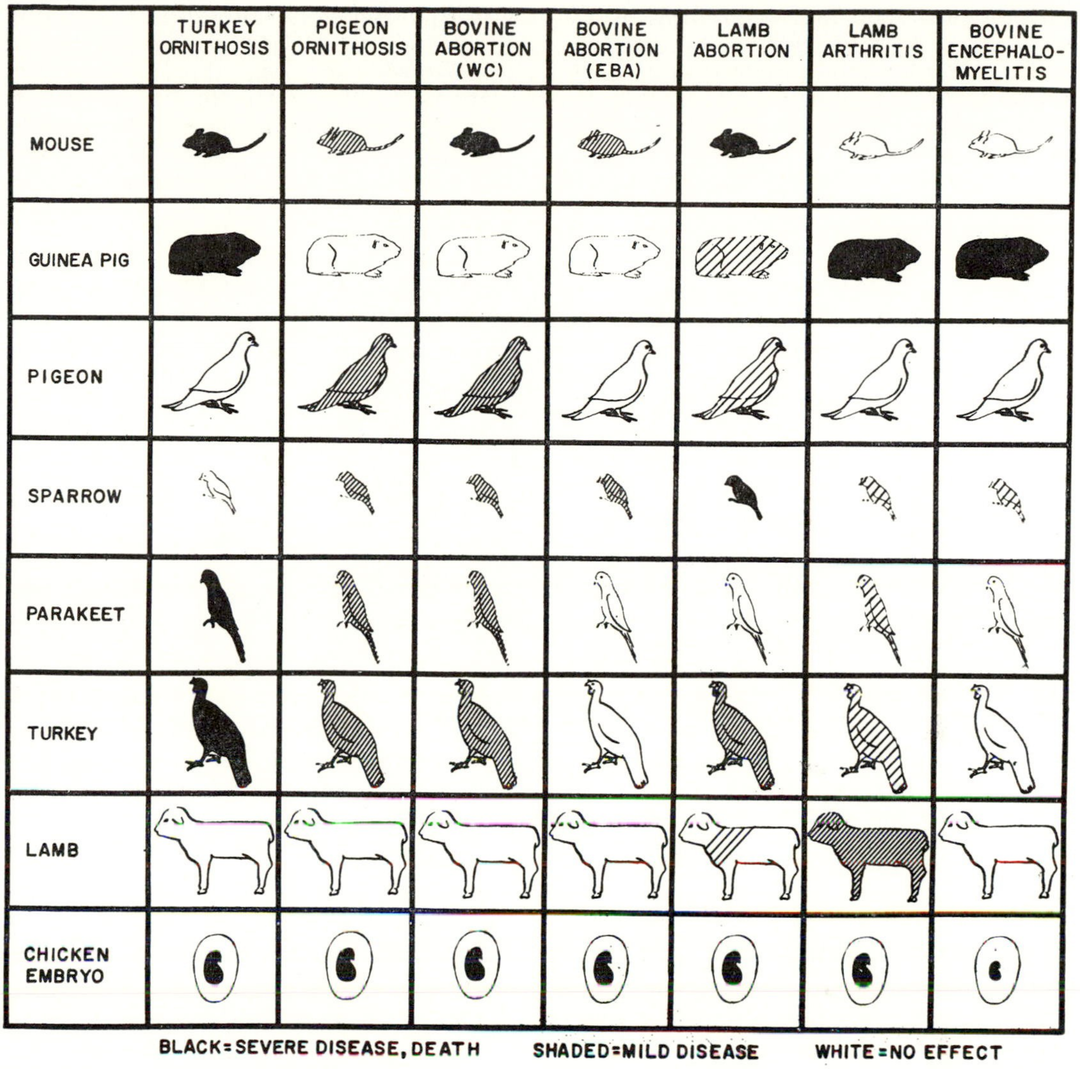

BLACK=SEVERE DISEASE, DEATH   SHADED=MILD DISEASE   WHITE=NO EFFECT

FIG. 13.8—Schematic chart representing effects of 7 strains of C. psittaci *in 8 species of wild, domestic, and laboratory animals. Source host and disease are listed at top; experimental hosts are listed along side. (Page, 1967)*

animals indicate that these strains are highly infectious and lethal for mice, guinea pigs, turkeys, and parakeets but are inocuous to pigeons and sparrows. In contrast, strains of low toxigenicity have a high infectivity but low lethality for mice, pigeons, sparrows, and turkeys. Often they are not infectious for guinea pigs.

Since such experimental determinations do not take into account the organisms' communicability and mode of transmission between species under natural conditions, their interpretation relative to natural disease is limited. Nevertheless, they are useful in characterizing new chlamydial isolates, and their potential for revealing unsuspected epizootiologic relationships should not be underrated.

EPIZOOTIOLOGY

The epizootiology of ornithosis in each of the various species of domestic fowl is probably intertwined, because there appears to be a subtle but extensive interplay of chlamydiae of varying virulence between wild and domestic hosts and probably between different species of domestic hosts. Common reservoirs of chlamydiae include such wild and feral birds as sea gulls, ducks, herons, egrets, and pigeons, all of which readily intermingle with domestic birds. Gulls and egrets have been shown to carry and excrete highly virulent strains of chlamydiae without suffering apparent ill effects. Meyer (1967) has listed over 120 other wild avian species that have been transient hosts if not carriers of chlamydiae. It is possible that continuing interspecies transfers of chlamydiae have served to confound efforts to identify decisively the source or sources of these organisms to domestic hosts. One possible explanation of the rise and fall of explosive ornithosis epizootics in domestic birds in the midst of continuing mild infection of other reservoir hosts was unintentionally offered by an anonymous author in Lancet (1955):

How did all this ebb and flow of infection come about? . . . Mutation of the pathogen towards greater virulence with coincidental favorable host factors opens the way to its rapid proliferation and transfer for a time. But with the increasing slaughter of the hosts, the parasite, too, tends to perish, and its field of action is soon narrowed. Natural selection may thus be constantly acting in favor of a more comfortable ecology, a state of live-and-let-live with the host whereby both survive with only minor inconvenience. This would make the explosive (epidemic) phase short and the stabilized (endemic or symptomless) phase relatively long. If this be so, a constant flux in the epidemiological pattern of a disease is a natural phenomenon, and is likely to continue as new varieties, milder or more deadly, arise from ordinary pathogens or from nature's vast reservoir of feeble pathogens or non-pathogenic microorganisms.

Aside from the possibility of genetic variations affecting the pathogenicity patterns of the organisms, many questions remain concerning the maintenance of chlamydiae in nature and the transmission of these agents to domestic birds. Incubator hatching, prompt treatment (or elimination) of diseased individuals, and annual marketing are factors that combine to limit the survival of ornithosis agents in domestic hosts unless the organisms persist in holdover birds, bedding, or arthropods. In contrast, survival of the organisms in free-flying, nesting birds is assured where parent to offspring disease transmission is commonplace. Meyer (1965) has suggested that the questions remain because "poultry pathologists and epidemiologists have not studied the life history of large poultry flocks from incubator-hatched eggs through egg-laying maturity." This statement may be true except that such studies must be concerned basically with the ecology of chlamydiosis not only in the domestic birds but in other birds, mammals, and arthropods within the flock environment.

Another factor that seriously affects the final expression of ornithosis and its related economic loss is secondary or concurrent infection. While the large majority of ornithosis epizootics in turkeys in the United States have not been complicated with other disease agents, a significant number of epizootics in other bird species (ducks and pigeons) in which there was a high rate of bird mortality and human infection were those complicated by salmonellosis. Therefore, the investigator must also consider the role of enteric pathogens in epizootics of unusual virulence.

TURKEYS

Transmission

Careful examinations of hundreds of eggs from ornithosis-infected breeding flocks have indicated that transovarian passage of the agents of ornithosis does not occur (Davis et al., 1957; Page and Bankowski, 1959). Therefore, chlamydial infection of a flock of turkeys is likely to be initiated by exposure of a few birds to an exogenous source of organisms. Large numbers of chlamydiae are excreted in the droppings of ornithosis-infected birds, and their dried excrement can remain infectious for many months. Infectious dust in nest box debris or pens can produce infection in susceptible birds or mammals when it is inhaled. Thus the source of infection to a new flock of birds may be the dried excrement from (1) infected wild birds intermingling with the flock, (2) infected holdover or replacement turkeys introduced into the new flock, or (3) infected birds previously kept on the premises. While inhalation of infectious particles is probably the primary route of infection, a second means for introduction of chlamydiae into the new avian hosts may be contamination of a skin wound with chlamydiae carried on the bodies of nest mites or bird lice. According to Eddie et al. (1962), chlamydiae were recovered from homogenates of nest mites remaining in nest boxes of turkeys removed 3 months earlier from the premises. Whether the chlamydiae survived in or on the surfaces of the mites for this period of time is not known, but the relationship of these arachnids to the transmission of ornithosis in birds needs further investigation.

Once the organisms gain entrance to the host, they are engulfed by phagocytes in which they multiply and from which they are released to infect other tissues. When the organisms spill into the bloodstream, they are filtered out in the liver, spleen, and kidney and are returned to the environment in cloacal excrement. By repetition of this cycle the organisms are spread to other members of the flock. Intraflock communicability of the agents is high; serologic surveys of naturally exposed flocks indicate that by the time the disease becomes apparent, over 95% of the birds have circulating antibody titers. This process takes a variable time, depending on the number of organisms originally introduced and the susceptibility of the birds. Other factors may influence the development of disease. Ornithosis is detected more often in breeding flocks than in young birds raised for meat production. It may be that the physiological stress of active ovulation causes an increased susceptibility, or that laying hens are more likely to be exposed to organisms in the dust from contaminated nest boxes, or that breeding birds are often maintained longer than meat birds, thereby allowing more time for the infection to progress slowly through the flock.

Pathogenesis

The path of the organisms and their sites of multiplication have been studied in detail in experimental turkeys after exposure of the birds to measured doses of *C. psittaci* by the airborne or oral routes (Page, 1959a). In airborne infection experiments, young turkeys were exposed for 5 minutes to an infectious aerosol of the toxigenic NJ-1 turkey strain. Two birds were killed at 4, 8, 24, 36, 48, 72, 96, 120, and 336 hours after exposure. At necropsy, tissues of 14 separate organs were removed aseptically from each bird, homogenized, and titrated in mice to determine the number of mouse LD_{50} of chlamydiae present in each gram of tissue. This study revealed that small numbers of organisms had penetrated to the abdominal air sacs and mesentery

within 4 hours after infection and larger numbers of organisms were present in the lungs and thoracic air sacs. Within 24 hours, the numbers of organisms in the lungs and air sacs were more than 100 million per gram of tissue. Within 48 hours, chlamydiae were found in low levels in the blood, spleen, and kidney. They were present in high numbers in the turbinates and colon contents within 72 hours, and the numbers found on the surface of the heart gradually increased to a high level by the 4th day.

It was reasoned that the organisms multiplied in the lung, air sacs, and pericardial membrane and then were released into the blood and filtered out in the spleen, liver, and kidneys. Many organisms were returned to the environment via the nasal and intestinal excretions. The tissues of birds that succumbed to acute disease contained greater than 100 million organisms per gram, indicating that in the terminal stage an overwhelming spread of the organisms had occurred throughout the body.

In spite of protective clothing and equipment, two persons associated with this experiment contracted psittacosis from the infectious aerosol generated to expose the turkeys.

In another experiment, young turkeys were fed capsules containing a suspension of 40,000 mouse LD_{50} of *C. psittaci*. At the 1st, 2nd, and 5th days postinfection, two birds were killed and necropsied, and the major organs and 10 segments of tissues from various parts of the gastrointestinal tract were removed for homogenization and titration in mice. Examination of these birds at necropsy revealed no gross lesions, and the organisms were recovered in very low numbers from only one tissue sample—the jejunum content of one bird killed on the 5th day. The remaining capsule-fed birds were kept in the same quarters with unexposed control birds for the next 3 months. The course of the infection was followed in these birds by serologic tests and by isolation of chlamydia from the blood of each bird at regular intervals. Within 15 days, 3 of the capsule-fed birds developed a transient chlamydial bacteremia and a low level of circulating antibodies. By the 25th day, the organisms could not be found in their blood and their antibody titers had risen, but organisms were recovered from the blood of 8 other birds including 2 uninfected cage mates. By the 47th day, the infection had spread until every bird had experienced chlamydemia followed by development of serum antibodies. Periodic tests of bird droppings on the floor of the cage indicated that chlamydiae were present in excretions within a few days after the birds were initially fed the infectious suspension and were there in high concentration later. It appeared that the organisms in the first infectious feeding survived passage through the intestinal tract of the birds and then were spread by airborne means to the same birds. By this route of infection the birds were more susceptible. The organisms multiplied in these birds and were in turn spread to other cage mates in higher concentrations until all became infected, including 5 control birds. Of further epidemiologic interest is the fact that the animal caretaker for these turkeys also contracted psittacosis during this experiment.

Turkeys necropsied 35, 51, 54, or 78 days following the original oral instillation of chlamydiae still contained small numbers of organisms in their pericardial membrane, kidney, or liver, but none were isolated from major organs beyond the 78th day. This suggested that turkeys might retain virulent organisms for as long as 2 months after exposure to infection, but unless they suffered an overwhelming infection, they soon sterilized their tissues.

Incubation Period, Signs, Morbidity, Mortality

The incubation period of ornithosis in turkeys is variable, depending on number and toxigenicity of the organisms inhaled by the host. Experimentally the incubation period prior to the onset of definitive signs may range from 5 to 10 days in young turkeys infected with a toxigenic strain of C. psittaci. In birds exposed by natural means with small doses, or in older more resistant birds, the period may be longer. Strains of low virulence cause less severe signs, thereby making the incubation period less definable. In natural epizootics the spread of either type of organism among the birds of a flock occurs at the same rate but in any case may take 2–8 weeks to produce noticeable signs in a large number of birds. Once the organisms are propagating rapidly, the rate of their spread increases until virtually all birds of a flock within a given enclosure are exposed. At the peak of exposure and infection, 50–80% of the individuals in the flock will show clinical signs.

Turkeys exposed to toxigenic strains of C. psittaci become cachexic, anorexic, and hyperthermic and excrete yellow-green gelatinous droppings (Fig. 13.9). Egg production of severely affected hens drops rapidly and may cease temporarily or remain very low until complete recovery. On a flock basis, egg production may drop from a peak of 60% to 10–20%. Mortality ranges from 10 to 30%.

When a flock is infected with a less toxigenic strain of C. psittaci, only 5–20% of them may show signs of anorexia and loose greenish droppings. The rest may show transient mild signs. Egg production may drop rapidly to approximately a 40% rate but in time recovers. Mortality is low, ranging from less than 1% to 4%. Birds that die show all the signs and lesions of acute disease.

Gross Lesions

Less toxigenic strains cause the same basic lesions in turkeys as do the toxigenic strains, and the lesions caused by the former are less severe and less extensive and thereby less likely to be fatal. In overwhelming infections with toxigenic strains, the organisms multiply to a very high titer

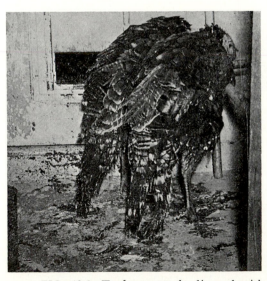

FIG. 13.9—Turkeys acutely diseased with ornithosis caused by toxigenic (NJ-1) strain of C. psittaci. Yellow-green gelatinous droppings cover floor. (Page, 1959a)

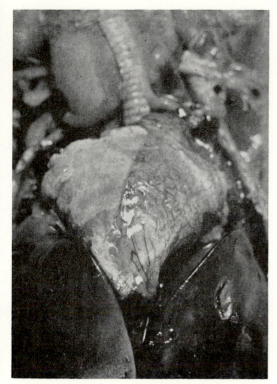

FIG. 13.10—*Gross lesions of acute fatal ornithosis in young turkey infected by airborne route. Thickened congested pericardial membrane was partially removed to show severe pericarditis and epicardial encrustation. Prominent also are cardiomegaly and hepatomegaly. (Page, 1959a)*

(10⁸ or more) in the lungs, air sac, and pericardium and spread via the blood to all parts of the body. The lungs show a diffuse congestion, and the pleural cavity may contain fibrinous exudate. In fatal cases a dark transudate may fill the thoracic cavity (Fig. 13.10). The pericardial membrane is thickened, congested, and coated with fibrinous exudate. The heart surface may be covered with thick fibrin plaques or encrusted with yellowish flaky exudate (Fig. 13.11). The heart may be enlarged. The severe damage to the lungs and heart undoubtedly is a major cause of death. The liver is enlarged and discolored and may be coated with a thick fibrin film. The air sacs are thickened and heavily coated with fibrinous exudate. The spleen becomes enlarged, dark, and soft. The peritoneal serosa and mesentery show vascular congestion and may be coated with foamy, white fibrinous exudate. All of these exudates

contain large numbers of mononuclear cells in whose cytoplasms numerous microcolonies of chlamydiae may be seen. The fibrinous exudates found on all the organs and tissues of the thoracic and peritoneal cavities reflect vascular damage as well as the increasing inflammatory response caused by the continued multiplication of the organisms.

In birds that survive infection with a strain of low toxigenicity, the lungs may not be seriously affected, but multiplication of the organisms on the epicardium may result in the formation of one or more fibrin plaques on the heart. Figure 13.12 illustrates the epicardial lesion in a turkey from a naturally infected flock. The air sacs of the bird were thickened and coated with fibrinous exudate, and the peritoneal cavity contained copious amounts of foamy, stringy exudate (Fig. 13.13). The spleen was enlarged 2–4 times and covered with gray-white spots representing areas of focal cellular proliferation. The liver was enlarged, mottled, and covered with a thick fibrin film. Other birds involved in the same epizootic had similar lesions, although the severity varied. In all cases, however, fibrinous exudates containing numerous chlamydiae-laden monocytes were present on the air sacs, viscera, and peritoneal serosa.

Histopathology

Beasley et al. (1959) studied the cellular changes in 500 turkeys of various ages injected intratracheally with suspensions of the toxigenic TT strain of *C. psittaci*. These authors found that the organisms produce both necrotizing and proliferative changes in the host's tissues comparable with those caused by other chlamydial strains in other species (with the exception of focal necrosis of the liver which is prominent in parrots and mice). However, the specific cellular changes and corresponding organ damage were decidedly more severe and extensive in young turkeys than in older turkeys. The age at which turkeys appear to be more resistant to standardized doses of *C. psittaci* is 15 weeks (Beasley, personal communication).

A majority of the birds that Beasley and his colleagues examined had tracheitis characterized by extensive infiltration of mononuclear cells, lymphocytes, and heterophils in the lamina propria and submucosa.

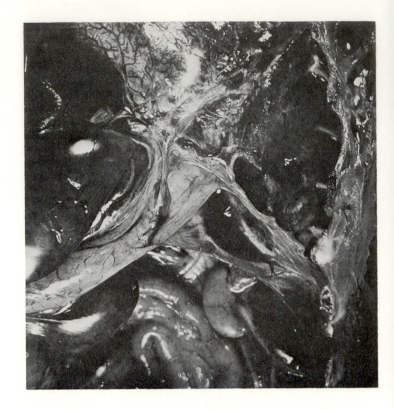

FIG. 13.11—Gross lesions of acute fatal ornithosis in young turkey infected by airborne route. Pericardial sac is thickened and congested. Lung is congested and thoracic cavity is filled with transudate fluid. Spleen is enlarged with dark blotches on surface. (Page, 1956)

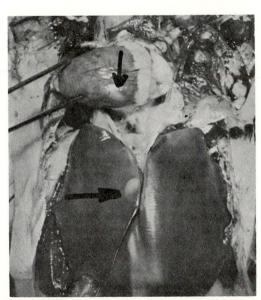

FIG. 13.12—Field case of ornithosis in turkey caused by C. psittaci strain of low virulence. Arrows point to fibrin plaques on heart and enlarged liver.

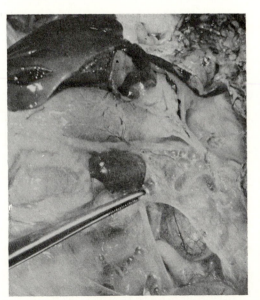

FIG. 13.13—Same turkey as in Fig. 13.12 but showing enlarged spleen and fibrinous, foamy exudate on thickened air sacs.

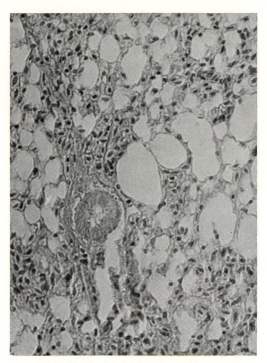

FIG. 13.14—Section of lung of normal turkey. Pollack's trichrome, ×500. (Page, 1956)

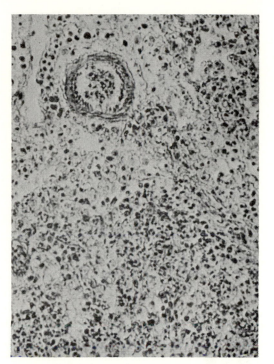

FIG. 13.15—Section of lung of turkey with acute fatal ornithosis showing diffuse pneumonitis. Functional air cells are absent or occluded with inflammatory cells. Pollack's trichrome, ×500. (Page, 1956)

Cilia were absent in severely damaged areas. This extensive tracheal damage is not necessarily characteristic of naturally infected birds but might be expected as a result of intratracheal inoculation of large numbers of organisms. Epithelioid pneumonitis in varying degrees was found in 80–100% of 10-week-old birds but less often (10–20%) in mature birds. The lungs of severely affected birds were congested and had extensive infiltration of the tertiary bronchi and respiratory tubules with large mononuclear cells and fibrin. There was necrosis of individual cells and of large areas of tissue; the parenchyma and stroma were equally affected. Normal and infected lungs in section are compared in Figures 13.14 and 13.15.

Beasley and his colleagues further found fibrinous to fibrinopurulent inflammatory exudates present on the respiratory and peritoneal surfaces in a majority of infected turkeys and a similar exudate on the epicardium. The pericardium and epicardium were thickened by the swelling of congested vessels and an inflammatory exudate containing fibrin, large mononuclear cells, and varying numbers of lymphocytes and heterophils. Sections of normal and infected turkey hearts from another study are shown in Figures 13.16 and 13.17.

These authors also found an infectious myocarditis in more than half of the infected birds, but arteritis was present in only 8% of the birds. Hepatitis was present in over 90% of the birds, and in severely affected individuals there was a diffuse dilation of sinusoids with infiltration of mononuclear cells, lymphocytes, and heterophils. Proliferated and swollen Kupffer cells were filled with debris and a yellowish pigment thought to be hemosiderin. Necrotic hepatic cells were scattered throughout the organ with little focal necrosis. The diffuse character of the infiltration seen in young birds was more focal. Acutely sick turkeys had a catarrhal enteritis. The spleens of a majority of the birds were altered with cellular proliferation and necrosis more marked in younger than in older birds. The proliferative response and necrosis explain the enlarged and mottled appearance of the spleen at necropsy.

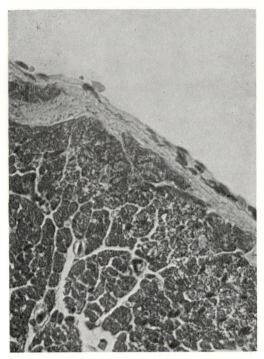

FIG. 13.16—Section of heart of normal turkey showing part of epicardium. Pollack's trichrome, ×500. (Page, 1956)

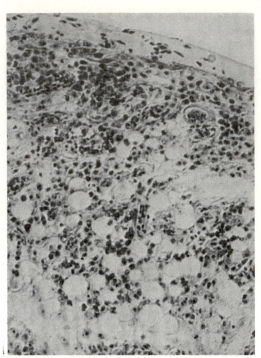

FIG. 13.17—Section of heart of young turkey with fatal ornithosis. Epicardium has thick crust of inflammatory exudate. For gross appearance of heart see Fig. 13.10. Pollack's trichrome, ×500. (Page, 1956)

Degenerative changes and cellular infiltration were observed in the kidneys of half of the infected birds, but similar lesions of less severity were also found in uninoculated birds.

The organisms also caused orchitis and epididymitis. Beasley et al. (1961) state that "the ornithosis agent seemed to have an affinity for the active germinal epithelium. . . . Fibrin and inflammatory cells appeared in association with the desquamated and necrotic epithelium filling the seminiferous tubules with eosinophilic exudate." It was also observed that often the immediate cause of death in adult males with ornithosis was rupture of testicular blood vessels followed by massive internal bleeding.

The brains of 6 infected birds were examined by Beasley and his associates; the organs were without significant changes.

The less toxigenic strains of C. psittaci also cause cellular proliferation and necrosis of major organs and vascular congestion in turkeys, but the lesions are less extensive and less severe (except in the air sacs) than those caused by more virulent strains. Pneumonitis is seen only in birds that suc-

cumb to the disease. Infections with strains of low virulence tend to produce chronic long-lasting infections with low mortality (Gale et al., 1960).

Immunity

As indicated by the aforementioned studies of Beasley et al. (1961), age apparently confers some degree of resistance to organ damage caused by C. psittaci infection. This moderate degree of resistance appears at the age of 15 weeks and probably increases slightly as the bird gets older.

The major breeds of commercially raised turkeys—Broad Breasted Bronze, Beltsville White, and their crosses—appear to be equally susceptible to experimental infection with C. psittaci.

The degree of active immunity to reinfection induced in turkeys by natural ornithosis has not been tested, nor has the resistance induced by experimental infection with organisms of low virulence been determined. That some postinfection immunity occurs in turkeys, however, was implied in the experiments of Page (1959a), described in the section on pathogenesis. In these tests the progress of infection which was initiated by an oral dose of chlamydiae and then spread by natural means through a group of 19 turkeys was followed by blood tests and clinical observations. At varying times over a period of 47 days, each bird developed chlamydemia, hyperthermia, and mild anorexia. The chlamydemia lasted up to 10 days in each bird but was followed by clinical normalcy and apparent resistance to further bloodstream infection, in spite of environmental contamination sufficient to infect all unexposed birds and the caretaker who fed and watered the birds daily.

Humans do not seem to have the same reinfection immunity. At least 2 research workers who conducted aerosol-infection experiments were simultaneously exposed for brief periods to aerosols of *C. psittaci* on 2 different occasions 4 months apart. Both workers developed clinical psittacosis 10–13 days after each exposure.

Vaccination immunity will be discussed in the section on Prevention and Control.

DUCKS

Epizootiology and Transmission

Ornithosis in domestic ducks in the United States is not an important problem since the epizootics in ducks have been rare and of low virulence (Korns, 1955). However, ornithosis in ducks is a serious economic and occupational health problem in Europe. The most damaging epizootics have occurred in Czechoslovakia and have been reviewed in detail by Strauss (1967). These epizootics occurred between 1949 and 1963 when the Czechoslovakian poultry industry was in a stage of postwar expansion toward mass production of meat fowl. According to Strauss, chlamydial organisms are widely distributed among wild and domestic bird populations in Czechoslovakia. The organisms have been isolated from wild ducks, gulls, and partridges as well as domestic ducks, chickens, turkeys, cattle, and swine. Transmission of the disease agent to ducks and between ducks is presumed to be primarily by the airborne route, since no definitive alternate route of the infection has been discovered. The reservoir source of the infection to ducks is not known.

Signs, Morbidity, and Mortality

Ornithosis in Czechoslovakian ducks is a severe, debilitating, often fatal disease. Acutely sick young ducks develop trembling, imbalanced gait, and cachexia. They become anorexic and diarrhetic; their intestinal excreta is greenish and watery. They develop a serous or purulent discharge around the eyes and nasal orifices. The discharge becomes encrusted in the feathers around the eyes (Fig. 13.18). Emaciation and muscle atrophy become marked as the disease progresses. In the terminal stage the infected duck usually dies in convulsions.

In serologic surveys of infected flocks, morbidity ranges between 10 and 80%. Mortality varies from 0 to 30%, depending on the age of the birds when they become infected (young birds are more susceptible)

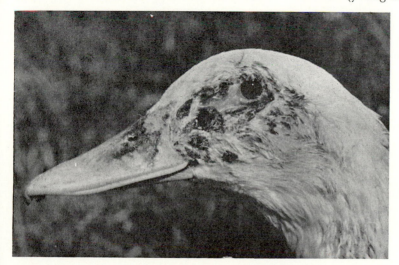

FIG. 13.18—Seropurulent discharge and encrustation of auricular and nasal areas of duck with ornithosis. (Meyer, 1965)

and whether concurrent salmonellosis is present.

Gross Lesions and Histopathology

Strauss (1967) described the overt disease in young ducks as producing lacrimation, conjunctivitis, rhinitis, occasional panophthalmitis, bulbar atrophy, and inflammation of the infraorbital sinuses. Dissection revealed atrophic pectoral muscles and a general polyserositis. Serous or serofibrinous pericarditis, hepatomegaly, perihepatitis, and splenomegaly were common. The liver and spleen occasionally had grayish or yellowish necrotic foci.

Laboratory Animal Susceptibility

The strains of *C. psittaci* isolated from ducks cause a fatal meningoencephalitis when inoculated intracerebrally into mice and rabbits, but fail to affect pigeons or chickens. According to Strauss (1967), the strains of *C. psittaci* from ducks produce only nonclinical "latent" ornithosis in experimentally inoculated ducks. This observation is difficult to reconcile with the obvious severity of ornithosis in naturally infected ducks unless other factors such as environmental stress caused by crowding, unsanitary conditions, and concurrent bacterial infection are taken into account.

Immunity

The resistance of ducks to reinfection has not been studied. The immunity derived from various vaccination attempts will be discussed under Prevention and Control.

PIGEONS

Epizootiology

The results of numerous serologic surveys indicate that pigeons are one of the most common reservoir hosts of chlamydial organisms. In the experience of this author, only 2 of 50 groups of feral pigeons tested were serologically negative for antibodies to the chlamydial group antigen. Over 1,000 birds from different flocks in California and Iowa were examined over a period of 10 years by the author. The average incidence of positive serology within each group was 50% and ranged from 30 to 90%. Meyer (1965) summarized the worldwide incidence determined by 50 investigators in 24 countries of the exposure and development of chlamydial antibody titers of feral and loft pigeons. Of 16,539 pigeons tested, 4,458 (26.9%) had positive serology as determined by complement fixation tests. As for the incidence of active carriers, 645 (19.9%) pigeons of 3,248 whose tissues were tested for the presence of chlamydiae carried the agents.

The common pigeon, derived originally from the European rock dove, has adapted to living in close association with human habitations. The common feral pigeon is a hardy, widely distributed bird that often intermingles with and nests and breeds near farm animals. Pigeons are also raised as poultry (squabs), showbirds, or racing birds. The fact that these birds are so widely distributed and utilized increases their significance as prime disseminators of chlamydial organisms into the domestic environment.

Transmission, Carriers, and Possible Vectors

There is strong evidence that an important factor in the perpetuation of ornithosis in pigeons is the parent-to-nestling transmission cycle (Meyer et al., 1942a; Davis, 1955). The organisms are shed in the nasal and intestinal excretions of infected parents and transferred to the young by inhalation and ingestion of dried excrement. As for other modes of transmission, passage through the egg has never been proven, but transmission of the organisms between hosts on or in bird lice remains a possibility.

Environmental factors such as crowding, unsanitary quarters, extreme variations in temperature, large numbers of chlamydiae in the immediate environment, and host susceptibility influence the spread of ornithosis and its outcome in individual birds. Under crowded, unsanitary, high-dose conditions, a majority of young birds may be overcome by ornithosis. Those that survive may become chronically infected. Such carriers may be lesionless shedders that continuously contaminate their environment. Other birds may show no serological or clinical evidence of infection and appear to be permanently resistant. Concurrent salmonellosis or trichomoniasis seriously affects the course of ornithosis and may cause high mortality in both young and old birds.

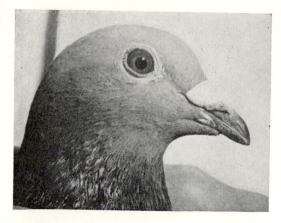

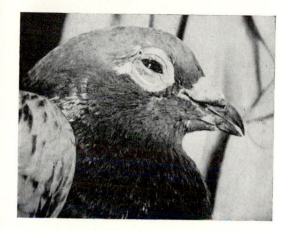

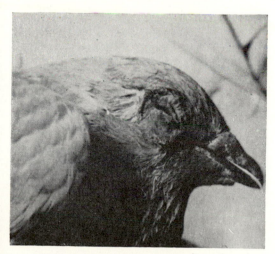

FIG. 13.19—*Signs of conjunctivitis in racing pigeons.* **Top:** *normal pigeon.* **Center and bottom:** *increasingly severe signs of disease caused by* C. psittaci. (*Courtesy Jac. Jansen, Utrecht, Netherlands*)

Signs

The clinical course of uncomplicated ornithosis in young pigeons or doves is variable, but those that develop acute disease are anorexic, unthrifty, and diarrhetic. Some birds develop conjunctivitis, swollen eyelids, and rhinitis (Fig. 13.19). Respiratory difficulties cause them to make creaking, rattling sounds. In time the birds become weak, thin, or emaciated. Survivors recover to become carriers. Other birds appear to pass through the infection to the carrier stage showing no signs or at best transient diarrhea. If such carrier birds then become infected with salmonellae or trichomonads, signs and lesions of acute disease develop. The most probable course of disease in uncomplicated ornithosis in pigeons is that of an inapparent infection followed by the development of a carrier state. Should environmental stress or secondary infection complicate the primary chlamydial infection, acute disease and fatality may follow.

Gross Lesions

Uncomplicated ornithosis in pigeons causes lesions somewhat similar to those in turkeys infected with a mildly virulent strain of *C. psittaci.* Fibrinous exudates are found on the thickened air sacs (Fig. 13.20), on the peritoneal serosa and mesentery, and occasionally on the epicardium. The liver is usually swollen, soft, and discolored (Fig. 13.21). The spleen may be enlarged, soft, and dark. If catarrhal enteritis occurs, more urates than normal appear in the cloacal contents. Less severe infections may involve only the liver or air sacs. Some heavily infected shedders show no lesions whatsoever (Page and Bankowski, 1959).

Immunity

The natural, acquired, or vaccination-induced immunity of pigeons to ornithosis has not been systematically studied. Since chlamydial infection is widespread among flocks of commercial, show, and feral pigeons, it is difficult to delineate genetic resistance from acquired immunity in these birds. Serologically negative pigeons have been tested numerous times for their susceptibility to various strains of *C. psittaci* (Meyer, 1965; Page, 1967). These tests indi-

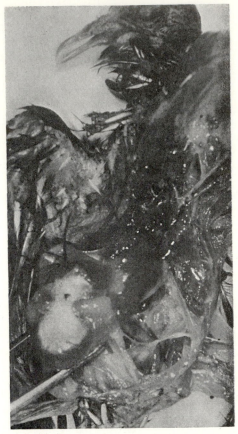

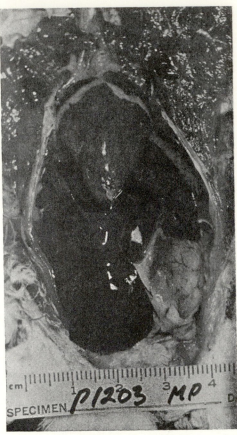

FIG. 13.20—*Field case of acute ornithosis in emaciated young dove. Viscera have been dislodged to show thickened air sacs covered with fibrinous exudate. Large fibrin plaque is present on epicardium.*

FIG. 13.21—*Field case of acute ornithosis in pigeon. Hepatomegaly is most pronounced gross abnormality, but air sacs (not shown) were thickened and coated with sticky, purulent exudate containing large numbers of chlamydiae.*

cate that pigeons are inherently insusceptible to intracerebral inoculations of large numbers of highly toxigenic chlamydial strains from turkeys and to other strains from domestic herbivores (see Fig. 13.8); yet they are very sensitive and susceptible to a variety of mildly virulent strains from pigeons, sparrows, and some mammalian strains. Resistance of these birds to virulent organisms introduced by a normally sensitive route must certainly imply that pigeons have some natural protective mechanisms that prevent certain types of chlamydial strains from multiplying and causing damage to their tissues.

CHICKENS

Epizootiologic and laboratory evidence indicates that chickens appear to be relatively resistant to disease caused by *C. psittaci*. While acute infection progresses to disease and fatality only in young birds, the incidence of actual epizootics is very low. Experimentally even young birds are resistant to many strains of *C. psittaci*. In acute cases the birds have fibrinous pericarditis and hepatomegaly. Most natural infections are inapparent and transient. Serologic surveys indicate that the incidence of infection among flocks is low.

GEESE

Incidental to studies of ornithosis in ducks, several investigators have observed the disease in geese and have isolated *C. psittaci* from diseased tissues (Trojan and Strauss, 1955; Strauss, 1967). Clinical and necropsy findings were similar to those in ducks.

PHEASANTS

Chlamydiae of low virulence have been isolated from tissues of sick pheasants raised on pheasant farms, but no large-scale epizootics of ornithosis in this species have been reported (Meyer, 1965). Serologic surveys of both wild and commercially raised pheasants in Illinois (Meyer, 1965) and Iowa (Page, 1964, unpublished data) indicate that the incidence of exposure to chlamydiae followed by development of antibody is very low in the Midwest. Strauss (1967), however, reported that humans have contracted psittacosis after contact with pheasants. It seems likely that both wild and domestic pheasants would have occasional exposures to chlamydiae excreted by other hosts, but the factors accounting for the lack of acute ornithosis in this species are not known.

DIAGNOSIS

A positive diagnosis of ornithosis in a bird can be made on the basis of isolation and identification of the etiologic agent from diseased tissues of the host, or upon demonstration of a fourfold rise in the host's circulating antibody titer against chlamydial group or specific cell wall antigens. Correlative with these positive indications should be the presence of gross or microscopic lesions (except in the case of certain carriers) and clinical signs typical of ornithosis.

A diagnosis of probable ornithosis in a flock of sick birds may be made upon the demonstration of a high incidence (greater than 50%) of the birds with circulating antibody titers of 1:64 or more.

A positive diagnosis of ornithosis cannot be made simply on the basis of "typical" gross lesions, cellular alterations, or clinical signs.

ISOLATION AND IDENTIFICATION OF *C. psittaci*

Specimen Collection

In cases of acute, severe ornithosis, the specimens to collect at necropsy for the isolation of *C. psittaci* are the inflammatory exudates appearing at the site of major tissue damage or the abnormal organs themselves—for example, fibrinous exudates in or on the lungs, air sacs, liver, spleen, or mesentery; samples of tissues of the lungs, spleen, liver, or kidney; auricular or nasal exudates; or blood, if chlamydemia is suspected.

Only a small amount of tissue is needed, but it is important to collect the tissues aseptically since contaminating bacteria interfere with the isolation of chlamydiae. If such contaminants are unavoidably present, the specimen may be homogenized in the antibiotic solution described in the paragraph under Inoculum Preparation. Whole blood may be collected for isolation attempts, but success in recovering the organisms depends upon whether a state of bacteremia existed at the time of bleeding.

In cases of mild or inapparent clinical signs in a suspect host, samples of liver, spleen, or kidney (especially those organs that are enlarged or off color) should be collected aseptically at necropsy for isolation attempts. When there is doubt as to which tissue should be collected, the tissue or organ showing inflammation, hyperemia, or petechial hemorrhages should be taken for examination.

In cases where it is desirable or necessary to keep the infected individual host alive, the following specimens should be taken for isolation of chlamydiae:

1. Whole heparinized blood taken during the febrile period.
2. Conjunctival scrapings if inflammation or exudate is present.
3. Peritoneal fluid if ascites is present.
4. Tracheal swabs if respiratory difficulties are present.
5. Intestinal excrement if diarrhea is present.

Blood for Serology

Serology may play an important role in diagnosis if the etiologic agent cannot be isolated. Ideally, blood should be taken during the acute and convalescent stages of the disease in an individual and serum saved for testing. If there is a substantial rise in titer of circulating chlamydial antibodies between consecutive bleedings, a positive diagnosis is affirmed. In the case of infected flocks, paired samples of sera from tagged birds are the most desirable for conclusive serodiagnosis; however, if serial bleedings are not possible, a single bleeding of at least 10% of the birds can be of assistance in making a tentative diagnosis.

Hazards to Humans in Handling Specimens

Most strains of *C. psittaci* recovered from birds may cause disease in man if the organisms are inhaled in sufficient quantities. Fine particles of dried excrement from infected birds or mammals, infectious aerosols from tracheal or nasal expulsions of infected animals, or those aerosols created in the laboratory by mechanical manipulations of suspensions of organisms in syringes and pipettes may be a source of infection for susceptible humans. Unheated sera from chlamydemic animals may be hazardous to serologists.

Direct Examination of Infected Hosts

Tissues infected with *C. psittaci* usually show vascular congestion, petechial hemorrhages, or surface deposits of sticky exudates. Spleens and livers may be enlarged, dark, soft, or mottled. The splenic surface may have numerous vaguely outlined white spots. The exudates on the surfaces of organs characteristically contain chlamydia-infected monocytes.

Microscopic Examination of Exudates

The cytoplasms of mononuclear cells in fibrinous exudates contain microcolonies of *C. psittaci* which are readily visible microscopically at ×800 or more magnification when fresh wet mounts of exudate are viewed with phase contrast optics (Fig. 13.6). While some cells contain granules that are part of their normal structures and which can be mistaken for chlamydiae, phase contrast microscopy of fresh exudates is a superior and more convenient method of direct examination for chlamydiae than any staining method. While a few small-sized spherical bodies in a few cells are not meaningful, the presence of numerous mononuclear cells, many of which contain spherical bodies 0.2–0.4μ in diameter, is suggestive of chlamydial infection—barring complication with mycoplasma organisms. But observation of such "typical" exudates is only the first step leading the investigator to determine the nature of the suspicious organisms.

The use of fluorescein-conjugated specific antibody preparations for the identification of intra- and extra-cellular chlamydiae is practical and of great value in assisting the specific diagnosis of chlamydiosis. Such preparations are not available commercially, however, so each diagnostic laboratory must prepare its own, and the potency and reliability of the preparations depend upon the care with which they are prepared. Suitable antibody for fluorescein conjugation may be prepared in rabbits, lambs, and pigeons but not calves. Specific fluorescence can be prevented by prior treatment of the cells with unconjugated specific antiserum. Conjugated antibody prepared against the chlamydial group antigen causes the cytoplasm of infected cells to fluoresce brightly under ultraviolet light (Fig. 13.22). Considerable experience with a given preparation and with chlamydiae-infected tissues from a variety of tissues and animals is necessary before a diagnosis of ornithosis can be made solely on evidence of a positive fluorescent antibody test. A positive diagnosis is usually correlated with positive serological, clinical, and necropsy findings.

Specimens for Histopathology

Specimens preserved for sectioning should be fixed in Zenker's solution so that adequate staining of chlamydiae by Giemsa's method may be performed. In general, sectioning of tissues for histopathology does not assist the rapid diagnosis of chlamydiosis, since the lesions are difficult to distinguish from those caused by mycoplasma organisms, but the study of sections is indispensable to the description of cellular changes caused by chlamydiae in any new form of chlamydiosis or in certain experimental work.

Inoculum Preparation

Tissues suspected of containing *C. psittaci* should be aseptically homogenized to approximately a 20% suspension in beef heart broth or saline buffered with phosphate to pH 7.2. If the original tissues are contaminated with bacteria other than chlamydiae, they should be homogenized in buffered diluent containing 1 mg/ml each of streptomycin sulfate, vancomycin, and kanamycin sulfate, centrifuged at 1,000 g for 10 minutes, the sediment discarded, and the supernatant fluid recentrifuged. The supernatant fluid is again recentrifuged. The final supernatant is then inoculated into experimental animals or cell cultures.

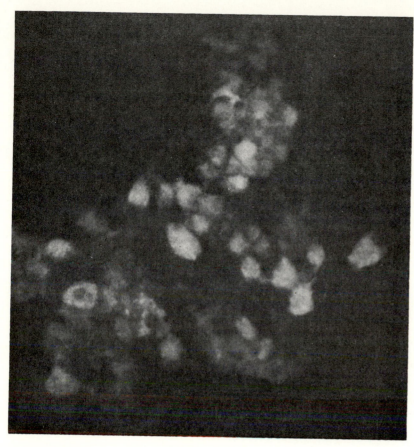

FIG. 13.22—Micrograph of air sac exudate of turkey naturally infected with C. psittaci stained with fluorescein-conjungated ornithosis antibody and photographed under ultraviolet light. Cytoplasm of infected cells fluoresces brightly. ×4,000.

Uncontaminated fluid exudates from infected animals may be inoculated directly into experimental hosts to isolate chlamydiae.

Experimental Hosts

CHICKEN EMBRYOS. The most convenient and readily available host for isolation of *C. psittaci* is the chicken embryo. The yolk sac membrane is the primary site of chlamydial growth and is the route of choice for inoculation. Up to 0.5 ml of fluid may be injected into the yolk sac of 6–7-day-old embryos. Growth and multiplication of chlamydiae may cause death of the embryo within 3–10 days after inoculation, depending upon the number of organisms inoculated and the temperature of incubation. Recent research has indicated that multiplication of *C. psittaci* is greatly stimulated by incubation of the inoculated embryos at 39° C instead of the traditional 37° C. The optimum temperature for many *C. psittaci* strains may be higher than 39° C, but at 39° C the organism's growth rate is acceler-ated with no detrimental thermal effect on the embryo. Use of 39° C may shorten by several days the time required for multiplication of the organisms to embryo lethal levels (Page, 1971). The vascular congestion typical of that seen in embryonic yolk sacs inoculated with *C. psittaci* is illustrated in Figure 13.23. For preservation of the strain, yolk sacs may be stored at −20 to −70° C indefinitely. For identification of the organisms in the yolk sac, the membrane must be prepared as an antigen for serologic tests described below.

MICE. Most strains of *C. psittaci* from birds may be isolated or propagated in laboratory mice 3–4 weeks of age, inoculated either by the intraperitoneal, intracerebral, or intranasal route. After intraperitoneal inoculation of the mouse, the organisms multiply in the peritoneal serosa, resulting in progressive inflammation leading to accumulation of large amounts of fibrinous exudate in the cavity. The ascites fluid volume may total several times the blood vol-

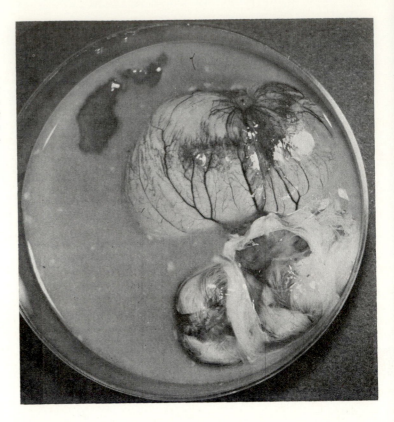

FIG. 13.23—Vascular congestion in yolk sac is prominent gross abnormality in chicken embryo inoculated 10 days earlier with C. psittaci. Organisms multiply to 10^9 organisms per gram yolk sac.

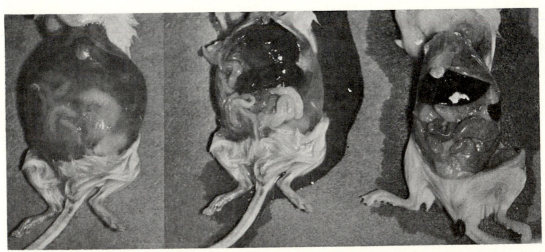

FIG. 13.24—Gross lesions of C. psittaci strain of low virulence in laboratory mice infected intraperitoneally. Swollen abdomen of mouse on left is caused by accumulation of ascites fluid in peritoneal cavity. Fluid contains numerous chlamydia-laden mononuclear cells. Same mouse in center showing enlarged spleen. Normal uninoculated mouse on right.

ume of the mouse and produces a swollen abdomen (Fig. 13.24). Some infected mice become so swollen they are unable to move about and in time succumb. Splenomegaly is a prominent gross lesion. Enlarged spleens are the organ of choice from which to recover the infectious agent or preserve for subpassage.

GUINEA PIGS. As previously indicated, many strains of chlamydiae, especially those of low virulence, do not multiply and cause gross lesions in guinea pigs; therefore, this host is not the one of choice for initial isolation of avian strains. However, chlamydial strains of high virulence multiply in guinea pigs and cause severe lesions and death (Fig. 13.25).

CELL CULTURES. Chlamydiae in bird tissues may be isolated and propagated in primary cultures of chicken embryo cells or in certain line cell cultures derived from mouse or human tissues. Cell monolayers immersed in standard culture medium with 10% mammalian serum are well suited for characterization of the organism's intracellular colonial morphology and glycogen production. Cell culture-propagated organisms also may be used for preparation of chlamydial antigens. Growth and multiplication of the organisms produce cell destruction and sloughing of monolayers. The time required for cytopathogenicity depends on the number and strain of organism inoculated, the strain of cell culture, and the temperature of incubation.

Identification of the New Isolant as Chlamydia psittaci

The organisms should have a typical intracellular morphology—spherical bodies 0.2–1.5μ in diameter distributed about the cytoplasm of the host cell (Fig. 13.3)—and the suspension must be free of all bacteria capable of colonization on lifeless bacteriological media. Secondly, the organisms must be shown by complement fixation or other serologic method to contain the chlamydial group antigen. The test for this is described in the section below on serology. Thirdly, microcolonies of the organisms in cell culture must be negative by the iodine test for glycogen, as described in the section on etiology (see also Fig. 13.5). Lastly, the multiplication of the organisms must be shown not to be inhibited by the

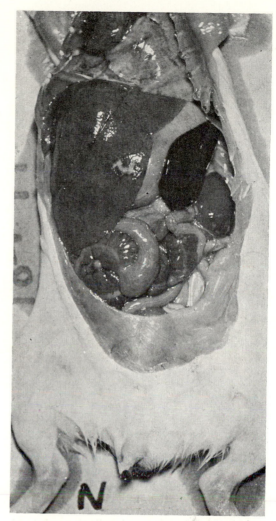

FIG. 13.25—*Gross lesions caused by C. psittaci strain of high virulence in guinea pig 10 days after intraperitoneal inoculation of organisms. Hepatomegaly, splenomegaly, and fibrinous serositis are the prominent lesions.*

presence of sodium sulfadiazine. In this test a suspension of the organisms is titrated in a duplicate series in chicken embryos, with one set of infected embryos inoculated with 1 mg sodium sulfadiazine per embryo and the other set inoculated with an equal volume of diluent instead of drug. The difference between the ELD_{50} determined for the two titration sets should not be greater than 10, indicating that the drug does not inhibit the growth of the chlamydial isolant.

However, if the new isolant forms compact intracellular microcolonies, contains the group antigen, is glycogen-positive, and is sensitive to sodium sulfadiazine, it is classified as *C. trachomatis*.

SEROLOGY

The chlamydial group antigen common to all strains of organisms of the genus *Chlamydia* is useful for serologic surveys, serodiagnosis for individuals, and identification of chlamydiae. Strain-specific antigens found in the cell walls of the organisms may be useful for epizootiologic or epidemiologic purposes in tracing the spread of certain strains, but specific cell wall antigens are laborious to prepare and are not in general use.

Methods

A variety of serologic methods have been studied for their use in detecting chlamydial antibodies in the sera of birds and mammals; the most common method used is one that involves a complement fixation system. Standard CF methods employing boiled and phenolized chlamydial antigens are used for titering antisera from pigeons and mammals. However, antisera from turkeys, chickens, ducks, geese, pheasants, sparrows, parakeets, and other birds do not normally fix guinea pig complement after reaction with homologous antigens. Since fowl antibody combines with antigen satisfactorily, Rice (1948) developed an indirect complement fixation (ICF) method whereby avian antibody could be detected. One CF unit of antiserum derived from mammals was added to each dilution of fowl antiserum being tested. In the presence of fowl antibody, antigen was taken up with none left over to react with mammalian antibody; therefore, complement was not fixed in tests of positive avian sera. Conversely, with negative fowl sera, antigen was taken up by the added mammalian antibody, and complement was fixed. Thus positive and negative sera had reactions that were the reverse of those found in normal direct CF tests on mammalian sera. The ICF method was first applied to testing avian sera for chlamydial group antibodies by Karrer et al. (1950); it is still used as a standard test although the method requires extraordinary care and precision in performance and standardization of reagents.

Because of these difficulties, alternative procedures using direct CF procedures were developed by Brumfield and Pomeroy (1957) and Benedict and McFarland (1956). Brumfield and Pomeroy found that the addition of normal rooster serum containing sufficient quantities of avian C'1 fraction of complement to each dilution of fowl test serum produced fixation of complement when the antigen was present. Thus a normal indicator system was established. The test worked well, but research soon proved that not all roosters contained the required component in sufficient quantities, and the difficulties in obtaining and testing potent rooster sera were nearly equal to the rigors of setting up a workable ICF system (Brumfield et al., 1961).

A second alternative method developed by Benedict and McFarland (1956) used a chlamydial antigen extracted from egg-propagated chlamydiae by sodium lauryl sulfate. The antigen was purified by acid precipitation followed by resolubilizing the antigen in buffered solutions of higher pH. This antigen combined with chlamydial group antibody and fixed complement in a normal direct CF method. Unfortunately this method of antigen preparation with resultant simplification of the CF method for the detection of ornithosis antibodies in fowl sera has never been commonly used; therefore, it suffers from the necessary widespread testing that is needed to establish its usefulness once and for all. Comparative tests on numerous fowl sera using Karrer's ICF, Benedict's direct CF, and other methods have shown that all tests are satisfactory for the detection of chlamydial group antibodies.

Other tests employing hemagglutination inhibition (HI), conglutinating complement absorption (CCA), and simple capillary tube agglutination (CTA) tests have been developed for detecting chlamydial antibodies. According to Gogolak and Ross (1955), the hemagglutinin is an antigenic phospholipoprotein. This fact was used by Hilleman (1955) to develop an HI procedure that was simple and sensitive. This was followed by the Benedict and O'Brien (1958) passive hemagglutination test which utilized tanned red cells coated with chlamydial antigen. All these tests lack the widescale testing at different laboratories necessary to prove their reliability and usefulness.

Agglutination methods have been tested

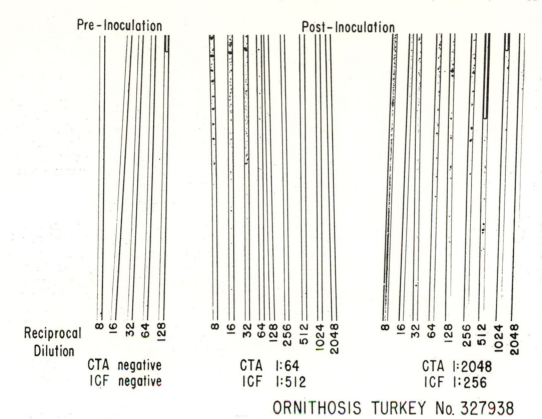

Pre-Inoculation   Post-Inoculation

Reciprocal
Dilution

| CTA | negative | CTA | 1:64 | CTA | 1:2048 |
| ICF | negative | ICF | 1:512 | ICF | 1:256 |

ORNITHOSIS TURKEY No. 327938

FIG. 13.26—Capillary tube agglutination test reactions on serial dilutions of three consecutive sera from a turkey before and after C. psittaci *infection. Second and third sera were from blood taken on 3rd and 8th weeks postinoculation. Giemsa-stained antigen is clumped in the presence of positive serum. Actual size.*

by many investigators. The most promising of these is one devised by Mason (1959) which employs a suspension of Giemsa-stained purified chlamydiae as antigen. The stained antigen is reacted with antiserum in a capillary tube (Fig. 13.26). The test is simple to do, direct, and highly sensitive for detecting agglutinins which appear in the sera of fowl prior to the development of CF detectable antibodies. Thus the CTA test is useful for the early serodiagnosis of ornithosis. Disadvantages to the test are that nonspecific agglutination occurs when serum dilutions lower than 1:8 are used, and special methods for dispersion of the antigen in suspension must be used to prevent autoagglutination.

Recent research has shown that the agglutination and ICF tests detect both the 19S and 7S types of antibody produced in turkeys and other animals (Page et al., 1967).

Interpretation of Results

The response of a host to an antigenic stimulus is governed by the amount and timing of the antigen introduced into the host as well as other factors, one of them being the length of the period elapsing between injection of antigen and appearance of detectable levels of circulating antibodies. Normally circulating agglutinins appear in detectable levels within 3–5 days after chlamydiae reach the bloodstream, and CF or ICF antibodies appear 5–10 days later. In birds exposed to large infective doses, antibodies appear earlier; if the dose is small, they appear later. When a bird is infected with a large dose of a highly virulent organism, rapid growth and multiplication of the organisms may overwhelm the host before detectable antibodies are produced. Birds chronically infected with chlamydiae of low virulence often develop unusually high titers because of the strong antigenic stimulus provided over a long period of time. In view of the variability of the antigenic stimulus, it is generally unwise to ascribe a certain titer of circulating antibody in individual hosts as an indicator of current disease. However, the demonstration of high titers in a majority of individuals of a flock showing clinical signs is presumptive evidence of current infection. Demonstration of at least a fourfold rise in circulating antibody titer in an individual bird, however, is diagnostic of current infection.

Details of the ICF procedure are given by Meyer and Eddie (1964), of the CTA test by Mason (1959), and comparisons of these tests on 635 sera taken at intervals from experimentally infected turkeys are reported by Page and Bankowski (1960).

Preparation of CF Antigen from Yolk Sac-Propagated Organisms

The antigen used in the ICF test of Karrer et al. and the direct CF test of Brumfield and Pomeroy is easily prepared by harvesting heavily infected yolk sacs of chicken embryos, homogenizing the membranes to make a 20–30% suspension by weight in buffered saline or beef heart infusion broth, and then boiling the suspension for 30 minutes. After the suspension has cooled, phenol is added to make a final dilution of 0.5% phenol. After storage at 4° C for 24 hours, the antigen is ready for testing. Serial dilutions of antigen are tested for potency in a CF test against serial dilutions of a high-titered chlamydial antiserum of mammalian origin and also against a negative serum as a control. Once the potency is ascertained, the antigen may be used to test sera at a dilution appropriate to the CF procedure being used for testing avian sera. The ICF test for fowl antisera utilizes 1 CF unit of antigen, 2 exact units of complement, and 1 CF unit of mammalian antibody. For pigeon or mammalian antisera, 4 CF units of antigen are usually used.

Identification of New Chlamydial Isolants by CF Tests

New isolants may be conclusively identified as members of the genus *Chlamydia* by propagating them in chicken embryos and preparing the infected yolk sacs as antigen by the method described above. The new antigen is titrated against a constant low dilution of positive antiserum in a direct CF test. Fixation of complement in such a test implies the presence of chlamydial group antigen. A minimum of 10,000 organisms per unit volume of antigen is necessary to produce one CF unit. Yolk sacs usually support the growth of chlamydiae to titers of 10^6–10^9 per gram of membrane, so most antigens prepared by this method have a titer of at least 1:64 against 4 units of antiserum.

TREATMENT

As mentioned before, *C. psittaci* is susceptible to penicillin, chloramphenicol, and the tetracyclines, but only the tetracyclines are both economically feasible and effective for large-scale treatment of poultry flocks. The most practical route of administration is incorporation of the drug into the feed or drinking water. Penicillin is not very effective by this route, and chloramphenicol has toxic side effects. Drug coated grain or composite mash is the most common vehicle for medicating birds.

TURKEYS

The treatment of turkeys infected with toxigenic chlamydiae by incorporating 100–300 g chlortetracycline per ton of feed for 2 weeks was shown by Davis and Delaplane (1955) to reduce the severe effects of ornithosis, but the medication did not completely eliminate the organisms from the birds' tissues; thus the processing of such birds for market remained a human health hazard. However, raising the drug levels to 400 or 800 g per ton for 3 weeks completely suppressed the infection (Davis and Delaplane, 1958; Davis and Watkins, 1959). In other epizootics in Oregon, treatment of turkeys infected with a highly virulent agent at levels of 200–400 g chlortetracycline per ton feed failed to sterilize the birds' tissues; later tests indicated that only levels as high as 2,800 g per ton were therapeutically successful, in spite of the inclusion of chelating agents to reduce the calcium levels at the site of drug absorption (Meyer, 1965).

Successful treatment of turkeys infected with chlamydiae of low virulence has been reported for epizootics in Minnesota, California, and New Mexico (Pomeroy, 1957, personal communication; Page and Bankowski, 1959; Francis, 1960). In these cases drug levels of 200–400 g per ton of feed given to the birds for periods of 1–3 weeks were effective in reducing clinical signs and in sterilizing the birds' tissues, thereby permitting the birds to be marketed without hazard to human health. But treatment at these levels, especially for periods as short as 7 days (California epizootic), did not allow sufficient time for resolution of gross lesions in the birds; when the turkeys were processed, gross lesions resulting from pericarditis, perihepatitis, airsacculitis, and splenitis were still prominent and caused a high rate of organ condemnation. A large number of these discarded hearts and other tissues were examined for the presence of chlamydiae and found to be free of viable organisms (Page and Bankowski, 1959).

For birds that are to be kept for an extended period after treatment, such as special breeding stock, an alternating treatment regime is recommended. The birds should be fed medicated feed for 2 weeks, regular feed for 2 weeks, and then medicated feed again for 2 weeks. At the end of another several weeks on regular feed the birds should be carefully examined clinically for hyperthermia, diarrhea, and rise in circulating antibody titer. In any case, treatment should be combined with disinfection of poultry houses and improvement in containment with respect to removing potential sources of reinfection.

Thorough professional judgment must be utilized in consideration of the treatment and disposition of ornithosis-infected birds. Upon diagnosis of the disease, turkeys should be immediately placed on medicated feed at levels at least as high as 400 g drug per ton followed by laboratory tests to ascertain the virulence of the disease agent in the birds. Based on a review of the clinical history of the flock and the results of laboratory tests, judgments have to be made in regard to the potential hazards to human health in future handling of the birds with respect to the economics of the appropriate treatment and probable condemnation rates of bird tissues at processing. Formation of these judgments requires the cooperation and combined talents of the flock owner, practicing veterinarian, veterinary and medical health officials, and their technical staffs.

DUCKS AND OTHER FOWL

Essentially the same principles of disease treatment and control of the disposition of infected turkeys apply also to ducks and other fowl. However, since chlamydial infection in these fowl is often complicated by secondary salmonellosis, it is important to apply an adequate treatment level of a drug or combination of drugs that will affect both infections. It is also necessary to confirm the efficacy of the treatment before release of the birds for marketing or continued survival for breeding purposes.

PIGEONS

Several reports testify to the difficulties in effectively treating chronic chlamydial infection in pigeons so as to eliminate the carrier state (Meyer and Eddie, 1955; Arnstein et al., 1964). While oral administration of chlortetracycline dramatically reduced mortality of squabs during acute epizootics, this method failed to suppress the infection entirely, thereby leaving carriers to reinfect survivors. Meyer (1965) suggests that alternating periods of treatment with periods of no treatment will eventually remove the carrier state.

PREVENTION AND CONTROL

MANAGEMENT PROCEDURES

The source of infection should be controlled. On the assumption that transmission of chlamydiae occurs principally by inhalation of dried excrement from infected birds, any new group of incubator-hatched, infection-free poults, ducklings, or young birds should be placed in an environment that is free of droppings, litter, feathers, and dust from other potentially infected birds. The new birds should be placed only in housing that has been thoroughly disinfected and/or steam cleaned. If possible, the new birds should be protected from having contact with holdover birds from previous flocks or with wild or feral birds, especially pigeons. Replacement birds, if any are to be introduced into a flock, should be blood-tested and accepted only if they are found serologically negative for chlamydial antibodies. It would also be advisable to restrict contact of the flock with any other farm animals, since cattle, sheep, cats, and rodents are known to be occasional reservoirs of chlamydial organisms.

Affected birds should be isolated. If a flock consists of several groups of birds maintained in separate but contiguous areas and one of the groups is suspected of having chlamydiosis, every effort should be made to prevent the diseased birds or their excretions from coming in contact with other groups of birds. Sick birds should be promptly isolated, and adequate professional assistance should be sought to ascertain a conclusive diagnosis. Once a positive diagnosis is made, the affected birds should immediately be given therapeutic levels of tetracyclines in their feed and kept under as sanitary conditions as possible to prevent spread of the disease. Serologic and clinical surveillance by periodic blood-testing and observation of nearby flocks should be conducted for several months to determine if the infection has spread. If positive titers or clinical signs appear in these birds, the flock should be promptly treated with medicated feed. All wild and feral birds should be prevented from intermingling with an infected flock if possible, since it is very likely that they will pick up the disease agents and excrete them among unexposed poultry or mammals.

Selective Breeding for Resistance

Every animal disease investigator has periodically observed that among any large group of animals exposed to a given dose of disease organisms, there often are a few individuals that appear to be unaffected by the exposure. When such observations are the result of scientific design, they can be used to select disease-resistant breeding stock. Such selective breeding is in fact practiced by the chicken breeding industry to develop stock that is resistant to respiratory disease. There is no theoretical reason why the principle cannot be applied to breeding for resistance to chlamydiosis.

VACCINATION AND IMMUNIZATION

Bacterins

Numerous preparations of killed chlamydiae, with and without adjuvants, have been used in attempts to immunize birds and laboratory animals against chlamydial infection. Formalin-inactivated concentrated suspensions of chlamydiae injected repeatedly by the intraperitoneal route into mice protect them against challenge by the same route with homologous or heterologous strains (Wagner et al., 1946). Apparently a large number of immunizing antibodies accumulate in the fluids of the peritoneal cavity. Duff and Mumford (1966) showed that mice immunized with killed chlamydiae and challenged by the intraperitoneal route with organisms of the same or other strains developed large quantities of ascitic fluid, each milliliter of which contained in excess of 100,000 mouse immunizing doses 50%. Other investigators have had similar results in immunizing mice against challenge with chlamydial agents, but the same success has not been achieved with birds. Ricebirds and parakeets inoculated with formalinized chlamydiae were immune to small challenge doses (100 MLD_{50}) but not larger ones (Meyer et al., 1942b). Pigeons vaccinated with similar preparations and then exposed 4 months later were as susceptible to reinfection by natural means as were nonvaccinated controls (Hughes, 1947). Formalinized bacterins mixed with adjuvants have not provided decisive immunity to chlamydiosis in domestic fowl or in psittacines. Meyer and Eddie (1962) sought by immunization procedures to prevent acute ornithosis in turkeys not only to reduce mortality and turkey meat condemnation losses but to reduce the risk of occupational infection among turkey handlers. They inoculated turkeys with formalinized chlamydiae mixed with homogenized oil adjuvants (e.g., "Bayol-F, Arlacel A"). Three intramuscular injections of vaccine one month apart induced some degree of immunity, for mortality in vaccinates after challenge with virulent chlamydiae by the intratracheal route was lower than that in the controls, but a single dose gave less protection. Among the controls, 50% of the birds had gross lesions, and the organisms were recovered from 47% of the surviving birds. Of the thrice vaccinated birds, gross lesions were present in one-third of them 30 days after challenge, and chlamydiae were recovered from 14% of them. These results indicate that only marginal protection in terms of mortality and lesion reduction was achieved by multiple vaccination. More importantly, triple vaccination was ineffective in preventing chronic infection and the carrier stage.

Arnstein (1967) used formalinized suspensions of chlamydiae with an adjuvant (which he did not describe) in attempts to immunize parakeets and parrots against psittacosis. Vaccinated parakeets had a 21% mortality compared with 80% in the controls when their immunity was challenged with 500 mouse LD_{50} of organisms. However, when vaccinated birds were challenged with 10,000 mouse LD_{50}, 95% of the vaccinates died compared with 100% mortality in the controls. Essentially the same results were obtained in parrots. In both cases, half of the vaccinated birds surviving the low dose challenge were infected carriers for at least 60 days.

Living Vaccines

In other tests, Arnstein immunized parrots with a vaccine containing over 10^7 egg LD_{50} of a strain of *C. psittaci* isolated from a cow with enteritis. The strain caused no clinical signs initially in the parrots, produced high antibody titers, and was recovered from the blood of the vaccinates at the 25th but not the 40th postvaccination day. The birds were then challenged with a virulent psittacosis strain. A significantly lower challenge mortality occurred in the vaccinated birds than in the controls (15% vs 69%), but the challenge organisms could be recovered equally well from both vaccinated and control birds at the 20th, 60th, and 90th days post challenge. Thus, while mortality was substantially reduced by vac-

cination, the chronic carrier stage could not be prevented. Therein lies the vexing problem in the effective immunization of domestic birds.

Outlook for Chlamydial Vaccines

Thus far all forms of vaccination against chlamydiosis have shown only marginal success in achieving the goals demanded of a method for preventing both acute and chronic disease in domestic birds. These difficulties, coupled with the high cost of producing and administering vaccine and the lessened need to immunize large segments of poultry populations, make it very unlikely that vaccination against ornithosis will play a large role in the control of disease in poultry in the near future.

FEDERAL REGULATIONS REGARDING CHLAMYDIOSIS

According to regulations of the USDA, the movement of poultry, carcasses, or offal from any premises where the existence of ornithosis has been proven by isolation of a chlamydial agent is prohibited. Both the Agricultural Research Service of the USDA and the Food and Drug Administration of the U.S. Department of Health, Education and Welfare forbid interstate movement of birds from infected flocks. There is no restriction of movement of eggs from an infected flock.

REFERENCES

Anderson, D. R., Hope E. Hopps, M. F. Barile, and B. C. Bernheim. 1965. Comparison of the ultrastructure of several rickettsiae, ornithosis virus, and mycoplasma in tissue culture. *J. Bacteriol.* 90:1387–1404.

Andrews, J. M. 1957. The importance of psittacosis in the United States. *J. Am. Vet. Med. Ass.* 130:109–16.

Anonymous. 1955. The ebb and flow of infection. *Lancet* II, p. 611.

Arnstein, P. 1967. Observations on chemotherapy and immunization of birds against psittacosis. *Am. J. Ophthalmol.* 63:1260–63.

Arnstein, P., D. H. Cohen, and K. F. Meyer. 1964. Medication of pigeons with chlortetracycline in feed. *J. Am. Vet. Med. Ass.* 145:921–24.

Banks, Joyce, B. Eddie, J. Schachter, and K. F. Meyer. 1970. Plaque formation by *Chlamydia* in L cells. *Infection and Immunity* 1:259–62.

Beasley, J. N., D. E. Davis, and L. C. Grumbles. 1959. Preliminary studies on the histopathology of experimental ornithosis in turkeys. *Am. J. Vet. Res.* 20:341–49.

Beasley, J. N., R. W. Moore, and J. R. Watkins. 1961. The histopathologic characteristics of diseases producing inflammation of the air sacs in turkeys. A comparative study in pure and mixed infections. *Am. J. Vet. Res.* 22:85–92.

Benedict, A. A., and C. McFarland. 1956. Direct complement-fixation test for diagnosis of ornithosis in turkeys. *Proc. Soc. Exp. Biol. Med.* 92:768–71.

Benedict, A. A., and E. O'Brien. 1958. A passive hemagglutination reaction for psittacosis. *J. Immunol.* 80:94–99.

Brumfield, Helene P., and Pomeroy, B. S. 1957. Direct complement fixation by turkey and chicken serum in viral systems. *Proc. Soc. Exp. Biol. Med.* 94:146–49.

Brumfield, Helene P., H. Benson, and B. S. Pomeroy. 1961. Procedure for modified complement fixation test with turkey or chicken serum antibody. *Avian Diseases* 5:270–82.

Coles, J. D. W. A. 1940. Psittacosis in domestic pigeons. *Onderstepoort J. Vet. Res.* 15:141–48.

Davis, D. E., and J. P. Delaplane. 1955. Ornithosis in turkeys. *Proc. Book, Am. Vet. Med. Ass., 92nd Ann. Meet.*, p. 296.

———. 1958. The effect of chlortetracycline treatment of turkeys affected with ornithosis. *Am. J. Vet. Res.* 19:169–73.

Davis, D. E., and J. R. Watkins. 1959. The effect of chlortetracycline on the immunological response of turkeys infected with ornithosis. *J. Infect. Diseases* 104:56–60.

Davis, D. E., J. R. Delaplane, and J. R. Watkins. 1957. The role of turkey eggs in the transmission of ornithosis. *Am. J. Vet. Res.* 18:409–13.

Davis, D. J. 1955. Psittacosis in pigeons, pp. 66–73. In Beaudette, F. R. (ed.), *Psittacosis: Diagnosis, Epidemiology and Control.* Rutgers Univ. Press, New Brunswick, N.J.

Dickinson, E. M., W. E. Babcock, and J. G. Kilian. 1957. Ornithosis in Oregon turkeys. *J. Am. Vet. Med. Ass.* 130:117–18.

Duff, J. T., and Altha C. Mumford. 1966. Antibody for psittacosis group agents in ascitic fluid of mice implanted with sarcoma 180. *Bacteriol. Proc.*, p. 121.

Eddie, B., and T. Francis, Jr. 1942. Occurrence of psittacosis-like infection in domestic and game birds of Michigan. *Proc. Soc. Exp. Biol. Med.* 50:291–95.

Eddie, B., K. F. Meyer, F. L. Lambrecht, and D. P. Furman. 1962. Isolation of ornithosis bedsoniae from mites collected in turkey quarters and from chicken lice. *J. Infect. Diseases* 110:231–37.

Eddie, B., F. J. Radovsky, D. Stiller, and N. Kumada. 1969. Psittacosis-lymphogranuloma venereum (PL) agents *(Bedsonia chlamydia)* in ticks, fleas, and native mammals in California. *Am. J. Epidemiol.* 90:449–60.

Francis, D. W. 1960. Case report—An outbreak of ornithosis in New Mexico. *Avian Diseases* 4:310–11.

Gale, C., V. L. Sanger, and B. S. Pomeroy. 1960. The gross and microscopic pathology of an ornithosis virus of low virulence for turkeys. *Am. J. Vet. Res.* 21:491–97.

Gimenez, D. F. 1964. Staining rickettsiae in yolk sac cultures. *Stain Technol.* 39:135–40.

Gogolak, F. M., and M. R. Ross. 1955. The properties and chemical nature of the psittacosis virus hemagglutinin. *Virology* 1:474–96.

Gordon, F. B., and A. L. Quan. 1965. Occurrence of glycogen in inclusions of the psittacosis-lymphogranuloma venereum-trachoma agents. *J. Infect. Diseases* 115:186–96.

Hilleman, M. R. 1955. Serologic procedure for detecting psittacosis infection in birds, pp. 74–79. In Beaudette, F. R. (ed.), *Psittacosis: Diagnosis, Epidemiology and Control.* Rutgers Univ. Press, New Brunswick, N.J.

Hughes, D. L. 1947. Ornithosis (psittacosis) in a pigeon flock. *J. Comp. Pathol. Therap.* 57:67–76.

Irons, J. V., M. L. Denley, and T. D. Sullivan. 1955. Psittacosis in turkeys and fowls as a source of human infection, pp. 44–65. In Beaudette, F. R. (ed.), *Psittacosis: Diagnosis, Epidemiology and Control.* Rutgers Univ. Press, New Brunswick, N.J.

Karrer, H., K. F. Meyer, and B. Eddie. 1950. The complement fixation inhibition test and its application to the diagnosis of ornithosis in chickens and ducks. I. Principles and technique of the test. *J. Infect. Diseases* 87:13–23.

Korns, R. F. 1955. Psittacosis in ducks and persons exposed to ducks, pp. 80–89. In Beaudette, F. R. (ed.), *Psittacosis: Diagnosis, Epidemiology and Control.* Rutgers Univ. Press, New Brunswick, N.J.

Manire, G. P., and A. Tamura. 1967. Preparation and chemical composition of the cell walls of mature infectious dense forms of meningopneumonitis organisms. *J. Bacteriol.* 94:1178–83.

Mason, D. M. 1959. A capillary tube agglutination test for detecting antibodies against ornithosis in turkey serum. *J. Immunol.* 83:661–66.

Mason, D. M., and J. V. Irons. 1954. Epidemiology and epizootiology of turkey ornithosis. *Proc. 58th Ann. Meet. U.S. Livestock Sanit. Ass.*, pp. 326–29.

Meyer, K. F. 1941. Pigeons and barnyard fowls as possible sources of human psittacosis or ornithosis. *Schweiz. Med. Wochschr.* 71:79–85.

———. 1955. Problems in the control of psittacosis and ornithosis. *Proc. Am. Vet. Med. Ass. 92nd Ann. Meet.*, pp. 412–19.

———. 1959. Some general remarks and new observations on psittacosis and ornithosis. *Bull. WHO* 20:101–19.

———. 1965. Ornithosis, pp. 675–770. In Biester, H. E., and L. H. Schwarte (eds.), *Diseases of Poultry*, 5th ed. Iowa State Univ. Press, Ames.

———. 1967. The host spectrum of psittacosis-lymphogranuloma venereum agents. *Am. J. Ophthalmol.* 63:1225–45.

Meyer, K. F., and B. Eddie. 1953. Characteristics of a psittacosis viral agent isolated from a turkey. *Proc. Soc. Exp. Biol. Med.* 83:99–101.

———. 1955. Chemotherapy of natural psittacosis and ornithosis. Field trial of tetracycline, chlortetracycline, and oxytetracycline. *Antibiot. Ann.* 1954–55:544–55.

———. 1962. Immunity against some bedsonia in man resulting from infection and in animals from infection and vaccination. *Ann. N.Y. Acad. Sci.* 98:288–313.

———. 1964. Psittacosis-lymphogranuloma venereum group (Bedsonia infections), pp. 603–39. In Lennette, E. H., and N. J. Schmidt (eds.), *Diagnostic Procedures for Viral and Rickettsial Diseases*, 3rd ed. Am. Public Health Ass., New York.

Meyer, K. F., B. Eddie, and H. Y. Yanamura. 1942a. Ornithosis (psittacosis) in pigeons and its relation to human pneumonitis. *Proc. Soc. Exp. Biol. Med.* 49:609–15.

———. 1942b. Active immunization to *Microbacterium multiforme psittacosis* in parakeets and ricebirds. *J. Immunol.* 44:211–17.

Moore, R. W., and J. R. Watkins. 1960. The comparative effects of chlortetracycline and oxytetracycline in the treatment of turkeys with ornithosis. *J. Am. Vet. Med. Ass.* 136:565–68.

Morange, A. 1895. De la psittacose, ou infection speciale determinee par des perruches. *These de Paris*, pp. 1–77.

Moulder, J. W. 1964. The psittacosis group as bacteria. *CIBA Lectures Microbial Biochem.* John Wiley and Sons, New York.

———. 1966. The relation of the psittacosis group *(Chlamydiae)* to bacteria and viruses. *Ann. Rev. Microbiol.* 20:107–30.

Neal, J. E., and D. E. Davis. 1958. A comparison of the indirect complement fixation test, the direct complement fixation test, and the macroscopic agglutination test for ornithosis antibodies in turkey serums. *Am. J. Vet. Res.* 19:200–203.

Page, L. A. 1956. Experimental ornithosis in turkeys. Thesis, Univ. Calif. Berkeley.

———. 1959a. Experimental ornithosis in turkeys. *Avian Diseases* 3:51–66.

———. 1959b. Thermal inactivation studies on a turkey ornithosis virus. *Avian Diseases* 3:67–79.

———. 1960. Ecologic considerations in turkey ornithosis. *Am. J. Vet. Res.* 21:618–23.

———. 1966. Revision of the family Chlamydiaceae Rake (Rickettsiales): Unification of the psittacosis-lymphogranuloma venereum-trachoma group of organisms in the genus *Chlamydia* Jones, Rake and Stearns, 1945. *Int. J. Syst. Bacteriol.* 16:223–52.

———. 1967. Comparison of "pathotypes" among chlamydial (psittacosis) strains recovered from diseased birds and mammals. *Bull. Wildlife Disease Ass.* 3:166–75.

———. 1968. Proposal for the recognition of two species in the genus *Chlamydia* Jones, Rake and Stearns, 1945. *Int. J. Syst. Bacteriol.* 18:51–66.

———. 1971. The influence of temperature upon the multiplication of chlamydiae in chicken embryos. *Excerpta Med. Proc. 1970 Trachoma Conf.* (In press.)

Page, L. A., and R. A. Bankowski. 1959. Investigation of a recent ornithosis epornitic in California turkeys. *Am. J. Vet. Res.* 20:941–45.

———. 1960. Factors affecting the production and detection of ornithosis antibodies in infected turkeys. *Am. J. Vet. Res.* 21:971–78.

Page, L. A., J. M. Patterson, M. H. Roepke, and F. O. Glaser. 1967. Studies on the biophysical characteristics of antibodies produced in birds and mammals in response to experimental chlamydial infection (psittacosis). *J. Immunol.* 98:732–38.

Piraino, F. 1969. Plaque formation in chick embryo fibroblast cells by *Chlamydia* isolated from avian and mammalian sources. *J. Bacteriol.* 98:475–80.

Rice, C. E. 1948. Inhibitory effects of certain avian and mammalian antisera in specific complement-fixation systems. *J. Immunol.* 59:365–78.

———. 1961. The use of complement fixation tests in the study and diagnosis of viral diseases in man and animals—A review. VII. The psittacosis-lymphogranuloma venereum group. *Can. J. Comp. Med. Vet. Sci.* 25:74–79.

Strauss, J. 1956. Virological demonstration of ornithosis in men and ducks in Czechoslovakia. (In Czech.) *Cesk. Epidemiol. Mikrobiol. Immunol.* 5:281–90.

———. 1967. Microbiologic and epidemiologic aspects of duck ornithosis in Czechoslovakia. *Am. J. Ophthalmol.* 63:1246–63.

Tamura, A., and G. P. Manire. 1967. Preparation and chemical composition of the cell membranes of developmental reticulate forms of meningopneumonitis organisms. *J. Bacteriol.* 94:1184–88.

Tarizzo, M. L., and B. Nabli. 1967. The effect of antibiotics on the growth of TRIC agents in embryonated eggs. *Am. J. Ophthalmol.* 63:1550–57.

Trojan, J. A., and J. Strauss. 1955. An outbreak of ornithosis among workers in a poultry processing combine and experimental proof of its viral etiology. (In Czech.) *Casopis Lekaru Ceskych* 94:423–36.

Volkert, M., and M. Matthiesen. 1956. An ornithosis related antigen from a coccoid bacterium. *Acta Pathol. Microbiol. Scand.* 39:117–33.

Wagner, J., G. Meiklejohn, L. C. Kingsland, and H. W. Hickish. 1946. Psittacosis vaccines prepared from chick embryo tissues. *J. Immunol.* 54:35–46.

Weiss, E. 1967. Comparative metabolism of Chlamydia with special reference to catabolic activities. *Am. J. Ophthalmol.* 63:1098–1101.

CHAPTER 14

FUNGAL INFECTIONS

❖

H. L. CHUTE

Department of Animal Pathology
University of Maine
Orono, Maine

❖

ADVANCES in the past decade in the control of bacterial and viral diseases of birds have been outstanding. Although much experimental work has been done on the growth of fungi in the chicken egg embryo, very little or no progress has been made in the control of fungous diseases of birds. Fungous diseases are not the most common diseases of birds, yet they are prevalent enough to warrant economic attention.

In addition to the three fungal diseases of poultry (aspergillosis, favus, and thrush), two other fungal infections (histoplasmosis and cryptococcosis) are discussed. While not apparent pathogens of poultry, these are of significance from the public health standpoint because of their occurrence in poultry or the environments of birds.

A bibliography of avian mycosis by Chute et al. (1962) lists 709 references to fungi in birds. This bibliography brings out rare cases of reported fungous infections as well as experimental studies relating to birds and chicken egg embryos.

❖

ASPERGILLOSIS

❖

ASPERGILLOSIS has been observed in many birds and mammals. Frequent reference is made to the relationship of the disease in man to occupation, particularly in the so-called *gaveurs des pigeons* (pigeon feeders).

INCIDENCE AND DISTRIBUTION

Aspergillosis is encountered in poultry in two main forms. Acute outbreaks in which there are high morbidity and high mortality may occur particularly in young birds. In adults especially, an occasional bird in a flock or aviary may become affected while the other birds remain healthy. The numerous reports in the literature suggest that nearly all species of birds may be affected. The incidence of the disease is not great, however, as evidenced by reports from diagnostic laboratories.

It is generally agreed that *Aspergillus fumigatus* Fresenius is the most pathogenic and frequently encountered in disease processes due to aspergilli. The spores are widely distributed in nature, and birds frequently come in contact with them through contaminated feed or litter.

The fungous flora of young broiler chicks up to 13 weeks of age has been extensively studied by Chute et al. (1956). These workers observed that *A. fumigatus* may be found frequently and is not always pathogenic. The following genera were found in the lungs and air sacs: *Aspergillus, Penicillium, Paecilomyces, Cephalosporium, Trichoderma, Scopulariopsis,* and *Mucor*.

Aspergillosis is quite common in turkey poults, having been described by Lignières and Petit (1898). Hinshaw (1937) again described the disease in turkeys.

ETIOLOGY

The fungus grows quite readily on ordinary laboratory culture media at room temperature, at 37° C, and higher. Czapek's solution agar or Sabouraud's agar may be used. The colonies are green to bluish green at first and darken with age so as to

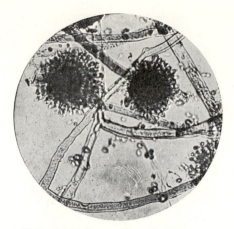

FIG. 14.1—*Aspergillus fumigatus.* ×250. *(Nowak,* Documenta Microbiologica, *courtesy Gustav Fischer)*

appear almost black. The colonies vary from velvety to floccose. The conidiophores are short, up to 300μ long by 2–8μ in diameter, the vesicles are apical flask-shaped up to 20–30μ in diameter, the sterigmata are 6–8 by 2–3μ, and the conidia are globose 2.5–3μ in diameter, in chains forming solid columns up to 400 by 50μ (Fig. 14.1) (Thom and Church, 1926).

TOXINS

Leber, according to Lucet (1897) and Van Heelsbergen (1929), succeeded in isolating toxins from cultures of *Aspergillus fumigatus.* Ceni and Besta (1902) were able to extract toxic materials from spores. A toxin reported by Bodin and Gautier (1906) was similar to bacterial toxins and produced clonicotonic convulsions, paralytic symptoms, and finally death. A toxin obtained by Henrici (1939) was toxic for rabbits, guinea pigs, mice, and chickens. This toxin was hemotoxic, neurotoxic, and histotoxic. Rabbits and dogs are very susceptible to aspergillus toxin. Pigeons, however, which are very susceptible to spontaneous infection, are very resistant to injected toxin.

Japanese workers Asakura et al. (1962) studied an allergic skin reaction against an alcoholic precipitate from a mycelial extract of *A. fumigatus.* Penguins showed a severe and prolonged skin sensitivity, whereas pigeons and ducks were quite resistant. Zoo penguins frequently die from *A. fumigatus* infections.

Forgacs and Carll (1955) selected strains of aspergillus, penicillium, and alternaria isolated from samples of feed associated with outbreaks of a hemorrhagic disease in poultry, and grew the cultures on grain which was fed to day-old chicks. Subsequently the chicks developed hemorrhages of the muscles, lungs, heart, gastrointestinal tract, and liver. Twenty chicks 6 weeks of age were given feed on which the species of alternaria had been cultured alone; they died and the necropsy revealed hemorrhages throughout the carcass.

PATHOGENICITY

Chute and O'Meara (1958) found the air sac inoculation route with spores to be a rapid and efficient method of screening fungi for pathogenicity in chickens. The following cultures isolated from chickens were used in experimental air sac infections and revealed both spores and mycelia in the tissue: *Paecilomyces varioti, Penicillium roqueforti, Penicillium brevi-compactum, Aspergillus glaucus* groups, *Trichoderma* spp., *Trichoderma koningi, Penicillium oxalicum, Aspergillus fumigatus, Alternaria* spp., *Penicillium islandicum, Stemphylium* spp., and *Penicillium cyclopium.*

PATHOGENESIS AND EPIZOOTIOLOGY

NATURAL AND EXPERIMENTAL HOSTS

Vigorous healthy birds apparently can withstand considerable exposure to aspergillus spores occurring under natural conditions. Inhalation of a considerable number of spores, as may occur when the litter or feed are heavily contaminated, may result in infection. The occasional bird which becomes infected in a flock which is otherwise healthy may do so because of lowered resistance or severe individual exposure. Aspergillosis can readily be produced experimentally by intrathoracic injection in chickens and pigeons. Schütz (1884), Bollinger (cited by Van Heelsbergen, 1929), and others observed that infection of the lungs was established following inhalation of spores. Walker (1915) reported that 5–7-day-old ostriches succumbed in 2–8 days to aspergillosis in the lungs and air sacs if spores were blown into the trachea. Intravenous inoculation resulted in pulmonary and hepatic aspergillosis. Young ostriches also developed the disease when kept on straw which had been artificially contaminated. Durant and Tucker (1935)

FIG. 14.2—Plaque from eye of chick with eye aspergillosis. ×2. (Chute, Univ. of Maine)

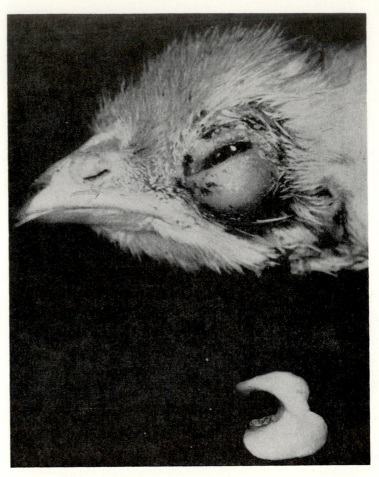

produced the disease in a poult by feeding mash from which *A. fumigatus* was isolated.

In recent years several reports have been made relative to aspergillus eye infections. Reis (1940) described a keratitis in chicks caused by *A. fumigatus*. He described the pathology and stated that usually only one eye was involved. Moore (1950) described ophthalmic aspergillosis which occurred in 5 widely separated flocks of young poults and in 3 breeding flocks (Fig. 14.2).

Systemic aspergillosis in poults has been reported by Witter and Chute (1952). Chute et al. (1955) also reported a systemic aspergillosis infection in 5-week-old cockerels which had been caponized. The authors considered that this resulted from a caponizing infection.

Aspergillus glaucus and *A. niger* may be encountered in some cases, particularly in cutaneous lesions. Lahaye (1928) discusses cutaneous aspergillosis in pigeons. Ainsworth and Rewell (1949) reported the isolation of 45 pure cultures of *A. fumigatus*, 3 of *A. flavus*, and 1 of *A. nidulans* from 78 cases of aspergillosis in captive wild birds. Jungherr and Gifford (1944) found fungal hyphae in the cerebellum of a poult which had exhibited nervous symptoms. In another outbreak in poults showing pneumomycosis and nervous manifestations, these workers recovered *A. fumigatus*, *A. niger*, and *Paecilomyces varioti* from the internal organs. *Paecilomyces varioti* was isolated also from the brain of one poult, but since fungal hyphae could not be demonstrated and the culture proved nonpathogenic, it was concluded that the symptoms and brain lesions had a toxigenic origin. Bullis (1950) recovered *A. fumigatus* from the cerebrums of poults which showed incoordination and later (unpublished) *Diplococcium* sp. from the cerebrums of similar poults. *Mucor* sp., *Penicillium* sp., and other fungi may be encountered in pulmonary mycosis, particularly in mixed infections (Thompson and Fabian, 1932; Baker et al., 1934).

A case of egg-borne aspergillosis was reported by Eggert and Barnhart (1953). They suggested that the fungus had penetrated through the eggshell during incubation and the recently hatched chicks were infected. Another case which was shown to be hatchery-borne was reported by Clark et al. (1954). From 21 ranches where 210,000 chicks were involved, there was mortality of 1–10%. The infection could not be traced to the hatching eggs but was readily found in the incubators, hatchers, incubator rooms, and intake ducts. Symptoms and lesions were noted in some day-old chicks, but generally classical lesions were observed in chicks 5 days of age.

O'Meara and Chute (1959) produced aspergillosis experimentally in hatching chicks. Chicks in the process of hatching and up to 2 days of age were easily infected with *A. fumigatus* spores by contaminating the forced draft incubator with wheat which had been seeded with *A. fumigatus*. Chicks older than 3 days of age were resistant to infection.

Chute and O'Meara (1961) reported some unusual cases of avian mycosis. Two cases of fungous tracheitis were observed, and in each case the mycelial growth extended through the cartilage.

Dyspnea, gasping, and accelerated breathing may be present. When these symptoms are associated with other respiratory diseases such as infectious bronchitis and infectious laryngotracheitis, they are usually accompanied by gurgling and rattling noises, whereas in aspergillosis there usually is no sound. Guberlet (1923) ascribed somnolence, inappetence, emaciation, increased thirst, and pyrexia to aspergillosis. Cases under his observation emaciated rapidly and showed a diarrhea in the later stages. Dysphagia was noted in cases in which the esophageal mucosa was involved. Mortality was as high as 50% in confined birds on some farms, whereas birds running outdoors were more resistant and escaped infection entirely on other farms. According to Van Heelsbergen (1929), some investigators have reported serous excretions from the nasal and ocular mucosa. Extreme

dyspnea was recorded by De Jong (1912) in canaries. In an outbreak in wild turkey poults reared in captivity, described by Durant and Tucker (1935), mortality began at 5 days, reached a peak at 15 days, and subsided at 3 weeks of age. Some affected poults died in convulsions within 24 hours. In two lots of poults 200 survived out of 785. Gauger (1941) reported an outbreak in adult chickens in which about 10% of the flock were affected with symptoms not unlike those shown by birds affected with laryngotracheitis and in which there was no abnormal mortality, but the egg production was temporarily lowered. Reis (1940) and Hudson (1947) have reported infection of the eyes in chicks 2–5 weeks of age. Infection in Reis's cases originated in sawdust litter and in Hudson's cases in bagasse litter. The outbreaks were characterized by the formation of a yellow cheesy pellet beneath the nictitating membrane which caused the lids to bulge (Fig. 14.2). There was some central ulceration of the cornea in the older chicks.

Raines et al. (1956) described an encephalitis including a torticollis and lack of equilibrium. Hubben (1958) reported meningoencephalitis in both turkeys and ducks.

The lesions depend considerably on the site of infection. Either localization or generalization may be observed. Individual lesions may be observed, for example, in the syrinx (Fig. 14.3) or in a single air sac. The lungs are most frequently involved. Pulmonary lesions vary from miliary nodules up to larger nodules (Fig. 14.4). In some cases there may be localized hepatization, and in others grossly visible mycelial masses may be present in the air passages and bronchi. There may be generalized involvement of the air sacs. Occasionally a circular disc-shaped necrotic mass with a concave surface, loosely attached to which there is a circular more or less flat or convex plaque, may be observed. Various manifestations of the disease have been described. Lange (1914) recorded nodules in the lungs and the thoracic and abdominal cavities of chickens, ducks, geese, and pigeons. These nodules varied from pinhead or millet seed size up to the size of a pea. They were yellow in color, of an elastically soft or cartilaginous consistency, and homogeneously caseous. Individual nodules

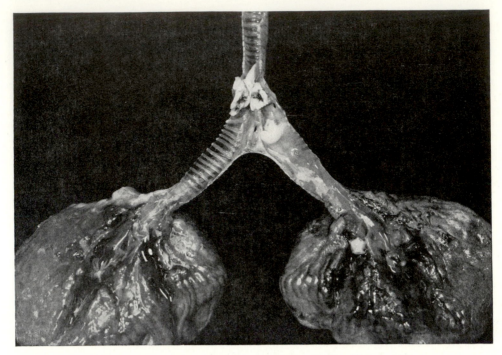

FIG. 14.3—Aspergillosis involving syrinx. (Bullis, Univ. of Mass.)

were noted on the intestinal serosa and in the parenchyma of the liver in a goose.

The nodules in the lungs of a turkey observed by Schlegel (1915) were pinhead to lentil size and were surrounded by an infiltrated or hemorrhagic corona with considerable hepatization. There were also grayish yellow, fibrinopurulent disc- or plate-shaped masses of exudate 2–5 mm thick on the pleura. Inflammation and detrital masses were present in the bronchi. The anterior thoracic, axillary, and cervical air sacs contained yellow caseous flat discs and masses consisting of inflamma-

tory exudate and mycelia. The left lower thoracic, upper posterior thoracic, and left abdominal air sacs were greatly distended. The walls of these air sacs were thickened and covered with a furlike growth of mold. Adjacent to the air sacs there were lentil-sized, knob-shaped, concentrically layered, turbid yellow, solid nodules composed of fibrin and mycelia. There were about 200 cc of reddish turbid fluid in the abdominal cavity.

There were no circumscribed yellowish foci in the outbreak in chicks reported by Savage and Isa (1933). There was a diffuse

FIG. 14.4—Aspergillosis nodules in lungs and plaquelike formations on the serous membranes. (Bullis, Univ. of Mass.)

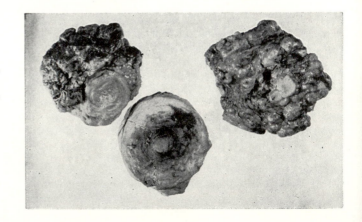

grayish yellow infiltration in the lungs, with about one-third of each lung involved. Mortality was 90% in this outbreak.

In pneumomycosis in a flamingo described by Mohler and Buckley (1904), the lungs were filled with nodules, and the mucosa of the bronchi was covered with membranous masses that consisted primarily of the fungous mycelium.

Archibald (1913) found gray round colonies of the fungus in the bronchioles in an ostrich, whereas in a case described by Jowett (1913) the lungs were covered with miliary foci.

Lahaye (1928) states that *Aspergillus glaucus* may be the cause of a disease of the skin in pigeons, particularly in young birds. Any part of the body may be affected with yellow scaly spots. The feathers in the affected areas are dry and easily broken.

Durant and Tucker (1935) observed yellowish white nodules up to 5×8 mm in the lungs of wild turkey poults being reared in captivity. The hyphae of the fungus also penetrated the tissue of the lung, and there was involvement of the adjacent air sacs.

In canaries observed by De Jong (1912) there were small whitish yellow, crusty coatings on the tongue, palate, and aditus laryngis and in the trachea and syrinx. Caseous foci in the lungs and caseous coatings on the pleura and peritoneum were also observed.

HISTOPATHOLOGY

The histological picture as described by Nieberle (1923) consists of focal pneumonia, multiple necrosis, and nodular formations which resemble tubercles. The diffuse pneumonic foci are indicative of fibrinous or catarrhal pneumonia. The alveoli, bronchioles, and bronchi are filled with mucus, stained fibrin, nuclear fragments, detritus, leucocytic and inflammatory cells, and mycelia. The mycelia penetrate the walls, and the surrounding pulmonary parenchyma shows an exudative cellular inflammation or necrosis. The tuberclelike nodules show in the center a radiating turf of hyphae surrounded by a reactive inflammatory wall which resembles granulation tissue. Foreign body giant cells are frequently observed. The fruiting organs (conidiophores, sterigmata, conidia) occur more frequently in the air sacs.

In turkey cases of ophthalmitis described by Moore (1953), the primary involvement was in the vitreous humor and the adjoining tissues. In one turkey he observed the presence of mycelia in the crystalline lens.

DIAGNOSIS

The fungus can be demonstrated by cultural methods if not in fresh microscopic preparations. Occasionally masses of the fungus are visible to the naked eye in the air passages of the lungs (Fig. 14.5), in the air sacs (Fig. 14.6), or in the abdominal cavity. The typical fruiting heads may be readily demonstrated in such lesions. Demonstration of the fungus by direct examination may be impossible in the small caseous nodules seen particularly in the lungs.

TREATMENT

Treatment of affected individuals is usually considered useless. They should be killed and the offending infective material removed. Lahaye (1928) reported favorable results in the treatment of aspergillosis of the skin in pigeons by the use of $HgCl_2$ solution, 1:500. The surface of the body was moistened or the birds dipped into the solution, following which they were rinsed in lukewarm water and dried.

In recent years many empirical treatments have been used, apparently with varying degrees of success. Quernhorst (1963) found that nystatin, amphotericin B, and trichomycin inhibited the growth of *A. fumigatus* cultures, whereas griseofulvin did not. The mortality rates in intra-abdominally infected day-old chicks were 60% for untreated controls but only 20% for those receiving 625 units of nystatin or 25 mg of amphotericin B intra-abdominally for 6 days. Necropsy showed fewer and less severe lesions in those treated with amphotericin B than in those treated with trichomycin.

Babras and Radhakrishnan (1967) administered hamycin (20 mg/ml in the drinking water) for one week to birds experiencing an acute outbreak of *A. fumigatus* and noted that it markedly reduced the mortality rate, compared to that in 7 similar but untreated infected flocks.

PREVENTION AND CONTROL

The avoidance of moldy litter or feed serves to prevent outbreaks of aspergillosis. An examination of the premises or materials used for feed or litter will usually re-

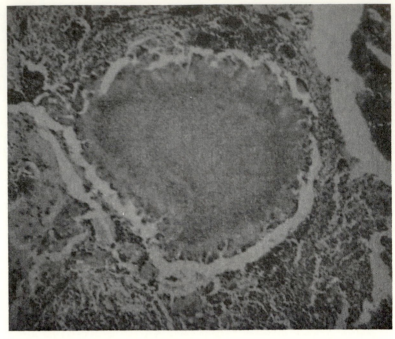

FIG. 14.5—Granuloma of lung from chick infected with A. fumigatus. (Chute, Univ. of Maine)

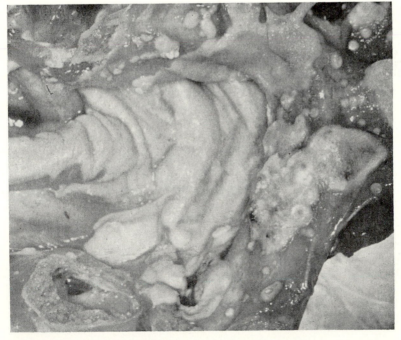

FIG. 14.6—Viscera and musculature with plaques from chicken experimentally infected in air sac with A. fumigatus. (Chute, Univ. of Maine)

veal the source of the infection. Careful selection of mash, grain, and litter is essential in preventing this disease. Access to musty, moldy strawstacks should be avoided.

Improperly kept drinking fountains used for dispensing milk have been found to be a source of infection. One outbreak was associated with contaminated milk cans. The inside of the lids of the cans used for transporting milk was found to be covered with a fine mold growth; the owner had washed and scalded the cans daily but thought it unnecessary to clean the lids. The storage barrels for the milk were also heavily infected.

The areas around feed hoppers and watering places are fertile fields for the growth of molds. Unless a permanent yard system is used, frequent moving of feed troughs and watering places is advisable. Placing feed containers and watering fountains on screened elevated platforms helps to prevent turkeys from picking up molds that develop in such places. Drainage is advisable for areas where water is liable to stand after rains.

Control is best accomplished by removing the cause. A careful search should be made for mold in the litter, the feed, and the feed and water containers. Daily cleaning and disinfection of feed and water utensils will aid in eliminating the infection. Spraying of the ground around the containers with chemical solutions may be advisable if it is impossible to change feeding areas frequently. In outbreaks, a 1:2,000 solution of copper sulfate in place of all drinking water may be used to aid in preventing the spread, though it should not be relied upon as a preventive to be used continually. The antifungal antibiotics as preventives for this disease should be considered.

REFERENCES

Ainsworth, G. C., and R. E. Rewell. 1949. The incidence of aspergillosis in captive wild birds. *J. Comp. Pathol. Therap.* 59:213–24.

Archibald, R. G. 1913. Aspergillosis in the Sudan ostrich. *J. Comp. Pathol. Therap.* 26:171–73.

Asakura, A., S. Nakagawa, M. Masui, and J. Yasuda. 1962. Immunological studies of aspergillosis in birds. *Mycopathol. Mycol. Appl.* 18:249–56.

Babras, M. A., and C. V. Radhakrishnan. 1967. Aspergillosis in chicks and a trial of hamycin in an outbreak. *Hindustan Antibiot. Bull.* 9:244–45.

Baker, A. Z., J. Courtenay-Dunn, and M. D. Wright. 1934. Observations on fungal pneumonia in the domestic fowl. *Vet. J.* 90: 385–89.

Bodin, E., and L. Gautier. 1906. Note sur une toxine producte par l'*Aspergillus fumigatus*. *Ann. Inst. Pasteur* 20:209–24.

Bullis, K. L. 1950. Poultry Disease Control Service. *Univ. Mass. Agr. Expt. Sta. Ann. Rept., Bull.* 459.

Ceni, C., and C. Besta. 1902. Ueber die Toxine von *Aspergillus fumigatus* und *A. flavescens* und deren Beziehungen zur Pellagra. *Zentr. Allgem. Pathol. Pathol. Anat.* 13:930–41.

Chute, H. L., and D. C. O'Meara. 1958. Experimental fungous infections in chickens. *Avian Diseases* 2:154–66.

———. 1961. Diagnosis of unusual cases of avian mycosis. *Can. Vet. J.* 2:383–87.

Chute, H. L., J. F. Witter, J. L. Rountree, and D. C. O'Meara. 1955. The pathology of a fungous infection associated with a capon-izing injury. *J. Am. Vet. Med. Ass.* 127: 207–9.

Chute, H. L., D. C. O'Meara, H. D. Tresner, and E. Lacombe. 1956. The fungous flora of chickens with infections of the respiratory tract. *Am. J. Vet. Res.* 17:763–65.

Chute, H. L., D. C. O'Meara, and E. S. Barden. 1962. A bibliography of avian mycosis (partially annotated). *Maine Agr. Expt. Sta. Bull.* 655.

Clark, D. S., E. E. Jones, W. B. Crowl, and K. F. Ross. 1954. Aspergillosis in newly hatched chicks. *J. Am. Vet. Med. Ass.* 124: 116–17.

De Jong, D. A. 1912. Aspergillosis der Kanarienvoegel. *Zentr. Bakteriol. Parasitenk. Abt. I. Orig.* 66:390.

Durant, A. J., and C. M. Tucker. 1935. Aspergillosis of wild turkeys reared in captivity. *J. Am. Vet. Med. Ass.* 86:781–84.

Eggert, M. J., and J. V. Barnhart. 1953. A case of egg-borne aspergillosis. *J. Am. Vet. Med. Ass.* 122:225.

Forgacs, J., and W. T. Carll. 1955. Preliminary mycotoxic studies on hemorrhagic disease in poultry. *Vet. Med.* 50:172.

Gauger, H. C. 1941. *Aspergillus fumigatus* infection in adult chickens. *Poultry Sci.* 20: 445–46.

Guberlet, J. E. 1923. An epizootic of aspergillosis in chickens. *J. Am. Vet. Med. Ass.* 63: 612–22.

Henrici, A. T. 1939. An endotoxin from *Aspergillus fumigatus*. *J. Immunol.* 36:319–38.

Hinshaw, W. R. 1937. Diseases of turkeys. *Calif. Agr. Expt. Sta. Bull.* 613.

Hubben, K. 1958. Case report—Aspergillus meningoencephalitis in turkeys and ducks. *Avian Diseases* 2:110–16.

Hudson, C. B. 1947. *Aspergillus fumigatus* infection in the eyes of baby chicks. *Poultry Sci.* 26:192–93.

Jowett, W. 1913. Pulmonary mycosis in the ostrich. *J. Comp. Pathol. Therap.* 26:253–57.

Jungherr, E., and R. Gifford. 1944. Three hitherto unreported turkey diseases in Connecticut, erysipelas, hexamitiasis, and mycotic encephalomalacia. *Cornell Vet.* 34:214–26.

Lahaye, J. 1928. *Maladies des Pigeons et des Poules, des Oiseaux de Basse-Cour et de Voliere.* Stemmetz-Haenen, Remouchamps.

Lange, W. 1914. Schimmelpilzerkankungen beim Gefluegel. *Deut. Tieraerztl. Wochschr.* 22:642–43.

Lignières, and G. Petit. 1898. Peritonite aspergillaire des dindons. *Rec. Med. Vet.* 75:145–48.

Lucet, A. 1897. Experimental and clinical study of *Aspergillus fumigatus*. *Vet. J.* 44:215–17, 285–88, 292–94; 45:226–31, 301–4.

Mohler, J. R., and J. S. Buckley. 1904. Pulmonary mycosis of birds with report of a case in a flamingo. *USDA BAI Circ.* 58:122–36.

Moore, Earl N. 1950. Ophthalmic aspergillosis in turkeys. *Proc. 22nd Ann. Meet. Northeast Conf. Lab. Workers in Pullorum Disease Control.*

———. 1953. *Aspergillus fumigatus* as a cause of ophthalmitis in turkeys. *Poultry Sci.* 32:796–99.

Nieberle, K. 1923. Die Lungenaspergillose, pp. 804–7. In Joest, E. (ed.), *Spezielle Pathologische Anatomie der Haustiere.* R. Schoetz, Berlin.

O'Meara, D. C., and H. L. Chute. 1959. Aspergillosis experimentally produced in hatching chicks. *Avian Diseases* 3:404–6.

Quernhorst, H. 1963. Treatment of experimental aspergillosis in poultry. Inaug. Dissertation, Hanover, Germany.

Raines, T. V., C. D. Kudas, F. H. Winkle, and B. S. Johnson. 1956. Encephalitic aspergillosis in turkeys—A case report. *J. Am. Vet. Med. Ass.* 129:435–36.

Reis, J. 1940. Queratomicose Aspergilica Epizootica em Pintos. *Arquiv. Inst. Biol.* (Sao Paulo) 48:437–50.

Savage, A., and J. M. Isa. 1933. A note on mycotic pneumonia of chickens. *Sci. Agr.* 13:341.

Schlegel, M. 1915. Schimmelpilzerkrankung (Aspergillose) in den Lungen bei Tieren. *Berlin. Muench. Tieraerztl. Wochschr.* 31:25.

Schütz. 1884. Eindringen von Pilzsporen in die Atmungswege und die dadurch bedingten Erkrankungen der Lungen und ueber den Pilz des Huehnergrindes. *Mitt. Kaiserl. Gesundheitsamt.* 2:208.

Thom, C., and Margaret B. Church. 1926. *The Aspergilli.* Williams & Wilkins Co., Baltimore.

Thompson, W. W., and F. W. Fabian. 1932. Molds in respiratory tract of chickens. *J. Am. Vet. Med. Ass.* 80:921–22.

Van Heelsbergen, T. 1929. *Handbuch der Gefluegelkrankheiten und der Gefluegelzucht.* Ferdinand Enke, Stuttgart. Pp. 312–22.

Walker, J. 1915. Aspergillosis in the ostrich chick. *Union S. Africa, Dept. Agr., Ann. Rept.* 3–4:535–74.

Witter, J. F., and H. L. Chute. 1952. Aspergillosis in turkeys. *J. Am. Vet. Med. Ass.* 121:387–88.

✤

FAVUS

✤

Favus is a chronic dermatomycosis affecting chickens, occasionally turkeys and some other birds, animals, and man. In the fowl the comb is almost always attacked, but other portions of the head may be affected; in severe cases the disease spreads to the feathered portions of the body.

INCIDENCE AND DISTRIBUTION

Favus occurs only infrequently in the United States. Possibly this is due to the lesser number of the heavier Asiatic breeds which are reported to be more susceptible. The disease is reported to be common in France.

ETIOLOGY

The causative fungus in the fowl is *Trichophyton megnini (Achorion gallinae).* Cultivation on Sabouraud's glucose agar is satisfactory. It is sometimes helpful to cover the inoculum with absolute alcohol and evaporate the alcohol to destroy the contaminating bacteria. Cultures grow slowly. Colonies develop as small round discs which are white and velvety and have small central cups and radial grooves. A reddish pigment varying from rose or strawberry red to a deep raspberry diffuses through the medium. Microscopically the branched mycelium is twisted, the septa are irregularly spaced, the spores are in clusters, and there are nodular organs and fuseaux. Typical lesions may be produced by inoculation of the scarified comb. Mice, rabbits, or guinea pigs may also be inoculated, although the lesions are not so typical in the guinea pigs (Jacobson, 1932; Dodge, 1935). Torres and Georg (1956) reported a case of *Trichophyton gallinae* in the scalp of a 4-year-old Puerto Rican girl. Experimental infections were produced in several chickens and guinea pigs.

SIGNS AND LESIONS

Lesions usually develop first on the comb. As the fungus spreads, white spots develop, the surface of which scales off, and the comb may appear as though sprinkled with flour (Fig. 14.7). Young birds with well-developed combs are most likely to be affected. The wattles and unfeathered portions of the head may be affected. As the disease progresses, the scaly deposits become thicker and form a wrinkled crust. Spontaneous recovery is reported in some cases. In other cases the fungus spreads to feathered portions of the body. The feathers fall out in patches. The skin becomes thickened in the affected areas and covered with scales and crusts, especially around the feather follicles. A moldy odor may be detected. Matruchot and Dassonville (1899) reported the appearance of favus simultaneously on feathered and nonfeathered portions of the body. Symptoms were not extensive in the cases observed by Sabouraud et al. (1909). Schlegel (1909) reported depression, weakness, emaciation, anemia, cachexia, and icterus in affected chickens. In some birds, in addition to the external lesions, there were necrotic foci, nodules, and yellowish caseous deposits on the mucosa of the upper respiratory tracts. Occasionally the bronchi and lungs were affected and necrotic caseous inflammation was observed in the crop and small intestine. The favus fungus could be demonstrated microscopically in these lesions. The fungus spreads slowly from bird to bird by direct contact and by the scales which become detached from affected individuals and contaminate the premises.

DIAGNOSIS

The characteristics of the gross lesions may be sufficient for diagnosis. If this is inconclusive, the fungus can be checked microscopically and culturally. Transmission of the disease to laboratory birds or animals or a study of the contagious nature of the disease in the flock may be helpful.

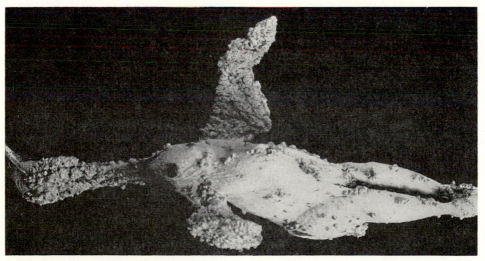

FIG. 14.7—Favus An unusual case affecting entire carcass. (L. D. Bushnell)

PREVENTION AND TREATMENT

Care should be exercised in adding new birds to the flock. Infected houses should be cleaned and disinfected. Badly affected birds should be killed. Mildly affected birds should be segregated, and treatment can be tried if desired. The majority of mildly affected birds will recover without treatment. Several individuals have been observed in which various treatments were used on one side of the head and the opposite side was left untreated; recovery was similar on each side. Van Heelsbergen (1929) suggests the following remedies: iodine and glycerine (tinct. iodine 1.0, glycerine 6.0); green soap and 5% phenol solution or bichloride of mercury (1:500), the latter to be used particularly on the body. Beach and Halpin (1918) found an oint-ment of formaldehyde and vaseline to be effective. This is prepared by melting vaseline in a jar in a water bath, adding 5% (by weight) of commercial formalin, tightening the cover, and shaking the mixture until the vaseline has solidified.

One or two applications well rubbed into the lesions usually suffice. Riedel (1950) observed recovery in a group of artificially infected chickens within 20 days following a single application of a 2% mixture of quaternary ammonium compounds consisting of equal parts of alkyl-dimethyl-benzyl-ammonium chloride and alkyl-di-methyl-dichlor-benzol-ammonium chloride.

Szecsenyi (1960) found that dipping infected hens in 0.5% pentachlorphenol controlled the infection.

REFERENCES

Beach, B. A., and J. C. Halpin. 1918. Observations on an outbreak of favus. *J. Agr. Res.* 15:415–18.

Dodge, C. W. 1935. *Medical Mycology.* C. V. Mosby Co., St. Louis. Pp. 554–55.

Jacobson, H. P. 1932. *Fungous Diseases.* Charles C Thomas, Springfield, Ill. Pp. 52–55.

Matruchot, L., and C. Dassonville. 1899. Recherches experimentales sur une dermatomycose des poules et sur son parasite. *Rev. Gen. Botan.* 11:429–44.

Riedel, B. B. 1950. Favus and its treatment with a quaternary ammonium compound. *Poultry Sci.* 29:741–42.

Sabouraud, R., A. Suis, and F. Suffran. 1909. La "crete blanche" (favus) de la poule et son parasite. *Rev. Vet.* 34:601.

Schlegel, M. 1909. Favuskrankheit (Huehner-grind). *Berlin. Muench. Tieraerztl. Wochschr.* 25:689.

Szecsenyi, I. 1960. Baromfi bor-es tollfavusa (Skin and feather favus in fowls). *Magy. Allatorv. Lapja* 15:129–32.

Torres, G., and L. K. Georg. 1956. A human case of *Trichophyton gallinae* infection contracted from chickens. *Proc. Soc. Am. Bacteriol. Meet.,* p. 84.

Van Heelsbergen, T. 1929. *Handbuch der Gefluegelkrankheiten und Gefluegelzucht.* Ferdinand Enke, Stuttgart. Pp. 322–27.

❖

THRUSH
(Mycosis of the Digestive Tract)

❖

STOMATITIS OIDICA, muguet, soor, moniliasis, iodiomycosis, candidiasis, and sour crop are other terms applied to mycotic infections of the digestive tract.

INCIDENCE

Mycosis of the digestive tract probably occurs rather frequently, but in many cases it does not appear to be of sufficient significance to be considered seriously. Numerous general discussions of poultry diseases fail to mention this disorder, and the paucity of diagnoses in reports from diagnostic laboratories suggests that it may not be of great consequence. However, serious outbreaks have been reported in many species of birds. Animals and man are also affected. Thrush has been observed in chickens, pigeons, geese, turkeys, pheasants, ruffed grouse, and quail.

Gierke (1932) reported an outbreak of a thrushlike disease occurring in turkeys in California. Hart (1947) reported the disease in turkeys and other fowl in New South Wales. A soluble endotoxin, toxic for mice, was isolated from *Candida albicans* by Salvin (1952). A review on the disease as it now exists in turkeys and chickens in California is recorded by Mayeda (1961).

ETIOLOGY

The etiological significance of yeastlike fungi in infections of the digestive tract of man was recognized by Langenbeck in 1839. Questions relating to the validity of species described and their generic nomenclature have retarded a proper understanding of this type of disease. Jungherr (1933b, 1934) found *Monilia albicans, Monilia krusei,* and *Oidium pullorum* n.s. to be associated with cases of thrush, but considered that *M. krusei* was not of etiological significance. *Mucor* sp. and aspergilli were also found in association with some cases. Hinshaw (1933) reported that *M. albicans* was found in most cases of thrush in turkeys and chickens which came to his attention. Both investigators considered that the mycotic infections were apt to be associated with unhygienic surroundings and perhaps secondary to other debilitating conditions. Eberth (1858) and Schlegel (1912) identified organisms observed by them as *Oidium albicans*.

The studies of Benham (1931), Worley and Stovall (1937), Martin and associates (1937), and others indicate the complexity of the problem. Stovall (1939) pointed out a means of improving the present uncertain status. He suggested a specific set of environmental conditions under which the biological characteristics of the organism were constant and could be demonstrated. Jungherr's (1934) characterization is as follows:

Monilia albicans: It is of widespread occurrence in gallinaceous birds, pathogenic to birds and also to rabbits on intravenous injection, and is indistinguishable from strains isolated from human sources. On Sabouraud's agar it produces a whitish, creamy, high-convex colony after incubation for 24 to 48 hours at 37° C. Young cultures consist of oval budding yeast cells, about 5½ by 3½μ in dimension. Older cultures show septate hyphae and occasionally spherical, swollen cells with thickened membrane, the so-called chlamydospores. In Dunham's peptone water containing 1 percent fermentable substance and 1 per cent Andrade's indicator, the organism produces acid and gas in dextrose, levulose, maltose, and mannose; slight acid in galactose and sucrose; and does not attack dextrin (variable according to brand), inulin, lactose, and raffinose. Gelatin stab cultures show short, villous to arborescent outgrowths without liquefaction of the medium.

The term "medical monilias" is frequently used in connection with the generic term Monilia since the term Monilia is also used for a separate group of fungi. Most workers have accepted the decision of an informal group meeting at the Third International Microbiological Congress in 1939 and use *Candida* as a generic name to replace the familiar but invalid *Monilia* (Skinner, 1947). *Candida albicans* is the most frequently isolated etiological agent associated with the disturbance commonly referred to as moniliasis.

SIGNS AND LESIONS

The signs are not particularly characteristic. Affected chicks show unsatisfactory growth, a stunted appearance, listlessness, and roughness of the feathers. Lesions occur most frequently in the crop (Figs. 14.8, 14.9 and 14.10) and consist of a thickening of the mucosa with whitish, circular, raised ulcer formations, the surfaces of which tend to scale off. Pseudomembranous patches and easily removed necrotic material over the mucosa are not uncommon. The mouth and esophagus may show ulcerlike patches. When the proventriculus is involved, it is swollen, the serosa has a glossy appearance, and the mucosa is hemorrhagic and may be covered with a catarrhal or necrotic exudate. Histologically, Jungherr (1933a) reported that crops "showed extensive destruction of the stratified epithelium deep in the Malpighian layer and quite often walled-off ulcers or extensive diphtheroid to diphtheritic membranes. The lesions were characterized by the absence of inflammatory reaction." Periportal focal necrosis in the liver in some cases suggested a toxic action upon the system.

The frequent association of mycosis of the digestive tract with other debilitating conditions such as gizzard erosions and intestinal coccidiosis must be considered. Gizzard erosions as such probably are not directly related to thrush. Likewise, the thickened intestine with watery contents

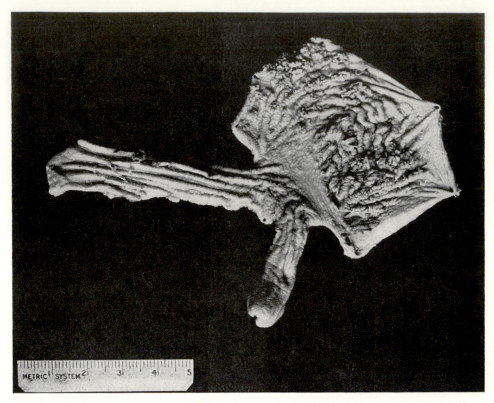

FIG. 14.8—Moniliasis (candidiasis) in crop of turkey. (Bullis, Univ. of Mass.)

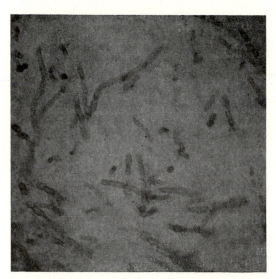

FIG. 14.9—Mycelia in stratified squamous epithelium of crop. Gridley. (Chute, Univ. of Maine)

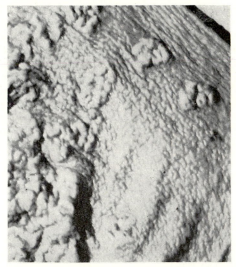

FIG. 14.10—Enlarged view of crop of turkey suffering from candidiasis. Note raised, piled-up exudate which tends to form roselike masses. (Hinshaw, Univ. of Calif.)

frequently noted in cases of thrush is probably due to coccidiosis or other protozoan infections.

In the case of thrush reported by Eberth (1858), the esophagus, crop (Figs. 14.8, 14.9), and proventriculus showed an ulcerated and scaly condition. The spores and hyphae of what he termed *Oidium albicans* could be readily demonstrated in the lesions. The proventriculus was the principle organ involved in the cases observed by Schlegel (1912). However, the mouth, pharynx, and crop were involved in some cases. Schlegel (1921) also observed the disease in geese. Diptheroid lesions were noted in the proventriculus and small intestine. Abscess formations were present under pulpy, soft, grayish white to brownish red necrotic masses. Hinshaw (1933) reported thrush in 12 flocks of turkeys, with lesions similar to those noted in chickens. Blaxland and Fincham (1950) studied 5 serious outbreaks in young turkeys. Their observations supported previous conclusions that moniliasis is likely to be associated with unhygienic surroundings and other debilitating conditions, but spread of infection appeared definite in many instances. Zürn (1882) and Klee (1899) described the disease in pigeons. Lehaye (1928) pointed out the similarity between thrush and pox in the pigeon. He demonstrated pox virus in many cases suspected of being thrush.

Tripathy (1965) considered that vascular damage in infected turkeys may be associated with *Candida* endotoxin. Atheromatous lesions were present on the intimal surface of the abdominal aorta in more than 50% of turkeys exposed to *C. albicans,* whereas there was only a 12.5% incidence of similar lesions in the uninfected controls.

DIAGNOSIS

Observation of the characteristic proliferative, relatively noninflammatory lesions, together with resultant heavy growth on primary cultures, serves to diagnose thrush. Because of the possibility of cultivation of *C. albicans* from apparently normal tissues, an original heavy growth is considered essential for diagnosis. The recognition of spores and more especially hyphae in fresh smear preparations is attended with some difficulty. Miliary abscesses are produced

in the kidneys of rabbits injected intravenously (Benham, 1931).

Underwood (1955) described an instrument known as McCarthy's foroblique panendoscope which was used to diagnose experimental crop moniliasis. This instrument was equipped with a viewing lens and an independent light source. Birds were starved for 12 hours in order to empty the crop to allow a clear view of the mucosa. A normal crop appeared to be light pink with a glistening smooth surface having numerous shallow convolutions, whereas a fungus-infected crop showed severe corrugations to mild whitish streaks, erosions, or diphtheritic formations and a deep red surrounding mucosa.

COURSE

Young birds are more susceptible to mycosis of the digestive tract than are older birds. Thus as infected birds grow older they tend to overcome the infection. Jungherr (1933a) observed an outbreak in which the losses amounted to 10,000 chicks out of 50,000 that were less than 60 days of age. He also reported (1934) that turkeys under 4 weeks of age succumbed rapidly to infection, but that outbreaks in birds 3 months of age resulted in a high percentage of recoveries.

TREATMENT AND CONTROL

Since mycosis of the digestive tract is apt to be related to unhygienic, unsanitary, overcrowded conditions, these conditions should not be allowed to exist or should be corrected. Jungherr (1933b) found that denatured alcohol and coal-tar derivatives were ineffective as disinfectants and suggested that iodine preparations be used. As a treatment he recommends that following an Epsom salt flush, one level teaspoonful of powdered bluestone (copper sulfate) be added to each 2 gallons of drinking water in nonmetal containers every other day during one week. Hinshaw recommends that a 1:2,000 solution of copper sulfate for turkeys be used as the sole source of drinking water during the course of the outbreak. Affected birds should be segregated. Lesions in the mouth can be treated by local application of a suitable antiseptic. The appearance of the disease in very young chicks suggests the surface of the egg as a source of infection. Such a possibility could be removed by dipping the eggs in an iodine preparation prior to incubation.

Kostin (1966) found that *C. albicans* organisms mixed with poultry droppings and applied to wooden boards could be controlled by exposure to 2% formaldehyde or 1% sodium hydroxide solution for one hour. Three hours treatment with a 5% solution of iodine monochloride in hydrochloric acid was also successful in disinfection.

Underwood et al. (1956), in experimental moniliasis produced in chicks and poults, found copper sulfate was ineffective for treating or preventing the disease.

Nystatin has been studied by Gentry et al. (1960) and by Kahn and Weisblatt (1963). One group reported that 220 mg nystatin per kg of diet was effective in eliminating moniliasis in a flock of turkeys. The other group found in experimental infections with *C. albicans* in both chickens and turkeys that crop score values appeared to be significantly reduced in the group fed the lowest level of nystatin (11 mg/kg). The highest level of nystatin (110 mg/kg) fed showed a very significant protection against mycotic infection.

Yacowitz et al. (1959) reported successful prevention of candidiasis in chickens by the addition of nystatin at a minimum level of 142 mg per kg of ration for a period of 4 weeks. Kahn and Weisblatt (1963) obtained similar results. Wind and Yacowitz (1960) successfully treated crop mycosis with nystatin by dispersing it in drinking water at levels of 62.5–250 mg per liter with sodium lauryl sulfate (7.8–25 mg per liter) for a 5-day period.

Tripathy (1965) found that the addition of Aureomycin (500 g/ton) to a vitamin A-deficient ration had no effect on the incidence or severity of crop candidiasis but increased the cells being shed in the feces. Turkeys fed on nystatin (100 g/ton) had a higher average weight and milder crop lesions than did untreated controls.

REFERENCES

Benham, R. W. 1931. Certain monilias parasitic on man. *J. Infect. Diseases* 49:183–215.

Blaxland, J. D., and I. H. Fincham. 1950. Mycosis of the crop (moniliasis) in poultry. *Brit. Vet. J.* 106:221–31.

Eberth, J. 1858. Einige Beobachtungen von pflanzlichen Parasiten bei Thieren. *Arch. Pathol. Anat. Physiol.* 13:522–30.

Gentry, R. F., G. R. Bubash, and H. L. Chute. 1960. *Candida albicans* in turkeys. *Poultry Sci.* 39:1252. (Abstr.)

Gierke, A. G. 1932. A preliminary report on a mycosis of turkeys. *Calif. Dept. Agr. Monthly Bull.* 21:229–31.

Hart, H. L. 1947. Moniliasis in turkeys and fowls in New South Wales. *Australian Vet. J.* 23:191–92.

Hinshaw, W. R. 1933. Moniliasis (thrush) in turkeys and chickens. *Proc. Fifth World's Poultry Congr.* 3:190–97.

Jungherr, E. 1933a. Observations on a severe outbreak of mycosis in chicks. *J. Agr. Res.* 46:169–78.

———. 1933b. Studies of yeast-like fungi from gallinaceous birds. *Storrs Agr. Expt. Sta. Bull.* 188.

———. 1934. Mycosis in fowl caused by yeast-like fungi. *J. Am. Vet. Med. Ass.* 84:500–506.

Kahn, S. G., and H. Weisblatt. 1963. A comparison of nystatin and copper sulfate in experimental moniliasis of chickens and turkeys. *Avian Diseases* 7:304–9.

Klee, R. 1899. Vergiftungen bei Gefluegel. (Poisoning of poultry.) *Jahresber. Vet. Med.* 19:236.

Kostin, V. V. 1966. Development of disinfection regime during candida mycosis in poultry. *Vses. Nauch. Issled. Inst. Vet. Sanit. Tr.* 25:157–62.

Lahaye, J. 1928. *Maladies des Pigeons et des Poules, des Oiseaux de Basse-Cour et de Voliere.* Stemmetz-Haenen, Remouchamps.

Martin, D. S., C. P. Jones, K. F. Yao, and L. E. Lee, Jr. 1937. A practical classification of the monilias. *J. Bacteriol.* 34:99–129.

Mayeda, B. 1961. Candidiasis in turkeys and chickens in the Sacramento Valley of California. *Avian Diseases* 5:232–43.

Salvin, S. B. 1952. Endotoxin in pathogenic fungi. *J. Immunol.* 69:89–99.

Schlegel, M. 1912. Soorkrankheit bei Huehnern. *Berlin. Muench. Tieraerztl. Wochschr.* 56:63. (Abstr.)

———. 1921. VII Soorkrankheit bei Gaensen. *Z. Infektionskr. Haustiere* 21:204. (Abstr.)

Skinner, C. E. 1947. The yeast-like fungi: Candida and Brettanomyces. *Bacteriol. Rev.* 11:227–74.

Stovall, W. D. 1939. Classification and pathogenicity of species of monilia. *Third Int. Congr. Microbiol.*, pp. 202–5.

Tripathy, S. B. 1965. Observations of changes in turkeys exposed to *Candida albicans*. *Dissertation Abstr.* 25:3187.

Underwood, P. C. 1955. Detection of crop mycosis (moniliasis) in chickens and turkey
poults with a panendoscope. *J. Am. Vet.
Med. Ass.* 127:229–31.

Underwood, P. C., J. H. Collins, C. G. Durbin,
F. A. Hodges, and H. E. Zimmerman, Jr.
1956. Critical tests with copper sulfate for
experimental moniliasis (crop mycosis) of
chickens and turkeys. *Poultry Sci.* 35:599–
605.

Wind, S., and H. Yacowitz. 1960. Use of Mycostatin in the drinking water for the treatment of crop mycosis in turkeys. *Poultry*

Sci. 39:904–5.

Worley, G., and W. D. Stovall. 1937. A study
of milk coagulation by monilia species. *J.
Infect. Diseases* 61:134–38.

Yacowitz, H., S. Wind, W. P. Jambor, N. P.
Willet, and J. F. Pagano. 1959. Use of
Mycostatin for the prevention of moniliasis
(crop mycosis) in chicks and turkeys. *Poultry Sci.* 38:653–60.

Zürn, F. A. 1882. Durch Schimmelpilze her-
vorgerufene Krankheiten des Gefluegels, p.
129. In *Die Krankheiten des Hausgefllue-
gels,* Weimar.

❖

HISTOPLASMOSIS

❖

HISTOPLASMOSIS is an infectious but
not contagious mycotic disease of man
and lower animals. It has been referred to as a reticuloendothelial disease caused by the fungus *Histoplasma capsulatum*. The organism
grows readily in culture media and
soil as a white to brown mold which
bears spores of two types: (1) spherical, minutely spiny *microconidia* 3–4
μ in diameter, and (2) spherical, or
rarely clavate, *macroconidia* 8–12μ in
diameter, with evenly spaced finger-
like projections over the surface.

HISTORY, INCIDENCE, AND
DISTRIBUTION

The disease was first described in 1906
by Darling while studying kala-azar in the
Canal Zone. The disease is widespread in
a variety of animals including dogs, cats,
rats, mice, woodchucks, skunks, opossums,
foxes, raccoons, and man.

It is not a common problem of birds, but
because of the public health aspects of the
disease, a constant monitoring of zoo birds
as well as chicken and turkey populations
should be available.

The geographical distribution appears to

be circumglobal. Reports have come from
United States, Central and South America,
Europe, Russia, Java, and Africa. There
are areas in the United States bordering
the Missouri, Ohio, and Mississippi rivers
in which the disease appears to be indigenous.

ETIOLOGY

Vanbreuseghem (1958) described in detail the growth of *Histoplasma capsulatum*
in the yeastlike and mycelial phase.

The yeastlike phase of the organism is
difficult to get and keep. At least four conditions for growth are necessary: (1) a temperature of at least 37° C, (2) a medium
rich in protein, preferably containing
blood, (3) a high degree of humidity (drying causes reversion to the mycelial phase),
and (4) a high concentration of CO_2. Frequent transfer of the culture on a solid
medium is necessary. Colonies appear
small, brilliant, and whitish.

The mycelial phase, which appears on
Sabouraud's medium, dextrose agar, potato, gelatin, or bread at any incubation temperature, is made up of segmented,
branched hyphae 2.5μ wide. They give
rise to ordinary chlamydospores, often in
chains, and also large round cells 20μ in
diameter. The colonies appear as a white
down which assumes a brownish color after 2 weeks. Brueck in 1951 found that *H.
capsulatum* grew well in the yolk sac of
embryonating eggs.

Wildervanck et al. (1953) found *H. capsulatum* in 3 sick fowls, 1 healthy fowl, 1
chick, and 3 of 4 pigeons in Surinam. His
work was related to an epidemiological
study. Menges (1954), with a histoplasmin

skin test, found 1% of fowls and no tur-keys positive of a small number tested in Kansas, Missouri, and Iowa. Menges and Habermann (1955) thought chickens un-likely to be carriers because, following in-tracardial inoculation of yeast phase into 24 chickens, only 1 died within 21 hours.

Schwarz et al. (1957) recovered *H. cap-sulatum* from the liver and spleen of 19 pi-geons within 14 days after intravenous in-oculation, and from 1 pigeon 45 days after inoculation. They also recovered the orga-nism from 5 chicks 7 days postinoculation.

Campbell et al. (1962) isolated the orga-nism from feathers of an old feather pillow which was brought from Hungary more than 30 years before and was used by an infant who had histoplasmosis. This refer-ence relative to the public health signifi-cance is further supported by Zeidberg et al. (1952), who found the organism in soil samples, chicken yards, and under dwell-ings where chickens had congregated.

Tewari and Campbell (1965) isolated *H. capsulatum* from feathers of chickens inoc-ulated intravenously and subcutaneously with the yeast phase of the organism. Schwarz et al. (1967) produced a granulo-matous lesion in the eyes of chickens exper-imentally infected with the organism.

Dodge et al. (1965) found positive sam-ples in a starling roost in Italy and soil samples from a school yard, and a high proportion of the schoolchildren were his-toplasmin-positive.

DIAGNOSIS

Diagnosis is based on three criteria: (1) culture of the organism, (2) histopa-thology, and (3) histoplasmin sensitivity. Most strains will grow on Sabouraud's agar at 30° C and at room temperature will re-vert to the hyphal type of growth.

The characteristic histopathology of his-toplasmosis is an extensive proliferation of reticuloendothelial cells, many of which contain yeast forms, either a few or so many that the cytoplasm is distended and en-larged. In some cases macrophages con-taining the organism can be seen in blood smears. Stains for bound glycogen (PAS, Bauer's, or Gridley stains) are helpful in differential staining of the organism.

Van Pernis et al. (1941) prepared histo-plasmin, a metabolic product of *H. cap-sulatum*. Its intradermal injection pro-duced a reaction similar to that induced by tuberculin. Apparently a diagnosis based on a reaction to histoplasmin is not un-equivocal as there may be cross-reactions with blastomycetin.

PREVENTION, CONTROL, AND TREATMENT

Recognized cases of histoplasmosis in man and animals have not been successfully treated. There is some evidence that the disease occurs in animals in a mild and un-recognized form.

REFERENCES

Brueck, J. W., and G. J. Buddingh. 1951. Prop-agation of pathogenic fungi in the yolk sac of embryonated eggs. *Proc. Soc. Exp. Biol. Med.* 86:258–61.

Campbell, C. C., G. B. Hill, and B. T. Falgout. 1962. *Histoplasma capsulatum* isolated from feather pillow associated with histoplasmosis of an infant. *Science* 136:1050–51.

Darling, S. T. 1906. A protozoan general in-fection producing pseudo-tubercles in the lungs and focal necrosis in the liver, spleen and lymph nodes. *J. Am. Med. Ass.* 46: 1283–85.

Dodge, H. J., L. Ajello, and O. K. Engelke. 1965. The association of a bird-roosting site with infection of school children by *Histo-plasma capsulatum*. *Am. J. Public Health* 55:1203–11.

Menges, R. W. 1954. Histoplasmin sensitivity in animals. *Cornell Vet.* 44:21–31.

Menges, R. W., and T. R. Habermann. 1955.

Experimental avian histoplasmosis. *Am. J. Vet. Res.* 16:314–20.

Schwarz, J., G. L. Baum, C. J. K. Wang, E. L. Bingham, and H. Rubel. 1957. Successful infection of pigeons and chickens with *His-toplasma capsulatum*. *Mycopathol. Mycol. Appl.* 8:189–93.

Schwarz, J., K. K. Sethi, and E. L. George. 1967. Experimental histoplasmic iridocylitis in chickens. *Arch. Pathol.* 83:461–65.

Tewari, R. P., and C. C. Campbell. 1965. Iso-lation of *Histoplasma capsulatum* from feathers of chickens inoculated intravenously with the yeast phase of the organism. *Sab-ouraudia* 4:17–22.

Vanbreuseghem, R. 1958. *Mycoses of Man and Animals*. Charles C Thomas, Springfield, Ill. Pp. 1–235.

Van Pernis, P., M. E. Benson, and P. Hollinger. 1941. Specific cutaneous reactions with his-toplasmosis. *J. Am. Med. Ass.* 117:436–37.

Wildervanck, A., W. A. Collier, and W. E. F. Winckel. 1953. Two cases of histoplasmosis on farms near Paramaribo (Surinam). *Doc. Med. Geograph. Trop.* 5:108–15.

Zeidberg, L. D., L. Ajello, A. Dillon, and L. C. Runyon. 1952. Isolation of *Histoplasma capsulatum* from soil. *Am. J. Public Health* 42:930–35.

❖

CRYPTOCOCCOSIS

❖

CRYPTOCOCCOSIS is a disease of man and animals which, in man, is characterized by a meningitis. Synonyms are torulosis, torula, yeast meningitis, and European blastomycosis.

HISTORY, INCIDENCE, AND DISTRIBUTION

The presence of an encapsulated yeast-like fungus in human lesions and pathological material was reported by Busse in 1894. In 1894 Sanfelice, in Italy, isolated the same organism (called *Saccharomyces neoformans*) from fruit juice. Since that time the disease has been found widely in man and has also been observed in horses, cattle, swine, cats, dogs, marmoset monkeys, and a cheetah. Although it has not been reported as a pathogen in birds, and epizootics have not occurred, its relationship to public health and its occurrence in birds' environments warrant discussion.

The disease is widely distributed around the world. An apparent geographical localization probably is due actually to recognition rather than to an actual limitation of distribution.

ETIOLOGY

The proper classification is a fungus of the imperfect yeast group under the name *Cryptococcus neoformans*. Skinner et al. (1945) and Vanbreuseghem (1952) gave complete descriptions of the organism. *C. neoformans* occurs as a saprophyte and has been found in wasps' nests, on grass, in the bodies of insects, and in butter and canned milk. It is a nonfilamentous yeast which does not form ascospores. It reproduces by budding; the cells are perfectly spherical and are surrounded by a thick mucilaginous capsule. The cell diameter is 4–6μ and the capsule is 1–2μ thick in cultured organisms. Fungus found in ulcerated lesions is 2–15μ in diameter.

It grows well in 48 hours at 37° C on glucose agar. Colonies are moist, shining, viscid, and whitish at first, then slightly brownish. It does not ferment sugars.

PATHOGENESIS AND EPIZOOTIOLOGY

In 1938 Bisbocci isolated a cryptococcus from a pheasant with enterohepatitis. Chickens were experimentally infected and developed the disease. Lesions consisted of granulomas and necrotic processes in the liver, intestines, lungs, and spleen.

Emmons in 1955 shocked the public health world by isolating *C. neoformans* from 16 of 19 premises and 63 of 111 specimens of pigeon droppings. The organism was found in the dropping sites but was not isolated from 20 pigeons examined. It appeared to grow as a saprophyte.

Bishop et al. (1960) confirmed those findings by isolating *C. neoformans* from 6 of 13 samples of pigeon nests and droppings obtained from Morgantown, West Virginia.

Staib (1961) isolated cryptococcus organisms from 28 fecal samples obtained from 201 species of birds at zoological gardens and pet shops in Germany. Twelve isolates were from canaries, one was from a wild pigeon, and the remainder were from psittacine and other birds.

Fragner (1962) isolated cryptococcus from the feces of the following: 48 pigeons, 13 fowls, 7 pheasants, 10 house martins, 4 jackdaws, and 3 chaffinches.

DIAGNOSIS

The organism can be cultured and is identified by the characteristics described above. Histopathology has proven extremely useful in the diagnosis of cases in mammals. The significant feature is the absence of an inflammatory reaction except in the late stages when the compression effects end and a chronic inflammatory reaction is produced. A stain called mucicarmine is specific and shows many budding spores with the thick capsule being darkly stained.

A culture of the organism may be tested experimentally in mice. An intracerebral injection of 0.05 ml of a suspension of the fungus produces typical gelatinous masses of budding cells in the meninges and causes death in 5–15 days.

TREATMENT

The prognosis is very grave for infected mammals, and to date no satisfactory treatment is known.

REFERENCES

Bisbocci, G. 1938. Infectious entero-hepatitis in fowls due to a cryptococcus. *Nuovo Ercolani* 43:290–314.

Bishop, R. H., R. K. Hamilton, and J. M. Slack. 1960. The isolation of *Cryptococcus neoformans* from pigeon nests. *W. Virginia Univ. Bull.* 26:31–32. (Abstr.)

Emmons, C. W. 1955. Saprophytic sources of *Cryptococcus neoformans* associated with the pigeon *(Columba livia)*. *Am. J. Hyg.* 62:227–32.

Fragner, P. 1962. Isolation of cryptococcus from bird feces. *Czech. Epidem. Mikrobiol. Immunol.* 11:135–39.

Skinner, Charles E., Chester W. Emmons, and Henry M. Tsuchuja. 1945. *Henrici's Molds, Yeasts and Actinomycetes.* John Wiley & Sons, Inc., New York.

Staib, F. I. 1961. *Cryptococcus neoformans* in bird feces. *Zentr. Bakteriol. Parasitenk. Abt. I. Orig.* 182:562–63.

Vanbreuseghem, R. (Transl. J. Wilkinson.) 1952. *Mycoses of Man and Animals.* Charles C Thomas, Springfield, Ill.

CHAPTER 15

NEOPLASTIC DISEASES

❖

INTRODUCTION

❖

B. W. CALNEK

Department of Avian Diseases
New York State Veterinary College
Ithaca, New York

❖

THIS CHAPTER deals with a variety of related and unrelated conditions possessing a single common denominator: neoplastic character. Some have been extensively studied because of their considerable economic importance. Others have served as highly suitable models for studying the various phenomena of neoplasia; indeed, medical research has found avian oncology an abundant resource. For presentation in this chapter, neoplasms are divided into two main categories, depending on whether or not the etiologic agent is known.

The virus-induced tumors are principally of mesodermal origin and are transmissible. Three diseases or disease complexes are described; each is afforded a separate subchapter because of its etiologic distinctness. One, Marek's disease, or neurolymphomatosis, is a lymphoproliferative disease affecting the peripheral nervous system and, to a greater or lesser degree, other tissues and visceral organs. Marek's disease (MD) is reported to be caused by a herpesvirus.

Second is a group of leukoses, sarcomas, and related neoplasms induced by a number of closely related RNA viruses (now called the leukosis/sarcoma group). Prominent in this group is lymphoid leukosis, another lymphoproliferative disease, affecting primarily the bursa of Fabricius and visceral organs. Also included are other neoplasms of hematopoietic origin, e.g., erythroblastosis, myeloblastosis, myelocytomatosis, and certain related neoplasms such as nephroblastoma, osteopetrosis. These conditions, along with the sarcomas and other connective tissue tumors, are etiologically related and are discussed as a group.

A third subchapter contains a brief description of a less well characterized condition, reticuloendotheliosis. This experimentally induced disease also is caused by an RNA virus (T-virus), one quite different from the leukosis/sarcoma viruses. The neoplastic nature of reticuloendotheliosis, while not firmly established, is considered probable or at least possible by a number of authors.

Tumors of unknown etiology of necessity are described only on the basis of morphologic characteristics and are discussed in a fourth subchapter. Included are a wide variety of benign and malignant neoplasms derived from muscle, epithelial, and nerve tissues; serous membranes; and pigmented cells.

The incidence and importance of neoplasms in poultry can be only generally estimated. Feldman and Olson (1965) quoted reports (1915–55) in which the incidence of tumors, excepting neurolymphomatosis and osteopetrosis, varied from 3 to 19%. In more recent years we have had the advantage of data accumulated by the USDA from federally inspected, slaughtered poultry (Table 15.1).

The incidence of "leukosis" as a cause for condemnation in young chickens (primarily broilers and roasters) increased markedly over a period of 8 years and in 1968 accounted for nearly 50% of all condemnations. In mature chickens, on the other hand, leukosis condemnations were fairly consistent and much lower than in the young birds. Condemnation rates with "other tumors" (nonleukotic) were relatively consistent and were much higher in mature chickens than in young birds. Many of the "other tumors" were leiomyomas of the mesosalpinx. While these data reflect the incidence of only those lesions prominent enough to be seen during a brief and cursory inspection, they point up the general seriousness of the problem in poultry

TABLE 15.1 ✍ Incidence of Neoplasms as Cause for Condemnation in Slaughtered Chickens

	Young Chickens*				Mature Chickens			
	Total inspected (millions)	Total condemned (millions)	Percent condemned		Total inspected (millions)	Total condemned (millions)	Percent condemned	
Year			Leukosis	Other tumors			Leukosis	Other tumors†
1961	1,736.8	34.6	5.7	0.2	119.8	3.6	9.0	9.3
1962	1,763.0	36.0	6.5	0.3	121.7	3.6	7.3	9.1
1963	1,835.0	39.9	10.2	0.3	129.0	4.0	7.3	9.2
1964	1,915.0	43.9	16.7	0.3	135.8	4.6	10.4	11.9
1965	2,057.6	49.4	21.9	0.4	134.7	5.1	9.1	19.6
1966	2,236.0	76.2	27.2	0.3	152.0	6.9	7.5	25.8
1967	2,319.4	83.2	35.6	0.3	170.2	8.1	5.9	22.1
1968	2,335.9	75.1	48.0	0.3	151.2	7.5	5.5	27.1

Summarized and compiled by B. R. Burmester from data distributed by Crops Reporting Board, Statistical Reporting Service, USDA, Washington, D.C.

    * Primarily broilers and roasters.

    † Other tumors were mostly leiomyomas of the mesosalpinx.

and support the concept that at least some neoplasms are increasing in frequency at an alarming rate. It is generally conceded that Marek's disease (the "leukosis" observed in young birds) is responsible for the increase and is one of the most serious disease problems confronting the poultry industry today. A USDA estimate of annual losses in the United States was placed at more than $150 million (AAAP Report, 1967) and, according to Biggs (1967), Kesteven estimated the losses from leukotic diseases (at least 50% of which are Marek's disease) in Great Britain to be about $40 million. The incidence of neoplasms other than lymphoid tumors appears to be low and of questionable economic significance.

Classification and nomenclature of the known transmissible neoplasms have presented a continuous problem. The dilemma is largely due to two factors. First, many virus strains appeared to have multipotent characteristics; i.e., they could sometimes induce a variety of neoplasms. Second, certain of the viruses induced some pathologic lesions which were indistinguishable (by available criteria) from those induced by another unrelated virus. The two prevalent lymphomatotic diseases, now called lymphoid leukosis and Marek's disease, were particularly confusing with regard to the latter point. The problem was compounded by the fact that most flocks and many birds (including those employed for experimental purposes) were infected with more than one agent, and it was virtually impossible to examine one virus strain without often also observing the ef-

fects of a second unrelated tumor virus. The prevalence of various unrelated (and related, but different) viruses in experimental birds used for passage of a given virus strain undoubtedly resulted in mixed virus populations in most cases, a factor which must be considered in arguments of the "multipotent character" of some viruses.

In general, terminology evolved along with an understanding of the pathologic changes associated with a given condition. Thus, while Marek (1907) described a "polyneuritis," Pappenheimer et al. (1926), who associated visceral lymphomata with the same disease, proposed the term neurolymphomatosis gallinarum. Few workers could decide what terminology was appropriate for each kind of lesion, and there was soon an abundant supply of choices (see synonyms in the following subchapters).

Trying to resolve the classification and terminology problem, and particularly to suggest uniform terminology, a committee (Jungherr, 1941) proposed a pathologic nomenclature. The scheme (which formed the basis of classification for a number of years) had two categories—*The Avian Leukosis Complex (ALC)* and *Other Tumors*. The ALC was divided to include: (1) lymphomatosis (visceral, neural, ocular, or osteopetrotic), and (2) leukosis (erythroblastic or myeloblastic). It was pointed out that the individual forms should be characterized as aleukemic, subleukemic, or leukemic. *Other Tumors* included myelocytomas and sarcomas. There was no attempt to infer etiologic unity by this classification. However, as Biggs (1967) pointed out, it turned out that both Marek's disease and lymphoid leukosis were classified together under the term lymphomatosis, and this no doubt contributed to the rather widespread conclusion that there was a single disease entity but with different manifestations. Biggs (1967) reviewed the development of our present concepts and terminology and observed that not all persons accepted this "unitarian" theory and further that Campbell, in 1954, had made a plea for clarification and a return to the earlier-held concept of two groups of diseases. Discussions toward that end culminated in the adoption by the World Veterinary Poultry Association of a classification and nomenclature scheme which clearly differentiated between the leukoses and Marek's disease (Biggs, 1962). Marek's disease was classified as neural, visceral, or ocular in type and the leukoses were divided into lymphoid, erythroid, and myeloid types. Many workers still adhered to the "unitarian" theory. However, it was soon obvious from studies on etiologic agents that a major division was warranted, and there is now rather universal acceptance of the separation (Burmester, 1966; AAAP, 1967).

Sevoian (1966) proposed a system in which each condition is classified first on pathologic character and second by etiologic criteria. Thus a lymphoid leukosis might be of Type I (if induced by a virus of the leukosis/sarcoma group), or Type II (if caused by the Marek's disease virus), or Type III, etc. Similarly, erythroid or myeloid leukosis would be subdivided into types. In this system two conditions, e.g. lymphoid leukosis (Type I) and erythroid leukosis (Type I), might be expressions of the same infection yet classified separately. Sevoian pointed out that this method has the advantage of being open-ended, facilitating the inclusion of both new pathologic manifestations caused by previously characterized agents and newly discovered agent types which cause lesions similar to those of other agents.

The choice of terminology for this chapter (Table 15.2) is based on that originally adopted by the World Veterinary Poultry Association and includes modifications in current use. It is not defended as the most suitable nomenclature. Rather it was selected because it is that most commonly employed today. The classification system which accompanies this nomenclature is especially suited to the mode of presentation which follows, i.e., categorization of diseases or disease complexes by agent type instead of by pathologic manifestation. Subdivision, within agent-type diseases, by pathologic expression has been employed where it seemed appropriate to the presentation.

TABLE 15.2 ❧ Transmissible Neoplasms

Nucleic Acid Type and Virus Classification of Etiologic Agent	Neoplastic Diseases

RNA, myxoviruses (possessing a group-specific antigen)	Leukosis/Sarcoma Group
	A. Leukoses
	  lymphoid leukosis
	  erythroblastosis
	  myeloblastosis
	  myelocytomatosis
	B. Sarcomas and other connective tissue tumors
	  fibrosarcoma, fibroma
	  myxosarcoma, myxoma
	  osteogenic sarcoma, osteoma
	  histiocytic sarcoma
	C. Related neoplasms
	  hemangioma
	  nephroblastoma
	  hepatocarcinoma
	  osteopetrosis

DNA, group B herpesvirus	Marek's disease
RNA, unclassified (T-virus)	Reticuloendotheliosis

REFERENCES

AAAP Report. 1967. Report of the American Association of Avian Pathologists-Sponsored Leukosis Workshop. *Avian Diseases* 11: 694–702.

Biggs, P. M. 1962. Some observations on the properties of cells from the lesions of Marek's disease and lymphoid leukosis. *Proc. 13th Symp. Colston Res. Soc.*, pp. 83–99.

———. 1967. Marek's disease. *Vet. Record* 81: 583–92.

Burmester, B. R. 1966. Report on Avian Leukosis Conference. *Poultry Sci.* 45:1411–15.

Campbell, J. G. 1954. Avian leucosis: A plea for clarification. Tenth World's Poultry Congr., pp. 193–97.

Feldman, W. H., and C. Olson. 1965. Neo- plastic diseases of the chicken, pp. 863–924. In Biester, H. E., and L. H. Schwarte (eds.), *Diseases of Poultry*, 5th ed. Iowa State Univ. Press, Ames.

Jungherr, E. 1941. Tentative pathologic no- menclature. *Am. J. Vet. Res.* 2:116.

Marek, J. 1907. Multiple Nervenentzuendung (Polyneuritis) bei Huehnern. *Deut. Tier- aerztl. Wochschr.* 15:417–21.

Pappenheimer, A. M., L. C. Dunn, and V. Cone. 1926. A study of fowl paralysis (neu- ro-lymphomatosis gallinarum). *Storrs Agr. Expt. Sta. Bull.* 143:187–290.

Sevoian, Martin. 1966. On the terminology and classification of the avian leukosis complex. *Avian Diseases* 11:98–103.

❖

MAREK'S DISEASE

❖

B. W. CALNEK

Department of Avian Diseases
New York State Veterinary College
Ithaca, New York

AND

R. L. WITTER

United States Department of Agriculture
Regional Poultry Research Laboratory
East Lansing, Michigan

❖

PROBABLY the most common of the lymphoproliferative diseases of chickens is Marek's disease (MD). This condition is characterized by a mononuclear infiltration of peripheral nerves and also (but less commonly and to a variable extent) the gonad, iris, various viscera, muscle, and skin. It is especially prevalent in chickens but has also been reported in several other avian species. Marek's disease is considered to be virus-induced, is transmissible, and can be distinguished etiologically from other lymphoid neoplasms of birds.

Terminology has been confusing. The wide variety of clinical signs and pathologic expressions, dependent primarily on the location of lesions, led to the promulgation of an equally wide variety of terms to identify the conditions. Mononuclear infiltration of peripheral nerves results in gross enlargement and causes paralysis. The inflammatory character of some of the peripheral nerve lesions prompted Marek (1907) to identify the disease as polyneuritis. Synonyms subsequently employed include neuritis (Doyle, 1926), neurolymphomatosis gallinarum (Pappenheimer et al., 1926), and range paralysis (Patterson et al., 1932). Mononuclear infiltration of the iris, which causes changes ranging from depigmentation to grayish opacity, is the basis for terms such as blindness, gray-eye, iritis, uveitis, and ocular lymphomatosis (Jungherr and Hughes, 1965). Leukotic lesions in various visceral organs and muscles were often referred to simply as visceral lymphomatosis; those in the skin have been identified as "skin leukosis." Biggs, in 1961, promoted the use of the term Marek's disease to clearly distinguish the condition from etiologically different lymphoproliferative diseases. He felt that in so doing there would be no prejudice against the inclusion of other lesions that might later be identified as expressions of the disease (Biggs,

1966). This term was adopted by the World Veterinary Poultry Association in 1960 (Biggs, 1962) and is in common usage today.

As already pointed out, Marek's disease is of immense economic significance to the poultry industry. In the United States annual losses attributable to "leukosis" (of which the majority is considered to be Marek's disease) have been estimated by the USDA to be in excess of $150 million (AAAP Report, 1967). Biggs (1967) quoted an estimated loss of at least $20 million per year in Great Britain. This, he calculated, constituted about 15% of the overall loss from disease in chickens and represented approximately 2.5% of all poultry income.

The public health significance of Marek's disease is not known.

HISTORY

A historical account of Marek's disease can be only partially complete. Until recently many workers who lumped this disease with other forms of the avian leukosis complex referred simply to "leukosis" or "lymphomatosis." Even those who insisted on separating Marek's disease from the "leukoses" could not distinguish between some kinds of lesions common to both conditions. Nonetheless, it is possible to identify certain studies, especially those in which neurolymphomatosis was reported as a prominent feature, as having dealt specifically with Marek's disease.

Pappenheimer et al. (1926) reviewed the literature of the period prior to their studies and considered the 1907 report by Marek from Hungary to be the first account of the disease. They recounted his detailed description of the clinical signs (paresis of legs and wings) of four roosters and the pathologic changes in one which was killed 5 weeks after signs were first noticed. It was that description of gross enlargement due to mononuclear infiltration of peripheral nerves and spinal nerve roots which encouraged the use of the term Marek's disease (Biggs, 1967).

Several outbreaks of the disease in the United States were reported by Kaupp (1921), whose observations dated to 1914. Studies by Van der Walle and Winkler-Junius 1924) indicated that the disease was in the Netherlands, and, according to Biggs (1967), Marek's disease was first recorded

in Great Britain by Galloway in 1929. It was subsequently noted in many other countries.

As observations by others were added to Marek's early description, it became apparent that lesions were not restricted to the spinal cord and peripheral nerves. Kaupp (1921) reported that blindness was frequently accompanied by paralysis; studies by Pappenheimer et al. (1926, 1929) revealed that extraneural lesions included visceral lymphomata, particularly in the ovary, and also infiltration of the iris and brain. The latter workers were of the opinion that neurolymphomatosis and the associated lymphomata were not related to the forms of leukosis reported by Ellerman, but that contention was not universally accepted until recent years. Outbreaks of the disease producing unusually high mortality have been observed at least since 1949 and are now quite common (Benton and Cover, 1957; Benton et al., 1962; Biggs et al., 1965; Dunlop et al., 1965). These are usually characterized by a preponderance of visceral lymphoid tumors, often without accompanying gross nerve enlargement. The visceral lesions, while in some cases simulating those of lymphoid leukosis, were considered by Biggs et al. (1965) to be forms of Marek's disease. Biggs (1966) has, for convenience, referred to this form as "acute Marek's disease," while the form described earlier (in which neural involvement predominates) was termed "classical Marek's disease."

Attempts to transmit the disease, along with descriptions of the gross and microscopic lesions, accounted for much of the research effort during the 1920s and 1930s. Transmission trials were often unsuccessful. Kaupp (1921) was unable to infect birds with blood and tissues from affected chickens, but he considered the condition infectious. Doyle (1926) was of the same opinion, but he too failed in transmission attempts. According to Jungherr and Hughes (1965), Van der Walle and Winkler-Junius reported the first positive transmission of the disease in 1924. However, interpretation of these and other early transmission trials is difficult since controls were usually inadequate and the facilities for housing experimental birds could not prevent the possibility of adventitious exposure. Pappenheimer and his associates (1926) induced the disease in about 25% of the chickens inoculated subdurally or intramuscularly with nerve tissue from affected birds. Olson (1940) observed that some workers encountered variable degrees of success at transmission while others failed. Indeed, it was not until the work of Sevoian et al. (1962) and Biggs and Payne (1963) that Marek's disease was experimentally transmitted with regularity. Their combined studies constituted a major breakthrough, especially as they pointed out that consistent assays of the agent could be done by intra-abdominal inoculation of susceptible day-old chicks. This permitted studies on agent characterization, pathogenesis, epizootiology, and genetic factors.

The importance of genetic constitution as it affects susceptibility to the disease was brought out by the classic work of Hutt and Cole (1947). Their studies, which began in the 1930s, laid the foundation for current efforts to control losses through genetic selection of breeding stocks, and their development of the S-line (susceptible strain) must be credited, in part, for the successful transmission studies by Sevoian and his co-workers.

It is especially significant that successful transmission was reported more frequently with cellular than with cell-free inocula. The avid cell association of the agent was particularly apparent when the use of chick assays permitted more critical studies (Biggs and Payne, 1967) and probably was the primary reason that the identity of the agent was so elusive. It was not until 1967 that nearly simultaneous, but independent, research in Great Britain (Churchill and Biggs, 1967) and the United States (Nazerian et al., 1968; Solomon et al., 1968) uncovered a group B herpesvirus as the probable etiologic agent.

INCIDENCE AND DISTRIBUTION

Marek's disease exists in poultry-producing countries throughout the world. Quite probably every flock of chickens raised in areas where poultry is prevalent experiences some loss. Because many reporting systems have not clearly differentiated between lymphoid leukosis and Marek's disease, it is difficult to determine the true incidence. Losses in affected flocks have been estimated to range from a few birds to 25 or 30% and occasionally as high as 60% of the birds (Jungherr and Hughes, 1965; Biggs, 1967).

A summary prepared by the American Association of Avian Pathologists (AAAP Report, 1967) stated that the incidence of the disease has increased sharply in the United States and other countries in recent years. Data compiled from reports of the USDA Statistical Reporting Service support this claim (see Table 15.1).

In the United States the incidence has not been uniform, largely due to the occurrence of acute explosive outbreaks in certain geographic areas. Losses have been especially high in areas where poultry (and more specifically broiler) raising is intensive. The uneven distribution may represent the existence of a more virulent form of the disease which occurs as an epizootic in certain areas (Biggs, 1967), but a satisfactory explanation is lacking. The AAAP Report (1967) pointed out that areas which have experienced severe outbreaks continue to be plagued with the acute disease.

ETIOLOGY

CLASSIFICATION

The etiological agent of Marek's disease was reported to be a herpesvirus following independent studies by workers in Great Britain (Churchill and Biggs, 1967) and the United States (Solomon et al., 1968; Nazerian et al., 1968). Each group observed areas of cytopathic effect (CPE) and found particles morphologically similar to herpesviruses in cultured chicken kidney cells or duck embryo fibroblasts inoculated with the MD agent. On the basis of morphogenesis, morphologic character, nucleic acid type, and cell-associated infectivity, both groups of workers identified their respective isolates as group B (cell-associated) herpesvirus.

Considerable circumstantial evidence gathered by these and other workers has implicated this herpesvirus in the etiology of MD:

1. Birds exposed to Marek's disease by a variety of means and with a variety of virus isolates invariably have yielded positive herpesvirus isolations, have detectable virus-associated antigens in their tissues, and develop antibodies against herpesvirus antigens (Chubb and Churchill, 1968; Churchill and Biggs, 1968; Spencer, 1969; Witter et al., 1969b; Purchase, 1969; Calnek and Hitchner, 1969). Exposed birds

which did not develop lesions had evidence of herpesvirus infection, but the incidence was lower than in those with lesions. Birds not exposed to Marek's disease virus and without lesions of the disease have been found consistently free of herpesvirus.

2. Cultures with herpesvirus plaques regularly induced MD in inoculated chicks whereas control cultures lacking these plaques were usually noninfectious. Furthermore, the plaque-inducing ability (in vitro) and the infectivity (in vivo) of an inoculum diluted out simultaneously and were equally sensitive to inhibitors of DNA replication (Churchill and Biggs, 1968; Spencer, 1969; Witter et al., 1969b).

3. Inocula which induced herpesvirus plaques in cell culture invariably induced Marek's disease when inoculated into chicks. Occasionally inocula which were infectious for chicks failed to infect cell cultures, probably because the chick assay was more sensitive than the cell culture assay (Witter et al., 1969b).

4. Both the infectivity of inocula for chicks and the plaque-forming ability of the herpesvirus in cell culture are closely cell-associated (Biggs et al., 1968a).

More recent studies made possible by the successful extraction of cell-free virus from the feather follicle epithelium (Calnek et al., 1970a; Nazerian and Witter, 1970) have provided direct evidence for the implication of the herpesvirus in the etiology of MD.

Unidentified cytopathogenic agents were isolated in chicken embryo fibroblast cultures from cases of Marek's disease by both Vindel (1964) and Kottaridis et al. (1968). Although characteristics of these agents in vitro were unlike those described for the herpesvirus, chicks inoculated with these agents developed MD lesions. However, in neither case were the experiments sufficiently described or controlled to unequivocally establish that these lesions were induced with the respective cytopathogenic agents. Other workers found chick embryo fibroblast cultures refractory to MD virus (Biggs and Payne, 1964; Witter et al., 1968a; Calnek et al., 1969). Evidence that the agents isolated by Vindel or Kottaridis may cause MD is not convincing; yet the possibility that these or other nonherpetic viruses may induce MD-like lesions in chickens has not been ruled out.

On the other hand, the etiologic role of the herpesvirus in MD appears amply supported by the evidence cited. Thus the early theory of Van der Walle and Winkler-Junius (1924) that MD was caused by a virus similar to that of herpes zoster in man seems to have been truly prophetic. Henceforth in this chapter, MD virus and herpesvirus will be considered as the same. It should be recognized, however, that many properties of MD virus have been determined by in vivo studies and thus are not dependent on this hypothesis for the etiology of Marek's disease.

MORPHOLOGY AND MORPHOGENESIS

The morphology and morphogenesis of this virus has been studied in detail (Churchill and Biggs, 1967; Nazerian et al., 1968; Nazerian and Burmester, 1968; Epstein et al., 1968; Ahmed and Schidlovsky, 1968). Hexagonal naked particles or nucleocapsids, 85–100 mμ, both with and without electron dense nucleoids, were found usually in the nucleus and occasionally in the cytoplasm of infected tissue culture cells or in extracellular fluids. The nucleocapsid apparently developed within the nucleus and obtained an additional membrane or envelope by budding from the nuclear membrane into the cytoplasm. The size of enveloped particles in thin-section preparations has been estimated at 150–170 mμ (Nazerian and Burmester, 1968) and 130 mμ (Epstein et al., 1968). Enveloped particles were principally associated with the nuclear membrane or in nuclear vesicles but have been observed in the cytoplasm. Virus particles observed in negatively stained preparations of lysed feather follicle epithelium had envelopes which measured 273–400 mμ and appeared as irregular amorphous structures (Calnek et al., 1970a). Thin-section preparations of the same tissue revealed large numbers of cytoplasmic enveloped herpesvirus particles which measured about 180–220 mμ (Calnek et al., 1970b) or 200–250 mμ (Nazerian and Witter, 1970). These were in keratinizing cells and often within cytoplasmic inclusion bodies composed of homogeneous amorphous material. Enveloped particles within nuclear vesicles or immediately outside the nucleus measured 150–170 mμ (Nazerian and Witter, 1970).

In negatively stained preparations the nucleocapsid was observed to have cubic,

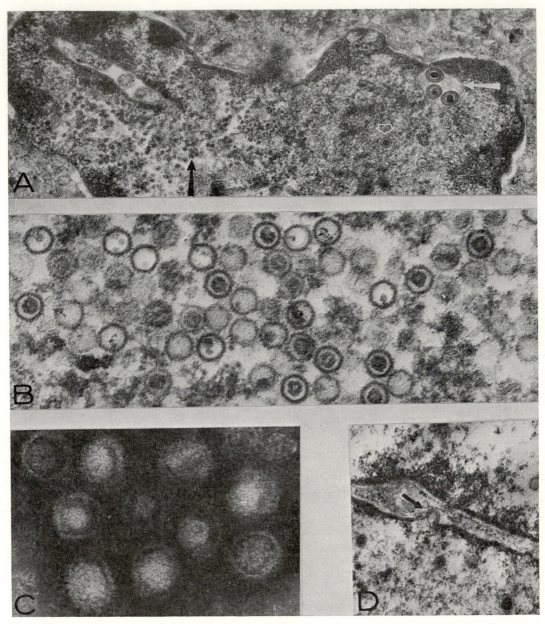

FIG. 15.1—Electron micrographs of Marek's disease herpesvirus and virus-infected cells. (A) Portion of infected duck embryo fibroblast showing 3 types of particles in nucleus: naked articles (**short white arrow**), enveloped particles (**long white arrow**), and aggregates of 35–40 mµ particles (**black arrow**). ×30,000. (B) Naked forms of the virus in nucleus of infected cell. Some particles have central nucleoids while others appear empty. ×69,000. (C) Negative contrast electron micrograph of typical herpesvirus particles from growth fluid of infected chicken embryo fibroblast cultures. ×126,000. (D) Portions of two adjacent nuclei in infected duck embryo fibroblast. Virus particle is budding from nucleus into the cytoplasm (**arrow**). ×30,000. (Courtesy K. Nazerian, USDA Regional Poultry Laboratory, E. Lansing, Mich.)

icosahedral symmetry and to possess 162 hollow-centered capsomeres. In some cells which contained typical herpesvirus particles, other smaller particles or ring-shaped structures 30–40 mμ were also seen. Their significance is not known, but similar particles have been observed associated with other herpesviruses (Morgan et al., 1959). Characteristic morphologic forms of intracellular and extracellular viruses are illustrated in Figure 15.1.

CHEMICAL COMPOSITION

The chemistry of the virus particle has not been studied directly. The inhibition of both cytopathic effect and infectivity in tissue cultures treated with 5-iododeoxyuridine or 5-bromodeoxyuridine suggested that the viral core contained DNA (Churchill and Biggs, 1967, 1968; Nazerian et al., 1968). This conclusion is further supported by cytochemical staining of the type A intranuclear inclusions which develop in infected cultured cells (Churchill and Biggs, 1967; Nazerian et al., 1968).

VIRUS REPLICATION

Virus spread in cell cultures appears to be largely cell-to-cell (Churchill and Biggs, 1967; Solomon et al., 1968) and may require active participation on the part of the donor cell (Calnek and Madin, 1969). There is, however, evidence that at least some cell-free, infectious virus is produced by infected cells. The reports of filtration of JM-infected plasma through a 0.3μ filter (Sevoian et al., 1962) and the consistent infectivity of plasma (centrifuged at 8,500 G for 20 minutes) obtained from chicks inoculated with the GA isolate (Eidson and Schmittle, 1968) were exceptional but supported this thesis. Furthermore, while early attempts to filter the GA isolate in plasma were unsuccessful (Eidson and Schmittle, 1968), some infectious cell-free virus was recently recovered from GA-infected chick kidney cultures (Eidson, personal communication). Similarly, Nazerian (1968) demonstrated small quantities of cell-free virus in fluids of cell cultures infected with the JM isolate.

The sites of virus replication in vivo are important to the epizootiology and pathogenesis of the disease. Virus infection can be associated with several tissues on the basis of finding viral-associated antigen with the fluorescent antibody and agar gel precipitin tests (Spencer, 1969; Calnek and Hitchner, 1969; Spencer and Calnek, 1970; Purchase, 1970; Calnek et al., 1970b; Von Bülow and Payne, 1970). Many cell types including those in lymphoid organs (bursa of Fabricius, thymus, spleen) and a variety of epithelial tissues have been found to contain viral antigen. Viral particles have been observed by electron microscopy in many of the tissues. Those in the keratinizing layers of the feather follicle epithelium have been mostly complete (enveloped) (Calnek et al., 1970a,b; Nazerian and Witter, 1970); naked virions have predominated in infected kidney tubules (Schidlovsky et al., 1969), bursa of Fabricius, leukotic gonad, and nerve plexus (Calnek et al., 1970b). Tumor cells generally have been found free of viral particles (Nakagawa, 1965; Nazerian et al., 1968; Ahmed and Schidlovsky, 1968; Schidlovsky et al., 1969; Wight, 1969), although they occasionally contain viral-associated antigen (Spencer, 1969; Calnek and Hitchner, 1969) and, as evidenced by their infectivity, must at least contain the viral genome. However, Ubertini and Calnek (1970), in the examination of a leukotic nerve plexus, were able to find herpesvirus particles (mostly naked) in immature lymphoid cells as well as in Schwann cells and degenerated lymphoblastoid cells (so-called "Marek's disease cells").

Enveloped virus is thought to be infectious in the cell-free state (Smith, 1964) and represents the "complete" virus. This concept is supported by the above observations, since the only infected tissues from which infectious cell-free virus preparations could be obtained were those in which enveloped virus was consistently observed (feather follicle epithelium) (Calnek et al., 1970a,b; Nazerian and Witter, 1970). Thus, virus replication apparently proceeds to different stages of completion in different tissues.

BIOLOGICAL PROPERTIES

The herpesvirus can infect cells in vitro and in vivo. In the former, infection may result in cytopathic effect, as with chicken kidney (CK) cells or duck embryo fibroblasts, or may be without observable effects. Witter et al. (1968a) reported that persistently infected cell cultures derived from a variety of tissues did not have noticeable differences from control cultures. Calnek and Madin (1969) found that, even with CK cells, infection did not commit a given cell to cytopathic change. In vivo, the effects of infection vary from degenerative (medulla of the bursa of Fabricius) to oncogenic (lymphoid tumor cells). Many common sites of infection detected with fluorescent antibody tests (e.g. kidney tubule epithelium, epithelium of the feather follicle) are apparently unaffected (Spencer, 1969; Calnek and Hitchner, 1969). The nature of the oncogenic response is not understood.

RESISTANCE TO CHEMICAL AND PHYSICAL AGENTS

Viral infectivity of blood cells or tumor cells was reduced or eliminated by treatments which either destroyed or removed viable cells from the inoculum; these included freeze-thaw (without stabilizer), sonication, lyophilization, centrifugation at 2,000 G, and filtration (Biggs and Payne, 1967; Churchill and Biggs, 1967; Biggs et al., 1968; Nazerian et al., 1968). Protection of cells during freezing by treatment with dimethyl sulfoxide preserved MD infectivity (Spencer and Calnek, 1967; Biggs and Payne, 1967). The infectivity of enveloped cell-free virus obtained from the feather follicle epithelium is not affected by most, or perhaps all, of the treatments found detrimental to blood or tumor cell infectivity (Calnek, unpublished data).

STRAIN CLASSIFICATION

Isolates of MD have been obtained and employed by many laboratories—e.g., JM (Sevoian et al., 1962), CONN-A (Chomiak et al., 1967), GA (Eidson and Schmittle, 1968), HPRS-14 (Biggs and Payne, 1963), and HPRS-16, -17, -18, -19, and -20 (Purchase and Biggs, 1967). These are not virus strains in the strict sense since their purity has not been ascertained. Differences between isolates are apparent, principally in virulence and in the tissue distribution of gross lesions. Isolates appear serologically indistinguishable (Purchase, 1969) except for cell culture attenuated isolates which lack an antigen demonstrable in virulent isolates (Churchill et al., 1969a).

LABORATORY HOST SYSTEMS

Marek's disease virus has been propagated and assayed in newly hatched chick, tissue cultures, and embryonated egg. Young chicks until recently have served

as the principal laboratory host for MD. Newly hatched chicks inoculated with MD virus develop lesions which can be detected histologically in the ganglia, nerves, and certain viscera after 2–4 weeks, or by gross examination after 3–6 weeks. The response is greatly dependent on the genetic susceptibility of the chicken and the virulence of the MD isolate. The presence of virus or antibody, which can be detected by in vitro tests, or the presence of viral associated antigen detected by FA tests on tissues are also specific host responses of inoculated chickens to MD infection.

Cultured duck embryo fibroblasts or chicken kidney cells are suitable for propagation of MD virus (Churchill and Biggs, 1967; Solomon et al., 1968). Infected cultures usually develop discrete focal lesions which, when mature, consist of clusters of rounded, refractile, degenerating cells. Foci are usually less than 1 mm in diameter and of variable cell density. Affected cells may contain two or more nuclei, and type A intranuclear inclusion bodies are commonly seen (Fig. 15.2). Despite the release of rounded cells into the medium as plaques mature, large areas of cell lysis are not seen. Plaques develop in 5–14 days on primary isolation and are usually enumerated by microscopic examination of the culture. Minor differences in the development and morphology of plaques in chick and duck cells have been described (Spencer, 1969; Witter et al., 1969a).

The development of virus pocks (Fig. 15.3) on the chorioallantoic membrane (CAM) of chick embryos following yolk sac inoculation with cellular MD virus preparations has been reported (Von Bülow, 1969). Inoculation into the yolk sac usually obviates the nonspecific graft-versus-host pocks which are common when immunologically competent cells are inoculated directly onto the CAM. The sensitivity of this procedure for detecting virus in blood or buffy coat cells is about equal to that of cell culture assay (P. M. Biggs, personal communication).

PATHOGENICITY

Virulence, as estimated from latent period and incidence of morbidity and mortality, is high for some virus isolates (JM, GA, and HPRS-16, -18, -19, and -20), whereas the CONN-A, HPRS-14, and HPRS-17 isolates are of significantly lower virulence.

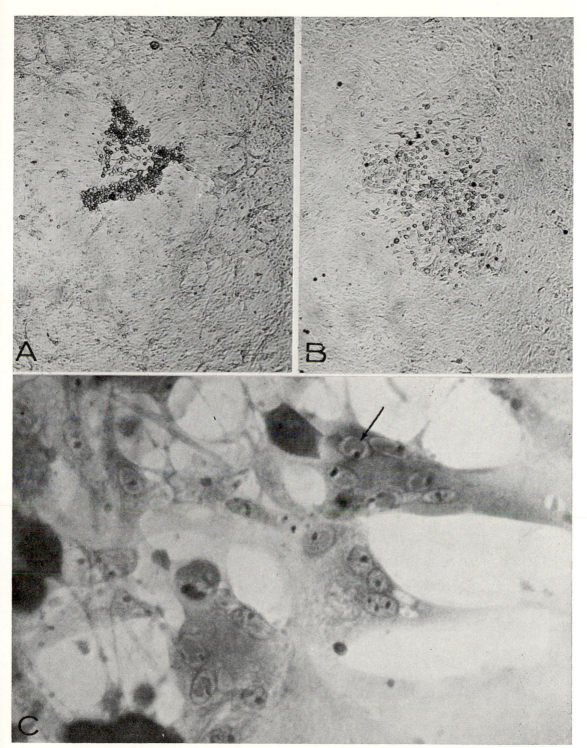

FIG. 15.2—*Cytologic changes in cultured cells infected with JM isolate of MD herpesvirus. (A) Focus of rounded, highly refractile cells in infected chicken kidney (CK) cell culture. Unstained, ×40. (B) Focus in infected culture of duck embryo fibroblasts. Unstained, ×40. (C) Syncytia in infected CK culture. Many of the nuclei in giant cells have inclusion bodies (arrow). H & E, ×860.*

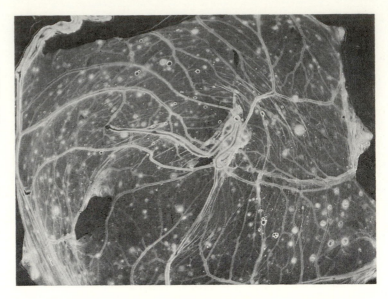

FIG. 15.3—*Chorioallantoic membrane from 19-day-old chicken embryo inoculated via yolk sac at 4 days old with blood from chickens infected with JM isolate.*

Tumors in the visceral organs, skin, and muscle are often induced by the highly virulent isolates. Isolates of low virulence may also induce visceral tumors, particularly in the gonad, but the incidence is often low. Enlargement of peripheral nerves and spinal ganglia is characteristic of infection induced by all isolates, but the incidence of these lesions may be higher with infection with low-virulence isolates. Since distribution of gross lesions can be influenced by the host chicken, this criterion may be of less value than virulence in characterizing and classifying isolates.

Churchill et al. (1969a) observed what was described as attenuation of MD herpesvirus following serial passage in chicken kidney cell culture. A change in the character of focal lesions and the loss of an antigenic component were accompanied by a decrease in pathogenicity or, in the author's opinion, a loss of oncogenicity.

PATHOGENESIS AND EPIZOOTIOLOGY

NATURAL AND EXPERIMENTAL HOSTS

In addition to the chicken, the turkey, pheasant, and perhaps quail may be natural hosts for Marek's disease. Nerve lesions characteristic of Marek's disease were observed in pheasants by Jungherr (1939). He reported extraneural lesions in the form of localized areas of muscle degeneration, particularly in the flexor leg muscles. These appeared as "tigering" grossly and as Zenker's degeneration microscopically. Similar

nerve and muscle lesions in turkeys were described by Andrewes and Glover (1939). Harriss (1939) and Johnson (1941) both claimed successful transmission of Marek's disease to pheasants, and Sevoian et al. (1963b) found turkey poults fully susceptible to the JM strain of virus. Witter et al. (1970b) also produced lymphoid tumors in turkeys with the JM isolate but were unable to reisolate the virus or detect antibody. On the other hand, herpesvirus, which was apparently nonvirulent but antigenically related to MD virus, was isolated from turkey flocks experiencing naturally occurring lymphoid tumors (Witter et al., 1970b). Kenzy and Cho (1969) isolated MD virus from a mature quail which had ocular MD lesions.

Evidence suggesting other natural hosts is more tenuous, although Wight (1963) quoted reports of the disease in several species including the pigeon, duck, goose, canary, budgerigar, and swan. His own observation of what appeared to be Marek's disease along with lymphoid leukosis in Japanese quail (*Coturnix coturnix japonica*) conflicted with Calnek's findings (unpublished data) in which newly hatched Japanese quail were refractory to inoculation with JM strain of virus. Kenzy and Cho (1969) failed to infect sparrows by contact exposure to infected chickens. Baxendale (1969) demonstrated precipitating antibody and reisolated virus from ducks experimentally infected with the HPRS-16 strain of virus; however, no clinical disease was observed. Reports of the use of other avian species as experimental hosts have not been noted, and there are no communications which suggest that nonavian species are susceptible. In a single trial Calnek (unpublished data) failed to induce disease in 12 Chinese hamsters inoculated with JM virus, either subcutaneously as newborns or in the cheek pouch at 1 month old. Churchill (1968) also was unsuccessful in attempts to produce tumors in hamsters with herpesvirus-infected CK cells inoculated subcutaneously or intracerebrally.

Naturally infected chickens are sometimes affected as early as the 3rd week of life, but the disease usually appears between the 2nd and 5th month. Often losses continue after the birds reach maturity, at which time ocular and visceral lesions become more apparent (Jungherr and Hughes, 1965). Biggs (1967) observed a tendency for the more acute disease to occur in younger groups.

TRANSMISSION

The mode of natural transmission has presented a baffling problem. The virus, as observed in tumor cells and in infected cell cultures, is avidly cell-associated; yet both the natural and experimental diseases are highly contagious. Either direct or indirect contact between birds effects virus spread (Biggs and Payne, 1963, 1967), and virus may be disseminated by the airborne route (Sevoian et al., 1963b; Colwell and Schmittle, 1968). Furthermore, Witter et al. (1968b) found that feces and litter from infected chickens remained infective up to 16 weeks at room temperature, and poultry house dust has been shown to be infective several weeks after collection (Beasley et al., 1970; Jurajda and Klimes, 1970). Thus it appears that in nature, infective virus must be independent of viable cells.

Several studies pointed to secreta and excreta as sources of virus. Oral or nasal washings have been consistently infectious (Witter and Burmester, 1967; Kenzy and Biggs, 1967; Eidson and Schmittle, 1968), but feces examined by the same workers were infectious only in the case of the studies by Witter and Burmester. These results are interesting in view of a study by Calnek and Hitchner (1969) in which JM-infected birds had viral associated antigen in the upper portions (esophagus, crop, and proventriculus) but never in the lower portions (intestine) of the alimentary tract. Also it should be pointed out that in the above studies, oral washings were infectious only upon intra-abdominal and, to a lesser degree, intranasal inoculation; per os administration was ineffective. Intact viable cells could have accounted for the infectivity of both the oral or nasal washings and the feces (Witter and Burmester obtained feces by cloacal swab) but not for the infectivity of litter stored for several months.

To determine where virus localizes in infected birds, Calnek and Hitchner (1969) applied a fluorescent antibody test to a variety of tissues. Viral associated antigen in the epithelial cells of the feather follicle (and occasionally in the feather barb cells) was prominent because it was the most consistent and persistent site of antigen, and antigen was often present in large concentrations (see Fig. 15.17D). The dermis and epidermis of the skin were always free of antigen. Affected follicular epithelial cells were stratified squamous epithelium, a cell type which sloughs off and probably also detaches with molted feathers and could therefore contaminate the environment. Calnek et al. (1970a) subsequently found enveloped herpesvirus in that location, and further found that cell-free filtrates of sonicated cells from that site contained infectious virus. For these reasons it is thought that the feather follicle epithelium (and perhaps feathers) may be the site most important to the transmission of the disease by providing the enveloped virus, either cell-free or within dead cells, which can survive in the environment or spread from bird to bird. Supportive evidence was provided by a study by Beasley et al. (1970) in which dander collected from infected birds was used to transmit MD.

Other potential means of spread include the darkling beetle *(Alphitobius diaperinus)* and possibly other vectors. Eidson et al. (1966) determined that beetles which had fed on infected carcasses transmitted the disease when fed to susceptible birds. Whether they might play a significant role in the epizootiology of the disease by preserving virus or can act only as a motile passive carrier of virus was not established. Other studies failed to demonstrate infectivity of these or other arthropods, such as free-living litter mites, in contact with infected chickens (Beasley, personal communication; Witter et al., 1968b; Brewer et al.,

1969a). Mosquitoes (*Culex quinquefasciatus* and *Culex pipiens*), after feeding on infected chickens, did not transmit MD by biting susceptible birds, and failed to infect birds to which they were fed (Brewer et al., 1969b). However, they were infectious when inoculated into chickens intra-abdominally. Whole or disrupted coccidial oocysts from birds naturally and experimentally infected with Marek's disease did not transmit the disease when inoculated into chicks (Long et al., 1968).

The existence of carrier birds has been established. It appears that many apparently normal birds may be infected (Sevoian and Chamberlain, 1962) and even viremic (Sevoian, personal communication); Kenzy and Cho (1969) found that such birds can act as a source of infection.

A factor of immense importance, but for which little information is available, is the role of egg transmission. Cole (1949) reviewed the literature and found that opinions varied regarding the likelihood of transovarian infection. His own observations led him to believe that this method of dissemination is insignificant in determining the incidence of disease among progeny. Further support for this contention was presented by Cole and Hutt (1951). Biggs (1966), on the other hand, considered circumstantial evidence to favor the likelihood of this means of dissemination. He cited instances in which the disease appeared in chicks hatched and raised in strict isolation. Similar observations by others have been common, but because of the extreme contagiousness of the virus it is impossible to draw definite conclusions. Biggs and Payne (1967) noted that virus-inoculated embryos survived and hatched normally but succumbed a few weeks later. In a preliminary report, Sevoian (1968a) claimed isolation of the agent from embryonated eggs. However, that has not been confirmed, and an extensive study by Solomon et al. (1970) failed to detect infection in over 5,000 embryos or chickens derived from known infected breeder flocks. It appears that egg transmission, if it occurs, must be at a very low rate.

Experimental transmission is effected most consistently by inoculation of day-old, genetically susceptible chicks with blood or tumor suspensions or by direct or indirect contact with infected birds. With inoculation of tumor cell suspensions there is always the hazard of inducing tumors by cell transplantation. Chromosome studies (Owen et al., 1966) in which the donor and recipient birds were of different sex indicated that transplantation is not the usual cause of lesions in experimental birds.

INCUBATION PERIOD

The incubation period for experimentally induced Marek's disease is rather well established. Chicks inoculated at 1 day of age excrete virus beginning at the 2nd or 3rd week postinoculation and develop microscopic lesions as early as 2 weeks postinoculation. Clinical signs and gross lesions, however, generally do not appear until between the 3rd and 4th weeks (Sevoian et al., 1962; Biggs and Payne, 1963, 1967; Vickers et al., 1967). When exposure is by contact with inoculated birds, the latent period is delayed by a period about equal to the time required before virus is excreted from the inoculates (Biggs and Payne, 1967). While the above figures represent the shortest incubation, there can be considerable variation. The same factors which influence the incidence of disease also affect the incubation period. These include virus strain, dosage, and route of infection as well as age, genetic strain, and sex of the host. The induction of tumors within 10 days postinoculation is suggestive of a transplantation response.

It is difficult to determine the incubation period of the disease under field conditions. While outbreaks sometimes occur in birds as young as 3–4 weeks, most of the serious cases begin after the 8th or 9th week, and it is usually impossible to determine the time and conditions of exposure.

CLINICAL SIGNS

The signs associated with Marek's disease have been described by numerous workers and well summarized by Sevoian and Chamberlain (1964), Jungherr and Hughes (1965), and Biggs (1966). In general, they are those associated with asymmetric, progressive paresis and later, complete paralysis of one or more of the extremities. Since any one or several of the nerves in the body may be affected, signs vary from one bird to another. Wing involvement is characterized by drooping of the limb. If nerves controlling the neck muscles are affected, the

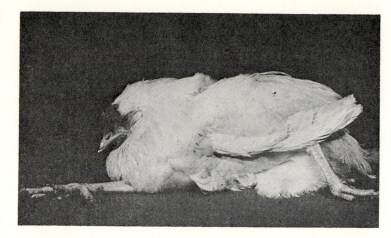

FIG. 15.4—Characteristic attitude in paralyzed chicken (note leg extension). (Courtesy H. G. Purchase, USDA Regional Poultry Laboratory, E. Lansing, Mich.)

head may be held low and there may be some torticollis. Vagal involvement can result in paralysis and dilatation of the crop and/or gasping. Because locomotory disturbances are easily recognized, incoordination or a stilted gait may be the first observed sign in an affected bird. A particularly characteristic attitude is that in which the bird has one leg stretched forward and the other backward as a result of unilateral paresis or paralysis of the leg (Fig. 15.4).

With acute outbreaks of Marek's disease, the syndrome is much more explosive and initially is characterized by a high proportion of birds with severe depression. A few days later some, but not all, birds develop ataxia and subsequently unilateral or bilateral paralysis of extremities. Others may die without extensive clinical disease. Many birds become dehydrated, emaciated, and comatose.

Blindness may result from involvement of the iris. Affected eyes gradually lose their ability to accommodate to light intensity. Clinical examination also reveals changes varying from concentric annular or spotty depigmentation or diffuse bluish fading to diffuse grayish opacity of the iris (Fig. 15.17 C). The pupil at first becomes irregular and at advanced stages is only a small pinpoint opening.

Nonspecific signs such as weight loss, paleness, anorexia, and diarrhea may be observed, especially in birds in which the course is prolonged. Under commercial conditions death often results from starvation and dehydration because of inability to reach food and water, or in many cases from trampling by pen mates.

MORBIDITY AND MORTALITY

As already pointed out, the incidence of Marek's disease is quite variable. A few of the birds which develop signs may recover from the clinical disease (Biggs and Payne, 1967), but in general, mortality is nearly equal to morbidity. A number of factors influence the extent of losses in affected flocks. These deal with either the infective agent or the host.

Those specifically related to the agent are virus strain, dosage, and route of exposure. Strains of virus associated with acute outbreaks of Marek's disease are more virulent and cause a higher disease incidence than do those associated with the so-called classical form of the disease (Biggs et al., 1965; Purchase and Biggs, 1967). Experimentally, and presumably also under natural conditions, the incidence is dose-dependent. Parenteral (intra-abdominal) administration of virus to susceptible chicks results both in a higher incidence and a shorter latent period than is observed following intranasal or oral instillation or contact exposure (Witter and Burmester, 1967).

Factors associated with the host which affect disease incidence include sex, genetic constitution, and age. Biggs and Payne (1967) and Cole (1968) observed that females experienced higher losses than males and agreed that the greater susceptibility of females was manifested in a shorter latent period. According to the former workers, the difference was apparently not due to sex hormones. Cole (1968) noticed that the difference was much less pronounced with relatively resistant strains than with susceptible strains of chickens, and Purchase and Biggs (1967) observed that the susceptibility differences between the sexes was apparent only in the case of infection with the highly virulent virus isolates. This variability would perhaps explain the fact that Pappenheimer et al. (1926) observed no association between disease incidence and sex.

Genetic factors play an important role in determining the outcome of exposure to virus and are evident in the case of both natural and experimental infection. It may be that the effects are mediated through susceptibility or resistance to infection itself, or through differences in response once infection is established, or both. Sevoian (personal communication) found the incidence of viremias in field flocks of various ages ranged from 25 to 80% and suggested that infection occurred at an early age and persisted, thus favoring the view that resistance or susceptibility is not at the level of infection. Data obtained by Spencer (1969) supported this hypothesis since differences in susceptibility of genetic lines of chickens to disease were not carried over to infection in vitro. He found kidney cell cultures from K-, C- (resistant), and S-line (susceptible) donor chickens equally susceptible to JM virus. However, Spencer (1969) and Calnek and Hitchner (1969) found that virus concentration in the kidney and the extent of distribution and concentration of viral associated antigen in a variety of tissues were directly proportional to known susceptibility to the disease. Further discussion of the role of genetic constitution is in the Prevention and Control section of this chapter.

Susceptibility to disease decreases with age, but the mechanism of this "age resistance" is unknown. Sevoian and Chamberlain (1963) titrated JM virus in three age groups of S-line chickens and found the infective dose for 14- and 26-month-old birds to be 1,000–10,000 times as great as that for day-old chicks. The pathologic response was also affected by age; neural lesions predominated in the younger birds while visceral lesions were most common in the older groups. Biggs and Payne (1967) inoculated 1-day-old and 50-day-old chickens with the B-14 isolate and observed respective incidences in the two groups of 73 and 6%. The effects of immunity and/or interference phenomena (resulting from prior infection with other viruses or relatively avirulent strains of Marek's disease virus) are not yet elucidated and could be responsible for the differences in susceptibility commonly associated with age. Field observations suggest that true age resistance either may not exist or may be overcome since severe outbreaks sometimes occur in flocks several months old.

The consistently high frequency of virus infection in commercial flocks (Sevoian, personal communication; Chubb and Churchill, 1968; Witter et al., 1969b), many of which have a low incidence of clinical disease, has led to speculation that severe outbreaks are precipitated by environmental stresses or other infectious diseases, especially coccidiosis. Thus far, no such secondary factor has been experimentally shown to influence the incidence of Marek's disease. Sublethal coccidial infection superimposed on Marek's disease-infected chicks did not increase overall mortality (Brewer et al., 1969a). Since immunological responsiveness is reduced with Marek's disease (Purchase et al., 1968), infected chickens may fail to develop immunity to other diseases. This appears to explain the association of Marek's disease with coccidiosis (Biggs et al., 1968b) and could also account for apparent relationships between Marek's disease and other diseases.

GROSS LESIONS

Nerve lesions are the most constant finding in affected birds. Macroscopic changes are not seen in the brain, but gross lesions can usually be found in one or more of the peripheral nerves and in the spinal roots and root ganglia. Lesion distribution appears to be similar for the natural and experimental diseases (Pappenheimer et al., 1926; Payne and Biggs, 1967). Goodchild (1969) made detailed macroscopic examinations of 502 birds with MD and found that certain of the autonomic nerves, as well as the more obvious nerves and plexuses, were commonly affected. Ninety-nine percent of the cases could have been diagnosed by examining only the following group: celiac, cranial mesenteric, brachial, and sciatic plexuses; the nerve of Remak; and the greater splanchnic nerve. The celiac plexus was most commonly involved; it was positive in 78% of the birds. Usually the plexuses of the sciatic and brachial nerves

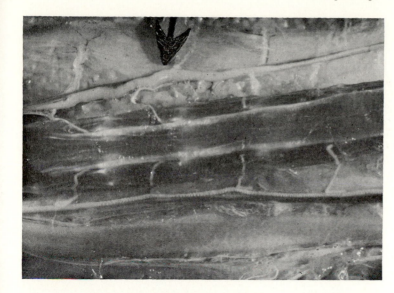

FIG. 15.5—*Enlarged leukotic cervical vagus. Affected trunk* (**arrow**) *is whitish and has lost the cross-striations evident in normal nerve trunk at bottom. (Courtesy M. C. Peckham, N.Y. State Veterinary College)*

are more enlarged than the respective trunks. Sevoian et al. (1962) found the dorsal root ganglia (DRG) consistently affected in chicks which had been inoculated with JM virus.

Affected peripheral nerves are characterized by loss of cross-striations, gray or yellow discoloration, and sometimes an edematous appearance. Localized or diffuse enlargement causes the affected portion to be 2–3 times normal size, in some cases much more. Because lesions are often unilateral, it is especially helpful to compare opposite nerves in the case of slight changes. Careful examination of the various nerve ramifications may be necessary to expose gross lesions in some birds, since enlargement can vary in degree from one portion of an affected nerve to another. Figures 15.5 and 15.6 illustrate characteristic gross changes in nerves.

Pappenheimer et al. (1926) described affected spinal root ganglia as enlarged, somewhat translucent, and of a slightly yellowish tinge. Enlargement was rarely symmetrical and lesions often extended into the contiguous tissue of the spinal cord. Ganglia may be exposed by removal of the dorsal part of the vertebral column.

Lymphoid tumors may occur in one or more of a variety of organs. The gonad (especially the ovary) is most often affected, but lymphomatous lesions can also be found in the lung, heart, mesentery, kidney, liver, spleen, adrenal, pancreas, proventriculus, intestine, iris, skeletal muscle, and skin. Probably no site is without occasion-

al involvement. Visceral tumors are especially common in the more acute forms of the disease and may be found in the absence of gross nerve lesions. Virus isolates from severe outbreaks tested by Purchase and Biggs (1967) induced visceral lesions in 62–89% of the inoculated birds. In contrast, an isolate from a milder ("classical") case of Marek's disease caused visceral lymphomata in only 5–7% of the inoculated birds.

Macroscopic changes in affected viscera, with the possible exception of the bursa of Fabricius, are indistinguishable from leu-

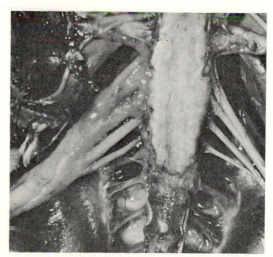

FIG. 15.6—*Leukotic sciatic plexus* (**left**) *and normal plexus* (**right**). *(Courtesy M. C. Peckham, N.Y. State Veterinary College)*

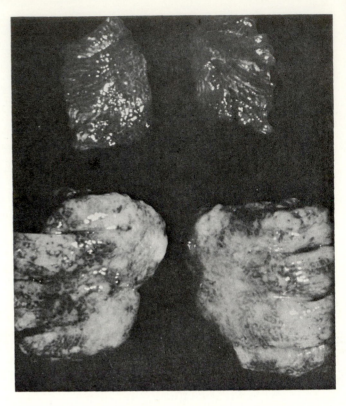

FIG. 15.7—(Top) Normal lungs. (Bottom) Lungs severely affected with Marek's disease tumors and composed mostly of leukotic tumor cells. (Courtesy H. G. Purchase, USDA Regional Poultry Laboratory, E. Lansing, Mich.)

kotic lesions induced by other agents (e.g., lymphoid leukosis virus). Enlargement, sometimes to several times normal size, is evident, and there is diffuse grayish discoloration. In some birds nodular tumorlike growths are found within and extending from the parenchyma of the organ. These are firm and smooth on cutting. Involvement of the lung results in solidification (Fig. 15.7). Diffuse infiltration of the liver causes the loss of normal lobule architecture and often gives the surface a coarse granular appearance. Lesions in the nonproducing ovary are observed as small to large grayish translucent areas. With large tumors the normal foliated appearance of the ovary is obliterated. Mature ovaries may retain function even though some follicles are tumorous (Fig. 15.8). Marked involvement is indicated by a cauliflowerlike appearance. The proventriculus becomes thickened and firm as a result of small to large leukotic areas within and between the glands. These areas may be seen through the serosal surface or on section. Affected hearts are pale from diffuse infiltration or have single or multiple nodular tumors in the myocardium (Fig. 15.9). Skin lesions

are usually associated with but not limited to feather follicles. They may coalesce. Distinct whitish nodules (Fig. 15.17A), especially evident in the dressed carcass, may become scablike with brownish crust formation in extreme cases (Benton and Cover, 1957). Muscle lesions may be in both superficial and deep layers and, according to Benton and Cover (1957), are most common in the pectoral muscles. Gross changes vary from tiny whitish streaks to nodular tumors. Affected areas are a lusterless whitish gray or may have a definite yellowish orange color (probably associated with necrosis).

The bursa of Fabricius, while usually atrophic when affected (Purchase and Biggs, 1967), may rarely develop tumors which appear as a diffuse thickening due to the interfollicular distribution of tumor cells. This lesion differs from the nodular tumor characteristic of lymphoid leukosis and may be easily differentiated histologically.

HISTOPATHOLOGY

The histopathologic changes associated with Marek's disease have been described

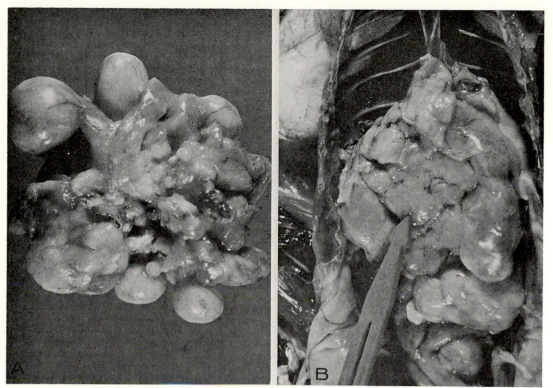

FIG. 15.8—Marek's disease tumors in mature ovary. (A) Early stage in which ovarian follicles are still present. (B) Advanced lesion in which ovary is no longer functional and is entirely replaced with tumor tissue. (Courtesy M. C. Peckham, N.Y. State Veterinary College)

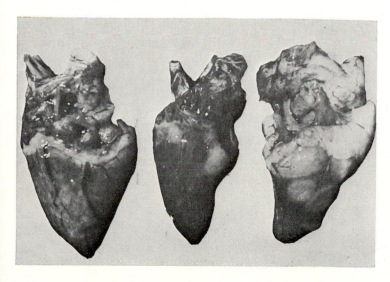

FIG. 15.9—Tumors in hearts of birds inoculated with HPRS-16 isolate of Marek's disease virus. (Courtesy H. G. Purchase, USDA Regional Poultry Laboratory, E. Lansing, Mich., and Blackwell Scientific Publications, Oxford, England)

by numerous workers who were in general agreement about the types of histologic lesions and the cell types involved (Pappenheimer et al., 1926, 1929; Furth, 1935; Campbell, 1956; Wight, 1962a,b; Payne and Biggs, 1967; Purchase and Biggs, 1967). However, the significance and interpretation of some of the histologic changes have not been so universally agreed upon.

Lesions in peripheral nerves consist of light to heavy infiltration of mononuclear cells, sometimes associated with edema, myelin degeneration, and Schwann cell proliferation. The term "infiltration" is not employed in the strict sense here because, as pointed out later, the origin of the cells is not clear. Axonal degeneration is rare. The offending cells are usually a mixture of several types including small and medium lymphocytes, plasma cells, and lymphoblasts. A few macrophages may be found. Payne and Biggs (1967) described an unusual cell with very basophilic, pyroninophilic, and vacuolated cytoplasm and a nucleus with little or no detail (Fig. 15.10D). The authors called it a "Marek's disease cell" and thought it to represent a degenerative process in a blast type cell. It was frequently seen in proliferative lesions.

Wight (1962b) quoted several reports which described the essential changes in affected nerves as an infiltration of inflammatory cells which are at first perivascular but subsequently increase in number until the nerve tissue is largely replaced by masses of cells. Wight himself classified the lesions into three types, two of which were essentially inflammatory or degenerative while the third was neoplastic. Type I lesions were characterized by cellular infiltration but relatively little edema. Most cells were small lymphocytes or plasma cells, but there were also some lymphoblasts in cases of massive infiltration. In Type II, edema was marked and only a few infiltrating cells (mostly plasma cells) were present. Fibrosis was occasionally seen. Type III was declared neoplastic because of massive infiltration with lymphoblastic cells and the observation of frequent mitoses. Sometimes there were also small lymphocytes, and some groups of these had germinal centers. All three types were considered histological variants of the same condition, but it was thought that the neoplastic changes followed the inflammatory lesions.

Payne and Biggs (1967) studied the pathogenesis of the experimental disease in chicks in order to examine the stages leading to advanced lesions. Chicks which had been inoculated at 1 day of age with the B-14 isolate developed microscopic changes which they categorized as A, B, or C type. Type A lesions were those first observed (14–21 days postinoculation) and consisted of proliferating lymphoid cells; in some cases there was demyelination and Schwann cell proliferation. "Marek's disease cells" were present. Type B lesions consisted of diffuse infiltration by plasma cells and small lymphocytes, usually with edema and sometimes with demyelination and Schwann cell proliferation. They were not seen until 28 or more days postinoculation and were sometimes mixed with A type lesions. A third lesion type (C), in which there was only a light infiltration by plasma cells and small lymphocytes, was observed in 4 of 6 clinically normal birds examined at 10 weeks. Thus, in contradiction to Wight (1962b) and others, Payne and Biggs considered the more inflammatory type changes to follow the proliferative lesions. Characteristic changes in nerves are illustrated in Figures 15.10A–C.

Histopathologic changes in the brain were described by Pappenheimer et al. (1926). Lesions were always focal in distribution and consisted of either compact perivascular cuffs of small densely staining lymphocytes (Fig. 15.11) or "submiliary nodules" composed of lymphocytes and paler elements. Jungherr and Hughes (1965) stated that the latter were probably of glial origin. The spinal cord had, in addition to

FIG. 15.10—*Microscopic lesions of Marek's disease in peripheral nerves. (A) Type A lesion characterized by marked cellular infiltration, numerous proliferating lymphoblastic cells, and no edema. H & E, ×530. (B) Type B lesion with edema, scattered infiltrating small and medium lymphocytes, plasma cells, and an occasional lymphoblast. H & E, ×530. (C) Minimal nerve lesion considered diagnostic of Marek's disease. Note very light scattering of darkly stained mononuclear cells. H & E, ×530. (D) "Marek's disease cell" (arrow) often seen in Type A lesions. H & E, ×1,600. (Fig. 15.10D courtesy C. F. Helmboldt, Univ. of Conn.)*

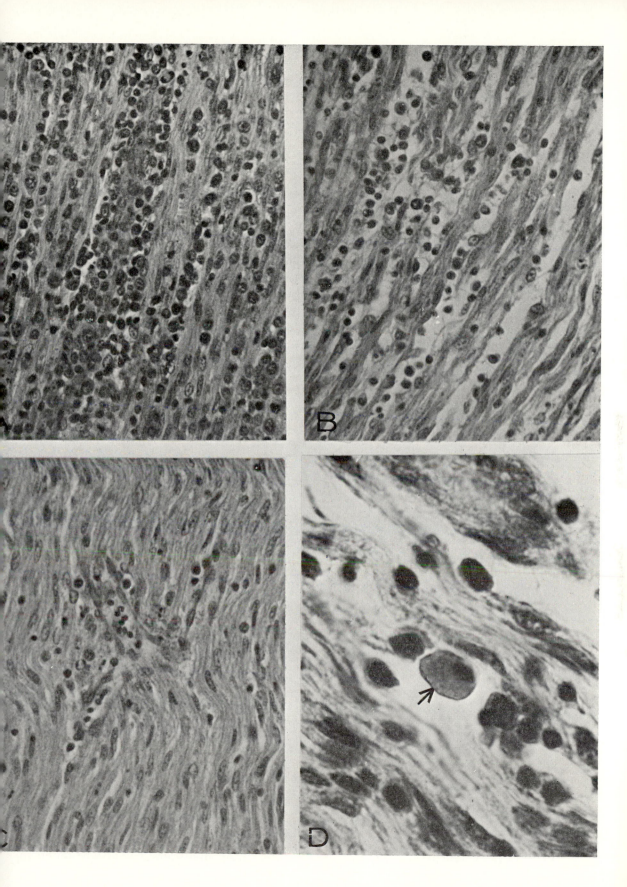

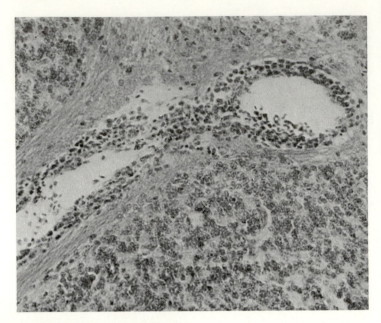

FIG. 15.11—Perivascular cuff of lymphocytes in white matter of cerebellum of MD virus-infected chicken. H & E, ×250. (Courtesy C. F. Helmboldt, Univ. of Conn.)

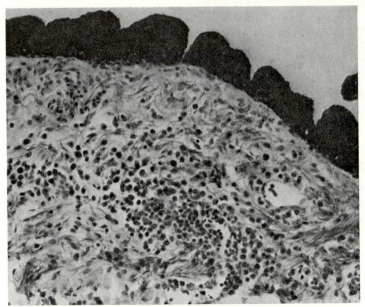

FIG. 15.12—Lymphoid cell infiltration in iris of bird with ocular lesions of Marek's disease. H & E, ×250. (Courtesy C. F. Helmboldt, Univ. of Conn.)

regional infiltrations, focal accumulations in the white matter and occasionally in the central gray matter. Root ganglia were intensely infiltrated but the ganglion cells were intact. Wight (1962a) found the central nervous system of affected birds often histologically normal or with only minimal lesions and concluded that Marek's disease is essentially a disease of peripheral nerves. He did not find plasma cells in the brain. Vickers et al. (1967) injected chicks with the CONN-A isolate of virus and noted

that central nervous system lesions, while apparent from the 2nd week postinoculation on, were most pronounced at 4–7 weeks when clinical manifestations were most severe. They observed mostly immature lymphocytes and only a few blast cells.

Jungherr and Hughes (1965) pointed out that the specific pathologic features of eye lesions are demonstrable only by histologic examination. The most constant change is mononuclear infiltration of the iris (Fig. 15.12), but infiltrates may also be found in

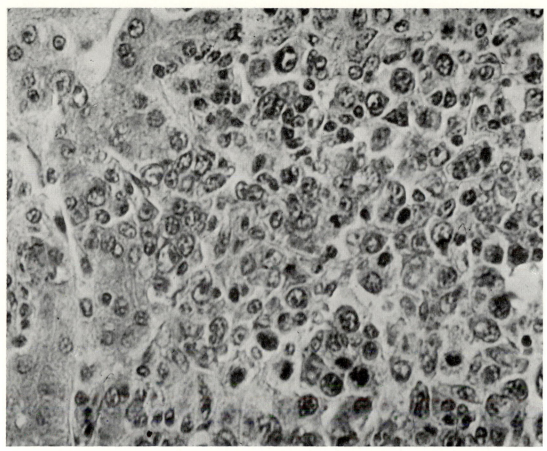

FIG. 15.13—*Liver tumor in bird with Marek's disease. Normal liver parenchymal cells may be seen on extreme left. H & E, ×3,000 (approx.). (Courtesy H. G. Purchase, USDA Regional Poultry Laboratory, E. Lansing, Mich.)*

the eye muscles, especially the *rectus lateralis* and *ciliaris*. Granular or amorphous material is sometimes present in the anterior chamber. Other but more rarely observed lesions involve the cornea (near Schlemm's canal), bulbar conjunctiva, pecten, and optic nerve. The iris and ciliary muscle lesions have been experimentally reproduced by Sevoian and Chamberlain (1962), who inoculated the JM isolate directly into the anterior chamber of the eye of day-old chicks.

Lymphomatotic lesions in the visceral organs are more uniformly proliferative in nature. The cellular composition is much like the A type lesions described for the nerves, consisting of diffusely proliferating small-to-medium lymphocytes, lymphoblasts, "Marek's disease cells," and activated and primitive reticulum cells (Payne and

Biggs, 1967). Plasma cells are rarely present (Purchase and Biggs, 1967). The composition of the tumors is the same from one organ to another even though the gross pattern of involvement may vary (Figs. 15.13, 15.14).

In contrast to the visceral lymphomas, lesions of the skin appear more inflammatory. In addition to the sometimes massive accumulations of mononuclear cells around the feather follicles, compact aggregates of proliferating cells (Fig. 15.15), often perivascular, and a few plasma cells and histiocytes are seen in the dermis (Helmboldt et al., 1963; Payne and Biggs, 1967). With small lesions the architectural integrity of the skin is maintained, but massive proliferative lesions may cause disruption of the epidermis resulting in an ulcer.

Changes in the bursa of Fabricius and

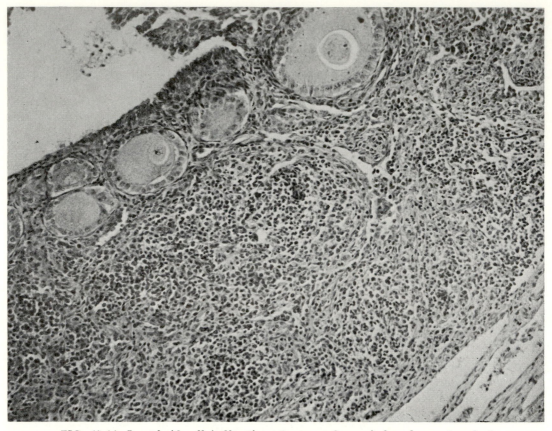

FIG. 15.14—Lymphoid cell infiltration of ovary. Organ is largely composed of tumor cells, but a few ovarian follicles can be seen in upper left portion. H & E, ×210.

FIG. 15.15—Dermal focal accumulations of mononuclear cells associated with Marek's disease. H & E, ×100. (Courtesy C. F. Helmboldt, Univ. of Conn.)

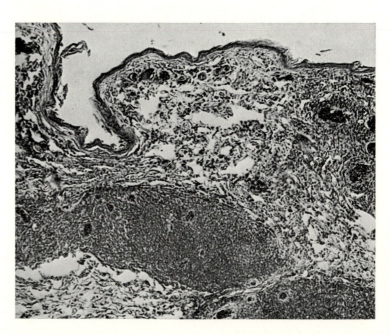

thymus of experimentally infected birds have been reported by Purchase and Biggs (1967) and Jakowski et al. (1969). In the bursa there were cortical and medullary atrophy, necrosis, cyst formation, and interfollicular lymphoid infiltration (Fig. 15.16). Atrophy of the thymus was sometimes severe and also involved both the cortex and medulla. In some cases there were areas of lymphoid proliferation in the thymus.

A number of reports quoted by Jungherr and Hughes (1965) described a mild leukocytosis in some affected birds, but this appeared neither of diagnostic significance (because of normal hematological irregularities) nor of statistical significance (when compared with the blood picture in nonaffected birds). Sevoian and Chamberlain (1964), in the course of their pathogenesis studies, found few changes in the blood. A slight decrease in the erythrocyte count occurred from the 7th to 12th days, and a transient leukopenia was observed at 2 days postinoculation. Some birds in terminal stages of the disease had elevated leukocyte counts (principally of the lymphoid series). Bone marrow changes in the form of multiple tumor nodules within the marrow were observed beginning at 10 days postinoculation. Purchase and Biggs (1967), on the other hand, observed no significant lesions in the bone marrow of affected birds.

Jakowski et al. (1970) observed that when chickens free of parental antibody were inoculated with MD virus at 1 day of age, necrosis and loss of architecture in the bursa of Fabricius and thymus were accompanied by a drastic reduction in packed cell volume and an aplasia of bone marrow.

The origin of the infiltrating cells is a point upon which there is not agreement. Biggs (1967) considered that Marek's disease was primarily a lymphoid disease with the infiltrating cells showing a predilection for nerve tissue, and Payne and Biggs (1967) pointed out that the earliest changes involved cells of the lymphoid series. They did, however, acknowledge that there might be primary changes in the nerves which cannot be seen with ordinary light microscopy but which stimulate lymphoid cells. Wight (1969), in a study of the ultrastructure of affected nerves, noted early and prominent changes in Schwann cells. Ubertini and Calnek (1970) likewise observed changes in those cells and also found them infected with herpesvirus. They supported

the hypothesis that infection of Schwann cells could result in an inflammatory response characterized by round cell infiltration. Sevoian and Chamberlain (1964) thought that the nerve changes resulted from proliferation of neurilemmal cells followed by differentiation to lymphoid cells. Proliferated cells originating from the primitive mesenchymal cells of the tunica adventitia of the arterioles and the lining cells of hepatic sinusoids also apparently differentiated to lymphoid cells and accounted for lesions in other organs.

Campbell (1956) and Wight (1962b) agreed with Marek's early interpretation of the inflammatory nature of the disease. Both recognized that some nerve lesions were neoplastic, but the latter author thought they represented only a rare sequel to the inflammatory lesions. Pappenheimer et al. (1926), on the other hand, considered the basic response to be neoplastic and thought there was some kind of transition between that and the inflammatory lesions. Furth (1935) supported that concept by regarding the inflammatory and degenerative changes as secondary to neoplastic infiltrations. Pathogenesis studies led Payne and Biggs (1967) to essentially the same conclusion, and they felt obliged to classify the pathological changes in birds which succumbed to A type nerve lesions and visceral lymphomata as neoplastic. In support they cited the following criteria: (1) progressive proliferation, (2) qualitative and quantitative differences in the lymphoid infiltrations as compared to those in lymphoid hyperplasia resulting from many other infections in fowl, (3) multifocal and diffuse origin, and (4) possibly abnormal cells. They further observed that the more virulent isolates of Marek's disease virus induced macroscopic lymphoid tumors in most birds. With the notable exception of Campbell (1956), who described the lymphoproliferative ovarian lesions as lymphogranulomas, there has been rather good agreement that the visceral lesions are neoplastic.

Wight and Siller (1965) compared paralyzed birds with apparently healthy birds and found them less susceptible to an inoculum which induced experimental allergic encephalomyelitis. They speculated that Marek's disease might be an autoimmune disease even though the initial excitant could be a virus. Ringen and Akhtar (1968)

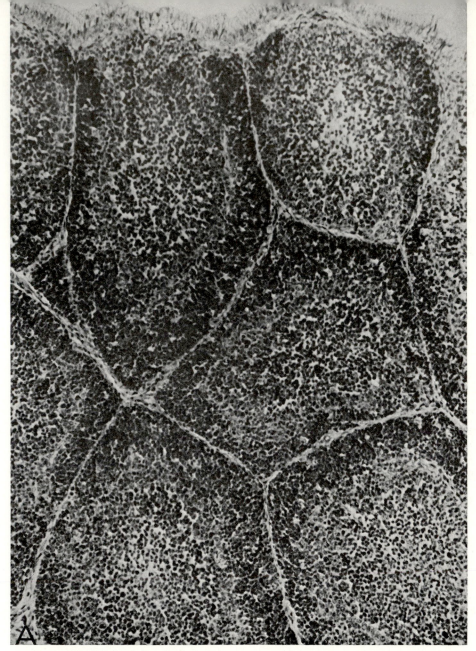

FIG. 15.16—Changes in bursa of Fabricius associated with Marek's disease. (A) Normal bursal follicles in chicken killed at 15 days of age. Note uniform architecture. (B) Cystic and necrotic follicles in atrophied bursa from chicken killed

observed that the presence of lymphocytes and plasma cells in affected nerves and remission of clinical signs following treatment with cortisone are also characteristics of other so-called autoimmune diseases. Furthermore, immunosuppression elicited by bursectomy or chemical means reduced the disease incidence in experimentally infected chickens (Payne and Biggs, 1967; Foster and Moll, 1968).

While little is actually known about the role of immunity in Marek's disease, it appears that an immune-type response does occur after exposure to the virus. Natural antibodies directed against herpesvirus-associated antigens have been demonstrated by several workers (Chubb and Churchill, 1968; Spencer, 1969; Purchase, 1969). The

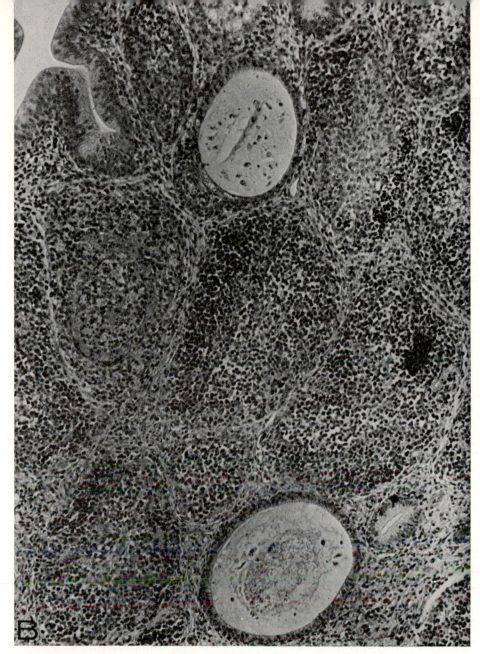

28 days after inoculation with HPRS-16 isolate of MD virus. H & E, ×200. (Courtesy H. G. Purchase, USDA Regional Poultry Laboratory, E. Lansing, Mich., and Blackwell Scientific Publications, Oxford, England)

presence of antibody in a large proportion of apparently normal birds from nearly all commercial flocks indicates that exposure is widespread and that most birds are competent to develop specific antibody. The same antibodies are observed in the blood of day-old chicks (probably acquired from the dam through the egg) but are depleted by about 3 weeks after hatching. Actively acquired antibodies may appear by 4–5 weeks of age in exposed birds (Chubb and Churchill, 1968; Purchase, 1969). Chubb and Churchill (1968) found that chicks with parental antibodies were not refractory to infection following contact exposure. However, the comparative susceptibility to tumor induction of chicks possessing or lacking parental antibody has not been reported.

Nonetheless, the phenomenon of "age resistance" (possibly a reflection of acquired immunity) and the observation that chicks reared in a contaminated environment may experience lower MD losses than chicks reared in a sanitary environment indirectly support the concept that an immune response may be influential. Further support came from Sevoian (personal communication), who inoculated dams with JM-infected cells and observed in their progeny some resistance to contact exposure. Churchill et al. (1969) determined that administration of a nonpathogenic MD virus to young chicks afforded measurable protection against later challenge with virulent virus. However, the basis for this protective effect was not clear.

Marek's disease has an effect on the bursal and thymic lymphoid systems (Payne and Biggs, 1967), both of which play a role in immunological competence in birds (Cooper et al., 1966). Bursal damage and thymic atrophy in severely affected birds are apparently the respective causes of reduced antibody production and delayed skin rejection (Purchase et al., 1968). Biggs et al. (1968) showed that Marek's disease infection could increase susceptibility to primary and secondary infection with coccidia, perhaps further evidence that the general immunologic function of birds is depressed. While there may be depression, there is certainly not a loss of function. Purchase et al. (1968) found that the ability to synthesize specific antibody (to bovine serum albumin) was decreased in infected birds, but there was no lowering in total levels of 7S or 19S gamma globulins. In fact, Ringen and Akhtar (1968), Howard et al. (1967), and Samadieh et al. (1969) all found elevated levels of gamma globulin associated with clinical signs of Marek's disease.

In connection with the observed effects of Marek's disease on the thymic and bursal systems, it is of interest to consider the influence of these organs on the development of the disease. According to Payne and Biggs (1967), who quoted the unpublished data of Payne, Witter, and Burmester, bursectomy coupled with X-irradiation reduced the incidence but did not eliminate the disease in exposed birds. This is in contrast to the situation with lymphoid leukosis wherein the bursa of Fabricius is requisite to the development of the disease. Thymectomy along with X-irradiation was of no influence on Marek's disease incidence.

DIAGNOSIS

ISOLATION AND IDENTIFICATION OF CAUSATIVE AGENT

The inoculation of chicks is the most sensitive method currently available for isolation and assay of virus. Due to variations among test chicks, housing facilities, and requirements for sensitivity, a standard technique has not been described. In general, test chicks from a susceptible source such as Regional Poultry Research Laboratory Line 7 or Cornell S-line should be exposed (by intraperitoneal inoculation or other suitable means) during the 1st week after hatching. Test lots should be strictly isolated to prevent infection from an adventitious source. After 2–10 weeks postinoculation the exposed chicks and appropriate positive and negative controls are examined for evidence of infection. Gross or microscopic lesions, virus isolation in cell culture, positive fluorescent antibody (FA) tests on tissues, or detection of antibody are all suitable criteria of infection in inoculated chicks. The specificity of all responses, particularly those based on microscopic lesions, should be ascertained, since lymphoid lesions which resemble those of MD may be induced by unrelated antigens including the ubiquitous virus of lymphoid leukosis (Calnek, 1968) and reticuloendotheliosis virus (Witter et al., 1970c).

Interpretation of minimal histologic lesions is highly subjective, and accurate guidelines have not been developed. Minor accumulations of lymphoid cells in peripheral nerves (Fig. 15.10C) and perivascular cuffs of lymphoid cells in the white matter of the cerebellar folia (Fig. 15.11) are considered useful diagnostic criteria by some workers. Specific bioassay procedures and their application in different laboratories have been described (Biggs and Payne, 1967; Spencer and Calnek, 1967; Kottaridis et al., 1968; Witter et al., 1968b, 1969b).

Tissue culture methods for isolation and assay of virus, although 40–1,000-fold less sensitive than chick inoculation (Biggs et al., 1968a; Witter et al., 1969a), are valuable by virtue of their relative simplicity. Cultures of duck embryo fibroblasts or chick kidney cells are prepared, incubated at 37° C, and inoculated when confluent.

Buffy coat cells, tumor cells, trypsinized kidney cells, or blood appear most suitable as inocula for isolation attempts. After 24–48 hours the inoculum is washed off and the culture maintained, usually without subculture. The development of typical MD herpesvirus plaques in inoculated cultures (Fig. 15.2) within 5–14 days, in the absence of such changes in comparable uninoculated control cultures, is evidence for the isolation of MD virus. Known infected inoculum should be used to determine the susceptibility of the test cultures.

Direct cultivation of kidney cells from a test chicken appears even more sensitive for herpesvirus isolation than inoculation of its blood onto a normal monolayer (Wit-

FIG. 15.17—(A) Leukotic tumors involving the feather follicles (skin leukosis). (Courtesy S. C. Schmittle, Vantress Farms, Duluth, Ga.) (B) Fluorescent antibody test in which herpesvirus infection of JM-inoculated chicken kidney cell culture is detected with fluorescein-conjugated antiserum. Infected cells appear bright green. ×640. (Courtesy H. G. Purchase, USDA Regional Poultry Laboratory, E. Lansing, Mich.) (C) Ocular lesions of Marek's disease. Note that normal eye on left has a sharply defined pupil and well-pigmented iris. Affected eye (right) has a discolored iris and very irregular pupil as a result of mononuclear cell infiltration. (Courtesy M. C. Peckham, New York State Veterinary College, Ithaca, N.Y.) (D) Virus-infected cells in the follicular epithelium lining of feather follicle. Cells containing herpesvirus-associated antigens fluoresce bright green after treatment with fluorescein-conjugated antiserum. ×640. (E) and (F) Methyl green pyronin stained smears of tumor cells from chickens with lymphoid leukosis (E) and Marek's disease (F). Lymphoid leukosis smear was from a bursal tumor in a bird inoculated 144 days earlier with RPL 12 isolate of lymphoid leukosis virus. Note the preponderance of uniformly large lymphoblastic cells (large nucleus, prominent nucleolus, abundant cytoplasm). The cells are characterized by the red staining (pyroninophilic, RNA-containing) cytoplasm. Marek's disease smear was from gonadal tumor in 6-week-old bird infected with JM isolate of MD virus. Note the varied cell population: lymphoblasts, small and medium lymphocytes. Only a few of the cells are characterized by pyroninophilic cytoplasm. Both smears ×700 approx. (Courtesy F. J. Siccardi, Campbell Soup, Fayetteville, Ark.)

ter et al., 1969a). The identity of a suspected isolate may be confirmed by the reproduction of Marek's disease in chicks inoculated with the infected culture. Further details on cell culture procedures are given by Churchill and Biggs (1968), Calnek and Madin (1969), and Witter et al. (1969a).

Identification of the causative agent may also be made by means of a fluorescent antibody test in which conjugated antiserum (directed against herpesvirus-associated antigen) is applied to frozen tissue sections from the test bird (Fig. 15.17B) (Spencer, 1969). This method appears to be sensitive and reliable and can detect virus infection in birds which are not considered positive by other criteria (Calnek and Hitchner, 1969). Examination of a single piece of deplumed skin from one of the feather tracts is particularly suitable, because antigen occurs most frequently and apparently persists in the cells lining the feather follicle (Fig. 15.17D).

SEROLOGY

Serologic evidence of MD infection can be obtained by the agar gel precipitin test (Chubb and Churchill, 1968), the indirect fluorescent antibody test (Spencer, 1969; Purchase and Burgoyne, 1970), or the indirect hemagglutination tests (Eidson and Schmittle, 1969). It is not known, however, whether the antibodies detected in these tests are directed toward the viral antigens or toward other virus-associated antigens produced by infected cells.

In the agar gel precipitin test, sera are reacted with antigen in an agar medium containing 8% sodium chloride. The antigen is prepared from heavily infected (nearly confluent MD virus plaques) chicken kidney or duck embryo fibroblast cultures. Cells from infected cultures are suspended ($1–4 \times 10^7$ cells/ml) and frozen and thawed 3 times. Development of precipitin lines (either single or multiple) between wells containing the reagents is evidence for the presence of antibody in the test serum. The specificity of the test should be ascertained through the use of positive and negative control serum and control antigen similarly made from uninoculated tissue cultures.

In the indirect fluorescent antibody test a suitable antigen (i.e., coverslip-cultured cells containing MD-virus plaques) is reacted with test serum and then with a suitable dilution of fluorescein-conjugated antiserum directed against chicken gamma globulin. Fluorescent staining, particularly of the round cells of the focal lesions (Fig. 15.17D), is evidence for antibody in the test serum—provided the antigen does not autofluoresce and the chicken anti-globulin conjugate does not stain the untreated antigen. Positive and negative control sera should be used.

The indirect hemagglutination test is carried out by reacting serum with tanned erythrocytes which have been treated with herpesvirus-associated antigen.

Since antigenic differences between isolates have not been reported, suitable antigens for both tests may apparently be made from any low-passage isolate. Purchase (1969) noted cross-reactivity of sera directed against various virus isolates.

DIFFERENTIAL DIAGNOSIS

Lymphoid leukosis is the principal disease to be considered in the differential diagnosis of MD, since these two etiologically distinct diseases are widespread and are characterized in part by similar gross lesions. Other diseases which may present confusing gross lesions or paralytic signs are riboflavin deficiency, myeloblastosis, erythroblastosis, reticuloendotheliosis, carcinoma of the ovary, other neoplasms, tuberculosis, histomoniasis, dermatitis, genetic gray eye, Newcastle disease, avian encephalomyelitis, perosis, and joint infections or injuries.

The inconsistency of pathognomonic gross lesions has necessitated consideration of other criteria in the postmortem diagnosis of MD, principally age and lesion distribution. Chickens may be diagnosed positive for Marek's disease if one or more of the following conditions are met: (1) leukotic enlargement of peripheral nerves or spinal ganglia; (2) iris discoloration and pupil irregularity, as in Figure 15.17C; (3) lymphoid tumors in various tissues (e.g., liver, heart, gonad, skin, muscle, proventriculus) in birds under 18 weeks of age; or (4) visceral lymphoid tumors in birds 18 weeks or older which lack neoplastic involvement of the bursa of Fabricius. Some assumptions critical to these criteria are the absence of bursal tumors in cases of MD in birds older than 18 weeks, the invariable presence of gross bursal tumors in cases of lymphoid leukosis, and the occur-

rence of lymphoid leukosis or other unrelated tumors only in birds older than 18 weeks. Although these assumptions are not invariably correct, diagnostic errors with these criteria should be infrequent provided that necropsies are done with care. Proper examination of the bursa is particularly important and requires incision of the organ with close inspection of the epithelial surface. Since gross lymphoproliferative lesions which are unrelated to MD have been observed in visceral tissues of young chickens (Calnek, 1968) and may also occur in other tissues such as the skin, care should be exercised in rendering diagnoses of MD based on minimal gross changes. However, specific guidelines are not available.

Diagnostic accuracy may be enhanced considerably by the employment of histological or cytological procedures. The mixed population of small to large lymphocytes, lymphoblasts, plasma cells, and "Marek's disease cells" differs substantially from the cell populations of lymphoid leukosis and reticuloendotheliosis tumors (composed largely of lymphoblasts and reticulum cells respectively). These diagnostic features may be seen in routine histologic sections stained with hematoxylin and eosin. However, examination of "touch" preparations taken directly from lesions of freshly killed birds and stained with methyl green pyronin or Shorr's stain gives better cytologic detail and can be prepared in a few minutes. Lymphoblasts of lymphoid leukosis tumors are uniformly pyroninophilic, whereas this is observed infrequently in cells of MD tumors (Siccardi and Burmester, 1970). Cytologic differences between MD and lymphoid leukosis tumors are illustrated in Figures 15.17E, F.

A summary of the essential pathologic differences between Marek's disease and lymphoid leukosis is found in Table 15.6 in the subchapter which deals with lymphoid leukosis.

TREATMENT

There is no effective, practical treatment for Marek's disease, either in flocks or in individual chickens. However, the ameliorative effect of immunosuppressant drugs on the disease (Foster and Moll, 1968) and the phenomenon of lesion regression (Wight, 1965; Payne and Biggs, 1967;

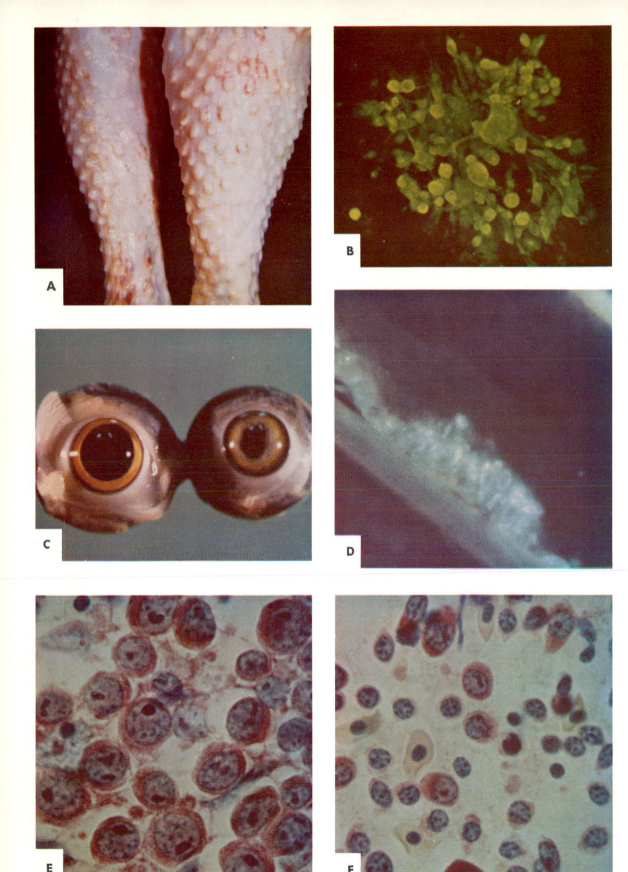

Schmittle and Aigster, personal communication), which has been particularly notable in cases of so-called "skin leukosis" under natural conditions, give some hope that future studies in this area could be fruitful.

PREVENTION AND CONTROL

No greater enigma in the study of Marek's disease has been encountered to date than the futility of procedures employed for practical control of the disease. This is amply supported by the remarkable increase in the incidence of MD in commercial flocks in recent years. Certain currently used or recommended procedures are described herein; however, more effective measures are urgently needed.

GENETIC RESISTANCE

Several lines of chickens with genetic resistance to MD have been selected and maintained experimentally (Hutt and Cole, 1948, 1957; Cole, 1968). Such chickens are relatively refractory to overt manifestations of MD (e.g., clinical signs, death, and gross lesions) but are apparently susceptible to virus infection. This resistance is effective against both natural exposure and inoculation with a wide spectrum of MD isolates. MD resistance appears independent of genetic factors which control production traits or resistance to lymphoid leukosis (Biggs et al., 1968c; Crittenden, 1968). The variation of MD susceptibility in single-sire families indicated that there was sufficient heterogeneity to warrant selection for resistance in commercial chickens (Cole, 1968; Biggs et al., 1968c). In fact, resistance of lines or families can be determined quantitatively (Sevoian, 1968b). Cole (1968) selected breeders (of a random-bred flock) through 2 generations by determining whose progeny were most refractory to inoculation with the JM isolate. This resulted in a "resistant line" from which only 13% of progeny were susceptible to JM challenge compared to 51% of the progeny of the unselected population. Similar selection procedures have been recently employed in commercial breeding operations, but as yet the resistance of commercial chicks has not been increased sufficiently to provide a satisfactory measure of control. Further progress can be expected but

undoubtedly will be less rapid than that achieved experimentally.

ISOLATION AND SANITATION

Isolation rearing and environmental sanitation have been widely advocated for the control of MD. These principles are founded on the assumption that virus-free chicks placed in a clean environment and isolated from subsequent exposure will remain free of disease. However, the application of these principles to commercial flocks has met with only limited success, probably because current procedures are inadequate for decontaminating the environment or preventing reintroduction of infection, particularly by the airborne route.

On the other hand, small groups of chicks from infected breeder flocks have been maintained free of infection for substantial periods using very strict isolation under laboratory conditions (Solomon et al., 1970). The practical value of this approach was emphasized by Drury et al. (1969) who successfully reared large groups of chickens free of MD in specially designed poultry houses ventilated with filtered air under positive pressure (FAPP). These FAPP houses were thoroughly cleaned, disinfected, and fumigated prior to use, and strict quarantine procedures were employed for all personnel. This procedure may have great potential value for the control or eradication of MD, but as yet its feasibility has not been established.

A modification of this procedure, employing FAPP rearing for the first 3 weeks, has been used experimentally to reduce condemnations in commercial broiler flocks (Eidson and Anderson, personal communication). Presumably this technique delays the onset of infection which under field conditions has been detected as early as the 9th day (Witter et al., 1970a).

VACCINATION

Despite the lack of direct evidence that chickens acquire a protective immunity through exposure, the isolation of the causative virus and the several aforementioned characteristics of MD which suggest an immune response to virus infection have stimulated considerable research on an MD vaccine. The first significant findings toward this end followed the apparent attenuation of an isolate of MD virus by continued cell culture passage. "Attenuated" virus (Churchill et al., 1969a) inoculated into young chicks rendered them less susceptible than uninoculated birds to challenge several weeks later with virulent virus from the same original isolate (Churchill et al., 1969b). Similarly, Kottaridis and Luginbuhl (1969) observed that chicken embryo fibroblasts, which had been inoculated in vitro with MD virus-infected bone marrow cells, induced a protective effect upon inoculation into young chicks. The nature of resistance in either case was undetermined.

Witter et al. (1970b) isolated a cell-associated herpesvirus from turkeys (HVT) which was found to be apathogenic for chickens but antigenically related to the MD herpesvirus. This virus, administered intraabdominally at 1 day of age, gave substantial protection against later challenge with MD virus (Okazaki et al., 1970). On the basis of these and other studies, HVT is presently considered as a strong candidate virus to serve as a vaccine for the control of MD.

REFERENCES

AAAP Report. 1967. Report of the American Association of Avian Pathologists-Sponsored Leukosis Workshop. *Avian Diseases* 11:694–702.

Ahmed, M., and G. Schidlovsky. 1968. Electron microscopic localization of herpesvirus-type particles in Marek's disease. *J. Virol.* 2:1443–57.

Andrewes, C. H., and R. E. Glover. 1939. A case of neurolymphomatosis in a turkey. *Vet. Record* 51:934–35.

Baxendale, W. 1969. Preliminary observations on Marek's disease in ducks and other avian species. *Vet. Record* 85:341–42.

Beasley, J. N., L. T. Patterson, and D. H. McWade. 1970. Transmission of Marek's disease by poultry house dust and chicken dander. *Am. J. Vet. Res.* 31:339–44.

Benton, W. J., and M. S. Cover. 1957. The increased incidence of visceral lymphomatosis in broiler and replacement birds. *Avian Diseases* 1:320–27.

Benton, W. J., M. S. Cover, and W. C. Krauss. 1962. The incidence of avian leukosis in broilers at processing. *Avian Diseases* 6:430–35.

Biggs, P. M. 1961. A discussion on the classification of the avian leucosis complex and fowl paralysis. *Brit. Vet. J.* 117:326–34.

———. 1962. Some observations on the properties of cells from the lesions of Marek's disease and lymphoid leukosis. *Proc. 13th Symp. Colston Res. Soc.*, pp. 83–99.

———. 1966. Avian leukosis and Marek's disease. Thirteenth World's Poultry Congr., Symp. Papers, pp. 91–118.

———. 1967. Marek's disease. *Vet. Record* 81:583–92.

———. 1968. Marek's disease—Current state of knowledge. *Current Topics Microbiol. Immunol.* 43:93–125.

Biggs, P. M., and L. N. Payne. 1963. Transmission experiments with Marek's disease (fowl paralysis). *Vet. Record* 75:177–79.

———. 1964. The relationship of Marek's disease (neurolymphomatosis) to lymphoid leucosis. *Nat. Cancer Inst. Monograph* 17:83–98.

———. 1967. Studies on Marek's disease. I. Experimental transmission. *J. Nat. Cancer Inst.* 39:267–80.

Biggs, P. M., H. G. Purchase, B. R. Bee, and P. J. Dalton. 1965. Preliminary report on acute Marek's disease (fowl paralysis) in Great Britain. *Vet. Record* 77:1339–40.

Biggs, P. M., A. E. Churchill, D. G. Rootes, and R. C. Chubb. 1968a. The etiology of Marek's disease—An oncogenic herpes-type virus. *Perspectives Virol.* 6:211–37.

Biggs, P. M., P. L. Long, S. G. Kenzy, and D. G. Rootes. 1968b. Relationship between Marek's disease and coccidiosis. II. The effect of Marek's disease on the susceptibility of chickens to coccidial infection. *Vet. Record* 83:284–89.

Biggs, P. M., R. J. Thorpe, and L. N. Payne. 1968c. Studies on genetic resistance to Marek's disease in the domestic chicken. *Brit. Poultry Sci.* 9:37–52.

Brewer, R. N., W. M. Reid, and H. Botero. 1969a. Studies on acute Marek's disease. The role of coccidia in transmission and induction. *Poultry Sci.* 47:2003–12.

Brewer, R. N., W. M. Reid, Joyce Johnson, and S. C. Schmittle. 1969b. Studies on acute Marek's disease. VIII. The role of mosquitoes in transmission under experimental conditions. *Avian Diseases* 13:83–88.

Calnek, B. W. 1968. Lesions in young chickens induced by lymphoid leukosis virus. *Avian Diseases* 12:111–29.

Calnek, B. W., and S. B. Hitchner. 1969. Localization of viral antigen in chickens infected with Marek's disease herpesvirus. *J. Nat. Cancer Inst.* 43:935–49.

Calnek, B. W., and S. H. Madin. 1969. Characteristics of the in vitro infection of chicken kidney cell cultures with a herpesvirus from Marek's disease. *Am. J. Vet. Res.* 30:1389–1402.

Calnek, B. W., S. H. Madin, and J. Kniazeff. 1969. Susceptibility of cultured mammalian cells to infection with a herpesvirus from Marek's disease and T-virus from reticuloendotheliosis of chickens. *Am. J. Vet. Res.* 30:1403–12.

Calnek, B. W., H. K. Adldinger, and D. E. Kahn. 1970a. Feather follicle epithelium: A source of enveloped and infectious cell-free herpesvirus from Marek's disease. *Avian Diseases* 14:219–33.

Calnek, B. W., T. Ubertini, and H. K. Adldinger. 1970b. Viral antigen, virus particles, and infectivity of tissues from chickens with Marek's disease. *J. Nat. Cancer Inst.* 45:341–52.

Campbell, J. G. 1956. Leucosis and fowl paralysis compared and contrasted. *Vet. Record* 68:527–28.

Chomiak, T. W., R. E. Luginbuhl, C. F. Helmboldt, and S. D. Kottaridis. 1967. Marek's disease. I. Propagation of the Connecticut A (Conn-A) isolate in chicks. *Avian Diseases* 11:646–53.

Chubb, R. C., and A. E. Churchill. 1968. Precipitating antibodies associated with Marek's disease. *Vet. Record* 83:4–7.

Churchill, A. E. 1968. Herpes-type virus isolated in cell culture from tumors of chickens with Marek's disease. I. Studies in cell culture. *J. Nat. Cancer Inst.* 41:939–50.

Churchill, A. E., and P. M. Biggs. 1967. Agent of Marek's disease in tissue culture. *Nature* 215:528–30.

———. 1968. Herpes-type virus isolated in cell culture from tumors of chickens with Marek's disease. II. Studies in vivo. *J. Nat. Cancer Inst.* 41:951–56.

Churchill, A. E., R. C. Chubb, and W. Baxendale. 1969a. The attenuation, with loss of oncogenicity of the herpes-type virus of Marek's disease (strain HPRS-16) on passage in cell culture. *J. Gen. Virol.* 4:557–64.

Churchill, A. E., L. N. Payne, and R. C. Chubb. 1969b. Immunization against Marek's disease using a live attenuated virus. *Nature* 221:744–47.

Cole, R. K. 1949. The egg and avian leucosis. *Poultry Sci.* 28:31–44.

———. 1968. Studies on genetic resistance to Marek's disease. *Avian Diseases* 12:9–28.

Cole, R. K., and F. B. Hutt. 1951. Evidence that eggs do not transmit leucosis. *Poultry Sci.* 30:205–12.

Colwell, W. M., and S. C. Schmittle. 1968. Studies on acute Marek's disease. VII. Airborne transmission of the GA isolate. *Avian Diseases* 12:724–29.

Cooper, M. D., R. D. A. Peterson, M. A. South, and R. A. Good. 1966. The functions of the thymus system and the bursa system in the chicken. *J. Exp. Med.* 123:75–102.

Crittenden, L. B. 1968. Avian tumor viruses: Prospects for control. *World's Poultry Sci. J.* 24:18–36.

Doyle, L. P. 1926. Neuritis in chickens. *J. Am. Vet. Med. Ass.* 68:622–30.

Drury, L. N., W. C. Patterson, and C. W. Beard. 1969. Ventilating poultry houses with filtered air under positive pressure to prevent airborne diseases. *Poultry Sci.* 48:1640–46.

Dunlop, W. R., S. D. Kottaridis, J. R. Gallagher, S. C. Smith, and R. G. Strout. 1965. The detection of acute avian leucosis as a contagious disease. *Poultry Sci.* 44:1537–40.

Eidson, C. S., and S. C. Schmittle. 1968. Studies on acute Marek's disease. I. Characteristics of isolate GA in chickens. *Avian Diseases* 12:467–75.

———. 1969. Studies on acute Marek's disease. XII. Detection of antibodies with a tannic acid indirect hemagglutination test. *Avian Diseases* 13:774–82.

Eidson, C. S., S. C. Schmittle, R. B. Goode, and J. B. Lal. 1966. Induction of leukosis tumors with the beetle *Alphitobius diaperinus. Am. J. Vet. Res.* 27:1053–57.

Epstein, M. A., B. G. Achong, A. E. Churchill, and P. M. Biggs. 1968. Structure and development of the herpes-type virus of Marek's disease. *J. Nat. Cancer Inst.* 41:805–20.

Foster, A. G., and T. Moll. 1968. Effect of immunosuppression on clinical and pathologic manifestations of Marek's disease in chickens. *Am. J. Vet. Res.* 29:1831–35.

Furth, J. 1935. Lymphomatosis in relation to fowl paralysis. *Arch. Pathol.* 20:329–428.

Goodchild, W. M. 1969. Some observations on Marek's disease (fowl paralysis). *Vet. Record* 84:87–89.

Harriss, S. T. 1939. Lymphomatosis (fowl paralysis) in the pheasant. *Vet. J.* 95:104–6.

Helmboldt, C. F., F. K. Wills, and M. N. Frazier. 1963. Field observations of the pathology of skin leukosis in *Gallus gallus. Avian Diseases* 7:402–11.

Howard, E. B., C. Jannke, J. Vickers, and A. J. Kenyon. 1967. Elevated gamma globulin levels in Marek's disease (neural lymphomatosis) of domestic fowl. *Cornell Vet.* 57:183–94.

Hutt, F. B., and R. K. Cole. 1947. Genetic control of lymphomatosis in the fowl. *Science* 106:379–84.

———. 1948. The development of strains genetically resistant to avian lymphomatosis. *Proc. 8th World's Poultry Congr.,* pp. 719–25.

———. 1957. Control of leukosis in fowl. *J. Am. Vet. Med. Ass.* 131:491–95.

Jakowski, R. M., T. N. Frederickson, R. E. Luginbuhl, and C. F. Helmboldt. 1969. Early changes in bursa of Fabricius from Marek's disease. *Avian Diseases* 13:215–22.

Jakowski, R. M., T. N. Fredrickson, T. W. Chomiak, and R. E. Luginbuhl. 1970.

Hematopoietic destruction in Marek's disease. *Avian Diseases* 14:274–85.

Johnson, E. P. 1941. Fowl leukosis—Manifestations, transmission, and etiological relationship of various forms. *Virginia Agr. Expt. Sta. Tech. Bull.* 76.

Jungherr, E. 1939. *Neurolymphomatosis phasianorum. J. Am. Vet. Med. Ass.* 94:49–52.

Jungherr, E., and W. F. Hughes. 1965. The avian leukosis complex, pp. 512–67. In Biester, H. E., and L. H. Schwarte (eds.), *Diseases of Poultry,* 5th ed. Iowa State Univ. Press, Ames.

Jurajda, V., and B. Klimes. 1970. Presence and survival of Marek's disease agent in dust. *Avian Diseases* 14:188–90.

Kaupp, B. F. 1921. Paralysis of the domestic fowl. *J. Am. Ass. Instructors Investigators Poultry Husbandry* 7:25–31.

Kenzy, S. G., and P. M. Biggs. 1967. Excretion of the Marek's disease agent by infected chickens. *Vet. Record* 80:565–68.

Kenzy, S. C., and B. R. Cho. 1969. Transmission of classical Marek's disease by affected and carrier birds. *Avian Diseases* 13:211–14.

Kottaridis, S. D., and R. E. Luginbuhl. 1969. Control of Marek's disease by the use of inoculated chicken embryo fibroblasts. *Nature* 221:1258–59.

Kottaridis, S. D., R. E. Luginbuhl, and T. N. Fredrickson. 1968. Marek's disease. II. Propagation of the Connecticut-A isolate in cell cultures. *Avian Diseases* 12:246–58.

Long, P. L., S. G. Kenzy, and P. M. Biggs. 1968. Relationship between Marek's disease and coccidiosis. I. Attempted transmission of Marek's disease by avian coccidia. *Vet. Record* 83:260–62.

Marek, J. 1907. Multiple Nervenentzuendung (Polyneuritis) bei Huehnern. *Deut. Tieraerztl. Wochschr.* 15:417–21.

Morgan, C., M. Rose, M. Holden, and E. Jones. 1959. Electron microscopic observations on the development of Herpes simplex virus. *J. Exp. Med.* 110:643–56.

Nakagawa, M. 1965. Pathological studies on fowl paralysis—the relationship between lesions in the nervous system and those in the visceral organs. *Japan. J. Vet. Res.* 13:55–56.

Nazerian, K. 1968. Electron microscopy of a herpesvirus isolated from Marek's disease in duck and chicken embryo fibroblast culture. *Proc. Electron Microscop. Soc. Am., 26th Ann. Meet.,* pp. 222–23.

Nazerian, K., and B. R. Burmester. 1968. Electron microscopy of a herpesvirus associated with the agent of Marek's disease in cell culture. *Cancer Res.* 28:2454–62.

Nazerian, K., and R. L. Witter. 1970. Cell-free transmission and in vivo replication of Marek's disease virus (MDV). *J. Virol.* 5:388–97.

Nazerian, K., J. J. Solomon, R. L. Witter, and B. R. Burmester. 1968. Studies on the etiology of Marek's disease. II. Finding of a herpesvirus in cell culture. *Proc. Soc. Exp. Biol. Med.* 127:177–82.

Okazaki, W., H. G. Purchase, and B. R. Burmester. 1970. Protection against Marek's disease by vaccination with a herpesvirus of turkeys. *Avian Diseases* 14:413–29.

Olson, C. 1940. Transmissible fowl leukosis. A review of the literature. *Mass. Agr. Expt. Sta. Bull.* 370.

Owen, J. J. T., M. A. S. Moore, and P. M. Biggs. 1966. Chromosome studies in Marek's disease. *J. Nat. Cancer Inst.* 37:199–203.

Pappenheimer, A. M., L. C. Dunn, and V. Cone. 1926. A study of fowl paralysis (neuro-lymphomatosis gallinarum). *Storrs Agr. Expt. Sta. Bull.* 143:187–290.

———. 1929. Studies on fowl paralysis (Neurolymphomatosis gallinarum). I. Clinical features and pathology. *J. Exp. Med.* 49:63–86.

Patterson, F. D., H. L. Wilcke, C. Murray, and E. W. Henderson. 1932. So-called range paralysis of the chicken. *J. Am. Vet. Med. Ass.* 34:747–67.

Payne, L. N., and P. M. Biggs. 1967. Studies on Marek's disease. II. Pathogenesis. *J. Nat. Cancer Inst.* 39:281–302.

Purchase, H. G. 1969. Immunofluorescence in the study of Marek's disease. I. Detection of antigen in cell culture and an antigenic comparison of 8 isolates. *J. Virol.* 3:557–65.

———. 1970. Virus-specific immunofluorescent and precipitin antigens and cell-free virus in tissues of birds infected with Marek's disease. *Cancer Res.* 30:1898–1908.

Purchase, H. G., and P. M. Biggs. 1967. Characterization of five isolates of Marek's disease. *Res. Vet. Sci.* 8:440–49.

Purchase, H. G., and G. H. Burgoyne. 1970. Immunofluorescence in the study of Marek's disease: Detection of antibody. *Am. J. Vet. Res.* 31:117–23.

Purchase, H. G., R. C. Chubb, and P. M. Biggs. 1968. Effect of lymphoid leukosis and Marek's disease on the immunological responsiveness of the chicken. *J. Nat. Cancer Inst.* 40:583–92.

Ringen, L. M., and A. S. Akhtar. 1968. Electrophoretic analysis of serum proteins from paralyzed chickens exposed to Marek's disease. *Avian Diseases* 12:4–9.

Samadieh, B., R. A. Bankowski, and E. J. Carroll. 1969. Electrophoretic analysis of serum proteins of chickens experimentally infected with Marek's disease agent. *Am. J. Vet. Res.* 30:837–46.

Schidlovsky, G., M. Ahmed, and K. E. Jensen. 1969. Herpesvirus in Marek's disease tumors. *Science* 164:959–61.

Sevoian, M. 1968a. Egg transmission studies of Type II leukosis infection (Marek's disease). *Poultry Sci.* 47:1644–46.

———. 1968b. Variations in susceptibility of three selected strains of chickens to cell suspensions of JM virus. *Poultry Sci.* 47:688–89.

Sevoian, M., and D. M. Chamberlain. 1962. Avian lymphomatosis. II. Experimental reproduction of the ocular form. *Vet. Med.* 57:608–9.

———. 1963. Avian lymphomatosis. III. Incidence and manifestations in experimentally infected chickens of various ages. *Avian Diseases* 7:97–102.

———. 1964. Avian lymphomatosis. IV. Pathogenesis. *Avian Diseases* 8:281–310.

Sevoian, M., D. M. Chamberlain, and F. T. Counter. 1962. Avian lymphomatosis. I. Experimental reproduction of the neural and visceral forms. *Vet. Med.* 57:500–501.

Sevoian, M., D. M. Chamberlain, and R. N. Larose. 1963a. Avian lymphomatosis. V. Air-borne transmission. *Avian Diseases* 7:102–5.

———. 1963b. Avian lymphomatosis. VII. New support for etiologic unity. *Proc. 17th World Vet. Congr.* 2:1475–76.

Siccardi, F. J., and B. R. Burmester. 1970. The differential diagnosis of lymphoid leukosis and Marek's disease. *USDA Tech. Bull.* 1412.

Smith, K. O. 1964. Relationship between the envelope and the infectivity of Herpes simplex virus. *Proc. Soc. Exp. Biol. Med.* 115:814–16.

Solomon, J. J., R. L. Witter, K. Nazerian, and B. R. Burmester. 1968. Studies on the etiology of Marek's disease. I. Propagation of the agent in cell culture. *Proc. Soc. Exp. Biol. Med.* 127:173–77.

Solomon, J. J., R. L. Witter, H. A. Stone, and L. R. Champion. 1970. Evidence against embryo transmission of Marek's disease virus. *Avian Diseases* 14:752–62.

Spencer, J. L. 1969. Cultivation of Marek's disease virus in cell culture and the application of immunofluorescence for virus detection. Ph.D. thesis, Cornell Univ.

Spencer, J. L., and B. W. Calnek. 1967. Storage of cells infected with Rous sarcoma virus or JM strain of avian lymphomatosis agent. *Avian Diseases* 11:274–87.

Spencer, J. L., and B. W. Calnek. 1970. Marek's disease: Application of immunofluorescence for detection of antigen and antibody. *Am. J. Vet. Res.* 31:345–58.

Ubertini, T., and B. W. Calnek. 1970. Marek's disease herpesvirus in peripheral nerve lesions. *J. Nat. Cancer Inst.* 45:507–14.

Van der Walle, N., and E. Winkler-Junius.

1924. De Neuritis-Epizootie bij Kippen te Barneveld in 1921. *Tijdschr. Vergel. Geneesk, Enz.* 10:34–50.

Vickers, J. H., C. F. Helmboldt, and R. E. Luginbuhl. 1967. Pathogenesis of Marek's disease (Connecticut A isolate). *Avian Diseases* 11:531–45.

Vindel, J. A. 1964. Cytochemistry of neurolymphomatosis virus reproduction in vitro. *Nat. Cancer Inst. Monograph* 17:147–57.

Von Bülow, V. V. 1969. Marek'sche Huehnerlaehmung: Reaktionen in experimentell infizierten embryonierten Ei. *Zentr. Veterinaermed.* 16:97–114.

Von Bülow, V. V., and L. N. Payne. 1970. Direkter Immunofluorescenzenz-Test bei der Marek'schen Krankheit. *Zentr. Veterinaermed.* 17:460–75.

Wight, P. A. L. 1962a. The histopathology of the central nervous system in fowl paralysis. *J. Comp. Pathol. Therap.* 72:348–59.

———. 1962b. Variations in peripheral nerve histopathology in fowl paralysis. *J. Comp. Pathol. Therap.* 72:40–48.

———. 1963. Lymphoid leukosis and fowl paralysis in the quail. *Vet. Record* 75:685–87.

———. 1965. The regenerative capacity of nerves affected by fowl paralysis. *Brit. Vet. J.* 121:278–82.

———. 1969. The ultrastructure of sciatic nerves affected by fowl paralysis (Marek's disease). *J. Comp. Pathol. Therap.* 79:563–70.

Wight, P. A. L., and W. G. Siller. 1965. Further studies of experimental allergic encephalomyelitis in the fowl. *Res. Vet. Sci.* 6:324–29.

Witter, R. L., and B. R. Burmester. 1967. Transmission of Marek's disease with oral washings and feces from infected chickens. *Proc. Soc. Exp. Biol. Med.* 124:59–62.

Witter, R. L., G. H. Burgoyne, and J. J. Solomon. 1968a. Preliminary studies on cell cultures infected with Marek's disease agent. *Avian Diseases* 12:169–85.

Witter, R. L., G. H. Burgoyne, and B. R. Burmester. 1968b. Survival of Marek's disease agent in litter and droppings. *Avian Diseases* 12:522–30.

Witter, R. L., J. J. Solomon, and G. H. Burgoyne. 1969a. Cell culture techniques for primary isolation of Marek's disease-associated herpesvirus. *Avian Diseases* 13:101–18.

Witter, R. L., G. H. Burgoyne, and J. J. Solomon. 1969b. Evidence for a herpesvirus as an etiologic agent of Marek's disease. *Avian Diseases* 13:171–84.

Witter, R. L., J. I. Moulthrop, Jr., G. H. Burgoyne, and H. C. Connell. 1970a. Studies on the epidemiology of Marek's disease herpesvirus in broiler flocks. *Avian Diseases* 14:255–67.

Witter, R. L., K. Nazerian, H. G. Purchase, and G. H. Burgoyne. 1970b. Isolation from turkeys of a cell-associated herpesvirus antigenically related to Marek's disease virus. *Am. J. Vet. Res.* 31:525–38.

Witter, R. L., H. G. Purchase, and G. H. Burgoyne. 1970c. Peripheral nerve lesions similar to those of Marek's disease in chickens inoculated with reticuloendotheliosis virus. *J. Nat. Cancer Inst.* 45:567–77.

❖

LEUKOSIS/SARCOMA GROUP

❖

H. GRAHAM PURCHASE

AND

BEN R. BURMESTER

United States Department of Agriculture Regional Poultry Research Laboratory East Lansing, Michigan

❖

THE LEUKOSIS/SARCOMA viruses have been grouped together because they possess several important characteristics in common. They induce in chickens, and to a much lesser extent in other avian species, a variety of transmissible benign and malignant neoplasms. Under natural conditions by far the most common is lymphoid leukosis, but the following may also occur: erythroblastosis, myeloblastosis, myelocytomatosis, endothelioma, nephroblastoma, hepatocarcinoma, fibrosarcoma, and osteopetrosis. A list of the neoplasms along with a summary of synonyms is given in Table 15.3 and is outlined by Burmester and Witter (1966). Viruses of this group have common physical and chemical characteristics, some of which are similar to those of the myxoviruses (thylaxoviruses) (Wilner, 1969). They also have a common group-specific complement fixing antigen.

Because of the interrelationships between these viruses and their similarity to one another, they are discussed as a group in most portions of this chapter. Sections of the chapter which reflect the host response (i.e., sections on clinical signs, pathology, hematology, pathogenesis, and differential diagnosis) are discussed under the pathological entities without regard for the virological properties of the inducing agent(s) other than their inclusion in the leukosis/sarcoma group. The nature of host response is determined by both the virus genome and the host cell.

HISTORY

Lymphoid leukosis as a disease appears to have been recognized for a long time. More than a century ago Roloff (1868) reported a case of "lymphosarcomata," and in 1896 Caparini described fowl leukemia. In 1905 Butterfield made a diagnosis of "aleukemic lymphoadenosis" in 3 hens in the United States. Ellermann (1921b) described the 3 classical types of leukemia; erythroid, myeloid, and lymphoid (in his terminology "intravasculäre Leukose," "myeloische," and "lymphatische Leukose" respectively). Comprehensive reviews of the conditions have been prepared (Olson, 1940; Engelbreth-Holm, 1942; Furth, 1946; Chubb and Gordon, 1957; Darcel, 1957a,b, 1960; Beard, 1963a,b; Biggs and Payne, 1964, 1967; Vogt, 1965; Purchase, 1966).

LYMPHOID LEUKOSIS

Lymphatic leukosis was the only extravascular form of leukosis represented in Ellermann's classification (1921b) of transmissible avian neoplasms. For a long time after Ellermann published his classification, many investigators still thought that lymphatic leukosis was not transmissible and referred to the aleukemic form as lymphocytoma or lymphadenoma. Jungherr (1941) designated the disease as visceral lympho-

TABLE 15.3 ❧ Neoplasms Caused by Viruses of Leukosis/Sarcoma Group

Neoplasm	Synonyms
Leukoses	
Lymphoid leukosis	Big liver disease, lymphatic leukosis (Ellermann, 1921a), visceral lymphoma (Pappenheimer et al., 1926), lymphocytoma (Feldman, 1932), lymphomatosis (Furth, 1933), visceral lymphomatosis (Jungherr, 1941), lymphoid leukosis (Campbell, 1961; Biggs, 1961).
Erythroblastosis	Leukemia (Warthin, 1907), intravascular lymphoid leukosis (Ellermann, 1921a), erythromyelosis (Bayon, 1929), erythroleukosis (Ellermann, 1923; Furth, 1931), erythroblastosis (Engelbreth-Holm and Rothe-Meyer, 1932).
Myeloblastosis	Leukemic myeloid leukosis (Ellermann, 1921b), leukomyelose (Kitt, 1931), myelomatosis (Furth, 1933), myeloblastosis (Nyfeldt, 1934), granuloblastosis (Jungherr, 1941), myeloid leukosis (Darcel, 1957a).
Myelocytoma(tosis)	Myelocytoma (Pentimalli, 1915), aleukemic myeloid leukosis (Ellermann, 1921a), leukochloroma (Mathews, 1929), myelomatosis (Furth, 1933).
Connective tissue tumors	
Fibroma and fibrosarcoma	
Myxoma and myxosarcoma	
Histiocytic sarcoma	
Osteoma and osteogenic sarcoma	
Related tumors	
Hemangioma	Hemangiomatosis, endothelioma (Furth, 1933, 1934), hemangioblastomas, hemangioendotheliomas.
Nephroblastoma	Embryonal nephroma (Feldman and Olson, 1933), renal adenocarcinoma (Carr, 1956), adenosarcoma (Thorell, 1958), nephroblastoma (Ishiguro et al., 1962; Walter et al., 1962), cystadenoma (Mladenov et al., 1967).
Hepatocarcinoma	
Osteopetrosis	Marble bone, thick leg disease, sporadic diffuse osteopetrosis (Pugh, 1927), osteopetrosis gallinarum (Jungherr and Landauer, 1938).

matosis, but this nomenclature has been superseded by those of Campbell (1961) and Biggs (1961) so that the disease is now called lymphoid leukosis.

Furth (1933) provided good evidence for the transmission of this neoplasm with filtrates, but unequivocal proof of the filterability of the agent or agents awaited the work of Burmester and his associates (Burmester, 1947; Burmester and Cottral, 1947; Burmester and Denington, 1947). The recent development of in vitro techniques for assay of lymphoid leukosis viruses has helped to characterize them and to elucidate their relationship to the sarcoma viruses. These are presented in other sections of this chapter and in comprehensive reviews (Oberling and Guerin, 1954; Beard, 1957, 1963b; Vogt, 1965).

ERYTHROBLASTOSIS

Ellermann and Bang (1908) were the first to report the experimental transmission of erythroblastosis. Subsequently numerous strains were established, and the viral etiology and pathologic nature of the disease were characterized in extensive studies (Ellermann, 1921a; Olson, 1940; Beard, 1963a). Many of the strains caused both erythroblastosis and myeloblastosis; others produced erythroblastosis and fibrosarcomas or erythroblastosis and lymphoid leukosis. In addition, recognized strains of virus which induce primarily lymphoid leukosis, myeloblastosis, or fibrosarcomas have also been reported to induce some cases of erythroblastosis (Burmester et al., 1959b; Burmester and Walter, 1961). However, mixtures of specific viruses have not yet been ruled out.

MYELOBLASTOSIS

Myeloblastosis was transmitted by Schmeisser in 1915; since then Furth (1931), Engelbreth-Holm and Rothe-Meyer (1932), and Nyfeldt (1934) have observed myeloblastosis in their transmission experiments. Early passages of the BAI strain A virus (Hall et al., 1941) caused both erythroblastosis and myeloblastosis; however, recent passages derived by selection of the original donor at Duke University have induced myeloblastosis alone (Eckert et al., 1953).

MYELOCYTOMATOSIS

The distinctive appearance and aleukemic character of this disease were first described by Pentimalli (1915); later Furth (1933) described some leukemic cases. Most "strains" or isolates causing myelocytoma also caused other neoplasms such as erythroblastosis, hepatocarcinoma, and renal carcinoma (Löliger and Schubert, 1966; Mladenov et al., 1967).

NEPHROBLASTOMA

Several viruses of the leukosis/sarcoma group have been found to induce kidney tumors. They include BAI strain A (myeloblastosis), ES4 strain (erythroblastosis sarcoma), MH2 strain (reticuloendothelioma), and MC29 strain (myelocytomatosis) (Carr, 1956, 1960; Burmester et al., 1959b; Mladenov et al., 1967).

OSTEOPETROSIS

Karschner (1926) was the first to use the term osteopetrosis for a human disease referred to colloquially as marble bone. It is now apparent that the hypertrophic osteopathies of fowl described in the 1920s were probably osteopetrosis (Besnoit and Robin, 1922; Ball and Auger, 1924; Pugh, 1927; Sanger, 1963). Jungherr and Landauer (1938) described the pathologic alterations in detail and suggested the term osteopetrosis gallinarium. They were the first to reproduce the disease, and they called attention to its frequent association with lymphoid leukosis. For this reason they suggested its inclusion in the avian leukosis complex. Burmester and his associates (Burmester, 1947; Fredrickson et al., 1965) also noticed that osteopetrosis was frequently associated with lymphoid leukosis. They found that osteopetrosis occurred during serial passage of 12 of 14 recently isolated strains of lymphoid leukosis virus. Others have reproduced the disease without lymphoid leukosis (Campbell, 1963); however, in their experiments soft tissue tumors were observed in addition to osteopetrosis.

CONNECTIVE TISSUE TUMORS

Fibrosarcomas and myxosarcomas were first transmitted with cell-free filtrates by Rous in 1911. They have been studied in many laboratories since then. Ellermann and Bang (1908) noticed this tumor in their early transmission studies.

INCIDENCE AND DISTRIBUTION

With few exceptions, leukosis/sarcoma virus infection occurs in all chicken flocks;

by sexual maturity most birds have been exposed. Nevertheless, the incidence of clinical disease is generally quite low and is estimated to be much less than that for Marek's disease.

DISEASE INCIDENCE

Lymphoid leukosis only occasionally is thought to produce heavy losses in commercial breeder flocks, although sporadic cases occur in most flocks of adult birds. It has been reported in the Japanese quail *(Coturnix coturnix japonica)* (Löliger and Schubert, 1967), turkey (Simpson et al., 1957), pheasant, pigeon, duck, goose, canary, and budgerigar (Reis and Nobrega, 1956); but once again there is no assurance that it was not Marek's disease. More recently Wight (1963) recorded 4 cases of lymphoid leukosis in a flock of quail and was able to distinguish them from Marek's disease.

Compared to lymphoid leukosis, erythroblastosis occurs infrequently under field conditions, but it has been found in most breeds of chicken. Exceptionally, it has been reported to occur in 5-week-old birds as an epizootic (Hamilton and Sawyer, 1939).

Except in the older literature there are very few reports of the natural occurrence of myeloblastosis. It would appear to be rare, especially when unassociated with erythroblastosis.

Sporadic cases of myelocytomatosis occur among young adult birds, but only very rarely are there multiple-case flocks. The disease was observed in about 1% of the birds in 2 consecutive broiler flocks on one farm (W. Mathey, personal communication).

Other than the leukotic tumors, hemangiomas appear to be the most frequently occurring tumors; however, the incidence is highly variable. Campbell and Appleby (1966) reported that they comprised 25% of all tumors in broilers. The skin was most often affected though tumors occurred in many other tissues and organs.

In adult chickens nephroblastomas may comprise 3–10% of all tumors exclusive of lymphoid leukosis and Marek's disease (Jackson, 1936; Olson and Bullis, 1942; Guillon et al., 1963). In broilers the proportion of nephroblastomas appears to be somewhat higher, i.e. 16% (Campbell and Appleby, 1966).

Osteopetrosis occurs less frequently than lymphoid leukosis, though it is also widespread and epizootics occur sporadically in broilers. In all types of chicken, males are more frequently affected than females. It occurs very rarely in turkeys.

There are very few good data on the incidence of the connective tissue tumors. These tumors are often slow growing and may not be the primary cause of death, so that most reports describe tumors found among cases that are brought to a diagnostic laboratory for other reasons. When birds with lymphoid leukosis or Marek's disease are omitted from the data, connective tissue tumors appear to comprise about 20% of the tumors found (Goss, 1940; Campbell and Appleby, 1966). The incidence of connective tissue tumors in chickens is probably less than 1 in 1,000, but epizootics have occurred. Perek (1960) reported an outbreak of histiocytic sarcoma in a flock of 600 1-year-old hens. Tumors were found in 90% of 400 birds examined during a 4-month period.

INCIDENCE OF VIRUS INFECTION

Viruses of the leukosis/sarcoma group are almost ubiquitous, and their occurrence in many flocks has been studied in detail (Purchase, 1966). The presence of different subgroups of viruses in field flocks has been studied by examining birds for the presence of antibody, by determining which viruses are shed in the eggs, and by examining field isolates. The tests indicate that subgroup A viruses are encountered more commonly than subgroup B viruses. In one study (Calnek, 1968a), 1.6–12.5% of the embryos from 8 commercial flocks representing a variety of sources contained subgroup A viruses, and there was significant shedding in every flock. Subgroup B viruses were relatively rare and were shed in the eggs much less frequently than subgroup A viruses. A similar preponderance of subgroup A viruses has been isolated from field outbreaks of leukosis (Payne et al., 1968; Churchill, 1968). Both subgroups of avian leukosis viruses were isolated from 3 egg-propagated vaccines (Churchill, 1968). Viruses of subgroup C have been isolated only from laboratory strains of leukosis virus (Duff, 1968).

ETIOLOGY

CLASSIFICATION

Viruses of the leukosis/sarcoma group have in common certain properties of the viral genome; i.e., they produce a characteristic pathologic response and contain the common group-specific complement fixing antigen. Further classification into subgroups and types depends on properties of the envelope, e.g., host range, interference spectrum, and antigenicity. Thus a virus can be a sarcoma or lymphoid leukosis virus and belong to any one of at least 4 subgroups.

Virus Group

In the type of nucleic acid they contain, in size, and in susceptibility to lipid solvents and low pH, members of the avian leukosis/sarcoma viruses group resemble the myxoviruses (thylaxoviruses) (Wilner, 1969). The resemblance is also apparent in their structure, viz. lack of cubic symmetry and possession of a limiting membrane with "spikes" at the surface and a filamentous element in the interior (Eckert et al., 1963). However, no internal helical substructure has yet been demonstrated. They all contain a characteristic group-specific antigen demonstrable by the complement fixation test. Except for some minor differences associated with the type of cell from which the virus originated, the viruses of this group are biophysically and biochemically indistinguishable from one another.

Virus Subgroups

Avian leukosis/sarcoma viruses have been divided into 4 subgroups on the basis of their host range in genetically different chick embryo fibroblast cultures (Vogt and Ishizaki, 1965), their interference with members of the same subgroup (Vogt and Ishizaki, 1966b), and viral envelope antigens detected by serum neutralization (Ishizaki and Vogt, 1966; Vogt and Ishizaki, 1966a; Duff and Vogt, 1969).

Genetic host range or cellular genetic resistance to infection by viruses of a particular subgroup is controlled by an autosomal locus called the avian tumor virus locus. Loci for subgroup A viruses (tva) and for subgroup B viruses (tvb) segregate independently (Payne and Biggs, 1966; Critten-

TABLE 15.4 ❧ Summary of Genotypic and Phenotypic Nomenclature Applied to the Two Genetic Systems and Susceptibility to 4 Subgroups Of Virus

Genotype	Phenotype	Subgroup Susceptibility			
		A	B	C	D
$a^sa^sb^sb^s$	C/O	S*	S	S	S
$a^sa^rb^sb^s$	C/O	S	S	S	S
$a^ra^rb^sb^s$	C/A	R†	S	S	S
$a^sa^sb^sb^r$	C/O	S	S	S	S
$a^sa^rb^sb^r$	C/O	S	S	S	S
$a^ra^rb^sb^r$	C/A	R	S	S	S
$a^sa^sb^rb^r$	C/B	S	R	S	S‡
$a^sa^rb^rb^r$	C/B	S	R	S	S‡
$a^ra^rb^rb^r$	C/A,B	R	R	S	S‡

Source: Modified from Crittenden (1968), Duff and Vogt (1969).
* Susceptible.
† Resistant.
‡ Susceptibility lower than with other genotypes.

den et al., 1967). The mode of inheritance of resistance to subgroup C and D viruses has not yet been examined. The alleles controlling susceptibility (a^s, b^s) are dominant over the alleles controlling resistance (a^r, b^r). Cells phenotypically resistant to the growth of subgroup A viruses are termed C/A cells and those resistant to subgroup B viruses, C/B (Table 15.4). C/AB cells are resistant to viruses of both subgroups; C/O cells are susceptible to viruses of all known subgroups (Vogt and Ishizaki, 1965).

Subgroup C viruses grow equally well in all cell types; subgroup D viruses grow better in C/O and C/A cells than in C/B and C/AB (Duff and Vogt, personal communication).

Interference between leukosis and sarcoma viruses has been well characterized (Vogt and Ishizaki, 1966b). Leukosis viruses do not produce a rapid cytopathic effect in cell culture, but infected cells are resistant to subsequent challenge with cytopathogenic sarcoma viruses of the same subgroup. This is the basis of the resistance inducing factor (RIF) test (Rubin, 1960a). They are, however, fully susceptible to challenge with sarcoma viruses of another subgroup (Vogt and Ishizaki, 1966b) and thus can be readily classified into at least 4 subgroups. A classification of the more common viruses is given in Table 15.5. There are indications that additional subgroups

TABLE 15.5 ❧ Classification of Leukosis/Sarcoma Viruses

Strain	Subgroups and Designation			
	A	B	C	D
Sarcoma				
Bryan Standard	BS-RSV-1			
Bryan High-Titer	BH-RSV-1			
Schmidt Ruppin	SR-RSV-1	SR-RSV-2		SR-RSV-D
Harris		HA-RSV		
Carr-Zilber	CZ-RSV-A	CZ-RSV-B		CZ-RSV-D
Prague	PR-RSV-A	PR-RSV-B	PR-RSV-C	
B77			B77	
Prc 2	Prc 2-A	Prc 2-B		
Leukosis				
LL—erythroblastosis	RPL12, F42			
Rubin strain LL	RIF-1	RIF-2		
Myeloblastosis BAI strain A	AMV-1	AMV-2		
Erythroblastosis strain R			AEV	
MC29—myelocytoma	MC29-A	MC29-B		
Sarcoma associated				
Bryan High-Titer	RAV-1, RAV-3	RAV-2		
Bryan Standard	RAV-4, RAV-5			
Schmidt Ruppin			RAV-7	
			RAV-49	RAV-50
Harris		RAV-6		
Carr-Zilber		CZAV		CZAV
Fujinami	FAV-1, FAV-2			
Other associated Myeloblastosis	MAV-1	MAV-2		
Rous sarcoma pseudotypes				
Bryan High-Titer (examples)	BH-RSV (RAV-1)	BH-RSV (RAV-2)		
Bryan Standard (examples)	BS-RSV (RAV-1)	BS-RSV (RAV-2)		
Fujinami pseudotypes (examples)	FS (FAV-1) FS (FAV-2)			

Source: Modified from Burmester (1966).

exist; however, their importance remains to be determined.

Virus Types

Antigenic relationships delineate different virus types. Neutralizing antisera produced in chickens are specifically directed against the type-specific envelope antigens of the virus. When monotypic antisera, prepared by immunization of chickens with purified virus stocks, are used for comparisons in the neutralization and fluorescent antibody tests, the different subgroups can be defined immunologically (Chubb and Biggs, 1968). Each subgroup consists of several distinct antigenic types. In general, subgroup B viruses appear more heterogeneous than those of subgroup A. Antisera react more strongly with homologous virus than with heterologous viruses of the same subgroup. With rare exceptions, antisera do not react with viruses of a different subgroup (Ishizaki and Vogt, 1966).

MORPHOLOGY

Ultrastructure

Viruses of the avian leukosis/sarcoma group cannot be distinguished on the basis of their ultrastructural characteristics. In size, shape, and ultrastructural detail the particles from the various diseases studied are identical and similar to other RNA tumor viruses (Beard, 1962).

Negatively stained preparations of lymphoid leukosis/sarcoma viruses reveal essentially spheroidal particles which are readily distorted into sperm, crescent, and other forms (Fig. 15.18) under some conditions of drying (Bonar et al., 1963a). Characteristic knoblike projections on the surface of these particles appear similar to those seen with myxoviruses. The inner nucleoid of the virus appears to be more firm and less easily distorted than the outer portion. When virus preparations are frozen and thawed, fixed in formaldehyde, or

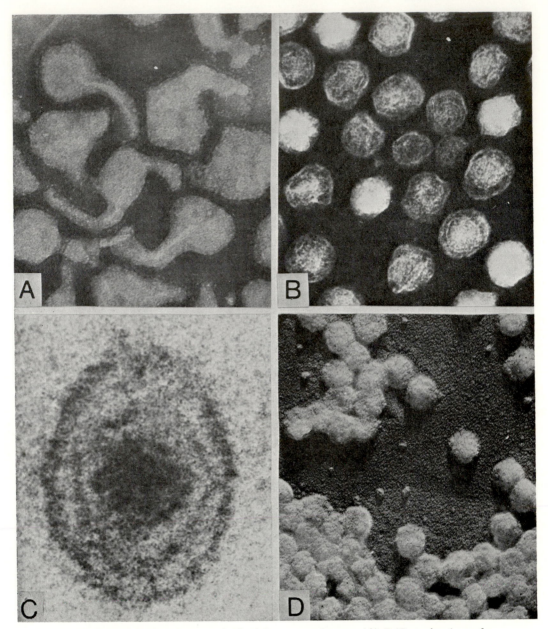

FIG. 15.18—Ultrastructure of leukosis/sarcoma viruses. (A) BAI strain A myeloblastosis virus, unfixed and negatively stained with neutralized phosphotungstic
acid. Peripheral fringe about particles is resolved in some places into discrete
"knobs." ×150,000. (B) Negative staining as for (A), but preparation was fixed in
formaldehyde before drying. Spheroidal shape is fairly well retained, and some
particles have been penetrated by stain revealing internal structure—outer membrane, inner membrane, and granular or filamentous nucleoid. ×150,000. (C)
Thin section of BAI strain A myeloblastosis virus sedimented from plasma, fixed
in osmium tetroxide, and stained with lead subacetate. Inner and outer membranes and granular character of nucleoid can be seen. The impression of granules might be derived from sectioning of filaments. Some granules appear to be
hollow. ×510,000. (D) Purified BAI strain A myeloblastosis virus fixed and
shadowed with chromium. ×50,000. (Courtesy R. A. Bonar, Duke Univ. Medical
Center, and J. Nat. Cancer Inst.)

treated with ether, Freon, or saponin, the inner structure is revealed as a granular or filamentous nucleoid surrounded by a thin membrane separated from an outer membrane by a relatively electron-lucent space (Fig. 15.18) (Bonar et al., 1963a). The filament in the interior is approximately 30–40 Å in diameter, of undetermined length, and arranged in the form of an intricate coil (Eckert et al., 1963; Bonar et al., 1964).

Thin sections prepared and stained by the usual techniques reveal an inner electron dense core which is about 35–45 mμ in diameter, an intermediate membrane, and an outer membrane (Fig. 15.18). The overall diameter of the particle is 80–120 mμ with an average of 90 mμ (Bernhard et al., 1956; Bonar et al., 1963a).

When purified virus preparations are fixed while the virus is in suspension, dried, and a collodion pseudoreplica prepared and shadowed with chromium, essentially spherical particles are seen (Fig. 15.18). If drying occurs after freezing and thawing and before fixation, the particles take on a "fried egg" appearance. The particle appears flattened with a thick rim and an eccentrically located spheroidal body which probably represents the nucleoid and inner membrane (Bonar et al., 1963a).

Size

The Rous sarcoma virus particle as determined by filtration through membranes of graded pore size is 75–100 mμ in diameter (Elford and Andrewes, 1935). Using similar methods, Young (1966) found the virus of osteopetrosis to be between 100 and 200 mμ. By ultracentrifugation, Kahler et al. (1954a,b) estimated the size of a Rous sarcoma virus particle in concentrated sucrose solution to be 90 mμ; Sharp and Beard (1954) found the avian myeloblastosis virus particle to be 144 mμ in diameter in bovine serum albumin. These figures are consistent with the electron microscopic measurements given above.

Density

Rous sarcoma virus density was estimated to be 1.15 and 1.18 g/ml in sucrose and rubidium chloride gradients respectively (Kahler et al., 1954a,b; Crawford, 1960). Values of 1.16–1.22 g/ml were obtained in sucrose by Robinson and Duesberg (1968). The increased density may have been due to the hypertonic nature of the solution in

which the virus particles are suspended; i.e., inorganic salts have a higher osmotic pressure than sucrose. However, there is apparently considerable buoyant density heterogeneity (Crawford, 1960). Hanafusa et al. (1964) reported that Rous-associated virus has the same density as Rous sarcoma virus, i.e. 1.20 g/ml in sucrose. However, Rous sarcoma virus particles from nonproducer cells were found to differ slightly from infectious Rous sarcoma virus in density and sedimentation velocity (Robinson et al., 1967).

Avian myeloblastosis virus was found to have a density of 1.06 g/ml in bovine serum albumin solution (Sharp and Beard, 1954). Since no controlled comparisons of the densities of avian myeloblastosis virus and Rous sarcoma virus have been made, it is probable that differences in estimates of density were due to the conditions employed in different laboratories.

CHEMICAL COMPOSITION

Considerable difficulty has been encountered in purifying avian tumor viruses sufficiently so that chemical analyses would be meaningful. Avian myeloblastosis virus has been studied most extensively; it contains 30–35% lipid, 60–65% protein, 2.2% RNA, and no DNA (Bonar and Beard, 1959; Beard, 1963a).

Viral RNA

The detergent sodium dodecyl sulfate disrupts leukosis/sarcoma viruses, liberating intact RNA which can then be purified by phenol extraction and alcohol precipitation. The RNA has a sedimentation coefficient (S_{20w}) of between 69S and 74S (Svedberg units) in 0.11 molar NaCl (Robinson et al., 1967; Robinson and Duesberg, 1968). Accurate determinations indicate that the RNAs of avian myeloblastosis virus, Rous sarcoma virus from nonproducer cells, and Rous-associated virus are indistinguishable; however there is considerable heterogeneity (Robinson and Duesberg, 1968). Bonar et al. (1967) described 4 distinct RNA components of avian myeloblastosis virus, all of which were intrinsic to the agent. Duesberg (1968) has presented evidence that the RNA of Rous sarcoma virus is an aggregate of smaller RNA molecules rather than a single polypeptide as reported by Blair and Duesberg (1968).

The molecular weight of the RNA has

been estimated to be $9.8 \times 10^6 - 10 \times 10^6$ (Crawford and Crawford, 1961; Bonar et al., 1963b; Granboulan et al., 1966).

The results of determinations of the base compositions of RNA for viruses of this group are summarized by Vogt (1965). These determinations were by various methods using different viruses, making comparisons difficult since analyses of the same virus by different workers did not agree. However, a recent study by Robinson and Duesberg (1968) indicated that the base compositions of the viral RNA of Rous sarcoma virus with its associated virus, avian myeloblastosis virus, and Rous sarcoma virus from nonproducer cells were almost identical. There was no similarity between the base compositions of leukosis/sarcoma viruses and fixed cell RNA.

Viral Lipid

The lipid composition of partially purified avian myeloblastosis virus is qualitatively similar to that of the host cell (Rao and Beard, 1964). However, distinct quantitative differences have been described (Rao et al., 1966). While it is probable that the viral lipids are "host specific" (Robinson and Duesberg, 1968) in that they are synthesized by the host cell, it is also clear that some process of selection is involved in the incorporation of lipid into the virus particle; its composition does not reflect that of the host cell as a whole or of its membrane.

Viral Protein

When avian myeloblastosis virus is disrupted by sodium dodecyl sulfate and the split products are subjected to Tiselius electrophoresis at pH 7.5, several components can be detected. The fastest migrating is viral RNA and the slowest is a protein antigen which reacts in the complement fixation test with sera from hamsters bearing Schmidt-Ruppin tumors and sera from rabbits immunized with unfractionated, disrupted avian myeloblastosis virus (Bauer and Schafer, 1965). This antigen inoculated into rabbits induces antibodies which react with a variety of leukosis/sarcoma viruses in the complement fixation test, indicating that this component is the group-specific antigen.

The group-specific antigen is considered to be an internal structural component of the virus. Thus, virus purified by ultracentrifugation does not react in the complement fixation test unless the group-specific antigen is released by chemical or physical procedures (Bauer and Schafer, 1966). Similarly, mammalian antisera will not react with the group-specific antigen in the indirect fluorescent antibody test unless the substrate containing the antigen is first fixed with a lipid solvent (Payne et al., 1966). Also, such sera will not neutralize the virus.

Robinson and Duesberg (1968) reported that 3 major and 2 minor viral protein bands can be distinguished by electrophoresis. Bands obtained with the Bryan and Schmidt-Ruppin strains of Rous sarcoma virus and particles from RSV-infected, nonproducer cells were indistinguishable. They estimated that at least 4–8 proteins or protein-containing macromolecules are present in avian tumor viruses.

Host Cell Contribution

Leukosis viruses mature by budding from the cell membrane, and the viral coat or envelope is derived, at least in part, from the cell membrane. Thus virus and host antigens may occur together on the viral envelope. There is serological evidence for the presence of host antigens on the surface of virus particles; substances that react with antiserum to normal chicken tissue and to Forssman antigens are inseparable from the virus by ultracentrifugation or electrophoresis. Furthermore, the above antisera may precipitate and neutralize leukosis viruses, particularly avian myeloblastosis virus and strain R (Eckert et al., 1955d; Beard et al., 1957). Rubin (1956), using Rous sarcoma virus, has shown that virus neutralization by antiserum prepared against normal chicken tissues is different in many ways from neutralization by virus-specific antisera. He concluded that the effect is due to the deleterious action of anti-chicken serum on the infected cells and not to direct neutralization of the virus itself.

In order to resolve these discrepancies, there should be a reexamination of the role of each of the factors in the different systems.

The enzyme activity of avian myeloblastosis virus has been studied in great detail. Virus obtained either from the peripheral blood of infected chickens or from myeloblast cell cultures contains a triphosphatase which will dephosphorylate adenosine triphosphate or inosine triphosphate but not adenosine diphosphate. The enzyme is present at the surface of the virus particle, presumably in the envelope. It is relatively stable under variations of pH or temperature which destroy the biological activity of the virus. The virus acquires enzyme activity during release from cells which possess high adenosine triphosphatase activity at their surface. Thus blast cells in the cortex of the thymus, myeloblasts in the blood of leukemic birds, and myeloblasts in culture all liberate virus particles, more than 90% of which have enzyme activity. On the other hand, cells without enzyme activity on their surface (e.g. chicken embryo fibroblasts and certain kidney tumors) release virus which is also devoid of activity. It appears that the adenosine triphosphatase activity of the cell membrane is incorporated into the envelope of the virus particle during maturation of the particle. The role of these cell components in the viral envelope is unknown (De Thé, 1964).

Other viruses examined, such as strain R and ES4, rarely exhibited adenosine triphosphatase activity. Since erythroblasts and other cells from which they mature do not have this enzyme, it is conceivable that the few enzyme positive particles were elaborated by cells other than erythroblasts (De Thé, 1964; De Thé et al., 1964).

Preparations of avian myeloblastosis virus may also contain a polynucleotide phosphorylase complex which is most active with guanosine diphosphate as substrate but which also acts on the diphosphates of adenosine, uridine, and cytidine. The specific activity of this enzyme is only about 1/10 of that of the triphosphatase (Riman and Thorell, 1960).

RESISTANCE TO CHEMICAL AND PHYSICAL AGENTS

Lipid Solvents and Detergents

All of the viruses of this group so far tested resembled the myxoviruses and arboviruses in that they contained essential lipids. Thus ethyl ether completely abolished their infectivity (Friesen and Rubin, 1961; Young, 1966). The detergent sodium dodecyl sulfate disrupts these lipid-containing

viruses and releases the RNA (Robinson et al., 1965; Robinson and Duesberg, 1968).

Thermal Inactivation

The half-life of various leukosis/sarcoma viruses at 37° C varies from 100 to 540 minutes (average around 260 minutes), depending on the composition of the medium in which the virus is suspended, the tissue of origin of the virus, and the strain of the virus (Vogt, 1965). Avian tumor viruses are inactivated rapidly at higher temperatures, thus the half-life for Rous sarcoma virus at 50° C is 8.5 minutes and at 60° C 0.7 minutes (Dougherty, 1961).

The thermal lability of these viruses is a critical factor in storage. Even at −15° C the half-life of avian myeloblastosis virus is less than a week (Eckert et al., 1955c), and it is only at temperatures below −60° C that avian tumor viruses can be stored for several years without loss of infectivity (Bryan et al., 1954). Virus is degraded by freezing and thawing (Robinson et al., 1965) and the group-specific antigen is released.

pH Stability

There is little change in the stability of viruses of this group between pH of 5 and 9; however, outside this range the inactivation rates are markedly increased (Bryan et al., 1950, 1951; Eckert et al., 1955b; Bonar et al., 1957).

Ultraviolet Irradiation

Rous sarcoma virus is 10 times more resistant than Newcastle disease virus to exposure to ultraviolet light, even though these viruses have similar size, structure, RNA content, and sensitivity to X-rays (Rubin and Temin, 1959; Rubin, 1960b). This is apparently typical of all viruses of this group, since it has also been found with certain field strains (Friesen and Rubin, 1961).

VIRUS REPLICATION

Virus Synthesis and Release

When Rous sarcoma virus is placed on the chorioallantoic membrane, it penetrates susceptible cells and becomes inaccessible to neutralizing antibody within 3 hours (Harris, 1954; Rubin, 1956). Virus entry is followed by an eclipse period of approximately 15 hours, at which time virus reap-

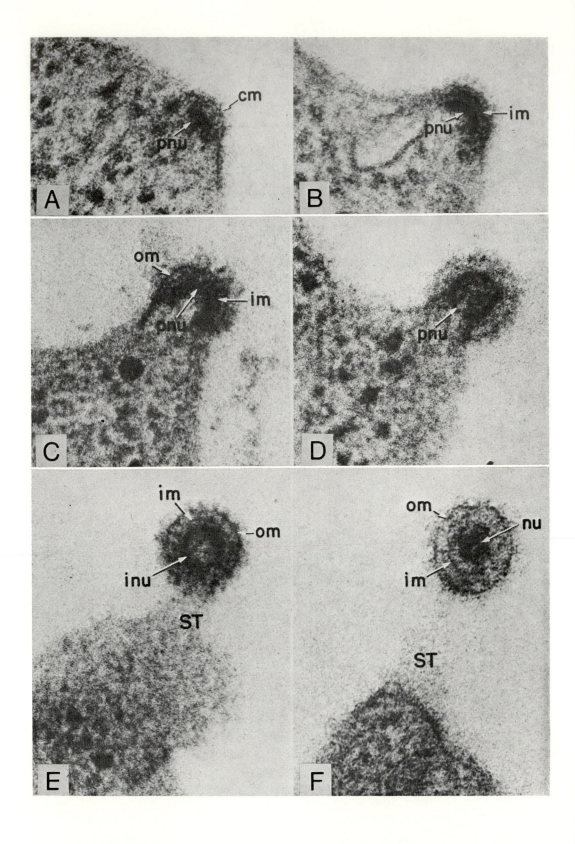

pears. The virus titer increases until a maximum is reached in about 6 days (Prince, 1958). Virus is released continuously from infected cells. In cultured chicken embryo fibroblasts, virus entry is rapid, occurring in a little more than an hour, and new virus synthesis can be demonstrated at 12–14 hours after infection.

Virus particles are formed and released from infected cells by a process of "budding" from the cell membrane (Fig. 15.19) (Haguenau et al., 1962; Heine et al., 1962). Initially there is a localized thickening of the cell membrane which is marked by high contrast at a specific point. The protrusion increases in size, and a second inner membrane is formed by condensation of micrographically undetectable precursors. As the protuberance grows, the prenucleoid is formed as a spherical shell which is electron dense in osmium tetroxide-fixed sections. A particle, of the dimensions of the virus enclosed within two distinct membranes, is formed and then pinched off from the cell membrane and freed into the extracellular space. The particles "mature" to the typical structure by rearrangement of the thick inner shell to form the dense central nucleoid after the particle has separated from the cell (Haguenau and Beard, 1962; Bonar et al., 1964). Not infrequently particles are formed by budding of the lining structure of cytoplasmic vacuoles. Such activity may be responsible for some of the osmiophilic cytoplasmic bodies packed with virus particles.

Biochemical studies of virus multiplication have not been performed because of the difficulties encountered in virus purification and/or the cumbersome nature of the tests for viral activity. However, much information, reviewed by Vogt (1965), has been obtained indirectly by the use of inhibitors of nucleic acid metabolism. Experiments indicated that there is an early stage in replication which is dependent on DNA synthesis and a later stage which is independent of this requirement. When cells are treated with actinomycin D early during the infectious cycle, there is a strong irreversible inhibition of virus production. Later in the infectious cycle only a temporary interruption in Rous sarcoma virus synthesis occurs. Functionally, intact DNA is necessary throughout the infectious cycle. The requirement for DNA synthesis during the replication of an RNA virus is unusual and occurs only in the leukosis/sarcoma viruses. Other RNA viruses may require DNA functions but not DNA synthesis.

Defectiveness

Some sarcoma viruses, particularly Bryan's standard and Bryan's high-titer strains of Rous sarcoma virus and Fujinami sarcoma virus, are defective. They lack the genetic information necessary to reproduce themselves. Infectious virus is not produced, probably because certain envelope antigens required for infection of most cells used for assay are not produced. (See reviews by Purchase, 1965; Vogt, 1965). The genome of the defective sarcoma virus controls: (1) replication of the viral RNA, (2) transformation of the infected cells, including both morphology of the transformed cell and character of focal lesions in cell cultures (Fig. 15.20), and (3) production of the group-specific complement fixing antigen. Thus morphologically altered cells from which no infectious virus is released may result from infection with defective virus. These have been termed nonproducer (NP) or converted non-virus-producing (CNVP) cells. (See review by Purchase, 1965.) Any one of the leukosis viruses or nondefective sarcoma viruses can act as "helper virus." By coinfecting the same cell with the defective virus, the complete helper virus genome complements that of the defective virus and both infec-

FIG. 15.19—Ultrastructure of leukosis/sarcoma virus release. Virus budding at cell membrane of different leukemic myeloblasts from either circulating blood or tissue culture after various periods in vitro. Micrographs show different stages in increased size of dense prenucleoid (pnu) beneath cell membrane (cm) in (A) and subsequent involvement of cell membrane in (B) and (C). Structures suggestive of outer (om) and inner particle membranes (im) are in buds in (B) and (C). A typical "immature" avian tumor virus particle before nucleoid (inu) condensation is shown in (E), and the dense nucleoid (nu) characteristic of "free" particles in (F). The surface of buds and particles peripheral to outer membrane is irregular and indistinct. ST = stalk. ×215,000. (Courtesy G. de Thé, Duke Univ. Medical Center, N.C., and J. Nat. Cancer Inst.)

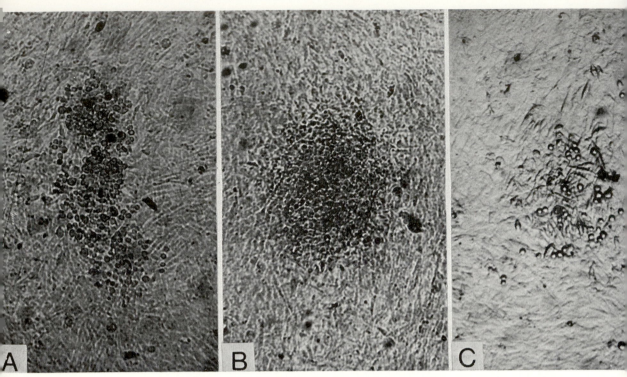

FIG. 15.20—Foci induced by Rous sarcoma virus in cell culture. (A) Unstained focus of transformed spherical, refractile chick embryo cells infected 6 days previously with Bryan's standard strain of Rous sarcoma virus. ×100. (B) Unstained focus of transformed, polygonal, opaque Rous sarcoma cells infected 6 days previously with Bryan's high-titer strain. ×100. (C) Unstained focus of transformed round and fusiform cells infected 6 days previously with Popken's preparation of Rous sarcoma virus. ×100.

tious Rous sarcoma virus and helper virus are produced simultaneously. Both viruses have identical complete envelope antigens. Even though this Rous sarcoma virus can infect cells, it has a defective genome and is therefore dependent upon helper virus for continued replication. All stocks of defective Rous sarcoma virus contain one or more helper viruses called Rous-associated viruses (RAV); many times, the titer of the helper virus is higher than that of the defective virus.

The characteristics determined by the helper virus are all functions of the viral envelope, namely: (1) infectivity and range of infectivity in genetically different cells, (2) interference patterns among and between subgroups, (3) type-specific antigenicity, and (4) rate of virus maturation. The Rous sarcoma virus produced from a dually infected cell is identical, with respect to the above characteristics, to the helper virus.

The first 3 characteristics determine the subgroup to which the virus belongs and have been discussed in detail under subgroup classification. The rate of maturation of Rous sarcoma virus is dependent upon that of the helper because virus assembly is rate-limiting for Rous sarcoma virus. Rous sarcoma viruses with the above properties determined by a specific helper virus are referred to as pseudotypes, and the helper virus is given in parentheses (Vogt and Ishizaki, 1966a), e.g. BH-RSV (RAV-1) (see Table 15.5).

Recent work has demonstrated that nonproducer cells may produce small quantities of virus which contain Rous sarcoma virus RNA (Vogt, 1967; Robinson et al., 1967). It has been called Rous sarcoma virus-zero, RSV (O). It will produce typical neoplastic transformation in cells of specific types—i.e. in cultures of all quail cells and in most C/A cells—but only in occasional C/O cells and then in very low titer. Hence Rous sarcoma virus-zero does not appear to belong to subgroup A, B, C, or D, though it may have some relationship to subgroup B viruses (Vogt, 1967). These results indicate that defectiveness of the sarcoma viruses may be quantitative and not absolute. It is possible that a similar situation may exist in vivo (Dougherty et al., 1967).

Most sarcoma virus strains (e.g., the Schmidt-Ruppin strain of RSV) are not defective. They do not need a helper virus in order to produce infectious progeny virus, and nonproducer cells cannot be prepared from them. However, phenotypic mixing with other leukosis/sarcoma viruses may still occur.

Advantages Derived from Defectiveness

Since the sarcoma virus activated from nonproducer cells by a leukosis virus can be detected directly in cell culture, this procedure of activation of nonproducer cells can be readily used as an assay for leukosis viruses (see nonproducer test). In addition this offers a method for preparing "tailor-made" Rous sarcoma viruses with envelope properties (i.e. host range, interference, and viral antigens) identical to the helper virus. Determinations of host range, interference pattern, and neutralization can be performed more easily with the "tailor-made" sarcoma viruses than with the leukosis viruses, since the former can be readily quantitated in cell culture, by inoculation of chorioallantoic membranes of embryonated eggs or by inoculation of chicks.

Nonproducer tumors may be induced in vivo when small amounts of stock virus are inoculated into chicks and cells become infected with the defective Rous sarcoma virus genome alone. By making use of this phenomenon Rous sarcoma virus pseudotypes can be prepared in vivo (Purchase and Okazaki, 1966). Since nonproducer cells can also be produced on chorioallantoic membranes (Harris, 1967), it is possible that Rous sarcoma virus pseudotypes could also be produced in this medium.

BIOLOGICAL PROPERTIES

When leukosis/sarcoma viruses infect susceptible cells in vitro or in vivo, the cells may be neoplastically transformed (undergo morphologic alteration), or there may be essentially no morphologic change at all.

In either case a persistent infection results and the cells elaborate virus continuously. Cells infected and morphologically altered in culture exhibit only a narrow spectrum of differences from their progenitor normal elements. Still less difference is evident between culture-altered chick embryo or bone marrow cells and the corresponding neoplastic cells induced in the host, e.g. fibroblasts (sarcoma), myeloblasts (myeloblastosis), myelocytes (myelocytomatosis), or erythroblasts (erythroblastosis). In contrast, there is a broad spectrum of neoplastic alterations in the chicken and intact embryo which do not have counterparts in cell culture.

In cell culture the basic characteristics of chicken embryo cells (fibroblasts) are usually altered by neoplasia to cells of structure more primitive than that of the fibroblasts. On the other hand, myeloid cells in bone marrow cultures when exposed to strain MC29 virus become more mature and differentiate to the level of granulated myelocytes. In the chicken, however, morphologic changes result predominantly in cell differentiation, as in myelocytomatosis and nephroblastoma, to forms and organization resembling but not attaining highly complex normal structures. It would appear that morphologic response in vitro may be largely related to the influence of the virus per se (Langlois et al., 1969), whereas the responses in the bird are the result of synergistic actions of both virus and microenvironmental factors in the host (De Thé et al., 1962).

The cell responds to virus infection by the production of infectious virus within 14–24 hours. In the initial stages of infection, synthesis and liberation of virus proceed without evident change in cell structure. Morphologic alteration occurs as a separate process at varying intervals after infection, e.g. in vitro in 3–5 days (RSV or strain MC29) or 10–21 days (strains RPL12, ES4, R, and BAI strain A), and in vivo in 5–7 days (RSV), 14–28 days (BAI strain A), or 8–10 weeks (RPL12 and lymphoid leukosis).

LABORATORY HOST SYSTEMS

Chick Inoculation

Rous sarcoma virus and other sarcoma viruses produce tumors when inoculated subcutaneously into the wing web, intramuscularly, intra-abdominally, or by contact with inoculated chickens. Subcutaneous inoculation into the wing web is most commonly used for titrations of stocks of Rous sarcoma virus (Bryan, 1956), and either this route or intramuscular inoculation is used for virus isolation and virus propagation (Purchase and Okazaki, 1964). Intracerebral inoculation of chicks can be employed for the detection of genetic resistance to the virus. On subcutaneous inoculation in the wing web with high doses of virus, tumors are first palpable after about 3 days and in susceptible chickens may grow rapidly, ulcerate, and metastasize. With low doses of virus, tumors may occur as late as 35 days after inoculation. There are extensive reviews on the methods and interpretation of results (Bryan, 1956). Following intracerebral inoculation of day-old chicks, specific deaths occur between 7 and 35 days postinoculation (Groupé et al., 1956). Tumors occur in the brain at the site of inoculation and metastases occur throughout the body. By intravenous inoculation of end point dilutions of Rous sarcoma virus preparations, Burmester and Walter (1961) were able to induce not only the expected disease but also lymphoid leukosis and erythroblastosis. These were presumed to have been caused by the Rous-associated lymphoid leukosis virus present as a helper (Burmester, 1964).

By inoculating the RPL12 strain of virus intra-abdominally into day-old susceptible line 15I chicks, Burmester and Gentry (1956) were able to obtain a lymphoid leukosis response in 200–270 days. This procedure was used by Burmester and Fredrickson (1964) for the initial isolation of virus from field cases. The time required for quantitative assay of certain strains passaged in the laboratory was shortened to 63 days by using the less sensitive erythroblastosis response (Burmester, 1956a) and to 43 days when embryos were inoculated intravenously (Piraino et al., 1963). In these transmission experiments all sources of virus that caused lymphoid leukosis also caused erythroblastosis. Osteopetrosis, hemangiomas, and fibrosarcomas were also observed in chickens of certain strains and passages. The host-virus interrelations have been studied in great detail by Burmester et al. (1959a, 1960a).

Avian myeloblastosis virus can be titrated in susceptible chicks by intravenous inoculation at 1–3 days of age (Eckert et al., 1951, 1953, 1954). Adenosine triphosphatase activity is closely associated with avian myeloblastosis virus particles. Plasmas with a high enzyme activity also contain large amounts of virus. The enzyme assay method (Beaudreau and Becker, 1958) is indispensable for routine and large-scale studies for assay of individual plasmas and myeloblast culture fluids. Osteopetrosis has been reproduced by intravenous inoculation of day-old chicks using certain preparations of RPL12 virus (Burmester et al., 1960a), although the response has not been used for quantitation of the virus. Holmes (1964) and Young (1966) were able to induce the disease by the intramuscular injection of infective whole blood or plasma.

Embryo Inoculation

Rous sarcoma virus induces pocks on the chorioallantoic membranes of susceptible embryos. When chorioallantoic membranes of 11-day-old embryos are inoculated by the technique of Dougherty et al. (1960), pocks can be counted 8 days later (Fig. 15.21). Tumors can also be produced by intravenous inoculation at 10–13 days incubation and by yolk sac inoculation at 5–8 days incubation. Some strains induce hemorrhages 7 days after intravenous inoculation into 11-day-old embryos, and this procedure has been used for quantitative measurements of virus concentration (Coates et al., 1968).

Leukosis viruses have been quantitated by the intravenous inoculation of 11-day-old embryos of susceptible line 15I chicks. Chicks that hatched did not have overt neoplasia; however, specific deaths began within a week of hatching. The rate of mortality increased rapidly so that by 2 weeks of age a high incidence was obtained. Most chicks died of erythroblastosis, although many also developed a variety of solid tumors including fibrosarcomas, endothelial tumors, nephromas, and chondromas. In addition there were numerous hemorrhages. When chicks were held for a postinoculation period of 46 days the responses were higher, by 1–2 $\log_{10}$ dilutions, than those observed in chicken inoculations. Most chickens that survived the neoplasms which appeared before 100 days postinoculation developed lymphoid leukosis after that time (Piraino et al., 1963).

Avian myeloblastosis virus produced a myeloblastosis response in a similar time

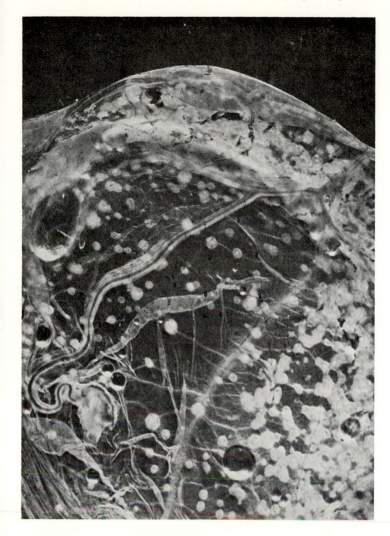

FIG. 15.21—Pocks induced by Bryan's high-titer strain of Rous sarcoma virus on chorio-allantoic membrane of chicken embryo. (Courtesy F. Piraino, City Health Dept., Milwaukee, Wis.)

when inoculated intravenously into susceptible embryos (Baluda and Jamieson, 1961).

Cell Culture

Most leukosis viruses replicate but do not produce a cytopathic effect in cell culture except after prolonged passage (Calnek, 1964). Sarcoma viruses, on the other hand, produce a characteristic rapid cytopathic effect (Fig. 15.20) in susceptible cultured cells, and they can be readily and accurately quantitated by this criterion (Manaker and Groupé, 1956). The properties of leukosis/sarcoma viruses in cell culture are described in more detail under the section on isolation and identification of the agents.

All leukosis viruses thus far studied in culture induce infection and morphologic change in chicken embryo cells marked by general shortening and rounding of spindle shapes to contours somewhat determined by the virus strain (Bernhard et al., 1956; Heine et al., 1962, 1969; Haguenau and Beard, 1962; Haguenau et al., 1962). Ultrastructural alterations, also somewhat dependent on virus strain (Heine et al., 1969), vary from slight abnormalities to considerable changes in the cytoplasm or nucleus or both. Cytoplasmic structural alterations, pronounced in chick embryo cells infected with strain MC29 virus, as an example (Heine, et al., 1969), are characterized by shortening and rounding of contours, smoothing of the cell membrane with fewer filiform processes, high concentration of ribosomes and polysomes, very limited rough endoplasmic reticulum with narrow lumina, few lysosomes and other analogous bodies, and infrequent vacuoles containing virus. Somewhat similar features characterize the cytoplasm of the myeloid cells growing in strain MC29 virus-infected bone marrow cultures (Langlois et al., 1969). An additional attribute was a gray-stained background matrix which, together with the abundant ribosomes and polysomes, imparted a "grainy" homogeneous appearance to the whole cytoplasm. This aspect of structure is of common occurrence in the cells of myelocytomatosis in the bird (Mladenov et al., 1967). Few granules develop in the tissue culture cells in contrast to numerous granules in myelocytoma (Mladenov et al., 1967) and frequently in myelocytomatosis also.

In the less pronounced and different changes in Rous sarcoma virus-infected chick embryo cells (Haguenau and Beard, 1962; Heine et al., 1962), the Golgi apparatus is often hyperplastic with a proliferation of the vesicular elements, and there is vacuolization of the cytoplasm and increased pseudopodial activity. Characteristic osmiophilic, gray-body inclusions occur in various stages of formation or vacuolization. These bodies, of the character of lysosomes (Heine et al., 1964), may be surrounded by a single or double membrane or be apparently without a membrane (Dmochowski et al., 1964) and linked to an indentation of the cell surface through a row of pinocytic vesicles (Haguenau and Beard, 1962). The amorphous, osmiophilic substance may occur alone or together with characteristic virus particles; some of the bodies may be packed with virus particles.

The bone marrow of young or adult birds responds to leukosis agents with virus liberation and growth of erythroid (Heine, et al., 1961; Beard, 1963a) or myeloid (Bonar et al., 1959, 1960; Langlois et al., 1969) cells, depending on the virus strain involved. Erythroblasts (Heine et al., 1961) and myeloblasts (Bonar et al., 1959) originating from leukosis virus infection of bone marrow cells in culture do not differ greatly from the respective elements in the bird with erythroblastosis or myeloblastosis, nor indeed from erythroblasts and myeloblasts in the normal bird. Relatively numerous pseudopodial and filiform processes in these elements suggest unusual activity of the cell membrane. Vacuoles, some containing virus, are relatively numerous. Also present in both erythroblasts and myeloblasts

are small numbers of osmiophilic or gray bodies (Fig. 15.22) containing virus and other materials similar to those described in Rous sarcoma virus altered cells. However, the bodies are very numerous in myeloblasts after transfer to culture from leukemic chickens and after various treatments of the cultures (Heine et al., 1964). When carbon particles (Heine et al., 1961) or colloidal gold (Heine et al., 1964) are added to cultures of infected erythroblasts or myeloblasts, the carbon or gold appears in these inclusions together with the osmiophilic material and virus particles. Such behavior indicates that at least some of the contents of the gray bodies are ingested from outside the cell. In addition, the bodies exhibit a variety of enzymatic activities and attributes characteristic of lysosomes (Heine et al., 1964).

The cytoplasm of a variety of avian virus-infected cells (Haguenau and Beard, 1962; Heine et al., 1968) may occasionally contain other anomalous structures (Fig. 15.23), as first described by Bernhard et al. (1956). These consist of densely massed osmiophilic particles shown to be RNA granules (Heine et al., 1968). Embedded within the mass are spherical bodies about 44 $m\mu$ in diameter, enclosed in a membrane and surrounded by an outer ring of ribonucleoprotein granules. The nature of these "clusters" (Haguenau and Beard, 1962) or "aberrant structures" (Heine et al., 1968) is not yet clear. Although the spheres resemble virus-particle nucleoids, there is no evidence that the structures participate in the regular processes of virus synthesis and liberation from the cell. It is possible, however, that the formations may represent aggregates of virus components not organized into particles because of the lack of external membrane envelope.

Nuclear changes likewise are prominent in some of the altered cells, particularly in chicken embryo cells infected with strain MC29 (Heine et al., 1969). The organelle, elongated in the normal spindle-shaped cell, becomes essentially spherical in the altered element. Striking attributes are the greatly enlarged nucleolus or nucleoli and the relatively homogeneous appearance of the nucleoplasm. Except for size the nucleolus is not structurally unusual. The appearance of the nucleoplasm is related primarily to the small proportion of condensed chromatin and the relatively large

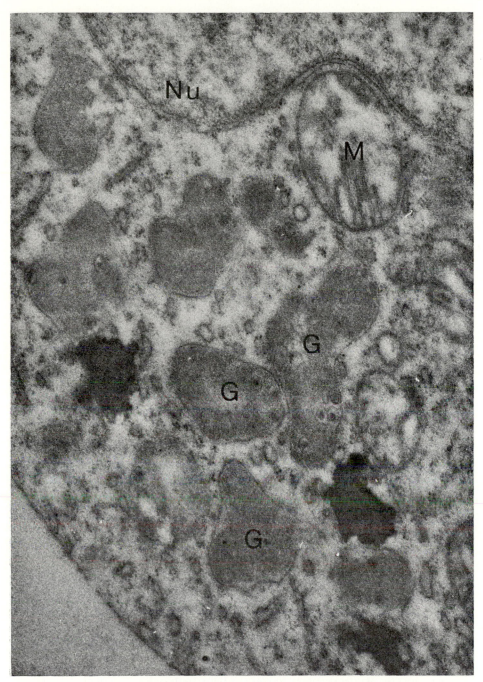

FIG. 15.22—Ultrastructural changes in leukosis/sarcoma virus-infected cells. A myeloblast obtained from the circulation and cultured in vitro 2 days in tissue culture medium containing 50% chicken serum. In general morphology it does not differ from myeloblasts taken directly from circulation. Gray bodies (G) of irregular shape contain amorphous material, embedded in which are virus particles of typical appearance (Nu = nucleus, M = mitochondrion). ×44,000. (Courtesy R. A. Bonar, Duke Univ. Medical Center)

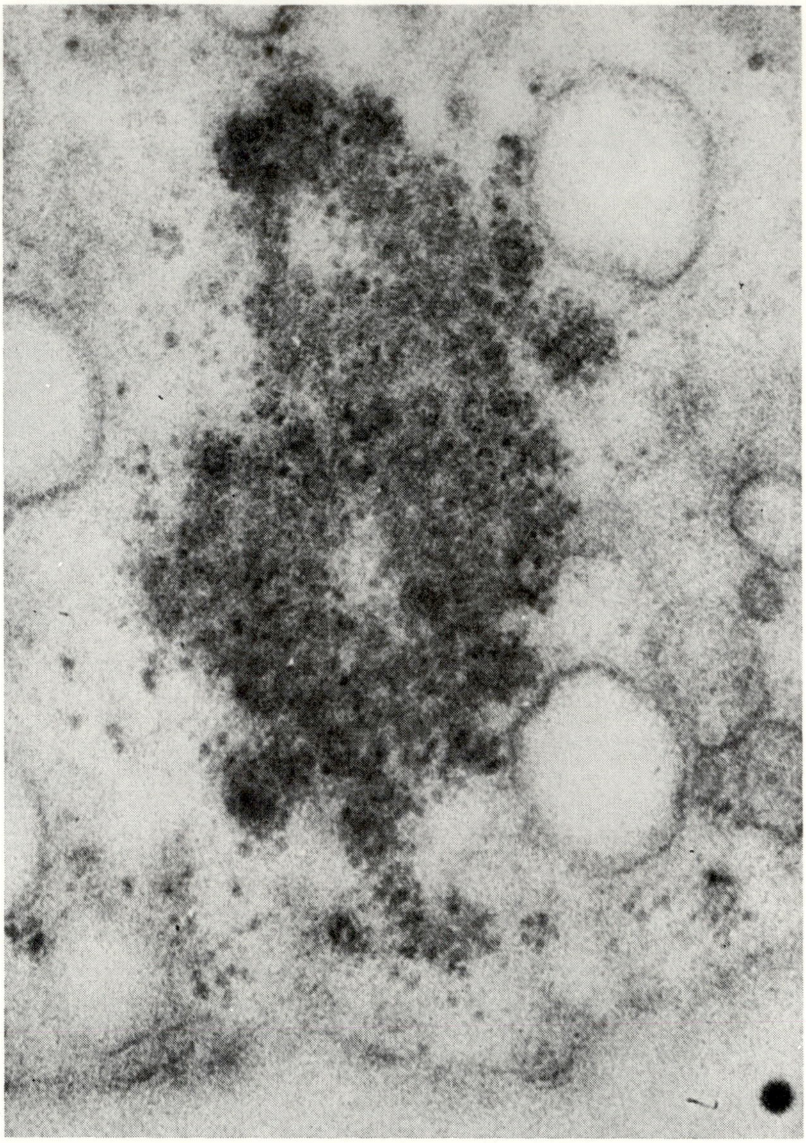

FIG. 15.23—Ultrastruc-
tural changes in leuko-
sis/sarcoma virus-infect-
ed cells. Cytoplasmic
structures in erythro-
blast of erythroblastic
leukemia induced by
strain R virus.
×143,000.

amount of chromatin in the diffuse or dispersed state which is highly characteristic
of these cells altered by strain MC29. Much
of the material is demonstrable as threads
of 30–125 Å in diameter, the smallest of
which approach the size of deoxyribonucle-
oprotein strands. Some nucleolar enlargement occurs also in Rous sarcoma virus-
infected cells. The *pars amorpha* may be
conspicuous, and there may be "unrolling"
of the nucleolonema not notable in other
altered cells. Chromatin is mostly of the
condensed form resembling that in the normal cells. Chicken embryo cells altered by

ES4 virus show no unusual features of nuclear structure.

Nucleoli are very large also in myeloid
bone marrow cells treated with strain
MC29 (Langlois et al., 1969), but the proportion of diffuse and dispersed chromatin
is far less than in the altered chicken embryo cells. The nucleus as a whole is relatively small in these cells in comparison
with the nuclei of myeloblasts induced by
BAI strain A. A conspicuous difference between strain MC29-induced myelocytes and
BAI strain A-induced myeloblasts is the relatively small nucleolus in the latter which

is scarcely larger than that in the normal cells. An additional difference is the relatively normal state of condensed chromatin in the myeloblast.

PATHOGENICITY

In early work it was quite evident that experimentally induced tumors in birds resembled the tumor from which the inoculum originated. This was observed especially with the "sarcoma" group of viruses which induced primarily solid tumors of the connective tissue. In some instances, particularly with the diseases of the hematopoietic organs, this was not the case. As research progressed and closer observations were made of the experimental chicken, isolates were found to produce more than one type of response and the situation became confusing.

When a leukosis strain was passaged successively from chicken to chicken in one laboratory under a given standard set of conditions, tumors of relatively consistent pathology were produced. Over the years these have been referred to as virus strains, but since they were not in any way genetically purified, there was no knowledge of the number of virus entities present. Thus, even though the viral etiology of many of the tumors has been conclusively proved, there is still no clear understanding of the etiologic relationships between the diseases. Two major opposing theories have been proposed. The first considers that a single viral entity is the cause of all the different neoplasms induced by one strain and that the different pathological entities produced reflect differences in response of the host systems involved; thus the hematopoietic system responds with erythroblastosis and the lymphopoietic system with lymphoid leukosis. In the alternative hypothesis, it is presumed that each pathological disease is caused by a different individual viral entity and therefore that most strains are mixtures of different entities. It is possible that the oncogenic properties of one strain will fit the first hypothesis and those of another strain will fit the second. Even though some evidence has accumulated to distinguish between these two possibilities, the situation has not yet been fully resolved.

Under standard conditions a given virus strain induces a relatively constant spectrum of tumors. Thus Rous sarcoma virus causes predominantly sarcomas at the site of inoculation, strain R infection results in erythroblastosis, and BAI strain A, myeloblastosis when large amounts of these viruses are inoculated. By various manipulations it has been possible to alter the spectrum of tumors produced, and when an understanding of the conditions is obtained, tumors of a particular type can be reproduced at will. A discussion of the effects of some of these manipulations follows.

Source or Origin of Virus

The strain of virus has a profound effect upon the tumor response obtained. In this respect the Bryan strain of Rous sarcoma virus has produced characteristic fibrosarcomata through many passages in many laboratories, and the BAI strain A of avian myeloblastosis has produced predominantly myeloblastosis ever since passages were made from the single chicken with myeloblastosis (Eckert et al., 1951). Many virus strains, including those from the field, when handled under identical conditions produce slightly different tumor spectrums; i.e., each strain has its own oncogenic spectrum (Fig. 15.24), with some neoplasms occurring frequently in chickens inoculated with one strain but rarely among those given another strain. During passage from donor birds with erythroblastosis, RPL28 (Strickland) consistently produced more sarcomas than RPL27 (Hickory) or RPL26 (Magadore), even though in 3 consecutive passages most of the birds were killed by all 3 strains (Fredrickson et al., 1965).

Within a particular strain, differences were obtained by using donor birds of different sources with different tumors. Initial isolation of virus from field cases in day-old line 15I chicks resulted in responses similar to those induced by a low dose of the RPL12 strain of avian tumor virus (Burmester and Fredrickson, 1964). Serial transfer from donors with lymphoid leukosis resulted primarily in lymphoid leukosis, but by selecting donor birds with erythroblastosis rather than lymphoid leukosis, the disease produced was predominantly erythroblastosis (Fredrickson et al., 1965). As will be explained later, this was almost certainly due to a dose effect. In another instance the selection of virus donors with hemangiomas resulted in a larger proportion of birds with hemangiomas than in the previous passage of the strain (Burmester

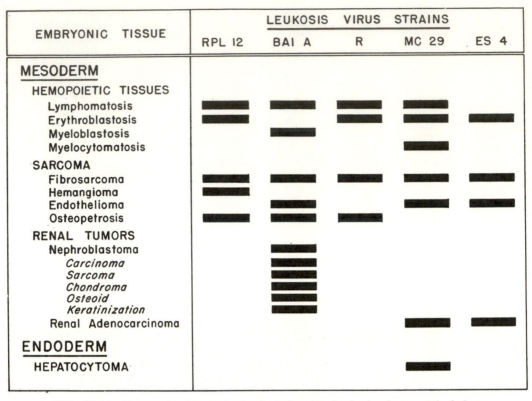

FIG. 15.24—Oncogenic spectrum of selected avian leukosis viruses. Black bars represent a response of that type. (Courtesy J. W. Beard, Duke Univ. Medica. Center)

et al., 1959a). Thus there is some heterogeneity in the virus strains themselves, related possibly to the presence of more than one virus, or perhaps to capacity for virus alteration in some way by growing in a particular tissue or culture. These factors can be exploited to produce a tumor spectrum which is close to the one desired.

Dose Influence

High doses of RPL12 virus induced primarily erythroblastosis, whereas doses closer to the end point induced predominantly lymphoid leukosis (Burmester et al., 1959a). Sarcomas, endotheliomas, and hemorrhages also appeared to be more common with high virus doses. The occurrence of osteopetrosis showed no dependency on dose (Fredrickson et al., 1964).

Route of Inoculation

The responses obtained after administration by routes which are less efficient portals of entry of the virus into the host reflected the decreased effective dose. Thus exposure of susceptible birds by contact with birds inoculated with a high dose of RPL12 resulted in a lymphoid leukosis response similar to that expected with 1/1,000 of the dose of RPL12 (Burmester et al., 1959a). On the other hand, intramuscular inoculation of RPL26 favored the induction of sarcomas, whereas intravenous inoculation produced mainly erythroblastosis and hemorrhages (Fredrickson et al., 1964). These differences may still reflect differences in the amounts of virus which reach the target cells by the different routes; thus one would expect more virus to reach the erythropoietic tissue when administered intravenously than when given intramuscularly.

Age of Host

In general, resistance of birds to development of neoplasms of all types increases with age. The rate of increase of age resistance varies with the route of inoculation. In this respect resistance increases very rapidly between 1 and 21 days of age with oral or nasal administration but relatively slowly when virus is inoculated intravenously (Burmester et al., 1960a). The types of tumors produced also reflect the decreased effective dose (Burmester et al., 1959a). However, the incidence of some tumors decreases more rapidly than one would expect from the dose effect alone. For example certain RPL12 virus preparations given intravenously at 1 day of age caused a high incidence of osteopetrosis; the proportion of chickens inoculated at 3 weeks of age and developing osteopetrosis was only 1/10 that of chickens inoculated at 1 day of age (Burmester et al., 1960a).

There is an interesting exception in that very young birds are somewhat less susceptible to strain R virus than are older birds (Beaudreau et al., 1956).

Breed and Sex of Recipient

The response of different lines of chickens to leukosis viruses varies greatly. Once again these variations can be partly explained on the basis of a variable level of effective virus; i.e., resistant chickens respond in the same manner as susceptible chickens inoculated with lower doses of virus. On the other hand, some responses are characteristic of the lines of chicken recipients (Burmester et al., 1959a, 1960b).

Females are more susceptible to lymphoid leukosis than males (Burmester, 1945). Castration of both males and females increased the incidence of lymphoid leukosis, and testosterone increased the resistance of males and capons (Burmester and Nelson, 1945). This may have been a direct effect of the hormone or an indirect effect of the hormone on the bursa of Fabricius.

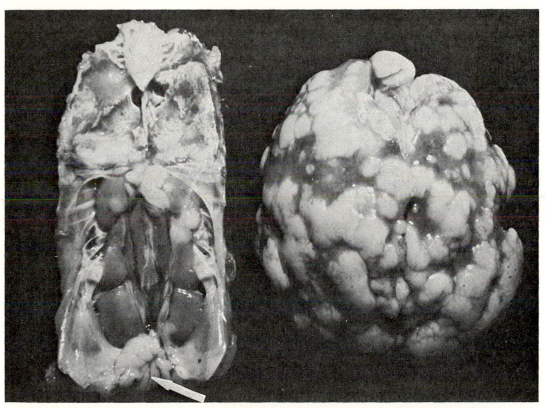

FIG. 15.25—*Lymphoid leukosis transplant. Bird died 14 days after inoculation at 1 day of age with suspension from lymphoid leukosis tumor induced by HPRS-2 Rous associated leukosis virus. A lymphoid tumor was also present in abdominal muscle at site of inoculation. Note metastases in liver, lung, and kidney and absence of tumor in bursa (arrow).*

HOMOTRANSPLANTATION

Many of the tumors induced by viruses of the leukosis/sarcoma group are homotransplantable. In some instances transplanted tumors can be readily differentiated from primary virus-induced tumors. Thus transplanted lymphoid leukosis tumors grow to a palpable size within 5–10 days and result in death shortly thereafter, whereas primary virus-induced tumors only develop 4 months after inoculation of day-old chicks. Other transplantable tumors also have a shorter incubation period than their virus-induced counterparts. Transplanted lymphoid leukosis tumors and nephroblastoma generally appear at the site of inoculation instead of in their originating organs; e.g., in lymphoid leukosis tumor transplants there is usually no bursal tumor (Fig. 15.25). Histologically transplanted tumors are generally more uniform and more anaplastic than the tumors from which they originate (compare Figs. 15.26 and 15.31). Thus transplanted lymphoid leukosis tumors are composed almost exclusively of large anaplastic lymphoblasts with a vesicular nucleus and several large nucleoli (Fig. 15.26). They do not contain any medium or small lymphocytes which may be present in the tumor in the original host.

Using the sex chromosome techniques, the fate of cells from donors of one sex can be accurately determined in recipients of the opposite sex (Vogt, 1965).

Rous sarcomas can be serially transplanted; however, by the 2nd generation only 0.05% of these cells are of donor origin (Ponten, 1962a). Even in histocompatible chickens, the proportion of cells in metaphase falls rapidly until there are no mitotic donor cells 6 days after cell inoculation (Ponten, 1964). Thus Rous sarcoma cells do not survive long in the recipient, and tumors in the recipient are formed largely from recruited cells.

Leukemic myeloblasts from donor birds inoculated with avian myeloblastosis virus (BAI strain A) failed to persist in the recipient when transplanted, and the leukemic cells had the karyotype of the recipient (Baluda, 1962).

Erythroblasts from donor birds inoculated with strain R, on the other hand, persisted for longer periods of time in the recipient—in highly inbred chickens up to the 5th transplant generation (Ponten, 1962c).

Lymphoid cells from some lymphoid leukosis tumors can be transplanted indefinitely. This is certainly true for the tumor from which the RPL12 strain of virus originated (Ponten, 1962b) and for many other virus-induced lymphoid leukosis tumors. However, some tumors are converted into neoplasms dominated by cells of recipient origin (Ponten and Burmester, 1967).

Nephroblastomas induced by avian myeloblastosis virus (BAI strain A) have been homotransplanted to the breast muscle (Walter et al., 1962; Ishiguro et al., 1962). Recipients have, in addition to tumors at the site of inoculation, metastatic tumors in the viscera and secondary tumors such as myeloblastosis and lymphoid leukosis. Since typical renal growths occurred at the site of inoculation, there is not much doubt that these tumors were of donor origin. However, it is likely that the secondary neoplasms were induced by virus elaborated by the transplant.

Investigations of tumor transplants have been of limited assistance in the understanding of virus-induced tumors. Thus immunity and genetic resistance to tumors resulting directly from the transplantation of neoplastic cells have no relation to the immunity or genetic resistance to virus infection or induction of tumors by virus.

PATHOGENESIS AND EPIZOOTIOLOGY

NATURAL AND EXPERIMENTAL HOSTS

The natural hosts for all viruses of this group are chickens; no viruses of this group have been isolated from other avian species. However, experimentally some viruses have a wide host range, and some can be adapted to grow in unusual hosts by passage in very young animals or by the induction of immunological tolerance prior to inoculation of the virus. Rous sarcoma virus has the widest host range. It will cause tumors in chickens, pheasants, guinea fowl, ducks, pigeons, Japanese quail, turkeys (Dunkel et al., 1964) and rock partridge (Ianconescu and Samberg, 1967). Smida et al. (1968) were unable to induce tumors in ducks with the Bryan strain of Rous sarcoma virus, but they were successful with the Praha and Schmidt-Ruppin strains, Fujinami sarcoma virus, and B77 sarcoma virus. MH2 virus did not induce tumors in

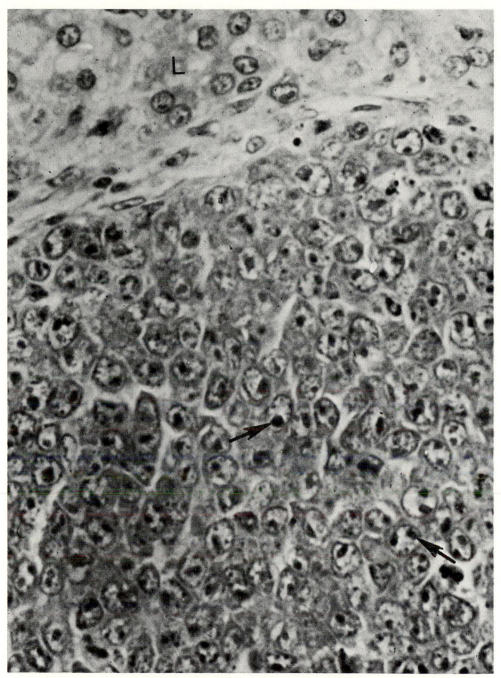

FIG. 15.26—Microscopic appearance of tumor in Fig. 15.25. Note homogeneous large anaplastic lymphoblasts with prominent nucleoli (**arrow**) compressing the liver cells (**L**). Compare these cells with those in Fig. 15.31 which resulted from infection with virus rather than cells. Cells from bird in Fig. 15.30 were transplanted to induce tumors shown in Figs. 15.25 and 15.26. ×1,000.

ducks. Some strains of sarcoma virus induce tumors in mammals (Vogt, 1965).

Osteopetrosis can be reproduced in turkeys by inoculation of fresh whole blood from affected chickens (Holmes, 1964). RPL12 strain of lymphoid leukosis virus did not produce lymphoid leukosis or erythroblastosis in Japanese quail (Crittenden and Purchase, unpublished data; Rauscher et al., 1964), and the virus did not multiply in the quail. These birds are, however, susceptible to myeloblastosis (Rauscher et al., 1964).

NATURAL TRANSMISSION

Leukosis/sarcoma viruses can be transmitted vertically from parent to offspring or horizontally from bird to bird. The latter is slow and inefficient, and close contact may be necessary for significant and rapid spread. Because of this and the lability of the virus, contact spread is not considered significant in most instances. On the other hand, egg transmission is of utmost importance in the perpetuation of virus infection.

Few parental flocks have been examined in detail for the presence of leukosis viruses by the resistance inducing factor (RIF) test (Rubin, 1960a) or for the presence of antibodies. In a flock selected for susceptibility to leukosis, Rubin detected evidence of infection in all birds; i.e., they had antibody or virus or both (Rubin et al., 1962). On the other hand, Levine and Nelsen (1964), in a similar study of a commercial egg-producing flock, found that 23% of the birds showed no evidence of infection. All 4 possible combinations of virus and antibody occur in mature birds but the ratios vary in different flocks. The relative frequencies also vary with the age of the birds.

In the epizootiology of this infection, the male plays only a minor role. Progeny from a viremic rooster do not have a higher incidence of viremia than progeny from a nonviremic rooster. On electron microscopic examination, viral budding has been seen in all structures of the reproductive organs of roosters except the germinal cells (Di Stefano and Dougherty, 1968), indicating that virus does not multiply in the sperm cells. The rooster therefore only acts as a carrier of the virus and a source of contact infection for other birds.

In the female the situation is different and more complicated. Viremic hens seldom have antibody, and the viremia appears to be of indefinite duration. Occasionally a bird may develop antibody and "overcome" the infection. Virus budding has been observed in hepatocytes (Beard, 1963a), in most of the cells in the ovary except the ovarian follicles, and in the connective tissue elements and the lining and glandular epithelial cells at all levels of the oviduct (Di Stefano and Dougherty, 1966). As in males, the germinal cells are not involved; however, virus can be isolated from most embryos from viremic hens.

In Rubin's studies, all nonviremic birds had antibody. Some also harbored virus, since they intermittently shed virus in their eggs. In Levine's flock, 75% of the birds with antibody shed virus, whereas in Rubin's flock only 1 out of 7 antibody positives were shedders. Calnek (1965) detected virus in the embryos of approximately 25% of the antibody-positive dams; some of the shedder hens laid only an occasional infected embryo (less than 1/10 of their total production). On the whole, birds with circulating antibody shed less frequently (intermittent shedders) than those without antibody but with circulating virus (continuous shedders). Up to 18 months of age, birds that shed virus in their eggs did so more consistently and at a higher level than birds of 2 or 3 years of age (Burmester and Waters, 1956; Bamberger, 1964); i.e., there was a general reduction in the rate of shedding as the birds got older. The amount of shedding was also dependent on the genetic line of chickens (Burmester et al., 1955).

There was a group of birds in each of the flocks studied by Rubin and Levine which had antibody and no evidence of virus in the circulation or being shed through the eggs. It is unknown whether these birds were carrying a cryptic infection somewhere in their body.

Electron micrographs have revealed virus particles in many organs from infected chick embryos (Fig. 15.27). Virus has also been recovered from many of these in cell culture (Rubin et al., 1961). Virus has been observed to bud from the pancreatic acinar cells of embryos from naturally or artificially infected hens which shed the virus, and there are masses of particles in the pancreatic lumen (Heine et al., 1963; Zeigel et al., 1964). Extracts of pancreas containing virus particles inoculated into susceptible

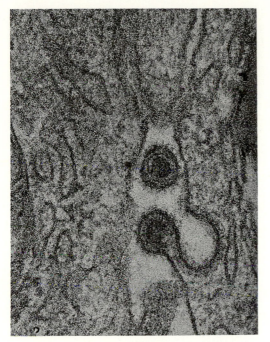

FIG. 15.27—*Elaboration of leukosis/sarcoma viruses in chicken embryo. Mature extracellular viral particle and viral bud at surface of medullary cord cell in ovary of 20-day chicken embryo congenitally infected with avian leukosis virus. Uranyl acetate and lead citrate, ×127,600. (Courtesy R. M. Dougherty, State Univ. of N.Y.)*

chickens resulted in much lymphoid leukosis (Zeigel et al., 1964). The large numbers of particles observed in the lumen of pancreatic ducts of embryos were not observed 2–3 days after hatching, suggesting that the particles were flushed out during the initiation of pancreatic activity at the first stimulus of feeding. They are then excreted in the droppings (which then are highly infectious). Infected chicks also have a high level of viremia, and virus probably enters the salivary glands early since oral washings from very young chicks have been shown to be infective (Burmester, 1956b; Rubin et al., 1961). These viremic chicks show no symptoms, are immunologically tolerant to the leukosis virus, and do not develop antibody (Rubin et al., 1962). Throughout their lives they act as a continuous source of virus for dissemination to the surroundings and thereby to susceptible birds. On reaching maturity, females become continuous shedders.

IMMUNITY

Most day-old chicks have maternal antibody ranging in titer from 1/10 to 1/100 of the titer in their respective dams; i.e., the efficiency of passive transfer is low. This gradually decreases until between 4 weeks (Rubin et al., 1961) and 7 weeks (Witter et al., 1966) when all the antibody is lost. The higher the level of antibody in the dam, the longer it persists in the progeny. After losing their maternal antibody, most chicks become infected from pen mates or from the surroundings and, after a transient viremia, develop antibodies which rise to high titer and can be detected for long periods or throughout the life of the bird.

Laboratory studies have shown that antibody which is actively acquired and detectable in the serum after vaccination is passed on to the progeny. It protects the progeny from occurrence of neoplasms on challenge with the homologous virus (Burmester, 1955; Burmester et al., 1957). In an experimental flock (Witter et al., 1966) and in field studies (Purchase et al., 1969), there was a definite indication that the presence of passively acquired maternal antibody in chicks delays the onset of actively acquired antibody. From this it would appear that infection with the homologous virus is also delayed. This delay may affect tumor formation since the rapid acquisition of "age resistance" to some avian oncogenic viruses has been shown repeatedly (Eckert et al., 1955a; Burmester et al., 1959a, 1960a). Thus there is little doubt that maternal antibody will give some protection against tumors caused by the homologous virus.

PATHOLOGY

One or more of the specific neoplasms induced by viruses of the leukosis/sarcoma group may occur in a given flock of chickens. The presence of a tumor similar to that produced under experimental conditions is only provisional evidence that the bird was infected with a virus of this group at some previous time. Some tumors do not yield virus, so it has not been possible to show that all tumors of a given type are caused by a virus of this group. In this section the pathology of the different neoplasms will be discussed without regard for the virological properties of the inducing agent(s). Only those entities which have been reproduced with viruses of the leukosis/sarcoma group will be described.

LYMPHOID LEUKOSIS

Incubation Period

After inoculation of susceptible embryos or 1–14-day-old susceptible chicks (e.g. line 15I) with a standard strain of virus (e.g. RPL12 [Burmester et al., 1959a], B15, or F42 [Biggs and Payne, 1964]), lymphoid leukosis appears between the 14th and 30th weeks of age. Very rarely do cases occur in chickens under 14 weeks old. In field outbreaks cases can occur any time after 14 weeks of age; however, the incidence is usually highest at about sexual maturity.

Clinical Signs

The outward signs of disease are not specific. The comb may be pale, shriveled, and occasionally cyanotic. Inappetance, emaciation, and weakness occur frequently. The abdomen is often enlarged and feathers are sometimes spotted with urates and bile pigments. Enlargement of the liver, bursa of Fabricius, and/or kidneys can often be detected on palpation, and the nodular nature of liver tumors can at times be detected. There is some indication that tumors are often of long standing; yet, once clinical signs begin to develop, the course may be quite rapid.

Morphologic Pathology

Grossly visible tumors occur after about 4 months of age and almost invariably involve the liver (Figs. 15.28, 15.36A), spleen, and bursa of Fabricius (Fig. 15.29). The size of tumors and number of organs affected are highly variable, but involvement is usually extensive in the liver and spleen. Many other organs such as the kidney, lungs, gonad, heart, bone marrow, and mesentery may also be affected, and occasionally massive tumors occur in these organs.

The tumors are soft, smooth, and glistening; a cut surface appears slightly grayish to creamy-white and seldom has areas of necrosis. The growth may be nodular (Fig. 15.28), miliary, or diffuse (Fig. 15.36A),

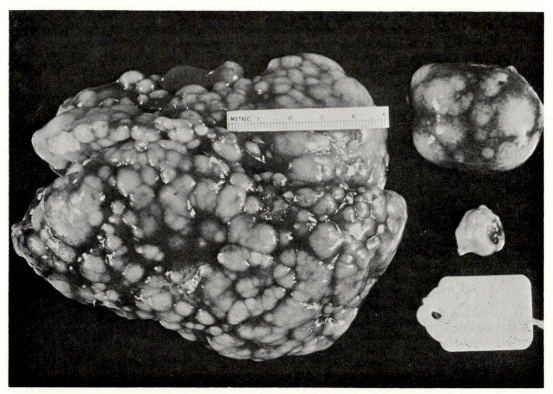

FIG. 15.28—Lymphoid leukosis. Nodular lesions in liver and spleen of bird inoculated at 1 day of age with RPL12-L31 virus.

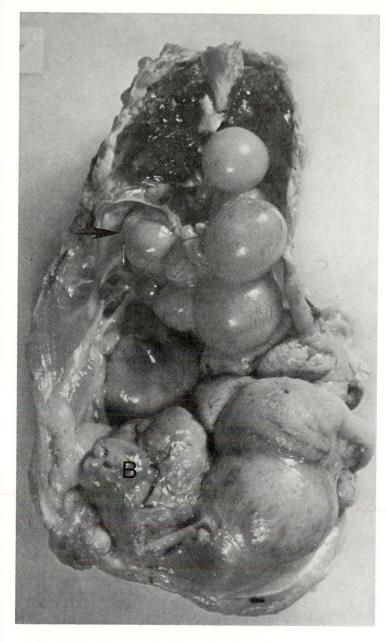

*FIG. 15.29—Lymphoid leukosis. Large tumor of bursa of Fabricius (**B**) and kidneys (**arrow**) in naturally occurring case of lymphoid leukosis in adult hen.*

or a combination of these forms. This is particularly evident in the liver and spleen. In the nodular form the lymphoid tumors vary from the size of a pinhead to that of a hen's egg, and may occur singly or in large numbers. They are generally spherical but may be flattened when they are close to the surface of an organ. The granular or miliary form, which is most obvious in the liver, consists of numerous small nodules, less than 2 mm in diameter, uni-formly distributed throughout the parenchyma. In the diffuse form the organ is uniformly enlarged, slightly grayish in color, and usually very friable. Occasionally, however, the liver is firm, fibrous, and almost gritty.

Microscopically all tumors are focal and multicentric in origin. Even in organs which appear diffusely involved when examined grossly, the microscopic pattern is one of coalescing foci. As the tumor cells

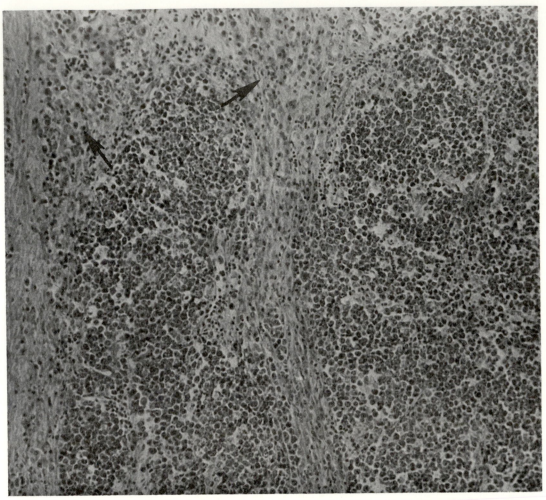

FIG. 15.30—Lymphoid leukosis. Liver tumor from bird which died 207 days after inoculation at 1 day of age with HPRS-2 Rous associated leukosis virus. Note displacement and compression of hepatic parenchyma (arrows). ×250.

proliferate, they displace and compress the cells of the organ rather than infiltrating between them (Fig. 15.30). Nodules in the liver are usually surrounded by a band of fibroblastlike cells which have been shown to be remnants of sinusoidal endothelial cells (Gross et al., 1959).

Tumors consist of aggregates of large lymphoid cells which may vary slightly in size but are all at the same primitive developmental stage. They have a poorly defined cytoplasmic membrane, much basophilic cytoplasm, and a vesicular nucleus in which there is margination and clumping of the chromatin and one or more conspicuous acidophilic nucleoli (Fig. 15.31). In properly fixed tissues the nucleoli may be so prominent that they resemble nuclear inclusion bodies found in some other viral diseases. The cytoplasm of most of the tumor cells contains a large amount of RNA which stains red with the methyl green pyronine stain, indicating that the cells are immature and rapidly dividing (Cooper et al., 1968). The predominant cell is considered to be a lymphocyte precursor or immature cell of the lymphocytic developmental series and has been referred to as a lymphoblast, hemocytoblast, and reticulolymphocyte. Characteristic features of the cell can best be seen in wet-fixed smears of fresh specimens which have been stained with May-Grünwald Giemsa, methyl green pyronine, or other cytologic stains.

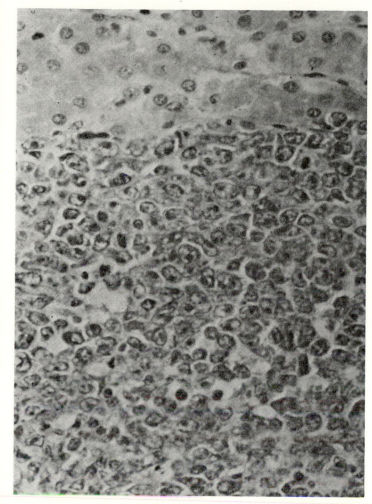

FIG. 15.31—Lymphoid leukosis in liver of RPL12 virus-inoculated bird. Note compression of hepatic parenchyma by proliferation of extravascular, primitive, lymphoid cells. ×1,000.

Somewhat different lesions have been described in young chickens. Calnek (1968b) infected day-old chickens and examined them 4–10 weeks later. He observed no clinical signs of disease but found gross lesions in the spleen (Fig. 15.32), heart, and testis and microscopic lesions in the liver and other visceral organs as well as the dorsal root ganglia. The spleen was slightly or moderately enlarged and usually mottled; the testis and heart had one or more small (up to 1 mm diameter) grayish, translucent areas. Microscopically the lesions were either small discrete foci or larger diffuse areas of lymphoblasts (Fig. 15.33). These lesions were transitory, since they were not grossly visible in birds over 10 weeks of age and the microscopic accumulations were also markedly reduced. Whether the lesions described were neoplastic or reactive was not determined.

ULTRASTRUCTURE. Vacuoles are found infrequently in the lymphoid cells of birds with lymphoid leukosis, but occasional virus particles have been observed budding from the plasma membranes of lymphoblasts (Dmochowski et al., 1964).

HEMATOLOGY. There are no consistent or significant changes in the cellular elements of the circulating blood. In occasional cases, the circulating large lymphocytes or lymphoblasts have more "buds" or pseudopods than usual. Rarely are there frank leukemic cases in which lymphoblasts predominate. Lymphoblasts are characterized by their large size, large eccentric nucleus with spongy chromatin, and moderate amount of intensely basophilic cytoplasm. Horiuchi et al. (1960) described granule-containing cells (G. cells) associated with the development of clinical lymphoid leu-

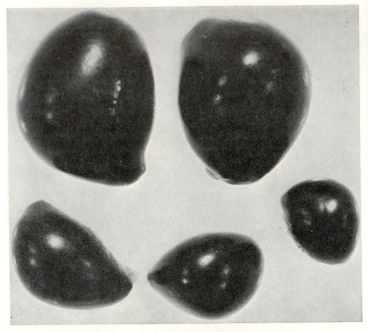

FIG. 15.32—Lesions in young chickens induced by leukosis virus. Note enlargement of 2 spleens from 4-week-old birds inoculated with RIF-1 at 1 day of age. Three smaller spleens are from comparable but uninoculated controls. (Courtesy B. W. Calnek, N.Y. State Veterinary College)

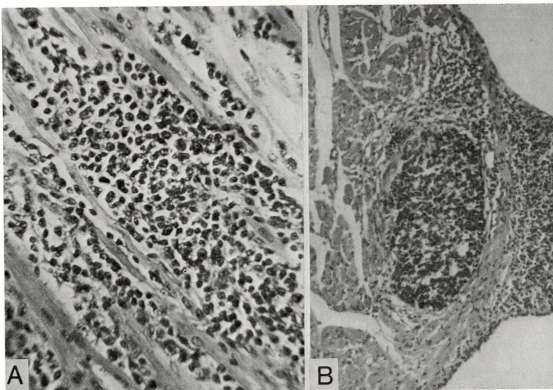

FIG. 15.33—Lesions in young chickens induced by a leukosis virus. (A) Heart from 4-week-old RIF-3 infected chick. Diffuse accumulations of lymphoid cells among myocardial fibers. ×430. (B) Endocardial surface, 6-week-old RIF-1 infected chick. Two circumscribed foci of lymphoid cells are visible; one protrudes from myocardium. ×100. (Courtesy B. W. Calnek, N.Y. State Veterinary College)

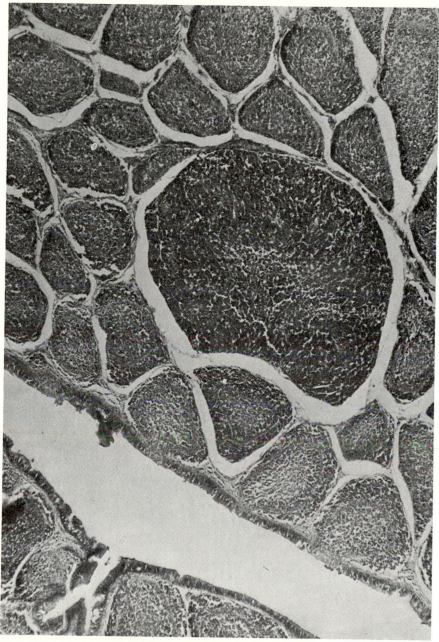

FIG. 15.34—*Lymphoid leukosis. Lymphoblastic transformation in single bursal follicle. All surrounding follicles are histologically normal in this and other sections from 16-day-old chicken infected with RPL12 virus at hatching. Methyl green pyronin,* ×40. (*Courtesy P. B. Dent, McMaster Univ. and* J. Nat. Cancer Inst.)

kosis. The cells appeared to be early forms of myelocytes except that their nuclei showed degenerative changes. In blood smears they were never numerous and were not easily identified.

Pathogenesis

There are two lines of evidence that lymphoid leukosis is a malignancy of the bursa-dependent lymphoid system. The first is that surgical or hormonal removal of the bursa of Fabricius from chickens infected at hatching with RPL12 strain of leukosis virus reduces or eliminates the incidence of the malignancy. In fact, surgical bursectomy at any time between 1 day and 5 months of age results in a significant reduction in deaths from lymphoid leukosis (Peterson et al., 1966). In addition, hormonally induced atrophy of the bursa has a similar effect (Burmester, 1969). Thymectomy has no effect on the course of the disease.

Detailed histopathological examination of the bursa has provided the second line of evidence. Changes in isolated bursa follicles can be observed as early as 8 weeks of age; by 16 weeks abnormal follicles are present in the bursas of most infected chickens (Fig. 15.34). Affected follicles become engorged with uniform blastlike cells with a pyroninophilic cytoplasm, and there is a loss of distinction between the cortex and the medulla. The abnormal follicles expand and displace the adjacent normal bursal follicles until by 16–24 weeks of age at the earliest, a gross tumor of the bursa is visible (Fig. 15.35). The constituent cells of the abnormal follicles are similar to those in lymphoid leukosis tumors of the bursa and the other visceral organs. Autopsies performed on chickens dying with lymphoid leukosis have revealed macroscopic tumors of the bursa in almost every case (Dent et al., 1967; Cooper et al., 1968; Burmester, 1969).

Thus it appears that even though lymphoid leukosis viruses multiply in almost all organs of the body, the cells of the bursa of Fabricius are the target cells in which neoplastic transformation takes place. As the bird grows older, cells of the bursa-dependent system leave the bursa and the bursa involutes. The tumor cells also migrate from the bursa and initiate metastatic foci in other visceral organs. At about the time of sexual maturity (16–24 weeks of age) the tumor involvement is so extensive that birds succumb to the disease.

Differential Diagnosis

Lymphoid leukosis and Marek's disease can be differentiated from one another only with great difficulty, since similar lymphoid tumors may occur in both diseases in the same visceral organs during the same age period. The visceral lesions of these two diseases cannot be distinguished by gross examination. Diagnosis is possible in most instances on careful microscopic examination; however, considerable experience is necessary. In coming to a decision, the history, symptoms, gross and microscopic lesions, and cytology should all be considered. The following points should

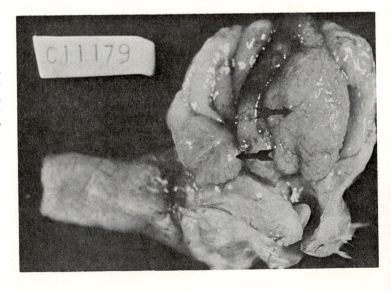

FIG. 15.35—Lymphoid leukosis. Earliest visible multiple tumors of bursa (**arrows**). *(Courtesy F. J. Siccardi, Regional Poultry Research Laboratory, E. Lansing, Mich.)*

receive special attention (Carr and Campbell, 1958; Siccardi and Burmester, unpublished data).

Ordinarily, lymphoid leukosis does not occur before 16 weeks of age, and most of the mortality occurs between 24 and 40 weeks. Marek's disease, on the other hand, may occur as early as 6 weeks, and the peak of mortality varies from 10 to 20 weeks. Occasionally losses continue after this age and may reach a peak even after 20 weeks.

Characteristic signs of paralysis and "gray eye" are specific for Marek's disease. Nodular tumors of the bursa can often be palpated through the cloaca in birds affected with lymphoid leukosis.

Gross lesions in the autonomic and peripheral nervous systems and the iris are specific for Marek's disease. Nodular lymphoid skin lesions as well as lymphoid tumors of the skeletal muscles have not been associated with lymphoid leukosis, and preliminary investigations point to a relation with Marek's disease.

As explained in the section on pathogenesis, the bursa of Fabricius plays a central role in the development of lymphoid leukosis. When distinct focal lymphoid tumors are present in the bursa, a diagnosis of lymphoid leukosis can be made. Such tumors are often quite small and may be overlooked. In some birds Marek's disease induces a premature nonspecific atrophy of the bursa. In others the bursa may be tumorous, in which case the walls and the plica may be thickened due to interfollicular infiltration and proliferation of the lymphocytes.

The microscopic lymphoid infiltration in the nerves, cuffing around the small arterioles in the white matter of the cerebellum, and follicular pattern of lymphoid cell infiltration in the skin which are characteristic of Marek's disease are not seen with lymphoid leukosis. The enlarged bursal follicles of tumors of the bursa consisting of uniform large lymphocytes which are usual with lymphoid leukosis are not associated with Marek's disease in which atrophy of the follicles and an interfollicular infiltration with pleomorphic lymphocytes are characteristic.

Cytologically, lymphoid leukosis tumors are generally composed of a homogeneous population of lymphoblasts (Fig. 15.31). In contrast, the growths of Marek's disease contain lymphoid cells that vary in size and maturity from lymphoblasts to small lymphocytes, and plasma cells may also be present. Special stains such as methyl green pyronin are very helpful for cytology (see Fig. 15.17E,F, Marek's disease subchapter). The immature lymphoblasts characteristic of lymphoid leukosis tumors are highly pyroninophilic, whereas the medium and small lymphocytes which predominate in tumors of Marek's disease do not stain with pyronin.

TABLE 15.6 ❧ Comparison of Epizootiological and Pathological Differences between Lymphoid Leukosis and Marek's Disease

	Lymphoid Leukosis	Marek's Disease
Age of onset	>16 weeks of age	>4 weeks of age
Clinical signs		
Paralysis or paresis	Absent	Usually present
Gross lesions		
Peripheral nerve and ganglion involvement	Absent	Usually present
Bursa of Fabricius	Nodular tumor	Diffuse enlargement or atrophy
Skin and muscle tumors	Usually absent	May be present
Microscopic lesions		
Peripheral nerve infiltration	Absent	Usually present
Cuffing in white matter of cerebellum	Absent	Usually present
Skin infiltration with follicular patterns of lymphoid cells	Absent	Often present
Cell proliferation in bursa of Fabricius	Intrafollicular	Interfollicular
Cytology of lymphoid cells	Uniform "blast" cells	Pleomorphic mature and immature cells

Some guidelines for differentiating between lymphoid leukosis and Marek's disease are given in Table 15.6.

Other diseases which may at times be confused with lymphoid leukosis are erythroblastosis, myeloblastosis, myelocytomatosis, Pullorum disease, tuberculosis, enterohepatitis, Hjärre's disease, and fatty degeneration of the liver.

ERYTHROBLASTOSIS

Incubation Period

The incubation period is influenced by the virus source, the dose and route of inoculation, and the age and genetic constitution of the host. After intra-abdominal inoculation of RPL12 strain virus into susceptible day-old chicks, the incubation period varies from 21 to 110 days (Burmester et al., 1959a). On intravenous inoculation of 11-day-old embryos, chicks have occasionally been found to have erythroblastosis on hatching (Purchase, unpublished data). Strain R produces a much more rapid response, and in some experiments, birds inoculated with high doses have all died between 7 and 12 days postinoculation (Beard, 1963a). Field strains and viruses passaged in cell culture induce erythroblastosis after a longer incubation period (Burmester and Fredrickson, 1964; Burmester, 1966). Passage from donors with erythroblastosis greatly shortens the incubation period (Fredrickson et al., 1965).

Other strains of virus which produce erythroblastosis include F42 (Biggs, 1964), ES4, and strain 13 (Beard, 1963a). Field cases usually occur in birds over 3 months of age.

Clinical Signs

Two forms of erythroblastosis have been described. The blastic or proliferative form is more commonly observed than the anemic form. It is characterized by the presence of many erythroblasts in the blood, whereas in the anemic form, there are relatively few immature cells in the circulating blood and the predominant feature is a marked anemia. Results of transmission experiments have suggested a close etiologic relationship between the two forms (Stubbs and Furth, 1932).

The earliest signs of either form are lethargy, general weakness, and either a slight paleness or cyanosis of the comb. As the condition advances, the combs of chickens with the anemic form become paler until they are light yellow to almost white. Chickens with the proliferative form may become pale or cyanotic. There is usually weakness, emaciation, diarrhea, and there may be profuse hemorrhage from one or more of the feather follicles. The course varies from a few days to several months; the anemic form is usually of shorter duration.

Morphologic Pathology

In birds that die with either form of the disease there is usually a general anemia which is often accompanied by petechial hemorrhages in various organs such as the muscles, the subcutis, and the viscera. Thrombosis, infarction, and rupture of the liver or spleen may be observed. There may be a subcutaneous edema of the lungs, hydropericardium, ascites, and a fibrinous clot on the ventral surface of the liver (Fig. 15.36B).

The most characteristic gross alteration in the proliferative form is diffuse enlargement of the liver and spleen and to a lesser extent the kidneys (Fig. 15.36B). These organs are usually cherry red to dark mahogany and are soft and friable. The liver may be finely mottled due to degeneration around the central veins of the lobules. The marrow is hyperplastic, very soft or watery, dark blood red or cherry red, and often has hemorrhages.

In the anemic form there is usually an atrophy of the visceral organs, particularly the spleen. The bone marrow is pale and jellylike and the marrow spaces may be

FIG. 15.36—Comparison of leukoses. **(A)** Lymphoid leukosis. Diffuse form affecting the liver. This lesion is grossly indistinguishable from those in Marek's disease. **(B)** Erythroblastosis. Enlarged cherry red liver and spleen. Note the fibrinous exudate. **(C)** Myeloblastosis. Note enlarged grayish red liver. **(D)** Erythroblastosis. Note the basophilic cytoplasm and perinuclear halo. Blood smear, Giemsa, ×1,300. **(E)** Myeloblastosis. Myeloblasts are slightly smaller than erythroblasts, the cytoplasm is not as basophilic, the nucleus is less vesicular, and nucleoli are not as frequent or conspicuous. Blood smear, Giemsa, ×1,300. **(F)** Myelocytomatosis. Note myelocytes packed with acidophilic granules. Section of tumor, Giemsa, ×1,300.

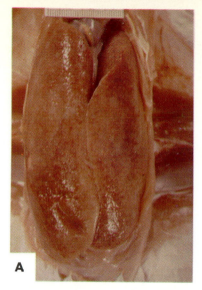

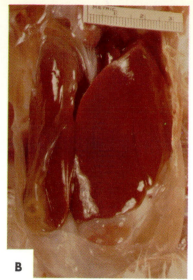

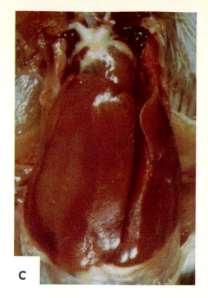

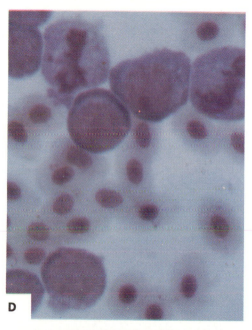

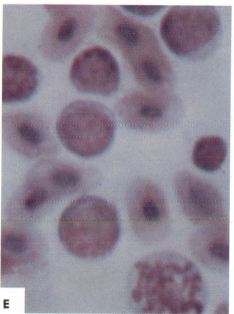

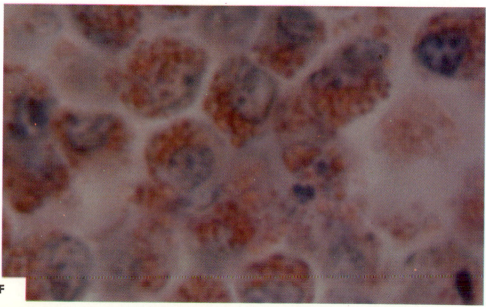

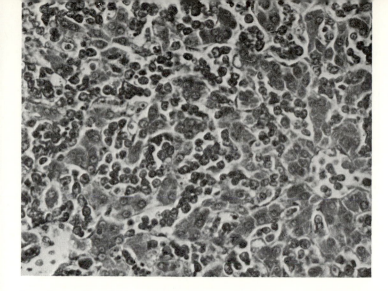

FIG. 15.37—*Erythroblastosis. Liver sinuses permeated with erythroblasts in bird 40 days after inoculation with strain MC29 leukosis virus. ×280. (Courtesy J. W. Beard, Duke Univ. Medical Center)*

largely replaced by spongy bone as seen in osteodystrophia fibrosa (Stubbs and Furth, 1932).

Microscopic examination of the marrow in early cases reveals blood sinusoids filled with rapidly proliferating erythroblasts which fail to mature. In advanced cases the marrow consists of sheets of homogeneous erythroblasts with small islands of myelopoietic activity and little or no adipose tissue. In contrast, in the aplastic form there may be a decreased erythropoietic activity, and in advanced cases the marrow is almost acellular.

The alterations in the visceral organs in the proliferative form are primarily due to a hemostasis which results in an accumulation of erythroblasts in the blood sinusoids and capillaries (Fig. 15.37). This results in dilation of the sinusoids which is particularly evident in the liver, spleen, and bone marrow. As this process continues the sinusoids become greatly distended, resulting in pressure atrophy of the parenchyma. In the liver there may also be a terminal degeneration and even a necrosis of the hepatic cells around the central veins due to local anoxia. Even though the accumulations of erythroblasts may be very extensive, they always remain entirely intravascular. This is in contrast to lymphoid leukosis and myeloblastosis.

In the anemic form the liver often has accumulations of small lymphocytes and granulocytes indicative of a reactive center; however, careful search will reveal localized areas of erythropoietic activity.

The primary cell involved is the erythroblast. The early (with a nucleolus) and late erythroblast (without a nucleolus) (Lucas and Jamroz, 1961) correspond to the proerythroblast and erythroblast of Bensis and the rubriblast and prorubricle of A.M.A. nomenclature respectively (Lucas, 1959). The cell has a large round nucleus with very fine chromatin and 1 or 2 nucleoli and a large amount of cytoplasm which is basophilic. There are a perinuclear halo, vacuoles, and occasionally fine granules. The cell is irregular in shape and often has pseudopodia.

ULTRASTRUCTURE. Numerous studies have been made of the primitive cells in erythroblastosis induced by different strains of virus including strain R (Heine et al., 1961) and RPL12 (Dmochowski et al., 1964). Neoplastic erythroblasts in the tissues, spleen, and bone marrow are, for the most part, indistinguishable from the corresponding cells of the normal bird, except that virus particles may be present in the extracellular spaces and within vacuoles inside the cells. In erythroblasts in the circulating blood, as in cell culture, there is much increase in membrane activity with vacuolization of the cytoplasm and budding of virus particles from the cell membrane. Only occasionally are the aberrant structures seen in erythroblasts (Heine et al., 1961; Dmochowski et al., 1964).

HEMATOLOGY. Changes in the blood reflect those occurring in other organs such as liver, spleen, and bone marrow and depend largely on the extent of anemia or leukemia. When there is severe anemia, the blood is watery, light red, and clots slowly. In contrast, acute cases may show no grossly apparent changes, though usually the blood appears dark red with a smoky overcast. Properly stained blood smears reveal a variable number of erythroblasts (Fig. 15.36D). These vary in maturity from the early erythroblast, which is the predominant cell, to the various stages of polychrome erythrocytes. The more mature cells often appear early in the course of the disease or during remission, if and when it occurs.

The thrombocytic series of cells may be somewhat increased in number and immaturity. Similarly, in most naturally occurring cases, immature cells of the myelocytic series appear in the peripheral circulation. Occasionally they are as prominent as the erythroblasts.

Pathogenesis

When birds are artificially exposed to a strain causing erythroblastosis, the first alterations are found in 3 days as foci of proliferating erythroblasts in the bone marrow sinusoids. By the 7th day the primitive cells reach the circulating blood, and occasional foci of erythropoiesis are present in the sinusoids of the liver and spleen. Erythroblasts continue to accumulate in the hepatic sinusoids until death of the host. This may occur within a few days of the appearance of erythroblasts in the blood, though in most naturally occurring cases the disease proceeds much more slowly (Ponten and Thorell, 1957).

Differential Diagnosis

Although the gross lesions of the liver, spleen, and bone marrow provide the basis for a presumptive diagnosis, a firm diagnosis must be based on finding large numbers of erythroblasts by microscopic examination of a blood smear and sections or smears of the liver and bone marrow. Chickens in the early stages of disease or without obvious signs may easily be missed unless microscopic examination is made.

The anemic form is often very difficult to differentiate from anemia due to nonneoplastic causes. In erythroblastosis there is usually a defect in the maturation of the erythroblasts, resulting in the presence of large numbers of erythroblasts and very few polychrome erythrocytes. In anemia the reverse usually occurs. Extramedullary erythropoiesis and stasis of erythroblasts in the sinusoids are usually more prominent in erythroblastosis than in anemia.

The proliferative form of erythroblastosis can be distinguished from myeloblastosis on the following grounds. In myeloblastosis the liver is usually pale red and the marrow is whitish, whereas in erythroblastosis the liver and marrow are usually cherry red. In myeloblastosis the cells accumulate intra- and extravascularly, whereas in erythroblastosis they are always intravascular. The erythroblast and the myeloblast may be difficult to distinguish. Erythroblasts have a basophilic cytoplasm and a perinuclear halo; myeloblasts often have some granules.

Erythroblastosis can be distinguished from lymphoid leukosis by the nature and distribution of the lesions. Microscopically the cytoplasm of lymphoblasts is somewhat less basophilic than that of erythroblasts, and there is also a larger nuclear-cytoplasmic ratio than in the latter cells. Lymphoblasts are more variable in size and shape than erythroblasts, but they are all at the same primitive developmental stage. Lymphoblasts tend to have an ovoid rather than spherical nucleus and a finer, more delicate-looking chromatin network.

Myelocytomas are easily distinguished from erythroblastosis.

MYELOBLASTOSIS

Incubation Period

The only strain of virus which induces predominantly myeloblastosis and is in general use is BAI strain A. After inoculation of susceptible day-old chicks with large doses of virus, changes in the blood can be observed in 10 days and birds die a few days thereafter. Mortality continues for about 1 month and only occasional deaths occur after this (Eckert et al., 1953, 1954; Burmester et al., 1959b). Löliger (1964) described strains of virus (EII and CMII) which produced myeloblastosis, myelocytoma, and other tumors.

Clinical Signs

The signs are similar to those of erythroblastosis. At first there is a lethargy, general weakness, and slight paleness of the comb. As the condition develops, these signs become marked and there is inappetance, pronounced dehydration, emaciation, and diarrhea. There may be hemorrhage from one or more of the feather follicles due to a blood clotting deficiency.

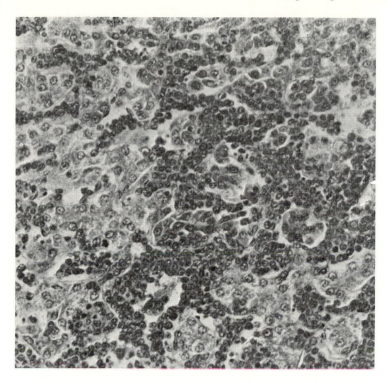

FIG. 15.38—Myeloblastosis. Distribution of myeloblasts in liver of bird with myeloblastic leukemia 19 days after inoculation with BAI strain A virus. ×280. (Courtesy A. J. Langlois, Duke Univ. Medical Center)

The course is highly variable but is generally longer than that for erythroblastosis.

Morphologic Pathology

There is usually an anemia. The parenchymatous organs are enlarged and friable, but in chronic cases the liver may be firm. Gray diffuse tumor nodules may occur in the liver and occasionally in other visceral organs. The bone marrow is usually firm and reddish gray to gray. In advanced cases the liver, spleen, and kidneys have grayish infiltrations which are usually diffuse but often give the organ a mottled or even granular appearance (Fig. 15.36C).

Microscopic examination of parenchymatous organs reveals massive intravascular and extravascular accumulations of myeloblasts with a variable proportion of promyelocytes (Fig. 15.38). Infiltration and proliferation are particularly extensive outside the sinusoids and around the portal tracts in the liver lobules. There is, therefore, a marked replacement of the original tissues by the pathologic cells. This is in contrast to the fairly uniform intravascular leukostasis encountered in erythroblastosis. The bone marrow shows intensive myeloblastic activity which is confined to the extrasinusoidal areas.

The pathologic and hematologic features of both erythroblastosis and myeloblastosis overlap in many naturally occurring cases.

ULTRASTRUCTURE. In circulating myeloblasts from birds with myeloblastosis induced by BAI strain A, virus particles are only rarely found and then in small numbers in clear vacuoles (Bonar et al., 1959, 1960; Beard, 1963a; Dmochowski et al., 1964; Langlois et al., 1969). However, reticular and phagocytic elements of the spleen and bone marrow are frequently packed with virus particles. When myeloblasts are transferred to cell culture, large numbers of lysosomes appear in the cytoplasm (Heine et al., 1964) (Fig. 15.22). After some time in cell culture, virus particles can be seen in both lysosomes and vacuoles and budding at the cell membrane. No other changes can be observed in these cells.

HEMATOLOGY. Myeloblastosis is characterized by a spectacular leukemia (Fig. 15.36E). Up to 2 million myeloblasts per cu mm (Eckert et al., 1951) may be found in the peripheral blood. They may comprise 75% of all the cells in the blood; thus, on centrifugation, there may be more "buffy coat" than red cells. The myeloblasts are large cells with slightly basophilic clear cytoplasm and a large nucleus containing 1–4 acidophilic nucleoli which do not usually stain prominently. Often promyelocytes and myelocytes are also present, and they can easily be identified by their specific granulation which in the early forms is primarily basophilic.

The disease may result in a secondary anemia. When this occurs, polychrome erythrocytes and reticulocytes are usually present. Such a secondary anemia is easily distinguished from the condition in which erythroblastosis and myeloblastosis occur together, since in the latter case blast forms of both cell series are in the circulating blood.

Pathogenesis

The target organ of the causative virus is the bone marrow, and the first neoplastic alteration is in the form of multiple foci of proliferating myeloblasts in the extrasinusoidal areas. These grow rapidly, overtake the normal bone marrow elements, and spill over into the sinusoids. This is followed, perhaps within 1 day, by a leukemia and invasion of other organs by myeloblasts (Lagerlof and Sundelin, 1963).

Differential Diagnosis

As in erythroblastosis, a tentative diagnosis may be made based on gross lesions; however, these are often so similar to those of lymphoid leukosis that specific diagnosis cannot be made without examination of a blood smear. Examination of liver or bone

marrow sections is very helpful when there is some doubt as to the identity of the cell type. The myeloblast is, on the average, smaller than the erythroblast or lymphoblast; its cytoplasm is more acidophilic and is polygonal or angular. The nucleus is less vesicular and the nucleolus, while present, is not nearly as frequently seen nor as conspicuous as in the other two leukoses.

MYELOCYTOMATOSIS

Incubation Period

On inoculation of MC29 intravenously into young chicks, myelocytomas were obtained in 3–11 weeks (Mladenov et al., 1967). The incubation period in field cases is unknown, but most cases are observed in immature birds. Mathey (personal communication) observed an outbreak in a 6-week-old broiler flock.

Clinical Signs

The general signs are similar to those of myeloblastosis. In addition, skeletal growths of myelocytes may result in abnormal protruberances of the head (Fig. 15.39) and, to a lesser extent, the thorax and shank. The course is highly variable and usually prolonged.

Morphologic Pathology

The tumors are distinctive and can be recognized on gross examination with some degree of certainty. Characteristically they occur on the surface of bones in association

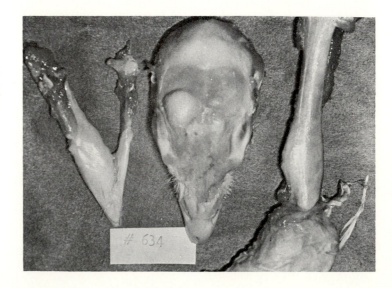

FIG. 15.39—Myelocytoma of mandible, skull, and tibia of 8-week-old chicken. (Courtesy W. J. Mathey, Wash. State Univ.)

with the periosteum and near cartilage, though any tissue or organ may be affected. Tumors often develop at the costochondral junctions of the ribs, the posterior sternum, and the cartilaginous bones of the mandible and nares. The flat bones of the skull are also often affected (Fig. 15.39). Myelocytomas are dull, yellowish white in color, soft and friable or cheesy, and diffuse or nodular. They sometimes have a thin layer of bone over them which is easily broken. Multiple tumors are common and are usually bilaterally symmetrical.

The tumors consist of compact masses of strikingly uniform myelocytes with very little stroma (Fig. 15.36F). The tumor cells are similar to the normal myelocytes found in the bone marrow. Their nuclei are large, vesicular, and usually eccentrically located, and a distinct nucleolus is commonly present. The cytoplasm is tightly packed with acidophilic granules which are usually spherical. When imprint preparations of fresh tumors are stained with May-Grünwald Giemsa, the granules appear brilliant red (see Fig. 15.36F) (Mladenov et al., 1967). However, in some flocks, tumors with cells containing basophilic granules have been reported (Löliger and Schubert, 1966). In the liver, myelocytes crowd the sinuses, invade the acinar cords, and destroy and re-place the hepatocytes (Fig. 15.40). A principal attribute of the neoplastic myelocytes is the formation of cohesive, organized, and invasive growths in parenchymatous organs.

ULTRASTRUCTURE. Ultrastructural features of myelocytoma and myelocytomatosis cells (Mladenov et al., 1967) vary from those of well-differentiated myelocytes to those of undifferentiated, nongranulated myelocytes (Langlois et al., 1969). Myelocytes with granules staining red with May-Grünwald Giemsa do not differ notably in ultrastructure from their normal myelocyte counterparts. Cells without granules exhibit primitive structure similar to but not identical with that of the myeloid progenitor (hemocytoblast) cells. These myelocytes are essentially identical with the cells originating in cultures of bone marrow treated with virus strain MC29. The principal features are a singular "grainy" appearance of the cytoplasm related to high ribosome, polysome, and protein content; sparse rough endoplasmic reticulum; relatively small nucleus with nucleoplasm containing some (but not predominant) diffuse and dispersed chromatin; and a greatly enlarged nucleolus of usual structure. In structure and behavior these cells are greatly different from

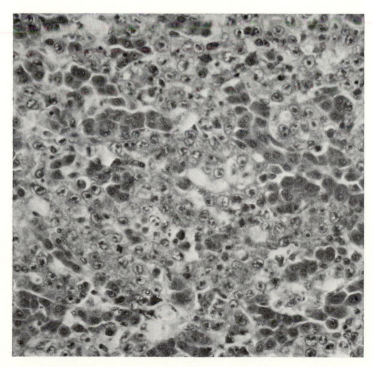

FIG. 15.40—Myelocytoma. Distribution of nongranulated myelocytes in liver of bird 30 days after inoculation with strain MC29 virus. Primitive cells with typical large nucleoli fill sinuses and actively invade parenchymal cell cords destroying and replacing hepatocytes. ×280. (Courtesy A. J. Langlois, Duke Univ. Medical Center)

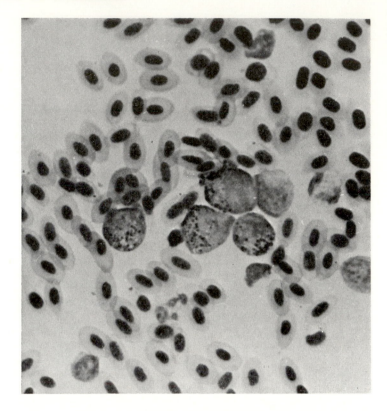

FIG. 15.41—*Myelocytoma. Granulated myelocytes in blood smear from bird 23 days after inoculation with strain MC29 leukosis virus. ×750. (Courtesy J. W. Beard, Duke Univ. Medical Center)*

the myeloblasts induced by BAI strain A virus.

HEMATOLOGY. The disease is essentially aleukemic but occasionally is associated with erythroblastosis. In some birds, especially in the laboratory disease, there may be a distinct leukemia of granulated or nongranulated myeloid cells (Fig. 15.41).

Pathogenesis

The earliest alterations occur in the bone marrow in which there is a crowding of the intersinusoidal spaces, principally by myelocytes, and a destruction of the sinusoid walls. Whereas in the normal bird the intersinusoidal spaces contain myeloid series cells in different stages of development, in myelocytomatosis the spaces contain essentially only 2 types of cells—the primitive hemocytoblast and the neoplastic cell, the myelocyte. The latter appears to arise directly from the hemocytoblast, and differentiation is arrested most often at the nongranulated but also at the granulated myelocyte level (Mladenov et al., 1967). The nongranulated myelocytes are distinctly different from myeloblasts both in morphology and in vitro growth potentials; myeloblasts proliferate enduringly in culture but myelocytes persist only a few days. Myelocytes proliferate and soon overgrow the bone marrow. Tumors form by expansion of the marrow growths so that in some cases large neoplasms may crowd through the bone and finally destroy and extend through the periosteum without involving it. Extramedullary tumors may arise by metastasis.

Differential Diagnosis

The distinctive character and location of the tumors provide the basis for a diagnosis, which can be verified by examination of a stained smear or tumor section. Gross tumors must be differentiated from myeloblastosis, lymphoid leukosis, osteopetrosis and necrotic and/or purulent processes which occur in tuberculosis, pullorum disease, and mycotic infections.

HEMANGIOMAS

Incubation Period

After experimental inoculation of young chicks with field strains of virus (Fredrick-

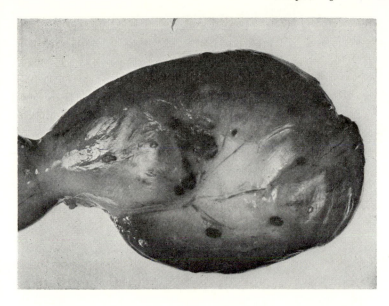

FIG. 15.42—*Hemangioma of gizzard serosa of RPL12 virus-inoculated bird. Note dark circumscribed and raised tumor nodules. (Courtesy M. A. Gross, Regional Poultry Research Laboratory, E. Lansing, Mich., and J. Nat. Cancer Inst.)*

son et al., 1965), hemangiomas appeared in 3 weeks to 4 months. Most isolates or virus strains have been found to cause hemangiomas (Olson, 1940; Burmester, 1947; Fredrickson et al., 1964). These tumors have been found in birds of various ages.

Clinical Signs

Hemangiomas usually occur singly in the skin though primary multiplicity is not uncommon. When the wall ruptures, profuse hemorrhage ensues. The feathers near the tumor are bloodstained, and the bird may become pale and die of exsanguination.

Morphologic Pathology

In the skin or on the surface of visceral organs hemangiomas can best be described as "blood blisters" (Fig. 15.42). Chickens with ruptured hemangiomas of the skin may be severely anemic. Blood clots are often found in visceral tumors. The cavernous form is characterized by greatly distended blood spaces with thin walls composed of endothelial cells (Fig. 15.43). Capillary hemangiomas are solid masses varying from gray-pink to red. The endothelium may proliferate into dense masses (hemangio endothelioma) leaving mere clefts for blood channels (Fig. 15.44), develop into a lattice with capillary spaces, or grow into collagen-supported chords with larger interspersed blood spaces. In general, skin tumors are more encapsulated and have more trabeculae than visceral tumors.

ULTRASTRUCTURE. There have been no reports of electron microscopic studies of hemangiomas.

HEMATOLOGY. The blood picture is normal in uncomplicated cases. When the tumor has ruptured, there may be signs of anemia. It should be borne in mind that hemangiomas often occur in conjunction with erythroblastosis and myeloblastosis.

Pathogenesis

Hemangiomas are tumors of the vascular system and as such usually involve all layers of the blood vessels. In some instances the endothelium may proliferate more than the supporting tissue. Occasionally the primitive anaplastic cells may differentiate to hemocytoblasts so that considerable erythropoiesis can occur in these growths (Fig. 15.45).

Differential Diagnosis

Hemangiomas on the skin should be differentiated from wounds, bleeding feather follicles, and cannibalism. Those in the visceral organs should be differentiated from hemorrhages and sarcomas.

NEPHROBLASTOMA

Incubation Period

BAI strain A (Burmester et al., 1959b), ES4 (Carr, 1956), MH2 (Carr, 1960), and the Murray-Begg sarcoma viruses induce a

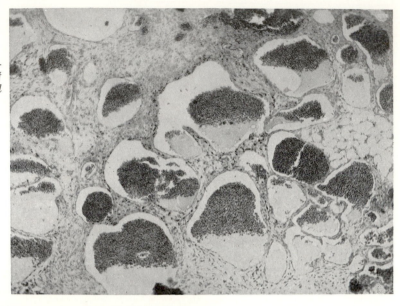

FIG. 15.43—Cavernous hemangioendothelioma of mesentery. (Feldman and Olson, 1965)

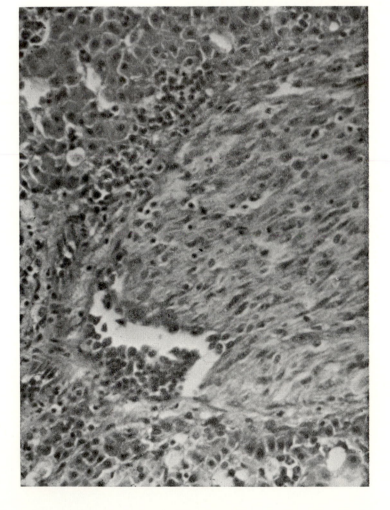

FIG. 15.44—Endothelioma in liver of bird inoculated with RPL30 leukosis virus. Occlusion of portal vein by inward growing spindle cells from blood vessel. ×250. (Courtesy T. N. Fredrickson, Regional Poultry Research Laboratory, E. Lansing, Mich., and J. Nat. Cancer Inst.)

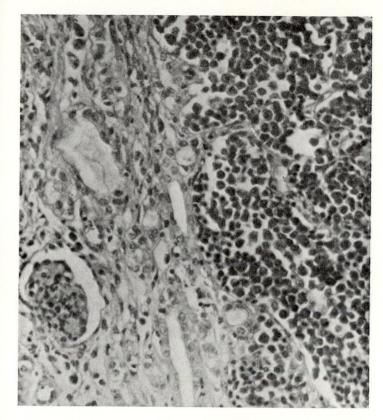

FIG. 15.45—*Hemangioma with erythropoiesis in kidney in bird 34 days after inoculation with field isolate of leukosis virus. Many erythroblasts within sinusoids appear to have budded off from sinusoidal walls.* ×250.

high incidence of nephroblastomas (Beard, 1963a). With BAI strain A, nephroblastomas occur in birds which survive the myeloblastosis; incidence may reach 60–85% of the birds inoculated (Burmester et al., 1959b). Most cases occur between 2 and 6 months of age. In the field, nephroblastomas are seen in chickens older than 5 weeks of age.

Clinical Signs

In uncomplicated cases there are no signs while the tumors are small. As the tumor increases in size, there is usually emaciation and general debility. Paralysis may result when the tumor exerts pressure on the sciatic nerve.

Morphologic Pathology

Nephroblastomas vary greatly in appearance from small, pinkish gray nodules which may be embedded in the kidney parenchyma to large, yellowish gray, lobulated masses that replace most of the kidney tissue (Fig. 15.46). Tumors are often pedunculated and may be connected to the kidney by only a thin fibrous and vascular stalk. Large tumors are often cystic, and sometimes huge cystic masses involve the whole of both kidneys.

The histological variation between different tumors or areas of the same tumor is striking (Fig. 15.47). There is usually a neoplastic proliferation of both epithelial and mesenchymal elements, though the proportion and differentiation of these elements vary widely. The epithelial structures vary from enlarged tubules with invaginated epithelium and malformed glomeruli, through irregular masses of distorted tubules, to groups of large, irregular, cuboidal, undifferentiated cells with little tubular organization. Tumors composed primarily of these elements have been referred to as adenocarcinomas (Mladenov et al., 1967). Sometimes cystic tubules predominate, in which case the term cystadenoma is more relevant (Mladenov et al., 1967). Particularly in tumors induced by BAI strain A avian myeloblastosis virus, the epithelial growths may be embedded in loose mesenchyma or frank sarcomatous stroma. There may be islands of keratinizing stratified squamous epithelial structures (pearls),

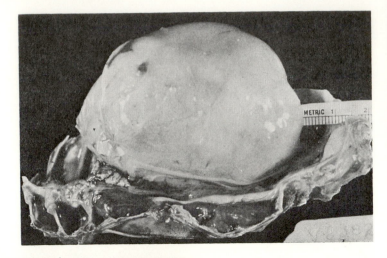

FIG. 15.46—Nephroblastoma. Bird was inoculated at 1 day of age with avian myeloblastosis virus (BAI strain A).

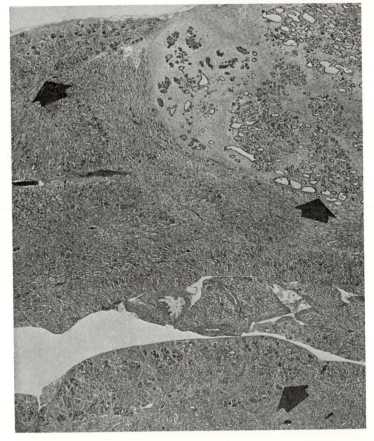

FIG. 15.47—Nephroblastoma. Bird was inoculated at 1 day of age with cloned preparation of avian myeloblastosis virus (BAI strain A). Note primary multiplicity since tumors in different areas are of two distinct types (arrows). ×20.

cartilage, or bone. Such growths have been referred to as nephroblastomas (Ishiguro et al., 1962).

Primary multiplicity of tumors may occur, but metastases are rare.

ULTRASTRUCTURE. In the epithelial ne-

phronic elements of nephroblastomas induced by BAI strain A virus (Beard, 1963a), cytoplasmic aberrant structures are occasionally seen in large or small aggregates. There is intensive budding of virus particles at the cell membrane and often large amounts of virus in the intercellular spaces. Occasional budding from the cytoplasmic membrane of the fibroblastic elements of the stroma has been observed. Numerous abnormal virus particles which bud from the chondrocytes contain segments of cartilage fibrils. The sarcomatous elements consist of cells similar in morphology to those in other avian sarcomas. Virus particles have been observed budding from the epithelial cells in cystadenomas and adenocarcinomas induced by strain MC29 myelocytomatosis virus (Mladenov et al., 1967). There were large accumulations of particles in the spaces in the cysts and tubules. Collection of such masses of particles was probably related to the lack of tubule and glomerular drainage and meager vascular communication. Particles were also present in vacuoles and dilated canaliculi of the kidney growths.

HEMATOLOGY. Uncomplicated cases are aleukemic.

Pathogenesis

There is some evidence that nephroblastomas originate from embryonic rests or nephrogenic buds in the kidneys (Ishiguro et al., 1962). These epithelial structures enlarge and become neoplastic. The supporting stroma of mesenchymal elements also proliferates and in turn may be altered. There is an extensive multiplication of the tumor cells (usually the convoluted tubules and/or stroma) and varying degrees of differentiation with some abnormal differentiation. In the most differentiated form, nephrogenic cells form glomeruli, tubules, or keratinized epithelium (pearls), whereas the cells of the stroma form sarcomas, cartilage, and bone. Anaplasia of the kidney cells can result in sheets of large epithelioid cells with almost no tubular organization. Malformed and blocked tubules result in cysts.

Differential Diagnosis

Nephroblastoma should be suspected when tumor nodules or large masses are found only in the kidney or are encountered suspended from the lumbar region. The diagnosis can be verified by microscopic examination. Tumors should be differentiated from other causes of kidney enlargement including hematomata, lymphoid leukosis, and accumulation of urates.

OSTEOPETROSIS

Incubation Period

After experimental inoculation of day-old chicks with RPL12-L29 (Sanger et al., 1966) or other viruses (Holmes, 1964), osteopetrosis may develop anytime after 1 month of age. It is most commonly seen in birds 8–12 weeks of age. The disease probably has a similar incubation period in the field.

In 1968 Dougherty et al. isolated a subgroup B virus from stocks of the Schmidt-Ruppin strain of Rous sarcoma virus. It produced almost exclusively osteopetrosis.

Clinical Signs

The long bones of the limbs are most commonly affected (Fig. 15.48). There is a uniform or irregular thickening of the diaphyseal or metaphyseal regions which can be detected by inspection or palpation. In active cases the affected areas are unusually warm. Birds in which the disease is advanced have a characteristic "bootlike" appearance of the shanks. Affected chickens are usually stunted, pale in the unfeathered regions, and walk with a stilted gait or limp.

Morphologic Pathology

The first grossly visible changes occur in the diaphysis of the tibia and/or tarsometatarsus. Alterations soon are seen in other long bones and bones of the pelvis, shoulder girdle, and ribs, but not the digits. The lesions are usually, but not always, bilaterally symmetrical. Lesions first appear as distinct pale yellow foci against the grayish white translucent normal bone. The periosteum is thickened and the abnormal bone is spongy and at first easily cut. The lesion is commonly circumferential and advances to the metaphysis, giving the bone a fusiform appearance (Fig. 15.49). Occasionally the lesion remains focal or is eccentric. The severity of the lesion varies from a slight exostosis to a massive asymmetrical enlargement with almost complete obliteration of the marrow cavity. In long-standing cases the periosteum is not as thickened as it was earlier; when it is removed, the porous irregular surface of the very hard osteopetrotic bone is revealed.

Osteopetrosis and lymphoid leukosis frequently occur together in the same bird.

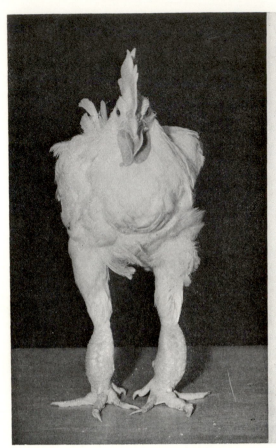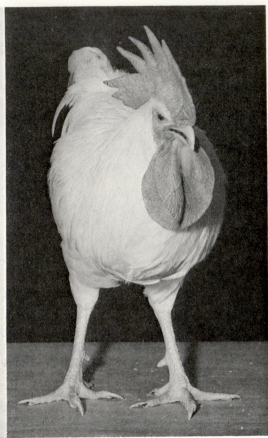

FIG. 15.48—Osteopetrosis. Both birds are 24 weeeks old. Chicken on left was injected with RPL12-L39 at 1 day of age and has advanced osteopetrotic lesions of the shanks. (Courtesy V. L. Sanger, Michigan State Univ.)

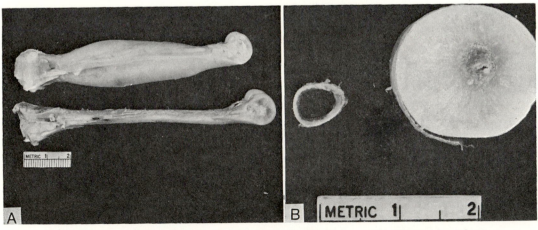

FIG. 15.49—Osteopetrosis of tibia in 10-week-old chicken. (A) Shorter length of bone is due to reduced growth and not necessarily to disease. Lower tibia is from control bird of same age. (B) Cross section of middle of shaft of bones in (A). (Courtesy V. L. Sanger, Mich. State Univ., and Can. J. Comp. Med. Vet. Sci.)

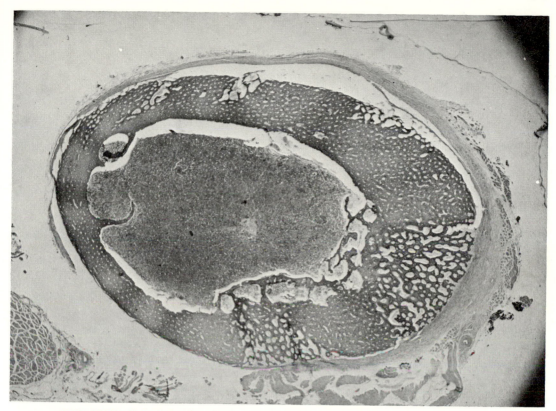

FIG. 15.50—*Osteopetrosis. A cross section of humerus from 8-week-old chicken. Six separate osteopetrotic foci are present, two of which extend from endosteum to periosteum. ×18. (Courtesy V. L. Sanger, Mich. State Univ., and* Am. J. Vet. Res.*)*

Other tumors have also been described (Campbell, 1961). When birds are not simultaneously affected with lymphoid leukosis, there is usually a general atrophy of the visceral organs, particularly the spleen.

Microscopically the periosteum over the lesion is greatly thickened due to an increase in number and size of the basophilic osteoblasts. Affected bones differ from normal bones in the following ways. Spongy bone converges centripetally toward the center of the shaft (Fig. 15.50). There is an increase in size and irregularity of the Haversian canals and an increase in the number and size and an alteration in position of the lacunae (Fig. 15.51). Osteocytes are more numerous, large, and eosinophilic, and the new bone is basophilic and fibrous.

ULTRASTRUCTURE. Virus particles are present in many of the tissues of birds infected with the osteopetrosis virus described by Young (1966). Virus particles were seen to bud from the cell membrane of cells from various tissues of the body.

HEMATOLOGY. The blood picture is ordinarily aleukemic, but sometimes there is a relative or an absolute lymphocytosis. There is often a secondary anemia, which no doubt reflects the progressive reduction of hematopoietic tissue as the marrow cavity becomes filled with bone. There is active erythropoiesis in the remaining bone marrow and sometimes in focal areas of the liver, but immature stages are not observed in the peripheral blood.

Pathogenesis

The osteopetrotic lesion is basically proliferative rather than osteolytic or degenerative, and there is some question as to whether it is neoplastic or not. Many investigators consider the lesion to be hypertrophic rather than neoplastic (Pugh, 1927;

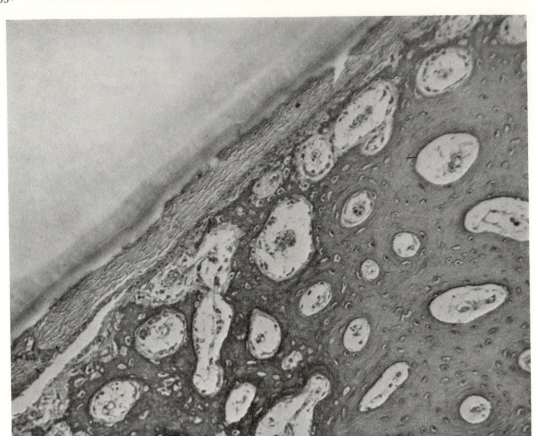

FIG. 15.51—Osteopetrosis. Early lesion under periosteum **(top)**. Spaces are large and irregular, lacunae are large and scattered, and fibrous bone is stained basophilic. Normal compact bone at lower right. ×220. (Courtesy V. L. Sanger, Mich. State Univ., and Am. J. Vet. Res.)

Moulton, 1961; Campbell, 1961; Sanger et al., 1966).

Differential Diagnosis

The bone lesions of advanced cases are sufficiently distinctive to present no difficulty in diagnosis. Cross and longitudinal sectioning of the long bones is helpful in detecting slight exostoses and endostoses, particularly in the early stages.

Among other osteopathies, rickets and osteoporosis can be differentiated from osteopetrosis by their epiphyseal formation of osteoid or porous bone. In perosis there is twisting and flattening of the shank while the bone structure itself remains normal.

CONNECTIVE TISSUE TUMORS

This section will deal with those connective tissue tumors for which there is some evidence of transmissibility and viral etiology. They include fibrosarcoma and fibroma; myxosarcoma and myxoma; histiocytic sarcoma, osteoma, and osteogenic sarcoma; and chondrosarcoma. All of the tumors of this group may occur as either benign or malignant growths. Benign tumors grow slowly, never invade the surrounding tissues, and remain almost indefinitely strictly localized processes. The malignant forms grow more rapidly, infiltrate, and are capable of metastasis.

Most strains or isolates which induce tumors of the connective tissues are multipotent; i.e., they induce a variety of tumors. Examples are Rous sarcoma virus (Burmester and Walter, 1961) and ES4 (Beard, 1963a), which also induce erythroblastosis and lymphoid leukosis. On the other hand, most strains of leukosis virus such as

RPL12 (erythroblastosis and lymphoid leukosis), BAI strain A (myeloblastosis), and strain R (erythroblastosis) also cause one or more of the solid tumors listed above. Even viruses isolated directly from field cases of lymphoid leukosis have produced fibrosarcomas, myxosarcomas, and histiocytic sarcomas as well as hemangiomas and nephroblastomas (Fredrickson et al., 1964, 1965). For review and references see Beard (1963a) and Vogt (1965).

Incubation Period

Tumors develop rapidly and are palpable within 3 days after inoculation of chicks with high doses of Rous sarcoma virus. With leukosis viruses, sarcomas may occur anytime after inoculation but are most frequently observed in the first 2–3 months. In field flocks connective tissue tumors may occur in birds at any age.

Clinical Signs

Until tumors become extremely large, affect the function of an organ, ulcerate, or metastasize, they do not affect the well-being of the host. Some tumors of the visceral organs and most of those affecting the muscles or integument are palpable. Death may be due to secondary bacterial infection, toxemia, hemorrhage, or dysfunction of an organ affected by the tumor. Benign tumors may never cause death, whereas malignant ones may follow a very rapid course resulting in death within a few days.

MORPHOLOGIC PATHOLOGY

The different connective tissues distributed throughout the body provide potential sources of a variety of tumors. Fibromas, myxomas, and sarcomas are most likely to arise in the integument or in the muscles; tumors composed of cartilage or bone or a mixture of these arise where these two tissues are normally found. Sometimes multipotent mesenchymal cells give rise to cartilage and bone where these tissues are not ordinarily present. Of all the connective tissue tumors, the histiocytic sarcoma is capable of the widest distribution. Secondary metastatic foci of malignant tumors occur most frequently in the lungs, liver, spleen, and intestinal serosa. Primary multiplicity may occur in both benign and malignant tumors; it is characteristic of histiocytic sarcomas.

Fibromas and fibrosarcomas are first noticed as firm lumps attached to the skin, in the subcutaneous tissue, or in the muscles (Fig. 15.52) and occasionally in other organs. As they grow, the overlaying skin often undergoes necrosis and thus results in ulceration and secondary infection. When they are cut, their fibrous nature is apparent.

Fibromas in their simplest form consist of mature fibroblasts interspersed with collagen fibers arranged in wavy parallel bands or in whorls. Slow-growing tumors are more differentiated and contain more

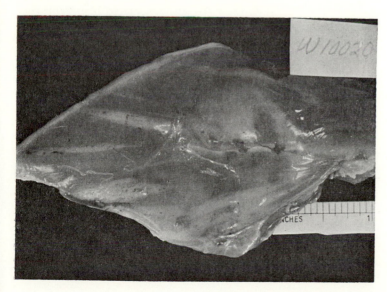

FIG. 15.52—*Fibrosarcomas in breast muscle of bird inoculated at 1 day of age with field isolate of leukosis virus.*

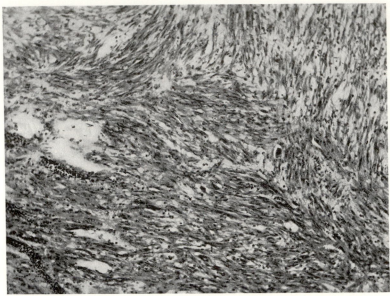

FIG. 15.53—Fibrosarcoma in musculature of breast. Neoplastic process was bilateral and had metastasized to lung. ×120. (Feldman and Olson, 1965)

collagen and fewer cells than those growing more rapidly. Some fibromas may have edematous areas, and these should not be confused with myxomas and myxosarcomas. If necrosis, ulceration, and secondary infection have occurred, various inflammatory and necrotic alterations may be observed in the tumor. Inflammatory changes may be so prominent that the tumor may be confused with a granuloma.

Fibrosarcomas are characterized by their aggressive and destructive growth, their cellular composition, and the immaturity of their constituent cells (Fig. 15.53). Large irregular and hyperchromic fibroblasts are abundant and mitosis is common. The tumors contain less collagen than fibromas, and this is concentrated in and near irregular septa which subdivide the tumor. Regions of necrosis often occur in rapidly growing tumors. Edema is sometimes present.

Myxoma and myxosarcoma are softer than fibromas and fibrosarcomas. They contain characteristic tenacious slimy material that pulls out into long strings.

Myxomas consist of stellate or spindle-shaped cells surrounded by a homogeneous, slightly basophylic, mucinous matrix. Long cytoplasmic processes may extend from the stellate cells and become fused with the sparse collagen fibrils. In the malignant form, the myxosarcoma, the mucinous matrix is less abundant and fibroblasts are proportionately more numerous and more immature than in myxomas (Fig. 15.54). The histogenesis and structure of the primary myxosarcomatous tumors are similar to those of the fibroblastic tumors. The essential difference is that in the myxomatous tumors, the fibroblastic cells are more specialized and are capable of producing large amounts of mucin in addition to the usual products, namely collagen and elastic fibrils.

Histiocytic sarcomas are firm fleshy tumors which consist of a mixture of two or more cell types that, while morphologically dissimilar, are closely related histogenically. The most striking microscopic feature is the highly varied nature of the cellular constituents (Fig. 15.55). The cells may be (1) spindle-shaped usually appearing in groups or bundles as in fibrosarcomas, (2) stellate reticulum-producing elements (fixed histiocytes), and/or (3) large phagocytic cells or macrophages (free histiocytes). In addition, there usually are numerous transitional forms, many of which are polymorphic. In the primary tumors spindle-shaped cells usually predominate, whereas in the metastatic foci primitive histiocytic forms are more numerous.

Osteomas and osteogenic sarcomas are hard tumors which may arise from the periosteum of any bone. Osteomas are structurally similar to bone except that much of the finer histologic detail is lack-

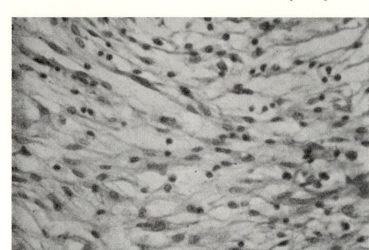

FIG. 15.54—Myxosarcoma induced by Rous sarcoma virus. ×240. (Courtesy C. F. Helmboldt, Univ. of Conn.)

FIG. 15.55—Histiocytic sarcoma of heart. Note varied character of cellular constituents. ×240. (Courtesy C. F. Helmboldt, Univ. of Conn.)

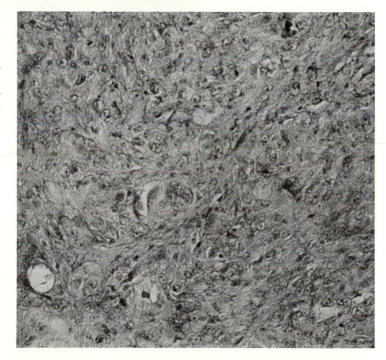

ing. They consist of a homogeneous acidophilic matrix of osseomucin containing collections of osteoblasts at irregular intervals. Osteogenic sarcomas are usually very cellular infiltrative growths which invade and destroy surrounding tissues. The cells are spindle-shaped, ovoid, or polyhedral, and many are in mitosis. The nuclei are prominent and the cytoplasm basophilic. Multi-

nucleated giant cells may be quite numerous. Although an osteogenic sarcoma is usually a rapidly growing, highly cellular neoplasm of mostly undifferentiated cells, there are usually areas in which there is sufficient differentiation for the production of osseomucin. The presence of osseomucin is usually sufficient to identify these tumors.

Chondromas and chondrosarcomas rarely

occur in chickens, although cartilage and bone are often found within fibro- or myxosarcomas. Such tumors may be designated as fibrochondro-osteosarcomas. Microscopically chondromas have a typical and unique structure, i.e., groups of two or more chondrocytes lying in a homogeneous matrix of chondromucin. Tumors may be separated into lobules by strands of fibrous connective tissue. In chondrosarcomas there is considerable cellular variation, ranging from the most immature to the fully mature chondrocyte. The former are undifferentiated and spindle-shaped while the latter are spheroidal. Those in the intervening zone are polymorphic.

ULTRASTRUCTURE. Only the sarcomas produced by Rous sarcoma virus have been examined in detail. Spindle-shaped cells, macrophagelike cells, and mast cells have been described (Bernhard et al., 1956; Haguenau and Beard, 1962; Heine et al., 1962). It is possible that all of these forms, as well as those seen in cultures of chick embryo cells treated with Rous sarcoma virus, are originally derived from fibroblasts or connective tissue cells. Tumor cells (Haguenau and Beard, 1962) are similar to the cells in culture in showing numerous pseudopodia and pronounced cytoplasmic vacuolization. Some of the vacuoles may contain virus particles. Structures similar though not identical to the gray bodies in myeloblasts have been described, and "clusters" (Haguenau and Beard, 1962) (aberrant structures) (Heine et al., 1968) may also occur in the cytoplasm. Cartilage and osteoid tissue occasionally occur in nephroblastomas, and their ultrastructure has been described. It is likely that chondrosarcomas and osteosarcomas will have many ultrastructural aspects in common with these tumors.

HEMATOLOGY. Anemia is common when tumors affect the bone marrow or when they ulcerate and hemorrhage occurs.

Pathogenesis

Connective tissue tumors probably originate from primitive mesenchymal cells of mesodermal origin. Their diverse structural forms reflect the direction and extent of differentiation. Thus the frequent occurrence of more than one tissue in a tumor is a reflection of the multipotency of the precursor cells. For example, chondrocytes are derived from primitive mesenchymal cells which have undergone a gradual process of change and maturation. Finally, mature chondrocytes, which produce chondromucin in addition to collagen and elastic fibrils, are evolved. An analogous differentiation occurs during the ontogeny of osteoblasts and fibroblasts. The more anaplastic tumors are composed of cells in which maturation has been arrested at an earlier stage.

Differential Diagnosis

These tumors are usually easy to distinguish from the leukoses. They should not be confused with granulomas, e.g. Hjärre's disease, tuberculosis, pullorum disease, results of trauma, myelocytomas, and leiomyomas.

DIAGNOSTIC TESTS

ISOLATION OF CAUSATIVE AGENT

Plasma, serum, or tumor are the best materials for virus isolation. Virus can also be isolated from most of the soft organs of the body and from oral washings and feces (Burmester, 1956b; Rubin et al., 1961). When it is important to determine whether dams are shedding virus in their eggs, 10-day-old embryos should be used (Burmester et al., 1955; Rubin et al., 1961). All viruses of this group are very thermolabile and can only be preserved for long periods at temperatures below −60° C (Hanafusa et al., 1964).

TESTS FOR VIRUS

The first successful procedure developed for virus isolation was the inoculation of susceptible chicks (see section on laboratory host systems). Some viruses (e.g. Rous sarcoma virus) produce pocks on the chorioallantoic membranes of embryonated eggs. These procedures have been largely superseded by the more rapid and less expensive cell culture techniques described below.

It should be noted that very few of the tests (the complement fixation test and possibly the nonproducer and fluorescent antibody tests) are suitable for all leukosis and sarcoma viruses. The resistance inducing factor test can be satisfactorily performed only on viruses which are not rapidly cytopathogenic (i.e. leukosis viruses). The other tests are highly specific for certain virus strains; thus adenosine triphosphatase activity and hematopoietic transformation are suitable only for avian myeloblastosis virus (BAI strain A), and rapid transformation of fibroblast cultures is produced only by certain sarcoma viruses.

Resistance Inducing Factor (RIF) Test

In general, leukosis viruses do not induce alterations in cultured cells except after prolonged passage (Calnek, 1964). However, when chicken embryo fibroblasts are infected with a leukosis virus, they become resistant to superinfection by a sarcoma virus of the same group. Only viruses of the same subgroup interfere with one another in this way. The property of interference has been used extensively for assay of leukosis viruses by the RIF test (Rubin, 1960a) and also in delineating the virus subgroups (Vogt and Ishizaki, 1966b). In the RIF test, known susceptible chicken embryo fibroblast cultures are inoculated with material suspected of containing a leukosis virus. Cells are subcultured at least 3 times at 3–4-day intervals, and at each passage a sample of the cells is tested for susceptibility to Rous sarcoma viruses of different subgroups. Alternatively, supernatant fluids may be transferred to new cell cultures every 4 days. In this case, cells may be challenged without subculture 4–6 days after inoculation (Calnek, 1965, and personal communication). Control cultures infected with known leukosis viruses and uninfected cultures are always included to establish the validity of the tests. The presence of a leukosis virus in a cell culture is indicated by a 10-fold or greater reduction in the number of foci produced by a standard stock of Rous sarcoma virus when compared with the number of foci on similarly challenged control cells. Several different challenge viruses, one for each subgroup, must be used to detect leukosis viruses belonging to different subgroups; each requires a separate cell culture plate for testing.

Complement Fixation Test for Avian Leukosis Viruses (COFAL Test)

The COFAL test is dependent upon a group-specific protein antigen of avian leukosis/sarcoma viruses (Sarma et al., 1964). The antigen is present in the supernatant fluid and in the cells of infected cultures and inside the virus particles themselves. It is not present on the surface of the virus particles. When hamsters are infected with Rous sarcoma virus (usually the Schmidt-Ruppin strain) a tumor develops, and some of the hamsters produce antibody to the group-specific antigen. Rabbit antiserum, prepared against the group-specific antigen liberated (with detergent) from purified virus preparations, can also be used (Bauer and Schafer, 1966). The mammalian antiserum is used in a complement fixation test to detect the group-specific antigen produced in infected chicken embryo fibroblast cultures. In executing the test, cells from the chicken embryo fibroblast test cultures are harvested, adjusted to a standard concentration, frozen and thawed, and used as antigen in the complement fixation test. Samples which fix complement in the presence of antiserum are considered positive. Suitable controls are necessary.

To obtain a suitable antigen from low titer inocula it is necessary to cultivate the inoculated fibroblasts for 12–28 days before they are harvested. Thus the test may take as long as the RIF test to achieve an end result. However, since the group-specific antigen is common to all viruses of the leukosis/sarcoma group, only one set of reagents is needed to detect all infections of this group. Occasionally antigens which are not present in the inocula may cause false reactions in this test (Payne and Chubb, 1968). The nature of these antigens has not been determined.

Nonproducer (NP) Test

NP cells can be activated to produce Rous sarcoma virus by agents of the leukosis/sarcoma group (Purchase, 1965; Vogt, 1965), and this property has been used in assaying for these agents (Rispens and Long, unpublished data).

To obtain NP cells, chicken embryo fibroblasts are infected with a defective strain of Rous sarcoma virus. Usually Bryan's high titer RSV (RAV-1) is employed. In order to preclude simultaneous infection with the helper virus (RAV-1), limiting dilutions of the stock preparation are used to infect chicken embryo fibroblasts which are then cultivated on a "feeder layer" of duck embryo fibroblasts or mouse embryo fibroblasts which are insusceptible to infection. To avoid virus spread, the cultures are maintained after infection under an agar overlay containing antiserum against RAV-1. These foci are picked from the cultures and propagated on fresh feeder layers. Stocks of cells which are neoplastically transformed but do not produce virus detectable on C/O (susceptible phenotype) cells (therefore, NP cells) can be frozen with dimethyl sulfoxide in liquid nitrogen and used later for detecting leukosis/sarcoma viruses (Kelloff and Vogt, 1966).

In the nonproducer activation test, mixtures of susceptible chicken embryo fibroblasts and nonproducer cells are inoculated with specimens suspected of containing leukosis viruses. Known positive (inoculated with known leukosis virus) and negative (uninoculated) controls are always included. After 5–9 days of cultivation, the supernatant fluids are removed and assayed for infectious Rous sarcoma virus by the inoculation of C/O (phenotype susceptible to viruses of all subgroups) cultures, embryos, or chickens. Since the infecting leukosis virus and the progeny sarcoma virus belong to the same subgroup, one can determine the subgroup of the infecting virus by the host range (Vogt and Ishizaki, 1965) or interference patterns (Vogt and Ishizaki, 1966b) of the progeny sarcoma virus.

Comparison of Tests (Table 15.7)

All three tests require a standard source of leukosis/sarcoma virus-free chick embryos of known phenotype for use in cell culture. Cells for use in the COFAL test must, in addition, be free of the genetically controlled antigen which reacts in the test (Payne and Chubb, 1968). In the RIF test, stocks of challenge virus of each subgroup are required; in the COFAL test, specific antiserum is a necessity; and in the NP test, quantities of nonproducer cells are a prerequisite. The RIF and COFAL tests should not be performed directly on cells obtained from embryos of unknown genetic origin, since the results may be confused by genetic resistance in the former case and the genetically controlled "nonspecific" antigen in the latter case; however, nonproducer cells can be cocultivated with the cells from the embryos to be tested. Both the RIF and COFAL tests require several subcultures to propagate the virus sufficiently; therefore, much more work is involved than in the NP test.

The indicator systems are different in the 3 tests. In the RIF test the number and appearance of Rous foci after challenge is highly dependent on the physiologic condition of the cells. Thus when cell cultures are not in optimal condition it is not possible to perform a RIF test. On the other hand, a cell extract is used in the COFAL test, and it can be stored frozen and tested on more than one occasion if necessary. Similarly, in the NP test the supernatant fluid of cell cultures can be stored and tested for virus by either the cell culture, chorioallantoic membrane, or chick inoculation techniques. The results are usually more clear-cut in the NP cell test than in the RIF or COFAL tests.

The subgroup of an infecting leukosis virus can be determined by any of the tests. In the RIF test, only Rous sarcoma virus (RSV) belonging to the same subgroup as the leukosis virus is subjected to interference. In the COFAL test, genetically resistant cells can be employed; thus a leukosis virus of subgroup A will not produce complement fixation antigens in cells of the C/A phenotype (resistant to subgroup A viruses). In the NP cell test, genetically resistant nonproducer cells can be prepared, or the supernate from the activated nonproducer cells (which contains Rous virus of the same subgroup as the leukosis virus) can be placed on genetically resistant cells or embryos or used in an interference test with a leukosis virus of known subgroup.

Fluorescent Antibody Tests

The direct (Kelloff and Vogt, 1966) and indirect (Payne et al., 1966) fluorescent antibody (FA) tests have been used to detect viral antigen in chicken embryo fibroblast cultures. When mammalian group-specific antisera are used and cells are fixed in acetone, the test becomes analogous to the COFAL test (Kelloff and Vogt, 1966; Payne et al., 1966). Avian sera are subgroup- or even type-specific (Payne et al., 1966).

Adenosine Triphosphatase (ATPase) Assay

Avian myeloblastosis virus has on its surface an enzyme which dephosphorylates adenosine triphosphate. This activity can be used as a quantitative assay to determine the amount of myeloblastosis virus present in the plasma of infected chickens or in supernates of myeloblast cultures (Beaudreau and Becker, 1958).

TABLE 15.7 ❧ Comparison of Methods for Assaying Leukosis Viruses

Method	Requirements	Response Measured	Additional Requirements for Subgroup Determination	Time Required (days)
In vivo				
Chick inoc 1 day ia	LL susceptible*	LL	Genetically resistant chickens	270
Chick inoc 1 day ia	Erythro susceptible†	Erythro	Genetically resistant chickens	63
Embryo inoc 11 days iv	Erythro susceptible	Erythro	Genetically resistant chickens	43
Cell culture				
RIF	RSV pseudotypes, C/O cells	Resistance to formation of RSV foci in CC	Challenge virus of known subgroup	12‡ + 6
COFAL	Hamster antiserum, C/O, COFAL antigen-free cells	Complement fixation	Genetically resistant cells	12 + 1
NP	NP cells	RSV foci in CC or on CAM, or tumors in chicks	Genetically resistant cells or RIF test with leukosis virus of known subgroup	8 + 6

Abbreviations: LL = lymphoid leukosis; Erythro = erythroblastosis; ia = intra-abdominal; iv = intravenous; RIF = resistance inducing factor; COFAL = complement fixation for avian leukosis viruses; NP = nonproducer; RSV = Rous sarcoma virus; C/O = cells phenotypically susceptible to infection by viruses of all subgroups; CC = cell culture; CAM = chorioallantoic membrane.

* Chickens susceptible to infection by the virus and to lymphoid leukosis tumor formation, e.g. line 151 chickens.
† Chickens susceptible to virus infection and to development of erythroblastosis (or myeloblastosis).
‡ Approximate number of days necessary to cultivate the virus plus the number of days to indicate presence of virus.

Hematopoietic Transformation

Avian myeloblastosis virus will infect cultures of avian hematopoietic tissue and induce focal transformation into myeloblasts. Assays are usually based on a quantal response in which individual cultures are scored as positive or negative (Baluda, 1963).

Transformation of Fibroblasts

In sensitive chick embryo fibroblast cultures, sarcoma viruses produce "foci" of morphologically transformed cells which can be seen microscopically after 4–5 days (Fig. 15.20) and grossly after about 10 days (Manaker and Groupé, 1956). The "foci" consist of rounded refractile cells which become multilayered. The morphology of the transformed cells and the shape of the focus produced is characteristic of the infecting virus. Sarcoma viruses also activate non-producer cells, produce the group-specific complement fixation antigen, and can be detected by the fluorescent antibody technique (Vogt and Luykx, 1963).

SEROLOGY

Serum or egg yolk are suitable for antibody determination, but heparinized plasma should not be used when tests are made in cell culture.

Tests

Neutralization of a Rous sarcoma virus pseudotype is an indication of current or past infection with a leukosis or sarcoma virus of the same subgroup and the same or similar type. A virus of one subgroup will not be neutralized by antibodies provoked by a virus of a different subgroup (Ishizaki and Vogt, 1966). Usually a 1:5 dilution of heat-inactivated (56° C for 30 minutes) serum is mixed with an equal quantity of a standard preparation of Rous sarcoma virus of a known pseudotype, and after incubation the residual virus is quantitated by any one of many procedures (Burmester and Okazaki, 1964); the cell culture assay is most commonly used (Rubin et al., 1962).

Serotypes

Viruses of the avian leukosis/sarcoma group have been divided into 4 subgroups— A, B, C, and D—on the basis of host range in genetically susceptible or resistant cells

(Vogt and Ishizaki, 1965), interference spectrum (Vogt and Ishizaki, 1966b), and viral envelope antigens (Ishizaki and Vogt, 1966; Duff and Vogt, 1969). A classification of the viruses most fully studied appears in Table 15.5 (Burmester, 1966; Vogt and Ishizaki, 1966a).

Within each subgroup different viruses can be distinguished by the ability of monovalent antisera to neutralize them and other viruses of the same subgroup. Even though there is usually some cross-neutralization between viruses belonging to the same subgroup, the kinetics of the neutralization vary (Chubb and Biggs, 1968) and the slopes of curves for heterologous systems differ from those of the homologous system. There are no common neutralization antigens among viruses of different subgroups. The diagnosis of infection by serological means requires that representatives of all serotypes be employed. Leukosis viruses themselves may be used, but more commonly Rous sarcoma virus pseudotypes are employed in the neutralization tests.

TREATMENT

In general, no practical therapeutic measures have been found for treatment of the diseases of the avian leukosis complex. In evaluating potentially therapeutic agents, it must be remembered that temporary remissions of clinical signs may occur spontaneously. All attempts to treat virus-induced neoplasia have resulted in negative or irreproducible results.

PREVENTION AND CONTROL
ERADICATION

It is most encouraging that leukosis viruses can be eliminated from flocks which subsequently show no evidence of diseases of the leukosis/sarcoma group. The present methods for achieving a virus-free flock are long, complicated, and expensive and are not yet applicable for large-scale use. Nevertheless, success with experimental flocks warrants some discussion here.

Those who have successfully eliminated leukosis viruses from such flocks have obtained progeny from dams which do not shed leukosis viruses. The chicks were reared in isolation. For reasonable assurance that hens are not shedding virus, several clutches of eggs must be tested immediately prior to those used for hatching.

Usually 3 pools of 4 embryos each are obtained from each hen and tested for virus by one of the accepted methods. Most hens which shed virus continuously or intermittently will be detected by this means, and negative findings will provide reasonable assurance that the progeny will be free of leukosis viruses. For confirmation, samples from the progeny taken during the growing period and again at sexual maturity should be tested for virus and antibody to all virus subgroups. Flocks from which leukosis viruses have been eradicated have been maintained free of virus without difficulty (Hughes et al., 1963; Levine and Nelsen, 1964).

Even though the elimination of vertical transmission is not practical at present, there are several procedures which can reduce or eliminate horizontal spread and thereby reduce the level of exposure, particularly during the period immediately after hatching. In order to reduce the infection remaining from previous populations, incubators, hatchers, brooding houses, and all equipment should be thoroughly cleaned and disinfected between each use. Chick boxes should not be reused, and each farm should have only one age group of chickens. The danger of introducing strains of virus which are not already present in the population can be eliminated if eggs or chicks from different sources are not mixed and chicks are reared under isolation conditions which will prevent cross-contamination of flocks.

HOST RESISTANCE

There are two levels at which blocks in the sequence of events which lead to tumor induction may have their effect. At either level the end result is that chickens appear to be resistant to the disease in question.

Blocks to Viral Envelope Functions

In order to replicate and/or produce neoplastic transformation, the avian leukosis/sarcoma virus must penetrate host cells. Thus factors which prevent penetration act as the first line of defense in the prevention of these diseases. Genetic resistance to cell penetration by the virus is highly efficient. There is ample evidence that this kind of resistance is expressed in vivo as resistance to disease. In this respect chickens homozygously resistant at the tva locus are more resistant to induction of

acute neoplasms and lymphoid leukosis by subgroup A viruses. Since most of the leukosis viruses isolated from the field are of the A subgroup, the locus is also effective in increasing resistance to field exposure. On the other hand, since resistance to infection is almost complete and thus homozygous resistant birds do not support virus replication, they do not produce antibody (Crittenden and Okazaki, 1966; Crittenden, 1968). Heterozygous progeny of these birds would not be protected by maternal antibody and would be more susceptible to disease.

Alleles for resistance and susceptibility to subgroups A, B, and C occur in almost all chicken populations. Among the flocks so far studied there have been some exceptions. One line of chickens, most of which were of the C/A phenotype (resistant to A subgroup virus), was observed by L. N. Payne (personal communication). Crittenden and Motta (1969) challenged chorioallantoic membranes of embryonated eggs from 25 comercial white egg lines, 17 meat lines, and 6 brown egg lines with Rous sarcoma viruses of different subgroups. One white egg line and 1 meat line appeared to be fully resistant to subgroup A, 1 white egg line and 3 brown egg lines to subgroup B, and 1 brown egg line to subgroup C viruses. In this study there was a high proportion of intermediate counts of pocks on the chorioallantoic membrane which could not be explained on the basis of the single gene for resistance. If resistance is controlled by the same genetic system, it may be that different alleles are present, or it may be that susceptibility is only partially dominant resulting in the intermediate resistance observed.

Blocks to Nucleoid Functions

The penetration and uncoating of the virus allows the nucleoid to enter the cell, to direct viral replication, and to induce neoplastic transformation. A block in the function of the nucleoid RNA may have origin in either the host cell or the virus and result in failure of transformation, production of viral progeny, or both. In addition, infected cells (whether they produce virus or not) and neoplastically transformed cells have new antigens on their surface. These antigens are similar to transplantation antigens and are foreign to the host. If the host develops cellular or humoral immunity to these antigens, the cells carrying them may be destroyed and thereby eliminated. These may be regarded as the second line of host defense.

The mechanism of genetic resistance at the second line of defense is undefined. Lines 15I and 6 (Burmester et al., 1960b) are inbred strains of chickens, both of which are susceptible to virus infection at the first line of defense. However, line 6 is apparently more effective in utilizing the second line of defense, since it is much more resistant to tumor development than line 15I (Crittenden, 1968).

Genetic Selection

Selection for resistance to subgroup A or B viruses by artificial exposure to Rous sarcoma virus of subgroup A or B respectively is a relatively simple procedure. However, Crittenden (1968) has discussed some of the problems raised by this approach. Mutant viruses are more likely to overcome resistance due to a single gene than that related to a multiple gene effect, and mutant subgroups may then be favored. In a host population resistant to virus penetration, there can be no effective selection for resistance to the development of neoplasms; for this reason mutant viruses may take over. It is probable that past selection for host viability has increased the resistance of infected birds to the development of neoplasms. This type of resistance is poorly defined but may be controlled by a number of genes and is consequently more difficult to overcome by viral mutation.

IMMUNIZATION

The possible use of antiviral vaccines to increase the host resistance at the first line of defense is very attractive. In a series of attempts to inactivate leukosis viruses by various means, Burmester (unpublished data) demonstrated that the ability of these virus preparations to produce antibody was destroyed at almost the same point as the virus was inactivated. Although some suc-cess has been obtained with inactivated virus (Beard, personal communication), the procedures are not suitable for field application. Crittenden's experiments provided evidence that multiplication of live virus is necessary to induce an immune response when the dose of inoculum is small (Crittenden and Okazaki, 1966). Attempts to produce attenuated strains of virus which do not induce disease have failed.

No attempts have been made to increase the resistance of the host by immunization with cell surface antigens of infected or transformed cells. Increase of host resistance would be induced at the second line of defense. The approach warrants further study.

REMOVAL OF THE BURSA OF FABRICIUS

Since the bursa of Fabricius plays such a central role in the pathogenesis of lymphoid leukosis, and since lymphoid leukosis is the most common of the diseases induced by this group of viruses, removal of the bursa of Fabricius offers some possibilities in the control of the disease. In experimentally infected chickens surgical removal before 5 months of age (Peterson et al., 1966) or treatment of embryos or young chicks with testosterone or corticosteroids has resulted in elimination of the malignancy. Unfortunately these procedures have had some undesirable side effects. In the case of surgical bursectomy there is a higher incidence of osteopetrosis and nonspecific deaths and a decrease in body weight. In addition to the increased nonspecific mortality and decrease in body weight caused by both of the above hormones, testosterone also produces a masculinization of the chicken which has a serious effect on egg production. Searches for androgen analogues which will control lymphoid leukosis without side effects are of no avail. Until some method is found for reducing the associated economic loss, artificial manipulations cannot be considered applicable under field conditions.

REFERENCES

Ball, V., and L. Auger. 1924. Osteopathic hypertrophiante apneumique. *Rev. Gen. Med. Vet.* 33:5–12.

Baluda, M. A. 1962. Properties of cells infected with avian myeloblastosis virus, pp. 415–25. In Frisch, L. (ed.), *Cold Spring Harbor Symposium Quantitative Biology 27,* Cold Spring Harbor Biological Lab., Long Island, N.Y.

———. 1963. Conversion of cells by avian myeloblastosis virus, pp. 118–37. In *Perspectives in Virology,* III. Academic Press, New York.

Baluda, M. A., and P. P. Jamieson. 1961. *In*

vivo infectivity studies with avian myelo-blastosis virus. *Virology* 14:33–45.

Bamberger, K. 1964. Survey on the experimental and literary basis of the control of avian leucotic complex in Hungary. *Acta Vet.* 14:253–65.

Bauer, H., and W. Schafer. 1965. Isolation of a group-specific antigen from avian myeloblastosis virus (BAI strain A). *Z. Naturforsch.* 20:815–17.

———. 1966. Origin of group-specific antigen of chicken leukosis viruses. *Virology* 29:494–97.

Bayon, H. P. 1929. The pathology of transmissible anaemia (erythromyelosis) in the fowl; its similarity to human haemopathies. *Parasitology* 21:339–74.

Beard, Dorothy, G. S. Beaudreau, R. A. Bonar, D. G. Sharp, and J. W. Beard. 1957. Virus of avian erythroblastosis. III. Antigenic constitution and relation to the agent of avian myeloblastosis. *J. Nat. Cancer Inst.* 18:231–59.

Beard, J. W. 1957. Nature of the viruses of avian myeloblastosis and erythroblastosis, pp. 336–44. In *Proc. 3rd Nat. Cancer Conf.*, Lippincott Co., Philadelphia, and Am. Cancer Soc., Inc.

———. 1962. Etiologic aspects of the avian leukemias. *Progr. in Hematol.* 3:105–35.

———. 1963a. Avian virus growths and their etiologic agents, pp. 1–127. In Haddow, A., and S. Weinhouse (eds.), *Advances in Cancer Research*. Academic Press, New York and London.

———. 1963b. Viral tumors of chickens with particular reference to the leukosis complex. *Ann. N.Y. Acad. Sci.* 108:1057–85.

Beaudreau, G. S., and Caroline Becker. 1958. Virus of avian myeloblastosis. X. Photometric microdetermination of adenosinetriphosphatase activity. *J. Nat. Cancer Inst.* 20:339–49.

Beaudreau, G. S., R. A. Bonar, Dorothy Beard, and J. W. Beard. 1956. Virus of avian erythroblastosis. II. Influence of host age and route of inoculation on dose response. *J. Nat. Cancer Inst.* 17:91–100.

Bernhard, W., C. Oberling, and P. Vigier. 1956. Ultrastructure de virus dans le sarcome de Rous, leur rapport avec le cytoplasme des cellules tumorales. *Bull. Cancer* 43:407–22.

Besnoit, C., and V. Robin. 1922. Contribution a l'etude clinique de la tuberculose aviaire (osteoperiostite diffuse sans localisation viscerale). *J. Med. Vet. Zootechnic* 68:741–49.

Biggs, P. M. 1961. A discussion on the classification of the avian leucosis complex and fowl paralysis. *Brit. Vet. J.* 117:326–34.

———. 1964. The avian leucosis complex. *World's Poultry Sci. J.* 20:78–91.

Biggs, P. M., and L. N. Payne. 1964. Relationship of Marek's disease (neural lymphoma-

tosis) to lymphoid leukosis. *Nat. Cancer Inst. Monograph* 17:83–98.

———. 1967. The avian leucosis complex. *Vet. Record* (Suppl.) 80:v–vii.

Blair, C. D., and P. H. Duesberg. 1968. Structure of Rauscher mouse leukaemia virus RNA. *Nature* 220:396–99.

Bonar, R. A., and J. W. Beard. 1959. Virus of avian myeloblastosis. XII. Chemical constitution. *J. Nat. Cancer Inst.* 23:183–97.

Bonar, R. A., Dorothy Beard, G. S. Beaudreau, D. G. Sharp, and J. W. Beard. 1957. Virus of avian erythroblastosis. IV. pH and thermal stability. *J. Nat. Cancer Inst.* 23:183–42.

Bonar, R. A., D. F. Parsons, G. S. Beaudreau, Caroline Becker, and J. W. Beard. 1959. Ultrastructure of avian myeloblasts in tissue culture. *J. Nat. Cancer Inst.* 23:199–225.

Bonar, R. A., D. Weinstein, J. R. Sommer, Dorothy Beard, and J. W. Beard. 1960. Virus of avian myeloblastosis. XVII. Morphology of progressive virus-myeloblast interactions *in vitro*. *Nat. Cancer Inst. Monograph* 4:251–90.

Bonar, R. A., Ursula Heine, Dorothy Beard, and J. W. Beard. 1963a. Virus of avian myeloblastosis (BAI strain A). XXIII. Morphology of virus and comparison with strain R (erythroblastosis). *J. Nat. Cancer Inst.* 30:949–97.

Bonar, R. A., R. H. Purcell, Dorothy Beard, and J. W. Beard. 1963b. Virus of avian myeloblastosis (BAI strain A). XXIV. Nucleotide composition of the pentose-nucleic acid and comparison with strain R (erythroblastosis). *J. Nat. Cancer Inst.* 31:705–16.

Bonar, R. A., Ursula Heine, and J. W. Beard. 1964. Structure of BAI strain A (myeloblastosis) avian tumor virus. *Nat. Cancer Inst. Monograph* 17:589–614.

Bonar, R. A., L. Sverak, D. P. Bolognesi, A. J. Langlois, Dorothy Beard, and J. W. Beard. 1967. Ribonucleic acid components of BAI strain A (myeloblastosis) avian tumor virus. *Cancer Res.* 27:1138–57.

Bryan, W. R. 1956. Biological studies on the Rous sarcoma virus. IV. Interpretation of tumor-response data involving one inoculation site per chicken. *J. Nat. Cancer Inst.* 16:843–63.

Bryan, W. R., M. E. Maver, J. B. Moloney, M. T. Wood, and C. L. White. 1950. Comparative stability of the agent of chicken tumor I in citrate and phosphate buffers at 37° C. *J. Nat. Cancer Inst.* 11:269–77.

Bryan, W. R., M. E. Maver, J. B. Moloney, D. Calnan, C. L. White, and M. Wood. 1951. Biological activity of the agent of chicken tumor I (Rous) in citrate buffers of various molar concentrations. *J. Nat. Cancer Inst.* 11:929–37.

Bryan, W. R., J. B. Moloney, and D. Calnan. 1954. Stable standard preparations of the

Rous sarcoma virus preserved by freezing and storage at low temperatures. *J. Nat. Cancer Inst.* 15:315–29.

Burmester, B. R. 1945. The incidence of lymphomatosis among male and female chickens. *Poultry Sci.* 24:469–72.

———. 1947. Studies on the transmission of avian visceral lymphomatosis. II. Propagation of lymphomatosis with cellular and cell-free preparations. *Cancer Res.* 7:786–97.

———. 1955. Immunity to visceral lymphomatosis in chicks following injection of virus into dams. *Proc. Soc. Exp. Biol. Med.* 88:153–55.

———. 1956a. Bioassay of the virus of visceral lymphomatosis. I. Use of short experimental period. *J. Nat. Cancer Inst.* 16:1121–27.

———. 1956b. The shedding of the virus of visceral lymphomatosis in the saliva and feces of individual normal and lymphomatous chickens. *Poultry Sci.* 35:1089–99.

———. 1964. Discussion. Transmission of virus from field cases of avian lymphomatosis. III. Variation in the oncogenic spectra of passaged virus isolates. *Nat. Cancer Inst. Monograph* 17:28.

———. 1966. Report on avian leukosis conference. *Poultry Sci.* 45:1411–15.

———. 1969. The prevention of lymphoid leukosis with androgens. *Poultry Sci.* 48:401–8.

Burmester, B. R., and G. E. Cottral. 1947. The propagation of filtrable agents producing lymphoid tumors and osteopetrosis by serial passage in chickens. *Cancer Res.* 7:669–75.

Burmester, B. R., and E. M. Denington. 1947. Studies on the transmission of avian visceral lymphomatosis. I. Variation in transmissibility of naturally occurring cases. *Cancer Res.* 7:779–85.

Burmester, B. R., and T. N. Fredrickson. 1964. Transmission of virus from field cases of avian lymphomatosis. I. Isolation of virus in line 15I chickens. *J. Nat. Cancer Inst.* 32:37–63.

Burmester, B. R., and R. F. Gentry. 1956. The response of susceptible chickens to graded doses of the virus of visceral lymphomatosis. *Poultry Sci.* 35:17–26.

Burmester, B. R., and N. M. Nelson. 1945. The effect of castration and sex hormones upon the incidence of lymphomatosis in chickens. *Poultry Sci.* 24:509–15.

Burmester, B. R., and W. Okazaki. 1964. Discussion of neutralization by antibody of strain RPL12 and Rous sarcoma (Bryan) viruses as measured by different methods. *Nat. Cancer Inst. Monograph* 17:509–22.

Burmester, B. R., and W. G. Walter. 1961. Occurrence of visceral lymphomatosis in chickens inoculated with Rous sarcoma virus. *J. Nat. Cancer Inst.* 26:511–18.

Burmester, B. R., and N. F. Waters. 1956. Variation in the presence of the virus of visceral lymphomatosis in the eggs of the same hens. *Poultry Sci.* 35:939–44.

Burmester, B. R., and R. L. Witter. 1966. An outline of the avian leukosis complex. *USDA Prod. Res. Rept.* 94.

Burmester, B. R., R. F. Gentry, and N. F. Waters. 1955. The presence of the virus of visceral lymphomatosis in embryonated eggs of normal appearing hens. *Poultry Sci.* 34:609–17.

Burmester, B. R., W. G. Walter, and A. K. Fontes. 1957. The immunological response of chickens after treatment with several vaccines of visceral lymphomatosis. *Poultry Sci.* 36:79–87.

Burmester, B. R., M. A. Gross, W. G. Walter, and A. K. Fontes. 1959a. Pathogenicity of a viral strain (RPL12) causing avian visceral lymphomatosis and related neoplasms. II. Host-virus interrelations affecting response. *J. Nat. Cancer Inst.* 22:103–27.

Burmester, B. R., W. G. Walter, M. A. Gross, and A. K. Fontes. 1959b. The oncogenic spectrum of two "pure" strains of avian leukosis. *J. Nat. Cancer Inst.* 23:277–91.

Burmester, B. R., A. K. Fontes, and W. G. Walter. 1960a. Pathogenicity of a viral strain (RPL12) causing avian visceral lymphomatosis and related neoplasms. III. Influence of host age and route of inoculation. *J. Nat. Cancer Inst.* 24:1423–42.

Burmester, B. R., A. K. Fontes, N. F. Waters, W. R. Bryan, and V. Groupé. 1960b. The response of several inbred lines of White Leghorns to inoculation with the viruses of strain RPL12 visceral lymphomatosis-erythroblastosis and of Rous sarcoma. *Poultry Sci.* 39:199–215.

Butterfield, E. E. 1905. Aleukaemic lymphadenoid tumors of the hen. *Folia Haematol.* 2:649–57.

Calnek, B. W. 1964. Morphological alteration of RIF-infected chick embryo fibroblasts. *Nat. Cancer Inst. Monograph* 17:425–47.

———. 1965. Studies on the RIF test for the detection of an avian leukosis virus. *Avian Diseases* 9:545–59.

———. 1968a. Lymphoid leukosis virus: A survey of commercial breeding flocks for genetic resistance and incidence of embryo infection. *Avian Diseases* 12:104–11.

———. 1968b. Lesions in young chickens induced by lymphoid leukosis virus. *Avian Diseases* 12:111–29.

Campbell, J. G. 1961. A proposed classification of the leucosis complex and fowl paralysis. *Brit. Vet. J.* 117:316–25.

———. 1963. Virus induced tumors in fowls. *Proc. Roy. Soc. Med.* 56:305–7.

Campbell, J. G., and E. C. Appleby. 1966.

Tumours in young chickens bred for rapid body growth (broiler chickens): A study of 351 cases. *J. Pathol. Bacteriol.* 92:77–90.

Caparini, U. 1896. Fetati leucemici nei polli. *Clin. Vet.* (Milan) 19:433–35.

Carr, J. G. 1956. Renal adenocarcinoma induced by fowl leukaemia virus. *Brit. J. Cancer* 10:379–83.

———. 1960. Kidney carcinomas of the fowl induced by the MH₂ reticuloendothelioma virus. *Brit. J. Cancer* 14:77–82.

Carr, J. G., and J. G. Campbell. 1958. Three new virus-induced fowl sarcomata. *Brit. J. Cancer* 12:631–35.

Chubb, L. G., and R. F. Gordon. 1957. The avian leucosis complex—A review. *Vet. Rev. Annotations* 3:97–120.

Chubb, R. C., and P. M. Biggs. 1968. The neutralization of Rous sarcoma virus. *J. Gen. Virol.* 3:87–96.

Churchill, A. E. 1968. Studies on the serological and interfering properties of avian leucosis virus isolates from field outbreaks of disease and from three vaccines. *Res. Vet. Sci.* 9:68–75.

Coates, H., T. Borsos, M. Foard, and F. B. Bang. 1968. Pathogenesis of Rous sarcoma virus in the chicken embryo with particular reference to vascular lesions. *Int. J. Cancer* 3:424–39.

Cooper, M. D., L. N. Payne, P. B. Dent, B. R. Burmester, and R. A. Good. 1968. Pathogenesis of avian lymphoid leukosis. I. Histogenesis. *J. Nat. Cancer Inst.* 41:373–89.

Crawford, L. V. 1960. A study of the Rous sarcoma virus by density gradient centrifugation. *Virology* 12:143–53.

Crawford, L. V., and E. M. Crawford. 1961. The properties of Rous sarcoma virus purified by density gradient centrifugation. *Virology* 13:227–32.

Crittenden, L. B. 1968. Avian tumor viruses: Prospects for control. *World's Poultry Sci. J.* 24:18–36.

Crittenden, L. B., and J. V. Motta. 1969. A survey of genetic resistance to leukosis-sarcoma viruses in commercial stocks of chickens. *Poultry Sci.* 5:1751–57.

Crittenden, L. B., and W. Okazaki. 1966. Genetic influence of the Rs locus on susceptibility to avian tumor viruses. II. Rous sarcoma virus antibody production after strain RPL12 virus inoculation. *J. Nat. Cancer Inst.* 36:299–303.

Crittenden, L. B., H. A. Stone, R. H. Reamer, and W. Okazaki. 1967. Two loci controlling genetic cellular resistance to avian leukosis-sarcoma viruses. *J. Virol.* 1:898–904.

Darcel, C. le Q. 1957a. A note on the classification of the leucotic diseases of the fowl. *Can. J. Comp. Med.* 21:145–59.

———. 1957b. Research on the fowl leucoses —An abridged review. *Can. J. Comp. Med.* 21:344–55.

———. 1960. The experimental transmission of avian leukosis: A review. *Cancer Res.* 20:2–17.

Dent, P. B., M. D. Cooper, L. N. Payne, R. A. Good, and B. R. Burmester. 1967. Characterization of avian lymphoid leukosis as a malignancy of the bursal lymphoid system, pp. 251–65. In Pollard, M. (ed.), *Perspectives in Virology*, Vol. 5. Academic Press, New York.

De Thé, G. 1964. Localization and origin of adenosine-triphosphatase activity of avian myeloblastosis virus. A review. *Nat. Cancer Inst. Monograph* 17:651–71.

De Thé, G., Ursula Heine, H. Ishiguro, J. R. Sommer, Dorothy Beard, and J. W. Beard. 1962. Biologic response of nephrogenic cells to avian myeloblastosis virus. *Federation Proc.* 21:919–29.

De Thé, G., Caroline Becker, and J. W. Beard. 1964. Virus of avian myeloblastosis (BAI strain A). XXV. Ultracytochemical study of virus and myeloblast phosphatase activity. *J. Nat. Cancer Inst.* 32:201–35.

Di Stefano, H. S., and R. M. Dougherty. 1966. Mechanisms for congenital transmission of avian leukosis virus. *J. Nat. Cancer Inst.* 37:869–83.

———. 1968. Multiplication of avian leukosis virus in the reproductive system of the rooster. *J. Nat. Cancer Inst.* 41:451–64.

Dmochowski, L., C. E. Grey, F. Padgett, P. L. Langford, and B. R. Burmester. 1964. Submicroscopic morphology of avian neoplasms. VI. Comparative studies on Rous sarcoma, visceral lymphomatosis, erythroblastosis, myeloblastosis and nephroblastoma. *Texas Rept. Biol. Med.* 22:20–60.

Dougherty, R. M. 1961. Heat inactivation of Rous sarcoma virus. *Virology* 14:371–72.

Dougherty, R. M., J. A. Stewart, and H. R. Morgan. 1960. Quantitative studies of the relationships between infecting dose of Rous sarcoma virus, antiviral immune response, and tumor growth in chickens. *Virology* 11:349–70.

Dougherty, R. M., H. S. Di Stefano, and F. K. Roth. 1967. Virus particles and viral antigens in chicken tissues free of infectious avian leukosis virus. *Proc. Nat. Acad. Sci. U.S.* 58:808–17.

Dougherty, R. M., R. H. Conklin, J. P. Whalen, and H. S. Di Stefano. 1968. Etiology of avian osteopetrosis. *Federation Proc.* 27:681.

Duesberg, P. H. 1968. Physical properties of Rous sarcoma virus RNA. *Proc. Nat. Acad. Sci. U.S.* 60:1511–18.

Duff, R. G. 1968. A new subgroup of avian tumor viruses. Ph.D. thesis. Univ. Colo.

Duff, R. G., and P. K. Vogt. 1969. Characteristics of two new avian tumor virus subgroups. *Virology* 39:18–30.

Dunkel, V. C., F. J. Rauscher, and V. Groupé. 1964. Further studies on Rous sarcoma virus. Experiences with virus-host-tumor interactions in turkeys. *Nat. Cancer Inst. Monograph* 17:179–200.

Eckert, E. A., Dorothy Beard, and J. W. Beard. 1951. Dose-response relations in experimental transmission of avian erythromyeloblastic leukosis. I. Host-response to the virus. *J. Nat. Cancer Inst.* 12:447–63.

———. 1953. Dose response relations in experimental transmission of avian erythromyeloblastic leukosis. II. Host response to whole blood and to washed primitive cells. *J. Nat. Cancer Inst.* 13:1167–84.

———. 1954. Dose-response relations in experimental transmission of avian erythromyeloblastic leukosis. III. Titration of the virus. *J. Nat. Cancer Inst.* 14:1055–66.

———. 1955a. Dose-response relations in experimental transmission of avian erythromyeloblastic leukosis. V. Influence of host age and route of virus inoculation. *J. Nat. Cancer Inst.* 15:1195–1207.

Eckert, E. A., I. Green, D. G. Sharp, Dorothy Beard, and J. W. Beard. 1955b. Virus of avian erythromyeloblastic leukosis. V. pH stability of the virus particles, the infectivity and the enzyme dephosphorylating adenosine triphosphate. *J. Nat. Cancer Inst.* 15:1209–15.

———. 1955c. Virus of avian erythromyeloblastic leukosis. VII. Thermal stability of virus infectivity; of the virus particle; and of the enzyme dephosphorylating adenosinetriphosphate. *J. Nat. Cancer Inst.* 16:153–61.

Eckert, E. A., D. G. Sharp, Dorothy Beard, I. Green, and J. W. Beard. 1955d. Virus of avian erythromyeloblastic leukosis. IX. Antigenic constitution and immunologic characterization. *J. Nat. Cancer Inst.* 16:593–643.

Eckert, E. A., R. Rott, and W. Schafer. 1963. Myxovirus-like structure of avian myeloblastosis virus. *Z. Naturforsch.* 18:339–40.

Elford, W. J., and C. H. Andrewes. 1935. Estimation of the size of a fowl tumour virus by filtration through graded membranes. *Brit. J. Exp. Pathol.* 16:61–66.

Ellermann, V. 1921a. Histogenese der uebertragbaren huehner leukose. II. Die intravaskulere lymphoide leukose. *Folia Haematol.* 26:165–75.

———. 1921b. The Leucosis of Fowls and Leukemia Problems. Gyldendal, London.

———. 1923. Histogenese der uebertragbaren Huehnerleukose. IV. Zusammenfassende Betrachtungen. *Folia Haematol.* 29:203–12.

Ellermann, V., and O. Bang. 1908. Experimentelle leukamie bei huhnern. *Zentr. Bakteriol. Parasitenk. Abt. I. Orig.* 46:595–609.

Engelbreth-Holm, J. 1942. *Spontaneous and Experimental Leukemia in Animals*. Oliver and Boyd, London.

Engelbreth-Holm, J., and A. Rothe-Meyer. 1932. II. Ueber den Zusammenhang zwischen den verschiedenen Huhnerleukoseformen (Anamie-erythroblastose-myelose). *Acta Pathol. Microbiol. Scand.* 9:312–32.

Feldman, W. H. 1932. *Neoplasms of Domesticated Animals*. W. B. Saunders Co., Philadelphia.

Feldman, W. H., and C. Olson. 1933. Keratinizing embryonal nephroma of the kidneys of the chicken. *Am. J. Cancer* 19:47–55.

———. 1965. Neoplastic diseases of the chicken, pp. 863–924. In Biester, H. E., and L. H. Schwarte (eds.), *Diseases of Poultry*. Iowa State Univ. Press, Ames.

Frederickson, T. N., H. G. Purchase, and B. R. Burmester. 1964. Transmission of virus from field cases of avian lymphomatosis. III. Variation in the oncogenic spectra of passaged virus isolates. *Nat. Cancer Inst. Monograph* 17:1–29.

Fredrickson, T. N., B. R. Burmester, and W. Okazaki. 1965. Transmission of virus from field cases of avian lymphomatosis. II. Development of strains by serial passage in 151 chickens. *Avian Diseases* 9:82–103.

Friesen, B., and H. Rubin. 1961. Some physicochemical and immunological properties of avian leukosis virus (RIF). *Virology* 15:387–96.

Furth, J. 1931. Erythroleukosis and the anemias of the fowl. *Arch. Pathol.* 12:1–30.

———. 1933. Lymphomatosis, myelomatosis and endothelioma of chickens caused by a filtrable agent. I. Transmission experiments. *J. Exp. Med.* 58:253–75.

———. 1934. Lymphomatosis, myelomatosis and endothelioma of chickens caused by a filtrable agent. II. Morphological characteristics of the endotheliomata caused by this agent. *J. Exp. Med.* 59:501–17.

———. 1946. Recent experimental studies on leukemia. *Physiol. Rev.* 26:47.

Goss, L. J. 1940. The incidence and classification of avian tumors. *Cornell Vet.* 30:75–88.

Granboulan, N., J. Huppert, and F. Lacour. 1966. Examen au microscope electronique du RNA du virus de la myeloblastose aviaire. *J. Mol. Biol.* 16:571–75.

Gross, M. A., B. R. Burmester, and W. G. Walter. 1959. Pathogenicity of a viral strain (RPL12) causing avian visceral lymphomatosis and related neoplasms. I. Nature of lesions. *J. Nat. Cancer Inst.* 22:83–101.

Groupé, V., F. J. Rauscher, A. S. Levine, and W. R. Bryan. 1956. The brain of newly hatched chicks as a host-virus system for biological studies on the Rous sarcoma virus (RSV). *J. Nat. Cancer Inst.* 16:865–75.

Guillon, J. C., I. Chouroulinkov, and L. Renault. 1963. Les tumeurs renales spontanees des gallinaces; A propos de 23 observations. *Bull. Assoc. Franc. Etude Cancer* 50:593–620.

Haguenau, Francoise, and J. W. Beard. 1962. The avian sarcoma-leukosis complex; its biology and ultrastructure, pp. 1–59. In Dalton and Haguenau (eds.), *Tumors Induced by Viruses.* Academic Press, New York, London.

Haguenau, Francoise, H. Febvre, and J. Arnoult. 1962. Mode de formation intra-cellulaire du virus du sarcome de Rous. Etude ultrastructurale. *J. Microscopie* 1:445–54.

Hall, W. J., C. W. Bean, and M. Pollard. 1941. Transmission of fowl leucosis through chick embryos and young chicks. *Am. J. Vet. Res.* 2:272–79.

Hamilton, C. M., and C. E. Sawyer. 1939. Transmission of erythroleukosis in young chickens. *Poultry Sci.* 18:388–93.

Hanafusa, H., T. Hanafusa, and H. Rubin. 1964. Analysis of the defectiveness of Rous sarcoma virus. I. Characterization of the helper virus. *Virology* 22:591–601.

Harris, R. J. C. 1954. Multiplication of Rous No. 1 sarcoma agent in the chorioallantoic membrane of the embryonated egg. *Brit. J. Cancer* 8:731–36.

———. 1967. The properties of non-virus-producing (NP) Rous sarcoma cells. *Biochem. Pharmacol.* 16:707–10.

Heine, Ursula, G. S. Beaudreau, Caroline Becker, Dorothy Beard, and J. W. Beard. 1961. Virus of avian erythroblastosis. VII. Ultrastructure of erythroblasts from the chicken and from tissue culture. *J. Nat. Cancer Inst.* 26:359–88.

Heine, Ursula, G. de Thé, H. Ishiguro, and J. W. Beard. 1962. Morphologic aspects of Rous sarcoma virus elaboration. *J. Nat. Cancer Inst.* 29:211–23.

Heine, Ursula, G. de Thé, Dorothy Beard, and J. W. Beard. 1963. Multiplicity of cell response to the BAI strain A (myeloblastosis) avian tumor virus. V. Elaboration of virus by pancreas of chickens inoculated with the agent. *J. Nat. Cancer Inst.* 30:817–35.

Heine, Ursula, R. A. Bonar, Caroline Becker, and J. W. Beard. 1964. Lysosome system of avian leukemic myeloblasts. *Nat. Cancer Inst. Monograph* 17:677–99.

Heine, Ursula, Dorothy Beard, and J. W. Beard. 1968. Ultracytochemical studies on aberrant structures in avian virus tumor cells. *Cancer Res.* 28:585–94.

Heine, Ursula, A. J. Langlois, J. Riman, and J. W. Beard. 1969. Ultrastructure of chick embryo cells altered by strain MC29 avian leukosis virus. *Cancer Res.* 29:442–58.

Holmes, J. R. 1964. Avian osteopetrosis. *Nat. Cancer Inst. Monograph* 17:63–79.

Horiuchi, T., M. Moriwaki, and R. Ishitani.

1960. Pathological studies on the visceral lymphomatosis in the chicken, especially the findings on the peripheral blood. *Japan. J. Vet. Sci.* 2:256–58.

Hughes, W. F., D. H. Watanabe, and H. Rubin. 1963. The development of a chicken flock apparently free of leukosis virus. *Avian Diseases* 7:154–65.

Ianconescu, M., and Y. Samberg. 1967. Experimental Rous sarcoma in the rock partridge *(Alectoris graeca). Refuah Vet.* 24:178–72.

Ishiguro, H., Dorothy Beard, J. R. Sommer, Ursula Heine. G. de Thé, and J. W. Beard. 1962. Multiplicity of cell response to the BAI strain A (myeloblastosis) avian tumor virus. I. Nephroblastoma (Wilms' tumor): Gross and microscopic pathology. *J. Nat. Cancer Inst.* 29:1–39.

Ishizaki, R., and P. K. Vogt. 1966. Immunological relationships among envelope antigens of avian tumor viruses. *Virology* 30:375–87.

Jackson, C. 1936. Neoplastic diseases in poultry. *J. S. African Vet. Med. Ass.* 7:1–69.

Jungherr, E. L. 1941. Tentative pathologic nomenclature for the disease complex variously designated as fowl leucemia, fowl leucosis, etc. *Am. J. Vet. Res.* 2:116.

Jungherr, E. L., and W. Landauer. 1938. Studies on fowl paralysis. III. A condition resembling osteopetrosis (marble bone) in the the common fowl. *Storrs Agr. Expt. Sta. Bull.* 222.

Kahler, H., W. R. Bryan, B. J. Lloyd, Jr., and J. B. Moloney. 1954a. The density of the Rous sarcoma virus in sucrose solutions. *J. Nat. Cancer Inst.* 15:331–36.

———. 1954b. The sedimentation of the Rous sarcoma virus. *J. Nat. Cancer Inst.* 15:337–39.

Karshner, R. G. 1926. Osteopetrosis. *Am. J. Roentgenol. Radium Therapy* 16:405–19.

Kelloff, G., and P. K. Vogt. 1966 Localization of avian tumor virus group-specific antigen in cell and virus. *Virology* 29:377–84.

Kitt, T. 1931. Die Leukomyelose der Huehner. *Ergeb. Mikrobiol. Immunitaetsforsch. Expt. Therap.* 12:15–29.

Lagerlof, B., and P. Sundelin. 1963. The histogenesis and haematology of virus-induced myeloid leukaemia in the fowl. *Acta Haematol.* 30:111–22.

Langlois, A. J., R. B. Fritz, Ursula Heine, Dorothy Beard, D. P. Bolognesi, and J. W. Beard. 1969. Response of bone marrow to MC29 avian leukosis virus *in vitro. Cancer Res.* 29:2056–74.

Levine, S., and Doris Nelsen. 1964. RIF infection in a commercial flock of chickens. *Avian Diseases* 8:358–68.

Löliger, H. C. 1964. Histogenetic correlations between the reticular tissue and the different types of avian leukosis and related neoplasms. *Nat. Cancer Inst. Monograph* 17: 37–61.

Löliger, H. C., and H. J. Schubert. 1966. Ubertragungsversuche mit aviaren Myelozytomen (tumorformige Chloroleukosis, s. Chlorome). *Pathol. Vet.* 3:492–505.

———. 1967. Investigations on the etiology and pathology of the lymphoid cell leucosis of Japanese quails. (English summary.) *Deut. Tieraerztl. Wochschr.* 74:154–58.

Lucas, A. M. 1959. A discussion of synonymy in avian and mammalian hematological nomenclature. *Am. J. Vet. Res.* 20:887–97.

Lucas, A. M., and C. Jamroz. 1961. Atlas of Hematology. USDA Monograph 25.

Manaker, R. A., and V. Groupé. 1956. Discrete foci of altered chicken embryo cells associated with Rous sarcoma virus in tissue culture. *Virology* 2:839–40.

Mathews, F. P. 1929. Leukochloroma in the common fowl. Its relation to myelogenic leukemia and its analogies to chloroma in man. *Arch. Pathol.* 7:442–57.

Mladenov, Z., Ursula Heine, Dorothy Beard, and J. W. Beard. 1967. Strain MC29 avian leukosis virus. Myelocytoma, endothelioma, and renal growths: Pathomorphological and ultrastructural aspects. *J. Nat. Cancer Inst.* 38:251–85.

Moulton, J. E. 1961. *Tumors in Domestic Animals.* Univ. Calif. Press, Berkeley and Los Angeles.

Nyfeldt, A. 1934. Etude sur les leucoses des poules. I. Une myeloblastose pure. *Sang* 8:566–84.

Oberling, C., and M. Guerin. 1954. The role of viruses in the production of cancer, pp. 353–423 In Greenstein, J. P., and A. Haddow, *Advances in Cancer Research*, Vol. II. Academic Press, New York.

Olson, C., Jr. 1940. Transmissible fowl leukosis. A review of the literature. *Mass. Agr. Expt. Sta. Bull.* 370.

Olson, C., Jr., and K. L. Bullis. 1942. A survey and study of spontaneous neoplastic diseases in chickens. *Mass. Agr. Expt. Sta. Bull.* 391.

Pappenheimer, A. M., L. C. Dunn, and V. Cone. 1926. A study of fowl paralysis (neuro-lymphomatosis gallinarum). *Storrs Agr. Expt. Sta. Bull.* 143.

Payne, F. E., J. J. Solomon, and H. G. Purchase. 1966. Immunofluorescent studies of group-specific antigen of the avian sarcomaleukosis viruses. *Proc. Nat. Acad. Sci. U.S.* 55:341–49.

Payne, L. N., and P. M. Biggs. 1966. Genetic basis of cellular susceptibility to the Schmidt-Ruppin and Harris strains of Rous sarcoma virus. *Virology* 29:190–98.

Payne, L. N., and R. C. Chubb. 1968. Studies on the nature and genetic control of an antigen in normal chick embryos which reacts in the COFAL test. *J. Gen. Virol.* 3: 379–91.

Payne, L. N., L. B. Crittenden, and W. Okazaki. 1968. Influence of host genotype on responses to four strains of avian leukosis virus. *J. Nat. Cancer Inst.* 40:907–16.

Pentamalli, F. 1915. Ueber die Geschwuelste bei Huehnern. I. Mitteilung. Allgemeine Morphologie der spontanen und der transplantablen Huehnergeschwuelste. *Z. Krebsforsch.* 15:111–53.

Perek, M. 1960. An epizootic of histocytic sarcomas in chickens induced by a cell-free agent. *Avian Diseases* 4:85–94.

Peterson, R. D. A., H. G. Purchase, B. R. Burmester, M. D. Cooper, and R. A. Good. 1966. The relationships among visceral lymphomatosis, bursa of Fabricius and bursa-dependent lymphoid tissue of the chicken. *J. Nat. Cancer Inst.* 36:585–98.

Piraino, F., W. Okazaki, B. R. Burmester, and T. N. Frederickson. 1963. Bioassay of fowl leukosis virus in chickens by the inoculation of 11-day-old embryos. *Virology* 21:396–401.

Ponten, J. 1962a. Homologous transfer of Rous sarcoma by cells. *J. Nat. Cancer Inst.* 29: 1147–59.

———. 1962b. Transplantation of chicken tumor RPL12 in homologous hosts. *J. Nat. Cancer Inst.* 29:1013–21.

———. 1962c. Transmission *in vivo* of chicken erythroblastosis by intact cells. *J. Cellular Comp. Physiol.* 60:209–15.

———. 1964. The *in vivo* growth mechanism of avian Rous sarcoma. *Nat. Cancer Inst. Monograph* 17:131–45.

Ponten, J., and B. R. Burmester. 1967. Transplantability of primary tumors of RPL12 virus-induced lymphoid leukosis. *J. Nat. Cancer Inst.* 38:505–13.

Ponten, J., and B. Thorell. 1957. The histogenesis of virus-induced chicken leukemia. *J. Nat. Cancer Inst.* 18:443–54.

Prince, A. M. 1958. Quantitative studies on Rous sarcoma virus. III. Virus multiplication and cellular response following infection of the chorioallantoic membrane of the chick embryo. *Virology* 5:435–57.

Pugh, L. P. 1927. Sporadic diffuse osteoperiostitis in fowls. *Vet. Rev.* 7:189–90.

Purchase, H. G. 1965. Rous sarcoma and its helper viruses (a review). *Avian Diseases* 9:127–45.

———. 1966. The epizootiology of the avian leukosis complex, pp. 209–20. In Winqvist, G. (ed.), *Comparative Leukemia Research*. Pergamon Press, Oxford and New York.

Purchase, H. G., and W. Okazaki. 1964. Morphology of foci produced by standard preparations of Rous sarcoma virus. *J. Nat. Cancer Inst.* 32:579–89.

————. 1966. *In vivo* replacement of the helper virus in Bryan's strain of Rous sarcoma virus by AMV and RPL12 viruses. *J. Nat. Cancer Inst.* 37:563–71.

Purchase, H. G., J. J. Solomon, and D. C. Johnson. 1969. Avian leukosis-sarcoma viruses and antibody in field flocks, and their relationship to "leukosis" mortality. *Avian Diseases* 13:58–71.

Rao, P. R., and J. W. Beard. 1964. Lipide composition of avian BAI strain A (myeloblastosis) virus and virus associated meyeloblasts. *Nat. Cancer Inst. Monograph* 17: 673–75.

Rao, P. R., R. A. Bonar, and J. W. Beard. 1966. Lipids of BAI strain of avian tumor virus and of the myeloblast host cell. *Exp. Mol. Pathol.* 5:374–88.

Rauscher, F. J., J. A. Reyniers, and M. R. Sacksteder. 1964. Response or lack of response of apparently leukosis-free Japanese quail to avian tumor viruses. *Nat. Cancer Inst. Monograph* 17:211–29.

Reis, J., and P. Nobrega. 1956. *Tratado de Doencas das Aves*, 2nd ed. Edicoes Melboramentos, Sao Paulo.

Riman, J., and B. Thorell. 1960. A nucleotide enzyme complex associated with fowl leukemia virus. *Biochem. Biophys. Acta* 40: 565–67.

Robinson, H. L. 1967. Isolation of noninfectious particles containing Rous sarcoma virus RNA from the medium of Rous sarcoma virus-transformed nonproduct cells. *Proc. Nat. Acad. Sci. U.S.* 57:1665–62.

Robinson, W. S., and P. H. Duesberg. 1968. The chemistry of RNA tumor viruses, pp. 306–31. In Frankel-Conrat (ed.), *Molecular Basis of Virology*. Reinhold Book Corp., New York.

Robinson, W. S., A. Pitkanen, and H. Rubin. 1965. The nucleic acid of the Bryan strain of Rous sarcoma virus: Purification of the virus and isolation of the nucleic acid. *Proc. Nat. Acad. Sci. U.S.* 54:137–44.

Robinson, W. S., H. L. Robinson, and P. H. Duesberg. 1967. Tumor virus RNA's. *Proc. Nat. Acad. Sci. U.S.* 58:825–34.

Roloff, F. 1868. *Mag. ges. Thierheilk* 34:190 (cited by Chubb and Gordon, 1957). The avian leukosis complex—A review. *Vet. Rev. Annotations* 32:97–120.

Rous, P. 1911. A sarcoma of the fowl transmissible by an agent separable from tumor cells. *J. Exp. Med.* 13:397–411.

Rubin, H. 1956. An analysis of the apparent neutralization of Rous sarcoma virus with antiserum to normal chick tissues. *Virology* 2:545–58.

————. 1960a. A virus in chick embryos which induces resistance in vitro to infection with Rous sarcoma virus. *Proc. Nat. Acad. Sci. U.S.* 46:1105–19.

————. 1960b. Growth of Rous sarcoma virus in chick embryo cells following irradiation of host cells or free virus. *Virology* 11:28–47.

Rubin, H., and H. M. Temin. 1959. A radiological study of cell-virus interaction in the Rous sarcoma. *Virology* 7:75–91.

Rubin, H., A. Cornelius, and Lois Fanshier. 1961. The pattern of congenital transmission of an avian leukosis virus. *Proc. Nat. Acad. Sci. U.S.* 47:1058–60.

Rubin, H., Lois Fanshier, A. Cornelius, and W. F. Hughes. 1962. Tolerance and immunity in chickens after congenital and contact infection with an avian leukosis virus. *Virology* 17:143–56.

Sanger, V. L. 1963. Pathogenesis of osteopetrosis in chickens. Ph.D. thesis. Michigan State University, East Lansing.

Sanger, V. L., T. N. Frederickson, C. C. Morrill, and B. R. Burmester. 1966. Pathogenesis of osteopetrosis in chickens. *Am. J. Vet. Res.* 27:1735–44.

Sarma, P. S., H. C. Turner, and R. J. Huebner. 1964. An avian leucosis group-specific complement fixation reaction. Application for the detection and assay of non-cytopathogenic leucosis viruses. *Virology* 23:313–21.

Schmeisser, H. C. 1915. Spontaneous and experimental leukemia of the fowl. *J. Exp. Med.* 22:820–38.

Sharp, D. G., and J. W. Beard. 1954. Virus of avian erythromyeloblastic leukosis. IV. Sedimentation, density and hydration. *Biochem. Biophys. Acta* 14:12–17.

Simpson, C. F., D. W. Anthony, and F. Young. 1957. Visceral lymphomatosis in a flock of turkeys. *J. Am. Vet. Med. Ass.* 130:93–96.

Smida, J., V. Thurzo, and V. Smidova. 1968. Susceptibility of ducklings to different strains of Rous sarcoma virus and to other avian tumor viruses. *Neoplasma* 15:329–36.

Stubbs, E. L., and J. Furth. 1932. Anemia and erythroleucosis occurring spontaneously in the common fowl. *J. Am. Vet. Med. Ass.* 81:209–22.

Thorell, B. 1958. Induktion von Nierentumoren durch Leukaemievirus. *Zentr. Allgem. Pathol. Pathol. Anat.* 98:314.

Vogt, P. K. 1965. Avian tumor viruses. Vol. 11:293–385. In Smith, K., and M. Lauffer (eds.), *Advances in Virus Research*. Academic Press, New York and London.

————. 1967. A virus released by "non-producing" Rous sarcoma cells. *Proc. Nat. Acad. Sci. U.S.* 58:801–8.

Vogt, P. K., and R. Ishizaki. 1965. Reciprocal patterns of genetic resistance to avian tumor viruses in two lines of chickens. *Virology* 26:664–72.

Vogt, P. K., and R. Ishizaki. 1966a. Criteria for the classification of avian-tumor viruses, pp. 71–90. In Burdett, W. J. (ed.), *Viruses Inducing Cancer.* Univ. Utah Press, Salt Lake City.

———. 1966b. Patterns of viral interference in the avian leukosis and sarcoma complex. *Virology* 30:368–74.

Vogt, P. K., and N. Luykx. 1963. Observations on the surface of cells infected with Rous sarcoma virus. *Virology* 20:75–87.

Walter, W. G., B. R. Burmester, and C. H. Cunningham. 1962. Studies on the transmission and pathology of a viral-induced avian nephroblastoma (embryonal nephroma). *Avian Diseases* 6:455–77.

Warthin, A. S. 1907. Leukemia of the common fowl. *J. Infect. Diseases* 4:369–80.

Wight, P. A. L. 1963. Lymphoid leucosis and fowl paralysis in the quail. *Vet. Record* 75: 685–87.

Wilner, B. I. 1969. *A Classification of the Major Groups of Human and Other Animal Viruses,* 4th ed. Burgess Publ. Co., Minneapolis.

Witter, R. L., B. W. Calnek, and P. P. Levine. 1966. Occurrence of lymphomatosis in chickens free of resistance-inducing factor (RIF) virus. *Avian Diseases* 10:32–42.

Young, D. 1966. Some characteristics of the virus responsible for osteopetrosis in chickens. *J. Comp. Pathol. Therap.* 76:45–50.

Zeigel, R. F., B. R. Burmester, and F. J. Rauscher. 1964. Comparative morphologic and biologic studies of natural and experimental transmission of avian tumor viruses. *Nat. Cancer Inst. Monograph* 17:711–31.

❖

RETICULOENDOTHE-LIOSIS

❖

B. W. CALNEK

Department of Avian Diseases
New York State Veterinary College
Ithaca, New York

❖

IN 1958 Tweihaus isolated a virus from adult turkeys with leukosis-like lesions (Zeigel et al., 1966). This virus which Sevoian et al. (1964a) called T-virus, caused a consistent, rapid, and marked reticuloendotheliosis following inoculation into young chickens, turkeys, and Japanese quail. There was a short incubation period and high mortality, and affected birds had markedly enlarged livers and spleens. There is no evidence that there is a naturally occurring disease associated with this virus, and there is no known economic or public heath significance.

A report by Aulisio and Shelokov (1969) indicated that virus infections in commercial flocks are prevalent. They found specific antibody in egg yolk of eggs from 41 of 92 flocks tested (located in 9 different states). In contrast, Sevoian et al. (1964b), Bose and Levine (1967), and Witter et al. (1970) all failed to detect antibody in commercial flocks. Witter et al. (1970) speculated that the antibodies found by Aulisio and Shelokov may have been directed against chicken syncitial virus, an immunologically related agent known to occur in some flocks (Cook, 1969).

Sevoian et al. (1964a) described the experimental disease as a lymphomatosis and considered the virus oncogenic. Others preferred to classify the lesions as a reticuloendotheliosis but have been unable to decide whether the condition is hyperplastic or neoplastic (Zeigel et al., 1966; Olson, 1967). Because most authors have at least entertained the possibility of oncogenicity of the virus, inclusion of a brief description of the disease in this chapter is warranted.

ETIOLOGY

Zeigel et al. (1966) found the T-virus (also called RE virus, strain T) basically similar to the RNA-containing viruses of the myxovirus group. Mature virus particles, which ranged from 85 to 110 mμ in diameter, typically possessed a diffuse, relatively dense nucleoid and a limiting membrane. They could be distinguished morphologically from representative avian leukosis viruses (RPL12, RIF, AMV) and a variety of common avian myxoviruses, par-amyxoviruses, and adenoviruses. Virus particles were observed budding from cells in the manner described for both avian leukosis and murine leukemia viruses.

Both cellular and cell-free preparations of virus have been found biologically active, but the virus titer was generally reduced in the latter. Cell-free virus retained activity following storage at −70° C for 4 months and was viable after 12 hours at 4° C or 2 hours at 37° C. Viral activity was destroyed after heating to 56° C for 30 minutes or after exposure to 25 or 50% ether (Theilen et al., 1966).

In vitro virus replication occurs in cultures of chicken, quail, and duck embryo fibroblasts and can persist for long periods without perceptible changes in the infected cells (Theilen et al., 1966; Bose and Levine, 1967; Calnek et al., 1969). Calnek et al. found a variety of mammalian cell types refractory to infection. Theilen et al. (1966) and Bose and Levine (1967) observed that cells infected with T-virus were not resistant to Rous sarcoma virus (A and B subgroups) and did not react in the COFAL test, thus affording evidence of the fundamental difference between T-virus and the avian leukosis viruses. Furthermore, T-virus was not neutralized by antisera against various sarcoma and leukosis virus strains (Theilen et al., 1966).

In addition to cell cultures, the chicken embryo may be considered a laboratory host. Sevoian et al. (1964b) infected embryos by yolk sac inoculation and observed embryo discoloration along with enlargement and transcoloration of the liver and spleen. The latter organ was sometimes 20 times normal size. Tumorous nodules were observed in some spleens, and the chorioallantoic membrane was occasionally thickened. High virus doses, especially with cellular inocula, caused sporadic mortality during the latter part of the incubation period. Theilen et al. (1966) inoculated embryos by the CAM route and considered mortality, large solitary pocklike lesions on the CAM, and greenish discoloration of the embryo as criteria of infection.

PATHOGENESIS AND EPIZOOTIOLOGY

The only reported natural infection was in the turkey flock from which the virus was originally isolated; thus only the experimental disease can be described. At least three species are suitable experimental hosts: chicken, turkey, and Japanese quail. The turkey poult appears most susceptible, but the character of the response is essentially similar in all three. Descriptions are provided by Sevoian et al. (1964a), Larose and Sevoian (1965), Theilen et al. (1966), and Olson (1967).

The incubation period is related to the virus dose and may be as short as 3 days or as long as 3 weeks—in most cases 1–2 weeks. The onset is either acute or peracute, and death occurs soon afterward. Clinical signs (depression and perhaps labored respiration) may be seen for 1–6 hours before death. Mortality depends on virus dose and to some extent the age at inoculation. Day-old chicks are more susceptible than birds 2 or more weeks of age. Most but not all infected birds succumb.

Affected birds manifest enlarged livers and spleens with infiltrative lesions ranging from pinpoint to large focal or even diffuse involvement. Subcapsular nodules are common in the spleen, and splenomegaly may be so marked as to cause rupture of the organ. Livers may be pale or yellowish brown. Distended gall bladders are characteristic of birds which succumb to the peracute disease. Nodular lesions may also be seen in other visceral organs including gonad, heart, kidney, and pancreas. Larger nodules have central necrosis. Witter et al. (1970) found that very low doses of virus may result in grossly enlarged (not more than twice normal size) peripheral nerves not unlike those seen in Marek's disease. The most noticeable enlargements were seen in the cervical portion of the vagus nerve.

Histologic changes are apparently similar in all species and are the same following infection with either cellular or cell-free inoculum. The primary lesion, regardless of organ, is one of rapid proliferation of mononuclear cells around blood vessels and in lymphoid follicles. The offending cells, which are apparently of the reticuloendothelial system, are characteristically primitive with large or oval nuclei; prominent nucleoli; and abundant, poorly defined, neutrophilic or basophilic cytoplasm (Fig. 15.56). Mitotic figures are common. More mature lesions may contain differentiated cells resembling those of the lymphoid series. Proliferation is most marked in the liver and spleen. According to Witter

FIG. 15.56—(A) Proliferated
reticuloendothelial (RE) cells
in liver of bird experimentally infected with T-virus. Microscopic lesions are characteristically around blood vessels. H & E, ×90. (B) Higher
magnification of RE cells in
affected liver. Note uniformly immature nature of cells
(e.g. large vesicular nuclei
with prominent nucleoli). A
mitotic figure may be seen at
right of center. H & E, ×380.

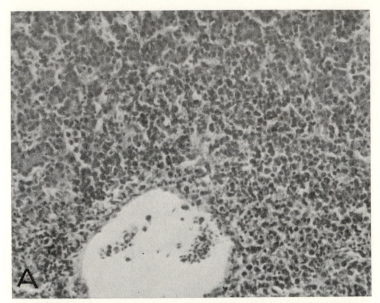
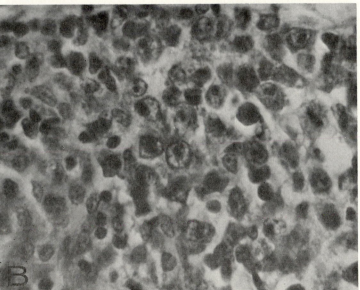

et al. (1970), there can be a diffuse infiltration of lymphocytes and plasma cells, sometimes with edema, in peripheral nerves.

Larose and Sevoian (1965) detected virus-
neutralizing antibody in the sera of birds
which survived inoculation or were exposed
by contact with infected birds. In the latter the percentage of positive sera was low,
suggesting inefficient horizontal transmission or low-grade infection. Significantly,
contact-exposed birds experienced neither
mortality nor morbidity. If natural infec-

tions do occur, it would seem likely that
they are subclinical.

DIAGNOSIS

Virus may be isolated and identified by
either embryo or bird inoculation. In either case it is desirable to employ cell-free inoculum. Four-day-old chicken embryos
should be inoculated via the yolk sac and
those dead after 12 days and all survivors
at 20 days examined for evidence of the described lesions. Chickens, turkeys, or Japa-

nese quail should be inoculated preferably at 1 day of age but older birds can be employed. Clinical-pathological evidence of infection with T-virus centers on a short (less than 3 weeks) incubation period, high mortality, and the development of characteristic gross lesions. Microscopic identification of proliferating reticuloendothelial cells is confirmatory, but ultimate identification of the virus should be on a serologic basis.

The pathologic response must be distinguished from other proliferative diseases. Lymphoid leukosis (LL) has a long (several months) incubation period but may cause infiltrative lesions in young chickens (Calnek, 1968). However, there is no mortality in young birds with LL, and gross lesions are restricted to the spleen, heart, and gonad. Marek's disease (MD) may cause tumorous enlargement of the liver and spleen within 3 weeks postinoculation, but, except in the occasional case of apparent tumor cell transplantation, MD isolates do not induce early mortality. The use of cell-free inocula obviates the transplantation problem. Various bacterial pathogens may cause enlargement of the liver and/or spleen. These can be identified by routine bacteriological examination and the pathologic changes identified as inflammatory on histologic examination. Because of the general lack of paralysis, mortality, and neoplasms in birds displaying reticuloendotheliosis virus-induced nerve lesions, there should be little confusion with Marek's disease. Nonetheless, serologic differentiation should be relied upon.

Serologic tests suitable for identifying specific viral antigens include virus neutralization (Larose and Sevoian, 1965) and fluorescent antibody (FA) (Calnek et al., 1969). Employment of known virus in the neutralization test or virus-infected cells in an indirect FA test may be used to identify specific antibody as evidence of infection in birds.

REFERENCES

Aulisio, C. G., and A. Shelokov. 1969. Prevalence of reticuloendotheliosis in chickens: Immunofluorescence studies. *Proc. Soc. Exp. Biol. Med.* 130:178–81.

Bose, H. R., Jr., and A. S. Levine. 1967. Replication of the reticuloendotheliosis virus (strain T) in chicken embryo cell culture. *J. Virol.* 1:1117–21.

Calnek, B. W. 1968. Lesions in young chickens induced by lymphoid leukosis virus. *Avian Diseases* 12:111–29.

Calnek, B. W., S. H. Madin, and A. J. Kniazeff. 1969. Susceptibility of cultured mammalian cells to infection with a herpesvirus from Marek's disease and T-virus from reticuloendotheliosis of chickens. *Am. J. Vet. Res.* 30:1403–12.

Cook, M. K. 1969. Cultivation of a filterable agent associated with Marek's disease. *J. Nat. Cancer Inst.* 43:203–12.

Larose, R. N., and M. Sevoian. 1965. Avian lymphomatosis. IX. Mortality and serological response of chickens of various ages to graded doses of T-strain. *Avian Diseases* 9:604–10.

Olson, L. D. 1967. Histopathologic and hematologic changes in moribund stages of chicks infected with T-virus. *Am. J. Vet. Res.* 28:1501–7.

Sevoian, M., R. N. Larose, and D. M. Chamberlain. 1964a. Avian lymphomatosis. VI. A virus of unusual potency and pathogenicity. *Avian Diseases* 8:336–47.

——. 1964b. Avian lymphomatosis. VIII. Pathological response of the chicken embryo to T virus. *Nat. Cancer Inst. Monograph* 17:99–119.

Theilen, G. H., R. F. Zeigel, and M. J. Twiehaus. 1966. Biological studies with RE virus (strain T) that induces reticuloendotheliosis in turkeys, chickens, and Japanese quail. *J. Nat. Cancer Inst.* 37:731–43.

Witter, R. L., H. G. Purchase, and G. H. Burgoyne. 1970. Peripheral nerve lesions similar to those of Marek's disease in chickens inoculated with reticuloendotheliosis virus. *J. Nat. Cancer Inst.* 45:567–77.

Zeigel, R. F., G. H. Theilen, and M. T. Twiehaus. 1966. Electron microscopic observations on RE virus (strain T) that induces reticuloendotheliosis in turkeys, chickens, and Japanese quail. *J. Nat. Cancer Inst.* 37:709–29.

❖

TUMORS OF UNKNOWN ETIOLOGY

❖

C. F. HELMBOLDT

AND

T. N. FREDRICKSON

Department of Animal Diseases
University of Connecticut
Storrs, Connecticut

❖

THIS CATEGORY includes a wide variety of neoplasms for which no etiologic agent has been found. This single limitation reduces the incidence of neoplasms to be dealt with to a rather low figure as viral-induced types are the overwhelming form.

From an economic and public health view, these tumors are of minor significance. No evidence exists as to their transmissibility to man, nor is their incidence a cause for concern in condemnation figures (Furrow, personal communication).

INCIDENCE

Actually the incidence of avian tumors of this category is an unknown figure surrounded by the impressive statistics concerning the viral neoplasms. Available figures are usually from limited populations. For example, a flock of 343,600 broiler birds had a tumor incidence of 0.69%, of which only 2 dysgerminomas, 2 thecomas, 4 granulosa cell tumors, and 2 arrhenoblastomas could be considered of unknown etiology (Campbell, 1967). The authors have personally seen over 100,000 sections of the domestic fowl; in addition many more specimens have been seen grossly. Nonleukotic tumors other than those of known viral etiology were only uncommonly seen.

The incidence of such tumors may also be distorted by casual necropsy procedures which could relegate the tumor to a classification of the viral type. Another explanation might be that poultry husbandry practices tend to kill most birds at a relatively young age before tumors have a chance to develop. Finally, it may be that many birds slaughtered or necropsied in fact do have tumors other than those of unknown etiology but that the tumors are microscopic and thus overlooked. As an example, the oviduct adenocarcinoma was reported at a 50% incidence in one flock when oviducts were examined histologically (Swarbrick et al., 1968). It becomes apparent that the economics of poultry husbandry dictate against determining the true potential incidence of neoplastic diseases.

ETIOLOGIC FACTORS

At the moment no etiologic factors are known. It would appear that this category can be characterized as similar to that of neoplasms of man and other higher mammals and be considered a riddle.

TUMOR CLASSIFICATION

None of the numerous classifications for the avian leukosis complex are appropriate. One may resort to any number of classification schemes (Jackson, 1936; Goss, 1940; Campbell, 1947; Feldman and Olson, 1959) which are based on cell type from which the tumor originates. No classification is entirely satisfactory, but neither is it extremely important. The name of most tumors immediately categorizes them as to origin, and this is sufficient since our knowledge is so limited.

The biologic characteristics of a neoplasm are of importance in coming to a decision of malignancy versus benignancy. Little clinical evidence is available for fowl, so this is not a significant aid in classification.

For the purposes of this discussion, tumors will be considered under the various organ systems.

CENTRAL NERVOUS SYSTEM

Avian Astrocytoma (avian glioma
[Jungherr and Wolf, 1939]; glioblastoma
multiforme [Jackson, 1954])

This is apparently a rare tumor; only 7 cases are known (Belmonte, 1935; Jungherr and Wolf, 1939; Jackson, 1954; Biering-Sørensen, 1956; Jortner, personal communication). However, in recent years two separate groups reported these in epizootic proportions (Ostendorf and Henderson, 1962; Wight and Duff, 1964).

SIGNS. Affected birds are chiefly adults, and signs of the affliction are not always present. There may be torticollis, retropulsion, incoordination, etc. The most suggestive point is the transitory nature of these signs; the bird at one moment seems to be in difficulty, suddenly it rights itself and acts perfectly normal.

GROSS PATHOLOGY. Although the tumor is rather small, usually no larger than 5 mm, it is not difficult to see. Fixed tissue offers the best view, and a sagittal cut is by far the best. The neoplasm appears as a sharply delineated whitish area. Those seen by Wight and Duff (1964) always appeared at the base of the cerebellum; in our series the neoplasm was always in the area of the thalamus.

HISTOPATHOLOGY. This is essentially a fibrillary astrocytoma which appears to arise in paraventricular areas. The cases studied by us were always in the neighborhood of the third ventricle (Fig. 15.57) but were definitely not of ependymal origin. In fact, the tumor when it began to encroach on the ventricle was covered by the characteristic single-layered ependyma. Demarcation from unaffected brain was fairly sharp (Fig.

15.58); there were no hemorrhages, giant cells, or areas of pressure necrosis as seen in glioblastoma multiforme; yet there was a marked perivascular reaction of lymphocytes in the brain bordering the tumor. The neoplastic cells varied considerably in morphology but remained within the confines of the term polygonal in character (Fig. 15.59). Fibrillar processes which are compatible with the astrocytic nature can be demonstrated; the processes and other cytoplasmic material are copious and dense. Lobulation by dense fibrous tissue is common. Special stains such as phosphotungstic acid-hemotoyxlin, Laidlaw connective, and Cajal's technique demonstrate that only the walls are fibrous tissue; the tumor itself is not but seems to consist entirely of ectodermal cells.

The neoplasm can be classified as benign astrocytoma. It does not metastasize but apparently continues to expand and eventually causes fatal pressures on the ventricular system.

ETIOLOGIC FACTORS. One theory proposed was that this tumor results from a former episode of encephalitis (Erichsen and Harboe, 1953). Although this idea is attractive, it is difficult to substantiate. If it were the case, the incidence of such a sequel would be very low, as numerous cases of avian encephalomyelitis and some cases of Marek's disease recover. Toxoplasmosis concomitant with astrocytomas has been

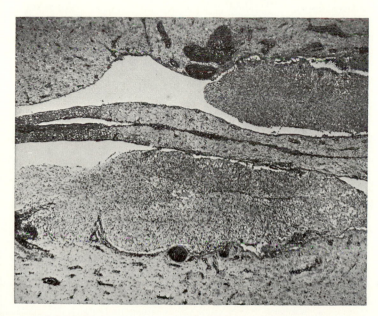

FIG. 15.57—*Astrocytoma from mature hen. Septum pellucidum divides tumor which is attached to fissura neopaleostriatica.* ×30.

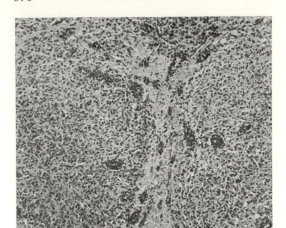

FIG. 15.58—Astrocytoma from thalamus of mature hen. Darker foci in and around neoplastic masses are perivascular infiltrates of lymphocytes. ×75.

seen by two separate investigators (Biering-Sørensen, 1956; Ostendorf and Henderson, 1962). All other observers have failed to note this, suggesting that the protozoa were coincidental or that they initiate the tumor and then die out.

INTEGUMENT

Neoplasms of the avian integument other than those of known viral etiology are rare. The two components, epithelium and derma, are the tissues of origin. Those of the derma are usually sarcomas and so-called "skin leukosis" (Marek's disease) which place them as viral types.

A review of the literature reveals only 2 types which can be considered here. A third, the trichoepithelioma, will be presented, but it may not be a tumor.

Hemangiopericytoma

This tumor was first reported in man (Stout and Murray, 1942) and later in the dog (Mulligan, 1955). The literature contains a report of 2 such avian tumors (Sastry et al., 1967), to which 4 unreported ones may be added (Department of Animal Diseases, University of Connecticut, Storrs, unpublished data).

GROSS PATHOLOGY. This is an easily overlooked tumor that is noted only if it as-

sumes any size. Often it is a small subcutaneous nodule about 1 cm in diameter which almost invariably occurs in the cervical region. It is fairly dense, white, and well delineated but firmly embedded in the subcutis.

HISTOPATHOLOGY. The histologic appearance is a spindle cell sarcoma with rather striking, concentrically arranged cells. Within the whorls an arteriole is invariably present. Any question of the characteristic concentric laminar structure can be readily clarified by subjecting the neoplasm to a silver stain which brings out the concentric arrangement of the supportive fibers (Fig. 15.60). The cells are monotonously similar, being spindle-shaped with a nucleus to conform to this morphology; the chromatin is not particularly impressive. The cytoplasm is abundant, but individual cells seem to merge into each other. A capsule is present.

The tumor is considered benign, as biologically it does not metastasize nor cause any problem except possibly because of size. Surgical removal has been successfully attempted in two cases.

ETIOLOGIC FACTORS. No evidence exists which could place this as a viral tumor.

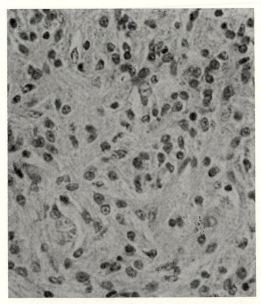

FIG. 15.59—Higher magnification of Fig. 15.58. Fibrous quality of astrocytoma is obvious. Nuclei are monotonous in their regularity. ×190.

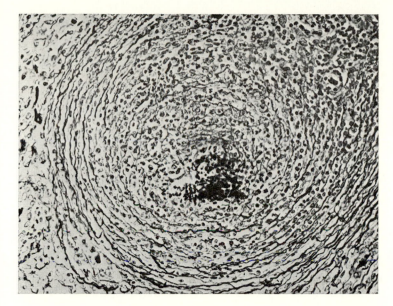

FIG. 15.60—*Hemangiopericy-toma from neck skin of imma-ture hen. Silver-stained sec-tion illustrates concentric ring of pericytes about a small ar-tery.* ×190.

Never has this occurred in experimental procedures employing the RPL series of viruses. One cannot clearly rule out the Marek's disease agent, but the high incidence of the disease versus the rarity of the tumor tends to make this a slim possibility.

Squamous Cell Carcinoma (epithelioma, epithelioblastoma, epidermoid)

A number of people have reported tumors of the integument. For example, Jackson (1936), Olson and Bullis (1942), and Furrow (personal communication) all saw a very few tumors of this category.

GROSS PATHOLOGY. The general appearance of this neoplasm gives the impression of trauma and is probably responsible for the relatively low estimates of incidence. The tumor seems to present a raw or bleeding surface which invariably forms an eschar of cellular debris mixed with dust. Thus the usual picture is a black rough area raised on the skin. The feet and legs are reported as the common site (Feldman and Olson, 1959), although the skin of the neck also seems to be a common area of involvement.

HISTOPATHOLOGY. The surface is composed of blood cellular elements, fibrin, dust, and often bacterial colonies. The eschar is underlaid by proliferating cells from squamous epithelium, but the cell layer of origin is difficult to determine. The cells form large irregular clumps and are deeply basophilic with some resemblance to the normal epidermis. The commonly present inflammatory reaction breaks up the continuity of the surface so that isolated cell groups are not unusual. Intercellular spines are not seen, and mitosis almost seems to be in the same category. Frequent keratin pearls are seen (Figs. 15.61, 15.62).

The tumor is difficult to classify as its appearance suggests malignancy, but evidence of metastasis is lacking (Feldman and Olson, 1959). In fact, one may be hard put even to designate a badly inflamed squamous cell tumor as neoplastic. Perhaps the best applicable criterion of neoplasia is the fact that the lesion persists and does not heal. The deep-staining basophilic characteristic, lack of metastasis, and formation of bizarre masses of cells suggest that the designation of squamous cell carcinoma might better be basal cell tumor.

Trichoepithelioma (benign cystic epithelioma)

From the standpoint of semantics this term describes an impossible tumor, as "tricho" refers to hair. Rather than introduce a new term, the word will be used here to describe a debatable neoplasm of the avian skin. Small discrete nodules, often solitary, are not an uncommon finding on the avian skin. Usually dismissed as inconsequential changes (such as trauma), these are overlooked.

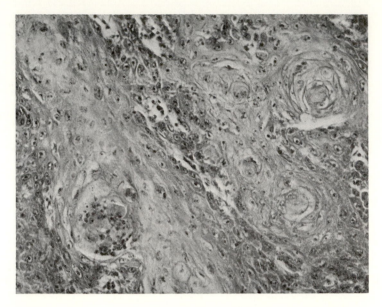

FIG. 15.61—Squamous cell carcinoma from skin of mature hen. Keratin masses or pearls are formed in neoplastic epithelium. ×190.

GROSS PATHOLOGY. One such neoplasm was an incidental finding while seeking carcinomas of the skin. The nodule is small, being only a matter of millimeters in diameter, and is smooth, glistening, and firm. No feather seems to be growing from the lesion and, in fact, it is not easily seen.

HISTOPATHOLOGY. The lesion is well circumscribed and is separated from the surrounding tissue by a pronounced fibrous

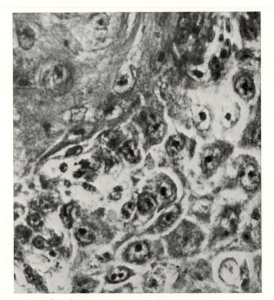

FIG. 15.62—Higher magnification of Fig. 15.61. Cells have lost their polarity and intercellular bridges are gone. ×480.

wall which appears to be the basal cell layer of the feather follicles except it is considerably exaggerated. The inner contents are layers of keratinized debris, probably a mixture of feather follicle and squamous epithelium. However, nothing is recognizable in the inner contents (Fig. 15.63).

ETIOLOGIC FACTORS. If this is an inflammatory lesion, we could think of trauma and infection as reasonable causes. These still might be considered etiologic factors if the lesion is neoplastic, as we believe.

UROGENITAL SYSTEM

Since the embryonal nephroma or nephroblastoma is without question a viral-induced neoplasm, one need not consider the kidney and other portions of the urinary tract in this section. However, the female reproductive tract is quite another matter. The ovary presents a problem in dealing with classification (by system) since it is an exocrine as well as an endocrine gland. In addition, the histogenesis of ovarian tumors has never been clearly determined.

Classification is probably best achieved by placing the genital tumors in categories by cellular origin. This has the additional advantage of also considering the physiologic aspects. Since the genital tumors of the hen do not seem to be greatly different from those of higher mammals, there is little point in establishing still another classification; thus, it is suggested that a recent

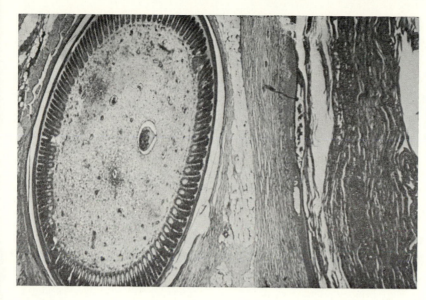

classification of human urogenital neoplasms be employed (Hertig and Gore, 1961). The following is adapted from their classification:

1. Gonadal stromal tumors
   a. granulosa-theca cell
   b. arrhenoblastoma
2. Germ cell tumors
3. Cystoma (germinal epithelial origin)
   a. ovarian carcinoma
   b. fallopian tube carcinoma

It should be pointed out that all statistical figures on occurrence as to sex are biased, as poultry husbandry practices result in large numbers of hens versus only a few males.

Ovarian Carcinoma (adenocarcinoma, carcinoma leiomyomatosum [Jackson, 1936], peritoneal carcinomatosis [Nobel et al., 1964], adenocarcinomata of fowls [Wilson, 1967])

This is by far the most common tumor of unknown etiology of the hen. The size and striking appearance of the tumor cannot fail to attract attention. In addition, its similarity to its human counterpart suggests the hen as a suitable animal model.

The incidence of this tumor is unknown. It apparently is associated with advancing age, which is not a common situation in poultry. Surveys of this tumor actually go back to 1906 (Nobel et al., 1964).

GROSS PATHOLOGY. The victim is invariably a mature hen, at least 1 year of age. Many affected birds are in fairly good condition but show nonspecific signs such as lethargy and general lack of alertness. Ascites is a frequent complication in advanced cases; the fluid is clear, amber, and viscid in consistency. Apparently fibrin is not a constituent as the fluid does not coagulate nor are fibrin tags seen.

The typical affected bird has countless white, firm, discrete, coalescing tumors on the serosal surfaces of the abdominal viscera (Fig. 15.64). These usually measure about 1 cm, but coalescing tumors measure up to several centimeters. It is sometimes not possible to determine the site of origin. A striking feature is the massive involvement of the duodenal loop and pancreas (Nobel et al., 1964) which anatomically are in contact with the affected ovary. Since this tumor spreads by transcoelomic implants, the pancreatic lesion is not surprising. This characteristic should be mentioned, however, as some pathologists are prone to designate the lesion as a pancreatic adenocarcinoma. Although impressive lesions are seen in the abdomen, they rarely are found on the thoracic surface despite the lack of an ineffective diaphragm.

HISTOPATHOLOGY. The tumor falls into two distinct groups, although basically they are the same. In the less common the adenomatous portion is pronounced. In the common type the glandular portions are scarce

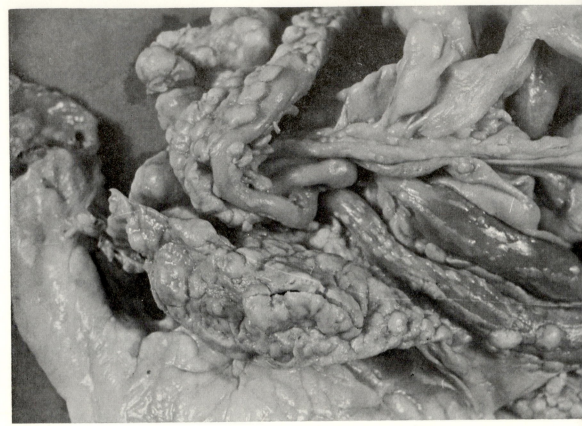

FIG. 15.64—Ovarian carcinoma in hen. Serosal surfaces of intestines and mesentery are covered by countless implants. Normal size.

FIG. 15.65—Ovarian adenocarcinoma, scirrhous type, from aged hen. Darker areas represent small islands of glandular tissue on background of leiomyoma (see Fig. 15.68). ×30.

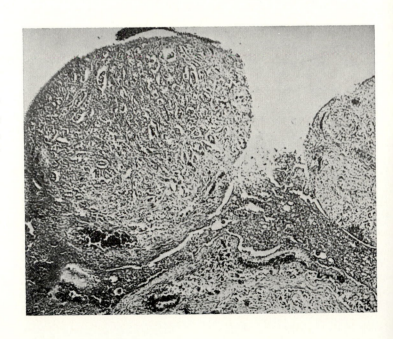

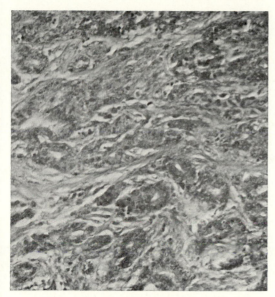

FIG. 15.66—Ovarian adenocarcinoma from aged hen. This minute tumor was found only on microscopic examination. ×190.

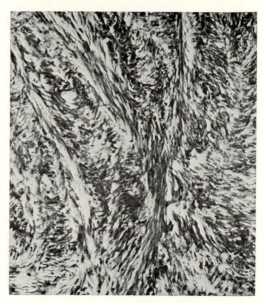

FIG. 15.68—Leiomyosarcoma from mature hen. Interlacing strains of smooth muscle are typical (see Fig. 15.65). ×190.

while the fibrous and muscular tissues predominate. This characteristic has led to the designation of medullary or scirrhous types (Figs. 15.65–15.67). While no serious objection to this differentiation can be raised, it is well to remember that the tumor may vary from place to place in the same bird.

The usual tumor presents oblong to cordlike acini lined by a single layer of cuboidal epithelium. Proteinaceous debris may be seen in larger glands but this is not common. The cells are normal in appearance; mitosis and anaplasia are rare. The acini may be crowded together or even compressed into the so-called medullary type. The nonacinous portion is chiefly muscle and connective tissue, so the designation carcinoma leiomyomatosum (Fig. 15.68) (Jackson, 1936) is a valid one.

The benign-appearing acini and leiomyoma belie the malignant character of this neoplasm. The muscular portion particularly can be seen invading and replacing tissue; this is best seen in the pancreas. Constriction of the intestine is seen but complete obstruction is probably rare.

ETIOLOGIC FACTORS. This is definitely an age-connected tumor. In our own experience, birds over 2 years of age have a high risk; in closely controlled flocks, birds began to die at $3\frac{1}{2}$ years of age, and all had

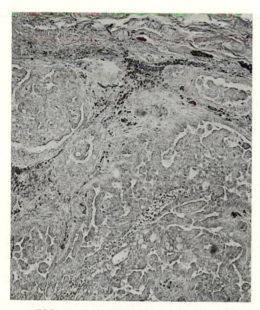

FIG. 15.67—Ovarian adenocarcinoma, medullary type, from aged hen. Tumor masses form irregular papillae and are highly cellular. ×30.

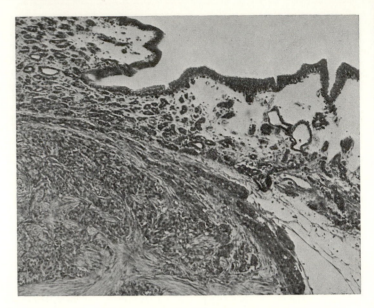

FIG. 15.69—Fallopian tube adenocarcinoma of aged hen. More active glandular portion is at lower left; mucin is lifting off surface epithelium. ×175.

died of ovarian carcinoma by 9 years of age. Manipulation of older birds by presenting additional light over the natural sources increased the incidence of the tumor, probably by pituitary stimulation. This brought out the significant feature that the tumor begins in active ovaries (Greenwood, 1967).

Fallopian Tube Carcinoma (oviduct carcinoma [Goodchild and Cooper, 1968], oviduct adenocarcinoma [Swarbrick et al., 1968])

This was considered a rare tumor until the report of Swarbrick et al. (1968) who saw an incidence of up to 50% when microscopic studies were made.

GROSS PATHOLOGY. Since this tumor apparently spreads by implantation, it may be confused with the ovarian carcinoma. Although the fallopian tube tumor is said to be far more mucoid than the ovarian carcinoma, this is not a reliable characteristic when viewed with the naked eye.

HISTOPATHOLOGY. This is a cystadenocarcinoma occurring in the epithelial portions of the infundibulum and magnum (Jackson, 1936; Goodchild and Cooper, 1968). The epithelial portions are the prominent features; the connective tissue seems supportive only. The epithelium is cuboidal and often piles up in what seems to be tortuous glandular structures. These fill with mucinous substance and coalesce, and the contents form cysts or sometimes merely

pools of mucin (Figs. 15.69, 15.70). No etiologic factors are known.

Granulosa Cell Tumor
(granulosa theca-cell tumor)

Although this tumor is relatively common in higher vertebrates, it seems virtually unknown in the domestic fowl. The

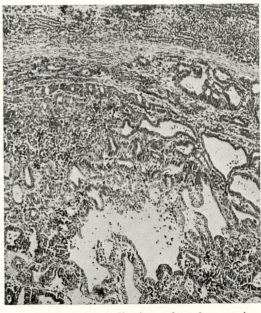

FIG. 15.70—Fallopian tube adenocarcinoma of aged hen. There is considerable cystic dilation of glandular portion while serosa (top) consists largely of undifferentiated cells. ×75.

literature contains 2 reports (Awadhiya and Jain, 1967; Campbell, 1967), which amount to 5 cases. Our own observations include one irrefutable instance of this neoplasm.

GROSS PATHOLOGY. The picture is identical to that of ovarian carcinoma and (in our case) occurred in a flock which had other instances of this tumor. This is another example of the necessity of histology in order to gain meaningful statistical figures.

HISTOPATHOLOGY. The folliculoid pattern consists of a definite stroma limiting the follicle which is lined by several layers of polygonal cells with fairly copious cytoplasm (Fig. 15.71). It is in this layer that rosettes (the so-called Call-Exner bodies [Fig. 15.72], which were prevalent in our case) are formed. This polygonal cell layer is abruptly ended to form a center of paler cells, the luteinized theca externa, which is responsible for the hormonal activity in mammals.

Arrhenoblastoma (masculinoma, androblastoma, arrhenoma)

This tumor is undoubtedly rare, as it is in other species (Hertig and Gore, 1961), but the startling clinical signs of masculinization are so impressive that many cases are brought to the attention of pathologists (Gupta and Langham, 1968).

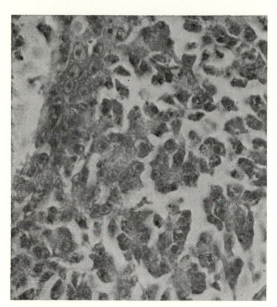

FIG. 15.72—Same as Fig. 15.71. Many Call-Exner cells (arranged in rosette pattern with their nuclei at right angles to central space) are present. ×190.

GROSS PATHOLOGY. The affected bird is invariably mature. The obvious masculinization, which is seen best in the comb and wattles is striking. The neoplasm is white and dense, and involves the ovary. Unlike the ovarian adenocarcinoma, it does not seem to implant on adjacent viscera. The benignancy of the lesion is well illustrated in mammals in which two ovaries are present but only one is affected.

HISTOPATHOLOGY. Tubules reminiscent of the testis are the prominent feature. The cytoplasm is usually one cell in depth, but the pronounced vacuolar cytoplasm gives a different first impression. The vacuoles and the cell morphology both suggest a Sertoli cell which is feminizing but which may act differently in this environment. The interstitium or Leydig cell area is positive for fat, but the cells are not as plentiful as one would expect from the masculine character of the bird (Figs. 15.73, 15.74).

ETIOLOGIC FACTORS. Although one proposal suggests that this is a teratogenous growth, the idea is not particularly attractive as age and previous egg production seem to be factors. A more palatable thesis is that this neoplasm evolves from a granulosa-theca cell tumor.

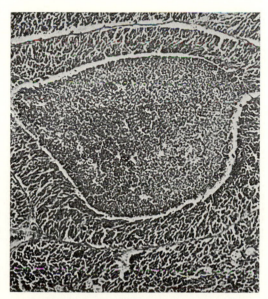

FIG. 15.71—Granulosa-theca cell tumor of mature hen. ×75.

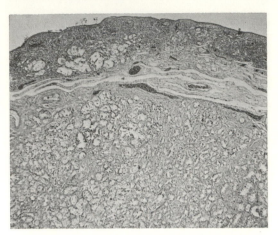

FIG. 15.73—*Arrhenoblastoma from ovary of mature hen. Testicularlike pattern of ovary is seen. ×30. (Courtesy Department of Pathology, Mich. State Univ.)*

DIGESTIVE SYSTEM

Apparently tumors occur chiefly in the accessory organs of digestion. Any reported in the tract itself may have been the result of an ovarian carcinoma (Feldman and Olson, 1959), and critical evaluation is required for proper classification. An adenocarcinoma of the ileocecal valve (Feldman and Olson, 1959), bile duct adenoma (Savage, 1926; Heim, 1931; Olson and Bullis, 1942), and hepatoma (Olson and Bullis, 1942) are the types reported in the literature.

Bile Duct Adenoma (cholangioma)

GROSS PATHOLOGY. A solitary liver nodule which can be almost any size should be looked upon as possibly a bile duct adenoma. The tumor is well circumscribed and firm. Since it might obstruct a major branch of the ductal system, an obstructive jaundice could conceivably result.

HISTOPATHOLOGY. There is a monotonous repetition of bile ducts on a background of connective tissue, all surrounded by a connective tissue capsule (Fig. 15.75). The ductal epithelium appears to be normal cuboidal. However, a malignant version may occur, and then the epithelium piles up to form irregularly obstructed ducts while the background connective tissue appears sarcomatous. In the one malignant tumor seen there were no metastases (Fig. 15.76).

Hepatoma

GROSS PATHOLOGY. This tumor at times causes changes so subtle that it is not easily detected. Any alteration in color or shape can be suspected. Unfortunately, most suspicious cases turn out to be cirrhoticlike conditions (an interesting observation since cirrhosis can be a prelude to a neoplasm). Hepatomas can be confused with bile duct adenomas, particularly when they are well developed. Since both types seem to arise

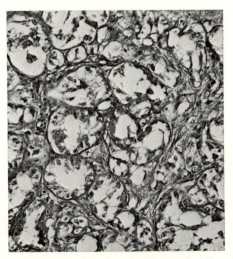

FIG. 15.74—*Same as Fig. 15.73. Pseudoseminiferous tubuli are seen. ×190. (Courtesy Department of Pathology, Mich. State Univ.)*

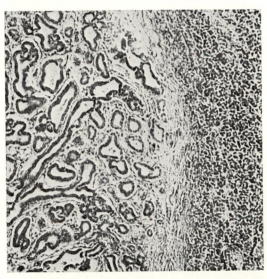

FIG. 15.75—*Bile duct adenoma from mature hen. Tumor is essentially a mass of proliferating bile ducts. ×75.*

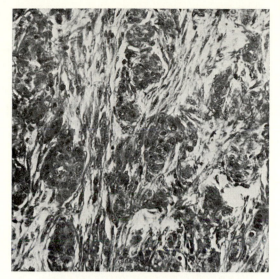

FIG. 15.76—Bile duct adenosarcoma from mature hen. This is malignant counterpart of Fig. 15.75. Ductal epithelium is forming dense epithelial structures which are contained by sarcomatous tissue. ×190.

from a common ancestral cell, this is not unusual.

HISTOPATHOLOGY. The normal hepatic architecture of lobulation and portal triads is lost. This abnormality may be difficult to ascertain in early lesions as the hen's liver has poor lobulation. The affected hepatic cell is larger than normal and is distorted with a larger than normal nucleus, which is also unusual in form. Two nuclei are not uncommon. The orderly arrangement of liver plates to central vein and triads is completely lost. Thus rather bizarre distortion and abnormal cells constitute the picture.

ETIOLOGIC FACTORS. Aflotoxicosis (Newberne et al., 1964) is possibly a cause of this tumor in ducks, but this is not a definite problem in chickens. In the latter, lymphoid leukosis virus may be involved, but consideration certainly should be given to metabolites of a toxic nature as possible etiologic factors.

MISCELLANEOUS

Primary tumors of unknown etiology occur which are not consistent to any organ. An example is the cystadenocarcinoma of the ovary (Feldman and Olson, 1959).

Carcinosarcoma

One type of tumor which we have seen (3 cases) can be classed as the rather controversial carcinosarcoma or adenosarcoma. The tumor exists as many small discrete nodules up to a few millimeters. These are yellowish, firm, and embedded in the lung. In some ways the gross appearance resembles the adult form of aspergillosis. The greater part of the tumor consists of rather innocuous appearing connective tissue (Fig. 15.77) which, however, invades the tertiary bronchi in a malignant fashion (Fig. 15.78). The cells have a plump, ovoid nucleus and copious but indistinct cytoplasm. The interlacing bundles of a typical sarcoma are lacking. Staining techniques do not reveal smooth muscle, nor does the cellular arrangement suggest it. Within the tumor, at the location of the tertiary bronchi, the adenomatous portion is present. This portion undoubtedly arises from the epithelium of the bronchus. The epithelial cells become basophilic and hyperplastic and arrange themselves in an acinar pattern. Because this portion is noninvasive, the term adenoma is more appropriate. No etiologic factors are known.

Mesothelioma

This tumor is unusually rare, according to other authors (Olson and Bullis, 1942;

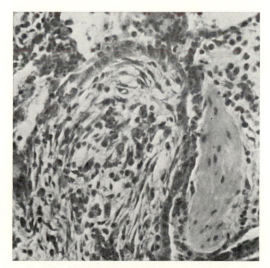

FIG. 15.77—Adenosarcoma of lung from immature hen. As lesion develops, copious amounts of mucin are secreted, resulting in a loosely arranged mass suggesting a myxofibroma. ×190.

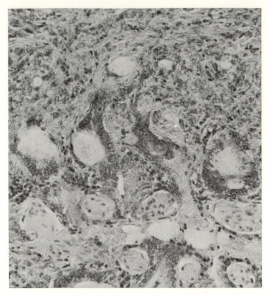

FIG. 15.78—Adenosarcoma of lung of mature hen. This may be terminal state of Fig. 15.77. ×190.

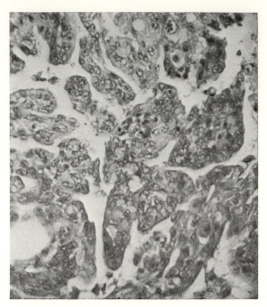

FIG. 15.80—Higher magnification of Fig. 15.79. Mesothelial cells make up most of this portion.

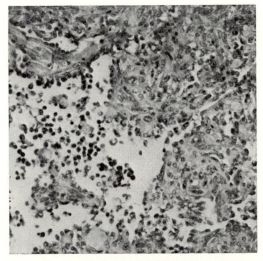

FIG. 15.79—Mesothelioma from abdomen of immature hen. Tumor consists of dense tissue of mesodermal origin upon which are formed mesothelial cells. ×75.

Feldman and Olson, 1959). It is a tumor of the mesothelial cells which are present on all serosal surfaces (Figs. 15.79, 15.80) and could probably be erroneously diagnosed as a granuloma or ovarian adenocarcinoma. The tumor is usually small, dark, smooth, and fairly dense. It is attached to a serosal surface by a stalk which is usually surprisingly small. Histopathologic characteristics include irregular fronds of fibrous tissue upon which is usually a single layer of mesothelial cells. The mesothelial layer faces a lumen which is approximately in the center of the mass. The neoplasm seems benign.

Melanoma

The melanoma can be considered a doubtful avian tumor. All reports (McGowan, 1928; Hoogland, 1929; Reinhardt, 1930) speak of this tumor as usually associated with the ovary. In fact, the mode of spread reported suggests an ovarian carcinoma. From one report, one gained the impression that trapped erythrocytes were the cause of the black color ascribed to the tumor. A small tumor of the base of the tongue (Olson and Bullis, 1942) is, of all those reported, the most likely to have been a true melanoma.

REFERENCES

Awadhiya, R. P., and S. K. Jain. 1967. Studies on the pathology of neoplasms of animals. I. Ovarian tumours in fowls. *Indian Vet. J.* 44:917–20.

Belmonte, V. 1935. Ueber ein Gliom beim Haushuhn. *Virchows Arch. Pathol. Anat. Physiol. Klin. Med.* 294:329–33.

Biering-Sørensen, U. 1956. On disseminated, focal gliosis ("multiple gliomas") and cerebral calcification in hens. *Nord. Veterinaermed.* 8:887–99.

Campbell, J. G. 1947. Neoplastic diseases in the fowl, pp. 350–86. In Blount, W. P. (ed.), *Diseases of Poultry*. Williams & Wilkins, Baltimore.

———. 1967. The epidemiology of tumours in intensively reared chickens. *Medical Monographs 2, Univ. Edinburgh,* pp. 241–49.

Erichsen, S., and A. Harboe. 1953. Toxoplasmosis in chickens. II. So-called gliomas observed in chickens infected with toxoplasmas. *Acta Pathol. Microbiol. Scand.* 33:381–86.

Feldman, W. H., and C. Olson. 1959. Neoplastic diseases of the chicken, pp. 863–924. In Biester, H. E., and L. H. Schwarte (eds.), *Diseases of Poultry,* 4th edition. Iowa State Univ. Press, Ames.

Goodchild, W. M., and D. M. Cooper. 1968. Oviduct adenocarcinoma in laying hens. *Vet. Record* 82:389–90.

Goss, L. J. 1940. The incidence and classification of avian tumors. *Cornell Vet.* 30:75–88.

Greenwood, A. W. 1967. Controlled environment and cancer incidence in the domestic fowl. *Medical Monographs 2, Univ. Edinburgh,* pp. 225–35.

Gupta, B. N., and R. F. Langham. 1968. Arrhenoblastoma in an Indian desi hen. *Avian Diseases* 12:441–44.

Heim, F. 1931. Huehnergeschwulste. *Z. Krebsforsch.* 33:76.

Hertig, A. T., and H. Gore. 1961. Tumors of the female sex glands, Pt. 3. Tumors of the ovary and fallopian tube. *Atlas of Tumor Pathology,* Section IX, Fascicle 33. Armed Forces Institute of Pathology, Washington, D.C.

Hoogland, H. J. M. 1929. Geschwuelste bei Huehnern, pp. 484–97. In van Heelsbergen, T. (ed.), *Handbuch der Gefluegelkrankheiten und der Gefluegelzucht.* Ferdinand Enke, Stuttgart.

Jackson, C. 1936. The incidence and pathology of tumours of domesticated animals in South Africa. A study of the Onderstepoort collection of neoplasms with special reference to their histopathology. *Onderstepoort J. Vet. Sci. Animal Ind.* 6:3–460.

———. 1954. Gliomas of the domestic fowl: Their pathology with special reference to histogenesis and pathogenesis and their relationship to other diseases. *Onderstepoort J. Vet. Sci. Animal Ind.* 26:501–97.

Jungherr, E. L., and A. Wolf. 1939. Gliomas in mammals. *Am. J. Cancer* 37:493–509.

McGowan, J. P. 1928. *On Rous, Leucotic and Allied Tumours in the Fowl: A Study in Malignancy.* Macmillan Co., New York.

Mulligan, R. M. 1955. Hemangiopericytoma in the dog. *Am. J. Pathol.* 31:773–79.

Newberne, P. N., W. W. Carlton, and C. N. Wogan. 1964. Hepatomas in rats and hepatorenal injury in ducklings fed peanut meal or *Aspergillus flavus. Pathol. Vet.* 1:105–32.

Nobel, T. A., F. Neumann, and M. S. Dison. 1964. A histological study of peritoneal carcinomatosis in the laying hen. *Avian Diseases* 8:513–22.

Olson, C., and K. L. Bullis. 1942. A survey and study of spontaneous neoplastic diseases in chickens. *Mass. Agr. Expt. Sta. Bull.* 291, Amherst.

Ostendorf, J., Jr., and W. Henderson. 1962. Toxoplasmosis in chickens. *Proc. 12th World's Poultry Congress,* pp. 385–87.

Reinhardt, R. 1930. Die pathologisch-anatomischen Veruenderungen bei den spontanen Krankheiten der Hausvogel. *Ergeb. Allgem. Pathol. Pathol. Anat.* 23:553.

Sastry, G. A., P. Rama Rao, J. Christopher, and N. R. Gopala Naidu. 1967. Haemangiopericytoma (a report of three cases). *Indian Vet. J.* 44:30–32, 44.

Savage, A. 1926. Adenocarcinoma of gallbladder in a hen. *Cornell Vet.* 16:66–68.

Stout, A. P., and M. R. Murray. 1942. Hemangiopericytoma. A vascular tumor featuring Zimmerman's pericytes. *Ann. Surg.* 116:26–33.

Swarbrick, O., J. G. Campbell, and D. M. Berry. 1968. An outbreak of oviduct adenocarcinoma in laying hens. *Vet. Record* 82:57–59.

Wight, P. A. L., and R. H. Duff. 1964. The histopathology of epizootic gliosis and astrocytoma of the domestic fowl. *J. Comp. Pathol. Therap.* 74:373–80.

Wilson, J. E. 1967. Adenocarcinomata in poultry. *Medical Monographs 2, Univ. Edinburgh,* pp. 238–40.

CHAPTER 16

AVIAN
INFECTIOUS BRONCHITIS

❖

M. S. HOFSTAD
Veterinary Medical Research Institute
Ames, Iowa

❖

AVIAN INFECTIOUS BRONCHITIS is an acute, highly contagious respiratory disease of chickens characterized by tracheal rales, coughing, and sneezing. In addition young chicks may have a nasal discharge, and in laying flocks there is usually a drop in production.

Infectious bronchitis is of economic importance to the poultry industry. In laying flocks the major loss is decreased production and poor quality of eggs. In young chickens there may be mortality and a loss in weight gain and feed efficiency. The highly transmissible nature of the disease makes it a constant threat to unvaccinated flocks. The immunizing program against the disease is a continuous yearly cost to the poultry producer. In broiler production the disease or the live virus vaccine may be a predisposing factor in outbreaks of *Mycoplasma gallisepticum* infection.

Infectious bronchitis appears to have no public health significance. The bronchitis-like agents isolated from human respiratory disease, while morphologically similar, are serologically distinct from avian infectious bronchitis virus (Almeida and Tyrrell, 1967; McIntosh et al., 1967). The finding of low neutralizing antibody titers against avian bronchitis virus in human sera from individuals associated with poultry has been reported by Miller and Yates (1968). However, the significance of these findings has yet to be evaluated.

HISTORY

The first report of avian infectious bronchitis was by Schalk and Hawn (1931), who had observed the disease in North Dakota in the spring of 1930. Within the next several years reports of the disease were made by others in the United States (Beaudette and Hudson, 1933; Bushnell and Brandly, 1933; Beach and Schalm, 1936).

Early reports indicated that infectious bronchitis was primarily a disease of young chicks. However, it was later observed that the disease was common in semimature and laying flocks as well. During the 1940s infectious bronchitis was a serious respiratory disease of laying flocks and caused marked losses in egg production. The prevalence and economic importance of the disease resulted in efforts to control it by immunization. By the middle 1950s vaccination programs had proved effective in reducing losses from infectious bronchitis.

Winterfield and Hitchner (1962) reported a nephrosis condition associated with some outbreaks of infectious bronchitis. This syndrome was also reported from Australia and appeared to be more severe than in the United States (Cumming, 1963).

INCIDENCE AND DISTRIBUTION

Avian infectious bronchitis has been reported from many countries (Estola, 1966). The disease probably occurs in most parts of the world where poultry is raised. Natural outbreaks of the disease in the United States have declined in the past decade due to widespread use of modified live virus vaccines. However, respiratory disease "breaks" do occur occasionally in bronchitis vaccinated flocks. Strains of bronchitis virus of different serotypes may be responsible for some of these outbreaks. Hitchner et al. (1966), in a study to determine the incidence of different serological types in the United States, concluded that a diversity of bronchitis virus types is prevalent in chicken flocks. However, the exact role of different virus serotypes in the epizootiology of infectious bronchitis is not fully understood.

ETIOLOGY

The causative agent of avian infectious bronchitis is a filterable virus capable of passing through the Selas 06 and Millipore 0.22μ filters. The virus usually does not pass through the 0.1μ filter. However, Estola (1966) reported the Finnish strain to pass through the 0.1μ filter but with considerable loss of titer. Inoculation of chickens via the respiratory tract with Millipore 0.22μ filtrate containing virus results in respiratory symptoms, and the virus can be readily recovered from tracheal swabs of the inoculated birds.

CLASSIFICATION

The group classification of infectious bronchitis virus (IBV) remains unsettled at the present time. The RNA nature, size, and ether sensitivity of the virus makes it similar to the myxoviruses, but morphologically it does not fit into this group. Avian IBV now appears to be a prototype for a previously unrecognized group which includes the mouse hepatitis virus and a virus isolated from humans with colds. Based on electron microscope studies of negatively stained virus particles, the name Coronavirus has been proposed for this group (Tyrrell et al., 1968).

MORPHOLOGY

Ultrastructure

Avian IBV particles tend to be circular, although some pleomorphism of the stained virus is observed. No filamentous or tailed forms are seen as with Newcastle disease virus. The virus particle has characteristic club-shaped projections uniformly distributed on its surface (Fig. 16.1). According to McIntosh et al. (1967), these are approximately 20 mμ long and 10 mμ wide at their outer edge with a narrow base. They are spaced loosely around the particle in contrast to the closely spaced, rod-shaped projections on myxoviruses.

Size and Density

Berry et al. (1964) reported the size of IBV to be 80–120 mμ in diameter including the projections. Cunningham (1966) found the sedimentation constant of IBV to be 344S, from which he estimated the diameter of the particle to be 80–100 mμ. He reported the size to be 80–100 mμ from electron microscopic studies. However, McIntosh et al. (1967) reported the size variation from 120 to 200 mμ. Cunningham (1966) reported the specific gravity of IBV to be 1.24 in cesium chloride and 1.19 in sucrose.

Symmetry

The internal structure of IBV has not been determined. Berry et al. (1964) stud-

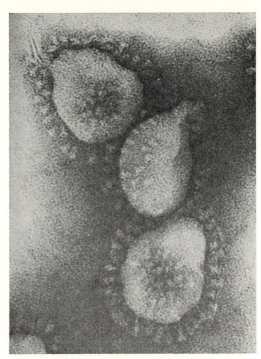

FIG. 16.1—*Virion of avian infectious bronchitis illustrating crownlike projections. Preparation negatively stained with phosphotungstic acid.* ×*300,000. (Berry and Almeida, 1968)*

ied ether-treated particles and found most of them disrupted, but no morphological pattern could be observed.

CHEMICAL COMPOSITION

Cunningham (1963) reported infectious bronchitis virus to contain ribonucleic acid (RNA). He and his co-workers found DL-parafluorophenyl-alanine (FPA), an inhibitor of viral RNA synthesis, to inhibit the development of infectious bronchitis virus in cell cultures. Akers and Cunningham (1968) confirmed these findings but found that at low concentrations of FPA, syncytia were produced and the titer of the virus was reduced; at a higher concentration of FPA both the formation of syncytia and released virus were inhibited. Aminopterin, a suppressor of DNA, had no effect on the growth of the virus. The susceptibility of the virus to ether indicates that the surface of the particle contains an essential lipid. Berry et al. (1964) were unable to demonstrate neuraminidase associated with bronchitis virus.

VIRUS REPLICATION

Becker et al. (1967) studied the morphogenesis of infectious bronchitis virus in infected embryonated eggs. The virus appears to develop in the cytoplasm by a process of budding into cisternae or vesicles, incorporating intracytoplasmic cellular membrane material into its outer coat. The club-shaped projections observed on the virus particle in negatively stained preparations were not observed on the surface of the virus in tissue sections of the infected chorioallantoic membrane. Nazerian and Cunningham (1968) confirmed these studies in chicken embryo cell cultures. The overall diameter of completed particles was 67–110 mμ. Lukert (1966a), using direct fluorescent antibody staining of infected kidney cell cultures, observed fluorescence in the perinuclear region as early as 4 hours postinoculation. The staining rapidly became diffuse in the cytoplasm, but at no time was fluorescence observed in the nucleus. The staining became granular as infection progressed and appeared to be associated with the cell membrane.

BIOLOGICAL PROPERTIES

Untreated infectious bronchitis virus does not agglutinate avian erythrocytes. However, Carbo and Cunningham (1959) found the virus to agglutinate chicken red blood cells after IBV-containing allantoic fluid had been treated with 1% trypsin for 3 hours at 37° C. This reaction was not specific since it could be inhibited by normal as well as immune serum. Muldoon (1960) reported that the hemagglutinin could be released after treatment of the virus with 1% trypsin for 30 minutes at 56° C. The treated virus could be stored for 3 weeks at −65° C without loss of activity. Before trypsin treatment the hemagglutinin was stable for 6½ hours at 56° C.

Cunningham (1966) separated the hemagglutinin, 60–70 mμ in diameter, from the infectious virus by diethylaminoethyl cellulose (DEAE) column chromatography. The hemagglutinin elutes and selectively destroys receptors on the erythrocytes for itself and for trypsin- or ether-modified virus, but not for Newcastle disease virus or influenza PR8 type A virus. The hemagglutinin was composed of 51% protein, 34% lipid, and traces of carbohydrate and RNA.

RESISTANCE TO CHEMICAL AND PHYSICAL AGENTS

Thermostability

Most strains of infectious bronchitis virus are inactivated after 15 minutes at 56° C. Using a dilution of infective allantoic fluid suspended in 20% horse serum, Hofstad (1956b) found only 8 of 60 strains to survive 30 minutes at 56° C. One strain survived for 45 minutes. DuBose and Grumbles (1959) have suggested thermostability tests at 56° C for 30–45 minutes to differentiate between infectious bronchitis virus and quail bronchitis virus, the latter being stable at 56° C for periods up to 60 and 90 minutes.

Hopkins (1967) found strains of infectious bronchitis virus to be more stable at 50° C in 1M $MgSO_4$, Na_2SO_4, Na_2HPO_4, and K_2SO_4 than in 1M NaCl, KCl, $CaCl_2$, and $MgCl_2$. The stabilizing effect was due to the anion, the trivalent anions being more protective than divalent anions.

Singh (1960) found a bimodal inactivation curve at 56° C indicating the existence of two phases—an O (original) phase which was relatively thermostable and a D (derivative) phase which was thermolabile. Virus strains in high embryo passage levels, such as Beaudette strain, are in the D phase.

Stability at Cold Temperatures

Avian infectious bronchitis virus stores well at −30° C in the form of infective allantoic fluid. Virus fluids kept at this temperature have remained viable for periods up to 17 years. Infected tissues stored in 50% glycerin are well preserved, and in this medium tissues can be shipped to a laboratory for diagnosis without refrigeration.

Lyophilization

Infectious bronchitis virus can be preserved for indefinite periods by lyophilization. Infective allantoic fluid lyophilized in glass ampules, sealed under vacuum, and stored in the refrigerator has remained viable for at least 24 years. Buthala (1956) found 10% glucose to give a stabilizing effect to bronchitis virus in the lyophilized and frozen states. Hofstad and Yoder (1963) found lyophilized bronchitis virus to be completely inactivated within 6 months when stored at 37° C. This compared with lyophilized Newcastle disease virus which was inactivated within 10 months and laryngotracheitis virus which survived for 3 years.

pH Stability

Quiroz and Hanson (1958) reported infectious bronchitis virus to resist 1% HCl at pH 2 for 1 hour at room temperature, a treatment which inactivated Newcastle disease, laryngotracheitis, and fowl pox viruses.

Ether and Sodium Deoxycholate

Petek and Corazzola (1958) reported 20% ether reduced the titer but did not completely inactivate the virus. The same was found by Quiroz and Hanson (1958). However, IBV is considered to be ether-labile in virus characterization studies.

Tevethia and Cunningham (1968) found that a 0.2% sodium deoxycholate solution completely inactivated the virus in allantoic fluid within 10 minutes at room temperature.

Disinfectants

Cunningham and Stuart (1946) found a laboratory strain of IBV to be destroyed by common disinfectants such as 1% liquor cresolis saponatus, 1:10,000 $KMNO_4$, 70% alcohol, and 1% formalin within a 3-minute contact period. Quiroz and Hanson (1958) found 1% phenol to have no effect on IBV exposed for 1 hour at room temperature, a treatment which inactivated the B_1 strain of Newcastle disease virus.

Ethylene Oxide (Carboxide)

Avian infectious bronchitis virus in the moist state and virus dried over anhydrous $CaCl_2$ was inactivated when exposed to 10% ethylene oxide gas in CO_2 for 16 hours. However, this period of time did not inactivate virus which had been lyophilized and exposed (Mathews and Hofstad, 1953).

Trypsin

Buthala (1956) reported IBV to be resistant to the action of trypsin. Up to 40 mg per ml for 1 hour at 37° C did not affect the infectivity of the virus.

SOLUBLE ANTIGENS ASSOCIATED WITH INFECTIOUS BRONCHITIS VIRUS

Tevethia and Cunningham (1968) found 3 soluble antigens in virus infective allantoic fluid and the chorioallantoic membrane by the agar-gel diffusion technique.

Antigen 1 line formed closest to the antibody well and was formed in 4 hours at room temperature. Antigen 2 line formed near line 1 but closer to the antigen well, and required 24–30 hours to form. Antigen 3 line formed nearest the antigen well and required 5–6 days to form. Antigen 1 was the smallest, passing through the Millipore 0.1μ filter. All antigens were sensitive to trypsin.

STRAIN CLASSIFICATION

Several different serological types of avian infectious bronchitis virus have been identified (Jungherr et al., 1956; Hofstad, 1956a, 1958). The usual field strain encountered is designated as the Massachusetts type. Several isolates commonly designated as the Massachusetts type are the pathogenic chicken strain (41), the Beaudette embryo lethal strain (42), and strain 33. The Connecticut strain (46) and two Iowa strains (97 and 609) represent additional serotypes.

More recently isolates of IBV have been reported which are serologically different from the previously recognized types. Winterfield et al. (1964) reported on the JMK strain. Von Bülow (1967) described a new field strain from Germany. Berry and Stokes (1968) studied antigenic variation between 8 English and 3 foreign IBV strains and concluded that the variation was minor and of subtype character. Their study did not include the American strains other than the Massachusetts type. The Australian "T" strain of IBV described by Cumming (1963) has some antigenic differences demonstrable in virus neutralization tests.

While it is possible to demonstrate marked serological differences between strains in virus neutralization tests using convalescent sera, the use of hyperimmune sera will usually demonstrate less antigenic variation.

Cross-immunity studies in chickens indicate some cross-protection to challenge between isolates even though virus neutralization tests indicate marked differences (Hofstad, 1961). The Massachusetts type stimulates greater protection against challenge with heterologous strains than do the other types. Cross-protection tests between the Australian "T" isolate and the Massachusetts type indicate cross-immunity when challenged soon after recovery.

LABORATORY HOST SYSTEMS

Chicken Embryos

The virus of infectious bronchitis grows well in the developing chicken embryo. Dwarfing of a few embryos with survival of 90% of the embryos through the 19th day of incubation is characteristic of IBV field material upon initial inoculation in 10–11-day embryonating chicken eggs. Embryo mortality and dwarfing increase as the number of serial passages increases, so that by the 10th passage most of the embryos are stunted and up to 80% may die by the 19th day of incubation.

EMBRYO CHANGES RESULTING FROM GROWTH OF VIRUS. The characteristic embryo changes are seen several days after inoculation of the virus. During candling only slight movement of a dwarfed embryo may be observed. Upon opening the air-cell end of the egg, the embryo is seen curled into a spherical form with the thickened amnion closely adherent to the embryo (Fig. 16.2).

The yolk sac appears shrunken, and an increased volume of usually clear allantoic fluid is present. A consistent internal lesion of the bronchitis-infected embryo is the persistence of the mesonephros containing urates. This lesion appears to be associated with the stunting of the embryo and is not specific for bronchitis infection. Another lesion found in embryonating eggs inoculated with nonlethal isolates of bronchitis virus is the thickened amnion and adjacent layer of the allantois covering the stunted embryo. The beginning of this lesion can usually be detected on the 3rd day after inoculation. It likewise is not a pathognomonic lesion since it can also be observed following inoculation of eggs with lentogenic strains of Newcastle disease virus.

MICROSCOPIC LESIONS IN INFECTED EMBRYOS. The microscopic lesions in the embryo have been studied by Loomis et al. (1950). They found congestion with perivascular cuffing and some necrosis of the livers by the 6th day after inoculation. All the lungs were pneumonic, characterized by congestion, cellular infiltration, and serous exu-

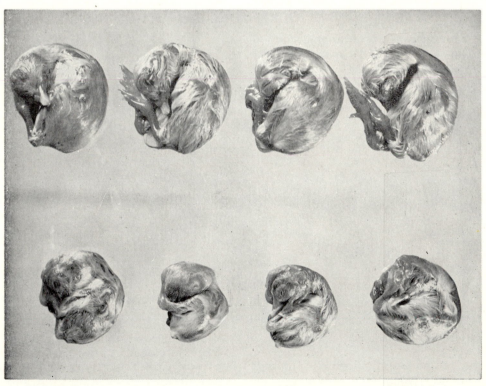

FIG. 16.2—Comparison of normal 16-day-old embryos (**above**) and dwarfed, infected embryos of same age (**below**). (Hofstad and Bauriedel, Iowa State Univ.)

date in the bronchial sacs. In the kidneys there was interstitial nephritis with edema and distention of the proximal convoluted tubules with casts. The glomeruli were not altered. The chorioallantoic and amniotic membranes were edematous. No inclusion bodies were found.

EFFECT OF TEMPERATURE ON VIRUS GROWTH. Simpson and Groupé (1959) found the incubation temperature to markedly alter the virus growth, virulence, and population stability in embryonated eggs. One recently isolated strain of virus reached the same maximum titer in eggs incubated at 34° C or 38° C, but it required at least 30 hours longer to attain this level at 34° C. The virus was lethal for embryos at 38° C, but only 20% were killed at 34° C.

DISTRIBUTION OF VIRUS IN THE EMBRYONATING CHICKEN EGG. Studies by Cunningham and El Dardiry (1948) showed that after the virus was inoculated into the allantoic sac, the highest concentration of virus is recovered from the chorioallantoic membrane, followed in order by the allantoic fluid, amnionic fluid, and liver. The highest concentration of virus, 10^7 embryo lethal doses, was detected 36 hours after inoculation. A decrease of titer resulted if eggs were left in the incubator after death of the embryo. Groupé (1949) detected an interfering substance in the allantoic fluid of such eggs. The substance was not present when infected eggs were removed immediately or not more than 2 hours after death of the embryo. Hitchner and White (1955) studied the growth curve of a vaccine strain (20–30 embryo passages) of infectious bronchitis virus in eggs and found maximum virus concentration 24–30 hours after allantoic route inoculation. The Beaudette embryo lethal strain (42) of virus was found to reach its maximum titer in 12 hours.

Turkey Embryo

DuBose (1967) found the Beaudette strain (42) of IBV to grow in turkey embryos for 11 serial passages. However, a low-passage chicken embryo strain, Massachusetts (41), could not be propagated serially in turkey embryos. By alternating passages in chicken and turkey embryos he succeeded in adapting the virus and continued propagating the virus for 17 serial passages in turkey embryos. However, the virus had not become markedly modified in its pathogenicity for chickens, its antigenic character, or its immunogenicity.

Cell Cultures

Avian infectious bronchitis virus has been grown in cultures of kidney cells, lung cells, and liver cells of the 15–18-day chicken embryo. The kidney cells are most often used in studies on IBV. Lukert (1966a) found that kidney and lung cells were most sensitive to IBV, liver cells 40–60 times less sensitive, and embryo fibroblast cells of low sensitivity.

Recent isolates of the virus in low embryo passage grow poorly or not at all in cell cultures. The same strains after 6–10 passages in chicken embryos will produce the usual cytopathic effect (CPE) in kidney cell cultures, according to Kawamura et al. (1961). These authors also found that some strains remained mildly cytopathic with low virus titers even after 10 serial cell culture passages, while most strains increased in CPE and virus titer. Akers and Cunningham (1968) studied the rate of virus growth in cell cultures of chicken embryo kidney cells. In cumulative growth studies a 4-hour eclipse was noted. Cell-associated virus reached a maximum of 10^5 at 24 hours, and extracellular or released virus of 10^6 cell culture infective doses at 36 hours.

The microscopic lesion observed in chicken embryo kidney cell cultures after inoculation of IBV is the formation of syncytia followed by necrosis (Cunningham, 1963). The syncytia are first observed 6 hours after inoculation, and by 18–24 hours large syncytia containing up to 100 nuclei are found. Syncytia may also be prominent in infected liver cell cultures but are usually smaller. In contrast syncytia are inconspicuous in lung cell cultures (Lukert, 1966a).

PLAQUE FORMATION BY IBV. The formation of plaques in chicken embryo kidney cells under agar has been reported by Wright and Sagik (1958). Cunningham and Spring (1965) confirmed these findings and found that it was necessary to use an atmosphere of 8% CO_2 and 85% relative humidity to obtain reproducible results. They found that a 90-minute adsorption period was optimum for the Beaudette strain of IBV. Plaque counts follow a linear relationship with dose, and plaques can be inhibited by specific immune serum.

Lukert (1966b) has found the plaque reduction technique to be an accurate method for assaying antibody levels in chicken sera and is comparable to the neutralization method in embryonating chicken eggs. However the neutralizing indexes are generally slightly higher when done in embryonating eggs.

PATHOGENICITY

Avian infectious bronchitis virus is pathogenic only for the chicken. When the virus is grown in chicken embryos it gradually loses its pathogenicity for chickens. This loss of pathogenicity for chickens occurred after 89 egg transfers with a Rhode Island strain mentioned by Delaplane and Stuart (1941). Hoekstra and Rispens (1960) found their strain of bronchitis virus to possess some pathogenicity after 120 embryo passages. (Additional information is given under attenuation of vaccine strains.)

PATHOGENESIS AND EPIZOOTIOLOGY

NATURAL HOSTS

The chicken is the only natural host for IBV. All ages are susceptible, but the disease is most severe in baby chicks where it causes some mortality. Following aerosol exposure of chickens to the virus there is rapid multiplication of the virus in the respiratory tract. Virus can be isolated from the trachea and lungs at 24 hours through the 8th day. Virus also multiplies in nonrespiratory tissues such as the kidney and bursa where it may persist longer than in the lung and trachea.

EXPERIMENTAL HOSTS

Turkeys do not respond to aerosol inoculations of IBV. Intravenous inoculation of turkeys may result in a viremia for varying periods up to 48 hours. Simpson and Groupé (1959) found suckling mice to be susceptible by intracerebral inoculation of the embryo-adapted Beaudette strain. However, a low passage embryo-propagated strain of IBV was not lethal for mice. Estola (1966) found the Finnish and several other strains of IBV in low embryo passage to readily adapt to suckling mice and suckling rabbits by intracerebral inoculation. However suckling guinea pigs were resistant.

TRANSMISSION

The virus spreads rapidly among chickens in a flock. Susceptible chickens placed in a room with infected chickens usually develop symptoms within 48 hours. Airborne transmission has been demonstrated experimentally (Levine and Hofstad, 1947). The distance a virus is transmitted through the outside atmosphere is not known, although it has been assumed, during epizootics, that the virus spreads between flocks where the farms are close and in the direction of the prevailing wind. The optimum climatic conditions necessary for airborne transmission between farms are not known.

CARRRIERS AND VECTORS

Attempts to demonstrate recovered carriers beyond 49 days have failed. Following inoculation of a group of chickens with bronchitis virus, Fabricant and Levine (1951) were unable to detect the presence of virus in tracheal swabs and in the yolk of eggs collected from recovered birds after 36 days. In 9 trials where bronchitis-recovered birds were placed in contact with susceptible chickens, Hofstad (1947) was unable to demonstrate the presence of virus longer than 35 days after recovery. Pette (1959) has recovered bronchitis virus from the cloacal contents up to 24 days after experimental oral infection. Cook (1968) was able to demonstrate virus up to 49 days after experimental infection when chickens were housed in strict isolation. Vectors do not appear to be a factor in the spread of IBV.

INCUBATION PERIOD

The incubation period of infectious bronchitis is 18–36 hours, depending on the dosage and route of inoculation. Chickens exposed to an aerosol of undiluted infective egg fluid regularly have tracheal rales within 24 hours. Natural spread requires about 36 hours or more.

SIGNS

Young Chickens

The characteristic respiratory signs in chicks are gasping, coughing, tracheal rales, and nasal discharge. Wet eyes may be observed, and an occasional chick may have swollen sinuses. The chicks appear depressed and many are seen huddled under the heat source. Prince et al. (1962) found feed consumption and weight gain significantly reduced by bronchitis infection.

Growing Chickens

The outstanding signs in chickens over 5–6 weeks of age are tracheal rales with some gasping and coughing. The disease may go unnoticed if the birds are on range and not observed carefully. Rales are usually not heard unless the chickens are handled or the caretaker listens to the flock at night when the birds are quiet. Temperatures of 12.6, 18.2, and 23.8° C did not influence the performance of bronchitis-infected chickens 4–8 weeks of age (Prince et al., 1967).

Adult Laying Flocks

The respiratory symptoms are tracheal rales, gasping, and coughing. In addition the flock usually drops in production. Generally the drop in production is one-half the predisease level, but this will vary with the period of lay. Flocks affected in the latter part of their laying year usually have a marked drop in egg production and a molt. Such flocks require long periods of time to recover production and usually become un-

profitable. Pullets in good condition may suffer only a slight drop in production and regain normal production within a few weeks after recovery from respiratory signs. Broadfoot and Smith (1954) found egg production reduced 25%, the number of unsettable hatching eggs increased 92%, and hatchability reduced 7% in outbreaks of bronchitis studied.

In addition to the decline in production, there may be soft-shelled, misshapen, and rough-shelled eggs (Fig. 16.3). Shell irregularities in recovered flocks may persist for an indefinite period of time.

Internal quality of eggs, as observed when breaking out eggs on a flat surface, may be inferior from a varying percentage of birds following bronchitis outbreaks. The albumen may be thin and watery without definite demarcation between the thick and thin albumen of the normal fresh egg (Fig. 16.4).

McDougall (1968) reported loss of internal quality of eggs in bronchitis-infected hens, but this was not apparent until 2

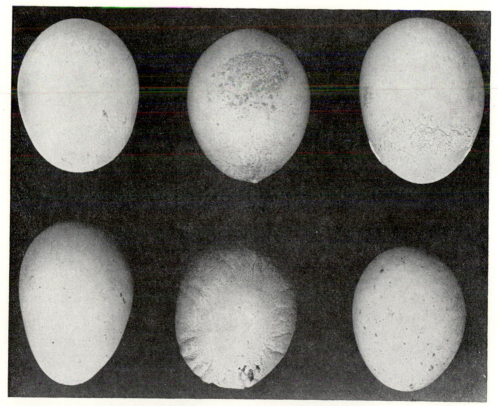

FIG. 16.3—*Thin-shelled, rough, and misshapen eggs laid by hens during an outbreak of infectious bronchitis. (Van Roekel, Univ. of Mass.)*

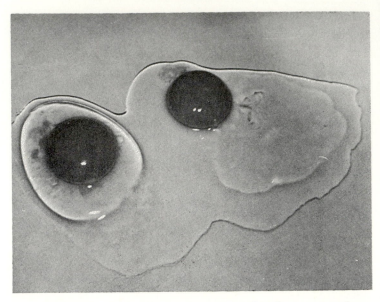

FIG. 16.4—Contents of two eggs. **(Left)** Normal egg. **(Right)** Egg from chicken exposed to infectious bronchitis virus at 1 day of age showing watery albumen and yolk separated from thick albumen. (Courtesy R. A. P. Crinion, Iowa State Univ.)

weeks after clinical symptoms had subsided and the birds were resuming production. Crinion (1969, personal communication), in trapnesting hens which had recovered from an experimental exposure to IBV at 1 day of age, found poor internal egg quality—watery albumen, yolk separating from the albumen, and albumen sticking to the inner shell membrane—to be correlated with poor shell quality.

HEMATOLOGY

Blood counts taken during the course of the disease reveal a leukopenia during the first 2 days followed by a leukocytosis which declines after the 7th day to reach normal by the 15th day (Machado, 1951).

MORBIDITY AND MORTALITY

All birds in the flock become infected, but mortality is observed only in young chicks. Death loss is variable depending on age of the chicks, presence or absence of passive antibodies, and environmental conditions. Mortality may be as high as 25% in young chicks but is usually negligible in chickens over 6 weeks of age. The Australian "T" strain, because of its predilection for the kidney, has been found to produce a greater mortality in chicks than the American strains.

GROSS LESIONS

Necropsy of affected chicks reveals a serous, catarrhal, or caseous exudate in the trachea, nasal passages, and sinuses. The air sacs may appear cloudy or contain a yellow caseous exudate. In chicks that die a caseous plug may be found in the lower trachea or bronchi. Small areas of pneumonia may be observed around the large bronchi.

Necropsy of infected chickens that are in production reveals fluid yolk material in the abdominal cavity. This is a nonspecific lesion and is found in other diseases causing a marked drop in production. The only gross lesion in the upper respiratory tract is a serous or catarrhal exudate in the trachea. Sevoian and Levine (1957) studied the gross lesions of the reproductive tract of bronchitis-infected chickens. Oviduct length and weight were markedly reduced and required 21 days to return to normal. Physiological stress of withholding feed and water produced the same effect but required only half the time to regain normalcy. Broadfoot et al. (1956) found evidence of permanent damage to the oviduct, resulting in false layers, following bronchitis infection in chicks under 2 weeks of age. Crinion (1969, personal communication) found IBV to cause severe lesions in the middle third of the oviduct following exposure of day-old White Leghorn chicks to IBV. The isthmus and magnum were the portions most seriously involved. Cumming (1963) has described a nephrosis associated with outbreaks of infectious bronchitis with the "T" strain. The kidneys are swollen and pale, with tubules and ureters often distended with uric acid crystals (Fig. 16.5).

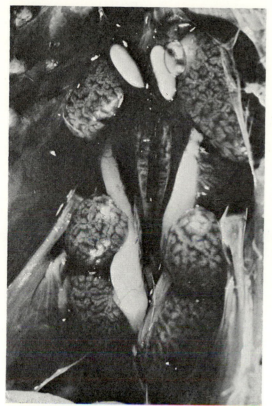

FIG. 16.5—*Kidney lesions associated with infectious bronchitis caused by "T" strain of virus. Note swollen kidneys with tubules and ureters extended with uric acid crystals. (Courtesy R. B. Cumming, Univ. of New England, Armidale, N.S.W., Australia)*

Similar findings have been reported by Winterfield and Hitchner (1962) and by Julian and Willis (1969).

HISTOPATHOLOGY

The principal microscopic lesions in the respiratory tract are cellular infiltration and edema of the mucosa and submucosa, vascular congestion, hyperplasia and vacuolation of the epithelium, and hemorrhage in the submucosa (Figs. 16.6, 16.7). There is usually no interruption of the continuity of the tracheal epithelium, and the lumen contains exudate in which cellular elements are usually sparse or absent (Fig. 16.8). Sevoian and Levine (1957) compared the microscopic changes of the oviducts from IBV-infected hens and from hens placed under stress by removing feed and water. Microscopically the height of the cellular epithelium lining the oviduct was sharply reduced and the cells became cuboidal in shape with some loss of cilia. Dilating of the glands occurred in half the oviducts studied. In the lamina propria and intertubular stroma of the oviducts, lymphocytic foci and cellular infiltration were present. Significantly fewer changes of a similar nature were seen in the group under stress from feed and water deprivation. Crinion (1969, personal communication) studied the microscopic lesions of oviducts exposed by aerosol when 1 day of age. He found lymphoid cell infiltration in the oviduct as early as the 2nd day. Focal areas of lymphocytes were first observed on the 11th day in the infected group but not until the 7th week in the controls. The main oviduct lesion appeared to be a localized hypoplasia first observed on the 23rd day. This lesion was found in 22% of the infected chicks necropsied. The localized hypoplasia, followed by continued growth of the remainder of the oviduct, caused a loss of patency, with a resulting cyst posterior to the area of hypoplasia (Fig. 16.9). An additional 21% of these birds with patent oviducts had localized areas of glandular hypoplasia in the caudal magnum and cranial isthmus at sexual maturity.

IMMUNITY

Active

Chickens that have recovered from the natural disease are resistant to intratracheal inoculations with the homologous strain as soon as symptoms have subsided. It requires about 3 weeks for chickens to reach a high level of antibodies following exposure to bronchitis virus. Flocks that have experienced an outbreak of bronchitis have some degree of immunity, and antibodies can be demonstrated for at least a year. However, observations by Van Roekel et al. (1950) have suggested that immunity to the disease may decline sufficiently for reinfection to occur in some flocks following exposure to the virus. The plurality of strains has complicated immunity studies with IBV.

Tissue

Local tracheal immunity appears to play an important part in resistance to bronchitis. If chickens have recovered from an aerosol exposure of high embryo passage IBV

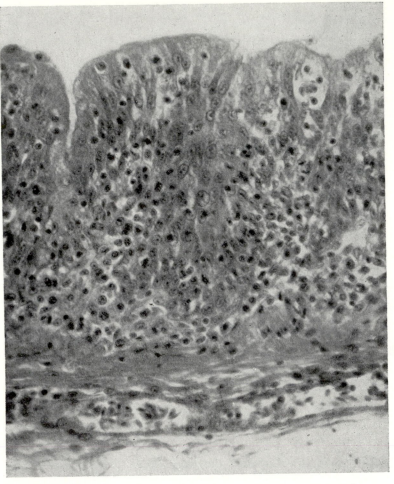

FIG. 16.6—Portion of trachea from experimentally infected bird 72 hours following inoculation showing thickened tracheal mucous membrane due to cellular infiltration and edema. ×450.

and subsequently challenged with a low embryo passage virus, they will be resistant for a relatively short period of time even though circulating antibodies are low or not demonstrable.

Passive

Eggs laid by recovered hens will carry antibodies which will later be absorbed by the hatched chick. The passive antibody levels are highest soon after hatching and decline steadily to negligible levels by 4 weeks. Passive antibodies serve to reduce the severity of the disease but do not prevent respiratory infection following exposure to the virus.

DIAGNOSIS

The diagnosis of infectious bronchitis must be based upon isolation of the virus or by demonstrating an ascending antibody titer against a known strain of bronchitis virus. Because of the plurality of strains it may be necessary to use strains other than the Massachusetts type in demonstrating bronchitis antibodies.

It is difficult to make a field diagnosis in the early stages of the disease because its early clinical manifestations are similar to those of Newcastle disease and laryngotracheitis. After the disease has progressed sufficiently, knowledge of the symptoms, mortality, and duration may make a presumptive diagnosis possible.

VIRUS ISOLATION

Infectious bronchitis virus may be isolated by intratracheal inoculation of susceptible chicks with a broth suspension of lung and trachea collected from an infected bird during early stages of the disease. Symptoms of tracheal rales will follow an incubation period of 18–36 hours. This short incubation period is characteristic of infec-

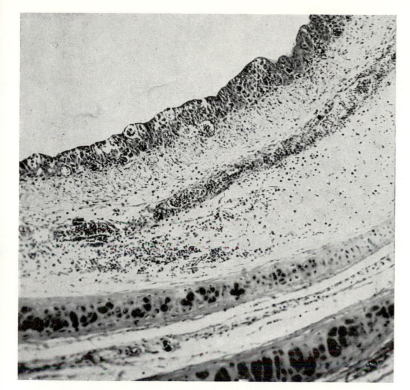

FIG. 16.7—Portion of trachea from field case of infectious bronchitis showing cellular infiltration and edema of mucosa and submucosa, vascular congestion, vacuolation of the epithelium, and hemorrhage in the submucosa.

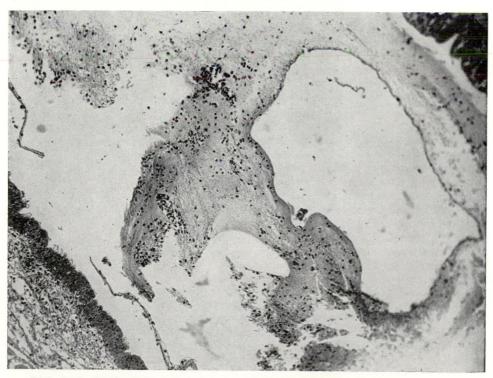

FIG. 16.8—Portion of trachea from field case of infectious bronchitis showing exudate containing scattered cellular elements in lumen of lower trachea. ×100.

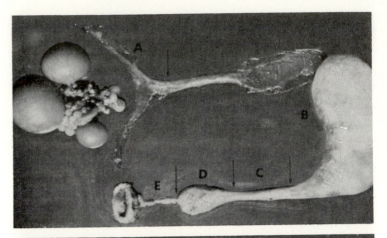

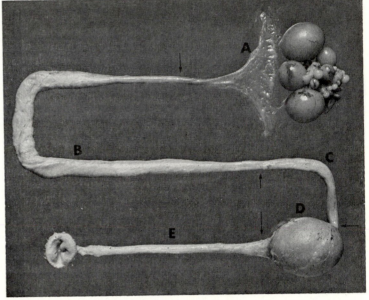

FIG. 16.9—Reproductive organs of two chickens. Both ovaries appear normal. Oviducts have been demarcated approximately by arrows into their five respective parts: infundibulum (A), magnum (B), isthmus (C), uterus (D), and vagina (E). Lower photograph represents normal oviduct with an egg in the uterus; upper photograph illustrates oviduct from a hen subsequent to exposure with infectious bronchitis virus, strain 33, at 1 day of age, showing area of localized hypoplasia in magnum and a cyst posterior to it but not involving the vagina. (Courtesy R. A. P. Crinion, Iowa State Univ.)

tious bronchitis. Inoculation of both susceptible and immune chickens would give definite information for a diagnosis. However, this procedure is not commonly carried out. Isolation of the virus is most frequently done in the embryonating chicken egg. This is achieved by inoculating a suspension of lung and trachea into the allantoic cavity of 9–11-day-old embryonating eggs. The eggs used may be from bronchitis-immune hens, but eggs from bronchitis-susceptible hens are preferred. The virus may also be found in other tissues to a lesser extent, such as the aqueous humor, spleen, kidney, bursa of Fabricius, and air sac. Contaminating bacteria may be controlled by filtration utilizing the Millipore series through 0.22 mμ or the Selas series

through 03. An easier method is to add a mixture of antibiotics such as penicillin (15,000 units) and dihydrostreptomycin (15 mg per ml). The presence of bronchitis virus in the embryonating egg following inoculation is somewhat difficult to discern in the initial passage since there is little change in the majority of the embryos inoculated. Dwarfing of a few embryos by some strains and survival of most of the embryos in the initial passage is characteristic of bronchitis virus. Its presence can be definitely detected, however, by the intratracheal inoculation of susceptible chicks with allantoic fluid collected after a postinoculation period of 48–96 hours. If bronchitis virus is present, the chicks will have tracheal rales after a period of 18–36 hours. No hemagglutinating properties should be demonstrable in the allantoic fluid.

The information obtained following the above procedures, together with a typical flock history and symptoms, would permit a diagnosis of infectious bronchitis within 3–4 days. Results of further egg passages of the isolated virus and the detection of antibodies in the serum collected from the inoculated chicks 3 weeks after recovery would positively confirm the diagnosis.

SEROLOGY

The diagnosis of avian infectious bronchitis by serological methods is based on demonstration of an ascending serum antibody level. The first sample of blood is collected during the initial stages of the disease and the second sample is taken in 2 or 3 weeks. Both samples of serum are tested for neutralizing antibodies against IBV. Demonstration of a negative or low antibody titer in the serum collected early and a higher titer after recovery constitutes a diagnosis of infectious bronchitis. The plurality of strains may necessitate using strains of IBV other than the Massachusetts type, the most frequently encountered strain.

Berry and Almeida (1968) have found a greater neutralizing capacity of serum by 2–3 log units when heat-labile components of fresh unheated serum are present in the virus-serum mixture. Thus it is important in comparing serum samples that they be treated the same. All sera should be inactivated at 56° C for 30 minutes, and if complement is to be used in the neutralization test, fresh chicken serum may be added to the serum dilution.

Stinski and Cunningham (1969) have studied the neutralizing antibody complex of IBV. When the complex was diluted, there was a slight but significant dissociation. The complex could be readily dissociated by acid with maximum separation occurring within 1 minute at pH 1.7 with a recovery of 60% of the virus. Antibody and virus could be reassociated at neutrality.

Virus Neutralization

VARYING VIRUS CONSTANT SERUM METHOD. The usual method of detecting antibodies is to set up tenfold dilutions in broth of a known embryo-adapted bronchitis virus, such as the Beaudette strain. The virus titer is determined by inoculating each tenfold dilution into a group of four or five 9–12-day-old embryonating eggs. Each egg receives 0.05 ml. When the virus dilutions are being made, a portion of each dilution of virus is mixed in a separate tube with an equal amount of suspect serum. The two portions are mixed by shaking the tubes. Each mixture of virus dilution plus serum is then inoculated into a set of four or five embryonating eggs, using 0.1 ml. Maximum neutralization occurs in 15 minutes, and neutralizing of the virus is exponential (Page and Cunningham, 1962).

Following inoculation the eggs are incubated and candled daily for 1 week to remove eggs containing dead embryos. The 50% end point of embryo mortality in each series can then be determined by the method of Reed and Muench (1938). The difference between these end points represents an index of the neutralizing capacity of the serum. For example, if the mortality end point of the virus titration was in the 10^{-6} dilution and the end point of the serum-virus mixture was in the 10^{-3} dilution, then the log neutralizing index of the serum is 3.0 or 1,000 neutralizing doses in 0.05 ml of serum. The neutralizing capacity of serum from bronchitis-recovered chickens should have 100 or more neutralizing doses (Fabricant, 1951).

CONSTANT VIRUS VARYING SERUM METHOD. This technique has not been used extensively for measuring antibody levels against IBV, but the method may have an advantage when using hyperimmune serum in that end points would be easier to obtain. In the test, between 100 and 1,000 embryo infective doses (EID_{50}) are used against twofold dilutions of serum starting with a 1:10 dilution. Five embryos are inoculated with each virus-serum mixture and the 50% end point calculated at the end of 8 days. The neutralizing capacity of the serum is that dilution of serum which protects half the embryos.

SURVIVING VIRUS IN SERUM-VIRUS MIXTURES. Berry and Almeida (1968) determined antibody levels in serum by mixing virus and serum and then diluting the mixture to determine the surviving virus. In their test 0.1 ml of serum was added to a 1:6 dilution of virus and the mixture incubated for 1 hour at 37° C and then left overnight at 4° C, after which tenfold dilutions were inoculated into 5 embryos each. This method is simple and may be useful in the study of serotypes of IBV.

PLAQUE REDUCTION METHOD. Lukert (1966b) found virus neutralization in cell cultures to be useful in measuring neutralizing antibodies. In the test, 0.4 ml of either virus control or virus serum mixture is inoculated onto monolayers of chicken embryo kidney cells and allowed to absorb for 90 minutes. Two plates are inoculated with each dilution. At 48 hours the plates are stained with a 0.001% solution of neutral red saline. The plaque-reduction neutralization index is determined as in the chicken embryo virus neutralization test.

INTERFERENCE SEROLOGICAL METHOD. Beard (1968) described a test in which IBV can be detected by its ability to block infection of cell cultures by Newcastle disease virus (NDV). In the test twofold serum dilutions are made in maintenance medium and mixed with equal amounts of a 1:10 dilution of IBV infective allantoic fluid. The mixtures are left at 4° C for 1 hour, and then 1 ml is added to the 4 ml of maintenance medium covering the monolayers in the 60-mm plastic plates. The cultures are held 20–30 hours at 37° C in a 5% atmosphere of CO_2, and then 10^6 embryo lethal doses of the B_1 strain of NDV are added in 0.5 ml of medium. When NDV has produced cytopathic lesions in the control plates, all dishes are stained with 0.5% crystal violet in 10% formalin for 5 minutes. If antibodies are present to neutralize the IBV, the cells remain susceptible to the action of NDV.

AGAR GEL PRECIPITATION TECHNIQUE. Woernle (1959) and Woernle and Brunner (1960) demonstrated bronchitis antibodies by the agar gel precipitation technique. This test is done by placing antigen (chorioallantoic membrane suspension from infected embryos in one well in the agar and antiserum in an adjacent well and observing the precipitin lines between the two. Woernle (1960) found no difference between German strains, the Beaudette strain, and the Connecticut and Massachusetts strains by the agar gel precipitin test. Witter (1962) found precipitins no earlier than 7 days, and they persisted for 20–94 days. Demonstration of a precipitin increment between early and later serum samples was suggested for diagnosis.

FLUORESCENT ANTIBODY PROCEDURE. Braune and Gentry (1965) found this technique to be useful in detecting IBV in tracheal smears of acutely affected chickens. Tracheal smears are air dried and flooded with specific fluorescein-conjugated gamma globulin for 30 minutes at room temperature. The stained smears are then washed in buffered saline at pH 7.25, mounted with buffered saline-glycerol, and examined under ultraviolet microscopy.

OTHER METHODS OF SEROLOGICAL DIAGNOSIS. Brumfield and Pomeroy (1957) applied the direct complement-fixation test to infectious bronchitis diagnosis. Jeon (1962) standardized the details of the test and studied the principal mechanism involved in the technique. Steele and Luginbuhl (1964) developed a direct complement-fixation test for IBV using infected allantoic fluid antigen concentrated by ultracentrifugation and guinea pig antiserum prepared against infected chicken kidney cell cultures. An indirect test was also developed for the titration of chicken antiserum against the Beaudette egg-adapted strain. However, results using antisera against the Massachusetts strain did not react with the Beaudette strain of virus in the indirect complement-fixation test. Brown et al. (1962) described an indirect hemagglutination test for infectious bronchitis. The virus is adsorbed onto tannic acid-treated horse red blood cells and after washing is mixed with the suspected serum. If the serum has antibodies it reacts with the antigen and causes clumping of the red cells. Vasington (1962) also described a similar indirect hemagglutination test; however, he used sheep erythrocytes instead of horse red cells.

DIFFERENTIAL DIAGNOSIS

Infectious bronchitis may resemble other acute respiratory diseases such as Newcastle disease, laryngotracheitis, and infectious coryza. Newcastle disease is generally more severe than infectious bronchitis. In baby chicks nervous signs may be observed in a few chicks, and in laying flocks the drop in production is greater than in infectious bronchitis.

Laryngotracheitis tends to spread more

slowly in the flock, but respiratory signs may be more severe than infectious bronchitis. However, some strains of laryngotracheitis produce a mild disease which may go unnoticed. Laryngotracheitis rarely occurs in young baby chick flocks, and infectious bronchitis is commonly seen in young chicks as well as in older flocks.

Infectious coryza can be differentiated on the basis of its facial swelling which rarely occurs in infectious bronchitis. A nasal discharge usually accompanies coryza; in infectious bronchitis a nasal discharge occurs only in young chicks. Tracheal rales may occur with coryza but are not as characteristic as for infectious bronchitis. A fetid odor may be detected in chronic cases of coryza.

TREATMENT

There is no specific treatment for infectious bronchitis. In flocks of young chicks it is helpful to increase the temperature of the room as well as of the brooder. Overcrowding should be corrected and drafts should be eliminated. Anything the poultryman can do to keep up feed consumption in the flock should be encouraged so as to avoid excessive loss in weight in the birds. Dusting or spraying so-called cold remedies is not worth the cost. Recovery takes place as the birds acquire an immunity to the virus. If the disease is complicated with chronic respiratory disease or air sac infection, treatment with the broadspectrum antibiotics may be indicated.

PREVENTION AND CONTROL

MANAGEMENT PROCEDURES

The best preventive is strict isolation of the flock, along with sound management practices such as adding only day-old chicks as replacement stock and rearing them in isolation. Even on farms with sound management practices, infectious bronchitis may occur, particularly in heavily populated areas. This has brought on the necessity of using immunization procedures in the control of the disease.

IMMUNIZATION

The first immunization procedure used was started about 1941 in the New England states (Van Roekel et al., 1950). It consisted of inoculating a small portion of the birds in a flock with a field strain of virus and al-

lowing natural spread to the rest of the flock. This was usually done at 7–15 weeks of age when the disease would produce the least economic loss to the poultryman. After recovery from the infection, the flock would be immune to bronchitis through the laying year.

This type of vaccination procedure using pathogenic field strains has been replaced with modified live virus vaccines.

Types of Vaccine

INACTIVATED VACCINE. No inactivated vaccines are produced commercially in the United States. However, in England 4 commercial inactivated bronchitis vaccines are available (McMartin, 1968). Woernle (1961) reported some success with an adsorbed bronchitis vaccine inactivated by 0.2% formalin. McDougall (1968) reported on a controlled experiment where a group had been vaccinated with inactivated vaccine. Two doses were given 10 weeks apart, and the immunity challenged 15 weeks after the second vaccination. Results of serology were negative, and the vaccinated flock dropped from 70 to 49% production after challenge while the unvaccinated controls dropped from 75 to 23%. Egg quality was also affected. McMartin (1968) found that inactivated vaccine induced some resistance in the reproductive tract but did not protect the respiratory system against challenge. Winterfield (1967) reported negative results using a commercial inactivated IBV vaccine.

MODIFIED LIVE VIRUS VACCINE. The commercial bronchitis vaccines available utilize strains of virus that have been modified by 25 or more chicken embryo serial passages. This reduces their pathogenicity and spreading ability to some extent, but it should be emphasized that these modified strains are still capable of spreading; in the very young chick without passive antibodies and in laying flocks in high production they may produce undesirable results.

Vaccine Virus Strains

In a field survey by Hitchner et al. (1966), antibodies against several bronchitis serotypes were demonstrated. Thus a vaccine strain should be selected having a broad spectrum of antigenic components. The Massachusetts type has been found to induce the best immunity against challenge with heterologous strains (Raggi, 1960; Hofstad, 1961; Winterfield, 1968).

While other vaccine strains (primarily the Connecticut type) have been used in modified live virus vaccines because of their lessened pathogenicity, they have not proven to be as effective as the Massachusetts type strains. Bivalent vaccines have come into use to obtain added protection against a diversity of bronchitis types. However, Winterfield (1968) has found a greater and more prolonged respiratory reaction to bivalent vaccines, and the Massachusetts type strain appeared to interfere with the development of Connecticut type antibodies.

Attenuation of Vaccine Strain

Modification of IBV for vaccine production has been accomplished by serial passages in chicken embryos. The greater the number of passages, the greater the reduction of pathogenicity for the chicken. Unfortunately there is also an accompanying reduction in immunogenicity.

Exactly at what embryo passage level a particular strain loses its pathogenicity for the chicken is difficult to ascertain and probably varies between strains and between procedures of embryo passage. Larose and Van Roekel (1961) observed strain 41 Massachusetts type to be pathogenic for chickens after 300 serial transfers in chicken embryos. The author found strain 33, after 144 embryo passages, to cause marked respiratory signs and a 50% drop in production in laying chickens following aerosol exposure. The same strain was capable of infecting day-old chicks after 168 embryo passages when given by aerosol exposure. Few respiratory signs were observed, but virus multiplication occurred in the trachea. Immunity to challenge was short-lived.

Degree of Strain Modification for Vaccines

Selection of the proper degree of modification of a strain of virus for vaccine production is difficult. Since broilers require early vaccination and not long-term immunity, the strain used for them should be selected on the basis of low pathogenicity but still capable of stimulating the desired short-term immunity. It is likely that such a strain could not be administered by way of the drinking water (because high embryo-passaged, attenuated strains have poor invasiveness) and probably would require

aerosol administration for the desired results (Hofstad and Yoder, 1966).

The strain needed for laying flocks and breeders should be selected on the basis of inducing an adequate long-term immunity, and this would require a less modified strain of virus than one used for broilers.

Age at Vaccination

Broilers require immunization at an early age. If chicks possess passive antibodies derived from the yolk, they can be vaccinated when a few days old with live attenuated IBV. Since most commercial chicks possess some passive antibodies, a common procedure is to vaccinate at 4–5 days of age and again at 4 weeks. However, optimum immune response is obtained in chickens 6 weeks or older as they become immunologically more mature. Replacement flocks should be vaccinated at 2–4 months.

Effect of Passive Antibodies on Immune Response

Chickens can be immunized against infectious bronchitis virus even though they possess congenital antibodies. The degree of immunity may be less than that obtained in fully susceptible chicks, since passive antibodies prevent a total infection of the bird. However, Raggi and Lee (1965) found that passive antibodies did not materially influence immune response to live virus vaccine as judged by challenge.

Methods of Vaccine Administration

Labor-saving methods of vaccinating chickens such as spraying, dusting, and placing the vaccine in the drinking water have become standard procedures. The immune response and the severity of the vaccination reaction may depend to some extent on the method of administration. Chickens exposed to an aerosol of IBV vaccine will generally have a more severe respiratory reaction than those exposed by the drinking water method. Likewise, aerosol-exposed chickens have a greater virus distribution in nonrespiratory tissue than chickens exposed by the drinking water (Hofstad and Yoder, 1966). The assumption that aerosol exposure induces a better immune response than drinking water exposure has not been confirmed experimentally.

The commonest and easiest procedure for bronchitis vaccination is to place the vaccine in the drinking water. The disadvantage of this method is that the virus is immediately exposed to a variety of conditions. Avian IBV is not a very resistant virus, and placing it in a variety of waters and watering containers leads to variable results. When this method of administration is used, it should be emphasized that the proper dilution be adhered to, that only clean watering containers be used, and that a stabilizing material such as powdered skim milk (3.2 oz packet per 10 gal) be added to help preserve the virus (Gentry, 1968, personal communication).

Combining Bronchitis Vaccine with Other Vaccines

Bronchitis vaccines have been combined with Newcastle disease vaccines as an added convenience and apparently without interference in immune response from each vaccine (Markham et al., 1956). However, interference has been demonstrated between these two viruses in certain combinations (Hanson et al., 1956; Raggi and Lee, 1964), and it would seem advisable that whenever possible and practical the bronchitis immunization should be administered separately.

REFERENCES

Akers, T. G., and C. H. Cunningham. 1968. Replication and cytopathogenicity of avian infectious bronchitis virus in chicken embryo kidney cells. *Arch. Ges. Virusforsch.* 25:30–37.

Almeida, June D., and D. A. J. Tyrrell. 1967. The morphology of three previously uncharacterized human respiratory viruses that grow in organ cultures. *J. Gen. Virol.* 1:175–78.

Beach, J. R., and O. W. Schalm. 1936. A filtrable virus distinct from that of laryngotracheitis, the cause of a respiratory disease of chicks. *Poultry Sci.* 15:199–206.

Beard, C. W. 1968. An interference type of serological test for infectious bronchitis virus using Newcastle disease virus. *Avian Diseases* 12:658–65.

Beaudette, F. R., and C. B. Hudson. 1933. Newly recognized poultry disease. *North Am. Vet.* 14:50–54.

Becker, W. B., K. McIntosh, Jane H. Dees, and R. M. Channock. 1967. Morphogenesis of avian infectious bronchitis virus and a related human virus (Strain 229E). *J. Virol.* 1:1019–27.

Berry, D. M., and June D. Almeida. 1968. The morphological and biological effects of various antisera on avian infectious bronchitis virus. *J. Gen. Virol.* 3:97–102.

Berry, D. M., and K. J. Stokes. 1968. Antigenic variations in isolates of infectious bronchitis virus. *Vet. Record* 83:157–60.

Berry, D. M., J. G. Cruickshank, H. P. Chu, and R. J. H. Wells. 1964. The structure of infectious bronchitis virus. *Virology* 23:403–7.

Braune, M. O., and R. E. Gentry. 1965. Standardization of the fluorescent antibody technique for the detection of avian respiratory viruses. *Avian Diseases* 9:535–45.

Broadfoot, D. I., and W. M. Smith, Jr. 1954. Effects of infectious bronchitis in laying hens on egg production, percent unsettable eggs and hatchability. *Poultry Sci.* 653–54.

Broadfoot, D. I., B. S. Pomeroy, and W. M. Smith, Jr. 1956. Effects of infectious bronchitis in baby chicks. *Poultry Sci.* 35:757–62.

Brown, W. E., S. C. Schmittle, and J. W. Foster. 1962. A tannic acid modified hemagglutination test for infectious bronchitis of chickens. *Avian Diseases* 6:99–106.

Brumfield, H. P., and B. S. Pomeroy. 1957. Direct complement fixation by turkey and chicken serum in viral systems. *Proc. Soc. Exp. Biol. Med.* 94:146–49.

Bushnell, L. D., and C. A. Brandly. 1933. Laryngotracheitis in chicks. *Poultry Sci.* 12:55–60.

Buthala, D. A. 1956. Some properties of the avian bronchitis virus. Ph.D. thesis, Iowa State Coll., Ames.

Carbo, L. J., and C. H. Cunningham. 1959. Hemagglutination by trypsin-modified infectious bronchitis virus. *Am. J. Vet. Res.* 20:876–83.

Cook, Jane K. A. 1968. Duration of experimental infectious bronchitis in chickens. *Res. Vet. Sci.* 9:506–14.

Cumming, R. B. 1963. Infectious avian nephroses (uraemia) in Australia. *Australian Vet. J.* 39:145–47.

Cunningham, C. H. 1963. Newer knowledge of infectious bronchitis virus. *Proc. 17th World Vet. Congr.* 1:607–10.

———. 1966. Newer information on the properties of infectious bronchitis virus. *Proc. 13th World's Poultry Congr.*, pp. 416–18.

Cunningham, C. H., and A. H. El Dardiry. 1948. Distribution of the virus of infectious bronchitis of chickens in embryonated chicken eggs. *Cornell Vet.* 38:381–88.

Cunningham, C. H., and M. P. Spring. 1965. Some studies of infectious bronchitis virus in cell culture. *Avian Diseases* 9:182–93.

Cunningham, C. H., and H. O. Stuart. 1946. The effect of certain chemical agents on the virus of infectious bronchitis of chickens. *Am. J. Vet. Res.* 7:466–69.

Delaplane, J. P., and H. O. Stuart. 1941. The modification of infectious bronchitis virus of chickens as a result of propagation in embryonated chicken eggs. *Rhode Island Univ. Agr. Expt. Sta. Bull.* 284:1–20.

DuBose, R. T. 1967. Adaptation of the Massachusetts strain of infectious bronchitis virus to turkey embryos. *Avian Diseases* 11:28–38.

DuBose, R. T., and L. C. Grumbles. 1959. The relationship between quail bronchitis virus and chicken embryo lethal orphan virus. *Avian Diseases* 3:321–44.

Estola, Timo. 1966. Studies on the infectious bronchitis virus of chickens isolated in Finland. *Acta Vet. Scand.* 7 (Suppl.) 18:1–111.

Fabricant. J. 1951. Studies on the diagnosis of Newcastle disease and infectious bronchitis of fowls. IV. The use of the serum neutralization test in the diagnosis of infectious bronchitis. *Cornell Vet.* 41:68–80.

Fabricant, J., and P. P. Levine. 1951. The persistence of infectious bronchitis in eggs and tracheal exudates of infected chickens. *Cornell Vet.* 41:240–46.

Groupé, V. 1949. Demonstration of an interference phenomenon associated with infectious bronchitis virus (IBV) of chickens. *J. Bacteriol.* 58:23–32.

Hanson, L. E., F. H. White, and J. O. Alberts. 1956. Interference between Newcastle disease and infectious bronchitis viruses. *Am. J. Vet. Res.* 17:294–98.

Hitchner, S. B., and P. G. White. 1955. Growth-curve studies of chick-embryo-propagated infectious bronchitis virus. *Poultry Sci.* 34: 590–94.

Hitchner, S. B., R. W. Winterfield, and G. S. Appleton. 1966. Infectious bronchitis virus types—Incidence in the U.S. *Avian Diseases* 10:98–102.

Hoekstra, J., and B. Rispens. 1960. Infectieuze bronchitis bij pluimvee. III. De ontwikkeling van een mild werkendvaccin. *Tijdschr. Diergeneesk.* 85:398–403.

Hofstad, M. S. 1947. A study of infectious bronchitis in chickens. IV. Further observations on the carrier status of chickens recovered from infectious bronchitis. *Cornell Vet.* 37:29–34.

———. 1956a. Infectious Bronchitis. *Progr. Rept. Vet. Med. Res. Inst., Ames, Iowa.* 1956:13–14.

———. 1956b. Stability of avian infectious bronchitis virus at 56° C. *Cornell Vet.* 46: 122–28.

———. 1958. Antigenic differences among isolates of avian infectious bronchitis virus. *Am. J. Vet. Res.* 19:740–43.

———. 1961. Antigenic and immunological studies on several isolates of avian infectious bronchitis virus. *Avian Diseases* 5:102–7.

Hofstad, M. S., and H. W. Yoder, Jr. 1963. Inactivation rates of some lyophilized poultry viruses at 37° C and 3° C. *Avian Diseases* 7:170–77.

———. 1966. Avian infectious bronchitis virus distribution in tissues of chicks. *Avian Diseases* 10:230–39.

Hopkins, S. R. 1967. Thermal stability of infectious bronchitis virus in the presence of salt solutions. *Avian Diseases* 10:261–67.

Jeon, Y. S. 1962. Modified complement fixation test of avian infectious bronchitis virus. Univ. Microfilm Inc., Ann Arbor, Mich. *Dissertation Abstr.* 34:400.

Julian, R. J., and N. G. Willis. 1969. The nephrosis-nephritis syndrome in chickens caused by a Holte strain of infectious bronchitis virus. *Can. Vet. J.* 10:18–19.

Jungherr, E. L., T. W. Chomiak, and R. E. Luginbuhl. 1956. Immunologic differences in strains of infectious bronchitis. *Proc. 60th Ann. Meet. U.S. Livestock Sanit. Ass.,* pp. 203–9.

Kawamura, H., S. Isogai, and H. Tsubahara. 1961. Propagation of avian infectious bronchitis virus in chicken kidney tissue culture. *Nat. Inst. Animal Health Quart.* 1:190–98.

Larose, R. N., and H. Van Roekel. 1961. The effect of rapid embryo passage upon the infectious bronchitis virus. *Avian Diseases* 5:157–68.

Levine, P. P., and M. S. Hofstad. 1947. Attempts to control airborne infectious bronchitis and Newcastle disease of fowls with sterilamps. *Cornell Vet.* 37:204–10.

Loomis, L. N., C. H. Cunningham, M. L. Gray, and F. Thorpe, Jr. 1950. Pathology of the chicken embryo infected with infectious bronchitis virus. *Am. J. Vet. Res.* 11:245–51.

Lukert, P. P. 1966a. Immunofluorescence of avian infectious bronchitis virus in primary chicken embryo kidney, liver, lung and fibroblast cell cultures. *Arch. Ges. Virusforsch.* 18:265–72.

———. 1966b. A plaque reduction method for the detection of neutralizing antibodies for infectious bronchitis virus. *Avian Diseases* 10:305–13.

McDougall, J. S. 1968. Infectious bronchitis in laying fowls—Its effect upon egg production and subsequent egg quality. *Vet. Record* 83:84–86.

Machado, A. V. 1951. The effect of infectious bronchitis and NDV on the blood cells of the chicken. Thesis. Cornell Univ., Ithaca, New York.

McIntosh, K., Jane H. Dees, W. B. Becker, A. Z. Kapikian, and R. M. Chanock. 1967. Recovery in tracheal organ cultures of novel viruses from patients with respiratory disease. *Proc. Nat. Acad. Sci.* 57:933–40.

McMartin, D. A. 1968. Preliminary investigation of methods for evaluating inactivated vaccines for infectious bronchitis virus. *Brit. Vet. J.* 124:36–42.

Markham, F. S., A. H. Hammar, E. B. Perry, and W. C. Tesar. 1956. Combined Newcastle disease-infectious bronchitis vaccines and the absence of the interference phenomena. *Cornell Vet.* 46:538–48.

Mathews, J., and M. S. Hofstad. 1953. The inactivation of certain animal viruses by ethylene oxide (carboxide). *Cornell Vet.* 43:452–61.

Miller, Louise T., and V. J. Yates. 1968. Neutralization of infectious bronchitis virus by human sera. *Am. J. Epidemiol.* 88:406–9.

Muldoon, R. L. 1960. Some characteristics of the hemagglutinating activity of IBV. Ph.D. thesis, Mich. State Univ. *Dissertation Abstr.* 22:2152.

Nazerian, K., and C. H. Cunningham. 1968. Morphogenesis of avian infectious bronchitis virus in chicken embryo fibroblasts. *J. Gen. Virol.* 3:469–70.

Page, C. A., and C. H. Cunningham. 1962. The neutralization test for infectious bronchitis virus. *Am. J. Vet. Res.* 23:1065–71.

Petek, M., and S. Corazzola. 1958. Azione inattivante dell' etere etilico e del siero fresco sul virus della bronchite infettiva. *Vet. Ital.* 9:515–20.

Pette, J. 1959. Zur Ausscheidung des Huehnerbronchitis virus im Kloakeninhalt. *Monatsh. Tierheilk.* 11:296–300.

Prince, R. P., L. M. Potter, R. E. Luginbuhl, and T. Chomiak. 1962. Effect of ventilation rate on the performance of chicks inoculated with IBV. *Poultry Sci.* 41:268–72.

Prince, R. P., J. H. Whitaker, R. E. Luginbuhl, and L. D. Matterson. 1967. Effect of environmental temperatures on healthy chicks and chicks inoculated with infectious bronchitis virus. *Poultry Sci.* 46:1098–1102.

Quiroz, C. A., and R. P. Hanson. 1958. Physical-chemical treatment of inocula as a means of separating and identifying avian viruses. *Avian Diseases* 2:94–98.

Raggi, L. G. 1960. A variant type of infectious bronchitis virus in a commercial vaccine. *Avian Diseases* 4:312–19.

Raggi, L. G., and G. G. Lee. 1964. Infectious bronchitis virus interference with growth of Newcastle disease virus. II. Interference in chickens. *Avian Diseases* 8:471–80.

———. 1965. Lack of correlation between infectivity, serological response and challenge results in immunization with an avian infectious bronchitis vaccine. *J. Immunol.* 94:538–43.

Reed, L. J., and H. Muench. 1938. A simple method of estimating fifty per cent endpoints. *Am. J. Hyg.* 27:493–97.

Schalk, A. F., and M. C. Hawn. 1931. An apparently new respiratory disease of baby chicks. *J. Am. Vet. Med. Ass.* 78:413–22.

Sevoian, M., and P. P. Levine. 1957. Effects of infectious bronchitis on the reproductive tracts, egg production, and egg quality of laying chickens. *Avian Diseases* 1:136–64.

Simpson, R. W., and V. Groupé. 1959. Temperature of incubation as a critical factor in the behavior of avian bronchitis virus in chicken embryos. *Virology* 8:456–69.

Singh, I. P. 1960. Some properties of IBV as determined by thermal and formalin inactivation. Ph.D. thesis. Univ. Microfilm Inc., Ann Arbor, Michigan. *Dissertation Abstr.* 22:2153.

Steele, F. M., and R. E. Luginbuhl. 1964. Direct and indirect complement-fixation tests for infectious bronchitis virus. *Am. J. Vet. Res.* 25:1249–55.

Stinski, M. F., and C. H. Cunningham. 1969. Neutralizing antibody complex of infectious bronchitis virus. *J. Immunol.* 102:720–27.

Tevethia, S. S., and C. H. Cunningham. 1968. Antigenic characterization of infectious bronchitis virus. *J. Immunol.* 100:793–98.

Tyrrell, D. A. J., June D. Almeida, D. M. Berry, C. H. Cunningham, D. Hamre, M. S. Hofstad, L. Mallucci, and K. McIntosh. 1968. Coronaviruses. *Nature* 220:650.

Van Roekel, H., K. L. Bullis, M. K. Clarke, O. M. Olesiuk, and F. G. Sperling. 1950. Infectious bronchitis. *Mass. Agr. Expt. Sta. Bull.* 460:1–47.

Vasington, P. J. 1962. Studies on passive hemagglutination with infectious bronchitis virus. Univ. Microfilm Inc., Ann Arbor, Michigan. *Dissertation Abstr.* 22:2949.

Von Bülow, V. 1967. Infektioese Bronchitis der Huehner. IV. Charakterisierung eines neuen Feldstammes des IB-Virus (IBV-10). *Zentr. Veterinaermed.* 14B:151–62.

Winterfield, R. W. 1967. Immunity response from an inactivated infectious bronchitis vaccine. *Avian Diseases* 11:446–51.

———. 1968. Respiratory signs, immunity response, and interference from vaccination with monovalent and multivalent infectious bronchitis vaccines. *Avian Diseases* 12:577–84.

Winterfield, R. W., and S. B. Hitchner. 1962. Etiology of an infectious nephritis- nephrosis syndrome of chickens. *Am. J. Vet. Res.* 23:1273–79.

Winterfield, R. W., S. B. Hitchner, and G. S. Appleton. 1964. Immunological characteristics of a variant of infectious bronchitis virus isolated from chickens. *Avian Diseases* 8:40–47.

Witter, R. L. 1962. The diagnosis of infectious

bronchitis of chickens by the agar gel precipitin test. *Avian Diseases* 6:478–92.

Woernle, H. 1959. Diagnose der Infektioesen Bronchitis der Huehner mit Hilfe der Praezipitationsreaktion im festen Agarmedium. *Monatsh. Tierheilk.* 11:154–67.

———. 1960. Ein Beitrag zur Infectioesen Bronchitis der Huehner. *Monatsh. Tierheilk.* 12:111–16.

———. 1961. Impfversuche mit Adsorbat-Vakzine bei der Infektioesen Bronchitis des Huhnes. *Monatsh. Tierheilk.* 13:136–42.

Woernle, H., and A. Brunner. 1960. Zur Epizootiologie der Infektioesen Bronchitis der Huehner. *Tierarztl. Umschau* 15:217–21.

Wright, B. S., and B. P. Sagik. 1958. Plaque formation in monolayers of chicken embryo kidney cells. *Virology* 5:573–74.

CHAPTER 17

LARYNGOTRACHEITIS

❖

LYLE E. HANSON

*Department of Veterinary Pathology
and Hygiene
University of Illinois
Urbana, Illinois*

❖

LARYNGOTRACHEITIS is an acute disease of chickens characterized by signs of respiratory depression, gasping, and expectoration of bloody exudate. The affected cells of the tracheal mucous membrane become swollen and edematous resulting in erosion and hemorrhages. Intranuclear inclusions are present in the early stages of the disease.

The disease has been identified as laryngotracheitis, infectious laryngotracheitis, and avian diphtheria. Although most articles refer to the disease as infectious laryngotracheitis, the term laryngotracheitis was used as early as 1930 (Beach, 1930; Graham et al., 1930). Some of the early investigators also referred to the disease as infectious bronchitis.

Laryngotracheitis is a serious disease of chickens in areas of large concentrations of poultry in the United States, Europe, and Australia. The disease is responsible for egg production and death losses.

The disease affects only poultry and therefore has no public health significance.

HISTORY

The disease was first described in 1925 (May and Tittsler). Some reports indicate it may have existed earlier (Beach, 1926; Hinshaw, 1931). The disease was referred to as infectious bronchitis by some of the early investigators. The name of infectious laryngotracheitis was later adapted by the special Committee on Poultry Diseases of the American Veterinary Medical Association in 1931.

INCIDENCE AND DISTRIBUTION

Laryngotracheitis has been identified in Canada (Gwatkin, 1925), Holland (Van Heelsbergen, 1929), Germany (Fritzsche and Gerriers, 1959), Great Britain (Dobson, 1935), Australia (Seddon and Hart, 1935), Sweden (Magnusson, 1940), Poland (Marek, 1948), and Finland (Rislakki, 1965).

ETIOLOGY

CLASSIFICATION

Laryngotracheitis (LT) virus has all the characteristics of the herpes group of virus. The virus is cuboidal shaped, enveloped, ether-sensitive, and contains a core composed of desoxyribonucleic acid.

MORPHOLOGY

Electron micrographs of laryngotracheitis-infected chicken embryo cell cultures contain cuboidal-shaped icosahedral viral particles similar to the structure of herpes simplex virus. Watrach et al. (1963) described the hexagonal-shaped virons to be 80–100 mμ. The capsids have icosahedral symmetry and are composed of 162 elongated hollow capsomeres (Fig. 17.1) (Watrach, et al., 1963; Cruickshank et al., 1963). The virons have nucleic acid cores composed of desoxyribonucleic acid (Goodheart, 1968, personal communication). The complete virus particle, which has an irregular envelope surrounding the nucleocapsid, has a diameter of 195–250 mμ. The surface of the envelope contains fine projections on the delimiting membrane.

CHEMICAL COMPOSITION

The nucleic acid core of the herpes group of viruses is composed of DNA. The buoyant density of LT viral DNA is 1.704 g/ml which is consistent with DNA values of some of the other herpes viruses (Goodheart, 1968, personal communication). The chemical values of LT virus have not yet been established. Studies of herpes simplex and pseudorabies virus have demonstrated the capsid to be a specific protein. The envelope which contains lipid is derived, at least in part, from the host nuclear membrane. Antigenic studies indicate that the envelope contains host antigens (Wildy and Watson, 1962).

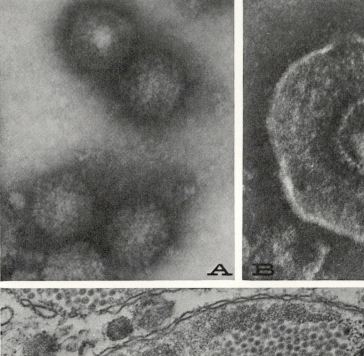

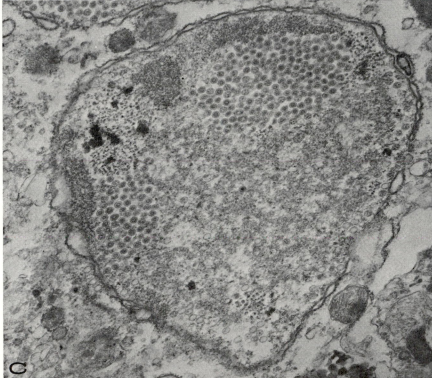

FIG. 17.1—Electron micrographs of infectious laryngotracheitis virus. (A) Group of "full" capsids, each of which has a hexagonal profile. Negative contrast technique, ×160,000. (B) "Empty" capsid contained in envelope. Notice hexagonal outline of capsid and projections at periphery of envelope. Negative contrast technique, ×160,-000. (C) Aggregates of virus particles forming an inclusion body in nucleus of chicken embryo kidney tissue culture cell. Notice peripheral accumulations of chromatin and centrally located amorphous material; the latter forms part of inclusion body. ×18,500. (Figs. A, B—Watrach et al., 1963; Fig. C—Watrach, Univ. of Ill.)

VIRUS REPLICATION

Replication of LT virus appears to be similar to herpes simplex and pseudorabies viruses.

Laryngotracheitis virus is adsorbed on the surface of the cell. Viral entry in the cell apparently occurs by pinocytoses. The rate of adsorption varies with volume of inoculum and the cell system. Holmes and Watson (1963) observed that enveloped particles of herpes simplex virus were more readily adsorbed than naked nucleocapsids.

The envelope and capsid are disrupted by host enzymes releasing DNA which migrates to the cell nucleus. The first evidence of new LT viral components is observed in the nucleus in approximately 10–12 hours (Reynolds et al., 1968).

The completed nucleocapsids migrate through the nuclear membrane of the cell which forms the envelope. The enveloped virus particles accumulate in a vacuolar membrane in the cytoplasm. Vacuoles containing the viral particles migrate to the plasma membrane and release the virus at the surface through disruption of the cell wall (Darlington and James, 1966; Nii et al., 1968).

RESISTANCE TO CHEMICAL AND PHYSICAL AGENTS

Laryngotracheitis viral particles are sensitive to lipolytic agents, heat, and various disinfectants. Fitzgerald and Hanson (1963) reported LT virus became noninfective after exposure to ether for 24 hours. Although LT virus will survive for extended periods when lyophilized or when held at —20 to —60° C (Webster, 1959; Goldhaft, 1961), it is destroyed in 10–15 minutes at 55° C (Schalm and Beach, 1935) and in 48 hours held in broth at 38° C (Brandly, 1934). Virus in tracheal tissue of a chicken carcass is destroyed in 44 hours at 37° C or in the chorioallantoic membrane in 5 hours at 25° C (Cover and Benton, 1958). A solution of 3% cresol or 1% lye will inactivate LT virus in less than 1 minute.

STRAIN CLASSIFICATION

Distinct immunologic strains have not been isolated, although some variations in neutralizing abilities have been demonstrated between strains of varying pathogenicity (Burnet, 1936; Pulsford, 1953, 1954). In studies by Pulsford and Stokes (1953), one strain of the virus was found to be almost completely resistant to neutralization by antisera prepared against a number of LT viral strains.

A number of workers have isolated and studied strains of LT virus that caused only mild signs of disease (Burnet, 1936; Satriano et al., 1957; Cover and Benton, 1958; Ahmed and Monreal, 1963; Mayr et al., 1964). Pulsford (1953, 1961) has postulated that LT virus may exist in some chicken populations in a subclinical form as an enteric orphan virus.

LABORATORY HOST SYSTEMS

Laryngotracheitis virus can be readily propagated in the embryonating chicken egg. The virus causes formation of opaque plaques due to proliferation and necrotic lesions (Fig. 17.2). The plaques which have opaque edges with depressed central areas of necrosis are observed as early as 48 hours and often extend linearly with increase in numbers and size. Embryo deaths occur in 2–12 days following inoculations with LT virus. Survival time of infected embryos decreases with additional egg passages (Burnet, 1934; Brandly, 1935, 1937).

LT virus can be readily propagated in chicken embryo cell cultures. The first cellular changes which can be observed as early as 4–6 hours are chromatin displacement and rounding of the nucleoli. Cytoplasmic fusion results in the formation of multinucleated cells. Intranuclear inclusion bodies can be detected as early as 12 hours with the concentration occurring 30–36 hours after inoculation (Fig. 17.3). Large cytoplasmic vesicles develop on the multinucleated cells and become more basophilic as the cells degenerate (Reynolds et al., 1968).

PATHOGENESIS AND EPIZOOTIOLOGY

NATURAL AND EXPERIMENTAL HOSTS

The chicken is the primary natural host affected by LT virus. Although the disease affects all ages of chickens, the most characteristic signs are observed in adult birds.

Several workers have described a form of LT in pheasants and pheasant-chicken crosses (Kernohan, 1931b; Hudson and Beaudette, 1932a). Recently Winterfield and So (1968) were able to infect young turkeys with laboratory propagated strains of LT virus. The lesions involved primarily the upper respiratory tract. Winterfield and So (1968) also reported an isolation of LT virus from the trachea of a peafowl. The previous negative attempts to infect turkeys (Brandly, 1936; Seddon and Hart, 1936) apparently indicate a definite age resistance. The species of birds which appear to be refractory to the virus of ILT are starlings, sparrows, crows, doves, ducks, pigeons, and guinea fowl (Beach, 1931; Brandly and Bushnell, 1934; Seddon and Hart, 1936). Rabbits, guinea pigs, and white rats were also refractory (Beach, 1931; Seddon and Hart, 1936).

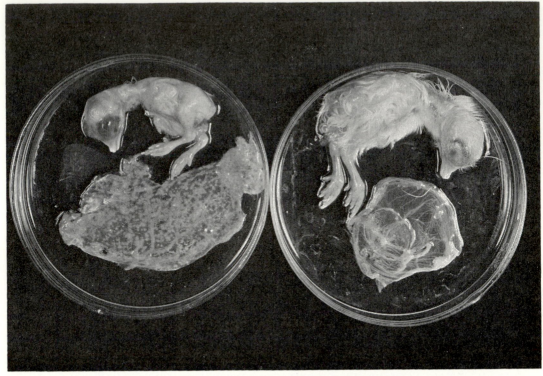

FIG. 17.2—*Chicken embryos at 14 days of age.* **(Right)** *Normal embryo and chorioallantoic membrane.* **(Left)** *LT virus-infected embryo is stunted and chorioallantoic membrane has numerous foci of proliferation. (Hanson, Univ. of Ill.)*

Embryonating eggs of turkeys and chickens are susceptible while those of duck, guinea fowl, and pigeons are unaffected (Brandly, 1936).

TRANSMISSION

The natural portals of entry of the virus are through the upper respiratory tract and intraocular route (Beaudette, 1930, 1937). Oral ingestion appears to be an unlikely mode of transmission (Gibbs, 1931). Transmission occurs more readily from acutely infected birds than through contact with clinically recovered carrier birds.

Virus has been isolated from tracheal tissues of recovered chickens for as long as 2 years (Komarov and Beaudette, 1932; Seddon, 1952). LT virus has been demonstrated in approximately 2% of the recovered birds (Beaudette, 1949; Seddon, 1952). Although LT virus has not been recovered from vaccinated birds longer than 11 days after inoculation (Brandly and Bushnell, 1934; Beach, 1935; Seddon, 1952; Hungerford, 1962), occurrence of field outbreaks

following contact between vaccinated and unvaccinated birds indicates LT virus is transmitted by some vaccinated hens for longer periods (Nicol et al., 1945). Laryngotracheitis infections may recur on a farm if the previously vaccinated LT birds are not isolated from susceptible pullets (Beaudette, 1937).

Mechanical transmission can occur by the use of contaminated equipment and litter (Gibbs, 1934a; Dobson, 1935; Beaudette, 1937; Kingsbury and Jungherr, 1957; Jordan, 1963).

Egg transmission of virus contained in the interior or on the exterior of the egg has not been demonstrated. LT virus-infected embryos die before hatching time. LT virus is inactivated in less than 24 hours at 37° C (Jordan, 1966).

INCUBATION PERIOD

Signs usually appear in 6–12 days following natural exposure (Kernohan, 1931a; Seddon and Hart, 1935). Intratracheal exposure results in a shorter incubation pe-

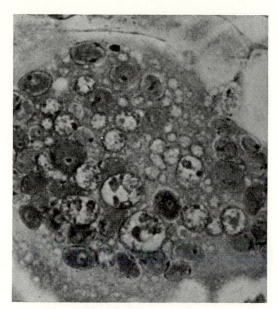

FIG. 17.3—Chicken embryo kidney cell monolayer 72 hours after inoculation with LT virus. Large giant cell with numerous nuclei containing inclusion bodies. May-Grünwald-Giemsa, ×320. (Fitzgerald and Hanson, Univ. of Ill.)

riod of 2–4 days (Seddon and Hart, 1935; Benton et al., 1958; Jordan, 1963).

The epizootic form of the disease which spreads rapidly in susceptible chickens affects up to 90–100% of the flocks. Mortal-

ity, which varies from 5 to 70%, usually averages between 10 and 20% (Beach, 1926; Hinshaw et al., 1931; Seddon and Hart, 1935).

SIGNS

The characteristic signs of an acute infection are nasal discharge and moist rales followed by coughing and gasping (Figs. 17.4, 17.5) (Beach, 1926; Kernohan, 1931b). Marked dyspnea and expectoration of blood-stained mucus is characteristic of the severe forms of the disease (Beach, 1926; Hinshaw, 1931; Hinshaw et al., 1931; Seddon and Hart, 1935; Jordan, 1958).

Mild enzootic forms of the disease have been described by workers in the United States, Australia, New Zealand, and Great Britain (Pulsford and Stokes, 1953; Webster, 1959; Cover and Benton, 1958; Seddon and Hart, 1935). In the mild forms, signs are unthriftiness, reduction in egg production, watery eyes, conjunctivitis, swelling of the infraorbital sinuses, persistent nasal discharge, and hemorrhagic conjunctivitis. The morbidity as indicated by clinical signs may be as low as 5% (Raggi et al., 1961).

The course of the disease varies with the severity of the lesions. Generally most chickens recover in 10–14 days, but extremes of 1–4 weeks have been reported (Beach, 1926; Hinshaw et al., 1931).

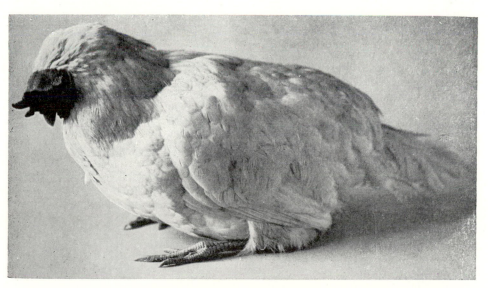

FIG. 17.4—Advanced case of laryngotracheitis. Attitude during expiration. (Beach and Freeborn, Univ. of Calif.)

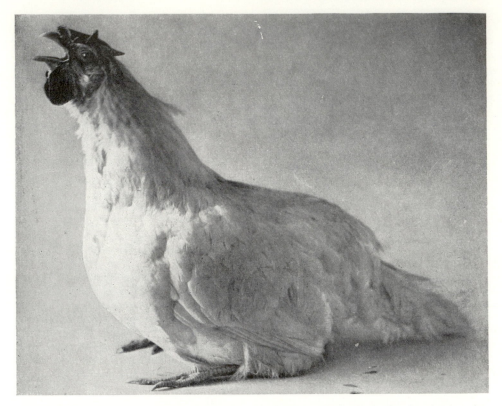

FIG. 17.5—Laryngotracheitis. Same fowl as Fig. 17.4. Attitude during inspiration.

GROSS LESIONS

Lesions occur most consistently in tracheal and laryngeal tissues. Tissue changes vary from mucoid inflammation early in the disease to degeneration of the mucosa resulting in necrosis and hemorrhages in later stages. Expulsion of desquamated epithelial tissue and blood clots may occur during violent coughing and convulsive respirations. Extension of the inflammation down the bronchi into the lungs and airsacs can occur. Edema and congestion of the epithelium of the conjunctiva and infraorbital sinuses may be the only lesion observed in some of the less pathogenic infections.

HISTOPATHOLOGY

The microscopic changes vary with the stage of the disease. Electron microscopic studies indicate the first cellular change occurs in the nucleus during the formation of viral capsids. Following migration of the virus through the nuclear membrane into the cytoplasm, the complete enveloped particles aggregate into large masses contained in a vascular structure. Large masses of viral particles in the cytoplasm result in the cloudy swelling observed in light microscopic studies of early cellular changes (Watrach et al., 1959; Reynolds et al., 1968).

As the cellular changes progress, the cells enlarge, lose cilia, and become edematous. Lymphocytes, histocytes, and plasma cells migrate into the mucosa and submucosa after 2–3 days. Later cellular destruction causes separation of the mucosa and submucosa and hemorrhages. As the disease progresses, cellular infiltration becomes more marked. Cellular infiltration and mucosal degeneration is most extensive in the trachea and larynx (Seifreid, 1931).

Intranuclear inclusion bodies occur in epithelial cells as early as 12 hours after infection. Watrach et al. (1963) reported that the fixative is important in demonstration of inclusions (Fig. 17.6).

IMMUNITY

The resistance of susceptible chickens to laryngotracheitis virus is altered following natural infections or vaccination. The du-

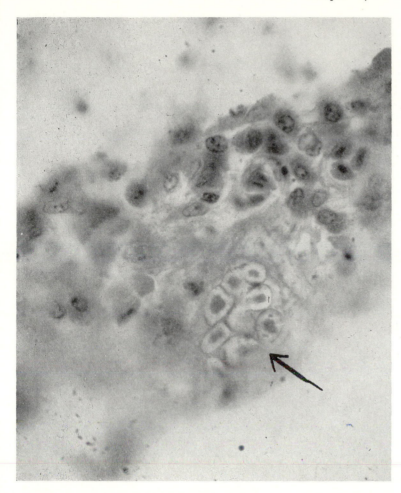

FIG. 17.6—Tracheal mucosa from chick killed on 5th day following intratracheal inoculation. Arrow points toward group of nuclei containing inclusion bodies characteristic of infectious laryngotracheitis. ×1,200.

ration of resistance induced from a natural infection is usually a year or more. The resistance may indicate an endemic infection in the flock as some birds remain carriers for extended periods. The resistance induced by vaccination varies from 6 weeks to as long as 1 year (Beaudette, 1949; Shibley et al., 1962; Raggi and Lee, 1965). The refractory period varies with virus strain, concentration of active virus in the vaccine, and route of application (Gibbs, 1933; Hitchner and Winterfield, 1960; Raggi and Lee, 1965). A number of workers have reported vaccine breaks occurring less than 5 months after vaccination (Oxer, 1945; Seddon, 1952; Jordan, 1964b; Raggi and Lee, 1965). Raggi and Lee (1965) concluded that laryngotracheitis vaccine must contain more than 10^2 embryo plaque-forming units per ml to be capable of inducing satisfactory immunity.

Virus neutralization tests are used to in-dicate satisfactory responses to vaccination (Hitchner et al., 1958). However, Shibley et al. (1962) stated they were unable to establish a satisfactory correlation between virus neutralizing indices and resistance to challenge.

Passive immunity can be induced by administration of hyperimmune serum (Gibbs, 1933). Immune serum given intratracheally as late as 44 hours after infection is capable of preventing signs of laryngotracheitis (Brandly, 1935). The cost of hyperimmune serum and application precludes the use in control of laryngotracheitis.

DIAGNOSIS

Laryngotracheitis, like many other diseases, cannot be reliably diagnosed by observation of signs and lesions. Although some acute signs of the disease are characteristic, many signs are similar to other respiratory diseases of poultry.

The acute disease with typical coughing, expulsion of blood and high mortality can be readily identified as laryngotracheitis (Delaplane, 1945; Van Roekel, 1955). In all other forms of the disease, laboratory confirmation should be obtained prior to use of control procedures. Virus can readily be isolated from tracheal and lung tissue by chicken embryo inoculation, by inoculation of trachea and infraorbital sinuses of susceptible chickens (Hitchner and White, 1958a), and by cell culture inoculation (Chomiac et al., 1960).

Demonstration of intranuclear inclusion bodies in tracheal or conjunctival tissues stained with Giemsa stain is also diagnostic of LT virus (Beveridge and Burnet, 1946; Cover and Benton, 1958). Inclusion bodies can be consistently demonstrated in birds only in early stages (1–5 days) of the disease, as necrosis and desquamation destroy the affected epithelial tissue. The action of the fixative of low pH is important in the formation of the inclusion body (Cover and Benton, 1958). The reliability of this procedure, as shown by Keller and Hebel (1962), indicated inclusion bodies could be observed in 57% of 60 specimens while virus was isolated from 72% of the same specimens.

A rapid diagnostic method was developed by Pirozok et al. (1957) in which tissues are embedded in a carbo-wax, sectioned, stained, and are available for examination in 3 hours. Sevoian (1960) developed a rapid procedure for identification of inclusion bodies in tissue by a simultaneous fixation and dehydration procedure. A rapid identification of virus in tracheal tissue can be made with the use of fluorescent antibody (Braune and Gentry, 1965).

Intratracheal inoculation of susceptible and immune chicks with tracheal exudate or tissue suspension from affected birds provides a reliable diagnostic procedure (Pulsford and Stokes, 1953).

The most common isolation procedure has been the inoculation of 9–12-day-old embryonating chicken eggs with tracheal exudate or tracheal and lung suspension (Gorham, 1957). The material is treated with antibiotic solutions (penicillin and streptomycin) and inoculated on the chorioallantoic (CA) membrane or into the allantoic sac. The CA route, the most sensitive method, results in a 2 log or greater titer than by other routes (Hitchner and White, 1958b; Jordan, 1964b).

Laryngotracheitis virus causes focal proliferation of the chorioallantoic membrane (Fig. 17.2). The lesions which appear as early as 3 days vary from a few scattered foci to large numbers involving the entire chorioallantoic membrane. Intranuclear inclusions can be readily demonstrated in cells of the proliferated tissue.

Changes consisting of giant cell formation, intranuclear inclusions, and necrosis are formed in chicken embryo kidney cell monolayers within 24 hours following inoculation (Pulsford, 1960; Chang et al., 1960; Fitzgerald and Hanson, 1963) (Fig. 17.3).

SEROLOGY

Virus neutralization has been used successfully to demonstrate the presence or absence of LT antibodies. Burnet (1936) observed that viral neutralization could be measured by utilizing the CAM pock counting technique. Viral neutralization tests can be conducted by mixing serial tenfold dilutes of the viral suspension with equal quantities of antiserum or by diluting the sera 1:2 or 1:5 (Hitchner et al., 1958). The serum-virus mixture should be held at room temperature for an hour before inoculating to insure adequate neutralization (Burnet, 1936; Hitchner et al., 1958).

TREATMENT

No drug has been effective in reducing the extent of lesions or relieving signs of the disease. If a diagnosis of laryngotracheitis is obtained early in a disease outbreak, vaccination of the unaffected birds may induce partial protection before the infection is extended to the remaining birds.

PREVENTION AND CONTROL

MANAGEMENT PROCEDURES

As LT infections often result in some carrier birds, it is extremely important to avoid mixing vaccinated or recovered chickens with susceptible chickens. Special precautions should be taken to obtain complete history when mixing breeding stock. The use of sound sanitation procedures will avoid exposing susceptible chickens by means of contaminated equipment or buildings as the virus will survive for 10 days at temperatures of 13–23° C (Schalm and Beach, 1935).

IMMUNIZATION

Vaccination has provided a method of developing resistance in a susceptible chicken population located in a geographic area where laryngotracheitis is endemic. Vaccination is recommended in flocks raised on farms where the disease has previously occurred. However, as vaccination can result in carrier birds, it is not recommended in a geographic area where the disease is not prevalent (Black and Beaudette, 1934; Nicol et al., 1945).

Immunization of chickens was first accomplished by deliberately exposing the birds through the introduction of infected chickens into the susceptible flocks. Hudson and Beaudette (1932b,c) discovered that LT virus could be propagated by applying the virus directly on the cloacal mucosa. The chickens inoculated by this method were found to resist intratracheal inoculation of the virus. Later Brandly and Bushnell (1934) recommended vaccination of cloacal tissue as it provided a more consistent immunity. Recent information concerning the role of bursa tissue in antibody production provides greater emphasis to this concept.

Effective vaccination has been measured by examination of the bursa of birds 4–5 days following vaccination for edematous catarrhal or hemorrhagic inflammation commonly referred to as "takes" (Gibbs, 1934b). Effective vaccination of chickens has been accomplished by exposure via infraorbital sinuses (Shibley et al., 1962), intranasal instillation (Benton et al., 1958), and feather follicle (Molgard and Cavett, 1947; Hunt, 1959). Cell culture attenuated strains are capable of inducing resistance when used as vaccines (Gelenczei and Marty, 1964).

Virus attenuated by cell culture passage (Gelenczei and Marty, 1964), feather follicle passage (Molgard and Cavett, 1947; Hunt, 1959, 1962; Hungerford, 1962), or mi'd enzootic strains (Pulsford and Stokes, 1953) all have been capable of inducing resistance in susceptible birds. Immunity apparently is enhanced in endemic areas by subclinical infections (Hungerford, 1962).

Vaccination has been accomplished with virulent and avirulent strains. The virulent vaccines should be used with caution and applied to the vent or cloacal tissues to avoid exposure of the respiratory tissues. Care should be taken to dip the brush into the vaccine before each application. Inoculation of the bursa of Fabricius provides a more consistent uniform method of exposure but is limited to the growing chick. The vaccinated birds should be examined for takes 4–5 days following application of the vaccine. Inflammation of the mucous membranes of the inoculated tissues indicates a take and usually signifies the birds will resist exposure. However, several Australian workers (Oxer, 1945; Seddon, 1952; Jordan, 1964a) have reported LT breaks even when a high percentage of takes was observed (Seddon, 1952). Exposure of the upper respiratory tissue to high concentrations of virulent LT virus following cloacal vaccination has resulted in some respiratory signs.

The availability of attenuated LT virus strains precludes the use of virulent strains in most areas. Attenuated virus vaccines applied by the feather follicle, eye drop, or intranasal routes have provided acceptable protection (Gelenczei and Marty, 1964).

REFERENCES

Ahmed, A. A. S., and G. Monreal. 1963. Ueber den Nachweis der latenten Formen der infektiosen Laryngotracheitis der Huhner mittels des Agar-gel-precipitationstestes. *Zentr. Veterinaermed.* 10:110–19.

Anonymous. 1963. Methods for the examination for poultry biologics. *Nat. Acad. Sci. Nat. Res. Council,* Publ. 1038.

Atherton, J. G., and Wilma Anderson. 1957. Propagation in tissue culture of the virus of infectious laryngotracheitis of fowls. *Australian J. Exp. Biol. Med. Sci.* 35:335–46.

Beach, J. R. 1926. Infectious bronchitis of fowls. *J. Am. Vet. Med. Ass.* 68:570–80.

———. 1930. The virus of laryngotracheitis of fowls. *Science* 72:633–34.

———. 1931. A filtrable virus, the cause of infectious laryngotracheitis of chickens. *J. Exp. Med.* 54:809–16.

———. 1935. The survival of the virus of infectious laryngotracheitis in the bursa of Fabricius and cloaca of chickens after "intrabursal" injection. *J. Infect. Diseases* 57:133–38.

Beaudette, F. R. 1930. Infectious bronchitis. *New Jersey Agr. Expt. Sta. Ann. Rept.* 51:286.

Beaudette, F. R. 1937. Infectious laryngotracheitis. *Poultry Sci.* 16:103–5.

———. 1949. Twenty years of progress in immunization against virus diseases of birds. *J. Am. Vet. Med. Ass.* 115:232–44, 367–77.

Benton, W. J., M. S. Cover, and L. M. Greene. 1958. The clinical and serological response of chickens to certain laryngotracheitis viruses. *Avian Diseases* 2:383–96.

Beveridge, W. I. B., and F. M. Burnet. 1946. *Med. Res. Council Spec. Rept. Ser.* No. 256.

Black, L. M., and F. R. Beaudette. 1934. Infectious bronchitis vaccination. *New Jersey Agr. Expt. Sta. Ext. Bull.* 123:1–8.

Brandly, C. A. 1934. Some studies on infectious laryngotracheitis—A preliminary report. Effect of infectious laryngotracheitis on fertility and hatchability. *J. Am. Vet. Med. Ass.* 84:588–95.

———. 1935. The continued propagation of the virus upon the CAM of the hen's egg. *J. Infect. Diseases* 57:201–6.

———. 1936. Studies on the egg-propagated viruses of infectious laryngotracheitis and fowl pox. *J. Am. Vet. Med. Ass.* 88:587–99.

———. 1937. Studies on certain filtrable viruses. (1) Factors concerned with the egg-propagation of fowl pox and infectious laryngotracheitis. *J. Am. Vet. Med. Ass.* 90:479–87.

Brandly, C. A., and L. D. Bushnell. 1934. A report of some investigations of infectious laryngotracheitis. *Poultry Sci.* 13:212–17.

Braune, M. O., and R. F. Gentry. 1965. Standardization of the fluorescent antibody technique for the detection of avian respiratory viruses. *Avian Diseases* 9:535–44.

Burnet, F. M. 1934. The propagation of the virus of infectious laryngotracheitis on the CAM of the developing egg. *Brit. J. Exp. Pathol.* 15:52–55.

———. 1936. Immunological studies with the virus of infectious laryngotracheitis of fowls using the developing egg technique. *J. Exp. Med.* 63:685–701.

Chang, P. W., V. J. Yates, A. H. Dardiri, and D. E. Fry. 1960. Some observations on the propagation of infectious laryngotracheitis in tissue culture. *Avian Diseases* 4:384–90.

Chomiac, T. W., R. E. Luginbuhl, and C. F. Helmboldt. 1960. Tissue culture and chicken embryo techniques for infectious laryngotracheitis. *Avian Diseases* 4:235–46.

Cover, M. S., and W. J. Benton. 1958. The biological variation of infectious laryngotracheitis virus. *Avian Diseases* 2:375–83.

Cruickshank, J. G., D. M. Berry, and B. Hay. 1963. The fine structure of infectious laryngotracheitis virus. *Virology* 20:376–78.

Darlington, R. W., and C. James. 1966. Biological and morphological aspects of the growth of equine abortion virus. *J. Bacteriol.* 92:250–57.

Delaplane, J. P. 1945. Differential diagnosis of respiratory diseases of fowl. *J. Am. Vet. Med. Ass.* 106:83.

Dobson, N. 1935. Infectious laryngotracheitis in poultry. *Vet. Record* 15:1467–71.

Fitzgerald, J. E., and L. E. Hanson. 1963. A comparison of some properties of laryngotracheitis and herpes simplex viruses. *Am. J. Vet. Res.* 24:1297–1303.

Fritzsche, K., and E. Gerriers. 1959. *Gefluegel Krankheiten.* Verlag. Paul Parey, Berlin-Hamburg. Pp. 77–81.

Gelenczei, E. F., and E. W. Marty. 1964. Studies on a tissue-culture modified infectious laryngotracheitis virus. *Avian Diseases* 8:105–22.

Gibbs, C. S. 1931. Infectious laryngotrachetitis. *Mass. Agr. Expt. Sta. Bull.* 280:241.

———. 1932. Chronic carriers of infectious laryngotracheitis. *J. Am. Vet. Med. Ass.* 81:651–54.

———. 1933. The Massachusetts plan for the eradication and control of infectious laryngotracheitis. *J. Am. Vet. Med. Ass.* 83:214–17.

———. 1934a. Infectious laryngotracheitis field experiments: Vaccination. *Mass. Agr. Expt. Sta. Bull.* 305:57–58.

———. 1934b. Infectious laryngotracheitis vaccination. *Mass. Agr. Expt. Sta. Bull.* 311:1–20.

Goldhaft, T. M. 1961. Viability of pox and laryngotracheitis vaccines. *Avian Diseases* 5:196–200.

Gorham, J. R. 1957. A simple technique for the inoculation of the chorioallantoic membrane of chicken embryos. *Am. J. Vet. Res.* 18:691–92.

Graham, R., F. Thorp, and W. A. James. 1930. Subacute or chronic infectious avian laryngotracheitis. *J. Infect. Diseases* 47:87–91.

Gwatkin, R. 1925. Some notes on avian diphtheria. *Ontario Vet. Coll. Rept.*, pp. 54–61.

Hinshaw, W. R. 1931. A survey of infectious laryngotracheitis of fowls. *Calif. Agr. Expt. Sta. Bull.* 520:1–36.

Hinshaw, W. R., E. C. Jones, and H. W. Graybill. 1931. A study of mortality and egg production in flocks affected with infectious laryngotracheitis. *Poultry Sci.* 10:375–82.

Hitchner, S. B., and P. G. White. 1958a. A comparison of the drop and brush methods for applying infectious laryngotracheitis vaccine. *American Scientific Laboratories Inc. Res. Rept.* 4.

———. 1958b. A comparison of embryo and bird infectivity using five strains of laryngotracheitis virus. *Poultry Sci.* 37:684–90.

Hitchner, S. B., and R. W. Winterfield. 1960. Revaccination procedures for infectious laryngotracheitis. *Avian Diseases* 4:291–303.

Hitchner, S. B., Catherine A. Shea, and P. G.

White. 1958. Studies on the serum neutralization test for the diagnosis of laryngotracheitis in chickens. *Avian Diseases* 2: 258–69.

Holmes, I. H., and D. H. Watson. 1963. An electron microscope study of the attachment and penetration of herpes virus in BHK 21 cells. *Virology* 21:112–23.

Hudson, C. B., and F. R. Beaudette. 1932a. The susceptibility of pheasants and a pheasant bantam cross to the virus of infectious bronchitis. *Cornell Vet.* 22:70–74.

———. 1932b. The susceptibility of cloacal tissue to the virus of infectious bronchitis. *Cornell Vet.* 23:63–65.

———. 1932c. Infection of the cloaca with the virus of infectious bronchitis. *Science* 76:34.

Hungerford, T. G. 1962. *Diseases of Poultry,* 3rd ed. Angus and Robertson, Ltd., Sydney, London, Melbourne, and Wellington.

Hunt, S. 1959. The feather follicle method of vaccinating baby chicks with laryngotracheitis vaccine. *Proc. Poultry Sci. Conv.,* pp. 29–30.

———. 1962. Field experience with feather follicle vaccination of day-old chickens for infectious laryngotracheitis. *Proc. 12th World's Poultry Congr.,* pp. 335–38.

Jordan, F. T. W. 1958. Some observations on infectious laryngotracheitis. *Vet. Record* 70:605–10.

———. 1963. Further observations of the epidemiology of infectious laryngotracheitis of poultry. *J. Comp. Pathol. Therap.* 73:253–64.

———. 1964a. The control of infectious laryngotracheitis. *Zentr. Veterinaermed. Ser. B* 11:15–32.

———. 1964b. Diagnosis of infectious laryngotracheitis by chick embryo inoculation. *J. Comp. Pathol. Therap.* 74:119–28.

———. 1966. A review of the literature on infectious laryngotracheitis (ILT). *Avian Diseases* 10:1–26.

Keller, K., and P. Hebel. 1962. Diagnostico de las inclusiones de laringotraqueitis infecciosa en frotis y cortes histologicos. *Zooiatria* (Chile) 4, 1:1.

Kernohan, G. 1931a. Infectious laryngotracheitis of fowls. *J. Am. Vet. Med. Ass.* 78: 196–202.

———. 1931b. Infectious laryngotracheitis in pheasants. *J. Am. Vet. Med. Ass.* 78:553–55.

Kingsbury, F. W., and E. L. Jungherr. 1957. Indirect transmission of infectious laryngotracheitis in chickens. *Poultry Sci.* 36: 1133. (Abstr.)

Komarov, A., and F. R. Beaudette. 1932. Carriers of infectious bronchitis. *Poultry Sci.* 11:335–38.

Magnusson, H. 1940. En ny honssjukdom (Inf. Inflaryngotrakeit). *Scand. Vet. Tidskr.* 30: 629–31.

Marek, K. 1948. Zakazny laryngotracheitis kur. *Med. Weterynar.* 4:767–70.

May, H. G., and R. P. Tittsler. 1925. Tracheolaryngitis in poultry. *J. Am. Vet. Med. Ass.* 67:229–31.

Mayr, A., P. Dorn, and H. Mahnel. 1964. An atypical mild form of infectious laryngotracheitis with special reference to diagnosis and differential diagnosis. *Zentr. Veterinaermed.* 11B:572–83.

Molgard, P. C., and J. W. Cavett. 1947. The feather follicle method of vaccinating with fowl laryngotracheitis vaccine. *Poultry Sci.* 26:563–67.

Nicol, G., D. T. Oxer, and C. J. R. Gorrie. 1945. The difficulty of differential diagnosis of infectious laryngotracheitis on clinical grounds from other respiratory diseases. *Australian Vet. J.* 21:49–50.

Nii, S., C. Morgan, and H. M. Rose. 1968. Electron microscopy of herpes simplex virus. II. Sequence of development. *J. Virol.* (Kyoto) 2:517–36.

Oxer, D. T. 1945. Vaccination against infectious laryngotracheitis. *Australian Vet. J.* 21:154–55.

Pirozok, R. P., C. F. Helmboldt, and E. L. Jungherr. 1957. A rapid histological technique for the diagnosis of infectious avian laryngotracheitis. *J. Am. Vet. Med. Ass.* 130: 406–8.

Pulsford, M. F. 1953. Possible P-Q type variation in infectious laryngotracheitis virus. *Nature* 172:1193–95.

———. 1954. Variation in the virus of infectious laryngotracheitis and its epizoological implications. *Proc. 10th World's Poultry Congr.,* pp. 242–44.

———. 1960. The growth of three strains of infectious laryngotracheitis virus of fowls in tissue culture. *Australian J. Exp. Biol. Med. Sci.* 38:153–62.

———. 1961. Epidemiology of infectious laryngotracheitis of poultry. *Australian Vet. J.* 37:97–99, 272–73.

Pulsford, M. F., and J. Stokes. 1953. Infectious laryngotracheitis in South Australia. *Australian Vet. J.* 29:8–12.

Pulsford, M. F., H. V. Chamberlain, and J. Topham. 1956. A preliminary note on laryngotracheitis vaccination with virus of low virulence. *Australian Vet. J.* 32:138–40.

Raggi, L. G., and G. G. Lee. 1965. Infectious laryngotracheitis outbreaks following vaccination. *Avian Diseases* 9:559–65.

Raggi, L. G., J. R. Brownell, and G. F. Stewart. 1961. Effects of infectious laryngotracheitis virus on egg production and quality. *Poultry Sci.* 40:134–40.

Reynolds, H. A., A. M. Watrach, and L. E. Hanson. 1968. Development of the nuclear inclusion bodies of infectious laryngotracheitis. *Avian Diseases* 12:332–47.

Rislakki, V. 1965. Case report: Infectious laryngotracheitis of poultry in Finland. *Avian Diseases* 9:339–42.

Satriano, S. F., R. E. Luginbuhl, C. F. Helmboldt, and E. L. Jungherr. 1957. Isolation of infectious laryngotracheitis virus from lachrymal fluid of chicks. *Poultry Sci.* 36: 1155. (Abstr.)

Schalm, O. W., and J. R. Beach. 1935. The resistance of the virus of infectious laryngotracheitis to certain physical and chemical factors. *J. Infect. Diseases* 56:210–23.

Seddon, H. R. 1952. Infectious laryngotracheitis, pp. 122–41. In Seddon, H. R. (ed.). *Diseases of Domestic Animals in Australia,* Part 4. Protozoan and Viral Diseases, Dept. Health, Serv. Publ. 8.

Seddon, H. R., and L. Hart. 1935. The occurrence of infectious laryngotracheitis in New South Wales. *Australian Vet. J.* 11:212–22.

———. 1936. Infectivity experiments with the virus of laryngotracheitis of fowls. *Australian Vet. J.* 12:13–16.

Seifried, O. 1931. Histopathology of infectious laryngotracheitis in chickens. *J. Exp. Med.* 56:817–26.

Sevoian, M. 1960. A quick method for the diagnosis of avian pox and I.L.T. *Avian Diseases* 4:474–77.

Shibley, G. P., R. E. Luginbuhl, and C. F. Helmboldt. 1962. A study of infectious laryngotracheitis strains. I. Comparison of serological and immunogenic properties. *Avian Diseases* 6:59–71.

Van Heelsbergen, T. 1929. *Handbuch der Gefluegelkrankheiten und der Gefluegelzucht.* Ferdinand Enke, Stuttgart. Pp. 262–64.

Van Roekel, H. V. 1955. Respiratory diseases of poultry. *Advan. Vet. Sci.* 2:64–97.

Watrach, A. M., A. E. Vatter, L. E. Hanson, M. A. Watrach, and H. E. Rhoades. 1959. Electron microscopic studies of the virus of avian infectious laryngotracheitis. *Am. J. Vet. Res.* 20:537–44.

Watrach, A. M., L. E. Hanson, and M. A. Watrach. 1963. The structure of infectious laryngotracheitis virus. *Virology* 21:601–8.

Webster, R. G. 1959. Studies on infectious laryngotracheitis in New Zealand. *New Zealand Vet. J.* 7:67–71.

Wildy, P., and D. H. Watson. 1962. Electron microscope studies on the architecture of animal virus particles. *Cold Springs Harbor Symp. Quant. Biol.* 27:25–47.

Winterfield, R. W., and I. G. So. 1968. Susceptibility of turkeys to infectious laryngotracheitis. *Avian Diseases* 12:186–90.

CHAPTER 18

NEWCASTLE DISEASE

❖

R. P. HANSON

*Departments of Veterinary Science
and Bacteriology
University of Wisconsin
Madison, Wisconsin*

❖

FOUR FORMS of Newcastle disease (ND)—Doyle's, Beach's, Beaudette's, and Hitchner's—have been described that are so clinically and pathologically distinctive that a discussion which treats of signs and lesions, economic significance, even of the epizootiology of the disease in only a general fashion becomes confusing and misleading.

All four pathologic forms are caused by true Newcastle disease viruses that are morphologically indistinguishable. All induce the production of antibodies that cross-protect, cross-neutralize, and inhibit the hemagglutinins of each other. Differences in titer that occur are attributable to quantitative differences in the antigens of the envelope and to antigenic avidity rather than distinctive antigens (Upton et al., 1953). The virus population that can be recovered from an infected individual suffering from a given form of the disease is not necessarily uniform and may, in fact, contain a number of genetically distinct subpopulations which are separable in culture. Nevertheless, the virus recovered from a given form of the disease with rare exceptions induces that form of the disease. Consequently the form of the disease has epizootiological as well as pathological significance.

An infectious, highly contagious, and destructive malady, Newcastle disease attacks chiefly chickens and turkeys. Various other birds as well as certain mammals, particularly man, may also be infected with the virus.

1. Doyle's form of the disease, first recognized in 1926 (Doyle, 1927), is an acute lethal infection of all ages of chickens. Hemorrhagic lesions of the digestive tract are a prominent pathologic feature. Some writers have called this form, which is caused by certain velogenic strains, Asiatic NDV.

2. Beach's form of the disease described 15 years later (Beach, 1942, 1946) is an acute and frequently lethal infection of chickens of all ages, characterized by lesions in the respiratory tract and nervous system. Hemorrhages are conspicuously absent from the digestive tract. It was initially called nervous respiratory disease or pneumoencephalitis and is caused by certain velogenic strains.

3. Beaudette's form of the disease recognized a few years later (Beaudette and Black, 1946) is an acute respiratory and sometimes lethal nervous infection of young chickens. In older birds mortality is rare. Some of the mesogenic strains which produce this form have been used as vaccines.

4. Hitchner's form of the disease, the last to be described (Hitchner and Johnson, 1948; Hitchner, 1950), is a mild or inapparent respiratory infection of chickens caused by lentogenic strains. Mortality is rare in birds of any age. Several lentogenic strains are widely used as vaccines.

Confusion over the identity of a disease that has several forms led to creation of local names, some of which have become synonyms (Beaudette, 1943; Brandly et al., 1946a): pseudo-fowl pest, pseudovogel-pest, atypische Geflugelpest, pseudo-poultry plague, avian pest, avian distemper, Ranikhet disease, and avian pneumoencephalitis.

High mortality of 50–100% among adult birds has characterized Doyle's form of the disease in many countries: Java (Kraneveld, 1926), England (Doyle, 1927; Reid, 1961), India (Sahai, 1937), Philippines (Coronel, 1948) and Africa (Kaschula, 1961a,b). Flocks were devastated and market operations upset. Less lethal forms of Beach and Beaudette have also been the source of major economic losses. Crippling as well as impaired growth and poor feed utilization often occur among surviving birds. The greatest loss among layers frequently results from reduced production and impairment of eggshell and albumen quality (Lorenz and Newlon, 1944; Berg et al., 1947).

Reduction of fertility and hatchability of eggs has also been reported, and additional losses have come from restrictions upon the export of eggs (both hatching and table eggs), of baby chicks, of breeding and other stock, and of dressed poultry (Rept. Comm. Fowl Pest, 1962).

Man exposed to Newcastle disease virus develops conjunctivitis (Lippman, 1952), usually mild and persisting for 1–2 days but on occasion quite severe and even leading to some lasting impairment of vision (Hanson and Brandly, 1958). A generalized disease has rarely been reported (Quinn et al., 1952). Most infections have occurred among laboratory workers who handle the virus, either in research or vaccine production laboratories (Brandly, 1951). Vaccinators and individuals who eviscerate and prepare poultry for market may become infected. On occasion this has led to compensation for industry-acquired infection. Infections have been very rare among individuals rearing poultry and preparing dressed poultry for the table (Evans, 1955, 1956).

HISTORY

Accounts of the various facets of the history of Newcastle disease, recognition of the disease, attempts to understand the nature of the etiological agent and the disease induced, and measures used in its control have been summarized and reviewed: Beaudette's reports to the U.S. Livestock Sanitary Association (Beaudette, 1943, 1948, 1949, 1950, 1951), the Huntington Laboratory reports (Brandly et al., 1946a,b), the University of Wisconsin Symposium (Hanson, 1964), and the Canadian Department of Agriculture Monographs (Lancaster, 1966).

From a review of the literature it would appear that Newcastle disease first occurred in and around seaports, apparently as a consequence of commerce moving by sea. Only much later in these countries did it appear in the interior. While this may be the correct reading of the situation, one must remember that individuals with training required to diagnose diseases of poultry are more apt to be located in or near the populous centers of commerce, where birds are moving to market and where it takes the least effort on the part of the grower to bring a sick bird to the attention of a pathologist. Secondly, it is in such situations that sea birds, several species of which have been found to be infected on some remote sea coasts (Wilson, 1950; Blaxland, 1951), would also be most likely to contaminate poultry if they are a natural reservoir.

The places at which a disease is recognized and the time at which it is recognized are as much dependent on the availability of individuals trained to recognize and distinguish disease as on the occurrence of the disease itself. That the most acute form of the disease was recognized first and that subsequently milder and milder forms were seen until the inapparent form was at last discovered some 20 years after the disease was first described should not be taken as an indication that these forms actually appeared in this sequence, but rather that recognition of the less virulent forms had to wait for the development of more sophisticated and sensitive methods.

ORIGIN

At least three alternative hypotheses exist for the origin of a virus that is the cause of a previously unrecognized disease. These hypotheses should be considered in an attempt to understand the history of Newcastle disease.

1. The virus originated at some point in time and place as a result of a major mutation or series of mutations from a related virus and then was disseminated from that location throughout the world.

2. The virus existed in essentially its present form in some other species, probably a vertebrate animal in which it induced an unrecognized disease. The contact of this species with the domestic chicken, the principal host of NDV, while infrequent, provided an occasional opportunity for introduction of the virus into this population.

3. The virus has always been present as an unrecognized and presumably mild virus disease of chickens. Changes in the nature of the host population in recent years have provided the opportunity for selection of viral mutants of greater virulence, thus giving rise to the present overt and distinctive disease.

While there is not enough evidence to substantiate any of these three theories, their relative probability can be weighed. There are two serious problems with the first hypothesis. Newcastle disease was recognized almost simultaneously in three widely separated places in 1926. This situation is not consistent with the idea of a single origin and subsequent dissemination of a new entity. Secondly, we know of no other instance of a new virus arising from another one by mutation, nor of a way to induce such a major change in the laboratory. Influenza A subtypes, which on the basis of our knowledge of their epidemiology have a point of origin, are the result of minor mutational changes in the influenza virion, a situation quite different from the birth of a distinctive antigenic entity.

Newcastle disease virus has been isolated from a rather wide range of wild birds, any one of which might provide the reservoir needed for the second hypothesis. Some of these birds associate directly with chickens, feeding and watering in the same pens and yards. Others feed on poultry offal or manure spread on fields, and still others are killed for sport or as vermin, and their viscera may be fed to poultry. It has never been clear, in instances in which wild birds have been found to be infected, whether they obtained their virus from chickens or the chickens obtained their virus from wild birds. To answer the question of a free-flying reservoir a determination must be made as to whether Newcastle disease virus infection can be maintained in a wild population which is not associated in any way with domestic fowl. It would be most unlikely that aerosol dissemination has been the primary means of spread in a wild dispersed population as it is in dense confined poultry populations. Alternative communication methods are known for such diseases as African swine fever and rabies which have a wildlife reservoir, and this may be true of ND. While Newcastle disease could have been introduced into chickens from a wild reservoir at any time in the past, the airborne infection we know today could not have persisted in chickens in Europe or North America before the rise of intensive year-round poultry production (Taylor, 1964). In the tropics where reproduction occurs throughout the year and live birds move from village to village, hawked by peddlers, a lesser population would presumably have sufficed for survival.

Existence of mild forms of Newcastle disease, such as one described from North Ireland by McFerran (personal communication) and one in Australia by Simmons (1967), would have gone unrecognized in the past, as they undoubtedly still go unrecognized in other parts of the world today. Such a virus, occurring as an enteric infection, would be a logical ancestral form of today's virus and meets the requirements of the third hypothesis. The changes necessary for the development of the several pathologic forms of the disease from such a source have been paralleled in laboratory studies (Estupinan, 1968). A Newcastle disease virus culture recovered in Delaware contained at least 6 genotypes which could be separated by suitable techniques and shown to differ in virulence and antigenic character. This family of genotypes contained 2 members that were of very low virulence and 2 that were highly virulent; yet all components were shown to have originated from a single, highly mutable member of the family. Selective influences could be provided by the major changes in poultry management which have taken place concomitant with the rise of Newcastle disease as a major problem. These include changes in nutrition, in the size and density of a flock, and in the genetics of the bird itself (earlier maturity, increased egg production, and loss of broodiness) (Bird, 1964).

The conjectured evolutionary scheme based on changes in the host is not a new idea. McKercher (1963) has proposed that infectious bovine rhinotracheitis, a recently recognized respiratory disease of cattle, is caused by the same virus as the centuries-old venereally transmitted coital vesicular exanthema of cattle. The earlier form of the disease could and did persist in small herds; the more recent respiratory form can exist only in the large feedlot populations that have been created in the past few decades by new methods of handling cattle—a situation which is analogous to the changes in management of poultry. However, it is still premature to decide which of the hypotheses best accounts for the origin of Newcastle disease virus.

RESEARCH MODEL

Newcastle disease virus has become a model, widely employed by virologists throughout the world who are interested in the nature of life itself. An immense and fascinating literature on substructure of the virion (Kingsbury and Darlington, 1968), steps in its replication (Wheelock, 1963), sequence of enzymatic processes and role of inhibitors (Kingsbury, 1962; Wilson, 1968), mechanism of interferon production (Baron, 1964) and its relevance to viral multiplication provides little at present of practical value to the individual concerned with control of Newcastle disease. The payoff will come in time, probably in some unexpected fashion. By providing new insights and new methods, these fundamental studies provide (as have others in the past) solutions to some problems now facing us.

INCIDENCE AND DISTRIBUTION

Newcastle disease was recognized in 1926 in three widely separated countries—England (Doyle, 1927), Java (Kraneveld, 1926), and Korea (Konno et al., 1929). Two other countries—India (Edwards, 1928) and the Philippines (Farinas, 1930)—were added within a year.

The epizootic described by Doyle spread over the northern English coast around Newcastle on Tyne (from which the common name of the disease was derived) and then disappeared after 9 months, leaving England free of the disease for about 7 years. Kraneveld's pseudo fowl plague of Java and Konno's new fowl pest of Korea persisted in those countries and soon became recognized in many areas of the Far East.

Within 10 years ND had been reported in Japan (Nakamura et al., 1933), East Africa (Hudson, 1937; Vandemaele, 1961), and Australia (Johnstone, 1931), usually persisting but sometimes disappearing as in Australia (Albiston and Gorrie, 1942). By the time of World War II it had appeared in several countries of the Middle East (Komarov, 1940; Berke and Golem, 1949). Italy was the first European nation to experience it (Wagener, 1948, Brandly et al., 1946a), but within a few years almost all other countries on the Continent had also recognized it (Eckert, 1957). Additional countries in Africa and Asia that had not previously reported Newcastle disease now also knew it (Lancaster, 1966).

Newcastle disease was first reported in the United States in 1944 (Minard and Jungherr, 1944; Beach, 1944), at a time when the disease was already established on both coasts. It had been present for 5 or 6 years in California in a pathologic form (Beach) that had not previously been recog-

nized as Newcastle disease and which had been known as respiratory nervous disease (Stover, 1942) and later as pneumoencephalitis (Beach, 1942). On the east coast it was initially inapparent (Minard and Jungherr, 1944). Beaudette later suggested (Beaudette and Hudson, 1956) that the disease may have existed in a mild form in the United States as early as 1938. By 1948 it was established over most of the country (Byerly, 1948).

Canada first reported the virus in 1948 (Walker, 1948). In South America the disease appeared in the fifties: Venezuela (Divo, 1950), Chile (Gallardo, 1951), and Colombia (Arenas, 1952). Argentina did not experience an epizootic until 1961 (Monteverde et al., 1962).

The disease recognized initially in all nations was either Doyle's type (reported from 1926 to 1944 in Asia and Europe) or Beach's type (which predominated in America from 1944 to the present). Later the milder forms initially reported from the United States by Beaudette and Black (1946) and Hitchner and Johnson (1948) were found to exist in other parts of the world—Japan (Kawashima et al., 1953), England (Reid, 1955), and France (Lissot, 1956; Fontaine et al., 1965). Some of the strains inducing these mild forms of disease may have been introduced from the United States through importations of poultry or poultry products as has been alleged, but other mild strains are clearly distinguishable from any recovered in the United States, Australia (French et al., 1967), Ireland (McFerran, 1969, personal communication), Russia, and Thailand (Hanson et al., 1967). Today one or more forms of ND are present in all poultry-producing nations of the world.

ETIOLOGY

The agent of Newcastle disease was recovered in 1926 by Doyle (1927) from diseased birds and shown to be filterable and distinguishable antigenically from the virus of fowl plague.

CLASSIFICATION

Newcastle disease virus (NDV) has been classed as a myxovirus. Characteristically this family of viruses contains ribonucleic acid and has a helical structure and an outer lipid-containing envelope. The myxoviruses have been further subdivided into an influenza group and a parainfluenza or paramyxovirus group. Newcastle disease virus belongs to the latter group along with several other avian and animal parainfluenza viruses.

At least 3 antigenically distinctive parainfluenza viruses have been recovered from chickens and turkeys. One isolated in chicken embryos from turkeys in Ontario which were dying of a severe respiratory disease has not yet been described in the literature (Lang, 1969, personal communication). Myxovirus Yucaipa, initially isolated in California from chickens exhibiting a mild respiratory disease and subsequently recovered from turkeys in Alberta and Ontario (Lange, 1969, personal communication), has been described by Bankowski and Corstvet (1960) and Dinter et al. (1964). Fowl parainfluenza 2, apparently distinct from Sendai, has been isolated from apparently normal chicken embryos in Germany (Waterson, 1964; Wagner and Enders-Ruckle, 1966). The other parainfluenza viruses produce disease in mammals (Dinter, 1964). Among them are parainfluenza of cattle, respiratory syncytial virus and mumps virus of man, and 3 antigenically related viruses—measles of man, distemper of the dog, and rinderpest of the cow (Chanock and Coates, 1964).

The true influenza viruses have a smaller virion (80–120 mμ across) and a smaller nucleocapsid (90 Å in diameter) (Andrewes et al., 1955). Influenza viruses affecting birds include fowl plague and a large number of antigenically distinguishable viruses isolated from ducks, turkeys, quail, pheasants, and several wild birds. The avian influenzas share an antigenic component with influenza A viruses of man, swine, and horses. The antigenically distinct influenza B virus affects only man.

MORPHOLOGY

Size and Ultrastructure

Burnet and Ferry (1934), by filtration data, estimated the size of the viral particle to be 80–120 mμ. On the basis of electron micrographs, Bang (1948) later calculated the diameter to be 112 mμ. The present and much more detailed picture of the morphology of Newcastle disease virus is based upon several methods of purification and on examination of negative stained preparations in the electron microscope (Rott and Schafer, 1961; Schafer, 1963; Waterson, 1964). The virion or mature virus unit, which varies in size from 120 to 300 mμ but is usually about 180 mμ (Waterson and Cruickshank, 1963), consists of an envelope and an internal component (Fig. 18.1). The ether-sensitive and osmotically deformable envelope (Bang, 1947) has a pattern of projections or spikes (80 Å long) and contains the antigenic components that stimulate the host to produce hemagglutinin-inhibiting and virus-neutralizing antibodies (Rott, 1964). The significance of great numbers of large and pleomorphic particles in some preparations of virus, particularly of certain clones, has not been established. The internal component or nucleocapsid, also known as the G-antigen or NP-antigen, consists of a long and much coiled tube which has a diameter of 180 Å (Schafer and Rott, 1959). The protein structural units of the tube are arranged in a helix around the central hollow axis; within them and determining the entire configuration is ribonucleic acid.

BIOLOGICAL PROPERTIES

Newcastle disease virus possesses a number of biological and physical characteristics by which it may be distinguished qualitatively or quantitatively from other myxoviruses and by which strains of NDV may be distinguished from each other. Among these properties are the abilities to agglutinate and to lyse erythrocytes, to induce toxic changes without multiplication, to enter certain cells and replicate, to infect and incite various signs and lesions in certain hosts and cause the death of some hosts, to be specifically neutralized by or to react with antibodies, and to be inactivated by selected chemical agents under defined conditions. If the procedures used in determining these properties are properly standardized and controlled, all the actions can be quantitated and the results obtained can be repeated with a considerable degree of exactness.

Hemagglutination

Foremost among the biological properties of NDV is its ability to adsorb to the surface of red cells and to induce their aggregation. Hemagglutination of NDV was first described by Burnet (1942), who also found this action to be inhibited by specific antiserum. The hemagglutinin is structurally identified with projections on the envelope

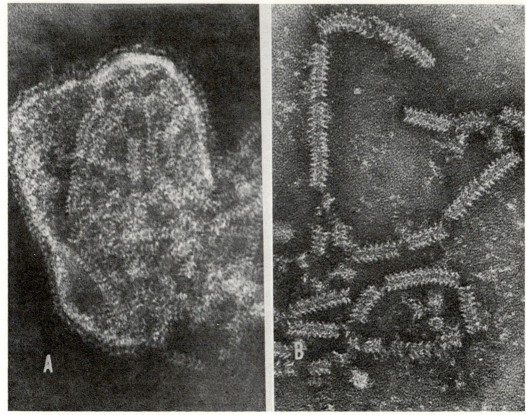

FIG. 18.1—Virion of Newcastle disease virus (Italian strain). (A) Rupture of envelope through which inner component is emerging. (B) Fragments of inner component. Preparation negatively stained with phosphotungstic acid. ✕300,-000. (Courtesy June D. Almeida and A. P. Waterson)

of the virus (Rott, 1964), and it has been chemically determined to be associated with the enzyme neuraminidase. Hemagglutination may be measured by the sedimentation rate of agglutinated red cells (Hirst and Pickels, 1942) or by the pattern which the aggregated cells form on a curved glass surface (Salk, 1944). The latter has been found to be the most practical method of quantitating the hemagglutinating activity of the virus. The process of hemagglutination consists of two stages: attachment of the virus to the receptor substance on the cell surface (agglutination) and destruction of the receptor substance by the enzyme neuraminidase (Ackermann, 1964). The second stage (McCollum and Brandly, 1955b; Sagik and Levine, 1957) is associated with the release of the virus from the surface of the cell (elution). The rate of elution may be measured by repeatedly resuspending cells until agglutination no longer takes place in any of a series of virus dilutions. It may be complete within 30 minutes or may take more than 12 hours, depending on the strain of virus. Rate of elution as measured in this fashion is not an exact index of neuraminidase activity. The latter is better measured by the destruction of a specially prepared substrate fetuin (Laver and Kilbourne, 1966; Estupinan, 1968).

While erythrocytes of all amphibia, reptiles, and birds are agglutinated to some degree by NDV (Clark and Nagler, 1943; Placidi and Santucci, 1956), some mammalian erythrocytes are inagglutinable. Man, mouse, and guinea pig erythrocytes are agglutinated by all strains of NDV; those of cattle, goat, sheep, swine, and horses are agglutinated by some but not all strains (Winslow et al., 1950b). The erythrocytes of certain individual cattle may be agglutinated by one Newcastle strain while cells of another individual are not. The sensitivity of any erythrocyte to agglutination, particularly such variably reactive cells as those of cattle, is dependent in part on ionic concentration of the salts and the pH of the suspending solution. Reported lack of agglutinability of certain mammalian cells by some NDV strains appears to be explained by their rapid elution, a process which occurs before small and slowly moving erythrocytes have had time to settle to form a pattern (Barahona, 1969).

Erythrocytes are not the only type of cell to which the virus adsorbs and which may be agglutinated as a result of this adsorption. Chu (1953) demonstrated that sperm cells may be agglutinated by the action of NDV. The adsorption of NDV to brain cells and other cells may be demonstrated by the reduction such adsorption induces in the ability of the virus preparation to subsequently agglutinate avian erythrocytes (Piraino and Hanson, 1960).

Approximately 100,000 virus-infective units equal 1 hemagglutinating unit. The number of viral particles in a preparation may be approximated on the basis of its hemagglutinating activity. However, the hemagglutinating activity of the virus is not necessarily inactivated at the same rate as is the infectivity of the virus preparation (Hanson et al., 1949; Tolba and Eskarous, 1962). Some strains of NDV which lose their hemagglutinating activity on treatment at 56° C within 5 minutes remain capable of infecting embryonated eggs or other suitable hosts even after a further period of 25 minutes of heating. Other strains retain their ability to hemagglutinate after treatment at 56° C for 180–240 minutes, although their ability to produce infection was lost within the first 90 minutes. In this respect NDV differs from the influenza viruses, all of which lose their ability to infect embryonated eggs before they lose their ability to hemagglutinate. The rate at which the hemagglutinin is destroyed by heat is characteristic of an ND strain and may be used as a property for differentiating it from other strains.

Hemolysis

Like other parainfluenzas, NDV possesses a hemolysin. The virus is capable of lysing those erythrocytes that it can agglutinate (Kilham, 1949; Burnet, 1950; Burnet and Lind, 1950). The hemolytic activity of virus preparations is enhanced by freezing and thawing, dialysis, sonic vibration, and osmotic shock (McCollum and Brandly, 1955a). The salt concentration and pH of the suspending solution and the temperature at which the reaction takes place are important (Granoff and Henle, 1954). Picken (1964) has suggested that the hemolytic capability of NDV can be separated from its hemagglutinative activity by chemical procedures.

REPLICATION

Replication of NDV has been studied in cell culture systems. The virion, on reaching a cell surface, presumably adsorbs to it as it does to erythrocytes. The virion was believed to pass through the cell membrane by viropexis (Silverstein and Marcus, 1964). More recent investigations suggest that the penetration of myxoviruses is more analogous to that of the phage in that the viral envelope remains on the cell membrane and only the inner components of the virion enter the cell (Morgan and Howe, 1968). On entry the virion loses its integrity, the envelope disappears, and it is supposed that the nucleoprotein core becomes a long filament. Infective virus cannot be found for the next 3 hours. During the eclipse period, NDV-specific antigen can be demonstrated by complement fixation and by use of fluorescent antibody. First to be detected is the NP antigen in the cytoplasm near the nucleus (Rott, 1964). Then the hemagglutinating antigen and neuraminidase can be found throughout the cytoplasm. The specific antigens accumulate, and structures identical in appearance to the mature virion appear just within the cell membrane 3–4 hours after infection (Kingsbury, 1962; Wheelock, 1963). Sometimes these particles pack the microvilli. If the cell is destroyed by sonic disruption, the particles are found to be infectious. In the usual course of events the virions are released as some microvilli are sloughed from the cell membrane (Bang, 1952). Liberation of virus starts 4 hours after infection and can continue for another 4 hours without destruction of vital processes of the infected cell. An excess of virus-specific substances, external NP antigen, viromicrosomes, and released hemagglutinin are produced within cells that are not incorporated into the virions (Rott, 1964).

There is some evidence that the virion may be produced either at the cell surface and incorporate cell membrane substance or within the cytoplasm and incorporate endoplasmic reticulum substance (Rott and Schafer, 1962). The first class of particles is sensitive to hydroxylamine and is usually avirulent for chickens. The second class is resistant to hydroxylamine treatment and is usually virulent for chickens.

NDV interferes with the multiplication and pathologic expression of certain other viruses and in turn is interfered with by certain viruses (Chanock, 1955; Morimoto et al., 1962; Raggi et al., 1963). Mixed infections in chickens can result in aborted disease and immunologically reduced response (Hanson et al., 1956). In cell cultures, interference induced by other viruses on multiplication of NDV has been utilized in the development of procedures to detect noncytopathic viruses (Shimizu et al., 1964). Conditions under which Newcastle disease virus induces the formation of interferon in many host systems has been extensively studied (Baron, 1964). Mixed infections consisting of NDV and influenza virus sometimes result in production of combined forms, a type of recombinant (Granoff and Hirst, 1954; Granoff, 1962).

RESISTANCE TO AGENTS

The stability of NDV can be measured on the basis of alterations in the ability of the virus to infect, to agglutinate cells, and to induce an immunogenic response. These abilities can be destroyed at varying rates by exposure to such physical and chemical treatments as heat, light, ultraviolet, x-ray, oxidation processes, pH changes, and chemical compounds. The rate at which the reactivity of the virus is destroyed varies with the strain of virus. It is also dependent on the time of exposure to treatment, the quantity of virus which is initially exposed, the nature of the suspending medium, and interactions among treatment variables.

Thermal

The sensitivity of the virus to thermal changes has been studied in greater detail than has any other environmental factor (Hanson et al., 1949; Foster and Thompson, 1957). All activity of the virus is destroyed within 1 minute at 100° C. At 56° C the destruction of infectivity, hemagglutinative activity, and immunogenicity occur within periods of 5 minutes to 6 hours. At 37° C, hours and days are required to in-

duce these changes; at 20° C and 8° C, months and years pass before all reactivity of the virus is lost.

Ultraviolet Rays and pH

NDV is destroyed by exposure to ultraviolet light rays in a similar fashion to that of other myxoviruses (Levinson et al., 1944). It has a rather broad stability in the presence of varying hydrogen ion concentrations. The infectivity is retained for many hours at a pH as low as 2 and as high as 10 (Moses et al., 1947).

Chemical

The inactivating effect of chemicals is very much dependent on substances in the suspending medium, large quantities of protein reducing the effect of chemicals and delaying the inactivation of the virus. Formalin (Brandly et al., 1946c), beta-propiolactone (Mack and Chotisen, 1955), and phenol have been used to destroy the infectivity without severely damaging the immunogenicity of the preparation. At low temperatures dilute formalin will destroy the infectivity without markedly affecting the hemagglutinin and without readily detectable effect upon the immunogenicity of the preparation. All known viricidal chemicals will destroy NDV with reasonable rapidity (Tilley and Anderson, 1947; Cunningham, 1948; Beamer and Prier, 1950).

Environmental

The stability of NDV in nature is greatly dependent on the medium in which the virus is present, e.g. decaying carcasses, feces (Zakomirdin, 1963; Mickalov and Vrtiak, 1963), drying or fermenting matter (Olesiuk, 1951; Boyd and Hanson, 1958), or mucous droplets in air. Proteinaceous matter may not only be protective but may nullify the action of the disinfectant (Walker et al., 1953). Environmental conditions, particularly warm temperature and solar radiation, facilitate the destruction by chemicals. Freezing temperatures suspend most inactivating procedures (Dobson and Simmins, 1951). When disinfection is desired it should follow physical cleaning and in winter should be carried out only in the presence of supplemental heat.

STRAIN CLASSIFICATION

A strain of NDV is a culture that has been recovered from a chicken or other ani-

TABLE 18.1. ✨ Characteristics of Some Representatives of Newcastle Virus Strains

Test System	NDV Strains							
	Bl	F	Roak-in	MK107	Hick.	GB	Herts	Milano
Chick embryo fibroblast monolayer								
Plaque types	C*	C*	C	C	C/R	C	C/R	C/R
Plaque sizes (mm)	1*	1*	0.5	0.5	0.5–4	1–2	0.5–4	0.5–4
Plaque populations (total of types and sizes)	1*	1*	1	1	6	2	2	3
Chicken embryo (10-day allantoic sac)								
Mean death time of minimum lethal dose in hours	128	168	70	65	40	50	56	40
Chicken (day-old, intracerebral inoculation)								
ICP index (no. dead and day of death)	0.1	0.1	0.8	1.5	1.9	1.8	1.7	2.0
Chicken (8-week old, IN, IM, or IV inoculation)								
LD_{50} (log base ten)	0	0	0	0	10^8	10^9	10^9	10^9
Lesion rating	R	R	R	R	R/N	R/N	R/N/D	R/N/D
Hemagglutinin								
Elution time (hours)	3	20	34	10	68	96	48	24
Thermostability								
Hemagglutinin in minutes	5	5	5	5	15	60	30	120
Mouse (intracerebral inoculation of weanlings)								
Toxicity index (no. dead and day of death)	0.1		0.6		0.1	3.7	2.2	4.0

Plaque types: C = clear, R = red. *Plaques formed only in presence of Mg and DEAE.
Lesion rating: R = respiratory tract lesions, N = central nervous system lesion, D = digestive tract lesions.

mal by inoculation of a suitable laboratory host system such as embryonated chicken eggs or cell cultures. Designating a culture as a strain does not by rules of nomenclature signify that it is necessarily distinct or different from any other culture or isolate, although almost all strains of NDV that have been characterized on the basis of their physical stability and biological properties have been shown to differ slightly or markedly from one another (Hanson, 1949; Hanson and Brandly, 1955) (Table 18.1). Among the strains that are almost avirulent (lentogenic) are Bl, F, and LaSota that have been extensively used as vaccines. Among the strains of highest virulence (velogenic) are Milano, Herts, and GB that have been used as challenge strains. From the latter and some of the milder strains, one can isolate sublines which are differentiable from the parent culture on the basis of plaque morphology (Granoff, 1964; Schloer and Hanson, 1968b). These lines

may be differentiable on the basis of their virulence for a selected host system, a physical characteristic, or a difference in antigenicity (Daniel and Hanson, 1968a). Sublines may also be separated by use of properties such as ability of a portion of a viral population to resist thermal shock (Goldman and Hanson, 1955), ability to propagate in a given host system (Komarov and Goldsmit, 1946; Brueckner et al., 1950), or ability to be adsorbed to certain cells (Piraino and Hanson, 1959). With few exceptions, strains are composed, on initial isolation, of heterogeneous populations that are separable on bases of plaque type or ability to surmount physical or biological hurdles. These population segments presumably arise through mutation (Granoff, 1964) and persist both in nature and in culture with varying degrees of success so that any population is the sum of the mutants surviving at that time.

LABORATORY HOST SYSTEMS

The ability of the viral preparation to provoke a pathogenic change in a host system in the absence of multiplication has been designated toxicity. Burnet (1942) first reported that NDV possesses this capability. The toxic response is elicited following intracerebral, intranasal, and intravenous administration of the virus in mice and intravenous injection in rabbits. When introduced into the brain of a mouse, the virus incites central nervous system disturbance with paralysis within 2 days and death in 3 days (Upton et al., 1953b; Groupé and Dougherty, 1956). Following nasal instillation, it may induce pneumonia and death of mice (Ginsberg, 1951); following intravenous injection in rabbits, it may cause lymphocytopenia (Evans and Melnick, 1950) and fever (French and Bennett, 1952).

Chickens

From the standpoint of economics, the most important property of NDV is its ability to produce disease and death of chickens—a property in which the strains differ markedly. Strains may be grouped for convenience into 3 classes of differing virulence for chickens: velogenic, mesogenic, and lentogenic (Hanson and Brandly, 1955). Irrespective of route of exposure, chickens receiving velogenic strains develop severe disease, exhibiting one or more types of lesions, and often die. Embryos receiving a minimal lethal dose of a velogenic strain die within 50 hours. Clear or both clear and red plaques, some of which are large, are produced in chicken embryo fibroblast (CEF) monolayers. When introduced by peripheral routes, mesogenic strains usually produce a mild disease which rarely results in death of the chicken. If the virus is introduced directly into the central nervous system, severe disease and death result. Chicken embryos are killed within 50–60 hours after receiving a minimum lethal dose of a mesogenic strain. These strains usually produce small clear plaques on CEF. Lentogenic strains produce a mild or inapparent disease in chickens irrespective of method of exposure. If the lentogenic virus is introduced directly into the central nervous system, it does not multiply and does not result in death of the bird. Embryos are not killed until 100 hours after receiving a minimal lethal dose of a lentogenic strain. Plaques are induced on CEF monolayers when magnesium and diethylaminoethyl are added to the medium, and only rarely when the additives are not present (Barahona and Hanson, 1968).

Cell Cultures

Newcastle disease virus is capable of producing changes in many cell culture systems. These changes are of two primary types: necrosis of the cell (Fig. 18.2) and alteration in form or physiology of the cell. The alterations may be characterized by increased permeability to dyes (Fig. 18.3) or by formation of giant cells (Fig. 18.4). Many types of primary cells (Bankowski, 1964), particularly of avian origin (Rubin et al., 1957; Goldwasser and Kohn, 1957; Morehouse et al., 1963b), and certain cell lines of mammalian origin are readily infected by NDV (Gelenczei and Bordt, 1960; Brandt, 1961). Lancaster (1966) in his review lists 18 primary and 11 cell lines as susceptible. On cell monolayers, NDV induces the formation of plaques (Granoff, 1964; Schloer and Hanson, 1968b). Plaques are circumscribed areas in a monolayer of cells in which the virus has multiplied and destroyed or altered the cells in such a manner that the modification is evident to the naked eye. The plaques produced by NDV can be grouped into two basic types—clear and red—as well as intermediate turbid forms, and into several size classes ranging from 0.5 to 4.0 mm in diameter. The degree of the cell destruction within these plaques varies in such a way that plaques can be described as clear if most or almost all of the cells are destroyed, turbid if only a few of the cells have been destroyed, and red if the only change is permeability of the cell to a dye. Thiry (1963) was the first to describe this last type of plaque. Some strains of the virus produce plaques with sharp margins; other strains produce plaques with a faint or indistinct margin. In the latter instance it is difficult to distinguish the boundary between plaque and monolayer. Syncytial formation is sometimes evident in red plaques (Schloer and Hanson, 1968a). Depending on temperature and nature of the monolayer, plaques develop within 2–6 days following inoculation of the virus. Since the morphology of a plaque changes with time, most descriptions of NDV plaques are based on observation at 96 hours.

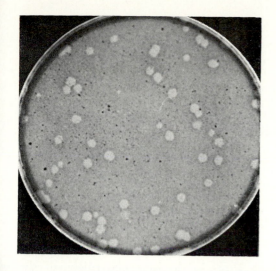

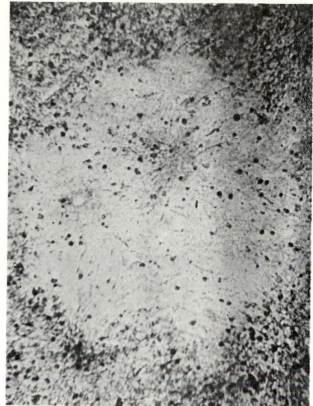

FIG. 18.2—(*Above*) *Large clear plaques of Newcastle disease virus (Milano strain LC clone) on chick embryo fibroblast monolayer stained with neutral red after 96 hours incubation.* (*Right*) *Enlargement (×25) of representative clear plaque. Ragged edges and presence of some viable cells within plaque are evident.* (*Courtesy Gertrude Schloer*)

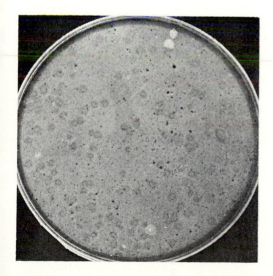

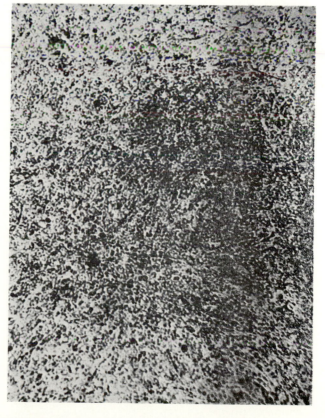

FIG. 18.3—(*Above*) *Large red plaques of Newcastle disease virus (Milano strain R clone) on chick embryo fibroblast monolayer stained with neutral red after 96 hours incubation.* (*Right*) *Enlargement (×25) of representative red plaque. Infected cells take up more stain than do normal cells. In most instances after prolonged incubation infected cells are destroyed and the plaque clears.* (*Courtesy Gertrude Schloer*)

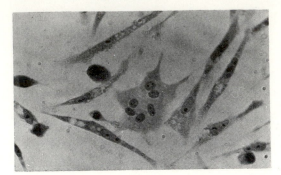

FIG. 18.4—Polykaryocyte formed by NDV in chick embryo fibroblast monolayer. Often observed in red plaques.

Velogenic and mesogenic strains are cytopathic and produce plaques in chicken embryo fibroblasts within 96 hours. Lentogenic strains are cytopathic but fail to produce plaques in chicken embryo fibroblasts within 96 hours in the absence of magnesium and DEAE (Barahona and Hanson, 1968). Many laboratory strains of NDV as well as new isolates contain more than one type of plaque and sometimes as many as 6 types differing in size and clarity or redness. Virus contained in a plaque may be suspended and inoculated onto another monolayer. The plaques which grow from such an inoculum will resemble the parent. Three successive transfers of well-separated plaques are usually carried out to establish a clone which with a few exceptions will breed true.

Chicken Embryos

All strains of NDV induce infection of chicken embryos which lead, with few exceptions, to death of the embryo. The lentogenic strains may fail to induce death of the embryo when antibodies are present in the yolk (Report of Poultry Disease Subcommittee, 1963) and may sometimes induce infections without death in embryos in the absence of antibodies (French et al., 1967). Velogenic and mesogenic strains produce such rapid infection that the yolk antibody is incapable of modifying it. The route of infection, the temperature at which the egg is incubated, the age of the embryo, and the quantity of virus introduced modify the infectious process (Hanson et al., 1947). Infection is more rapidly fatal when the inoculated embryos are young, when the quantity of virus introduced is large, and when the incubation temperature is above

37° C (Sinha, 1958). Yolk sac and intravenous inoculation result in more rapid fatality than do allantoic and chorioallantoic membrane inoculation. Even lentogenic strains when inoculated into the yolk sac kill embryos in 48 hours (Estupinan et al., 1968). The route of infection modifies the order in which tissues become infected and the rate at which the virus titer increases in them (Hanson et al., 1947). High titers of virus are found in the extra-embryonic fluids 24–48 hours before death of the embryo. The difference in time varies with the strain, being less than 24 with velogenic strains and more than 48 with lentogenic strains. However, development of high titers in the lung and spleen of the embryo itself precede death by only 2–6 hours. Presumably the presence of virus in these tissues is associated with changes that result in death. Consequently the rapidity with which these sites in the embryo are reached by the virus probably determines the length of the period between infection and death.

A measure of the virulence of a strain of NDV for the chicken embryo can be based on the number of hours that elapse between introduction of the minimal infective dose and death of the embryo (Hanson and Brandly, 1955). Lentogenic strains take over 100 hours; mesogenic and velogenic strains, 60 hours or less. The gross lesions induced by ND include petechial hemorrhage on the skin of the embryo over the extremities, with some strains, particularly over the cranial area (Bang, 1964).

PATHOGENICITY

The pathogenicity of NDV for chickens is determined largely by the strain of the virus (Sinha et al., 1952) but also in part by the dose (Karzon and Bang, 1951), route of administration (Kohn, 1955; Beard and Easterday, 1967c), age of the chicken (Vadlamudi, 1963), and certain environmental conditions (Sinha et al., 1952). The younger the chicken, the more virulent the virus. Breed or genetic stock of chicken has only a slight effect upon susceptibility to the virus (Cole and Hutt, 1961). At high ambient temperatures, chickens appear to be more susceptible and more frequently develop neurologic signs (Sinha et al., 1957). Some of the velogenic strains are capable of producing death following the introduction of only a few infective particles; other strains require a million or more infective units to induce death; some strains are nonfatal even in enormous doses. The route of infection modifies the nature of the pathogenic process. Natural routes of infection, such as intranasal, oral, and ocular, by which dusts and aerosols bearing virus reach the host, are most frequently associated with development of respiratory disease (Beard and Easterday, 1967c). Intramuscular, intravenous, and intracerebral administrations usually enhance the neurovirulence of the virus.

PATHOGENESIS AND EPIZOOTIOLOGY

NATURAL AND EXPERIMENTAL HOSTS

Newcastle disease virus has been isolated from such barnyard visitors as the starling (Gillespie et al., 1950), sparrow (Gustafson and Moses, 1953), pigeon and dove (Hanson and Sinha, 1952; Walker et al., 1954); from scavengers like crows and jackdaws (Shah and Johnson, 1959; Keymer, 1961); from predators like great horned owl (Ingalls et al., 1951) and osprey (Zuijdam, 1952; and from migratory waterfowl such as swan, ducks, geese (Asplin, 1947; Palmer, 1969), gannets, and shags (Blaxland, 1951). The individuals examined had either shown abnormal behavior or had died of an acute disease.

In most instances when investigators have attempted experimental infections of these species by natural routes the birds have suffered only transitory infection and shed virus for a short time in either nasal secretions or in feces (Spalatin et al., 1968). Following convalescence they have developed antibodies. Intracerebral route of inoculation has in many instances resulted in fatal infections. Lack of agreement among investigators over susceptibility of wild birds should be expected, as immune status of the subjects, origin of the virus strain, titer of the inoculum, and route of exposure have not always been known; when they have been known they have seldom been comparable. The rather contradictory experiences in zoological gardens—particularly among gallinaceous birds which in some instances have not been affected at all (Kloppel, 1963) and in other instances have suffered heavy mortality (Parnaik and Dixit, 1953)—are a good example of the difficulty in interpreting reports without knowledge of the immune status of the birds prior to exposure. Numerous investigators using several strains have shown that most species of gallinaceous birds known to be free of antibody (quail, pheasant, and partridge) will suffer lethal infection (Fenstermacher et al., 1946; Kaschula, 1950). Instances of death occurring among species which were reputed to have been naturally infected, but which subsequently have not been found to be experimentally susceptible, might be attributable to complicated infections.

There is no substantial evidence of seasonal differences in the prevalence of ND. The virus is known to be present in all seasons in both temperate and tropical regions, and both severe and mild disease has been reported in all seasons. There may be effects of weather on disease manifestation, as experimental studies suggest that environmental temperature and air pollution associated with poor winter ventilation can each modify the host response. Interaction of environmental factors and management procedures and rather inadequate means of measuring prevalence and severity of disease may have obscured some real effects.

TRANSMISSION AND CARRIERS

The primary mode of transmission of NDV within a flock is by aerosol. Approximately 2 days after exposure and a full day before showing clinical signs of disease, the infected bird begins to liberate virus in the air that leaves its respiratory tract and continues to do so for several days (Sinha et al., 1954). Coughing, gasping, and other disturbances of respiration are not required to generate an infective aerosol but probably enhance its production. Whenever birds are confined the population of infective virus builds up in the air (DeLay et al., 1948) and is maintained there by the turbulence induced by the normal activity of the birds. Larger particles settle at night when there is less activity but smaller particles remain airborne for days (Anderson et al., 1964). The ease of disseminating vaccines as sprays (Hitchner and Reising, 1953) and dusts (Price et al., 1955) corroborates the importance of aerosols in the infection of chickens. Even water vaccines probably enter the chicken as a drinking-induced aerosol.

The role of small particle aerosols which move many feet and stay airborne for many hours was questioned by Andrewes (1960). He demonstrated that chicks infected when

1 day of age transferred the virus to pen mates but not to chicks from which they were separated by only a wire screen. In experiments in which others have demonstrated small particle aerosol generation (Sinha et al., 1954), older chickens have been used and the donors had received their virus by aerosol. Liberation of virus from the respiratory tract in large amounts is dependent upon a number of factors, chiefly the initiation of the infection by aerosol (Beard and Easterday, 1967c). Others include the strain of virus, age of host (Sinha et al., 1952), and environmental situation (i.e. ambient temperature) (Sinha et al., 1957).

Dissemination between flocks over long distances has frequently been related to movement of apparently normal poultry (Jungherr and Terrell, 1946) and also may be accomplished by the introduction into feed of diseased tissues such as poultry offal (Dobson and Simmins, 1951) or by contamination of feed or water (Bolin, 1948; Jungherr, 1948; Kaschula, 1950; Gustafson and Moses, 1953). Man's clothing and foot gear and artifacts such as crates, feed sacks, and trucks undoubtedly act as mechanical vectors (Jungherr and Markham, 1962). Infection can occur through the digestive tract (Kohn, 1959), although differences in their ability to do this probably occur among strains of virus.

Proof is lacking that NDV can be transmitted from the hen through the egg to the hatchling. Nevertheless, in eggs laid by diseased hens, infection and death of embryos may occur, particularly during the first 4–5 days of incubation (Doll et al., 1950a; Prier et al., 1950; Bivins et al., 1950). The chicken embryo is susceptible to the virus of ND during all of the successive stages of development. The disease produced is modified by the age of the embryo (Blattner and Williamson, 1951; Williamson et al., 1956) and may be arrested by passive congenital antibodies (Brandly et al., 1946d) which, if present, enter the embryonic circulation about the 15th day (Buddingh, 1952). The lentogenic (vaccine) strains take 2–3 times as long to induce fatal infection of embryos when inoculated by conventional routes and may under some conditions not kill the embryo (French et al., 1967). On the other hand, if inoculated into the yolk sac of antibody-free eggs they kill quickly (Estupinan et al., 1968). There is growing evidence (DeLay, 1947; French et al., 1967) that the virus may under circumstances not yet defined pass through the egg to the hatchling.

Other domesticated fowl may serve to transport and perpetuate the disease. Turkeys, which usually suffer less severely than do chickens (Gray et al., 1954; Gale, 1964), have been suspected of being initial foci of epizootics in certain localities (Van Roekel, 1964). Ducks and geese infrequently develop clinical disease although they commonly possess antibodies (Asplin, 1947).

In some instances vaccine may have served to introduce the virus into flocks or into regions, either because it was not completely inactivated (Placidi, 1956; Spalatin and Hanson, 1968) or because it contained the active virus as a contaminant (Zarger and Pomeroy, 1950; Hanson et al., 1967).

INCUBATION PERIOD

The incubation period of ND after natural exposure has been reported to vary from 2 to 15 days or longer, with an average of 5–6 days. The incubation time as well as severity of the disease decreases gradually from hatching to maturity. The response of offspring of immune hens may be altered favorably by the passive protection afforded by antibodies derived from the yolk. However, with heavy exposure to virulent NDV, rapidly developing prostration and early death may be observed to the exclusion of other signs.

An outbreak of ND may be so acute and severe as to kill all or nearly all of the birds in a flock within 3 or 4 days. At the other extreme, the disease may be so mild that symptoms are scarcely noticeable, or they may be absent and the disease subclinical in nature. Natural and acquired differences in both the virus and the host, as well as known dosage and various environmental factors, largely appear to explain differences in the nature and course of the disease.

A sequence of events following introduction of NDV into the chicken is initiated by multiplication of the virus at the site of introduction (Asdell and Hanson, 1960). There follows liberation of virus into the blood stream, a second cycle of multiplication in visceral organs, a second release into the blood stream, and in some instances passage into the central nervous system. Signs of disease and liberation of virus into the environment are associated with the second release of the virus into the blood stream. The course of the disease is determined by the defense mechanisms that come into play at this time. The pathogenicity of NDV for chickens can be measured by the ability of the virus to produce death; to produce central nervous system signs such as paralysis, tremor, and torticollis; and to produce respiratory signs which may be marked or so slight as to become evident only upon a disturbance of the birds. Sometimes the only effect of the virus expressed is on the ability of the bird to lay or to maintain its rate of gain. The virulence of NDV for susceptible chickens presents a complete continuum from very rapid fatal infection to an inapparent disease.

SIGNS, MORBIDITY, AND MORTALITY

In Doyle's form disease appears suddenly, birds sometimes being found dead without having shown any signs (Iyer, 1943). More often the birds first appear listless, respiration is increased, weakness becomes more apparent, and death preceded by prostration occurs in 5–7 days. A watery greenish diarrhea, sometimes bloodstained, is not uncommon and may be profuse (Albiston and Gorrie, 1942). Diarrhea is usually accompanied by dehydration (Thompson and Osteen, 1952). A rise in temperature of 4–6° C occurs early in disease; before death it drops below normal. Clonic spasms, muscular tremors, torticollis, and opisthotonos appear in birds that survive the initial phase of disease (Fig. 18.5). Other central

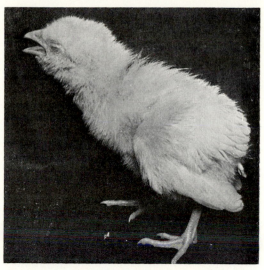

FIG. 18.6—Chick infected with NDV showing respiratory difficulty.

nervous system involvement is paralysis of the legs and occasionally the wings (Ressang, 1961). Mortality is usually 90% (Dobson, 1939).

Beach's form of disease appears suddenly and spreads rapidly. Respiratory distress, coughing, and gasping are marked (Beach, 1943) (Fig. 18.6). Appetite drops, egg production falls or stops. Diarrhea has not been observed with this form in America. Nervous signs may appear within a day or two or not until after a week or more. Paralysis of leg or wing and torticollis are not uncommon. Mortality is variable (Goldhaft and Wernicoff, 1948). More than 50% of adult birds have died in some instances (Binns et al., 1949; Boney, 1951), but 10% mortality is more common. Among immature chickens death loss is as high as 90%.

Beaudette's form is an acute respiratory disease of adult chickens marked by coughing but rarely gasping. There is a drop in appetite, and egg production falls and may cease. The pause may continue for 1–3 weeks (Biswal and Morrill, 1954), and occasionally birds do not return to normal production (Platt, 1948). Egg quality is affected (Knox, 1950).

Hitchner's form of disease may be inapparent in adult birds (Bankowski, 1961). In other instances respiratory signs (rales) may be detectable when birds are at roost (Asplin, 1952) or by listening at the breast of a disturbed bird. Death losses are usually negligible, although in young birds, partic-

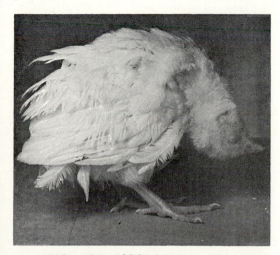

FIG. 18.5—Chick infected with NDV showing torticollis.

ularly when complicated by other infections, mortality of 30% may occur. Nervous signs have not been seen with this form in North America.

A review of the nature of virulence of NDV (Waterson and Pennington, 1967) considers differences both in the virion itself and its relationship to cells and in the relationship of host defenses to the virus.

GROSS LESIONS

The pathological changes found in Newcastle disease vary greatly from bird to bird, from flock to flock, and from one geographical region to another. Among the factors that create these differences are the virus strain involved, the route of exposure, the severity of exposure, the age and breed of bird, and environment. While the lesions found in the disease are not directly related to the severity of disease, there is a trend in that direction. Readily recognizable changes are seldom found in the inapparent forms of ND and almost invariably are found in birds that have died of the severe forms of the disease. A major pathological feature of the disease is variation.

Extensive literature has developed on ND, and not surprisingly there is disagreement among the reports on the pathological manifestations. Confusion has been introduced in some instances because some of the birds that have been described with ND were suffering from more than one disease. Finally, truly pathognomonic lesions have not been recognized as such in Newcastle disease. If gross lesions are to be useful in diagnosis it is important to remember that all the changes found in ND also occur in other diseases, and that the overall patterns encountered are more significant than are individual changes. This is especially true of the more severe forms of the disease. In the inapparent form, the finding of no gross lesions is suggestive of Newcastle disease. The chief sources of information on pathology have been the reports of Jungherr (1964) and of Jungherr in association with others (Jungherr and Minard, 1944; Jungherr et al., 1946). Critical review of current literature has been provided by S. H. McNutt (1968, personal communication).

In Doyle's form of the disease, an outstanding lesion is the dark red or purplish red hemorrhagic lesion associated with some necrosis in the intestinal wall, especially in the posterior half of the duodenum and in the jejunum and ileum. These lesions vary in size (increasing from those only a few millimeters across) and are recognized only when the intestine is opened, wherein they appear as small red areas having definite but somewhat irregular borders to large ones as much as 15 mm or more in length. The latter may be thick enough to bulge inwardly to the extent that the intestinal lumen is constricted, and they may also bulge outwardly. A process of this size and color can be readily detected on viewing the unopened intestine. These larger hemorrhagic necrotic areas may appear somewhat bleblike, perhaps because of the edema about them. The hemorrhagic necrotic areas that occur in the cecal tonsils are evidently of the same nature but less striking because there is less hemorrhage (Crawford, 1930; Orr and John, 1946). On occasion the diphtheroid necrotic inflammation of the intestinal mucosa simulates the "button" ulcers of hog cholera and is considered to be thoroughly suggestive of Newcastle disease. Hemorrhages are sometimes seen on the glandular surface of the proventriculus in the enteric form of the disease.

In other forms of ND the primary lesions are found in the respiratory tract. A serous or catarrhal exudate is present in the nasal passages, larynx, and trachea. Hemorrhages may occasionally be found in the trachea. The lungs are usually normal although the lower anterior portion may sometimes be pneumonic. Thickened membranes of one or more air sacs is a common finding, particularly in young birds. At times one or more air sacs may contain a catarrhal or caseous exudate. Necropsy of chickens and turkeys in production reveals fluid yolk material in the abdominal cavity and flaccid yolk follicles as a result of cessation of lay. The spleen may be enlarged in the early stages and shrunken in later stages.

In embryos the common changes are congestion and hemorrhages (Buddingh, 1952). Some strains of virus produce more hemorrhage than others. Occasionally there are particularly large cranial hemorrhages. Hemorrhage is also seen in the yolk sac (Bang, 1964).

HISTOPATHOLOGY

Histologically, hyperemia, edema, hemorrhages, and other blood vessel changes are found in various organs. The other vessel changes consist of hydropic degenerations of the media, hyalinization of capillaries and arterioles, development of hyaline thrombosis in the small vessels, and finally necrosis of the endothelial cells of the vessels. Regressive changes found in the lymphopoietic system consist of disappearance of lymphoid tissue, hyperplasia of reticulum, and plasmorrhagia of the spleen. Hyperplasia of the reticulohistiocytic cells in various organs, especially the liver, takes place in subacute cases. DeKock (1954) observed intranuclear inclusions in the reticulum cells of the spleen. Lesions of necrotizing nature are found throughout the organ. These have been designated hyaline necrosis or fibrinoid necrosis (Jungherr et al., 1946). These changes are seen mostly in Doyle's form of the disease.

The hemorrhagic-necrotic lesions in the intestine are believed by some to develop in the lymphoid aggregates or at least in association with such aggregates. It is a bit difficult in chickens to determine when a disease process develops in a lymphoid aggregate and when the lymphoid aggregate develops as a result of a disease process. Such aggregates develop in the chicken trachea in a matter of days following exposure by aerosol to Newcastle disease virus (Beard and Easterday, 1967c). When lesions in the proventriculus are examined histologically it is found that such hemorrhages are associated with minute ulcers (Montroni, 1961). Small focal areas of necrosis are seen in the liver. When lesions are present in the gall bladder and heart they are necrotic, sometimes with hemorrhage. Lymphocytic infiltration has been described in the pancreas.

Respiratory System

While the respiratory distress in Newcastle disease has been attributed to a number of things, including an effect on the respiratory center (De Moulin, 1951) or distension and damage of the capillaries (Potel, 1950; Obel et al., 1956), the effect on the membranes of the upper respiratory tract is very severe and most certainly contributes to such distress (Burnstein and Bang, 1957; Beard and Easterday, 1967c). This is obvious on examination of such affected tissues. Beard and Easterday (1967a) exposed individual groups of young chickens by aerosol and by intramuscular injection to a lentogenic strain (B1) and a velogenic strain (GB) of NDV. Neither strain produced much reaction in the mucosa of the upper respiratory passages when exposure was by intramuscular injection, but when exposure was by aerosol the microscopic changes in the mucous membrane of the trachea were truly astounding for both strains. The reaction reached its peak 4–5 days postexposure and was marked by pronounced congestion, edema, and dense cellular infiltration. Lymphocytes were the principal cells involved, but large phagocytes (foam cells) were abundant, especially in the exudate within the trachea. Infiltrating cells so packed the mucosa that it was surprising to discover that the surface epithelium was seldom lost. Beard and Easterday (1967c) also found that the process clears rapidly— as early as 6–8 days after exposure—so that birds dying of Newcastle disease at that time may have mucosa of the upper respiratory passages entirely free of inflammation. Various changes have been found in the lungs of birds suffering from ND, but birds dying of the most severe form of the disease may fail to have lung lesions. The changes in the lungs are reported to be proliferative and exudative—hyperplasia and hypertrophy of the cells of the alveolar walls, accumulations of fluid and cells (including leukocytes, erythrocytes, and foam cells) in the alveoli and air passages.

Inflammatory changes of the pericardium, especially of the air sacs, are interesting but not especially useful in diagnosis. Other infections that involve the air sacs may be superimposed on ND, and it is not improbable that other infections can cause a similar airsacculitis. Edema, cell infiltration, and increased thickness and density due to proliferation of connective tissue are seen in the air sacs of chickens affected with ND.

Nervous System

Encephalitis is not present in the inapparent forms of the disease and may not be present in some birds affected with more severe enteric forms. However, abnormalities in the central nervous system are a most significant feature of ND whenever they are present.

It is generally agreed that glia foci, neuronal degeneration, perivascular lymphocytic infiltration, and hypertrophy of endothelial cells are found in the central nervous system of chickens suffering from ND. Lesions are fairly well distributed throughout the central nervous system—the cord, medulla, midbrain, cerebellum; not much is reported in the cerebrum. There is nothing remarkable about this distribution. In reporting his observations on "functional localization of lesions in Newcastle disease," Auer (1952) stated that a principal lesion was "general invasion by lymphocytes" into the tissues of the central nervous system. Working with pigeons, Kaschula (1951) found evidence that NDV might travel by way of the nerves to the brain. A mild nonsuppurative neuritis has been observed in Newcastle disease (Kohler, 1953; Mohr, 1953.)

The microscopic lesions of ND can be differentiated from the lesions of vitamin E deficiency and from avian encephalomyelitis. Vitamin E deficiency is a degenerative lesion resulting in hemorrhages in the cerebellum. The differentiation between ND and avian encephalomyelitis will be discussed in Chapter 19. One of the main differentiating features is the central chromatolysis of neurones in the medulla in avian encephalomyelitis, which rarely occurs in ND.

Reproductive System

In a study of the reproductive tract, Biswal and Morrill (1954) found an oophoritis and salpingitis. Egg production ceased for 7–22 days, and shell weight and thickness were affected for as long as 56 days. Functionally the greatest damage was to the uterus or shell forming portion of the oviduct. There was nothing truly remarkable about the details of the changes in the female reproductive organs. These included atresia of the follicles together with infiltration of inflammatory cells and formation of lymphoid aggregates. Similar aggregates were prominent in the oviduct.

Other Systems

An exudative inflammation of the internal ear may develop which is said to be the cause of a tactic movement of the head and characteristic head posture. On rare occasions there is graying of the eyes due to infiltration of cells into the iris. Minor vesicles of the wattle skin have also been mentioned. As in many virus diseases, leukopenia develops shortly after artificial exposure—at about day 6 (Machado, 1951).

IMMUNITY

All NDV strains are capable of provoking an antibody response in chickens, rabbits, and other species into which they are introduced. The ND virion contains several antigens. The antigens that induce the virus-neutralizing antibody and the hemagglutinating antibody are associated with the envelope of the virus. When the latter is destroyed by ether, one of the gel-diffusion lines is eliminated. The NP antigen or soluble antigen is associated with the nucleoprotein portion of the virus. The NP antigen is detected in the complement-fixation test and is distinguishable from the HA antigen and the virion-associated antigen in the gel-diffusion test.

The virus-neutralizing antibody effectively blocks the ability of the virus to fatally infect chickens, chicken embryos, and cells in culture. Resistance to reinfection is usually associated with presence of moderate to high titer of neutralizing antibodies (Levine et al., 1950). The difference between the virus-neutralizing antibody, the hemagglutination-inhibiting antibody, and the refractivity of chickens to challenge becomes apparent on a temporal scale (Coleman, 1959). Antibodies appear in the serum of chickens within 6–10 days after introduction of infection while signs of clinical disease are still apparent. Peak titer is reached in 3–4 weeks. Decline is initially slow but becomes apparent in 3–4 months, and antibodies become undetectable in 8–12 months. Hemagglutination-inhibiting antibodies usually disappear first while virus-neutralizing antibody is still high (Coleman, 1959). Refractivity of chickens to a disabling reinfection sometimes persists after disappearance of detectable circulating antibody.

Minor antigenic differences exist among NDV strains (Upton et al., 1953a). Strains can be distinguished on the basis of the gel-diffusion test, the hemagglutination-inhibition test, and the virus-neutralization test. These differences are both qualitative and quantitative in nature (Schloer, 1964).

DIAGNOSIS

ISOLATION AND IDENTIFICATION

The unequivocal method of diagnosing ND is the isolation and identification of the causative agent. Serologic and pathologic examinations may suffice to confirm suggestive histories and signs in regions where ND is enzootic, but new foci or extension of new pathologic forms and recognition of new hosts require recovery and identification of the virus.

The more pathogenic and invasive strains are widely distributed in the host and present in high concentration in the many tissues and organs (Hofstad, 1951; Sinha et al., 1952; Baskaya et al., 1952). On the other hand, lentogenic strains may be limited to either the respiratory or digestive tracts (Karzon and Bang, 1951). In populations consisting of several ages, younger individuals are more likely to yield virus (Brandly et al., 1946b; Beaudette et al., 1949a).

Specimens for attempting isolation of the virus should be selected from cases in the incubative and early clinical stages of the disease as the virus rapidly disappears from the tissues of the host on the development of demonstrable circulating antibodies (Brandly et al., 1946b; Hofstad, 1951; Asdell and Hanson, 1960; Report of the Poultry Disease Subcommittee, 1963). Some segments of the viral population present in infected chickens disappear prior to development of immunity or death.

Chickens exposed by aerosol to a strain of virus containing several genetically distinguishable subpopulations yielded the entire complex on culture of tracheal exudates only during the incubative and early clinical stages of disease. During later stages of disease, particularly when the chicken was moribund or dead, only one component which was unrepresentative of the original culture could be isolated (Daniel and Hanson, 1968b; Estupinan, 1968). Even during earlier clinical stages of disease, cloacal swab cultures and tracheal cultures which were taken at the same time sometimes yielded different components. Heterogeneity of virus cultures recovered during epizootics is not uncommon and may always exist if sampling is adequately carried out. Since it is difficult or impossible to understand epizootiological events or host response with an unrepresentative culture of the virus which induced them, adequate sampling of both incubative and clinically affected individuals is necessary.

Virus has been isolated on rare occasions from the brain and excreta after circulating antibodies were present (Walker and McKercher, 1954). Explant procedures make possible replicable isolation of virus from tracheal and brain tissues as long as 2 months after antibodies become detectable (Heuschele, 1968).

Chicken Embryos

The embryonating chicken egg is preferred to the chicken or other animals for isolation of NDV. As a rule, fertile eggs (preferably from healthy nonimmune hens) which have been incubated for 9–11 days at 37–38° C are injected in the allantoic chamber with suspensions of suspected tissues. Antibiotic agents, usually either penicillin or streptomycin or more commonly a mixture of the two, are added to the inoculum to suppress or destroy bacteria which may be present (Brandly et al., 1946b; Thompson and Osteen, 1948; Beaudette et al., 1948). The injected eggs are returned to the incubator, candled once or twice daily for a 5-day period or until death of all or a large part of the embryos has occurred. Embryonic deaths during the 1st day are considered to be due to trauma or nonspecific causes. Examination of embryos dying subsequently may or may not reveal congestive or hemorrhagic changes, as these alterations may be poorly defined or absent during initial or early egg passages of NDV. If the clear, bacteria-free, allantoic fluids agglutinate a 1% suspension of chicken erythrocytes, ND virus should be suspected and the identity of the HA should be determined by inhibition with known ND immune serum. Identification of the isolate may be confirmed by specific neutralization of the infectivity by known immune serum.

The use of susceptible chickens for isolation and identification of NDV may be expedient and desirable under certain circumstances where adequate isolation can be maintained.

Cell Cultures

Newcastle disease virus can be readily propagated in primary cells of avian origin (Topacio, 1934; Fastier, 1954; Levine and Sagik, 1956; Rubin et al., 1957; Matewa, 1960; Morehouse et al., 1963b), in some mammalian primary cells (Chanock, 1955; Chaproniere and Pereira, 1955; Brandt, 1961; Wheelock and Tamm, 1961; Morehouse et al., 1963a), in some mammalian cell lines (Gelenczei and Bordt, 1960; Schloer, 1964), and even in primary cells of certain cold-blooded vertebrates (Schindarow and Todorov, 1962; Melendez et al., 1965). Most extensively used for isolation of the virus are either chicken embryo fibroblasts or chicken embryo kidney cells grown as monolayers on glass or plastic (Bankowski et al., 1959; Bankowski, 1964). Fibroblasts are prepared by mincing the torso of 8–9-day-old embryos, treating the suspension with trypsin to further separate the cells, washing the suspension, and then distributing a predetermined quantity of cells in a petri dish or flat-sided bottle (Schloer and Hanson, 1968a). The growth medium must contain a balanced salt solution, embryo extract (or lactalbumin hydrolysate, vitamins, and amino acids), and serum. Incubation in a moist atmosphere charged with CO_2 at a temperature of $37°$ C permits the cells to form a monolayer in approximately 24–48 hours.

The virus inoculum appropriately diluted in balanced salt solution is added and agitated, and then the monolayer is overlaid with a gel (usually 1% agar with nutrient medium). Once the agar is set the plate is inverted and incubated as before. Plaques develop in 2–7 days, depending on the genetic characteristics of the virus inducing them and the influence of environmental factors (Schloer and Hanson, 1968a). A second overlay containing neutral red (usually applied approximately 72 hours after inoculation of virus) is required to render the plaques visible.

The velogenic strains when grown on CEF monolayers usually exhibit large clear (2–4 mm) or large red plaques (2–4 mm) or both types and may also show small plaques (0.5–1.5 mm) of either type (Daniel and Hanson, 1968b). The large plaques, if cloned and subsequently inoculated into chickens, are almost invariably highly virulent for chickens. The small and tiny plaques are of moderate or low virulence. Virus from chickens infected with one of the mild forms of Newcastle disease usually has only a single small clear or turbid plaque when plated on CE fibroblasts. The avirulent form rarely produces plaques without the addition of magnesium and DEAE to the overlay medium (Barahona and Hanson, 1968).

SEROLOGY

The virus neutralization (VN) test is based on the ability of serum globulins, which have been induced in animals following infection with NDV, to render the virus noninfective when virus and serum are mixed in correct proportions. Rubin and Franklin (1957) concluded that since NDV is neutralized by immune serum in an exponential manner, only one antibody molecule is required for inactivation of a virus particle; and that while a single antibody molecule can inactivate the virus as far as its ability to produce infective progeny is concerned, the attachment of several molecules is required to prevent adsorption of the virus to the host cell. Therefore, dilutions of either or both the serum and virus in a series of tubes make the test quantitative as well as qualitative.

Virus Neutralization in Chicken Embryos

The procedure (Report of Poultry Disease Subcommittee, 1963) for a specific virus neutralization test is briefly as follows: Equal parts of serum from a recovered chicken suspected of having Newcastle disease are mixed with progressive tenfold dilutions of the virus. A similar series of normal serum and virus mixtures and a series of tenfold dilutions of virus alone serve as controls on virus titer and specificity of serum-virus reaction. The virus dilutions should extend beyond the highest dilution which proves infective or lethal. At least 4 and preferably 5 chicks or embryonating eggs are injected with a uniform quantity of the virus and serum-virus mixtures respectively.

Serum samples from chicken flocks that have no history of ND infection or vaccination will neutralize less than 100 infective units of the virus or no virus at all, while an equal volume of serum from a chicken infected 10–20 days previously will neutralize a thousand to a million more infective units of virus. If drawn prior to the 10th day after an outbreak of suspected ND in the flock, serum samples for VN or other serologic testing may give misleading negative results. Since antibodies persist for 6–9 months, the demonstration of antibody is not in itself sufficient to relate it to the clinical disease which the flock has just undergone. One must either isolate the virus or demonstrate an increase in antibody titer between the acute or early convalescent period and late convalescence. The serum of chicks of immune dams may contain significant antibodies derived passively from the yolk during the first 3 weeks of life (Brandly et al., 1946d). The relevance of antibody to infection during this period is demonstrable only if titer increases rather than wanes. Other virus diseases of chickens do not induce antibodies that cross-react with Newcastle disease virus in any way. However, mumps virus infection may cause human serum to give completely or partially positive HI, CF, and VN tests with NDV (Evans, 1956). The blood should be collected aseptically from chickens; if it is to undergo transit to a laboratory or be held for a period, the serum should be separated. The addition of merthiolate (1:50,000) to serum samples controls bacterial contamination and may render even contaminated serum samples suitable for VN testing in eggs. Yolk of eggs diluted at least 1:5 with saline may be used in VN and HI tests instead of blood to ascertain the ND status of a laying flock. Storage at low temperature (6° C) or in the frozen state favors preservation of the antibody titer for a protracted period.

The virus neutralization test in chicken embryos is usually performed by titrating the virus in parallel in the presence of normal serum (control) and the positive or unknown serum. The difference becomes the neutralization titer. Other methods of detecting the virus neutralizing potency of a serum may be used. Each requires a suitable dilution of serum and virus. Among them are inhibition of cytopathic effect, inhibition of acid production (metabolic inhibition test), blockage of hemadsorption, and zone inhibition of plaque formation induced by serum containing beads or discs.

The virus neutralization test employing known ND immune serum may serve for rapid identification of infective agents suspected yet not known to be NDV. In such tests qualitative antigenic differences (Bang and Foard, 1953) and heat-labile and -stable nonspecific inhibitors (Karzon, 1956) must be recognized and guarded against.

Plaque Neutralization

The plaque neutralization test is perhaps the most sensitive method of detecting neutralizing antibody. Serial dilutions of serum are mixed with a constant quantity of virus (50–100 pfu), incubated, and inoculated on prepared monolayers of CEF. Overlay is added and the culture incubated; at the appropriate time (72 hours) a second overlay with neutral red is added. The cultures are examined 24–48 hours later under suitable light conditions to count the number of plaques. Reduction of plaque count by given dilution of serum in reference to the control provides the measure of neutralizing activity of the serum.

Hemagglutination (HA) and Hemagglutination-Inhibition (HI) Tests

The finding by Burnet (1942) that NDV, like influenza, agglutinated the red blood cells of chicks and that such hemagglutination was specifically inhibited or neutralized by ND immune serum provided a simple and useful diagnostic method. The test for HA may serve as a rapid method for detecting NDV in the fluids or extracts of infected tissues of fowl as well as in the fluids of infected eggs (Monti, 1952; Mitscherlich and Gurturk, 1952; Clark et al., 1955). Hanson et al. (1947) showed that minimal NDV titers of at least 10^6 infective doses are required if the allantoic or amniotic fluids are to induce hemagglutination. Bronchitis and laryngotracheitis viruses, while infective for the chicken embryo, do not cause hemagglutination, thus providing a means of differentiation from the HA-positive NDV (Brandly et al., 1946b).

As with the test for neutralization of NDV infectivity by specific immune serum, the test for inhibition or neutralization of the hemagglutinative activity of the virus (HI) gives quantitative as well as qualitative information. In the alpha procedure the virus suspension in serial twofold dilutions beginning with 1:5 is mixed with equal volumes of the serum under test and a 0.5% suspension of chicken red cells. In the beta procedure the serum is serially diluted and admixed with the red cell suspension and a constant quantity (10 HA units) of the virus (Report Poultry Disease Subcommittee, 1963). The test, with adequate control (serum alone, cells alone, known positive serum, known negative serum), is incubated at room temperature for 30 minutes and the results read on the basis of the agglutination pattern. Typical complete HA ($+ + + +$) is represented by a continuous layer of cells covering the entire rounded bottom of the tube; a thicker layer, irregular in outline, covering a portion of the bottom is a partial or $+ + +$ reaction; a small central disc with a narrow granular fringe of agglutinated cells, a $+ +$ reaction; and a larger button or disc of cells with a narrow ring of agglutinated cells is classed as a $+$ reaction. Complete inhibition of the HA reaction, like the normal unimpaired settling of cells as in the control tubes, leaves a central compact button with a sharp edge. The highest dilution of virus giving a $+ +$ or higher reaction represents the titer of the virus, and the quantity of virus involved is considered a unit. Elution of virus from the cells and their subsequent release from the agglutinated layer causes a cascading or sliding of the cells to the bottom of the tube with the formation of a disc or button, such as occurs when erythrocytes sediment normally. Rapid serum and whole blood HI tests have been devised and used with satisfactory results (Luginbuhl and Jungherr, 1949; Zargar and Pomeroy, 1949; Walker, 1952; Raggi, 1960).

The HI test, although simpler and faster than the VN test and also a measure of the immune response, cannot be directly equated with the latter. The "VN antibody" persists longer than "HI antibody," and serum fractionation studies have revealed physical differences (Brandly et al., 1947; Hanson et al., 1950). An HI titer value of 10 obtained by the beta procedure has been considered as of marginal diagnostic significance, one of 20 or higher as definitely indicating prior infection of the bird. On the basis of their studies, Doll et al. (1950b) concluded that time of development, persistence, and HI titer reached are determined in part by strain of virus and route of infection. After several routes of infection, a titer of 10 or 20 was obtained in 5–6 days. More than 90% of the experimentally exposed chickens showed positive titers at the 10th day, and all were positive on the 12th day. Direct and indirect complement-fixation tests have been utilized and found highly specific for serologic diagnosis of ND (Boulanger and Rice, 1953; Nitzschke, 1954; Brumfield and Pomeroy,

1957). Since a specific immune response is rarely demonstrable until 7 days after NDV infection, the detection of hemagglutinins in tissues such as the lung may be utilized as an early diagnostic test, particularly when known immune serum is used to show specific inhibition (McClurkin et al., 1954).

Challenge Tests

Definitive diagnosis of prior ND infection may be accomplished by inoculating virulent titered NDV into suitable individuals from flocks suspected of having been infected at least a week previously. Susceptible controls should be inoculated simultaneously. Resistance to infection indicates immunity.

Other Tests

The fluorescent antibody procedure allows more rapid detection of NDV infection than HI or regular egg inoculation, according to Maestrone and Coffin (1961). The procedure has been used in studies of pathogenesis (Beard and Easterday, 1967c).

DIFFERENTIAL DIAGNOSIS

History of rapid contagion is suggestive but in no way distinguishes ND from certain other diseases and may not always be apparent.

The clinical manifestation of ND in chicks can be confused with those of many other infections and even poisonings. Infectious bronchitis, laryngotracheitis, fowl plague, avian influenza, coryza, mycoplasmosis—all have some respiratory manifestations that are similar to those of ND. The disturbances of the central nervous system resemble some features of avian encephalomyelitis, Marek's disease, and certain poisonings.

No gross or histological changes can be considered pathognomonic.

Diagnosis requires laboratory tests, either isolation and identification of the virus or demonstration of a specific increase in antibody between the acute and convalescent stages of disease.

PREVENTION AND CONTROL

The simplest and most logical measure against Newcastle disease is to prevent contact of the virus with the susceptible bird. A second is vaccination which gives the animal a degree of protection against infection in the event of exposure. The third and least satisfactory and least economical procedure is to attempt treatment of the animal after it is exposed or has become affected.

A combination of sanitary management (to reduce chance of exposure) and a vaccination program is required to combat a highly contagious disease such as ND when it has become widely established in a community, region, or country. However, both measures must be systematically carried out on an area basis if control is to be reasonably effective. A minimum of 70% of the flocks in an area of high population must be included at the outset in the sanitary program, combined with a satisfactory twice-a-year or oftener vaccination program.

Risk of exposure to and spread of ND generally increases in proportion to the size of the flock, the rearing and maintaining of birds of different ages on the premises, and the proximity of the housing units.

General compliance with a sanitary program prevents ND where the poultry population is not too great and flocks are some distance apart. Vaccination may be used with sanitation in less concentrated production areas as a means toward eradication of ND.

A regional program to eliminate NDV, based on rigid sanitation, has been implemented in Maine and found acceptance and reasonable success (Chute and O'Meara, 1963). On the other hand, continuous application of the slaughter policy against ND in Great Britain in the face of reintroduction of infection and the prevalence of mild or subclinical infection has fallen short of success while imposing serious financial burdens on breeding and research stock perpetuation (Report of the Committee on Fowl Pest Policy, 1962).

Natural selection toward development of greater genetic resistance is said to take place when ND becomes enzootic in a poultry population (Knox, 1950; Francis and Kish, 1955; Takamatsu et al., 1956). The statistically significant differences in resistance to ND among 6 families as well as 2 strains of White Leghorn chickens which support early observations of such variability have been reported by Cole and Hutt (1961). Mortality among 7,000 pullets following Roakin strain wing web vaccination in successive years was 3.2 and 7.2% in strain K compared to 0.7 and 0.8% among

strain C birds. The practicality of intentional exposure to ND as the basis of a breeding program toward controlling ND has not been demonstrated.

PREVENTION BY SANITARY MANAGEMENT

Basic specific precautions are necessary to exclude ND infection from the poultry operation and to prevent its spread.

Hatchery

The hatchery must be isolated from broiler, dressing, or other poultry operations or plants. The following precautions should be observed: use separate buildings for brooding "started" chicks; use separate labor for work outside the hatchery; follow a policy of selling only day-old chicks; inspect production records of the supply flocks weekly in order to avoid use of eggs from flocks showing a significant drop in egg production; exclude used chick boxes and feed sacks; dispose of hatchery wastes properly; keep visitors and nonessential personnel from the hatching and brooding areas.

The Farm Flock

Sources of infection must be kept away from the flock by changing clothing and disinfecting footwear after visiting possible sources of contamination; insisting that blood-testing crews or other essential service personnel change their clothes and disinfect equipment; buying replacement stock as day-old chicks from reliable hatcheries (preferably local) to minimize the chances of disease exposure during transit by means other than the personal vehicle of the buyer; rearing the replacement flock on clean premises entirely apart from the adult flock; preventing the return or introduction of used poultry crates, feed sacks, or other equipment, materials, or vehicles; disposing of manure properly; disposing of dead birds by burning or deep burial; replacing contaminated or unfit deep litter; and annually or oftener, routinely cleaning and disinfecting the laying and brooder houses and range shelter.

Broiler Plant

Strict sanitary precautions as already defined must be observed.

Produce Plant

Care must be taken to guard against the purchase of poultry in the active stages of

ND. The gross contamination of crates and vehicles which results may carry the infection to birds in hatcheries and in broiler plants of clients. Frequent periodic cleaning and disinfection of facilities, equipment, and materials and proper disposal of offal and wastes will reduce the hazard.

Feed Dealer and Processor

The reuse of feed sacks should be discouraged unless properly cleaned and sterilized; proper measures to avoid spreading infection to and from farms should be practiced and encouraged.

Veterinarian

The local veterinarian can be active in disseminating knowledge on basic sanitation and providing advice to the poultryman on general and specific disease prevention problems. With laboratory assistance he can supply an early diagnosis and, if necessary, institute a proper vaccination service and control program (Pomeroy and Brandly, 1953).

Experience with the extensive application of triethylene glycol aerosol as a means of controlling spread of ND in a large broiler plant led Ellis et al. (1952) to the conclusion that while the air treatment appeared to reduce the incidence of ND, as estimated by the prevalence of high HI titers, it did not prevent the spread of benign ND infection or have a significant effect upon the weight of birds at slaughter. The hazards and means of sanitizing used burlap feed bags contaminated with NDV and other agents have been clarified by Jungherr (1950).

PREVENTION BY VACCINATION

Both types of Newcastle disease vaccines (inactivated virus and living virus) are now in use generally. If properly prepared, handled, and administered, they may be expected to stimulate a substantial degree of immunity in a large proportion of healthy vaccinated fowl (Levine and Fabricant, 1952). However, even the more pathogenic living NDV vaccines fail to engender permanent or lifelong protection in healthy, immunologically mature chickens against clinical or subclinical infection. Immunologic capacity is weak at hatching but strengthens substantially so as to equal that of the mature bird at about 6 weeks of age (Wolfe and Dilks, 1948). However, vaccina-

tion at an early age is frequently necessary where ND is enzootic (Ellis and Crook, 1952).

Inactivated Vaccines

Inactivated or killed NDV vaccines are prepared by growing suitably antigenic strains of virus in embryonating eggs; harvesting the dead or dying embryos and tissues (Hanson et al., 1951; Hofstad et al., 1963); and inactivating the virus, usually by chemical agents such as formaldehyde (Brandly et al., 1946c; Hofstad, 1953), crystal violet (Doyle and Wright, 1950; Osteen et al., 1961), or beta-propriolactone (Mack and Chotisen, 1955; LoGrippo, 1960; Keeble and Wade, 1963). Growth of virus in tissue cultures for vaccine production is also being practiced (Bankowski and Corstvet, 1960). Adjuvants such as alumina gel are added to increase and prolong the immunizing effect (Traub, 1944). The vaccines must be tested for safety and potency and given a "use expiration" date before release.

Each dose of the vaccine contains a relatively large quantity of killed virus, the normal reaction to which governs directly the degree and duration of the immunity which the bird can develop.

Inactivated ND vaccine affords some protection by a blocking or "interference" effect within several days after injection. Specific immunity against ND develops within a week after vaccination; it is well advanced after 2 weeks in healthy birds 10 days of age or older when vaccinated. All individuals in a flock may not develop a substantial immunity, and the immunity may wane considerably 2–6 months after vaccination. The degree to which protection is enhanced by revaccination depends upon the residual immunity, either active or passive, which is present at the time of revaccination. Critical work (Hofstad, 1953, 1954, 1955) has demonstrated that a minimal period of 9 weeks is required between initial vaccination and revaccination with killed vaccine if a maximal degree and duration of immunity to the "booster" dose is to be stimulated. Satisfactory reinforcement of immunity with living virus vaccine has been reported with intervals as short as 1–3 weeks (Geurden et al., 1950; Zuijdam, 1953; Lancaster, 1964).

The titer and persistence of immunity evoked by inactivated vaccines are usually less than those by the living vaccines. Yet only the former may be relied upon to prevent some undesirable effects of vaccination in laying flocks or in stock suffering from other diseases (Gross, 1961; Hoekstra, 1961) or devitalizing factors (Pomeroy and Brandly, 1953; Garside, 1962).

Live Virus Vaccines

Living NDV vaccines are usually prepared by growing in embryonating eggs modified or "weakened" strains of the virus (Brandly et al., 1946c; Hitchner, 1964; Lancaster, 1964). Avian cell cultures have also served as a source of ND vaccine (Bankowski and Boynton, 1948; Bankowski, 1950). Cultures of mammalian cells as a substitute for those of chicken origin are suggested in order to avoid contamination with chicken latent or orphan agents (Bankowski, 1957). Usually the infected embryo material is dried to powder from the frozen state. Further refrigeration before it is used as a reconstituted liquid or as a dust and proper care during its use are required to keep the vaccine virus alive and capable of producing satisfactory results.

The living ND vaccines now available from commercial sources are administered by different routes: the "stick" or wing web puncture (Beaudette et al., 1949b; Van Roekel, 1955), intramuscular injection (Bankowski, 1957), "drop" intranasal (Doll et al., 1950c) or conjunctival sac instillation, and by spraying or nebulizing (Johnson and Gross, 1952; Crawley, 1954) as well as dusting (Markham et al., 1955) for inhalation. Mechanical spraying of liquid vaccine and dispersion of micronized dry virus vaccine, as well as adding the virus to the drinking water (Gagliardi, 1953; Winterfield and Seadale, 1956, 1957), were designed to permit vaccination exposure and infection of entire lots or flocks (i.e. mass vaccination), thus saving the time and labor required for individual administration of the vaccine.

The trend toward the mass method of vaccination (i.e. aerosol, dust, or drinking water administration) is indicated by the fact that over 90% of the ND vaccine either alone or combined with bronchitis vaccine has been of this type in the United States for some years (Hitchner, 1964). The saving of time, labor, and vaccine cost by mass vaccination (Hitchner and Reising, 1953; Van Waveren and Zuijdam, 1955; Markham et al., 1957; Larose and Van Roekel, 1959) is not without sacrifice in uniform immunity resulting from vaccination of each bird of the flock (Lancaster, 1964). Obvious disadvantages are lack of uniformity in dosage, particularly with very young and devitalized birds (underexposure and overexposure) or in birds of any age as a result of variation in environment (humidity and temperature fluctuations and the presence of viricidal factors in air and water) and likely exposure of vaccinating personnel and dissemination to other fowl and mammals (Bankowski and Hill, 1954; Dardiri et al., 1962).

VACCINE STRAINS. The NDV strains employed in living vaccines are of reduced or modified pathogenicity (Hanson and Brandly, 1955). The least pathogenic (lentogenic) strains—B1 (Hitchner and Johnson, 1948), LaSota (Winterfield et al., 1957), and F (Asplin, 1952; Rouseff and Miteff, 1956)—are employed in birds of all ages for intranasal or intraocular instillation, admixture with the drinking water, or dusting and spraying. The moderately pathogenic (mesogenic) strains—Roakin (Beaudette et al., 1949b), MK 107 (Van Roekel et al., 1948), Mukteswar (Haddow and Idnani, 1946; Bornstein et al., 1949), H (Hertfordshire) (Iyer and Dobson, 1940; Ceccarelli, 1954), Haifa (Komarov and Goldsmit, 1946)—have been commonly used for wing web (intradermal), intramuscular, or feather follicle vaccination of stock older than 4 weeks, of nonlaying birds, and of other disease-free vigorous stock.

Chicks less than 3 weeks of age possess globulins received from the hen through the yolk. If the hen had antibodies to ND, the chick will be passively immune for a short period and protected to a degree against debilitating infection (Brandly et al., 1946d; Beaudette and Bivins, 1953). Since the antibody wanes rapidly at a rate that varies among individuals, it is not surprising that considerable controversy has existed concerning the protection afforded the chicks, particularly whether such individuals could be successfully immunized (Levine and Fabricant, 1950; Winterfield and Seadale, 1957; Bankowski and Corstvet, 1962; Keeble and Wade, 1963). Further complicating the picture is the immaturity of the immune mechanism of chickens less than 6 weeks of age (Bankowski and Rosenwald, 1956). The respiratory tracts of congenitally immune chicks can usually be infected, but the resulting immune response may be poor. In other instances it has been reported to be reasonably good (Hitchner et al., 1950; Doll et al., 1951; Lancaster et al., 1960).

Tests applicable to identification and safety of vaccine strains of ND have been devised (Hanson and Brandly, 1955; Hanson, 1956; Lancaster, 1964). The need for rigid requirements of ND vaccine purity (Johnson et al., 1954) is emphasized by the demonstration of NDV in some lots of commercial pox and laryngotracheitis vaccines (Zargar and Pomeroy, 1950; Hanson et al., 1967) and of the possibility of vaccine contamination with lymphomatosis via the eggs of carrier hens used for ND vaccine production (Burmester et al., 1956).

The quantity of virus introduced as living vaccine is so small that unless infection is established and multiplication ensues there is not enough viral antigen present to stimulate a satisfactory degree of immunity. Some degree of protection resulting from an interference develops quickly (Watanabe et al., 1968). The specific immunity engendered by living vaccine infection should appear within 5–7 days after vaccination and be of substantial degree after the 2nd week. The duration of immunity from living vaccine may vary greatly from flock to flock and among individuals. It may wane appreciably within 2 months, and revaccination is usually recommended within 2 months to a year (Doll et al., 1950c; Lancaster, 1964).

Immunity can be determined by exposing the vaccinates to infection and ascertaining both the qualitative and quantitative aspects of the response. Among the first are: (1) freedom from impairment of growth, activity, or productiveness; (2) freedom from signs of disease and lesions; (3) refractivity to multiplication of the organism. The three can be measured as increments or can be scored as intensity indices. The response is seldom one of a state of complete refractivity. Infection of the respiratory tract with virus multiplication can be established in chickens that have high levels of circulating antibody (Beard and Easterday, 1967b). Such individuals may show some mild sign of disease or none and may suffer mild or severe impairment of such activities as egg laying. In some instances they may shed the virus and infect susceptible individuals.

Beard and Easterday (1967a) determined that route of administration of the immunizing antigens played a major role in establishing the nature of refractiveness of the individual to reinfection. Unless the live virus vaccine was introduced into the respiratory tract, this tract developed only a poor and transitory resistance to infection by a challenge virus. Nasal drop and ocular instillation were less satisfactory than an aerosol that penetrated the lower reaches of the respiratory tract. Birds that had received the vaccinating virus in such a manner could not be reinfected for many weeks. The respiratory tract refractivity appeared to be due to localized immunity. Histologically a marked increase occurred in small lymphoid nodules within the submucosa, and the tracheal mucus contained a neutralizing substance. With explants from such birds Heuschele (1968) demonstrated the continuing production over a period of 2–3 weeks of NDV neutralizing substances.

Adequate and reliable information on the maximal and average duration of a serviceable immunity to ND resulting from a single or repeated vaccination is limited (Lancaster, 1964). Age and individual immunologic capacity as well as environmental and other factors affecting the host animal all mitigate against uniformity of its immune response to vaccination. Inapparent infection from repeated exposure can be ascertained with reasonable but not unequivocal accuracy by testing for antibody titer before, and at intervals after, challenge. Persistence of high antibody titer in some field flocks following a single vaccination may be the result of inapparent reinfection. That reported failure to induce a lasting immunity is not characteristic of only lentogenic strains of virus was illustrated by a study of a mesogenic Indian (Mukteswar) vaccine (Bornstein et al., 1949). These workers concluded in consequence of ND "breaks" following vaccination that the immunity engendered by it could not be depended upon for longer than a year.

Breaks due to antigenic inadequacy of the vaccine are probably of lesser importance than breaks associated with improper handling and use of the vaccine (Jungherr and Markham, 1962).

Simultaneous vaccination against ND

and bronchitis or ND and fowl pox has been further exploited toward saving labor and handling of birds. However, pox vaccination, either with chicken or pigeon source virus, requires manipulating the individual birds. Although a mixture of pigeon pox and ND viruses has been applied by the feather follicle method (Richter, 1956), a commercial product has not been offered.

The saving in time and expense of simultaneous vaccination invites the risk of interference with development of maximal immunity against one of the diseases (Hanson et al., 1956; Bankowski and Rosenwald, 1956; Hitchner and White, 1956) or of exalting one of the agents (Hanson, 1957). Some investigators report, however, that no diminution in response followed simultaneous vaccination with ND and bronchitis (Markham et al., 1956). There are various reports of the activation or aggravation of latent infections or parasitic effects and other devitalizing influences from the use of vaccines (Placidi, 1956; Rouseff, 1956; Markham et al., 1957). Vaccines have made it possible to raise large flocks of chickens relatively free of disease in a region with a high chicken population and a history of enzooticity. However, the infection has not been eliminated and remains widely distributed. Problems continue to occur through failure to vaccinate properly, failure of the vaccine, or concurrent and debilitating disease.

REFERENCES

Ackermann, W. Wilbur. 1964. Cell surface phenomena of Newcastle disease virus, pp. 153–65. In Hanson, R. P. (ed.), *Newcastle Disease Virus: An Evolving Pathogen.* Univ. Wisconsin Press, Madison.

Albiston, H. E., and C. J. R. Gorrie. 1942. Newcastle disease in Victoria. *Australian Vet. J.* 18:75–79.

Anderson, D. P., R. P. Hanson, and F. Cherms. 1964. Studies on measuring the environment of turkeys raised in confinement. *Poultry Sci.* 43:305–18.

Andrewes, C. H. 1960. Viruses of the common cold. *Sci. American* 203:88–100.

Andrewes, C. H., F. B. Bang, and F. M. Burnet. 1955. A short description of the myxovirus group (influenza and related viruses). *Virology* 1:176–84.

Arenas, J. D. 1952. Contribucion al estudio de la enfermadad de Newcastle. *Ann. Rept. Univ. Nac. Colombia Fac. Med. Vet. Zoot. Rev.*

Asdell, Mary K., and R. P. Hanson. 1960. Sequential changes in the titer of Newcastle disease virus in tissues—a measure of the defense mechanisms of the chicken. *Am. J. Vet. Res.* 21:128–32.

Asplin, F. D. 1947. Newcastle disease in ducks and geese. *Vet. Record* 59:621–23.

———. 1952. Immunization against Newcastle disease with a virus of low virulence (Strain F) and observations on sub-clinical infection in partially resistant fowls. *Vet. Record* 64:245–49.

Auer, J. 1952. Functional localization of lesions in Newcastle disease. I. General survey. *Can. J. Comp. Med. Vet. Sci.* 16:277–84.

Bang, F. B. 1947. Newcastle virus. Conversion of spherical form to filamentous forms. *Proc. Soc. Exp. Biol. Med.* 64:135–37.

———. 1948. Studies on Newcastle disease virus. I. An evaluation of the method of titration of the virus in the embryo. II. Behavior of the virus in the embryo. III. Characters of the virus itself with particular reference to electron microscopy. *J. Exp. Med.* 88:233–66.

———. 1952. Development of Newcastle disease virus in cells of the chorio-allantoic membrane as studied in thin sections. *Bull. Johns Hopkins Hosp.* 92:309–29.

———. 1964. Pathogenesis in the embryo, pp. 247–56. In Hanson, R. P. (ed.), *Newcastle Disease Virus: An Evolving Pathogen.* Univ. Wisconsin Press, Madison.

Bang, F. B., and M. Foard. 1953. The serology of Newcastle disease virus infection. I. The reaction between various sera and the virus. *J. Immunol.* 76:342–47.

Bang, F. B., and A. Warwick. 1957. The effect of an avirulent and a virulent strain of Newcastle virus (Myxovirus multiforme) on cells in tissue culture. *J. Pathol. Bacteriol.* 73:321–30.

Bankowski, R. A. 1950. Further studies on *in vitro* cultivated pneumoencephalitis (Newcastle disease) virus and its use as a vaccine. *Vet. Med.* 45:322–27.

———. 1957. A modified live Newcastle disease virus vaccine. *Proc. Soc. Exp. Biol. Med.* 96:114–18.

———. 1961. A study of asymptomatic Newcastle disease in a breeding flock. *Res. Vet. Sci.* 2:193–201.

———. 1964. Cytopathogenicity of Newcastle disease virus, pp. 231–46. In Hanson, R. P. (ed.), *Newcastle Disease Virus: An Evolving Pathogen.* Univ. Wisconsin Press, Madison.

Bankowski, R. A., and W. H. Boynton. 1948. Preliminary report on the propagation of avian pneumoencephalitis virus (Newcastle disease) *in vitro. Vet. Med.* 43:305–6.

Bankowski, R. A., and R. Corstvet. 1960. Immunity and the reproductive tract of laying hens vaccinated with the tissue culture Newcastle disease virus. *Am. J. Vet. Res.* 21: 610–17.

———. 1961. Isolation of hemagglutinating agent distinct from Newcastle disease from the respiratory tract of chickens. *Avian Diseases* 5:253–69.

———. 1962. Nature of immunity to Newcastle disease in vaccinated chickens. I. Influence of residual resistance upon the level and duration of immunity following revaccination. *Avian Diseases* 6:333–48.

Bankowski, R. A., and R. W. Hill. 1954. Factors influencing the efficiency of vaccination of chickens against Newcastle disease by the air-borne route. *Proc. Am. Vet. Med. Ass. 91st Ann. Meet.*, pp. 317–27.

Bankowski, R. A., and A. S. Rosenwald. 1956. Poultry vaccination, why and how. *Univ. Calif. Exp. Sta. Circ.* 455:1–19.

Bankowski, R. A., R. Corstvet, and J. Fabricant. 1958. A tissue culture-modified Newcastle disease virus. II. Immunogenicity of the live tissue culture-modified Newcastle disease virus in chickens. *Avian Diseases* 2: 227–40.

Bankowski, R. A., H. Izawa, and J. Hyde. 1959. Tissue culture—A diagnostic tool—with particular reference to Newcastle disease and vesicular exanthema viruses. *Proc. Ann. Meet. U.S. Livestock Sanit. Ass.* 63:377–88.

Barahona, H. H. 1969. Plaque enhancement and effect of magnesium and diethylaminoethyl dextran on replication of Newcastle disease virus lentogenic strains. Ph.D. thesis. Univ. Wisconsin, Madison.

Barahona, H. H., and R. P. Hanson. 1968. Plaque enhancement of Newcastle disease virus (lentogenic strains) by magnesium and diethylaminoethyl dextran. *Avian Diseases* 12:151–58.

Baron, Samuel. 1964. Relationship of interferon and temperature to virulence of Newcastle disease virus, pp. 205–20. In Hanson, R. P. (ed.), *Newcastle Disease Virus: An Evolving Pathogen.* Univ. Wisconsin Press, Madison.

Baskaya, H., H. E. Burd, C. B. Hudson, and J. A. Bivins. 1952. A comparison of Newcastle disease virus recovery from bone marrow and from pools of respiratory tract and spleen. *Am. J. Vet. Res.* 13:405–6.

Beach, J. R. 1942. Avian pneumoencephalitis. *Proc. Ann. Meet. U.S. Livestock Sanit. Ass.* 46:203–23.

———. 1943. Avian pneumoencephalitis. *North Am. Vet.* 24:288–92.

———. 1944. The neutralization *in vitro* of avian pneumoencephalitis virus by Newcastle disease immune serum. *Science* 100: 361–62.

———. 1946. The status of avian pneumoencephalitis and Newcastle disease in the United States. *J. Am. Vet. Med. Ass.* 108: 372–76.

Beamer, P. D., and J. E. Prier. 1950. Studies on Newcastle disease. III. Resistance of Newcastle disease virus to certain chemical agents. *Cornell Vet.* 40:57–60.

Beard, C. W., and B. C. Easterday. 1967. The influence of the route of administration of Newcastle disease virus on host response. I. Serological and virus isolation studies. II. Studies on artificial passive immunity. III. Immunofluorescent and histopathological studies. *J. Infect. Diseases* 117:55–61, 62–65, 66–70.

Beaudette, F. R. 1943. A review of the literature on Newcastle disease. *Proc. Ann. Meet. U.S. Livestock Sanit. Ass.* 47:122–77.

———. 1948. The immunization of birds against Newcastle disease. *Proc. Ann. Meet. U.S. Livestock Sanit. Ass.* 52:254–65.

———. 1949. An addendum to a review of the literature on Newcastle disease. *Proc. Ann. Meet. U.S. Livestock Sanit. Ass.* 53:202–20.

———. 1950. Recent literature on Newcastle disease. *Proc. Ann. Meet. U.S. Livestock Sanit. Ass.* 54:132–53.

———. 1951. Current literature on Newcastle disease. *Proc. U.S. Livestock Sanit. Ass.* 55: 108–74.

Beaudette, F. R., and J. A. Bivins. 1953. The influence of passive immunity on the response to intramuscular and intranasal administration of Newcastle disease virus. *Cornell Vet.* 43:513–31.

Beaudette, F. R., and J. J. Black. 1946. Newcastle disease in New Jersey. *Proc. Ann. Meet. U.S. Livestock Sanit. Ass.* 49:49–58.

Beaudette, F. R., and C. B. Hudson. 1956. Evidence of Newcastle disease in eastern United States as early as 1938. *Cornell Vet.* 46:227–44.

Beaudette, F. R., J. A. Bivins, and B. R. Miller. 1948. Use of antibiotic agents for bacterial sterilization of respiratory exudates from naturally infected cases of Newcastle disease. *Am. J. Vet. Res.* 9:97–101.

———. 1949a. A comparison of filtration and antibiotic treatment for the recovery of Newcastle virus from spontaneous cases. *Am. J. Vet. Res.* 10:92–95.

———. 1949b. Newcastle disease immunization with live virus. *Cornell Vet.* 39:302–34.

Berg, L. R., G. E. Bearse, and C. M. Hamilton. 1947. The effect of Newcastle disease on egg production and egg quality. *Poultry Sci.* 26:614–22.

Berke, Z., and S. B. Golem. 1949. (Newcastle

disease in Turkey). *Turk Ijiyen Tecrubi Biyol. Dergisi* 9:132–49.

Binns, W., H. M. Nielsen, and M. L. Miner. 1949. Severe Newcastle disease outbreak causes serious losses to Utah poultry industry. *Utah Farm Home Sci.* 10:1–2, 17.

Bird, H. R. 1964. The changing environment of the chicken, pp. 35–46. In Hanson, R. P. (ed.), *Newcastle Disease Virus: An Evolving Pathogen.* Univ. Wisconsin Press, Madison.

Biswal, G. 1954. Additional histological findings in the chicken reproductive tract. *Poultry Sci.* 33:843–51.

Biswal, G., and C. C. Morrill. 1954. The pathology of the reproductive tract of laying pullets affected with Newcastle disease. *Poultry Sci.* 33:880–97.

Bivins, J. A., Barbara R. Miller, and F. R. Beaudette. 1950. Search for virus in eggs laid during recovery post inoculation with Newcastle disease virus. *Am. J. Vet. Res.* 11:426–27.

Blattner, R. J., and A. P. Williamson. 1951. Developmental abnormalities in the chick embryo following infection with Newcastle disease virus. *Proc. Soc. Exp. Biol. Med.* 77:619–21.

Blaxland, J. D. 1951. Newcastle disease in shags and cormorants and its significance as a factor in the spread of this disease among domestic poultry. *Vet. Record* 63:731–33.

Blood, B. D. 1950. Epidemiology of Newcastle disease. *Bull. Pan Am. Sanit. Bur.* 29:28–49.

Bolin, F. M. 1948. Isolation of Newcastle disease virus from feces of the domestic cat and the common chicken louse. *Proc. 48th Ann. Meet. Soc. Am. Bacteriol.,* p. 43. (Abstr.)

Boney, W. A. 1951. The isolation of a neurotropic strain (GB) of Newcastle disease virus. *Southwestern Vet.* 5:19–21.

Bornstein, S., A. Rautenstein, and H. E. Moses. 1949. A large-scale vaccination breakdown with "Mukteswar" Newcastle vaccine, and its investigation by means of the haemagglutination inhibition test. *Refuah Vet.* 6:155–58.

Boulanger, P., and Christine E. Rice. 1953. A study of complement-fixation methods as applied to the demonstration of antibodies in birds. *Proc. Am. Vet. Med. Ass.* 90:316–21.

Boyd, R. J., and R. P. Hanson. 1958. Survival of Newcastle disease virus in nature. *Avian Diseases* 2:83–93.

Brandly, C. A. 1951. Poultry diseases as public health problems. *Public Health Rept.* 66:668–72.

Brandly, C. A., H. E. Moses, E. Elizabeth Jones, and E. L. Jungherr. 1946a. Epizootiology of Newcastle disease of poultry. *Am. J. Vet. Res.* 7:243–49.

Brandly, C. A., H. E. Moses, E. L. Jungherr, and E. Elizabeth Jones. 1946b. The isolation and identification of Newcastle disease virus. *Am. J. Vet. Res.* 7:289–306.

Brandly, C. A., H. E. Moses, E. Elizabeth Jones, and E. L. Jungherr. 1946c. Immunization of chickens against Newcastle disease. *Am. J. Vet. Res.* 7:307–32.

Brandly, C. A., H. E. Moses, and E. L. Jungherr. 1946d. Transmission of antiviral activity via the egg and the role of congenital passive immunity to Newcastle disease in chickens. *Am. J. Vet. Res.* 7:333–42.

Brandly, C. A., R. P. Hanson, S. H. Lewis, Nancy S. Winslow, W. R. Pritchard, H. H. Hoyt, and C. M. Nerlinger. 1947. Variables and correlations in laboratory procedures for Newcastle disease diagnosis. *Cornell Vet.* 37:324–36.

Brandt, C. D. 1961. Cytopathic action of myxoviruses on cultivated mammalian cells. *Virology* 14:1–10.

Brueckner, A. L., R. L. Reagan, D. M. Schenck, H. O. Werner, and J. W. Hickman. 1950. Mammalian adaptations of Newcastle disease virus. *Proc. Am. Vet. Med. Ass. Ann. Meet.* 87:163–65.

Brumfield, H. P., and B. S. Pomeroy. 1957. Direct complement fixation by turkey and chicken serum in viral systems. *Proc. Soc. Exp. Biol. Med.* 94:146–49.

Buddingh, G. J. 1952. The pathological effects of viruses on the chick embryo. *Ann. N.Y. Acad. Sci.* 55:248–53.

Burmester, B. R., C. H. Cunningham, G. E. Cottral, R. C. Belding, and R. F. Gentry. 1956. The transmission of visceral lymphomatosis with live virus Newcastle disease vaccines. *Am. J. Vet. Res.* 17:283–89.

Burnet, F. M. 1942. The affinity of Newcastle disease virus to the influenza virus group. *Australian J. Exp. Biol. Med. Sci.* 20:81–88.

———. 1950. The haemolytic action of Newcastle disease virus. I. Two types of interaction between virus and red cells. *Australian J. Exp. Biol. Med. Sci.* 28:299–309.

Burnet, F. M., and J. D. Ferry. 1934. The differentiation of the viruses of fowl plague and Newcastle disease: Experiments using the technique of chorio-allantoic membrane inoculation of the developing egg. *Brit. J. Exp. Pathol.* 15:56–64.

Burnet, F. M., and P. E. Lind. 1950. Haemolysis by Newcastle disease virus. II. General character of the haemolytic action. *Australian J. Exp. Biol. Med. Sci.* 28:129–50.

Burnstein, T., and F. B. Bang. 1957. Infection of the upper respiratory tract of the chick with a mild (vaccine) strain of Newcastle disease virus. I. Initiation and spread of the infection. II. Studies on the pathogenesis of the infection. *Bull. Johns Hopkins Hosp.* 102:127–57.

Byerly, T. C. 1948. Report of the committee on incidence of Newcastle disease. *J. Am. Vet. Med. Ass.* 12:125–26.

Cairns, H. J. F. 1951. The growth of influenza viruses and Newcastle disease virus in mouse brain. *Brit. J. Exp. Pathol.* 32:110–17.

Ceccarelli, A. 1954. Il Vaccino "H" (ceppo Hertfordshire) nella profilassi della pseudopeste aviare. *Zooprofilassi* 9:421–28, 431.

Chanock, R. M. 1955. Cytopathogenic effect of Newcastle disease virus in monkey kidney cultures and interference with poliomyelitis viruses. *Proc. Soc. Exp. Biol. Med.* 89:379–81.

Chanock, R. M., and Helen V. Coates. 1964. Myxoviruses—A comparative description, pp. 279–98. In Hanson, R. P. (ed.), *Newcastle Disease Virus: An Evolving Pathogen.* Univ. Wisconsin Press, Madison.

Chaproniere, D. M., and H. G. Pereira. 1955. Propagation of fowl plague and of Newcastle disease viruses in cultures of embryonic human lung. *Brit. J. Exp. Pathol.* 36:607–10.

Chu, H. P. 1953. The agglutination of spermatozoa by viruses in influenza, mumps and Newcastle disease. *Proc. 6th Int. Congr. Microbiol.* 2:413–14.

Chute, H. L., and D. C. O'Meara. 1963. The development of chickens free of common poultry diseases. *Maine Agr. Expt. Sta. Bull.* 613.

Clancy, C. F., H. R. Cox, and C. A. Bottorff. 1949. Laboratory experiments with living Newcastle disease vaccine. *Poultry Sci.* 28:58–62.

Clark, D. S., E. E. Jones, and F. K. Ross. 1955. The use of aqueous humor for early diagnosis of Newcastle disease. *Am. J. Vet. Res.* 16:138–40.

Clark, E., and F. P. O. Nagler. 1943. Haemagglutination by viruses. The range of susceptible cells with special reference to agglutination by vaccinia virus. *Australian J. Exp. Biol. Med. Sci.* 21:103–6.

Cole, R. K., and F. B. Hutt. 1961. Genetic differences in resistance to Newcastle disease. *Avian Diseases* 5:205–14.

Coleman, P. H. 1959. Studies of the antigenic nature of the myxoviruses. Ph.D. thesis. Univ. Wisconsin, Madison.

Coronel, A. B. 1948. Newcastle disease in the Philippines with special reference to immunization. *Int. Congr. Trop. Vet. Med. Malaria* 4:1366–73.

Crawford, M. 1930. Ranikhet Disease. *Ann. Rept. Gov. Vet. Surgeon.* Colombo, Ceylon.

Crawley, J. F. 1954. Immunization of chickens against infectious bronchitis and Newcastle disease by the spray method. *Proc.*

10th World's Poultry Congr. 2:234–37.

Cunningham, C. H. 1948. The effect of certain chemical agents on the virus of Newcastle disease of chickens. *Am. J. Vet. Res.* 9:195–97.

Daniel, M. D., and R. P. Hanson. 1968a. Differentiation of representative Newcastle disease virus strains by their plaque-forming ability on monolayers of chick embryo fibroblasts. *Avian Diseases* 12:423–33.

———. 1968b. Isolation and characterization of three plaque type clones of the Hickman strain of Newcastle disease virus. *Avian Diseases* 12:434–40.

Dardiri, A. H., V. J. Yates, and T. D. Flanagan. 1962. The reaction to infection with the B1 strain of Newcastle disease in man. *Am. J. Vet. Res.* 23:918–21.

DeKock, G. 1954. Studies on the histopathology and pathogenesis of Newcastle disease of fowls in South Africa, with special reference to the lymphoid tissue. (A preliminary report.) *Onderstepoort J. Vet. Res.* 26:599–620.

DeLay, P. D. 1947. Isolation of avian pneumoencephalitis (Newcastle disease) virus from the yolk sac of four-day old chicks, embryos, and infertile eggs. *Science* 106:545–46.

DeLay, P. D., K. B. DeOme, and R. A. Bankowski. 1948. Recovery of pneumoencephalitis (Newcastle) virus from the air of poultry houses containing infected birds. *Science* 107:474–75.

Dinter, Z. 1964. Avian myxoviruses, pp. 299–312. In Hanson, R. P. (ed.), *Newcastle Disease Virus: An Evolving Pathogen.* Univ. Wisconsin Press, Madison.

Dinter, Z., S. Hermodsson, and L. Hermodsson. 1964. Studies on myxovirus Yucaipa: Its classification as a member of the paramyxovirus group. *Virology* 22:297–304.

Divo, A. 1950. La enfermedad de Newcastle en Venezuela. *Bol. Venezuela Inst. Invest. Vet.* Caracas 3:547–75.

Dobson, N. 1939. Newcastle disease. *Proc. Seventh World's Poultry Congr.* 7:250–53.

Dobson, N., and G. B. Simmins. 1951. The introduction of Newcastle disease by means of frozen poultry carcasses. *Off. Rept. Ninth World's Poultry Congr.* 3:18–21.

Doll, E. R., M. E. Wallace, and W. H. McCollum. 1950a. Preincubation inoculation of eggs with Newcastle disease virus. *Poultry Sci.* 29:582–85.

———. 1950b. Interpretation of serologic procedures for the diagnosis of Newcastle disease. *Am. J. Vet. Res.* 11:265–71.

———. 1950c. Reinfection of chickens vaccinated by the intranasal method with live B1 Newcastle disease virus. *Am. J. Vet. Res.* 11:437–40.

Doll, E. R., W. H. McCollum, and M. E. Wallace. 1951. Susceptibility to Newcastle disease infection of chickens from hens immunized with live virus vaccines. *Am. J. Vet. Res.* 12:232–71.

Doyle, T. M. 1927. A hitherto unrecorded disease of fowls due to a filter-passing virus. *J. Comp. Pathol. Therap.* 40:144–69.

Doyle, T. M., and E. C. Wright. 1950. An inactivated vaccine against Newcastle disease. *Brit. Vet. J.* 106:139–61.

Eckert, J. 1957. (Epizootiology and epidemiological map of fowl pest in Europe.) Inaugural dissertation, Univ. Hanover.

Edwards, J. T. 1928. A new fowl disease. *Ann. Rept. Imp. Inst. Vet. Res. Mukteswar,* 1928. pp. 14–15.

Ellis, C. C., and E. Crook. 1952. Sanitation and vaccination in the control of Newcastle and other diseases in a large broiler plant. *Proc. Ann. Meet. U.S. Livestock Sanit. Ass.* 56:284–88.

Ellis, P., C. A. Brandly, and R. P. Hanson. 1952. The influence of triethylene glycol aerosol on the growth, morbidity and mortality rates of a broiler flock. *Poultry Sci.* 31:394–98.

Estupinan, J. 1968. The heterogeneity of a virulent strain of Newcastle disease virus. Ph.D. thesis. Univ. Wisconsin, Madison.

Estupinan, J., J. Spalatin, and R. P. Hanson. 1968. Use of yolk sac route of inoculation for titration of lentogenic strains of NDV. *Avian Diseases* 12:135–38.

Evans, A. S. 1955. Pathogenicity and immunology of Newcastle disease virus in man. *Am. J. Public Health* 45:742–45.

———. 1956. The laboratory diagnosis of Newcastle disease in man. *Am. J. Clin. Pathol.* 26:163–65.

Evans, C. A., and D. L. Melnick. 1950. Attempts to produce lymphocytopenia in rabbits following intravenous inoculation of certain viruses. *J. Infect. Diseases* 86:223–25.

Farinas, E. C. 1930. Avian pest, a disease of birds hitherto unknown in the Philippine Islands. *Philippine J. Agr.* 1:311–66.

Fastier, L. B. 1954. Infectivity titrations of the viruses of western equine encephalomyelitis and Newcastle disease by tissue culture methods. *J. Immunol.* 72:341–47.

Fenstermacher, R., B. S. Pomeroy, and W. A. Malmquist. 1946. Newcastle disease in Minnesota. *Proc. Ann. Meet. U.S. Livestock Sanit. Ass.* 50:151–57.

Fontaine, M. P., M. Fontaine, D. Chabas, and A. J. Brian. 1965. Presence of a Newcastle disease-like virus agent in chicken embryo cells. *Avian Diseases* 9:1–7.

Foster, N. M., and C. H. Thompson, Jr. 1957. The comparative thermolability of four strains of Newcastle disease virus of widely varying virulence. *Vet. Med.* 52:119–21.

Francis, D. W., and A. F. Kish. 1955. Familial resistance to Newcastle disease in a strain

of New Hampshires. *Poultry Sci.* 34:331–36.

French, E. L., and Joan Bennett. 1952. The pyrogenic effect of the influenza mumps group of viruses in the laboratory rabbit. *Australian J. Exp. Biol. Med. Sci.* 30:479–88.

French, E. L., T. D. St. George, and J. J. Percy. 1967. Infection of chicks with recently isolated Newcastle disease virus of low virulence. *Australian Vet. J.* 43:404–9.

Gagliardi G. 1953. La vaccinazione per via orale contro la pseudo peste dei polli. *Atti. Soc. Ital. Sci. Vet.* 7:911–17.

Gale, G. 1964. Recognition of Newcastle disease as a new disease. Discussion, p. 99. In Hanson, R. P. (ed.), *Newcastle Disease Virus: An Evolving Pathogen,* Univ. Wisconsin Press, Madison.

Gallardo, Koch E. 1951. Estudio experimental de la enfermedad de Newcastle en Chile. *Rev. Soc. Med. Vet. Chile* 3:5–8.

Garside, J. S. 1962. Newcastle disease vaccination. *Vet. Record* 74:1497–99.

Gelenczei, E., and D. Bordt. 1960. Studies of Newcastle disease virus strains in various cell cultures. *Am. J. Vet. Res.* 21:987–92.

Geurden, L. M. G., A. Devos, and J. Mortelmans. 1950. Immunisatieproeven tegen Pseudovogelpest. *Vlaams Diergeneesk. Tijdschr.* 19:177–94.

Gillespie, J. H., B. Kessel, and J. Fabricant. 1950. The isolation of Newcastle disease virus from a starling. *Cornell Vet.* 40:93–94.

Ginsberg, H. D. 1951. Mechanics of production of pulmonary lesions in mice by Newcastle disease virus (NDV). *J. Exp. Med.* 94:191–211.

Goldhaft, T. M., and N. Wernicoff. 1948. High mortality associated with a widespread outbreak of Newcastle disease. *Cornell Vet.* 38:181–85.

Goldman, E. C., and R. P. Hanson. 1955. The isolation and characterization of heat-resistant mutants of the Najarian strain of NDV. *J. Immunol.* 74:101–5.

Goldwasser, R., and A. Kohn. 1957. Neutralization and titration of Newcastle disease virus in chicken embryo tissue cultures. *Am. J. Vet. Res.* 18:390–95.

Granoff, A. 1962. Heterozygosis and phenotypic mixing with Newcastle disease virus. *Cold Spring Harbor Symp. Quant. Biol.* 27:319–26.

———. 1964. Nature of the Newcastle disease virus population, pp. 107–18. In Hanson, R. P. (ed.), *Newcastle Disease Virus: An Evolving Pathogen.* Univ. Wisconsin Press, Madison.

Granoff, A., and W. Henle. 1954. Studies on the hemolytic activity of Newcastle disease virus (NDV). *J. Immunol.* 72:322–28.

Granoff, A., and G. K. Hirst. 1954. Experimental production of combination forms of virus. IV. Mixed influenza A-Newcastle disease virus infections. *Proc. Soc. Exp. Biol. Med.* 86:84–89.

Gray, J. E., G. H. Snoeyenbos, and H. A. Peck. 1954. Newcastle disease in turkeys. Report of a field outbreak. *J. Am. Vet. Med. Ass.* 124:302–7.

Gross. W. B. 1961. *Escherichia coli* as a complicating factor of Newcastle disease vaccination. *Avian Diseases* 5:132–34.

Groupé, V., and R. M. Doughtery. 1956. Neuropathic effect of Newcastle disease virus in mice and modification of host response by receptor destroying enzyme, vital interference, and xerosin. *J. Immunol.* 76: 130–37.

Gustafson, D. P., and H. E. Moses. 1953. The English sparrow as a natural carrier of Newcastle disease virus. *Am. J. Vet. Res.* 14: 581–85.

Haddow, J. R., and J. A. Idnani. 1946. Vaccination against Newcastle (Ranikhet) disease. *Indian J. Vet. Sci.* 16:45–53.

Hanson, L. E. 1957. Some factors responsible for variations in viral immunity. *J. Am. Vet. Med. Ass.* 130:505–8.

Hanson, L. E., F. H. White, and J. O. Alberts. 1956. Interference between Newcastle disease and infectious bronchitis viruses. *Am. J. Vet. Res.* 17:294–98.

Hanson, R. P. 1949. Characteristics of certain strains of Newcastle disease virus. Ph.D. thesis. Univ. Wisconsin, Madison.

———. 1956. An intracerebral inoculation test for determining the safety of Newcastle disease vaccines. *Am. J. Vet. Res.* 17: 16–17.

Hanson, R. P. (ed.). 1964. *Newcastle Disease Virus: An Evolving Pathogen.* Univ. Wisconsin Press, Madison. Pp. 1–352.

Hanson, R. P., and C. A. Brandly. 1955. Identification of vaccine strains of Newcastle disease virus. *Science* 122:156–57.

———. 1958. Newcastle disease. Symposium on animal disease and human health. *Ann. N.Y. Acad. Sci.* 70:585–97.

Hanson, R. P., and S. K. Sinha. 1952. Epizootic of Newcastle disease in pigeons and studies on transmission of the virus. *Poultry Sci.* 31:404–8.

Hanson, R. P., Nancy S. Winslow, and C. A. Brandly. 1947. Influence of the route of inoculation of Newcastle disease virus on selective infection of the embryonating egg. *Am. J. Vet. Res.* 8:416–20.

Hanson, R. P., Elizabeth Upton, C. A. Brandly, and Nancy S. Winslow. 1949. Heat stability of hemagglutinin of various strains of Newcastle disease virus. *Proc. Soc. Exp. Biol. Med.* 70:283–87.

Hanson, R. P., Nancy S. Winslow, C. A. Brandly, and Elizabeth Upton. 1950. Antiviral activity of Newcastle disease immune sera. *J. Bacteriol.* 60:557–60.

Hanson, R. P., E. Crook, and C. A. Brandly. 1951. Comparisons of immunogenicity of five strains of Newcastle disease virus as formalinized vaccines. *Vet. Med.* 46:451–52.

Hanson, R. P., J. Spalatin, and E. M. Dickinson. 1967. Criteria for determining the validity of a virus isolation. *Avian Diseases* 11:509–14.

Heuschele, W. P. 1968. Local immunity and virus persistence in the trachea of chickens following infection with Newcastle disease virus. Ph.D. thesis. Univ. Wisconsin, Madison.

Hirst, G. K., and E. G. Pickels. 1942. A method for the titration of influenza hemagglutinins and influenza antibodies with the aid of a photo electron densitometer. *J. Immunol.* 45:273–83.

Hitchner, S. B. 1950. Further observations on a virus of low virulence for immunizing fowls against Newcastle disease. *Cornell Vet.* 40:60–70.

———. 1964. Control of Newcastle disease in the United States by vaccination, pp. 85–98. In Hanson, R. P. (ed.), *Newcastle Disease Virus: An Evolving Pathogen.* Univ. Wisconsin Press, Madison.

Hitchner, S. B., and E. P. Johnson. 1948. A virus of low virulence for immunizing fowls against Newcastle disease (avian pneumoencephalitis). *Vet. Med.* 43:525–30.

Hitchner, S. B., and G. Reising. 1953. Results of field tests on spraying a commercially prepared Newcastle disease vaccine. *Proc. Am. Vet. Med. Ass. 90th Ann. Meet.,* pp. 350–55.

Hitchner, S. B., and P. G. White. 1956. An immunologic study of various modifications of a vaccination program for Newcastle disease and infectious bronchitis. *Am. Scientific Lab. Inc. Res. Rept.* 3.

Hitchner, S. B., G. Reising, and H. Van Roekel. 1950. The intranasal vaccine—its role in a Newcastle disease control program. *Proc. Ann. Meet. U.S. Livestock Sanit. Ass.* 54: 154–60.

Hoekstra, J. 1961. Control of Newcastle disease and infectious bronchitis by vaccination. *Brit. Vet. J.* 117:289–95.

Hofstad, M. S. 1951. A quantitative study of Newcastle disease virus in tissues of infected chickens. *Am. J. Vet. Res.* 12:334–39.

———. 1953. Immunization of chickens against Newcastle disease by formalin-inactivated virus. *Am. J. Vet. Res.* 14:586–89.

———. 1954. The secondary immune response in chickens revaccinated with inactivated Newcastle disease virus vaccine. *Am. J. Vet. Res.* 15:604–6.

———. 1955. The immune response in chickens following the use of three different types of inactivated Newcastle disease vaccine. *Am. J. Vet. Res.* 16:608–12.

Hofstad, M. S., J. C. Picken, K. E. Collins, and and H. W. Yoder. 1963. Immunogenicity of inactivated Newcastle disease virus preparations. *Avian Diseases* 7:435–45.

Hudson, J. R. 1937. Observation on a highly fatal virus disease of fowls from East Africa. *Vet. J.* 93:356–68.

Ingalls, W. L., R. W. Vesper, and A. Mahoney. 1951. Isolation of Newcastle disease virus from the great horned owl. *J. Am. Vet. Med. Ass.* 119:71.

Iyer, S. G. 1943. Studies on Newcastle (Ranikhet) disease virus. *Indian J. Vet. Sci.* 13:1–26.

Iyer, S. G., and N. Dobson. 1940. A successful method of immunization against Newcastle disease of fowls. *Vet. Record* 52:889–94.

Johnson, E. P., and W. B. Gross. 1952. Vaccination against pneumoencephalitis (Newcastle disease) by atomization of nebulization in incubators and chick boxes with the B1 virus. *Vet. Med.* 47:364–66, 371.

Johnson, E. P., R. P. Hanson, A. S. Rosenwald, and H. Van Roekel. 1954. The responsibility of state and federal agencies in the improvement of poultry vaccines. *J. Am. Vet. Med. Ass.* 125:441–46.

Johnstone, R. N. 1931. Pseudo poultry plague, symptoms and precautions recommended. *J. Dept. Agr., Victoria* 29:25–28.

Jungherr, E. L. 1948. Report of the Committee on modes of spread of Newcastle disease. *J. Am. Vet. Med. Ass.* 112:124–25.

———. 1950. Studies on sanitizing used feed bags. *J. Am. Vet. Med. Ass.* 117:324–28.

———. 1964. Pathogenicity of Newcastle disease virus for the chicken, pp. 257–72. In Hanson, R. P. (ed.), *Newcastle Disease Virus: An Evolving Pathogen.* Univ. Wisconsin Press, Madison.

Jungherr, E. L., and F. S. Markham. 1962. Relationship between a Puerto Rican epizootic and the B-1 strain of Newcastle disease virus. *Poultry Sci.* 41:522–28.

Jungherr, E. L., and E. L. Minard. 1944. The pathology of experimental avian pneumoencephalitis. *Am. J. Vet. Res.* 5:125–34.

Jungherr, E. L., and N. Terrell. 1946. Observations on the spread of Newcastle disease. *Proc. Ann. Meet. U.S. Livestock Sanit. Ass.* 50:158–71.

Jungherr, E. L., E. E. Tyzzer, C. A. Brandly, and H. E. Moses. 1946. The comparative pathology of fowl plague and Newcastle disease. *Am. J. Vet. Res.* 7:250–88.

Karzon, D. T. 1956. Non-specific viral inactivating substance (VIS) in human and mammalian sera. Natural antagonists to the inactivator of Newcastle disease virus and observations on the nature of the union between the inactivator and virus. *J. Immunol.* 76:454–63.

Karzon, D. T., and F. B. Bang. 1951. The pathogenesis of infection with a virulent (CG 179) and an avirulent (B) strain of Newcastle disease in the chicken. I. Comparative rates of viral multiplication. *J. Exp. Med.* 93:267–84.

Kaschula, V. R. 1950. The epizootiology of Newcastle disease and its control by vaccination. *J. S. African Vet. Med. Ass.* 21:134–40.

———. 1951. An observation on the pathogenesis of infection of artificial Newcastle disease in pigeons. *J. S. African Vet. Med. Ass.* 22:143–95.

———. 1961a. A comparison of disease in village and in modern poultry flocks in Nigeria. *Bull. Epiz. Diseases Africa* 9:397.

———. 1961b. The pattern of distribution of lesions in Newcastle disease in Northern Nigeria. *J. Comp. Pathol. Therap.* 71:343–49.

Kawashima, H., T. Sato, and T. Hanaki. 1953. The latest outbreak of Newcastle disease in Japan. *Rept. Govt. Exp. Sta. Animal Hyg.* (Japan) 27:151–67.

Keeble, S. A., and J. A. Wade. 1963. Inactivated Newcastle disease vaccine. *J. Comp. Pathol. Therap.* 72:186–200.

Keeble, S. A., P. G. Box, and D. W. Christie. 1963. Vaccination against Newcastle disease. *Vet. Record* 75:151–52.

Keymer, I. F. 1961. Newcastle disease in the jackdaw *(Corvus monedula)*. *Vet. Record* 73:119–22.

Kilham, L. 1949. A Newcastle disease virus (NDV) hemolysin. *Proc. Soc. Exp. Biol. Med.* 71:63–66.

Kingsbury, D. W. 1962. Use of actinomycin D to unmask RNA synthesis induced by Newcastle disease virus. *Biochem. Biophys. Res. Commun.* 9:156–61.

Kingsbury, D. W., and R. W. Darlington. 1968. Isolation and properties of Newcastle disease virus nucleocapsid. *J. Virol.* 2:248–55.

Kloppel, G. 1963. (Newcastle disease in ostriches.) *Kleintier-Praxis* 8:10–11.

Knox, C. W. 1950. The effect of Newcastle disease on egg production, egg weight and mortality rate. *Poultry Sci.* 29:907–11.

Kohler, H. 1953. Die Bedeutung der Encephalitis bei der Diagnose der Newcastle-Krankheit der Huehner. *Deut. Tieraerztl. Wochschr.* 60:261–67.

Kohn, A. 1955. Quantitative aspects of Newcastle disease virus infection—effect of route of infection on the susceptibility of chicks. *Am. J. Vet. Res.* 16:450–57.

———. 1959. The role of the alimentary tract and the spleen in Newcastle disease. *Am. J. Hyg.* 69:167–76.

Komarov, A. 1940. Newcastle disease in Palestine. *Palestine Vet. Bull.* 1:107–11.

Komarov, A., and L. Goldsmit. 1946. Preliminary observation on the modification of a strain of Newcastle disease virus by intracerebral passage through ducklings. *Vet. J.* 102:212–18.

Konno, T., Y. Ochi, and K. Hashimoto. 1929. Neve Gefluegelseuhe in Korea. *Deut. Tieraerztl. Wochschr.* 37:515–17.

Kraneveld, F. C. 1926. Over een in Ned-Indie heerschende Ziekte onder het Pluimves. *Ned. Indisch Bl. Diergeneesk.* 38:448–50.

Lancaster, J. E. 1964. Newcastle disease control by vaccination. *Vet. Bull.* 34:57–76.

———. 1966. Newcastle disease, a review 1926–1966. *Can. Dept. Agr. Monograph* 3. Queen's Printer, Ottawa.

Lancaster, J. E., M. Merriman, and A. A. Reinzi. 1960. The intranasal Newcastle disease vaccination of chicks from immune parents. *Can. J. Comp. Med. Vet. Sci.* 24:52–55.

Larose, R. N., and H. Van Roekel. 1959. Response of chicken flocks to commercial Newcastle disease and infectious bronchitis vaccines. *Poultry Sci.* 38:1221. (Abstr.)

Laver, W. O., and E. D. Kilbourne. 1966. Identification in a recombinant influenze virus of structural proteins derived from both parents. *Virology* 30:493–501.

Levine, P. P., and J. Fabricant. 1950. Susceptibility to Newcastle infection of chicks with congenital serum antibodies. *Cornell Vet.* 40:213–25.

———. 1952. Efficacy of Newcastle disease vaccines under controlled conditions. *Cornell Vet.* 42:449–56.

Levine, P. P., J. Fabricant, J. H. Gillespie, C. I. Angstrom, and G. B. Mitchell. 1950. The results of pen contact exposure of susceptible chickens to chickens recovered from Newcastle disease. *Cornell Vet.* 40:206–10.

Levine, S., and B. P. Sagik. 1956. The interactions of Newcastle disease virus (NDV) with chick embryo tissue culture cells: Attachment and growth. *Virology* 2:57–68.

Levinson, S. O., A. Milzer, H. Shaughnessy, J. Neal, and F. Oppenheimer. 1944. Production of potent inactivated vaccines with ultraviolet irradiation. *J. Am. Med. Ass.* 125:531–32.

Lippmann, O. 1952. Human conjunctivitis due to the Newcastle disease virus of fowls. *Am. J. Ophthalmol.* 35:1021–28.

Lissot, G. 1956. Peste aviaire, variete maladie de Newcastle, a virus faible. *Bull. Acad. Vet. France* 29:43, 45.

LoGrippo, G. A. 1960. Investigations of the use of beta-propiolactone in virus inactivation. *Ann. N.Y. Acad. Sci.* 83:578–94.

Lorenz, F. W., and W. E. Newlon. 1944. Influence of avian pneumoencephalitis on subsequent egg quality. *Poultry Sci.* 23:193–98.

Luginbuhl, R. E., and E. Jungherr. 1949. A plate hemagglutination-inhibition test for Newcastle disease antibodies in avian and human serums. *Poultry Sci.* 28:622–24.

McClurkin, A., S. K. Sinha, and R. P. Hanson. 1954. Rapid diagnosis of Newcastle disease using lung extract. *Am. J. Vet. Res.* 15:314–15.

McCollum, W. H., and C. A. Brandly. 1955a. Hemolytic activity of Newcastle disease virus. *Am. J. Vet. Res.* 16:584–92.

———. 1955b. Destruction of virus hemagglutination inhibitor of eggwhite by Newcastle disease virus. *Proc. Soc. Exp. Biol. Med.* 90:158–62.

Machado, A. V. 1951. The effect of infectious bronchitis and Newcastle disease on the blood cells of chickens. Ph.D. thesis, Cornell Univ., Ithaca.

Mack, W. N., and A. Chotisen. 1955. Betapropriolactone as a virus altering agent for a Newcastle disease vaccine. *Poultry Sci.* 34:1010–13.

McKercher, D. G. 1963. Studies of the etiologic agents of infectious bovine rhinotracheitis and Blaschenausschlag (coital vesicular exanthema). *Am. J. Vet. Res.* 24:501–8.

Maestrone, G., and D. C. Coffin. 1961. Study of Newcastle disease by the fluorescent antibody technique. I. Infection of chick embryos. II. Experimental infections in chicks. *Arch. Vet. Ital.* 12:97–105, 193–99.

Markham, F. S., A. H. Hammar, P. Gingher, H. R. Cox, and J. Storie. 1955. Vaccination against Newcastle disease and infectious bronchitis. I. Preliminary studies in mass vaccination with liver virus dust vaccines. *Poultry Sci.* 34:442–48.

Markham, F. S., A. H. Hammar, E. B. Perry, and W. C. Tesar. 1956. Combined Newcastle disease-infectious bronchitis vaccines and the absence of interference phenomenon. *Cornell Vet.* 46:538–48.

Markham, F. S., W. H. Patton, A. H. Hammar, C. A. Bottorff, P. E. Gingher, E. D. Perry, and W. C. Tesar. 1957. A second flock history after immunization against Newcastle disease and infectious bronchitis and observations on chronic respiratory disease. *Poultry Sci.* 36:150–59.

Matewa, V. 1960. Vergleichende versuche der Isolierung von Newcastle virus auf Gewebekulturen von Huhnerembryonen und bebruteten Huhnereieren. *Zentr. Bakteriol. Parasitenk. Abt. I. Orig.* 178:8–14.

Medina Blanco, M. 1949. Aportaciones et estudio de la immunizacion y de las causas que la rebajan en la enfermedad de Newcastle en Espana. *Bol. Inform. Col. Vet. Esp. Supl. Cient.* 3:355–66.

Melendez, L., J. Spalatin, and R. P. Hanson. 1965. Influence of temperature on induction by Newcastle disease virus of polykaryocytes in garter snake cells. *Am. J. Vet. Res.* 26:1451–56.

Mickalov, J., and O. J. Vrtiak. 1963. (Survival

of the virus of Newcastle disease in deep litter.) *Slovak Veterinarstvi* 1:9–10.

Minard, E. L., and E. Jungherr. 1944. Neutralization tests with avian pneumoencephalitis virus. *Am. J. Vet. Res.* 5:154–57.

Mitscherlich, E., and S. Gürtürk. 1952. Die serologische Untersuchung von Organextrakten gestorbener Huhner auf klassische und atypische Gefluegelpest (Newcastle-Krankheit). *Deut. Tieraerztl. Wochschr.* 59: 371–72.

Mohr, F. 1953. Die Huhnerpestneuritis. Ein Beitrag zur Differential-diagnose: Atypische Gefluegelpest-Mareksche Gefluegellahme. *Berlin. Muench. Tieraerztl. Wochschr.* 66: 205–8.

Monteverde, J., D. Hector Simeone, M. Rodrequez-Leiva, and E. J. Chialvo. 1962. Enfermedades de Newcastle. I. Su hallazo en la Republica Argentine. *Cienc. Vet.* (Mex.) 7:154–66.

Monti, G. 1952. La Diagnosi postmortale della pseudopeste aviare mediante la reazione di Hirst. *Arch. Vet. Ital.* 3:215–26.

Montroni, L. 1961. Pseudopeste aviare. Stomaco ghiandolare e intestino. *Zooprofilassi* 16: 133–35.

Morehouse, L. G., D. P. Gustafson, and H. E. Moses. 1963a. Growth of Newcastle disease virus in cell cultures derived from swine embryo lymph nodes. *Am. J. Vet. Res.* 24: 588–94.

Morehouse, L. G., H. E. Moses, and D. P. Gustafson. 1963b. Newcastle disease virus in tissue culture cells derived from chickens. *Am. J. Vet. Res.* 24:580–87.

Morgan, C., and C. Howe. 1968. Structure and development of viruses as observed in the electron microscope 1X entry of parainfluenza 1 (Sendai) virus. *J. Virol.* 2:1122–32.

Morimoto, T., T. Omori, and M. Matumoto. 1962. Interference of Russian spring-summer encephalitis virus with Newcastle disease virus in cell culture of bovine embryonic kidney. *Japan. J. Exp. Med.* 32:163–83.

Moses, H. E., C. A. Brandly, and E. Elizabeth Jones. 1947. The pH stability of viruses of Newcastle disease and fowl plague. *Science* 105:477–79.

Moulin, F. de. 1951. Pathologische-histologisch onderyoek van pseudopest by Kippen in Nederland. *Tijdschr. Diergeneesk.* 76:389–407.

Nakamura, J., S. Oyama, F. Fukushio, and N. Tomonoga. 1933. Vergleichende immunbiologische Untersuchungen der Korea, Huhnerseuchenvirus und des japanischen Gefluegelpestvirus, zugleich ueber die Beziehung zum Virus der Newcastle disease. *Jap. Soc. Vet. Sci.* 12:135–45.

Nitzschke, E. 1954. Zur Frage des Vorkommens von Virustragern und Spaetausscheidern bei der atypischen Gefluegelpest. *Berlin. Muench. Tieraerztl. Wochschr.* 67:335–38.

Obel, A. L., K. Bakos, and O. T. Sundberg. 1956. Untersuchungen ueber die Ursache der Dyspnoe bei experimentellen Newcastle-Krankheit der Huehner. *Nord. Vet. Med.* 8:243–49.

Olesiuk, O. M. 1951. Influence of environmental factors on viability of Newcastle disease virus. *Am. J. Vet. Res.* 12:152–55.

Orr, W., and K. T. John. 1946. A Malayan virus disease of fowls. *Vet. Record* 58:117–19.

Osteen, O. L., L. O. Mott, and E. Gill. 1961. The use of killed virus vaccine to control Newcastle disease. *Proc. Ann. Meet. U.S. Livestock Sanit. Ass.* 64:232–34.

Palmer, S. 1969. Some infectious diseases of Canada geese. Ph.D. thesis, Univ. Wisconsin, Madison.

Parnaik, D. O., and S. G. Dixit. 1953. Ranikhet disease in Indian partridges. *Indian Vet. J.* 30:145–47.

Picken, J. C. 1964. Themolability of Newcastle disease virus, pp. 167–88. In Hanson, R. P. (ed.), *Newcastle Disease Virus: An Evolving Pathogen.* Univ. Wisconsin Press, Madison.

Piraino, F. P., and R. P. Hanson. 1959. Isolation of a non-neurotropic line of Newcastle disease virus from a neurotropic parental type. *Virology* 8:383–85.

———. 1960. An *in vitro* method for the identification of strains of Newcastle disease virus. *Am. J. Vet. Res.* 21:125–27.

Placidi, L. 1956. Accidents consecutifs a la vaccination contre la maladie de Newcastle. Influence de la temperature ambiante. Roles respectifs du vaccin et l'hote. *Bull. Off. Int. Epiz.* 45:393–408.

Placidi, L., and J. Santucci. 1956. Agglutination comparee des hematies de la poule, du chameau et des equides par les virus de la maladie de Newcastle et de la peste aviaire. *Ann. Inst. Pasteur* 90:528–29.

Platt, C. S. 1948. Some observations on the effect of Newcastle disease upon laying fowl. *Poultry Sci.* 27:201–6.

Pomeroy, B. S., and C. A. Brandly. 1953. Facts about Newcastle disease. *Univ. Minn. Agr. Expt. Sta., North Central Regional Publ.* 34:1–22.

Potel, K. 1950. Zur Histopathologie der Pneumo-Encephalitis (Newcastle disease). *Exp. Veterinaermed.* 1:31–44.

Price, R. J., C. A. Bottorff, K. Seeger, A. W. Sylstra, and F. S. Markham. 1955. Vaccination against Newcastle disease and infectious bronchitis. 2. Field trials in mass vaccination with live virus dust vaccines. *Poultry Sci.* 34:449–55.

Prier, J. E., T. W. Millen, and J. O. Alberts. 1950. Studies on Newcastle disease. IV. The presence of NDV in eggs of hens vaccinated with live vaccine. *J. Am. Vet. Med. Ass.* 116:54–55.

Quinn, R. W., R. P. Hanson, J. W. Brown, and C. A. Brandly. 1952. Newcastle disease virus in man. Clinical and virus isolation studies in 3 cases. *J. Lab. Clin. Med.* 40:736–43.

Raggi, L. G. 1960. A rapid macroscopic plate agglutination test for Newcastle disease—A preliminary report. *Avian Diseases* 4:320–23.

Raggi, L. G., G. G. Lee, and V. Sohrab-Haghighat. 1963. Infectious bronchitis virus interference with growth of Newcastle disease virus. I. Study of interference in chicken embryos. *Avian Diseases* 7:106–22.

Reid, J. 1955. Fowl pest. *Agriculture* London 61:465–70.

———. 1961. The control of Newcastle disease in Great Britain. *Brit. Vet. J.* 117:275–88.

Report of the Committee on Fowl Pest Policy. 1962. Her Majesty's Stationery Office, London, Command Paper 1664, pp. 1–108.

Report of Poultry Disease Subcommittee on Animal Health, Agr. Bd., Div. Biol. Agr., Nat. Acad. Sci., Nat. Res. Council, Washington, D.C. 1959. *Methods for the Examination of Poultry Biologics,* 1st ed. Publ. 705, pp. 1–108.

Report of Poultry Disease Subcommittee on Animal Health, Agr. Bd., Div. Biol. Agr., Nat. Acad. Sci., Nat. Res. Council, Washington, D.C. 1963. *Methods for the Examination of Poultry Biologics,* 2nd ed. (rev.). Publ. 1038, pp. 1–158.

Ressang, A. A. 1961. (Newcastle disease in Indonesia. Part II. Its symptomatology, gross and microscopic anatomy.) *Commun. Vet.* (Bogor, Indonesia) 5:16–37.

Richter, J. H. M. 1956. Een gekombineerde enting tegen kippenpokken en pseudo-vogelpest. *Tijdschr. Diergeneesk.* 81:763–67.

Rodriguez, J. E., V. ter Menlen, and W. Henle. 1967. Studies on persistent infections of tissue cultures. VI. Reversible changes in Newcastle disease virus populations as a result of passage in L cells or chick embryos. *J. Virol.* 1:1–9.

Rott, R. 1964. Antigenicity of Newcastle disease virus, pp. 133–46. In Hanson, R. P. (ed.), *Newcastle Disease Virus: An Evolving Pathogen.* Univ. Wisconsin Press, Madison.

Rott, R., and W. Schafer. 1961. Fine structure of subunits isolated from Newcastle disease virus (NDV). *Virology* 14:298–99.

———. 1962. Hydroxylamin—Empfindlichkeit des Newcastle Disease Virus (NDV). *Z. Naturforsch.* 17b:861–62.

Rouseff, C. G. 1956. Mengenabhangigkeitsverhaltnis zwischen interferierendun Virusstammen der atypischen Gefluegelpest bei Versuchen an Huhnern. *Arch. Exp. Veterinaermed.* 10:207–10.

Rouseff, C. G., and G. Miteff. 1965. Preparation d'un vaccin contre la maladies de Newcastle avec la souche "F" et verification de son innocuite. *Bull. Off. Int. Epiz.* 45:409–14.

Rubin, H., and R. M. Franklin. 1957. On the mechanism of Newcastle disease virus neutralization by immune serum. *Virology* 3:84–95.

Rubin, H., R. M. Franklin, and M. Baluda. 1957. Infection and growth of Newcastle disease virus (NDV) in cultures of chick embryo lung epithelium. *Virology* 3:587–600.

Sagik, B. P., and S. Levine. 1957. The interaction of Newcastle disease virus (NDV) with chicken erythrocytes: Attachment, elution, and hemolysis. *Virology* 3:401–16.

Sahai, L. 1937. Doyle's disease of fowls: Its diagnosis and control. *Agr. Livestock India* 7:11–17.

Salk, J. E. 1944. A simplified procedure for titrating hemagglutinating capacity of influenza virus and the corresponding antibody. *J. Immunol.* 49:87–98.

Schafer, W. 1963. Structure of some animal viruses and significance of their components. *Bacteriol. Rev.* 27:1–17.

Schafer, W., and R. Rott. 1959. Untereinheiten des Newcastle Disease und Mumps-Virus. *Z. Naturforsch.* 14b:629–31.

Schindarow, L., and S. Todorov. 1962. (Growth of Newcastle disease virus in tortoise kidney tissue culture.) *Zentr. Bakteriol. Parasitenk. Abt. I. Orig.* 186:495–501.

Schloer, Gertrude. 1964. Plaque characteristics of Newcastle disease virus. Ph.D. thesis. Univ. Wisconsin, Madison.

Schloer, Gertrude, and R. P. Hanson. 1968a. Plaque morphology of Newcastle disease virus as influenced by cell type and environmental factors. *Am. J. Vet. Res.* 29:883–95.

———. 1968b. Relationship of plaque size and virulence for chickens of 14 representative Newcastle disease virus strains. *J. Virol.* 2:40–47.

Scott, G. R., M. A. Gibson, and D. Danskin. 1956. The reappearance of Newcastle disease in Kenya. *Bull. Epiz. Diseases Africa* 4:65–68.

Shah, K. V., and H. N. Johnson. 1959. Isolation of Ranikhet (Newcastle) virus from a fledgeling koel *(Eudynamis scolopaceus)* by intracerebral inoculation of mice. *Indian J. Med. Res.* 47:604–8.

Shimizu, T., T. Kumagai, S. Ideda, and M. Matumoto. 1964. A new *in vitro* method (END) for detection and measurement of hog cholera virus and its antibody by means of effect of HC virus on Newcastle disease virus in swine tissue culture. III. END neutralization test. *Arch. Ges. Virusforsch.* 14: 215–26.

Silverstein, Samuel C., and Philip I. Marcus. 1964. Early stages of Newcastle disease virus-

Hela cell interaction: An electron microscopic study. *Virology* 23:370–80.

Simmons, G. C. 1967. The isolation of Newcastle disease virus in Queensland. *Australian Vet. J.* 43:29–30.

Sinha, S. K. 1958. Influence of temperature of incubation of embryonating eggs following inoculation of Newcastle disease virus. *Avian Diseases* 2:138–47.

Sinha, S. K., R. P. Hanson, and C. A. Brandly. 1952. Comparison of the tropisms of six strains of Newcastle disease virus in chickens following aerosol infection. *J. Infect. Diseases* 91:276–82.

———. 1954. Aerosol transmission of Newcastle disease in chickens. *Am. J. Vet. Res.* 15:287–92.

———. 1957. Effect of environmental temperature upon facility of aerosol transmission of infection and severity of Newcastle disease among chickens. *J. Infect. Diseases* 100:162–68.

Spalatin, J. S., and R. P. Hanson. 1968. Recovery of an NDV strain indistinguishable from Texas GB. *Avian Diseases* 10:372–74.

Spalatin, J. S., J. Estupinan, and R. P. Hanson. 1968. The significance of age of the chick in establishing the ICP index. *Avian Diseases* 12:139–41.

Stover, D. E. 1942. A filterable virus, the cause of a respiratory nervous disorder of chickens. *Am. J. Vet. Res.* 3:207–13.

Takamatsu, Y., T. Miyamoto, K. Zaizen, A. Kawakubo, and H. Nagashima. 1956. Outbreaks of Newcastle disease in Tokyo in the spring of 1951. *Nippon Inst. Biol. Sci. Bull. Biol. Res.* 1:63–69.

Taylor, L. W. 1964. The chicken as an evolving host, pp. 23–24. In Hanson, R. P. (ed.), *Newcastle Disease Virus: An Evolving Pathogen.* Univ. Wisconsin Press, Madison.

Thiry, L. 1963. Chemical mutagenesis of Newcastle disease virus. *Virology* 19:225–36.

Thompson, C. H., Jr., and O. L. Osteen. 1948. A technique for the isolation of Newcastle disease virus using streptomycin as a bacterial inhibitor. *Am. J. Vet. Res.* 9:303–5.

———. 1952. Immunological and pathological findings on a highly virulent strain of Newcastle disease virus from Mexico. *Am. J. Vet. Res.* 13:407–16.

Tilley, F. N., and W. A. Anderson. 1947. Germicidal action of certain chemicals on the virus of Newcastle disease (Avian pneumoencephalitis). *Vet. Med.* 42:229–30.

Tolba, M. K., and Eskarous, J. K. 1962. Effect of temperature on the hemagglutination activities and infectivity of chick embryos of different strains of Newcastle disease and fowl plague viruses. *Arch. Kreislaufforsch.* 38:234–40.

Topacio, T. 1934. Cultivation of avian pest virus (Newcastle disease) in tissue culture. *Philippine J. Sci.* 53:245–52.

Traub, E. 1944. Weitere Mitteilungen ueber die Aktive-Immunisierung mit Absorbat-Impfstoffen gegen die atypische Gefluegelpest. *Z. Infektionskrankh. Haustiere* 60:367–79.

Upton, Elizabeth, R. P. Hanson, Nancy W. Tepley, and C. A. Brandly. 1951. Neurotoxicity of Newcastle disease virus (NDV) for hamsters and mice. *Proc. 51st Ann. Meet. Soc. Am. Bacteriol.,* p. 87. (Abstr.)

Upton, Elizabeth, R. P. Hanson, and C. A. Brandly. 1953a. Antigenic differences among strains of Newcastle disease virus. *Proc. Soc. Exp. Biol. Med.* 84:691.

Upton, Elizabeth, R. P. Hanson, Dorothy Dow, and C. A. Brandly. 1953b. Studies on intracerebral inoculation of Newcastle disease virus (NDV) into mice. I. Response of weanling mice to 25 strains of NDV. *J. Infect. Diseases* 92:175–82.

Vadlamudi, Srikrishnan. 1963. Studies on the blood-brain barrier in chickens to Newcastle disease virus. Ph.D. thesis. Univ. Wisconsin, Madison.

Vandemaele, F. P. 1961. The epizootiology of Newcastle disease in Africa south of the Sahara. *Bull. Epiz. Diseases Africa* 9:371–81.

Van Roekel, H. 1946. *Proc. Conf. Newcastle Disease,* USDA.

———. 1955. An evaluation of Newcastle disease-wing-web vaccine. *Proc. 92nd Ann. Meet. Am. Vet. Med. Ass.,* p. 324. (Abstr.)

Van Roekel, H., F. G. Sperling, K. L. Bullis, and Olga M. Olesiuk. 1948. Immunization of chickens against Newcastle disease. *J. Am. Vet. Med. Ass.* 112:131–32.

Van Waveren, G. M., and D. M. Zuijdam. 1955. Vaccinatie tegen pseudo vogelpest (Newcastle disease) door het mengen van entstof door het drinkwater. *Tijdschr. Diergeneesk.* 80:685–96.

Wagener, K. 1948. Die Kriegsverseuchung Deutchlands mit Gefluegelpest in epizootologischer Betrachtung. *Berlin. Muench. Tieraerztl. Wochschr.* 61 (6): 61–65.

Wagner, K., and G. Enders-Ruckle. 1966. Ein im Huhnerei vorkommendes Parainfluenza-Virus. *Zentr. Veterinaermed.* 13B:215–18.

Walker, R. V. L. 1948. Newcastle disease. *Can. J. Comp. Med. Vet. Sci.* 12:172–76.

———. 1952. Studies in Newcastle disease. IV. Rapid methods of diagnosis. *Can. J. Comp. Med. Vet. Sci.* 16:333.

Walker, R. V. L., and P. D. McKercher. 1954. Studies in Newcastle disease. IX. Further investigation of the carrier problem. *Can. J. Comp. Med. Vet. Sci.* 18:431–32.

Walker, R. V. L., R. Gwatkin, and P. D. McKercher. 1953. Efficiency of a quaternary ammonium-glycol mixture against Newcastle disease virus and *Salmonella pullorum. Can. J. Comp. Med. Vet. Sci.* 17:225–29.

Walker, R. V. L., P. D. McKercher, and G. L. Bannister. 1954. Studies in Newcastle disease. VII. The possible role of the pigeon as a carrier. *Can. J. Comp. Med. Vet. Sci.* 18:244–45.

Watanabe, M., T. Furutani, and Y. Nishimura. 1968. Resistance of chicken to Newcastle disease virus after inoculation with Bl and Mukteswar strains and prior to production of neutralizing antibody. *Nat. Inst. Animal Health Quart.* 8:112–13.

Waterson, A. P. 1964. The morphology and composition of Newcastle disease virus, pp. 119–32. In Hanson, R. P. (ed.), *Newcastle Disease Virus: An Evolving Pathogen.* Univ. Wisconsin Press, Madison.

Waterson, A. P., and J. G. Cruickshank. 1963. The effect of ether on Newcastle disease virus. A morphological study of eight strains. *Z. Naturforsch.* 18b:114–18.

Waterson, A. P., and T. H. Pennington. 1967. Virulence in Newcastle disease virus, a preliminary study. *Brit. Med. Bull.* 23:138–43.

Wheelock, E. F. 1963. Intracellular site of Newcastle disease virus nucleic acid synthesis. *Proc. Soc. Exp. Biol. Med.* 114:56–60.

Wheelock, E. F., and I. Tamm. 1961. Biochemical basis for alterations in structure and function of Hela cells infected with Newcastle disease virus. *J. Exp. Med.* 114:617–32.

Wilcox, W. C. 1959. Quantitative aspects of *in vitro* virus-induced toxic reaction. I. General aspects of the reaction of Newcastle disease virus with L cells. *Virology* 9:30–44.

Williamson, A. P., R. J. Blattner, and L. Simonsen. 1956. Mechanism of the teratogenic action of Newcastle disease virus on the chicken embryo. *J. Immunol.* 76:275–80.

Wilson, D. E. 1968. Inhibition of host- cell protein and ribonucleic acid synthesis by Newcastle disease virus. *J. Virol.* 2:1–6.

Wilson, J. E. 1950. Newcastle disease in a gannet, *Sula bassana.* A preliminary note. *Vet. Record* 62:33–34.

Winslow, N. S., R. P. Hanson, Elizabeth Upton, and C. A. Brandly. 1950. Agglutination of mammalian erythrocytes by Newcastle disease virus. *Proc. Soc. Exp. Biol. Med.* 74:174–78.

Winterfield, R. W., and E. H. Seadale. 1956. Newcastle disease immunization studies. I. Viability of Newcastle disease virus administered as a vaccine in the drinking water. *Am. J. Vet. Res.* 17:5–11.

———. 1957. Newcastle disease immunization studies. 3. The immune response of chickens vaccinated at an early age with B₁ Newcastle disease virus administered through the drinking water under field conditions. *Poultry Sci.* 36:65–70.

Winterfield, R. W., C. L. Goldman, and E. H. Seadale. 1957. Newcastle disease immunization studies. 4. Vaccination of chickens with B₁, F and LaSota strains of Newcastle disease virus administered through the drinking water. *Poultry Sci.* 36:1076–88.

Wolfe, H. R., and E. Dilks. 1948. Precipitin production in chickens. III. The variation in the antibody response as correlated with the age of the animal. *J. Immunol.* 58:245–50.

Zakomirdin, A. A. 1963. (Biothermaldisinfection of manure from poultry with Newcastle disease and infectious laryngotracheitis.) *Veterinariya* 40:64–66.

Zargar, S. L., and B. S. Pomeroy. 1949. A rapid whole blood plate test for the diagnosis of Newcastle disease. *J. Am. Vet. Med. Ass.* 115:354.

———. 1950. Isolation of Newcastle disease from commercial fowlpox and laryngotracheitis vaccines. *J. Am. Vet. Med. Ass.* 116:304–5.

Zuijdam, D. M. 1952. Isolation of Newcastle disease virus from the osprey and the parakeet. *J. Am. Vet. Med. Ass.* 120:88–89.

———. 1953. Vaccination against Newcastle disease. *Proc. XV Int. Vet. Congr.* 1:252–56.

CHAPTER 19

AVIAN ENCEPHALOMYELITIS

❖

R. E. LUGINBUHL

AND

C. F. HELMBOLDT

Department of Animal Diseases
University of Connecticut
Storrs, Connecticut

❖

AVIAN ENCEPHALOMYELITIS (AE) is a viral infection which affects primarily young chickens and is characterized by ataxia and tremor, especially of the head and neck. Jones (1932) first named the disease epidemic tremor; later, infectious avian encephalomyelitis was suggested by Van Roekel et al. (1938, 1939). In 1939, the binomial avian encephalomyelitis was recommended by the Committee on Poultry Disease Nomenclature of the American Veterinary Medical Association (Beach, 1939).

Prior to 1962 this disease was of great economic importance to the poultry industry. Since that time it has been reasonably well controlled by vaccination. Up to the present time no public health significance has been attached to this disease.

HISTORY

Jones (1932, 1934) first encountered the disease in 1930 in 2-week-old Rhode Island Red chicks from a commercial flock. Tremor but no ataxia was observed in this outbreak. In 1931 two additional outbreaks were observed in 1- and 4-week-old chicks

We are indebted to Dr. H. Van Roekel for permitting the use of material from the previous edition as the basis for parts of this chapter.

raised on different farms but originating from the same breeding flock. Tremor and ataxia were noted in these outbreaks. During the next two years an increasing number of outbreaks was observed in Connecticut, Maine, Massachusetts, and New Hampshire, which led to AE being tagged the "New England disease."

Jones (1934) first propagated the causative agent in susceptible chicks by intracerebral (IC) inoculation with brain material from spontaneous cases. Experimental infections in chicks resulted in signs of disease within 6–44 days, most often between 12 and 28 days, after IC inoculation. The disease was produced more often after serial passage of the agent in chicks.

INCIDENCE AND DISTRIBUTION

This disease has been reported from virtually all areas of the world where poultry is raised on a commercial basis (Seddon, 1952; Markson and Blaxland, 1955; D. Coles, personal communication; Lindgren et al., 1957; Anon., 1958; C. K. Lee, personal communication; J. E. Wilson, personal communication; Animal Health Branch, 1963; N. Kuba, personal communication; Dorn and Kronthaler, 1964; Hemsley, 1964; McLachlan, 1965; Odagiri et al., 1965; Riggenbach, 1965; Willemart, 1965).

The virus (AEV) is embryo-transmitted and hence the disease may be disseminated via the egg or through young chicks. The disease behavior is very similar wherever it occurs; the sudden appearance and unpredictable duration are reasons for great concern to the breeder, hatcheryman, and grower.

ETIOLOGY

CHARACTERISTICS OF THE VIRUS

Jones (1934) passed the agent through Seitz and Berkefeld N filters and preserved the virus in brain tissue in 50% glycerin for at least 69 days. Van Roekel et al. (1938) confirmed the filterability of the agent through Seitz and celloidin filters, and Olitsky (1939) reported the agent capable of passing through Seitz 1 and 2 disc filters and Berkefeld V and N candles. Later, by gradocol membrane filtration, the virus was found to have a diameter of 20–30 mμ (Olitsky and Bauer, 1939). This size estimate was essentially confirmed by studies in which the virus was shown to pass a 50-

mμ Millipore filter membrane but was retained by a 10-mμ membrane (Butterfield, 1967). In ultracentrifugation and density gradient studies (Butterfield, 1967), the virus layered visibly at the median point of tubes containing a cesium chloride gradient with a specific gravity of 1.33 gm/cm^3. This suggests the virus is of RNA composition.

Studies of the chemical properties of AEV reveal that it is resistant to chloroform, acid, trypsin, pepsin, and deoxyribonuclease and is protected against the effects of heat by divalent magnesium ions (Von Bülow, 1964; Butterfield, 1967).

Physical, chemical, and serologic tests demonstrate no significant differences between the Van Roekel laboratory strain of AEV and 19 field isolates of the virus (Butterfield, 1967).

BIOLOGICAL PROPERTIES

Thus far no serologic differences have been detected between the various isolates of avian encephalomyelitis; however, a distinction should be made between the natural strains and those that have been embryo-adapted.

Natural Strains (Field Isolates)

The pathogenicity of these isolates varies. All are enterotropic; they infect young chicks readily via the oral route and are shed in the feces. However, some tend to be more neurotropic than others and produce severe central nervous system lesions, with signs in young chicks. Usually the field isolates are nonpathogenic for embryos until adapted to the embryo by rapid passage.

Embryo-Adapted Strains (Van Roekel Strain)

The Van Roekel strain is highly neurotropic, causes signs of disease in chickens of all ages by parenteral inoculation, but cannot easily infect via the oral route. Oral infection requires very high dosage, and rarely does the disease spread. This strain is pathogenic for embryos from susceptible flocks and produces a muscular dystrophy (Fig. 19.1) and decreased movement. Live embryos examined after 18 days of age may show a persistent heartbeat, but the voluntary muscles may be partially or completely immobilized (Jungherr et al., 1956; Calnek and Jehnich, 1959). The use of eggs from a susceptible flock is essential for isolation and propagation of the virus in embryos. The virus was detected in the brains of inoculated embryos 3–4 days postinoculation, and peak titers were found 6–9 days postinfection (Calnek and Jehnich, 1959; Burke et al., 1965). Histopathological changes in embryos infected with egg-adapted virus have been described as uniform in character but variable in intensity and location, consisting of encephalomalacia and muscular dystrophy (Jungherr et al., 1956). Neural lesions were characterized by severe local edema, gliosis, vascular proliferation, and pyknosis (Figs. 19.2, 19.3). The muscular changes consisted primarily of eosinophilic swelling and necrosis, fragmentation, and loss of striations of affected fibers with rare sarcolemmal proliferation and heterophil infiltration.

LABORATORY HOST SYSTEMS

The baby chick, chicken embryos from susceptible flocks (Van Roekel et al., 1939, 1941; Jungherr et al., 1956; Wills and Moulthrop, 1956; Sumner et al., 1957a), cell cultures of neuroglial cells (Mancini and Yates, 1967), chicken embryo kidney (Mancini and Yates, 1968b), and chicken embryo fibroblast cells (Mancini and Yates, 1968a) have been used to propagate the virus. Virus was successfully propagated in embryonating eggs inoculated via the yolk sac, allantoic sac, and intraocular routes (Jungherr et al., 1956; Wills and Moulthrop, 1956; Sumner et al., 1957a; Burke et al., 1965). The yolk sac route of inoculation for chicken embryos has been adopted by most investigators as the route of choice.

PATHOGENESIS AND EPIZOOTIOLOGY

NATURAL AND EXPERIMENTAL HOSTS

Avian encephalomyelitis virus appears to have a limited host range. The chicken, pheasant (Phasianus torquatus), and coturnix quail (Coturnix japonica) have all succumbed to natural infection. Hill and Raymond (1962) were able to produce clinical signs of AE in quail chicks inoculated at 1–14 days of age. The experimental chicks were maintained in the same room with the adult breeding quail. Fifteen days after the chicks were inoculated, the adult flock manifested a decline in egg production and hatchability. Clinical signs of AE and mortality were observed among the chicks

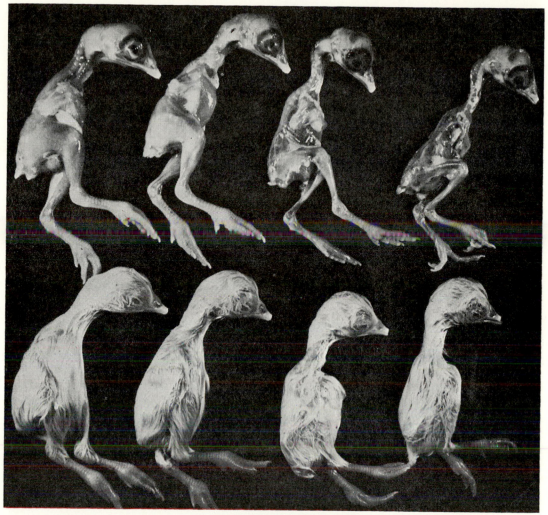

FIG. 19.1—Embryos inoculated via yolk sac with Van Roekel strain of AE virus at 6 days incubation. Examined at 18 days incubation. Top and bottom rows are the same except top row embryos are skinned. Embryo on left uninoculated. Remaining embryos left to right inoculated with progressively greater doses of virus. (Courtesy B. W. Calnek, Cornell Univ.)

hatched from eggs collected during the outbreak of the disease. Ducklings, turkey poults, young pigeons, and guinea fowl have been infected experimentally. Mice, guinea pigs, rabbits, and monkeys were refractory to virus introduced intracerebrally (Van Roekel et al., 1939, 1940; Olitsky and Van Roekel, 1952; Mathey, 1955; Mohanty and West, 1968).

TRANSMISSION

The intracranial route of inoculation has given the most consistent results in reproducing the disease in chickens. Other routes

by which infection has been experimentally established are intraperitoneal, subcutaneous, intradermal, intravenous, intramuscular, intrasciatic, intraocular, oral, and intranasal inoculation (Olitsky, 1939; Van Roekel et al., 1939; Jungherr and Minard, 1942; Feibel et al., 1952; Schaaf and Lamoreux, 1955; Calnek et al., 1960; Butterfield et al., 1969).

The disease may be observed in all seasons of the year. In young chicks the disease can nearly always be traced to a parent stock that has experienced a recent infection. In such parent stock, one may find

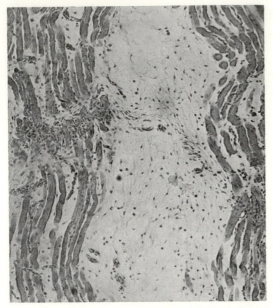

FIG. 19.2—Bivicenter cervicis muscle of 18-day-old chicken embryo infected with AE virus. Muscle fibers are fragmented and separated by edema. H & E, ×30.

in retrospect a decline in egg production that usually was transient and may or may not have been observed. Taylor and Schelling (1960) reported that some breeding flocks which were susceptible at 5 months of age did not encounter the infection for a subsequent period of 13 months. The source and mode of spread of the infection to adult breeding flocks is not understood at present. However, it has been observed that chickens in flocks on farms with multiple age groups usually are immune when they come into production. Birds in isolated flocks of a single age group are usually still susceptible at production age. Chickens of all ages are susceptible to the infection by experimental inoculation (Olitsky, 1939; Van Roekel et al., 1939; Feibel et al., 1952) if they do not contain antibodies.

For some time natural transmission of the disease presented a baffling problem. Early investigations failed to demonstrate the disease in progeny hatched from eggs obtained from breeders that survived a natural infection (Jones, 1934; Bottorff et al., 1936; Van Roekel et al., 1941). Considerable field evidence and some experimental results show rather conclusively that the infection is egg-borne (Van Roekel et al., 1941; Jungherr and Minard, 1942; Schaaf and Lamoreux, 1955; Taylor et al., 1955; Calnek et al., 1960).

Transmission of the disease by direct or indirect contact, either with naturally or experimentally infected chickens, has been reported. Calnek et al. (1960) suggested that AE is an enteric infection in growing and adult birds. The virus may be eliminated in the droppings in sufficient concentration to infect young susceptible chicks by the oral route. Chicks placed in a wire battery in a contaminated poultry house became infected but at a much lower rate

FIG. 19.3—Cerebellum of infected 18-day-old chicken embryo. There is marked lack of development of internal granular layer, cerebellar white matter, and N. cerebellaris. Brain should be almost complete at this stage. H & E, ×30.

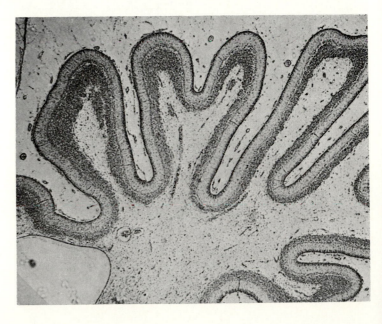

than did chicks placed in direct contact with infected chicks 11 days after hatching. The minimum incubation period following oral administration of the virus-contaminated feces was 11 days. Attempts to show transmission of infection by aerosol yielded negative results. It was suggested that in the field, most of the chicks hatched from susceptible dams may become infected as the result of contact with a few congenitally infected chicks. Richey (1962) incriminated a ready-to-lay pullet flock housed in the same building but in a separate pen as the source of the infection for outbreaks that occurred in several susceptible breeding flocks 45 weeks of age. The pullet flock had experienced an acute outbreak of the disease at 3 weeks of age. It was suggested that a "carrier" existed in the pullet flock. While certain aspects of transmission of the disease have been well established, other phases remain unknown.

Schaaf and Lamoreux (1955) stated that incubator transmission of the disease does not occur, and Jungherr and Minard (1942) reported that hatchability was not affected. On the contrary, Taylor et al. (1955) reported a high embryo death pattern during the last 3 days of incubation. The percentage of embryos which hatched declined from a 78.6% preinfection level to 59.6% during the clinical stage and increased to 75.4% postinfection. Eggs produced just prior to and during the period of depressed egg production showed a decreased hatchability and an increased embryo mortality during the last 3 days of incubation. Furthermore, only the chicks from the group with depressed hatchability showed signs of the disease; the chicks hatched prior to and after the affected hatch appeared normal. Similar observations have been reported by other workers (Calnek et al., 1960; Richey, 1962).

Calnek et al. (1960) demonstrated that transmission of the infection can occur in the incubator. Three groups of susceptible eggs were selected. One group was inoculated at 6 days incubation; a second group was uninoculated, but the two groups were incubated and hatched in the same incubator. Another uninoculated group was hatched in a separate incubator. The chicks from the inoculated group manifested signs on the 1st day of age; by the 6th day, 49 of 52 showed clinical evidence of the disease. The chicks from the uninoculated group hatched with the infected birds first manifested signs on the 10th day, and 15 of 18 chicks exhibited clinical evidence. The isolated control group of 19 chicks remained negative.

INCUBATION PERIOD

In studies concerning the epizootiology of AE conducted by Calnek and co-workers (1960), it was demonstrated that the incubation period for this disease in chicks infected by embryo transmission was 1–7 days, whereas chicks infected by contact transmission or by oral administration had a minimum incubation period of 11 days.

SIGNS

This disease presents an interesting syndrome which may be characterized as follows. In natural outbreaks the disease usually makes its appearance when the chicks are 1–2 weeks of age, although affected chicks have been observed at the time of hatching. Affected chicks, as a rule, first show a slightly dull expression of the eyes, followed by a progressive ataxia due to incoordination of the muscles. This ataxia may be detected readily by exercising the chicks. As the ataxia grows more pronounced, the chicks show an inclination to sit on their haunches. When disturbed, such chicks may move about, exhibiting little control over their speed and gait; finally they come to rest on their haunches or fall on their sides. Some chicks may refuse to move, or they may walk on their hocks and shanks. The dull expression becomes more pronounced and is accompanied by a weakened cry or inability to cry. Fine tremors of the head and neck may become evident, the frequency and magnitude of which may vary. Exciting or disturbing the chick may bring on the tremor, which may continue for variable periods of time and recur at irregular intervals. The ataxic signs usually, but not always, appear before the tremor. In some cases only tremor has been observed. Jungherr (1939) stated that of histologically positive field cases, 36.9% showed ataxia, 18.3% showed tremor, and 35% showed both; 9.2% showed no clinical signs. The ataxia usually progresses until the chick is incapable of moving about, and this stage is followed by inanition, prostration, and finally death. Chicks with marked ataxia and prostration are frequently trampled upon by their pen mates, thus hastening death. Some chicks with definite signs of AE may survive and grow to maturity, and in some instances the signs may disappear completely. Among 83 naturally infected chicks reared at the laboratory, only 24 survived after a period of 8 months. Seven of the 24 survivors developed a blindness as the result of an opacity or bluish discoloration of the lens of one or both eyes. A few progeny from these survivors, as they became mature, developed an eye condition that resembled the condition observed in the naturally infected dams. The gross pathology consisted of an apparent enlargement of the eyeball, a marked opacity of the lens, seemingly fixed pupil, and total blindness in some cases. No characteristic signs of AE were detected in these progeny (Van Roekel et al., 1936, 1937). Somewhat similar observations have been reported by other workers (Peckham, 1957; Bridges and Flowers, 1958).

While the natural disease is known to occur in adult flocks (as substantiated by a decline in egg production, positive serologic evidence, and presence of the disease in progeny), it is of interest that neurologic signs of AE as seen in chicks do not occur in mature birds.

MORBIDITY AND MORTALITY

Morbidity from the natural disease has been observed only in young stock, although inapparent infections do occur in mature flocks. The usual morbidity rate is 40–60% if all of the chicks come from the infected flock. The mortality rate averages 25% and may exceed 50%. These rates are considerably lower if many of the chicks comprising the flock originate from breeder flocks of immune birds.

GROSS LESIONS

The only gross lesions that have been associated with AE in chicks are whitish areas (due to masses of infiltrating lymphocytes) in the muscularis of the ventriculus. These are subtle changes and require favorable conditions to be discerned. No changes have been described for infected adult birds.

HISTOPATHOLOGY

The principal changes are in the central nervous system and some viscera. The peripheral nervous system is not involved—a point of importance in differential diagnosis.

In the central nervous system the lesions are those of a disseminated, nonpurulent encephalomyelitis and a ganglionitis of the dorsal root ganglia. The most frequently encountered addition is a striking perivascular infiltrate which seems to occur in all portions of the brain and spinal cord (Fig. 19.4) except the cerebellum where it is confined to the N. cerebellaris. The infiltrating small lymphocytes may pile up several layers to form an impressive cuff.

Microgliosis occurs both as diffuse and as nodular aggregates. The glial lesion is seen chiefly in the cerebellar molecular layer where it tends to be compact (Fig. 19.5). A loose gliosis is usually found in the N. cerebellaris, brain stem, midbrain, optic lobes, and less often in the corpus striata. In the midbrain, two nuclei—N. rotundus and N. ovoidalis—are invariably affected with a loose microgliosis which can be considered pathognomonic (Fig. 19.6). Another lesion of pathognomonic significance is central chromatolysis (axonal reaction) of the neurones in the nuclei of the brain stem, particularly those of the medulla oblongata (Fig. 19.7). If several sagittal sections are made, one can almost always find this alter-

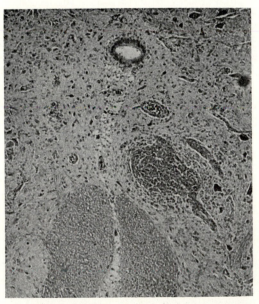

FIG. 19.4—Spinal cord at lumbar level of chick. In gray matter are large glial nodule and several perivascular infiltrates of lymphocytes. Central canal is at top of picture. H & E, ×75.

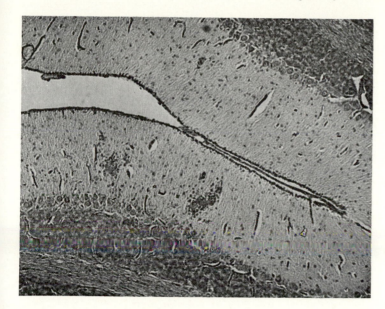

FIG. 19.5—Cerebellum of chick. In molecular layer are glial foci which are common in avian encephalomyelitis. H & E, ×75.

ation. The dying neurone is surrounded by satellite oligodendroglia, and later microglia phagocytize the remains; the central chromatolysis is never seen without an attending cellular reaction.

Lesions in the spinal cord are identical to those of the brain. Although no detailed study of the spinal cord has been made, random sampling of the various levels suggest that all levels are involved.

The dorsal root ganglia often contain rather tight aggregates of small lymphocytes amid the neurones. The lesion is always confined to the ganglion and never enters the nerves (Fig. 19.8).

In general, the signs cannot be correlated with the severity of the lesions or the distribution in the central nervous system.

The visceral lesions appear to be hyperplasia of the lymphocytic aggregates which are scattered in a random fashion throughout the bird. In the proventriculus there are normally a few small lymphocytes in the muscular wall; in AE these are obvious dense aggregates which are certainly pathognomonic (Fig. 19.9). In the ventriculus muscle similar lesions occur, but unfortunately they also occur in Marek's disease. In the pancreas circumscribed lymphocytic follicles are normal (Lucas, 1951), but in AE the number increases several times (Fig. 19.10). In the myocardium and particularly the atrium there are aggregates of lymphocytes considered to be the result of AE (Springer and Schmittle, 1968). However,

lymphocytes in the myocardium of young chicks are not unusual; one may consider them a lesion only if widespread and accompanied by the previous noted alterations.

There appears to be an excellent correlation between clinical signs and histologic lesions. In one study 11% had signs but no lesions while 8% had lesions but no

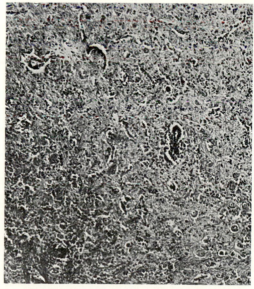

FIG. 19.6—Nucleus ovoidalis of chick. Diffuse gliosis and small perivascular infiltrates are seen. This lesion is seen only in avian encephalomyelitis. H & E, ×75.

FIG. 19.7—Medulla oblongata of chick. There is diffuse gliosis, and in center a neurone is undergoing central chromatolysis. H & E, ×75. Inset shows tigrolysis and loss of nucleus. ×480.

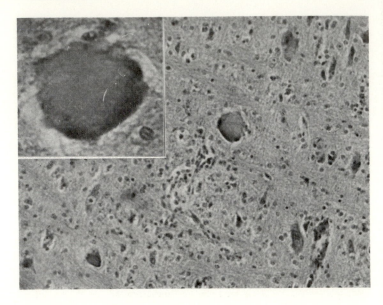

signs (Jungherr and Minard, 1942). Later Jungherr believed that all birds with clinical signs had histologic lesions. This was based on more intensive research which in turn was based on multiple sections of the brain and viscera. Experimentally inoculated chicks killed in sequential fashion invariably yield lesions 1–2 days before clinical signs. As a matter of fact, recovered birds free of signs have central nervous system lesions for at least a week, probably much longer.

IMMUNITY

Birds recovered from natural and experimental infection develop circulating antibodies capable of neutralizing the virus (Olitsky, 1939; Jungherr and Minard, 1942; Feibel et al., 1952; Sumner et al., 1957a; Calnek and Jehnich, 1959; Moore and

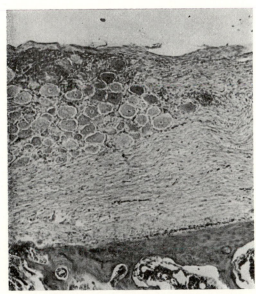

FIG. 19.8—Dorsal root ganglion of lumbar level of chick. Dense infiltrate of lymphocytes confined to ganglion. Sciatic nerve is unaffected. H & E, ×75.

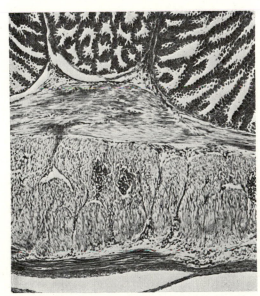

FIG. 19.9—Proventriculus of chick. Dense lymphocytic foci are in muscular wall. This lesion is pathognomonic. H & E, ×30.

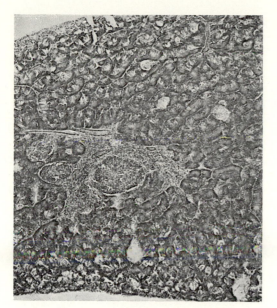

FIG. 19.10—*Pancreas of young chick. Several follicles of lymphocytes are present. This lesion is significant only when abnormal numbers of follicles are present. H & E, ×30.*

Flowers, 1959; Taylor and Schelling, 1960). Antibodies also appear in the yolk of eggs from immune hens and may render embryonating eggs resistant to virus inoculated via the yolk sac. In a flock survey for embryo susceptibility to the virus, Sumner et al. (1957b) found a wide range in the titration end points of the AE virus in eggs received from 119 flocks. A majority of the tested flocks had no history of AE but produced embryos resistant to the virus, suggesting that they had undergone a mild infection. It was suggested that in an exposed flock, not all hens become immune to a degree measurable by the test. Olitsky and Van Roekel (1952) reported that chicks inoculated with an active virus which fail to show clinical signs of the disease may not be rendered resistant.

Active

The serologic response in AE is relatively slow in developing and usually is not detectable until about 4 weeks after infection. Serum neutralization indices of unexposed birds are less than 1.1, whereas those of exposed birds usually range between 1.8 and 3.4. Birds with positive neutralization indices have been reported capable of resisting an intracerebral challenge with 10,000 EID_{50} of AE virus (Calnek and Jehnich, 1959).

Flocks of chickens containing birds with positive neutralization indices or positive embryo susceptibility tests rarely have recurrent outbreaks of AE.

Passive

Antibodies transferred to the progeny from the dam via the embryo do occur in this disease. These antibodies can be demonstrated in the egg yolk (Sumner et al., 1957b). Birds from immune dams were not fully susceptible to oral inoculation until 8–10 weeks of age, and antibodies were demonstrated in the serum until 4–6 weeks of age (Calnek et al., 1961).

DIAGNOSIS

ISOLATION AND IDENTIFICATION OF CAUSATIVE AGENT

The most sensitive system for the assay of virus is to inoculate embryos (obtained from a susceptible flock) via the yolk sac when 5–7 days of age, allow these to hatch, and observe the chicks for signs of disease during the first 10 days of life (Hoekstra, 1964; Von Bülow, 1965). When clinical signs appear, brain, proventriculus, and pancreas should be sectioned and examined for lesions as described in the histopathology section.

The brain is the best source of virus for isolation, although other tissues and organs induce the disease when inoculated into chicks (Van Roekel et al., 1938; Jungherr and Minard, 1942).

SEROLOGY

Chickens that have been exposed to the live virus will manifest an immunologic response that can be measured with the standard virus neutralization test (Sumner et al., 1957b; Calnek and Jehnich, 1959). The Van Roekel embryo-adapted strain is recommended to determine the neutralizing capacity of the serum or plasma. Undiluted serum or plasma is mixed with tenfold dilutions of the virus and the resulting mixtures are inoculated via the yolk sac into susceptible 6-day-old embryonating chicken eggs. The embryos are examined for characteristic lesions 10–12 days postinoculation. The neutralization index is calculated as the log difference between EID_{50} virus titer and EID_{50} virus-serum titer. An index of 1.1 or greater is considered as positive evidence of previous exposure to the virus. Among samples from a recently exposed flock, the neutralization index may vary from 1.5 to 3.0. Antibodies may be detected as early as the 2nd week after exposure and remain at significant levels for at least several months. Calnek and Jehnich (1959) reported that in many instances, birds having no detectable neutralizing antibodies (NI less than 1.1) would resist intracerebral challenge with as many as 10,000 EID_{50} of virus. The inconsistent availability of susceptible eggs has been a deterrent in the wider usage of the virus neutralization test.

Another method used to determine the immunity of a flock is the embryo susceptibility test. Sumner et al. (1957b) first employed this test as a means to determine which breeding flocks had experienced the infection. A sample of fertile eggs is selected from each flock and the eggs are incubated. After 6 days of incubation, each embryo is inoculated via the yolk sac with 100 EID_{50} of the egg-adapted virus. The embryos are examined 10–12 days postinoculation for characteristic lesions. If 100% of the embryos are affected, the flock is considered susceptible; less than 50% affected indicates immunity. Intermediate figures should be considered nondefinitive and may indicate recent exposure. Adequate controls should be included in conducting the embryo susceptibility test. This test serves as a useful tool to determine the immune status of breeder flocks.

DIFFERENTIAL DIAGNOSIS

In spontaneous cases a tentative, and frequently a definite, diagnosis of disease can be made when a complete history of the flock and typical specimens are provided for histopathology.

Histopathologic evidence of gliosis, lymphocytic perivascular infiltration, axonal type of neuronal degeneration in the central nervous system, and hyperplasia of the lymphoid follicles in certain visceral tissues usually can be considered as a basis for a positive diagnosis. Virus isolation or positive serology (virus neutralization test) gives a more specific diagnosis.

This disease should not be confused with other avian diseases manifesting similar clinical signs, such as Newcastle disease, equine encephalomyelitis infection, nutri-tional disturbances (rickets, encephalo-malacia, and riboflavin deficiency), and Marek's disease.

AE is predominantly a disease of 2–3-week-old chicks. Since Newcastle disease may strike at this time, a problem of differential diagnosis can arise. Certain lesions are peculiar to AE: (1) central chromatolysis as opposed to peripheral chromatolysis of Newcastle disease; (2) gliosis in the N. rotundus and N. ovoidalis which are not affected by Newcastle disease; (3) lymphocytic foci in the muscular wall of the proventriculus; and (4) circumscribed lymphocytic follicles in the pancreas whereas Newcastle disease causes only rarely an interstitial pancreatitis.

Encephalomalacia (EM) generally appears 2–3 weeks later than AE and from the standpoint of clinical history and signs should be no problem. Histologically EM causes severe degenerative lesions in no way similar to AE.

Marek's disease, which occurs still later, presents little difficulty owing to its negative characteristics. The peripheral nerve involvement and the state of lymphomatosis of the viscera are two criteria not seen in AE. Furthermore, the lymphocytes of AE are mature and lymphoblasts characteristic of MD are not seen.

PREVENTION AND CONTROL

No satisfactory treatment is known for acute outbreaks in young chicks. It is advisable to check the management in order that the chicks will receive adequate nutrition and a suitable environment. The removal and segregation of affected chicks may be indicated under certain conditions, but generally it is advisable to kill them since they will not develop into profitable stock. It appears that once a flock has experienced an outbreak of the disease no further evidence of the disease is likely to be observed (Schaaf and Lamoreux, 1955).

Effective immunization procedures have been developed to protect breeding flocks against outbreaks of the disease and in turn prevent the spread of the virus to the progeny via the egg-borne route (Schaaf, 1958, 1959; Calnek and Taylor, 1960; Calnek et al., 1961; Butterfield et al., 1961; Van Roekel et al., 1961). Schaaf (1958) first recognized that chickens exposed to the virus developed an immunity and that such birds did not produce infected progeny. This observation formed the basis for a program of vaccinating growing birds by the wing-web method. No evidence of avian encephalomyelitis was observed in progeny produced by more than a million chickens vaccinated with live virus.

Calnek et al. (1961) and Von Bülow (1965) were successful in immunizing immature birds by using a satisfactory vaccine strain which was administered by the oral route or in the drinking water. As a result of natural spread, oral vaccination of only a small percentage of the birds resulted in satisfactory immunity in the entire flock. Since progeny from vaccinated or naturally infected flocks may retain passive antibodies for approximately 8 weeks, they should not be vaccinated until 10 weeks of age or older. It is recommended that all replacement stock for breeding flocks be immunized against the disease. Commercial vaccines are available. An effective immunization program applied to all breeding stock should eliminate clinical outbreaks of the disease in the chick population.

Effective inactivated vaccines for AE have also been produced (Schaaf, 1959; Calnek and Taylor, 1960; Butterfield et al., 1961; Macleod, 1965). At the present time, the inactivated vaccine may be applicable for susceptible breeding flocks that are in production and for breeding flocks located in areas where the disease incidence is low.

AVIAN ENCEPHALOMYELITIS IN TURKEYS

In 1968, AE was encountered in turkey flocks in Minnesota (Pomeroy, 1970). The disease in turkeys resembles the disease in chickens. A drop in egg production occurs in laying flocks which is of economic concern to the flock owner. In young poults the signs are primarily paralytic and the mortality and microscopic pathology are similar to that observed in chicks. The vaccines used in controlling the disease in chickens could presumably be used for turkeys if such vaccines are approved for use in turkeys.

REFERENCES

Animal Health Branch. 1963. *Animal Health Yearbook.* Food and Agriculture Organization of the United Nations. Printed in Italy.

Anonymous. 1958. Report of the committee on nomenclature and reporting of diseases. *Proc. 30th Ann. Meet. N.E. Conf. on Avian Diseases.*

Beach, J. R. 1939. Poultry diseases. *J. Am. Vet. Med. Ass.* 95:613–16.

Bottorff, C. A., A. E. Tepper, C. L. Martin, T. B. Charles, and F. D. Reed. 1936. Epidemic tremors (trembling chick disease). *New Hampshire Agr. Expt. Sta. Circ.* 51:1–8.

Bridges, C. H., and A. I. Flowers. 1958. Iridocyclitis and cataracts associated with an encephalomyelitis in chickens. *J. Am. Vet. Med. Ass.* 132:79–84.

Burke, C. N., H. Krauss, and R. E. Luginbuhl. 1965. The multiplication of avian encephalomyelitis virus in chicken embryo tissues. *Avian Diseases* 9:104–8.

Butterfield, W. K. 1967. Characterization of the virus of avian encephalomyelitis. Ph.D. thesis, Univ. Conn.

Butterfield, W. K., R. E. Luginbuhl, C. F. Helmboldt, and F. W. Sumner. 1961. Studies on avian encephalomyelitis. III. Immunization with an inactivated virus. *Avian Diseases* 5:445–50.

Butterfield, W. K., C. M. Helmboldt, and R. E. Luginbuhl. 1969. Studies on avian encephalomyelitis. IV. Early incidence and longevity of histopathologic lesions in chickens. *Avian Diseases* 13:53–57.

Calnek, B. W., and H. Jehnich. 1959. Studies on avian encephalomyelitis. I. The use of a serum-neutralization test in the detection of immunity levels. II. Immune responses to vaccination procedures. *Avian Diseases* 3:95–104, 225–39.

Calnek, B. W., and Patricia J. Taylor. 1960. Studies on avian encephalomyelitis. III. Immune response to beta-propiolactone inactivated virus. *Avian Diseases* 4:116–22.

Calnek, B. W., Patricia J. Taylor, and M. Sevoian. 1960. Studies on avian encephalomyelitis. IV. Epizootiology. *Avian Diseases* 4:325–47.

———. 1961. Studies on avian encephalomyelitis. V. Development and application of an oral vaccine. *Avian Diseases* 5:297–312.

Dorn, P., and O. Kronthaler. 1964. Observations on the spread of avian encephalomyelitis in breeding flocks. *Arch. Gefluegelk.* 28:49–56.

Feibel, F., C. F. Helmboldt, E. L. Jungherr. and J. R. Carson. 1952. Avian encephalomyelitis—Prevalence, pathogenicity of the virus, and breed susceptibility. *Am. J. Vet. Res.* 13:260–66.

Hemsley, L. A. 1964. The incidence of infectious avian encephalomyelitis ("epidemic tremors") in broiler breeding flocks and its economic effect. *Veterinarian* 2:193–201.

Hill, R. W., and R. G. Raymond. 1962. Apparent natural infection of Coturnix quail hens with the virus of avian encephalomyelitis. Case report. *Avian Diseases* 6:226–27.

Hoekstra, J. 1964. Experiments with avian encephalomyelitis. *Brit. Vet. J.* 120:322–35.

Jones, E. E. 1932. An encephalomyelitis in the chicken. *Science* 76:331–32.

———. 1934. Epidemic tremor, an encephalomyelitis affecting young chickens. *J. Exp. Med.* 59:781–98.

Jungherr, E. L. 1939. Pathology of spontaneous and experimental cases of epidemic tremor. *Poultry Sci.* 18:406.

Jungherr, E. L., and E. L. Minard. 1942. The present status of avian encephalomyelitis. *J. Am. Vet. Med. Ass.* 100:38–46.

Jungherr, E. L., F. Sumner, and R. E. Luginbuhl. 1956. Pathology of egg-adapted avian encephalomyelitis. *Science* 124:80–81.

Lindgren, N. O., A. Nilsson, and K. Bakos. 1957. Infektiose aviare encephalomyelitis beim kucken in Schweden. *Nord. Veterinarmed.* 9:801–21.

Lucas, A. M. 1951. Lymphoid tissue and its relationship to so-called normal lymphoid foci and to lymphomatosis. I. Qualitative study of dove and pigeon. *Poultry Sci.* 30:116–24.

McLachlan, I. 1965. South Australia. The Institute of Medical and Veterinary Science. Twenty-fifth Annual Report of the Council, 1962–63, p. 74, The Institute; Adelaide. *Vet. Bull.* 35:326. (Abstr.)

Macleod, A. J. 1965. Vaccination against avian encephalomyelitis with a betapropialactone inactivated vaccine. *Vet. Record* 77:335–38.

Mancini, L. O., and V. J. Yates. 1967. Cultivation of avian encephalomyelitis virus *in vitro*. I. In chick embryo neuroglial cell culture. *Avian Diseases* 11:672–79.

———. 1968a. Cultivation of avian encephalomyelitis virus *in vitro*. II. In chick embryo fibroblastic cell culture. *Avian Diseases* 12:278–84.

———. 1968b. Cultivation of avian encephalomyelitis virus in chicken embryo kidney cell culture. *Avian Diseases* 12:686–88.

Markson, L. M., and J. D. Blaxland. 1955. Suspected infectious avian encephalomyelitis in poultry in Britain. *Vet. Record* 67:131.

Mathey, W. J., Jr. 1955. Avian encephalomyelitis in pheasants. *Cornell Vet.* 45:89–93.

Mohanty, G. C., and J. L. West. 1968. Some observations on experimental avian encephalomyelitis. *Avian Diseases* 12:689–93.

Moore, R. W., and A. I. Flowers. 1959. The development of a chicken embryo lethal strain of avian encephalomyelitis virus. *Avian Diseases* 3:239–44.

Odagiri, Y., S. Yoshimura, Y. Yomo, H. Mochizuki, and N. Funabashi. 1965. Observations on an avian encephalomyelitis-like disease. *J. Japan. Vet. Med. Ass.* 18:589–93.

Olitsky, P. K. 1939. Experimental studies on the virus of infectious avian encephalomyelitis. *J. Exp. Med.* 70:565.

Olitsky, P. K., and J. H. Bauer. 1939. Ultrafiltration of the virus of infectious avian encephalomyelitis. *Proc. Soc. Exp. Biol. Med.* 42:634–36.

Olitsky, P. K., and H. Van Roekel. 1952. Avian encephalomyelitis (epidemic tremor), pp. 619–28. In Biester, H. E., and L. H. Schwarte (eds.), *Diseases of Poultry,* 3rd ed. Iowa State Univ. Press, Ames.

Peckham, M. C. 1957. Lens opacities in fowls possibly associated with epidemic tremors. Case report. *Avian Diseases* 1:247–55.

Pomeroy, B. S. 1970. Avian encephalomyelitis in turkeys is a new disease on the horizon. *Gobbles* 25 (Mar.): 9, 22.

Richey, D. J. 1962. Avian encephalomyelitis (epidemic tremor). Case report. *Southeastern Vet.* 13:55–57.

Riggenbach, C. 1965. Avian encephalomyelitis in western Switzerland. *Schweiz. Arch. Tierheilk.* 107:18–21.

Schaaf, K. 1958. Immunization for the control of avian encephalomyelitis. *Avian Diseases* 2:279–89.

———. 1959. Avian encephalomyelitis immunization with inactivated virus. *Avian Diseases* 3:245–56.

Schaaf, K., and W. F. Lamoreux. 1955. Control of avian encephalomyelitis by vaccination. *Am. J. Vet. Res.* 16:627–33.

Seddon, H. R. 1952. Avian encephalomyelitis, pp. 147–48. In Seddon, H. R. (ed.), *Diseases of Domestic Animals in Australia,* Pt. 4. Protozoan and Viral Diseases, Dept. Health, Serv. Publ. 8. Canberra.

Springer, W. T., and S. C. Schmittle. 1968. Avian encephalomyelitis. A chronological study of the histopathogenesis in selected tissues. *Avian Diseases* 12:229–39.

Sumner, F. W., E. L. Jungherr, and R. E. Luginbuhl. 1957a. Studies on avian encephalomyelitis. I. Egg adaption of the virus. *Am. J. Vet. Res.* 18:717–19.

Sumner, F. W., R. E. Luginbuhl, and E. L. Jungherr. 1957b. Studies on avian encephalomyelitis. II. Flock survey for embryo susceptibility to the virus. *Am. J. Vet. Res.* 18:720–23.

Taylor, J. R. E., and E. P. Schelling. 1960. The distribution of avian encephalomyelitis in North America as indicated by an immunity test. *Avian Diseases* 4:122–33.

Taylor, L. W., D. C. Lowry, and L. G. Raggi. 1955. Effects of an outbreak of avian encephalomyelitis (epidemic tremor) in a breeding flock. *Poultry Sci.* 34:1036–45.

Van Roekel, H., K. L. Bullis, O. S. Flint, and

M. K. Clarke. 1936. "Epidemic tremors" in chickens. *Mass. Agr. Expt. Sta. Ann. Rept., Bull.* 327:75.

———. 1937. "Epidemic tremor" in chicks. *Mass. Agr. Expt. Sta. Ann. Rept., Bull.* 369:89.

Van Roekel, H., K. L. Bullis, and M. K. Clarke. 1938. Preliminary report of infectious avian encephalomyelitis. *J. Am. Vet. Med. Ass.* 93:372–75.

———. 1939. Infectious avian encephalomyelitis. *Vet. Med.* 34:754.

Van Roekel, H., K. L. Bullis, O. S. Flint, and M. K. Clarke. 1940. Avian encephalomyelitis. *Mass. Agr. Expt. Sta. Ann. Rept., Bull.* 369:94.

Van Roekel, H., K. L. Bullis, and M. K. Clarke. 1941. Transmission of avian encephalomyelitis. *J. Am. Vet. Med. Ass.* 99:220.

Van Roekel, H., B. W. Calnek, R. E. Lugin-buhl, and P. D. McKercher. 1961. Committee report on a tentative program for the control of avian encephalomyelitis. *Avian Diseases* 5:456–60.

Willemart, J. P. 1965. Infectious avian encephalomyelitis in France. *Rec. Med. Vet.* 141:845–56.

Wills, F. K., and I. M. Moulthrop. 1956. Propagation of avian encephalomyelitis virus in the chick embryo. *Southwestern Vet.* 10:39–42.

Von Bülow, V. 1964. Physico-chemical properties of the virus of avian encephalomyelitis with special reference to purification and preservation of virus suspensions. *Zbl. Veterinaermed.* 11B:674–86.

———. 1965. Avian encephalomyelitis. Cultivation, titration, and handling of the virus for live vaccines. *Zbl. Veterinaermed.* 12B:298–311.

CHAPTER 20

AVIAN INFLUENZA

❖

B. C. EASTERDAY

Department of Veterinary Science
University of Wisconsin
Madison, Wisconsin

AND

BELA TUMOVA

Institute for Epidemiology
and Microbiology
Prague, Czechoslovakia
(Visiting Department of Veterinary Science
University of Wisconson, 1968–70)

❖

MANY TYPE A influenza viruses have been isolated from several avian species in various parts of the world, and a variety of disease syndromes are associated with infections of these viruses. The avian influenza viruses have been considered an especially significant group because of their relationships to human, swine, and equine influenza viruses and the very complex antigenic relationships which have been found.

The economic importance of these infections has not been defined. It is relatively easy to describe the magnitude of loss when mortality rates are high, as in the case of infection with fowl plague, Chicken/Scot/59, Turkey/Eng/63, Tern/S. Africa/61, and Duck/Czech/56 viruses (Stubbs, 1965; Becker, 1966; Wells, 1963; Pereira et al., 1965; Koppel et al., 1956). However, there are many other infections in which mortality rates are low and the losses as a result of sinusitis, other respiratory involvement, and retarded growth are more insidious (Roberts, 1964; Rinaldi et al., 1965, 1966a,b, 1967a,b, 1968a,b). In the United States and Canada the greatest losses have

probably been due to loss of breeding and laying efficiency in turkey hens (Bankowski and Mikami, 1964; Bankowski and Conrad, 1966; Lang et al., 1965, 1968a,b).

The public health significance of these infections remains speculative. Several of the viruses are antigenically related to the human A_2 influenza viruses, and antibodies against some have been found in human serum. Whether these viruses circulate from one avian species to another or between avian and mammalian species is not known. A virus closely related to the "Dutch strain" of fowl plague virus was isolated from the blood of a man suffering from an undiagnosed illness after he had visited the Far East and Middle East (De-Lay et al., 1967). There are no reports of infections of laboratory personnel working with avian influenza viruses. This is in contrast to the frequent infection of individuals working with Newcastle disease virus (see Chapter 18).

HISTORY, INCIDENCE, AND DISTRIBUTION

More than 80 avian influenza viruses are associated with different infections among several domestic and wild avian species in several parts of the world (Table 20.1). There is little information on the incidence in various geographic locations, but limited serological surveys indicate that infections are not widespread with regard to individual birds.

The earliest description of an avian influenza virus was that of fowl plague virus. This disease was first reported by Perroncito in Italy in 1878 and was shown to be due to "filterable virus" in 1900 by Centanni and Savonuzzi (Stubbs, 1965). The virus causes high mortality among chickens, turkeys, and other species. While fowl plague was long considered a separate disease entity, Schafer (1955) showed that the virus contained the soluble antigen common to type A influenza viruses, and it has subsequently been considered one of the highly pathogenic members of that group. Fowl plague virus has been reported in many countries throughout the world including most of Europe, Great Britain, Russia, North Africa, Middle East, Far East, South America, and North America. Infections have not been reported in the United States since 1929, but the disease is probably endemic in some countries of the

TABLE 20.1 ❧ Chronology of Avian Influenza Viruses

Virus Strain[a] (other designation)	Host of Origin	Country of Origin	Year Isolated	Nature of Disease	Reference
Fowl plague (Dutch strain)	domestic and wild birds	Indonesia	1927	[b]	Stubbs, 1965
Virus N (Dinter strain) (N/Germany/49)	adult and young chickens	Germany	1949	ND-like[c] sudden death 20% mortality	Dinter, 1949, 1964
D/Can/53 (F.A. Duck/Can)	ducklings	Canada	1953	ND-like[c] sinusitis high morbidity 20% mortality	Walker & Bannister, 1953; Mitchell et al., 1967
D/Czech/56 (A-Anatis/Kosice/56)	ducklings	Czechoslovakia	1956	sinusitis, high morbidity high mortality	Koppel et al., 1956; Blaskovic et al., 1959
D/Eng/56	ducklings	England	1956	resp. dis. sinusitis	Simmins & Asplin, 1956; Pereira et al., 1965
Ch/Scot/59 (Smith strain)	adult chickens	Scotland	1959	fowl plague-like high morbidity high mortality	Wison, 1960; Pereira et al., 1965
D/Ukraine/1/60 (Jalta-60)	ducklings	Ukraine (USSR)	1960	sinusitis	Tsimokh, 1961; Prokofeva & Tsimokh, 1966
D/Ukraine/2/60 (Borki-60)	ducklings	Ukraine	1960	sinusitis	
D/Ukraine/3/60 (Sartana)	ducklings	Ukraine	1960	sinusitis	
D/Ukraine/1/61	ducklings	Ukraine	1961	sinusitis	
Tern/South Africa/61	common tern Sterna hirundo	South Africa	1961	fowl plague-like	Rowan, 1962; Becker, 1963, 1966, 1967
D/Eng/62	ducks	England	1962	sinusitis	Roberts, 1964
Ty/Eng/63 (Langham strain)	turkeys	England	1963	fowl plague-like sudden death	Wells, 1963
D/Ukraine/1/63	ducklings	Ukraine	1963	sinusitis	V. A. Isachenko, 1968[d]
Ty/Can/63 (Ty/Ontario/3724/63 Wilmot strain)	turkeys	Canada	1963	resp. dis.	Lang et al., 1965; Lang & Wills, 1966
Ty/Calif/64 (M. meleagrium)	turkeys	USA	1964	mild resp. dis.	Bankowski & Mikami, 1964; Bankowski & Conrad, 1966

TABLE 20.1 ❧ (continued)

Virus Strain[a] (other designation)	Host of Origin	Country of Origin	Year Isolated	Nature of Disease	Reference
Ty/Ontario/5510/64 5614/64	turkeys	Canada	1964	sinusitis	G. Lang, 1968[d]
Ty/Calif/3/65 (AC #3)	adult turkeys	USA	1965	resp. disease 0.5% morbidity low mortality	Bankowski, 1967
Ty/Mass/65 (3740)	young turkeys	USA	1965	resp. disease sudden death low mortality low morbidity	Pereira et al., 1966; Olesiuk et al., 1967
Ty/Ontario/5050/65	turkeys	Canada	1965	[b]	G. Lang, 1968[d]
D/It/858/65	ducklings	Italy	1965	sinusitis high morbidity low mortality	
Ty/It/741/65 811/65 983/65 1031/65	young turkeys	Italy	1965	sinusitis high mortality	Rinaldi et al., 1965; Pereira et al., 1967a
Q/It/1117/65 1655/65	quail	Italy	1965	resp. dis. 45–95% morbidity 15–75% mortality	
D/It/574/66 946/66 1671/66	ducklings	Italy	1966	sinusitis high morbidity low mortality	
Ph/It/647/66	young pheasants	Italy	1966	resp. dis. 80% morbidity 15–35% mortality	
Q/It/54/66	young quail	Italy	1966	resp. dis. 45–95% morbidity 15–75% mortality	Rinaldi et al., 1965; Pereira et al., 1967a
Ch/It/1166/66	broiler chickens	Italy	1966	chron. resp. dis.	
D/Yugo/446/66	ducks	Yugoslavia	1966	[b]	H. G. Pereira, 1968[d]
Ty/Eng/1/66	turkeys	England	1966	[b]	Wannop, 1966
Ty/Calif/5142/66 (5142)	young turkeys	USA	1966	sinusitis low mortality	Bankowski, 1967
Ty/Wis/1/66	adult turkeys	USA	1966	sinusitis high morbidity low mortality	Pereira et al., 1967b; Smithies et al., 1969a

TABLE 20.1 ❧ (continued)

Virus Strain[a] (other designation)	Host of Origin	Country of Origin	Year Isolated	Nature of Disease	Reference
Ty/Alberta/6962/66	turkeys	Canada	1966	ill-defined	[b]
Ty/Ontario/6213/66 7732/66	turkeys	Canada	1966	[b]	Lang et al., 1968a, b
Ty/Ontario/ 25/66 5265/66 5379/66 5412/66 5447/66	turkeys	Canada	1966	[b]	G. Lang, 1968[d]
Ty/Minn/67	turkeys	USA	1967		B. S. Pomeroy, 1967[d]
D/It/1209/67 1425	ducks	Italy	1967	sinusitis	
Ty/It/ 928/67 665/67 708/67 1076/67 1393/67	turkeys	Italy	1967	sinusitis	A. Rinaldi, 1968[d]
Q/It/ 335/67 504/67 534/67 1441/67 180/67 181/67 1662/67 1712/67	quail	Italy	1967	sinusitis	H. G. Pereira, 1968[d]
D/Germany/210/67	ducks	Germany	1967	[b]	J. Glystorff, 1968[d]
D/Germany/210/67	ducks	Germany	1967	[b]	J. Glystorff, 1968[d]
Ty/Wash/67	turkeys	USA	1967	[b]	W. J. Mathey 1968[d]
Ch/It/1173/67	chickens	Italy	1967	sinusitis 60–80% morbidity 5% mortality	Rinaldi et al., 1968b
Ph/It/907/67	pheasants	Italy	1967	[b]	[b]
Ty/Ontario/6118/67 6828/67	turkeys	Canada	1967	[b]	G. Lang, 1968[d] (9 strains of same origin under study)
[b]	quail	Italy	1968	[b]	A. Rinaldi, 1968[d] (14 strains under study)

TABLE 20.1 ❧ (continued)

Virus Strain[a] (other designation)	Host of Origin	Country of Origin	Year Isolated	Nature of Disease	Reference
Chukar/It/1026/68	partridges	Italy	1968	rhinosinusitis 60% morbidity 20% mortality	Rinaldi et al., 1968a
D/Germany/1868/68	ducks	Germany	1968	[b]	J. Glystorff, 1968[d]
Ty/Wash/68	turkeys	USA	1968	[b]	W. J. Mathey 1968[d]
D/Manching/68	ducklings	Germany	1968	20% mortality	J. Glystorff, 1968[d]
[b]	ducks	Germany	1968	[b]	Schettler, 1968[d]
[b]	pigeons	Germany	1968	[b]	H. G. Pereira, 1968[d]
Ty/Wis/68	turkeys	USA	1968	[b]	Smithies et al., 1969b
D/Penn/486/69	ducks	USA	1969	[b]	Florence S. Lief, 1969[d]
Ty/Minn/70	turkeys	USA	1970	[b]	Bela Tumova 1970[d]

Abbreviations: Ty = turkey, D = duck, Ph = pheasant, Ch = chicken, Q = quail.
[a] Names of strains are given as follows: Species/country of origin/serial/year of isolation.
[b] Specific information unavailable.
[c] Newcastle disease-like.
[d] Personal communication.

Middle and Far East (DeLay et al., 1967).

A virus, virus N, with similarities to fowl plague virus, was isolated from chickens in Germany in 1949 (Dinter, 1949, 1964). It was considered to be a variant of fowl plague virus (Dinter and Bakos, 1950) and subsequently shown to be a type A influenza virus (Rott and Schafer, 1960).

A virus (Duck/Canada/53) isolated from ducklings suffering central nervous system derangement in Manitoba in 1952 (Walker and Bannister, 1953) was also later identified as a type A influenza virus (Mitchell et al., 1967). In 1956 type A influenza viruses were isolated from ducks in Czechoslovakia and England (Koppel et al., 1956; Roberts, 1964). In 1959 a virus was isolated in Scotland from chickens with a fowl plaguelike disease. An antigenically related virus was isolated from terns with fowl plaguelike disease in South Africa, and viruses have been isolated from ducks with respiratory disease and sinusitis in the Ukraine and other regions of the USSR since 1960 (Kornilova, 1960; Prochorov and Feoktistov, 1960; Tsimokh, 1961; Prokofeva et al., 1963; Prokofeva and Tsimokh, 1966).

Since 1963 a great number of type A influenza viruses have been isolated with increasing frequency from various species with different disease syndromes. It cannot be determined whether this represents an absolute increase in infection rate or an increasing awareness of the presence of these disease entities and improved techniques for detection of viruses and/or antibody. An example of this may be the Duck/Canada/53 influenza virus which was isolated in 1952 and remained unidentified until 1967. Because of the increasing awareness of influenza virus infections among avian and other species the "filterable agent" isolated in 1952 (Walker and Bannister, 1953) was reexamined and identified as being a type A influenza virus and related to the fowl plague virus (Mitchell et al., 1967).

ETIOLOGY

CLASSIFICATION

Avian influenza viruses are classified as myxoviruses. This term designates a group of related viruses carrying RNA in the core of an enveloped pleomorphic virion, sensitive to ether and with the original members having a special affinity for certain mucins (Andrewes et al., 1955). Waterson (1962) divided the myxoviruses into two groups—*Myxovirus influenzae* and *M. parainfluenzae*—based on differences in certain physical and biological properties, size of nucleocapsid, and mode of multiplication (Table 20.2).

The largest and epizootiologically (or epidemiologically) probably most important group is that of *M. influenzae*, the so-called true influenza viruses. To date three types—A, B, and C—are known, based on differences in type-specific ribonucleoprotein antigen. While B and C influenza viruses have been reported to cause disease only among humans, type A viruses cause respiratory disorders in man, swine, horses, and several avian species (see Strain Classification and Antigenic Relationship).

Newcastle disease virus, Yucaipa virus, and *M. parotitidis* (mumps) are placed

TABLE 20.2 ❊ Differences between *Myxovirus influenzae* and *M. parainfluenzae*

	Myxovirus influenzae	*Myxovirus parainfluenzae*
Particle size	80–120 mμ	150–200 mμ
Diameter of nucleocapsid	9 mμ	19 mμ
Molecular weight of RNA	2×10^6	7.5×10^6
Filaments	usual	unusual
Formation of S antigen in	nucleus	cytoplasm
Formation of incomplete virus	+	0
Eosinophilic cytoplasmic inclusion	0	+
Multiplicity reactivation	+	0
Hemolysis	unusual	usual
Inactivation by hydroxylamine	+	0

Source: Modified from Waterson (1962).

among the parainfluenza viruses as their biological properties are similar and because of some antigenic overlapping. Viruses in the third myxovirus group have typical morphology and internal virion structure, although they do not have the typical properties of hemagglutination or hemadsorption. Included are measles, distemper, rinderpest, and respiratory syncytial virus.

The system for naming isolants of influenza viruses as provisionally adopted by the World Health Organization is as follows: type/species (other than human)/country or place of origin/serial number (if known or important)/year of isolation—e.g., A/Turkey/Wis/1966. Two viruses, fowl plague and virus N, are exceptions to this system.

MORPHOLOGY

The infective particles of freshly isolated strains are usually filamentous, and the filaments may be as long as 4 mμ. In egg-adapted laboratory strains the particles are usually short rods or nearly spherical forms 80–120 mμ in diameter. According to Dawson and Elford (1949), the rods appear to be composed of partially fused spheres.

The spherical forms seen in negatively stained preparations show a tubular nucleocapsid surrounded by a lipoprotein coat (envelope) with numerous spikes (peplomeres) 3 mμ thick and 10 mμ long. Disruption of envelope by ether or sodium dodecylsulfate releases both hemagglutinin (which is probably identical with peplomeres) and neuraminidase that is attached to hemagglutinin and lies between spikes (Fenner, 1968). Hemagglutinin together with neuraminidase forms the so-called envelope or V-antigen specific for each strain. A virion with a partially disrupted envelope (from ether treatment) releases the nucleocapsid carrying helically arranged subunits, protein and single-stranded RNA. Ribonucleoprotein, 9 mμ in diameter, is arranged in the form of a firmly packed coil (Apostolov and Flewett, 1965). This internal part of the virus is known as the soluble, G (gebundenes), or internal antigen and is the same for all strains of one type.

Characteristics similar to those originally observed with human influenza virus have been reported for several of the avian viruses: Duck/Czech/56 (Frano et al., 1958), Duck/Eng/56 (Waterson et al., 1963), Tern/S. Africa/61 (Becker, 1963), fowl plague and virus N (Waterson et al., 1961; Almeida et al., 1966), Turkey/Ontario/3724/63 and Turkey/Ontario/6213/65 (Lang and Wills, 1966; Lang et al., 1968a).

Electron microscopic examination of Turkey/Ontario/7732/66 revealed pleomorphic structure with rounded and filamentous forms with diameters of 67–186 mμ and lengths of 30–880 mμ (Lang et al., 1968b).

CHEMICAL COMPOSITION

Most of the work on chemical composition was done with the viruses of human origin, fowl plague, and virus N (Schafer, 1957, 1963; Rott and Schafer, 1960). With several strains the infective virion was shown to consist of 0.9% RNA (traces of DNA were probably impurities), 18.5% lipids, 7% polysaccharides, and about 70% protein (Ada and Perry, 1956; Kates et al., 1961).

The RNA consisted of several distinct pieces of single-stranded RNA with a characteristic base composition (adenine, guanine, cytosine, uracil). The sedimentation coefficient, estimated by density gradient centrifugation of detergent-phenol extracts, was between 9S and 18S (Ada, 1957). Although the amount of RNA in influenza virus is rather small, it is considered to be sufficient to code for hemagglutinin, neuraminidase, and ribonucleoprotein, all of which are currently recognized as components important for virus replication. Efforts to demonstrate infectious RNA from influenza viruses have given equivocal results.

Influenza viruses, like other enveloped riboviruses, contain large amounts of lipids synthesized by the infected cell and are considered to be a building component of the viral envelope. According to Zillig et al. (1955), 24% of fowl plague virus consists of lipids having the same composition as the host cell lipids.

Several carbohydrates (including ribose, galactose, mannose, fructose, glucosamine) have also been demonstrated as an integral part of the envelope contributed by the host cell in the final stage of virus multiplication (Ada and Gottschalk, 1956). The viral envelope contains host-cell specific material (Harboe, 1963; Harboe et al., 1966), apparently carried in a carbohydrate associated with the viral coat protein (Laver and Webster, 1966).

Most of the viral components are associated with protein; 38% of the viral protein is ribonucleoprotein (internal or S antigen) which is responsible for the type specificity, e.g. type A, B, or C. However, Davenport et al. (1960) reported that there may be minor but important differences in the ribonucleoprotein within a given type, and Laver (1964) showed that a difference in ribonucleoprotein of two type A strains may be due to a difference in amino acid sequences. These findings are of theoretical importance and do not affect the standard techniques for diagnostic serology.

Hemagglutinating subunits, the most important components known on the surface of the virion, are probably complex protein containing hemagglutinin and viral neuraminidase. They are known as "envelope antigen" and are responsible for strain specificity. Hemagglutinin has a sedimentation coefficient of 15S, is composed of a number of polypeptide chains (Laver, 1964; Fenner, 1968), is noninfectious, and has hemagglutinating ability. Antibodies formed against hemagglutinin are protective and are detectable in the hemagglutination-inhibition test, virus-neutralization test, or the strain-specific complement-fixation test (Fabiyi et al., 1958) (see Diagnosis).

Neuraminidase deserves special attention. It is associated with a protein with a sedimentation coefficient of 9S (Fenner, 1968) accounting for 5–15% of the total viral protein. Enzymatic activity of neuraminidase was found to be identical to that of receptor destroying enzyme (RDE) of *Vibrio cholerae* by Gottschalk (1957), who proposed its name and defined its activity. It has no hemagglutinating ability and is distinct from the host neuraminidase demonstrated in avian and mammalian tissue (Ada et al., 1963). Both neuraminidase and hemagglutinating subunits are virus-coded products.

VIRUS REPLICATION

Multiplication of influenza viruses has been studied by many workers who employed electron microscopic examination of thin sections of infected organs, immunofluorescence, autoradiography, and a variety of biological techniques. Fowl plague virus frequently has been used as a model (Breitenfeld and Schafer, 1957; Zimmerman and Schafer, 1960; Fraser, 1967a,b; Fedova and Tumova, 1968; Fenner, 1968).

Infection is initiated by attachment of virus to the cell (a process similar to adsorption of virus to red blood cells) and then penetration into the cytoplasm. In this first stage, viral envelope hemagglutinin is involved. Neuraminidase plays no role in either attachment or entry. After penetration the envelope is stripped off the viral core and neither is detectable for a period of time (the eclipse phase). Synthesis of RNA begins soon after the infection. Ribonucleoprotein antigen is detectable after 3 hours in the nucleus (where it is assembled) and after 6 hours in the cytoplasm (Fig. 20.1). Hemagglutinin has not been found in the nucleus. It is observed first at 4 hours after the infection throughout the cytoplasm, but it is more concentrated in certain areas near the nuclear membrane. Later, hemagglutinin antigen accumulates at the cell periphery and in protruding filaments.

The virion is completed in the cytoplasm, and maturation occurs by budding from a cytoplasmic membrane. This final stage, release from the cell, is helped by neuraminidase and may be blocked by anti-neuraminidase serum. In the course of maturation, lipids, carbohydrates, and other host materials are incorporated into the viral envelope.

The character of multiplication when fully infectious virus particles are released from the cell is called *infectious;* i.e., virus can infect another cell. Under certain conditions S antigen remains in the nucleus, and envelope antigens fail to concentrate at the periphery of the cell. In such cases the multiplication cycle is called *abortive;* only noninfectious hemagglutinin (unable to infect another cell) may be produced (Franklin and Breitenfeld, 1959; Rott and Scholtissek, 1963). Other types of imperfect virus replication are called defective, delayed, or persistent and are described in detail in a review by Fraser (1967b).

The infection of cells with a high multiplicity input leads to the production of incomplete virus (Von Magnus, 1954). Incomplete virus contains an excess of hemagglutinin and only a very small amount of ribonucleoprotein and may be avoided by inoculation of diluted virus.

Genetic Interaction

Influenza viruses were the first animal viruses shown to be capable of genetic inter-

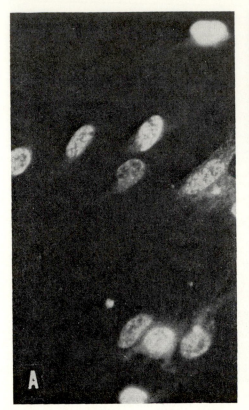

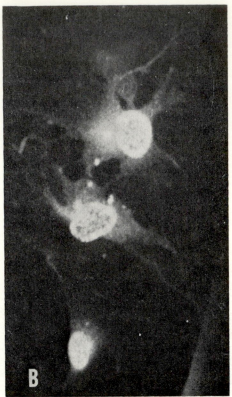

FIG. 20.1—Growth of fowl plague virus in diploid cells (WI-38) as studied with immunofluorescence. (A) S-antigen in nuclei 17 hours after infection. (B) S-antigen in transit from nucleus to cytoplasm. Note concentration in region of perinuclear membrane and fluorescent granules in cytoplasm near nucleus. (A and B stained with anti-S serum conjugated with fluorescein isothiocyanate.) (C) V-antigen in cytoplasm. Specific fluorescence is observed in cytoplasm and there is no fluorescence in nucleus. (Stained with anti-V serum conjugated with fluorescein isothiocyanate.) ×400.

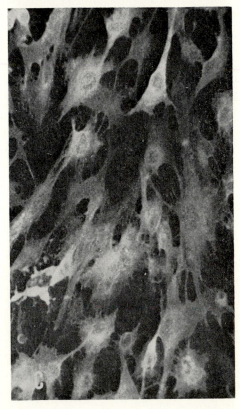

action. The studies of Burnet and others, who investigated the combination of a large number of strains under different experimental conditions, are reviewed by Kilbourne (1963) and Fenner and Sambrook (1964). Most of the early genetic studies employed recombination of human influenza viruses in mice or chicken embryos. Simpson and Hirst (1961) were the first using plaque technique and cross-reactivation to demonstrate genetic interaction between human and porcine influenza viruses. Tumova and Pereira (1965) observed cross-reactivation between two plaque-forming avian influenza viruses and a number of non-plaque-forming strains of human, porcine, and equine origin. Cross-reactivation of ultraviolet light-inactivated fowl plague virus and active A_2/Singapore/57 virus resulted in recombinant virus having the envelope antigens of both parents. Laver and Kilbourne (1966) and Easterday et al. (1969) have shown that such hybrids contain in their envelope neuraminidase of one and hemagglutinin of the other parental strain.

The recombination studies have become especially interesting because of the increasing number of isolations of avian influenza strains which share either hemagglutinin or neuraminidase antigen with human, swine, or equine influenza viruses (see Antigenic Relationship). However, it remains speculative whether recombination can occur under natural conditions.

BIOLOGICAL PROPERTIES

The biological properties of the avian influenza viruses have not been studied extensively, but in general they are similar to those of the well-known human influenza strains. However, differences do exist, and even those strains isolated from the same locality may differ in such characteristics as pathogenicity for birds, plaque-producing ability, and lethality for chicken embryos (Pereira et al., 1967a; Lang et al., 1968a,b).

Hemagglutination

All influenza viruses agglutinate fowl and certain mammalian erythrocytes. Erythrocytes from a wide range of species have been agglutinated by avian influenza viruses (Frano and Kapitancik, 1959; Blaskovic et al., 1959; Tsimokh, 1961; Lang et al., 1968b).

Adsorption of virus to mucoprotein receptors on the erythrocytes results in hemagglutination and is followed under appropriate conditions by elution. Gottschalk (1957) has shown that the reaction which occurs by means of neuraminidase is based on splitting the N-acetyl-neuraminic acid side chain of the receptor mucoproteins. Adsorption and elution rates vary with different virus strains. Most elute readily at 37° C. Following elution the erythrocytes cannot be agglutinated again with the homologous virus.

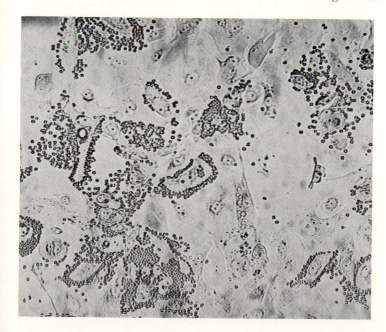

FIG. 20.2—*Hemadsorption due to influenza virus infection. Monkey kidney cell cultures infected with mammalian origin influenza virus with guinea pig erythrocytes adsorbed to surface of infected cells.*

A phenomenon similar to hemagglutination can be demonstrated in tissue culture cells infected with influenza virus. In this reaction, called hemadsorption (Vogel and Shelokov, 1957), erythrocytes adsorb to cells in which virus has replicated (Fig. 20.2). Both hemagglutination and hemadsorption are used widely for diagnostic purposes.

Nonspecific Inhibitors

The serum of many animal species contains inhibitory substances of varied chemical nature called nonspecific inhibitors. They react with the hemagglutinin units of the viral envelope and prevent hemagglutination, thus simulating specific hemagglutination-inhibiting antibodies. They differ in sensitivity to thermoinactivation and are active especially against influenza viruses.

The α inhibitor (Francis, 1947) is active against heated influenza viruses A_0 and A_1 and can be destroyed effectively by RDE and trypsin (Sampaio and Isaacs, 1953). The β inhibitor (Chu, 1951) is a thermolabile (destroyed by heating at 56° C for 30 minutes) protein active against A_1 virus. The γ inhibitor, a thermolabile mucoprotein (Cohen and Dorman, 1965) active against A_2 viruses, is inactivated by treatment with KIO_4 or RDE (Expert Committee, 1959). The γ inhibitor is present in high levels in many samples of serum from horses, cattle, guinea pigs, and man.

Most of the avian viruses are believed to be insensitive to nonspecific inhibitors. However, some sharing common hemagglutinin antigen with human or swine viruses may ultimately be shown to be sensitive. Therefore, serum samples tested against relatively unknown avian virus should be treated to remove inhibitors.

RESISTANCE TO CHEMICAL AND PHYSICAL AGENTS

Influenza viruses are readily inactivated by ultraviolet irradiation (UV), although different strains may require different exposure times to reach the same effect. They are relatively stable at pH 7–8 but labile at low pH (Lang et al., 1968a). Viral infectivity and hemagglutinin may be stabilized by the addition of protein (10% calf serum or 0.5% gelatin) to the medium used for dilution or storage.

Hemagglutinating and infectious capacity can usually be maintained for several years at —60° C and for several weeks at 4° C. Hemagglutinin is more stable than infectivity. Other successful methods for virus storage include lyophilization of buffered suspension and refrigeration (4° C) of infected tissue in 50% glycerol-saline.

Both the infectivity and hemagglutinating activities are retained when carried down on the precipitate with protamine, alum, or calcium phosphate or when treated with 35% methanol at —5° C (Andrewes and Pereira, 1967). The method of precipitation with calcium phosphate has been widely used in the production of influenza vaccines for humans and equines.

Infectivity is rapidly destroyed by formaldehyde, detergents, oxidizing agents (iodine), dilute acids, ether, sodium desoxycholate, hydroxylamine, sodium dodecylsulfate, and ammonium ions (Franklin and Wecker, 1959; Laver, 1963). Lang et al. (1968a,b) reported decreased infectivity of the Turkey/Ontario/7732/66 and Turkey/Ontario/6213/66 viruses at 4° C 48 hours after treatment of allantoic fluid with 0.05–0.1% formalin; hemagglutinating activity remained stable for 4 weeks.

Thermoinactivation rates differ among antigenically related and unrelated strains isolated in the same geographical area from the same species. Lang et al. (1968a,b) found differences in inactivation rates at 56° C. Turkey/Ontario/3724/63 virus at 56° C lost its infectivity after 15 minutes, but hemagglutinin remained active more than 120 minutes. Homme and Easterday (1970) found that 6 hours were necessary to destroy infectivity of Turkey/Wis/66 virus at 56° C. Fowl plague virus survived after 15 minutes at 55° C but was destroyed after 5 minutes or less at 60° C (Moses et al., 1948). Mitchell et al. (1968) reported that 8 strains of avian influenza were more stable in aerosols than were 6 strains of human influenza A_0, A_1, A_2.

STRAIN CLASSIFICATION AND ANTIGENIC RELATIONSHIP

The type A viruses are divided into subtypes on the basis of differences in the envelope antigen.

Those of human origin comprise 3 subtypes—A_0, A_1, A_2. The strains of A_2 subtypes are the most interesting as they have very definite relation to some animal influenza viruses, particularly those of avian origin.

TABLE 20.3 ❧ Subtypes of Avian Influenza Viruses

Subtype 1	Subtype 2	Subtype 3	Subtype 5	Subtype 6	Subtype 7
Fowl plague	Virus N	D/Eng/56	Ch/Scot/59	Ty/Canada/63	D/Ukraine/2/60
Ty/Eng/63	D/Canada/53	D/Ukraine/1/60	Tern/S. Africa/61	Ty/Calif/64	D/Ukraine/1/63
	D/It/858/65		Ty/Ontario/7732/66	Ty/Mass/65	
	Ty/It/983/65		Ty/Ontario/6213/66	Ty/Wis/66	Subtype 8
	Q/It/1117/65[a]	Subtype 4	Ty/Ontario/6828/67	Ty/Eng/66	Ty/Ontario/6118/68
	Q/It/544/66	D/Czech/56	Ty/Wis/68	Ty/Minn/67	
	Ph/It/647/66	D/Eng/62		D/Manching/68	
	D/It/574/66[b]				
	Ch/It/1173/67[b]				
	Chukar/It/1026/68[a]				

N. B. Only a limited number of the most well known strains are listed.

Source: Adapted from Pereira et al. (1966, 1967a); Rinaldi et al. (1968a,b); Mitchell et al. (1967); Tumova et al. (1970); Glystorff (1968); Pereira (1968); Smithies et al. (1969b).

[a] Virus reacts also with subtypes 4 and 6.
[b] Virus reacts with subtype 6.

Four subtypes were described in the first attempt to provide a classification of avian influenza viruses (Pereira et al., 1965). Subsequently 6 subtypes were described (Pereira et al., 1966), and 2 viruses recently studied may represent 2 more subtypes (Tumova, unpublished data) (Table 20.3). With the rapidly increasing number of new isolates, antigenic overlapping (antigenic bridges) between strains was observed and classification into subtypes has become more complicated (Pereira et al., 1967a).

The continued isolation of new viruses suggests that avian viruses are widespread and that their number and classification is far from definitive.

While the ribonucleoprotein antigen of all influenza viruses remains stable, changes can occur in envelope antigen. These may be either gradual changes within a given subtype (such an altered strain is referred to as an antigenic variant) or sharp changes leading to a novel subtype. It is a peculiarity of avian and equine viruses in contrast to human influenza virus that strains with different properties may coexist in the same population when new variants appear.

The origin and evolution of antigenic changes have not been clarified, and several hypotheses proposed do not satisfactorily explain the appearance of either the variant or a novel subtype.

The hypothesis of a common origin of type A influenza viruses, presumably in an animal carrier, has received considerable support in recent years with the recovery of a number of new viruses from different animal species related to human influenza strains by envelope antigens.

Relationships among strains are commonly determined by analysis of the envelope (surface) antigens by 3 methods: (1) The hemagglutination-inhibition test detects similarities and differences in the hemagglutinin among strains. (2) The strain-specific complement-fixation test employing V-antigen detects similarities and differences in the hemagglutinin and/or neuraminidase. (3) The neuraminidase inhibition test determines the antigenic character of the neuraminidase.

Strains closely related by hemagglutinin may have differences in their neuraminidase. Some strains related by either or both of the envelope antigens form antigenic bridges between subtypes (Fig. 20.3). There are also antigenic bridges to the porcine, equine, and human A_2 influenza viruses.

The antigenic relationships shown are those that had been determined by late 1969. With the isolation of new strains, new techniques, and continued antigenic analyses new and additional relationships have since been described.

Considerable attention has been directed to the relationship between the neuraminidases or hemagglutinin of avian and human influenza strains in connection with the possibility of interspecies transfer and virus recombination in nature (Laver and Kilbourne, 1966; Kilbourne et al., 1967; Pereira et al., 1967b). The relationship of avian to human A_2 strains is especially interesting and presents many questions with respect to the role of animals in the ecology and possible interspecies transfer of influenza viruses (Pereira, 1969).

LABORATORY HOST SYSTEMS

Chicken Embryos

All strains grow readily in embryonating hens' eggs. Some viruses, when inoculated into the allantois, cause death of the embryo with dark red skin, petechial hemorrhages, congested muscles, and lesions in internal organs. Lang et al. (1968b) observed the death of embryos 20–24 hours after inoculation with a high multiplicity input of Turkey/Ontario/7732/66.

Cell Cultures

Some avian strains grow in chicken and monkey kidney cell cultures (Pereira et al., 1965). Others that have been grown in chicken embryos produce in certain cell culture systems one cycle of infection (either with or without cytopathic effect) terminated by the production of noninfectious virus. Such was observed with fowl plague virus in L cells (Franklin and Breitenfeld, 1959) and with several avian influenza strains in human diploid cell strain WI-38 (Tumova and Fedova, 1968). The fowl plague virus was adapted to the WI-38 cell strain without difficulty, and infectious virus was produced in the course of 15 passages (Fedova and Tumova, 1968). Fowl plague virus also was successfully grown in myeloblasts (obtained from chickens inoculated with avian myeloblastosis virus) (Zavada and Rosenbergova, 1968) and in pri-

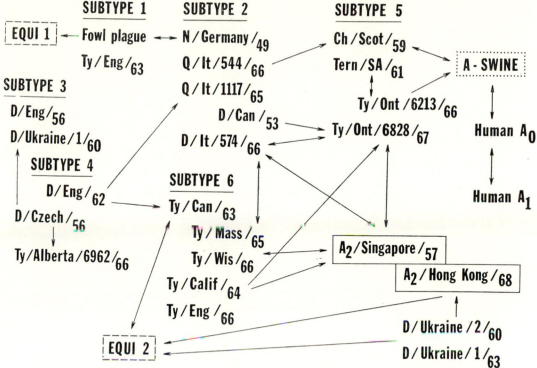

FIG. 20.3—*Schema of envelope antigen relationships among A influenza viruses. (Results of hemagglutination-inhibition and strain-specific complement fixation tests.) Arrow → indicates reactions of antibody X vs antigen Y, and arrow ⟷ indicates antibody X vs antigen Y and antigen X vs antibody Y. (Tumova, unpublished data)*

mary human embryonic lung cell cultures (Chaproniere and Pereira, 1955).

Most of the strains induce plaques on primary chicken fibroblast monolayers, but there are considerable strain differences in size, type, and time of appearance of the plaques (Fig. 20.4). This characteristic permits purification of viral progeny (the method of choice), and characteristic strain differences constitute a useful marker in genetic studies (Pereira et al., 1965, 1967a). Plaque production with the following strains has not been reported: Duck/Czech/56, Quail/Italy/1655/65, Quail/Italy/54/66, Quail/Italy/1577/66, Duck/Italy/946/66, Duck/Italy/1671/66.

Laboratory Animals

RABBITS AND GUINEA PIGS. Rabbits and guinea pigs inoculated intravenously with Turkey/Ontario/6213/65 did not show signs of disease (Lang et al., 1968a). However, death and severe lung lesions developed in guinea pigs infected with fowl plague virus (Tu-

mova, unpublished data). Guinea pigs intranasally exposed to Duck/Eng/56, Duck/Czech/56, and fowl plague viruses produce anti-S antibody with considerable individual variation.

MICE. Mice intranasally exposed to the Duck/Eng/56 virus had no signs of disease, and virus was not recovered; but serial passage (intranasal inoculation) of Duck/Czech/56 virus in mice caused lung lesions (Andrewes and Worthington, 1959).

FERRETS. Ferrets were apparently refractory to intranasal inoculation with Duck/Eng/56, Duck/Czech/56, or Duck/Ukraine/1/60 virus (no signs of disease and no antibody response) (Andrewes and Worthington, 1959; Tumova et al., 1970). However, intranasal exposure with fowl plague, Duck/Ukraine/2/60, or Duck/Ukraine/1/63 virus caused overt signs of disease accompanied by elevated body temperature 24–48 hours after exposure (Tumova et al., 1970).

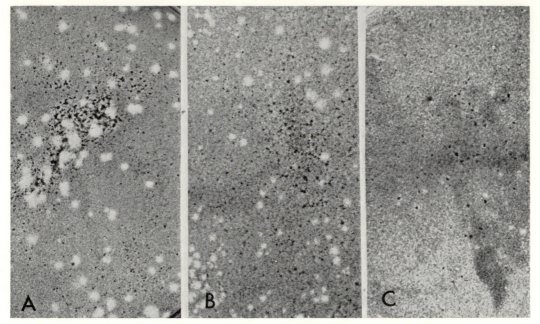

FIG. 20.4—*Plaques in chicken embryo fibroblast cultures 72 hours after infection with* (A) *Turkey/England/63,* (B) *Tern/S. Africa/61,* (C) *Chicken/Scotland/59. All with agar overlay, stained with neutral red. Note differences in size and morphology.*

PATHOGENICITY

There is a considerable range of pathogenicity among the avian influenza viruses. The fowl plague, Turkey/Eng/63, Chicken/Scot/59, and Tern/S. Africa/61 viruses, which are generally considered the most pathogenic of the avian influenza viruses, all result in high morbidity (up to 100%) and mortality (up to 100%) under natural conditions (Lang et al., 1968b). The Duck/Czech/56 virus was also reported to cause a high mortality rate (approximately 40%) (Koppel et al., 1956).

Several viruses with various degrees of antigenic relatedness have been isolated from the quail (Rinaldi et al., 1967b; Mandelli et al., 1968) and can cause severe disease among quail during the first 2 weeks of life. The Turkey/Ontario/7732/66 virus has been described as highly pathogenic (Lang et al., 1968b), although under natural conditions it causes mortality rates of only 2–13%. Experimentally inoculated chickens and turkeys, however, usually develop severe lesions and die within a few days.

Morbidity rates are high following infection with several of the other avian influenza viruses. However, mortality rates are usually low and the signs of disease (respiratory, enteric and reproductive) are of variable degrees of severity. Inapparent infections have been described primarily under experimental conditions (Homme et al., 1970).

The effect of age susceptibility to infection and severity of disease varies with the host species and the virus. Higher morbidity and mortality rates are observed in newly hatched battery-reared quail (Coturnix) than in adults (Rinaldi et al., 1967b; Mandelli et al., 1968). Homme et al. (1970) showed that turkeys of any age could be infected by contact with infected turkeys or exposure with aerosols of virus. Lang et al. (1968a) reported that under experimental conditions the Turkey/Ontario/6213 virus was pathogenic to very young turkey poults but not to older turkeys or to chickens of any age. In other instances, adult breeding turkeys have been severely involved with high morbidity and low mortality rates (Lang et al., 1965, 1968a,b).

PATHOGENESIS AND EPIZOOTIOLOGY

NATURAL AND EXPERIMENTAL HOSTS

Several species, including chickens, turkeys, ducks (wild and domestic), quail *(Co-*

turnix coturnix japonica), pheasants *(Phasianus colchicus L.),* partridge *(Alectoris chukar),* terns *(Sterna hirundo),* pigeons, and geese (domestic and wild), are natural and/ or experimental hosts for avian influenza viruses (Table 20.1).

Chickens and occasionally other species have been involved in outbreaks of fowl plague in North America (Stubbs, 1965). In recent years, however, the influenza viruses have been isolated only from turkeys and ducks (Walker and Bannister, 1953; Mitchell et al., 1967; Lang, 1968, personal communication). Avian influenza antibodies have been demonstrated in serum collected from North American migratory waterfowl *(Branta canadensis* and *Chen hyperborea)* (Easterday et al., 1968a).

On the European and African continents, type A influenza viruses have been isolated from a variety of avian species. In recent years most of the isolated viruses have been from ducks, quail, turkeys, chickens, and pheasants.

Although several of the avian influenza viruses are antigenically related to those of mammalian origin (Fig. 20.4), there is no evidence that the avian viruses circulate in mammalian hosts under natural conditions.

TRANSMISSION

There are indications that close contact is necessary for the transmission of the disease. Infections may or may not transfer, depending upon the intimacy of the contact. For example, Narayan et al. (1969a) reported contact transmission among turkeys kept together on the floor, but not to turkeys housed in cages 1 meter above the floor of the same room. Bankowski and Conrad (1966), to the contrary, noted experimental contact infections among turkeys in adjacent pens. Homme et al. (1970) studied the rate of contact spread in 15-week-old turkeys; 97 susceptible turkeys placed in contact with 3 infected turkeys were all infected within 13 days (Fig. 20.5). In another experiment involving 4 adjacent flocks of turkeys, they observed that the infection was self-limiting and did not spread to all flocks even though the flocks were in close proximity and no precautions were taken to prevent spread by the caretakers. Chicken-to-chicken transmission has also been described (Becker and Uys, 1967; Narayan et al., 1969a).

The possibility of vertical transmission

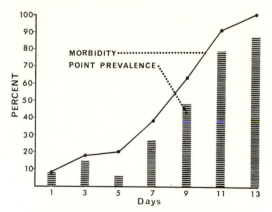

FIG. 20.5—*Graphic illustration of spread of Turkey/Wis/1/66 virus through flock of 100 turkeys. Three infected turkeys were placed with 97 susceptible turkeys on day 0. Point prevalence bars indicate percentage of turkeys from which virus was isolated on day indicated. Morbidity line indicates accumulated percentage of turkeys from which virus was isolated.*

must be considered. Narayan et al. (1969a) reported the isolation of virus from eggs produced by infected turkeys, and Lang et al. (1968b) cited an outbreak in an isolated flock of 8,800 turkeys imported to Canada as fertile eggs (7,000 birds) and day-old poults (1,100 birds). There are other examples of outbreaks in which the source of infection is elusive. In North America infected turkey breeding flocks are common; thus infected eggs are likely used for hatching purposes.

Successful experimental routes of exposure include aerosol, intranasal, intrasinus, intratracheal, oral, conjunctival, intramuscular, intraperitoneal, intravenous, and intracranial administration of the various viruses.

There is no evidence to suggest that invertebrate hosts are involved in the interepizootic maintenance or transmission of these viruses.

EPIZOOTIOLOGY

The epizootiology of avian influenza is not well understood. It has been suggested that wild birds are involved in the dissemination of virus (Wells, 1963; Easterday et al., 1968). However, there is only one report of an isolation from wild birds. In that case the virus was shown to be the cause of an epizootic with a high mortality rate among terns in South Africa (Becker,

1966). Easterday et al. (1968) examined serum from 9 species of wild North American birds and found antibodies against several of the avian influenza viruses in serum from two species—Canada goose (*Branta canadensis*) and snow goose (*Chen hyperborea*). Wells (1963) suggested that the Turkey/Eng/63 virus, highly pathogenic and closely related to the fowl plague virus, was introduced into Great Britain by migratory birds.

Becker (1966) indicated that the Chicken/Scot/59 and Tern/S. Africa/61 viruses may have epizootiologic as well as antigenic relationships. He postulated that seabirds might suffer latent influenza virus infections which could change to overt disease under conditions of stress such as poor feeding and unfavorable weather conditions. In 1959 Wilson (cited by Becker, 1966) observed that seabirds were driven inland by weather conditions and were present on the farm where the Chicken/Scot/59 virus was isolated.

Fowl plague virus can be spread by wild birds and can be carried downstream in running water. Although fowl plague can spread very rapidly among various species, it may be that only a single species on a farm is involved in an outbreak (Stubbs, 1965). Walker and Bannister (1953) reported that on a farm where there were chickens, turkeys, geese, and ducks, only the ducks were involved in a disease from which a hemagglutinating virus (subsequently shown to be related to virus N) was isolated.

One of the striking features of disease outbreaks is that the source of the causative virus is usually unknown. Equally puzzling may be the disappearance of the disease and the virus after an outbreak. The source of the infection in Wisconsin turkeys in 1966 was not determined (Smithies et al., 1969a). Lang et al. (1965) also failed to learn the source of infection in 5 flocks in 3 locations approximately 100 miles apart. There was no known communication among flocks.

In other situations the disease has become enzootic. Rinaldi et al. (1967b) and Mandelli et al. (1968), who described the disease in quail (*Coturnix*) reared under confinement conditions, found it was perpetuated by the constant introduction of newly hatched susceptible birds.

There is an indication that birds may be persistently infected with selected viruses; however, the duration of time that birds may be infected has not been defined. Homme et al. 1970) could isolate virus from turkeys for at least 21 days after exposure. They presented serological evidence which suggested that the virus persisted for 3 months. Bankowski and Conrad (1966) isolated virus from the trachea of a chicken 36 days after exposure, and Lang et al. (1968a) reported that virus could be isolated from some tissues of turkey poults found dead 22 days after exposure. Although there is direct and indirect evidence that virus is present in birds for a considerable time, the importance of such with regard to virus dissemination is not understood. The duration of virus persistence and the conditions under which the virus is disseminated need definition.

INCUBATION PERIOD

The incubation periods for the various diseases caused by these viruses is extremely variable. It may range from a few hours to a few days and is dependent upon the dose of virus, the route of exposure, and the species exposed. With viruses which do not cause overt disease, the incubation (based on the reisolation of virus) may be a matter of a few hours or as long as 2–3 days.

SIGNS

The signs of disease are extremely variable and depend on the species affected, age, sex, concurrent infections, infecting virus, environmental factors, etc. Those re-

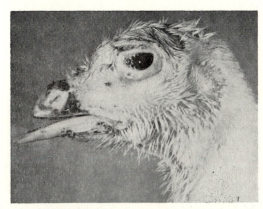

FIG. 20.6—*Five-week-old turkey naturally infected with Turkey/Calif/64 virus. Note eye involvement and swollen sinus. (Courtesy R. A. Bankowski)*

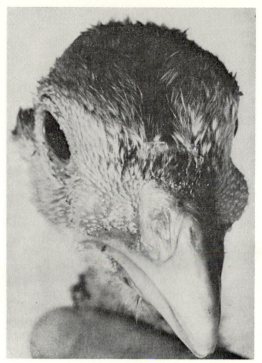

FIG. 20.7—Turkey poult experimentally infected with Turkey/Calif/64 virus 35 days postinoculation. Note swollen sinus. (Courtesy R. A. Bankowski)

ported include decreased activity, decreased feed consumption, emaciation, increased broodiness of hens, decreased egg production, mild to severe respiratory signs, coughing, sneezing, rales, excessive lacrimation, huddling, ruffled feathers, sinusitis, edema of head and face, cyanosis of unfeathered

skin, nervous disorder, and diarrhea. Any of these signs may occur singly or in various combinations (Figs. 20.6–20.9). In some cases, the disease is rapidly fulminating and birds are found dead without previous signs. Thus the two extremes of the disease, fatal infections and inapparent infections, are without overt signs of disease.

The specific signs of fowl plague have been described by several authors (Jungherr et al., 1946; Stubbs, 1965), and many variations of clinical signs have been noticed. There is usually a sudden onset with the birds being dull, inappetent, and ruffled. In mature birds there is a cessation of egg production. Some birds die without showing signs. Signs may reflect abnormalities of the respiratory, enteric, or nervous systems. Cutaneous changes in the form of cyanosis and edema may be observed. Wells (1963) described an outbreak of fowl plague in a flock of about 1,600 turkeys in England. There were sudden deaths in regularly mounting numbers, and egg peritonitis was common in laying hens. Ill birds were in a comatose state, often with the head nearly touching the litter. The only other external signs of disease were edematous faces in 2 turkeys.

In 1961 mass mortality among European common terns was described in South Africa (Rowan, 1962). In addition to the large numbers of terns found dead, many were unable to fly and had severe diarrhea. The disease spread rapidly along 1,000 miles of South African coast from Port Elizabeth to Lambert Bay over a period of about 3 weeks. There were no overt signs of dis-

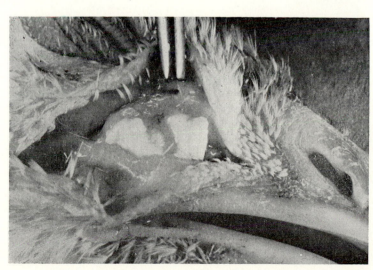

FIG. 20.8—Turkey poult experimentally infected with Turkey/Calif/64 virus 31 days postinoculation. Note caseous exudate in sinus. (Courtesy R. A. Bankowski)

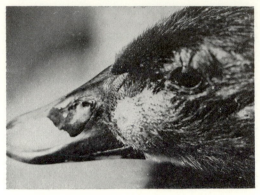

FIG. 20.9—Swollen sinus and nasal discharge in duck infected with influenza virus related to virus N. (Courtesy G. Mandelli)

ease in any other species associated with the terns.

<h3>MORBIDITY AND MORTALITY</h3>

Both morbidity and mortality rates with influenza virus infections are extremely variable. The mortality rate may vary depending on the virus and species involved. The conditions of exposure may also be important. While losses have rarely exceeded 10% in natural outbreaks among turkeys on the North American continent, the mortality rate under experimental conditions has been extremely high with some of the viruses isolated (Lang et al., 1968a,b). In other cases under experimental conditions, both morbidity and mortality rates have been at or near zero (Lang et al., 1965; Olesiuk et al., 1967; Homme and Easterday, 1970c; Homme et al., 1970).

Morbidity rates generally are poorly defined, largely because of the very large size of flocks involved (thousands of birds) and the ill-defined signs of disease in many of the outbreaks. It is obvious that in cases where the mortality rate has been high the morbidity rate has also been high. There are some examples, however, where morbidity has been high and mortality low (Roberts, 1964).

<h3>GROSS LESIONS</h3>

The gross lesions observed in several avian species have been extremely varied with regard to their location and severity, depending at least partly on the strain of the infecting virus. The lesions described in experimental infections have been similar to those observed in natural infections but may be more or less severe involving the same or different tissues.

A variety of congestive, hemorrhagic, transudative, and necrobiotic changes have been described with those infections (fowl plague, Chicken/Scot/59, Tern/S. Africa/61, Turkey/Eng/63) in which the mortality rates were high (Jungherr et al., 1946; Wells, 1963; Uys and Becker, 1967). The congestive, hemorrhagic, and necrotic changes may be observed first in the skin, comb, and wattles. As the disease progresses other organs may be involved. Yellow-gray foci were frequently observed in the liver, spleen, kidneys, and lungs in experimental fowl plague infections in chickens (Jungherr et al., 1946). On the contrary, Rowan (1962) described the lungs, liver, kidneys, spleen, and heart as normal in the highly fatal disease of terns. Yellow-gray exudates on the air sacs, peritoneum, and in the oviducts and fibrinous pericarditis have been commonly observed with these highly fatal infections. Similar lesions were reported in ducks in Manitoba infected with a type A influenza virus (Walker and Bannister, 1953; Mitchell et al., 1967).

Two viruses (Turkey/Ontario/6213/65 and Turkey/Ontario/7732/66), related to the Chicken /Scot/59 virus, isolated from turkeys in Ontario have caused similar congestive, hemorrhagic, and transudative changes (Lang et al., 1968a,b). Severe lesions were produced experimentally in turkeys and chickens with the Turkey/Ontario/7732/66 virus, but the lesions were not striking in experimental infections with the Turkey/Ontario/6213/65 virus (Lang et al., 1968a,b; Narayan et al., 1969a,b; Rouse et al., 1968). The most marked lesions in both turkeys and chickens were observed in the urogenital system (Turkey/Ontario/7732/66 infection).

Sinusitis of variable severity and character has been described by several authors in several species including ducks, turkeys, chickens, quail (Coturnix), partridge, and pheasants (Figs. 20.6–20.9). Sinusitis has been especially common among ducks (Koppel et al., 1956; Tsimokh, 1961; Roberts, 1964; Prokofeva and Tsimokh, 1966). In one of the outbreaks described by Roberts (1964), both influenza virus and mycoplasma were isolated from sinus exudates. Sinusitis has not been commonly reported in turkeys in North America. In Italy the most common lesion reported among infected quail, pheasants, ducks, chickens, and turkeys has been sinusitis with mucopurulent to caseous exudates. Fibrinous or fibrinopurulent pericarditis and/or airsacculitis have also been observed (Rinaldi et al., 1965, 1966a,b, 1967a,b, 1968a,b).

HISTOPATHOLOGY

Histopathologic descriptions of avian influenza infection have been limited primarily to those conditions in which there have been severe overt disease and obvious gross changes: i.e., fowl plague in Europe, the Middle East, and the Orient and the more recent episodes of influenza among various avian species in Great Britain, Europe, South Africa, and North America.

Classic naturally occurring fowl plague was characterized by edema, hyperemia, hemorrhages, and foci of perivascular lymphoid cuffing—chiefly in the myocardium, spleen, lungs, brain, wattles, and to lesser extent liver and kidney (Gerlach and Michalka, 1926). Parenchymal degeneration and necrosis were present in the spleen, liver, and kidney. Early emphasis was placed on brain lesions (Seifried, 1931; Findlay et al., 1937) which included foci of necrosis, perivascular lymphoid cuffing, glial foci, vascular proliferation, and neuronal changes.

Chickens dying of experimental fowl plague due to the intravenous inoculation of Dutch East Indies strain—in addition to widespread edema, hyperemia, and hemorrhage—had foci of necrosis in spleen (75%), liver, lung, kidney, intestine, and pancreas in that decreasing order of frequency (Jungherr et al., 1946). Necrotic foci were random, seldom confluent, and predisposed to locations with terminal capillary circulation (i.e. lacteal tissue of intestinal villi). In the spleen, necrosis occurred in the periarteriolar lymphoid sheaths and was often surrounded by a halo of fibrinoid material. Necrotic foci in the visceral organs were first detected by acidophilic changes and heterophil infiltration. Swollen parenchymal cells with small marginated nuclei degenerated in focal areas to necrosis. Although eosinophilic cytoplasmic globules or granules, probably nonspecific, have been described by most authors, no valid inclusion bodies have been reported. Small necrotic foci were found in the brain at 24 hours postinoculation and at later times were larger in size. Advanced lesions in the central nervous system were accompanied by signs of encephalitis (i.e. perivascular lymphoid cuffing, vascular-glial reactions, and neuron degeneration). Rarely secondary foci of encephalomalacia were found.

Immunized birds which were challenged and developed subacute or chronic disease had the same basic lesions as the acute disease. These lesions (termed the "immune-challenge" reaction) were often exaggerated and were associated with well-developed lymphoid follicles in the parenchymatous organs. Lesions in the chicken embryo included hemorrhages in muscle and nerve tissue; the severity and location depended on route of inoculation.

The lesions produced in 6-week-old chickens by the intranasal and intraconjunctival inoculation of the Tern/S. Africa/61 and Chicken/Scot/59 viruses have been examined sequentially and compared by Uys and Becker (1967). Most of the chickens infected with the "tern virus" did not survive beyond 6 days. Foci of necrosis and lymphoid infiltration were seen in spleen, myocardium, brain, eyes, ocular muscles, comb, and skeletal muscle. Splenic lesions were chiefly proliferation of reticular cells in the red pulp accompanied by heterophil accumulation; a small number had necrotic foci with fibrin exudation. Curiously, the periarteriolar sheath remained nonreactive. Edema and hydropic degeneration of myocardial fibers seen 4 days postinoculation rapidly developed into severe myocarditis with focal areas of necrotic muscle. Despite high virus titers, there were no lesions in the lung (and no respiratory signs). After 5 or 6 days a diffuse encephalitis developed in both the cerebrum and cerebellum of the chickens infected with the "tern virus." There was widespread perivascular cuffing with mononuclear cells, necrosis of neuronal cells, "edema and a diffuse cellularity," and in some chickens hemorrhage. The lesions in the chickens infected with the Chicken/Scot/59 virus were much less severe.

The distinguishing features between the lesions caused by these 2 viruses were the degree of cardiac, brain, ocular, and cutaneous involvement, being less severe or absent with the Chicken/Scot/59 virus.

There are several descriptions of changes associated with natural and experimental infections with the viruses isolated in North America and Italy (Figs. 20.10–20.15).

The histological lesions seen in the sinus in the experimental disease were similar to those described for duck sinusitis by Rinaldi et al. (1966a,b), e.g. cell degeneration, epithelial hyperplasia, infiltration of heterophils, and acute inflammation of the lamina propria. Rinaldi et al. (1966a,b) reported squamous metaplasia of the epithelium and fibrosis of lamina propria which were not prominent in the experimental infections of the poults with the Turkey/Ontario/6213/66 virus (Rouse et al., 1968). Sinusitis was not a conspicuous sign in the natural disease from which the "6213 virus" was isolated.

One of the most striking lesions observed in experimental infections with the Turkey/Ontario/6213/66 and Turkey/Ontario/7732/66 viruses was pancreatitis with extensive necrosis of acinar cells (Rouse et al., 1968; Narayan et al., 1969b) (Fig. 20.10).

Degenerative and necrotic changes have been observed in other organs including the liver (Fig. 20.11) (Lang et al., 1965; Naray-

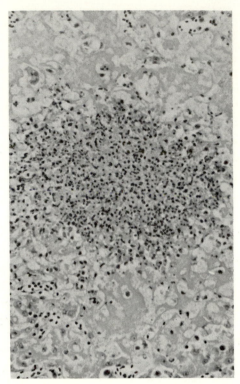

FIG. 20.11—*Hepatic focal necrosis following infection with Turkey/Ontario/7732/66 virus.* ×400. *(Courtesy G. Lang)*

an et al., 1969b), brain and meninges (Figs. 20.12, 20.13) (Narayan et al., 1969b), myocardium (Fig. 20.14) (Narayan et al., 1969b), and cutaneous tissues (Fig. 20.15) (Narayan et al., 1969b).

The lesions caused by at least 5 influenza viruses considered to be pathogenic share some similarities but have some distinctive features. For example, multiple focal necrosis was characteristic with infection with the Turkey/Ontario/7732/66 virus but not with the Turkey/Ontario/6213/66 virus. The pancreatic necrosis was the noteworthy lesion with the latter virus infection. Myocarditis, as described for the Tern/S. Africa/61 virus infection, was not observed in the Chicken/Scot/59 infection but was found with the Turkey/Ontario/7732/66 virus infection.

DIAGNOSIS

It has been suggested that some of the histologic changes described are sufficiently characteristic to permit a diagnosis of certain avian myxovirus infections (Jungherr et al., 1946; Uys and Becker, 1967). How-

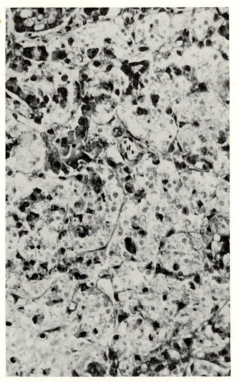

FIG. 20.10—*Pancreatic focal necrosis following infection with Turkey/Ontario/7732/66 virus.* ×400. *(Courtesy G. Lang)*

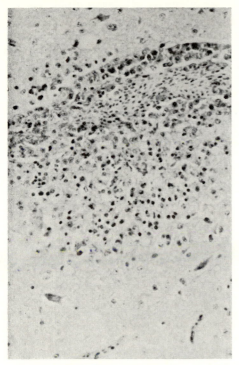

FIG. 20.12—Focal necrosis in forebrain following infection with Turkey/Ontario/7732/66 virus. ×250. (Courtesy G. Lang)

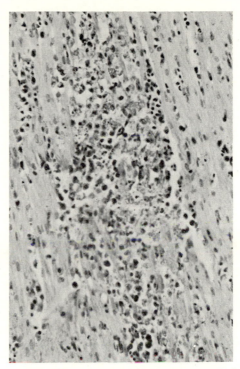

FIG. 20.14—Myocardial focal necrosis following infection with Turkey/Ontario/7732/66 virus. ×250. (Courtesy G. Lang)

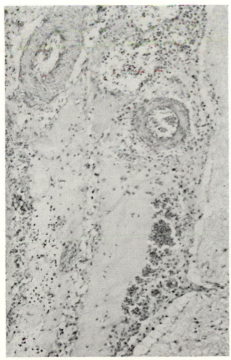

FIG. 20.13—Acute meningitis following infection with Turkey/Ontario/7732/66. ×160. (Courtesy G. Lang)

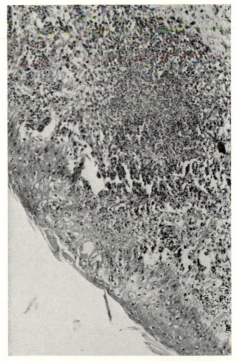

FIG. 20.15—Focal necrosis, congestion, and edema in comb following infection with Turkey/Ontario/7732/66 virus. ×250. (Courtesy G. Lang)

ever, because there is considerable variability in both the kind and degree of lesions associated with different infections, the combination of virologic and serologic procedures must be employed for a definitive diagnosis of avian influenza virus infection. Every possible precaution must be taken to avoid contamination of diagnostic materials, especially with laboratory strains of influenza and Newcastle disease. Materials collected for virus isolation and identification attempts should be divided into aliquots (one or more frozen at —60° C) to later permit confirmation of the identity of recovered agents.

ISOLATION AND IDENTIFICATION OF CAUSATIVE AGENT

Materials suitable for virus isolation include swabs from the respiratory tract, aspirated sinus exudate, or tissue (including blood) from dead birds or birds killed in extremis. Dry cotton swabs used for swabbing the nasal passages and/or trachea are placed in sterile broth containing antibiotics (penicillin, streptomycin, and mycostatin) and incubated at 37° C for 1 hour (to allow the antibiotics to act on contaminating bacterial and mycotic agents). The material may be kept at 4° C if inoculation of eggs is possible within 4–6 hours of collection; otherwise it should be frozen (—60° C). Tissues are ground with sufficient broth to make a 10% suspension and the particulate matter removed by low speed centrifugation. Filtration of the tissue or swab suspensions may be necessary if gross bacterial or mycotic contamination is a problem. Membrane filters with an average pore diameter of 0.22μ may be used for this purpose.

Methods for the isolation of influenza viruses are outlined and described adequately by several authors (Expert Committee, 1959; Jensen, 1961; Davenport and Minuse, 1964). Embryonated chicken eggs incubated 10–11 days are the most common medium for isolation. Usually each of 4–6 eggs is inoculated via the allantoic chamber with 0.1–0.2 ml of material. In some cases virus isolation is difficult unless the amniotic route of inoculation is employed. Allantoic and amniotic routes of inoculation may be used on the same egg to increase the probability of growth of virus. Inoculated eggs are incubated at 35° C for 48 hours. Some of the avian influenza viruses grow rapidly,

and the embryo may die in less than 48 hours. In other cases the virus may grow poorly and/or the embryo may not die even after a longer period. Eggs should be candled at least daily. Those containing dead embryos should be removed from the incubator as soon as they are detected and the allantoic and amniotic fluids collected and tested with chicken erythrocytes for the presence of hemagglutinin.

Embryos alive after 48 hours should be cooled at 4° C for 8–12 hours (to kill the embryo and clot the blood) and the allantoic and amniotic fluids collected for testing. If there is an insufficient cooling period there may be bleeding and the collected fluids will contain considerable amounts of erythrocytes. In such cases fluids should be kept at 37° C for 45–60 minutes to allow elution of virus from the erythrocytes before testing for hemagglutinin. The escape of erythrocytes into the allantoic fluid should be avoided, because some of the avian influenza viruses do not elute well from the erythrocytes (Homme and Easterday, 1970a).

Virus Identification

Standard methods for testing for the presence of hemagglutinin by macro- or microtechniques may be employed. Fluids from each egg should be tested individually. Those which contain hemagglutinin (virus) may be pooled and divided into aliquots. At least one aliquot should be kept for future reference and testing. A second passage in eggs is usually made before identification procedures are initiated. If hemagglutinin is not then detected, a sample of the collected fluid should again be inoculated into eggs. Most laboratories consider 3 passages a practical limit for detection of avian influenza virus (a sample may be considered negative if hemagglutinins are not detected after 3 passages). However, some influenza viruses may require more than 3 passages to allow sufficient virus growth to be detected by the hemagglutination test.

The first step in the identification of the hemagglutinin as belonging to an influenza virus is to confirm, with the type-specific complement fixation (CF) test, the presence of the type A specific antigen (Expert Committee, 1959). For this test any A influenza postinfection serum of mammalian origin and containing a known level of antibodies may be used. The gel diffusion technique described by Schild and Pereira (1969) and Beard (1970) may also be used to determine the presence and type of S antigen and/or anti-S antibody.

The hemagglutination-inhibition (HI) test may also be employed in an initial identification, but the diversity of antigenic reactivity of the avian influenza viruses should be kept in mind. If one has available only a limited number of test antigens or antisera, the HI test may lead to false negative results. Certain antigens and antisera with especially broad reactivity may be utilized for this test. The World Health Organization (WHO) has provided to reference laboratories a set of such antigens and antisera for preliminary identification of the avian influenza viruses. The materials in the set have especially broad reactivity and are adequate for the detection and a preliminary identification of most of these viruses. The antigens (and their antisera) included are fowl plague, Duck/Eng/56, Duck/Eng/62, Turkey/Wis/66, Quail/Italy/1117/65, Chicken/Scot/59, and Newcastle disease virus.

For laboratories not familiar with identification techniques and not having several influenza reference antigens and antisera on hand, final identification is best done by a laboratory such as the World Influenza Center or one of the WHO regional influenza virus laboratories. Identification of the hemagglutinating agent as a myxovirus may be done on the basis of physical and biochemical properties as described by Horstmann and Hsiung (1965).

SEROLOGY

Serological diagnosis with avian serum may be accomplished by HI, virus neutralization (VN), and gel diffusion tests. Serum should be collected from affected birds as soon as possible after the onset of the disease (acute phase serum). Second and third samples of serum (convalescent phase serum) should be collected on the 14th and 28th days after onset (Homme and Easterday, 1970b). One convalescent serum sample collected on the 21st day may be sufficient. However, in some animal influenza infections, antibody may not be detected until after 21 days. It is imperative that paired serum samples (i.e. acute and convalescent serum samples) be used for serological testing and the levels of antibody in

the two samples compared. Serum should be kept frozen ($-20°$ C) until tested. Details of the performance of the HI and VN tests are adequately described (Expert Committee, 1959; Jensen, 1961; Davenport and Minuse, 1964).

Inhibitors in the serum may interfere with the specificity of the HI test. The serum should therefore be treated before testing to reduce or destroy their activity. Heat and receptor-destroying enzyme (RDE) will remove most inhibitors (Expert Committee, 1959). The use of trypsin and sodium periodate is also recommended, but no one treatment is completely satisfactory. These treatments may also reduce the level of specific antibody. Some nonchicken sera (turkey, goose, etc.) contain nonviral substances which agglutinate the chicken erythrocytes used in the HI test. It is often necessary to remove such hemagglutinins by pretreatment of the serum with chicken erythrocytes (Nakamura and Easterday, 1967). The quantity of these hemagglutinins may be such as to mask low levels of specific antibody. It is generally considered that avian serum is unsatisfactory for use in the direct CF test.

Immunofluorescence techniques have been used for rapid diagnosis of influenza in human beings (Liu, 1961; Hers, 1962), but there have been no reports of the use of these techniques for the diagnosis of influenza virus infections in avian species. Becker (1967) employed immunofluorescence to demonstrate the sites of virus replication in experimentally infected terns.

DIFFERENTIAL DIAGNOSIS

Because of the broad spectrum of signs and lesions reported with infections of avian influenza viruses in several species, a definitive diagnosis must be made by virological and/or serological methods. Other infections which must be considered in the differential diagnosis include Newcastle disease virus, Yucaipa virus, reo viruses, chlamydial organisms, and mycoplasma. Concurrent infections with the avian influenza viruses and mycoplasmal agents have been described (Roberts, 1964).

TREATMENT

Presently there is no practical specific treatment for avian influenza virus infections. Rinaldi (1968, personal communication) has employed "amantadine" for treatment of infection in a large flock of quail (*Coturnix*) in Italy. The mortality rate in quails 17–20 days of age was reduced by approximately 50%, but the treatment did not appear to reduce the rate of infection. All other treatments which have been used have been of a supportive nature to relieve respiratory distress. Antibiotic treatment has been employed to reduce the effects of concurrent mycoplasma and/or bacterial infections.

PREVENTION AND CONTROL

There are no unique recommendations for the prevention and control of the avian influenza virus infections. There is a paucity of information on the epizootiology of these infections. As already indicated, the source of the virus for most of the outbreaks is unknown, and while there is circumstantial evidence to suggest vertical transmission of these viruses, infections in many cases appear to be self-limiting. Experimental evidence indicates that transmission requires relatively close contact.

Homme et al. (1970) observed overt signs of disease in experimental infections only when the turkeys were chilled, and they suggested that stressful environmental conditions should be avoided to prevent disease in infected birds. Since some turkeys and probably other species may carry these viruses for long periods of time, the introduction of recovered birds into susceptible flocks or the introduction of susceptible birds into recovered flocks should be avoided.

Eradication procedures have always been employed against outbreaks of fowl plague in the United States. Narayan et al. (1969b) suggested that "the terms plague or pest should be discarded because they do not connote a precise etiology." Although there are elaborate procedures available for the eradication of fowl plague in the United States, it should be kept in mind that other type A influenza virus infections may also cause or have the potential to cause high mortality rates among various avian species.

Stubbs (1965) reported that various kinds of vaccines have been employed against fowl plague, and Rinaldi (1968, personal communication) vaccinated quail hens with virus inactivated with β-propriolactone in an effort to provide maternal antibody to newly hatched birds. In the latter trial there was good correlation between levels of antibody in the serum of the hens and the yolk and serum of the newly hatched chicks. Critically controlled vaccination trials, however, have not been conducted with the avian influenza viruses. The diversity of subtypes and lack of antigenic relationships (see Fig. 20.4) will complicate the development of effective vaccines.

ECOLOGY OF *M. INFLUENZAE*: ROLE OF AVIAN SPECIES

The hypothesis that animals play an important role in the ecology of influenza viruses and may serve as a possible source of new subtypes which infect human beings is not new. Until recently there was a paucity of factual support for such a hypothesis. The demonstration of antibodies against A_2/Singapore/57 virus in animal serum (Kaplan and Payne, 1959) and of swine and equine influenza antibodies in the serum from aged persons (Schild and Stuart-Harris, 1965; Masurel and Mulder, 1966; Davenport et al., 1967; Tumova et al., 1968) has given indirect evidence of possible animal-human influenza relationships. There are no reports of the direct demonstration of natural infection of animals with influenza viruses of human origin or vice versa, which exclude the possibility of laboratory contamination. The only possible exception has been the report of the isolation of a fowl plaguelike virus from a human (De-Lay et al., 1967).

However, the interesting fact remains that the new variants appearing in recent years—A_2/Singapore/1/57 and A_2/Hong Kong/1/68—were detected first in the Far East. These viruses differed from preceding ones, and both have been shown to be related to avian and/or horse influenza viruses by the hemagglutinin and/or neuraminidase antigens (see Antigenic Relationship and Fig. 20.4).

The antigenic relationships between the human and avian viruses suggest the possibility that human A_2 subtype might have originated in an avian population (Pereira et al., 1967b; Tumova and Pereira, 1968; Webster and Pereira, 1968; Tumova and Easterday, 1969; Tumova et al., 1970). The fact that the neuraminidase of A_2 influenza virus is quite unrelated to the neuraminidase of A_1 strains provides strong support that A_2 virus could not have been derived from A_1 subtype (Paniker, 1968). Webster and Pereira (1968) compared 3 avian influenza viruses related to A_2/Singapore/57 and found that they all shared a common or similar neuraminidase. Furthermore, these avian viruses were similar to a virus produced in the laboratory by means of recombination between an avian and A_2 virus, which contained the hemagglutinin of the avian parent and neuraminidase of the A_2 parent. They speculated on the potentially large reservoir of avian influenza viruses in nature with which human strains could recombine to give rise to new pandemic strains. It must be pointed out that under natural conditions, recombination is likely to be only a chance occurrence. One could further speculate that this recombination could take place either in the avian or human host and the resulting virus might be infectious and cause an epidemic or epizootic either in the host in which the recombination occurred or in another host.

It is also possible that the cycles of animal and human influenza infections are independent of one another and that there is no need to speculate on the interspecies transfer of influenza viruses.

Any of these interpretations may ultimately be shown to be incorrect because of our present lack of knowledge about the natural history of many of these and other viruses and their hosts. Many questions remain to be explained concerning the ecology of influenza viruses including, but not limited to, the following: (1) What is the world distribution of avian and other animal influenzas and the species involved? (2) What is the role of wild birds in the dissemination of these viruses? (3) What is the significance of finding identical strains in two or more distant foci?

The distribution of the viruses and species involved have been described for relatively limited areas of the world. Wild birds have been incriminated for the intro-duction of viruses into Great Britain (Wells, 1963), but only one virus has been isolated from wild species (Becker, 1966). Antibodies have been demonstrated in the serum from wild birds in North America, but the significance of these antibodies remains unknown (Easterday et al., 1968). It remains to explain the significance of finding antigenically identical or similar viruses in two distant places, as for example Chicken/Scot/59 — Tern/SA/61 — Turkey/Ontario/6213/66; Duck/Eng/56 — Duck/Ukraine/1/60; Duck/Italy/574/65 — Turkey/Ontario/6828/67–Turkey/Massach/65.

Insufficient attention is being devoted to the study of avian influenza. The ever new isolations of avian strains suggest that these viruses are widely spread, probably still spreading and producing considerable economic loss among avian species. Furthermore, there is need and adequate justification to understand the role of avian species in the ecology of type A influenza viruses regardless of the host involved.

ADDENDUM

Several viruses have been isolated from various avian species since completion of this manuscript. Further antigenic analyses have been done employing especially the viral enzyme and its antibody. Schild and Newman (1969) have provided more evidence about various antigenic relationships among avian influenza viruses and viruses of human (A_2/Hong Kong) and swine (A/Sw/15) origin. Additionally, the Duck/Penn/486/69 virus (Florence S. Lief, 1969, personal communication), the only avian influenza virus from other than turkey origin in the United States, has been shown to have enzyme related to Chicken/Scot/59 and the Swine/15 viruses (Tumova and Easterday, unpublished data).

REFERENCES

Ada, G. L. 1957. Ribonucleic acid in influenza virus, pp. 104–15. In Wolstenhohme, G. E. W., and E. C. P. Millar (eds.), *Ciba Foundation Symposium: The Nature of Viruses*. J. A. Churchill Ltd., London.

Ada, G. L., and A. Gottschalk. 1956. The component sugars of the influenza virus particle. *Biochem. J.* 62:686–89.

Ada, G. L., and B. T. Perry. 1956. Influenza virus nucleic acid: Relationship between biological characteristics of the virus particle and properties of the nucleic acid.

J. Gen. Microbiol. 14:623–33.

Ada, G. L., Patricia E. Lind, and W. G. Laver. 1963. An immunological study of avian, viral and bacterial neuraminidase based on specific inhibition of enzyme by antibody. *J. Gen. Microbiol.* 32:225–33.

Almeida, June D., F. Himmelweit, and A. Isaacs. 1966. Studies on the intracellular haemagglutinin component of fowl plague virus and other myxoviruses. *J. Gen. Microbiol.* 45:153–58.

Andrewes, C. H., and H. G. Pereira. 1967.

Viruses of Vertebrates, 2nd ed. Bailliere, Tindall, and Cassell Ltd., London. Pp. 162–76.

Andrewes, C. H., and Griselda Worthington. 1959. Some new or little-known respiratory viruses. *Bull. World Health Organ.* 20: 435–43.

Andrewes, C. H., F. B. Bang, and G. M. Burnet. 1955. A short description of the myxovirus group. *Virology* 1:176–84.

Apostolov, K., and T. H. Flewett. 1965. Internal structure of influenza virus. *Virology* 26:506–8.

Bankowski, R. A. 1967. Two new myxoviruses complicating respiratory disease diagnosis. *Calif. Poultry Health Symp.,* Univ. Calif., Davis.

Bankowski, R. A., and R. D. Conrad. 1966. A new respiratory disease of turkeys caused by virus. *Proc. 13th World's Poultry Congr.,* pp. 371–79.

Bankowski, R. A., and T. Mikami. 1964. An apparently new respiratory disease of turkeys. *Proc. 68th Ann. Meet. U.S. Livestock Sanit. Ass.,* pp. 495–517.

Beard, C. W. 1970. Agar Gel-diffusion test for the detection of influenza virus anti-S antigen antibody in avian and mammalian serum. *Bull. World Health Organ.* 42:779–86.

Becker, W. B. 1963. The morphology of tern virus. *Virology* 20:318–27.

———. 1966. The isolation and classification of tern virus: Influenza virus A/Tern/South Africa/1961. *J. Hyg.* 64:309–20.

———. 1967. Experimental infection of common terns with tern virus: Influenza virus A/Tern/South Africa/1961. *J. Hyg.* 65:61–65.

Becker, W. B., and C. J. Uys. 1967. Experimental infection of chickens with influenza A/Tern/South Africa/1961 and Chicken/Scotland/1959 viruses. I. Clinical picture and virology. *J. Comp. Pathol. Therap.* 77:159–65.

Blaskovic, D., V. Rathova, and L. Borecky. 1959. Antigenic relationships to myxoviruses of a virus isolated from a respiratory infection in ducks. *Acta Virol.* 3:17–24.

Breitenfeld, P. M., and W. Schafer. 1957. The formation of fowl plague virus antigens in infected cells as studied with fluorescent antibodies. *Virology* 4:328–45.

Chaproniere, Donna M., and H. G. Pereira. 1955. Propagation of fowl plague and Newcastle disease viruses in culture of embryonic human lung. *Brit. J. Exp. Pathol.* 36:607–10.

Chu, C. M. 1951. The action of normal mouse serum on influenza virus. *J. Gen. Microbiol.* 5:739–57.

Cohen, A., and J. Dorman. 1965. Non-specific

inhibitors of A₂ influenza virus in human sera. *Acta Virol.* 9:519–25.

Davenport, F. M., and Elva Minuse. 1964. Influenza viruses, pp. 455–69. In Lennette, E. H., and N. J. Schmidt, *Diagnostic Procedures for Viral and Rickettsial Diseases,* 3rd ed. Am. Pub. Health Ass., New York.

Davenport, F. M., R. Rott, and W. Schafer. 1960. Physical and biological properties of influenza virus components obtained after ether treatment. *J. Exp. Med.* 112:765–82.

Davenport, F. M., A. V. Hennessy, and Elva Minuse. 1967. Further observation on the significance of Equine-2/63 antibodies in man. *J. Exp. Med.* 126:1049–61.

Dawson, I. M., and W. J. Elford. 1949. The investigation of influenza and related viruses in the electron microscope by a new technique. *J. Gen. Microbiol.* 3:298–311.

DeLay, P. D., Helen L. Casay, and Haskell S. Tobiash. 1967. Comparative study of fowl plague virus and a virus isolated from man. *Public Health Rept.* 82 7:615–20.

Dinter, Z. 1949. Eine Variante des Virus der Gefluegelpest in Bayern? *Tieraerztl. Umschau* 4:185–86.

Dinter, Z. 1964. Avian myxoviruses, pp. 299–311. In Hanson, R. P. (ed.), *Newcastle Disease Virus: An Evolving Pathogen.* Univ. Wisconsin Press, Madison.

Dinter, Z., and K. Bakos. 1950. Ueber die Beziehungen des Virus N zu dem Virus der klassischen Gefluegelpest. *Berlin. Muench. Tieraerztl. Wochschr.* 63:101–5.

Easterday, B. C., D. O. Trainer, Bela Tumova, and H. G. Pereira. 1968. Evidence of infection with influenza viruses in migratory water fowl. *Nature* 219:523–24.

Easterday, B. C., W. G. Laver, H. G. Pereira, and G. C. Schild. 1969. Antigenic composition of reactivant virus strains produced from human and avian influenza A viruses. *J. Gen. Virol.* 5:83–91.

Expert Committee on Respiratory Virus Diseases. 1959. *World Health Organ. Tech. Rept. Ser.* 170.

Fabiyi, A., Florence S. Lief, and W. Henle. 1958. Antigenic analysis of influenza viruses by compliment fixation. II. The production of antisera to strain specific V antigens in guinea pigs. *J. Immunol.* 81:467–77.

Fedova, Dagmar, and Bela Tumova. 1968. Propagation of type A myxovirus influenzae in diploid cell strain WI-38. II. The S and V antigens of fowl plague and A₂/Singapore/57 viruses as studied by immunofluorescence. *Acta Virol.* 12:331–39.

Fenner, F. 1968. Molecular and cellular biology. In *The Biology of Animal Viruses,* Vol. I. Academic Press, New York and London.

Fenner, F., and J. F. Sambrook. 1964. The genetics of animal viruses. *Ann. Rev. Microbiol.* 18:47–94.

Findlay, G. M., R. D. MacKenzie, and Ruby O. Stern. 1937. The histopathology of fowl pest. *J. Pathol. Bacteriol.* 45:589–96.

Francis, T., Jr. 1947. Dissociation of hemagglutinating and antibody measuring capacities of influenza virus. *J. Exp. Med.* 85:1–7.

Franklin, R. M., and P. M. Breitenfeld. 1959. The abortive infection in Earle's L cells by fowl plague virus. *Virology* 8:293–307.

Franklin, R. M., and E. Wecker. 1959. Inactivation of some animal viruses by hydroxylamine and the structure of ribonucleic acid. *Nature* 184:343–45.

Frano, J., and B. Kapitancik. 1959. Influenza virus A anatis isolated from ducks with a respiratory disease. II. Haemagglutinating properties. *Vet. Casopis* 8:244–54.

Frano, J., V. Bystrický, and J. Vrtiak. 1958. Influenza virus A anatis, isolated from ducks with a respiratory disease. I. Morphological study. *Vet. Casopis* 7:411–18.

Fraser, K. B. 1967a. Immunofluorescence of abortive and complete infections by influenza A virus in hamster BHK-21 cells and mouse L cells. *J. Gen. Virol.* 1:1–12.

———. 1967b. Defective and delayed myxovirus infections. *Brit. Med. Bull.* 23 2:178–84.

Gerlach, F., and J. Michalka. 1926. Ueber die in Jahre 1925 in Oesterreich beobachtete Gefluegelpest. *Deut. Tieraerztl. Wochschr.* 34:897–902. Cited by Jungherr et al., 1946.

Gottschalk, A. 1957. Neuraminidase: The specific enzyme of influenza virus and vibrio cholerae. *Biochem. Biophys. Acta* 23:645–46.

Harboe, A. 1963. The normal allantoic antigen which neutralizes the influenza virus HI-antibody to host material. *Acta Pathol. Microbiol. Scand.* 57:488–92.

Harboe, A., R. Schoyen, and A. Bye-Hansen. 1966. Haemagglutination-inhibition by antibody to host material of fowl plague virus grown in different tissue of chick chorioallantoic membrane. *Acta Pathol. Microbiol. Scand.* 67:573–78.

Hers, J. F. P. 1962. Fluorescent antibody technique in respiratory viral disease. *Am. Rev. Respirat. Diseases* 88:316–32.

Homme, P. J., and B. C. Easterday. 1970a. Avian influenza virus infections. I. Characteristics of influenza A/Turkey/Wisconsin/1966 virus. *Avian Diseases* 14:66–74.

———. 1970b. Avian influenza virus infections. III. Antibody response in turkeys to influenza A/Turkey/Wisconsin/1966 virus. *Avian Diseases* 14:277–84.

———. 1970c. Avian influenza virus infections. IV. Influenza A/Turkey/Wisconsin/1966

virus in pheasants, ducks, and geese. *Avian Diseases* 14:285–90.

Homme, P. J., B. C. Easterday, and D. P. Anderson. 1970. Avian influenza virus infections. II. Epizootiology of influenza A/Turkey/Wisconsin/1966 virus in turkeys. *Avian Diseases* 14:240–47.

Horstmann, Dorothy M., and G. D. Hsiung. 1965. Principles of diagnostic virology. In Horsfall, F. L., and I. Tamm (eds.), *Viral and Rickettsial Diseases of Man,* 4th ed. J. B. Lippincott Co., Philadelphia.

Jensen, K. E. 1961. Diagnosis of influenza by serologic methods. *Am. Rev. Respirat. Diseases* 83:120–24.

Jungherr, E. L., E. E. Tyzzer, C. A. Brandly, and H. E. Moses. 1946. The comparative pathology of fowl plague and Newcastle disease. *Am. J. Vet. Res.* 7:250–88.

Kaplin, M. M., and A. M. M. Payne. 1959. Serological survey in animals for type A influenza in relation to the 1957 pandemic. *Bull. World Health Organ.* 20:465–88.

Kates, M., A. C. Allison, D. A. J. Tyrrell, and A. T. James. 1961. Lipids of influenza virus and their relation to those of the host cell. *Biochem. Biophys. Acta.* 52:455–66.

Kilbourne, E. D. 1963. Influenza virus genetics. *Progr. Med. Virol.* 5:79–126.

Kilbourne, E. D., Florence S. Lief, J. L. Schulman, R. I. Jahiel, and W. G. Laver. 1967. Antigenic hybrids of influenza viruses and their implications. *Perspectives Virol.* 5:87–106.

Koppel, Z., J. Vrtiak, M. Vasil, and St. Spiesz. 1956. Mass illness of ducklings in Eastern Slovakia with a clinical picture of infectious sinusitis. *Veterinarstvi* 6:267–68.

Kornilova, A. L. 1960. Infectious catarrh of respiratory tract of ducks. (In Russian.) *Veterinariya* 3:40–41.

Lang, G., and C. G. Wills. 1966. Wilmot virus, a new influenza A virus infecting turkeys. *Arch. Ges. Virusforsch.* 19:81–90.

Lang, G., A. E. Ferguson, M. C. Connell, and C. G. Wills. 1965. Isolation of an unidentified hemagglutinating virus from the respiratory tract of turkeys. *Avian Diseases* 9:495–504.

Lang, G., B. T. Rouse, O. Narayan, A. E. Ferguson, and M. C. Connell. 1968a. A new influenza virus infection in turkeys. I. Isolation and characterization of virus 6213. *Can. Vet. J.* 9:22–29.

Lang, G., O. Narayan, B. T. Rouse, A. E. Ferguson, and M. C. Connell. 1968b. A new influenza A virus infection in turkeys. II. A highly pathogenic variant, A/Turkey/Ontario/7732/66. *Can. Vet. J.* 9:151–60.

Laver, W. G. 1963. The structure of influenza viruses. II. Disruption of the virus particle and separation of neuraminidase activity. *Virology* 20:251–62.

——. 1964. Structural studies on the protein subunits from three strains of influenza virus. *J. Mol. Biol.* 9:109–24.

Laver, W. G., and E. D. Kilbourne. 1966. Identification in a recombinant influenza virus of structural proteins derived from both parents. *Virology* 30:493–501.

Laver, W. G., and R. G. Webster. 1966. The structure of influenza viruses. IV. Chemical studies of the host antigen. *Virology* 30:104–15.

Liu, C. 1961. Diagnosis of influenzal infection by means of fluorescent antibody staining. *Am. Rev. Respirat. Diseases* 83:130–32.

Mandelli, G., A. Rinaldi, L. Nardelli, G. Cervio, D. Cessi, and A. Valeri. 1968. Osservazioni epidemiologiche su di un focolaio di influenza A della quaglia domestics *(Coturnix coturnix japonica). Proc. Soc. Ital. Sci. Vet. Grado,* 26–29 Settembre 1968.

Masurel, N., and J. Mulder. 1966. Studies on the content of antibodies for equine influenza viruses in human sera. *Bull. World Health Organ.* 34:885–93.

Mitchell, C. A., L. F. Guerin, and J. Robillard. 1967. Myxovirus influenza A isolated from ducklings. *Can. J. Comp. Med. Vet. Sci.* 31:103–5.

——. 1968. Decay of influenza A viruses of human and avian origin. *Can. J. Comp. Med. Vet. Sci.* 32:544–46.

Moses, H. E., C. A. Brandly, Elizabeth Jones, and E. L. Jungherr. 1948. The isolation and identification of fowl plague virus. *Am. J. Vet. Res.* 9:314–28.

Nakamura, R. M., and B. C. Easterday. 1967. Serological studies of influenza in animals. *Bull. World Health Organ.* 37:559–67.

Narayan, O., G. Lang, and B. T. Rouse. 1969a. A new influenza A virus infection in turkeys. IV. Experimental susceptibility of domestic birds to virus strain Turkey/Ontario/7732/1966. *Arch. Ges. Virusforsch.* 26:166–82.

——. 1969b. A new influenza A virus infection in turkeys. V. Pathology of the experimental disease by strain Turkey/Ontario/7732/1966. *Arch. Ges. Virusforsch.* 26:149–65.

Olesiuk, O. M., G. H. Snoeyenbos, and D. H. Roberts. 1967. An influenza A virus isolated from turkeys. *Avian Diseases* 11:203–8.

Paniker, C. K. J. 1968. Serological relationship between the neuraminidases of influenza viruses. *J. Gen. Virol.* 2:385–94.

Pereira, H. G. 1969. Influenza: Antigenic spectrum. *Progr. Med. Virol.* 11:46–79.

Pereira, H. G., Bela Tumova, and V. G. Law. 1965. Avian influenza A viruses. *Bull. World Health Organ.* 32:855–60.

Pereira, H. G., G. Lang, O. M. Olesiuk, G. H. Snoeyenbos, D. H. Roberts, and B. C. Easterday. 1966. New antigenic variants of avian influenza A viruses. *Bull. World Health Organ.* 35:799–802.

Pereira, H. G., A. Rinaldi, and L. Nardelli. 1967a. Antigenic variation among avian influenza A viruses. *Bull. World Health Organ.* 37:553–58.

Pereira, H. G., Bela Tumova, and R. G. Webster. 1967b. Antigenic relationship between influenza A viruses of human and avian origin. *Nature* 215:982–83.

Prochorov, A. V., and P. I. Feoktistov. 1960. Study of duck sinusitis. (In Russian.) *Sb. Ref. V.I.E.V.,* 1.

Prokofeva, M. T., and P. F. Tsimokh. 1966. Virus influenza of ducks, pp. 95–106. (In Russian.) In *Poultry Diseases.* Kolos Moscow.

Prokofeva, M. T., E. I. Gurova, and P. F. Tsimokh. 1963. Virus influenza of ducks. (In Russian.) *Veterinariya* 10:33–35.

Rinaldi, A., G. Cervio, and G. Mandelli. 1965. Observazioni ed isolamento del virus N (Dinter 1949) da un focolaio di sinusite infettiva nelle anatre. *Estratto Selezione Vet.* 6:430–34.

——. 1966a. Sinusite degli anatroccoli causata primitivamente da unagente filtrabile sierologicamente riferibile al virus N (Dinter 1949). *Bull. Inst. Sieroterapico Milanese* 45:255–72.

——. 1966b. Infezione respiratoria dei tacchinotti causatta da un agente filterabile strettamente affine al virus N (Dinter 1949). *Estratto Selezione Vet.* 7:336–39.

Rinaldi, A., L. Nardelli, H. G. Pereira, G. C. Mandelli, R. Gandolfi, and G. Cervio. 1967a. Focolaio di influenza A nel fagiano (Phasianus colchicus L). *Atti Soc. Ital. Sci Vet.* 21:867–72.

Rinaldi, A., L. Nardelli, H. G. Pereira, G. C. Mandelli, D. Cessi, and G. Cervio. 1967b. Focolai di influenza A nella quaglia domestics *(Coturnix coturnix japonica). Atti Soc. Ital. Sci. Vet.* 21:872–77.

Rinaldi, A., L. Nardelli, H. G. Pereira, G. C. Mandelli, G. Cervio, and R. Gandolfi. 1968a. Focolaio di influenza A nella coturnice orientale *(Alectoris chukar). Proc. Soc. Ital. Sci. Vet. Grado,* 26–29 Settembre 1968.

Rinaldi, A., L. Nardelli, H. G. Pereira, G. C. Mandelli, G. Cervio, and A. Valeri. 1968b. Isolamento di virus del tipo influenza A dal pollo. *Proc. Soc. Ital. Sci. Vet. Grado* 26–29 Settembre 1968.

Roberts, D. H. 1964. The isolation of an influenza A virus and a mycoplasma associated with duck sinusitis. *Vet. Record* 76:470–73.

Rott, R., and W. Schafer. 1960. Physikalish-chemische und biologische Eigenschaften des virus N und seine Beziehungen zur Influenza A Untergruppe der Myxoviren. *Zentr. Veterinaermed.* 7:237–48.

Rott, R., and C. Scholtissek. 1963. Investigation about the formation of incomplete forms of fowl plague virus. *J. Gen. Microbiol.* 33:303–12.

Rouse, B. T., G. Lang, and O. Narayan. 1968. A new influenza A virus infection in turkeys. *J. Comp. Pathol. Therap.* 78:525–33.

Rowan, M. K. 1962. Mass mortality among European common terns in South Africa in April–May 1961. *Brit. Birds* 55:103–14.

Sampaio, A. A. de C., and A. Isaacs. 1953. The action of trypsin on normal serum inhibitors of influenza virus agglutination. *Brit. J. Exp. Pathol.* 34:152–58.

Schafer, W. 1955. Vergleichende sero-immunologische Untersuchungen ueber die Viren der Influenza und klassischen Gefluegelpest. *Z. Naturforsch.* 106:81–91.

———. 1957. Units isolated after splitting fowl plague virus, pp. 91–103. In Wolstenholme, G. E. W., and E. C. P. Millar (eds.), *Ciba Foundation Symposium: The Nature of Viruses,* J. A. Churchill Ltd., London.

———. 1963. Structure of some animal viruses and significance of their components. *Bacteriol. Rev.* 27:1–17.

Schild, G. C., and H. G. Pereira. 1969. Characterization of the ribonucleoprotein and neuraminidase of influenza A viruses by immuno-diffusion. *J. Gen. Virol.* 4:355–64.

Schild, G. C., and R. W. Newman. 1969. Immunological relationships between the neuraminidases of human and animal influenza viruses. *Bull. World Health Organ.* 41:437–45.

Schild, G. C., and C. H. Stuart-Harris. 1965. Serological epidemiological studies with influenza A viruses. *J. Hyg.* 63:479–90.

Seifried, O. 1931. Gefluegelpest-Encephalitis. Pathologische Histologic. Lubarsch-Ostertag Ergebnisse der allgemeinen Pathologic und Pathologischen. *Anat. Menschen Tiere* 24:661–65.

Simpson, R. W., and G. K. Hirst. 1961. Genetic recombination among influenza viruses. I. Cross reactivation of plaque-forming capacity as a method for selecting recombinants from the progeny of crosses between influenza A strains. *Virology* 15:436–51.

Smithies, Lois K., D. B. Radloff, R. W. Friedell, G. W. Albright, V. E. Misner, and B. C. Easterday. 1969a. Two different type A influenza virus infections in turkeys in Wisconsin. I. 1965–66 outbreak. *Avian Diseases* 13:603–6.

Smithies, Lois K., F. G. Emerson, S. M. Robertson, and D. D. Ruedy. 1969b. Two different type A influenza virus infections in turkeys in Wisconsin. II. 1968 outbreak. *Avian Diseases* 13:606–10.

Stubbs, E. L. 1965. Fowl plague, pp. 813–22. In Biester, H. E., and L. H. Schwarte (eds.), *Diseases of Poultry,* 5th ed. Iowa State Univ. Press, Ames.

Tsimokh, P. F. 1961. Haemagglutination reaction in infectious sinusitis of ducks. *Veterinariya* 38:63–65.

Tumova, Bela, and B. C. Easterday. 1969. Relationship of envelope antigens of animal influenza viruses to human A₂ influenza strains isolated in the years 1957–1968. *Bull. World Health Organ.* 41:429–35.

Tumova, Bela, and Dagmar Fedova. 1968. Propagation of type A myxovirus influenzae in diploid cell strain WI-38. I. Adaptation experiments with strains of human and animal origin. *Virol. Prague* 12:324–30.

Tumova, Bela, and H. G. Pereira. 1965. Genetic interaction between influenza A viruses of human and animal origin. *Virology* 27:253–61.

———. 1968. Antigenic relationship between influenza A viruses of human and animal origin. *Bull. World Health Organ.* 38:415–20.

Tumova, Bela, Eva Svandova, and G. Stumpa. 1968. Findings of antibodies to animal influenza viruses in human sera and their significance for the study of interviral antigenic relationship. *J. Hyg. Epidemiol. Microbiol. Immunol. Prague* 12:284–95.

Tumova, Bela, Valentine Isachenko, and B. C. Easterday. 1970. Antigenic relationships of duck influenza strains isolated to avian, equine, and A₂/Hong Kong/1/68 viruses. To be published.

Uys, C. J., and W. B. Becker. 1967. Experimental infection of chickens with influenza A/Tern/South Africa/1961 and Chicken/Scotland/1959 viruses. II. Pathology. *J. Comp. Pathol. Therap.* 77:167–73.

Vogel, J., and A. Shelokov. 1957. Adsorption-hemagglutination test for influenza virus in monkey kidney tissue culture. *Science* 126:358–59.

Von Magnus, P. 1954. Incomplete forms of influenza virus. *Advan. Virus Res.* 2:59–78.

Walker, R. V. L., and G. L. Bannister. 1953. A filterable agent in ducks. *Can. J. Comp. Med. Vet. Sci.* 17:248–50.

Waterson, A. P. 1962. Two kinds of myxoviruses. *Nature* 193:1163–64.

Waterson, A. P., R. Rott, and W. Schafer. 1961. The structure of fowl plague virus and virus N. *Z. Naturforsch.* 16b:154–56.

Waterson, A. P., J. H. V. Hurrel, and K. W. Jensen. 1963. The fine structure of influenza A, B and C viruses. *Arch. Ges. Virusforsch.* 12:487–95.

Webster, R. G., and H. G. Pereira. 1968. A common surface antigen in influenza viruses from human and avian sources. *J. Gen. Virol.* 3:201–8.

Wells, R. J. H. 1963. An outbreak of fowl plague in turkeys. *Vet. Record* 75:783–86.

Zavada, J., and Marta Rosenbergova. 1968. Double neutralization of fowl plague virus reproduced in chick myeloblasts. *Acta Virol. Prague* 12:282–84.

Zillig, W., W. Schafer, and S. Ullmann. 1955. Ueber den Aufbau des Virus-elementarteilchens der klassischen Gefluegelpest. *Z. Naturforsch.* 10:199–206.

Zimmerman, W. T., and W. Schafer. 1960. Effect of p-fluorophenylalanine on fowl plague in turkeys. *Vet. Record* 75:783–86. 676–98.

CHAPTER 21

ARBOVIRUS INFECTIONS

❖

PHILIP H. COLEMAN

Department of Microbiology
Medical College of Virginia
Richmond, Virginia

AND

ROBERT E. KISSLING

Center for Disease Control
Health Services and Mental
Health Administration
U.S. Department of Health,
Education and Welfare
Atlanta, Georgia

❖

AN ARBOVIRUS has been defined as one "which in nature, can infect hematophagous arthropods by their ingestion of infected vertebrate blood. It multiplies in their tissues and is transmitted by bite to susceptible vertebrates" (World Health Organization, 1961).

Of 204 viruses currently catalogued as arboviruses, 21 involve avian species as natural and sometimes essential vertebrate hosts (Catalogue of Arthropod-Borne Viruses of the World, 1967). Although birds play an important role in the ecology of many arboviruses, in most instances the bird-virus relationship is probably a commensalistic one where the virus does not produce disease in the bird.

Only a few arboviruses are known to produce avian disease, particularly in domestic and game fowl. Of the 204 catalogued arboviruses, only 2—Eastern equine encephalitis and Western equine encephalitis— have been repeatedly reported as producing clinically evident, naturally occurring disease in economically important birds.

❖

EASTERN AND WESTERN EQUINE ENCEPHALITIS VIRUSES IN BIRDS

❖

THE WESTERN EQUINE ENCEPHALITIS (WEE) VIRUS was first isolated in 1930 from infected horses in California (Meyer et al., 1931). Isolation of Eastern equine encephalitis (EEE) virus followed two years later from infected horses in the eastern United States (Ten Broeck and Merrill, 1933; Giltner and Shahan, 1933). Today we know that these viruses occur endemically throughout the tropical and temperate zones of the Western Hemisphere.

A few years after the etiology of EEE was established, Fothergill and Dingle (1938) reported the isolation of this virus from a pigeon in Massachusetts during investigation of an epidemic in 1938 which involved both man and horses. Concurrently, ring-necked pheasants in Connecticut were found to be naturally infected with the eastern virus (Tyzzer et al., 1938). During the same year, Van Roekel and Clarke (1939) isolated the eastern virus from a ring-necked pheasant submitted to them by a game breeder in New Jersey. Other epornitics of EEE in pheasants have been recognized in the Atlantic coast states from New Jersey to Massachusetts (Beaudette et al., 1952; Luginbuhl et al., 1958; Dougherty and Price, 1960; Faddoul and Fellows, 1965; and Goldfield and Sussman, 1968). Other pheasant epornitics have been reported in Florida by Simpson (1959) and in Maryland and Delaware (Morbidity and Mortality Report, 1968).

In addition to pheasants, pen-raised chukar partridges have suffered severe epornitics of EEE in Maryland (Moulthrop and Gordy, 1960) and in Florida (Ranck et al., 1965). Clinical outbreaks have occurred in young White Pekin ducklings (Dougherty and Price, 1960) and in turkeys (Spalatin et al., 1961).

Although WEE virus does not produce naturally occurring clinically recognized disease in domestic poultry or game birds as frequently as EEE virus, several WEE outbreaks are on record. Severe losses in a turkey flock were attributed to WEE infection by Woodring (1957). Outbreaks have been reported in pheasants (Faddoul and Fellows, 1965) and in chukars (Ranck et al., 1965).

ETIOLOGY

Although EEE and WEE viruses are easily distinguishable by serodiagnostic methods, they share minor antigenic components and for this reason are classified together in the Group A arboviruses. The virus particles are spherical and 40–50 nm in diameter. Their chemical composition consists primarily of ribonucleic acid, proteins, and lipids. They are readily inactivated by a number of chemical agents such as ether, chlorine, and phenol and by heating at 60° C for 30 minutes. They are most stable in a menstruum containing serum or plasma albumin, a low salt concentration, and buffered to pH 7.6–9.0. They may be preserved in 50% glycerin buffered to pH 7.6 for short periods, wet-frozen at −70° C or in liquid nitrogen for several years, or in the lyophilized state at 4° C almost indefinitely.

Both viruses readily infect most laboratory animals when inoculated intracerebrally. Mice and guinea pigs are especially susceptible. They die of encephalitis within 2–5 days when inoculated with the eastern virus, and in 4–7 days when inoculated with the western virus. In mammals the eastern virus is more infective than the western virus by peripheral routes of inoculation. Newly isolated strains of WEE virus vary in their pathogenicity and may have to be host-adapted by serial passage in laboratory animals to increase virulence and produce deaths consistently.

Both viruses cause death of chicken embryos within 18–72 hours after inoculation by any route. Embryos dying of infection present a purplish hemorrhagic appearance. A number of cell cultures show cytopathic changes when infected with these viruses. Chicken and duck embryo fibroblast and hamster kidney cell cultures have been used in laboratory studies more than other cultures.

PATHOGENSIS AND EPIZOOTIOLOGY

Both EEE and WEE viruses infect a wide variety of hosts including many species of birds, mammals, reptiles, and arthropods.

TRANSMISSION

Both viruses are transmitted among wild birds principally by mosquito vectors, but only certain species of mosquitoes are capable of serving as effective transmitters. Virus is circulated in the blood of infected birds for 2–5 days, and during this time the mosquitoes have the opportunity to become infected by feeding on the birds. High concentrations of virus are more infectious for mosquitoes than low concentrations. Therefore, small passerine birds which tend to have higher concentrations of virus in their blood than larger birds are potentially the most important hosts for mosquito infection.

Under epidemic conditions, a swamp-breeding mosquito, *Culiseta melanura*, is the most important transmitter of EEE virus among the wild birds (Chamberlain, 1958). Although its biology is not known completely, it is thought to be preferentially a bird feeder. During epidemic periods, other mosquitoes which are susceptible, such as *Mansonia* spp. and *Aedes* spp., may become important transmitters of the virus (Chamberlain et al., 1954b). Various species of the mosquito genus *Culex* in the eastern United States are poor transmitters of the eastern virus, however. The fact that members of the *Culex pipiens* complex are generally the commonest mosquitoes found in poultry houses may explain the low incidence of antibody to EEE found in chickens. Pheasant farms, on the other hand, are frequently located on submarginal land adjacent to swamps, favored sites for the breeding of the primary bird vector *Culiseta melanura*. These facts can explain the occasional outbreaks noted in pheasant flocks.

There is ample evidence that direct transmission of EEE may occur among pheasants through feather picking and cannibalism. The virus is present in the blood, feather quills, and mouth secretions of infected pheasants. A beak covered with infected blood as a result of pecking can transmit the infection to other birds pecked upon. Pheasants may also be infected experimentally by oral administration of the virus (Holden, 1955; Satriano et al., 1958).

The chief vector of WEE virus in the western part of the United States is *Culex tarsalis*. In the eastern United States, however, this virus shares the same habitat as EEE virus and appears to be transmitted by the same vectors. There is little doubt that *C. melanura* is the main transmitter of WEE virus to wild birds in the east, just as it is of EEE virus.

Undoubtedly both EEE and WEE viruses can occasionally be transmitted mechanically by biting insects through the medium of contaminated mouth parts. A biting gnat or deerfly, for example, might take a partial feeding from a viremic animal and shortly thereafter complete its feeding upon a normal one. This type of transmission, however, is merely supplementary to the main mechanism, which is by the feeding of biologically infected mosquitoes. The virus infects first the gut tissue, then various tissues of the body, including the salivary glands of the mosquito. Generally 1–2 weeks are required for this cycle. Thereafter the mosquito can remain infected for life.

CLINICAL FEATURES

The clinical disease produced in birds by these viruses usually is evidenced by a central nervous system syndrome; the clinical signs and pathology vary only slightly for the different avian species.

Chickens

Although naturally occurring outbreaks have not been reported in chickens, newly hatched chickens are very susceptible to both EEE and WEE viruses. Day-old chickens succumb rapidly to infection without showing signs of central nervous system involvement; instead they exhibit a diarrhea (sometimes with a bloody discharge) and extreme prostration (Chamberlain et al., 1954a). Histologically, myocarditis is the outstanding lesion (Tyzzer and Sellards, 1941). Chickens more than 3 weeks of age, on the other hand, show no clinical signs of disease when infected by these viruses. The effect of infection upon egg production is not known, but it is probably negligible, since chickens of laying age generally respond with only a low-grade or nondetectable viremia, and antibody response may be variable.

Pheasants

Comprehensive clinical and histopathological studies of EEE virus infection in ring-necked pheasants have been reported by Jungherr et al. (1958) and Faddoul and Fellows (1965). In this species the outstanding signs of infection are referrable to central nervous system involvement and consist of leg paralysis, torticollis, and tremors. No prominent gross lesions are seen upon postmortem examination. Histopathologic lesions consist of vasculitis, microgliosis, focal meningitis, and neuronal degeneration.

The mortality among clinically ill pheasants is approximately 75%. Birds recovering from the acute phase of the disease may develop sequelae consisting of incoordination or muscular weakness. Pheasants may also experience clinically inapparent infections.

Chukars

Clinical signs of EEE virus infection in chukars have been described as similar to those in avian encephalomalacia—that is, ruffled feathers and somnolence followed by prostration and death (Moulthrop and Gordy, 1960). Gross pathological lesions are not prominent. Histopathological lesions are those normally associated with viral encephalitis: gliosis, satellitosis, and perivascular lymphocytic infiltration. Mortality varies from 30 to 85% (Ranck et al., 1965).

Turkeys

Clinical signs in turkeys include drowsiness, tremors, progressive weakness, and leg paralysis. Spalatin et al. (1961) indicated that EEE virus did not produce gross pathologic changes, but histopathologic examination revealed encephalitis and degenerative changes.

Ducks

In the one reported epornitic in ducks, Dougherty and Price (1960) reported that the most consistent sign of EEE infection was a bilateral, posterior paresis followed by paralysis. Characteristic gross pathological lesions were not seen, and the most consistent microscopic lesion was edema of the white matter of the spinal cord. Mortality ranged from 2 to 60%, and mortality was not observed in birds older than 18 days.

Wild Birds

Stamm (1963) reported that 52 species of wild birds were susceptible to EEE virus infection and 51 species were susceptible to WEE infection. However, native wild birds usually experience inapparent infections with these viruses (Kissling et al., 1954), although clinical disease and death may result in introduced species such as the English sparrow (Stamm and Kissling, 1956) and domestic pigeon (Fothergill and Dingle, 1938).

DIAGNOSIS

Since pathological examination reveals no pathognomonic lesions and clinical signs may be confused with other avian diseases, definitive diagnosis must be made by isolating and identifying the virus.

Although a variety of laboratory hosts are suited for isolation of EEE or WEE virus, chicken embryos, freshly hatched chickens, newborn mice, and chicken or duck embryo tissue culture systems are most widely used. Chicken embryos 9–14 days of age are satisfactory when inoculated into the amniotic cavity. Freshly hatched chickens should be no more than 1/2 day old, since an age resistance develops rapidly; the subcutaneous route of inoculation should be used. Newborn mice should be inoculated intracerebrally. Virus can usually be isolated from the brain of clinically ill birds, but in subclinically infected species the acute serum, liver, spleen, and heart may be more likely to contain virus in detectable quantities. Bacterial contaminants in the serum or tissue emulsions may be controlled by the addition of 1,000 units of sodium penicillin G and 2 mg of streptomycin sulfate per ml. When the inoculum contains virus, it will generally kill chicken embryos, newborn mice, or 1/2-day-old chickens within 18–72 hours. Avian tissue culture fluid systems will usually show cytopathic effects in 24–48 hours, and in agar overlay systems plaques can be readily observed in 36–48 hours.

Specific identification is made by serological methods, preferably by neutralization test, but the complement-fixation (CF) test can also be used. Applicable detailed procedures are given by Work (1964). The allantoic fluid from infected embryos, infected tissue culture fluid, or an alkaline suspension of brain material from infected mice serves adequately as antigen for either of these tests. In the CF test the antigen is tested against both EEE and WEE antisera known to contain complement-fixing antibodies. Appropriate controls to determine anticomplementary and nonspecific reactions are necessary. The CF reactivity of allantoic fluid is usually rather low, with expected titers generally in the range of 1:2–1:8; the CF reactivity of infected newborn mouse brain is usually much higher, however, with titers of 1:16–1:128.

For the neutralization test the virus dilution-constant serum method is used. Tenfold virus dilutions are mixed in equal parts with specific immune serum and incubated at 37° C for 2 hours before inoculation of the test hosts. Infected allantoic fluids or mouse brains usually contain 10^6–10^8 LD_{50} of virus per 0.1 ml. Chicken embryos, mice, or tissue cultures may be used as hosts in the neutralization test. Appropriate controls, using normal serum in place of the immune serum, are necessary.

Birds recovering from infection develop specific neutralizing and hemagglutinin-inhibiting antibodies against the virus.

PREVENTION AND CONTROL

Protection against mosquitoes will prevent the introduction of EEE virus into bird flocks. Fine mesh screening, particularly for young birds, is the best protection. In pheasant outbreaks, debeaking or other methods of preventing cannibalism and feather pulling will check the spread of virus in the flock.

Prophylactic immunization of pheasants, using products designed for equine inoculation but diluted 1:5, will lower the mortality rate should the virus be introduced (Sussman et al., 1958).

Where possible, rearing pens for game birds should be located away from the margins of freshwater swamps, since in areas such as these the virus is found endemically in wild birds and infection rates in mosquitoes tend to be especially high.

❖

ARBOVIRUSES OF UNKNOWN SIGNIFICANCE

❖

As INDICATED ABOVE, many arboviruses are capable of infecting birds, but very few produce clinical disease in domestic or peridomestic birds.

ST. LOUIS ENCEPHALITIS (SLE) VIRUS

St. Louis encephalitis virus is a Group B arbovirus found throughout tropical and temperate areas of the Western Hemisphere. This virus has been isolated from chickens and geese but has not been shown to produce disease in these hosts. Gainer et al. (1964) were able to isolate SLE virus

from the brain and blood of domestic pigeons during an outbreak of illness in a flock. However, they could not reproduce the disease in pigeons in laboratory trials.

ISRAEL TURKEY MENINGO-ENCEPHALITIS

Israel turkey meningo-encephalitis virus was isolated in Israel in 1959 from domestic turkeys clinically ill with a neurological syndrome. This virus is a Group B arbovirus and related antigenically to St. Louis encephalitis virus. Present information indicates that the virus is not widespread and has produced disease on only the one occasion (Komarov and Kalmar, 1959).

OTHERS

Arboviruses known to infect birds in the United States but which have not yet been incriminated in producing avian disease include Turlock, Hughes, Buttonwillow, Flanders, Hart Park, Venezuelan equine encephalitis, and Mermet.

REFERENCES

Beaudette, F. R., J. J. Black, C. B. Hudson, and J. A. Bivine. 1952. Equine encephalomyelitis in pheasants from 1947 to 1951. *J. Am. Vet. Med. Ass.* 121:478–83.

Catalogue of Arthropod-Borne Viruses of the World. 1967. Compiled by R. M. Taylor. U.S. Government Printing Office, Washington, D.C.

Chamberlain, R. W. 1958. Vector relationships of the arthropod-borne encephalitides in North America. *Ann. N.Y. Acad. Sci.* 70: 312–19.

Chamberlain, R. W., R. K. Sikes, and R. E. Kissling. 1954a. Use of chicks in Eastern and Western equine encephalitis studies. *J. Immunol.* 73:106–14.

Chamberlain, R. W., R. K. Sikes, D. B. Nelson, and W. D. Sudia. 1954b. Studies on the North American arthropod-borne encephalitides. VI. Quantitative determinations of virus vector relationships. *Am. J. Hyg.* 60: 278–85.

Dougherty, E., III, and J. I. Price. 1960. Eastern encephalitis in White Pekin ducklings on Long Island. *Avian Diseases* 4:247–58.

Faddoul, G. P., and G. W. Fellows. 1965. Clinical manifestations of Eastern equine encephalomyelitis in pheasants. *Avian Diseases* 9:530–35.

Fothergill, L. D., and J. H. Dingle. 1938. A fatal disease of pigeons caused by the virus of the Eastern variety of equine encephalomyelitis. *Science* 88:549–50.

Gainer, J. H., W. G. Winkler, A. L. Lewis,

W. L. Jennings, and P. H. Coleman. 1964. Isolations of St. Louis encephalitis virus from domestic pigeons, *Columba livia. Am. J. Trop. Med. Hyg.* 13:472–74.

Giltner, L. T., and M. S. Shahan. 1933. The 1933 outbreak of infectious equine encephalomyelitis in the eastern states. *North Am. Vet.* 14:25–27.

Goldfield, M., and O. Sussman. 1968. The 1959 outbreak of Eastern encephalitis in New Jersey. I. Introduction and description of the outbreak. *Am. J. Epidemiol.* 87:1–10.

Holden, P. 1955. Transmission of Eastern equine encephalomyelitis in ring-necked pheasants. *Proc. Soc. Exp. Biol. Med.* 88: 607–10.

Jungherr, E. L., C. F. Helmboldt, S. F. Satriano, and R. E. Luginbuhl. 1958. Investigation of Eastern equine encephalomyelitis. III. Pathology in pheasants and incidental observations in feral birds. *Am. J. Hyg.* 67:10–20.

Kissling, R. E., R. W. Chamberlain, R. K. Sikes, and M. E. Eidson. 1954. Studies on the North American arthropod-borne encephalitides. III. Eastern equine encephalitis in wild birds. *Am. J. Hyg.* 60:251–65.

Komarov, A., and E. Kalmar. 1959. A hitherto undescribed virus disease—turkey encephalitis. Proc. Israel Microbiol. Soc., Bull. Res. Council, Israel. *Exp. Med.* 8(E):64.

Luginbuhl, R. E., S. F. Satriano, C. F. Helmboldt, A. L. Lamson, and E. J. Jungherr.

1958. Investigation of Eastern equine encephalomyelitis. II. Outbreaks in Connecticut pheasants. *Am. J. Hyg.* 67:21–34.

Meyer, K. F., C. M. Haring, and Beatrice Howitt. 1931. The etiology of epizootic encephalomyelitis in horses in the San Joaquin Valley, 1930. *Science* 74:227–28.

Morbidity and Mortality Weekly Report 17: 371. 1968. U.S. Dept. Health, Education and Welfare, Public Health Serv., National Communicable Disease Center, Atlanta.

Moulthrop, I. M., and Betty Anne Gordy. 1960. Eastern viral encephalomyelitis in chukar *(Alectoris graeca). Avian Diseases* 4:380–83.

Ranck, F. M., Jr., J. H. Gainer, J. E. Hanley, and S. L. Nelson. 1965. Natural outbreak of Eastern and Western encephalitis in pen-raised chukars in Florida. *Avian Diseases* 9:8–20.

Satriano, S. F., R. E. Luginbuhl, R. C. Wallis, E. L. Jungherr, and L. A. Williamson. 1958. Investigation of Eastern equine encephalomyelitis. IV. Susceptibility and transmission studies with virus of pheasant origin. *Am. J. Hyg.* 67:21–34.

Simpson, C. F. 1959. Case report—Equine encephalomyelitis in pheasants in Florida. *Avian Diseases* 3:89–91.

Spalatin, J., L. Karstad, J. R. Anderson, L. Lauerman, and R. P. Hanson. 1961. Natural and experimental infections in Wisconsin turkeys with the virus of Eastern encephalitis. *Zoonoses Res.* 1:29–48.

Stamm, D. D. 1963. Susceptibility of bird populations to Eastern, Western, and St. Louis encephalitis viruses. *Proc. 13th Int. Ornith. Congr.,* pp. 591–603.

Stamm, D. D., and R. E. Kissling. 1956. Influence of season on EEE infection in English sparrows. *Proc. Soc. Exp. Biol. Med.* 92:374–76.

Sussman, O., D. Cohen, J. Gerende, and R. E. Kissling. 1958. Equine encephalitis vaccine studies in pheasants under epizootic and pre-epizootic conditions. *Ann. N.Y. Acad. Sci.* 70:328–41.

Ten Broeck, C., and M. H. Merrill. 1933. A serological difference between Eastern and Western equine encephalomyelitis virus. *Proc. Soc. Exp. Biol. Med.* 31:217–20.

Tyzzer, E. E., and A. W. Sellards. 1941. The pathology of equine encephalomyelitis in young chickens. *Am. J. Hyg.* 33(B):69–81.

Tyzzer, E. E., A. W. Sellards, and B. L. Bennett. 1938. The occurrence in nature of "equine encephalomyelitis" in the ring-necked pheasant. *Science* 88:505–6.

Van Roekel, H., and M. K. Clarke. 1939. Equine encephalomyelitis virus (Eastern type) isolated from ring-necked pheasants. *J. Am. Vet. Med. Ass.* 94:466–68.

Woodring, F. R. 1957. Naturally occurring infection with equine encephalomyelitis virus in turkeys. *J. Am. Vet. Med. Ass.* 130: 511–12.

Work, T. H. 1964. Isolation and identification of arthropod-borne viruses. In *Diagnostic Procedures for Viral and Rickettsial Diseases,* 3rd ed. Am. Public Health Ass., Inc., New York, N.Y., pp. 312–55.

World Health Organization. 1961. Arthropod-borne viruses—Report of a study group. *WHO Tech. Rept. Ser.* 219, pp. 1–68.

CHAPTER 22

AVIAN POX

❖

CHARLES H. CUNNINGHAM

*Department of Microbiology and
Public Health
Michigan State University
East Lansing, Michigan*

❖

Pox of birds is a viral disease characterized by a pronounced transitory inflammatory process, hyperplasia of the epidermis and feather follicles with intracytoplasmic inclusions, and terminating with the formation of scabs and desquamation of the degenerated epithelium. In some cases diphtheritic membranes may develop in the mouth and esophagus.

Synonyms are bird pox, *Geflügelpocken* (German), *variole aviaire* (French), *viruela aviar* (Spanish), *bouba* (Portuguese).

Flock mortality is usually low in natural infections. It may be high if a virulent virus is present or if the disease is complicated by parasitism, other infections, or poor condition of the flock. The greatest economic losses are usually from retardation of development of the affected bird and impaired egg production.

Pox of birds is not of public health significance as mammals are not affected.

HISTORY

Pox has long been observed in avian species. There was early concern that the disease of birds was related to the pox disease and diphtheria of man until investigations proved otherwise. The term "fowl pox" first included all pox diseases of birds, but it now designates the disease of chickens and the type species of the avian poxviruses. It is unfortunate that the term "chicken pox" was not originally used to designate the disease of chickens instead of a term to describe a disease of man which is now known not to be caused by a poxvirus.

Bollinger (1873) differentiated between the histologic lesions and inclusions of fowl pox and variola, and Borrel (1904) discovered minute coccoid components or elementary bodies within the inclusion. Inclusions have since been known as Bollinger bodies and the elementary bodies as Borrel bodies.

Bollinger considered the inclusions to be protozoan parasites, and some investigators incriminated various bacteria and fungi as the etiologic agents. Filterability of the now known virus was first demonstrated by Marx and Sticker (1902). Carnwarth (1908) determined that the virus was responsible for the cutaneous and diphtheritic forms of the disease. Woodruff and Goodpasture (1929, 1930, 1931) presented conclusive evidence for the first time that the virus was not only intimately associated with the inclusion but was resident within it as the elementary body or etiologic viral agent of fowl pox.

INCIDENCE AND DISTRIBUTION

Pox is prevalent worldwide, and birds of all ages, sexes, and breeds are susceptible to the virus.

ETIOLOGY

CLASSIFICATION

The avian poxviruses—fowl, turkey, pigeon, and canary—are one of the subgroups of the poxviruses which are the largest and most complex of the viruses of vertebrates (Joklik, 1966; Andrewes and Pereira, 1967; Fenner, 1968; Woodson, 1968; Wilner, 1969).

MORPHOLOGY

Fowl poxvirus, the type species and best-studied of the avian poxviruses, serves as the descriptive model for the subgroup.

In infected dermal epithelium of the chicken and the ectodermal chorioallantoic membrane (CAM) of the chicken embryo, the virus, in various stages of maturation, is contained in a cytoplasmic inclusion body which is an oval to round structure varying from 5 to 30μ in its greatest diameter (Randall, Gafford, and Arhelger, 1961), surrounded by a membrane, and composed of a matrix of finely granular material (Arhelger et al., 1962; Arhelger and Ran-

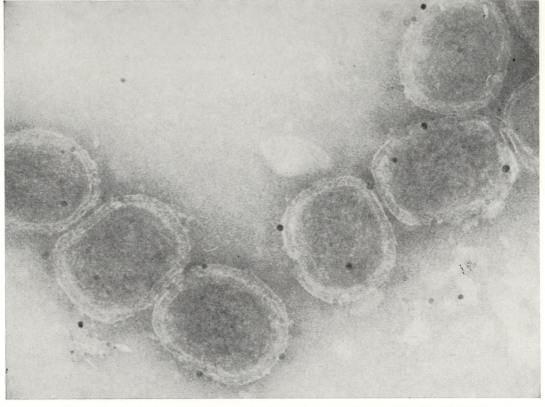

FIG. 22.1—*Purified preparation of fowl poxvirus negatively stained with PTA, pH 7.0. ×84,000. (Hyde et al., 1965)*

dall, 1964; Randall et al., 1964; Cheville, 1966; Tajima and Ushijima, 1966).

Fowl poxvirus is brick-shaped or rectangular and its structure is demonstrable by a variety of electron microscope techniques. Shadowed preparations of the virus have average dimensions of 258×354 mμ (Randall et al., 1964) and mean dimensions of $3,220 \pm 902$ Å length and $2,640 \pm 739$ Å width, axial ratio of 1.22 (Fenner, 1968).

Virus negatively stained with phosphotungstic acid (PTA) has average dimensions of 265×334 mμ (Randall et al., 1964). When stained with neutral PTA, the virus has a conspicuous capsularlike material without evidence of external surface structures (Fig. 22.1), but pseudoreplicas have an arrangement of rodlets or tubules on the surface (Fig. 22.2) (Hyde et al., 1965).

When combined uranyl acetate and platinum shadowing is used, irregularly spaced and arranged surface knobs varying from 300 to 400 Å are evident. Treatment of the

virus with trypsin appears to unwind the outer layer of the membrane of the virus resulting in twisted ropelike structures. The knobby surface is not present after this treatment. The inner layer of the membrane is about 200–300 Å thick (Hyde et al., 1965).

Sodium laurel sulfate (SLS) removes an outer lipoprotein coat of the virus and releases the deoxyribonucleic acid (DNA) without completely destroying the virus. Virus treated with SLS and DNase and stained with PTA has subunits approximately 40 Å on an inner layer (Hyde et al., 1965).

A typical poxvirus on thin section is composed of an outer membrane enclosing the lateral bodies and the biconcave genome-containing core or nucleoid which have also been identified in the avian poxviruses (Fig. 22.3C) (Arhelger and Randall, 1964; Cheville, 1966; Tajima and Ushijima, 1966).

The average dimensions of thinly sec-

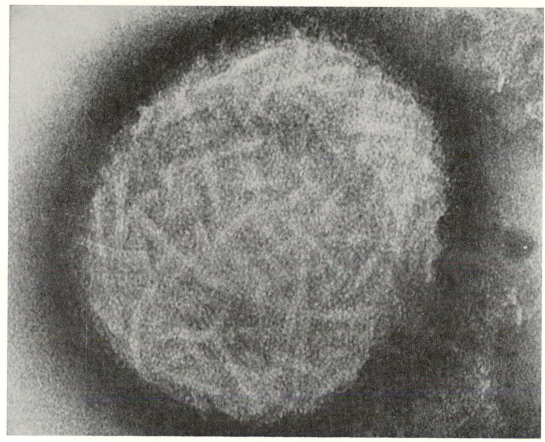

FIG. 22.2–*Pseudoreplicas of impure preparation of fowl poxvirus negatively stained with PTA, pH 7.0. Surface covered with rodlets or hollow tubules. ×200,000. (Hyde et al., 1965)*

tioned fowl, canary, and pigeon poxviruses grown in host cells of different types are similar although there are individual variations. In the dermal epithelium of the chicken, fowl poxvirus is $164 \times 252 \times 284$ mμ (Tajima and Ushijima, 1966).

CHEMICAL COMPOSITION

Inclusion bodies containing virus can be isolated free of cellular debris by digesting the infected cells with 1% trypsin in phosphate buffered saline solution (PBS), pH 7.6, followed by differential centrifugation and washing with PBS. The average weight of an inclusion body is 6.1×10^{-7} mg, of which approximately 50% is extractable lipid. The average weight of protein per inclusion is 7.69×10^{-8} mg and of DNA 6.64×10^{-9} mg (Randall et al., 1962).

Rupture of the inclusion by sonic treatment releases the virus and matrix which may be separated by differential centrifugation for physical and chemical analyses. Virus may be purified by chromatography on methylated albumin-kieselguhr columns (Randall et al., 1966). The fowl poxvirus genome is a double-stranded DNA molecule (Gafford and Randall, 1967) extractable by detergent or phenol, but higher yields are obtained by SLS, chloroform-butanol methods. The extracted DNA is infectious for cells of the CAM of the chicken embryo but not for the chicken skin (Randall et al., 1966).

The particle weight of the virus is 2.04×10^{-14} g, but this may be high because of bound water. About 47% of the weight of the virus and 83% of the matrix are extractable by chloroform-methanol. On the average, the virus contains 7.51×10^{-15} g of protein, 4.03×10^{-16} g of DNA, and 5.54×10^{-15} g of lipid. The lipid compositions of virus and matrix are very similar: total cholesterol—virus 22.0%, matrix 20.5%; glycerol—virus and matrix each 3.9%; and free fatty acid—virus 31.5%; matrix 25.5%. The phospholipid content of the matrix is 8.4%, about 2.2 times that of virus, 3.8%. Ribonucleic acid and carbohydrate are not present (Randall et al., 1964).

The four main constitutive bases—adenine (A), thymine (T), guanine (G), and cytosine (C)—are paired. The base ratio of AC to GC is 1.8. The GC content of the DNA is approximately 35%. The molar ratio of purines to pyrimidines is approximately unity (Randall et al., 1962). Approximately 15% of the DNA molecules have the unusual property of renaturation, suggesting that this may be due to cross-linking. The melting point of the DNA in 7.2 M $NaClO_4$ is 39.1° C indicating 34.6% GC, and the density in CsCl is 1.6945 indicating 35% GC (Szybalski et al., 1963).

The molecular weight of the viral DNA, 200–240×10^6 daltons, by physicochemical methods represents the largest viral DNA molecule yet isolated and is a reasonable approximation of the viral genome (Gafford and Randall, 1967). The average contour length of a single molecule is about 100μ and represents essentially the total DNA of a single virion. This is equivalent to a possible minimum of 192×10^6 daltons (Hyde et al., 1967).

REPLICATION

Although basic information concerning the avian poxviruses is not as extensive or complete as that for the poxviruses in general and vaccinia virus in particular, there is a considerable fund of knowledge of the biosynthesis and morphogenesis of fowl poxvirus.

Replication of the avian poxviruses and the inclusion body appears to be similar in dermal or follicular epithelium of the chicken and the ectodermal cells of the CAM of chicken embryos.

After adsorption to and penetration of the cell membrane by fowl poxvirus, 1 hour after infection of dermal epithelium (Arhelger et al., 1962) and 2 hours after infection of the CAM (Arhelger and Randall, 1964), there is a dissolution or uncoating of the virus prior to synthesis of new virus from precursor material.

Biosynthesis of fowl poxvirus in dermal epithelium involves two almost distinct phases: host response during the first 72 hours and synthesis of infectious virus from 72 to 96 hours (Cheevers and Randall, 1968; Cheevers et al., 1968).

Beginning at 36–48 hours, synthesis of host DNA is accompanied by hyperplasia of the epithelium. The host DNA declines sharply from 60 to 72 hours, but the hyperplasia ends at 72 hours with a 2.5-fold increase in the number of cells.

Replication of viral DNA begins between 12 and 24 hours, but only 0.1% of the maximum is attained during the first 60 hours. Between 60 and 72 hours there is an exponential rate of synthesis of viral DNA. From 72 to 96 hours the ratio of viral DNA to host DNA progressively increases to a maximum of greater than 2:1, and the maximum titer of virus is attained after cell proliferation has ceased.

During morphogenesis of the virus, incomplete forms and intermediate or developmental forms in transitional stages leading to mature forms or virions have been described (Arhelger et al., 1962; Arhelger and Randall, 1964; Cheville, 1966; Tajima and Ushijima, 1966).

The latent period is relatively long. At about 48 hours, areas of viroplasm with incomplete membranes around them are present in the cytoplasm (Arhelger and Randall, 1964; Cheville, 1966). The membranes close to form particles which consist of a dense viroplasm surrounded by a double membrane and containing a nucleoid. Viroplasmic particles condense and acquire an additional outer membrane to become incomplete virions. The incomplete virions migrate to lipid-containing vacuoles or inclusion body vacuoles which are derived from lipid granules of the cytoplasm, contain a matrix and rodlike structures, and are surrounded by a lipid membrane. Inclusion bodies are present at 72 hours after infection of dermal epithelium of the chicken (Arhelger et al., 1962) and at 96 hours after infection of the CAM (Arhelger and Randall, 1964). The incomplete virion then penetrates the inclusion body vacuole and thereby acquires a membrane coat (Cheville, 1966). The probable function of the inclusion body is to provide and localize precursor material for the lipid coat of the virion.

The mechanism of release of virions from the inclusion body is unknown. Separation of the virion from the dermal epithelium of the chicken is probably the result of necrosis and desquamation of the cell (Arhelger et al., 1962).

Fowl poxvirus emerges from the cells of the CAM by a budding process resulting in the acquisition of an additional outer membrane obtained from the cell membrane (Fig. 22.3) (Arhelger and Randall, 1964). The fowl pox virion is considered to be composed of a core, core membrane, 2 inner membranes, an intermediate membrane, an outer membrane, and a dense outer coat (Cheville, 1966).

There is some evidence that the classical inclusion body (Bollinger body) observable by light microscopy is not always a structure indispensable for the development and maturation of avian poxviruses. Matrix inclusion bodies consisting of aggregates of finely granular and fibrillar material have also been described. They are about 3μ long and are best examined by electron microscopy (Tajima and Ushijima, 1966).

The significance and relationship of matrix inclusion bodies to the classical inclusion and synthesis of infectious virus have not been resolved. Infectious virus may be produced by cells in which matrix inclusion bodies only are present. Classical and matrix inclusion bodies develop in the dermal epithelium of chickens infected with fowl and canary poxviruses and in the CAM infected with fowl, canary, and pigeon poxviruses. Classical inclusion bodies do not develop in chicken embryo cell cultures infected with canary poxvirus, but matrix inclusion bodies do develop (Tajima and Ushijima, 1966). Classical inclusion bodies are not produced by fowl poxvirus in epithelial or fibroblast cells derived from chicken embryos and examined by light microscopy (Bang et al., 1951).

An avian poxvirus isolated from *Junco hyemalis* produces nuclear as well as cytoplasmic inclusion bodies concomitantly in the same cell of dermal epithelium of the chicken and of the CAM. Junco pox in many respects resembles fowl pox. The cytoplasmic inclusion bodies are similar to the classical inclusion bodies of fowl poxvirus, but the nuclear inclusion body is devoid of viral particles (Beaver and Cheatham, 1963). Mature virus has been observed in nuclei of the CAM infected with fowl poxvirus, but its significance in the infective process is unknown (Arhelger and Randall, 1964).

RESISTANCE TO CHEMICAL AND PHYSICAL AGENTS

With few exceptions, experiments on the effect of environmental influences on avian poxviruses have been conducted with preparations containing extraneous cellular and tissue material, and the results are only relative.

One of the characteristics of the avian poxviruses is their resistance when desiccated. Generally, chemical agents such as ethyl alcohol, sodium hydroxide, and liquor cresolis saponatus in concentrations

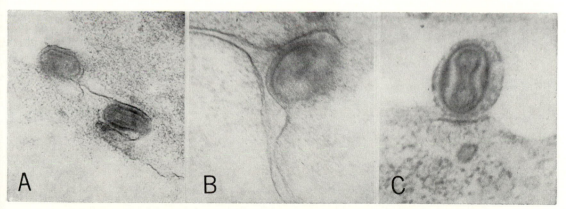

FIG. 22.3—Emergence of fowl poxvirus from cells of CAM. (A) and (B) Particles appear to be budding from surface, and cell membrane appears to be surrounding virus. (C) Virus is separated from cell and completely enclosed by an outer layer obtained from cell membrane. (A) ×43,000; (B) and (C) ×62,000. (Arhelger and Randall, 1964)

commonly used for disinfection inactivate fowl poxvirus in about 10 minutes.

Deoxyribonucleic acid extracted from fowl poxvirus by phenol at 25° C and 50° C, by SLS, and by modifications of these methods is infectious for the CAM of chicken embryos but not for chicken skin. Whole virus infects both the CAM and the chicken skin with equal efficacy. Extracted DNA is stabile at 100° C for 10 minutes, but whole virus is inactivated. Strands of DNA are destroyed when treated with DNase for 10–15 minutes at room temperature or 37° C, but whole virus is not affected. Chloroform-butanol inactivates the virus but not the DNA. Trypsin is without effect on the DNA or the whole virus (Randall et al., 1966).

There are conflicting reports as to the sensitivity of fowl poxvirus to ether and to chloroform. Some authors (Andrewes and Pereira, 1967) state that the virus is resistant to ether but sensitive to chloroform; others (Randall et al., 1964) state that the virus is sensitive to both ether and chloroform. One author (Fenner, 1968) considers the sensitivity to ether to be negligible.

STRAIN CLASSIFICATION

Members of the avian poxvirus subgroup are antigenically and immunologically distinguishable from each other to a degree, but varying cross-relationships do exist. There is the unresolved question whether members of the subgroup should be regarded as naturally or artificially host-modified variants of fowl poxvirus.

Complement-fixation, hemagglutination-inhibition, neutralization, and fluorescent antibody tests distinguish fowl poxvirus from other subgroups of the poxvirus group. Alkaline digests of vaccinia and myxoma virus, however, contain a nucleoprotein precipitinogen which is common to all viruses, including fowl poxvirus, of the poxvirus group (Woodroofe and Fenner, 1962).

Present knowledge does not allow further differentiation of the individual members of the avian poxviruses into separate strains.

An experimentally induced mutant of fowl poxvirus resulting from intracerebral passage of the virus in chicks has been described (Goodpasture, 1959). The mutant is capable of infecting immature epithelium of renal tubules following intravenous or direct intrarenal inoculation. An adenomatous hyperplasia results from the latter route. Basophilic cytoplasmic inclusion bodies resembling those of vaccinia virus and acidophilic inclusion bodies typical of fowl poxvirus are present in the same cell. The mutant produces soft, pliable gross lesions on the CAM differing from the firm, opaque hyperplastic lesions typical of fowl poxvirus infection. It has been proposed that the original fowl poxvirus has undergone a number of mutations which determined the cytotropism.

LABORATORY HOST SYSTEMS

Birds, avian embryos, and cell cultures derived from avian embryos are employed for study of the avian poxviruses.

Birds

The avian poxviruses affect a wide range of birds of various families by natural or artificial infection. They form a subgroup of viruses of varying degrees of cross-relationship which may be the result of host modification. Differentiation of the viruses is based on their pathogenicity for the host

TABLE 22.1 ❧ Host Spectrum of Canary, Turkey, Fowl, and Pigeon Poxviruses

Virus	Day-Old Chicks cut.	iv	Chickens cut.	iv	Turkeys cut.	iv	Pigeons cut.	iv	Ducks cut.	iv	Canaries cut.	iv
Canary	±	0	+	0	+	0	+G	+G	+	0	+D	+D
Turkey	+G	+G	+	+G	+	+G	+G	+G	+	+G	0	0
Fowl	+G	+G	+G	+G	+G	+G	+	+	0	0	0	0
Pigeon	+	0	+	0	+	0	+G	+G	0	0	0	0

Source: Modified from Mayr (1963) and Gelenczei and Lasher (1968).
Abbreviations: cut. = cutaneous; iv = intravenous; + = local pox lesions; +G = local pox lesions and generalized infection; +D = local pox lesions and death; 0 = no signs.

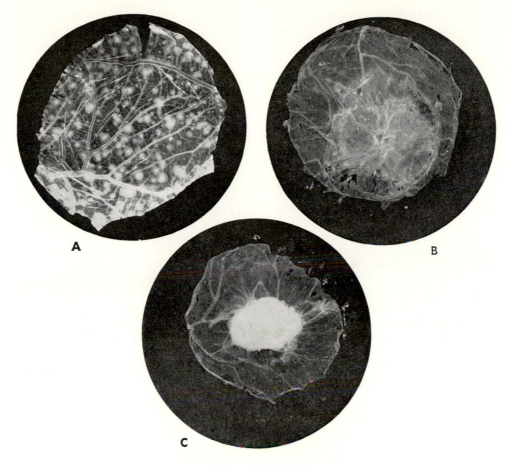

FIG. 22.4—*Fowl and pigeon pox lesions on CAM. (A) Metastatic fowl pox lesions. (B) Diffuse fowl pox lesions. (C) Focal pigeon pox lesions. (Brandly, Univ. of Ill.)*

spectrum (Table 22.1). Inoculation by the scarified skin, feather follicle, and intravenous routes is used. Interpretation of infection is based on the formation of a typical pox lesion, generalized infection, or death.

Avian Embryos

Chicken embryos 10–12 days old are commonly employed for propagation of avian poxviruses on the CAM by the artificial air cell route (Woodruff and Goodpasture, 1931; Cunningham, 1966). Duck and turkey embryos have been used as well as other species of avian embryos.

Typical infection of the CAM of the chicken embryo is a compact, proliferative pock lesion which may be focal or diffuse (Fig. 22.4). For the best macroscopic examination of the lesions, the inoculum should be dilute enough so that individual lesions are produced rather than an overwhelming infection of the entire membrane. Macroscopic lesions considered to be characteristic of those produced by the respective viruses are described below (Mayr, 1963).

The lesion produced by fowl poxvirus on the 6th day is compact and gray, about 5 mm thick with a central necrotic area. Secondary lesions are small and flat with a ring zone.

Pigeon poxvirus is less virulent than fowl poxvirus, and the lesions are not as pronounced or generalized. On the 8th day the lesion is 5–6 mm thick without necrosis, and there is considerable variation in the ring zone. Secondary lesions appear at about 8–10 days.

Canary poxvirus lesions on the 8th day

are similar to those of pigeon poxvirus but are smaller with primary and secondary lesions.

Turkey poxvirus behaves similarly to fowl poxvirus but is less virulent for the embryo. The main difference from fowl poxvirus is that on the 6th day the ring zones are more turbid; there is edema of the membrane and a greater inclination to proliferation and necrosis. Incubation is shorter than that of pigeon poxvirus.

Titration of virus is performed by inoculating the CAM of each of 5 chicken embryos per serial 10-fold dilution of virus with at least 0.1 ml via the artificial air cell. Embryos dead during the 1st day postinoculation are not included in the final results.

After 5–7 days incubation all embryos are examined for lesions on the CAM (Fig. 22.4). The results are expressed as the embryo infective dose$_{50}$ (EID$_{50}$) per ml based on the quantal dose-response (Cunningham, 1966). A single pock lesion on the CAM is considered to be a positive response for that embryo.

The enumerative dose-response, or "pock-counting" method (Cunningham, 1966), based on the number of pocks per CAM may be used, but the difficulties of technique and interpretation make it impractical for routine titration.

Cell Culture

Avian poxviruses can be propagated in chicken embryo fibroblast cell cultures (Bang et al., 1951; Mayr, 1963; Hyde et al., 1965; Tajima and Ushijima, 1966) and in duck embryo fibroblast cell cultures (Gelenczei and Lasher, 1968).

CYTOPATHIC EFFECTS. Characteristic cytopathic effects (CPE) produced by the virus in chicken embryo fibroblasts are an initial phase of rounding of the cells followed by a second phase of degeneration and necrosis. The time sequence of these events varies with the virus (Mayr, 1963).

Canary poxvirus-induced changes are present 2 days after infection. The cells are granular, not as rounded as with the other viruses, and destruction occurs by the 3rd day (Mayr, 1963) or 5th day (Tajima and Ushijima, 1966).

Pigeon poxvirus causes rounding of the cells 3–4 days after infection and necrosis at 8–9 days (Mayr, 1963).

Fowl and turkey poxviruses act similarly in that the CPE begin on the 2nd day and rounding of the cells is complete on the 4th or 5th day. Subsequent changes proceed rather slowly, and the cells are not completely destroyed until the 8th or 9th day (Mayr, 1963).

Other authors (Gelenczei and Lasher, 1968) report that fowl, turkey, and pigeon poxviruses induce CPE of chicken embryo fibroblasts with complete destruction of the cells 3–4 days after inoculation. Degeneration of duck embryo fibroblasts occurs 4–5 days after inoculation.

Titration of virus by the quantal dose-response is performed by preparing serial 10-fold dilutions of the virus and using at least 0.1 ml of inoculum for each of 5 tubes of cell culture per dilution. The results may be expressed as the cell culture dose$_{50}$ (CCD$_{50}$) per ml based on the CPE per tube of cell culture (Cunningham, 1966).

Cell cultured virus may also be assayed on the CAM of the chicken embryo for comparative purposes.

PLAQUE FORMATION. Plaque formation in monolayers of chicken embryo fibroblast cell cultures in petri dishes with agar overlay is another method for study of the avian poxviruses. The plaques are best examined on the 11th day of incubation after a vital strain has been applied to the monolayers of cells (Mayr, 1963).

Plaques formed by the respective viruses are sufficiently characteristic to be considered as an aid in differentiation (Mayr, 1963). Ring zones occur similar to those of pocks on the CAM.

Fowl poxvirus produces a clear central plaque with a less clear peripheral zone. The plaques vary from small (about 2 mm) to large (up to 9 mm). In the latter the central plaque is about 4 mm in diameter.

Plaques produced by turkey poxvirus resemble those of fowl poxvirus, but they develop more slowly and are smaller at a given period of incubation.

Pigeon poxvirus produces small plaques (1–3 mm in diameter) with a characteristic lysis not present in plaques produced by the other viruses.

Canary poxvirus produces plaques larger than those of pigeon poxvirus. The central plaque is not clear due to vacuolization of the cells, but ring zones are present.

Titration of virus by the enumerative dose-response uses 0.5 ml of serial 10-fold dilutions of virus for each petri dish of cell culture per dilution. Four cultures per dilution are generally used. After a suitable period for adsorption of virus, agar overlay is applied. The cultures are then incubated for several days (11 days, Mayr, 1963), a vital stain such as neutral red is applied, and the plaques are counted. The results are expressed as plaque-forming units (PFU) per ml (Cunningham, 1966). There is a linear relationship between the number of PFU and the amount of virus.

According to one author (Mayr, 1963), the titer of the virus by the enumerative dose-response of PFU is higher than that by pock counts on the CAM but lower than the quantal dose-response of CPE.

PATHOGENESIS AND EPIZOOTIOLOGY

NATURAL AND EXPERIMENTAL HOSTS

Chickens and turkeys are the most economically important domestic fowl as natural hosts of pox infection, although the disease is of importance in squab-raising plants. Pigeons and canaries are of special importance to bird fanciers. Experimental hosts may be any of the avian species.

Pox may occur in birds of any age, even as young as a few days or weeks old. The disease occurs most commonly in chickens during the fall and winter months when they are housed and in the laying flock during later periods. The disease may occur in broilers particularly during the summer season. Turkeys are usually affected a few days or weeks before marketing or later at breeding time. Squabs may become infected while in the nest, but the disease is encountered more often in older pigeons. Canaries are affected at any age.

TRANSMISSION

Poxvirus infection occurs through mechanical transmission of the virus to the injured or lacerated skin as the virus is unable to penetrate intact epithelium. There is a transient viremia during natural or artificial infection, but a true carrier status does not exist (Pilchard et al., 1962).

Blood-sucking arthropods, especially numerous species of mosquitoes of the genera *Culex* and *Aedes,* are capable of the extrinsic transmission of avian poxviruses from bird to bird and have been responsible for widespread outbreaks during the summer months. There is no evidence of a latent period or of multiplication of the virus within the vector. Mosquitoes can remain infective for several weeks and produce consecutive infections. Intermediate feedings on nonavian species do not impair the effectiveness of transmission (DaMassa, 1966).

INCUBATION PERIOD

The incubation period of the natural disease in chickens, turkeys, and pigeons varies from about 4 to 10 days and is about 4 days in canaries.

SIGNS

Individual signs of typical pox infection may be in one of three forms or in a combination: (1) cutaneous lesions of the head region and perhaps on the featherless areas such as the legs, feet, and vent (Figs. 22.5, 22.6); (2) diphtheritic lesions of the mouth region (Fig. 22.7); and (3) infection of the nasal chambers with accompanying coryza-like signs. In some cases of pox in broilers, the lesions may be found primarily on the feet. There are no internal lesions characteristic of the natural disease.

MORBIDITY AND MORTALITY

The morbidity rate of pox in chickens and turkeys varies from a few birds being infected to involvement of the entire flock if a virulent virus is present and no control measures are taken. Birds affected with the cutaneous form of the disease are more likely to recover than those with the diphtheritic form involving the respiratory tract. Concomitant infections, parasitism, and poor husbandry complicate the disease.

Effects of the disease in chickens usually involve emaciation and poor weight gain; egg production is temporarily retarded if layers are infected. The course of the disease is about 3–4 weeks, but if complications are present the duration may be considerably longer.

In turkeys retardation of weight development of market birds is of greater financial importance than losses by death. Blindness and starvation cause most of the losses. If the disease occurs in breeding birds, decreased egg production and impaired fertility are the result. In uncomplicated, mild infections the course of the disease may be

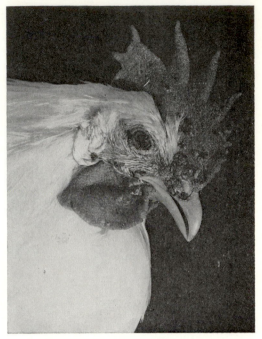

FIG. 22.5—Fowl pox. (Hofstad, Iowa State Univ.)

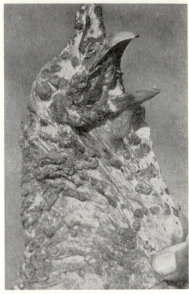

FIG. 22.6—Fowl pox in turkey 3 weeks after lesions first appeared. (Hinshaw, Univ. of Calif.)

2–3 weeks. Severe outbreaks often last for 6, 7, or even 8 weeks.

Flock mortality in both chickens and turkeys is usually low but in severe cases may be as high as 50%. In pigeons the morbidity and mortality rates are similar to those with chickens. Pox in canaries is usually a fatal disease.

GROSS LESIONS

The characteristic lesion of the cutaneous form of pox in chickens is a local epithelial hyperplasia involving both epidermis and underlying feather follicles, with the formation of nodules which first appear as small white foci and then rapidly increase in size and become yellow. Adjoining lesions may coalesce and become rough and gray or dark brown (Fig. 22.5). After about 2 weeks, sometimes sooner, the lesions have areas of inflammation at the base and become hemorrhagic. Formation of a scab, which may last for another week or possibly 2 weeks, ends with desquamation of the degenerated epithelial layer. If the scab is removed early in its development, there is a moist, seropurulent exudate underneath covering a hemorrhagic, granulating surface. When the scab drops off naturally, a smooth scar may be present; in

FIG. 22.7—Fowl pox lesion in mouth and esophagus of turkey. (Hinshaw, Univ. of Calif.)

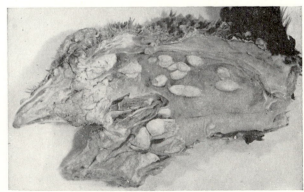

mild cases of the disease there may be no noticeable scar.

In the diphtheritic form slightly elevated, white, opaque nodules develop on the mucous membranes. The nodules rapidly increase in size and often coalesce to become a yellow, cheesy, necrotic pseudo- or diphtheritic membrane. If the membranes are removed they leave bleeding erosions. The inflammatory process may extend into the sinuses, particularly the infraorbital sinus, resulting in swollen sinuses, and also into the pharynx resulting in respiratory disturbances of the host.

The first indication of pox in turkeys are the minute yellowish eruptions on the dewlap, snood, and other head parts. They are soft and, in this pustular stage, easily removed, leaving an inflamed area covered with a sticky serous exudate. The corners of the mouth, eyelids, and oral membranes are commonly affected. The lesions enlarge and become covered with a dry scab or a yellow-red or brown wartlike mass (Fig. 22.6). In young poults the head, legs, and feet may be completely covered with pustules. The disease may even spread to the feathered parts of the body.

The mouth parts, tongue, esophagus, and occasionally the crop may be covered with masses of soft, yellow, diphtheritic ulcers, closely adhering to the mucous membranes (Fig. 22.7). These diphtheritic ulcers of pox must be differentiated from the small,

deep-seated, irregular, diphtheritic ulcers or cankers often found in the mouths of turkeys and not associated with typical head lesions. These latter cankers are common in turkeys vaccinated against pox or recovered from an outbreak. Their cause is not known.

Frequently during the breeding season atypical cases of pox appear in adult turkeys vaccinated with fowl pox vaccine several months previously. In these outbreaks, which usually involve only a small percentage of the birds, the mucous membranes of the eyes and mouth are the principal parts affected. Externally no lesions in the eyes may be visible, but the inner surfaces of the lids may have soft yellow diphtheritic ulcers causing increased lacrimation and inflammation of the eye.

HISTOPATHOLOGY

The most important feature of infection of cells of the skin and mucous membrane of birds and of cells of the CAM is hyperplasia of the epithelium, with associated inflammatory changes and the characteristic eosinophilic cytoplasmic inclusion body observable by light microscopy (Fig. 22.8). Other cellular alterations are considered to be nonspecific (Jennings, 1967; Fenner, 1968).

Inclusion bodies may be present in various stages of development, depending upon the time after infection. During develop-

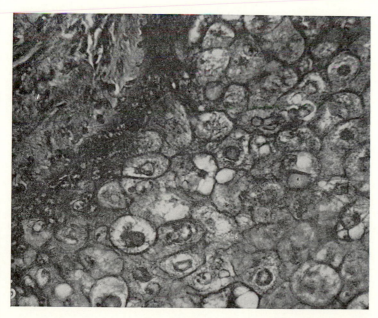

FIG. 22.8—*Epithelial changes in fowl pox.* ×460. *(Biester, Iowa State Univ.)*

ment there is disorganization of the cellular structure, and the lipid-containing inclusion bodies increase in size and number. In some cases the inclusion body may occupy almost the entire cytoplasm with resulting necrosis of the cell. Until 72 hours, inclusion bodies are Feulgen-equivocal, but after this time they are Feulgen-positive following lipid extraction (Todd and Randall, 1958).

IMMUNITY

Actively acquired immunity against the avian poxviruses results from recovery of the bird from natural infection or vaccination.

Passively acquired immunity is not of consequence with the avian poxviruses.

DIAGNOSIS

CLINICAL

Cutaneous lesions typical of avian pox (Figs. 22.5, 22.6) usually are sufficient for diagnosis of the disease. The diphtheritic form of the disease (Fig. 22.7) follows the cutaneous form and should not cause confusion unless complicating infections are present.

MICROSCOPY

Wet mount preparations for examination for cytoplasmic inclusion bodies by light microscopy (direct, phase contrast, dark field) may be made by scraping material lightly from the base of a well-formed papular lesion of the dermal epithelium and placing it on a glass slide, adding a few drops of water, and pressing gently with a cover slip. Inclusion bodies of varying size and shape with refractile, granular, internal components can be observed at magnifications of 300–400 diameters. Inclusion bodies might occupy almost all the cytoplasm.

Cellular debris can be digested by placing the scrapings on a concave slide and adding a few drops of 1% solution of trypsin in 0.2% sodium bicarbonate. After a few minutes of incubation at room temperature, prepare a wet mount on a flat glass slide and examine for inclusion bodies. Cells are digested by the trypsin but the lipid membrane of the inclusion body is not affected.

Scrapings from a lesion can also be fixed in Zenker's or Bouin's fluid, mordanted with potassium permanganate solution, stained with carbol-anilin-fuchsin, counterstained with methylene blue solution, and decolorized in absolute ethyl alcohol for light microscopy. The virus within the inclusion body stains pink (Goodpasture, 1928).

Stained tissue sections (Fig. 22.8) may be processed by conventional methods (Cheevers and Randall, 1968) or by using a solution which fixes and dehydrates the tissues simultaneously (Sevoian, 1960). With the latter method sections can be examined in about 3 hours.

ISOLATION AND IDENTIFICATION OF VIRUS

Bird Inoculation

Avian poxviruses can be transmitted by applying a suspension of the lesion material from infected birds to susceptible birds by scarification of the comb or by the "stick" and "feather follicle" methods. Fowl poxvirus can be transmitted readily from chicken to chicken, with typical cutaneous lesions developing in 5–7 days (Figs. 22.5, 22.11, 22.12). In atypical cases microscopy of lesion specimens may be advisable in addition to bird inoculation.

Identity of the avian poxviruses is usually based on differential susceptibility of the host spectrum (Table 22.1).

Avian Embryos

A specimen from a dermal lesion should be ground in a mortar and pestle with an abrasive, and then about 5 ml of a diluent such as nutrient broth or saline solution is added to prepare a suspension. After adding penicillin (1,000 units per ml) and streptomycin (1 mg per ml) the coarse material in the suspension should be sedimented by centrifugation. The supernatant fluid is then inoculated into 10–12-day-old chicken embryos on the CAM via the artificial air cell (Cunningham, 1966); 5–7 days after inoculation, the CAM is examined for pock lesions (Fig. 22.4).

Cell Culture

Cell cultures are not generally employed for initial isolation of the avian poxviruses.

Fowl poxvirus added to a suspension of trypsinized chicken embryo fibroblasts and then examined microscopically 24–48 hours later for cell agglutination may be used for quantitative titration with the results expressed as cell agglutination units. The test is reported (Kangude and Hanson, 1961) to be relatively simple to perform, economical, accurate, and less time-consuming than the CAM pock-counting method.

IMMUNOLOGY AND SEROLOGY

Immunity Tests

These tests are generally used to determine the immunogenicity of fowl and pigeon pox vaccines. At least 5 susceptible birds are vaccinated according to the directions of the manufacturer. An additional 5 nonvaccinated and isolated birds of the same source and age are kept as controls. At least 10 days after vaccination, the vaccinated and control birds are challenged with a different strain of fowl poxvirus capable of causing clinical signs of pox in at least 80% of the control birds. The challenge virus may be applied on the comb or by the wing web stick or feather follicle methods at a site opposite from that used for vaccination. The birds should be examined for "takes." For satisfactory immunization, at least 80% of the controls should have lesions of fowl pox and at least 80% of the vaccinated birds should not have lesions of fowl pox.

Cross-immunity tests for the antigenic relationship of the avian poxviruses are not generally practical for routine diagnosis but may be utilized for experimental purposes.

Immunodiffusion

Immunodiffusion may be used as a routine diagnostic test for differential identification of fowl and pigeon pox viruses or antibody from those of other avian viral diseases (Woernle, 1966). The test is simple to perform and results may be obtained within about 24 hours. Properly prepared high-potency antigen and antibody must be used for best results.

Soluble antigen from CAM stock virus or from CAM virus isolated from infected chickens is extracted by chloroform from the homogenized CAM of the chicken embryo and then concentrated with ammonium sulfate.

Stock precipitating antiserum collected from chickens 15–20 days after inoculation with the virus is defatted with chloroform and then concentrated with ammonium sulfate.

Concentrated antigen and antiserum may be stored at −20° C.

Good quality, clear agar containing 8% NaCl, pH 7.0–7.2, is required. After the reagent wells are cut in the agar in petri dishes, the bottom of each well is sealed with a drop of liquid agar. The reagents are then placed in the appropriate wells. The dishes are incubated at room temperature in a humidity chamber and examined daily.

Precipitating antibodies occur early and disappear rapidly after infection of birds, and serum must be collected at the appropriate time, usually 15–20 days after known infection.

Hemagglutination

Direct hemagglutination (HA) by a soluble antigen of fowl poxvirus has been described, but specific antibody does not inhibit HA (Mayr, 1956).

A passive HA test using tannic acid-treated horse erythrocytes coated with partially purified, fluorocarbon-treated fowl poxvirus has been reported to detect HA antibodies in serum of chickens by the 3rd week after inoculation (Tripathy et al., 1970). The test appears to be sensitive and capable of detection of antibodies for at least 15 weeks. Further studies are necessary to determine the practical importance of this test for routine diagnosis of fowl pox.

Neutralization

Virus neutralization in cell culture or chicken embryos (Cunningham, 1966) is not practical as a routine diagnostic test because of the usually low concentration of neutralizing antibody in chickens recovered from a natural infection. The test is applicable, however, when a high concentration of antibody can be produced under experimental conditions.

TREATMENT

There is no specific medicinal treatment for birds infected with avian poxviruses. Proper husbandry should be practiced to alleviate environmental stress.

PREVENTION AND CONTROL

IMMUNIZATION

Two types of live virus vaccines are used for immunization of birds against pox: fowl pox vaccine and pigeon pox vaccine. These vaccines contain the respective poxviruses at a minimum concentration of 10^4 EID_{50}

per ml (Winterfield and Hitchner, 1965; Gelenczei and Lasher, 1968). Fowl pox and pigeon pox vaccines labeled "chick embryo origin" are prepared from the infected CAM. Fowl pox vaccine labeled "tissue culture origin" is prepared from chicken embryo fibroblast cultures.

The success of a vaccination program depends upon the potency and purity of the vaccine and its application under the conditions for which it is specifically intended. Vaccination is equivalent to producing a mild form of the disease. Directions for use of a vaccine as supplied by the producer should be followed explicitly. Vaccine should not be used in a flock affected with other diseases or in a generally poor condition. All birds within a house should be vaccinated on the same day. Other susceptible birds on the premises should be isolated from the birds being vaccinated. If

pox appears in a flock in an initial outbreak with a few birds affected, the nonaffected birds should be vaccinated.

A vaccine vial should not be opened before immediate use of the contents. Only one vial should be opened at a time, and the entire contents should be used within about 2 hours. After the vaccine is prepared, the person's hands should be washed thoroughly. The vaccine should be applied to the bird only at the site for vaccination. Extreme precautions should be taken not to contaminate other parts of the bird, the premises, or miscellaneous equipment.

All contaminated vaccine equipment, unused vaccine, empty vials, etc. should be decontaminated, preferably by incineration. No prepared vaccine should be saved for later use.

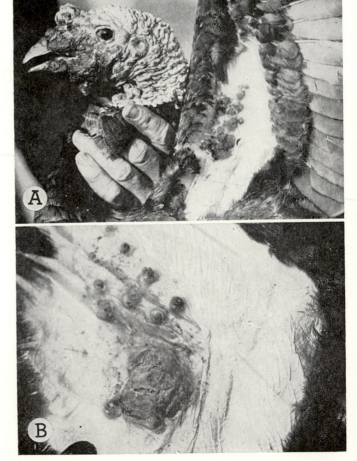

FIG. 22.9—(A) Wing web about 6 weeks after vaccination on this area. Virus spread from vaccination area to other areas on wing and head. Turkey died within few days after picture was taken. (B) Close-up of A at somewhat earlier stage. (Hinshaw, Univ. of Calif.)

Fowl Pox Vaccine

The "chick embryo origin" vaccine contains live, nonattenuated fowl poxvirus capable of producing infection in a flock if used improperly.

Fowl pox vaccine is applied by the wing web stick method to 4-week-old chickens and to chickens about 1–2 months before egg production is expected to start. It is also used to revaccinate chickens held for the 2nd year of egg production. The vaccine is not to be used on laying birds.

Turkeys may be vaccinated by the wing web stick method, but the virus may spread to and infect the head region (Fig. 22.9). The site of choice for vaccination is about midway on the thigh (Fig. 22.10). Initially, turkeys are vaccinated when they are 2–3 months old, but those to be used as breeders should be revaccinated before production. Revaccination at 3–4-month intervals during the laying season might be of some advantage, depending upon circumstances.

Fowl pox vaccine is not to be used on pigeons.

Pigeon Pox Vaccine

Pigeon pox vaccine contains live, nonattenuated, natural virus for pigeons. If used improperly the vaccine can cause a severe reaction in these birds. The virus is less pathogenic for chickens and turkeys.

Pigeon pox vaccine has been commonly applied by brush to the denuded feather follicles on the leg. However, newer pigeon pox vaccines may be applied by the wing web stick method and can be used on chickens of any age. It is generally used, however, on 4-week-old chickens and on chickens about 1 month before egg production is expected to start. When birds younger than 4 weeks old are vaccinated, they should be revaccinated before production. Birds held for the 2nd year of production should be revaccinated.

Turkeys can be vaccinated at any age by

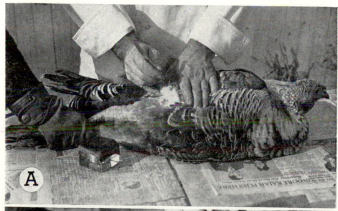

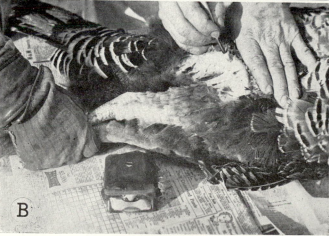

FIG. 22.10—Vaccinating on thigh. Long tuft of feathers that normally covers area is being held back by vaccinator's left hand. (Hinshaw, Univ. of Calif.)

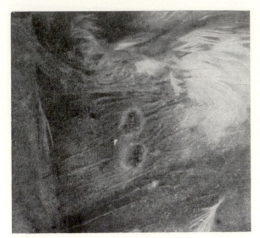

FIG. 22.11—*Wing web of chicken. Six-day "takes," fowl pox vaccine. (Brunett, Cornell Univ.)*

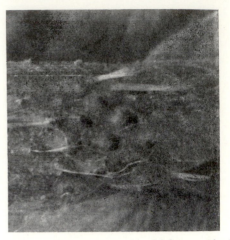

FIG. 22.12—*Leg of chicken. Six-day "takes," fowl pox vaccine, feather follicle method. (Brunett, Cornell Univ.)*

the wing web or thigh stick methods. Day-old poults can be vaccinated if necessary, but it is better to wait until they are about 8 weeks old for a better immune response. Revaccination may be necessary and advisable during the growing period. Turkeys retained as breeders should be revaccinated.

Pigeons can be vaccinated by the wing web stick method. The vaccine can be applied by the feather follicle method, but this is not generally employed.

"Takes"

The flock should be examined about 7–10 days after vaccination for evidence of "takes." A "take" consists of swelling of the skin or a scab at the site where the vaccine was applied and is evidence of a successful vaccination (Figs. 22.11, 22.12). Immunity will normally develop in 10–14 days after vaccination. If the vaccine was properly applied to susceptible birds, the majority should have "takes." In large flocks at least 10% of the birds should be examined for "takes."

The lack of a "take" could be the result of vaccine being applied to an immune bird, use of a vaccine of inadequate potency (one used after the expiration date or subject to deleterious influences), or improper application of the vaccine.

Prophylactic Vaccination

Immunization against pox consists of vaccinating susceptible birds prior to the time when the disease is likely to occur. This is usually done during the spring and summer months in those areas where the disease occurs in the fall and winter months. In tropical climates where the disease may occur throughout the year, vaccination may be done at any time when warranted without regard to seasonal periods.

Vaccination is indicated in 3 types of flocks:

1. Vaccination is indicated in a flock infected the previous year. All young stock produced on the premises or introduced from other sources should receive fowl pox vaccine. When several lots of birds are raised each year, each lot should be vaccinated at the appropriate age. Vaccinated birds should be isolated to prevent possible spread of infection to nonvaccinated birds.

2. If pox was present the previous year and pigeon pox vaccine was used, birds should be revaccinated with fowl pox vaccine as the immunity from pigeon pox vaccine is not of long duration.

3. In areas where pox is prevalent, fowl pox vaccine should be used to protect the flock against infection from neighboring flocks.

REFERENCES

Andrewes, C. H., and H. G. Pereira. 1967. *Viruses of Vertebrates,* 2nd ed. Williams & Wilkins Co., Baltimore.

Arhelger, R. B., and C. C. Randall. 1964. Electron microscopic observations on the development of fowlpox virus in chorioallantoic membrane. *Virology* 22:59–66.

Arhelger, R. B., R. W. Darlington, L. G. Gafford, and C. C. Randall. 1962. An electron microscopic study of fowlpox infection in chick scalps. *Lab. Invest.* 11:814–25.

Bang, F. B., Ellen Levy, and G. O. Gey. 1951. Some observations on host-cell-virus relationships in fowlpox. I. Growth in tissue culture. II. The inclusion produced by the virus on the chick chorioallantoic membrane. *J. Immunol.* 66:329–45.

Beaver, D. L., and W. J. Cheatham. 1963. Electron microscopy of Junco pox. *Am. J. Pathol.* 42:23–40.

Bollinger, O. 1873. Ueber Epithelioma contagiosum beim Haushuhn und die sogenannten Pocken des Gefluegels. *Arch. Pathol. Anat. Physiol.* 58:349–61.

Borrel, A. 1904. Sur les inclusions de l'epithelioma contagieux des oiseaux (molluscum contagiosum). *Compt. Rend. Soc. Biol.* 2:642–43.

Carnwarth, T. 1908. Zur Aetiologie der Huehnerdiphtherie und Gefluegelpocken. *Arb. Kaiserl. Gesundh.* 27:388–402.

Cheevers, W. P., and C. C. Randall. 1968. Viral and cellular growth and sequential increase of protein and DNA during fowlpox infection in vivo. *Proc. Soc. Exp. Biol. Med.* 127:401–5.

Cheevers, W. P., D. J. O'Callaghan, and C. C. Randall. 1968. Biosynthesis of host and viral deoxyribonucleic acid during hyperplastic fowlpox infection in vivo. *J. Virol.* 2:421–29.

Cheville, N. F. 1966. Cytopathologic changes in fowlpox (turkey origin) inclusion body formation. *Am. J. Pathol.* 49:723–37.

Cunningham, C. H. 1966. *A Laboratory Guide in Virology,* 6th ed. Burgess Publ. Co., Minneapolis.

DaMassa, A. J. 1966. The role of *Culex tarsalis* in the transmission of fowl pox virus. *Avian Diseases* 10:57–66.

Fenner, F. 1968. *The Biology of Animal Viruses,* Vol. I. Academic Press, New York.

Gafford, L. G., and C. C. Randall. 1967. The high molecular weight of the fowlpox virus genome. *J. Mol. Biol.* 26:303–10.

Gelenczei, E. F., and H. N. Lasher. 1968. Comparative studies of cell-culture-propagated avian pox viruses in chickens and turkeys. *Avian Diseases* 12:142–50.

Goodpasture, E. W. 1928. Virus diseases of fowls as exemplified by contagious epithelioma fowl pox of chickens and pigeons, pp.

235–77. In Rivers, T. M., *Filterable Viruses.* Williams & Wilkins Co., Baltimore.

———. 1959. Cytoplasmic inclusions resembling Guarnieri bodies and other phenomena induced by mutants of the virus of fowlpox. *Am. J. Pathol.* 35:213–31.

Hyde, J. M., L. G. Gafford, and C. C. Randall. 1965. Fine structure of the coat and nucleoid material of fowlpox virus. *J. Bacteriol.* 89:1557–69.

———. 1967. Molecular weight determination of fowlpox virus DNA by electron microscopy. *Virology* 33:112–20.

Jennings, A. R. 1967. Cellular and tissue reactions, pp. 211–67. In Betts, A. O., and C. J. York (eds.), *Viral and Rickettsial Infections of Animals,* Vol. I. Academic Press, New York.

Joklik, W. K. 1966. The poxviruses. *Bacteriol. Rev.* 30:33–66.

Kangude, G. M., and L. E. Hanson. 1961. "Cell agglutination" technique for quantitative titration of fowlpox virus. *Avian Diseases* 5:139–43.

Marx, E., and A. Sticker. 1902. Untersuchungen ueber das Epithelioma contagiosum des Gefluegels. *Deut. Med. Wochschr.* 28:893–95.

Mayr, A. 1956. Arbeiten ueber das haemagglutinierende Prinzip bei den Tierpockenviren. *Arch. Ges. Virusforsch.* 6:439–71.

———. 1963. Neue Verfahren fuer die Differenzierung der Gefluegelpoxkenviren. *Berlin. Muench. Tieraerztl. Wochschr.* 76:316–24.

Pilchard, E. I., Jr., L. E. Hanson, and J. O. Alberts. 1962. Fowlpox virus neutralization antibody and viremia in turkeys. *Avian Diseases* 6:396–402.

Randall, C. C., L. G. Gafford, and R. B. Arhelger. 1961. Electron microscopic examination of isolated fowlpox inclusions. *Virology* 14:381–82.

Randall, C. C., L. G. Gafford, and R. W. Darlington. 1962. Bases of the nucleic acid of fowlpox virus and host deoxyribonucleic acid. *J. Bacteriol.* 83:1037–41.

Randall, C. C., L. G. Gafford, R. W. Darlington, and J. M. Hyde. 1964. Composition of fowlpox virus and inclusion matrix. *J. Bacteriol.* 87:939–44.

Randall, C. C., L. G. Gafford, R. L. Soehner, and J. M. Hyde. 1966. Physiochemical properties of fowlpox virus deoxyribonucleic acid and its anomalous infectious behavior. *J. Bacteriol.* 91:95–100.

Sevoian, M. 1960. A quick method for the diagnosis of avian pox and laryngotracheitis. *Avian Diseases* 4:474–77.

Szybalski, W., R. L. Erikson, G. A. Gentry, L. G. Gafford, and C. C. Randall. 1963. Unusual properties of fowlpox virus DNA. *Virology* 19:586–89.

Tajima, M., and T. Ushijima. 1966. Electron microscopy of avian pox viruses with special reference to the significance of inclusion bodies in viral replication. *Japan. J. Vet. Sci.* 28:107–18.

Todd, W. M., and C. C. Randall. 1958. The Feulgen reaction of fowlpox inclusions after lipid extraction. *Arch. Pathol.* 66:150–53.

Tripathy, D. N., L. E. Hanson, and W. L. Myers. 1970. Passive hemagglutination test with fowlpox virus. *Avian Diseases* 14:29–38.

Wilner, B. I. 1969. *A Classification of the Major Groups of Human and Other Animal Viruses,* 4th ed. Burgess Publ. Co., Minneapolis.

Winterfield, R. W., and S. B. Hitchner. 1965. The response of chickens to vaccination with different concentrations of pigeon pox and fowl pox vaccines. *Avian Diseases* 9:237–41.

Woernle, H. 1966. The use of the agar-gel diffusion technique in the identification of certain avian virus diseases. *Veterinarian* 4:17–28.

Woodroofe, Gwendolyn M., and F. Fenner. 1962. Serological relationships within the poxvirus group: an antigen common to all members of the group. *Virology* 16:334–41.

Woodruff, Alice M., and E. W. Goodpasture. 1931. The susceptibility of the chorio-allantoic membrane of chick embryos to infection with fowl-pox virus. *Am. J. Pathol.* 7:209–22.

Woodruff, C. E., and E. W. Goodpasture. 1929. The infectivity of isolated inclusion bodies of fowl-pox. *Am. J. Pathol.* 5:1–10.

———. 1930. The relation of the virus of fowl-pox to the specific cellular inclusions of the disease. *Am. J. Pathol.* 6:713–20.

Woodson, B. 1968. Recent progress in poxvirus research. *Bacteriol. Rev.* 32:127–37.

Journal Article No. 4701 from Mich. Agr. Expt. Sta.

CHAPTER 23

DUCK VIRUS HEPATITIS

❖

P. P. LEVINE

Department of Avian Diseases
New York State Veterinary College
Cornell University
Ithaca, New York

❖

THIS DISEASE is a highly fatal, rapidly spreading viral infection of young ducklings characterized primarily by a hepatitis. It is of economic importance to all duck-growing farms because of the high potential mortality if not controlled by immune serum therapy or vaccination. The virus of duck hepatitis is not known to have any public health significance.

HISTORY AND DISTRIBUTION

An acute disease of ducklings, characterized by enlarged livers mottled with hemorrhages, was observed in the spring of 1945 by Levine and Hofstad (1945). The disease affected ducklings during the 1st week of age, and death was rapid after signs were observed. While the disease could be transmitted in ducklings, no agent was isolated. During the spring of 1949, Levine and Fabricant (1950) studied a highly fatal disease of young White Pekin ducks on Long Island, New York. The disease spread rapidly; before the summer was over practically all of the 70-odd duck farms in the area had suffered losses. At first, ducks 2–3 weeks of age were affected; gradually the disease attacked younger birds until ducklings less than a week old were succumbing. On severely affected farms, mortalities up to 95% were not uncommon in some broods. Successive lots of ducks almost invariably be-

came infected. Later, occasional broods would escape with little mortality. It was estimated that 15% of the total number of ducklings started for that year died from the disease—a total of 750,000 birds. In the United States the disease has been diagnosed in Massachusetts, Illinois (Hanson and Alberts, 1956), and Michigan. It has also been reported from Canada (Macpherson and Avery, 1957), England (Asplin and McLauchlan, 1954; Asplin, 1956), Germany and Egypt (Shehata and Reuss, 1957), the Netherlands (Smits, 1957), Belgium (Schyns, 1957), Italy (Rossi and Pini, 1957; Agrimi, 1958), Russia (Prokofiva and Doroshko, 1960), and Hungary (Derzsy, cited by Reuss, 1959a). Tauraso et al. (1969), in their review of literature, mention the disease having been reported also from Brazil, India, Czechoslovakia, Israel, France, Thailand, and Japan.

ETIOLOGY

Duck hepatitis is caused by a filterable virus which was first isolated in chicken embryos by Levine and Fabricant (1950). No serological relationship was demonstrated between this virus and the virus causing duck plague, and likewise no neutralization of the duck hepatitis virus occurred when tested with convalescent serum from cases of human and canine virus hepatitis (Fabricant et al., 1957). The virus of duck hepatitis contains RNA and has been tentatively classified as a picornavirus by Tauraso et al. (1969).

MORPHOLOGY

Size

Duck hepatitis virus (DHV) has been estimated to be 20–40 mμ in size by Reuss (1959a). Richter et al. (1964) observed 30 mμ particles in thin liver sections under the electron microscope. Tauraso et al. (1969) confirmed the size to be less than 50 mμ by filtration of the agent through Millipore filters.

BIOLOGICAL PROPERTIES

Fitzgerald and Hanson (1966) were unable to demonstrate hemagglutination of washed erythrocytes of the chicken, duck, sheep, horse, guinea pig, mouse, snake, swine, and rabbit using cell-cultured DHV. Cell cultures infected with DHV failed

Revised by M. S. Hofstad, Veterinary Medical Research Institute, Ames, Iowa.

to hemadsorb red cells of green and rhesus monkeys, hamster, mouse, rat, rabbit, guinea pig, human O, goose, duck, and day-old chicks. High-titered virus suspensions would not hemagglutinate red cells of the same species when tested at a pH range of 6.8–7.4 and at temperatures of 4°, 24°, and 37° C (Tauraso et al., 1969).

RESISTANCE TO CHEMICAL AND PHYSICAL AGENTS

Heating the virus at 50° C for 1 hour had no effect on the titer of the virus (Tauraso et al., 1969). Hanson et al. (1964) found that most of the virus was inactivated at 56° C after 30 minutes. However, Asplin (1961) reported it to survive 56° C for 60 minutes, but it was inactivated when heated at 62° C for 30 minutes. Hanson et al. (1964) found active virus at 7 days but not at 9 days when held at 37° C. Pollard and Starr (1959) found the virus to survive storage in cell-free culture medium for 21 days at 37° C. The virus-infected embryonic fluids remained viable for 28 days at 25° C and remained infective for as long as 9 years at −20° C storage (Hanson et al., 1964).

Pollard and Starr (1959) reported the virus to resist treatment with ether and fluorocarbon. The virus was found to be resistant to chloroform, pH 3.0, and trypsin (Tauraso et al., 1969). Hanson et al. (1964) found DHV resistant to treatment with 30% methanol, ammonium sulfate, protamine sulfate, and Freon 112 Heptane.

Asplin (1961) reported the virus to survive for at least 10 weeks in uncleaned infected brooders, and for longer than 37 days in moist feces stored in a cool shed. The virus was still active in embryonic fluid after 700 days in a refrigerator at 2–4° C. The virus was not inactivated when exposed to 2% lysol at 37° C for 1 hour nor by 0.1% formalin at 37° C for 8 hours.

LABORATORY HOST SYSTEMS

Chicken Embryos

Levine and Fabricant (1950) were the first to demonstrate propagation of the virus in the allantoic sac of 9-day-old chicken embryos. From 10 to 60% of the embryos died by the 5th or 6th day and were stunted or edematous (Figure 23.1). Hwang and Dougherty (1964) passaged a DHV strain as two lines in 10-day-old chicken embryos.

The serially passaged lines became nonpathogenic for newly hatched ducklings at the 20th and 26th transfers. The virus titer in chicken embryos was 1–3 logs lower than when grown in ducklings.

Hwang (1965a) reported on the development of a chicken embryo lethal strain of DHV by serial embryo passages. Using a homogenate of dead embryos and chorioallantoic membrane in embryonic fluid, the embryo mortality reached 100% at the 63rd passage. More consistent results were obtained when 5–7-day-old embryos were inoculated via the yolk sac.

Cell Cultures

Pollard and Starr (1959) reported propagation of DHV through 25 serial passages in cell cultures prepared with chicken embryo explants. However, the virus did not grow in cultures of trypsinized chicken embryo cells or in mammalian cells. Kaeberle et al. (1961) were able to demonstrate some growth of virus in chicken embryo liver cells, but no cytopathogenic effect could be demonstrated. The titer of the virus decreased over 7 passages.

Fitzgerald et al. (1963) reported cell alterations in stained duck embryo kidney cell cultures associated with growth of the virus. They observed small focal areas of degeneration and necrosis as early as 16 hours after inoculation, with most cells affected by 72 hours. The cytopathic effect was first noticed at the 8th passage and occurred consistently from the 16th through the 26th passage. They were unable to induce cytopathic effect in chicken embryo kidney cell cultures using infected fluid from the 25th duck embryo kidney cell culture passage.

Fitzgerald and Hanson (1966) determined the growth curve of DHV in duck embryo kidney cell cultures. The latent phase was approximately 2–4 hours. The first measurable amount of virus released was between 4 and 8 hours after inoculation. The virus titer continued to increase until a peak was reached in 24 hours and remained at that titer for 96 hours after inoculation.

Hwang (1966) attempted to grow DHV in duck embryo liver cells but found this system unsuitable for virus propagation.

PATHOGENICITY

Asplin (1958) and Reuss (1959b) reported loss of pathogenicity for ducklings after

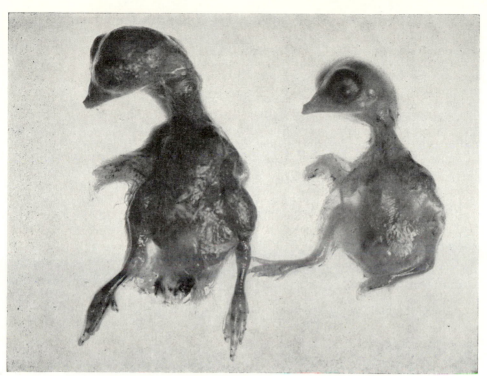

FIG. 23.1—*(Left) Normal 15-day-old chick embryo. (Right) Fifteen-day-old chick embryo inoculated with duck virus 6 days previously. Note small size and edema, especially around thigh and abdomen. (Courtesy Cornell Veterinarian)*

chicken embryo passages. Hwang (1965a) found one virus strain to have lost its pathogenicity for ducklings after 20 or more passages in chicken embryos. He also found that the same strain had lost its pathogenicity for ducklings after the 6th passage in duck embryo fibroblasts, but the virus retained its pathogenicity for chicken embryos (Hwang, 1965b).

Hwang and Dougherty (1964) reported chicken embryo passaged strains, while nonpathogenic for ducklings, did multiply in the tissues but at a lower titer than field strains. Field strains were found in fairly high concentrations in the brain of ducklings; the chicken embryo passaged strains could not be detected or were present in low concentrations in the brain.

PATHOGENESIS AND EPIZOOLIOLOGY

NATURAL AND EXPERIMENTAL HOSTS

In outbreaks duck hepatitis occurred only in young ducklings. Adult breeders on infected premises did not become infected and continued in full production.

Field observations indicated that chickens and turkeys were resistant. However, Rahn (1962) found that day-old and week-old poults exposed to DHV developed signs, lesions, and neutralizing antibody. Poults after either oral or intraperitoneal exposure had mottled livers and enlarged gall bladders and spleens. DHV was isolated from livers up to 17 days after oral exposure of day-old poults. Schoop et al. (1959) and Reuss (1959a) failed to infect chickens experimentally. The latter worker could not transmit the disease to rabbits, guinea pigs, white mice, or dogs. Asplin (1961) reported that young chickens can contract an inapparent infection and pass it on by contact to other chicks.

TRANSMISSION

Under field conditions the disease spreads rapidly to all susceptible ducklings in the flock. Although the high mortality and rapid spread of the disease on farms indicated extreme contagiousness, occasional exceptions were observed. In one pen 65% of the ducks died, while in an adjoining pen separated only by a 14-inch curb, the mortality was negligible.

The first efforts to transmit the disease to small groups of 3 or 4 caged ducklings by injection and feeding of egg-propagated virus were not successful. In another experiment, with tissues from a natural outbreak, some of the ducklings became infected. Transmission was most easily accomplished by intramuscular injection and by feeding egg-propagated virus and infected organs to larger groups of ducklings (10–20) kept on litter under a hover. The incubation period was 24 hours in most experiments, and nearly all the deaths took place by the 4th day. Uninoculated ducklings placed in the same pens with the inoculated birds contracted the disease and died somewhat later than the injected ducks.

Egg transmission presumably does not take place. Newly hatched ducklings produced by breeders on infected premises remained well when taken to premises where no ducks were being kept. Asplin (1958) confirmed this finding.

CARRIERS AND VECTORS

Reuss (1959a) reported that recovered ducks may excrete virus in the feces for up to 8 weeks after infection. Asplin (1961) stated that there is strong field evidence to incriminate wild birds as mechanical carriers of the virus over short distances. He also suggested that the possibility of an unknown host, acting as a healthy carrier, might be responsible for new outbreaks at great distances. Vectors are not known to be a factor in transmission of the disease.

SIGNS

The onset and spread of the disease are very rapid, with practically all the mortality occurring within 3–4 days. Affected ducklings at first fail to keep up with the brood. Within a short time the birds stop moving and squat down with eyes partially closed. The ducklings fall on their sides, kick spasmodically with both legs, and die with heads drawn back (Fig. 23.2). Death occurs within an hour or so after signs are noted. During the height of severe outbreaks, the rapidity with which ducklings die is astonishing.

MORBIDITY AND MORTALITY

The morbidity is 100% and mortality is variable. In some broods less than a week old the mortality may reach 95%. In ducklings 1–3 weeks of age the mortality may be 50% or less. In ducklings 4–5 weeks old the mortality is low or negligible.

GROSS LESIONS

The principal lesions are found in the liver which is enlarged and contains punctate or ecchymotic hemorrhages (Fig. 23.3). Frequent reddish discoloration or mottling of the liver surface is seen. The spleen is sometimes enlarged and mottled. In numerous cases the kidneys are swollen and the renal blood vessels injected. These lesions were reproduced in young ducks by inoculation and feeding of egg-propagated virus.

HISTOPATHOLOGY

The microscopic changes in uncomplicated, experimentally induced infections have been studied (Fabricant et al., 1957). The primary changes consisted of necrosis of the hepatic cells and proliferation of the bile duct epithelium. Varying degrees of inflammatory cell response and hemorrhage occurred. Regeneration of the liver parenchyma was observed in ducklings that did not die.

IMMUNITY

Recovery from the disease results in a solid immunity and neutralizing antibodies in the serum. Active immunity can be induced in adult ducks by injection of certain strains of virus (Asplin, 1961). Some strains of virus require repeated injections to obtain high levels of antibody (Reuss, 1959b). Passive immunity can be conferred to ducklings by injection of serum from recovered or immunized birds. Passive antibodies may also be transferred through the yolk to the hatched duckling to protect the bird for a few weeks.

DIAGNOSIS

ISOLATION AND IDENTIFICATION OF THE VIRUS

The virus may be isolated by inoculating infective liver suspensions or blood into the allantoic sac of 9-day-old chicken embryos. Stunted and edematous embryos are observed in those that die on the 5th or 6th day. Edema may be noted especially around the thigh and abdomen. The amniotic sac contains an excess of fluid. The yolk sac is reduced in size and the contents are more

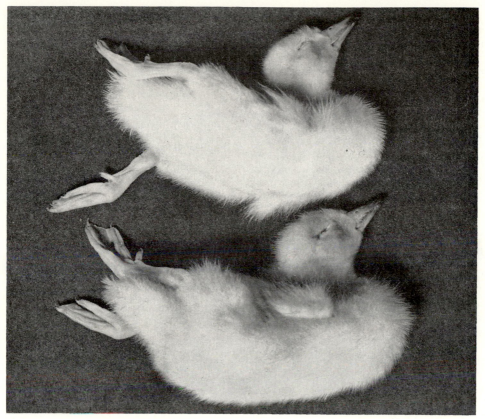

FIG. 23.2—*Ducklings dead from infection with virus hepatitis. Note typical opisthotonus.*

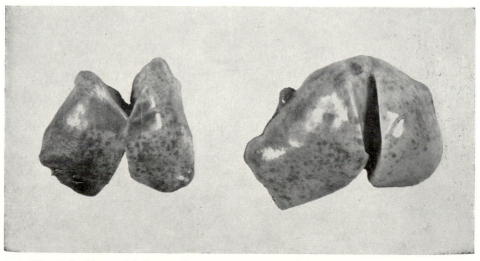

FIG. 23.3—*Liver with hemorrhagic lesions caused by duck virus hepatitis infection.*

viscous than usual. A greenish discoloration of the embryonic fluid and yolk sac is often found and may be detected on candling of the eggs. The livers of the embryos often are greenish in color and frequently have whitish yellow necrotic foci, varying from pinhead in size to larger areas involving considerable portions of the parenchyma. Allantoic fluids from these embryos and from infected duck tissues contain the virus and will kill 10–60% of the embryos by the 6th day. Identification of the virus can be made by virus neutralization tests with specific immune serum.

SEROLOGY

Serological tests have not been useful in diagnosing outbreaks of the disease. However, the virus neutralization test is useful in virus identification. Murty and Hanson (1961) described the use of the agar gel diffusion precipitin test for the identification of the virus.

DIFFERENTIAL DIAGNOSIS

The sudden onset, rapid spread, and acute course of this disease are characteristic. Lesions in the livers of young ducklings up to 3 weeks of age are practically pathognomonic. Duck virus hepatitis may be differentiated from duck plague on the basis of lesions and age of birds affected. In duck plague adult birds are commonly affected and hemorrhagic lesions occur in all organs and muscles. Necrotic plaques may be observed throughout the gut.

TREATMENT

Serum therapy in the field has proved to be highly successful. This requires a bank storage of antiserum so that it is readily available when needed. The Duck Disease Laboratory at Eastport, Long Island, keeps such a bank of antiserum processed from blood collected from recovered birds at the time of slaughter.

When the first deaths in an outbreak of the disease occur, 0.5 ml of the duck hepatitis antiserum is injected intramuscularly into all ducklings of the brood. If the antiserum is of sufficient potency, one treatment will usually suffice.

PREVENTION AND CONTROL

MANAGEMENT PROCEDURES

The disease can be prevented by strict isolation, particularly during the first 4–5 weeks. However, in areas where the disease is prevalent, it is very difficult to obtain the degree of isolation necessary to prevent the disease.

IMMUNIZATION

Resistance against duck hepatitis may be conferred to ducklings by three methods: (1) injection of immune serum from recovered or hyperimmunized ducks as described under treatment; (2) immunization of breeding stock to insure high levels of antibody in the yolk of the hatching egg and thus transfer immunity by way of the yolk to the hatched duckling; (3) active immunization of the ducklings directly with live avirulent strains of DHV.

Immunization of Breeders

Asplin (1958) developed an attenuated strain of virus (TN) which was used successfully to immunize breeders. The method was to inoculate 0.5 ml of undiluted egg-propagated virus intramuscularly 2–4 weeks before collecting hatching eggs. Reuss (1959b) found it necessary with the strain of virus he used to make repeated injections in breeders to obtain sufficient antibody levels to protect hatched ducklings against challenge with virulent virus. The optimum age, dosage, route of inoculation, strain of virus, and interval between initial and subsequent vaccinations are not known (Asplin, 1961).

Immunization of Ducklings

Asplin (1958) demonstrated loss of pathogenicity of one strain (TN) of DHV for young ducklings after cultivation of the virus in chicken embryos. Similarly, other workers have found a reduction of the pathogenicity of the virus by serial passage in chicken embryos (Schoop et al., 1959; Reuss, 1959b; Hwang and Dougherty, 1962).

This led Asplin (1958) to use his strain of virus to vaccinate young ducklings by foot web puncture with a needle which had been dipped in egg-propagated virus. Reuss (1959b) also reported successful immunization experiments with his attenuated strain. The degree of attenuation of the virus is of importance (Asplin, 1961). Asplin found that virulence of the attenuated strain increased after 24 passages of the virus through ducklings. The TN strain passaged 104 times in chicken embryos failed to immunize.

REFERENCES

Agrimi, P. 1958. L'epatitie virale delle anatre (Levine e Fabricant 1950). Signalazione di un episodio. Idientificazione del virus e prove di transmissione sperimentale. *Zooprofilassi* 13:541–51.

Asplin, F. D. 1956. The production of ducklings resistant to virus hepatitis. *Vet. Record* 68:412–13.

———. 1958. An attenuated strain of duck hepatitis virus. *Vet. Record* 70:1226–30.

———. 1961. Notes on epidemiology and vaccination for virus hepatitis of ducks. *Office Int. Epizooties Bull.* 56:793–800.

Asplin, F. D., and J. D. McLauchlan. 1954. Duck virus hepatitis. *Vet. Record* 66:456–58.

Fabricant, J., C. G. Rickard, and P. P. Levine. 1957. The pathology of duck virus hepatitis. *Avian Diseases* 1:256–74.

Fitzgerald, J. E., and L. E. Hanson. 1966. Certain properties of a cell-culture modified duck hepatitis virus. *Avian Diseases* 10:157–61.

Fitzgerald, J. E., L. E. Hanson, and M. Wingard. 1963. Cytopathic effects of duck hepatitis virus in duck embryo kidney cell cultures. *Proc. Soc. Exp. Biol. Med.* 114:814–16.

Hanson, L. E., and J. O. Alberts. 1956. Virus hepatitis in ducklings. *J. Am. Vet. Med. Ass.* 128:37–38.

Hanson, L. E., H. E. Rhoades, and R. L. Schricker. 1964. Properties of duck hepatitis virus. *Avian Diseases* 8:196–202.

Hwang, J. 1965a. A chicken-embryo-lethal strain of duck hepatitis virus. *Avian Diseases* 9:417–22.

———. 1965b. Duck hepatitis virus in duck embryo fibroblast cultures. *Avian Diseases* 9:285–90.

———. 1966. Duck hepatitis virus in duck embryo liver cell cultures. *Avian Diseases* 10:508–12.

Hwang, J., and E. Dougherty, III. 1962. Serial passage of duck hepatitis virus in chicken embryos. *Avian Diseases* 6:435–40.

———. 1964. Distribution and concentration of duck hepatitis virus in inoculated ducklings and chicken embryos. *Avian Diseases* 8:264–68.

Kaeberle, M. L., J. W. Drake, and L. E. Hanson. 1961. Cultivation of duck hepatitis virus in tissue culture. *Proc. Soc. Exp. Biol. Med.* 106:755–57.

Leibovitz, L., and J. Hwang. 1968. Duck plague on the American continent. *Avian Diseases* 12:361–78.

Levine, P. P., and J. Fabricant. 1950. A hitherto-undescribed virus disease of ducks in North America. *Cornell Vet.* 40:71–86.

Levine, P. P., and M. S. Hofstad. 1945. Duck disease investigation. *Ann. Rept. N.Y.S. Vet. Coll.,* Ithaca, pp. 55–56.

Macpherson, L. W., and R. J. Avery. 1957. Duck virus hepatitis in Canada. *Can. J. Comp. Med.* 21:26–31.

Murty, D. K., and L. E. Hanson. 1961. A modified microgel diffusion method and its application in the study of the virus of duck hepatitis. *Am. J. Vet. Res.* 22:274–78.

Pollard, M., and T. J. Starr. 1959. Propagation of duck hepatitis virus in tissue culture. *Proc. Soc. Exp. Biol. Med.* 101:521–24.

Prokofiva, M. T., and I. N. Doroshko. 1960. Virus hepatitis of ducklings. *Veterinariya* 37:38–40.

Rahn, D. P. 1962. Susceptibility of turkeys to duck hepatitis virus—Serological comparison of duck hepatitis virus and turkey hepatitis virus. Master's thesis. Univ. Illinois.

Reuss, U. 1959a. Virusbiologische Untersuchungen bei der Entenhepatitis. *Zentr. Veterinaermed.* 6:209–48.

———. 1959b. Versuche zur aktiven und passiven Immunisierung bei der Virushepatitis der Entenkueken. *Zentr. Veterinaermed.* 6:808–15.

Richter, W. R., E. J. Rodzok, and S. M. Moize. 1964. Electron microscopy of viruslike particles associated with duck viral hepatitis. *Virology* 24:114–16.

Rossi, C., and A. Pini. 1957. L'epatite da virus degli anatroccoli. Osservazioni e ricerche. *Vet. Ital.* 8:1175–89.

Schoop, G., H. Staub, and K. Ergüney. 1959. Ueber Virushepatitis der Enten. 5. Mitteilung: Versuche zur Adaptation des Virus und embryonierte Huehnereier. *Monatsh. Tierheilk.* 11:99–106.

Schyns, P. 1957. L'hepatite a virus du caneton. *Ann. Med. Vet.* 101:264–71.

Shehata, H., and V. Reuss. 1957. Virus-Hepatitis der Enten in Deutschland. *Deut. Tieraertzl. Wochschr.* 64:27–29.

Smits, W. H. 1957. Voorlopige Mededeling betreffende een Virusziekte bij Eendenkuikens. *Tijdschr. Diergeneesk.* 82:177–83.

Tauraso, N. M., G. E. Cogill, and M. J. Klutch, 1969. Properties of the attenuated vaccine strain of duck hepatitis virus. *Avian Diseases* 13:321–29.

CHAPTER 24

DUCK PLAGUE
(Duck Virus Enteritis)

❖

LOUIS LEIBOVITZ

Cornell University
New York State Veterinary College
Department of Avian Diseases
Duck Research Laboratory
Eastport, New York

❖

DUCK PLAGUE is an acute contagious herpesvirus infection of ducks, geese, and swans that is characterized by vascular damage with tissue hemorrhages and free blood in the body cavities, enanthematous digestive mucosal lesions, lesions of lymphoid organs, and retrograde changes of the parenchymatous organs.

Synonyms for the disease are eendenpest (Dutch), peste due canard (French), entenpest (German), and duck virus enteritis (USDA, 1967). Although Bos (1942) first employed the term duck plague, it was proposed as the official title by Jansen and Kunst (1949).

In the duck-producing areas of the world where the disease has been reported, duck plague has produced significant economic losses. Prior to 1959 the disease frequently resulted in mortalities up to 100%, but death losses have been somewhat fewer in more recent outbreaks (Jansen, 1968). Where severe outbreaks occur in breeder ducks, the associated loss of egg production and replacement ducklings may halt duck production. If the disease occurs at the time of marketing, a high rate of carcass condemnation can be expected. Since the first reported American outbreak of the disease in the concentrated duck-producing area of Long Island, New York (Leibovitz and Hwang, 1968a), duck plague has resulted in a loss estimated in excess of $1 million for a 1-year period for this small industry.

Due to the paucity of information relative to anatine diseases, no appraisal can be made of other possible outbreaks in the many geographically dispersed small flocks of domestic ducks and geese.

While the disease has been detected in wild, free-flying Anseriformes (ducks, geese, and swans) (Leibovitz and Hwang, 1968b; Leibovitz, 1968; Peckham, 1968, personal communication; Locke, 1968, personal communication), the importance of the disease for wild waterfowl has not been established. More evidence is needed to define these currently detected outbreaks as either emerging exotic or preexisting undetected infections on the American continent. Conversely, investigation of possible infection of wild waterfowl should be undertaken on those continents where the disease has been reported only in domestic ducks and geese.

Although the virus has been adapted to grow in embryonating chicken eggs and chicks under 2 weeks of age (Jansen, 1968), natural infection has been limited to Anseriformes. The infection has not been reported in other species of birds, mammals, or man.

HISTORY

Baudet (1923) reported an outbreak of an acute hemorrhagic disease of domestic ducks in the Netherlands. Bacterial cultures were negative, and he reproduced the disease experimentally in domestic ducks by the injection of liver suspensions which were filtered through a Chamberland L_3 candle. Although he presented his findings as a previously unreported viral infection of ducks that failed to infect chickens, he concluded that the disease was due to a specific duck-adapted strain of fowl plague virus.

Subsequent similar outbreaks were reported in the Netherlands. Fortunately each formed a segment of a continuous commentary and reappraisal of the etiology of a disease that clinically and pathologically resembled fowl plague. DeZeeuw (1930) substantiated Baudet's findings and again indicated the specificity of the virus for ducks. Although he found chickens, pigeons, and rabbits refractory to experimental infection, he also believed the agent to be a specific duck-adapted strain of fowl plague. DeZeeuw suspected that wild waterfowl were carriers of the disease, since they were found within the areas of the outbreak.

Bos (1942) reexamined the findings of the above workers and observed new outbreaks. He further characterized the lesions, clinical course, and immune response of ducks by experimental study and was unable to experimentally infect chickens, pigeons, rabbits, guinea pigs, rats, and mice. Bos concluded that the disease was not due to fowl plague virus, but rather was a new distinct viral disease of ducks which he termed duck plague. He based this conclusion on the high degree of specificity of the agent for ducks both in experimental and natural infection, the persistence of the disease as a uniform entity within the Netherlands, and the longer incubation period. He differentiated the disease from Newcastle disease (pseudo-fowl pest). These observations were further supported by more detailed studies of Jansen and Kunst (1949). Since recognition of the disease, Jansen (1961, 1963, 1964a,b, 1968), Jansen and Kunst (1949, 1964), and Jansen and Wemmenhove (1965) have published extensively on their observations, experimental studies, virus propagation, incidence and distribution of the disease, its pathology, and immunity.

INCIDENCE AND DISTRIBUTION

In addition to the Netherlands, duck plague has been suspected in France (Lucam, 1949) and China (Jansen and Kunst, 1964) and has been confirmed in Belgium (Devos et al., 1964) and India (Mukerji et al., 1963, 1965). In 1967 the first reported outbreak on the American continent was observed in White Pekin ducks in the concentrated duck-producing area of Long Island (Leibovitz and Hwang, 1968a). Since this report the disease has been detected on 12 other commercial duck farms on Long Island (Urban, 1968). In addition, outbreaks in wild, free-flying waterfowl on Long Island have occurred at 7 different locations (Leibovitz and Hwang, 1968b; Leibovitz, 1968). The disease has also been detected at 3 localities in central New York State (Peckham, 1968, personal communication), 1 in Pennsylvania, and 1 in Maryland (Locke, 1968, personal communication). Whether these reports represent extension of an emerging exotic infection or previous unreported enzootic infection on the Amer-

ican continent is unknown and poses a problem to government regulatory agencies.

The maintenance of concentrated large numbers of susceptible domestic ducks and geese enhances the probability of the detection of the disease. In contrast, the dearth of information relative to the disease in wild waterfowl, small domestic flocks, ornamental bird collections, and zoos is probably due to the more limited veterinary surveillance and inadequate sampling. Accordingly, the reported incidence of the disease in domestic ducks may be misleading when compared to natural occurrence in other species of Anseriformes.

In the Netherlands a higher incidence was noted in the spring of the year (Jansen, 1963); however, in the concentrated White Pekin duck-producing area of Long Island, no marked seasonal increase was noted. A higher incidence in wild, free-flying Anseriformes on Long Island was noted in the fall of the year 1967 (Leibovitz, 1968).

ETIOLOGY

The causative agent of duck plague is a filterable virus belonging to the herpesvirus group.

MORPHOLOGY

Electron microscopy of thin sections of virus-infected cell cultures 48 hours after inoculation revealed virus particles in both the nucleus and cytoplasm of the cell (Breese and Dardiri, 1968). In the nucleus the particles were approximately 91 mμ in diameter with a core approximately 48 mμ in diameter. Smaller dense particles of approximately 32 mμ in diameter were also observed in some nuclei. Larger particles of approximately 181 mμ in diameter with densely stained cores of 75 mμ were observed in the cytoplasm (Fig. 24.1). These had a less densely stained envelope. The capsid structure of the virion has not been resolved (Breese and Dardiri, 1968).

Hess and Dardiri (1968) estimated the size of the virus within this range by filtration studies. Virus suspensions passed through Millipore membranes of 0.22μ porosity, but infectious virus was retained by membranes of 0.1μ porosity.

CHEMICAL COMPOSITION

The virion of duck plague contains deoxyribonucleic acid (DNA), as determined

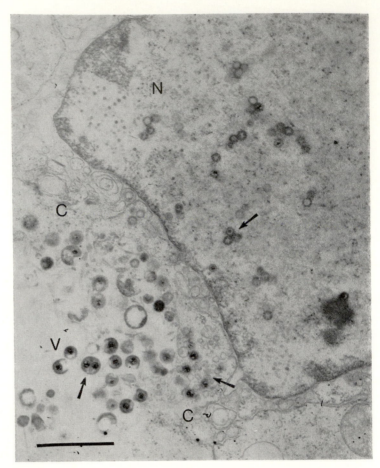

FIG. 24.1—Thin section of Epon-embedded cells infected 48 hours with Long Island isolate of duck plague virus. Virus particles (arrows) appear in several forms in the nucleus (N), cytoplasm (C), and cytoplasmic vacuole (V). Magnification mark = 1μ. (Breese and Dardiri, 1968)

by Breese and Dardiri (1968). They demonstrated by electron microscopy of thin sections that ribonuclease had no effect on the morphology of the virus, while exposure to deoxyribonuclease led to removal of the central core of the virus without affecting the envelope.

Fluorescence of intranuclear inclusion bodies in cell cultures stained with acridine orange was also indicative of the presence of DNA (Hess and Dardiri, 1968). The virion also contains an essential lipid, as indicated by its inactivation with pancreatic lipase (Hess and Dardiri, 1968).

REPLICATION

Breese and Dardiri (1968) studied the development of the virus in cell cultures by electron microscopy of thin sections and by growth curves of intracellular and extracellular virus. Examination of thin sections revealed developmental forms only in the nucleus 12 hours after inoculation. By 24 hours, in addition to viral forms in the nu-

cleus, larger particles with an envelope were observed in the cytoplasm.

Virus titrations of similar cell cultures demonstrated new cell-associated virus 4 hours after inoculation, with a maximum titer reached at 48 hours. Extracellular virus was first detected 6–8 hours after inoculation and reached a maximum titer at 60 hours.

BIOLOGICAL PROPERTIES

The virus of duck plague is nonhemagglutinating (Jansen, 1961) and nonhemadsorbing (Dardiri and Hess, 1968). The virus causes intranuclear inclusions in infected chicken and duck embryo cell cultures (Hess and Dardiri, 1968) (Fig. 24.2). Dardiri and Hess (1968) demonstrated plaque-forming ability of the virus in cell cultures.

RESISTANCE TO CHEMICAL AND PHYSICAL AGENTS

Toth (1968, personal communication) and Hess and Dardiri (1968) found the vi-

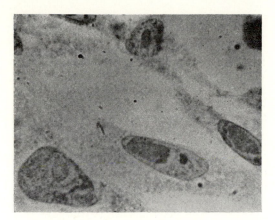

FIG. 24.2—*Inclusion bodies in duck embryo fibroblasts infected with duck plague virus.* ×25,000. *(Courtesy Plum Island Animal Disease Laboratory)*

rus to be sensitive to ether and chloroform. Exposing the virus for 18 hours at 37° C to trypsin, chymotrypsin, and pancreatic lipase markedly reduced or inactivated the virus. However, papain, lysozyme, cellulase, DNase, and RNase had no effect.

Thermal Stability

Thermal inactivation studies by Hess and Dardiri (1968) revealed the virus to be destroyed after heating for 10 minutes at 56° C. It required 90–120 minutes to inactivate the virus at 50° C. At room temperature (22° C) the infectivity was lost after 30 days. Drying over calcium chloride at 22° C resulted in inactivation after 9 days.

pH Stability

Exposure of the virus for 6 hours at pH levels of 7, 8, and 9 resulted in no loss of titer, but a measurable titer reduction was noted at pH 5, 6, and 10. At pH 3 and 11 the virus was rapidly inactivated. A marked difference in inactivation rates was noted between pH 10 and 10.5 (Hess and Dardiri, 1968).

STRAIN CLASSIFICATION

While differences in virulence between strains of duck plague virus have been noted, all strains appear immunologically identical (Jansen, 1968; Dardiri and Hess, 1968). The virus is immunologically distinct from all other known avian viruses, including fowl plague, Newcastle, and duck hepatitis virus (Bos, 1942; Jansen and Kunst, 1949;

Levine and Fabricant, 1950; Dardiri and Hess, 1968).

LABORATORY HOST SYSTEMS

Primary isolations of the virus can best be obtained by propagation on the chorioallantoic membrane of embryonating duck eggs (Jansen, 1961); 9–14-day-old embryonating duck eggs may be employed. While the virus can be adapted to grow in embryonating chicken eggs (Jansen, 1961), eggs are unsatisfactory for primary isolation. The virus has been propagated in duck embryo cell cultures (Kunst, 1967; Dardiri and Hess, 1968) and chicken embryo cell cultures (Dardiri and Hess, 1968). Kunst reported a cytopathic effect of the virus in cell cultures. Dardiri and Hess (1968) demonstrated plaque-forming ability of the virus and developed a cell culture plaque assay method for titrating duck plague viral concentrations and plaque inhibition by neutralizing antisera.

PATHOGENESIS AND EPIZOOTIOLOGY

NATURAL AND EXPERIMENTAL HOSTS

To date, the reported natural susceptibility to duck plague has been limited to members of the family Anatidae (ducks, geese, and swans) of the order Anseriformes. The fact that the virus can be adapted by serial passage to grow in embryonating chicken eggs and even in chickens up to 2 weeks of age (Jansen, 1964b) suggests a wider host range than reported. Natural outbreaks of the disease have been noted in a variety of domestic ducks (*Anas platyrhynchos domesticus*), including the White Pekin, Khaki Campbell, Indian Runner, hybrids, and native ducks of mixed breeding. Grey Call ducks have been found resistant to lethal infection (Van Dorssen and Kunst, 1955). Outbreaks have been noted in Muscovy ducks (*Cairina moschata*) (Jansen, 1961; Leibovitz and Hwang, 1968b; Peckham, 1968, personal communication) and domestic geese (*Anser anser domesticus*) (Jansen and Wemmenhove, 1965).

Domesticated Anseriformes, principally domestic ducks and to a lesser extent domestic geese, are maintained in large numbers in concentrated duck- and goose-producing areas. The producers maintain a continuous surveillance for the presence and diagnosis of anseriform disease. Accordingly the reported incidence of duck plague in domesticated Anseriforms compared to that of the relatively unobserved wild waterfowl may be misleading. An appraisal of the importance of this disease to wild waterfowl has not been made; however, outbreaks of the disease in domestic ducks are frequently associated with aquatic environments that are cohabited by wild waterfowl (DeZeeuw, 1930; Leibovitz and Hwang, 1968b).

Van Dorssen and Kunst (1955) studied the experimental susceptibility of various species of Anseriformes to duck plague. In addition to the domesticated species, they found mallards *(Anas platyrhynchos platyrhynchos)*, Garganey teal *(Anas querquedula)*, gadwall *(Anas strepera)*, European widgeon *(Anas penelope)*, wood ducks *(Aix sponsa)*, shovelers *(Spatula clypeata)*, sheldducks *(Tadorna tadorna)*, tufted ducks *(Aythya fuligula)*, common pochards *(Aythya ferina)*, common eiders *(Somateria mollissima)*, white-fronted geese *(Anser albifrons)*, bean geese *(Anser fabalis)*, and mute swans *(Cygnus olor)* susceptible to lethal infection. European teal *(Anas crecca)* and pintails *(Anas acuta)* were resistant to the lethal effects but produced antibodies against the virus as a result of experimental exposure. Mallards were more resistant to the lethal effects, and Van Dorssen and Kunst considered this species as a possible natural reservoir of infection.

Of the order Charadriiformes, herring gulls *(Larus argentatus)* and black-headed gulls *(Larus ridibundus)* were not susceptible to experimental infection and failed to produce antibodies against the virus (Van Dorssen and Kunst, 1955).

The first reported outbreaks of the spontaneous disease in wild waterfowl were noted in the state of New York on Long Island (Leibovitz and Hwang, 1968a; Leibovitz, 1968). The disease was detected in mallards, black ducks *(Anas rubripes)*, a Canada goose *(Branta canadensis)*, a bufflehead *(Bucephala albeola)*, a greater scaup *(Aythya marila)*, and a mute swan *(Cygnus olor)*. In addition, the disease has been detected in domestic Muscovy ducks *(Cairina moschata)* and wild mute swans in central New York State, in Canada geese *(Branta canadensis)* and Egyptian geese *(Alopochen aegyptiacus)* in Pennsylvania, and in a black duck in Maryland.

Day-old chicks can be infected with the virus; after serial passages through day-old chicks, infection has been produced in chicks up to 2 weeks of age (Jansen, 1968).

TRANSMISSION

Duck plague can be transmitted directly by contact between infected and susceptible birds and indirectly by contact with a contaminated environment. Since waterfowl are dependent upon an aquatic medium that provides a common vehicle for feeding, drinking, and body support, water appears to be the natural medium of transmission of the virus from infected to susceptible individuals. Support of this concept is found in the history of new outbreaks of the disease in domestic ducks which have been limited to birds having access to open bodies of water cohabited by wild, free-flying waterfowl. Once infection is established, however, it can be maintained in the absence of open water or infected birds if susceptible populations are moved into recently contaminated premises.

New loci of infection may be established by the movement of infected waterfowl onto bodies of water previously free of virus contamination. Once virus dispersion occurs, environmental contamination can be increased and sustained by the recycling of infection through new susceptible populations that arrive at the infected aquatic premises. Accordingly the course and duration of the infection is defined by population densities and the rate of transmission between infected and susceptible waterfowl. Population densities in concentrated duck-producing areas encourage rapid spread of the disease with high mortality. Breeder ducks are usually selected and placed in a defined area and maintained in the same location for the balance of their productive life. Once a breeder population is exposed, the disease is self-limiting. In contrast, market ducks are progressively moved as they mature and are relocated in quarters formerly occupied by the next oldest age group. Thus infection in market ducklings tends to be a continuous recycling of infection as susceptible ducklings are moved into the recently contaminated environment.

Experimentally the disease can be transmitted via the oral, intranasal, intravenous, intraperitoneal, intramuscular, and cloacal routes of administration. Potential transmission by blood-sucking arthropods is suggested by the viremic character of the disease.

While the virus has been recovered from an egg removed from the cloaca of an infected domestic duck (Jansen, 1964b), the virus has not been recovered from eggs which have been laid.

While the carrier state has been suspected in wild ducks (DeZeeuw, 1930; Van Dorssen and Kunst, 1955), specific evidence to support this concept has not been reported. Contact between domestic and wild Anseriformes is common and frequently mediated by the use of open bodies of water for duck production.

INCUBATION PERIOD AND AGE

In domestic ducks the incubation period ranges from 3 to 7 days. Once overt signs of the disease appear, death usually follows within 1–5 days. Since natural infection has been observed in ages ranging from 7-day-old ducklings to mature breeder ducks, all ages are susceptible.

SIGNS

In domestic breeder ducks, sudden high and persistent flock mortality is often the first reported observation. Mature ducks die in good flesh. Prolapse of the penis may be evident in dead mature male breeders. In laying flocks a drop in egg production of 25–40% may be noted during the period of greatest mortality.

As the disease progresses within a flock, more signs are observed. Photophobia, associated with half-closed pasted eyelids, inappetence, extreme thirst, droopiness, atax-

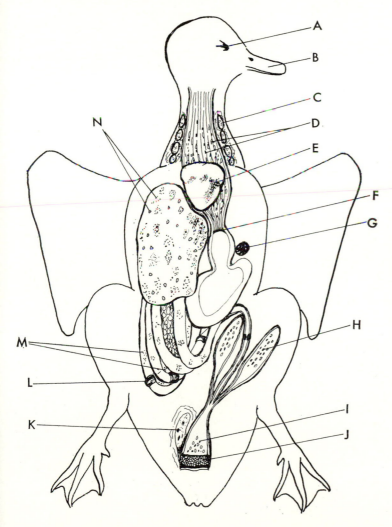

FIG. 24.3—Sketch of duck plague lesions observed in domestic ducks. (A) Sticky half-closed eyes. (B) Blue beak. (C) Pinpoint hemorrhages on thymus and discoloration of adjacent tissues. (D) Hemorrhagic macules and crusty plaques in esophagus. (E) "Paint-brush" hemorrhages on heart. (F) Hemorrhagic esophageal-proventricular sphincter. (G) Dark mottled spleen. (H) Cecal mucosal lesion. (I) Rectal mucosal lesion. (J) Cloacal lesion. (K) Bursal hemorrhages and discoloration of surrounding tissues. (L) Lesion of intestinal annular band. (M) Mesenteric and serosal hemorrhages. (N) Hemorrhages and white spots on liver.

ia, ruffled feathers, nasal discharge, soiled vents, and a watery diarrhea appear. Affected ducks are unable to stand; they maintain a posture with drooping outstretched wings and head down, suggesting weakness and depression. Sick ducks forced to move may evidence tremors of the head, neck, and body.

Young market ducklings 2–7 weeks of age evidence dehydration, loss of weight, blue beaks, and often a bloodstained vent.

MORTALITY

Total mortality in outbreaks in domestic ducks has ranged from 5 to 100%. Morbidity based on the observation that sick birds usually die approaches closely the percentage of mortality. Adult breeder ducks tend to experience greater percentage of mortality than young ducks.

GROSS LESIONS

The specific pathologic response to duck plague virus is dependent upon the species affected (Leibovitz, 1968); age, sex, and susceptibility of the affected host; stage of infection; and virulence and intensity of virus exposure (Leibovitz and Hwang, 1968a,b).

The lesions of duck plague are those of vascular damage (as expressed in tissue hemorrhages and the presence of free blood in body cavities), enanthematous lesions in specific locations on the mucosal surface of the gastrointestinal tract, lesions of lymphoid organs, and retrograde sequelae in parenchymatous organs (Fig. 24.3). These collective lesions, when present, are pathognomonic of duck plague.

Tissue hemorrhages in the form of petechiae, ecchymoses, or larger extravasations may be found on or in the myocardium, other visceral organs, and their supporting structures, including the mesentery and the serosal investments. On the visceral pericardium of the heart, especially within the coronary grooves, closely packed petechiae give the surface a red "paint-brushed" appearance. The latter lesion is observed more frequently in mature breeder ducks than in young market ducklings. When the heart chambers are exposed, endocardial mural and valvular hemorrhages also may be observed.

The surface of the liver, pancreas, intestines, lungs, and kidney may be covered with petechiae. In mature laying females, hemorrhages may be observed in the deformed discolored ovarian follicles (Fig. 24.4), and massive hemorrhages from the ovary may fill the abdominal cavity. The lumina of the intestines and gizzard are often filled with blood. The esophageal-proventricular sphincter appears as a hemorrhagic ring at the junction of the two organs.

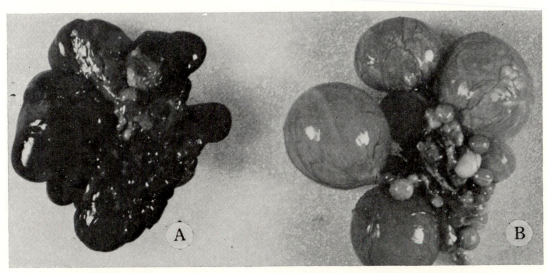

FIG. 24.4—(A) Free hemorrhage in deformed discolored ovarian follicles of mature White Pekin duck affected with duck plague. (B) Ovary of normal mature breeder duck.

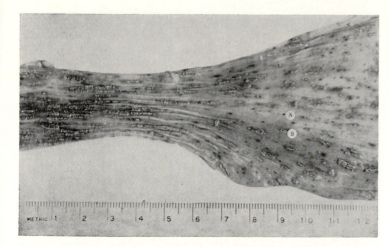

FIG. 24.5—Mucosal lesions on longitudinal folds of esophagus of mature White Pekin duck infected with duck plague. (A) Hemorrhagic macular lesions. (B) Supplemental crusty necrotic plaques appearing later in course of disease.

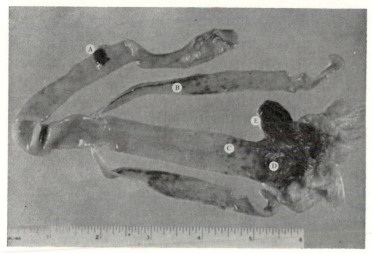

FIG. 24.6—Mucosal lesions of posterior digestive tract of 4-week-old White Pekin duckling. (A) Dark (red) posterior ileal annular band. (B) Hemorrhagic macular cecal lesions. (C) Hemorrhagic macular rectal lesions. (D) Cloacal lesions composed of dark (green) closely packed crusty plaques. (E) Thin-walled dark (red) bursa of Fabricius.

Specific digestive enanthematous mucosal lesions are found in the esophagus (Fig. 24.5), ceca, rectum, and cloaca (Fig. 24.6). Each of these lesions undergoes progressive alterations during the course of the disease. Initially, macular surface hemorrhages appear, which are later covered by elevated yellowish white crusty plaques. This type of lesion subsequently becomes organized into a green superficial scab devoid of its former hemorrhagic base. These lesions range in size from approximately 1 mm to 1 cm in length. In the esophagus and cloaca these lesions may become confluent; however, close inspection will reveal their composite structure. In the esophagus the macules occur parallel to the longitudinal folds. When the macular concentrations are great, the smaller lesions may merge to form larger ones, suggesting a patchy diphtheritic membrane. In young ducklings individual lesions of the esophagus are less frequent; sloughing of the entire mucosa tends to occur, and the lumen becomes lined with a thin yellowish white membrane.

In the ceca the macular lesions are singular, separated, and well defined between the folds of the mucosal surface. The external surface of the affected ceca presents a barred and congested appearance.

Rectal lesions are usually few in number with greatest concentration at the posterior portion of the rectum, adjacent to the cloaca.

In the cloaca (Fig. 24.6) macular lesions are densely packed, and initially the entire mucosa appears reddened. Later the individual plaquelike elevations become green in color and form a continuous scalelike band lining the lumen of the organ.

All lymphoid organs are affected. The

spleen tends to be normal or smaller in size, dark in color, and mottled (Fig. 24.8). The thymus has multiple petechiae and yellow focal areas, both on the surface and when sectioned. These are surrounded by a zone of clear yellow fluid which infiltrates and discolors the subcutaneous tissues of the adjacent cervical region, i.e. from the thoracic inlet to the upper third of the neck. The latter lesion is of importance in meat inspection and is easily detected as the opened neck of the carcass is observed on the processing line. The bursa of Fabricius during early infection is intensely reddened (Fig. 24.6). The exterior becomes surrounded by a clear yellow fluid that discolors the adjacent tissue of the pelvic cavity. When the lumen of the bursa is opened, pinpoint yellow areas are found on an intensely reddened surface. Later during the course of the infection, the walls of the bursa become thin and dark in color, and the bursa cavity is filled with a white coagulated exudate. The intestinal annular bands (Fig. 24.7) appear as intensely reddened rings visible both from the external surface and the internal surface of the intestines. Yellow pinpoint areas can be observed on the mucosal surface, and later during infection the entire band becomes a dark brown color and tends to separate at its margins from the internal surface of the intestines. (The annular bands are 4 normal, regularly spaced lymphoid organs that are located in the anterior and posterior portions of those regions of the avian intestines commonly referred to in mammals as the jejunum and ileum. The bands are approximately 1 cm wide. When viewed from the serosal surface, they give the appearance of ringlike transverse dilations of the intestinal wall. Inside the lumen of the organ they form slight elevations of the mucosal circumference. The posterior ileal annular band can be found on that portion of the ileum located between the 2 attached ceca and is usually an incomplete ring. The anterior ileal and posterior jejunal annular bands are well-defined, complete rings, while the anterior jejunal band is faint and poorly defined.)

Of the parenchymatous organs, the liver offers the greatest surface area for examination. During early stages of infection, the entire liver surface is a pale copper color with the admixture of irregularly distributed pinpoint hemorrhages and white focal areas, which give the surface a heterogeneous speckled appearance (Fig. 24.8). Late stages of infection are characterized by dark bronze or bile-stained livers without the previously noted hemorrhages, and the white focal areas on the surface are larger and more distinct on this darkened background.

While the above lesions are representative of the general findings of duck plague, each age group responds distinctively. In

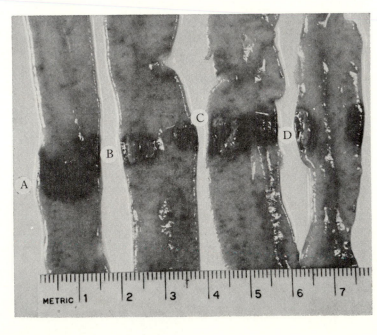

FIG. 24.7—Lesions of intestinal annular bands of 4-week-old White Pekin duckling infected with duck plague. (A) Anterior jejunal annular band. (B) Posterior jejunal annular band. (C) Anterior ileal annular band. (D) Posterior ileal annular band. Note dark (red) bands with lighter (yellow) plaques and pinpoint hemorrhages on intestinal mucosa.

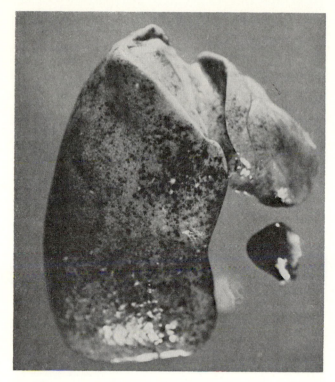

FIG. 24.8—Liver and spleen of 5-week-old White Pekin duckling affected with duck plague. Note pale (copper) liver surface marked by pinpoint to larger hemorrhages and irregular white focal areas representative of early stages of infection. Spleen is slightly smaller than normal with dark mottling.

ducklings tissue hemorrhages are less pronounced and lymphoid lesions are more prominent. In mature domestic ducks with regressed bursa of Fabricius and thymus, the tissue hemorrhages and reproductive tract lesions predominate.

In geese the intestinal lymphoid discs (ILD) (Leibovitz, 1969b) are analogous to the annular bands found in ducks. In a single Canada goose, lesions of the ILD resembled "buttonlike ulcers" (Leibovitz, 1969a). Similar intestinal lesions have been observed by Locke (1968, personal communication) in an outbreak of duck plague in Canada geese and Egyptian geese.

HISTOPATHOLOGY

The initial injury produced by duck plague virus is an alteration of the walls of the blood vessels. Although some alterations can be noted in the larger blood vessels, the smaller blood vessels, venules, and capillaries are more markedly involved. The endothelial lining is broken, and the connective tissue elements of the wall become less compact, with visible separations at those points where extravasations of the blood elements pass from the lumen through the thin ruptured wall into the tissue proper. As a result of vascular damage, the dependent tissues undergo progressive retrograde changes. Accordingly, tissue changes proceed from those of hemorrhage to necrosis. Such microscopic changes can be found within any of the visceral organs, including those that are free of gross lesions.

The specific gross digestive enanthematous lesions are represented microscopically by areas of hemorrhage and subsequent necrosis of the mucosal surface, adjacent to superficial concentrations of small blood vessels in the submucosa. Such collections of blood vessels can be found in the longitudinal esophageal mucosal folds; at the proventricular-esophageal sphincter; and within the small intestinal, cecal, rectal, and cloacal mucosa.

In addition to the vascular damage described, a selective tissue destruction is noted in all lymphoid organs. This includes the thymus, the bursa of Fabricius, the spleen, the intestinal annular bands, and other focal collections of lymphoid tissue within the digestive tract (esophageal-proventricular sphincter and posterior margins of the cloaca). Within these lymphoid organs, lymphocytes and the reticular syncytium are destroyed.

Although inclusion bodies have been reported in affected tissues (Dardiri et al., 1967; Leibovitz and Hwang, 1968a), the specific significance of these inclusion bodies has not as yet been established.

On the basis of histopathologic findings, the lesions of duck plague are noninflammatory and degenerative in character. The distribution of gross and microscopic lesions suggests this virus to be reticuloendotheliotrophic. However, more work is needed to characterize the histopathologic findings.

IMMUNITY

Recovered birds are immune to reinfection by duck plague virus. An active immunity has been demonstrated following use of a modified live virus vaccine (Jansen, 1964b). Parental (egg-transmitted) immunity has been demonstrated in ducklings and may interfere with the response to live virus vaccine (Toth, 1968, personal communication). Passive immunization has not been reported.

DIAGNOSIS

The complete gross lesions seen at necropsy are diagnostic of duck plague. Histopathologic studies can further support these findings. The isolation and identification of the virus provide a confirmation, even in the absence of diagnostic morphologic alterations. The isolation of a virus that fails to propagate in chicken embryos, that grows when inoculated on the chorioallantoic membrane of 9–14-day-old embryonating duck eggs, and that produces the characteristic lesions and mortality when inoculated into susceptible day-old ducklings is highly suggestive of the duck plague virus. The neutralization of such an isolate by known duck plague antisera confirms the identification. An increase in the serum neutralization titer following convalescence from the disease would demonstrate the progress of the disease within a flock. A virus neutralization index of 1.75 and more indicates infection experience with the duck plague virus (Dardiri and Hess, 1967). A virus neutralization index of 0.0–1.5 log 10, ELD_{50} was found in sera of domestic and wild waterfowl that had reportedly not been exposed to the disease. The use of chicken embryo-adapted duck plague virus in chicken eggs for serum neutralization studies would be more conveni-

ent and safer than the use of field strain viruses inoculated onto the chorioallantoic membrane of duck eggs (Dardiri and Hess, 1967).

Differential diagnosis requires consideration of other diseases that produce hemorrhagic and necrotic lesions in Anseriformes. In domestic ducks the common diseases that produce such alterations are duck virus hepatitis, pasteurellosis, necrotic and hemorrhagic enteritis, trauma, drake damage, and specific intoxications. While Newcastle disease, fowl pox, and fowl plague are reported to produce similar changes in Anseriformes, these diseases have been infrequently reported.

PREVENTION AND CONTROL

There are no reported treatments for duck plague infection. Prevention is achieved by maintaining susceptible birds in environments free of exposure to the duck plague virus. These measures include the addition of stock known to be free of duck plague and avoiding contact and traffic with possible contaminated material. The introduction of the disease by wild, free-flying Anseriformes and contaminated aquatic environments must be prevented. Once the disease has been introduced, control can be effected by depopulation, removal of the birds from the infected environment, sanitation, and disinfection. All possible measures should be taken to prevent dissemination of the virus by free-flowing water. If authorized by government agencies, all susceptible ducklings should be vaccinated with a chicken embryo-adapted duck plague vaccine.

If the disease is not an enzootic infection and is truly exotic, measures should be taken to further prevent the entry and dissemination into geographic areas known to be free of the disease. This would include specific examination to prevent the importation of infected Anseriformes. Accordingly, a surveillance would be made of ornamental bird collectors, zoos, and domestic growers of Anseriformes. Efforts should be made to increase the efficiency of detection of this disease by laboratory workers and waterfowl specialists, in order that its presence, status, and importance be better defined.

IMMUNIZATION

Immunization has been employed as a

preventive measure and also in controlling disease outbreaks.

Inactivated Vaccine

Butterfield and Dardiri (1968) have studied the effectiveness of inactivated vaccine. Field experience suggests that inactivated vaccines currently employed are not as efficacious as the modified live virus vaccine.

Live Virus Vaccine

A chicken embryo-adapted strain of duck plague virus that is avirulent for domestic ducks has been developed by Jansen (1964b) and has been extensively employed with good success in the Netherlands. This vaccine strain has been employed with limited success in outbreaks of the disease on commercial duck farms on Long Island. Jansen (1964a) has reported an interference phenomenon following vaccination. Vaccinated birds acquired a resistance to infection as early as the 1st day following vaccination. In Long Island outbreaks on commercial duck farms, the protection afforded by the interference phenomenon has not been as dramatic; persistent field infections have been observed in vaccinated flocks.

To date, the modified chicken embryo-adapted vaccine has been limited to experimental use and has not been authorized for general distribution in the United States. The vaccine was administered in 0.5-ml doses by the subcutaneous route in domestic ducklings over 2 weeks of age. The vaccine strain does not spread among contacts. Apparently vaccinated ducklings do not excrete the inoculated virus to a degree that would be sufficient to bring about contact immunization (Jansen, 1968).

REFERENCES

Baudet, A. E. R. F. 1923. (Mortality in ducks in the Netherlands caused by a filtrable virus; fowl plague.) *Tijdschr. Diergeneesk.* 50:455–59.

Bos, A. 1942. (Some new cases of duck plague.) *Tijdschr. Diergeneesk.* 69:372–81.

Breese, S. S., Jr., and A. H. Dardiri. 1968. Electron microscopic characterization of duck plague virus. *Virology* 34:160–69.

Butterfield, W. K., and A. H. Dardiri. 1968. Serologic and immunologic response of ducks to inactivated and attenuated duck plague virus. *Proc. Ann. Meet. Am. Soc. Microbiol.,* p. 161. (Abstr.)

Dardiri, A. H., and W. R. Hess. 1967. The incidence of neutralizing antibodies to duck plague virus in serums from domestic ducks and wild waterfowl in the United States of of America. *Proc. 71st Ann. Meet. U.S. Livestock Sanit. Ass.,* pp. 225–37.

———. 1968. A plaque assay for duck plague virus. *Can. J. Comp. Med. Vet. Sci.* 32: 505–10.

Dardiri, A. H., W. R. Hess, S. S. Breese, Jr., and H. R. Seibold. 1967. Characterization of duck plague virus from a duck disease outbreak in the United States. *Proc. 39th N.E. Conf. on Avian Diseases,* p. 14. (Abstr.)

Devos, A., N. Viaene, and H. Statelens. 1964. (Duck plague in Belgium.) *Vlaams Diergeneesk. Tijdschr.* 33:260–66.

DeZeeuw, F. A. 1930. Nieuwe gevallen van eendenpest en de specificiteit van het virus. *Tijdschr. Diergeneesk.* 57:1095–98.

Hess, W. R., and A. H. Dardiri. 1968. Some properties of the virus of duck plague. *Arch. Ges. Virusforsch.* 24:148–53.

Jansen, J. 1961. Duck plague. *Brit. Vet. J.* 117:349–56.

———. 1963. (About the incidence of duck plague.) *Tijdschr. Diergeneesk.* 88:1341–43.

———. 1964a. The interference phenomenon in the development of resistance against duck plague. *J. Comp. Pathol. Therap.* 74: 3–7.

———. 1964b. Duck plague (a concise survey). *Indian Vet. J.* 41:309–16.

———. 1968. Duck plague. *J. Am. Vet. Med. Ass.* 152:1009–16.

Jansen, J., and H. Kunst. 1949. Is duck plague related to Newcastle disease or to fowl plague? *Proc. XIV Int. Vet. Congr.* 2:363–65.

———. 1964. The reported incidence of duck plague in Europe and Asia. *Tijdschr. Diergeneesk.* 89:765–69.

Jansen, J., and R. Wemmenhove. 1965. (Duck plague in domesticated geese [*Anser anser*].) *Tijdschr. Diergeneesk.* 90:811–15.

Kunst, H. 1967. Isolation of duck plague virus in tissue cultures. *Tijdschr. Diergeneesk.* 92: 713–14.

Leibovitz, L. 1968. Progress report: Duck plague surveillance of American Anseriformes. *Bull. Wildlife Disease Ass.* 4:87–90.

———. 1969a. Comparative pathology of duck plague in wild Anseriformes. *J. Wildlife Management* 33:294–303.

———. 1969b. Duck plague, pp. 22–33. In Davis, J. W., R. C. Anderson, Lars Karstad, and D. O. Trainer (eds.), *Infectious and Parasitic Diseases of Wild Birds.* Iowa State Univ. Press, Ames.

———. 1971. Gross and histopathologic changes of duck plague (duck virus enteritis). *Am. J. Vet. Res.* 32:275–90.

Leibovitz, L., and J. Hwang. 1968a. Duck plague on the American continent. *Avian Diseases* 12:361–78.

———. 1968b. Duck plague in American Anseriformes. *Bull. Wildlife Disease Ass.* 4: 13–14.

Levine, P. P., and J. Fabricant. 1950. A hitherto-undescribed virus disease of ducks in North America. *Cornell Vet.* 40:71–86.

Lucam, F. 1949. La peste aviaire en France. *Rept. 14th Int. Vet. Congr.* 2:380–82.

Mukerji, A., M. S. Das, B. B. Ghosh, and J. L.

Ganguly. 1963. Duck plague in West Bengal. I and II. *Indian Vet. J.* 40:457–62,

———. 1965. Duck plague in West Bengal. III. *Indian Vet. J.* 42:811–15.

Urban, W. D. 1968. Current status of duck virus enteritis (duck plague). *Proc. 40th N.E. Conf. Avian Diseases*, p. 69. (Abstr.)

USDA. 1967. *Duck Virus Enteritis.* Federal Register 32 (89):7012–13.

Van Dorssen, C. A., and H. Kunst. 1955. (Susceptibility of ducks and various other waterfowl to duck plague virus.) *Tijdschr. Diergeneesk.* 80:1286–95.

CHAPTER 25

TRANSMISSIBLE ENTERITIS OF TURKEYS (BLUECOMB) AND HEMORRHAGIC ENTERITIS

❖

B. S. POMEROY

Department of Veterinary Bacteriology and Public Health College of Veterinary Medicine St. Paul, Minnesota

❖

TRANSMISSIBLE ENTERITIS OF TURKEYS (BLUECOMB)

❖

TRANSMISSIBLE ENTERITIS (bluecomb disease) is an acute highly infectious disease affecting turkeys of all ages. It is characterized by loss of appetite, weight loss, and wet droppings.

Synonyms are mud fever of turkeys (Peterson and Hymas, 1951) and bluecomb disease of turkeys (Pomeroy and Sieburth, 1953).

Surveys of turkey growers conducted by the State-Federal Crop and Livestock Reporting Service in Minnesota in 1951, 1956, 1961, and 1966 indicate that transmissible enteritis was the most costly disease encountered by the turkey industry in that state. In 1966 it was estimated that 19% of the flocks experienced loss from the disease. Previous reports indicated that flocks involved varied from a low of 14% in 1951 to 31% in 1961. In 1968 the number of flocks involved was lower than in 1966. This reduction resulted from changes in production in areas that have had a constant problem with the disease. The estimated value of the birds lost in 1966 was $519,000, and morbidity losses would greatly increase that figure. It has been established from cost of production studies of field outbreaks that 2–4 cents per pound is added to the cost of production in flocks experiencing the disease. In Minnesota in 1966 the disease alone accounted for 23% of turkey death losses from all causes. Because of the change in turkey production to a year-round operation on many farms, the disease is encountered frequently in young birds before they are placed on ranges. This is particularly true in areas that have heavy concentrations of turkeys and the disease is enzootic the year around.

HISTORY

Peterson and Hymas (1951) described an unfamiliar disease of turkeys, observed in the state of Washington for the previous 7 years and known locally as "mud fever," which had the general characteristics of pullet disease in chickens. Pomeroy and Sieburth (1953) reported on an extensive outbreak of the disease that occurred in Minnesota in 1951. A similar condition had been recognized as occurring sporadically in turkey flocks on range for several years. In the 1951 outbreak severe losses were recognized in young turkeys for the first time. In the earlier outbreaks the disease has been designated as trichomoniasis of the lower intestinal tract because of the presence of increased numbers of trichomonads in the ceca and rectum. E. I. Boyer (1953, personal communication) reported on the disease in New York as having a similar pattern to that described in Minnesota. The disease was recognized in Virginia as a serious disease problem in young turkeys (Sieburth and Johnson, 1957). Ferguson (1961) reported the disease had occurred in Ontario for several years and in 1959 had become a serious problem.

INCIDENCE AND DISTRIBUTION

Published and personal reports indicate that the disease is widely distributed in the United States and Canada, particularly in highly concentrated turkey-producing areas. The more severe outbreaks are noted in areas that practice multiple brooding and essentially have year-round turkey production. Until the etiologic agent is identified and diagnostic tests are available, the true distribution of the disease in the United States will not be known.

ETIOLOGY

The exact cause of transmissible enteritis has not been fully characterized. Pomeroy and Sieburth (1953) demonstrated the infectious nature of the disease and were able to reproduce the disease with unfiltered intestinal contents. Tissues other than the intestinal tract did not harbor the transmissible agent. Sieburth (1954) studied various bacterial isolates from the intestinal tract of infected poults but was unable to reproduce the disease with various types of microorganisms. The agent failed to pass Seitz EK, Berkefeld N, and sintered glass UF filters. Sieburth and Pomeroy (1955) reported additional studies on the etiology but were unsuccessful in isolating a specific agent. Tumlin et al. (1957) established that the agent readily passed Berkefeld and Selas filters of the smallest pore size but would not pass through a Seitz EK filter. Sieburth and Johnson (1957) reported similar findings. Tumlin and Pomeroy (1958b) found that 1:2 dilutions of serum from recovered field cases completely neutralized Selas 02 filtrates of agent-bearing intestinal contents, but no evidence of measurable passive immunity was found in their progeny. Truscott et al. (1960) isolated a small gram-negative anaerobic pleomorphic rod from the intestinal tract which they considered to be the etiologic agent. Truscott and Morin (1964) further characterized the agent as a member of the genus *Vibrio* and reproduced the disease with vibrio cultures. Vibrio isolations were made from the liver and bile as well as intestinal tract. Serological studies suggested that at least 3 serological types were isolated. The relationship of these vibrios to the vibrio associated with avian hepatitis was not established. Truscott (1968) further reported on studies using vibrio cultures and reproduced transmissible enteritis by the inoculation of vibrios via the oral, intravenous, or intraperitoneal routes of inoculation; transmission was accomplished with intestinal suspensions from affected poults. Sharma (1968) studied 5 strains of microaerophilic vibrios isolated from bluecomb-infected turkeys in-

cluding an isolate from Truscott. Serial passages in poults and turkeys did not enhance the virulence of any strain. Vibrios were noninfective to day-old poults when given alone by oral or intraperitoneal route. The disease was reproduced with bacteria-free filtrates of intestinal contents of bluecomb-infected turkeys in both conventional and germ-free reared poults. His results did not support the findings of Truscott. C. T. Larsen (1964, unpublished data) has also investigated extensively the role of vibrios isolated from field outbreaks. He consistently isolated an enterovirus on the chorioallantoic membrane of embryonating chicken eggs from filtrates of intestinal material but failed to reproduce the disease with the isolated virus, whereas the filtrates inoculated orally into day-old poults reproduced the disease. Deshmukh et al. (1969) recovered 9 viral isolates from intestinal specimens of suspected outbreaks from widely separated geographical areas. Five of these isolates were characterized and classified: one was a papovavirus, two were reoviruses, and two were enteroviruses. Pathogenicity and immunogenicity studies revealed no etiologic association between the viruses and transmissible enteritis. Wooley and Gratzek (1969) isolated from field outbreaks of bluecomb disease in Georgia 5 viral isolates on chicken embryonic kidney cells. The viruses appeared to be either reo- or picornavirus. Fujisaki et al. (1969) reported on the recovery of several virus isolates from the intestinal tracts of infected turkeys. The isolates belonged to the reovirus group. The results of inoculation and immunoserologic studies suggested that these viruses were involved in the bluecomb syndrome. Hofstad et al. (1969) were not able to reproduce the disease with pure cultures of vibrios but were able to reproduce the disease with filtrates passed through Millipore 0.3μ or 0.22μ filters. Iowa and Minnesota isolates were studied and found to be immunologically similar. The etiologic agent was not successfully cultivated in embryonating chicken and turkey eggs or cell cultures.

PATHOGENESIS

HOSTS

The disease affects turkeys of all ages. Various attempts to infect chickens have met with failure (Pomeroy and Sieburth,

1953; Sieburth and Johnson, 1957). C. T. Larsen (1968, unpublished data) was unable to infect chickens, pheasants, and seagulls. Hofstad et al. (1969) were unable to transmit the disease to Coturnix quail and hamsters.

TRANSMISSION

The disease is readily transmitted by unfiltered and filtered intestinal material by the oral or rectal route. Filtrates given intraperitoneally will reproduce the disease, but intramuscular and subcutaneous routes fail to infect the poults. Suspensions of heart, liver, spleen, kidney, and pancreas from infected turkeys did not cause the disease when administered orally to day-old poults.

Under natural conditions the disease spreads rapidly through a flock and from flock to flock on the same farm. Circumstantial evidence indicates that the disease is spread from farm to farm by personnel, equipment, and vehicles. Free-flying birds may serve as mechanical vectors.

There is no evidence that the disease is egg-transmitted, but the infection may be introduced into started poults in a hatchery battery room and then transmitted to poults shipped from the hatchery.

The agent is eliminated in the droppings of turkeys recovered from the disease for several months and will remain viable in intestinal tracts stored at $-20°$ C or lower for over 5 years. It is readily destroyed under laboratory conditions in cages and batteries by cleaning and sanitizing and allowing 4 days or more of depopulation. Under field conditions in turkey brooder buildings that can be cleaned and sanitized and allowed 3–4 weeks or more of depopulation, there is a die-off of the agent. However, in pole barns, yards, and ranges the agent may survive in frozen feces from one year to the next even though the farm is depopulated of turkeys (Pomeroy and Sieburth, 1953; Larsen and Pomeroy, 1968, unpublished data).

INCUBATION PERIOD

The incubation period is 48–72 hours but may be as short as 24 hours or as long as 5 days. The feed intake usually drops within 24 hours, loss of body weight occurs within 48 hours, and lower body temperature is noted within 48 hours, with watery droppings correlated with drop in feed intake (Pomeroy and Sieburth, 1953; Larsen and Pomeroy, 1968, unpublished data).

SIGNS

In young poults the disease appears suddenly; there is depression, subnormal body temperature, anorexia, loss of body weight, and frothy or watery droppings. There is constant chirping and poults seek heat. In growing turkeys the appearance of the disease is sudden with a concurrent drop in feed and water consumption with watery droppings, subnormal body temperature, and loss of body weight. The flock is depressed and sick birds show darkening of the head and skin with a sunken crop (Fig. 25.1). The droppings may contain mucous threads and casts and may be greenish to brownish in color. As the disease progresses in a flock and water and feed consumption continues depressed, the droppings contain primarily urates. In turkeys in production a pattern similar to that in growing turkeys is encountered; in addition there is a rapid drop in egg production and eggshells are chalky (Pomeroy and Sieburth, 1953; Larsen and Pomeroy, 1968, unpublished data).

Dziuk et al. (1969a) reported on extensive studies on physiological effects of fasting and bluecomb disease in turkeys. Medium white 8–10-week-old turkeys were used in the studies. During bluecomb disease, reductions occurred in body weight, ingestion and excretion of dry matter and water, and rectal temperature which were comparable to those seen in control-fasted turkeys.

MORBIDITY AND MORTALITY

Nearly 100% of the flock shows evidence of infection, with loss of weight varying on the degree to which individual birds go off feed and water. Environmental conditions play an important role on the loss that may be sustained in a flock under natural conditions. Under experimental conditions in young poults the loss may vary from 50 to 100%. In older birds (6–8 weeks) the loss may approach 50%, whereas under field conditions the losses may vary from 5 to 50% with higher losses occasionally encountered. In young turkeys 4–8 weeks of age the death loss may be kept to a minimum if supplemental heat is provided. In range turkeys 8 weeks or older, the loss may be low but is dependent on environmental

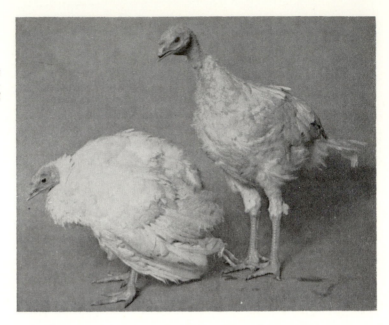

FIG. 25.1—*Turkey on left with signs of transmissible enteritis (bluecomb). Normal mate on right.*

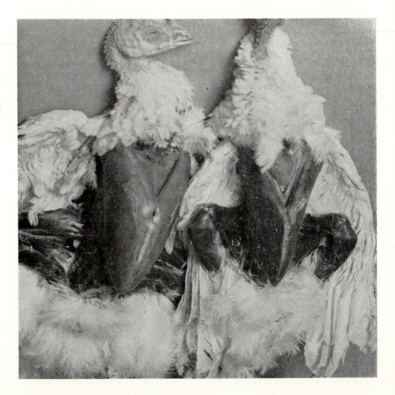

FIG. 25.2—*Exposed breast of normal turkey on left. Breast on right from affected turkey shows dehydration and loss of flesh.*

conditions. If adverse weather conditions prevail, the loss may be as high as 25–50%.

The course of the disease may extend over a period of 10 days to 2 weeks and may require several weeks for the birds to regain lost weight. In mature birds, particularly males, some never regain satisfactory weight, and there is a general unevenness in the flock. The morbidity loss may be high because of the loss of weight, stunted birds, and inability of the flock to mature at a normal rate.

GROSS LESIONS

The gross lesions are confined primarily to the intestinal tract. The contents of the duodenum, jejunum, and ceca are watery and gaseous. There may be a gelatinous mucus and occasionally casts. The ceca are distended and filled with watery, yellowish brown contents having a fetid odor. Small petechial hemorrhages may be noted on the surface of the intestinal mucosa.

The breast muscle usually appears dehydrated, and the carcass is generally emaciated (Fig. 25.2). The internal organs are usually normal, but abnormalities are noted occasionally. The pancreas may have a chalky appearance with numerous whitish areas. Urate deposits may occasionally be present in the kidneys and ureters. The spleen is frequently smaller than normal (Pomeroy and Sieburth, 1953; Sieburth, 1954; Sieburth and Pomeroy, 1955).

HISTOPATHOLOGY

Hilton (1954) examined tissues from experimentally and spontaneously infected turkeys. With the exception of the adrenals and intestinal tract none of the organs showed significant changes. The adrenals revealed a complete obliteration due to large numbers of round cells with hyperchromatic nuclei. The pancreas showed numerous foci of acinar cells revealing a hydropic degeneration. Lymphoid foci were numerous. In the cytoplasm of many cells an eosinophilic inclusion, varying in size up to twice the diameter of the nucleus, was noted. Giemsa-stained sections revealed that the pancreatic inclusions probably originated as aggregates of intracytoplasmic granules.

A time sequence study of intestinal lesions showed that at 2 days postinfection there was a prominent concentration of goblet cells on the tips of the villi (N. R. Adams, 1969, personal communication). Epithelial cells were more cuboidal and lost their microvilli. The lamina propria was infiltrated with mononuclear cells and was separated from the epithelium. At 3 days postinfection nearly all goblet cells had disappeared, and epithelial cells appeared washed out. Lesions were most distinct in the jejunum but were also seen in the duodenum, ileum, and cecum. Over the following 2 weeks goblet cells reappeared, and epithelial cells regained their microvilli and normal density. The infiltration of lamina propria gradually subsided.

It was also noted that argentaffin cell numbers decreased gradually until the 7th day postinfection. The argentaffin cells were normal by the 21st day.

HEMATOLOGY

Hilton (1954) found a marginal hemoconcentration and a definite monocytosis which occurred on the 8th and 9th days of the infection and was preceded by a transitory heterophilia and a lymphocytosis.

CHEMICAL PATHOLOGY

Dziuk et al. (1969a) reported that infected turkeys had a negative balance for both Na^+ and K^+. Additionally, plasma Na^+, K^+, Cl^-, and osmolality were significantly reduced in infected turkeys. Dziuk and Evanson (1969) continued these studies and found that there were differences in balances and body concentrations of Na^+ and K^+ between the control-fed group and infected and fasted groups. Negative Na^+ and K^+ balances were similar in both fasted groups (control and infected) while the noninfected control-fed group had a positive balance. Duke et al. (1969) used the transit times of 51_{Cr} as a means of estimating characteristics of gastrointestinal motility in turkeys. Turkeys having severe signs of the disease had longer transit time, less frequent excretion, and smaller recovery of 51_{Cr}.

Active

Turkeys that have recovered from experimental infections of transmissible enteritis have been challenged 3–4 weeks later or longer and have resisted challenge. Field observations have indicated that flocks recovering from the disease do not suffer a second attack (Pomeroy and Sieburth, 1953; Sieburth, 1954; Larsen and Pomeroy, 1968, unpublished data).

Passive

Serum from birds that had recovered from the disease was filtered and 1 ml was given subcutaneously to day-old poults, and then the poults were exposed to experimental infections. The serum gave no protection (Pomeroy and Sieburth, 1953). Additional studies indicated that parental immunity was lacking completely or was very low when poults from recovered and susceptible breeding flocks were challenged with filtrates of infected intestinal material (Tumlin and Pomeroy, 1958b).

DIAGNOSIS

Since the causative agent has not been isolated, there are no specific laboratory procedures to identify the disease. History, signs, and lesions are very helpful, but to verify the clinical observations, unfiltered and filtered intestinal material may be inoculated orally into day-old poults. Weight gains, rectal temperature, mortality, and lesions in the inoculated poults should be compared to a control group. To further verify the transmission of the disease, serial passage may be made using filtered intestinal material.

DIFFERENTIAL DIAGNOSIS

In young poults the disease must be differentiated from inanition (starve-outs), water deprivation, hexamitiasis, salmonellosis, and related infections. Flocks that have been medicated may have complicating infection of moniliasis. In growing and mature birds increased numbers of trichomonads are found in the contents of the ceca and rectums. Their role in natural outbreaks is not known. The possibility of known specific infections such as erysipelas, fowl cholera, and enterohepatitis must be eliminated by laboratory studies.

TREATMENT

Various types of treatments have been tried under controlled laboratory and field conditions—antibiotics, drugs, chemicals, vitamin supplements, immune serum, and clostridial antitoxin. No regime has been found that will completely prevent the disease. Antibiotics and other drugs may be helpful in reducing the mortality. The effectiveness may be related to the control of secondary infections such as *E. coli* and salmonellae. Peterson and Hymas (1951) reported success in individual oral treatment of turkeys with penicillin, chlortetracycline, and oxytetracycline. At 500 g per ton in the feed or 1.0 g per gallon of drinking water, penicillin, chlortetracycline, oxytetracycline, and streptomycin were effective in reducing death loss but had little effect on morbidity (Pomeroy and Sieburth, 1953; Sieburth and Pomeroy, 1956; Pomeroy, 1956a,b; Larsen and Pomeroy, 1968, unpublished data). Tumlin and Pomeroy (1958a) reported the prophylactic value of 3 nitrofurans in experimental infections that resulted in reduced mortality but had no effect on morbidity. Truscott et al. (1960) found the organism they considered the causative agent of bluecomb disease resistant to penicillin, streptomycin, tetracycline, erythromycin, chloromycetin, and spotein but sensitive to neomycin. They recommended 0.7 g of neomycin per gallon of drinking water as a treatment.

The treatment that is commonly used is as follows:

1. In the brooder house, additional heat is provided until the birds are comfortable and then decreased gradually as the flock improves. Birds on range need additional protection from the weather.

2. Calf milk replacer, 25 lb per 100 gallons of drinking water, is commonly used and mixed fresh each day.

3. Potassium chloride, 450 g per 100 gallons of drinking water, is added to milk suspension.

4. An antibiotic, 100 g per 100 gallons of drinking water, is then added. Neomycin, oxytetracycline, chlortetracycline, streptomycin, penicillin, or bacitracin may be used.

5. Because of secondary intestinal mycosis that usually occurs following high levels of antibiotics, Mycostatin may be used in the feed.

6. A mixture of milk replacer, potassium chloride, and antibiotic in the drinking water is used for 4–5 days, then untreated water is given for 1 day and medication repeated for an additional 4–5 days. It is usually about 10 days before the flock begins to return to improved feed and water consumption.

MANAGEMENT PROCEDURES

Prevention is the only answer to the problem at the present time. Farms that have had outbreaks of the disease should be completely depopulated of all turkeys and other fowl, followed by a cleanup and sanitizing of the house, equipment, and area around the permanent buildings. A period of depopulation for a few weeks is highly desirable before repopulation. Since feces from carrier birds are the primary source of infection, the die-off of the agent in feces and litter probably will occur faster in summer than in winter. Sieburth and Johnson (1957) studied the viability of the infection in Horsfall-Bauer cages and found that a thorough cleaning with water, use of sanitizing agents, and 4 days vacancy readily killed the agent. In the laboratory at Minnesota where the disease has been under study since 1951, the cycle of infection is easily broken by depopulation and cleaning, sanitizing, and resting the equipment for a few days. Under field conditions depopulation of a farm has not always been successful in preventing recurrence of the disease. This procedure has been tried on many farms with partial success. However, the application of strict isolation and control of personnel has demonstrated that the introduction of the disease into a brooder building can be prevented. One farm that has had a continuous problem with the disease for almost 20 years because of year-round production depopulated and, with a rest period of several weeks before restocking with day-old poults, has gone 18 months without recurrence. Also helpful was the elimination of active infection on neighboring turkey farms at the same time.

As stated earlier, the infection may be introduced on a turkey farm from outside sources. Observations point to processing trucks, equipment, and personnel that move from one farm to another without proper precautions. Other vectors may be involved in the transmission from active infections to new flocks in the area.

IMMUNIZATION

The disease must be prevented in the brooding period in order to avoid serious losses. Two procedures have been used on farms that continually have the problem.

1. Poults 5–6 weeks of age are transferred to a growing building equipped with supplemental heat and controlled environment. Birds from a flock on the same farm that have gone through the disease are placed in an adjacent pen to provide exposure. As soon as the flock breaks out with the disease, the birds are placed on treatment.

2. Intestines from a recovered flock (collected at the processing plant) are ground, stored in plastic bags, and frozen at $-20°$ C. For exposure the frozen material is thawed and used at the rate of 1 lb ground intestinal material to 1,250 gal drinking water (1:10,000 dilution). The drinking water is treated with neomycin at a rate of 1 g per gal. One day's supply of drinking water is treated. Within 3–5 days the flock will start to show signs of disease; at this time the flock is treated and the environment controlled.

The exposure programs are recommended after all other programs have failed and only on farms and areas that have a continual problem. Depopulation and strict isolation procedures should be tried first, because there are risks attached to the exposure program. The program was tried on over 500,000 turkeys; maximum mortality was 17.5%, minimum was 0%, and average loss was 5%.

REFERENCES

Bergersen, R. A. 1952. Minnesota turkey death losses—1951, *Bull. State-Federal Crop and Livestock Reporting Serv., Minnesota,* May, 1952.

Deshmukh, D. R., C. T. Larsen, S. K. Dutta, and B. S. Pomeroy. 1969. Characterization of pathogenic filtrate and viruses isolated from turkeys with bluecomb. *Am. J. Vet. Res.* 30:1019–26.

Duke, G. E., H. E. Dziuk, and Linda Hawkins. 1969. Gastrointestinal transit-times in normal and bluecomb diseased turkeys. *Poultry Sci.* 48:835–42.

Dziuk, H. E., and O. A. Evanson. 1969. Balances of Na$^+$ and K$^+$ in normal and bluecomb diseased turkeys. *Poultry Sci.* 48:961–63.

Dziuk, H. E., O. A. Evanson, and C. T. Larsen. 1969a. Physiologic effects of fasting and bluecomb in turkeys. *Am. J. Vet. Res.* 30:1045–56.

Dziuk, H. E., G. E. Duke, O. A. Evanson, D. E. Nelson, and Patricia N. Schultz. 1969b. Force-feeding turkeys during bluecomb disease. *Poultry Sci.* 48:843–46.

Erlandson, V. A., and D. O. Mesick. 1957.

Minnesota's turkey industry—1956, *Bull. State-Federal Crop and Livestock Reporting Serv., Minnesota,* May, 1957.

———. 1962. Minnesota's turkey industry—1961, *Bull. State-Federal Crop and Livestock Reporting Serv., Minnesota,* June, 1962.

Ferguson, A. E. 1961. Bluecomb—Transmissible enteritis in turkeys. *Can. Poultry Rev.* 85:74–76.

Fujisaki, Yujiro, H. Kawamura, and D. P. Anderson. 1969. Reoviruses isolated from turkeys with bluecomb. *Am. J. Vet. Res.* 30:1035–43.

Hilton, F. E. 1954. The pathology of blue comb of turkeys. M.S. thesis, Univ. Minnesota.

Hofstad, M. S., Norman Adams, and M. L. Frey. 1969. Studies on a filtrable agent associated with infectious enteritis (bluecomb) of turkeys. *Avian Diseases* 13:386–93.

Larsen, C. T. 1968. Progress in research on bluecomb disease and long range research needs. *Nat. Turkey Federation Ann. Meet.* Jan. 9, 1968.

Mesick, D. O. 1967. Minnesota's turkey industry—1966, *Bull. State-Federal Crop and Livestock Reporting Serv., Minnesota,* June, 1967.

Peterson, E. H., and T. A. Hymas. 1951. Antibiotics in the treatment of an unfamiliar turkey disease. *Poultry Sci.* 30:466–68.

Pomeroy, B. S. 1956a. High level use of antibiotics. *Proc. 1st Int. Conf. on the Use of Antibiotics in Agr.* Nat. Acad. Sci., Nat. Res. Council, Publ. 397, pp. 56–67.

———. 1956b. Use of furazolidone and antibiotics in bluecomb disease of turkeys. *Proc. 1st Nat. Symp. on Nitrofurans in Agr.,* pp. 75–78.

Pomeroy, B. S., and J. M. Sieburth. 1953. Bluecomb of turkeys. *Proc. Am. Vet. Med. Ass., Ann. Meet.,* pp. 321–28.

Sharma, T. S. 1968. Characterization and comparative studies of vibrios associated with

bluecomb (transmissible enteritis) of turkeys. Ph.D. thesis. Univ. Minnesota.

Sieburth, J. M. 1954. Bluecomb disease of turkeys: Antibiotic prophylaxis and etiology. Ph.D. thesis. Univ. Minnesota.

Sieburth, J. M., and E. P. Johnson. 1957. Transmissible enteritis of turkeys (blue comb). *Poultry Sci.* 36:256–61.

Sieburth, J. M., and B. S. Pomeroy. 1955. Bluecomb disease of turkeys. III. Preliminary studies on etiology. *Proc. Am. Vet. Med. Ass., Ann. Meet.,* pp. 301–6.

———. 1956. Bluecomb disease of turkeys. II. Antibiotic treatment of poults. *J. Am. Vet. Med. Ass.* 128:509–13.

Truscott, R. B. 1968. Transmissible enteritis of turkeys—Disease reproduction. *Avian Diseases* 12:239–45.

Truscott, R. B., and E. W. Morin. 1964. A bacterial agent causing bluecomb disease in turkeys. II. Transmission and studies of the etiological agent. *Avian Diseases* 8:27–35.

Truscott, R. B., M. C. Connell, A. E. Ferguson, and C. G. Wills. 1960. A bacterial agent causing bluecomb disease in turkeys. I. Isolation and preliminary laboratory investigation. *Avian Diseases* 4:391–401.

Tumlin, J. T., and B. S. Pomeroy. 1958a. The prophylactic effect of nitrofurans in feed on bluecomb disease mortality and weight gains in day-old poults. *Proc. 2nd Nat. Symp. on Nitrofurans in Agr.,* p. 144.

———. 1958b. Bluecomb disease of turkeys. V. Preliminary studies on parental immunity and serum neutralization. *Am. J. Vet. Res.* 19:725–28.

Tumlin, J. T., B. S. Pomeroy, and R. K. Lindorfer. 1957. Bluecomb disease of turkeys. IV. Demonstration of a filterable agent. *J. Am. Vet. Med. Ass.* 130:360–65.

Wooley, R. E., and J. B. Gratzek. 1969. Certain characteristics of viruses isolated from turkeys with bluecomb. *Am. J. Vet. Res.* 30:1027–33.

❖

HEMORRHAGIC
ENTERITIS

❖

HEMORRHAGIC ENTERITIS is an acute disease of growing turkeys, characterized by short-term depression with bloody droppings followed by sudden death.

The disease when first reported in Minnesota caused an average mortality of about 10% in turkeys ranging from 7 to 12 weeks of age (Pomeroy and Fenstermacher, 1937). Gross and Moore (1967) reported that in Virginia as well as some other states the disease has become a serious economic problem, with flock mortality ranging from less than 1% to over 60%.

HISTORY

Pomeroy and Fenstermacher (1937) first described the condition of hemorrhagic enteritis in turkeys. It was encountered during the summer months, and the flocks involved had been reared on wire porches for 6–8 weeks and then transferred to field ranges. The losses occurred 10–14 days after the poults were put on range. The outbreaks occurred when the ranges were very poor because of severe heat and drouth. Since then the disease has been encountered in fryer-roaster type turkeys raised under complete confinement. It has a tendency to repeat in successive groups raised in the same buildings. Gale and Wyne (1957) described two outbreaks in 7–11-week-old turkeys reared in confinement, with 1.6 and 3.5% mortality.

INCIDENCE

The disease has been reported from many of the turkey raising areas of the United States. Eastern, north central, and western states have reported losses from the disease.

ETIOLOGY

Earlier attempts to reproduce the disease met with failure, although *E. coli* had been isolated from some of the birds dying from the disease (Pomeroy and Fenstermacher,

1937; Gale and Wyne, 1957). Gross and Moore (1967) were able to reproduce the disease by the cloacal route with 10% suspension of intestinal contents obtained from a turkey naturally infected with hemorrhagic enteritis. The etiology apparently involves a filterable agent (0.22μ or less) which can be passed serially in a culture of streptococci from the intestinal tracts of normal turkeys. They speculated that the filterable agent might be a bacteriophage that grows in streptococci. The transmissible agent survived at $-40°$ C in intestinal material and at $4°$ C in 10% suspension of gut contents in tryptose broth for several months.

PATHOGENESIS

HOSTS

The disease has been described only in turkeys. Gross and Moore (1967) reported that chickens and possibly other birds might be a reservoir of infection for turkeys since their intestines contained the agent 5 days after inoculation even though they had no outward signs of infection and few lesions. Young turkeys less than 4 weeks appear to be resistant. It usually affects turkeys to 14 weeks of age but has been reported in older turkeys.

TRANSMISSION

Under natural conditions the disease is transmitted via the oral route. Gross and Moore (1967) had no difficulty transmitting the disease by cloacal route. The disease has a tendency to recur on certain farms. There is little known about carriers and vectors of the disease.

INCUBATION PERIOD

Gross and Moore (1967) reported the incubation period to be approximately 5 days. At the onset of signs of blood droppings there is a drop in feed and water consumption and body weight.

SIGNS

The first sign of the disease in a flock is sudden death; blood may be seen oozing from the anus of the dead bird, or the feathers around the anus may be soiled with dark-colored blood. If the flock is examined carefully, some birds will show depression and bloody droppings. The disease may be observed from 10 to 20 days in a flock. Gross and Moore (1967) in experimental infections noted that birds passed bloody droppings only over a 24-hour period after 5–6 days incubation period. The drop in feed and water consumption lasted for a few days and then returned to normal. Birds that hemorrhage almost always die.

MORBIDITY AND MORTALITY

The average loss was about 10% in the early studies on the disease in Minnesota. Gross and Moore (1967) reported that flock mortality ranged from less than 1% to over 60%. Birds that did not show clinical signs of the disease did not exhibit any effect on weight gain or water and feed consumption. The authors indicated there was little evidence of loss from morbidity.

GROSS LESIONS

The skin of birds dying from hemorrhagic enteritis usually has an anemic appearance. The carcass is in good physical condition; there may be feed in the crop, indicating an illness of short duration. Numerous capillary hemorrhages are found in the breast and thigh muscles. Petechial hemorrhages on the apex of the heart, on the auricular fat, and on the auricles are not uncommon. The lungs appear pale and edematous. The liver usually presents no gross lesions, but petechial and ecchymotic hemorrhages may be seen along the border and upon the surface of the liver. Splenomegaly is not found, but a dark discoloration is more or less regularly present. The kidneys are pale; occasionally a few petechial hemorrhages are observed on the surface. Ecchymoses are present in the mucosa at the junction of the proventriculus and gizzard and in the region of the pyloric opening. These hemorrhages often extend to the serosa. Occasionally the cornified epithelium of the gizzard contains hemorrhages. The entire intestinal tract is distended, extremely cyanotic, and filled with sanquineous material. The mucosa is markedly congested. The inflammatory changes are most prominent in the duodenal portion; other parts of the tract are less seriously involved. Abnormal changes of the ceca are not regularly found. In some cases these appendages are filled with blood and the mucosa shows evidence of inflammation. The larynx, trachea, esophagus, and crop show no gross changes (Pomeroy and Fenstermacher, 1937).

HISTOPATHOLOGY

The initial stage consists of an infiltration of the lamina propria with numerous erythrocytes and round cells and edema. The villi very often become distended and resemble club-shaped structures as the core fills with cells. There is separation of the epithelial layer from the tip of the villi and desquamation of the epithelium from the surface of the villi, with heterophil infiltration at the junction between necrotic and living tissue. As the mucosa heals in recovered cases, the epithelium again becomes attached to the villi. Macrophages containing hemosiderin are common. By the 10th day, all major signs of the infection have disappeared. Microscopic lesions in the liver vary; in some cases slight congestion is found and in others a considerable degree of hemorrhage is present. Occasionally the changes are more marked and consist of cellular degeneration and destruction (Pomeroy and Fenstermacher, 1937; Gross, 1967).

HEMATOLOGY

In experimental infections the hematocrit values are normal until the 6th day when there is a marked drop, followed by a gradual return to the normal range by the 15th day. Lymphocyte counts drop on the 6th day and return to the normal by the 8th day. Heterophil counts drop on the 7th day, are about 160% normal on the 11th day, and return to normal by the 15th day (Gross and Moore, 1967).

IMMUNITY

There is little information on the length of immunity. Since the course of the disease is 10–20 days and there is rarely recurrence after the flock has recovered, these observations suggest that an immunity has developed. Serum from recovered birds appears to have antibodies or antitoxin since it has some protective effect in acute cases.

DIAGNOSIS

The history and lesions of hemorrhagic enteritis are highly suggestive of the disease. Since the etiology of the disease is not clearly defined, the causative agent cannot be isolated and identified.

DIFFERENTIAL DIAGNOSIS

Acute bacterial infections such as colibacillosis, erysipelas, and fowl cholera should be eliminated. Overdose of sulfaquinoxaline and other drugs may produce toxic effect with a plastic bone marrow and be confused with hemorrhagic enteritis. Toxic fungi may be a possibility as a contributing factor. The role of toxic fungi causing enteric disorders in turkeys must be considered. Occasionally there is confusion in the use of the terms hemorrhagic enteritis and internal hemorrhage; the latter is related to rupture of the aorta.

TREATMENT

Various medication programs have been tried with little success. The disease runs its course no matter what drugs are used. Evidence from field trials has indicated that serum from recovered turkeys has value in stopping an outbreak.

PREVENTION AND CONTROL

Since the etiologic agent has not been clearly defined, there is no suggestive program that can be used on a preventive basis. Management programs must be watched closely to provide adequate water supply, feed, and shade while on range.

REFERENCES

Gale, C., and J. W. Wyne. 1957. Preliminary observations on hemorrhagic enteritis of turkeys. *Poultry Sci.* 36:1267–70.

Gross, W. B. 1967. Lesions of hemorrhagic enteritis. *Avian Diseases* 11:684–93.

Gross, W. B., and W. E. C. Moore. 1967. Hemorrhagic enteritis of turkeys. *Avian Diseases* 11:296–307.

Pomeroy, B. S., and R. Fenstermacher. 1937. Hemorrhagic enteritis in turkeys. *Poultry Sci.* 16:378–82.

CHAPTER 26

MISCELLANEOUS VIRAL INFECTIONS

VIRAL ARTHRITIS

N. O. OLSON

Division of Animal and Veterinary Sciences
West Virginia University
Morgantown, West Virginia

VIRAL ARTHRITIS is a widespread poultry infection which involves the synovial membrane, tendon sheaths, and myocardium. In England the infection has been called tenosynovitis by Dalton and Henry (1967) in order to distinguish from infectious synovitis. The economic importance of this disease to the poultry industry is not known; however, in acutely affected flocks, mortality, poor growth, poor feed efficiency, and condemnations are significant factors. The disease has been recognized only in chickens.

HISTORY

The disease was first recognized by Olson et al. (1957). The arthritis virus was first isolated from a field case in which *Mycoplasma synoviae* was also isolated. Later, virus was isolated from the tibiofemoral joint of a chicken showing no gross lesions and in 1967–68 from birds in two field outbreaks (Olson and Solomon, 1968). The disease was reported from England (Dalton and Henry, 1967) and, as observed by the present author, resembles the disease in the United States.

INCIDENCE AND DISTRIBUTION

The incidence of infection is not known; in many cases the disease has been confused with infectious synovitis. Widespread infections in a flock may go unrecognized. The condition has been seen primarily in broiler birds in the eastern and southern parts of the United States.

ETIOLOGY

The disease is caused by an RNA reovirus with a particle size of 75 mμ and shows a common precipitin antibody with the Crawley virus (Walker, 1971). The virus is heat-resistant and has withstood 60° C for 8–10 hours, 56° C for 22–24 hours, 37° C for 15–16 weeks, 22° C for 48–51 weeks, 4° C for over 3 years, —20° C for over 4 years, and —63° C for over 10 years. It is not sensitive to ether but is slightly sensitive to chloroform. It is resistant to pH 3.0. Chlortetracycline, tylosin, and erythromycin have no effect on the virus (Olson and Kerr, 1966).

The virus grows well in cultures of primary chicken embryo fibroblasts (Taylor et al., 1966). Inoculation with infected allantoic fluid causes a cytopathic effect (CPE) seen starting on the 3rd day. Small holes develop in the cell sheet, and individual cells shrink and develop cytoplasmic extensions. By the 7th day, only a few cells remain attached. Staining with acridine orange reveals green-staining cytoplasmic inclusions presumed to contain RNA.

No hemagglutinating activity, hemadsorption, or neutralizing activity of the virus has been demonstrated (Taylor et al., 1966).

The virus grows readily in the embryonating chicken egg following inoculation via the yolk sac or chorioallantoic membrane (CAM). Mortality in CAM-inoculated embryos usually occurs on the 7th or 8th day postinoculation; embryos are slightly dwarfed, and enlarged liver and spleen with necrotic foci are common. The latter lesion is pronounced in embryos that survive to 20 days. Small, discrete, slightly raised, white lesions may be found on the CAM. Histologically, areas of necrosis of the ectoderm with only a moderate stimulation of the epithelial cells are seen. The mesoderm adjacent to a plaque is edematous and contains numerous inflammatory cells. Edema alone may be found. Mortality following yolk sac inoculation occurs on the 3rd to 4th day. Affected embryos show a marked purplish discoloration, and internal organs are hemorrhagic. Embryos which survive to the 20th day exhibit lesions as described for the CAM-inoculated embryos. Embryo mortality generally does not occur following inoculation via the allantoic sac.

There may be variation in the pathogenicity of the virus for chickens; 2-week-old chickens are more susceptible than chickens 5–20 weeks old (Kerr and Olson, 1964). Clinical disease may occur in contact-exposed birds (Olson and Solomon, 1968).

PATHOGENESIS AND EPIZOOTIOLOGY

NATURAL AND EXPERIMENTAL HOSTS

The chicken is the only known natural or experimental host. Attempts to establish active infection in the canary, pigeon, turkey, guinea pig, rat, mouse, hamster, and rabbit failed.

TRANSMISSION

Horizontal transmission occurs between birds in direct contact. Whether indirect contact results in virus spread is not known. Chickens hatched from known naturally infected hens and reared in isolation have shown evidence of infection; in an unreported experiment conducted by the author, 1 of 500 chickens from artificially infected breeders showed clinical signs of viral arthritis at 8 weeks but no virus was isolated. The inapparent infection in many flocks makes estimates of egg transmission rates difficult. Carrier chickens may be a problem, since virus has been shown to persist in a bird for at least 289 days (Olson and Kerr, 1967).

INCUBATION PERIOD

The incubation period in inoculated 2-week-old chickens varies from 1 day (footpad inoculation) to 11 days (intramuscular, intravenous, sinus) (Olson, 1959). The incubation period following intratracheal inoculation and contact exposure is 9 and 13 days respectively (Olson and Solomon, 1968).

SIGNS, MORBIDITY, AND MORTALITY

In most field cases the infection is inapparent. In acute infections lameness is present and some chickens are stunted. With chronic infection lameness is more pronounced, and in a small percentage of the infected chickens the hock joint is immobilized. In a flock of 36,000 broilers, the infection, first diagnosed as infectious synovitis, appeared in 8 of 16 pens when the chicks were 3–4 weeks old. Approximately 550 birds died or were removed because of lameness by 7–8 weeks. Another 4,500 birds were stunted.

In another flock of approximately 15,000 broilers, no clinical signs of viral arthritis were observed, but approximately 5% of the birds had enlargement in the area of the gastrocnemius tendon or in the digital flexor tendon when observed on the processing line. At 9 weeks, birds from this flock had an average weight of only 3.66 pounds, feed conversion was 2.45, mortality totaled 5%, and the condemnation rate was 2.6%. Virus was isolated from 2 birds condemned for toxemia, and of 80 serum samples obtained from this flock, 89% had antibodies detected in a precipitin test. This inapparent infection probably caused the poor performance of these broilers.

GROSS LESIONS

The gross lesions in naturally infected chickens are observed as swellings of digital flexor tendons and metatarsal extensor tendons. The latter lesion is evident by palpation just above the hock and may be readily observed when the feathers are removed. Swellings of the foot pad and elbow joint are less frequent. The hock or elbow joint usually contains a small amount of straw-colored or blood-tinted exudate; in a few cases, there is a considerable amount of purulent exudate resembling that seen with infectious synovitis. Early in the infection there is marked edema of the tarsal and metatarsal tendon sheaths. Petechial hemorrhages are frequent in the synovial membranes above the hock (Fig. 26.1).

The inflammation of the tendon areas progresses to a chronic type lesion characterized by hardening and fusion of the tendon sheaths. Small pitted erosions develop in the articular cartilage of the distal tibiotarsus. These erosions enlarge, coalesce, and extend into the underlying bone. An overgrowth of fibrocartilaginous pannus develops on the articular surface. The condyles and epicondyles are frequently involved (Kerr and Olson, 1969). In experimentally inoculated chickens, the diaphesis of the proximal metatarsal of the affected limb is enlarged.

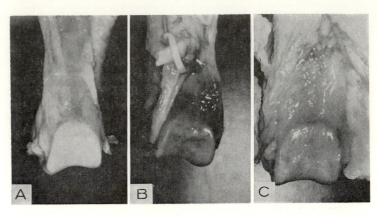

FIG. 26.1—Viral arthritis lesions in distal posterior tibia of inoculated chickens. (A) Normal. (B) Cartilage erosions and hemorrhages of synovial membrane 35 days postinoculation. (C) Erosions of cartilage and marked thickening of synovial membrane 212 days postinoculation.

HISTOPATHOLOGY

The histologic changes have been described by Kerr (1965) and Kerr and Olson (1969). In general, they are the same for natural and experimental infections. During the first 7 days following foot-pad inoculation, edema, coagulation necrosis, heterophil accumulation, and perivascular infiltration are seen. There also is hypertrophy and hyperplasia of synovial cells, infiltration of lymphocytes and macrophages, and a proliferation of reticular cells. These last lesions cause the parietal and visceral layers of the tendon sheaths to become markedly thickened. The synovial cavity is filled with heterophils, macrophages, and sloughed synovial cells. A periostitis characterized by increased osteoclasts develops.

Subsequent inflammatory changes are more chronic. There is an increase in the amount of fibrous connective tissue and a pronounced infiltration or proliferation of reticular cells, lymphocytes, macrophages, and plasma cells. The synovial membrane develops villous processes, and lymphoid nodules are seen by 15 days postinoculation.

The same general inflammatory changes develop in the tarsometatarsal area and in the area of the hock joint. The development of sesamoid bones in the tendon of the affected limb is inhibited. Some tendons are completely replaced by irregular granulation tissue, and large villi form on the synovial membrane.

The linear growth of cartilage cells in the proximal tarsometatarsal bone becomes narrow and irregular. Erosions on the cartilage of the hock joint are accompanied by a granulation pannus. Osteoblasts become active and lay down a thickened layer of bone beneath the erosion. Osteoblastic activity is present on the condyles, epicondyles, and accessory tibia producing osteoneogenesis and subsequent exostosis (Kerr and Olson, 1969).

The lesions found in the heart have been described in detail (Kerr and Olson, 1967). An infiltration of heterophils between myocardial fibers is a constant finding. In some cases it is accompanied by proliferating mononuclear cells, probably reticular cells.

Erythrocyte, hematocrit, and total leukocyte determinations are generally within normal range, though there may be a rise in the heterophil percentage and a decrease in the lymphocyte percentage (Kerr, 1965).

IMMUNITY

Immunity to viral arthritis has not been demonstrated; the ability to recover the agent 289 days after exposure indicates that immunity, if present, may be incomplete (Olson and Kerr, 1967). Precipitating antibodies develop and are discussed under serology.

DIAGNOSIS

A presumptive diagnosis may be made on the basis of signs and lesions. The involvement of primarily the metatarsal extensor and digital flexor tendons (Fig. 26.2) and the heterophil infiltration in the heart aid in differentiating the infection from bacterial and mycoplasmal synovitis. Since the lesions resulting from infectious (mycoplasmal) synovitis are similar, a positive diagnosis based on lesions would not be made unless serum from the affected chicken was negative for *Mycoplasma synoviae* (MS). If the agglutination test is positive for MS, demonstration of the agent either by the fluorescent antibody (FA) technique or virus isolation is essential.

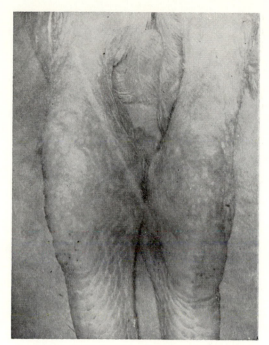

FIG. 26.2—An 8-week-old broiler showing marked swelling of digital flexor and metatarsal extensor tendons. Diagnosis can frequently be made based on this lesion.

A direct FA technique, described by Corstvet and Sadler (1964), gives excellent results. Tissue sections stained with conjugated antiserum are examined with a UV microscope; the antigen is seen as bright green masses in the tendon sheaths.

Virus isolation may be accomplished by using part of the affected tendon along with the sheaths. Tissues diluted approximately 1:10 with nutrient broth are ground. Part of the resulting mixture is treated with penicillin and streptomycin, and part is left untreated for aerobic and anaerobic cultivation on blood agar.

The antibiotic-treated materials are inoculated into the yolk sacs of 5–7-day-old embryonating chicken eggs. On first passage, infected embryos should die in 4–15 days. Many surviving embryos should show typical pathologic changes as described previously. Yolk harvested from dead embryos, if free of bacteria and fungi, may be inoculated into additional embryos and 2-week-old chickens for further propagation of the isolate. After sufficient virus is obtained, tentative identification may be made by heating virus samples to 60° C for

1, 2, and 4 hours. Virus survival, determined by the yolk sac inoculation of 5–7-day-old embryos, suggests the presence of the arthritis agent.

A further test for identification is made by using the double gel diffusion technique as described by Crowle (1961). The agar for the gel diffusion test is dissolved in 0.01 M phosphate buffer at pH 7.2 containing 8% salt. For antigen, the portion of a CAM showing plaques is removed, rinsed three times in physiological saline or Hanks balanced salt solution, and ground. Usually the CAM is edematous so that additional fluid is not needed for grinding. Each individual CAM is checked separately against known antiserum.

A variety of designs of wells for use in the agar gel plates was described by Crowle (1961). For viral arthritis, wells approximately 3 mm in diameter and 3 mm apart, 1 centered within a circle of 6, have given satisfactory results. To test suspect or known sera, the known antigen is placed in the center well and sera are placed in the outside wells. If antigens are to be compared, the reverse procedure is used with the antigens in the outside wells.

One or two lines are usually produced within 24 hours at room temperature. This method may be used to identify either virus or antibody. Following inoculation of chickens, serum precipitin antibodies develop in 2–3 weeks and in contact controls in 3–4 weeks. In naturally infected flocks serum from 85–100% of the chickens reacts. In experimentally inoculated flocks usually 100% of the birds react.

TREATMENT, PREVENTION, AND CONTROL

No treatment for affected birds is known.

The generally recommended procedures for control of infectious diseases must be followed for viral arthritis. For broilers, an all-out, all-in procedure should be followed. It is known that virus spread occurs from bird to bird and possibly between houses on the same farm. The resistance of the virus to environmental factors would indicate that it may be carried mechanically.

Disinfectants have not been adequately tested, but lye is thought to be effective in killing the virus.

It has been possible to raise flocks free of infection, based on signs and gel diffusion tests, following removal of an infected flock from the premises.

Egg transmission, contaminated vaccines, or both as a source of contamination of clean flocks cannot be ruled out at this time.

REFERENCES

Corstvet, R. E., and W. W. Sadler. 1964. The diagnosis of certain diseases with the fluorescent antibody technique. *Poultry Sci.* 43:1280–88.

Crowle, A. J. 1961. *Immunodiffusion.* Academic Press, New York and London.

Dalton, P. J., and R. Henry. 1967. "Tenosynovitis" in poultry. *Vet. Record* 80:638.

Kerr, K. M. 1965. Three synovitis agents in chickens. M.S. thesis, West Virginia Univ., Morgantown.

Kerr, K. M., and N. O. Olson. 1964. Control of infectious synovitis. 14. The effect of age of chickens on the susceptibility to three synovitis agents. *Avian Diseases* 8:256–63.

———. 1967. Cardiac pathology associated with viral and mycoplasmal arthritis in chickens. *2nd Conf. Biol. Mycoplasma.* N.Y. Acad. Sci. 143:204–17.

———. 1969. Pathology in chickens experimentally inoculated or contact infected with an arthritis producing virus. *Avian Diseases* 13:729–45.

Olson, N. O. 1959. Transmissible synovitis of poultry. *Lab. Invest.* 8:1384–93.

Olson, N. O., and K. M. Kerr. 1966. Some characteristics of an avian arthritis viral agent. *Avian Diseases* 10:470–76.

———. 1967. The duration and distribution of synovitis producing agents in chickens. *Avian Diseases* 11:578–85.

Olson, N. O., and D. P. Solomon. 1968. A natural outbreak of synovitis caused by the viral arthritis agent. *Avian Diseases* 12:311–16.

Olson, N. O., D. C. Shelton, and D. A. Munro. 1957. Infectious synovitis control by medication-effect of strain differences and pleuropneumonia-like organisms. *Am. J. Vet. Res.* 18:735–39.

Taylor, D. L., N. O. Olson, and R. G. Burrell. 1966. Adaptation of an avian arthritis viral agent to tissue culture. *Avian Diseases* 10:462–70.

Walker, E. R. 1971. An electron microscopic study of an avian reovirus that causes arthritis. Thesis, West Virginia Univ., Morgantown.

❖

INFECTIOUS BURSAL DISEASE

❖

S. B. HITCHNER

Department of Avian Diseases
New York State Veterinary College
Ithaca, New York

❖

THE RECOGNITION of a specific disease entity affecting the bursa of Fabricius of chickens was reported by Cosgrove (1962). He called the disease avian nephrosis because of the extreme kidney damage in birds that succumbed to infection. Since outbreaks were first observed on farms in the neighborhood of Gumboro, Delaware, Gumboro disease became a synonym for the condition.

The disease is prevalent in the concentrated poultry-producing areas of the United States and may account for considerable losses in individual flocks. However, the direct economic loss from mortality and retarded growth is not proportional to the incidence of infection; most flocks are exposed at an age when resistance is fairly high. Whether there may be subclinical or secondary effects resulting from altered function of the bursa of Fabricius is not known.

HISTORY

Confusion as to the etiology of the avian nephrosis syndrome developed when attempts were made to isolate the causative agent. Winterfield and Hitchner (1962) described an isolate (Gray) of infectious bronchitis virus obtained from the kidney of a field case of avian nephrosis. A small percentage of the chicks experimentally inoculated with this virus died and exhibited a nephrosis not unlike that seen in the newly reported syndrome. Because of the similarity between the kidney lesions induced by Gray virus and those seen in avian nephrosis as described by Cosgrove (1962), it was first believed that that virus was the causative agent. Later studies, however, revealed that birds immune to the Gray virus could still be infected with the infectious bursal disease agent and would develop changes in the bursa specific for that disease. In subsequent studies with chickens affected with the bursal disease, Winterfield et al. (1962) succeeded in isolating an agent in embryonating eggs. The mortality pattern was irregular and the agent was difficult to maintain on serial passage. This isolate was shown to be the true cause of infectious bursal disease; the Gray virus was considered to be an isolate of infectious bronchitis virus with nephrotoxic tendencies.

INCIDENCE AND DISTRIBUTION

Infectious bursal disease has been reported from all major poultry-producing areas in the United States and has also been recognized in Great Britain, Italy, Israel, West Germany, and the Netherlands. In addition, Winterfield (1969) has shown by serologic evidence that the disease is present in Brazil, Venezuela, and Chile.

From extensive field surveys Landgraf et al. (1967) in West Germany, Meroz (1966) in Israel, and Parkhurst (1964a) in the United States all concluded that disease incidence is greatest in chicks 3–6 weeks of age. The earliest outbreaks were reported in 11-day-old chicks, and the latest in birds 84 days of age. The average mortality rate noted in these three reports ranged from 4 to 8.8%, with the highest single-flock mortality rate at 37.6%. The duration of clinical signs in a flock was 5–7.5 days.

ETIOLOGY

CLASSIFICATION AND MORPHOLOGY

Numerous studies have proven the causative agent to be a virus. Mandelli et al. (1967) and Petek and Mandelli (1968) have suggested that it be classified as a reovirus. It would seem desirable that this be considered a tentative classification until con-

firmed by additional studies. According to electron microscopic studies (Mandelli et al., 1967; Cheville, 1967) the virus has a particle size of 58–65 mμ.

RESISTANCE TO CHEMICAL AND PHYSICAL AGENTS

Benton et al. (1967b) studied the physico-chemical properties of the virus and found it resistant to ether and chloroform, inhibited at pH 12.0 but unaffected at pH 2.0, and still viable after 5 hours at 56° C. The virus was unaffected by exposure for 1 hour at 30° C to a 0.5% phenol or 0.125% merthiolate concentration. There was a marked reduction in virus titer when exposed to 0.5% formalin for 6 hours. The virus was treated with various concentrations of three disinfectants—an iodine complex, a phenolic derivative, and a quaternary ammonium compound—for a period of 2 minutes at 23° C. Only the iodine complex had any deleterious effects upon the virus.

Landgraf et al. (1967) found that virus survived at 60° C but not at 70° C for 30 minutes; chloramine in 0.5% concentration killed the virus after 10 minutes' exposure.

LABORATORY HOST SYSTEMS

Chicken Embryos

In the initial attempts, most workers had difficulty in making a virus isolation, or if successful, in serial propagation. Landgraf et al. (1967) reported a typical experience using the allantoic sac route of inoculation. On the 1st passage all inoculated embryos died; on the 2nd passage 30% died; and on the 3rd passage there was no embryo mortality.

Continued studies (Hitchner, 1970) uncovered three factors that could explain these earlier difficulties: (1) Embryonating eggs that originated from flocks recovered from the disease were highly resistant to the growth of the virus. (2) In early virus passage the allantoamnionic fluid (AAF) had a very low virus content, while the chorioallantoic membrane (CAM) and embryo each had a much higher, and nearly equal, virus content. (3) Comparison of the allantoic sac, yolk sac, and CAM as routes of inoculation showed the allantoic sac to be the least desirable route, giving embryo infective dose$_{50}$ (EID$_{50}$) virus titers of 1.5–2.0 logs lower than by the CAM route. The yolk sac route gave titers that were intermediate. With the allantoic fluid having the lowest virus concentration and the allantoic sac being the least efficient route of inoculation, it is understandable that virus propagation may have failed with this combination of factors.

Embryo adaptation of the virus by serial passage apparently can result in increased virus concentration in the AAF (Winterfield, 1969). Virus isolate 2512, obtained from Winterfield after 46 embryo passages, was selected for a growth curve study (Hitchner, 1970); virus concentrations in the embryo, CAM, and AAF (titrated by the CAM route) all reached a peak 72 hours postinoculation.

Inoculation of the virus into 10-day-old embryonating eggs resulted in embryo mortality usually beginning the 3rd day, with the bulk of the mortality occurring by the 5th day. Embryos rarely died after the 7th postinoculation day. Gross lesions observed in the embryo were: (1) edematous distension of the abdominal region, (2) cutaneous congestion and petechial hemorrhages, particularly along the feather tracts, (3) occasional hemorrhages on toe joints and in the cerebral region, (4) mottled-appearing necrosis and ecchymotic hemorrhages in the liver (latter stages), (5) a pale "parboiled" appearance of the heart, (6) congestion and some mottled necrosis of the kidneys, (7) extreme congestion of the lungs, (8) pale spleen, occasionally with small necrotic foci.

The CAM had no plaques but at times had small hemorrhagic areas. The bursa of Fabricius did not undergo any marked changes in infected embryos.

Cell Culture

Landgraf et al. (1967) reported the propagation of infectious bursal disease virus in chicken embryo fibroblasts, and Petek and Mandelli (1968) reported cytopathic effects due to the virus in chicken embryo kidney cell cultures. In neither of these reports was there any indication that the cytopathogenic agents were inoculated into susceptible chickens to confirm that they were the infectious bursal disease virus.

PATHOGENESIS AND EPIZOOTIOLOGY

NATURAL AND EXPERIMENTAL HOSTS

The chicken is the only species in which natural infection has been reported. All breeds may be infected, but it has been observed that White Leghorns show a more severe reaction to the virus than do heavy breeds. There are no reports that other avian species have been tested for susceptibility.

The age of greatest susceptibility is between 3 and 6 weeks. However, chickens of older ages have been infected, and it would appear that because of the high specificity of the virus for the bursa of Fabricius, clinical infection is possible as long as that organ is functional. In two attempts to infect adult laying birds, no clinical signs of infection were observed (Hitchner, 1970). Young chicks exposed at 1–14 days of age also showed little in the way of clinical signs, indicating an early-age resistance.

TRANSMISSION, CARRIERS, VECTORS

Infectious bursal disease is highly contagious; once infection has been introduced into a pen or house, other birds on the same premises may soon show signs of the disease. The appearance of this disease in successive broods of chicks on a farm once it has appeared is one of the peculiar traits of this infection. The highly stable character of the virus undoubtedly contributes to this factor. Benton et al. (1967a) found that houses which had contained infected birds were still infective for other birds 54 and 122 days respectively after removal of the infected birds. They also demonstrated that water, feed, and droppings taken from infectious pens remained infectious for 52 days. Although air-borne virus has been suspected as a means of transmission, their studies failed to prove air transmission to be a factor; however, this study was not considered conclusive.

Whether or not a true carrier state exists in recovered birds has not been determined. Snedeker et al. (1967) demonstrated that the lesser mealworm (*Alphitobius disperinus*), taken from a house 8 weeks after an outbreak, was infectious for susceptible chickens when fed as a ground suspension.

INCUBATION PERIOD AND SIGNS

The incubation period is very short. Helmboldt and Garner (1964) inoculated 21-day-old chickens in the eye and were able to detect histological evidence of infection in the bursa of Fabricius 24 hours later. Clinical signs were detected 2–3 days postinoculation.

One of the earliest signs of infection in a flock is the tendency for some birds to pick at their own vent. Cosgrove (1962), in his original report, mentioned soiled vent feathers, whitish or watery diarrhea, anorexia, depression, ruffled feathers, trembling, severe prostration, and finally death. Affected birds became dehydrated and, in the terminal stages of the disease, had a subnormal temperature.

MORBIDITY AND MORTALITY

In fully susceptible flocks the disease appears suddenly, and there is a high morbidity rate, approaching 100%. The ruffled feathers and droopy appearance of the birds is the predominant sign and would be suggestive of an acute outbreak of coccidiosis. Mortality usually begins on the 3rd day postinfection and will peak and recede in a period of 5–7 days. The actual mortality may be nil, but the rate can reach levels of 20–30%. Striking features of this disease are the sudden and high rate of morbidity, the spiking death curve, and the rapid flock recovery.

The initial outbreaks on a farm are usually the most acute. Recurrent outbreaks in succeeding broods are less severe and frequently go undetected. This probably results from exposure of the chicks at an earlier age when they are less susceptible, or from the protective influence of parental antibodies at the time of exposure.

GROSS LESIONS

Birds that succumb to the infection are dehydrated with darkened discoloration of the pectoral muscles. Frequently hemorrhages are present in the thigh and pectoral muscles. There is increased mucus in the intestine, and renal changes are prominent (Cosgrove, 1962); the latter occur only in birds that die or are in advanced stages of the disease. At such times the kidneys are somewhat enlarged, the tubules are clearly evident due to distension with accumulated urates, and the ureters are likewise distended. In birds killed and examined during the course of the infection, the kidneys appear essentially normal.

The bursa of Fabricius appears to be the primary target of this virus. Cheville (1967) made a detailed study of bursal weights for the 12 days following infection. It is important that the sequence of changes be understood when examining birds for the diagnosis of the disease. On the 3rd day postinfection, the bursa begins to increase in size and weight due to edema and hyperemia. It is approximately double its normal weight by the 4th day and then begins to recede in size. By the 5th day it has returned to its normal weight; but the bursa then continues to atrophy rapidly, and from the 8th day onward it is approximately 1/3 of its original weight.

By the 2nd or 3rd postinfection day, bursas have a gelatinous, yellowish transudate covering the serosal surface. The longitudinal striations on the surface become prominent, and instead of the normal white color, the bursa appears cream-colored. When the bursa recedes to its normal size, the transudate disappears, and during the period of atrophy the organ becomes more gray in appearance.

Infected bursas often show necrotic foci and at times petechial or ecchymotic hemorrhages on the mucosal surface. Occasionally extensive hemorrhage throughout the entire bursa has been observed; in these cases the birds may void blood in the droppings.

The spleen may be slightly enlarged and very often has small gray foci uniformly dispersed on the surface (Rinaldi et al., 1965). Occasionally hemorrhages are observed in the mucosa at the juncture of the proventriculus and gizzard.

HISTOPATHOLOGY

The histopathology of infectious bursal disease has been studied by Helmboldt and Garner (1964), Cheville (1967), Mandelli et al. (1967), and Peters (1967). Helmboldt and Garner (1964) regarded the condition as an infectious lymphocidal disease with histologic lesions appearing in lymphoid structures—the bursa of Fabricius, spleen, thymus, and cecal tonsil. In the bursa histologic changes appeared as early as 1 day postinoculation. The normal follicular structure was altered by degeneration and necrosis of lymphocytes in the medullary area (Cheville, 1967). The lymphocytes were replaced by heterophils, pyknotic debris, and hyperplastic reticuloendothelial cells. Hemorrhages often appeared but were not a consistent lesion. By the 3rd and 4th days postinoculation all lymphoid follicles were affected. The weight increase at this time was due to severe edema, hyperemia, and marked accumulation of heterophils.

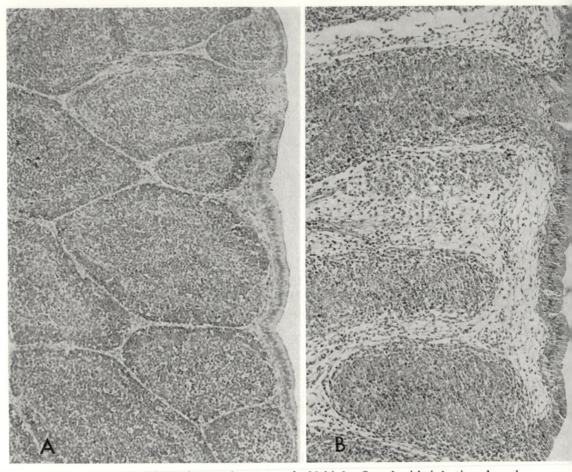

FIG. 26.3—*Photomicrographs of 6-week-old birds affected with infectious bursal agent. Tissues are bursa of Fabricius fixed in 10% buffered saline and stained with H & E. (A) Normal tissue. Large active follicles consist of lymphoid cells which form discrete follicles with little interfollicular tissue. Covering epithelium is simple columnar. ×40. (B) Bursa approximately 24 hours after disease began. Note interfollicular edema mixed with phagocytic cells, many of which are heterophils. Follicles are already beginning to degenerate. ×40. (C) Single*

As the inflammatory reaction declined, cystic cavities developed in the medullary areas of the follicles, necrosis and phagocytosis of the heterophils and plasma cells occurred, and there was a fibroplasia in the interfollicular connective tissue (Cheville, 1967). Proliferation of the bursal epithelial layer produced a glandular structure of columnar epithelial cells containing globules of mucin. During the reparative stage, scattered foci of lymphocytes appeared but did not form healthy follicles during the observation period of 18 days postinoculation (Helmboldt and Garner, 1964). Figure 26.3 shows some of the histologic changes observed in the bursa of Fabricius.

In the early stages of infection, there is hyperplasia of the reticuloendothelial cells around the adenoid sheath arteries of the spleen. By the 3rd day there is lymphoid necrosis in the germinal follicles and the periarteriolar lymphoid sheath. The spleen recovers from the infection rather rapidly with no sustained damage to the germinal follicles.

The thymus and cecal tonsils show some cellular reaction in the lymphoid tissues in the early stages of infection, but as in the spleen, the damage is less extensive than in the bursa, and recovery is more rapid.

Helmboldt and Garner (1964) found lesions in the kidney in less than 5% of the

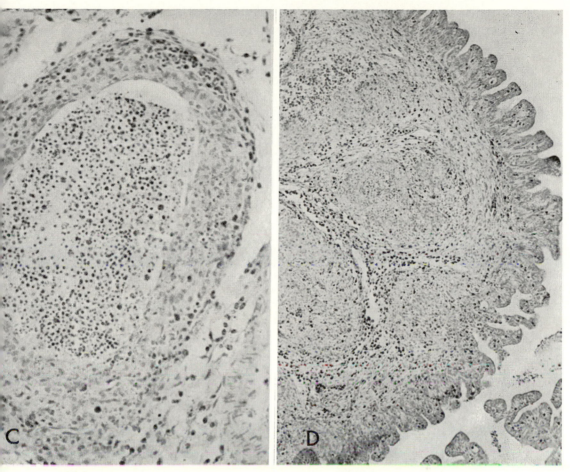

follicle approximately 60 hours after disease began. Medullary portion is now a mass of cellular debris surrounded by cortical remnants. Only reticular cells exist in any number, but scattered among them are a few lymphocytes which will later regenerate. ×250. (D) Terminal phase of severe infection. Only ghosts of follicles remain while heterophils (scattered dark cells) are actively engaged in phagocytosis. ×40. (Courtesy C. F. Helmboldt, Univ. of Conn.)

birds examined, but it should be pointed out that the birds examined were killed at intervals postinfection and did not succumb to the disease. In the affected birds, large casts of homogeneous material infiltrated by heterophils were observed in the kidney. Peters (1967) remarked that the kidneys reacted only nonspecifically, despite their being grossly affected.

The liver may have slight perivascular infiltration of monocytes (Peters, 1967).

IMMUNITY

Active

A good serologic response results when young susceptible birds are exposed to the virus. Winterfield (1969) assessed neutralizing antibodies in chickens 3 weeks after vaccination at 3 days and 4 weeks of age respectively. He used chicken embryo-adapted virus for both the vaccination and neutralization tests. The birds vaccinated at 4 weeks of age had virus-neutralizing $\log_{10}$ titers of 3.5, whereas the antibody response in the 3-day-old-vaccinated chicks was in a much lower range—1.5–2.0 logs.

Hitchner (1970), in a study of birds inoculated at 12 weeks of age, found antibody $\log_{10}$ titers of 3.0 or greater at 26 days postinoculation. Five birds tested at 27 weeks postinoculation had virus neutralizing titers of >3.8 each. Adult birds apparently do not respond as well to the antigen, probably due to the absence of an active bursa of Fabricius. In one trial an adult laying flock showed no serologic response when tested 49 days after virus exposure. In another trial in laying birds, low serologic titers were evident 38 days postinoculation; these increased to highly significant levels by 70 days.

Passive

Dams which possess significant levels of antibody transmit these antibodies through the yolk of the egg. They inhibit virus growth in embryonating eggs regardless of the route of inoculation (Hitchner, unpublished data). The transfer of parental antibodies to the chick similarly protects the chick from infection. In one study to determine the persistence of parental antibodies, chicks from immune dams were exposed to virulent virus at various intervals after hatching. It was found that all chicks up to 4 weeks of age were completely protected (0/20 became infected), and some were protected (2/5 infected) at 5 weeks posthatching. Chicks hatched from a susceptible flock and exposed to virus at the same intervals showed a 100% (25/25) infection rate.

DIAGNOSIS

In acute outbreaks in fully susceptible flocks, the high morbidity, the rapidity of onset and recovery from clinical signs (5–7 days), and the spiked mortality curve should lead one to suspect infectious bursal disease. Confirmation of the diagnosis can be made at necropsy by examination for the characteristic grossly visible changes in the bursa of Fabricius. It should be remembered that during the course of the infection the bursa undergoes distinctive changes in size and color (see Gross Lesions).

In very young chicks or in chicks partially protected by parental antibodies, the disease could be subclinical. In such cases the infection might be identified at necropsy by observing gross changes in the bursa.

ISOLATION AND IDENTIFICATION OF THE CAUSATIVE AGENT

To isolate the virus from dead birds submitted for examination, broth suspensions of either the bursa of Fabricius or the kidney can be used as inoculum. The kidney may be less subject to bacterial contamination and for this reason is the organ of choice. Kidney tissue can be collected on the end of a sterile cotton swab and suspended in antibiotic-treated broth, either directly or after maceration. After thorough suspension and centrifugation to sediment the large tissue particles, the supernatant fluid is inoculated by the CAM route into 9–11-day-old embryonating eggs that originated from a fully susceptible breeding flock. Infected embryos usually die 3–5 days postinoculation. For subsequent passage the entire embryo or affected organs and the CAM of dead embryos should be harvested.

To identify the isolate as infectious bursal disease virus, a neutralization test should be conducted with known positive serum. If embryos are available from known immune and nonimmune flocks, titration of the unknown virus suspension in embryos from the two sources could be used as a screening procedure.

SEROLOGY

Suspensions of infected tissues can be expected to have EID_{50} titers in the range of 10^5–10^6/ml and are suitable for use in virus neutralization tests. Unless the strain used has been adapted for the allantoic sac route, the CAM route of inoculation should be employed. Fully susceptible embryos are required. To help avoid nonspecific embryo mortality, eggs with dropped CAMs should not be turned after inoculation. Aside from these points, the routine procedure for conducting virus neutralization tests may be used.

DIFFERENTIAL DIAGNOSIS

Birds that die from infectious bursal disease usually show an acute nephrosis. Because of the many other conditions which may cause nephrosis, the kidney changes alone are not sufficient cause for a diagnosis of bursal disease. A critical examination of the bursa of Fabricius along with the flock history will usually distinguish infectious bursal disease from other nephrosis-causing conditions.

Birds that die from water deprivation may have kidney changes and even gray, atrophied bursa closely resembling those seen with bursal disease infection. However, unless this occurs as a flock condition, such changes would be seen in relatively few birds. A history of the flock would be essential in aiding in the diagnosis of these cases.

Certain nephrotoxic strains of infectious bronchitis virus cause nephrosis (Winterfield and Hitchner, 1962). These cases can be differentiated from infectious bursal disease by the fact that there are no changes in the bursa of Fabricius, and usually deaths from this infection are preceded by respiratory signs. However, the possibility that the two diseases may occur simultaneously in a flock should not be overlooked.

The muscular hemorrhages and the mucosal hemorrhages seen at the juncture of the proventriculus and gizzard are similar to those reported for hemorrhagic syndrome and could be differentiated by the accompanying changes in the bursa in infectious bursal disease. It is not unlikely that before the bursa was recognized as the primary organ affected in this infection, some cases were diagnosed as hemorrhagic syndrome.

Jakowski et al. (1969) reported bursal atrophy in experimentally induced infection with 4 isolates of Marek's disease. The atrophy was observed 12 days postinoculation, but the histologic response was distinctly different from that found in infectious bursal disease.

TREATMENT

Numerous treatments have been used to try to ameliorate the course of the infection, but none has proved successful. Cosgrove (1962) treated field flocks with antibiotics, large doses of vitamin A, sulfonamides, and furazolidone without success. Parkhurst (1964b) used erythromycin, multiple vitamins, molasses, and sulfamethazine and reported that no treatment was consistently successful. It should be pointed out that due to the rapid spontaneous recovery of the flock, treatments might appear highly effective if nontreated controls were not maintained for comparison.

PREVENTION AND CONTROL

The epizootiology of this infection is not fully understood, but it is known that contact with infected birds and contaminated fomites readily spread the infection. Therefore, the sanitary precautions that are applied to prevent the spread of most poultry infections should be used in the case of infectious bursal disease.

MANAGEMENT PROCEDURES

Once the infection occurs on premises, control is usually naturally accomplished by exposure of the chicks to infection at an early age when they are not highly susceptible to the disease or still carry parental antibody. On some farms the cleanup between broods is not too thorough, and the persistence of the virus provides this exposure by natural means. On other farms, because of effective disinfection procedures, the birds do not acquire this early infection but are exposed at a later age when they are highly susceptible.

IMMUNIZATION

Bursal Tissue Vaccine

To assure the infection of the flock at a desirable age, birds may be exposed using a tissue suspension prepared from infected bursas. Edgar and Cho (1965) used such a procedure to "vaccinate" 3 million chickens, mostly broilers. The inoculum, applied ocularly or via the drinking water at 3–7 days of age, was used on farms that had histories of previous outbreaks that averaged 5% mortality at 4–5 weeks of age. Losses from the disease in the vaccinated flocks averaged less than 0.7%.

Embryo-propagated Vaccine

When the means for propagation of the virus in embryonating eggs became known, the crude tissue vaccines were replaced by virus produced in embryos. Snedeker et al. (1967) made eight serial passages in embryos inoculated via the allantoic sac. A vaccine prepared from suspensions of embryos from the eighth passage had a titer of $10^{3.25}$ EID$_{50}$/ml and was administered to 7–10-day-old chicks with apparently good results. Such a vaccine is recommended for use only on premises that have had a previous outbreak of infectious bursal disease.

Winterfield (1969) studied the immunizing potential of a virus strain that had undergone 50 serial passages in chicken embryos. Virus from the 27th and 41st passages induced no clinical signs in susceptible chickens but resulted in good protection when immunity of the birds was challenged 3 weeks postvaccination.

A commercial lyophilized vaccine is available for use on those premises which previously have experienced infectious bursal disease.

REFERENCES

Benton, W. J., M. S. Cover, and J. K. Rosenberger. 1967a. Studies on the transmission of the infectious bursal agent (IBA) of chickens. *Avian Diseases* 11:430–37.

Benton, W. J., M. S. Cover, J. K. Rosenberger, and R. S. Lake. 1967b. Physico-chemical properties of the infectious bursal agent (IBA). *Avian Diseases* 11:438–45.

Cheville, Norman F. 1967. Studies on the pathogenesis of Gumboro disease in the bursa of Fabricius, spleen and thymus of the chicken. *Am. J. Pathol.* 51:527–51.

Cosgrove, A. S. 1962. An apparently new disease of chickens—Avian nephrosis. *Avian Diseases* 6:385–89.

Edgar, S. A., and Yung Cho. 1965. Avian nephrosis (Gumboro disease) and its control by immunization. *Poultry Sci.* 44:1366.

Helmboldt, C. F., and E. Garner. 1964. Experimentally induced Gumboro disease (IBA). *Avian Diseases* 8:561–75.

Hitchner, S. B. 1970. Infectivity of infectious bursal disease virus for embryonating eggs. *Poultry Sci.* 49:511–16.

Jakowski, R. M., T. N. Frederickson, R. E. Luginbuhl, and C. F. Helmboldt. 1969. Early changes in bursa of Fabricius from Marek's disease. *Avian Diseases* 13:215–22.

Landgraf, H., E. Vielitz, and R. Kirsch. 1967. Untersuchungen ueber das Auftreten einer infektioesen Erkrankung mit Beteiligung der Bursa Fabricii (Gumboro disease). *Deut. Tieraerztl. Wochschr.* 74:6–10.

Mandelli, G., A. Rinaldi, A. Cerioli, and G. Cervio. 1967. Aspetti ultrastrutturali della borsa di Fabrizio nella malattia di Gumboro del pollo. *Atti Soc. Ital. Sci. Vet.* 21:1–5.

Meroz, M. 1966. An epidemiological survey of Gumboro disease. *Refuah Vet.* 23:235–37.

Parkhurst, R. T. 1964a. Pattern of mortality in avian nephrosis. *Poultry Sci.* 43:788–89.

———. 1964b. On-the-farm studies of Gumboro disease in broilers. *Avian Diseases* 8:584–96.

Petek, M., and G. Mandelli. 1968. Proprieta biologiche di un reovirus isolato da un focalaio di malattia di Gumboro. *Atti Soc. Ital. Sci. Vet.* 22:875–79.

Peters, G. 1967. Die Histologic der Gumboro-Krankheit. *Berlin. Muench. Tieraertzl. Wochschr.* 80:394–96.

Rinaldi, A., G. Cervio, and G. Mandelli. 1965. Aspetti epidemiologici, Anatomo-clinici ed istologici di una forma morbosa dei polli verosimilmente identificabile con la considdetta "malattia di Gumboro." *Atti Conv. Patol. Aviare*, pp. 77–83.

Snedeker, Carol, F. K. Wills, and I. M. Moulthrop. 1967. Some studies on the infectious bursal agent. *Avian Diseases* 11:519–28.

Winterfield, R. W. 1969. Immunity response to the infectious bursal agent. *Avian Diseases* 13:548–57.

Winterfield, R. W., and S. B. Hitchner. 1962. Etiology of an infectious nephritis-nephrosis syndrome of chickens. *Am. J. Vet. Res.* 23:1273–79.

Winterfield, R. W., S. B. Hitchner, G. S. Appleton, and A. S. Cosgrove. 1962. Avian nephrosis, nephritis and Gumboro disease. *L & M News and Views.* 3:103.

TURKEY VIRAL HEPATITIS

❖

G. H. SNOEYENBOS

*Department of Veterinary and
Animal Science
University of Massachusetts
Amherst, Massachusetts*

❖

TURKEY VIRAL HEPATITIS (TVH) is an acute, highly contagious, typically subclinical disease of turkeys which produces lesions of the liver and less frequently of the pancreas.

The disease was first described simultaneously by Mongeau et al. (1959) from Ontario, Canada, and by Snoeyenbos et al. (1959) from Massachusetts. Diagnostic summaries indicate that the disease has been observed in a number of states. Mandelli et al. (1966) recognized the disease in Italy and suggested hepatopancreatitis as a more appropriate designation. The true incidence and distribution is unknown due to the transient usually subclinical nature of the infection and the lack of serological means to detect previous infection.

ETIOLOGY

The etiologic agent is a virus which passes a 0.1μ membrane filter and is resistant to ether, chloroform, phenol, and creoline but not to formalin. In a yolk menstruum it survived for 6 hours at $60°$ C, 14 hours at $56°$ C, and 4 weeks at $37°$ C. It retained viability for 1 hour at pH 2 but not at pH 12 (Tzianabos and Snoeyenbos, 1965a).

The virus may be propagated in the yolk sac of chicken and turkey embryos injected not later than 7 and 10 days of age respectively. Mandelli et al. (1966) found the 6-day-old chicken embryo much superior to older embryos. Viral replication has been demonstrated 66 hours after injection, and the virus titer peaked at approximately 90 hours. Rapid embryo passage did not great-

ly enhance the final titer which was seldom greater than EID_{50} of 3.5 (Tzianabos, 1965). Other routes of embryo injection did not always result in viral replication. A variety of tissue culture systems has failed to support viral replication (Tzianabos and Snoeyenbos, 1965b). A one-way antigenic relationship has been reported between TVH rabbit antiserum and duck hepatitis virus in an agar gel diffusion test (Tzianabos and Snoeyenbos, 1965b).

PATHOGENESIS AND EPIZOOTIOLOGY

Infection has been recognized only in the turkey. White Pekin ducks, chickens, pheasants, and coturnix quail were refractory to experimental exposure. Transmission readily occurs by direct or indirect contact. Transmission via the egg has been suggested on a basis of field observations and isolation of virus from an ovum of an artificially infected turkey hen. The virus has been consistently isolated from the liver and feces of infected birds and less frequently from bile, blood, and kidneys during the first 28 days after infection. After that time the virus apparently disappears (Snoeyenbos and Basch, 1960; Tzianabos and Snoeyenbos, 1965b).

Based on the time of appearance of lesions, the incubation period in poults injected intraperitoneally with TVH virus was as short as 48 hours and usually no longer than 7 days in either injected or contact poults.

SIGNS

The disease is usually subclinical and is thought to become apparent only in the presence of other stressor agents. Variable degrees of flock depression and sudden death of apparently normal birds are usually noted in clinical cases. There is suggestive evidence that affected breeder flocks may exhibit decreased production, fertility, and hatchability. Morbidity and mortality appear to be largely determined by the severity of concurrent stressor agents. Nearly 100% morbidity has been reported by some flock owners. A mortality rate of 25% in one flock was reported, but usually mortality is very low and occurs during a 7–10 day period. Mortality in birds over 6 weeks of age has not been reported.

PATHOLOGY

Distinct gross lesions have been observed only in the liver and pancreas. Mandelli et al. (1966) also observed catarrhal enteritis, bronchopneumonia, and peritonitis or airsacculitis in specimens which may have had intercurrent infections. Hepatic lesions consist of focal gray, sometimes slightly depressed areas ranging to several millimeters in diameter. Lesion distribution is variable. Birds which die usually exhibit very extensive lesions, often coalescing, which may be partially masked by vascular congestion and focal hemorrhage. Bile staining is not uncommon. Pancreatic lesions, less consistently observed than hepatic lesions, are often prominent and consist of roughly circular gray-pink areas, often extending across a lobe.

Histopathologic lesions have not been extensively studied. Pronounced lesions have been reported only in the liver and pancreas. Early fatty metamorphosis in the liver is followed by focal necrosis, hemorrhage, and mononuclear foci (Snoeyenbos et al., 1959; Mongeau et al., 1959; Mandelli et al., 1966). Lesions are most severe at about the 7th day postinfection. Focal parenchymal necrosis of the pancreas also occurs, but these lesions are less consistently observed than those of the liver.

Some immunity develops following infection. Exposure of recoverd birds resulted in less frequent and less extensive lesions than in initially infected controls (Snoeyenbos and Basch, 1960). Antibodies have not been demonstrated in turkey serum using direct or indirect complement fixation, virus neutralization, or agar gel diffusion tests. Progeny of recovered breeders developed extensive lesions following exposure (Tzianabos and Snoeyenbos, 1965b).

DIAGNOSIS

Presence of lesions in both the liver and pancreas is almost pathognomonic, as no other disorder is known to produce comparable lesions in both organs. Bacterial infections which produce hepatic lesions can be identified by appropriate bacteriological examination. Histomoniasis, particularly if suppressed by medication, may produce confusing hepatic lesions without cecal involvement. These cases can be diagnosed by demonstration of the histomonad (see Chapter 31).

Virus may be demonstrated by injecting 0.2 ml of ground liver suspension into the yolk sac of 5–7-day-old chicken embryos. Most embryos die between 4 and 10 days postinoculation and exhibit marked cutaneous congestion and hemorrhage. Low dosage results in delayed mortality; embryos are stunted and show less cutaneous congestion. Embryonic fluids are nonhemagglutinating. Isolates may be further characterized by yolk sac or intraperitoneal injection of turkey poults with 0.2 ml yolk harvest and examination for lesions 5–10 days postinoculation.

TREATMENT

There is no effective treatment. The virus is unaffected by antibiotics. Secondary bacterial invasion does not appear to be an important problem. Prevention of stress, including treatment of concurrent diseases, is indicated.

REFERENCES

Mandelli, G., A. Rinaldi, and C. Giulio. 1966. Hepato-pancreatitis of a probable viral nature in the turkey. *Giorne. Pollicoltori* 16: 101–4.

Mongeau, J. D., R. B. Truscott, A. E. Ferguson, and M. C. Connell. 1959. Virus hepatitis in turkeys. *Avian Diseases* 4:388–96.

Snoeyenbos, G. H., and H. I. Basch. 1960. Further studies of virus hepatitis of turkeys. *Avian Diseases* 4:477–84.

Snoeyenbos, G. H., H. I. Basch, and M. Sevoian. 1959. An infectious agent producing hepatitis in turkeys. *Avian Diseases* 4:377–88.

Tzianabos, T. 1965. Turkey viral hepatitis: Some clinical, immunological, and physiochemical properties. Ph.D. thesis. Univ. Mass.

Tzianabos, T., and G. H. Snoeyenbos. 1965a. Some physiochemical properties of turkey hepatitis virus. *Avian Diseases* 9:152–56.

——. 1965b. Clinical, immunological, and serological observations on turkey virus hepatitis. *Avian Diseases* 9:578–91.

QUAIL BRONCHITIS
AND INFECTIONS WITH
CHICKEN EMBRYO
LETHAL ORPHAN VIRUS

❖

R. T. DU BOSE

*Department of Veterinary Science
Virginia Polytechnic Institute
Blacksburg, Virginia*

❖

QUAIL BRONCHITIS (QB) is an acute, highly contagious, respiratory disease of bobwhite quail (*Colinus virginianus* Linne). The economic importance of the disease in wild quail or in captive quail is not well known, and public health significance has not been established. The disease has been reviewed in detail by DuBose (1967, 1971).

Chicken embryo lethal orphan virus (CELO)—closely related to quail bronchitis virus (QBV)—occurs as a usually inapparent infection in a number of avian species, and, with the exception of quail bronchitis, no avian disease entity has been ascribed to it. The question has been raised as to whether CELO virus infection may exacerbate infections with other pathogens already present in chickens. As an endogenous contaminant of embryonating eggs and cell cultures used in diagnosis, vaccine production, and research, CELO virus is of definite economic and public health significance. The report by Rinaldi et al. (1968) includes an extensive review of the literature on CELO virus.

After comparing QBV isolated from quail with bronchitis and CELO virus isolated from endogenously infected chicken embryos by Yates and Fry (1957), DuBose and Grumbles (1959) considered QBV and CELO virus to be the same agent. The term *orphan* is not appropriate for an agent that causes a recognized and named disease entity. On the other hand, the vast majority of the CELO isolates described in the literature have not been tested for pathogenicity in bobwhite quail, and CELO generally has been used to designate the isolates from sources other than quail.

In the following, the term *quail bronchitis virus* (QBV) will be used for the pathogenic agents isolated from bobwhite quail and the term *chicken embryo lethal orphan virus* (CELO) for the agents isolated from other sources and so designated in their original descriptions. CELO and QBV will be discussed together except when pathogenic differences merit separate headings. Under headings in which no work on QBV has been reported, QBV will not be mentioned.

HISTORY, INCIDENCE, AND
DISTRIBUTION

QUAIL BRONCHITIS

Quail bronchitis was first described by Olson (1950) from a 1949 outbreak in West Virginia. Subsequent descriptions were from occurrences in Texas in 1956–57 (DuBose et al., 1958, 1960) and in Virginia in 1959 (DuBose, 1967). Circumstantial evidence indicated transmission of QBV from inapparently infected chickens or captive game birds other than quail to the affected bobwhite quail. The disease was reproduced in quail by experimental infection with QBV (Olson, 1950; DuBose and Grumbles, 1959) and with CELO (DuBose and Grumbles, 1959; Yates, 1960). QBV and CELO were shown to be similar to infectious bronchitis virus of chickens (IBV) in their effect on inoculated chicken embryos and in inability to agglutinate washed chicken red blood cells; they were differentiated from IBV by virus neutralization tests and by their greater resistance to heat.

Since 1960 diagnostic reports from many states in which bobwhite quail are raised in captivity have noted at least sporadic incidence of the disease. The incidence and distribution in wild quail is not known, but high mortality in young quail and immunity in survivors suggest that the disease is self-limiting.

CELO VIRUS INFECTIONS

CELO virus was first isolated in 1952 from chicken embryos inoculated with unrelated materials (Yates et al., 1954), then from uninoculated chicken embryos (Du-Bose and Grumbles, 1959). Yates and Fry (1957) reported that it was serologically related to QBV but distinct from other well-known viruses of chickens, and that it readily adapted to serial propagation in chicken embryos; their suggestion that a latent, endogenous infection of embryonating eggs followed ovarian transfer from inapparently infected dams was later supported by preincubation inoculation of eggs and reisolation of the virus from the 19-day-old embryos and day-old chicks (Yates, 1960; Yates et al., 1960). The warning by Yates and Fry (1957) that CELO virus might prove to be a problem as a contaminant in vaccine production, diagnosis of viral diseases, and other procedures was substantiated by its isolation from the enteric systems of both healthy and diseased chickens (Taylor and Calnek, 1962), by its detection as an endogenous infection in chicken embryo kidney cell cultures (Chomiak et al., 1961; Yates et al., 1962; Burke et al., 1965), and by demonstration of its persistence in laboratory aerosols (Yates, 1960). A number of other viruses isolated in the United States in a variety of circumstances, including the GAL-3 and -4 strains of Gallus, adenolike virus (Sharpless, 1962), were later shown to be essentially indistinguishable from CELO virus by Burke et al. (1968).

Serologic tests indicated that CELO virus was widespread in chickens and present in turkeys and some wild birds in the United States (Yates et al., 1960). Rinaldi et al. (1968) cited reports on its isolation since 1963 in England, continental Europe, Japan, and India.

ETIOLOGY

CLASSIFICATION AND MORPHOLOGY

Rinaldi et al. (1968) noted that CELO virus conformed in characteristics to the adenoviruses. Wilner (1969) placed CELO and QBV together in the *avian* adenovirus group; and Burke et al. (1968), in a study subsequent to those cited by Wilner (1969), proposed a system for classifying the avian adenoviruses and suggested CELO (Phelps strain) as the prototype for an avian adenovirus subgroup. Although Wilner (1969) listed 9 avian adenovirus serotypes distinct from that represented by CELO and QBV, Burke et al. (1968) reported new evidence that 2 of them belong in the CELO serotype.

The morphology was described for CELO by Petek et al. (1963), and for CELO and QBV by Dutta and Pomeroy (1963, 1967). Both agents were within 69–76 mμ in diameter, were regular icosahedrons (cubic symmetry) with 252 capsomeres, and were without envelopes. The significance of smaller particles seen in the QBV preparations was not definitely established.

CHEMICAL COMPOSITION

Deoxyribonucleic acid (DNA) has been reported to be the structural nucleic acid of CELO virus. Kawamura et al. (1964) inhibited replication of CELO virus in chicken kidney cell cultures with 5-iododeoxyuridine (IUDR), which interferes with formation of DNA. The staining reaction of intranuclear inclusion bodies with acridine orange also indicated the presence of DNA. Burke et al. (1968) found 5-bromodeoxyuridine (BUDR) a better DNA inhibitor than IUDR in chick kidney cell cultures; both inhibited replication of 5 CELO isolates, including the proposed Phelps strain prototype. In the primary cell cultures, 5-fluorodeoxyuridine (FUDR) was not effective as a DNA inhibitor. Burke et al. (1968) confirmed the DNA specificity of cytochemical staining of CELO inclusion bodies by treatment with DNA-hydrolyzing enzyme (DNase) which reduced the number of Feulgen-positive (intensely pink) nuclei and removed the brilliant yellow fluorescence caused by acridine orange. RNase had no effect.

VIRAL REPLICATION

CELO virus multiplies in the nucleus of the host cell. Reports by Chomiak et al. (1961) and Kawamura et al. (1963) on the multiplication cycle after infection of chicken or chicken embryo kidney cell cultures were in general agreement with the findings of Burke et al. (1968) that the eclipse period was 7–10 hours, replication of viral DNA 7 hours or more, and maturation at least 7 hours. This approximate 21-hour minimum cycle is essentialy the same as the 20–22 hours noted by Kawamura et al. (1963) as needed for first manifestation of extracellular virus with the Ote and Phelps strains. Extracellular virus titers peaked at from 40 to 96 hours, according to the latter two reports.

From electron micrographs, Maeda et al. (1967) described two types of intranuclear inclusion bodies—reticular and aggregate—formed in chicken kidney cells by avian adenoviruses of different serotypes. They stated that CELO (Ote strain) gave rise to a number of the reticular bodies which they considered similar to the CELO-induced inclusions pictured earlier by Petek et al. (1963).

BIOLOGICAL PROPERTIES

Heat Stability

Many of the reports on biological properties were listed by Rinaldi et al. (1968). Heat stability at 56° C was noted in early work on CELO and QBV (Yates and Fry, 1957; DuBose and Grumbles, 1959) and in differentiating CELO or QBV from infectious bronchitis virus (DuBose et al., 1960), but the method described by Burke et al. (1968) in testing 5 isolates of the CELO serotype at 50° C in several different suspending fluids was suggested for use until a uniform procedure is agreed upon.

All 5 CELO isolates, plus 2 avian adenoviruses (GAL-1, -2) not of the CELO serotype, were stable at 50° C in cell culture maintenance medium and in medium diluted 1:1 with 60% glycerine in water, or with distilled water, or with 2 M NaCl. Loss of infectivity was less than 1 log dilution in 5 hours. Although monovalent cations have increased the heat resistance of the DNA viruses of vaccinia, herpes simplex and certain human adenoviruses, this effect was not noted with the avian adenoviruses tested with NaCl. In the presence of divalent cations—2 M MgCl$_2$ or CaCl$_2$ (1:1)—the 7 isolates became sensitive to 50° C, losing more than 1 log dilution of activity with MgCl$_2$ and more than 4 log dilutions with CaCl$_2$ in less than 1 hour.

The observation time for cell cultures inoculated with heat-treated virus suspensions should be noted in reports on heat sensitivity trials. Clemmer (1964) found that cytopathogenic effect (CPE) from an avian adenovirus held at 60° C for 40 minutes was delayed for approximately 14 days, and that a CELO serotype (strain 93), apparently inactivated by 80° C for 30 minutes,

was detected by CPE in a 2nd passage in cell cultures.

Hemagglutination

CELO virus agglutinates red blood cells of rats but not of sheep or chickens. Clemmer (1964) supported specificity of the hemagglutination (HA) by hemagglutination inhibition (HI) tests and correlated HA activity with infectivity titer of extracellular virus. Burke et al. (1968) reported HA in tubes in 90–120 minutes at 37° C with 5 CELO isolates. In the above, avian adenoviruses not of the CELO serotype were negative in HA tube tests with rat red blood cells, and all of the serotypes tested were negative on plate tests.

RESISTANCE TO PHYSICAL AND CHEMICAL AGENTS

Rinaldi et al. (1968) cited many of the earlier reports on this subject. From the point of view of possible classification as an adenovirus, stability at acid pH and in ether and chloroform are probably the most significant.

Yates (1960) demonstrated essentially complete stability of CELO at pH 3.0–9.0 and relative susceptibility to higher pH levels; stability at low pH was confirmed by Burke et al. (1965) and Adlakha (1966) with other CELO isolates. In parallel with criteria for mammalian adenoviruses, Burke et al. (1968) demonstrated that 5 CELO and 2 non-CELO serotype isolates from several laboratories lost no infectivity during 1 hour at pH 3.0 and 25° C.

Stability in ether and/or chloroform was reported by Petek et al. (1963) and subsequently by many others. Burke et al. (1968) demonstrated resistance of the 7 isolates above to chloroform and suggested chloroform for determining stability to lipid solvents. Clemmer (1964) noted a less than 1 log loss of infectivity with a nonpolar lipid solvent, trifluorotrichloroethane (Genetron 226—Allied Chemical Corp.), used for removing part of the nonviral proteins from a CELO virus suspension.

Reports on resistance of CELO to sodium desoxycholate, trypsin, saponins, and pentane were noted by Rinaldi et al. (1968); varying degrees of resistance to ethyl alcohol, phenol, and merthiolate and susceptibility to formaldehyde and iodine were reported by Petek et al. (1963), Clemmer

(1964), and Adlakha (1966). CELO virus was much more resistant to ultraviolet irradiation than the viruses of Newcastle disease or infectious laryngotracheitis, but it was 10 times as susceptible to photodynamic inactivation as Newcastle disease virus (Petek et al., 1963; Adlakha, 1966).

LABORATORY HOSTS AND PATHOGENICITY

In considering any laboratory host system for isolation or study of CELO or QBV, it should be noted that these agents and/or other adenoviruses have been detected as endogenous agents in avian embryos, in cell cultures, and in inapparent infections of both birds and mammals (Davis et al., 1967).

Avian Embryos

Both CELO and QBV propagated readily in chicken embryos inoculated via the chorioallantoic sac (CAS) at 9–12 days of incubation (Olson, 1950; Yates and Fry, 1957; DuBose et al., 1958). Early embryo mortality was sometimes observed in the 1st passage, seldom later than the 3rd. Characteristic changes included excess allantoic fluid, thickening and opacity of the amnion, decrease in amnionic fluid, stunting and curling of the embryo (also termed dwarfing), and necrotic foci or mottling in the liver. Some embryos were erythematous, particularly in the tarsal and metatarsal regions; others were engulfed to a great degree in the yolk sacs. Similar lesions may result from inoculation with the unrelated infectious bronchitis virus of chickens. Embryo infectivity titer of allantoic fluid from infected embryos may increase with serial passages to a level of 10^6–10^{11} chicken embryo lethal doses (CELD$_{50}$) per ml. Inoculations at 6–13 days of incubation via the yolk sac or chorioallantoic membrane were successful but not preferred (Yates and Fry, 1957; Yates, 1960).

Chomiak et al. (1961) found that inoculation of the chorioallantoic membrane (CAM) in 9-day-old chicken embryos with a high dose of CELO resulted within 2 days in gross lesions that progressed along the blood vessels, were often confluent by 6 days postinoculation, and were similar to but more localized than those of infectious laryngotracheitis (ILT). Histological studies showed ectodermal hyperplasia with concomitant mesodermal reaction of mesenchymal elements and prominent basophilic granular intranuclear inclusion bodies with hematoxylin and eosin staining; ILT virus caused acidophilic intranuclear inclusions. Ectodermal necrosis followed. Neither gross lesions of the CAM nor appearance of basophilic inclusion bodies differentiated infections with CELO from those with other serotypes of the avian adenovirus group (Kawamura et al., 1964).

After Rinaldi et al. (1968) inoculated chicken embryos with CELO by a combination CAS-CAM route (Fabricant's method, cited by Rinaldi et al.), they observed changes in the embryos similar to those described above for the CAS route, gross and microscopic lesions of the CAM similar to those reported by Chomiak et al. (1961), and in addition lesions of the liver which included intranuclear inclusions in the hepatic cells.

Ablashi et al. (1965) reported that latent infection of chicken embryos with CELO virus interfered with the propagation of Newcastle disease and influenza viruses. Viruses of QB, CELO, and infectious bronchitis were propagated in embryonating turkey eggs inoculated via the CAS but could not thereby be differentiated (DuBose and Grumbles, 1959).

Propagation after inoculation and/or detection of CELO or QBV in embryonating eggs may be interfered with by antibodies deposited in the yolk by immune hens (Yates et al., 1960, 1962).

Cell Cultures

CELO virus propagates readily in primary cultures of either chicken embryo kidney cells (Yates, 1960; Chomiak et al., 1961) or chicken kidney cells (Yates et al., 1962; Kawamura et al., 1963) with similar cytopathogenic effects. Taylor and Calnek (1962) termed it the "round type CPE." Significant differences are not found in the CPE caused by CELO and that caused by other serotypes of the avian adenoviruses (Kawamura et al., 1964; Burke et al., 1968). Characteristic changes include swelling, rounding, and increased refractivity of the cells as seen under low power. About 18 hours postinoculation the nuclei become much enlarged, with the nucleoli eccentric and sometimes against the margin of the nuclear membrane. Hematoxylin and eosin staining (H & E) may show early signs of intranuclear inclusion bodies as fine, light pink granules which later become deeper pink or bluish pink and coarser. Fully developed basophilic inclusion bodies (bluish) usually are apparent at 30–72 hours postinoculation or at about the time detachment of cells begins. Replication time and the Feulgen and acridine orange staining reaction were noted under Chemical Composition and Viral Replication herein.

Plaques in chicken embryo kidney cells overlaid by agar could be counted at 5 days postinoculation, increased from 0.5–1.0 mm to 10–11 mm in diameter at 28 days, and had continuous regular edges, whereas those produced by ILT virus had irregular edges (Chomiak et al., 1961).

In duck kidney cell cultures, CELO produced CPE similar to that in chicken kidney cells—including death and peeling away of cell sheets (Burke et al., 1959b). According to Mancini and Yates (1968), CELO virus replicated in both neuroglial and fibroblastic cell cultures from chicken embryos. In the fibroblasts round-type CPE and detachment of the cells occurred, but this effect was overcome and a sheet of healthy cells was reestablished. The authors suggested that this study should be repeated with methods that would decrease the possibility of cell types other than fibroblasts being in the culture. In the neuroglial cells no CPE was observed. Attempts to propagate CELO virus in monkey or bovine kidney cells were unsuccessful (Burke et al., 1959a; Yates, 1960). No CPE was produced in FL human amnion cells (Clemmer, 1964).

Other Laboratory Hosts

Newborn hamsters inoculated subcutaneously with CELO virus developed fibrosarcomas which could be transferred serially in weanlings by implant of the tumors or by inoculation with tumor homogenates (Sarma et al., 1965; Jasty et al., 1968). Although infectious CELO virus was not recovered from such tumors nor from early tumor cell cultures, a specific tumor antigen was demonstrated by complement fixation and by immunofluorescence in tumor cells subcultured in vitro at least 50 times and in hamster-born tumors induced by CELO virus (Potter and Oxford, 1969).

Suckling mice, rabbits, guinea pigs, pi-

geons, and Japanese quail inoculated with CELO virus showed no evidence of infection (Yates and Fry, 1957; Kawamura et al., 1963).

PATHOGENESIS AND EPIZOOTIOLOGY

NATURAL AND EXPERIMENTAL HOSTS

Because bobwhite quail are infected by natural transmission and develop a recognized disease—quail bronchitis (Olson, 1950; DuBose and Grumbles, 1959), and because inapparent infections in chickens are both widespread and naturally transmitted (Yates and Fry, 1957; Yates, 1960), we may for practical purposes consider them both as natural hosts for QBV or CELO virus. Bobwhite quail usually are affected by acute quail bronchitis at 8 weeks of age or less; the incidence of mild forms of the disease or possible inapparent infections is not known (DuBose, 1967, 1971). CELO virus infections are known to occur in adult chickens, but the incidence of isolations was highest from the 4–12-week age group in a study by Taylor and Calnek (1962).

Natural infections in turkeys, pheasants, redwing blackbirds, swan (Yates, 1960), goshawk, and "scolopacidi" (reports cited by Rinaldi et al., 1968) were indicated either by isolations of the agent or by detection of CELO-QBV antibodies in serum; the frequency of such infections and the status of such species as *natural hosts* are not really known.

Experimental hosts—in addition to quail, chickens, and those noted under laboratory hosts—have been investigated primarily to the extent of studying their susceptibility. No clinical signs were observed in pheasants inoculated with CELO by several routes, although their preinoculation serum contained no CELO antibodies; nestling starlings and sparrows also did not show specific reactions, but CELO was reisolated from the respiratory tracts and livers of the sparrows (Yates, 1960). Ducklings inoculated orally or intratracheally showed no respiratory signs, but CELO was reisolated from the feces, liver, spleen, and kidney during a viremic phase (Greuel, 1966, cited by Rinaldi et al., 1968). Turkeys inoculated with QBV or CELO have shown either transient respiratory signs or no signs; QBV was reisolated in some instances (Olson,

1950; Yates and Fry, 1957; DuBose et al., 1958).

In trials to determine susceptibility of a species, it should be kept in mind that infections achieved by artificial routes of exposure and with high doses of virus do not necessarily indicate that the species is generally susceptible to infection by natural means of exposure.

TRANSMISSIONS, CARRIERS, AND VECTORS

Quail Bronchitis

Quail bronchitis is apparently highly contagious (Olson, 1950; DuBose, 1967, 1971, and unpublished observations). Signs are usually seen in all susceptible young quail in contact with each other within 3–7 days of the signs first being noticed; transmission from pen to pen is rapid; and, unless stringent precautions are taken, the disease occurs in succeeding hatches during the year on the same game bird farm. Although not proved experimentally, airborne transmission is probable in addition to mechanical transmission. Circumstantial evidence indicates that QBV may be transmitted to bobwhite quail from a variety of other avian species not showing overt signs of disease.

CELO Infections in Chickens

Mechanical transmission of CELO in fecal material between flocks or pens, as well as within pens, is suggested by the demonstrated excretion of the virus in fecal or cloacal material (Taylor and Calnek, 1962; Clemmer, 1964). That airborne transmission also may be a factor is suggested by isolation of the agent from the respiratory tract (Kawamura et al., 1963) and the widespread incidence of infections. Transovarian transmission has been demonstrated beyond any reasonable doubt (Yates et al., 1960), but its importance compared to other modes of infection is not established.

INCUBATION PERIOD, SIGNS, MORBIDITY, AND MORTALITY

Quail Bronchitis

The incubation period of 2–7 days in experimentally infected quail (Olson, 1950; DuBose and Grumbles, 1959) is consistent with the rapid onset of signs noted in natural outbreaks (DuBose et al., 1958; Du-

Bose, 1967). In quail under 4 weeks of age, tracheal rales, coughing, and sneezing are characteristic, sometimes accompanied by huddling and depressed attitudes. Lacrimation and conjunctivitis may be observed, but nasal exudate is not a usual feature. Neural signs are infrequent but have appeared in both natural and experimental infections. The course of the disease is 1–3 weeks, morbidity may be 100%, and mortality ranges from 10 to 100%—frequently over 50%. Rapidity of spread and severity of the disease may be markedly less in older quail.

CELO Infections in Chickens

The incubation period in natural infections is not known, but Yates (1960) reisolated CELO from the intestines and other tissues 2 days after inoculation of 5–6-week-old chickens; Cook (1968) observed Feulgen-positive intranuclear inclusion bodies in tracheal epithelial cells 3 days after intratracheal inoculation; and Berry (1969) reported a drop in egg production apparent in the 1st week after inoculation with an "adenovirus" of the same serotype as a CELO virus (Isolate EV-89) studied by Burke et al. (1968). Circumstantial evidence indicates that CELO virus may be in the eggs within 8 days after natural infection of the hen (DuBose and Grumbles, 1959).

Signs of infection as a rule have been absent in uncomplicated cases of either natural or experimental infections with CELO or other avian adenovirus serotypes, an exception being the neural signs following intracerebral inoculation of CELO virus (Rinaldi et al., 1968). The infection apparently occurs in all or nearly all exposed chickens, and duration of the active infection (based on the periods during which CELO was excreted from individual birds) probably does not exceed 2 months and may be less than 1 month (Khanna, 1966; Burke et al., 1959a,b).

Combination Infections

Although increasing attention is being, and should be, paid to possible pathogenic effects of CELO infections, many instances in which signs have been noted may have been caused by other pathogens present (Rinaldi et al., 1968) or by large experimental doses or unusual routes of infection, or they have been noted in a very small percentage of the birds naturally infected (Kawamura et al., 1963). In addition to reports cited by Rinaldi et al. (1968) suggesting a potentiating effect by CELO infection on respiratory problems involving *Mycoplasma gallisepticum, Escherichia coli,* and IBV, studies by Berry (1969) indicate that experimental combinations of adenovirus (apparently CELO) with *M. gallisepticum* or *M. gallisepticum* plus IBV have a marked depressant effect on egg production.

GROSS LESIONS AND HISTOPATHOLOGY

Quail Bronchitis

Excess mucus in the trachea and/or bronchi and cloudy air sac membranes, sometimes with mucoid exudate, have been observed (Olson, 1950; DuBose et al., 1958; DuBose, 1967). Cloudy corneas, conjunctivitis, and congestion of nasal or infraorbital sinuses may occur. A few young quail may be infected but present no signs or gross lesions. Histopathology has not been reported.

CELO Infections in Chickens

Information on lesions in natural infections is scanty. Kawamura et al. (1963) observed a slight swelling of the upper trachea of 2 chickens and, microscopically, a slight proliferation of small round cells in the trachea mucosa. No bacterial assay was done, but the flock was negative for antibodies against IBV, *Hemophilus gallinarum,* and *M. gallisepticum.* The general lack of reports of gross lesions in uncomplicated natural infections and following experimental administration of CELO via natural routes—trachea, cloaca, or orally—supports the general view of CELO virus infection in chickens as an inapparent infection. Clemmer (1965), for instance, inoculated chicks orally and recovered CELO for at least 10 days from 14 levels of the gastrointestinal tract and a variety of other organs; yet all organs appeared normal grossly. Cook (1968) detected Feulgen-positive intranuclear inclusion bodies in tracheal epithelial cells following intratracheal inoculation but made no comment on gross lesions.

Severe hepatic and pancreatic lesions resulted from intravenous (IV) or intracerebral (IC) inoculations of CELO virus in young chickens; intranuclear inclusion bodies appeared in the hepatic cells and pancreatic acinar epithelial cells (Rinaldi et al., 1968). Lesions of the central nervous system following IC inoculations also were reported.

IMMUNITY

In quail bronchitis the duration of immunity is not known, but survivors of both natural and experimental infections were refractory up to 6 months later to challenge with QBV, and significant antibody levels developed in serum of quail following infection (Olson, 1950; DuBose and Grumbles, 1959; DuBose, 1967). DuBose (1971) suggested a procedure for determining degree and duration of immunity and for demonstrating possible inapparent infections in adult quail.

The general degree of acquired immunity in flocks of chickens that have recovered from natural infection with CELO virus is not known. Chickens inoculated orally at 22 days of age have developed detectable antibody levels in 10 days which peaked at 20 days postinoculation (Kawamura et al., 1963). Not all chicks in groups inoculated at 1 day of age were refractory to later challenge, but maternal antibody may have affected the uniformity of initial infections (Clemmer, 1965). Maternal antibody detectable in serum of chicks 4 days of age was not detected at 42 days. Antibody induced by prior injection of inactivated CELO (formaldehyde 1:10,000; 37° C for 4 days) inhibited pharyngeal but not cloacal excretion of virus after challenge with infectious virus.

DIAGNOSIS

QUAIL BRONCHITIS

Bases for a diagnosis have been reviewed by DuBose (1967, 1971). In quail chicks a sudden onset of rales, sneezing, or coughing spreading rapidly through the group and resulting in mortality suggests quail bronchitis. Excess mucus in tracheas, bronchi, and air sacs is added evidence of the disease. As noted previously, severity of signs, rapidity of spread, and presence of lesions probably would be less marked in older quail. Isolation and identification of an agent indistinguishable from QBV (or CELO) would confirm the diagnosis.

Inoculation of 9–11-day embryonating chicken eggs via the CAS with suspensions of aqueous humor, trachea, air sacs, and/or lungs has been used for isolation of the agent. Up to 3 blind passages are made with allantoic fluid harvested from chilled eggs at 6 days postinoculation, earlier if excess allantoic fluid or stunting is observed in daily candling. (Characteristic embryo lesions were noted under Laboratory Hosts.) Embryo mortality within 3 passages, stunting, thickening of the amnion, necrotic foci or mottling of the liver, and accumulation of urates in the mesonephros are typical changes caused by QBV or CELO (or by IBV, but there are no reports of IBV infection in quail). Neutralization of the isolated virus by specific QBV or CELO antiserum would confirm identification of the virus and the diagnosis.

The use of cell culture systems described for isolation of CELO and neutralization tests to determine serotype should prove useful in diagnosis of quail bronchitis, but such use has not been described.

Pulmonary aspergillosis may be differentiated from quail bronchitis by the presence of caseous nodules in the lungs or deposits in the air sacs with pockets of grayish or greenish spore accumulations. Although bacterial infections might complicate the disease, none is known to cause the rapid development of the signs, lesions, and mortality of quail bronchitis. DuBose (1967) suggested that Newcastle disease might present a clinical picture similar in part to quail bronchitis, but clinical Newcastle disease has not been described in bobwhite quail.

CELO INFECTIONS OTHER THAN QUAIL BRONCHITIS

A specific pattern of signs and/or lesions has not been established in avian species other than bobwhite quail; therefore, a diagnosis of CELO virus infection depends primarily on isolation and identification of the agent. The methods outlined below would also indicate the presence of avian adenoviruses other than the CELO-QBV serotype.

Isolation

Both the gastrointestinal tract and the respiratory system should be tested for presence of the virus. After centrifugation and treatment with antibiotic, supernatant fluid from suspensions of rectal or cloacal swabbings and from pharyngeal or tracheal swabbings is used as the inoculum for the host system.

Chick or chicken embryo kidney cell cultures have come into general use for propagation of CELO (see Laboratory Host Systems). CELO or other avian adenoviruses will cause the round type CPE and intranuclear inclusion bodies (H & E-basophilic, Feulgen-positive, or acridine orange-bright yellow or greenish fluorescence) usually within 30–72 hours. Fully developed inclusion bodies are usually present at the time CPE is evident and the cell sheet is beginning to peel. Cultures should be held at least 8 days and blind passages made in case of negative results. Parallel control cell cultures will help in detecting adventitious agents in the cell culture system. Cloning by subculturing from individual plaques in an agar overlay cell culture may be used to insure against mixtures of adenovirus serotypes in subsequent virus neutralization tests.

Chicken embryos may be inoculated at 9–11 days of incubation via the CAS or with a large dose on the CAM. Lesions consistent with infection of the embryo by CELO were noted under Laboratory Hosts and under diagnosis of quail bronchitis above. The pathogenic effects of non-CELO adenovirus serotypes in chicken embryos have not been sufficiently studied to be certain they might not induce similar effects. Intranuclear inclusion bodies in the CAM with the cytochemical staining reactions noted in cell cultures above would be consistent with isolation of an avian adenovirus.

Serology and Differential Diagnosis

Specific identification of CELO virus (or QBV) depends at present on determining the serotype (Kawamura et al., 1964; Burke et al., 1968) by neutralization with antiserum against CELO. Preparation of antiserum in rabbits as described by Burke et al. (1968) and with a cloned CELO virus would decrease chances of working with a multivalent antiserum. The virus neutralization tests described by Burke et al. (1968) for assay in cell cultures, or by Cunningham (1963) for assay in chicken embryos, are satisfactory for identification of the CELO-QBV serotype. Agglutination of rat (but not chicken or sheep) red blood cells would support identification of the agent and indicate that Newcastle disease virus

(HA-positive with chicken red blood cells) was not present.

Group (avian) complement-fixing and agar gel precipitin antigens are possessed by the avian adenoviruses (Kawamura et al., 1964; Burke et al., 1968) but have not been reported to definitely differentiate the serotypes.

TREATMENT, PREVENTION, AND CONTROL

QUAIL BRONCHITIS

There is no specific treatment for quail bronchitis. Prevention and control were described in more detail by DuBose (1967, 1971).

Slightly increased warmth in the brooder or house, adequate ventilation but no drafts, and avoidance of crowding are suggested supportive measures during an outbreak. Prevention is based on protecting susceptible quail from all possible sources of QBV or CELO. In addition to the usual sanitation procedures and measures to prevent entry of infectious agents onto the premises, care should be taken to keep adult quail away from young quail and other avian species from all the quail. Control measures on a farm should be started immediately when even a tentative diagnosis of quail bronchitis is made. In addition to general measures to prevent transmission from group to group, hatching operations may be deferred until 2 weeks after signs have disappeared in order to provide a break in the presence of the highly susceptible young quail.

CELO INFECTION IN CHICKENS

Probably because it has been generally considered an inapparent infection and comparatively innocuous, no emphasis has been given to prevention of CELO infections in chickens other than in flocks providing fertile eggs for diagnostic or research work. If the report by Berry (1969) and those cited by Rinaldi et al. (1968) on possible involvement of CELO in disease processes are confirmed, more interest should be raised in this area.

Inactivated CELO virus vaccine has had only a limited effect (Clemmer, 1965). Use of live virus as a vaccine should be viewed with extreme caution because of the possibility of inadvertently spreading CELO or other serotypes into areas where they are not extant.

REFERENCES

Ablashi, D. V., P. W. Chang, and V. J. Yates. 1965. The effect of a latent CELO virus infection in the chicken embryo, on the propagation of Newcastle disease and influenza viruses. *Avian Diseases* 9:407–17.

Adlakha, S. C. 1966. Effect of certain physical and chemical agents on chick embryo lethal orphan (CELO) and infectious laryngotracheitis (ILT) viruses. *Indian J. Vet. Sci.* 36:237–42.

Berry, D. M. 1969. Egg production and disease: Adenovirus. *Vet. Record* 84:397–98.

Burke, C. N., R. E. Luginbuhl, and E. L. Jungherr. 1959a. Avian enteric cytopathogenic viruses. I. Isolation. *Avian Diseases* 3:412–18.

———. 1959b. Avian enteric cytopathogenic viruses. II. Characteristics of a prototype. *Avian Diseases* 3:419–27.

Burke, C. N., R. E. Luginbuhl, and C. F. Helmboldt. 1965. The isolation of a latent adenolike virus from chicken kidney cell cultures. *Avian Diseases* 9:31–43.

Burke, C. N., R. E. Luginbuhl, and L. F. Williams. 1968. Avian adeno-like viruses—Characterization and comparison of seven isolates. *Avian Diseases* 12:483–505.

Cabasso, V. J. 1967. An interim scheme for virus nomenclature. *Am. J. Vet. Res.* 28:539–48.

Chomiak, T. W., R. E. Luginbuhl, and C. F. Helmboldt. 1961. Tissue culture propagation and pathology of CELO virus. *Avian Diseases* 5:313–20.

Clemmer, D. I. 1964. Characterization of agents isolated from market chickens in a quest for enteric viruses. *J. Infect. Diseases* 114:386–400.

———. 1965. Experimental enteric infection of chickens with an avian adenovirus (strain 93). *Proc. Soc. Exp. Biol. Med.* 118:943–48.

Cook, J. K. A. 1968. Isolation of a CELO virus from fertile chicken eggs. *Vet. Record* 82:294.

Cunningham, C. H. 1963. *Laboratory Guide in Virology*, 5th ed. Burgess Publ. Co., Minneapolis.

Davis, B. D., R. Dulbecco, H. N. Eisen, H. S. Ginsberg, and W. B. Wood. 1967. (Reprinted with corrections, 1968.) *Microbiology*. Harper & Row, New York.

DuBose, R. T. 1967. Quail bronchitis. *Bull. Wildlife Disease Ass.* 3:10–13.

———. 1971. Quail bronchitis. In Davis, J. W., R. C. Anderson, Lars Karstad, and D. O.

Trainer (eds.), *Infectious and Parasitic Diseases of Wild Birds.* Iowa State Univ. Press, Ames.

DuBose, R. T., and L. C. Grumbles. 1959. The relationship between quail bronchitis virus and chicken embryo lethal orphan virus. *Avian Diseases* 3:321–44.

DuBose, R. T., L. C. Grumbles, and A. I. Flowers. 1958. The isolation of a nonbacterial agent from quail with a respiratory disease. *Poultry Sci.* 37:654–58.

———. 1960. Differentiation of quail bronchitis virus and infectious bronchitis virus by heat stability. *Am. J. Vet. Res.* 21:740–43.

Dutta, S. K., and B. S. Pomeroy. 1963. Electron microscopic structure of chicken embryo lethal orphan virus. *Proc. Soc. Exp. Biol. Med.* 114:539–41.

———. 1967. Electron microscopic studies of quail bronchitis virus. *Am. J. Vet. Res.* 28: 296–99.

Jasty, V., L. T. Miller, and V. J. Yates. 1968. Histopathology of avian adenovirus (CELO) induced hamster tumors. *J. Am. Vet. Med. Ass.* 152:1346.

Kawamura, H., T. Sato, H. Tsubahara, and S. Isogai. 1963. Isolation of CELO virus from chicken trachea. *Nat. Inst. Animal Health Quart.* 3:1–10.

Kawamura, H., F. Shimizu, and H. Tsubahara. 1964. Avian adenovirus: Its properties and serological classification. *Nat. Inst. Animal Health Quart.* 4:183–93.

Khanna, P. N. 1966. Studies on cytopathogenic avian enteroviruses. II. Influence of age on virus excretion and incidence of certain serotypes in a colony of chicks. *Avian Diseases* 5:27–32.

Maeda, M., A. Okaniwa, and H. Kawamura. 1967. Morphological studies on intranuclear inclusion bodies in chicken kidney cell culture infected with avian adenovirus. *Nat. Inst. Animal Health Quart.* 7:164–77.

Mancini, L. O., and V. J. Yates. 1968. Growth of chicken-embryo-lethal-orphan (CELO) virus in chicken embryo neurological and chicken embryo fibroblastic cell cultures. *Avian Diseases* 12:348–53.

Olson, N. O. 1950. A respiratory disease (bronchitis) of quail caused by a virus. *Proc. 54th Ann. Meet. U.S. Livestock Sanit. Ass.,* pp. 171–74.

Petek, M., B. Felluga, and R. Zoletto. 1963. Biological properties of CELO virus: Stability to various agents, and electron-microscopic study. *Avian Diseases* 7:38–49.

Potter, C. W., and J. S. Oxford. 1969. Specific tumor antigen induced by chicken embryo lethal orphan (CELO) virus. *J. Gen. Virol.* 4:287–89.

Rinaldi, A., G. Mandelli, D. Cessi, A. Caleri, and G. Cervio. 1968. Proprieta' di un ceppo di virus CELO isolato dal pollo in Italia. *Clin. Vet.* 91:382–404.

Sarma, P. S., R. J. Heubner, and W. T. Lane. 1965. Induction of tumors in hamsters with an avian adenovirus (CELO). *Science* 149: 1108.

Sharpless, G. R. 1962. GAL virus. *Ann. N.Y. Acad. Sci.* 101:515–19.

Taylor, P. J., and B. W. Calnek. 1962. Isolation and classification of avian enteric cytopathogenic agents. *Avian Diseases* 6:51–58.

Wilner, B. I. 1969. *A Classification of the Major Groups of Human and Other Viruses,* 4th ed. Burgess Publ. Co., Minneapolis.

Yates, V. J. 1960. Characterization of the chicken-embryo-lethal-orphan (CELO) virus. Ph.D. thesis, Univ. Wisconsin.

Yates, V. J., and D. E. Fry. 1957. Observations on a chicken embryo lethal orphan (CELO) virus. *Am. J. Vet. Res.* 17:657–60.

Yates, V. J., D. E. Fry, and B. Wasserman. 1954. *Proc. 26th Ann. Meet. N.E. Conf. Lab. Workers in Pullorum Disease Control.*

Yates, V. J., P. W. Chang, A. H. Dardiri, and D. E. Fry. 1960. A study in the epizootiology of the CELO virus. *Avian Diseases* 4:500–505.

Yates, V. J., D. V. Ablashi, P. W. Chang, and D. E. Fry. 1962. The chicken-embryo-lethal-orphan (CELO) virus as a tissue-culture contaminant. *Avian Diseases* 6:406–11.

❖

AVIAN MONOCYTOSIS

❖

R. T. DU BOSE

*Department of Veterinary Science
Virginia Polytechnic Institute
Blacksburg, Virginia*

❖

Two APPARENTLY unrelated conditions, one in chickens and the other in turkeys, have been called avian monocytosis as a result of hematological findings. This subchapter will be concerned with only a brief description of the chicken disease. Transmissible enteritis (bluecomb) of turkeys is covered in Chapter 25.

In chickens avian monocytosis (pullet disease, bluecomb) was first described by Beaudette (1929) under the term X disease. It has been characterized as a transient disease with high morbidity; low mortality; and congestive, hemorrhagic, inflammatory, and necrotic lesions. After discussing various names that had been applied to the syndrome, Jungherr and Matterson (1944) pointed out that monocytosis apparently was associated with most of its pathologic expressions and suggested the scientific name "avian monocytosis."

Although it was mainly a problem in pullets during the first few months of lay, it has been observed in chicks as young as 4 weeks and in hens at 2 years of age. Lack of definitive criteria has hindered diagnostic classification, but occurrence has been reported in England, Europe, Japan, Australia, Pakistan, and India. Avian monocytosis was of great economic importance in sections of the United States in the second quarter of this century. Since then the incidence apparently has decreased to an almost negligible level, according to most state diagnostic reports.

Portions of this subchapter are from Chapter 31 of the previous edition by Drs. E. Jungherr (deceased) and B. S. Pomeroy and are used here with permission of Dr. Pomeroy.

ETIOLOGY

No definite causative agent has been established for avian monocytosis of chickens. Waller (1942, 1944), Watanabe (1952), and Watanabe et al. (1952) reported on the isolation of filterable agents, presumably viruses, in chicken embryos from cases of avian monocytosis. These reports were never confirmed by others. Noninfectious causes such as sudden temperature changes (Maas and Voute, 1961), nephrotoxic substances in new wheat (Quigley, 1943, 1944), and water deprivation (Fisher et al., 1961) have been incriminated in some outbreaks.

PATHOGENESIS

SIGNS, MORBIDITY, AND MORTALITY

Reviews were provided by Jungherr and Matterson (1944) and Jungherr and Pomeroy (1965). In a typical outbreak, a large proportion of an apparently healthy flock may suddenly develop inappetence, depression, and a watery or whitish diarrhea, sometimes with soiling of the vent feathers by urate accumulations. Cyanosis and wilting of the comb and wattles (bluecomb), sunken eyes, and dehydrated shanks are observed. In many birds the crop is distended with sour-smelling material. In laying birds a marked drop in egg production is typical, and recovery in production lags beyond the time when other signs of the disease have disappeared. Mortality may range from 0 to 50% but generally averages about 5% of the flock. The disease usually runs a course of 1–2 weeks, followed by a rapid clinical recovery, particularly in well-cared-for flocks.

GROSS LESIONS

In typical cases, chickens affected with avian monocytosis usually are in good flesh. The birds are dehydrated, and occasionally whitish gray streaks of degenerative areas are observed in the breast muscles. The crop is usually filled with sour-smelling feed and the intestines contain an accumulation of mucus. The liver is congested and the pancreas usually has a chalky appearance. The spleen appears normal. The kidneys are swollen with varying degrees of urate deposits. Occasionally typical cases of visceral gout are observed. In birds that are in production, the abdominal cavity is filled with slimy yolk material and the ovary contains broken or flabby yolk follicles.

HISTOPATHOLOGY

Microscopic lesions of diagnostic significance are found primarily in the kidney. In fresh necropsy material, extensive cloudy swelling, pyknosis, and desquamation of the epithelium of the proximal convoluted tubuli are observed. Other renal changes reported by Jungherr and Pomeroy (1965) consist of dilatation of tubuli associated with flattening of the epithelium and formation of hyaline casts (Fig. 26.4) and pseudogiant cells (Fig. 26.5) from infolding epithelium. The larger of these foci may show crystalloid radiating centers considered to be pathognomonic for uric nephritis (Siller, 1959). In protracted cases the tubuli show many cellular casts composed of disintegrating heterophils. The glomeruli may show thickening of the basement membrane and dilatation of the glomerular space containing desquamated cells (Fig. 26.6).

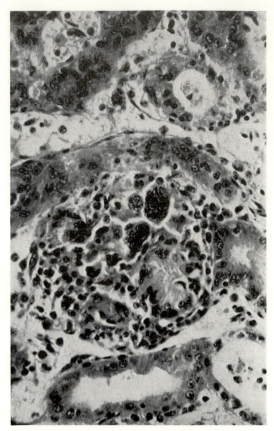

FIG. 26.5—Avian monocytosis. Section of kidney with pseudogiant cells in tubuli. ×500.

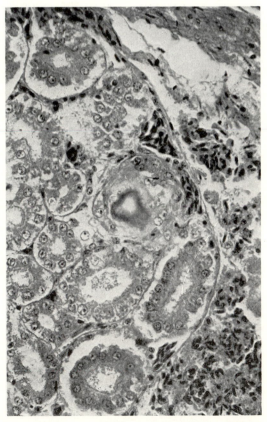

FIG. 26.4—Avian monocytosis. Section of kidney with large cast in center. ×500.

The intestinal changes are chiefly those of a catarrhal enteritis. There may be desquamation of the epithelium with the subepithelial zones showing marked increase in cellularity. The inflammatory cells are composed chiefly of mononuclears, lymphocytes, and histiocytes. It is not uncommon to find many cystic crypts containing inspissated mucus (Jungherr and Matterson, 1944).

The chalkiness in the pancreas appears to be brought about by cloudy swelling in the center of the acinar lobules, according to Jungherr and Pomeroy (1965). In addition, there appears to be an increase in the size of the Langerhans' islets.

The liver usually shows congestion and, according to Jungherr and Pomeroy (1965), there may occasionally be focal areas of necrosis, a lesion which when observed must be differentiated from vibrionic hepatitis.

The skeletal muscle of the breast may

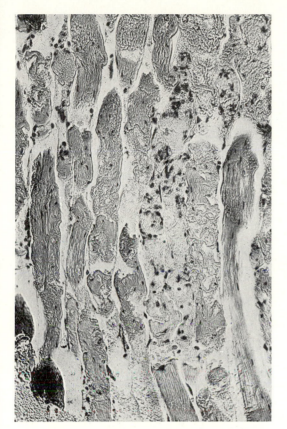

FIG. 26.6—Avian monocytosis. Section of kidney with dilated glomerular space containing desquamated cells. ×150.

show degenerative change typical of Zenker's degeneration (Fig. 26.7). The myofibers are either in a state of granular disintegration separated by interstitial edema or, more characteristically, show loss of striation, fragmentation, and hyaline swelling, associated with mild polynuclear infiltration and incipient regeneration (Jungherr and Pomeroy, 1965).

HEMATOLOGY

Jungherr and Pomeroy (1965) observed a relative and absolute monocytosis of about 20% or 8,000 per cu mm compared to the normal of 8.9% or 1,700. Blood changes varied in intensity with the clinicopathologic picture and seemed more marked when the kidneys were involved. A moderate but consistent leukocytosis averaging 40,000 per cu mm was observed. The chemicopathologic picture was believed to be "in keeping with a uremic concept of pullet disease."

DIAGNOSIS AND DIFFERENTIAL DIAGNOSIS

Widespread sudden morbidity associated with cyanosis and diarrhea, monocytosis, high uric acid content, hepatic necrosis, and uric nephrosis were considered diagnostic points by Jungherr and Matterson (1944), as long as fowl typhoid, pullorum disease, fowl cholera, and lymphomatosis involving the kidneys had been eliminated. Appropriate steps also should be taken to rule out avian vibriosis (Chapter 9), infectious bursal disease (this chapter), infections with nephrotropic infectious bronchitis virus (Chapter 16), and the fatty liver/kidney syndrome ("pink" disease, fat nephrosis) described by Barron et al. (1966).

In the absence of the above and other known disease entities, a diagnosis of avian monocytosis may be made on the basis of high monocytosis and the signs, lesions, and flock history described for the syndrome.

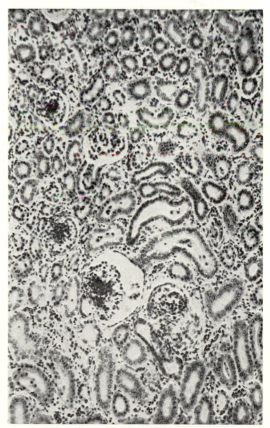

FIG. 26.7—Avian monocytosis. Zenker's degeneration in section of breast muscle.

TREATMENT, PREVENTION, AND CONTROL

Reports suggesting supplementation of the diet with potassium (supplied as molasses or as muriate of potash) and administration of oxytetracycline were cited by Jungherr and Pomeroy (1965), but efficacy of these treatments has not been generally confirmed. In the absence of known specific etiology, only general supportive measures can be recommended. For treatment or as a possible aid in prevention, provision should be made for adequate water, shade, ventilation, and protection from extreme heat or cold or other stress. Methods that bar transmission of infectious agents to or between groups of birds should be applied.

REFERENCES

Barron, N. S., B. S. Hanson, W. G. Siller, L. A. Hemsley, M. H. Fussell, D. McK. Fraser, and A. H. Sykes. 1966. The kidney/liver syndrome in chickens. *Vet. Record* 78: 624–26.

Beaudette, F. R. 1929. X disease. *New Jersey Agr. Expt. Sta., Poultry Pathol. Notes* 1:6–7.

Fisher, H., P. Griminger, H. S. Weiss, and C. B. Hudson. 1961. Observations on water deprivation and blue comb disease. *Poultry Sci.* 40:813.

Jungherr, E., and J. M. Levine. 1941. The pathology of so-called pullet disease. *Am. J. Vet. Res.* 2:261.

Jungherr, E., and L. D. Matterson. 1944. Avian monocytosis, so-called pullet disease. *Proc. 48th Ann. Meet. U.S. Livestock Sanit. Ass.,* pp. 185–96.

Jungherr, E., and B. S. Pomeroy. 1965. Avian monocytosis, pp. 455–56. In Biester, H. E., and L. H. Schwarte (eds.), *Diseases of Poultry,* 5th ed. Iowa State Univ. Press, Ames.

Maas, H. J. L., and E. J. Voute. 1961. Een praktijkonderzoek over de blauwe kam ziekte bij hoenders in "het land von Weert." *Vlaams Diergeneesk. Tijdschr.* 30:106.

Quigley, G. D. 1943. Is blue comb of fowls produced by wheat? *Poultry Sci.* 22:267.

———. 1944. The effect of wheat upon the incidence of pullet disease or blue comb. *Poultry Sci.* 23:386.

Siller, W. G. 1959. Avian nephritis and visceral gout. *Lab. Invest.* 8:1319.

Waller, E. F. 1942. Isolation of a filtrable virus from chickens affected with "blue comb" disease. *Science* 95:560.

———. 1944. Blue comb disease. *Proc. 48th Ann. Meet. U.S. Livestock Sanit. Ass.,* pp. 171–76.

Watanabe, M. 1952. Avian infectious diarrhea. I. Clinical, hematologic and histopathologic findings. *Japan. J. Vet. Sci.* 14:263–67.

Watanabe, M., T. Yamano, R. Mifune, and T. Oochi. 1952. Avian infectious diarrhea (similar to so-called pullet disease). *Virus* 2:99.

RABIES

❖

R. T. DU BOSE

Department of Veterinary Science
Virginia Polytechnic Institute
Blacksburg, Virginia

❖

RABIES is an acute infectious viral encephalitis characterized by symptoms of a central nervous system disturbance, progressive paralysis, and, in most species, termination by death. Most if not all warm-blooded animals are susceptible to infection. The virus is present in the saliva of infected mammals and in nature is usually transmitted by their bite. In birds naturally transmitted rabies is apparently rare, and not until recently has the overall pathogenesis of rabies in an avian species been adequately studied (Schneider and Burtscher, 1967).

No important public health significance has been established for rabies in birds. Schweinberg (1928) reported a case in which a patient had been injured by a rabid hen, and Schneider and Burtscher (1967) cited a report describing a clinically diagnosed case of rabies in a boy after being bitten by a goose. However, from a total of 100 countries reporting rabies surveillance data for 1967 to the World Health Organization, there were only 2 instances reported in which exposures of humans were associated with avian species considered positive for rabies (R. K. Sikes, 1969, personal communication). In spite of this comparative lack of economic or public health significance, susceptibility of birds to infection with rabies virus should be kept in mind by those concerned with diagnosis of avian diseases.

Portions of this subchapter are from Chapter 29 of the previous edition and are used here with permission of the author, Dr. L. H. Schwarte.

HISTORY

According to Schneider and Burtscher (1967), rabies in fowl was described in 1882 and even earlier, but the disease is not economically important in domestic poultry, and birds do not seem to play a role in sylvatic enzootics.

Gibier (1884) transmitted the disease to chickens, and Kraus and Clairmont (1900) studied the susceptibility of chickens, geese, and pigeons. Kraus and Clairmont (1900) and Von Löte (1904) reported on the susceptibility of several birds of prey. Von Löte considered chickens and pigeons more resistant than predatory birds to experimental infection. Remlinger and Bailly (1929a,b) transmitted the disease to the chicken by bites inflicted on the comb by a rabid dog, but they considered the occurrence of rabies in chickens under natural conditions to be comparatively rare. They also transmitted rabies to the stork (*Ciconia ciconia*) by intracerebral inoculation (Remlinger and Bailly, 1936). Jacotot (1938) reported experimental transmission to the pheasant (*Diardigallus diardi* B. P.).

INCIDENCE AND DISTRIBUTION

Rabies is almost worldwide in distribution as judged by its incidence in mammals (Tierkel, 1959), but the occurrence in birds has been so rarely proved that the incidence of the naturally transmitted clinical disease in avian species is almost nil.

ETIOLOGY

Rabies virus is one of the RNA-helical-enveloped viruses, a major group of agents with somewhat similar morphology but with differences in biological, physical, and fine-structure characteristics, and leads a subgroup termed the "rabieslike viruses" (Wilner, 1969). The virions of the rabieslike viruses are cylindrical, bullet-shaped particles approximately 60×175 mμ. Some round forms $80–200$ mμ in diameter have been reported, and surface projections have been seen. The nucleocapsids appeared to be complex helices formed of a strand $4–8$ mμ wide, the helical capsids being $10–20$ mμ in diameter. Buoyant density was $1.19–1.20$ g/cm^3 in CsCl.

Rabies virus contains RNA, is sensitive to ether and acid pH, is slowly inactivated in tissues stored in neutral glycerol, and is stable in frozen or lyophilized tissue extracts. These and other biological, chemical, and physical properties have been reviewed by Tierkel (1959), Davis et al. (1967), and Wilner (1969).

A complete virion apparently is formed by budding from the cell membranes (Wilner, 1969), but formation of the complete particle is preceded by the development of an intracytoplasmic ground substance or matrix which constitutes the Negri body (Hummeler et al., 1968). The strands which make up the matrix may be the nucleoprotein of the virion. In spite of isolations from various sources and attenuation by a variety of means, all rabies viruses appear to be of a single immunological type (Davis et al., 1967).

In chickens, Schneider and Burtscher (1967) found that fixed virus (Novi Sad strain) was lowest in pathogenicity, street virus was intermediate, and Flury virus (adapted to chicken embryos) was highest.

Mice, guinea pigs, rabbits, hamsters, and dogs have been employed to establish laboratory infections with rabies virus (Tierkel, 1959; Davis et al., 1967). The virus also has been propagated in chicken and duck embryos. Hamster kidney, human diploid, and chicken embryo cell cultures support viral multiplication, but cytopathogenic changes usually are not seen.

PATHOGENESIS AND EPIZOOTIOLOGY

NATURAL AND EXPERIMENTAL HOSTS

The susceptibility to infection of a number of species of birds has been amply demonstrated experimentally; but the evidence that many avian subjects do not develop clinical rabies after experimental inoculation or exposure (Kraus and Clairmont, 1900; Von Löte, 1904; Marie, 1904; Schneider and Burtscher, 1967), that some avian subjects recover after showing symptoms (Von Löte, 1904; Schneider and Burtscher, 1967), that virus does not necessarily appear in the saliva of all affected birds (Remlinger and Bailly, 1929a; Schneider and Burtscher, 1967), and that infection may take a closed form in which virus proliferation is restricted to and limited in the central nervous system (Schneider and Burtscher, 1967) all suggest that birds may be considered an atypical rather than a natural host.

Experimental avian hosts for rabies have included chickens, turkeys, geese, ducks, pigeons, peafowl, pheasants, storks, owls, hawks, songbirds, ravens, and falcons (Schneider and Burtscher, 1967); the numbers inoculated were not sufficient to establish a definite pattern of outcome for some of these species.

TRANSMISSION AND CARRIERS

Most of the natural infections in birds probably occur as the result of bites by rabid mammals. Schneider and Burtscher (1967) noted a report of a chicken farm in an endemic rabies region which has been frequently visited by foxes. Rabies in some of the chickens was diagnosed on the basis of increased irritability and paralytic symptoms and confirmed by detection of rabies antigen with fluorescent antibody (FA) in the brain of one chicken sent in for testing. Remlinger and Bailly (1929a,b) successfully simulated natural transmission to the chicken by bites on the comb by a rabid dog. In one instance they demonstrated transmission from bird to bird. After a fight between a healthy and an experimentally infected rooster, additional injuries were produced with the tip of the beak of the rabid bird in the comb of the former, and these wounds were brushed with saliva from the sick rooster. The raging form of rabies developed in 14 days. In similar attempts with other roosters and with guinea pigs, they were unable to show transmission from bird to bird or from bird to mammal. From their work with chickens and from their review of earlier reports, Schneider and Burtscher (1967) formed the opinion that natural transmission of rabies infection to birds was unlikely unless the virus was implanted in the central nervous system or in organs rich in vessels and nerves (combs and wattles), and that, in chickens at least, only massive doses would be likely to produce typical courses of infection. They also concluded that chickens and other birds were of only minor importance as carriers of the disease.

INCUBATION PERIOD, SIGNS, MORBIDITY, AND MORTALITY

Information on the incubation period and course of rabies in birds is predominantly from experimental studies. Considerable variation in the incubation period— from 2 weeks in owls and geese to 40 days or more in chickens—was recorded by Kraus and Clairmont (1900). They observed gradual cessation of signs and slow recovery in some instances. Signs in chickens included incoordination, paresis, paralysis, and in some emaciation and death. Von Löte (1904) infected predatory birds and chickens. Eleven days after subdural inoculation, a mouse hawk *(Buteo vulgaris)* showed inappetance, then disturbance of the central nervous system, and later convulsions of short duration. On the 3rd day after appearance of signs, the hawk was prostrate and on the 4th day died. On the other hand, 2 eagle-owls exhibited no appreciable signs of infection but died 2½ and 9 months respectively after inoculation. Guinea pigs inoculated with brain tissue from the 2 birds developed rabies. Of 3 cockerels inoculated with rabies virus, only 1 contracted the disease. After a 43-day incubation period, the affected bird refused food and showed incoordination for 3 days, returned to normal for 2 weeks, showed severe signs for 1 week, then recovered. A similar course was observed in a hen which completely recovered. After surveying the reports published from 1900 to 1938, Schneider and Burtscher (1967) concluded that the signs and course of experimental rabies in geese, ducks, storks, peacocks, and pheasants approximately resemble those in the chicken.

From their observations of the reactions of chicks and roosters to 3 strains of rabies viruses, Schneider and Burtscher (1967) tabulated the course of rabies in chickens as follows: (1) incubation period of 12–40 days, duration depending on the strain of virus; (2) paroxysmal excitations of varying severities for 1–2 days; (3) somnolence and lack of appetite for 1–5 days; and (4) a further course classified by group as: (a) loss of weight, loss of strength, and early death; or (b) paresis, paralysis, relapses, deterioration, and death; or (c) apparent recovery, aggressive relapses (usually after several months) with rapidly developing paralysis and death; or (d) with or without relapses, a final recovery.

GROSS LESIONS AND HISTOPATHOLOGY

As in mammals (Tierkel, 1959; Smith and Jones, 1966), no gross lesions have been reported for rabies in birds.

The histopathology of chicken rabies described by Schneider and Burtscher (1967) is of particular value because parallel observations were made on the clinical course of the disease and on the presence or absence of infectious virus in the central nervous system and various other organs, of noninfectious rabies-specific antigen in the central nervous system, of antibodies in the serum, and of virus-neutralizing substances in the central nervous system. At 7 days after intracranial inoculation with street virus, chicks showed an almost insignificant nonsupporative inflammation in the brain. The reaction increased in intensity and extent with time, reaching at 30–50 days postinoculation, a climax which coincided with the peak in clinical symptoms. The inflammatory reaction consisted mainly of vascular infiltration of histiocytes, lymphocytes, and plasma cells, with the latter two types predominating. Perivascular infiltrates and glial cell proliferation also were observed, as well as local edema and decay of the medullary sheath. Ganglion cells in the region of the inflammatory infiltrates showed degeneration. At 109 days postinoculation the infiltrates and cell proliferation had decreased considerably, and at 233 days could still be observed but were regressive in nature. During the course of the disease, the degree and extent of the inflammatory changes in the brain and spinal cord were about the same, and the amounts of rabies antigen detected by FA in the brain and spinal cord were similar, but virus infectious for mice was never reisolated from the spinal cord. Negri bodies, considered the only pathognomonic microscopic finding for rabies in mammals (Davis et al., 1967), were not found, although the street virus used possessed good Negri-body-forming properties. Schneider and Burtscher (1967) noted that this was in agreement with the experiences of other authors: that Negri bodies could only rarely be found in chicken brains and then only in small numbers, and that in the majority of cases they were absent.

IMMUNITY

The observations of Schneider and Burtscher (1967) suggest that an active immune mechanism rapidly develops in the central nervous system of chicks inoculated intracerebrally with street virus. A virus-neutralizing substance appears in the cell-free brain and spinal cord extracts and, as with serum antibody, can be titrated in a virus neutralization test. The substance was first detected at 18 days postinoculation, 3 days after the last successful reisolation of infectious virus, and increased in titer as the degree of histopathological reaction in the central nervous system increased. Although CNS-bound antibody was detected before and generally remained higher in titer than serum antibody, the two followed a somewhat parallel course (Schneider and Burtscher, 1967).

In a limited trial on acquired immunity, Schneider and Burtscher (1967) reinoculated 2 chickens which had received street virus 7 months previously and which had shown typical signs and then recovered. Three controls developed signs of rabies at 20 days postinoculation, but the reinoculated birds remained healthy. Thirty days after the 2nd inoculation, virus infectious for mice could not be reisolated and specific antigen could not be detected by FA, but a mild nonsuppurative encephalitis was observed and the antibody content of both brain and serum was high.

The reports of individual birds within several species being refractory to experimental infection and of the recovery of others after showing signs of rabies (Gibier, 1884; Kraus and Clairmont, 1900; Von Löte, 1904; Marie, 1904; Remlinger and Bailly, 1929a,b; Schneider and Burtscher, 1967) indicate that at the time of infection, birds already have an available defense mechanism over and above that found in the highly susceptible mammals.

DIAGNOSIS

Clinical signs in rabid birds vary to such a degree that they do not constitute a reasonable basis for diagnosis. The signs indicating a central nervous system involvement cannot be differentiated definitely from those seen in Newcastle disease, Marek's disease, avian encephalomyelitis, encephalomalacia, and some forms of chlorinated hydrocarbon intoxication.

The histopathological changes noted by Schneider and Burtscher (1967) are not pathognomonic, and Negri bodies may not be seen in the avian species. Isolation of the virus from the brain and its identification in a laboratory host such as the mouse is diagnostic, but infectious virus may not be obtainable from the bird once clinical signs have appeared. For a long period after infection, however, rabies-specific antigen in the central nervous system may be detected by FA and a rabies virus-neutralizing substance in cell-free brain extracts may be titrated.

Because of the unusual danger to humans, reisolation of infectious virus and other methods that might involve live rabies virus should not be attempted except under the guidance of qualified personnel who routinely perform such work or by those who first familiarize themselves with the necessary precautions. Wachendorfer (1967) has demonstrated that slide-smear preparations from infected brains are potentially infective for laboratory personnel regardless of the type of fixative and also after treatment with fluorescein-conjugated specific antibody material.

Each state has at least one laboratory with personnel and facilities for the diagnosis of rabies. Should rabies in a bird be suspected (particularly if there is reason to believe it has been bitten by a rabid animal), the bird should be killed and its head removed, placed in a water-tight container, chilled rapidly, and kept cold. Instructions should be obtained from the state laboratory for their preferred method of further packaging and shipping. Since submission of avian brains for rabies examination is extremely rare, the suggestion should be made to the receiving laboratory that Negri bodies may not necessarily be found in rabies-infected birds.

TREATMENT, PREVENTION, AND CONTROL

As is typical for viral infections, no effective treatment has been described. A program for prevention and control of rabies in domestic fowl presumably would be needed only in an area where rabies was enzootic in mammals and logically would include penning or housing that would preclude any contact between poultry and mammals. Schneider and Burtscher (1967) believed that it was not necessary to include poultry in laws concerning control of rabies in domestic animals, that it was sufficient to eliminate those which had been bitten, and that only birds that were obviously sick and suspected to be infected with rabies virus needed to be killed and submitted for laboratory examination.

Although attenuated rabies virus might be used for immunization of poultry, there seems to be no economic or public health grounds for such action.

REFERENCES

Davis, B. D., R. Dulbecco, H. N. Eisen, H. S. Ginsberg, and W. B. Wood. 1967. (Reprinted with corrections, 1968.) *Microbiology*. Harper & Row, New York.

Gibier, P. 1884. Recherches experimentales sur la rage. *Compt. Rend. Acad. Sci.* 98:531. (Abstr.)

Hummeler, K., N. Tomassini, F. Sokol, E. Kuwert, and H. Koprowski. 1968. Morphology of the nucleoprotein component of rabies virus. *J. Virol.* 2:1191–99.

Jacotot, H. 1938. Transmission de la rage au faisan (*Diardigallus diardi* B. P.). *Compt. Rend. Soc. Biol.* 127:131–32.

Kraus, R., and P. Clairmont. 1900. Ueber experimentelle Lyssa bei Voegeln. *Zeitschr. Hyg. Infektionskrankh.* 34:1–30.

Marie, M. A. 1904. Note sur la rage chez les oiseaux. *Compt. Rend. Soc. Biol.* 56:573–75.

Remlinger, P., and J. Bailly. 1929a. La rage du coq. *Ann. Inst. Pasteur* (Paris) 43:153–67.

———. 1929b. Nouvelles observations relatives a la rage du coq. *Bull. Acad. Vet. France* 82:286.

———. 1936. Transmission de la rage a la cignone (*Ciconia ciconia*). *Compt. Rend. Soc. Biol.* 123:383–85.

Schneider, L. G., and H. Burtscher. 1967. Untersuchungen ueber die Pathogenese der Tollwut bei Huehnern nach intracerebraler Infektion. *Zentr. Veterinaermed.* 14B:598–624.

Schweinberg, F. 1928. Seuchenbekaempfung. *Jahresber. Vet. Med.* 48:930.

Smith, H. A., and T. C. Jones. 1966. *Veterinary Pathology*, 3rd ed. Lea & Febiger, Philadelphia.

Tierkel, E. S. 1959. Rabies, pp. 183–226. In Brandly, C. A., and E. L. Jungherr (eds.), *Advances in Veterinary Science*, Vol. 5. Academic Press, New York and London.

Von Löte, J. 1904. Beitraege zur Kenntnis der experimentellen Lyssa der Voegel. *Zentr. Bakteriol. Parasitenk. Abt. I. Orig.* 35:741–44.

Wachendorfer, G. 1967. Zur Frage der Ueberlebensdauer des Tollwutvirus in fixierten und mit fluoresceinmarkierten Antikoerpern "gafaerbten" Praeparaten. *Berlin. Muench. Tieraerztl. Wochschr.* 80:127–30.

Wilner, B. I. 1969. *A Classification of the Major Groups of Human and Other Animal Viruses*, 4th ed. Burgess Publ. Co., Minneapolis.

❖

FOOT-AND-MOUTH DISEASE

❖

R. T. DU BOSE

*Department of Veterinary Science
Virginia Polytechnic Institute
Blacksburg, Virginia*

❖

FOOT-AND-MOUTH DISEASE (FMD) is a viral disease of both domestic and wild cloven-footed mammals and is characterized by production of vesicular lesions in and around the mouth and on the feet.

Synonyms for FMD are aphthous fever, fiebre aftosa, fievre aphtheuse, febre aphthose, and Maul-und-Klauenseuche. Its extremely infectious nature and its plurality of immunogenic types make it one of the most difficult diseases to control. Economic losses can be quite high in areas where FMD becomes enzootic in cattle, swine, sheep, or goats, not only because of direct effects on the infected animals, but also because import of animal products from infected areas is usually prohibited in those free of the virus. Birds are not considered natural hosts, but information on FMD merits attention because experimental infections in birds have been described, because the virus has been modified by propagation in chicks and avian embryos, and because circumstantial evidence that birds mechanically transmit the virus has been reported (Henderson, 1960). Beveridge (1968) suggested that future research be done on the importance of birds and their movements in relation to FMD outbreaks.

Reviews on the disease by Henderson (1960) and Callis et al. (1968); on the virus by Brooksby (1958), Shahan (1962), and

Wilner (1969); and on the evolution of FMD by Davidson (1968) note its occurrence on all of the major land masses of the world with the current exceptions of North America, Australia, and New Zealand and give details on the classification (RNA–Picornavirus group), morphology, properties, serology, pathogenesis, transmission, and other characteristics of the virus and on control of the disease. Smith and Jones (1966) described the histopathology of FMD in mammals.

Reports in the first third of the century on the clinical occurrence of FMD in fowl were described in earlier editions of this book by Olitsky (1945) and by Schwarte (1965), but they noted that the clinical diagnoses had been questioned because the lesions described resembled those of fowl pox and the occurrences were in areas known to be free from FMD. Olitsky and Schwarte also cited early unsuccessful attempts to experimentally transmit FMD virus to chickens, ducks, seagulls, sparrows, and martins.

EXPERIMENTAL INFECTION OF BIRDS

Galloway (1937) transmitted FMD virus through 8 serial transfers in wild ducks by inoculations of the foot pads and digits which resulted in the appearance of vesicles on the upper web surfaces. Following this, Gillespie (1954a, 1955a) propagated the virus in chickens. Day-old chicks inoculated intravenously developed macroscopic lesions of the gizzard muscle and occasionally of the heart during the 35, 24, and 20 serial passages made with types A, O, and C virus, respectively. Gizzard lesions also appeared in 6-week-old chickens inoculated intravenously and in day-old chicks inoculated subcutaneously, intraperitoneally, or into the foot pads with type A virus from the 12–13th chick passage. Bovine-propagated type O, but not A and C, could be transferred in chicks by intravenous inoculation.

Skinner (1954) inoculated newly hatched chicks intramuscularly with type O virus from mouse passages instead of from tissue culture. During a series of 12 alternate passages in chicks and mice, the hearts and inoculated muscle from chicks were used as inocula for the mice, but virus also could be recovered from the blood of chicks at 3–5 days postinoculation and, with the highest titer, from the tongues. Macroscopic lesions appeared on the tongues of chicks

after the 8th alternate passage of the above series and in newly hatched chicks inoculated intramuscularly with the original type O cattle strain. Local lesions developed in 2–4-month-old birds inoculated directly on the tongue epithelium during 6 serial passages with the original cattle strain. Regardless of age of the chickens, severe systemic disturbances did not occur, and lesions of the tongue healed in a few days without blemishes. In subsequent work (cited by Shahan, 1962), Skinner inoculated the tongues or foot pads in bantams, chickens, ducks, geese, guinea fowl, and turkeys and observed lesions similar to those that occur in naturally affected mammals.

In the hope that a rapid loss of pathogenicity for cattle would occur with additional transfers, Zahran (1961a) carried types A, O, and C in chicks of gradually increasing ages—1–29 days old—for 55, 84, and 50 passages respectively. However, these attempts to produce satisfactory vaccine strains for FMD have not produced results that are as promising as those obtained with some of the other laboratory systems.

MODIFICATION IN AVIAN EMBRYOS

The reports by Zahran (1961b) and De-Lay and Rozemeyer (1961) on propagation of FMD virus in embryonating eggs cite many of the previous references to work in this field. Traub and Schneider (1948) adapted type O guinea pig propagated FMD virus to chicken embryos by alternation with guinea pigs. Subsequently other investigators also adapted types A, O, and C to chicken embryos, but usually after alternating transfers with either guinea pigs or mice. FMD virus previously propagated in chicks was then adapted to chicken embryos by Skinner (1954) with type O from alternating mouse-chick passages, and by Gillespie (1955b) with type C from serial chick passages.

Propagation of type C virus in 14-day chicken embryos was initiated by inoculation of the chorioallantoic membrane (CAM) with heart and gizzard muscle suspension from the 6th chick passage (Gillespie, 1955b). The virus was maintained through 30 transfers in the same manner, using pooled suspensions of embryo hearts and gizzards collected at 3 days postinoculation as the inoculum. Embryo mortality was less than 50% from the 3rd to the 15th passage but greater thereafter. After the

1st passage, edema and hemorrhages of the skin of the head, breast, and abdominal regions; hemorrhage of the livers and kidneys; serous or bloody ascitic and pericardial fluid; and, occasionally, white and swollen areas in heart muscle were observed. The hearts had a higher infective titer in mice than other organs.

Of 2 oxen inoculated with type O virus from the 11th chicken embryo passage, neither developed the typical generalized signs of FMD; of 2 receiving 25th passage virus, neither developed any signs of infection. All 4, however, were immune to later challenge with type O virus that caused the generalized disease in control cattle. Gillespie considered the results encouraging but suggested that tests should be made in larger numbers of cattle before concluding that the chick and chicken embryo passaged virus was attenuated.

Skinner (1954) used the intravenous route for injection of muscle and heart suspensions into 14-day chicken embryos incubated at 35° C. At this lower than usual temperature, the embryos were more susceptible to infection, and type O virus was passaged in chicken embryos without intermediate serial transfers in chicks. Marked macroscopic lesions in cardiac muscles were observed.

The immunization of cattle with chicken embryo modified strains of FMD virus by Gillespie (1955b), and subsequent progress by others in this field, led Zahran (1961b) to propagate and modify types A, O, and C in 14-day chicken embryos following transfer in chicks. All three types showed a marked loss of pathogenicity for cattle after 20–28 passages in embryonating eggs but retained the ability to induce immunity. In the same year DeLay and Rozemeyer (1961) reported transfers of type C from the 28th (from Gillespie, 1955b) to the 44th chicken embryo passage. Six steers inoculated with virus from the 40th serial passage in chicken embryos did not develop generalized infections and were refractory to later challenge.

The outlook for the production in chicken embryos of effective modified live-virus vaccines against FMD is quite promising; but Zahran (1961b) appropriately warns that more information is needed on the duration of immunity, possible interference between modified viruses, excretion of virus from vaccinated animals, and possible transmission from vaccinated to nonvaccinated cattle.

Research on FMD in this country is under strict supervision by the federal government, and import of the virus into the United States is prohibited.

REFERENCES

Beveridge, W. I. B. 1968. Spread of foot-and-mouth disease. *Vet. Record* 82:143–44.

Brooksby, J. B. 1958. The virus of foot-and-mouth disease, pp. 1–37. In Smith, K. M., and M. A. Lauffer (eds.), *Advances in Virus Research*, Vol. 5. Academic Press, New York.

Callis, J. J., P. D. McKercher, and J. H. Graves. 1968. Foot-and-mouth disease—A review. *J. Am. Vet. Med. Ass.* 153:1798–1802.

Davidson, R. M. 1968. Evolution of some major epizootic virus diseases. *New Zealand Vet. J.* 16:56–63.

DeLay, P. D., and H. Rozemeyer. 1961. Foot-and-mouth disease virus—Its behavior in cattle after serial passages in chicken embryos and chicks. *Am. J. Vet. Res.* 22:533–36.

Galloway, I. A. 1937. *Fifth Progress Report of the Foot-and-Mouth Disease Research Committee*, pp. 29, 364, 369. H. M. Stationery Office, London.

Gillespie, J. H. 1954. The propagation and effects of type A foot-and-mouth virus in the day-old chick. *Cornell Vet.* 44:425–33.

———. 1955a. Further studies with foot-and-mouth disease viruses in day-old chicks. *Cornell Vet.* 45:160–69.

———. 1955b. Propagation of type C foot-and-mouth disease virus in eggs and effects of the egg-cultivated virus on cattle. *Cornell Vet.* 45:170–79.

Henderson, W. M. 1960. Foot-and-mouth disease and related vesicular diseases, pp. 19–77. In Brandly, C. A., and E. L. Jungherr (eds.), *Advances in Veterinary Science*, Vol. 6. Academic Press, New York and London.

Olitsky, P. K. 1945. Foot-and-mouth disease in fowl, pp. 503–5. In Biester, H. E., and L. Devries (eds.), *Diseases of Poultry*, 1st ed. Iowa State Univ. Press, Ames.

Schwarte, L. H. 1965. Foot-and-mouth disease in fowl, pp. 834–37. In Biester, H. E., and L. H. Schwarte (eds.), *Diseases of Poultry*, 5th ed. Iowa State Univ. Press, Ames.

Shahan, M. S. 1962. The virus of foot-and-mouth disease. *Ann. N.Y. Acad. Sci.* 101:444–54.

Skinner, H. H. 1954. Infection of chickens and chick embryos with the viruses of foot-

and-mouth disease and vesicular stomatitis. *Nature* 174:1052–53.

Smith, H. A., and T. C. Jones. 1966. *Veterinary Pathology,* 3rd ed. Lea & Febiger, Philadelphia.

Traub, E., and B. Schneider. 1948. Zuechtung des Virus der Maul- und Klauenseuche im bebrueteten Huehnerei. *Z. Naturforsch.* 3B:178.

Wilner, B. I. 1969. *A Classification of the Major Groups of Human and Other Animal Viruses,* 4th ed. Burgess Publ. Co., Minneapolis.

Zahran, G. E. D. 1961a. Foot-and-mouth disease virus. I. Propagation of 3 immunologic types of virus in chicks. *Am. J. Vet. Res.* 22:518–26.

————. 1961b. Foot-and-mouth disease virus. II. Propagation and modification of 3 immunologic types of virus in embryonating chicken eggs. *Am. J. Vet. Res.* 22:527–32.

CHAPTER 27

EXTERNAL PARASITES

❖

JOHN G. MATTHYSSE

*Department of Entomology and
Limnology
Cornell University
Ithaca, New York*

❖

THE EXTERNAL PARASITES of poultry to be considered in this chapter are arthropods that live on and in the skin and feathers. For convenience, the few arthropod parasites of internal organs, such as air sacs, will be included. Also important to poultry production are insects that breed in poultry manure, causing sanitary and public relations problems. Because of the large number of species of external parasites of bird hosts and of other arthropods related to poultry production, this discussion will emphasize those of the domesticated chicken, turkey, guinea fowl, duck, goose, and pigeon of the mainland of North America. Most recent texts on these parasites and their biologies are Soulsby (1968) and La-page (1968).

Certain ectoparasites of birds actually eat the dead cells of the skin and its appendages (e.g. lice). However, for many of them the skin merely serves as a convenient medium through which they draw blood or lymph and from which they obtain warmth and shelter.

Ectoparasites may be closely confined to their hosts during the entire life cycle (bird lice), with transmission taking place by host contacts. Others wander freely from bird to bird. Some are highly host specific, which contradicts the viewpoint that chicken lice, for example, propagate on horses or other animals. On the other hand, some species may maintain a rather loose relationship to their food supply. Adapted as they are to living on birds, they do not always confine their activities to one particular host species or even to birds as a group. Such forms include certain of the host-cosmopolitan insects: gnats, mosquitoes, bed bugs, and fleas. Other external parasites (fowl tick and chicken mite) attack birds only at night, hiding in surrounding shelters during the daytime.

Variations in habits such as noted above are important when control measures are to be considered. Mites as a group cannot be successfully controlled by any single method of attack because of habit variations among species. This indicates the necessity for accurate identifications as a preliminary. In case of doubt the various state and national diagnostic services may be called upon for assistance.

CLASSIFICATION

The parasites to be considered are members of the animal phylum Arthropoda, characterized by possession of externally segmented bodies, jointed appendages, and chitinous exoskeleton. However, adaptation to the parasitic mode of life frequently involves such modification in form and reduction in characters that recognition is difficult. The U.S. Public Health Service Pictorial Keys (Anon., 1967) is most useful for determining specific ectoparasites and flies.

Lice, flies, bugs, and fleas are members of the class Insecta, characterized by possession of a body divided into 3 regions (head, thorax, abdomen), 1 pairs of antennae attached to the head, 3 pairs of legs attached to the thorax, and trachea (air tubes) for breathing. Some adult insects have wings.

Insects undergo metamorphosis whereby immature stages may appear totally different from adults and not show the characteristics of the class Insecta. Examples are some fly maggots which possess no legs, antennae, or obvious body divisions. Lice, on the other hand, are easily recognized as insects regardless of stage. For classification of insects, see Comstock (1940) and Borror and DeLong (1964).

Mites are members of the class Arachnida, the order Acarina, characterized by closely fused body divisions, no antennae, and 4 pairs of legs (the first motile stage, larva, has 3 pairs of legs). Ticks are very large mites, contrasting sharply with the majority of mites which are much smaller than most insects. Acarina never possess wings. For classification of mites, see Baker and Wharton (1952), Baker et al. (1956), Strandtman and Wharton (1958), and Krantz (1970).

The common names and scientific binomials used are those accepted by the Entomological Society of America (Blickenstaff, 1965).

EXTERNAL PARASITES IN MODERN POULTRY PRODUCTION

The external parasite problem has changed completely with evolution of the poultry industry to intensive production. Host-specific parasites that spend their entire life on birds are now of minor importance. For example, incubating eggs and isolation of chicks from older birds has broken the normal cycle of louse infestation. Chicken lice are seldom seen in modern egg or broiler producing units. Dermanyssid mites, on the other hand, do not depend on transmission from older birds to chicks as they can live for long periods in poultry houses and do live on wild birds. As a result, mites remain major problems. The type of housing can be a deciding factor mitigating against some species of mites and flies. The poultry mite *Dermanyssus gallinae* seldom infests caged layer houses as there are no appropriate hiding places, such as manure-coated roosts, in which it can complete its life cycle. Instead, the crowding of birds favors the northern fowl mite *Ornithonyssus sylviarum* which completes its life cycle on the birds and moves freely among them. The housefly *Musca domestica* is seldom a problem inside climate-controlled layer houses in the North. Ingress is difficult and excess moisture in the manure prevents breeding. On the other hand, manure cones under outdoor caged poultry results in severe fly problems in the South. Modern broiler plants seldom have ectoparasite problems, as the chicks arrive with few or no parasites, and there is not enough time for parasites to increase to damaging numbers before the birds are slaughtered. MacCreary and Catts (1954) surveyed ectoparasites on Delaware poultry and gave relative importance and some biological notes on the various species. Simco and Lancaster (1965) discuss lice and mites in modern poultry practice in Arkansas and experiments on control.

It is evident that management should stress sanitary measures to utilize these advantages of modern poultry systems. External parasite problems will be minimized by thorough cleaning of houses between batches of birds, whole flock replacement rather than partial culling and replacement, smooth house construction and mesh to keep out wild birds, keeping manure too dry or too wet for fly breeding, and regular manure disposal.

Little has been written on ectoparasites of pigeons. Barker (1960) reviewed mites and lice affecting pigeons and their control.

DETECTION

Poultry seriously infested with the usual external parasites exhibit irritation and react by scratching, preening, and rubbing. Incipient infestations may be less obvious. Any unexplained production drop is cause to look for external parasites. Lice and northern fowl mites can be found by examining the skin after parting the feathers and also looking along the feathers. The skin and feathers around the vent as well as on the legs, wings, head, neck, breast, and back should be inspected. Good light and good eyes are needed to see these small parasites. An adequate light is a battery pack lamp held on the head by its elastic band, leaving the hands free to ruffle the feathers of the bird. Specific identity of the parasite requires examination under a microscope. Bloodsucking parasites that come to the birds only to feed are more difficult to detect. It is necessary to examine bedding, roosts, walls, cracks and crevices, and beneath manure clods. Nighttime examination of the birds may detect those parasites which feed on the birds at night. Specific locations are described subsequently under each parasite. Laboratory diagnosis is required for parasites in internal organs.

GENERAL CONTROL PROCEDURES

Although specific control will be given under each parasite, general information on insecticides, tolerances and residues, methods of application, and recommended treatments will be presented here to avoid repetition.

INSECTICIDES

The modern organophosphorous and carbamate insecticides are the main ectoparasite and fly control measures in use for direct application to poultry, litter, or buildings. A few older materials are still in use for combined disinfecting and pest control treatment of houses prior to introducing the flock. There is little reason to use the relatively ineffective older inorganic insecticides such as sulfur and lime. Application methods for many older insecticides require too much labor to be pertinent to modern poultry production. Among the botanical insecticides, pyrethrum remains very effective against flies and is a main ingredient of mist and aerosol fly sprays, particularly with synergists. Although nicotine sulfate (Black Leaf 40) remains effective against lice and mites, laborious individual bird application is required for cage birds, and mammalian and avian toxicity is relatively high.

Insecticides for use on poultry must be accepted by the Environmental Protection Agency (EPA) as causing no hazardous residues in eggs, meat, or other edible poultry products. The EPA has set tolerances in poultry products for only a very few insecticides and has declared only a few more safe to apply because of lack of toxicity or no residue produced. The Pesticides Regulation Division of the EPA has registered labels for only a few insecticides for application to poultry or to poultry premises, and only after these insecticides were accepted by EPA as causing no residues in food that could be hazardous to the consumer.

The chlorinated hydrocarbon insecticides in general are banned from use on poultry or in poultry houses because of residues caused in eggs and meat. Under no circumstances should DDT, benzene hexachloride (BHC), toxaphene, chlordane, aldrin, dieldrin, endrin, or heptachlor be used on poultry, in poultry houses, or on poultry feeds. Chlordane, lindane, and toxaphene are labeled for outdoor use against chiggers, but such treatments are likely to produce illegal residues in poultry (Liska et al., 1964).

Among the many organophosphorous and carbamate compounds that could be considered for poultry pest control are many that are too hazardous to the birds or to the applicator (Foulk and Matthysse, 1963; Radeleff, 1964; Sherman et al., 1964, 1965, 1967b). Others are ineffective. The remaining compounds that can be em-

ployed successfully and safely on the birds are the organophosphorous compounds malathion, coumaphos (Co-Ral), Rabon, and naled (Dibrom) and the carbamate compound carbaryl (Sevin). A few more organophosphorous compounds that may be used are: in the air for fly control while the birds are in the house—dichlorvos (Vapona); on the walls while the birds are in the house—ronnel (Korlan); on the walls with no birds in the house—dimethoate (Cygon) and Compound 4072; on manure which birds cannot contact—ronnel (Korlan), dimethoate (Cygon), dichlorvos (Vapona), and Zytron. Sugar baits for fly control may be used in poultry houses provided the birds cannot get at the bait. These baits may contain malathion, naled, ronnel, dichlorvos, or the carbamate dimetilan.

Many organophosphorous compounds such as parathion, methyl parathion, diazinon, and fenthion (Baytex) are very toxic to poultry and must never be allowed near birds.

Tolerances and Residues

Listed in Table 27.1 are residue tolerances for the common pesticides used for the control of poultry pests and the number of days that must elapse between application and slaughter or sale of eggs to remain under this legal residue tolerance.

All other insecticide uses (except for sulfur and lime-sulfur which require no tolerances) must be accepted as having no tolerance, thus no allowable residue. The fly spray ingredients—pyrethrins and synergists (piperonyl butoxide, MGK 264)—may be used on poultry or in poultry houses with no interval required between treatment and slaughter or gathering of eggs. Naled (Dibrom) and dichlorvos (Vapona) may also be used, but with specific restrictions (see page 797). Cygon (dimethoate) and Korlan (ronnel) may be used for fly control only if no contamination of birds, feed, or water occurs.

Insecticides should not be used on poultry or in poultry houses without reading the label carefully. All precautions on the label must be observed. Illegal insecticide residues in eggs and meat will result if the wrong insecticides are used, the wrong concentration or volume is used, or the application method is wrong. In all poultry treatment one must avoid contamination of

TABLE 27.1 ❧ Tolerances and Withdrawal Periods for Insecticides Used on Poultry

Insecticide	Specific Poultry Products	Tolerance in PPM	Required Withdrawal in Days before Slaughter
Malathion	Meat and meat by-products from poultry	4	0
	Eggs	0.1	—
Carbaryl (Sevin)	Meat and fat from poultry	5	7
	Eggs	0	—
Coumaphos (Co-Ral) (Plus oxygen analog)	Meat, fat, and meat by-products from poultry	1	0
	Eggs	0.1	—
Rabon	Meat and meat by-products from poultry	0.1	—
	Fat of meat from poultry	0.75	—
	Eggs	0.1	—

feed and water as well as feeding troughs and watering devices. All eggs should be picked up and removed to the egg room before starting to treat with insecticides. Application should be made late in the day or at night to avoid contaminating eggs. Off-flavors in eggs can be caused by direct contamination of eggshells. Ventilation should be supplied during dusting, spraying, or misting.

Pesticide residues may occur in eggs or meat from contaminants in feed, water, litter, or soil. Persistent chlorinated hydrocarbons, particularly DDT and dieldrin, have been found in poultry feeds, even though infrequently, causing illegal residues. Residue levels in eggs approximate levels in feed, and contaminated eggs continue to be produced long after pesticide ingestion ceases (Cummings et al., 1966). It is most important that feed manufacturers attempt to buy pesticide-free feed ingredients and that poultrymen take care not to use contaminated local ingredients nor keep birds in a known contaminated environment.

Grain fumigants can be hazardous to chickens. Ethylene dibromide residues will depress growth of chicks, egg production, and egg size (Caylor and Laurent, 1959; Bierer and Vickers, 1959; and Morris and Fuller, 1963). Fumigated grain should be thoroughly aerated before feeding to poultry.

Application

Laborious individual bird application methods are inappropriate to modern poultry production. For caged layer chickens, methods of choice include hydraulic spraying, mist spraying, and dusting from outside the cages as the birds mill around. Electric mist sprayers have the advantages of rapid treatment, minimum wetting of birds and house, light portable equipment, and concentrate application but require knowledgeable operators. Birds on litter can be treated efficiently by dust applied to the litter with consequent self-application as the birds scratch and scatter the litter. Residual fumigants such as dichlorvos in closed houses are most promising for the future but are not as yet labeled for general use on poultry. Eventually, systemic insecticides will be dispensed in feed and water, but progress is slow because of questions of residues and safety to the birds. No per os treatment is currently registered for commercial use.

DUSTING. Direct dusting of individual birds is laborious and too slow for large operations. A crank type rotary hand duster is very practical to blow dust at birds in cages or onto and over birds on the floor. *For conventional houses the easiest way to use dust is to apply to the litter.* Figure the square footage of floor area first; then weigh out the amount of dust necessary for this area; then scatter by means of a grain scoop or large can, attempting to cover the floor area evenly, including under roosts, feeders, and nest boxes. Dust bath boxes may be used for either conventional or caged birds. Put dilute insecticide in a shallow (3-inch) dusting box, about $1 \times 1\frac{1}{2}$ feet in size. For each 30 floor birds use 1 box, or put 1 box in each colony cage, but for economy's sake it is not necessary to have dusting boxes in all cages simultaneously.

SPRAYING. The usual cylindrical compressed air sprayers are satisfactory, although slow, for birds in cages or for treating roosts and walls. Knapsack sprayers (continuously pumped during spraying) giving a continuous spray are more efficient. *For cage birds be sure to spray from underneath* as well as tops and sides to give complete bird coverage. Power sprayers are much more rapid and efficient, particularly for large operations. When spraying houses with insecticide or disinfectant, high-pressure and large-volume output is most desirable to drive spray into all cracks and crevices.

MISTING. Electric mist machines are efficient, rapid, and labor-saving (Fig. 27.1). These are ideal for cage birds, and with a little thought and care can be used efficiently on birds in conventional houses. These machines are called mechanical "foggers," although as used they are really producing a coarse, wetting mist. Included are the Halaby Klip-on Fogger, Root-Lowell Atomist, Challenger, Microsol, and others. Most treatment has been done with the Halaby using the largest nozzle (4 gal/hr output). This machine will spray water suspensions of insecticide wettable powders and flowable formulations as well as emulsions and oil solutions. In the summer the mist machines can be used efficiently to dispense fly spray. *Mist machines are concentrate applicators and do not use the same mixtures as ordinary sprayers.* Generally they use 5–10 times the concentration and 1/5–1/10 the volume. Care must be taken not to overdose individual birds with such a strong spray. A good rate is 1 gal to 750 birds, requiring 15 minutes with a 4 gal/hr machine.

In general, it is best to use emulsions in mist machines, but Sevin "sprayable" and "flowable" formulations are very satisfactory. In all "fog" work, shake the container frequently during spraying to keep the insecticide from settling out.

Recommended Treatments

In using the treatments given in Table 27.2, observe the general precautions of not contaminating feed, water, utensils, feed troughs, and eggs and of not spraying in a confined, nonventilated area. Specific precautions include:

Coumaphos (Co-Ral)—Do not use more often than once a week, nor within 10 days of vaccination or other stress influence or in conjunction with other organic phosphates. Provide thorough ventilation while treating.

Carbaryl (Sevin)—Do not spray birds except with a water mist spray. Do not treat nest litter. Ventilate while spraying. Do not repeat treatment within 4 weeks. Do not keep birds on treated litter within 7 days of sale for slaughter.

Rabon—Do not repeat more often than every 14 days.

Other insecticides which may be used for specific purposes include 0.3% naled (Dibrom) emulsion at 1 gal/100 birds applied as a light mist to the birds (except for the heads) against lice and northern fowl mite (do not apply directly on chickens

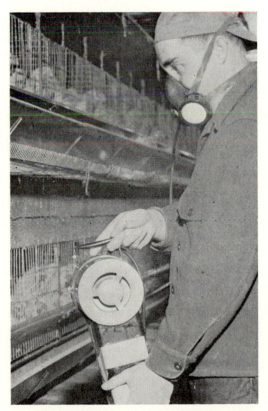

FIG. 27.1—*Electric mist spraying caged laying hens. (J. G. Matthysse, Cornell Univ.)*

TABLE 27.2 ✄ Appropriate Insecticides for Poultry

	Mala-thion	Couma-phos	Car-baryl	Ra-bon
Dust applied to birds	4–5%	0.5%	5%	—
Lb/100 birds	1	1	1	—
Dust applied to litter	4–5%	0.5%	5%	50%
Lb/100 sq ft	1.7–2	5	2.5	0.16
Spray applied to birds	0.5%	0.25%	0.5%	0.5%
Gal/100 birds	1	0.8–1	1	1
Concentrate mist applied to birds	—	—	4%	—
Gal/1,000 birds	—	—	1.3	—
Spray applied to house (walls, boxes, pits, etc.)	2%	0.25%	0.5%	0.5%
Gal/1,000 sq ft	1–2	1	1–2	1–2
Paint applied to roosts	3%	—	—	1%
Pt/150 lin ft	1	—	—	1.5

under 6 weeks old nor on turkeys less than 3 months old); 0.5% dichlorvos (Vapona) spray at 1 qt/1,000 sq ft of manure surface, window sills, outside of penned enclosures, and floor of feed storage rooms for control of flies, gnats, and mosquitoes; 100% sulfur dust or 1–2 oz wettable sulfur/gal as a dust or dip against deplumping mite.

New methods of poultry external parasite control are in the offing but not as yet labeled for use. Fumigation by the organophosphorous insecticide dichlorvos (Vapona) is most promising as a labor-saving efficient method, using gaseous evolution from sprays, treated surfaces, or slow release polymer formulations (Simco and Lancaster, 1965). Systemic insecticides in feed or water are promising for ectoparasite control and also for indirect prevention of fly breeding by excretion in poultry feces. Sherman (1965) reviews this method and summarizes his extensive work. Loomis et al. (1968) and Simco and Lancaster (1966) found this method effective in large-scale trials. Chemosterilants such as apholate have been effective in baits in poultry houses (Labrecque and Meifert, 1966) for fly control but are not as yet labeled for use because of toxicological hazards. Also, chemosterilants reduce fly populations slowly, a feature not likely to be a good selling point to poultrymen. "Inert" desiccating materials containing silica were

found effective by Tarshis (1967) and Lamina and Kruner (1966) but have not found general acceptance.

Simco and Lancaster (1965) summarize materials and methods appropriate for poultry pest control in commercial chicken flocks and give experimental results against most of the common pests. Race et al. (1969) give detailed directions for poultry pest control in New Jersey, and Furman et al. (1969a,b) detail control of external parasites of chickens, turkeys, and pigeons in California.

INSECTS

LICE

These insects are common and widespread external parasites of birds. Bird lice belong in the order Mallophaga, the chewing lice. Mallophaga are characterized by possession of chewing type mandibles located ventrally on the head, slight metamorphosis, no wings, dorsoventrally flattened body, and short antennae with 3–5 segments. There are more than 40 species of lice reported from domesticated fowls. Fortunately as far as the veterinarian and the poultry raiser are concerned, the various species of bird lice are at present all controlled by the same methods. Birds frequently harbor several species of lice at the same time. See Emerson (1956, 1962a) for keys and illustrations of the lice on chickens and turkeys.

The following list of lice of North American poultry is from Emerson (1956, 1962a,b) and Dalgleish (personal communication), with common names according to Entomological Society of America usage. The more important species are those with common names.

Chicken lice:
Cuclotogaster heterographa, chicken head louse (Fig. 27.3)
Goniocotes gallinae, fluff louse (Fig. 27.4)
Goniodes dissimilis, brown chicken louse (Fig. 27.5)
Goniodes gigas, large chicken louse
Lagopoecus sinensis
Lipeurus caponis, wing louse
Lipeurus lawrensis
Menacanthus cornutus
Menacanthus pallidullus (common, frequently confused with *M. stramineus*)

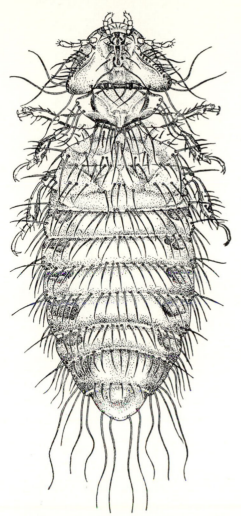

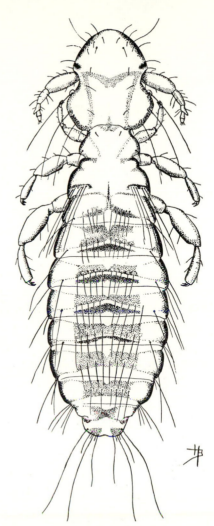

FIG. 27.2—Menopon, *probably* gallinae, *shaft louse.* ×55. *(Reis and Nobrega, 1956)*

FIG. 27.3—Cuclotogaster heterographa, *chicken head louse. (USDA)*

Menacanthus stramineus, chicken body louse
Menopon gallinae, shaft louse (Figs. 27.2, 27.7, 27.8)
Oxylipeurus dentatus
Turkey lice:
  Chelopistes meleagridis, large turkey louse
  Colpocephalum tausi
  Menacanthus stramineus, chicken body louse (probably turkey is original host)
  Oxylipeurus polytrapezius, slender turkey louse
  Oxylipeurus corpulentus (common on wild turkeys)
Guinea fowl lice:
  Amyrsidea desonsai
  Clayia theresae
  Goniocotes maculatus

Goniodes gigas, large chicken louse
Goniodes numidae, guinea feather louse
Lipeurus lawrensis
Lipeurus numidae, slender guinea louse
Menacanthus numidae
Menacanthus stramineus, chicken body louse
Menopon gallinae, shaft louse
Numidicola antennatus
Somaphantus lusius
Duck and goose lice:
  Anaticola anseris, slender goose louse
  Anaticola crassicornis, slender duck louse
  Anatoecus dentatus
  Anatoecus icterodes
  Ciconiphilus pectiniventris
  Holomenopon transvaalense
  Ornithobius mathisi
  Trinoton anserinum, goose body louse
  Trinoton querquedulae, large duck louse

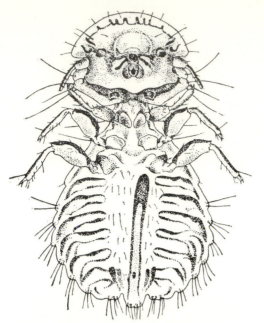

FIG. 27.4—Goniocotes, *probably* gallinae, fluff louse. ×20. (Reis and Nobrega, 1956)

Pigeon lice:
Bonomiella columbae
Campanulotes bidentatus compar, small pigeon louse
Coloceras damicorne
Colpocephalum turbinatum
Columbicola columbae, slender pigeon louse (Fig. 27.6)
Hohorstiella lata
Physconelloides zenaidurae

Lice will occasionally straggle from one bird species to another if these hosts are in close contact. However, only those lice included in the host-parasite list for any one species of bird are likely to become established. Others are of no economic importance.

Lice are cosmopolitan, at least some species occurring wherever domestic birds are raised. They are less frequently found on modern intensive chicken farms.

Lousiness (pediculosis) of birds is diagnosed by finding the straw-colored lice on the skin or feathers of the birds (Fig. 27.7). In size, lice of domestic birds vary from somewhat less than 1 mm in length to over 6 mm. Mallophaga up to 10 mm long occur on wild birds.

Lice spend the entire life cycle on the host. Eggs are attached, often in clusters, to the feathers and require 4–7 days to hatch (Fig. 27.8). The entire life cycle takes

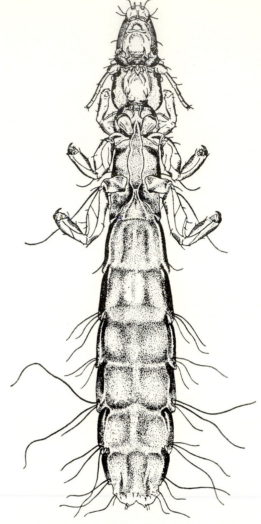

FIG. 27.5—Goniodes, *probably* dissimilis, brown chicken louse. ×42. (Reis and Nobrega, 1956)

about 3 weeks for completion. Stockdale and Raun (1965), working with the chicken body louse, give the incubation period as 4–5 days and each of the 3 nymphal instars 3 days. One pair of lice may produce 120,000 descendants within a period of a few months. Their normal life span is several months, but away from the birds they can remain alive only 5 or 6 days.

Although bird lice ordinarily eat feather products, it has been shown by Wilson (1933) that *Menacanthus stramineus,* the chicken body louse, may puncture soft quills near the bases and consume the blood that oozes out. This was confirmed by Crutchfield and Hixson (1943); in addition, they stated that the body louse draws

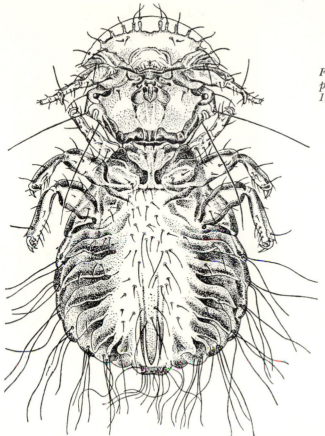

FIG. 27.6—Columbicola columbae, *slender pigeon louse.* ×48. *(Reis and Nobrega, 1956)*

blood by gnawing through the covering layers of the skin itself.

Severe lousiness in poultry originally was thought to follow malnutrition and lead to weight loss as well as to low production. There is conflicting evidence on these hypotheses. Warren et al. (1948) found no effect on laying records even following rather heavy louse infestation. Tower and Floyd (1961b) studied the effect of the body louse on egg production in New Hampshire pullets; they found no significant differences between infested and noninfested birds. Kartman (1949) concluded that lousiness is not necessarily an expression of malnutrition of the host; indeed the contrary appeared to be true. He also noted that debeaking the birds increased the number of lice present. Edgar and King (1950), studying the effect of moderate infestation by the chicken body louse, concluded that louse-free hens averaged about 11% greater egg production than did those infested, a difference in net income of 75–85 cents per

bird. Differences in body weight and in mortality between the two groups were not significant. A study by Gless and Raun (1959) revealed that an average of 23,000 chicken body lice per chicken reduced egg production by inbred hens an average of 15% to a maximum of 84% during a 14-week period. The number of birds used was very small. Stockdale and Raun (1960) could not demonstrate an effect of chicken body lice on egg production by hybrid hens. Further research is needed to quantify economic effect and to determine difference in effect according to the louse species involved. Also, breeding lines of chickens vary in louse susceptibility (Quigley, 1965).

It might be concluded that lice are not highly pathogenic to mature birds. However, there appears to be clinical evidence that lice irritate nerve endings, thus interfering with the rest and sleep so necessary to immature animals. Louse-infested chicks may die. Also, lousiness frequently accom-

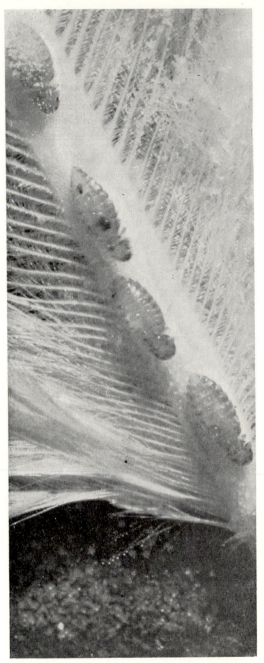

FIG. 27.7—Menopon gallinae, *shaft louse, on feather. (H. H. Schwardt, Cornell Univ.)*

panies manifestations of poor husbandry such as internal parasitisms, infectious diseases, malnutrition, and insanitation.

Howitt et al. (1948) isolated the virus of equine encephalomyelitis from chicken body louse *(Menacanthus stramineus).*

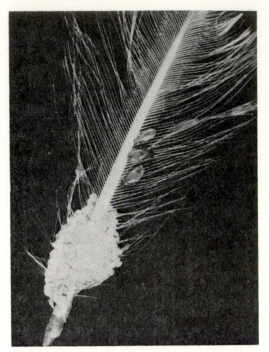

FIG. 27.8—Shaft louse eggs at base of feather. (R. Kriner, Rutgers Univ.)

More recently Meyer and Eddie (1960) and Eddie et al. (1962) isolated the virus of ornithosis from *Menopon gallinae,* the shaft louse, and from mites on chickens and turkeys.

Turkeys

Turkeys may be infested with the common chicken body louse *(Menacanthus stramineus),* the large turkey louse *(Chelopistes meleagridis),* and the slender turkey louse *(Oxylipeurus polytrapezius).* All are probably native to the turkey. *Oxylipeurus corpulentus* is occasionally found on wild turkeys. The large turkey louse is the most common turkey louse, according to Emerson (1962a), although Kellogg et al. (1969) found *M. stramineus* to be the most common louse on wild turkeys. Rearing turkeys in close confinement and unsanitary quarters favors lice more than does range rearing. It is important that breeding males and females be examined frequently for lice since parasites may be a very important cause of infertility. A common method of introducing lice to an uninfested ranch is the use of infested shipping crates that have been brought on the ranch by buyers. Growers should insist that buyers clean and disinfect all crates and equipment used to transfer stock to killing plants.

Control

Lice should be prevented by buying louse-free birds and never adding lousy birds to a clean flock. Galliform wild or domestic birds should never be allowed to contact chicken flocks. Lice tend to increase during the autumn and winter, so flocks should be examined for lice and treated before cold weather. Birds on the floor are most easily treated by scattering malathion, carbaryl, Rabon, or coumaphos dust on the litter. Roost painting with malathion or nicotine sulfate is pertinent to slatted floor operations but will not be completely effective if many birds roost on the floor. For caged layers, spraying is best using malathion, carbaryl, Rabon, or coumaphos. Lice can be controlled on caged birds by placing dust bath boxes (containing 1 lb of 4–5% malathion dust) in the cages (Rodriguez and Riehl, 1960a). For most complete control, repeat floor area treatment in 1 month and direct bird treatment in 10 days to 2 weeks. Some poultrymen apply an effective preventive spray to the whole interior of conventional houses soon after birds are first introduced, using 2% malathion in a high-pressure wetting spray. Simco and Lancaster (1965) reported on effectiveness of these louse control measures and also on dichlorvos fumigation. Against chicken body lice, dichlorvos (Vapona) as a spray or as vapor generated from resin strands or granules was found to be effective by Simco and Lancaster (1965). A new material very promising for poultry louse control is Ciodrin (Simco and Lancaster, 1965).

Rodriguez and Riehl (1959b) controlled lice on pigeons by 1% malathion dust on the birds or in the nests. Barker (1960) suggests malathion and pyrethrum sprays to control pigeon lice.

BUGS

The family Cimicidae in the order Hemiptera includes several bloodsucking parasites of birds. These insects are flattened dorsoventrally, thus allowing them to creep into crevices where they hide in the daytime. The adults measure about 2–5 mm in length by 1.5–3 mm in width. The color varies according to species from brown to yellow or red. Adults have small padlike wing remnants. The piercing-sucking mouthpart structure or "beak" is attached far forward on the head and is jointed, folding under the head and part of the thorax when not in use. Deeply pigmented eyes are prominent on the head. The abdomen has 8 segments. Stink glands provide the common bed bug and its surroundings with an unpleasant odor.

If attacked by large numbers of bugs, young birds especially may be seriously depleted of blood. The bites are usually followed by swelling and itching due to the injection of saliva into the wound.

Bed Bugs

The most widespread of these bugs is *Cimex lectularius,* the common bed bug (Fig. 27.9), which attacks man and most other mammals and poultry. It is most prevalent in temperate and subtropical climates. Poultry houses and pigeon lofts may become heavily invaded.

The female bed bug lays several 1-mm eggs per day in crevices until about 200 have been deposited. The eggs hatch in 4–20 days depending on temperature. There are 5 nymphal stages, the nymphs feeding at each stage and hiding to digest the meal of blood and to molt their skins. From egg hatching to adulthood requires 1–3 months depending on temperature. Nymphs may withstand starvation for about 70 days, and the adults may live without food from about 1 month at very warm temperatures to 1 year at cold tem-

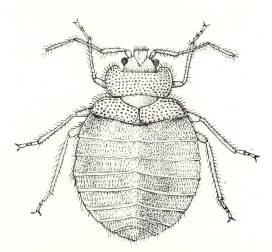

FIG. 27.9–Cimex lectularius, *common bed bug. (USDA)*

peratures. Feeding usually occurs at night, the bugs becoming engorged with blood within 10 minutes.

In the tropics and subtropics the closely related bed bugs *Cimex hemipterus* and *C. boueti* will also attack poultry. *C. columbarius* attacks pigeons in Europe.

Bird Bugs

The most important bird bug is the poultry bug *Haematosiphon inodorus,* also known as the Mexican chicken bug, adobe bug, or "coruco." It occurs in southern and western United States and in Central America. Usinger (1947) has found it in the nests of the California condor and of the great horned owl in Oklahoma. An account of its biology is given by Lee (1955a), and he mentions the turkey as a new host in New Mexico and Arizona (Lee, 1955b). It also attacks man.

Oeciacus vicarius, the swallow bug, is commonly found in the nests of swallows (particularly barn swallows) whence it may spread to poultry and to man (Myers, 1928).

Other cimicid bugs may be found occasionally on poultry in various countries outside the United States. *Ornithocoris toledoi* is a South American poultry pest known as the "Brazilian chicken bug." *Ornithocoris pallidus,* another South American species, has been found on chickens in Florida and Georgia (Usinger, 1966). Hicks (1959) summarizes occurrence of insects, including cimicids, in bird nests.

Assassin Bugs

The family Reduviidae in the order Hemiptera includes many predaceous bugs, but a few are minor bloodsucking pests of poultry. These are also known as cone-nose bugs (Fig. 27.10).

The body is cylindrical in shape, provided with wings in the adult. The narrow head bears a stout beak which is curved back into a groove in the prosternum. They are larger than true bed bugs, being up to 25 mm in length, and they have well-developed wings; otherwise their morphology, life cycles, and behavior are somewhat similar. Species of reduviid bugs reported as attacking poultry in the United States include *Triatoma sanguisuga*, the bloodsucking cone-nose, in Maryland, Florida, California, and Texas and *T. protracta*, the western bloodsucking cone-nose, in Utah and California. It is of interest to note that

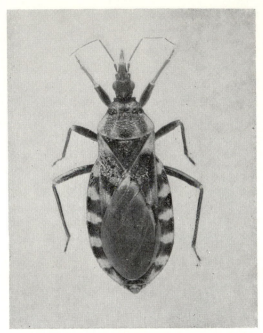

FIG. 27.10—Triatoma, *probably* lecticularia, *cone-nose assassin bug. (USDA)*

T. sanguisuga was found to harbor the virus of equine encephalomyelitis in Kansas by Kitselman and Grundmann (1940). This virus has also been found in natural infections in pigeons and pheasants.

CONTROL. Treatment should be directed against daytime hiding places of the bugs, in cracks and crevices of the walls and floors, under roosts, nest boxes, feeders, etc. A thorough spraying with malathion should be effective, preferably raised to the fowl tick dosage of 3%. Fumigation with hydrogen cyanide or sulfur dioxide can be resorted to in stubborn cases. Assassin bugs are more likely than bed bugs to invade poultry houses from the surrounding countryside and may be more difficult to control.

FLEAS

Fleas, order Siphonaptera, are parasites in the adult stage but free-living as larvae. The adults are characterized by possession of a tough laterally compressed body, piercing-sucking mouthparts, short antennae in grooves, simple or no eyes, long legs adapted for leaping, complete metamorphosis with larvae legless and wormlike and pupae in tiny cocoons.

Many species of fleas have been found

on birds, but only 6 species have been reported from poultry in this country. However, fleas are very adaptable bloodsucking
insects and may attack various host species.
They are cosmopolitan in distribution although more abundant in temperate and
warm climates.

They may be recognized as brown to
black insects running rapidly along the
skin and propelling themselves into the
open by leaping. In size they vary from
1.5 to 4 mm in the adult stage. The adults
suck blood one or more times during the
day, although some species are nocturnal.
The sticktight flea usually remains attached
to the host for days or weeks at a time.
Female fleas deposit several eggs per day
which roll off the host into surrounding
litter where they incubate. Dampness is
essential for further development. The
eggs are white nearly spherical bodies less
than 1 mm in diameter. Within one to
several weeks, depending upon species and
climate, the eggs hatch, liberating tiny maggotlike larvae that feed partly on organic
matter found in dust and litter; but their
principal food is flea feces deposited conveniently by the adult fleas. This flea feces
is rich in host blood-products, thus providing a highly nutritious diet for the larvae.
Flea larvae of nesting birds also utilize the
sheaths of feathers and epidermal scales
of young birds for food.

After the larvae have grown and shed
their skins (usually twice in a period varying from one to several weeks), they proceed to spin silken cocoons, entangling the
thread with various particles of dust and
dirt. Then follows the inactive pupal stage
for a period varying from one week to
months, depending upon the temperature.
During this period the pupae transform
into white, then yellow, then brown fleas.
Emerging from the pupal cocoons, the
young fleas seek a host, suck blood, and are
ready to reproduce within a few days.

Immature fleas may live for weeks or
months without food. Adult fleas may also
live for weeks without feeding, but when a
host is available their life span may extend
over many months to a year or more. The
total length of the life cycle is thus seen to
vary greatly depending upon such factors
as temperature, humidity, exposure, and
host availability. Dormant adults, disturbed by the slightest vibration, are activated and leave the cocoon to seek a host.

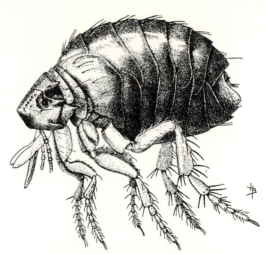

FIG. 27.11--Echidnophaga gallinacea,
sticktight flea. (USDA)

Birds returning to old haunts can become
infested with fleas that have remained
quiescent for long periods.

The fleas of domestic poultry in North
America include the following species:
Echidnophaga gallinacea, the sticktight flea;
Ceratophyllus gallinae, the European chick-
en flea; *C. niger,* the western chicken flea;
Ctenocephalides felis, the cat flea; *Pulex ir-
ritans,* the human flea; and *Orchopeas how-
ardii,* a squirrel flea. To determine fleas
and for distributional data see Fox (1940),
Hubbard (1947), Holland (1949), and
Geary (1959).

Sticktight Flea

Echidnophaga gallinacea (Fig. 27.11), the
cosmopolitan sticktight flea, more often
occurs in southern United States, although
occasionally it is found as far north as New
York. The adult is about 1.5 mm long and
is reddish brown in color. These fleas usually attach to the skin of the head, often
in clusters of a hundred or more. The
mouthparts are deeply embedded in the
skin so it is difficult to dislodge them. The
sticktight and chigoe fleas are unique
among poultry fleas in that the adults become sessile parasites unable to move on
the skin. The adult females forcibly eject
their eggs so that they reach surrounding
litter, 1–4 eggs per day being produced.
Incubation takes 4–14 days; the larval period lasts from 14 to 31 days; the pupal
period 9–19 days; and the newly emerged
fleas mature in 11–18 days.

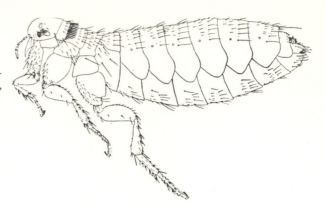

FIG. 27.12—Ceratophyllus gallinae, *European chicken flea. (Reis and Nobrega, 1956)*

The sticktight flea has been reported from the following hosts: chicken, turkey, pigeon, blackbird, bluejay, hawk, owl, pheasant, quail, sparrow; also man, horse, cattle, swine, dog, fox, cat, badger, coyote, deer, ground squirrel, lynx, mouse, opossum, rabbit, raccoon, rat, ring-tailed cat, and skunk.

This flea has not been accused of carrying infectious disease agents to chickens. The irritation and blood loss attributed to it may damage poultry seriously, especially young birds, in which death may occur. Production is lowered in older birds. Alicata (1942) experimentally transferred the rickettsia which causes human endemic (murine) typhus from infected rats to guinea pigs through the agency of sticktight fleas, thus indicating a possible public health importance of this parasite.

European Chicken Flea

Ceratophyllus gallinae (Fig. 27.12), the European chicken flea, has been reported from Maine, Massachusetts, Connecticut, New York, Delaware, Michigan, and Iowa. Undoubtedly it has a much wider distribution. The hosts include chicken, pigeon, bluebird, sparrow, and tree swallow; also man, dog, chipmunk, rat, and squirrel. The adult female measures 3–3.5 mm in length. This flea behaves like most fleas in that it stays on birds only long enough to feed, its breeding activities occurring in the nests and other surroundings.

Others

Ceratophyllus niger, the western chicken flea, is reported mainly from the Pacific Coast area, although Bigland (1955) found it in Alberta, Canada. It may attack various birds and mammals including chicken, turkey, cormorant, gull, magpie, sparrow, and woodpecker; also man, mouse, and rat. Its principal breeding place is in birds' nests. It resembles *C. gallinae* in appearance and biology.

Ctenocephalides felis, the cat flea, has also been reported from the chicken, pheasant, dog, fox, man, bobcat, coyote, opossum, rabbit, raccoon, rat, shrew, squirrel, and woodchuck. This flea is only an incidental pest of poultry in North America. The adult female is about 3 mm in length.

Pulex irritans, the human flea, attacks primarily man but may attack chickens. Other hosts are swine, dog, fox, cat, badger, coyote, deer, ground squirrel, guinea pig, lynx, mountain lion, opossum, prairie dog, rabbit, raccoon, rat, skunk, squirrel, weasel, wild swine, and burrowing owl. The adult female is about 4 mm long.

Orchopeas howardii, a flea ordinarily found on squirrels, has been noted to attack chickens in Massachusetts, according to Shaw and Clark (1953). Other hosts include dog, fox, cat, man, bobcat, chipmunk, coyote, mink, mole, mouse, opossum, rabbit, raccoon, rat, shrew, squirrel, weasel, woodchuck, owl, and swallow. The adult female is about 2.5 mm in length.

In the tropics the chigoe flea *Tunga penetrans* attacks poultry, becoming embedded in the skin but not congregating in masses as does the sticktight flea.

CONTROL. Most important are removal of infested litter and thorough house spraying to kill the immature fleas. Two percent malathion should be used as a spray on the floor and walls and in all cracks and crevices. Fresh litter should be put in the house and dusted with 4–5% malathion dust to kill the adult fleas on the birds and those that drop into the litter. Malathion dust in the nests should control fleas on pigeons and other poultry.

Control of the sticktight flea was reported by Rodriguez and Riehl (1961) using 4% malathion dust. This was applied twice at 28-day intervals, and effective control lasted for 150 days after the second application. The malathion dust was placed in dusting boxes or in soil wallows at the rate of 15 lb/100 chickens. In addition, the floors were covered with 4% malathion dust at the rate of 1 lb/20 sq ft.

Poultry, dogs, cats, and rats should be screened from under buildings, as they may serve to perpetuate flea invasions. Sunlight, hot dry weather, excessive moisture, and freezing hinder the development of fleas; darkness, coolness, dampness, and warmth favor them.

BEETLES

The beetles, insect order Coleoptera, possess chewing mouthparts, 2 pairs of wings with the first pair modified to horny wing covers or elytra and the second pair folded under the wing covers except during flight, and complete metamorphosis with a worm-like grub stage followed by the resting pupal stage. No beetles are true parasites of birds, but a few may occasionally feed on living skin if they contact it. Poultry will feed on beetles they find in litter or on the range, providing an opportunity for ingestion of parasites or inoculum associated with the beetles. The following tapeworms can be transmitted by beetles: *Raillietina cesticillus, R. magninumida, Choanotaenia infundibulum, Hymenolepis carioca, H. diminuta,* and *H. cantaniana.* (See Chapter 29 for specific host-parasite relationships.)

A few bacterial and virus infections are probably transmitted by beetles, particularly through prior feeding by beetles on infected carcasses. Theodorides (1949) lists past records on the beetles injurious to domestic birds and mammals.

Lesser Mealworm

The lesser mealworm *Alphitobius diaperinus* has been implicated in transmission of avian leukosis (including Marek's disease), but its importance in relation to incidence of the disease is debatable. Harding and Bissell (1958) found a heavy infestation of these beetles and their larvae in ground

corncobs used as litter for baby chicks. Healthy chicks were not molested, but the mealworm larvae had bored into the tissues of those that were dying. This damage might be mistaken for an attack on the living chicks. Eidson et al. (1966) demonstrated transmission of leukosis by ingestion of lesser mealworms, showing that the beetles may provide an important means of residual contamination of the environment and possibly a means by which contamination may be spread from one environment to another.

Lancaster and Simco (1967) found the life cycle of the lesser mealworm averaged 70 days, of which 48 were spent as larva, with temperature and diet affecting length of the cycle. They found these beetles in every one of 98 Arkansas poultry houses examined, sometimes in tremendous numbers. They did not obtain leukosis transmission in preliminary type experiments. Harris (1966) found the lesser mealworm in all 50 broiler houses he examined in northern Georgia, and MacCreary and Catts (1954) found it to be the commonest insect in poultry litter in Delaware.

Others

Tenebrio molitor, the yellow mealworm, is ordinarily found in the adult and grub stages consuming grain products stored in mills, warehouses, bakeries, and groceries. The beetles are shiny brown to almost black in color and about 15 mm long. They may infest setting hens, attacking mainly the feet where loss of skin may be followed by severe hemorrhage. The larvae or grubs, known as flour, meal, or bran "worms," are smooth, hard, yellow, cylindrical, wormlike creatures up to 30 mm long. These grubs have been found to erode the skin of young pigeons. According to Levi (1957), other related mealworm beetle larvae may produce similar damage.

Dermestes lardarius, the larder beetle, and related species ordinarily destroy stored grain products and meats (especially ham and bacon) or feed on hides, skins, furs, museum specimens, or decaying animal matter, notably the accumulated droppings in pigeon lofts. The adult larder beetle is about 7 mm long and black in color; the basal half of each wing cover is brownish yellow crossed by a band of three black spots. The larvae are up to 12 mm long, dark brown above, gray below, and covered with brown hairs. The larvae may attack the skin of nestling pigeons.

Silpha thoracica, S. opaca, Necrophorus vestigator, and possibly other species of the beetle family Silphidae (carrion beetles) may also breed in pigeon droppings. The larvae, which are up to 15 mm long and black, are reported to invade the skin of squabs; the wounds produced may be secondarily infested by fly maggots.

Macrodactylus subspinosus, the rose chafer, is a leaf-chewing beetle that, according to Lamson (1922), is highly poisonous when ingested in quantity by chicks, ducklings, goslings, poults, and young game birds. These beetles are found mainly from the Atlantic Coast through the midwestern states. Symptoms of poisoning appear about 4–5 hours after ingestion; birds become sleepy, wings droop, and muscular weakness develops. Death may occur in 5–24 hours. The condition is diagnosed by finding the beetles in the crop. No specific treatment for affected birds is available.

CONTROL. In general there is little point in attempting control of beetles on poultry ranges. Cleanliness of houses and lofts including proper manure and carcass disposal should prevent the problem in poultry houses. Stored grains and feeds should not be allowed to become infested with insects. Infested storages should be fumigated.

Lesser mealworms, and possibly other beetles in litter, can be controlled by dusting the litter and spraying walls and furnishings with carbaryl (Sevin) as recommended for poultry lice and mites. Harding and Bissell (1958) controlled adult and larval lesser mealworms in brooder house litter by spraying with 0.7% malathion emulsion. Lancaster et al. (1969) obtained control by using rice hulls treated with carbaryl, coumaphos, malathion, or Dursban as litter.

FLIES

The insect order Diptera, or flies, includes several families whose members annoy or suck blood from birds as well as mammals. All Diptera have 2 wings in the adult stage (except degenerate wingless forms) and pass through a complete metamorphosis including a maggotlike larva and a puparium resting stage. Mouthparts of the adults are of the piercing-sucking or sponging types. The intermittent nature of their feeding and excellent flight ability render adult flies ideal vectors of disease. For current information on bloodsucking flies and their control see Travis (1967, 1969). Certain species breed in poultry manure and may become so numerous as to create a health and public relations problem. For current information on manure-breeding flies see Anderson et al. (1968) and Anon. (1970).

Mosquitoes

Although mosquitoes are not as important to poultry as they are to man and other mammals, many species will feed on poultry and transmit disease. Some 140 species have been described from North America. How many of these suck blood from poultry is not known.

Mosquitoes belong to the family Culicidae. Most species are about 5 mm in length, and the wings are characteristically veined and scaled. The legs and abdomen are long and slender, and the small spherical head of the female is provided with elongated mouthparts for piercing the skin (Fig. 27.13). The male does not suck blood but feeds on plant juices, nectar, and other fluids.

Mosquitoes deposit their eggs on pools of water in which the larval and pupal stages are passed, or on moist soil subject to flooding. The adults emerge from the pupal cases and then seek a host. In warm weather the life cycle is completed in about 10–16 days for the more common species. The adults are most active on dull quiet days, especially toward evening and at night.

That mosquitoes may attack poultry in swarms is stated by Bishopp (1933), who reported the deaths of numerous chickens in Florida. The offending species was *Psorophora confinnis.* Besides losing blood, the birds appeared to show toxicity from the bites. Edgar and Williams (1948) and Edgar et al. (1951) found that over 99% of the mosquitoes in or near chicken houses in Alabama were *Culex pipiens quinquefasciatus,* the southern house mosquito. Others belonged in the genera Culex, Anopheles, and Aedes. Mosquito attacks appeared to reduce egg production.

Yates (1953) stated that although the mosquitoes *Culiseta incidens* and *C. inornata* bite man in the Pacific Northwest,

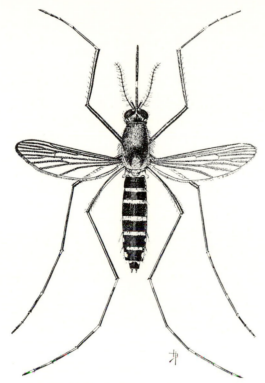

FIG. 27.13—Aedes taeniorhynchus, *black salt-marsh mosquito. (USDA)*

they were more important as pests of live-stock, including poultry. Dow et al. (1957) noted a host preference for birds, includ-ing chickens, by *Culex tarsalis.* MacCreary and Catts (1954) noted loss of blood and restlessness of roosting chickens when poul-try houses were invaded by *Aedes sollici-tans,* the salt-marsh mosquito, in Delaware. They also remarked on the large numbers of other species of mosquitoes seen in poul-try houses, notably *Culex pipiens pipiens,* the northern house mosquito, and *C. salinarius* and *Anopheles crucians.*

Fowl pox virus is transmitted by the mos-quitoes *Aedes stimulans, A. aegypti,* and *A. vexans,* according to Brody (1936) and Matheson et al. (1931). The first-named species harbored the virus for 2 days, whereas the last-named species continued to infect birds up to 39 days after contact-ing the virus of fowl pox and pigeon pox. Mosquitoes also transmit avian malaria caused by *Plasmodium* spp., as reviewed by Huff (1963, 1968). For the most part the birds affected are the smaller wild species and canaries. Davis (1940) called attention to the relationship of birds and mosquitoes

as hosts for the virus of eastern equine en-cephalomyelitis. Smith et al. (1948) infected 7 species of mosquitoes with the virus of St. Louis encephalitis of man by feeding them on infected chickens. The mosquitoes transferred the virus back to chickens. Morgante et al. (1969) found sera from many chickens positive to western enceph-alomyelitis (WE) virus in Alberta, Canada, with annual and seasonal coincidence to clinical illness in horses and man and to virus isolations from mosquitoes. Reeves (1965) reviewed avian (including chicken) virus reservoirs and mosquito vectors and their relation to human disease. In Sprad-brow's (1966) summary of arboviruses in domestic animals he notes a mosquito-borne turkey meningoencephalitis in Israel.

CONTROL. The best control of mosquitoes for housed poultry is complete screening of all openings. Screen doors should be equipped with spring closures. Mosquitoes landing on surfaces inside or outside the house will be killed by residual insecticide deposits of the type recommended for fly control. Poultry not in houses are most dif-ficult to protect from mosquitoes. Some al-leviation may be obtained by spraying all vegetation in the area with malathion, but this deposit is very short-lived, requiring frequent repetition at a cost which may be uneconomic. Pyrethrum fly spray can be fogged in houses or on ranges to kill mos-quitoes in an outbreak, but control will not last more than a few hours. Dichlorvos (Vapona) 0.5% spray may be applied at 1 qt/1,000 sq ft of surface of manure, win-dow sills, and outside of pens to give a lit-tle longer lasting control. Methoxychlor residual spray can be applied outdoors to vegetation from which poultry are ex-cluded.

In general, prevention of mosquito breeding is the best attack. The farm should be surveyed for all wet areas in which breeding may occur, including swamps, ponds, stagnant pools, and water-filled containers of all types. Breeding can be stopped by removal of such containers, covering cisterns and water barrels, clear-ing pool and pond edges of emergent vege-tation, drainage operations, and area treat-ment with insecticide. Currently, methoxy-chlor, malathion or Abate is recommended. Area treatment with insecticides is fraught with danger of water contamination and

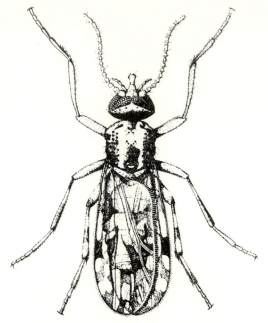

FIG. 27.14—Culicoides furens, *biting midge*. (USDA)

wildlife and fish kill. Only treatments currently approved should be used. In many states a permit must be obtained to treat stream and pond drainage basins. Consult your Extension Service and local public health authorities prior to outdoor use of pesticides. Promotion of communty-wide mosquito control is usually necessary as breeding areas may be far from the poultry farm. Up-to-date information is published annually by the U.S. Public Health Service (Anon., 1970) and by state extension services (Travis, 1969).

Biting Midges (Ceratopogonidae)

Culicoides spp. are biting midges, "punkies," or "no-see-ums," some 35 species of which have been reported from North America (Fig. 27.14). These are extremely small flies, though easily seen as small blackish specks moving on the skin. They attack birds and mammals. In Virginia some 20 species have been taken in chicken coops, with *Culicoides obsoletus* group (*C. obsoletus* and *C. sanguisuga*) and *C. crepuscularis* most abundant (Messersmith, 1965a). Hair and Turner (1968) record 10 *Culicoides* species feeding on chickens and turkeys, with *C. sanguisuga, C. haematopotus,* and *C. furens* taken in greatest abundance in their Virginia studies. The infec-

tive agent of avian infectious synovitis remains alive in *C. variipennis* for at least 24 hours, but transmission by bites has not been proven for any *Culicoides* species (Turner et al., 1963). Fallis and Wood (1957) report them as intermediate hosts for *Haemoproteus nettionis,* a blood protozoon of domesticated ducks in Canada. MacCreary and Catts (1954) found *Culicoides canithorax* on chickens near salt marshes in Delaware, but they could not determine its relationship to disease. Hori et al. (1964) reported on *Culicoides arakawae* as a vector of *Leucocytozoon caulleryi* in Japan, and on its control. Huff (1963, 1968) summarized transmission of these bird malarias.

CONTROL. Controlling biting midges is very difficult. They will pass through ordinary screen mesh. Screen treated with 6–7.7% malathion solution will continue to kill midges for more than 3 weeks (Jamnback, 1963). Fogging with pyrethrum fly spray or use of a dichlorvos surface spray may alleviate the problem. Residual deposits as applied for fly control will also help. The measures recommended against mosquito breeding will be found useful, as biting midges breed in wetlands though exact habitats are different.

Blackflies

Flies of the family Simuliidae (Fig. 27.15) are known as blackflies, turkey gnats, or buffalo gnats. They are similar in size to mosquitoes but dark, short, chunky, and hump-backed, with short legs. They have no ocelli, the compound eyes are excised at

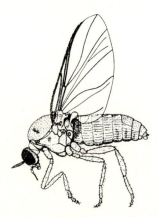

FIG. 27.15—Blackfly, family Simuliidae. (B. V. Travis, Cornell Univ.)

the antennae, the first tergum of the abdomen is modified into a basal scale usually bearing long hairs, and the wing venation is distinctive. More than 20 species have been reported to attack domesticated poultry in North America. At times they may cause serious damage to man and livestock. Swarms of blackflies may attack poultry, depleting the bird's blood volume and injecting toxic material. They also transmit certain blood protozoa belonging to the genus *Leucocytozoon*. Twinn (1936), Stone and Jamnback (1955), and Stone (1964) summarize blackfly species of eastern United States and eastern Canada.

The females are vicious bloodsuckers during daylight hours. They breed in running water from which they may travel several miles in search of blood. Eggs are laid on rocks, sticks, and other objects in the water; on floating vegetation; or dropped into streams. They may hatch in a few days, but some remain through the summer or even until the following spring. The larvae (Fig. 27.16) attach to stones or other objects. After 3–10 weeks or longer during which the larvae molt 6 times, the pupal stage is reached. This stage also occurs under water, lasting from a few days to a week or more. The adult flies of some species emerge in the spring, others during summer or early fall. Hibernation occurs in the egg or larval stage. Most temperate zone species have 1 generation a year.

Simuliids are most troublesome in the northern part of the temperate zone and the subarctic, but some important species are found even in the tropics. Reports of their occurrence in this country date back to the early part of the last century when buffalo gnats seriously interfered with homesteading operations in the South. It was noted then that they would swarm on poultry, forcing setting chickens and turkeys to leave their nests; they killed young birds by forcing their way in large numbers under the wings where they sucked blood.

Walker (1927) reported that *Simulium bracteatum* fatally attacked goslings in Canada, and Gibson (1930), also of Canada, found that *Simulium* sp. caused losses to chickens and turkeys. Underhill (1939) stated that *Simulium jenningsi* (syn. *S. nigroparvum*) and *S. slossonae* attacked turkeys in Virginia as far as 15 miles away from their breeding places. In 1928 heavy losses in chicks occurred in western Iowa.

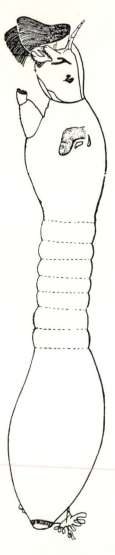

FIG. 27.16—Blackfly larva. (B. V. Travis, Cornell Univ.)

Swarms of gnats produced severe anemia, leaving a hemorrhage at each skin area punctured. The chicks ingested enormous numbers of the gnats so that their crops were distended with them. Edgar (1953) in Kansas studied the effects of the turkey gnat *Simulium meridionale* on egg production of chickens. Production dropped from 70% to 20% in 8 days. One hen died, but production became normal shortly after the flies disappeared.

It was not until 1932 that disease transmission by gnats to poultry was proved. Skidmore (1932a) of Nebraska found that *Simulium occidentale (meridionale)* could transmit *Leucocytozoon smithi*, a blood protozoon of turkeys. O'Roke (1934) showed that *S. venustum* (probably a misidentification, actually *S. rugglesi* [Shewell, 1955]) transmitted *L. simondi* to tame and wild ducks in Michigan. Johnson et al. (1938) showed *S. jenningsi* to transmit *L. smithi.* Fallis et al. (1956) in Canada reported the transmission of *L. simondi* to ducks by the black flies *S. croxtoni, S. euryadminiculum,* and *S. rugglesi.* Jones and Richey (1956) added *S. slossonae* to the list of vectors of *Leucocytozoon* to turkeys. Huff (1963, 1968) reviewed this bird malaria transmission. Anderson (1956), also in Canada, found that 6 species of blackflies transmitted the blood microfilariae of the nematode *Ornithofilaria fallisensis* to domesticated and wild ducks. Today ducks are not commercially produced in these localities.

CONTROL. This is difficult because these pests breed in streams, often some distance from the poultry farm, where insecticide treatment may be harmful to fish. The drifting smoke of smudge fires will repel the adult flies. Birds may be kept within screened enclosures during the daytime, using screen of 24 mesh per inch or smaller. The measures recommended for mosquito control, as well as cautions on watershed contamination by pesticides, are pertinent to blackfly control.

Stable Fly

Stomoxys calcitrans, the stable fly, attacks most mammals and birds. This fly is similar in size and appearance to the common housefly but possesses a piercing beak on the underside of the head. The bite is very irritating. The stable fly breeds in manure with high straw content or in wet crop refuse such as straw left in the field after grain harvest. Near the sea coast they can be very annoying because of breeding in windrows of wet seaweed.

Stable flies can be controlled by the same measures used against houseflies. Prevention of breeding requires cleanup of crop and other plant matter refuse and proper manure management to prevent production of moist manure mixed with bedding. For control in poultry houses use the measures recommended against houseflies.

Housefly and Its Relatives

Nonbiting flies breeding on poultry farms are a health and sanitation problem to the poultryman and his neighbors. Public pressure against poultry enterprises can force poultrymen out of business if odor and flies are not controlled. Intensive modern chicken farms produce a tremendous amount of manure that must be disposed of in a rapid and sanitary manner without allowing fly breeding.

The common nonbiting flies on poultry farms in the United States include housefly *(Musca domestica),* little housefly *(Fannia canicularis), F. femoralis,* latrine fly *(F. scalaris),* false stable fly *(Muscina stabulans),* and several species of blow flies (Calliphoridae) and flesh flies (Sarcophagidae). Throughout the world fecal breeding flies are a problem on poultry farms, with many other species of *Musca,* other genera, and indigenous Calliphoridae and Sarcophagidae involved. The manual by Scott and Littig (1962) is most useful for identifying flies and gives importance and biology of both biting and nonbiting flies.

These flies lay eggs in manure (some sarcophagids deposit living larvae) or on dead bird carcasses. Temperature determines development time. In hot weather the housefly can complete its life cycle in $1\frac{1}{2}$ weeks, but in colder weather it may require over $1\frac{1}{2}$ months. The maggots develop if there is adequate moisture in the manure, then worm their way to drier parts of the manure for pupation. The housefly does not diapause and survives northern winters by slow breeding in warm indoor locations such as dairy barns and in towns and cities. Part of the springtime northern housefly population probably originates from a northward breeding migration. Other filth-breeding flies survive northern winters by hibernation as diapausing adult or immature stages.

Flies have been incriminated as vectors of many mammalian as well as avian gastrointestinal diseases, largely through the flies' habit of feeding on inoculum in excrement and regurgitating onto food or feeds (West, 1951). Houseflies and maggots are readily snapped up by birds, affording transmission of helminths. They are intermediate hosts for the tapeworm *Choanotaenia infundibulum* of chicken and turkey. Skidmore (1932b) reports that common houseflies that have fed on infected fowl cholera blood can transmit this disease when fed to turkeys. The common housefly as well as *Lucilia* sp. (Calliphoridae) was capable of carrying eggs of the cecal worm

Heterakis gallinae, which contained the protozoan cause of histomoniasis of turkeys (Frank, 1953).

Certain fly larvae are of interest because, by breeding on decomposing cadavers, they may ingest toxins of the bacterium *Clostridium botulinum,* according to Bishopp (1923). If poultry eat such maggots, the disease botulism may occur. This has been called "limberneck," a term descriptive of one symptom but not characteristic of botulism alone. The larvae of the following species of flies have been incriminated as transmitters of botulinus toxins, types A and C: *Lucilia illustris* and *Phaenicia sericata* (Calliphoridae); sarcophagid larvae; and larvae of *Cochliomyia macellaria* (Calliphoridae), the secondary screwworm fly. Prompt burial, burning, or use of disposal pits for animal cadavers will do much to prevent botulism from these sources.

Schalk (1928) noted that "fly larvae" developing on tuberculous chicken cadavers could transmit *Mycobacterium tuberculosis* when fed to nontuberculous chickens.

Invasion of birds by fly larvae (maggots) is not as common as in mammals. Knipling and Rainwater (1937) mention that *Cochliomyia hominivorax,* the screwworm, will deposit eggs in wounds on chickens, turkeys, and geese. Maggots hatching from these eggs actively destroy living tissue. Stewart (1929) reported a case of cloacal invasion of a hen by screwworm larvae. Invaded wounds in valuable birds may be treated with 5% coumaphos (Co-Ral) dust or 0.25% coumaphos as a wash.

The nests of wild birds may become infested by the maggots of various species of fleshflies and blowflies, with disastrous effects on the nestlings.

CONTROL. Control must be based on proper management of manure and prompt disposal of dead bird carcasses. Houseflies are largely eliminated in caged layer houses by liquid manure systems. Conversely houseflies can be eliminated by keeping litter dry under birds in conventional floor houses. It is important to prevent overflow of watering devices, to repair water leaks, and to keep roofs in good condition. It is important to keep manure cones dry under birds on wire in southern and western United States. Dry sand or sawdust should be used as a base on which to grow new cones. Manure should be disposed of on schedule, remembering that the housefly maggot stage lasts less than a week in hot weather. Composting manure or covering with a black polyethylene tarpaulin will prevent fly breeding (Eastwood et al., 1966, 1967). Blowflies and flesh flies usually originate from carcasses.

Manure may be insecticide-treated if the management system prevents birds from contacting the manure. Effective treatments include 0.25% ronnel (Korlan), 0.25% dimethoate (Cygon), 0.5% dichlorvos (Vapona), 0.7% Zytron, 1% Rabon, and special larvicide calcium arsenate formulation. Use kerosene or fuel oil as the vehicle rather than water to prevent liquifying of the manure. About ½–1 gallon, depending on the insecticide, should be sprinkled over 100 sq ft of manure. Higher concentrations can be used including up to 2% ronnel or 1.25% dimethoate. Dichlorvos (Vapona) (0.5%) granules can be used at 2½ lb/650 sq ft of litter, repeated monthly. Eversole et al. (1965a) reported on manure treatment against the little housefly and on administration as a feed additive larvicide (Eversole et al., 1965b). A strong argument against larviciding manure is the possibility of causing resistance to these insecticides, rendering them useless for adult fly control. Also, manure treatment kills parasites and predators of flies, allowing for a rapid fly buildup as soon as the treatment is no longer effective. Calcium arsenate (Kilmag) may be preferred for larviciding manure as arsenicals are never used against adult flies and are less toxic to parasites and predators. One pound of 83% calcium arsenate in 2 gal of water may be applied to 500 sq ft of droppings at least once a week. Burton et al. (1965) found manure management costs related to fly control in California averaged 6.5 cents per bird per year and that fly control was directly related to efficiency of manure disposal.

Where practical, the adult flies should be screened out of poultry houses or prevented entry by tight house construction as in good cage houses. Bramhall et al. (1966) give directions for screening for fly control. Flies that gain entry can be killed by pyrethrum, dichlorvos (Vapona), or naled (Dibrom) space sprays or fogs. For large farms electric mist sprayers (foggers) are practical, but frequent use is necessary. Dichlorvos (Vapona) in resin strands or strips is effective but somewhat expensive.

Residual insecticide sprays applied to walls, ceilings, beams, and posts are effective depending on the resistance status of the flies involved. In many areas of the United States, flies are resistant to malathion, and there is some resistance to ronnel. This situation is likely to worsen. The several species of flies that are troublesome on poultry farms develop varying degrees of resistance under the same control procedures, but all species are capable of developing resistance to insecticides (Georghiou et al., 1967). Nevertheless, residual sprays are recommended as practical treatments because a single application may last for 1–2 months. The local extension service or state university entomology department should be consulted for the current insecticides considered to be most effective and safe. With birds in the house, 2.5% malathion or 1% ronnel (Korlan) may be used; 1% dimethoate (Cygon) may be used only when no birds are in the house. A promising new residual spray effective against some strains of resistant flies is 1% Rabon (SD8447) (Mathis and Schoof, 1968).

Axtell (1970) suggests an integrated fly control program for caged poultry houses, including early season manure removal and adult fly control by bait stations plus residual insecticide spraying of selected areas in the houses.

Liberal use of dry or liquid fly baits will alleviate the fly problem. Kilpatrick et al. (1962) used plastic chicken waterers as dispensers for dichlorvos (Vapona) liquid sugar bait and obtained good fly control. The waterers should be refilled every 3 weeks. Hansens and Vasvary (1964) give condensed directions for fly control on poultry farms. The annual summary of fly control experiments and recommendations of the U.S. Public Health Service (Anon., 1970) should be consulted for up-to-date information. Also see Anderson et al. (1968) for complete information on poultry ranch fly control.

Pigeon Fly

Pseudolynchia canariensis, the pigeon fly, is a rather important parasite of domesticated pigeons in warm or tropical areas (Fig. 27.17). It has been known since 1896 in the southern half of the United States and also occurs in many other countries. The pigeon fly is a member of the rather odd parasitic fly family Hippoboscidae, or louse flies. The body is dorsoventrally flattened and the head is provided with a short, stout beak. The life cycle is unusual as the larva matures inside the female and pupates immediately on being ejected from the mother. The pupa is white initially but quickly hardens and blackens.

The adult pigeon fly is dark brown and about 6 mm in length. The two transpar-

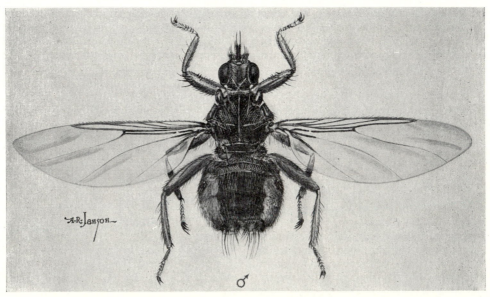

FIG. 27.17—Pseudolynchia canariensis, *pigeon fly. (Drake and Jones, 1930)*

ent wings are somewhat longer than the body. These flies move rapidly through the feathers and suck blood, particularly from nestling pigeons 2–3 weeks of age. They may also bite man, inflicting a painful skin wound that persists for several days. The pupal stage requires about 30 days; the adults live about 45 days and deposit 4 or 5 young.

Infested pigeons suffer from blood loss and irritation. Also, the pigeon fly may transmit a protozoan blood-cell parasite *Haemoproteus columbae,* the cause of a malarialike disease of pigeons.

CONTROL. Because these flies breed in pigeon nests, it is essential to clean the nests and surroundings at 15–20-day intervals and to burn or bury the cleanings. Pigeon lofts may be rid of adult flies by using a pyrethrum-containing fly spray (1 part pyrethrum extract to 2 parts of kerosene)

(Levi, 1957). This should not be sprayed on unhatched eggs. Pigeons may be freed from the flies by applying several pinches of fresh pyrethrum, rubbing it into the skin. A treatment worth trying would be several pinches of 4–5% malathion dust on each bird and into the nest.

MITES

The common free-living ectoparasitic mites of poultry belong to the family Dermanyssidae, including the chicken mite, northern fowl mite, and tropical fowl mite. These mites possess relatively well sclerotized free dorsal and ventral plates, claws and caruncles on the tarsi, one lateroventral sitgmata near each third coxa with a long peritreme extending almost to the gnathosoma, and small chelicerae on long sheathed bases. They are able to run rapidly on the skin and feathers. These mites are bloodsuckers, causing anemia when

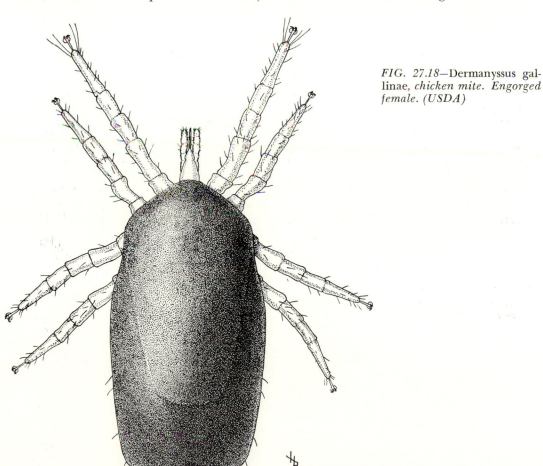

FIG. 27.18—Dermanyssus gallinae, *chicken mite. Engorged female. (USDA)*

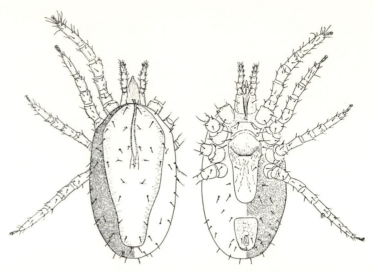

FIG. 27.19—Dermanyssus gallinae, *chicken mite. (Baker et al., 1956)*

abundant and killing chicks. Of lesser importance are members of many other mite families that bore into the skin or infect various internal passages and organs.

DERMANYSSIDAE

Chicken Mite

The chicken mite *Dermanyssus gallinae* (Fig. 27.18) is also known as the red mite, roost mite, or poultry mite. It is the commonest mite on poultry, being particularly serious in houses with roosts in warmer parts of the temperate zone. It is rare in caged layer operations. It can be identified (Fig. 27.19) by shape of the dorsal plate and by the long whiplike chelicerae which appear to be stylets, although very high magnification proves them chelicerate (like a

lobster claw). The adult female measures about 0.7×0.4 mm, varying in color from gray to deep red, depending on its blood content. Wisseman and Sulkin (1947) and Harrison (1962) have described the life cycle which may be completed in as little as 7 days. Adult females lay eggs in the hosts' surroundings 12–24 hours after their first blood meal. Eggs hatch in 48–72 hours when warm. The 6-legged larvae, without feeding, molt in 24–48 hours, becoming first-stage bloodsucking nymphs; they then molt to second-stage nymphs in another 24–48 hours, soon afterward molting to the adult stage. Chicken mites have lived up to 34 weeks without food (Kirkwood, 1963).

Chickens are the commonest hosts, but turkeys, pigeons, canaries, several wild birds, and man may be attacked. English

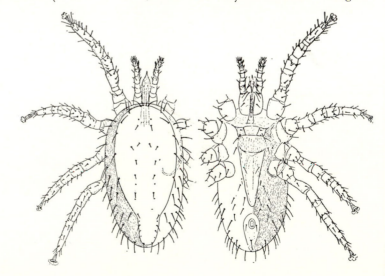

FIG. 27.20—Ornithonyssus sylviarum, *northern fowl mite. (Baker et al., 1956)*

sparrows frequently transmit this parasite because of the habit of lining their nests with chicken feathers. These mites may not only produce anemia, thereby seriously lowering production, but may actually kill birds through extraction of blood. This is particularly true of young birds and of setting and laying hens. Birds in production may refuse to lay in infested nests. This symptom indicates that poultry houses should be examined for mites. Often these mites can be found by looking under loose clods of manure on roosts. They are evident as tiny red to blackish dots, often clustered together. Inspection during the night is necessary for finding mites on the birds.

The chicken mite has been reported by Hertel (1904) and Plasaj (1925) as a transmitter of fowl cholera organisms, and by Hart (1938) of the fowl spirochete *Borrelia anserina*. Sulkin (1945) showed this mite to harbor the virus of equine encephalitis, western type; Howitt et al. (1948) showed it to harbor the virus of the eastern type. Smith et al. (1944) isolated human St. Louis encephalitis virus from the chicken mite, but Baker et al. (1956) believe the reported transmission of St. Louis encephalitis virus of man by the chicken mite to be inconclusive. Later studies with bird mites, including the chicken mite, from natural sources failed to demonstrate their role as vectors of the virus of St. Louis encephalitis or of the eastern and western strains of equine encephalitis virus (Chamberlain and Sikes, 1955; Reeves et al., 1955; and Sulkin et al., 1955). Thus the virus of St. Louis encephalitis was isolated from the chicken mite in the St. Louis area but not subsequently in other areas of the United States. Chamberlain (1968) considers the evidence of mite transmission of encephalitides to be unconvincing.

Northern Fowl Mite

The northern fowl mite *Ornithonyssus sylviarum* (Fig. 27.20) is most troublesome in the northern part of the temperate zone but can be a serious pest in southern United States and throughout the temperate zone. It is our most troublesome pest in modern caged layer houses, and can be a

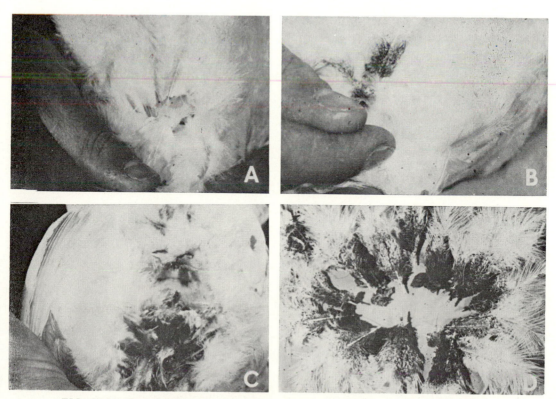

FIG. 27.21—*Four levels of feather blackening and soiling by northern fowl mite.*
(*J. G. Matthysse, Cornell Univ.*)

pest on range turkeys (Lancaster and Simco, 1968). It has been reported from many species of birds, including domesticated poultry and English sparrows, and also from rats and accidentally from man. Foulk and Matthysse (1965) and Hicks and Brown (1963) present most recent studies on wild bird hosts.

The northern fowl mite is often confused with the chicken mite but can be distinguished by possession of easily visible chelicerate chelicerae and shape of dorsal and anal plates. Unlike the chicken mite, the northern fowl mite can be found easily on birds in the daytime as well as at night as it breeds continuously on the birds. In heavy infestations the feathers are blackened (Fig. 27.21) and the skin scabbed and cracked, particularly around the vent. When infested birds are handled, the mites quickly crawl over the examiner's hands and arms. Parting the feathers reveals the mites, their eggs, cast-off skins, and excrement on the body surface and feathers. Poultrymen often diagnose a northern fowl mite infestation by seeing the mites crawling on eggs. These mites are vicious bloodsuckers. The scabs formed injure the appearance of dressed poultry (Payne, 1930). Although the northern fowl mite is the commonest and most important external parasite of caged layers in the United States, recent data throw doubt on economic importance. Loomis et al. (1970) could not detect an effect on egg production in chickens.

Reeves et al. (1947) recovered western type equine encephalitis virus from the northern fowl mite obtained from the nests of English sparrows and yellow-headed blackbirds. Hammon et al. (1948) isolated from the northern fowl mite from wild birds a virus or mixture of viruses from which the St. Louis and western equine encephalitis viruses were obtained. It is doubtful that the northern fowl mite plays any important role in epidemiology of encephalitides (Chamberlain, 1968). Hofstad (1949) and Brody (1938) respectively found that the northern fowl mite harbored the viruses of Newcastle disease (pneumoencephalitis) and fowl pox of poultry after feeding on infected chickens, but proof of transmission is lacking. Meyer and Eddie (1960) isolated the virus of ornithosis (*Bedsonia* sp.) from fowl mites (*Ornithonyssus* sp.) and also from nonparasitic mites found

in the nests of turkeys 2½ months after the nests had been abondoned because of ornithosis in the flock.

In the case of chickens, the life cycle of the northern fowl mite is completed on the birds. Eggs are laid mainly on the feathers and hatch in a day or so. The larval and two nymphal instars can be completed in less than 4 days, and the complete cycle in less than a week. In the north these mites increase during the autumn, becoming most serious in the winter, and usually drop to low numbers by summertime. Occasionally, however, infestations are found in the summer. This contrasts with the chicken mite which is a pest during warm weather in northern United States and is inactive in cold houses during the winter. Sikes and Chamberlain (1954) give the most complete study of the life history of the northern fowl mite. Combs and Lancaster (1965) give biological data on the mite, and Kirkwood (1963) found it to survive less than a month when no poultry were available.

The northern fowl mite appears to be introduced into laying hen flocks by four main methods (Foulk, 1964): (1) Hatchery and contract-started pullet farms may be infested, resulting in infested started pullets being put into laying houses. (2) Trucks and crates used to carry old birds or infested pullets may harbor infestations, resulting in new birds becoming infested. (3) Mites may be transported on personnel, equipment, or egg dividers and crates traveling from farm to farm. (4) Wild birds may bring mites into hen houses. Sparrows, pigeons, and phoebes nesting in or near poultry houses are suspected, although Foulk (1964) could not infest chicks with northern fowl mites taken from sparrows.

Tropical Fowl Mite

The tropical fowl mite *Ornithonyssus bursa* (Fig. 27.22) is distributed throughout the warmer regions of the world and possibly replaces the northern fowl mite in these regions. Roberts (1952) gives details on life history, damage, and control in Australia where it is an important poultry pest. It is a much less important pest in the United States. Hosts include poultry, pigeons, sparrows, myna birds, and even man. The tropical fowl mite closely resembles the northern fowl mite but can be distinguished by the shape of the dorsal plate and the pattern of setae. This mite can

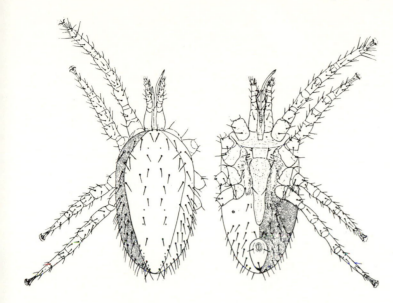

FIG. 27.22—Ornithonyssus bursa, *tropical fowl mite. (Baker et al., 1956)*

pass its entire life cycle on chickens. Its biology and habits are similar in general to those of the northern fowl mite, although a greater proportion of mite eggs are laid in the nests.

Sulkin and Izumi (1947) recovered the virus of western equine encephalomyelitis from the tropical fowl mite. This was confirmed by Miles et al. (1951).

CONTROL. The three species of dermanyssid mites can be controlled by the same insecticides applied to the birds and to litter. Carbaryl (Sevin), Rabon, and coumaphos (Co-Ral) are effective as dusts or sprays in most regions of the United States. However, Furman and Lee (1969) and Riehl (personal communication) report carbaryl failing in California, and Reid (personal communication) states that coumaphos has not been too effective and that there are reports of resistance to carbaryl in Georgia. Malathion has proven generally effective against the poultry mite but has failed against northern fowl mite in New York and California, probably because of resistance (Reid and Botero, 1966; Foulk and Matthysse, 1963; Rodriguez and Riehl, 1963). The problem may not be resistance engendered by use of malathion, as Reid et al. as early as 1956 reported malathion as only partially effective against northern fowl mite in Georgia. Nelson and Bertun (1965) supported the resistance theory by finding synergists that greatly increased malathion toxicity to northern fowl mite.

Northern fowl mite infestations on caged layer hens can be controlled satisfactorily by concentrated application of carbaryl by electric mist sprayer (Foulk and Matthysse, 1963). Rodriguez and Riehl (1960c) controlled northern fowl mite with dust bath boxes placed inside laying hen cages. The new organophosphorous compound Rabon (SD8447) has been found effective against northern fowl mite by Nelson et al. (1969).

For poultry mite control, the inside of the house should be sprayed with malathion, carbaryl, Rabon, or coumaphos, treating all hiding places of mites such as roosts, behind nest boxes, and in cracks and crevices. Nicotine sulfate or malathion roost painting will reduce the infestation but may not result in eradication. Kirkwood (1965) controlled chicken mite with 0.5 g 50% carbaryl inside 2.1 meters of a special hollow trap perch. Poultry houses should be cleaned thoroughly and disinfected before introducing a new flock.

In modern poultry practice the pest control goal should be eradication on the whole farm. Thorough insecticide application, repeated if necessary, can eradicate dermanyssid mites. Many poultrymen in the North practice preventive treatment of new flocks and annual treatment of the whole farm in the fall of the year. External parasites in general are prevented from causing economic damage. Ingress of mites from wild birds is prevented by controlling the size of ventilation openings, by screening, and by removal of wild bird nests. Holes should be patched with ¾″ chicken wire mesh. Started pullets should come from mite-free suppliers in crates and on trucks that are cleaned regularly and not used to haul old birds.

Sulfaquinoxaline in feed has proven effective against northern fowl mites in California (Furman and Stratton, 1964). However, use of sulfaquinoxaline in the necessary regimen may cause reduced egg production and mortality by internal hemorrhaging.

Simco and Lancaster (1965) compared several of the aforementioned treatments against dermanyssid mites and also found dichlorvos (Vapona) spray or fumigation from dichlorvos resin strands to be effective. They also reported best control of chicken mite by dimethoate (Cygon) house spray, with dichlorvos (Vapona) very effective and fenthion (Baytex) also effective. Dichlorvos spray (0.25%) applied twice to the roosting area of range turkeys controlled northern fowl mite (Lancaster and Simco, 1968). Dichlorvos appears to have inadequate penetration into crevices to control the chicken mite (Kirkwood, 1967).

LAELAPTIDAE

Occasionally mites of the family Laelaptidae will infest chickens, as for example *Haemolaelaps casalis* (Cwilich and Hadani, 1965); the same mite has been found on pigeons (Strandtman and Wharton, 1958).

CHIGGERS

Chiggers are larval mites of the family Trombiculidae. The nymphs and adults are free-living, usually in or on the soil. Although over 700 species are known, only a very few attack poultry. The larval chigger is 6-legged and possesses a single dorsal plate bearing a pair of sensillae and 4–6 setae. The legs are 7-segmented and bear 2 claws and an empodial bristle. Unfed chigger larvae are 0.1–0.45 mm in diameter, hence hardly visible unless they are engorged when they appear as minute red dots. The adults breed on the ground, especially along fencerows or in undisturbed wooded or brushy areas. The larvae attach to the skin, often in groups, and inject a highly irritant substance into the wound. The host forms a stylostome or feeding tube through which the larva feeds on liquified host tissue but not blood (Jones, 1950; Wharton and Fuller, 1952). Itching

vesicles or even abscesses may form at the points of attachment, surrounded by a zone of hyperemia and edema. Apparently a toxemia may occur, as indicated by the mortality that follows infestation of chicks, especially quail.

Chigger infestations are sporadic and localized; a heavily infested site may adjoin a habitat that appears similar to it in all respects but is free of these mites (Baker et al., 1956). Chiggers affect poultry mainly in the southern states.

Turkeys

The most important poultry chigger in the United States is *Neoschongastia americana* (Fig. 27.23), which is a serious pest of turkeys and wild birds such as quail (Ewing, 1929) and a minor pest of chickens all across southern United States, particularly Georgia, the Carolinas, Texas, Alabama, Arkansas, and Kentucky. This chigger also occurs in Central America and the West Indies. A subspecies *N. americana solomonis* occurs on several Pacific islands and Japan (Baker et al., 1956). *N. americana* was unimportant in past years when turkeys were marketed almost exclusively for the Thanksgiving and Christmas holidays in contrast to current marketing throughout the year, including the summertime period of chigger activity. Kunz et al. (1969) note that lesions on market-age turkeys cause a loss in value of about $1 per bird. Reid and Botero (1966) state that chiggers cost southeastern turkey growers 20 cents to $1 per bird because of downgrading at market time. The lesions resemble human pimples with a reddened area surrounding a white or yellow center which may be scabbed. Up to 100 mites or more may be found in a single sore, and 25–30 such lesions per turkey were commonly found on untreated birds during periods of peak infestations in Texas (Kunz et al., 1969). Kunz also notes that one lesion 3 mm in diameter or larger is sufficient cause for downgrading if its location is conspicuous on a freeze-packaged turkey.

Kunz et al. (1969) gives the following information on this turkey chigger in Texas: The larvae are abundant on tight, heavy clay soils that crack open when dry, and are most abundant if there is natural shade. They become active in central Texas in May and can be found on turkeys as late as mid-October, with peak infestation dur-

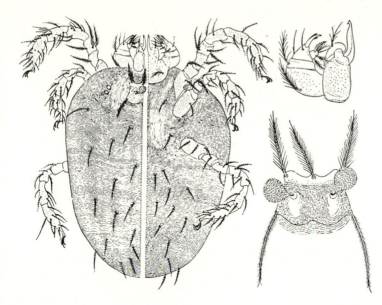

FIG. 27.23—Neoschöngastia americana *larva, chigger of chickens and turkeys. (Baker et al., 1956)*

ing June, July, and August. Number of generations per year is not known. Clusters of chiggers are observed on turkeys within 24 hours of placing the birds on infested ranges. Most chiggers leave the lesions within 8–10 days but a few remain up to 15 days. Approximately 3 weeks are required for most of the wounds to heal completely. Thus, in order for a control procedure to prevent downgrading it must protect turkeys for at least 4 weeks prior to marketing the birds. Unused ranges may remain infested for several years.

Others

Trombicula alfreddugesi is a widespread chigger that infests man and other mammals as well as birds. Heavily parasitized birds become droopy, refuse to feed, and may die from starvation and exhaustion. The larvae may be found in clusters in the anal area, on the inner aspects of the thighs, and under the wings (Baker et al., 1956). *Trombicula batatas* attacks chickens, turkeys, and many other birds and mammals as well as man from southern United States to Brazil (Baker et al., 1956). *Acomatacarus galli,* a chigger usually found on the rabbit, rat, and mouse, may be a pest of the chicken (Loomis, 1956). *Trombicula autumnalis* is the important European harvest mite which does attack poultry.

Certain chiggers transmit rickettsiae of human scrub typhus, but in the United States chiggers that attack poultry are not known to be involved in transmission of disease.

CONTROL. Currently only malathion is registered for use to control chiggers attacking poultry. Ranges should be treated with 0.25% malathion spray at 50 gal per acre or 4% malathion dust at 25 lb per acre 1 day before putting turkeys on. Weekly treatment may be necessary. Malathion spray (0.5%) may be applied to the birds also at weekly intervals. Treatment must commence 4–6 weeks prior to marketing.

These procedures are too laborious and costly for general practicality. Price and Kunz (1970), Price et al. (1970), and Dishburger et al. (1969) have found Dursban (Dow Chemical Co.) most promising for effective chigger control by a single application to turkey ranges. Price et al. (1970) state that 4 lb Dursban per acre prevented downgrading type lesions on turkeys for 6 weeks after the birds were placed on treated ranges. The spraying rate was 300 gal per acre; possibly rather high for maximum practicality. Diazinon, ethion, and Geigy GS-13005 were found effective by Kunz et al. (1971), but these insecticides as well as Dursban are not yet registered for this purpose.

Other chiggers, including *Trombicula alfreddugesi,* have been controlled with sulfur, toxaphene, lindane, coumaphos (Co-Ral), and other materials as area treatments to prevent attacks on man. The chlorinated hydrocarbon insecticides must *not* be used on poultry ranges, as excessive residues will result in the meat and fat.

FEATHER MITES

Most mites in the families Analgesidae, Pterolichidae, and Proctophyllodidae and a few in Cheyletidae live on the feathers of birds or in the quills. These feather mites are rather host specific so that only a few of the many known species are found on poultry. None is a major pest. Feather mites are rarely found on modern chicken farms as the cycle is broken by separation of the hatchery from producing flocks. Betke et al. (1963) found *Megninia cubitalis* and/or *Syringophilus bipectinatus* on almost half of feather samples from ducks in Germany but noted little or no pathogenicity.

Feather mites (except *Syringophilus*) belong to the superfamily Analgesoidea of the suborder Sarcoptiformes—characterized by absence of stigmata, possession of apodemes and usually strong chelae, and strong sclerotization of the body plates. Many species have one or more pairs of legs very oddly formed, and many possess anal suckers and odd posterior protuberances. Roveda and Boero (1962) give good figures and descriptions of most of the feather mites to be found on poultry.

Syringophilus bipectinatus (Fig. 27.24) is

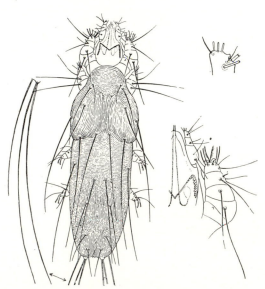

FIG. 27.24—Syringophilus bipectinatus, quill mite of poultry. (Baker et al., 1956)

commonly known as the quill mite. It belongs in the family Cheyletidae (in Myobiidae by some authors) bearing M-shaped peritremes, simple palpi without thumbclaw complex, needlelike chelicerae, short stubby legs with tarsal claws and brushlike pulvilli, and no dorsal body plates. These mites are elongate, with long setae on the body. *S. bipectinatus* was originally described in Europe in 1880, but it was not until 1932 that it was reported in the United States by Rebrassier and Martin from the chicken, turkey, and golden pheasant in Ohio. Schwabe (1956) found this mite on chickens in New Jersey. Hwang (1959) reported *S. bipectinatus* on chickens in Maryland and Pennsylvania. The mites occur inside the quills. A similar mite, *S. columbae,* has been described from pigeons by Hirst (1922). Lavoipierre (1953) described the female and male pigeon quill mite. Wild birds harbor related species. *S. bipectinatus* females measure up to 0.09 mm in length and 0.15 mm in width. The mites appear to cause partial or complete loss of feathers. The remaining quill stumps contain a powdery material in which the mites may be detected under low-power magnification. No specific method for control has yet been described. It would appear advisable to dispose of affected birds, then disinfect and clean their quarters.

Falculifer rostratus (family Pterolichidae) (Fig. 27.25), another feather-damaging mite, occurs principally between the barbs of the large wing feathers of pigeons. Although reported mainly in Europe, this mite has been noted in the United States, and it may be more or less widespread. In size the mite may be 0.8 mm long (Hollander, 1956). Levi (1957) states that he has not found the feathers to be harmed. There is some evidence that the nymphal stage of the mite may occur in the subcutis or the internal organs. *Falculifer cornutus* is also known from pigeons.

Pillers (1927) and others recommend that infested pigeons be fumigated with sulfur dioxide gas. This appears to be a tedious and rather dangerous procedure. Yager and Gleiser (1946) treated a group of Signal Corps pigeons for infection by *Falculifer rostratus,* using 10% DDT in talc. Slight control was achieved in 24 hours, with great reduction of the mites in 3 days;

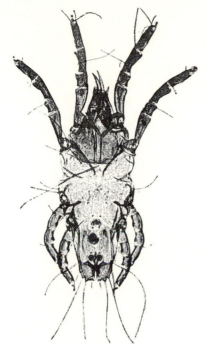

FIG. 27.25—Falculifer rostratus, *feather mite of pigeons.* ×68. *(Reis and Nobrega, 1956)*

there was no evidence of toxicity to the pigeons.

Freyana (Microspalax) *chanayi,* also a feather-inhabiting mite of the family Pterolichidae, has been reported from turkeys in Maryland by Chapin (1925). Its prevalence in Texas and Louisiana is mentioned by Bushnell and Twiehaus (1945). These mites congregate in the grooves on the undersides of the shafts of the wing feathers. *Dermoglyphus minor* and *D. elongatus* (Pterolichidae) have been reported from inside chicken and turkey quills.

Pterolichus obtusus (Pterolichidae) is found on flight and tail feathers of chickens, causing a grayish cast when very abundant and possibly reducing bird vigor. Alicata et al. (1946) tested dusts for control of this mite as well as *Megninia cubitalis* (see below).

Megninia cubitalis is the commonest analgesid mite of chickens in the United States, but reports of economic damage are rare. Turkeys are also attacked. Cwilich and Dison (1968) observed reduced egg production caused by these mites and obtained control by a malathion spray. Zumpt (1966) noted malnutrition as a contributing factor to *M. cubitalis* infestation and damage. Alicata et al. (1946) reported control by Lethane, sodium fluoride, sodium fluosilicate, and DDT dusts. DDT should not be used on chickens.

Megninia gallinulae is a rarely reported mite, found by Wickware (1921) in Canada. Apparently it is associated with loss of scales from the lower legs of chickens and a crusty dermatitis in the head region. Alwar et al. (1958) described depluming itch of fowls in India caused by *Megninia ginglymura* (Fig. 27.26). They found this mite on chickens, turkeys, geese, ducks, pigeons, and guineas. Levi (1957) states that pigeons in South Carolina may have the feathers of the neck and body infested by

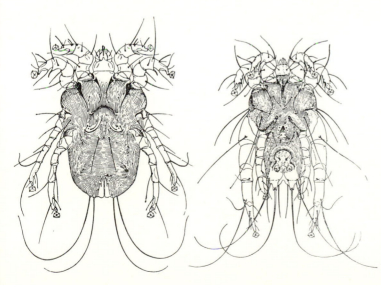

FIG. 27.26—Megninia ginglymura, *feather mite of poultry.* *(Baker et al., 1956)*

Megninia columbae. Tongson and Manuel (1965) reported on species of *Megninia* on turkeys, pigeons, and chickens. Hiepe et al. (1962) controlled *Megninia velata* on ducks with DDT and BHC, but these insecticides could be used only on breeders never to be sold as food.

Pterophagus strictus (family Proctophyllodidae) attacks pigeons. *P. obtusus* can be found on almost all poultry farms in the Philippines (Manuel and Siores, 1967).

OTHER MITES

Skin lesions of poultry can be caused by ectoparasitic mites of the families Sarcoptidae and Epidermoptidae of the suborder Sarcoptiformes. These mites differ from the feather mites in the absence of heavily sclerotized body plates (there is a single lightly sclerotized propodosamal shield on female epidermoptids), and they are much smaller.

Scaly-leg Mites

Scaly-leg mite *Knemidocoptes mutans* (Sarcoptidae) (Fig. 27.27) and related species occur on various birds. They are most commonly found on older birds that should ordinarily be culled from flocks. The mites are almost spherical in shape, short-legged, with strongly striated epidermis, and the dorsal striations are not interrupted. Adult

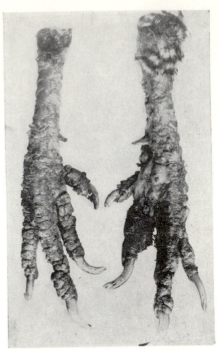

FIG. 27.28—*Lesions caused by scaly leg mites. (Benbrook and Sloss, 1961)*

females are about 0.5 mm in diameter; males are less than half that size, and the legs are longer. Lesions are produced on the unfeathered portions of the host's legs and occasionally on the skin of the comb and wattles. Tunnels are bored into the epithelium, causing proliferation and formation of scales and crusts (Fig. 27.28). This type of mite invasion of birds corresponds to sarcoptic mange of mammals. Affected birds may be crippled if the infestation is severe. The mites pass through their entire life cycle in the skin. Transmission to uninfested birds progresses slowly by contact with those infested and with their surroundings.

Control of scaly-leg mites should begin by culling or by isolating the affected birds. Additions to the flock should be inspected for lesions. Houses should be cleaned frequently, especially the roosts, which should be sprayed as recommended for the chicken mite. Repeated dipping in 0.5% malathion could be tried but no experimental work has been reported.

Depluming Mites

Knemidocoptes gallinae, the depluming mite, resembles the scaly-leg mite in general

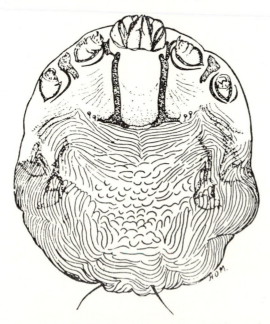

FIG. 27.27—*Knemidocoptes mutans, scaly leg mite. (Soulsby, 1968)*

structure although it is smaller, the adult female being about 0.3 mm in diameter. The striations are interrupted on the dorsal surface to form raised sculpturings. It invades the feathered areas of the epidermis of chickens, pigeons, and pheasants, especially around the feather bases, and burrows into the shafts. Intense irritation induces the host to pull out body feathers. The mites are more prevalent in spring and summer, at which time the infestation may spread rapidly by contact. Depluming mites produce injury by interfering with the control of body heat. Some of the affected birds will lose weight and show lowered production. *Knemidocoptes pilae* causes a serious mange of budgerigars (Ballarini, 1964).

Control of depluming mites is not easily accomplished. Prompt isolation of affected birds and disinfestation of houses as recommended for chicken mites should come first. Treatments recommended for individual birds include:

1. Dipping in mixture of sulfur (2 oz), soap (1 oz), and warm water (1 gal). This mixture should be thoroughly soaked into the skin, especially into the feet of cockerels. The birds may also be thoroughly dusted with 100% sulfur.

2. Use of ointments consisting of sulfur (1 part) and petrolatum (4 parts) or caraway oil (1 part) and petrolatum (5 parts).

3. Moistening affected areas with soapy water, then applying powdered pyrethrum or powdered sulfur with a powder blower.

4. Possibly malathion dip would be effective, but experimental testing is needed.

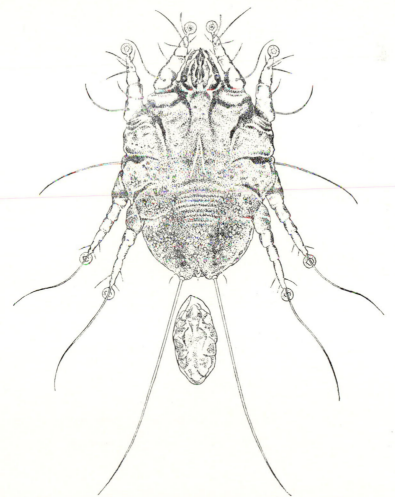

FIG. 27.29—Epidermoptes bilobatus, *epidermoptic scabies mite.* ×200. (*Reis and Nobrega, 1956*)

Freytag and Bendheim (1965) found Ody-len (Bayer Fabriken dimethyl diphenyl en-disulphide) effective for *Knemidocoptes pilae* mange of budgerigars.

Skin Mites

Epidermoptes bilobatus (Epidermopti-dae) (Fig. 27.29) is a skin mite frequently reported from Europe and more rarely from South and North America (James et al., 1930). It occurs on chickens and apparently may or may not produce lesions but has been described as a cause of pityriasis. The adult female is about 0.17–0.22 mm long. When lesions are produced, they consist first of a fine scaly dermatitis. This may be followed by the formation of thick, brownish, sharply edged scabs. Neveu-Lemaire (1938) suggests that the more severe lesions may be due partly to a concomitant fungus infection by *Lophophyton gallinae;* also that birds affected with epidermoptid mites often have depluming mites at the same time. Epidermoptic scabies may at times result in emaciation and even death. Pruritus is a common symptom.

Treatment of infested birds is recommended as for depluming scabies. In addition, Neveu-Lemaire (1938) suggests the use of balsam of Peru and alcohol (equal parts) applied to the skin.

Rivoltasia bifurcata, a mite similar to *Epidermoptes,* has been reported on chickens in Europe (Neveu-Lemaire, 1938), in Brazil (Reis, 1939), and in the United States (Bushnell and Twiehaus, 1945). In size it is said to be 0.25 × 0.15 mm. Only slight damage to feathers has been noted.

INTERNAL PARASITIC MITES

Internal passages of the respiratory system, air sacs, and subcutaneous tissue can be infested with sarcoptiform mites of the families Cytoditidae and Laminosioptidae, the mesostigmatid family Rhinonyssidae, and the prostigmatid family Speleognathidae. These mites are of odd occurrence on modern poultry farms but may be more common than reports would indicate as diagnostic procedures seldom include a search for these mites. Hyland (1963) comments on the species of endoparasitic mites of vertebrates.

Cyst Mites

The fowl cyst mite *Laminosioptes cysti-cola* (Laminosioptidae) (Fig. 27.30) has

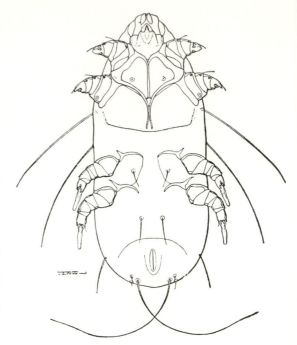

FIG. 27.30—Laminosioptes cysticola, *fowl cyst mite. ×376. (Hirst, 1922)*

been reported mainly from chickens and from turkeys, pheasants, geese, and pigeons in many parts of the world. It is most frequently noticed in the loose subcutaneous connective tissue. It has even been reported as occurring in the muscles, abdominal viscera, and lungs (pigeons) and on the peritoneum. Initial infestation is on the skin (Patyk, 1963). Ordinarily, subcutaneous mites do not appear to influence the health of infested birds, although the lesions produced may make carcasses unpalatable as food for man. If detected by the inspection service, the carcass is condemned.

The female mite measures about 0.25 × 0.11 mm. The gnathosoma is reduced and not visible from above, and the body bears a few long setae. The life cycle is unknown except that the female lays embryonated eggs. Neveu-Lemaire (1938) states that the mite will pass through all stages of its development even in the deeper tissues of the host.

Attention is most often called to subcutaneous mites by the occurrence of yellowish nodules up to several millimeters in diameter in the subcutis. These areas are often mistaken for tuberculous lesions. The nodules appear to be caseocalcareous deposits formed by the bird so as to enclose the mites after they die in the tissues. Large numbers of nodules are most often found in aged emaciated birds. Kasparek (1907) reported *L. cysticola* in pigeons in which the mites were surrounded by nodules in the lungs, causing death.

Perhaps more careful examination of the skin and subcutis of birds under a dissecting microscope might reveal the presence of this parasite more frequently. Otherwise, diagnosis will depend upon finding the characteristic nodular lesions and by seeing the mites or their remains in nodules that have been crushed under a cover glass in a drop of acidulated water (Lindquist and Belding, 1949).

Apparently no attempt has been made to control subcutaneous mites except by the destruction of affected birds.

Air Sac Mites

Respiratory system mites of poultry include the air sac mite *Cytodites nudus* (Cytoditidae) (Fig. 27.31), found in the bronchi, lungs, air sacs, and bone cavities connected therewith in birds. Air sac mites have been found in chickens, turkeys, pheasants, pigeons, canaries, and ruffed grouse from many parts of the world. Although not of common occurrence, these mites are often overlooked because of their small size and peculiar habitat.

The adult female mites are whitish specks, measuring about 0.6 × 0.4 mm. The mites appear nude because they bear but a few short setae. The gnathosoma is reduced, with minute chelicerae in a tube formed by coalescence of the palpi and gnathosoma. No details are known of the life cycle, although the usual speculation is that the mites lay eggs in the lower air passages, that these are coughed up and probably swallowed, reaching the ground in the droppings. The mode of infection is not known.

There is considerable conflict among observers as to the damage done by air sac mites. Some are of the opinion that they are practically harmless because their presence has been noted in apparently healthy birds. Others state that the mites are responsible for emaciation, peritonitis, pneumonia, and obstruction of air passages and that they are predisposing factors for tuberculosis. Heavy invasions have definitely been associated with weakness and grave loss in weight, so that affected birds resemble clinical cases of tuberculosis. Lindt and Kutzer (1965) found *C. nudus* to cause granulomatous pneumonia, which can be fatal.

Close inspection of the opened cadaver of an affected bird soon after death will show whitish dots moving slowly over the transparent air sac surfaces. Identification may easily be made by placing mites in a drop of water on a slide, applying a coverglass, and examining under magnification of 100 diameters. Little information has been published as to control of air sac mites. Most writers recommend destruction of the cadavers of affected birds, followed by disinfection and cleaning of the poultry house.

Other Respiratory System Mites

Other respiratory system mites of poultry and pigeons include a few members of the genera *Neonyssus, Rhinonyssus,* and *Sternostoma* of the family Rhinonyssidae, and *Speleognathus* of the Speleognathidae. None is an important pest of commercial poultry. *N. columbae* and *N. melloi* are nasal mites from pigeons (Crossley, 1950, 1952), *Sternostoma tracheacolum* is the canary lung mite (Fain and Hyland, 1962), and *R. rhinolethrum* is from ducks and geese. These mites are about 0.5 mm long, oval, bear no setae, possess two dorsal plates, and have stigmata without peritremes. *S. tracheacolum* occurs in the trachea, air sacs, bronchi, and parenchyma of

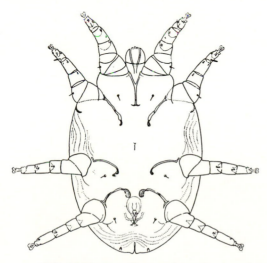

FIG. 27.31—Cytodites nudus, *air sac mite.* (Baker et al., 1956)

the lungs and on the surface of the liver. Murray (1966) controlled this mite in Gouldian finches with 0.04 g carbaryl (Sevin) on 50 g millet and 1 ml cod liver oil fed 3 times within 18–24 hours at weekly intervals. Mathey (1967) found these mites to be virulent parasites of budgerigars and suggested malathion, lindane, DDT, or sulfaquinoxaline therapy.

Speleognathus striatus, a third nasal mite of pigeons, was first found in Texas by Crossley (1952). The mite is white and 0.5 mm in length. The skin is soft and has no plates. There are a few short setae on the body and a pair of long sensory setae on the propodosoma. The legs are short with netlike sclerotization, and the coxae are divided into two groups. Clark (1957) reviewed the avian nasal mites belonging to the family Speleognathidae, stating that no pronounced lesions had been found in the hosts.

In addition to the mites listed, numerous other species have been noted on birds in various parts of the world. No doubt some of these will be found invading domestic poultry. For the present they may be considered of minor importance.

TICKS

Ticks are large mites belonging to the superfamily Ixodoidea of the Acarina, characterized by possession of a pair of stigmata posterior or lateral to the coxae and associated with a roundish or kidney-shaped stigmal plate; the hypostome is modified as a piercing organ provided with recurved teeth, and there is a pitlike sensory organ on the tarsi of the first pair of legs (Haller's organ). Unengorged adults of most common ticks are 2–4 mm long, but fully engorged females may reach more than 10 mm. However, unengorged larvae are similar in size to large mites. Ticks inhabiting poultry houses belong to the soft tick family Argasidae. These ticks have no scutum (dorsal shield) and may feed intermittently in all stages. The integument is leathery, wrinkled, and granulated in appearance. The capitulum (head) is ventrally placed near the anterior margin of the body (Fig. 27.32). Many hard ticks, family Ixodidae, will feed on poultry on ranges. These ticks possess a scutum in all stages and feed only once in each stage, remaining on the host for several days. The scutum usually appears shiny, and the capitulum is terminal at the anterior of the tick (Fig. 27.33). The *Manual on Livestock Ticks* (Diamant and Strickland, 1965) is most useful to determine North American tick species.

Losses caused by ticks may be of three general types. Foremost is the loss of host blood, which may cause death. Secondly, there is reduced production, no doubt associated with blood loss but also possibly due to tick-produced toxic substances. Thirdly, ticks in general are notorious transmitters of disease such as avian spirochetosis, tularemia, piroplasmosis, anaplasmosis, dirofilariasis, and certain rickettsial diseases (notably Rocky Mountain spotted fever)

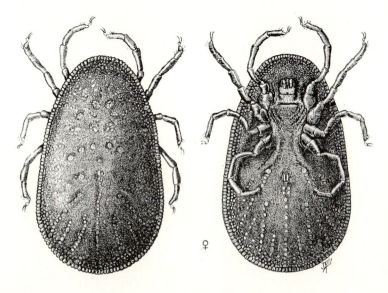

FIG. 27.32—Argas persicus group, fowl tick. Dorsal view on left, ventral view on right. (USDA)

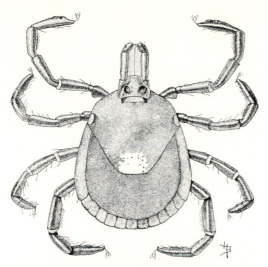

FIG. 27.33–Amblyomma americanum, lone star tick. (USDA)

and many viruses including encephalitis. The first two diseases are of particular interest to poultry raisers. Philip (1963) summarized recent contributions on ticks as vectors of disease.

FOWL TICKS

Soft ticks (Argasidae) are the most important ticks of poultry. The tick previously known as *Argas persicus* (Oken) (common name: fowl tick) is a group of species including *Argas sanchezi* Duges and *Argas radiatus* Raillet on chickens in the United States (Kohls et al., 1970). *A. persicus* is known, sensu strictu, from Pennsylvania, Maryland, Georgia, and California. It is present in Paraguay also. *A. sanchezi* is recorded from Arizona, California, Nevada, New Mexico, Texas, Utah, and Mexico. *A. radiatus* is recorded from Florida, Iowa, Texas, and Mexico. *Argas miniatus*, a member of this group, is known from Central and South America but not from the United States. Each species may have wide distribution in the world, but an accurate picture awaits more extensive tick collecting from poultry and critical examination of collections. Medley and Ahrens (1970) showed that the life cycles of *A. radiatus* and *A. sanchezi* were about equal in length but that temperature sensitivity limited *A. sanchezi* to 2–3 generations per year in south Texas. These authors also give data on reproductive potential and longevity for these two species.

Argas robertsi is found on chickens in Australia, along with *A. persicus* (Hoogstraal et al., 1968). *Argas walkerae* is the common tick on chickens in southern Africa (Kaiser and Hoogstraal, 1969).

These fowl ticks, sometimes called chicken ticks, blue bugs, tampans, or adobe ticks, are distributed mainly in those states along the Gulf of Mexico and the Mexican border. They are also established in many other tropical and temperate areas of the world. Although primarily parasites of birds, they may be found on mammals. In North America they have been reported from the following hosts: chicken, turkey, duck, dove, hawk, magpie, owl, quail, sparrow, thrush, vulture, and wild turkey; also from cattle, dog, and man. They have been reported on geese, guinea fowl, pigeons, canaries, and ostriches.

The mature blood-engorged female measures about 10×6 mm, and the mature male is about half that size. These ticks are relatively easily recognized by their flattened ovoid shape and reddish brown color.

The female may lay a total of 500–875 eggs in 4 or 5 separate batches (Chaudhury, 1960). Between layings she seeks a host for a meal of blood. The eggs are laid in sheltered crevices, including the bark of trees. They hatch in from 6–10 days in warm weather to 3 months during cool periods. The almost microscopic larvae or seed ticks become hungry in 4–5 days and seek a host, although they may live for several months without eating. After feeding on blood for 4–5 days, the larvae leave the host for a hiding place nearby, and generally in 3–9 days they reach the first nymphal stage. These nymphs become hungry in another 5–15 days but can do without food for as long as 15 months. Nymphs are active and feed only at night. The first instar nymphs feed in 10–45 minutes, leave the birds and hide for 5–8 days, shed their skins, and reach a second nymphal stage which is ready to feed in 5–15 days. After feeding for 15–75 minutes and hiding for 12–15 days, the adult ticks emerge from the nymphal skins ready to engorge with blood and, after about a week, to mate. A small number of the ticks pass through 3 nymphal instars. Oviposition commences 3–5 days after mating. The adult fowl tick in isolation may live for more than 4 years. Loomis (1961), working under laboratory conditions, found the complete life cycle required 7–8 weeks. During cold weather fowl ticks remain inactive in cracks and crevices. Hooker et al. (1912) gave a detailed study of life history of *Argas persicus*(?) in the southern United States.

Birds suffer to the greatest degree from attacks of these ticks during the warm, dry season. The loss of blood may reach proportions of a fatal anemia. At least there may be emaciation, weakness, slow growth, and lowered production. Ruffled feathers, poor appetite, and diarrhea are symptoms suggesting tick infestation.

The fowl tick is the most important poultry ectoparasite in many tropical countries, being a limiting factor in successful rearing of standard breeds of poultry (Reid, 1956; Chaudhury, 1960). Turkeys usually suffer even more than chickens, and recently hatched poults and chicks show the highest mortality. These ticks cause skin blemishes on turkeys, reducing market price.

The fowl tick is capable of transmitting the highly pathogenic spirochete *Borrelia anserina* in many parts of the world. Burroughs (1947) found tick-borne avian spirochetosis in chickens in the United States, and Hoffman et al. (1946) found it in turkeys. Burroughs allowed fowl ticks to feed on an apparently normal chicken, which in 6 days was positive for *Borrelia anserina* in blood smears. Apparently Brazil is the area nearest the United States in which avian spirochetosis commonly occurs. Rokey and Snell (1961) described epizootics of avian spirochetosis in Arizona associated with infestations by the fowl tick. Pavlovsky (1966) described natural nidi of avian spirochetosis in tree groves with wild bird rookeries infested by fowl ticks from which chickens, turkeys, geese, ducks, and several wild birds could be infected.

Fowl ticks also transmit *Aegyptianella pullorum* and fowl cholera *Pasteurella multocida*, according to Chaudhury (1960). However, Dimov (1966) could not transmit fowl cholera by the fowl tick even though ticks harbored *P. multocida* for 25 days. Gothe (1967) showed that all postembryonal stages of the fowl tick may be infected with *Aegyptianella pullorum* and transmit in the following stage. Aegyptianellosis has not been reported from the Americas. Howell et al. (1943) reported that occasionally fowl ticks may transmit the protozoan parasite causing anaplasmosis of cattle. There

is evidence that the fowl tick transmits salmonella.

Tick paralysis in chickens, a flaccid, afebrile motor paralysis, may result from attacks by the fowl tick. Etiology of this sporadic disease is poorly understood. Most likely tick paralysis is a reaction to salivary secretions, which may include a specific toxin. Ranck (personal communication) notes that the clinical signs may be confused with botulism or the neural signs of Marek's disease and also with transient paralysis, Newcastle disease, and possibly other bacterial or chemical toxins. However, Brown and Cross (1941) suggested fowl paralysis to be a virus disease, transmitted by fowl ticks.

Ticks of the *Argas persicus* group commonly attack chickens and other fowl but are rare on pigeons. The pigeon tick *Argas reflexus* is not in the *persicus* group. The subspecies *A. reflexus reflexus* attacks pigeons in Europe and Asia; *A. reflexus hermanni* is the pigeon tick of Africa (Hoogstraal and Kohls, 1960a,b). In most areas these pigeon ticks are not pests of chickens, but *A. r. hermanni* and *A. persicus* are found together on chickens in West Africa. *A. neghmei* is a pest of both chickens and pigeons in Chile. These *Argas* ticks, except *A. r. hermanni*, have been reported as pests of man (Hoogstraal, 1962). Probably both subspecies of *A. reflexus* are important vectors of fowl spirochetosis. *A. r. hermanni* in Egypt is suspected of transmitting West Nile virus, Chenuda virus, and the Quaranfil virus group among pigeons (Taylor et al., 1966) and is implicated in transmission of the Q fever rickettsia.

Control

Control requires treatment of the premises because the ticks are on their hosts only a short time and then hide in the bird's surroundings. The litter, walls, floors, and ceilings must be sprayed thoroughly, forcing spray into cracks and behind nest boxes. Outdoor runs and tree trunks should also be sprayed, using 1% Rabon, 3% malathion, 2% carbaryl (Sevin), or 0.3% naled (Dibrom) at 1–2 gal/1,000 sq ft of surface (Kraemer, 1959; Anon., 1966). Rodriguez and Riehl (1959c) controlled fowl ticks on turkeys by spraying feed troughs with 1% malathion.

Other methods for control of fowl ticks include use of metal construction, elimination of tree roosting, using roosts suspended from the ceiling, and converting to cage operation. Frequent inspection is necessary in order to combat ticks before their number has increased to a harmful extent.

Another soft tick *Ornithodoros hermsi* is one of the ticks that may transmit a spirochete of relapsing fever to man. It has also been found on fowl, bat, chipmunk, deer, and mouse.

HARD TICKS

Hard ticks (Ixodidae) of many species will feed on poultry as well as wild ground birds. Birds are preferred hosts of larvae and nymphs of some species of *Hyalomma* (Old World only) and *Amblyomma* ticks that are common in the adult stage on mammals. Ixodid tick females attach to hosts, mate, feed to repletion, then drop off and oviposit several thousand eggs in a single batch on the ground. The female dies after oviposition. The eggs hatch 1–2 months after the female leaves a host, and the 6-legged larvae climb up on the vegetation to await a new vertebrate host. There is only one larval and one nymphal instar, and each feeds but once to repletion. One-host ticks moult on the host (e.g. *Boophilus*), two-host tick larvae usually moult on the host and the nymphs on the ground, and three-host ticks drop from the host as soon as each stage is replete and moult on the ground. In the temperate zone many ixodid ticks have but one generation a year, spending the winter in diapause as eggs or immature or mature ticks. Even in the tropics some ticks require a year to complete their life cycle. Others may complete the cycle in 2–4 months. Ticks that do not find a host will live for a long period (over 2 years has been recorded), so that the cycle may be very prolonged. Also, premises and ranges will remain infested for long periods even when unoccupied.

Haemaphysalis leporispalustris, the rabbit tick, is found mainly on rabbits and hares, but also on dogs, cats, horses, and (rarely) man. The larvae and nymphs may infest chicken, quail, and various other wild birds.

Haemaphysalis chordeilis, the bird tick, has been recorded from the turkey in North America as well as from many wild birds, various domesticated mammals, and man (Cooley, 1946).

Haemaphysalis punctata nymphs cause tick paralysis of chicks in Europe (Pavlov, 1963).

Amblyomma americanum, the lone star tick, has been found on chickens and turkeys, although it is usually a parasite of the horse, cattle, many other mammals, and several wild bird hosts. Kellogg et al. (1969) found it to be common on wild turkeys.

Amblyomma tuberculatum, the gopher-tortoise tick, has been found on the chicken. Other hosts include cattle, dog, several species of wild birds, and the gopher-tortoise.

Ixodid ticks are more important poultry parasites in the tropics. *Haemaphysalis hoodi* has been reported to kill chickens in Uganda (Lucas, 1954).

REFERENCES

Alicata, J. E. 1942. Experimental transmission of endemic typhus fever by the sticktight flea *Echidnophaga gallinaceae*. *J. Wash. Acad. Sci.* 32:57.

Alicata, J. E., F. G. Holdaway, J. H. Quisenberry, and D. D. Jensen. 1946. Observations on the comparative efficacy of certain old and new insecticides in the control of lice and mites of chickens. *Poultry Sci.* 25:376.

Alwar, V. S., C. M. Lalitha, and H. N. Achuthan. 1958. Depluming itch in fowls caused by the feather mite *Megninia ginglymura* (Megnin)—A preliminary note. *Indian Vet. J.* 35:621–23.

Anderson, J. R., A. S. Deal, E. F. Legner, E. C. Loomis, and M. H. Swanson. 1968. Fly control on poultry ranches 1968–69. *Univ. Calif. Agr. Ext. Serv.* AXT–72 Rev.

Anderson, R. C. 1956. The life cycle and seasonal transmission of *Ornithofilaria fallisensis* Anderson, a parasite of domestic and wild ducks. *Can. J. Zool.* 34:485.

Anonymous. 1967. Pictorial keys to arthropods, reptiles, birds and mammals of public health significance. U.S. Public Health Serv., Atlanta, Ga.

———. 1968. Suggested guide for the use of insecticides to control insects affecting crops, livestock, households, stored products, forests, and forest products—1968. *USDA Agr. Handbook* 331.

———. 1970. Public health pesticides. *Pest Control* 40 (3): 15–54.

Arnold, H. L., Jr., and H. L. Arnold, Sr. 1943. The diagnosis and management of bird-mite bites (in man). *Proc. Staff Meet. Clin., Honolulu* 9:41–44.

Axtell, R. C. 1970. Integrated fly control program of caged poultry houses. *J. Econ. Entomol.* 63 (2): 400–405.

Baker, A. D. 1933. Some studies of the dipterous fauna of the poultry yard in Quebec in relation to parasitic troubles. *Poultry Sci.* 12:42–45.

Baker, E. W., and G. W. Wharton. 1952. *An Introduction to Acarology.* Macmillan Co., New York.

Baker, E. W., T. M. Evans, D. J. Gould, W. B. Hull, and H. L. Keegan. 1956. *A Manual of Parasitic Mites of Medical or Economic Importance.* National Pest Control Ass., Inc., New York.

Ballarini, G. 1964. *Cnemidocoptes pilae* in budgerigars and *Ornithonyssus sylviarum* in canaries. *Nuovo Vet.* 40:104–14.

Barger, E. H., L. E. Card, and B. S. Pomeroy. 1958. *Diseases and Parasites of Poultry,* 5th ed. Lea & Febiger, Philadelphia.

Barker, T. W. 1960. An inquiry into the control of pests of racing pigeons. *Pest Technol.* 2:203–8.

Beaudette, F. R. 1946. Common mosquito-borne diseases of birds. *Proc. 33rd Ann. Meet. New Jersey Mosquito Exterm. Ass.,* p. 31.

Benbrook, E. A. 1963. *Outline of Parasites Reported for Domesticated Animals in North America,* 6th ed. Iowa State Univ. Press, Ames.

Benbrook, E. A., and M. W. Sloss. 1961. *Veterinary Clinical Parasitology,* 3rd ed. Iowa State Univ. Press, Ames.

Bequaert, J. C. 1954. The Hippoboscidae or louse-flies (Diptera) of mammals and birds. Part II. Taxonomy, evolution and revision of American genera and species. *Entomologica Americana* N.S. 34:1–232.

Betke, P., J. Danailov, and G. Gräfner. 1963. Incidence, morphology and biology of the feather mites *Megninia* and *Syringophilus* in ducks. *Monatsh. Veterinaermed.* 18:218–21.

Bierer, B. W. 1954. Buffalo gnats and Leucocytozoon infections of poultry. *Vet. Med.* 49:107–10, 115.

Bierer, B. W., and C. L. Vickers. 1959. The effect on egg size and production of fungicide-treated and fumigated grains fed to hens. *J. Am. Vet. Ass.* 134:452–53.

Bigland, C. H. 1955. Chicken infestation with *Ceratophyllus niger* (black hen flea) in Alberta. *Can. J. Comp. Med. Vet. Sci.* 19:99.

Bigley, W. S., A. R. Roth, and G. W. Eddy. 1960. Laboratory and field tests against mites and lice attacking poultry. *J. Econ. Entomol.* 53:12–14.

Bishopp, F. C. 1923. Limberneck of fowls produced by fly larvae. *J. Parasitol.* 9:170–73.

———. 1929. The pigeon fly, an important pest of pigeons in the United States. *J. Econ. Entomol.* 22:974–80.

———. 1933. Mosquitoes kill livestock. *Science* 77:115.

Blickenstaff, C. C. 1965. Common names of insects. *Bull. Entomol. Soc. Am.* 11:287–320.

Borror, D. J., and D. M. De Long. 1964. *An Introduction to the Study of Insects.* Holt, Rinehart & Winston Inc., New York.

Bramhall, E. L., E. C. Loomis, and R. R. Parks. 1966. Poultry house screening for fly control. *Univ. Calif. Agr. Ext. Serv.* AXT-223.

Brennan, J. M. 1951. Two new species of Neoschongastia with a key to the species of the world (Acarina: Trombiculidae). *J. Parasitol.* 37:577–82.

Brody, A. L. 1936. The transmission of fowl pox. *Cornell Univ. Agr. Expt. Sta. Mem.* 195.

Brown, A. W. A. 1951. *Insect Control by Chemicals.* John Wiley and Sons Inc., New York.

Brown, J. C., and J. C. Cross. 1941. A probable agent for the transmission of fowl paralysis. *Science* 93:528.

Brown, R. L. 1966. *Pesticides in Clinical Practice.* Charles C Thomas, Springfield, Ill.

Burroughs, A. L. 1947. Fowl spirochaetosis transmitted by *Argas persicus* (Oken), 1818 from Texas. *Science* 105:577.

Burton, V. E., J. R. Anderson, and W. Stanger. 1965. Fly control costs on northern California poultry ranches. *J. Econ. Entomol.* 58:306–9.

Bushnell, L. D., and M. J. Twiehaus. 1945. Poultry diseases, their prevention and control. *Kans. Agr. Expt. Sta. Bull.* 326.

Busvine, J. R. 1966. *Insects and Hygiene,* 2nd ed. Methuen, London.

Cameron, D. 1938. The northern fowl mite *(Liponyssus sylviarum).* Investigations at MacDonald College, Quebec, with a summary of previous work. *Can. J. Res.* 16:230–54 (Sect. D).

Cassamagnaghi, A., Jr., A. Bianchi Bazesgue, and H. Ferrando. 1950. Sobre las endoacariasis de las gallinas y palomas domesticas. *Dir. Ganad. Bol. Mens.* 31:275–80.

Caylor, J. F., and C. K. Laurent. 1959. The effect of a grain fumigant on egg size of White Leghorn hens. *Poultry Sci.* 38:1194–95.

Chamberlain, R. W. 1968. Insect viruses, pp. 38–58. In Maramorosch, K. (ed.), *Current Topics in Microbiology and Immunology,* Vol. 42. Springer-Verlag, Berlin.

Chamberlain, R. W., and R. K. Sikes. 1950. Laboratory rearing methods for three common species of bird mites. *J. Parasitol.* 36:461–65.

———. 1955. Laboratory investigations on the role of bird mites in the transmission of eastern and western equine encephalomyelitis. *Am. J. Trop. Med. Hyg.* 4:106–18.

Chandler, A. C., and C. P. Read. 1961. Introduction to parasitology, 10th ed. John Wiley and Sons, New York.

Chapin, E. A. 1925. *Freyana (Microspalax)*

chaneyi from a turkey, *Meleagris gallopavo.* *J. Parasitol.* 12:113.

Chaudhury, R. P. 1960. Life-history, habits and control of fowl tick *Argas persicus* (Oken) under Indian conditions. *Indian J. Vet. Sci.* 29:124–34.

Clark, G. M. 1957. Observations on the acarine family Speleognathidae, including two previously unreported forms in native game birds. *J. Parasitol.* 43, Sec. 2:34.

Cleland, J. W. 1953. A preliminary note on the control of *Cnemidocoptes mutans* Robin. *New Zealand Entomologist* 1:17–18.

Coatney, G. R. 1931. On the biology of the pigeon fly, *Pseudolynchia maura* Bigot. *Parasitol.* 23:525–32.

Combs, R. L., Jr., and J. L. Lancaster, Jr. 1965. The biology of the northern fowl mite. *Univ. Arkansas Agr. Exp. Sta. Rept. Ser.* 138.

Comstock, J. H. 1940. *An Introduction to Entomology,* 9th ed. Comstock Publ. Co., Ithaca, N.Y.

Cooley, R. A. 1946. The genera *Boophilus, Rhipicephalus* and *Haemaphysalis* (Ixodidae) of the New World. *Nat. Inst. Health Bull.* 187.

Cooley, R. A., and G. M. Kohls. 1944. *The Argasidae of North America, Central America and Cuba.* The Univ. Press, Notre Dame.

Cotton, R. T., and R. A. St. George. 1929. The meal worms. *USDA Tech. Bull.* 95.

Creighton, J. T., G. W. Dekle, and J. Russell. 1943. The use of sulfur and sulfur compounds in the control of poultry lice. *J. Econ. Entomol.* 36:413–19.

Cross, H. F. 1962. In vivo studies of tissue reaction in chicks resulting from the feeding by larvae of *Trombicula splendens. J. Econ. Entomol.* 55:22–26.

Cross, R. F., and G. C. Folger. 1956. The use of malathion on cats and birds. *J. Am. Vet. Med. Ass.* 129:65–66.

Crossley, D. A., Jr. 1950. A new species of nasal mite. *Neonyssus columbae* from the pigeon. (Acarina, Mesostigmata, Rhinonyssidae). *Proc. Entomol. Soc. Wash.* 52:309–12.

———. 1952. Two new nasal mites from columbiform birds. *J. Parasitol.* 38:385–90.

Crutchfield, C. M., and H. Hixson. 1943. Food habits of several species of poultry lice, with special reference to blood consumption. *Florida Entomologist* 26:63–66.

Cummings, J. G., K. T. Zee, V. Turner, and F. Quinn. 1966. Residues in eggs from low level feeding of five chlorinated hydrocarbon insecticides to hens. *J. Ass. Offic. Agr. Chemists* 49:354–64.

Cunningham, H. B., C. D. Little, S. A. Edgar, and W. G. Eden. 1955. Species and relative abundance of flies collected from chicken manure in Alabama. *J. Econ. Entomol.* 48:620.

Cwilich, R., and M. S. Dison. 1968. Infestation of chickens by the mite *Megninia cubitalis* (Robin and Megnin) 1877. *Refuah Vet.* 24:125–26, 166–67.

Cwilich, R., and R. Hadani. 1965. Infestation of chicks with mites of the genera *Haemolaelaps* and *Cheyletus. Refuah Vet.* 22:55.

Davis, W. A. 1940. A study of birds and mosquitoes as hosts for the virus of eastern equine encephalomyelitis. *Am. J. Hyg.,* Sec. C, 32:45–59.

De Oliveira Castro, G. M. 1930. The transmission of epithelioma contagiosa by mosquitoes (trans. title). *Compt. Rend. Soc. Biol.* 105:316–18.

De Zayas, F. 1941. Los malophagos de las aves domesticas en Cuba. *Univ. Havana, Mem. Soc. Cub. Hist. Nat.* 15:201–10.

Diamant, G., and R. K. Strickland. 1965. *Manual on Livestock Ticks.* USDA ARS 91–94.

Dietrich, A. 1925. *Laminosioptes cysticola* und *Cytoleichus sarcoptoides* bei Huehnern. *Berlin. Muench. Tieraerztl. Wochschr.* 41:486–88.

Dimov, Iv. 1966. (Role of *Argas persicus* in the epizootiology of fowl cholera.) *Nauchni Trudove Visshiya Vet. Med. Inst.* 16:7–12.

Dishburger, H. J., J. R. Rice, W. S. McGregor, and J. Pennington. 1969. Residues of Dursban insecticide in tissues from turkeys confined on soil treated for chigger control. *J. Econ. Entomol.* 62:181–83.

Doetschman, W. H., and D. P. Furman. 1949. A tropical chigger, *Eutrombicula batatas* (Linn.) attacking man in California. *Am. J. Trop. Med.* 29:605–8.

Dorough, H. W., U. E. Brady, Jr., J. A. Timmerman, Jr., and B. W. Arthur. 1961. Residues in tissues and eggs of poultry dusted with Co-Ral (Bayer 21/199). *J. Econ. Entomol.* 54:25–30.

Dow, R. P., W. C. Reeves, and R. E. Bellamy. 1957. Field tests of avian host preference of *Culex tarsalis* Coq. *Am. J. Trop. Med. Hyg.* 6:294–303.

Downe, A. E. R., and P. E. Morrison. 1957. Identification of blood meals of blackflies (Diptera: Simuliidae) attacking farm animals. *Mosquito News* 17:37–50.

Drake, C. J., and R. M. Jones. 1930. The pigeon fly and pigeon malaria in Iowa. *Iowa State Coll. J. Sci.* 4:253–61.

Dubinin, V. B. 1953. Analgesoidea. II. Families Epidermoptidae and Freyanidae (trans. title). *Faunna SSSR* 57:1. (*Biol. Abstr.* 31 no. 36566, 1957.)

Eads, R. B. 1946. Control of the sticktight flea on chickens. *J. Econ. Entomol.* 39:659–60.

Eastwood, R. E., J. M. Kada, and R. B. Shoenburg. 1966. Plastic tarpaulins for controlling flies in stockpiled poultry manure fertilizer. *J. Econ. Entomol.* 59:1507–11.

Eastwood, R. E., J. M. Kada, R. B. Schoenburg, and H. W. Brydon. 1967. Investigations on fly control by composting manure. *J. Econ. Entomol.* 60:88–98.

Eddie, B., K. F. Meyer, F. L. Lambrecht, and D. P. Furman. 1962. Isolation of ornithosis bedsoniae from mites collected in turkey quarters and from chicken lice. *J. Infect. Diseases* 110:231–37.

Edgar, S. A. 1953. A field study of the effect of black fly bites on egg production of laying hens. *Poultry Sci.* 32:779–80.

Edgar, S. A., and D. F. King. 1948. Comparative efficiency of several old and new insecticides in the control of lice on poultry and the effect of the body louse, *Eomenacanthus stramineus,* on egg production. *Poultry Sci.* 27:659–60.

———. 1950. Effect of the body louse, *Eomenacanthus stramineus,* on mature chickens. *Poultry Sci.* 29:214–19.

Edgar, S. A., and B. D. McAnnally. 1955. Control of the northern feather mite, *Bdellonyssus sylviarum,* on chickens in cages and on litter. *Poultry Sci.* 34:91–96.

Edgar, S. A., and O. M. Williams. 1948. Effect of mosquitoes on poultry. *Poultry Sci.* 27:660.

Edgar, S. A., W. L. Walsh, and L. W. Johnson. 1949. Comparative efficacy of several insecticides and methods of application in the control of lice on chickens. *Poultry Sci.* 28:320–38.

Edgar, S. A., O. M. Williams, and E. F. Hester. 1951. Feeding habits of mosquitoes and their effect on poultry. *Poultry Sci.* 30:911–12.

Edgar, S. A., C. D. Little, and J. F. Herndon. 1953. Control of the fowl tick, *Argas persicus* (Oken), on an Alabama poultry farm. *J. Am. Vet. Med. Ass.* 123:446–47.

Eidson, C. S., S. C. Schmittle, R. B. Goode, and J. B. La. 1966. Induction of leukosis tumors with the beetle *Alphitobius diaperinus. Am. J. Vet. Res.* 27:1053–57.

Emerson, K. C. 1956. Mallophaga (chewing lice) occurring on the domestic chicken. *J. Kansas Entomol. Soc.* 29:63–79.

———. 1962a. Mallophaga (chewing lice) occurring on the turkey. *J. Kansas Entomol. Soc.* 35:196–201.

———. 1962b. *A Tentative List of Mallophaga for North American Birds (North of Mexico).* U.S. Army Dugway Proving Ground, Dugway, Utah.

———. 1964. *Checklist of the Mallophaga of North America (North of Mexico).* Pt. I and II. U.S. Army Dugway Proving Ground, Dugway, Utah.

Emmel, M. W. 1942. Field experiments in the use of sulfur to control lice, fleas, and mites of chickens. *Florida Agr. Exp. Sta. Bull.* 374.

Eversole, J. W., J. H. Lilly, and F. R. Shaw. 1965a. Comparative effectiveness and persistence of certain insecticides in poultry droppings against larvae of the little house fly. *J. Econ. Entomol.* 58:704–9.

———. 1965b. Toxicity of droppings from coumaphos-fed hens to little house fly larvae. *J. Econ. Entomol.* 58:709–10.

Ewing, H. E. 1911. The English sparrow as an agent in the dissemination of chicken and bird mites. *Auk* 28:335–40.

———. 1921. Studies on the biology and control of chiggers. *USDA Bull.* 986:1–9.

———. 1923. The dermanyssid mites of North America. *Proc. U.S. Nat. Museum,* 62, Art. 13:1–26.

———. 1929. Birds as hosts for the common chigger. *Am. Naturalist* 63:94–96.

———. 1936. A short synopsis of the North American species of the mite genus Dermanyssus. *Proc. Entomol. Soc. Wash.* 38:47–54.

———. 1944. The trombiculid mites (chigger mites) and their relation to disease. *J. Parasitol.* 30:339–65.

Ewing, H. E., and I. Fox. 1943. The fleas of North America. *USDA Misc. Publ.* 500.

Fain, A., and K. E. Hyland. 1962. The mites parasitic in the lungs of birds. The variability of *Sternostoma tracheacolum* Lawrence, 1948, in domestic and wild birds. *Parasitology* 52:401–24.

Fallis, A. M., and D. M. Wood. 1957. Biting midges (Diptera: Ceratopogonidae) as intermediate hosts for Haemoproteus of ducks. *Can. J. Zool.* 35:425–35.

Fallis, A. M., R. C. Anderson, and G. F. Bennett. 1956. Further observations on the transmission and development of *Leucocytozoon simondi. Can. J. Zool.* 34:389–404.

Faust, E. N., P. C. Beaver, and R. C. Jung. 1968. *Animal Agents and Vectors of Human Disease,* 3rd ed. Lea & Febiger, Philadelphia.

Floyd, E. H., and B. A. Tower. 1956. Insecticide-impregnated litter for control of chicken body lice *(Eomenacanthus stramineus)* on poultry. *Poultry Sci.* 35:896–900.

Foulk, J. D. 1964. Dissemination of the northern fowl mite, *Ornithonyssus sylviarum* (Acarina: Mesostigmata) and experiments on its control. Doctoral thesis, Cornell Univ., Ithaca, N. Y.

Foulk, J. D., and J. G. Matthysse. 1963. Experiments on control of the northern fowl mite. *J. Econ. Entomol.* 56:321–26.

———. 1965. *Ornithonyssus sylviarum* (Acarina: Mesostigmata) from wild birds and their nests. *J. Parasitol.* 51:126.

Fox, Irving. 1940. *Fleas of Eastern United States.* Iowa State Univ. Press, Ames.

Frank, J. F. 1953. A note on the experimental transmission of enterohepatitis of turkeys by arthropods. *Can. J. Comp. Med. Vet. Sci.* 17:230–32.

Frear, D. E. H. 1955. *Chemistry of the Pesticides,* 3rd ed. D. Van Nostrand Co., New York.

———. 1961. *Pesticide Index.* College Science Publishers, State College, Pa.

———. 1962. *Pesticide Handbook,* 14th ed. College Science Publishers, State College, Pa.

Freytag, U., and U. Bendheim. 1965. Symptomatology and treatment of cnemidocoptic mange of budgerigar. *Vet. Med. Rev. Bayer Leverkusen* 2:125–31.

Furman, D. P. 1953. Comparative evaluation of control procedures against the northern fowl mite *Bdellonyssus sylviarum* (Can. and Franz.) *J. Econ. Entomol.* 46:822–26.

———. 1957. Revision of the genus *Sternostoma* Berlese and Trouessart (Acarina: Rhinonyssidae). *Hilgardia* 26:473–95.

Furman, D. P., and R. A. Bankowski. 1949. Absorption of benzene hexachloride in poultry. *J. Econ. Entomol.* 42:980–82.

Furman, D. P., and W. S. Coates. 1957. Northern fowl mite control with malathion. *Poultry Sci.* 36:252–55.

Furman, D. P., and D. Lee. 1969. Experimental control of the northern fowl mite. *J. Econ. Entomol.* 63 (5): 1246–49.

Furman, D. P., and G. R. Pieper. 1962. Systemic acaricidal effects of Sevin in poultry. *J. Econ. Entomol.* 55:355–57.

Furman, D. P., and V. S. Stratton. 1964. Systemic activity of sulfaquinoxaline in control of northern fowl mite *Ornithonyssus sylviarum. Poultry Sci.* 43:1263–65.

Furman, D. P., and C. J. Weinmann. 1956. Toxicity of malathion to poultry and their ectoparasites. *J. Econ. Entomol.* 49:447–50.

Furman, D. P., E. C. Loomis, L. A. Riehl, and A. S. Rosenwald. 1969a. External parasites of turkeys. *Univ. Calif. Agr. Ext. Serv.* AXT-292 Rev.

———. 1969b. External parasites of chickens and pigeons. *Univ. Calif. Agr. Ext. Serv.* AXT-293 Rev.

Gallagher, B. A. 1920. Rose chafer poisoning poultry. *J. Am. Vet. Med. Ass.* 57:692–95.

Geary, J. M. 1959. The fleas of New York. *N.Y. State Coll. Agr.* Cornell Mem. 355.

Georghiou, G. P., M. K. Hawley, and E. C. Loomis. 1967. A progress report on insecticide resistance in the fly complex of California poultry ranches. *Calif. Agr.* 21:8–11.

Gibson, A. 1930. Insect and other external parasites of poultry in Canada. *Sci. Agr.* 11:208.

Gless, E. E., and E. S. Raun. 1958. Insecticidal control of the chicken body louse on range turkeys. *J. Econ. Entomol.* 51:229–32.

———. 1959. Effects of chicken body louse infestation on egg production. *J. Econ. Entomol.* 52: 358–59.

Godfrey, G. F., D. E. Howell, and F. Graybill. 1953. Effect of lindane on egg production. *Poultry Sci.* 32:183–84.

Gothe, R. 1967. Development of *Aegyptionella pullorum* Carpano, 1928, in the soft tick *Argas* (Persicargas) *persicus* (Oken, 1818) and transmission. *Z. Parasitenk.* 29:103–18.

Gould, G. E., and H. E. Moses. 1951. Lesser mealworm infestation in a brooder house. *J. Econ. Entomol.* 44:265.

Graesser, F. E. 1943. Scabies in a turkey. *Can. J. Comp. Med.* 7:13–14.

Griffiths, R. B., and F. J. O'Rourke. 1950. Observations on the lesions caused by *Cnemidocoptes mutans* and their treatment with special reference to the use of "Gammexane." *Ann. Trop. Med. Parasitol.* 44:93–100.

Guberlet, J. E., and H. H. Hotson. 1940. A fly maggot attacking young birds, with observations on its life history. *Murrelet* 21: 65–67.

Guilhon, J. 1952. Gale epidermoptique de la poule. *Bull. Acad. Vet. France* 25:83–86.

Hair, J. A., and E. C. Turner. 1968. Preliminary host preference studies on Virginia *Culicoides* (Diptera: Ceratopogonidae). *Mosquito News* 28:103–7.

Hall, M. C. 1929. Arthropods as intermediate hosts of helminths. *Smithsonian Inst. Misc. Collections* 81:1–77.

Hall, W. J. 1953. Diseases and parasites of poultry. *USDA Farmers' Bull.* 1652:91.

Hammon, W. McD., W. C. Reeves, R. Cunha, C. Espana, and G. Sather. 1948. Isolation from wild bird mites *(Liponyssus sylviarum)* of a virus or mixture of viruses from which St. Louis and western equine encephalitis viruses have been obtained. *Science* 107: 92–93.

Hansens, E. J., and L. M. Vasvary. 1964. Fly control on poultry farms. *Ext. Serv. Rutgers Univ. Leaflet* 217A.

Harding, W. C., Jr. 1955. Malathion to control the northern fowl mite. *J. Econ. Entomol.* 48:605–6.

Harding, W. C., Jr., and T. L. Bissell. 1958. Lesser mealworms in a brooder house. *J. Econ. Entomol.* 51:112.

Harding, W. C., Jr., and G. D. Quigley. 1956. Litter treatment with malathion to control the chicken body louse. *J. Econ. Entomol.* 49:806–7.

Harris, F. 1966. Observations on the lesser worm: *Alphitobius diaperinus* (Panz.). *J. Georgia Entomol. Soc.* 1:17–18.

Harrison, I. R. 1962. The biology of poultry red mite *(Dermanyssus gallinae)* and its control with contact and systemic insecticides. *Proc. 11th Int. Congr. Entomol.,* Vol. 2:469–73.

Hart, L. 1938. A short note on the transmission

of the fowl spirochaete *(Treponema anserinum)* by red mite *(Dermanyssus gallinae)*. *Vet. Res. Rept. Dept. Agr. N.S. Wales,* no. 7:74.

Harwood, P. D. 1948. Benzene hexachloride and poultry meat. *Science* 107:113.

Hearle, E. 1938. Insects and allied parasites injurious to livestock and poultry in Canada. *Can. Dept. Agr. Publ.* 604.

Herman, C. M. 1938a. Mosquito transmission of avian malaria parasites *(Plasmodium circumflexum* and *P. cathemerium)*. *Am. J. Hyg.* Sect. C., 27:345–50.

———. 1938b. Occurrence of larval and nymphal stages of the rabbit tick, *Haemaphysalis leporis-palustris,* on wild birds from Cape Cod. *Bull. Brooklyn Entomol. Soc.* 33:133–34.

Hertel, M. 1904. Gefluegelcholera und Huhnerpest. *Arb. Gesundh.* 20:453.

Hicks, E. A. 1959. *Check-List and Bibliography on the Occurrence of Insects in Birds' Nests.* Iowa State Coll. Press, Ames.

Hicks, E. A., and R. T. Brown. 1963. Acarine fauna of wild bird nests. *Iowa Acad. Sci.* 70:504–10.

Hiepe, T., D. Ebner, and R. Buchwalder. 1962. (Control of *Megninia* infestation in ducks). *Monatsh. Veterinaermed.* 17:605–10.

Hipolito, O., and M. G. [de] Freitas. 1943. Notas ornitopatologicas. Observacoes sobre alguns acarinos parasitos de *Gallus gallus domesticus,* em Minas. *Arquiv. Escola Super. Vet. Univ. Estado de Minas Gerais* 1:81–82.

Hirst, S. 1922. Mites injurious to domestic animals. *Brit. Mus. Econ. Ser.* 13:1–107.

Hoffman, R. A. 1956. Control of the northern feather mite and two species of lice on poultry. *J. Econ. Entomol.* 49:347–49.

———. 1960. The control of poultry lice and mites with several organic insecticides. *J. Econ. Entomol.* 53:160–62.

———. 1961. Experiments on the control of poultry lice. *J. Econ. Entomol.* 54:1114–17.

Hoffman, R. A., and R. O. Drummond. 1961. Control of lice on livestock and on parasites of poultry with General Chemical 4072. *J. Econ. Entomol.* 54:1052–53.

Hoffman, R. A., and R. E. Monroe. 1957. Further tests on the control of fly larvae in poultry and cattle manure. *J. Econ. Entomol.* 50:515.

Hoffman, H. A., T. W. Jackson, and J. C. Rucker. 1946. Spirochetosis in turkeys (a preliminary report). *J. Am. Vet. Med. Ass.* 108:329.

Hofstad, M. S. 1949. Recovery of Newcastle disease (pneumoencephalitis) virus from mites, *Liponyssus sylviarum,* after feeding upon Newcastle-infected chickens. *Am. J. Vet. Res.* 10:370–71.

Holland, G. P. 1949. The Siphonaptera of Canada. *Can. Dept. Agr. Publ.* 817, *Tech. Bull.* 70.

Hollander, W. F. 1956. Acarids of domestic pigeons. *Trans. Am. Microscop. Soc.* 75:461–80.

Hoogstraal, H. 1962. A brief review of tick, bird, and pathogen inter-relationships, pp. 55–71. In *Rept., Second Meet. FAO/OIE Expert Panel on Tick-borne Diseases of Livestock.* Mimeo.

Hoogstraal, H., and G. M. Kohls. 1960a. Observations on the subgenus *Argas* (Ixodoidea, Argasidae, *Argas)*. 1. Study of *A. reflexus reflexus* (Fabricius, 1794), the European bird argasid. *Ann. Entomol. Soc. Am.* 53 (5): 611–18.

———. 1960b. Observations on the subgenus *Argas* (Ixodoidea, Argasidae, *Argas)*. 3. A biological and systematic study of *A. reflexus hermanni* Audouin, 1827 (revalidated), the African bird argasid. *Ann. Entomol. Soc. Am.* 53 (6): 743–55.

Hoogstraal, H., M. N. Kaiser, and G. M. Kohls. 1968. The subgenus *Persicargas* (Ixodoidea, Argasidae, *Argas)*. 4. *Argas (P.) robertsi,* new species, a parasite of Australian fowl, and keys to Australian argasid species. *Ann. Entomol. Soc. Am.* 61 (2): 535–39.

Hooker, W. A., F. C. Bishopp, and H. P. Wood. 1912. The life history and bionomics of some North American ticks. *Bull. U.S. Bur. Entomol.* no. 106.

Hopkins, G. H. E., and T. Clay. 1952. A Check List of the Genera and Species of Mallophaga. *Brit. Mus. (Nat. Hist.) London.*

Hori, S., T. Toriumi, and A. Tanabe. 1964. Studies on the prevention of *Leucocytozoon* infection in the chicken. 1. The behaviour of *Culicoides arakawae* to an insecticide, DA-14-7. *Sci. Rept. Fac. Agr. Okayama Univ.* no. 24, 47–54.

Howell, D. E., G. W. Stiles, and L. H. Moe. 1943. The fowl tick *(Argas persicus),* a new vector of anaplasmosis. *Am. J. Vet. Res.* 4:73–75.

Howitt, B. F., H. R. Dodge, L. K. Bishop, and R. H. Gorrie. 1948. Virus of eastern equine encephalomyelitis isolated from chicken mites *(Dermanyssus gallinae)* and chick lice *(Eomenacanthus stramineus)*. *Proc. Soc. Exp. Biol. Med.* 68:622–25.

Hoyle, W. L. 1938. Transmission of poultry parasites by birds, with special reference to the "English" or house sparrow and chickens. *Trans. Kansas Acad. Sci.* 41:379–84.

Hubbard, C. A. 1947. *Fleas of Western North America.* Iowa State. Univ. Press, Ames.

Huff, C. G. 1932. Further infectivity experiments with mosquitoes and bird malaria. *Am. J. Hyg.* 15:751–54.

———. 1963. Experimental research on avian malaria. *Advan. Parasitol.* 1:1–67.

————. 1968. Recent experimental research on avian malaria. *Advan. Parasitol.* 6:293–312.

Hungerford, T. G. 1938. Field observations on spirochaetosis *(Spirochaeta anserina)* of poultry, transmitted by the red mite *(Dermanyssus avium)* in New South Wales. *Vet. Res. Rept. Dept. Agr. N.S. Wales* 7:71–73.

Hwang, J. C. 1959. Case report of the quill mite, *Syringophilus bipectinatus,* in poultry. *Proc. Helminthol. Soc. Wash.* 26:47–53.

Hyland, K. E. 1963. Current trends in the systematics of acarines endoparasitic in vertebrates, pp. 365–74. In Naegele, J. A. (ed.), *Advances in Acarology,* Vol. I. Cornell Univ. Press, Ithaca, N.Y.

Illingworth, J. F. 1915. Notes on the habits and control of the chicken flea. *(Echidnophaga gallinacea* Westwood). *J. Econ. Entomol.* 8:492–95.

Ivey, M. C., R. H. Roberts, H. D. Mann, and H. V. Claborn. 1961. Lindane residues in chickens and eggs following poultry house sprays. *J. Econ. Entomol.* 54:487–88.

James, W. A., R. Graham, and F. Thorp. 1930. Epidermoptic scabies in a hen. *J. Am. Vet. Med. Ass.* 76:93–95.

Jamnback, H. 1963. Further observations on the effectiveness of chemically treated screens in killing biting midges, *Culicoides sanguisuga* (Diptera: Ceratopogonidae). *J. Econ. Entomol.* 56:719–20.

Johnson, E. P., G. W. Underhill, J. A. Cox, and W. L. Threlkeld. 1938. A blood protozoon of turkeys transmitted by *Simulium nigroparvum* (Twinn). *Am. J. Hyg.* 27:649–65.

Jones, B. M. 1950. The penetration of the host tissue by the harvest mite, *Trombicula autumnalis* Shaw. *Parasitology* 40:247–60.

Jones, C., and D. J. Richey. 1956. Biology of the blackflies in Jasper County, South Carolina, and some relationships to a *Leucocytozoon* disease of turkeys. *J. Econ. Entomol.* 49:121–23.

Jones, L. M. 1965. *Veterinary Pharmacology and Therapeutics,* 3rd ed. Iowa State Univ. Press, Ames.

Judd, W. W. 1956. Dermatitis of humans caused by the fowl mite, *Dermanyssus gallinae* (Deg.) at London, Ontario. *Can. Entomol.* 88:109.

Kadner, C. G. 1941. Pigeon malaria in California. *Science* 93:281.

Kaiser, M. N., and H. Hoogstraal. 1969. The subgenus *Persicargus* (Ixodoidea, Argasidae, *Argas).* 7. *A. (P.) Walkerae,* new species, a parasite of domestic fowl in southern Africa. *Ann. Entomol. Soc. Am.* 62 (4): 885–90.

Kartman, L. 1949. Preliminary observations on the relation of nutrition to pediculosis of rats and chickens. *J. Parasitol.* 35:367–74.

Kaschula, V. R. 1950. "Scaly-leg" of the canary *(Serinus canaria* [L.]). *J. South Africa Vet. Med. Ass.* 21:117–19.

Kaschula, V. R., and S. A. R. Stephan. 1947. Mites, hitherto unrecorded in South Africa, collected in Natal from fowls, pigeons, turkeys, guinea-fowls, wild birds, and rabbits. *Onderstepoort J. Vet. Sci. Animal Ind.* 22: 51–57.

Kasparek, A. 1907. Bericht ueber die 79. Versammlung Deutscher Naturforscher und Aerzte in Dresden. *Deut. Tieraerztl. Wochschr.* 15:623–24.

Kaura, R. L., and S. G. Iyer. 1937. The occurrence of the air-sac mite, *Cytoleichus nudus* (Vizioli, 1870) in fowls in India. *Indian J. Vet. Sci.* 7:299–301.

Keler, S. 1938. Uebersicht ueber die gesamte Literatur der Mallophagen (1668–1938). *Z. Angew. Entomol.* 25:487–524.

Keller, J. C., and H. K. Gouck. 1957. Small-plot tests for the control of chiggers. *J. Econ. Entomol.* 50:141–43.

Kellogg, F. E., A. K. Prestwood, R. R. Gerrish, and G. L. Doster. 1969. Wild turkey ectoparasites collected in the southeastern United States. *J. Med. Entomol.* 6 (3): 329–30.

Kilpatrick, J. W., D. R. Maddock, and J. W. Miles. 1962. Modification of a semiautomatic liquid-poison bait dispenser for house fly control. *J. Econ. Entomol.* 55:951–53.

Kirkwood, A. C. 1963. Longevity of the mites *Dermanyssus gallinae* and *Liponyssus sylviarum. Exp. Parasitol.* 14:358–66.

————. 1965. A trap perch for the control of the poultry red mite *(Dermanyssus gallinae). Brit. Poultry Sci.* 6:73–78.

————. 1967. Control of poultry mites. *Brit. Poultry Sci.* 8:75–80.

Kitselman, C. H., and A. W. Grundmann. 1940. Equine encephalomyelitis virus isolated from naturally infected *Triatoma sanguisuga* Le Conte. *Kansas Agr. Expt. Sta. Tech. Bull.* 50:15.

Kligler, I. J., R. S. Muckenfuss, and T. M. Rivers. 1929. Transmission of fowl pox by mosquitoes. *J. Exp. Med.* 49:649–60.

Knapp, F. W. 1962. Co-Ral as a litter and nest dust to control the chicken body louse. *J. Econ. Entomol.* 55:571–72.

Knapp, F. W., and G. F. Krause. 1960. Control of the northern fowl mite, *Ornithonyssus sylviarum* (C. and F.) with ronnel, Bayer L13/59 and Bayer 21/199. *J. Econ. Entomol.* 53:4–5.

Knapp, F. W., C. J. Terhaar, and C. C. Roan. 1958. Dow ET-57 as a fly larvicide. *J. Econ. Entomol.* 51:361–62.

Knipling, E. F., and H. T. Rainwater. 1937. Species and incidence of dipterous larvae concerned in wound myiasis. *J. Parasitol.* 23:451–55.

Kohls, G. M., H. Hoogstraal, C. M. Clifford, and M. N. Kaiser. 1970. The subgenus *Persicargas* (Ixodoidea, Argasidae, *Argas*). 9. Redescription and new world records of *Argas (P.) persicus* (Oken), and resurrection, redescription, and records of *A. (P.) sanchezi* Duges, and *A. (P) miniatus* Koch, new world ticks misidentified as *A. (P.) persicus*. *Ann. Entomol. Soc. Am.* 63 (2): 590–606.

Kotlan, A. 1923. Ueber die Blutaufnahme als Nuhrung bei den Mallophagen. *Zool. Anz.* 56:231–33.

Kraemer, P. 1959. Relative efficacy of several materials for control of poultry ectoparasites. *J. Econ. Entomol.* 52:1195–99.

Kraemer, P., and D. P. Furman. 1959. Systemic activity of Sevin in control of *Ornithonyssus sylviarum* (C. and F.). *J. Econ. Entomol.* 52:170–71.

Krantz, G. W. 1970. *A Manual of Acarology.* Oregon State Univ. Press, Corvallis.

Kunz, S. E., M. A. Price, and O. H. Graham. 1969. Biology and economic importance of the chigger *Neoschongastia americana* on turkeys. *J. Econ. Entomol.* 62 (4): 872–75.

Kunz, S. E., M. A. Price, and R. Everett. 1971. Evaluation of insecticides to control the chigger *Neoschongastia americana* on turkeys. *J. Econ. Entomol.* 64(4):900–901.

Labrecque, G. C., and D. W. Meifert. 1966. Control of house flies (Diptera: Muscidae) in poultry houses with chemosterilants. *J. Med. Entomol.* 3:323–26.

Lamina, J., and N. Kruner. 1966. (Insecticidal action of a highly dispersed silicic acid on poultry ectoparasites). *Deut. Tieraerztl. Wochschr.* 73:124–29.

Lamson, G. H., Jr. 1922. The rose chafer as a cause of death of chickens. *Storrs Agr. Expt. Sta. Bull.* 110:117–34.

Lancaster, J. L., Jr., and J. S. Simco. 1967. Biology of the lesser mealworm, a suspected reservoir of avian leucosis. *Arkansas Agr. Expt. Sta. Rept. Ser.* 159:11.

———. 1968. Northern fowl mite control on mature turkeys on range. *J. Econ. Entomol.* 61:1471–72.

Lancaster, J. L., Jr., J. S. Simco, and R. Everett. 1969. Pre-treated rice hull litter for the control of the lesser mealworm. *Arkansas Agr. Expt. Sta. Rept. Ser.* 174:13.

Lapage, G. 1968. *Veterinary Parasitology,* 2nd ed. Oliver and Boyd, Edinburgh.

Lavoipierre, M. M. J. 1953. The undescribed male and female of the pigeon quill mite, *Syringophilus columbae* Hirst, 1920. *Trans. Roy. Soc. Trop. Med. Hyg.* 47:7.

Lee, R. D. 1955a. The biology of the Mexican chicken bug, *Haematosiphon inodorus* (Duges) (Hemiptera: Cimicidae). *Pan-Pacific Entomologist* 31:47–61.

———. 1955b. New locality records and a new host record for *Haematosiphon inodorus*

(Hemiptera: Cimicidae). *Pan-Pacific Entomologist* 31:137–38.

Le Roux, A. C. 1956. The safe, economical and practical destruction of *Argas persicus,* fowl tick, tampan, blue "bug," chicken tick or adobe tick. *World's Poultry Sci. J.* 12: 285–86.

Levi, W. M. 1957. *The Pigeon,* 2nd ed. Levi Publ. Co. Sumter, S.C.

Lindquist, W. D., and R. C. Belding. 1949. A report on the subcutaneous or flesh mite of chickens. *Mich. State Coll. Vet.* 10:20–21.

Lindt, S., and E. Kutzer. 1965. Air-sac mite *Cytodites nudus* as a cause of granulomatous pneumonia in fowl. *Pathol. Vet.* 2:264–76.

Linduska, J. P., F. A. Morton, and W. C. McDuffie. 1948. Tests of materials for the control of chiggers on the ground. *J. Econ. Entomol.* 41:43–47.

Linkfield, R. L., and W. M. Reid. 1958. Newer acaricides and insecticides in the control of ectoparasites of poultry. *J. Econ. Entomol.* 51:188–90.

Liska, B. J., G. C. Mostert, B. E. Langlois, and W. J. Stadelman. 1964. Problems resulting from the misuse of lindane for chigger control on turkey ranges as related to residues in edible tissues. *J. Econ. Entomol.* 57:682–83.

Loomis, E. C. 1961. Life histories of ticks under laboratory conditions (Acarina: Ixodoidea and Argasidae). *J. Parasitol.* 47:91–99.

Loomis, E. C., A. S. Deal, and W. R. Bowen. 1968. The relative effectiveness of coumaphos as a poultry feed additive to control synanthropic fly larvae in manure. *J. Econ. Entomol.* 61:904–8.

Loomis, E. C., E. L. Bramhall, J. A. Allen, R. A. Ernst, and L. L. Dunning. 1970. Effects of the northern fowl mite on white leghorn chickens. *J. Econ. Entomol.* 63(6):1885–89.

Loomis, R. B. 1956. The chigger mites of Kansas (Acarina: Trombiculidae). *Univ. Kansas Sci. Bull.* 37 (2): 1195–1443.

Lucas, J. M. S. 1954. Fatal anemia in poultry caused by a heavy tick infestation. *Vet. Record* 66:573–74.

MacCreary, D., and E. P. Catts. 1954. Ectoparasites of Delaware poultry including a study of litter fauna. *Univ. Delaware Agr. Expt. Sta. Bull.* 307:22.

Madden, A. H., A. W. Lindquist, and E. F. Knipling. 1944. Tests of repellents against chiggers. *J. Econ. Entomol.* 37:283–86.

Manuel, M. F., and F. Siores. 1967. *Pterolichus obtusus,* Robin, 1868, a common feathermite of chickens in the Philippines. *Indian Vet. J.* 44:1032–35.

Martin, M. 1934. Life history and habits of the pigeon louse *Columbicola columbae* (Linn.). *Can. Entomol.* 66:6–16.

Matheson, R., E. L. Brunett, and A. L. Brody.

1931. The transmission of fowl pox by mosquitoes. Preliminary report. *Poultry Sci.* 10:211–23.

Mathey, W. J. 1967. Respiratory acariasis due to *Sternostoma tracheacolum* in the budgerigar. *J. Am. Vet. Med. Ass.* 150:777–80.

Mathis, W., and H. F. Schoof. 1968. Chemical control of house flies in dairy barns and chicken ranches. *J. Econ. Entomol.* 61:1071–73.

Matthysse, J. G. 1970. 1971 poultry external parasite control recommendations for New York State. Mimeo. *Cornell Univ. Entomol. Dept.*

Medley, J. G., and E. Ahrens. 1970. Life history and bionomics of two American species of fowl ticks (Ixodoidea, Argasidae, *Argas*) of the subgenus *Persicargas*. *Ann. Entomol. Soc. Am.* 63 (6): 1591–94.

Mégnin, P. 1879. Les acariens parasites du tissue cellulaire et des reservoirs aeriens chez les oiseaux. *J. Anat. Physiol.* 15:123–53.

Menon, P. B., C. M. Sen Gupta, and B. C. Basu. 1951. Studies on the feeding of insecticides for the control of ectoparasites. *Indian Vet. J.* 27:430–37.

Messersmith, D. H. 1965a. *Culicoides* (Diptera: Ceratopogonidae) associated with poultry in Virginia. *Mosquito News* 25:321–24.

———. 1965b. Avian infectious synovitis: A review of the literature. *World's Poultry Sci. J.* 21:358–64.

———. 1965c. Report of a collection of *Culicoides* (Diptera: Ceratopogonidae) from western Virginia. *Virginia J. Sci.* 17 n.s. (2):83–104.

Metcalf, R. L. 1955. *Organic Insecticides: Their Chemistry and Mode of Action.* Interscience Publications, Inc., New York.

———. 1957. *Advances in Pest Control Research,* Vols. 1–8 (1957–62). Interscience Publications, Inc., New York.

Metz, K. 1911. *Argas reflexus,* die Taubenzecke. *Monatsh. Tierheilk.* 22:481–510.

Meyer, K. F., and B. Eddie. 1960. Feather mites and ornithosis. *Science* 132:300.

Michener, C. D. 1946. Observations on the habits and life history of a chigger mite, *Eutrombicula batatas* (Acarina: Trombiculinae). *Ann. Entomol. Soc. Am.* 39:101–18.

Micks, D. W. 1951. The laboratory rearing of the common fowl tick, *Argas persicus* (Oken). *J. Parasitol.* 37:102–5.

Miles, V. I., B. F. Howitt, R. Gorrie, and T. A. Cockburn. 1951. Encephalitis in Midwest. V. Western equine encephalitis virus recovered from mites, *Dermanyssus americanus* Ewing. *Proc. Soc. Exp. Biol. Med.* 77:395–96.

Moffatt, B. W. 1955. The stickfast flea of poultry. *Queensland Agr. J.* 81:239–41.

Morgante, O., J. A. Shemanchuk, and R. Windsor. 1969. Western encephalomyelitis virus infection in "indicator" chickens in southern Alberta. *Can. J. Comp. Med.* 33(3):227–30.

Morris, G. K., and H. L. Fuller. 1963. Effect of ethylene dibromide in the diet on the growth of chicks. *Poultry Sci.* 42:15–20.

Mullen, M. A. 1967. Studies on the biology of *Neoschongastia americana* (Hirst) (Acarina: Trombiculidae) on turkeys. M.S. thesis. Univ. Georgia.

Murray, M. D. 1966. Control of respiratory acariasis of Gouldian finches caused by *Sternostoma tracheacolum* by feeding carbaryl. *Australian Vet. J.* 42:262–64.

Myers, L. E. 1928. The American swallow bug, *Oeciacus vicarius* Horvath. *Parasitology* 20:159–72.

Najera, L., and H. F. Mayer. 1951. Action of some insecticides on *Argas persicus*. (Trans. title.) *Rev. Iberica Parasitol.* 11:61–74.

Nelson, C. B., E. L. Bramhall, W. V. Miller, and H. G. Simkover. 1969. Control of the northern fowl mite on laying hens with Shell SD–8447. *J. Econ. Entomol.* 62:47–49.

Nelson, T. E., and K. M. R. Bertun. 1965. Synergism of malathion against northern fowl mite. *J. Econ. Entomol.* 58:1117–18.

Neveu-Lemaire, M. 1938. *Traite d'Entomologie Medicale et Veterinaire.* Vigot Freres, Paris.

Olson, C. 1935. The effect of certain ectoparasites on the cellular elements and hemoglobin of the blood of the domestic chicken. *J. Am. Vet. Med. Ass.* 87:559–61.

O'Roke, E. C. 1930. The morphology, transmission, and life history of *Haemoproteus lophortyx* O'Roke, a blood parasite of the California valley quail. *Univ. Calif. (Berkeley) Publ. in Zool.* 36:1–50.

———. 1934. A malaria-like disease of ducks, caused by *Leucocytozoon anatis* Wickware. *Univ. Mich. School of Forestry and Conserv. Bull.* 4.

Parman, D. C. 1923. Biological notes on the hen flea, *Echidnophaga gallinacea*. *J. Agr. Res.* 23:1007–9.

Patyk, S. 1963. (Experimental infestation of fowls with *Laminosioptes cysticola*). *Weterynaria* 15:197–206.

Pavlov, P. 1963. Studies on tick paralysis observed among chicks in Bulgaria and caused by nymphs of *Haemaphysalis punctata*. *Ann. Parasitol. Human. Comp.* 38:459–61.

Pavlovsky, E. N. 1966. Natural nidality of transmissible diseases. Univ. Illinois Press, Urbana. (Translation.)

Payne, L. F. 1930. Feather mites and their control. Proc. 21st Ann. Meet., Poultry Sci. Ass. *Alabama Polytech. Inst. Bull.* 25 (1):61–63.

Peterson, E. H. 1949. Field tests of some insecticides in the control of the common red mite of poultry and of the northern fowl mite. *Poultry Sci.* 28:411–14.

Philip, C. B. 1963. Ticks as purveyors of animal ailments: A review of pertinent data and of recent contributions, pp. 285–325. In Naegele, J. A. (ed.), *Advances in Acarology,* Vol. I. Cornell Univ. Press, Ithaca, N.Y.

Pillers, A. W. N. 1921. *Notes on Mange, and Allied Mites for Veterinarians.* Bailliere, Tindall, and Cox, London.

——. 1927. Perforations in pigeons' feathers due to the mite, *Falculifer rostratus* (Buchholz). *Vet. J.* 83:410–13.

Pinto, C. 1930. *Arthropodos Parasitos e Transmissores de Doencas.* Mello e C., Rio de Janeiro 2v.

Plassaj, S. 1925. Sur la transmission du cholera aviaire par les *Dermanyssus.* Jugoslav. *Vet. Glasn.,* Livr. 1–6. (Rev. in *Rev. Gen. Med. Vet.* 34:654.)

Price, M. A., and S. E. Kunz. 1970. Insecticidal screening for chemicals to control the chigger *Neoschongastia americana* on turkeys. *J. Econ. Entomol.* 63 (2): 373–76.

Price, M. A., S. E. Kunz, and J. J. Matter. 1970. Use of Dursban to control *Neoschongastia americana,* a turkey chigger, in experimental pens. *J. Econ. Entomol.* 63 (2): 377–79.

Prouty, M. J., and G. R. Coatney. 1934. Further studies on the biology of the pigeon fly, *Pseudolynchia maura* Bigot. *Parasitology* 26:249–58.

Quigley, G. C. 1965. Family differences in attractiveness of poultry to the chicken body louse, *Menacanthus stramineus* (Mallophaga). *J. Econ. Entomol.* 58:8–10.

Race, S. R., E. J. Hansens, P. Granett, and R. R. Kriner. 1969. Poultry insect control recommendations for New Jersey. *Ext. Serv. Rutgers Univ.,* New Brunswick, N.J.

Radeleff, R. D. 1964. *Veterinary Toxicology.* Lea & Febiger, Philadelphia.

Raun, E. S. 1956. Chicken louse and mite control with malathion formulations. *J. Econ. Entomol.* 49:628–29.

Raun, E. S., and C. L. Nelson. 1956. How to delouse 4000 toms in 100 minutes. *Turkey World* 31 (May): 12.

Readio, P. A. 1927. Studies on the biology of the Reduviidae of America north of Mexico. *Univ. Kansas Sci. Bull.* 17:5.

Rebrassier, R. E., and E. D. Martin. 1932. *Syringophilus bipectinatus,* a quill mite of poultry. *Science* 76:128.

Reeves, W. C. 1965. Ecology of mosquitoes in relation to arboviruses. *Ann. Rev. Entomol.* 10:25–46.

Reeves, W. C., W. McD. Hammon, D. P. Furman, H. E. McClure, and B. Brookman. 1947. Recovery of western equine encephalomyelitis virus from wild bird mites *(Liponyssus sylviarum)* in Kern County, California. *Science* 105:411–12.

Reeves, W. C., W. McD. Hammon, W. H. Doetschman, H. E. McClure, and G. Sather. 1955. Studies on mites as vectors of western equine and St. Louis encephalitis viruses in California. *Am. J. Trop. Med. Hyg.* 4:90–105.

Reid, W. M. 1956. Incidence and economic importance of poultry parasites under different ecological and geographical situations in Egypt. *Poultry Sci.* 35:926–33.

Reid, W. M., and J. E. Ackert. 1937. The cysticercoid of *Choanotaenia infundibulum* (Bloch) and the housefly as its host. *Trans. Am. Microscop. Soc.* 56:99–104.

Reid, W. M., and H. Botero. 1966. How to beat the chigger problem. *Poultry Meat,* June A10–A12.

Reid, W. M., and R. L. Linkfield. 1957. New distribution record and economic importance of *Menacanthus cornutus* (Schoemmer) on Georgia broilers. *J. Econ. Entomol.* 50:375–76.

Reid, W. M., R. L. Linkfield, and G. Lewis. 1956. Limitations of malathion in northern fowl mite and louse control. *Poultry Sci.* 35:1397–98.

Reis, J. 1939. Alguns parasitas de *Gallus gallus* (L.) verificados em Sao Paulo. *Arquiv. Inst. Biol.* (Sao Paulo) 10:147–52.

Reis, J., and P. Nobrega. 1956. *Tratado de Doencas das Aves,* 2nd ed. Comp. Melhoramentos de Sao Paulo, Industrias de Papel.

Richardson, H. H. 1943. Studies of methyl bromide, chloropicrin, certain nitriles and other fumigants against the bedbug. *J. Econ. Entomol.* 36:420–26.

Richter, P. O., and W. M. Insko, Jr. 1948a. External parasites of chickens and their control. *Kentucky Agr. Expt. Sta. Bull.* 517.

——. 1948b. Control of the northern fowl mite, *Liponyssus sylviarum* (C. and F.). *J. Econ. Entomol.* 41:123–24.

Roberts, F. H. S. 1952. *Insects Affecting Livestock.* Angus and Robertson, Sydney and London. P. 267.

Roberts, F. H. S., P. J. O'Sullivan, P. Rumball, and A. W. McLauchlan. 1947. Observations on the value of DDT for the control of the poultry stickfast flea, *Echidnophaga gallinacea* Westwood. *Australian Vet. J.* 23:148–52.

Roberts, I. H., and C. L. Smith. 1956a. Poultry lice. In *Animal Diseases.* USDA Yearbook, pp. 490–93.

——. 1959b. Mites on poultry. In *Animal Diseases.* USDA Yearbook, pp. 493–96.

Rodriguez, J. L., Jr., and L. A. Riehl. 1956. Four pesticides tested against the fowl tick infesting turkeys in feed lots. *J. Econ. Entomol.* 49:713–14.

——. 1957a. Control of the chicken body louse on hens by self-treatment with malathion dust. *J. Econ. Entomol.* 50:64–67.

————. 1957b. Malathion spray for fowl tick control. *J. Econ. Entomol.* 50:41–43.

————. 1958. Malathion for control of chicken mites on hens in wire cages. *J. Econ. Entomol.* 51:158–60.

————. 1959a. Spot treatments with malathion dust for control of the northern fowl mite on hens in individual wire cages. *J. Econ. Entomol.* 52:13–14.

————. 1959b. Malathion dust for the control of two species of pigeon lice. *J. Econ. Entomol.* 52:772.

————. 1959c. Fowl tick on turkeys. *Calif. Agr.* 13:11.

————. 1960a. The malathion dust-bath for control of five species of lice on chickens. *J. Econ. Entomol.* 53:328.

————. 1960b. Malathion dust for chicken mite control. *J. Econ. Entomol.* 53:328–29.

————. 1960c. Control of northern fowl mite in community wire cages with malathion in special dust-bath boxes. *J. Econ. Entomol.* 53:701–4.

————. 1961. Sticktight flea control on chickens with malathion dust self-treatment. *J. Econ. Entomol.* 54:1212–14.

————. 1962. Control of flies in manure of chickens and rabbits by cockerels in Southern California. *J. Econ. Entomol.* 55:473–77.

————. 1963. Northern fowl mite tolerant to malathion. *J. Econ. Entomol.* 56:509–11.

Rokey, N. W., and V. N. Snell. 1961. Avian spirochetosis *(Borrelia anserina)* epizootics in Arizona poultry. *J. Am. Vet. Med. Ass.* 138:648–52.

Roth, L. M., and E. R. Willis. 1961. Biotic associations of cockroaches. *Smithsonian Inst. Misc. Collections* 141:1–470.

Roveda, R. J., and J. J. Boero. 1962. Acaros de las plumas. *Rev. Fac. Agron. Vet., Univ. Buenos Aires* 15:53–76.

Russell, E. L., and R. S. Stone. 1967. *Fly Control Research on Poultry Ranches,* Vols. I and II. Orange County Health Dept., Santa Ana, Calif.

Schalk, A. F. 1928. Results of some avian tuberculosis studies. *J. Am. Vet. Med. Ass.* 72:852–64.

Schwabe, O. 1956. A quill mite of poultry, a case report. *(Syringophilus bipectinatus.)* *J. Am. Vet. Med. Ass.* 129:481–82.

Scott, H. G., and K. S. Littig. 1962. Flies of public health importance and their control. *Training Guide—Insect Control Series.* Pt. V. Publ. 772. U.S. Dept. HEW, Communicable Disease Center, Atlanta, Ga.

Shane, S. M. 1965. Report on the occurrence of *Speleognathus striatus* in the domestic pigeon. *J. S. African Vet. Med. Ass.* 36:575–76.

Shaw, F. R., and G. Clark. 1953. Notes on certain ectoparasites in Massachusetts. *J. Econ. Entomol.* 46:1093–94.

Sherman, M. 1965. The effectiveness of insecticides administered orally to the fowl as a deterrent to the breeding of flies in droppings. *Proc. Hawaiian Entomol. Soc.* 19 (1):111–17.

Sherman, M., and G. H. Komatsu. 1963. Maggot development in droppings from chicks fed organophosphorus insecticide-treated rations. *J. Econ. Entomol.* 56:847–50.

Sherman, M., and E. Ross. 1960. Toxicity to house fly larvae of droppings from chickens fed insecticide treated rations. *J. Econ. Entomol.* 53:429–32.

————. 1961. Toxicity to house fly larvae of droppings from chicks administered insecticides in food, water, and as single oral dosages. *J. Econ. Entomol.* 54:573–78.

Sherman, M., E. Ross, and M. T. Y. Chang. 1964. Acute and subacute toxicity of several organophosphorus insecticides to chicks. *Toxicol. Appl. Pharmacol.* 6:147–53.

————. 1965. Acute and subacute toxicity of several insecticides to chicks. *Toxicol. Appl. Pharmacol.* 7:606–8.

Sherman, M., G. H. Komatsu, and J. Ikeda. 1967a. Larvicidal activity to flies of manure from chicks administered insecticide treated feed. *J. Econ. Entomol.* 60:1395–1403.

Sherman, M., R. B. Herrick, E. Ross, and M. T. Y. Chang. 1967b. Further studies on the acute and subacute toxicity of insecticides to chicks. *Toxicol. Appl. Pharmacol.* 2:49–67.

Shewell, G. E. 1955. Identity of the black fly that attacks ducklings and goslings in Canada (Diptera: Simuliidae). *Can. Entomol.* 87:345–49.

Sikes, R. K., and R. W. Chamberlain. 1954. Laboratory observations on three species of bird mites. *J. Parasitol.* 40:691–97.

Simco, J. S., and J. L. Lancaster, Jr. 1965. Control of common external parasites of commercial layers and hatchery flocks. *Arkansas Agr. Expt. Sta. Bull.* 703.

————. 1966. Field test to determine the effectiveness of coumaphos as a feed additive to control house fly larvae under caged layers. *J. Econ. Entomol.* 59:671–72.

Simco, J. S., B. N. McPherson, and J. L. Lancaster, Jr. 1962a. Controlling the chicken body louse. *Arkansas Farm Res.* 11:7.

————. 1962b. Control of the northern fowl mite. *Arkansas Farm Res.* 11:10.

Skidmore, L. V. 1932a. *Leucocytozoon smithi* infection in turkeys and its transmission by *Simulium occidentale* Townsend. *Zentr. Bakteriol. Parasitenk. Abt. I. Orig.* 125:329–35.

————. 1932b. The transmission of fowl cholera to turkeys by the common house fly (*Musca domestica* Linn.) (with brief notes on the viability of fowl cholera microorganisms). *Cornell Vet.* 22:281–85.

Smith, C. N. 1951. Compounds more toxic to fleas than DDT. *Am. J. Trop. Med.* 31:252.

Smith, C. N., and H. K. Gouck. 1944. DDT, sulfur and other insecticides for the control of chiggers. *J. Econ. Entomol.* 37:131–32.

———. 1947. The control of chiggers in woodland plots. *J. Econ. Entomol.* 40:790–95.

Smith, M. G., R. J. Blattner, and F. M. Heys. 1944. The isolation of the St. Louis encephalitis virus from chicken mites *(Dermanyssus gallinae)* in nature. *Science* 100:362–63.

———. 1945. Further isolation of St. Louis encephalitis virus; congenital transfer of virus in chicken mites *(Dermanyssus gallinae)*. *Proc. Soc. Exp. Biol. Med.* 59:136–38.

———. 1946. St. Louis encephalitis: Infection of chicken mites *Dermanyssus gallinae,* by feeding on chickens with viremia; transovarian passage of virus into the second generation. *J. Exp. Med.* 84:1–6.

———. 1947. St. Louis encephalitis: Transmission of virus to chickens by infected mites, *Dermanyssus gallinae,* and resulting viremia as source of virus for infection of mites. *J. Exp. Med.* 86:229–37.

Smith, M. G., R. J. Blattner, F. M. Heys, and A. Miller. 1948. Experiments on the role of the chicken mite, *Dermanyssus gallinae,* and the mosquito in the epidemiology of St. Louis encephalitis. *J. Exp. Med.* 87:119–38.

Smyth, H. F., Jr. 1956. The literature of pesticide toxicology. *J. Agr. Food Chem.* 4:644–46.

Snyder, F. M., and F. A. Morton. 1947. Benzyl benzoate-dibutyl phthalate mixture against chiggers. *J. Econ. Entomol.* 40:586–87.

Soloveichik, L. L. 1962. Infestation of poultry with the itch mite *(Laminosioptes cysticola)* (translated title). *Veterinariya* 39:50.

Soulsby, E. J. L. 1968. *Helminths, Arthropods and Protozoa of Domesticated Animals.* (6th ed. Moennigs Veterinary Helminthology and Entomology.) Bailliere, Tindall, and Cassell, London.

Spradbrow, P. 1966. Arbovirus infections of domestic animals. *Vet. Bull.* 36:55–61.

Stenram, H. 1956. The ecology of *Columbicola columbae* L. (Mallophaga). *Opuscula Entomologica* 21:170–90.

Stewart, M. A. 1929. A case of cloacal myiasis in a hen and its treatment. *Cornell Vet.* 19:49–51.

———. 1932. Dispersal of the sticktight flea of hens *(Echidnophaga gallinacea* Westw.). *J. Econ. Entomol.* 25:164–67.

Stockdale, H. J., and E. S. Raun. 1960. Economic importance of the chicken body louse. *J. Econ. Entomol.* 53:421–23.

———. 1965. Biology of the chicken body louse, *Menacanthus stramineus. Ann. Entomol. Soc. Am.* 58:802–5.

Stone, A. 1964. Guide to the insects of Connecticut part VI. The Diptera or true flies of Connecticut ninth fascicle Simuliidae and Thaumaleidae. *Conn. State Geol. Nat. Hist. Surv. Bull.* 97.

Stone, A., and H. A. Jamnback. 1955. The black flies of New York State (Diptera: Simuliidae). *N.Y. State Mus. Bull.* 349:1–44.

Strandtman, R. W., and G. W. Wharton. 1958. *A Manual of Mesostigmatid Mites.* Univ. Maryland Acarology Inst., Contrib. No. 4.

Strayer, J. 1966. External parasites of poultry. *Univ. Florida Agr. Ext. Serv. Circ.* 302.

Sulkin, S. E. 1945. Recovery of equine encephalomyelitis virus (western type) from chicken mites. *Science* 101:381–83.

Sulkin, S. E., and E. M. Izumi. 1947. Isolation of western equine encephalomyelitis virus from tropical fowl mites, *Liponyssus bursa* (Berlese). *Proc. Soc. Exp. Biol. Med.* 66:249–50.

Sulkin, S. E., C. L. Wisseman, Jr., E. M. Izumi, and C. Zarafonetis. 1955. Mites as possible vectors or reservoirs of equine encephalitis in Texas. *Am. J. Trop. Med. Hyg.* 4:119–35.

Tarshis, I. B. 1967. Silica aerogel insecticides for the prevention and control of arthropods of medical and veterinary importance. *Parasitology* 8:210–37.

Taylor, R. M., H. S. Hurlbut, T. H. Work, J. R. Kingston, and H. Hoogstraal. 1966. Arboviruses isolated from *Argas* ticks in Egypt: Quaranfil, Chenuda, and Nyamanini. *Am. J. Trop. Med. Hyg.* 15 (1): 76–86.

Theodoridès, J. 1949. Les Coleopteres nuisibles aux animaux domestiques. *Ann. Parasitol. Human Comp.* 24:116–23.

Thompson, R. P., and W. F. Hosking. 1957. A count of Mallophaga on a heavily infested hen. *Poultry Sci.* 36:213–14.

Tongson, M. S., and M. F. Manuel. 1965. A report on some feather-eating mites *(Megninia* spp.) infesting fowls in the Philippines. *Philippine J. Animal Ind.* 21:263–67.

Torres, C. M., H. Kent, and L. F. Moreira. 1951. Acarinose das respiratorias do canario ("*Serinuscanarius*" L.) por "*Sternostoma tracheacolum*" Lawrence, 1948. *Rev. Brasil. Biol.* 11:399–406.

Tower, B. A., and E. H. Floyd. 1961a. Consumer and organoleptic tests with broilers grown on lindane-impregnated litter. *Poultry Sci.* 40:234–38.

———. 1961b. The effect of the chicken body louse, *Eomenacanthus stramineus* on egg production in New Hampshire pullets. *Poultry Sci.* 40:395–98.

Travis, B. V. 1967. Biology and control of biting flies in New York State. *N.Y. State Coll. Agr. Cornell Ext. Bull.* 1186.

———. 1969. Recommendations to communities for chemical control of biting flies in

New York State. *N.Y. State Coll. Agr. Cornell Ext. Bull.* 1188.

Turner, C. C., Jr., N. L. Wehrheim, and D. H. Messersmith. 1963. Transmission studies of avian infectious synovitis by selected arthropod vectors. *Poultry Sci.* 42:1434–41.

Twinn, C. R. 1936. The blackflies of eastern Canada (Simuliidae, Diptera). *Can. J. Res. Sect. D., Zool. Sci.* 14:97–150.

Underhill, G. W. 1939. Two simuliids found feeding on turkeys in Virginia. *J. Econ. Entomol.* 32:765–68.

———. 1944. Blackflies found feeding on turkeys in Virginia *(Simulium nitroparvum* Twinn and *S. slossonae* Dyar and Shannon). *Virginia Agr. Expt. Sta. Tech. Bull.* 94.

USDA. 1964a. Fleas: How to control them. Leaflet 392.

———. 1964b. Poultry mites: How to control them. Leaflet 383.

———. 1965. Stored grain pests. *Farmers' Bull.* 1260.

———. 1966. The fowl tick: How to control it. Leaflet 382.

———. 1968a. Chiggers: How to fight them. Leaflet 403.

———. 1968b. Controlling mosquitoes in your home and on your premises. *Home Garden Bull.* 84.

———. 1969. Bed bugs: How to control them. Leaflet 453.

Usinger, R. L. 1947. Native hosts of the Mexican chicken bug, *Haematosiphon inodora* (Duges) (Hemiptera, Cimicidae). *Pan-Pacific Entomologist* 23:140.

———. 1966. Monograph of Cimicidae. Thomas Say Foundation Vol. 7. *Entomol. Soc. Am.* College Park, Maryland.

Van Heelsbergen, T. 1929. *Handbuch der Gefluegelkrankheiten und der Gefluegelzucht.* F. Enke, Stuttgart.

Vincent, L. E., D. L. Lindgren, and H. E. Drohne. 1954. Toxicity of malathion to the northern fowl mite. *J. Econ. Entomol.* 47:943–44.

Walker, G. P. 1927. A blackfly *(Simulium bracteatum)* fatal to goslings. *Can. Entomol.* 59:123.

Ware, G. W. 1961. BHC contamination of chicken eggs from treated litter. *J. Econ. Entomol.* 54:802–3.

Ware, G. W., and E. C. Naber. 1961. Lindane in eggs and chicken tissues. *J. Econ. Entomol.* 54:675–77.

Warren, D. C., R. Eaton, and H. Smith. 1948. Influence of infestations of body lice on egg production in the hen. *Poultry Sci.* 27:641–42.

West, L. S. 1951. *The Housefly: Its Natural History, Medical Importance and Control.* Comstock Publ. Co., Ithaca, N.Y.

Wharton, G. W., and H. S. Fuller. 1952. *A Manual of the Chiggers. Mem. Entomol. Soc. Wash.*, no. 4.

Whitehead, W. E. 1942. Lice and some other external parasites of domestic animals and poultry in the province of Quebec. *Macdonald College, McGill Univ., Farm Bull.* 7.

Whitlock, J. H. 1960. *Diagnosis of Veterinary Parasitisms.* Lea & Febiger, Philadelphia.

Wickware, A. B. 1921. An unusual form of scabies in fowls. *J. Parasitol.* 8:90–91.

Wilkins, S. D., and R. A. Dutcher. 1920. Limberneck in poultry. *J. Am. Vet. Med. Ass.* 57:653–85.

Wilson, F. H. 1933. A louse feeding on the blood of its host. *Science* 77:490.

———. 1934. The life-cycle and bionomics of *Lipeurus heterographus* Nitzsch. *J. Parasitol.* 20:304–11.

———. 1939. The life-cycle and bionomics of *Lipeurus caponis* (Linn.). *Ann. Entomol. Soc. Am.* 32:318–20.

———. 1941. The slender lice of American pigeons and doves, with descriptions of two new species. *J. Parasitol.* 27:259–64.

Wilson, H. G., and J. B. Gahan. 1957. Control of house fly larvae in poultry houses. *J. Econ. Entomol.* 50:613–14.

Wisseman, C. L., Jr., and S. E. Sulkin. 1947. Observations of the laboratory care, life cycle, and hosts of the chicken mite, *Dermanyssus gallinae. Am. J. Trop. Med.* 27:463–69.

Wolford, J. H., R. K. Ringer, T. H. Coleman, and H. C. Zindel. 1962. Nicotine sulfate treatment of turkey breeder hens housed in individual cages. *Mich. Agr. Expt. Sta. Quart. Bull.* 44:759.

Wright, W. H. 1944. The bedbug, its habits and life history and methods of control. *U.S. Public Health Serv., Public Health Rept. Suppl.* 175.

Yager, R. H., and C. A. Gleiser. 1946. *Trichomonas* and *Haemoproteus* infections and the experimental use of DDT in control of ectoparasites in a flock of Signal Corps pigeons in the Territory of Hawaii. *J. Am. Vet. Med. Ass.* 109:204–7.

Yates, W. W. 1953. Notes on the ecology of Culiseta mosquitoes found in the Pacific Northwest. *Mosquito News* 13:229–32.

Zumpt, F. 1966. The feather mite, *Megninia cubitalis* (Megnin), as a cause of "depluming itch," pp. 1027–28. In *1st Int. Congr. Parasitol.*, Vol. II. Pergamon Press, Oxford.

CHAPTER 28

NEMATODES AND ACANTHOCEPHALANS

❖

EVERETT E. WEHR

*Animal Disease and Parasite
Research Division
Agricultural Research Service
United States Department of Agriculture
Beltsville, Maryland*

❖

NEMATODES

❖

NEMATODES or roundworms are usually elongated, cylindrical, and unsegmented worms. The body is covered with a tough noncellular layer known as the cuticle. These worms have a well-developed alimentary tract and, in contrast to the tapeworms, are usually bisexual.

The class Nematoda is divided into a number of orders, the members of which are parasitic, semiparasitic, and free-living. In this chapter, only those forms that are parasitic in poultry are discussed.

The following key will aid in differentiating the 8 families containing species of poultry-parasitic nematodes.

1. Worms with free-living adult generation, that is, males and females developing outside of body; in digestive tract, hermaphroditic females only . . Strongyloididae
   Worms without a free-living generation, that is, incapable of producing males and females outside of body 2
2. Worms hairlike or threadlike; esophagus tubular and capillary, the tube embedded in or otherwise in relation to a single row of cells; in crop and small intestine . .
   . . . . Trichuridae

Worms thick as compared with above; esophagus well developed and muscular and with definite triangular lumen, not in relation to a single row of cells . . . 3

3. Cordons or other cephalic ornamentations present . . . . . . Acuariidae
   Cordons or other cephalic ornamentations absent 4
4. Preanal sucker present 5
   Preanal sucker absent 6
5. Esophagus with distinct posterior bulb containing a valvular apparatus . Heterakidae
   Esophagus without a distinct posterior bulb . . . . Ascarididae
6. Bursa present 7
   Bursa absent 8
7. Buccal capsule well developed and containing at least 6 teeth at base; oral opening hexangular . . . . . Syngamidae
   Buccal capsule reduced and containing not more than 3 teeth at base or none . .
   . . . . . . Trichostrongylidae
8. Pseudolabia absent . . . Thelaziidae
   Pseudolabia present . . . Spiruridae

GENERAL MORPHOLOGY

In general the body of a nematode is spindle-shaped with the anterior and posterior ends attenuated. The body covering or cuticle is usually marked by transverse grooves, and sometimes longitudinal folds or alae may be present. These alae may be confined to the anterior end of the body, in which case they are termed cervical alae; or they may be confined to the posterior part of the body, being then termed caudal alae (*Ascaridia galli*) (Fig. 28.1). The latter are found on the tail of the male worm and, in the case of certain groups, are modified to form a bursa (see Fig. 28.24B). Cuticular ornamentations are occasionally found on the anterior extremities of certain small groups of roundworms. These ornamentations may take the form of spines, cordons, or shields (see Fig. 28.11A).

The mouth opening is located at the extreme tip of the anterior end of the body and is usually surrounded by lips bearing sensory organs. In the more generalized type of nematodes, the mouth leads directly into a mouth cavity. This cavity may be considerably reduced or absent in the more specialized groups of nematodes. Directly posterior to the mouth cavity is the esophagus. This part of the intestinal tract may be simple, i.e. consisting of one undivided part; or it may be more complex, consisting

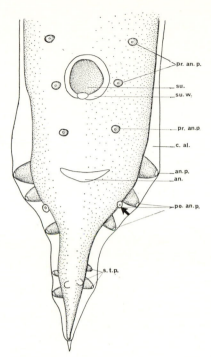

FIG. 28.1—Ascaridia galli. *Ventral view of posterior end of male* (an., *anus;* an. p., *anal papillae;* c. al., *caudal alae;* po. an. p., *postanal papillae;* pr. an. p., *preanal papillae;* s. t. p., *subterminal papillae;* su., *sucker;* su. w., *sucker wall*).

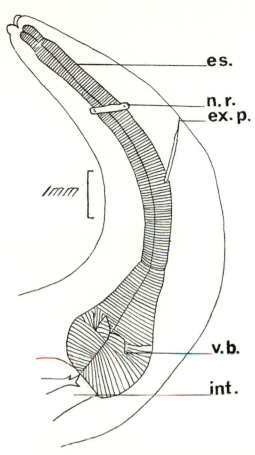

FIG. 28.2—Heterakis gallinarum. *Anterior end showing valvular bulb* (es., *esophagus;* ex. p., *excretory pore;* int., *intestine;* n. r., *nerve ring;* v. b., *valvular bulb*).

of a short anterior muscular part and a long posterior glandular part. A bulb may or may not be present at the posterior end of the esophagus (*Heterakis gallinarum*) (Fig. 28.2). Following the esophagus is the intestine which is connected with the anal or cloacal opening in the posterior end of the body by a short rectum.

The nematodes are, with very few exceptions, sexually distinct. The male can usually be distinguished from the female by the presence of two (sometimes only one) chitinous structures known as spicules which are located in the posterior end of the body. The spicules have been considered as intromittent organs for use during copulation. That the spicules do take an active part in copulation has been observed many times. They have been observed to withdraw and insert alternately over extended periods during coitus. It has been reported that the primary functions of the spicules is to keep the vulva and vagina open and, to some extent, to guide the sperm into the female. The female repro-

ductive products are discharged through the vulva, the position of which varies considerably in different groups of nematodes.

Sexual dimorphism is remarkably demonstrated by some species of nematodes. One of the most striking examples of this interesting phenomenon is *Tetrameres americana,* a nematode occurring in the proventriculus of certain kinds of poultry. The globular-shaped females enter the glands of the proventriculus or glandular stomach when very young, and as they begin to swell with eggs, their bodies assume the shape of the lumen of the glands. The adult male worm of this species is very much smaller than the female and retains the usual elongated nematode shape and usually lives free in the lumen of the proventriculus.

Nematodes are found in a variety of locations within the bodies of their hosts. The eyes, air sacs, thoracic and abdominal cavities, and tracheae are some of the unusual places that nematodes occur as parasites of avian hosts. The intestinal tract is of course the habitat of the largest number of species of roundworms.

DEVELOPMENT

Nematodes have both a direct (monoxenous) and an indirect (heteroxenous) type of development. Those worms with life histories of the first type require no invertebrate intermediate hosts to complete their life cycles and constitute approximately one-third of all the nematode species infecting poultry. However, the majority of the species of roundworms found in poultry are of the second type and depend upon such intermediate hosts as insects, snails, and slugs for the early stages of their development.

TABLE 28.1 ❧ Nematodes and Hosts from Poultry in United States

Nematodes	Location	Intermediate Hosts	Definitive Hosts
Oxyspirura mansoni	Eye	Cockroaches	Chicken, turkey, peafowl, ducks
Syngamus trachea	Trachea	None	Chicken, turkey, guinea fowl, goslings, pheasant
Cyathostoma bronchialis	Trachea	Unknown	Geese
Capillaria annulata	Esophagus, crop	Earthworms	Chicken, turkey, guinea fowl, pheasant, bobwhite quail
Capillaria contorta	Esophagus, crop	None	Turkey, duck, bobwhite quail, Hungarian partridge, ring-necked pheasant
Gongylonema ingluvicola	Crop	Unknown	Chicken, turkey, bobwhite quail
Dispharynx nasuta	Proventriculus	Sowbugs Pillbugs	Guinea fowl, turkey, chicken, pigeon, bobwhite quail
Seurocyrnea colini	Proventriculus	Cockroaches	Turkey, bobwhite quail, sharp-tailed grouse, prairie chicken
Tetrameres americana	Proventriculus	Grasshoppers Cockroaches	Chicken
Cheilospirura hamulosa	Gizzard	Grasshoppers Beetles Sandhoppers Weevils	Chicken, turkey
Amidostomum anseris	Gizzard	None	Duck, goose
Ascaridia galli	Small intestine	None	Chicken, turkey
Ascaridia columbae	Small intestine	None	Pigeon
Ascaridia numidae	Small intestine	Unknown	Guinea fowl
Ascaridia dissimilis	Small intestine	None	Turkey
Capillaria obsignata	Small intestine	None	Pigeon, chicken, turkey
Capillaria caudinflata	Small intestine	Earthworms	Chicken, turkey
Ornithostrongylus quadriradiatus	Small intestine	None	Pigeon, mourning dove
Heterakis gallinarum	Cecum	None	Chicken, turkey
Strongyloides avium	Cecum	None	Chicken, turkey
Trichostrongylus tenuis	Cecum	None	Chicken, duck, goose, guinea fowl
Subulura brumpti	Cecum	Grasshoppers Beetles Mealworms	Chicken, turkey, bobwhite quail
Subulura strongylina	Cecum	Unknown	Chicken, guinea fowl, bobwhite quail

Regardless of the type of development a certain species of nematode may have, it normally passes through four developmental stages before it becomes an adult, which is the final or fifth stage. Beginning with the second stage, each succeeding developmental stage in the life cycle is preceded by a molt. A molt is usually referred to as a shedding of the skin. In the case of some nematodes the loosened skin or cuticle may sometimes be retained for a short time as a protective covering, while in others it is shed at once.

Aside from the fact that certain nematodes require intermediate hosts to complete their development and others do not, the life histories of most nematodes infecting poultry are essentially the same. The eggs, which are deposited in the location in which the female worms are found, ultimately reach the outside in the droppings. This excorporal existence is apparently essential in order that the eggs may be rendered infective for the next host, be it avian or arthropod. The conditions existing within the body of the definitive host are usually inimical to the development of the eggs. However, once outside the body of the bird host and in the presence of optimum moisture and temperature requirements, these eggs undergo development. The time required for the eggs to embryonate depends somewhat upon the species of parasite, since, under similar environmental conditions, the eggs of some nematodes require only a few days to complete embryonation while others require several weeks. In the case of nematodes with a direct life cycle, the final host becomes infected by eating the embryonated eggs or the freed larvae. On the other hand, in the case of nematodes with an indirect life cycle, the intermediate host ingests the embryonated eggs or free larvae and retains the larvae within its body tissues. When a suitable final host eats the infested intermediate host containing infective larvae, it will become infected.

IMPORTANCE

Nematodes as a whole constitute the most important group of helminth parasites of poultry. Both in number of species affecting poultry and in the amount of damage done, this group of parasites far exceeds the flukes and cestodes.

Some of our most important individual worm parasites of poultry are found in this group. One species, *Heterakis gallinarum*, plays an important role in the transmission of the protozoan disease known as blackhead. Although considered of little economic importance as parasites of the domestic fowl, this species apparently has caused serious and enormous losses to the poultry industry in the role of a carrier of the blackhead organisms. The gapeworm is perhaps the most serious nematode parasite of young poultry, particularly chickens and turkeys. Until recently this worm was responsible for considerable losses among young birds both in this country and in Europe. Before changed poultry husbandry practices and other effective control measures reduced its devastating losses, this parasite was dreaded as much as blackhead. Despite all our efforts to control this worm, serious outbreaks of epidemics among pheasants continue to be reported as due to the poultry gapeworm. Needless to say, most of the nematodes parasitic in poultry and closely related birds may inflict serious injury to their respective hosts if infections are sufficiently large.

Table 28.1 shows species of nematodes found in poultry of this country, their intermediate hosts, usual locations, and kinds of poultry affected.

EYE

OXYSPIRURIASIS (THELAZIIDAE)

In the United States *Oxyspirura mansoni* is the causative agent of this disease in poultry. This roundworm is found beneath the nictitating membrane, conjunctival sacs, and nasolacrimal ducts of poultry in Florida, Louisiana, and possibly other southern states. This nematode belongs to the family Thelaziidae. Members of this family have a buccal capsule which may be well developed or rudimentary, and the vulva may be anterior or posterior to middle of body.

Oxyspirura mansoni (Cobbold 1879) (Manson's Eyeworm)

SYNONYM. *Filaria mansoni* Cobbold 1879.

DESCRIPTION. Mouth circular, surrounded by a 6-lobed chitinous ring (Fig. 28.3A). Two pairs of subdorsal and 1 pair of subventral teeth in mouth cavity.

Male 8.2 mm to 1.6 cm long by 350μ

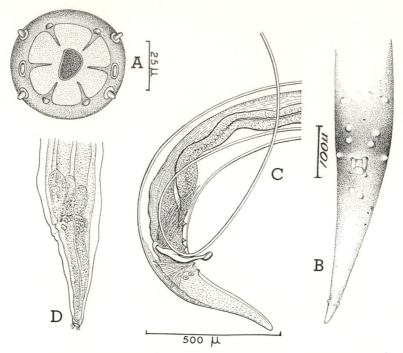

FIG. 28.3—Oxyspirura mansoni. *(A) Front view of head. (B) Ventral view, and (C) lateral view of male tail. (After Ransom, 1904) (D) Tail of second-stage larva. (After Fielding, 1928)*

wide. Tail curved ventrally, without alae. Four pairs of preanal and 2 pairs of post-anal papillae (Fig. 28.3B). Spicules unequal (Fig. 28.3C); one is 3–4.55 mm long and the other 180–240μ long.

Female 1.2–2 cm long by 270–430μ wide. Vulva 780μ to 1.55 mm from tip of tail. Eggs embryonated when deposited.

LIFE HISTORY. Sanders (1929) found that an intermediate host was necessary for the successful transmission of this parasite from one bird host to another.

The complete life cycle of the eyeworm as worked out by Sanders is as follows: The eggs of the mature female worm are deposited in the eyes of the bird host. They are then washed down the tear ducts, swallowed, and passed to the exterior in the droppings. The cockroach, *Pycnoscelus (Leucophaea) surinamensis,* which is an omnivorous feeder, ingests the nematode eggs deposited in the droppings of infected birds. Within approximately 50 days following ingestion of the infective eggs under experimental conditions, the cockroach contains in its body cavity mature larvae, which are capable of infecting a susceptible

host. The mature larvae are often contained within cysts which are located deep in the adipose tissue or along the course of the alimentary tract of the insect host. Some of the larvae release themselves from the capsules and are found free in the body cavity and legs of the cockroach. When an infected cockroach is swallowed by a chicken or other susceptible host, the infective larva is freed in the crop of the bird host, from which it later passes up the esophagus to the mouth and through the nasolacrimal duct to the eye.

Experimental evidence indicates that various wild birds are capable of becoming infected with the eyeworm of poultry and, as a result, may serve as sources of infection for domestic birds. Such birds as blackbird *(Agelaius phoeniceus),* bobolink *(Dolichonyx oryzivorus),* wild pigeon *(Columba livia),* loggerhead shrike *(Lanius ludovicianus),* and blue jay *(Aphelocoma cyanea)* have been experimentally infected with the eyeworm of poultry. Schwabe (1951) reported the eyeworm to occur naturally in English sparrow, mynah, Chinese dove, Japanese quail, and pheasant *(Phasianus torquatus torquatus and P. versicolor versi-*

color) in Hawaii. During the course of an investigation as to the role of natural reservoir hosts in the spread of the eyeworm in Hawaii, Schwabe decided that the local wild birds are of little importance in the dissemination of this poultry parasite.

PATHOLOGY. Birds harboring eyeworms show a peculiar ophthalmia. They appear uneasy and continuously scratch at the eyes, which are usually watery and show much inflammation. The nictitating membrane becomes swollen and projects slightly beyond the eyelids at the corners of the eyes and is usually kept in continual motion as if trying to remove some foreign object from the eye. The eyelids sometimes become stuck together, and a white cheesy material collects beneath them. If left untreated, severe ophthalmia may develop; as a result the eyeball may be destroyed. The worms are seldom if ever found in the eyes when severe symptoms are manifested, presumably due to unfavorable conditions existing there.

TREATMENT. The various therapeutic treatments—removal of nictitating membrane, anesthetizing the eyes with cocaine or butyn solution—are impractical and should not be resorted to except in rare and isolated instances. Proper housing of birds, strict sanitation, and use of insecticides for control of the intermediate host *Pycnoscelus*

surinamensis are the most practical and effective means for control of this parasite.

RESPIRATORY TRACT

SYNGAMIASIS (SYNGAMIDAE)

In the United States *Syngamus trachea* is the causative agent of "gapes" (labored breathing due to parasites) in chickens, turkeys, peacocks, and pheasants; *Cyathostoma bronchialis* is the causative agent of this disease in geese. They parasitize the trachea and less frequently the bronchi of these birds (Fig. 28.4).

Ershov (1956) states that syngamiasis of the domestic fowl in Russia is caused by *Syngamus skrjabinomorpha* and is limited to western Georgia (Russia).

Only in artificial rearing of pheasants is gapes a serious menace among these birds in the United States. Due to changes in hatching and rearing of young birds, gapeworms are not as serious a problem in poultry as they were a few years ago. However, it is said that this parasite continues to present something of a problem with turkeys raised on range in Tennessee and Kentucky.

Members of this family are characterized by having the vulva in the anterior part of the body, stoma (mouth cavity) well developed and hexagonal in cross section, and corona radiata (crown of spines around head) reduced or absent.

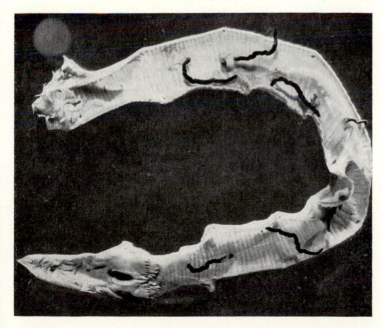

FIG. 28.4—*Syngamus trachea. Trachea showing attached gapeworms.*

FIG. 28.5—Syngamus trachea. (A) En-larged egg showing fully developed em-bryo. (B) Drawing of male and female gapeworms.

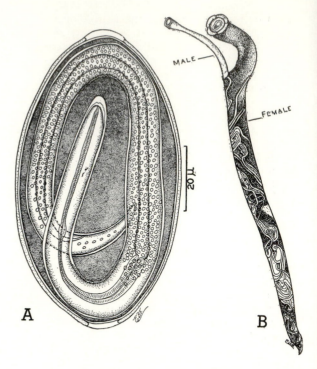

A   B

Syngamus trachea (Montagu 1811) (Gapeworm)

SYNONYMS. *Fasciola trachea* Montagu 1811; *Syngamus trachealis* Siebold 1836.

DESCRIPTION. Red worms, the color more pronounced in female. Mouth orbicular, with a hemispherical chitinous capsule, usually with 8 sharp teeth at the base. Mouth surrounded by a chitinous plate, the outer margin of which is incised to form 6 festoons opposite each other. Male permanently attached in copula to female, forming a Y (Fig. 28.5B).

Male 2–6 mm long by 200μ wide. Bursa obliquely truncated, provided with rays, sometimes with strikingly asymmetrical dorsal rays. Spicules equal, slender, short, 57–64μ long.

Female 5 mm to 2 cm long (longer in the turkey) by 350μ wide. Tail end conical, bearing a pointed process. Vulva promi-nent, about one-fourth of body length from anterior end, but the position varies with age. Eggs 90μ long by 49μ wide, ellipsoidal, operculated (Fig. 28.5A).

The gapeworm *Syngamus trachea* is sometimes designated as the "red-worm" or "forked-worm" because of its red color and because the male and female are joined together so that they appear like the letter Y. This parasite is cosmopolitan in distri-bution.

LIFE HISTORY. The life history of the gape-worm is peculiar in that transmission of this parasite from bird host to bird host may be successfully accomplished either di-rectly (by the feeding of embryonated eggs or infective larvae) or indirectly (by the ingestion of earthworms containing free or encysted gapeworm larvae which they had obtained by feeding on contaminated soil). The female gapeworm deposits its eggs through the vulvar opening under-neath the bursa of the attached male into the lumen of the trachea. The eggs reach the mouth cavity, are swallowed, and pass to the outside in the droppings. Following a period of incubation of approximately 8–14 days under optimum conditions of moisture and temperature, these eggs be-come embryonated. Soon after embryona-tion some of the eggs may hatch, the larvae living free in the soil. Should specimens of the earthworms *Eisenia (H) foetidus* and *Allolobophora (H) caliginosus*, and perhaps others, be present in the soil which has been contaminated with feces containing the eggs of gapeworms, these annelids will become infected with gapeworm larvae. Within the earthworm the larvae penetrate the intestinal wall, enter the body cavity, and finally invade the body musculature in which they may encyst for an indefinite period. Taylor (1938) stated that gapeworm larvae may remain infective to young chickens in the earthworm for as long as $4\frac{1}{3}$ years. This author also found that slugs and snails may also serve as transfer hosts of *Syngamus trachea* larvae and that live gapeworm larvae were obtained from snails over a year after infection. These mollusks are not essentially true intermediate hosts in the strict sense of the word, since they are not absolutely necessary for the successful transfer of the gapeworm to other susceptible bird hosts.

Clapham (1934) and other investigators have observed that strains of *Syngamus trachea* taken from various wild and domestic birds were more readily transferred to young chickens and with a greater degree of success if the earthworm was employed as an intermediary.

The exact path of migration of the gapeworm larva after it has once entered the intestinal tract of the avian host until it reaches the lung is not known. Walker (1886) believed that the larvae, after being swallowed by the definitive host, passed through the esophageal wall and entered the lungs directly from the outside. More recent observations have indicated that the path of migration may be via the blood stream. However, convincing evidence which tends to show the true path of migration is still lacking.

Observations by Wehr (1937) have shown that the infective larvae reach the lungs in an apparently unchanged condition within at least 6 hours after they have been ingested by the bird. By the 3rd day following inoculation, the larvae have developed to the fourth stage, and by the 7th day several fourth-stage larvae and a few immature adults—one pair of the latter in copula—were found in the lungs; five pairs of immature adults in copula were found in the trachea. It is evident from these and other observations that the male and female of *Syngamus trachea* may copulate as young adults while in the lungs sometime between the 3rd and 7th days following infection, and that the worms reach the trachea about the 7th day after ingestion of the embryonated eggs and larvae. These findings differ from those of Ortlepp (1923), who believed that the fourth stage

was the final stage in the development of this nematode, and that the second-stage larvae represented the infective stage. This latter observation is obviously an error, since the gapeworm embryo has been observed to molt twice inside the egg.

Approximately 2 weeks are required for the infective larvae to reach sexual maturity and for eggs to appear in the droppings. About half of this time is spent in the lungs and the other half in the trachea.

The role played by the wild birds in the spread of gapeworm disease is still undecided. So far as is known at the present time, wild birds probably are not an important factor in the spread of gapeworm disease in this country.

PATHOLOGY. Young birds are most seriously affected with gapeworms. The rapidly growing worms soon obstruct the lumen of the trachea and cause the birds to suffocate and die. Turkey poults, baby chicks, and pheasant chicks are very susceptible to infection with gapeworms, whereas the young of the other species of poultry which have been experimentally inoculated with infective eggs and larvae of gapeworms are not so seriously affected. Turkey poults usually develop gapeworm symptoms earlier and begin to die sooner following gapeworm infection than young chickens. Experimentally infected guinea fowls, pigeons, and ducks do not exhibit characteristic symptoms of gapeworm infections. Young pheasants, however, suffer from the disease to an extent comparable to that of young chicks and turkey poults. Fullgrown birds rarely show characteristic gapeworm symptoms unless heavily infected.

Young birds infected with gapeworms show symptoms of weakness and emaciation and usually spend much of their time with eyes closed and head drawn back against the body. From time to time they throw their heads forward and upward and open the mouth wide to draw in air. It is not uncommon to see an infected bird give its head a convulsive shake in an attempt to remove the obstruction from the trachea so that normal breathing may be resumed. Little or no food is taken by birds in the advanced stages of infection, and death is usually the end result.

An examination of the trachea of infected birds shows that the mucous membrane is extensively irritated and inflamed;

coughing is apparently the result of this irritation to the mucous lining. Lesions are usually found in the trachea of turkeys and pheasants but seldom if ever in the trachea of young chickens and guinea fowls. Observations have shown that these lesions or nodules are produced as a result of an inflammatory reaction set up at the site of attachment of the male worm. Since lesions have been observed only at the point of attachment of the male worm and observations have shown that the head of the male is deeply embedded in the nodular tissue, it is believed that the male worm usually remains permanently attached to the tracheal wall throughout the duration of its life. The female worms apparently detach and reattach from time to time in order to obtain a more abundant supply of food.

AGE OF HOST. Although young chicks are easily parasitized, investigators in this country have indicated that chickens 10 weeks or older are very difficult to infect experimentally with gapeworms. However, Crawford (1940) reported that gapeworms occurred commonly in the trachea of fowls of all ages, even in 3-year-old hens, in Ceylon. He stated that the number of worms found in the trachea of each fowl was usually small and that adult hens not infrequently were seen to exhibit typical symptoms of gapeworm disease. He considered the adult fowl to be an important factor in the perpetuation of gapeworm disease in Ceylon. Olivier (1943) reported the occurrence of *Syngamus trachea* in mature chickens in Maryland. One of these birds was heavily infected and exhibited typical clinical symptoms.

DIAGNOSIS. The inability of affected birds to breathe normally causes them to "gape" which is one of the early symptoms of the disease (Fig. 28.6). Affected birds constantly emit short whistling sounds and jerk their heads as if to free themselves of some obstruction that had become lodged in their throats.

It must be remembered, however, that there are other diseases which may cause birds to gape, such as bronchitis and laryngotracheitis. In order that one may be sure just what is the cause of the gaping, it is necessary to make a postmortem examination of one or more affected birds. If gapeworms are not present in the trachea, bronchitis or laryngotracheitis or some other disease causing similar symptoms must be diagnosed.

The detection of eggs of the gapeworm in the feces is one of the most reliable methods of determining the presence of gapeworms.

TREATMENT. Recently several workers have reported thiabendazole to be effective against the gapeworm when administered in the feed to naturally and experimentally infected birds. The drug was added to the feed at levels of 0.05–0.5% for 4–14 days. In those experiments in which necropsies and worm counts were made, the drug proved to be remarkably effective in removing the parasite.

Wehr and Hwang (1967) fed a mash containing 0.5% thiabendazole to 4-week-old turkey poults for 9–20 days. The drug removed in the aggregate 98% of the gapeworms from 117 birds. A total of 2,114 worms was recovered at necropsy from the 44 untreated birds. Generally the drug appeared effective, whether treatment was initiated on postinfection day 30 or started on day of infection.

Previous work by Sharpe (1964) has shown that thiabendazole fed at 0.1% of the feed would prevent pheasants from con-

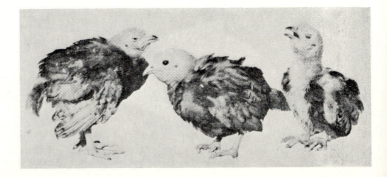

FIG. 28.6—*Birds affected with* Syngamus trachea.

tracting gapeworms. However, to feed this amount for an extended period—6 weeks or more until the birds are released to the wild—has proved to be expensive and not economical.

Although thiabendazole has proved to be highly effective in treating infected birds for gapeworms, more work is needed to determine the proper method, prophylactically or therapeutically, and the optimum dose in each case.

Cyathostoma bronchialis (Muehlig 1884)

SYNONYM. *Syngamus bronchialis* Muehlig 1884.

DESCRIPTION. Very similar to Syngamus, but larger and less firmly united in copula. Buccal capsule somewhat wider than deep, usually 6 but occasionally 7 triangular buccal teeth.

Male 8–12 mm long by 200–600μ wide. Spicules long and slender, 540–700 mm long, with tips slightly incurved.

Female 16–30 mm long by 750μ to 1.5 mm wide. Vulva with fairly prominent lips, situated in posterior part of anterior third of body. Tail acute. Eggs 68–90μ long, 43–60μ wide, with slight operculum in mature ones.

LIFE HISTORY. The life history is unknown but is probably similar to *Syngamus trachea*. This species of gapeworm is apparently widespread in domestic geese in Europe and to some extent in wild geese of the United States. The following record of its appearance in domestic geese of this country appears to be the only one.

PATHOLOGY. Griffiths et al. (1954) reported a morbidity of 80% with a mortality of about 20% in a flock of domestic geese near Duluth, Minnesota. The course of the disease extended over a period of 5 months, during which time the birds showed symptoms of respiratory distress as evidenced by throwing back their heads and gaping for air. Severely affected birds died soon after the appearance of respiratory disturbances. The symptoms exhibited were similar to those of laryngotracheitis. Recovered birds showed growth retardation. Cram (1928) reported infections of this gapeworm in Young Blue, Cackling, Snow, and Canada geese in Illinois.

CROP

At least three species of nematodes, commonly referred to as crop worms, occur in the crop of domestic fowls. Two of these are commonly known as capillarid worms or hairworms and belong to the family Trichuridae; the third is designated as the gullet worm and is a member of the family Thelaziidae.

CAPILLARIASIS (TRICHURIDAE)

Capillariasis is a parasitic disease caused by a group of roundworms known as hairworms, threadworms, or capillarids. These roundworms, although they belong to a single genus Capillaria, constitute a diversified group of parasites. The development and habits of some of the species vary greatly. The adult worms not only inhabit the digestive tract of man and of different kinds of animals, including birds, but they have been found in such unusual places as the urinary bladder and liver.

The esophagus and crop are the preferred sites of habitation by *Capillaria contorta* and *C. annulata*, while the small intestine is preferred by *C. obsignata*.

Capillariasis in poultry has long been recognized as a possible source of economic loss, and with the use of more intensive methods of rearing these birds, the problem has assumed even greater importance.

Members of this family are characterized by having the body more or less clearly divided into an esophageal portion and a posterior portion, the latter containing the other organs. The esophagus is a cuticular tube embedded in one side of a single or double row of esophageal glands. The male possesses a single spicule. The vulva is located at junction of esophageal and posterior portions of body.

Capillaria annulata (Molin 1858) (Annulated Threadworm)

Capillaria annulata occurs naturally in bobwhite quail, domestic chicken and turkey, pheasant, and Hungarian partridge. Worms of this species are similar in appearance to those of *Capillaria contorta* but may easily be differentiated by the presence of a cuticular swelling just back of the head (Fig. 28.7A).

Male usually 1–2.5 cm long by 52–74μ wide. Tail ends in two inconspicuous round lateral flaps, united dorsally by a cuticular flap. Spicule sheath beset with

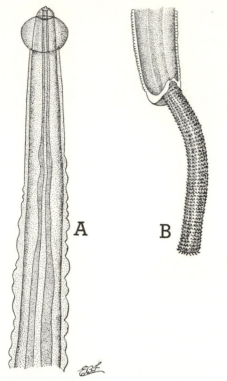

FIG. 28.7–Capillaria annulata. *(A) Head end.* *(B) Male tail. (After Ciurea, 1914)*

fine spines (Fig. 28.7B). Spicule 1.12–1.63 mm long.

Female usually 2.5–6 cm long by 77–120μ wide. Posterior portion of body (posterior to vulva) about 7 times as long as anterior portion. Vulva circular, located about opposite the termination of the esophagus. Eggs operculated, 55–66μ long by 26–28μ wide.

Madsen (1951) synonymized *Capillaria annulata* (Molin, 1858) with *Capillaria contorta* (Creplin, 1839). Because of the presence of a cuticular inflation around the head and experimental evidence which points to the necessity of an intermediate host for its complete development, *Capillaria annulata* has been recognized as a distinct species.

LIFE HISTORY. Eggs of this parasite pass out in the droppings of infected birds. They develop very slowly; a period of 24 days to over 1 month is sometimes necessary before they have reached the stage at which they contain an active embryo. Wehr (1936) discovered that the earthworm is required in

order to successfully transmit *C. annulata* from one bird host to another. He demonstrated that under both natural and artificial conditions two species of earthworms, *Eisenia (H) foetidus* and *Allolobophora (H) caliginosus,* served as intermediate hosts of this crop worm. Chickens and other susceptible hosts become infected with this worm by swallowing infected earthworms.

PATHOLOGY. Cram (1926c) reported this worm as being associated with deaths of turkeys in Maryland. The habit of burrowing into the crop mucosa causes a thickening of the crop wall and enlargement of the glands in the areas in which the worms are located. Usually there is slight or severe inflammation of the crop and esophageal walls, depending upon the severity of the infection. In heavy infections, the inner surface of the crop is immensely thickened, roughened, and badly macerated, with masses of worms concentrated primarily in this sloughing tissue (Fig. 28.8).

In pheasants, quail, and other gallinaceous game birds, infections with this parasite often prove fatal. In these birds the symptoms reported are principally malnutrition and emaciation, associated with severe anemia. Allen and Gross (1926) reported severe anemia in an infected ruffed grouse shortly before death.

HISTOPATHOLOGY. Hung (1926) made a histopathological study of three cases of varying intensity and reported the following changes:

On the basis of the above observations it is quite evident that the pathological changes caused by *C. annulata* may be divided into three stages. The first stage is the hyperemic stage in which only hyperemia and lymphocytic infiltrations are present. In the second stage the yellowish white nodules are present, and the lymphatic apparatus is enlarged and sometimes necrotic. The enlargement of the lymph follicles gives the appearance of nodules. The third stage is that of the formation of the pseudomembrane, in which the mucosa is covered with a membrane containing fibrin.

Capillaria contorta (Creplin 1839) (Contorted Threadworm)

Capillaria contorta has been reported from a large number of hosts, including duck, turkey (both domestic and wild), pheasant, quail, and ruffed grouse.

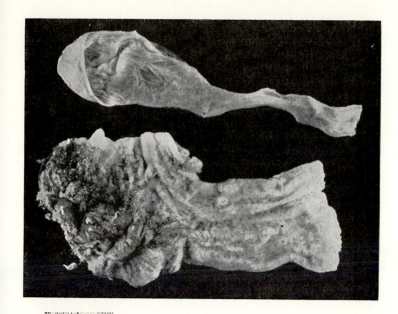

FIG. 28.8—Capillaria annulata. *Damage done to crop of quail compared with thin-walled normal crop.*

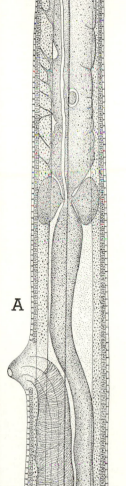

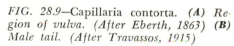

FIG. 28.9—Capillaria contorta. *(A) Region of vulva. (After Eberth, 1863) (B) Male tail. (After Travassos, 1915)*

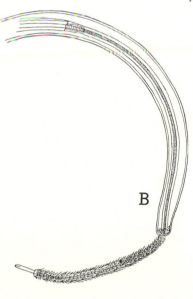

A

B

SYNONYMS. *Trichosoma contortum* Creplin 1839; *Thominx contorta* (Creplin 1839) Travassos 1915.

DESCRIPTION. Body threadlike, attenuated anteriorly and posteriorly.

Male 8 mm to 1.7 cm long by 60–70μ wide. Two terminal laterodorsal prominences on tail end. Spicule very slender and transparent, about 800μ long, according to Travassos. Spicule sheath covered with fine hairlike processes (Fig. 28.9B).

Female 1.5–6 cm long by 120–150μ wide. Vulva prominent, circular, 140–180μ posterior to beginning of intestine (Fig. 28.9A).

LIFE HISTORY. Eggs are apparently deposited in tunnels in the crop mucosa and escape into the lumen of crop and esophagus with the sloughed mucosa. They are found abundantly in droppings from infected birds. Approximately 1 month or slightly longer is required for embryos to develop within the eggs. Worms mature and pass another generation of eggs which pass to the outside in the droppings of susceptible avian hosts 1–2 months after feeding on the embryonated eggs. Attempts to experimentally infect chickens, guinea fowls, and pigeons were unsuccessful.

PATHOLOGY. When present in large numbers these worms are highly dangerous. In light infections the wall of the crop and esophagus become slightly thickened and inflamed. In heavy infections there is a marked thickening and inflammation, with a flocculent exudate covering the mucosa and with more or less sloughing of the mucosa (Fig. 28.10).

Affected birds become droopy, weak, and emaciated. Many deaths due to infection with this worm have been observed among wild turkeys and Hungarian partridges in this country.

The author visited a flock of domestic turkeys in Virginia, among which several birds were reported to have died from heavy infections with this crop worm. A number of visibly affected birds had been segregated from the main flock and were held in a pen by themselves. These birds moved only when disturbed, and then very slowly and with an unsteady gait. Occasionally a bird was seen to fall back on its hock joints and assume a penguinlike position. Others extended and retracted their heads and necks as if attempting to relieve an obstruction in their throats. The crops of the most severely affected birds were filled with a fetid liquid. Emmel (1939) observed that infection with this crop worm appeared first in the older birds; later those of all ages became affected. Affected birds appeared indisposed, weak, and droopy, with the forepart of the body slightly elevated. The birds were not inclined to move unless forced to do so. He also observed that the birds occasionally assumed a penguinlike posture, with the head drawn close to the body, and that affected birds frequently swallowed and in doing so always extended and "ducked" their heads.

GONGYLONEMIASIS (THELAZIIDAE)

This disease in poultry is caused by a single species, *Gongylonema ingluvicola*. It has been reported from chicken, turkey, and quail in the United States.

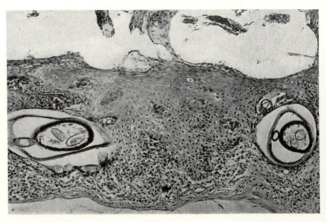

FIG. 28.10—*Section of crop of bobwhite quail showing* Capillaria contorta *and damage produced by it. Experimental infection.* ×114.

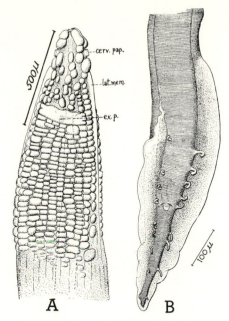

FIG. 28.11—Gongylonema ingluvicola. *(A)*
Head (cerv. pap., *cervical papillae;* lat.
mem., *lateral membrane;* ex. p., *excretory*
pore). *(B) Male tail. (After Ransom,*
1904)

Gongylonema ingluvicola Ransom 1904
(Gullet Worm)

DESCRIPTION. Anterior end of body with
a zone of shieldlike markings, few and scattered near head, numerous and arranged
in longitudinal rows farther back (Fig.
28.11A).

Male 1.7–2 cm long by 224–250μ wide.
Cervical papillae about 100μ from head
end. Tail with two narrow bursal asymmetrical membranes. Genital papillae variable in number and asymmetrical; preanal
papillae up to 7 on left side and up to 5
on right side (Fig. 28.11B). Left spicule as
long or nearly as long (1.7–1.9 cm) as body
and 7–9μ wide, with a barbed point; right
spicule 100–120μ long and 15–20μ wide.

Female 3.2–5.5 cm long by 320–490μ
wide. Vulva 2.5–3.5 mm from tip of tail.

LIFE HISTORY. Cram (1931a) fed larval
roundworms collected from the beetle *Cop-*
ris minutus to a chicken and recovered a
single male specimen of a species of *Gon-*
gylonema, tentatively identified as *G. in-*
gluvicola. Cram subsequently infected cockroaches by feeding embryonated eggs of *G.*
ingluvicola derived from mountain quail.

Some of the larvae recovered from the cockroaches were fed to a chicken. No worms
were found when the chicken was killed
79 days later.

PATHOLOGY. The only damage that has
been associated with these worms is the
local lesions in the form of burrows in the
mucosa of the crop.

STOMACH

Nematodes inhabiting the proventriculus
of domestic poultry belong to two families,
Acuariidae and Spiruridae.

DISPHARYNXIASIS (ACUARIIDAE)

The acuariids are characterized by having well-developed pseudolabia and cuticular ornamentations on the anterior part of
the body.

Dispharynx nasuta (Rudolphi 1819)
(Spiral Worm)

This parasite has been encountered in
the proventriculus of chicken, turkey,
guinea fowl, pigeon, pheasant, ruffed
grouse, bobwhite quail, Hungarian partridge, and other gallinaceous birds. In
addition it has been found in a number of
passerine birds in the United States. Yeatter (1934) found the incidence of this parasite among Hungarian partridge in the
Great Lakes region to be 31.6%. Bump
(1935) stated that this worm was the most
important parasite recovered from ruffed
grouse in New York State.

SYNONYMS. *Spiroptera nasuta* Rudolphi
1819; *Dispharagus spiralis* Molin 1858; *Acu-*
aria spiralis (Molin 1858) Railliet, Henry,
and Sisoff 1912. Goble and Kutz (1945)
concluded that all forms of *Dispharynx* recently recorded from galliform, columbiform, and passiform birds in the Western
Hemisphere are nonspecific and that a
morphological study of these forms indicates their identity as *Dispharynx nasuta*
(Rudolphi 1819) Stiles and Hassall 1920.
Dispharynx nasuta (Rudolphi 1819) Stiles
and Hassall 1920 has priority over *Disphar-*
ynx spiralis (Molin 1858) Skrjabin 1916.

DESCRIPTION. Four wavy cuticular cordons
on anterior end, originating at base of lips,
recurrent, the distal extremity of the cordons turning forward and extending anteriorly a short distance (Fig. 28.12A). Post-

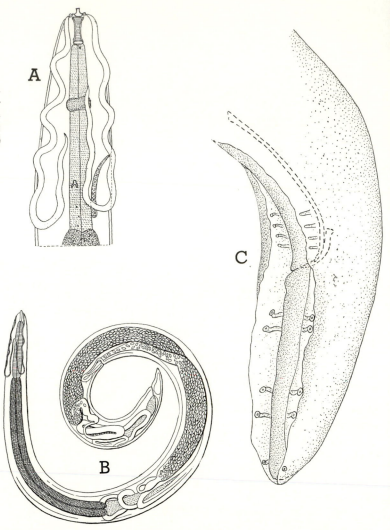

FIG. 28.12—Dispharynx nasuta. (A) Head end. (After Seurat, 1915) (B) Female, enlarged. (After Piana, 1897) (C) Male tail. (After Cram, 1928)

cervical papillae small, bicuspid, situated between the recurrent branches of the cordons. Body usually rolled in a spiral (Fig. 28.12B).

Male 7–8.3 mm long by 230–315μ wide. Five pairs of postanal and 4 pairs of preanal papillae (Fig. 28.12C). Long spicule 400μ long, slender and curved; short spicule 150μ long, navicular.

Female 9–10.2 mm long by 360–565μ wide. Small mucro on tip of tail. Vulva in posterior portion of body. Eggs embryonated when oviposited.

LIFE HISTORY. The pillbug (*Armadillidium vulgare*) and the sowbug (*Porcellio scaber*) were demonstrated to serve as intermediate hosts in experimental infections by Cram (1931b). The writer has repeatedly confirmed Cram's studies, using pigeons as definitive hosts. Within 4 days after ingestion of the embryonated eggs by these isopods, the larvae have escaped from the eggs and are found among the tissues of the body cavity of the crustacean. The larva completes its development in the isopod within approximately 26 days; it has then reached the third or infective stage.

The definitive host becomes infected with this nematode by swallowing infected pillbugs or sowbugs with food or water. According to Cram (1931b), the female worms become sexually mature and are depositing eggs 27 days after ingestion by a susceptible vertebrate host.

PATHOLOGY. These roundworms are usually seen with their heads buried deep into the mucosa. Formations of ulcers are often observed in the proventriculi of infected birds. In a heavy infection the wall of the proventriculus becomes tremendously thickened and macerated, tissue layers are indistinguishable, and the parasites become almost completely concealed beneath the proliferating tissue.

Allen (1924) believed that *D. nasuta (D. spiralis)* was the chief cause of "grouse disease" in northeastern United States. Heavy infections of this parasite resulted in the death of many carrier pigeons of the Signal Corps of the United States Army at Fort Sam Houston, Texas, a number of years ago (Cram, 1928). Several wild pigeons trapped at the Balboa Zoological Park, San Diego, California, and examined by the writer were found to be heavily infected with this parasite.

CYRNIASIS (SPIRURIDAE)

Cyrnea colini (Cram 1927))

SYNONYM. *Seurocyrena colini* (Strand 1929).

Cyrnea colini is of common occurrence in the bobwhite quail of southeastern states and has occasionally been collected from this same host and closely related birds in some northeastern states. It has also been reported from turkey in Georgia, prairie chicken in Wisconsin, and sharp-tailed grouse in Wisconsin and Montana.

The preferred location of this nematode is in the wall of the proventriculus at its junction with the gizzard.

DESCRIPTION. Slender yellowish white worms similar in appearance to *Cheilospirura hamulosa* but smaller and lack the so-called cordons or cuticular ornamentations on anterior part of the body. The head structures are quite complicated, and the tail of the male has winglike expansions or alae (Fig. 28.13).

Head with 4 lips, dorsal and ventral lips prominent and bearing 4 conspicuous projecting papillae and a prominent thumb-like projection. Lateral lips very large, each bearing 2 digitiform processes on inner surface and 2 winglike expansions on lateral surface. There are 2 obscure lateral papillae near base of lateral lips.

Male 6 mm long by 250μ wide. Buccal cavity 58μ deep; esophagus 2 mm long. Caudal alae nearly circular, with 10 pairs of pedunculated papillae, the anterior ones larger than posterior. Spicules very unequal, the left 2 mm long and the right 365μ.

Female 14–18 mm long by 315μ wide. Buccal cavity 75μ deep. Esophagus about 2.8 mm long. Vulva slightly salient, 915μ anterior to anus. Eggs 40.5 $\times$ 22.5μ.

LIFE HISTORY. The life history of this nematode is indirect, requiring the cockroach *Blatella germanica* as a temporary host. Since this intermediate host has been incriminated in an experimental role only, it is not known whether it actually serves in this same capacity under natural conditions.

PATHOLOGY. There has been little or no pathological change observed in connection with infections of this parasite.

TETRAMERIASIS (SPIRURIDAE)

The spirurids are characterized by having well-developed pseudolabia, cephalic papillae usually posterior to pseudolabia, and interlabia present or absent. The only member of this family found in poultry of this country has interlabia, and the sexes are distinctly dimorphic.

Tetrameres americana Cram 1927 (Globular Nematode)

SYNONYM. *Tropisurus americana* (Cram 1927).

The female of this species occurs in the glandular stomach of chickens and bobwhite quail (Fig. 28.14). At necropsy these bright red worms are often observed through the wall of the unopened proventriculus. The male of this species is very small, almost microscopic in size, and resembles other nematodes in shape. It is very seldom observed elsewhere than on the surface of the mucosa of the proventriculus. However, the males of some of the species of Tetrameres occurring in wild birds have been found on several occasions together with the females in the same glands. From all indications, it seemed that the two sexes in the cases cited were permanent residents of the glands in which they were found. When the male of *T. americana* enters the glands of the proventriculus, it apparently does so only long enough to mate with the female.

Cram (1931a) found this parasite to be common in quail which had been raised in

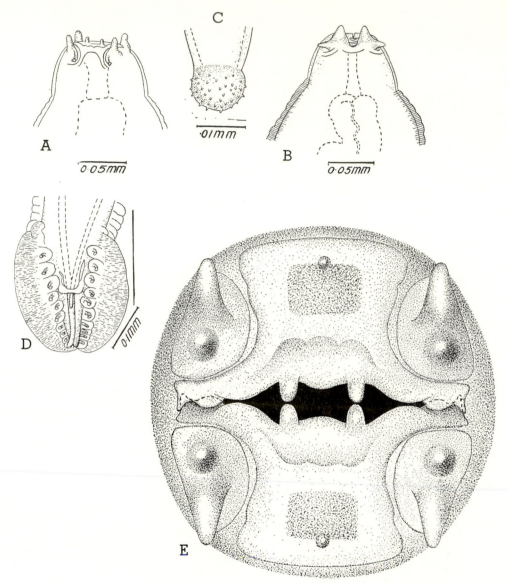

FIG. 28.13—*Cyrnea colini.* **(A)** *Head, oblique lateral view.* **(B)** *Head, ventral view.* **(C)** *Tail of third-stage larva.* **(D)** *Male tail.* **(E)** *Head, face view, semidiagrammatic. (After Cram, 1927)*

captivity and in close proximity to poultry in Virginia. Stoddard (1931) reported *T. americana* as being found occasionally in quail captured in its natural habitat in southeastern United States.

Swales (1933) described *T. crami* from the proventriculus of a domestic duck in Canada. He stated that this species, of which the female only is known, differs from *T. americana* chiefly in the shorter muscular esophagus and the relative positions of the anus and vulva.

Another species of Tetrameres, *T. fissispina,* closely related to *T. americana,* has been reported from wild and domestic ducks and chickens in Europe. Sugimoto and Nishiyama (1937) stated that this round worm was fairly common in chickens in Formosa.

DESCRIPTION. Mouth surrounded with 3 small lips; buccal cavity present.

Male 5–5.5 mm long by 116–133μ wide. Two double rows of posteriorly directed

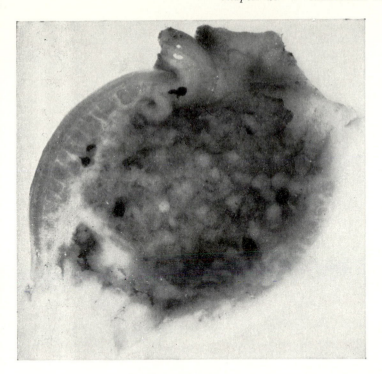

FIG. 28.14—Tetrameres americana. *Proventriculus showing female worms in glands.* (*After Cram, 1930*)

spines extend throughout whole body length in the submedian lines. Cervical papillae present. Tail long and slender. Two unequal spicules, 100μ and 290–312μ long respectively.

Female 3.5–4.5 mm long by 3 mm wide. Body globular, blood red in color, with 4 longitudinal furrows (Fig. 28.15). Uteri and ovaries very long, their numerous coils filling the body cavity.

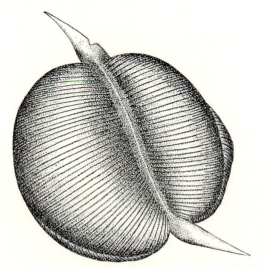

FIG. 28.15—Tetrameres americana. *Enlarged drawing of female.*

LIFE HISTORY. Cram (1931b) discovered that *T. americana* required an intermediate host for its complete development. She fed embryonated eggs of this worm to two species of grasshoppers (*Melanoplus femurrubrum* and *M. differentialis*) and a species of cockroach (*Blatella germanica*) and recovered infective larvae from the body cavities of these insects about 42 days after ingestion of the eggs. When the grasshopper or cockroach is swallowed by a suitable bird host and digested in its stomach, the larvae escape; they remain in the proventriculus and develop into adults within a few days. The complete life cycle of *T. fissispina* involves such intermediate hosts as the amphipod *Gammarus pulex;* the cladoceran *Daphnia pulex;* and several species of grasshoppers, cockroaches, and earthworms.

PATHOLOGY. According to Sugimoto and Nishiyama (1937), infected chickens become emaciated and anemic as a result of heavy infections. Cram (1931a) reported that *T. americana* has not been observed to produce any damage in quail. Barber (1916) stated that this proventricular worm was the cause of a serious catarrhal condition in chickens in Guam. In his report he mentioned that the walls of the proventriculus were so thickened that the lumen was almost entirely obliterated; as many as 47 worms were found embedded in the wall.

GIZZARD

Gizzard nematodes belong to two families, Acuariidae and Trichostrongylidae.

CHEILOSPIRURIASIS (ACUARIIDAE)

The disease is caused by species of the genus Cheilospirura which normally occur beneath the horny lining of the gizzard, usually in the cardiac and/or pyloric regions where the lining is soft and pliable. It occurs in the chicken and has occasionally been reported from the turkey. It is widely distributed in the United States.

Cheilospirura hamulosa (Diesing 1851) (Gizzard Worm)

SYNONYM. *Spiroptera hamulosa* Diesing 1851.

DESCRIPTION. Two large, triangular, lateral lips. The 4 cuticular cordons double, irregularly wavy, and extending almost to posterior extremity; not anastomosing or recurring anteriorly (Fig. 28.16A).
Male 9 mm to 1.9 cm long. Spicules very unequal and dissimilar, the left long and slender, the right short and curved. Tail tightly coiled; 2 very wide caudal alae present. Ten pairs of caudal papillae (Fig. 28.16B).
Female 1.6–2.5 cm long. Vulva slightly posterior to middle of body. Tail pointed. Eggs embryonated when deposited.

LIFE HISTORY. Investigations have shown that grasshoppers, beetles, weevils, and sandhoppers serve as intermediate hosts of *C. hamulosa* under natural as well as experimental conditions. Chickens and other susceptible avian hosts become infected with the adults of this roundworm by ingesting grasshoppers, beetles, weevils, and sandhoppers which are infected with larvae of this worm.
The infective or third stage larva may be recognized easily by the 2 prominent lip-like structures at the anterior end of the body, the dorsal curvature of the posterior portion of the body, and the presence of 4 digitiform processes at the tip of the tail.

PATHOLOGY. When present in small numbers, these worms cause no evident effect

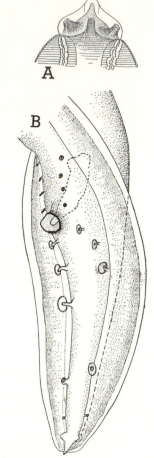

FIG. 28.16—Cheilospirura hamulosa. (*A*) Head. (*After Drasche, 1884*) (*B*) Male tail. (*After Cram, 1931b*)

on the health of the birds. In such infections the lining of the gizzard may show small local lesions which may also involve the muscular tissue. Soft nodules enclosing parasites may be found in the muscular portion of the gizzard. In heavy infections the wall of the gizzard may be seriously damaged. Le Roux (1926) reported that this parasite may weaken the wall to such an extent as to cause it to rupture, with ultimate formation of a sac or pouch.

TREATMENT. No drugs are thus far known which will affect these parasites in their usual location under the lining of the gizzard or in the muscular tissue.

PREVENTION AND CONTROL. Control measures involve prevention of fowls from eating the intermediate hosts (beetles, grasshoppers, and other insects) and general control measures for arthropods on poultry farms.

AMIDOSTOMIASIS (TRICHOSTRONGYLIDAE)

This disease may be caused by several species of the genus Amidostomum. They localize in the gizzard and inhibit growth and development of infected birds, particularly young birds, causing considerable mortality.

Members of this family are characterized by having reduced or rudimentary mouth cavity, no corona radiata, and usually a well-developed bursa.

Amidostomum anseris (Zeder 1800) (Gizzard Strongyle)

In the United States it has been reported from domestic geese in New York, Delaware, Pennsylvania, and Washington. No doubt this parasite has a much wider distribution than present records indicate.

SYNONYMS. *Strongylus anseris* Zeder 1800 in part; *Amidostomum nodulosum* (Rudolphi 1803) Seurat 1918.

DESCRIPTION. Worms slender and reddish. The short wide buccal capsule has 3 pointed teeth at its base (Fig. 28.17A).

Male 10–17 mm long by 250–350μ wide. Bursa with 2 large lateral lobes and a small median lobe (Fig. 28.17C). Dorsal ray short, bifurcating posteriorly, and the bifurcations forked and terminating in 2 tips. Spicules 200μ long, slender, and cleft near their middle. Gubernaculum slender and 95μ long.

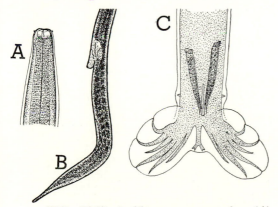

FIG. 28.17—Amidostomum anseris. *(A) Head end. (After Railliet, 1893) (B) Vulva and tail of female. (After Reinhardt, 1922) (C) Male tail. (After Railliet, 1893)*

Female 12–24 mm long, 300–400μ wide at vulva, thinning toward both extremities. Vulva transverse, in posterior part of the body (Fig. 28.17B). Eggs thin-shelled.

LIFE HISTORY. Eggs pass out in the droppings of infected birds in a partly developed stage, active embryos developing within a few hours and hatching taking place within a few days. Susceptible bird hosts become infected by swallowing with food or drinking water these infective larvae. Adult worms are recovered within approximately 40 days after the feeding of infective larvae.

PATHOLOGY. In the United States, Cram (1926a) reported an outbreak of amidostomiasis in a flock of geese in New York in which a large number of deaths occurred. Heavy losses among geese in Europe have been attributed to this nematode. Young birds show symptoms of loss of appetite, dullness, and emaciation. At necropsy the lining of the gizzard of a heavily parasitized bird appears necrotic, loosened, often sloughed in places, and dark brown or black in color in areas adjacent to the site of the worms.

HISTOPATHOLOGY. Bunyea and Creech (1926) found a very noticeable leukocytic invasion of the mucosa propria, with eosinophilic cells strikingly predominant.

DIAGNOSIS. Infected birds cannot, as a rule, be detected by their physical appearance. A general depression and listlessness, accompanied by a partial or complete inappetance, may be the common symptoms following infection. Laboratory diagnosis consists of detecting the eggs in the feces. A postmortem examination of ailing birds for the presence of worms in the gizzard is the most reliable diagnostic method.

TREATMENT. Ershov (1956) has recommended carbon tetrachloride for control of amidostomiasis in domestic geese. The dosage is 1 ml for goslings 21 days old, 4 ml for birds 3–4 months old, 5–10 ml for adults. The dehelminthization process is carried out in a confined area. After treatment the birds are kept in the enclosed area for at least 3 days. The excreta is collected and sterilized or disposed of properly. Following this procedure the birds are transferred to clean quarters while the vacated quarters are thoroughly cleaned and sterilized. At the most, treatment is inadequate and unsatisfactory.

INTESTINAL TRACT

ASCARIASIS (ASCARIDIDAE)

The members of this family are characterized by having 3 prominent lips, valvulated bulb absent, and preanal sucker sometimes present.

Ascaridia galli (Schrank 1788) (Common ascarid of chicken)

This large roundworm is one of the most common nematode parasites of chicken in the United States and elsewhere. It occurs occasionally in turkeys, but no serious pathologic effects have been reported from its presence in that host.

Specimens of this parasite have been recovered on a number of occasions from broken eggs. The worms had presumably wandered up the oviduct from the intestine via the cloaca with subsequent inclusion in the developing egg.

SYNONYMS. *Ascaris galli* Schrank 1788; *Heterakis lineata* Schneider 1866; *Heterakis inflexa* (Zeder 1800) Schneider 1866.

DESCRIPTION. Worms large, thick, yellowish white (Fig. 28.18). Head with 3 large lips.

Male 5–7.6 cm long by 490μ to 1.21 mm wide. Preanal sucker oval or circular,

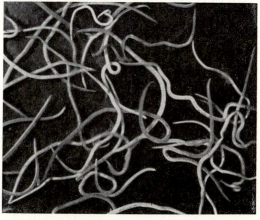

FIG. 28.18—Roundworms (Ascaridia galli) from small intestine of chicken. (Ackert, 1931)

with strong chitinous wall with a papilliform interruption on its posterior rim. Tail with narrow caudal alae or membranes and 10 pairs of papillae. Spicules equal and narrow.

Female 6–11.6 cm long by 900μ to 1.8 mm wide. Vulva in anterior part of body. Eggs elliptical, thick-shelled, not embryonated at time of deposition (Fig. 28.19).

LIFE HISTORY. The life history is simple and direct. According to Itagaki (1928), the infective eggs which are swallowed by the susceptible host hatch in either the proventriculus or the duodenum. Ackert (1931) observed that the young larvae, after hatching from the eggs, live free in the lumen of the posterior portion of the duodenum for the first 9 days, following which they penetrate the mucosa and cause hemorrhages. The young worms have again entered the lumen of the duodenum by the 17th or 18th day and remain there until maturity, which is reached within approximately 50 days after ingestion of the embryonated eggs. Tugwell and Ackert (1952) reported studies which showed that the Ascaridia larvae may enter the tissues as early as the 1st day and remain there as late as the 26th day after infection. The authors stated, however, that the large majority of larvae spend from the 8th to the 17th day in the intestinal mucosa.

Under optimum conditions of temperature and moisture, eggs in the droppings will develop to infectivity in 10–12 days; under less favorable conditions a longer time is necessary. The eggs are quite resistant to low temperatures. Ackert (1931) found that in the early stages of development, eggs survived freezing at $-12°$ to $-8°$ C for 15 hours but not for 22 hours; fertile eggs kept at $0°$ C for 1 month were unable to reach the infective stage subsequently, whereas eggs from the same culture, kept concurrently at $10°$ C for a month, developed normally to the infective stage when incubated at a higher temperature. Farr (1956) recovered *Ascaridia galli* larvae from experimental birds fed embryonated eggs of this worm which had been exposed continuously to outdoor conditions at Beltsville, Maryland, for 66 weeks. As regards high temperatures, 12 hours exposure to $43°$ C proved lethal for eggs in all stages of development.

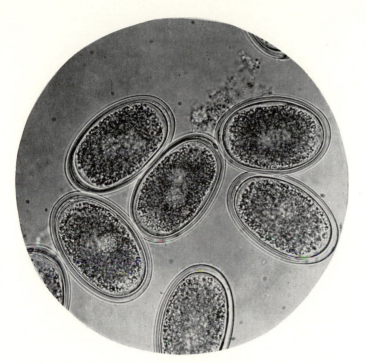

FIG. 28.19—Ascaridia galli *ova.* ×400. (Benbrook, 1928)

PATHOLOGY. Ackert (1940) found that chickens infected with a large number of ascarids suffer from loss of blood, reduced blood sugar content, increased urates, shrunken thymus glands, retarded growth, and greatly increased mortality. Droopiness, emaciation, and diarrhea are the common clinical symptoms manifested by heavily parasitized birds.

IMMUNITY. Experimental evidence is available to show that chickens 3 months or older manifest considerable resistance to infection with *Ascaridia galli*. Ackert et al. (1939) reported that the increased number of goblet cells found in the epithelial lining of the duodenum of chickens at 3 months or older may in some measure be responsible for the greater resistance to this nematode developed by these birds. The age at which the peak of goblet cell formation occurred was found to correspond very closely to the development of maximum resistance of the chickens to the growth of the nematodes.

Ackert and Beach (1933) showed that diets consisting chiefly of animal proteins and with little or no plant protein were important in aiding the chicken to build up resistance to infection with ascarids, and that diets consisting chiefly or wholly of vegetable proteins lowered the resistance to ascarid invasion. Alicata (1938) likewise observed that birds given a diet consisting principally of animal protein concentrates developed fewer worms than those which were given a diet low in animal protein. Diets high in vitamins A and B (complex) have been shown to increase the fowl's resistance to *Ascaridia galli*, and diets low in these vitamins definitely favor parasitism.

Experiments conducted by Ackert et al. (1935), which extended over a period of years and involved 1,351 chickens, showed that the heavier breeds such as Rhode Island Reds and White and Barred Plymouth Rocks were more resistant to ascarid infections than the lighter White Leghorns and White Minorcas.

Large roundworms similar in size and appearance to *Ascaridia galli* occur in the small intestines of pigeons, guinea fowls, wild turkeys, and other game farm species. *Ascaridia numidae* of the guinea fowl and *Ascaridia columbae* (Fig. 28.20) of the pigeon are shorter and somewhat thicker than *A. galli* of the chicken. The guinea fowl ascarid is the smallest of the three species. *Ascaridia dissimilis* (Fig. 28.21) has been found commonly both in domestic and wild turkey of this country and has

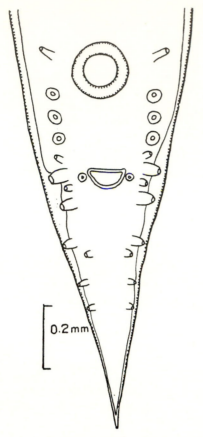

0.2 mm

FIG. 28.20—Ascaridia columbae. *Ventral view of posterior end of male worms showing arrangement of papillae (see Fig. 28.1 for terminology).* (J. Parasitol. *50:134*)

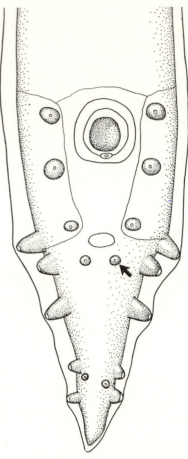

FIG. 28.21—Ascaridia dissimilis. *Ventral view of posterior end of male. Arrow denotes postanal papillae (see Fig. 28.1 for terminology).*

been reported by Vigueras (1931) from domestic turkey in Cuba. This ascarid is very similar in appearance to *A. galli* but is somewhat smaller. The relative position of the second pair of postanal papillae furnishes the most distinctive characteristics in separation of *A. dissimilis* from *A. galli*. They are located close to the anus in *A. dissimilis* but marginally and some distance from the anus in *A. galli* as well as in *A. columbae*. Shillinger (1942) reported *Ascaridia compar* as a parasite of the small intestine of bobwhite quail in the United States.

The life history of all the above ascarids has been elucidated, with the exception of *A. numidae* and *A. compar,* and found to be similar to that of *A. galli.*

PATHOLOGY. Birds heavily infected with

either *A. dissimilis, A. columbae,* or *A. numidae* are probably affected in a similar manner to those heavily infected with *A. galli.*

TREATMENT. Piperazine compounds have been widely adopted as a method of treatment for ascaridiasis. Since they are practically nontoxic, they have almost completely replaced the nicotine compounds which are somewhat toxic.

Bradley (1955) and Shumard and Eveleth (1955) reported that piperazine citrate administered at the rate of 8, 10, and 16 g/gal of drinking water for 1–4 days effectively removed all Ascaridia but not Heterakis.

Horton-Smith and Long (1956) tested

three piperazine compounds (piperazine carbon bisulphide, piperazine adipate, and piperazine citrate) against *A. galli* in chickens and reported that all adult worms were completely eliminated. The compounds were administered as single doses of 100–500 mg/kg body weight.

Colglazier et al. (1960) reported that a single 1-g dose of a 7:1 mixture of phenothiazine and piperazine removed 94% of the Heterakis and 100% of the Ascaridia. Comparable results were obtained against both species with a 0.75-g dose of a 12:1 mixture of the two chemicals.

Edgar et al. (1957) reported that a high percentage of all stages of *A. galli* or *A. dissimilis* larvae were eliminated by the higher concentrations of piperazine in drinking water, which is the most practical method of application for commercial flocks; its use against Heterakis was erratic.

Leiper (1954) pointed out that a high concentration of piperazine in contact with worms at a given time was very important in causing greatest elimination. Therefore, to be most effective, piperazine should be consumed by birds in a period of a few hours. A much smaller dosage administered over an extended period will remove fewer worms. Overnight water starvation seems to assist by bringing a higher concentration of the drug into contact with the worms at one time.

Since piperazine is available on the market as a wide variety of salts, it should be recognized that only the piperazine ingredient has efficacy, and the level should be calculated on the basis of milligrams of active piperazine per bird (Edgar et al., 1957).

None of the piperazine compounds is especially dangerous to the administrator or its recipients. Skin contact over a long period of time may produce a mild irritation, but washing of the exposed areas with copious amounts of water will alleviate the condition.

On Ascaridia these piperazine compounds exert a narcotizing effect, thus enabling the worms to be removed by means of natural peristalsis. The worms are expelled alive and may be seen wriggling if observed soon after expulsion. If the worms are mature and the eggs are well developed, reinfection may occur. Therefore, cleaning and disinfecting the quarters after treatment or removing the birds to clean quarters should be considered if practical.

Thienpont et al. (1966) and Bruynooghe et al. (1968) effectively removed the three common nematodes of the chicken—*Ascaridia galli, Heterakis gallinarum,* and *Capillaria obsignata*—with 40 mg/kg of body weight of dl-tetramisole. Kates et al. (1969) reported that levo-tetramisole given to turkeys naturally infected with *Ascaridia dissimilis, Heterakis gallinarum,* and *Capillaria obsignata* at the rate of 30 mg/kg of body weight was effective in the removal of these worms. However, further experimental work is needed on this and similarly related drugs to establish their usefulness and proper dosage in the control of these parasites.

PREVENTION AND CONTROL. With the advent of large poultry flocks, the whole question of prevention as well as treatment has been changed. Labor costs are high, and in order to curtail expenses it is necessary that more birds come under the supervision of one man.

In certain sections of the country poultrymen, particularly those that are interested in egg production, are switching to cages. When birds are confined to cages, one man can take better care of twice as many birds as when on the floor, and they apparently require less food. The birds are raised on the floor for the first few weeks, or until artificial heat is no longer needed. They are then transferred to grower cages which may accommodate 6–8 birds each. When about 20 weeks old, the birds are placed in layer cages.

Parasite control is often cited as reason for the current shift to cage operation. Undoubtedly this is true in many cases, but parasitism seems to be a problem even in cage birds in certain sections of the country. Worming, if necessary, is done at the time of transfer of birds from grower cages to layer cages. It may also be necessary to treat for worms at the time the birds are taken from the floor and placed into grower cages. The worms no doubt are picked up while the birds are on the floor and carried over when transferred to the grower cages. The worms grow to maturity in these birds, pass eggs, and, in some instances, are picked up by the noninfected birds in droppings from contaminated waterers or feeders.

CECUM

HETERAKIASIS (HETERAKIDAE)

Heterakis gallinarum (Schrank 1788) (Cecal worm of chicken)

H. gallinarum has been reported from the ceca of chickens, turkeys, guinea fowls, bobwhite quail, pheasants, and many other birds.

SYNONYMS. *Ascaris gallinae* Gmelin 1790; *Heterakis papillosa* Railliet 1885; not *Ascaris papillosa* Bloch 1782.

DESCRIPTION. Worms small, white. Head end bent dorsally. Mouth surrounded by 3 small, equally sized lips. Two narrow lateral membranes extend almost entire length of body. Esophagus ending in a well-developed bulb containing a valvular apparatus.

Male 7 mm to 1.3 cm long. Tail straight, ending in a subulate point; 2 large lateral bursal wings. Preanal sucker well developed, with strongly chitinized walls and small semicircular incision in posterior margin of wall of sucker. Twelve pairs of caudal papillae; 4 pairs distinctly postanal, 4 pairs of raylike papillae and 2 pairs of sessile papillae adanal, and 2 pairs of raylike papillae in vicinity of sucker (Fig. 28.22A). Spicules dissimilar, the long one 2–2.17 mm long, the short one 700μ to 1.1 mm long.

Female 1–1.5 cm long. Tail long, narrow, and pointed (Fig. 28.22B). Vulva not prominent, slightly posterior to middle of body. Eggs thick-shelled, ellipsoidal, unsegmented when deposited (Fig. 28.22C).

LIFE HISTORY. The eggs pass out in the feces in an unsegmented state. In approximately 2 weeks or less, under favorable conditions of temperature and moisture, these eggs will have reached the infective stage. When these are swallowed by a susceptible host, the embryos hatch from the eggs and develop to adult worms in the ceca. Roberts (1937) stated that the eggs hatched in the upper part of the intestine, and at the end of 24 hours the majority of the young worms have reached the ceca. Aside from a short period in the cecal mucosa—2–5 days, according to Uribe (1922)—the entire life of the cecal worm is spent in the lumen of the cecum. At necropsy the majority of the adult worms are found in the tips or blind ends of the ceca. Earthworms may ingest the eggs of the cecal worm and may be the means of causing an infection in poultry, as the latter are very fond of earthworms.

PATHOLOGY. Riley and James (1922) observed that the ceca of experimentally infected birds showed marked inflammation and thickening of the walls.

The chief economic importance of the cecal worm lies in its role as a carrier of the blackhead organism, *Histomonas meleagridis*. Graybill and Smith (1920) demonstrated by experimental methods that blackhead may be produced in susceptible birds by feeding embryonated eggs of *Heterakis gallinarum* taken from blackhead-infected birds. These authors were of the opinion that the cecal worms

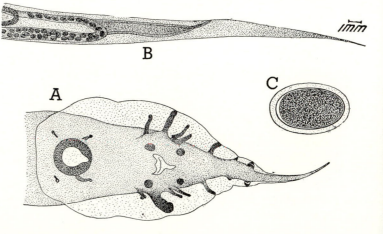

FIG. 28.22—Heterakis gallinarum. *(A) Male tail. (B) Female tail. (After Lane, 1917) (C) Egg. (After Cram, 1931a)*

lowered the resistance of the host to such a degree that the protozoan parasites already present were able to multiply to disease-producing proportions. Tyzzer (1926) presented evidence which indicated that the protozoan parasite is incorporated in the worm egg; however, he was unable to demonstrate the presence of the protozoan parasite within the egg. Kendall (1959) saw organisms which resembled Histomonas in a young larval *Heterakis gallinarum* worm. Gibbs (1962) identified the Histomonas organism in the gut wall and in the reproductive systems of the male and female and in the developing eggs of this cecal worm. Farr (1956) recovered Histomonas organisms from experimental birds fed droppings containing *Heterakis gallinarum* and other nematode eggs that had been exposed continuously on soil to natural weather conditions for 17–66 weeks. Several of the test birds which had been fed this material died of blackhead disease.

Two other species of cecal worms, *Heterakis beramporia* and *Heterakis isolonche,* occur in the ceca of chickens and pheasants respectively. So far as is known, the former species does not occur in birds of the United States. However, the latter species has been found in pheasants in Pennsylvania and Connecticut. Both of these heterakids produce nodules in their respective hosts.

TREATMENT. According to Colglazier et al. (1960), phenothiazine in 1-g doses removed 94% of the heterakids from 5 birds and only 24% of the ascarids; piperazine citrate, given by capsule in single doses containing 200 mg of piperazine, removed 66% of the heterakids and was completely effective against the ascarids. However, single 1-g doses of a 7:1 mixture or a 12:1 mixture of phenothiazine and piperazine removed 94% of the heterakids and 91% of the ascarids. It seems, therefore, that the combination of the two drugs is more effective against these roundworms than either alone.

SUBULURIASIS (HETERAKIDAE)

Subulura brumpti (Lopez-Neyra 1922) (Pinworm)

Several species of the genus Subulura have been reported from birds, but at pres-

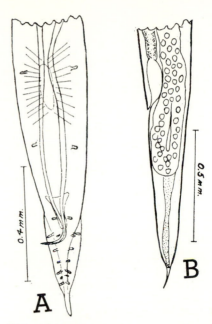

FIG. 28.23—*Subulura brumpti.* *(A) Posterior end of male, ventral view. (B) Posterior end of female, lateral view. (Cuckler and Alicata, 1944)*

ent more information is known about *S. brumpti* than the others. This species has been reported by Alicata (1939) to be a common pinworm of chickens in the Hawaiian Islands. Cram (1926b) and Dikmans (1929) reported this pinworm as occurring in turkey in Puerto Rico. Foster (1939) collected it from fowl in Panama, and Ward (1945) listed it as a parasite of quail in Mississippi (Fig. 28.23).

Another cecal worm, *Subulura strongylina,* has been reported by Venard (1933) from the bobwhite quail in Ohio; by Cram (1927) from the chicken and guinea fowl in Puerto Rico; by Dikmans (1929) from the guinea fowl and by Van Volkenberg (1938) from poultry in Puerto Rico.

SYNONYMS. *Allodapa brumpti* Lopez-Neyra 1922; *Allodapa suctoria* (Molin 1860) Seurat 1914; *Heterakis suctoria* Molin 1860; *Subulura suctoria* (Molin 1860) Railliet and Henry 1914.

DESCRIPTION. Small nematodes with anterior end curved dorsally. Mouth hexagonal, surrounded by 6 weakly developed lips, each with median papillae. Two pairs of larger papillae located dorsally and ventrally; well-developed amphids laterally. Anterior portions of esophageal wall cuticularized, forming 3 teethlike structures. Cephalic alae extending to anterior portion of intestine.

Male 8–10 mm long by 25–31μ wide. Esophagus 0.98–1.1 mm long. Tail curved ventrally and ending in prolongation. Caudal papillae (Fig. 28.23) consist of 3 pairs preanal, 2 pairs adanal, and 5 pairs postanal. Caudal alae narrow and not well developed. Caudal sucker 17–23μ long. Spicules similar and equal, 1.22–1.31 mm long. Gubernaculum 15–19μ long.

Female 12–15 mm long by 35–40μ wide. Esophagus 1–1.3 mm long. Tail straight and conical, ending in sharp point. Vulva anterior to middle of body. Eggs almost spherical, thin-shelled, 82–86μ by 66–76μ, fully embryonated when deposited.

LIFE HISTORY. Eggs pass from definitive hosts in cecal droppings. At this time they contain embryos which are infective to the intermediate host. Beetles (*Alphitobius disperinus, Trilobium castaneum, Dermestes vulpinus, Gonocephalum seriatum, Ammorphorus insulares*), grasshoppers (*Gonocephalus saltator, Oxya chinensis*), and earwig (*Euborella annulipes*) have been reported as intermediate hosts (Cuckler and Alicata, 1944). When the eggs are ingested by a susceptible host, the larvae hatch in 4–5 hours, penetrate the intestinal wall, and enter the body cavity. Further development occurs in the body cavity of the intermediate host. The first larval molt occurs on the 4th or 5th day after infection, and by the 7th or 8th day the larva encapsulates on the intestinal wall. The molt to the second stage occurs between the 13th and 15th days after ingestion, and shortly thereafter the larva contracts in length and coils up within the capsule. It is now in the third or infective stage. When the definitive host swallows an infected intermediate host, the larva migrates to the ceca and proceeds to develop to the fourth stage within about 2 weeks. The final molt takes place on about the 18th day after infection. The young adults continue to grow and develop, and eggs appear in the feces in about 6 weeks after infection (Cuckler and Alicata, 1944).

Abdou and Selim (1957) found the beetles *Ocnera hispida* and *Blaps polycreata* as intermediate hosts of *Subulura suctoria* in Egypt.

PATHOLOGY. Cuckler and Alicata (1944) reported that sections of the cecum showed no evidence of larval penetration or any extensive inflammatory reactions. Cram (1931a) did not observe any noticeable lesions produced by this worm in the ceca of the quail.

CAPILLARIASIS (TRICHURIDAE)

Species of Capillaria inhabit the lumen of the intestinal tract as well as the crop and esophagus. *Capillaria obsignata* is one of the principal ones of poultry in the United States, occurring in the small intestine of domestic and wild pigeon, chicken, and turkey.

Capillaria obsignata Madsen 1945 (Intestinal threadworm)

SYNONYMS. *Capillaria dujardini* Travassos 1915, nec Travassos 1914; *Capillaria columbae* (Rudolphi 1819) of Graybill 1924.

DESCRIPTION. Worms hairlike.

Male 8.4 mm to 1.2 cm long by 49–53μ wide. Cloacal aperture almost terminal, with a small bursal lobe on either side, the two lobes connected dorsally by a delicate bursal membrane (Fig. 28.24A). Spicule sheath with transverse folds; spicule 1.1–1.58 mm long.

Female 1–1.8 cm long by approximately 80μ wide. Vulva on slight prominence, slightly posterior to union of esophagus and intestine (Fig. 28.24C). Eggs slightly brownish, lemon-shaped, thick-shelled.

This hairworm occurs in the small intestine of domestic and wild pigeon, chicken, and turkey in the United States.

LIFE HISTORY. *Capillaria obsignata* has a direct development. The freshly deposited eggs are unsegmented and require 6–8 days to develop completely formed embryos. The embryos do not escape from the eggs until after they have been swallowed by a susceptible host. The larvae enter the mucosa of the duodenum and apparently complete their development there. A few sexually mature adults were removed by the author from the small intestine of a pigeon necropsied 19 days after ingestion of embryonated eggs, and a

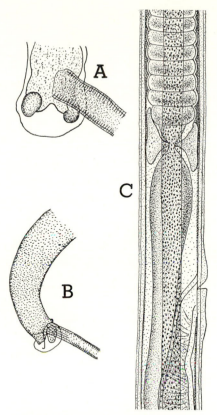

FIG. 28.24—Capillaria obsignata. *(A) Ventral view and (B) lateral view of male tail. (After Graybill, 1924) (C) Region of vulva. (After Eberth, 1863, slightly modified)*

large number of similarly developed adults were removed from the small intestine of a pigeon necropsied 26 days after infection. Fecal examination of the latter pigeon at the time of necropsy showed the presence of eggs.

It has been experimentally demonstrated that pigeons, once infected with *C. obsignata* and held under conditions designed to preclude reinfection, will remain infected for about 9 months.

C. obsignata has been reported from the small intestines of chickens and turkeys raised under natural conditions. Graybill (1924) stated that as a result of many necropsies of chickens and turkeys, this roundworm was never observed in these birds in large numbers. Wehr (1939a) was successful in obtaining natural infections in chickens and turkeys, but no heavy infections were encountered in the latter.

Another threadworm, *Capillaria caudinflata*, has occasionally been found in chickens, turkeys, and pheasants in the United States. This species of capillarid worm may be differentiated easily from other species of the same genus found in poultry of this country by the presence on the male tail of 2 large lateral transparent membranes just anterior to the cloacal aperture, and on the female of a flaplike valvular projection in the region of the vulva. The female of *C. phasianina* is differentiated from the female of *C. caudinflata* by the barrel-shaped valvular appendage and by the very small caudal alae in the male of the former (Kellogg and Prestwood, 1968).

Allen and Wehr (1942) experimentally infected turkeys with *C. caudinflata* by feeding to them earthworms of the species *Allolobophora caliginosa* which were removed from poultry yards in which were confined turkeys known to harbor this threadworm. Morehouse (1944) demonstrated that the above earthworm was an essential intermediate host for the successful transmission of *C. caudinflata* from turkey to turkey. Attempts by Wehr to transmit this threadworm by using species of the earthworm *Eisenia foetida* and *Lumbricus terrestris* were unsuccessful. Wehr and Allen (1945) introduced directly into the alimentary tracts of several earthworms (*Eisenia foetida*) embryonated eggs of *C. caudinflata*, and later adults of this worm were recovered at necropsy from turkeys to which these earthworms had been fed.

PATHOLOGY. Birds heavily infected with *C. obsignata* spend much of their time apart from the rest of the flock, huddled on the ground, underneath the roosts, or in some corner of the room. Such birds show definite symptoms of emaciation and diarrhea. The feathers around the vent frequently appear ruffled and soiled, and the skin and visible mucous membranes are more or less pale. Death is often the result of heavy infections. Levine (1938) reported that the first clinical symptoms of infection in chickens appeared on the 12th day after experimental inoculation of embryonated eggs. At this time the feces contained much pinkish material composed of mucus, necrosed epithelial cells, and numerous erythrocytes, granulocytes, and lymphocytes. From the

12th to the 16th days the feces of the birds were watery and contained large quantities of epithelium and inflammatory exudate which were being eliminated from the intestinal tract. Following this period most of the infected birds regained their normal appearance, and the feces became normal. However, many of the birds lost weight steadily, became extremely emaciated, and either died or were destroyed because of a weakened condition. In fatal and advanced cases of infection, the intestines show extensive destruction of the mucosa, often with complete sloughing of the mucous membrane. The intestines usually contain a large quantity of fluid. In nonfatal experimental cases the intestinal wall is thickened considerably owing to edematous infiltration.

Barile (1912) found these worms in turkeys showing hemorrhagic, croupous enteritis but was unable to state positively whether the worms were responsible for this pathological condition. Baker (1930), in connection with frequent findings of this worm in the province of Quebec, noted that the worms were associated with ulcerous patches varying in size from pinpoint areas to greatly extended and hardened areas. An infected chicken observed by Graham et al. (1929) in Illinois showed weakness, anemia, and emaciation before death. At necropsy the intestine just anterior to the ceca was markedly dilated, with a follicular diphtheritic enteritis present.

TREATMENT. Thienpont and Mortelmans (1962) reported that capillariasis in pigeons and chickens due to *Capillaria obsignata* could be controlled by administration of 1 cc of 10% methyridine solution subcutaneously in the pectoral region or into the leg (pigeon) and dorsal region between the wings (chickens). These authors stated that this drug must be administered with great care as (1) spilling of the drug on the skin may produce a small lesion; (2) nausea, slight ataxia, and incoordination were observed to some degree even with subeffective doses; and (3) death may sometimes result. The drug had no marked effect in coccidiosis and trichomoniasis and was only slightly effective against Ascaridia.

Hendricks (1962, 1963) has shown that methyridine is an excellent drug for the removal of *C. obsignata* from chickens.

The results of recent studies by Wehr et al. (1967) indicated that methyridine injected subcutaneously beneath the wing as a 5% aqueous solution was an effective anthelmintic for the removal of *C. obsignata* from the pigeon. Doses ranged from 23 mg (0.5 ml) to 45 mg (1.0 ml) per bird. There was a slight edema at the site of injection, and a transitory incoordination was observed in some of the treated birds. However, this failure of muscular incoordination disappeared within 2–3 hours and the birds returned to normal. Injections of 35–45 mg methyridine per bird were 99–100% effective against *C. obsignata* in naturally infected birds, but doses of 23 mg per bird removed only 62% of the worms. The anthelmintic action of the drug was relatively rapid, as indicated by elimination of the majority of the worms within 24 hours after treatment.

Clarke (1962), following a number of investigations in the use of haloxon against Capillaria infection in chickens, reported that individual doses of 25 and 50 mg per kg body weight practically eliminated all the worms. However, it was necessary to remove the birds from the infected environment immediately after dosing to prevent reinfection. It was suggested that the most suitable time to treat was immediately prior to movement from the rearing to the laying quarters.

In controlled anthelmintic tests, Colglazier et al. (1967) reported that haloxon was apparently 46–100% effective against *Capillaria contorta* in quail when administered at levels of 0.05–0.5% of the feed for 5–7 days. Results were best at the 0.075–0.5% levels. The highest concentration, however, was toxic, and one-fourth of the birds died. Single oral doses of the drug were not uniformly effective and produced undesirable side effects, primarily ataxia.

The necessity of handling each bird separately for treatment seems to reduce the practicability of these drugs except in cases of a small flock or a few birds.

Hygromycin B has been used extensively in controlling combinations of ascaridiasis, heterakiasis, and capillariasis. It shows greatest efficacy against *Heterakis gallinarum* and may completely eliminate this nematode when fed at the rate of 8–12 g per ton of feed for a period of 2 months or longer. Reductions in worm numbers of *A. galli* and *C. obsignata* are less dramatic, but users have found that continuous use in successive flocks grown in the same house may drastically reduce worm numbers and in some cases improve egg production in layers. Economic benefits which must include drug costs have not been fully demonstrated, but the product has been found most useful in flocks experiencing capillariasis where few other drugs are cleared for treatment or prevention. Hygromycin B has found some acceptance on pen-raised game bird farms where losses due to intestinal nematodes had resulted in severe losses.

Butynorate (dibutyltin dilaurate) sold as one of four constituents in a commercial coccidiostat, has been cleared for use in controlling roundworms as well as tapeworms. Although more costly than new highly efficacious coccidiostats, some broiler producers have continued to use this combination of four drugs because of the supplementary anthelmintic benefits.

ORNITHOSTRONGYLIASIS
(TRICHOSTRONGYLIDAE)

Many worm infections are chronic in nature, but ornithostrongyliasis caused by *Ornithostrongylus quadriradiatus* usually appears suddenly in a highly acute form, with many fatalities. The etiologic agent of this disease normally occurs in the upper part of the small intestine and is a blood-sucking parasite. The disease is common in pigeons of this country.

Ornithostrongylus quadriradiatus (Stevenson 1904) (Pigeon strongyle)

SYNONYMS. *Strongylus quadriradiatus* Stevenson 1904; *Trichostrongylus quadriradiatus* (Stevenson 1904) Shipley 1909; *Cephalostrongylus quadriradiatus* (Stevenson 1904) Irwin-Smith 1920.

DESCRIPTION. Worms delicate, slender, red when freshly collected, apparently from ingested blood in intestine. Cuticle about head inflated to form vesicular enlargement (Fig. 28.25A).

Male 9 mm to 1.2 cm long. Bursa bilobed, with no distinct dorsal lobe. Dorsal ray much shorter than other rays, not extending halfway to bursal margin, bifurcating near its tip to form 2 short tips; a stumpy process present on each side near base of ray. Spicules equal, 150–160μ long, somewhat curved, each terminating in 3 pointed processes (Fig. 28.25B). Telamon 57–70μ long, with 2 longitudinal processes extending backward and forward along dorsal wall of cloaca, and 2 lateral processes forming a partial ring through which the spicules protrude.

Female 1.8–2.4 cm long. Vulva near end

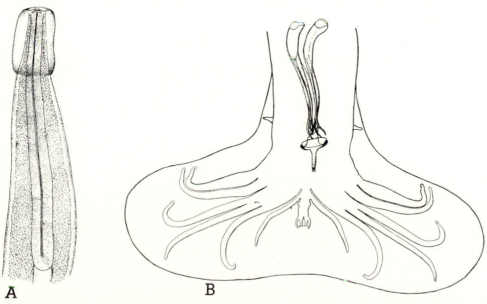

A   B

FIG. 28.25—Ornithostrongylus quadriradiatus. *(A) Anterior end. (B) Caudal bursa of male. (After Stevenson, 1904)*

of tail. Vagina short, followed by 2 powerful muscular ovejectors. Tail tapers to a narrow blunt end, bearing a short spine. Eggs segmenting when deposited.

This bloodsucking nematode occurs in the small intestine of pigeons and mourning doves in the United States.

LIFE HISTORY. The oval, thin-shelled eggs are voided in the droppings and hatch in approximately 19–24 hours under favorable conditions of moisture and temperature. After escaping from the egg, the young larva molts twice within the next 3 or 4 days. It has now reached the infective stage. When the infective larva is swallowed by a pigeon or other susceptible host, it grows to maturity in the small intestine. The female worm begins to deposit eggs in 5–6 days following ingestion of the larva.

PATHOLOGY. Stevenson (1904) observed that this parasite was the cause of many deaths among a flock of fancy pigeons in Washington, D.C. Le Roux (1930) mentioned this roundworm as having caused serious losses in a flock of valuable imported pigeons. Vigueras (1929) reported similar losses among pigeons in Cuba, and Komarov and Beaudette (1931) attributed large numbers of deaths among squabs as having been due to this bloodsucking parasite. These investigators agree that deaths among the birds were attributable principally to a ca-tarrhal enteritis and loss of blood due to hemorrhage.

Birds heavily infected with *Ornithostrongylus quadriradiatus* behave much the same as birds heavily parasitized with other bloodsucking parasites. They become droopy, remain squatted on the ground or floor, and if disturbed try to move but usually tip forward on the breast and head. Food is eaten sparingly and is frequently regurgitated, along with bile-stained fluid. There is a pronounced greenish diarrhea, and the bird gradually wastes away. Symptoms of difficult and rapid breathing usually precede death. The intestines of fatally infected birds are markedly hemorrhagic and have a greenish mucoid content with masses of sloughed epithelium (Fig. 28.26).

TRICHOSTRONGYLIASIS (TRICHOSTRONGYLIDAE)

Two species of nematodes belonging to the genus Trichostrongylus have been described from the ceca of birds—*T. pergracilis* and *T. tenuis*. A study of a large number of these species, however, has revealed that only one species is involved, and that *T. pergracilis* must be considered as a synonym of *T. tenuis*. *T. pergracilis* was originally described from the red grouse in England by Cobbold, and the possibility that he overlooked the description of *T. tenuis* cannot be ruled out.

T. tenuis was reported for the first time in the United States as a parasite of the

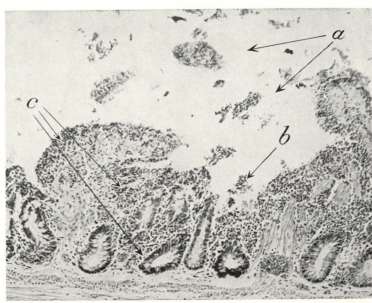

FIG. 28.26—Section of duodenum of pigeon during late stage of infection with Ornithostrongylus quadriradiatus showing (a) sloughing of mucosa, (b) necrotic areas, (c) lymphocytic infiltration. ×150. (After Cuvillier, 1937)

bobwhite quail *Colinus virginianus* by Cram (1925). Since then it has been collected from the pheasant *(Phasianus colchicus)*, blue goose *(Chen caerulescens)*, Canadian goose *(Branta canadensis)*, domestic goose *(Anser anser domesticus)*, guinea fowl *(Numida meleagridis)*, chicken *(Gallus domesticus)*, turkey *(Meleagridis gallopavo)*, and experimentally in other gallinaceous birds.

Trichostrongylus tenuis (Mehlis 1846) (Cecal trichostrongyle)

SYNONYMS. *Strongylus tenuis* Mehlis 1846 (in Creplin, 1846); *Strongylus pergracilis* Cobbold 1873; *Trichostrongylus pergracilis* (Cobbold 1873) Railliet and Henry 1909.

DESCRIPTION. Worms small and slender. Body gradually attenuated in front of genital opening. Mouth surrounded by 3 small, inconspicuous lips. Cuticle of anterior end of body lacking conspicuous striations for a distance of about 200–250μ from extremity, then with distinct serrated appearance for a distance of about 1–2 mm more.

Male 5.5–9 mm long by 48μ wide near center of body. Cuticle inflated on ventral surface just anterior to bursa. Bursa with one dorsal and two lateral lobes, the dorsal one not distinctly marked off from the lateral. Each lateral lobe supported by 6 rays (Fig. 28.27A). The dorsal ray bifid at its distal third, and each of these divisions again bifid and very finely pointed (Fig. 28.27B). Spicules dark brown in color, slightly unequal in length, the longest 120–164μ and the shortest 104–150μ; both much twisted, especially at distal ends, and provided with an earlike structure on proximal end (Fig. 28.27C). Both spicules apparently surrounded in distal two-thirds by a thin membrane extending for a short distance beyond distal ends. Gubernaculum strongly cuticularized along margins, spindle-shaped in ventral and dorsal views (Fig. 28.27D and E).

Female 6.5 mm to 1.1 cm long by 77–100μ wide at level of vulva. Vulva in posterior part of body, with crenulated edges. Uteri divergent. Eggs thin-shelled.

LIFE HISTORY. This worm has a direct life history. The eggs hatch within 36–48 hours after they have been passed in the droppings of the infected bird. The larvae become infective within approximately 2

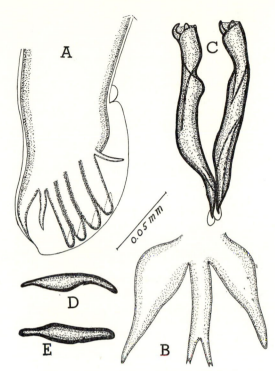

FIG. 28.27—Trichostrongylus tenuis. *(A) Bursa, lateral view, semidiagrammatic. (B) Dorsal and externodorsal rays of bursa showing variation which may occur in length of latter. (C) Right and left spicule, ventral view. (D) Gubernaculum, lateral view. (E) Gubernaculum, dorsal view. (A and B from European partridge, C to E from red grouse. Scale refers to camera lucida drawings B to E inclusive.) (After Cram and Wehr, 1934)*

weeks following expulsion of the eggs in the droppings. Within this time the larvae have molted twice. When the latter are picked up by a susceptible host, the infective larva molts twice more within the ceca of the bird before finally becoming an adult.

T. tenuis from pheasants has been successfully transmitted to domestic turkey, guinea fowl, and chicken.

PATHOLOGY. Cobbold (1873) discovered that *T. tenuis* was associated with the disease which decimated the red grouse population in Scotland. Clapham (1935) stated that typical lesions were noticed in certain birds and a fatal dose was as low as 500 infective larvae. The ceca were distended, and the blood vessels showed congestion. The cecal contents were solid and normal activity ceased. The mucosa of the ceca was inflamed and the ridges were greatly thickened. Symptomatic of severe Trichostrongylus infection are loss of weight and anemia. Cram and Cuvillier (1934) found some evidence that *T. tenuis* can be fatal to young goslings under certain conditions. The trichostrongyles were present in large numbers in the ceca, and the mucosa of the ceca was ulcerated and darkly stained with blood pigments.

Heavy mortality occurs usually in the fall, mainly in the young birds of that year's hatching, and again in the spring. Indications are that these two seasons are not isolated epidemics but rather are the peaks of a disease which continues in a chronic form the entire year.

DIAGNOSIS. A postmortem examination of a diseased bird and the presence of the worm in the ceca is necessary to establish the extent of infection and the damage done. The detection of eggs in the feces is evidence of infection.

TREATMENT. None is available.

STRONGYLOIDIASIS (STRONGYLOIDIDAE)

This disease in poultry is caused by *Strongyloides avium*. Cram (1929) reported the occurrence of this extremely small roundworm from the ceca of chickens in Louisiana. Later (1936b) she reported this species from the ceca and small intestine of chickens in Puerto Rico. The junco *Junco hyemalis* in Virginia and the coot *Fulica americana* in North Carolina have been found to harbor natural infections of this parasite.

Members of this family are characterized by having an alternation of generations, the free-living generation consisting of males and females while the parasitic generation consists of hermaphroditic females only.

Strongyloides avium Cram 1929

DESCRIPTION. Parasitic generation consisting of parthenogenetic females only in intestine of avian host; free-living generation consisting of both males and females, in soil.

Parasitic adult. 2.2 mm long by 40–45μ wide. Vulva with projecting lips, located 1.4 mm from head end. Uteri divergent from vulva; ovaries recurrent in simple "hairpin bends," their course not sinuous.

Eggs with very thin shells, segmenting when deposited.

LIFE HISTORY. The eggs hatch soon after being passed in the droppings, sometimes as soon as 18 hours. The young worms develop in the soil to adult males and females. Shortly thereafter the females give rise to young which feed, molt, and develop into other adult free-living males and females, or they may transform into another type of larvae known as the infective larvae. When these infective larvae are swallowed by a susceptible host, infection results. Unlike most species of nematodes, the parasitic cycle of *Strongyloides avium* consists of females only, no parasitic males having been found.

PATHOLOGY. During the early or acute stage of infection the walls of the ceca are greatly thickened; typical pasty cecal contents almost disappear, the discharge being thin and bloody. If the fowl survives this acute stage, the ceca gradually become functional again, and the thickening of the walls decreases. Young birds suffer most from infections with this worm. If infection is light or the birds are adults, little if any clinical effect has been noted.

PREVENTION AND CONTROL

Preventive measures for the control of poultry roundworms have been developed along the lines of sanitation, hygiene, and management; it is along these lines that the greatest progress has been made.

The proper selection of a permanent site for poultry runs is one of the first essentials to maintenance of health among the birds. The land should be sloping and of a sandy or gravelly nature to provide for proper drainage. If the soil is heavy or the lay of the land is such as to render natural drainage impossible, artificial drainage should be provided. The nonparasitic stages of helminth parasites require moisture for their proper development. Therefore, the presence of surface water, which birds are apt to drink, must be regarded as unhealthful; provisions should be made to eliminate it as soon as possible. Damp places and water holes are ideal breeding places for many of the intermediate hosts of poultry nematodes.

The practice of rotating birds from one area of land to another to reduce parasitism has been followed with reasonably good success in some sections of the country. The four-yard system is most widely advocated and probably best suited for general use. A given area of land—the amount depending upon the number of birds raised—is cross-fenced so that it is divided into four equal lots. The shelter or house is placed in the center of the plot and so constructed that a door opens into each pen. The birds are rotated from one pen to another, keeping them in each pen not longer than 2–3 months. After removing the birds from one of the pens, the ground in that pen may be prepared for planting to some green crop or left undisturbed to undergo self-sterilization by exposing the infected droppings to direct action of the sun, wind, and cold. The planting of the yards to a permanent or temporary crop serves a twofold purpose: (1) It furnishes abundant green food for the growing birds. (2) There is some evidence to indicate that birds are less likely to pick up contaminated soil when plenty of green food is available, thus reducing parasitism in the birds. The house and adjacent grounds should be cleaned as often as necessary to maintain good sanitation. The practice of removing the soil about the house to a depth of 6–8 inches and replacing it with sand or coarse ashes has sometimes been followed. During the summer months, birds spend a great deal of their time in the shade of the house, and it is necessary that extra precautions be taken to improve the sanitary conditions around the house.

Since the source of nematode infection is derived directly from eggs in the droppings or intermediate hosts associated with litter, methods of manure disposal or treatment need full consideration. Cleanout before putting in new flocks may be economically beneficial if heavy worm burdens occurred in previous flocks. (See also Chapter 29 for cestode control.)

The raising of different species of birds together or in close proximity is a dangerous procedure as regards parasitism. Ransom (1921) showed by careful investigations that adult turkeys served as carriers of gapeworms in transmitting gapeworm disease to little chicks and that older chickens were almost entirely insusceptible to infection with this species of worm. Adult turkeys carrying natural infections of gapeworms apparently suffer only slightly, while young chicks and turkey poults suffer very severely from infections with gapeworms.

Tyzzer (1928) established the fact that blackhead occurs in young and old chickens, the latter usually recovering from the disease without suffering a great deal. However, this same investigator also demonstrated that the recovered chickens remained carriers of the blackhead organism for an indefinite period, and that turkeys contract blackhead by exposure to infected poultry or runs occupied by the latter.

It follows from the work of Ransom, Tyzzer, and others that anyone wishing to raise poultry would do well to decide in the beginning to raise turkeys or chickens but not both on the same land or in close proximity to each other. Should a person desire to raise both chickens and turkeys, he should keep them on ranges well separated from one another.

It is dangerous too for turkeys and chickens to associate with guinea fowls. Wehr (1939b) showed experimentally that the guinea fowl is susceptible to infection with the poultry gapeworm *Syngamus trachea* at any age, and that this bird may carry the parasites for as long as 98 days.

Large poultry enterprises which contract production of broilers often require that the grower dispose of any "yard hens." This is a sound management practice since these older birds have frequently introduced parasites into a more susceptible young stock.

✤

ACANTHOCEPHALANS

✤

THE ACANTHOCEPHALA or thorny-headed worms are parasites occurring as adults in the intestinal tract of vertebrates.

In form they are elongate, roughly cylindrical, or spindle-shaped. Several distinct body regions are recognizable: retractile proboscis armed with hooks, a neck, and a body proper. The retractile proboscis always bears a considerable number of recurved hooks arranged in rows. The number, form, and arrangement of the hooks are valuable diagnostic characters. The body proper forms the major portion of the worm. It is usually unarmed but may bear small spines of definite form and arrangement on some portion of the external surface. This group of worms is deprived of a digestive tract. Nutrition is provided for entirely by absorption through the body wall. The sexes are separate in all cases. The male is smaller and more slender than the female and often distinguished externally by a bell-shaped bursa that surrounds the genital pore.

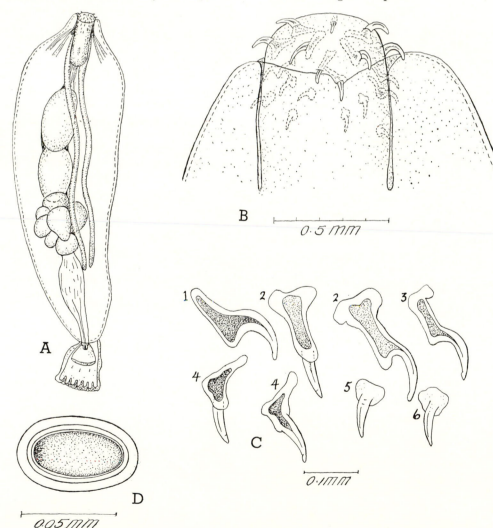

FIG. 28.28—Oncicola canis. (A) Male showing reproductive organs. (B) Proboscis. (C) Hooks from proboscis (numerals indicate row). (D) Egg. (Price, 1926)

So far as known, all species of Acantho-cephala require one or more intermediate hosts before reaching a stage of development where they are infective for the final host. Various arthropods, snakes, lizards, and amphibians serve as hosts of the larval stages of these parasites.

Only three species of thorny-headed worms have been reported as parasites of domestic poultry in North America, two of these as immature forms.

Oncicola canis (Kaupp 1909)

Oncicola canis (Kaupp 1909) was found in about 10% of the young turkeys around San Angelo, Texas, by Price (1929). The worms were encysted under the epithelial lining of the esophagus in numbers varying from a few to 100 or more. They were reported as the possible cause of death (Fig. 28.28).

The adults of this parasite occur in the dog and coyote. The presence of larval forms of this parasite in young turkeys suggests that such occurrences are accidental,

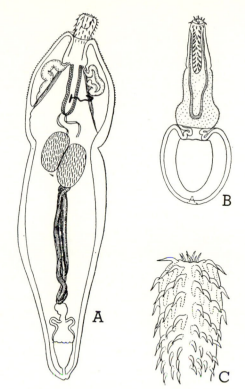

FIG. 28.30—Polymorphus boschadis. **(A)** *Male.* **(B)** *Larva from* Gamarus pulex. **(C)** *Proboscis of larvae.* (Lühe, 1911)

the young worms encysting when taken into an unsuitable host.

Plagiorhynchus formosus Van Cleave 1918

An immature male and two female specimens of *Plagiorhynchus formosus* Van Cleave 1918 were reported by Jones (1928) from the small intestine of a chicken collected at Vineland, New Jersey. Other bird hosts from which this species has been reported are the flicker (Bowie, Maryland), crow (Washington, D.C.), and robin (New Jersey) (Fig. 28.29).

Polymorphus boschadis (Schrank 1788)

Wickware (1922) reported *Polymorphus boschadis* (Schrank 1788) from the duck in Canada. This parasite is reported as causing serious injury and death among domesticated waterfowl, especially in young birds. It causes an inflammation of the intestine with subsequent anemia and cachexia. According to Schlegel (1921), the birds are sick only a short time, the gait is staggering, and the head and wings droop (Fig. 28.30).

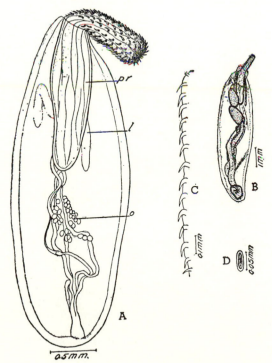

FIG. 28.29—Plagiorhynchus formosus. **(A)** *Young female (l, lemniscus; o, ovary; pr, proboscis receptacle).* (Jones, 1928) **(B)** *Male.* **(C)** *Hooks from proboscis.* **(D)** *Egg.* (Van Cleave, 1918)

REFERENCES

Abdou, A. H., and M. K. Selim. 1957. On the life cycle of *Sublura suctoria,* a cecal nematode of poultry in Egypt. *Z. Parasitenk.* 18: 20–23.

Ackert, J. E. 1931. The morphology and life history of the fowl nematode *Ascaridia lineata* (Schneider). *Parasitology,* 23:360.

Ackert, J. E. 1940. The large roundworm of chickens. *Vet. Med.* 35:106–8.

Ackert, J. E., and T. D. Beach. 1933. Resistance of chickens to the nematode, *Ascaridia lineata,* affected by dietary supplements. *Trans. Am. Microscop. Soc.* 52:51–58.

Ackert, J. E., L. L. Eisenbrandt, J. H. Wilmonth, B. Glading, and I. Pratt. 1935. Comparative resistance of five breeds of chickens to the nematode *Ascaridia lineata* (Schneider). *J. Agr. Res.* 50:607–24.

Ackert, J. E., S. A. Edgar, and L. P. Frick. 1939. Goblet cells and age resistance of animals to parasitism. *Trans. Am. Microscop. Soc.* 58:81–89.

Alicata, J. E. 1938. Studies on poultry parasites. *Hawaii Agr. Exp. Sta. Rept.* (1937), pp. 93–96.

Alicata, J. E. 1939. Preliminary note on the life history of *Subulura brumpti,* a common cecal nematode of poultry in Hawaii. *J. Parasitol.* 25:179–80.

Allen, A. A. 1924. The grouse disease in 1924. *Am. Game Protect. Ass. Bull.* 13:12–14.

Allen, A. A., and A. O. Gross. 1926. Report of the ruffed grouse investigations; Season of 1925–26. *Am. Game Protect. Ass. Bull.* 15:81, 86.

Allen, R. W., and E. E. Wehr. 1942. Earthworms as possible intermediate hosts of *Capillaria caudinflata* of the chicken and turkey. *Proc. Helminthol. Soc. Wash. D.C.* 9:72–73.

Baker, A. D. 1930. The internal parasites of poultry in Quebec. *Sci. Agr.* 11:150–58.

Barber, L. B. 1916. Livestock disease investigations. *Ann. Rept., Guam Agr. Expt. Sta.* (1915), pp. 25–41.

Barile, C. 1912. Sur une espece de trichosome signalee chez le dindon *(Meleagridis gallopavo domestica)* (L). *Bull. Soc. Zool.* 37:126–33.

Benbrook, E. A. 1928. Fecal examination for evidence of parasitism in domestic animals. *Vet. Med.* 23:392–97.

Bradley, R. E. 1955. Observations on the anthelmintic effect of piperazine citrate in chickens. *Vet. Med.* 50:444–46.

Bruynooghe, D., D. Thienpont, and O. F. J. Vanparijs. 1968. Use of Tetramisole as an anthelmintic in poultry. *Vet. Record* 82: 701–6.

Bump, G. 1935. Ruffed grouse in New York State during the period of maximum abundance. *Trans. 21st Am. Game Conf.,* pp. 364–69.

Bunyea, H., and G. T. Creech. 1926. The pathological significance of gizzard-worm disease of geese. *North Am. Vet.* 7:47–48.

Ciurea, I. 1914. Nematodes aus dem Pharynx und Oesophagus des Haushuhnes. *Z. Infektionskr. Haustiere* 15:49–60.

Clapham, P. A. 1934. Experimental studies on the transmission of gapeworm *(Syngamus trachea)* by earthworms. *Proc. Roy. Soc. (London),* Ser. B, 115:18–29.

———. 1935. Some helminth parasites from partridges and other English birds. *J. Helminthol.* 13:139–48.

———. 1950. On sterilizing land against poultry parasites. *J. Helminthol.* 24:137–44.

Clarke, M. L. 1962. Capillariasis in poultry. *Vet. Record* 74:1431–32.

Cobbold, T. S. 1873. The grouse disease. A statement of facts tending to prove the parasitic origin of the epidemic.

Colglazier, M. L., A. O. Foster, F. D. Enzie, and D. E. Thompson. 1960. The anthelmintic action of phenothiazine and piperazine against *Heterakis gallinae* and *Ascaridia galli* in chickens. *J. Parasitol.* 46:267–70.

Colglazier, M. L., E. E. Wehr, R. H. Burtner, and L. M. Wiest, Jr. 1967. Haloxon as an anthelmintic against the cropworm, *Capillaria contorta,* in quail. *Avian Diseases* 11: 257–60.

Cram, Eloise B. 1925. New records of economically important nematodes in birds. *J. Parasitol.* 12:113–14.

———. 1926a. A parasitic nematode as the cause of losses among domestic geese. *North Am. Vet.* 7:27–29.

———. 1926b. *Subulura brumpti* from the turkey in Puerto Rico. *J. Parasitol.* 12:164.

———. 1926c. A parasitic disease of the esophagus of turkeys. *North Am. Vet.* 7:46–48.

———. 1927. New records of distribution of various nematodes. *J. Parasitol.* 14:70.

———. 1928. Nematodes of pathological significance found in some economically important birds in North America. *USDA Tech. Bull.* 49:1–9.

———. 1929. A new roundworm parasite, *Strongyloides avium,* of the chicken, with observations on its life history and pathogenicity. *North Am. Vet.* 10:27–30.

———. 1930. The life histories of some roundworms parasitic in poultry. *Conf. Papers, Fourth World's Poultry Congr.,* Sect. C (Diseases and Their Control), pp. 529–34.

———. 1931a. Internal parasites and parasitic diseases of the bobwhite. Nematodes (roundworms) in quail, pp. 240–96. In Stoddard, H. L. (ed.), *The Bobwhite Quail: Its Habits,*

Preservation, and Increase. Charles Scribner's Sons, New York.

———. 1931b. Developmental stages of some nematodes of the Spiruroidea parasitic in poultry and game birds. *USDA Tech. Bull.* 227:27.

———. 1936a. Species of *Capillaria* parasitic in the upper digestive tract of birds. *USDA Tech. Bull.* 516:27.

———. 1936b. Notes concerning internal parasites of poultry in Puerto Rico. *Puerto Rico Agr. Expt. Sta., USDA, Agr. Notes* 70, May 15. Mimeo. leaves.

Cram, Eloise B., and Eugenia Cuvillier. 1934. Observations on *Trichostrongylus tenuis* infestations in domestic and game birds in the U.S. *Parasitology* 26:340–45.

Cram, Eloise B., and E. E. Wehr. 1934. The status of species of *Trichostrongylus* of birds. *Parasitology* 26:335–39.

Crawford, M. 1940. Infection of adult fowls with *Syngamus trachealis*. *Indian J. Vet. Sci.* 10:293–94.

Cuckler, A. C., and J. E. Alicata. 1944. The life history of *Subulura brumpti*, a cecal nematode of poultry in Hawaii. *Trans. Am. Microscop. Soc.* 63:345–57.

Cuvillier, E. 1937. The nematode, *Ornithostrongylus quadriradiatus*, a parasite of the domesticated pigeon. *USDA Tech. Bull.* 569.

Dikmans, G. 1929. Report of the parasitologist. *Puerto Rico Agr. Expt. Sta. Rept.* 1927, pp. 27–28.

Eberth, C. J. 1863. Untersuchungen ueber Nematoden Wurgh. *Nature Zeitschr.* 3:46–50.

Edgar, S. A., D. C. Davis, and J. A. Frazier. 1957. The efficacy of some piperazine compounds in the elimination of helminths from experimentally and naturally infected poultry. *Poultry Sci.* 36:495–510.

Emmel, M. W. 1939. Observations on *Capillaria contorta* in turkeys. *J. Vet. Med. Ass.* 94:612–15.

Ershov, V. S. 1956. *Parasitology and Parasitic Diseases of Livestock.* State Publ. House, Moscow.

Farr, M. M. 1956. Survival of the protozoan parasite *Histomonas meleagridis*, in feces of infected birds. *Cornell Vet.* 46:178–87.

Fielding, J. W. 1928. Additional observations on development of the eye worm of poultry. *Australian J. Exp. Biol. Med. Sci.* 5:1–8.

Foster, A. O. 1939. Some helminthic parasites recovered from domesticated animals (excluding equines) in Panama. *Proc. Helminthol. Soc. Wash. D.C.* 6:101–2.

Gibbs, B. J. 1962. The occurrence of the protozoan parasite *Histomonas meleagridis* in the adults and eggs of the cecal worm *Heterakis gallinae*. *J. Protozool.* 9:288–93.

Goble, F. C., and H. L. Kutz. 1945. The genus

Dispharynx (Nematoda: Acuariidae) in galliform and passeriform birds. *J. Parasitol.* 31:323–31.

Graham, R., F. Thorp, and R. L. Hectorne. 1929. Capillaria in chickens. *J. Am. Vet. Med. Ass.* 74:1060–63.

Graybill, H. W. 1924. *Capillaria columbae* (Rud.) from the chicken and turkey. *J. Parasitol.* 10:205–7.

Graybill, H. W., and T. Smith. 1920. Production of fatal blackhead in turkeys by feeding embryonated eggs of *Heterakis papillosa*. *J. Exp. Med.* 31:647–55.

Griffiths, H. J., R. M. Leary, and R. Fenstermacher. 1954. A new record for gapeworm (*Cyathostoma bronchialis*) infection of domestic geese in North America. *Am. J. Vet. Res.* 15:298–99.

Hendriks, J. 1962. The use of promintic as an anthelmintic against experimental infections of *Capillaria obsignata* Madsen, 1945, in chickens. *Tijdschr. Diergeneesk.* 87:314–22.

———. 1963. Methyridine in the drinking water against *Capillaria obsignata* Madsen, 1945, in experimentally infected chickens. *Tijdschr. Diergeneesk.* 88:418–24.

Horton-Smith, C., and P. L. Long. 1956. The anthelmintic effect of three piperazine derivatives on *Ascaridia galli* (Schrank, 1788). *Poultry Sci.* 35:606–14.

Hung, S. L. 1926. Pathological lesions caused by *Capillaria annulata*. *North Am. Vet.* 7:49–50.

Itagaki, S. 1928. On the life history of the chicken nematode, *Ascardia perspicillum*. *Proc. Third World's Poultry Congr.* pp. 339–44.

Jones, M. F. 1928. An acanthocephalid, *Plagiorhynchus formosus*, from the chicken and robin. *J. Agr. Res.* 36:773–75.

Kartman, L., Y. Tanada, F. G. Holdaway, and J. E. Alicata. 1950. Laboratory tests to determine the efficacy of certain insecticides in the control of arthropods inhabiting poultry manure. *Poultry Sci.* 29:336–46.

Kates, K. C., M. L. Colglazier, and F. D. Enzie. 1969. Comparative efficacy of levo-tetramisole, parbendazole, and piperazine citrate against some common helminths of turkeys. *Trans. Am. Microscop. Soc.* 88:142–48.

Kelley, G. W. 1962. Removal of *Syngamus trachea*, gapeworm, from pheasants with subcutaneously injected disophenol. *Poultry Sci.* 41:1358–60.

Kellogg, F. E., and A. K. Prestwood. 1968. Case report and differentiating characteristics of *Capillaria phasianina* from pen-raised pheasants of Maryland. *Avian Diseases* 12:518–22.

Kendall, S. B. 1959. The occurrence of *Histomonas meleagridis* in *Heterakis gallinae*. *Parasitology* 49:169–72.

Komarov, A., and F. R. Beaudette. 1931. *Orni-*

thostrongylus quadriradiatus in squabs. *J. Am. Vet. Med. Ass.* 79:393–94.

Lane, C. 1917. *Gireterakis girardi* (n. g., n. sp.) and other suckered nematodes. *Indian J. Med. Res.* 4:754–65.

Leiper, J. W. D. 1954. The piperazine compound v. 19 for the removal of *Ascaris* and *Oesophagostomum* from the pig. *Vet. Record* 66:596–99.

Le Roux, P. L. 1926. Helminths collected from the domestic fowl *(Gallus domesticus)* and the domestic pigeon *(Columba livia)* in Natal. *11th and 12th Rept. Dir. Vet. Educ. Res., Union S. Africa, Dept. Agr.* Pt. 1, pp. 209–17.

———. 1930. Helminthiasis of domestic stock in the Union of South Africa. *J. S. African Vet. Med. Ass.* 1:43–65.

Levine, P. P. 1938. Infection of the chicken with *Capillaria columbae* (Rud.). *J. Parasitol.* 24:45–52.

Lühe, M. 1911. Acanthocephalen. Register der Acanthocephalen und parasitischen Plattwuermer, geordnet nach ihrem Wirten. *Suesswasserfauna Deut. (Bauer)*, Heft 16, pp. 1–116.

Madsen, H. 1945. The species of *Capillaria* parasitic in the digestive tract of Danish gallinaceous and anatine game birds. *Danish Rev. Game Biol.* 1:1–112.

———. 1951. Notes on the species of *Capillaria* Zeder, 1800 known from gallinaceous birds. *J. Parasitol.* 37:257–65.

Morehouse, N. F. 1944. Life cycle of *Capillaria caudinflata*, a nematode parasite of the common fowl. *Iowa State Coll. J. Sci.* 18:217–53.

Olivier, L. J. 1943. The occurrence of *Syngamus trachea* in mature chickens. *Proc. Helminthol. Soc. Wash. D.C.* 10:87.

Ortlepp, R. J. 1923. The life-history of *Syngamus trachealis* (Montagu) v. Siebold, the gapeworm of chickens. *J. Helminthol.* 1:119–40.

Piana, G. P. 1897. Osservazioni sul *Dispharagus nasutus* Rud. dei polli e sulle larve nematoelmintiche della mosche e dei porcellioni. *Atti Soc. Ital. Sci. Nat. Museo Civico Storia Nat. Milano* 36:239–62.

Price, E. W. 1926. A note on *Oncicola canis* (Kaupp), an acanthocephalid parasite of the dog. *J. Am. Vet. Med. Ass.* 69, N.S. 22:704–10.

———. 1929. Acanthocephalid larvae from the esophagus of turkey poults. *J. Parasitol.* 15:290.

Railliet, A. 1893. *Traite de Zoologie Medicale et Agricole*, ed. 2 (fasc. 1).

Ransom, B. H. 1904. A new nematode *(Gongylonema ingluvicola)* parasitic in crops of chickens. *USDA BAI Circ.* 64.

———. 1921. The turkey an important factor in the spread of gapeworms. *USDA Bull.* 939:1–13.

Reinhardt, R. 1922. Handbuch der Gefluegel Krankheiten.

Riedel, B. B. 1951. Group treatment with caricide for ascariasis in poultry. *J. Parasitol.* 37:318–19.

Riley, W. A., and L. James. 1922. Life history and methods of control of the chicken nematode *(Heterakis papillosa* Bloch). *Minn. Agr. Expt. Sta. 30th Ann. Rept.* (1921–22): 70–71.

Roberts, F. H. S. 1937. Studies on the life history and economic importance of *Heterakis gallinae* (Gmelin, 1790; Freeborn, 1923), the cecal worm of fowls. *Australian J. Exp. Biol. Med. Sci.* 15:429–39.

Sanders, D. A. 1929. Manson's eyeworm of poultry. *Florida Agr. Exp. Sta. Bull.* 206:565–85.

Schlegel, M. 1921. *Echinorhynchus polymorphus* Brems., seuchenhaftes Entensterben verursachen. *Arch. Wiss. Prakt. Tierheilk* 47:216.

Schwabe, C. W. 1951. Studies on *Oxyspirura mansoni*, the tropical eyeworm of poultry. 11. Life history. *Pacific Sci.* 5:18–35.

Seurat, L. G. 1916. Sur un nouveau dispharage des palmipedes. *Compt. Rend. Soc. Biol.* 79:785–88.

Sharpe, G. I. 1964. Effects of thiabendazole on *Syngamus trachea* in pheasants. *Nature* 201:315–16.

Shillinger, J. E. 1942. *Diseases of Farm-Raised Game Birds.* USDA Yearbook, pp. 1226–31.

Shumard, R. F., and D. F. Eveleth. 1955. A preliminary report on the anthelmintic action of piperazine citrate on *Ascaridia galli* and *Heterakis gallinae* in hens. *Vet. Med.* 50:203–5.

Stevenson, E. C. 1904. A new parasite *(Strongylus quadriradiatus* n. sp.) found in the pigeon. *USDA BAI Circ.* 47:1–6.

Stoddard, H. L. 1931. *The Bobwhite Quail: Its Habits, Preservation, and Increase.* Charles Scribner's Sons, New York.

Sugimoto, M., and S. Nishiyama. 1937. On the nematode, *Tropisurus fissispinus* (Diesing, 1861), and its transmission to chickens in Formosa. *J. Japan. Soc. Vet. Sci.* 16:305–13.

Swales, W. E. 1933. *Tetrameres crami* sp. nov., a nematode parasitizing the proventriculus of a domestic duck in Canada. *Can. J. Res.* 8: 334–36.

Tanada, Y., F. G. Holdaway, and J. H. Quisenberry. 1950. DDT to control flies breeding in poultry manure. *J. Econ. Entomol.* 46:30.

Taylor, E. L. 1938. An extension to the longevity of gapeworm infection in earthworms and snails. *Vet. J.* 94:327–28.

Thienpont, D., and J. Mortelmans. 1962. Methridine in the control of intestinal capillariasis in birds. *Vet. Record* 74:850–52.

Thienpont, D., O. F. J. Vanparijs, A. H. M. Raeymaekers, J. Vanderberk, P. J. A. Demoen, R. P. H. Marsboom, C. J. E. Niemegeers, K. H. L. Schellekens, and P. A. J. Janssen. 1966. Tetramisole (R8299)—A new potent broad spectrum anthelmintic. *Nature* 209:1084–86.

Travassos, L. 1915. Contribuicoes para o conhecimento de fauna helminthologica brasileira. V. Sobre as species brasileiras do genero *Capillaria* Zeder, 1800. *Mem. Inst. Oswaldo Cruz* 7:146–72.

Tugwell, R. L., and J. E. Ackert. 1952. On the tissue phase of the life cycle of the fowl nematode *Ascaridia galli* (Schrank). *J. Parasitol.* 38:277–88.

Tyzzer, E. E. 1926. *Heterakis vesicularis* Froelich, 1791: A vector of an infectious disease. *Proc. Soc. Exp. Biol. Med.* 23:708–9.

———. 1928. Entero-hepatitis in turkeys and its transmission through the agency of *Heterakis vesicularis*. *Proc. Third World's Poultry Congr.*, pp. 286–90.

Uribe, C. 1922. Observations on the development of *Heterakis papillosa* Bloch in the chicken. *J. Parasitol.* 8:167–76.

Van Cleave, J. H. 1918. The Acanthocephala of North American birds. *Trans. Am. Microscop. Soc.* 37:19–47.

Van Volkenberg, H. L. 1938. Check list of parasites found among principal domestic animals in Puerto Rico. *Proc. Helminthol. Soc. Wash. D.C.* 5:7–8.

Venard, C. 1933. Helminths and coccidia from Ohio bobwhite. *J. Parasitol.* 19:205–8.

Vigueras, P. 1931. Nota sobre Algunos Helmintos de *Meleagris gallopavo*, Econtrados en Cuba, con Descripcionde una Nueva Especie. Habana, Cuba.

Von Drasche, R. 1883. Revision der in der Nematoden-Sammlung des k. k. zoolischen Hofcabinets befindlichen Original-Examplare Diesing's und Molin's. *Verhandl. Zool. Botan. Ges. Wien* (1882) 32:117–38.

Walker, H. D. 1886. The gapeworm of fowls *(Syngamus trachealis)*: The earthworm *(Lumbricus terrestris)* its original host. *Bull. Buffalo Soc. Nat. Sci.* 5:47–71.

Ward, J. W. 1945. A new locality record for five species of helminth parasites of the bobwhite quail. *Proc. Helminthol. Soc. Wash. D.C.* 12:71–72.

Wehr, E. E. 1936. Earthworms as transmitters of *Capillaria annulata*, the "cropworm" of chickens. *North Am. Vet.* 17:18–20.

———. 1937. Observations on the development of the poultry gapeworm, *Syngamus trachea*. *Trans. Am. Microscop. Soc.* 56:72–78.

———. 1939a. Studies on the development of the pigeon capillarid, *Capillaria columbae*. *USDA Tech. Bull.* 679:1–19.

———. 1939b. Domestic fowls as hosts of the poultry gapeworm. *Poultry Sci.* 18:432–36.

———. 1941. Controlling gapeworms in poultry. *USDA Leaflet* No. 207:1–6.

Wehr, E. E., and R. W. Allen. 1945. Additional studies on the life cycle of *Capillaria caudinflata*, a nematode parasite of chickens and turkeys. *Proc. Helminthol. Soc. Wash. D.C.* 12:12–14.

Wehr, E. E., and J. C. Hwang. 1967. Anthelmintic activity of thiabendazole against the gapeworm *(Syngamus trachea)* in turkeys. *Avian Diseases* 11:44–48.

Wehr, E. E., P. D. Harwood, and J. M. Schaffer. 1939. Barium antimonyl tartrate as a remedy for the removal of gapeworms from chickens. *Poultry Sci.* 18:63–65.

Wehr, E. E., M. L. Colglazier, R. H. Burtner, and L. M. Weist, Jr. 1967. Methyridine, an effective anthelmintic for intestinal threadworm, *Capillaria obsignata*, in pigeons. *Avian Diseases* 11:322–26.

Whitney, L. F. 1957. Practical test of the efficacy of piperazine citrate in pigeons. *Vet. Med.* 52:298–99.

Yeatter, R. E. 1934. The Hungarian partridge in the Great Lake region. *Univ. Mich. School of Forestry and Conserv. Bull.* 5:1–92.

CHAPTER 29

CESTODES

❖

EVERETT E. WEHR

Animal Disease and Parasite
Research Division
Agricultural Research Service
United States Department of Agriculture
Beltsville, Maryland

❖

THE CESTODES or tapeworms are flattened, ribbon-shaped, usually segmented worms. As adults they are found principally in the intestines of their hosts. These worms are hermaphroditic and lack both a mouth and an alimentary canal.

The class Cestoda has been subdivided into fourteen orders by Wardle and McLeod (1952). The tapeworms which occur in poultry of this country have been grouped by these authors into one order, Cyclophyllidea. The Cyclophyllidea or taenioid cestodes are, as adults, parasitic chiefly in the higher vertebrates and are of considerable economic and medical importance. These tapeworms are characterized by having a scolex with 4 cup-shaped suckers and with or without a rostellum.

The taenioid cestodes are grouped into a number of families, four of which contain species infecting poultry. The worms of the family Anoplocephalidae possess neither rostellum nor hooks. The proglottids are usually wider than long, and each proglottid contains one or two sets of genital organs. The genital pores are marginal, and the eggs frequently contain "pyriform" bodies. The species *Aporina delafondi* belongs to this family. The family Davaineidae is composed of tapeworms having a scolex with a simple rostellum which is armed with one or more rows of numerous hammer-shaped hooks. The suckers are usually also provided with hooks. Each pro-

glottid contains one or two sets of genital organs. The uterus is persistent and saclike or replaced by either numerous egg capsules or a paruterine body which later becomes transformed into a single egg capsule. Poultry tapeworms of the genera Davainea and Raillietina belong to this family. In the family Dilepididae, the rostellum is usually armed, but the suckers are unarmed. The genital pores are marginal, one or two in each segment. The uterus is saclike or resolved into egg capsules—uterus with or without paruterine body. The poultry tapeworms *Amoebotaenia sphenoides* and *Choanotaenia infundibulum* belong to this family. The Hymenolepididae is characterized by having a scolex with rostellum usually armed with a single row of hooks; the suckers are unarmed. The genital pores are usually unilateral, rarely two in each segment. The uterus is usually persistent and saclike. The eggs are enclosed in three envelopes. The species of poultry tapeworms belonging to the genus Hymenolepis belong to this family.

The species of cestodes parasitizing poultry of the United States belong to four families which may be differentiated by the following key:

1. Head armed with numerous hammer-shaped hooks . . . . Davaineidae
   Head armed with hooks not hammer-shaped, or unarmed 2

2. Testes few, 1 to 4, rarely more . . . .
   . . . . Hymenolepididae
   Testes numerous, more than 4 . . . 3

3. Head lacking rostellum; no paruterine organs in species occurring in poultry . . .
   . . . . . . Anoplocephalidae
   Head with retractile rostellum, usually armed, rarely unarmed; rarely without rostellum; with or without paruterine organs . . . . . . Dilepididae

GENERAL MORPHOLOGY

Structurally, a complete tapeworm consists of a head, neck or growth zone, and a variable number of segments or divisions. The head or scolex of a taenioid tapeworm consists of 4 cuplike organs or suckers which may surround a terminal retractile organ known as the rostellum. Hooks may or may not be found on the rostellum, and deciduous spines often arm the suckers. The number, size, and shape of the rostellar hooks vary as to species, and these variations are used by systematists in differentiating species and even genera of tapeworms. The term "neck" or "growth zone" is applied to the narrowed and unsegmented region located just back of the head and in some cestodes is not macroscopically distinct from the head. The segments or divisions of a tapeworm when taken collectively are generally spoken of as the strobila, and each segment or division as a proglottid. The size, shape, and development of proglottids vary tremendously even in the same individual worm. The anterior segments are usually broader than long and contain few if any recognizable internal organs. Those segments near the middle of the body of the tapeworm may have the antero-posterior diameter proportionately greater than that of the anterior segments. These segments are spoken of as mature segments, since in these proglottids both the male and female reproductive organs are distinctly differentiated. Eggs are not usually found in segments of this part of the body. The terminal or gravid segments are variable in shape and usually contain the uteri and eggs, or only eggs with the uterus either partly or wholly obliterated.

Since tapeworms lack an alimentary canal, food is absorbed through the surface of the body.

A tapeworm grows from the neck backwards, and segments are continually being budded off from the proliferating tissue found in this region. Therefore, the segments farthest removed from the growing region are the oldest from the standpoint of development. The newly formed segment contains no distinguishable organs, while the terminal segments of a completely formed tapeworm may be nothing more than egg sacs. The latter are known as gravid segments and are the ones usually found in the droppings of infected birds.

All adult tapeworms of poultry are found usually in the small intestines of their hosts. However, *Hymenolepis megalops,* the large-headed tapeworm of ducks, occurs in the cloaca and bursa of Fabricius of these birds. Each species of tapeworm usually shows some predilection for a particular portion of the small intestine to which to attach. The species *Hymenolepis carioca,* *H. cantaniana,* *Amoebotaenia*

sphenoides, and *Davainea proglottina* are usually found in the duodenal region of the small intestine; *Raillietina cesticillus,* *Choanotaenia infundibulum,* and *Metroliasthes lucida* in the jejunal region; and *Raillietina tetragona* and *R. echinobothrida* in the distal portion or ileum. However, in heavy infections, tapeworms may be found in portions of the small intestine other than their more normal locations.

Adult tapeworms of poultry differ considerably as to length and number of proglottids or segments. *Davainea proglottina* and *Amoebotaenia sphenoides* are two of the smallest tapeworms found in poultry. Mature specimens of the former species measure up to 4 mm in length and have a range of segments from 4 to 9; those of the latter species reach a length of 2–3.5 mm and possess approximately 30 proglottids. *Raillietina echinobothrida* and *R. tetragona,* on the other hand, are two of the largest tapeworms infecting poultry. Mature specimens of both of these may attain a length of approximately 25 cm and possess large numbers of proglottids.

DEVELOPMENT

In the case of every tapeworm of poultry in which the life history is known, an intermediate host is necessary for completion of the life cycle. Investigations have shown invariably that intermediate hosts of tapeworms have been invertebrates such as beetle, fly, snail, slug, or crustacean. Tapeworm segments are devoured by dung-feeding insects either along with their normal food or because they are attracted to the attention of the invertebrates by their movements.

The type of intermediate host that serves a particular tapeworm in its successful transference from one bird host to another depends to a large degree on the habits of the avian host. In the case of terrestrial birds (chickens, turkeys, guinea fowls, etc.) which deposit their body wastes principally away from ponds and streams, the intermediate hosts must necessarily have to be forms of animal life that lead a terrestrial life, or at least an amphibious one. On the other hand, tapeworms inhabiting water birds (ducks and geese) usually have aquatic invertebrates as natural intermediate hosts.

Invertebrates which serve as intermediate hosts of poultry tapeworms become infected with larval tapeworms by ingesting, along with their food, the free eggs or egg-bearing segments voided by the infected birds. Following ingestion the eggs hatch in the digestive tract; the embryos or larvae penetrate the intestinal wall, enter the body cavity, and after a few days become transformed into small, white, bladderlike, spherical bodies known as cysticercoids (small cysts). These cysts are distinctly visible to the unaided eye when placed in water after removal from the body of the intermediate host. Under proper magnification the head of the tapeworm may be seen near the center of the cyst.

Approximately 3 weeks are required for the embryos to develop into the cysticercoid stage after the eggs have been ingested by the intermediate host. No further development of the tapeworm takes place in the invertebrate host. The cysticercoids may remain alive in the invertebrate host and infective to the bird host for many months.

Poultry become infected with tapeworms by swallowing insects, snails, slugs, and other forms of animal life that may serve as intermediate hosts of these parasites. The cysticercoid is freed from the body of the intermediate host by the action of the digestive juices. Soon after the cysticercoid is liberated, the head evaginates and becomes attached to the intestinal wall. New segments or proglottids begin to form immediately at the neck region, and within approximately 3 weeks a mature tapeworm is formed. The entire life cycle, therefore, takes about 6 weeks for completion; under unfavorable conditions a longer period of time may be necessary.

IMPORTANCE

Chickens in this country may be infected with one to as many as seven species of tapeworms. With the exception of one or two of these species, all are of common occurrence. A few years ago the list of intermediate hosts of poultry tapeworms was small, but investigations within the last few years have been responsible for an alarming increase in the number of invertebrate intermediate hosts that tapeworms of poultry may utilize for the development of their larvae.

Control of poultry tapeworms involves treatment for removal of the tapeworms themselves and reduction of the numbers of intermediate hosts by sanitary measures. Since treatment of fowl taeniasis is still in an unsatisfactory state, sanitation has almost wholly been relied upon to prevent tapeworm infection. This method of control involves primarily the proper disposal of poultry manure containing eggs of tapeworms so that intermediate hosts cannot become infected with the larval stages of these parasites. Many of the intermediate hosts are flying insects, and once the latter have become infected with larval tapeworms they may be responsible for the spread of the disease to distant flocks. Recent investigations have indicated that clean birds held in close proximity to infected birds will invariably become infected with tapeworms within a relatively short time.

Table 29.1 lists the species of tapeworms found in poultry of this country, with their primary and secondary hosts, usual location, and kinds of poultry affected.

CLASSIFICATION

The tapeworms of poultry belong to the general group designated as taenioid cestodes, which are characterized primarily by the presence of 4 cup-shaped suckers on the head. The following key will aid in the differentiation of the genera of tapeworms found in poultry of this country:

1. Rostellum absent 2
   Rostellum present 3

2. Paruterine organ present . Metroliasthes
   Paruterine organ absent . . . Aporina

3. Mature worms small, usually not longer than 4–5 mm 4
   Mature worms large, longer than above . 5

4. Strobila consisting of 2–9 segments . . .
   . . . . Davainea
   Strobila consisting of numerous segments .
   . . . . Amoebotaenia

5. Testes 3 in number 6
   Testes more than 3 in number . . . 7

6. With a well-developed pseudo-holdfast organ, in addition to a small, true holdfast organ, containing no genital primordia . .
   . . . . Fimbriaria
   With only a true holdfast organ . . . .
   . . . . Hymenolepis

7. Rostellum armed with a single row of 16–20 hooks, each 20–30μ long . Choanotaenia
   Rostellum armed with either a single row or double row of 100 or more hooks, each 6–15μ long . . . . . Raillietina

TABLE 29.1   Tapeworms and Hosts from Poultry in United States

Tapeworms	Location	Intermediate Hosts	Definitive Hosts
Davainea proglottina	Duodenum	Slugs, snails	Chicken
Davainea meleagridis	Duodenum	Unknown	Turkey
Amoebotaenia cuneata	Duodenum	Earthworms	Chicken, turkey
Hymenolepis carioca	Duodenum	Stable fly Dung beetles	Chicken, turkey Bobwhite quail
Hymenolepis cantaniana	Duodenum	Beetles	Chicken, turkey Peafowl Bobwhite quail
Raillietina cesticillus	Jejunum	Beetles	Chicken, turkey Guinea fowl Bobwhite quail Gray jungle fowl
Choanotaenia infundibulum	Jejunum	Housefly, beetles	Chicken, turkey
Raillietina tetragona	Ileum	Ants	Chicken, turkey Guinea fowl, peafowl Bobwhite quail
Raillietina echinobothrida	Ileum	Ants	Chicken, turkey
Metroliasthes lucida	Ileum	Grasshoppers	Turkey, chicken Guinea fowl
Hymenolepis compressa	Intestine	Unknown	Duck, goose
Hymenolepis introversa	Intestine	Unknown	Duck
Hymenolepis megalops	Cloaca and bursa of Fabricius	Unknown	Duck
Hymenolepis tritesticulata	Intestine	Unknown	Duck
Hymenolepis coronula	Small intestine	Crustaceans Snails	Duck
Hymenolepis lanceolata	Small intestine	Crustaceans	Goose
Hymenolepis tenuirostris	Small intestine	Crustaceans Crayfish	Duck, goose
Raillietina magninumida	Small intestine	Beetles	Guinea fowl, chicken, turkey
Raillietina ransomi	Small intestine	Unknown	Wild turkey
Raillietina williamsi	Small intestine	Unknown	Wild turkey
Raillietina georgiensis	Small intestine	Ants	Wild turkey Domestic turkey
Aporina delafondi	Small intestine	Unknown	Pigeon
Fimbriaria fasciolaris	Small intestine	Water flea	Chicken

DESCRIPTIONS

The various species of poultry tapeworms will be listed and described according to family. The common names of most of the tapeworms listed in this chapter have been supplied, but in a few cases they are not known.

AMOEBOTAENIASIS (DILEPIDIDAE)

Members of the family Dilepididae are characterized by having a single set of reproductive organs in each proglottid. The uterus is saclike and more or less lobed or reticulate. Paruterine bodies are present or absent.

Amoebotaenis cuneata (Linstow 1872) (Wedge-shaped tapeworm of poultry)

This tapeworm, which usually occurs in the duodenal region of the small intestine, is apparently not a common parasite of poultry in the United States. It has been reported from chickens in Texas by Adams and Geiser (1933), in Kansas by Ferry (1934), in Tennessee by Todd (1946), in

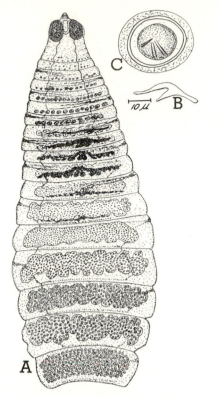

FIG. 29.1—Amoebotaenia cuneata. (A) Entire worm. (Monnig, 1926) (B) Rostellar hook. (C) Egg.

Alabama by Edgar (1956); and from chickens and turkeys in Michigan by Stafseth (1940).

SYNONYMS. *Taenia cuneata* von Linstow 1872, not Batsch 1786; *Taenia sphenoides* Railliet 1892; *Dicranotaenia sphenoides* (Railliet 1892) Railliet 1896.

DESCRIPTION. Mature worms 2–3.5 mm long, triangular or roughly fusiform in shape (Fig. 29.1A). Suckers unarmed; rostellum armed with single row of 12–14 hooks, 25–32μ long (Fig. 29.1B). Genital pores usually regularly alternate, located at extreme anterior point of segment margin. Testes 12–15 in number, usually in a transverse row across posterior part of segment. Eggs (Fig. 29.1C) not contained in capsules.

LIFE HISTORY. The intermediate host of this tapeworm is the earthworm. The earthworms *Eisenia (Helodrilus) foetida, Pheretina pequana, Ocnerodrilus (Ilyogenia) africanus,* and *Allolobophora chloritica* have

been found to serve as intermediate hosts. Mönnig (1926) grew the cysticercoids in earthworms *(Ocnerodrilus [Ilyogenia] africanus)* in 14 days. Four weeks were then required for the cysticercoids to develop into adult tapeworms in chickens. Cysticercoids from earthworms were identified as this species by Grassi and Rovelli (1889) and Meggitt (1916). Chickens become infected by eating earthworms which carry the infective larvae or cysticercoids of this cestode parasite.

PATHOLOGY. The damage done by this tapeworm is comparatively slight, according to Meggitt (1926). However, deaths in poultry due to this parasite have been reported.

CHOANOTAENIASIS (DIEPIDIDAE)

Choanotaenia infundibulum (Bloch 1779) (Funnel-shaped tapeworm of poultry)

This species may be readily distinguished from other poultry tapeworms by the rostellum, which is armed with a single row of relatively few and very large hooks, and bipolar egg filaments.

This cestode inhabits principally the jejunal region of the small intestine of chickens and turkeys and is widely distributed among these birds in the United States.

SYNONYMS. *Taenia infundibulum* Bloch, 1779; *Drepanidotaenia infundibuliformis* (Goeze, 1782) Railliet, 1893; *Choanotaenia infundibuliformis* (Goeze, 1782) Railliet, 1896.

DESCRIPTION. Mature worms attain a length of 23 cm. Suckers unarmed (Fig. 29.2A); rostellum armed with a single row of 16–20 hooks (occasionally 22) 20–30μ long (Fig. 29.2B). Genital pores irregularly alternate. Testes 25–40, occasionally as many as 55–60, grouped in posterior part of segment (Fig. 29.2C). Eggs with elongated filaments, not contained in capsules (Fig. 29.2D).

LIFE HISTORY. Birds become infected with adults of *C. infundibulum* by eating houseflies, grasshoppers, and several species of beetles. Cysticercoids have been found in houseflies and in some species of beetles as natural infections, and also after the insects have been fed eggs of this tapeworm. Horsfall and Jones (1937) reported that at a

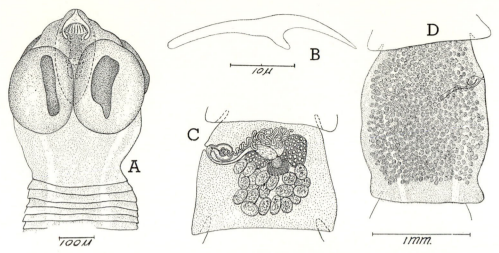

FIG. 29.2–Choanotaenia infundibulum. **(A)** *Scolex.* **(B)** *Rostellar hook.* **(C)** *Mature segment.* **(D)** *Gravid segment.* (Ransom, 1905)

temperature of 75–90° F, 17–20 days is the minimum time for development of the cysticercoids to the infective stage in the grasshopper *Melanoplus femurrubrum.* At a temperature of 60–75° F, 48 days is the minimum time for development of the cysticercoids in the beetle *Aphodius granarius.* The adult worm in the chicken requires 2–3 weeks for development to maturity.

PATHOLOGY. Probably similar to *R. cesticillus.*

METROLIASTHIASIS (DILEPIDIDAE)

Metroliasthes lucida Ransom 1900 (Transparent tapeworm of poultry)

This species is a very common tapeworm of turkeys in this country. It was reported from a chicken by Ransom (1905), but he evidently doubted the validity of the host record since he stated that the occurrence of *Metroliasthes lucida* in chickens is doubtful. However, the occurrence of this species in chickens has been reported more recently by Rietz (1930) from West Virginia, by Southwell (1921) from India, and by Schwartz (1925) from South Africa. It is readily recognized by the large unarmed head and the prominent spherical egg capsule, which is easily seen in the posterior part of each of the transparent segments in the posterior part of the body.

DESCRIPTION. Mature worms about 20 cm long. Suckers unarmed, rostellum lacking

(Fig. 29.3A). Genital pores irregularly alternate, near middle of or in gravid segments, definitely posterior to middle of segment margin. Uterus, when fully developed, consists of 2 sacs lying side by side very close together in posterior part of segment (Fig. 29.3D). Paruterine organ, a conical structure, develops anterior to uterus, eventually becoming a heavy-walled egg capsule for retention of eggs (Fig. 29.3E).

LIFE HISTORY. Cysticercoids were obtained by Jones (1930b) from grasshoppers several weeks after feeding them gravid segments of *M. lucida;* both laboratory-bred grasshoppers and those collected in the field became infected. Jones (1936a) infected turkeys and guinea fowls with *M. lucida* by feeding them cysticercoids from grasshoppers (*Melanoplus* species, *Chorthippus curtipennis,* and *Paroxya clavuliger*); chicks and quail remained negative for tapeworms after being fed cysticercoids of *M. lucida* from grasshoppers or beetles. The time required for development of cysticercoids in the insect host varies from 2 to 6 weeks. Approximately 3 weeks are required for development of the adult worm to maturity in the avian host.

PATHOLOGY. Probably similar to that of *R. cesticillus.*

DAVAINIASIS (DAVAINEIDAE)

Tapeworms of the family Davaineidae have a scolex with a simple rostellum which

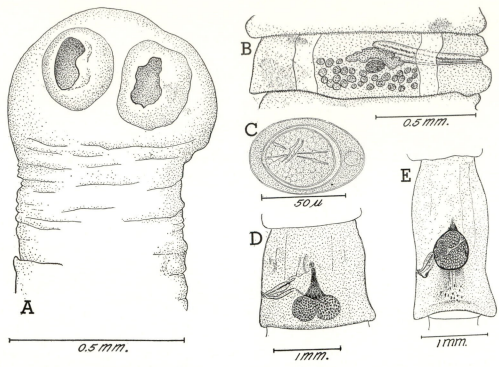

FIG. 29.3—Metroliasthes lucida. *(A)* Scolex. *(B)* Mature segment. *(C)* Egg. *(D)* Segment showing two-part uterus and developing paruterine organ. *(E)* Gravid segment. (Ransom, 1900)

is armed with one or more rows of numerous hammer-shaped hooks. The suckers may be armed or unarmed. One or two sets of reproductive organs may be present in each segment. The uterus is persistent and saclike, or replaced either by numerous egg capsules or by a paruterine body transforming later into a single egg capsule.

Davainea proglottina (Davaine 1860) (Tonguelike tapeworm of poultry)

In the United States this tapeworm has not been found to be as cosmopolitan in distribution as some of the other cestodes of poultry, being found chiefly in the moister parts. It has been reported from both eastern and western coastal states and from Tennessee and Alabama.

SYNONYM. *Taenia proglottina* Davaine 1860.

DESCRIPTION. Mature worms attain a length of about 4 mm (Fig. 29.4A). The strobila consists of 2–5 segments, rarely as many as 9. Each succeeding segment gradually increases in length and breadth, the last segment often being larger than the remainder of the parasite. Suckers armed with 3–6 rows of small hooklets, 5–8μ long. Genital pores usually regularly alternate, located at extreme anterior point of segment margin. Testes 12–21 in number (Fig. 29.4B). One egg in each egg capsule.

LIFE HISTORY. Cysticercoids of this tapeworm develop in approximately 3 weeks in several species of snails and slugs. Levine (1938) experimentally infected the garden slug (*Agriolimax agrestis*) with cysticercoids of *D. proglottina* and in turn infected chickens by feeding them garden slugs containing mature cysticercoids. When infected slugs or snails are eaten by chickens, the infective larva or cysticercoid develops to the adult worm with 4 segments in approximately 8 days.

PATHOLOGY. This tapeworm has been considered to be one of the obviously dangerous tapeworms of poultry. It has been observed that infected birds become emaci-

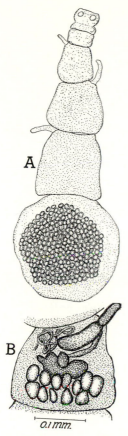

FIG. 29.4—Davainea proglottina. *(A)* Entire worm, with eggs in last segment. *(B)*
Mature segment. *(Meggitt, 1926)*

DESCRIPTION. Mature specimens up to 5 mm
long, composed of 17–22 segments. Suckers
armed with 4–6 rows of hooklets, the longest about 5μ long; rostellum with a double
row of about 100–130 hooks, 8–10μ long.
Genital pores usually regularly alternate,
located in extreme anterior point of segment margin. Testes 20–26 in number, in
posterior half of segment. One egg in each
capsule.

LIFE HISTORY. Unknown.

PATHOLOGY. Unknown.

RAILLIETINIASIS (DAVAINEIDAE)

Raillietina cesticillus (Molin 1858) (Broad-headed tapeworm of poultry)

The most distinctive feature of this tapeworm is the unusually broad and flattened
rostellum, with 2 rows of hooks near its
base.

This cestode is probably one of the most
common species occurring in poultry. It
is a rather large species, and its habitat is
the duodenal and jejunal regions. Southwell (1930) reported *R. cesticillus* from *Gallus sonnerati*, the gray jungle fowl, in the
Zoological Gardens of Calcutta.

SYNONYMS. *Taenia cesticillus* Molin 1858;
Raillietina cesticillus (Molin 1858) Joyeux
1923.

DESCRIPTION. Mature worms may attain a
length of 12 cm. Suckers unarmed; rostellum armed with 2 rows of hooks, about
300–500 in number (Fig. 29.5A and B).
Genital pores irregularly alternate, located
anterior to middle of segment margin. Testes 16–30 in number, in posterior part of
segment (Fig. 29.5C). Uterus divided into
egg capsules, each capsule containing a
single egg.

LIFE HISTORY. Birds become infected with
R. cesticillus after being fed various infected ground beetles and dung beetles. Cysticercoids have been observed in such beetles
as *Anisotarsus* spp., *Amara* spp., *Anaferonia*
spp., *Harpalus* spp., *Pterostichus* spp., and
other ground and dung beetles after they
have been given experimental feedings of
gravid segments of *R. cesticillus;* they also
have been observed in natural infections

ated and dull and lose weight, the plumage
becomes dry and ruffled, the movements
become slow, and the breathing becomes
rapid. At necropsy the intestinal mucosa
appears thickened, which may be hemorrhagic, and the intestine may contain a
large quantity of mucus which tends to be
fetid. Crawley (1922) has reported this
worm as killing chickens in Pennsylvania.
Rietz (1930) has reported paralysis associated with the presence of this worm. However, the true relationship of leg weakness
to this disease is still unknown.

Davainea meleagridis Jones 1936 (Turkey tapeworm)

This parasite was described from the duodenum of the domestic turkey by Jones
(1936b) in the vicinity of Washington,
D.C., and from the wild turkey by Gardiner
and Wehr (1949) in Maryland.

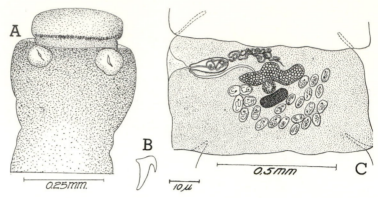

FIG. 29.5—Raillietina cesticillus. *(A) Head. (B) Hook from rostellum. (C) Mature segment. (Ransom, 1905)*

in some of these beetles. Larvae in beetles apparently require 2–4 weeks to develop to a stage infective for chickens. Adult worms in primary host usually require 2–3 weeks to develop to maturity.

PATHOLOGY. This worm has been reported to cause degenerations and inflammations of the villi of the intestine at the point of attachment by the rostellum. Heavy infections in young birds may cause emaciation. However, Stoddard (1931) noted no serious inflammation of the intestinal walls, nor was stoppage of the intestines found to result from the presence of the worms in quail. Ackert and Reid (1937) and Ackert (1932) demonstrated experimentally that chickens 2½–5 months of age are more resistant to infection with this species of tapeworm than younger birds, and that a reduction in the blood sugar and hemoglobin contents of the blood resulted from such infections. Harwood and Luttermoser

(1938) reported that growth rates of Rhode Island Red and White Leghorn chicks were retarded by infections with *R. cesticillus.*

Raillietina echinobothrida (Megnin 1881) (Spiny-headed or nodular tapeworm of poultry)

Raillietina echinobothrida is apparently widely distributed among poultry.

SYNONYMS. *Taenia echinobothrida* Megnin 1881; *Raillietina echinobothrida* (Megnin 1881) Fuhrmann 1924.

DESCRIPTION. Mature specimens measure up to 25 cm long. Suckers armed with 8–15 rows of hooks, 5–15μ long; rostellum armed with 2 rows of 200–240 hooks, 10–14μ long (Fig. 29.6A,C). Genital pores almost unilateral or definitely irregularly alternate, located at middle or usually posterior to middle of segment margin (Fig. 29.6B). Testes 20–30, occasionally as many

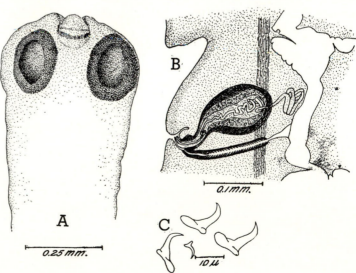

FIG. 29.6—Raillietina echinobothrida. *(A) Scolex. (B) Section through region of genital pore showing cirrus pouch and part of vagina. (Lang, 1929) (C) Hooks from suckers.*

as 45 in number. Uterus ultimately forming egg capsules, each capsule usually containing a single egg. Posterior segments of
strobila frequently becoming constricted
longitudinally through median line to
form windows in the center of the segments. However, this appearance of the
gravid segments is not constant in all specimens.

LIFE HISTORY. Jones and Horsfall (1935)
reported that the ants *Tetramorium
caespitum* and *Pheidole vinelandica* naturally harbored bladder worms or cysticercoids of *R. echinobothrida* and also those
of another closely related species *Raillietina tetragona*. The cysticercoids of the
two species were fed to laboratory-reared
chickens. Three weeks after ingesting the
cysticercoids, adults of the two species of
tapeworms were recovered postmortem
from the experimentally fed birds; the
controls were negative. All attempts to
produce experimental infections in ants
were unsuccessful. Large numbers of un-
dissected ants collected from infected poultry runs were fed to 23 chickens; 19 of the
chickens later became infected. Joyeux
and Baer (1937) reported finding cysticercoids of *R. echinobothrida* in naturally in-

fected ants *(Tetramorium semileave)* in the
region of Marseilles, France.

PATHOLOGY. This worm causes the formation of tubercles on the intestinal wall of
infected birds (Fig. 29.7). This condition
resembles tuberculosis and therefore must
be differentiated from that disease.

Gage and Opperman (1909) reported
losses of 50% in affected flocks in Maryland. They noted emaciation and a mucoid diarrhea as early symptoms, and later
listlessness, loss of appetite, and a tendency to huddle; some birds are weak and
epileptic. Death comes suddenly, accompanied by convulsions.

Raillietina tetragona (Molin 1858) (Four-gonad or oval-suckered tapeworm of poultry)

This worm is morphologically very similar to *Raillietina echinobothrida*. It is of
common occurrence but is rarely associated with the distinct tuberculosislike lesions produced by *R. echinobothrida*.

SYNONYMS. *Taenia tetragona* Molin 1858;
Raillietina tetragona (Molin 1858) Joyeux
1927.

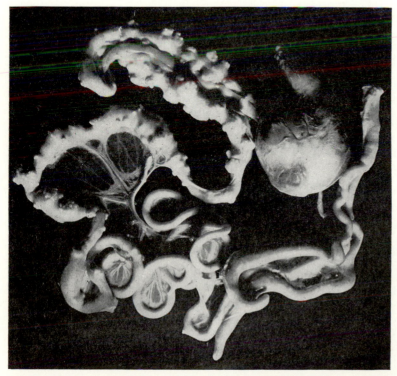

FIG. 29.7—*Nodular disease
of intestine of chicken
caused by tapeworms* Raillietina echinobothrida. *(After Bushnell and Brandly,
1929)*

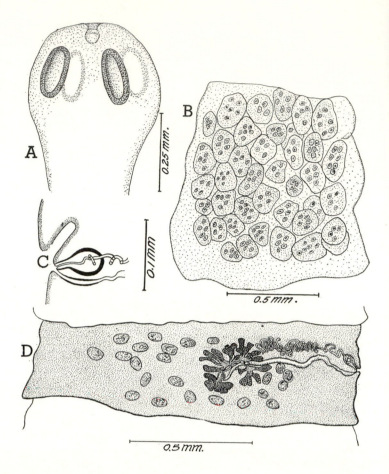

FIG. 29.8—Raillietina tetragona. *(A) Scolex. (B) Gravid segment. (C) Pore region showing cirrus pouch and vagina. (After Lang, 1929) (D) Mature segment. (After Ransom, 1905)*

DESCRIPTION. Worms measure as much as 25 cm long. Suckers armed with 8–12 rows of small hooks, 3–8μ long; rostellum armed with about 90–130 hooks, 6–8μ long, arranged in 1 or 2 rows (Fig. 29.8A). Genital pores usually unilateral, rarely irregularly alternate, located anterior to middle of segment margin. Testes 18–35 in number (Fig. 29.8D). Uterus eventually breaks up into egg capsules, 6–12 eggs in each capsule (Fig. 29.8B).

LIFE HISTORY. See life history of *R. echinobothrida*.

PATHOLOGY. Lopez-Neyra (1931) reported a single case in which he found small nodules in the intestine due to this species. In quail, Stoddard (1931) observed that this species may be the principal or only cause of death in cases of heavy infections. Of 25 birds, the deaths of which were attributed to infection with this species, the youngest was 17 days old and the oldest 60 days; the greatest mortality occurred between the ages of 25 and 40 days. Although many birds may recover if they survive to 2 months of age, they are almost certain to be undersized. Quail heavily infected with specimens of this tapeworm almost invariably have their crops and gizzards filled with food. That portion of the intestine occupied by these tapeworms sometimes becomes so distended that it is reduced to nearly one-half its length, being thrown into ridges of a purplish red color. The lining of the intestine frequently sloughs off in cases of heavy infections. In several instances Stoddard observed that bobwhites heavily infected with this species moved with difficulty, a partial paralysis being evident.

Raillietina magninumida Jones 1930 (Large guinea fowl tapeworm)

This tapeworm is a common parasite of guinea fowl in the United States. Hudson (1934) considered *R. magninumida* as a

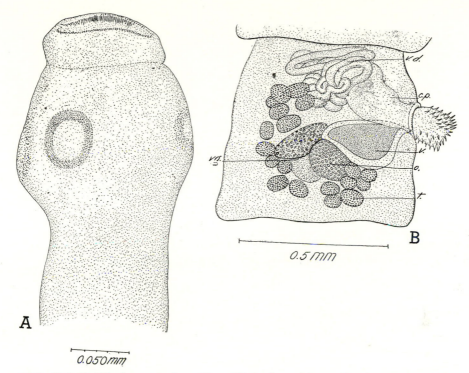

FIG. 29.9—Raillietina magninumida. *(A) Scolex with rostellum extended. (B) Mature segment (c.p., cirrus pouch; o., ovary; t., testes; v., vagina; f.g., vitelline gland; v.d., vas deferens).*

synonym of *R. numida* (Fuhrmann 1912). The latter species occurs in the guinea fowl of Africa.

SYNONYM. *Raillietina (Paroniella) magninumida* Jones 1930.

DESCRIPTION. Mature worms about 6–15 cm long. Suckers armed with about 10 rows of hooks, the largest 7–8μ long; rostellum armed with 2 rows of about 150–170 hooks, 8–11μ long (Fig. 29.9A). Genital pores unilateral. Testes 12–20 in number (Fig. 29.9B). Egg capsules containing 1 egg each.

LIFE HISTORY. Guinea fowl become infected with this species by ingesting beetles carrying cysticercoids of this tapeworm. Cysticercoids have been found in beetles both as a result of experimental feeding of gravid tapeworm segments and in natural infections. Approximately 3 weeks are required for the larva to develop to the infective stage in the beetle, and 3 weeks more are necessary for the cysticercoid to develop to the adult form in the guinea fowl.

PATHOLOGY. Adult birds seem little affected by this species, but younger birds appear to be considerably weakened by heavy infections. Detailed pathology of this species has not been studied.

Raillietina ransomi (Williams 1931) (Ransom tapeworm of poultry)

This species of tapeworm was reported by Williams (1931) and Wehr and Coburn (1943) from the eastern wild turkey.

SYNONYM. *Davainea ransomi* Williams 1931.

DESCRIPTION. Mature worms from 4 mm to 1.4 cm long by 650μ to 1.14 mm wide. Total number of segments varying from 24 to 61, usually between 30 and 40. Suckers unarmed, round or slightly oval, 85–100μ in diameter (Fig. 29.10A and B). Rostellum well developed, 53–91μ long and 150–206μ wide, hooks 500–520, in 2 rows, 8.8–9.6μ long and 11.2–12μ long (Fig. 29.10D). Genital pores irregularly alternate, anterior to middle of segment margin. Testes 15–25 in number (Fig. 29.10C).

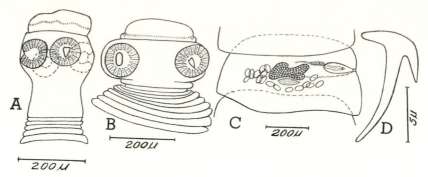

FIG. 29.10—Raillietina ransomi. **(A)** Head fully extended. **(B)** Head partially contracted. **(C)** Mature segment. **(D)** Hook. (Williams, 1931)

Uterus at first saclike, then branched, and finally disintegrating, the "embryos" being scattered through the parenchyma.

LIFE HISTORY. Unknown.

PATHOLOGY. Unknown.

Raillietina williamsi Fuhrmann 1932 (Williams' tapeworm of poultry)

This tapeworm occurs commonly in wild turkey.

SYNONYMS. *Davainea fuhrmanni* of Williams 1931, not Southwell 1922; *Raillietina (Raillietina) williamsi* Fuhrmann 1932.

DESCRIPTION. Mature specimens about 14.3–36.7 cm long by 3.5–4.25 mm wide. Suckers ellipsoidal, 150–190μ long by 135–170μ wide, armed with instable hooks, very deciduous, in 12–13 rows, those of the outer row being largest (Fig. 29.11A). Rostellum hemispherical, 200–214μ in diameter, armed with double crown of 152–156 hooks, larger and smaller hooks alternating (Fig. 29.11B). Genital pores unilateral, in anterior third of segment margin (Fig. 29.11C). Uterus breaking up into 75–100 egg capsules, each with 8–13 eggs (Fig. 29.11D).

LIFE HISTORY. Unknown.

PATHOLOGY. Unknown.

Raillietina georgiensis Reid and Nugara 1961 (Georgian tapeworm of poultry)

This tapeworm is most closely related to *R. williamsi, R. tetragona,* and *R. echinobothrida* from which it is differentiated by the size and number of rostellar hooks and the location of genital pores. It has

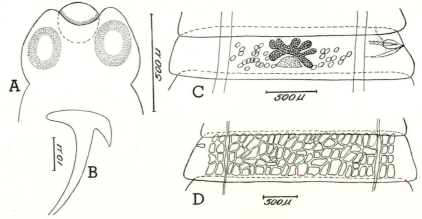

FIG. 29.11—Raillietina williamsi. **(A)** Head with rostellum partially retracted. **(B)** Rostellar hooks. **(C)** Mature segment. **(D)** Gravid segment showing single layer of egg capsules. (Williams, 1931)

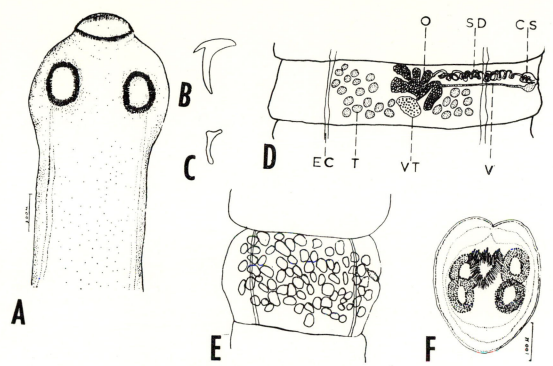

FIG. 29.12—Raillietina georgiensis. (**A**) Scolex. (**B**) Rostellar hook. (**C**) Acetabular hook. (**D**) Mature segment. (**E**) Gravid segment. (**F**) Cysticercoid. (Reid and Nugara, 1961)

been reported from the wild turkey in Alabama, Florida, Georgia and Tennessee and from the domestic turkey in Georgia.

DESCRIPTION. Fully developed worms 150–380 mm long. Suckers approximately round, with hooks 8–13μ long (Fig. 29.12 C); arranged in 8–10 circles. Rostellum armed with 220–268 hooks, each 17–23μ long and 12–16μ wide (Fig. 29.12B); arranged in 2 rows. Genital pores unilateral, rarely irregularly alternate, situated in middle third of body (Fig. 29.12D). Testes 23–29 in number; distributed in two groups, 7–9 poral and 16–20 aporal; lying between excretory canals. Gravid proglottids longer than broad, each containing 80–130 egg capsules, each capsule with 8–10 eggs.

LIFE HISTORY. The ant *Pheidole vinelandica* has been found naturally infected with cysticercoids (Fig. 29.12F). Domestic turkeys fed cysticercoids recovered from this ant became positive for tapeworms after about 20 days.

PATHOLOGY. Reid (1962) reported that a mild enteritis may develop in birds heavily infected with this tapeworm.

ANOPLOCEPHALIDOSIS (ANOPLOCEPHALIDAE)

These worms lack both rostellum and hooks. The proglottids are usually wider than long, and each contains one or two sets of reproductive organs. The testes are numerous. The uterus may persist or be replaced by egg capsules, or the eggs may pass into one or more paruterine organs. Eggs contain "pyriform bodies."

Aporina delafondi (Railliet 1892) (Poreless tapeworm)

This is a common tapeworm of pigeons in several parts of the world. In the United States it has been collected from pigeons in Iowa, Texas, Pennsylvania, and District of Columbia.

The genus Aporina was established by Fuhrmann (1902) for tapeworms of the parakeet. The distinguishing feature was seen by Fuhrmann as the absence of genital pores.

In 1927 Meggitt established the genus Killigrewia, but Fuhrmann (1932) reduced this genus to a synonym of Aporina.

Baer (1927) included in this genus *Taenia delafondi* Railliet 1892, which with rare exceptions possesses well-expressed genital pores.

SYNONYMS. *Taenia delafondi* Railliet 1892; *Bertiella delafondi* (Railliet 1892) Railliet and Henry 1909. Yamaguti (1961) transferred this species to the genus *Killigrewia* Meggitt 1927.

DESCRIPTION. Mature worms 7–16.5 cm long. Suckers unarmed; rostellum absent. Genital pores irregularly alternate, located in anterior third of segment margin. Testes about 100 in number. Eggs not contained in capsules.

LIFE HISTORY. Unknown.

PATHOLOGY. Unknown.

HYMENOLEPIASIS (HYMENOLEPIDIDAE)

The hymenolepid tapeworms have a scolex with rostellum that is armed with 1 row of hooks, rarely with a double row, or unarmed. The number of testes is rarely more than 4. The uterus is saclike, rarely reticulate. The eggs are enclosed in 3 envelopes.

Several species of the genus Hymenolepis have been transferred to other genera by the Russian helminthologists. The present writer has retained the following species in the genus Hymenolepis, pending a wider acceptance of the new classification.

Hymenolepis carioca (Magalhaes 1898) (Long hairlike tapeworm of poultry)

This tapeworm is readily recognizable by its very slender and threadlike form. Complete specimens are very difficult to obtain on account of the fragility of the worm; the head is usually broken off and lost. Several thousands of these worms have been found in a single chicken.

This is one of the most common tapeworms of the duodenum of chickens and turkeys in the United States. Stafseth (1940) reported this species as a parasite of quail in Michigan. Ward (1946) listed *H. carioca* as a parasite of the quail in Mississippi.

SYNONYMS. *Davainea carioca* Magalhaes 1898; *Weinlandia carioca* Mayhew 1925. This species has been placed in the

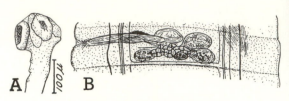

FIG. 29.13—Hymenolepis carioca. *(A)* Scolex. *(B)* Mature segment. *(After Ransom, 1902)*

genus *Echinolepis* Spassiky and Spasskaja 1954.

DESCRIPTION. Mature specimens 3–8 cm long, composed of many hundreds of segments; segments 3–5 times broader than long. Suckers and rostellum unarmed (Fig. 29.13A). Genital pores unilateral, located anterior to middle of segment margin. Testes 3 in number, usually in a more or less straight row across the segment (Fig. 29.13B).

LIFE HISTORY. Guberlet (1919) observed that chickens became infected with this tapeworm after they had been fed stable flies caught around poultry yards. It has been demonstrated by Jones (1929) and Cram and Jones (1929) that dung beetles act as intermediate hosts.

Horsfall (1938) successfully grew cysticercoids of this species in *Tribolium castaneum* and *T. confusum*. When flour beetles containing cysticercoids of *H. carioca* were fed to young chickens, the latter became infected with the adults of this worm. Cysticercoids develop in beetles to a stage which is infective for chickens within approximately 3 weeks. Development of the adult worm in the chicken to the time when gravid segments are passed requires 2–4 weeks.

PATHOLOGY. This tapeworm sometimes occurs in large numbers in chickens and turkeys, but it has very little if any effect on the growth rate of the birds (Luttermoser, 1940).

Hymenolepis cantaniana (Polonio 1860) (Branching tapeworm)

This species has been reported from poultry in the United States, Puerto Rico, Europe, and Asia. It is reported from quail collected in Maryland.

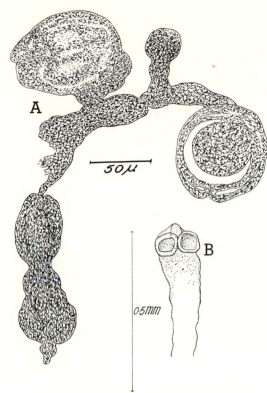

FIG. 29.14—Hymenolepis cantaniana. *(A) Developing larvae. (B) Head.*

SYNONYM. *Taenia cantaniana* Polonio 1860. This species has been placed in the genus *Staphylepis* Spassky and Oshmarin 1954.

DESCRIPTION. Mature specimens about 2 cm long. Rostellum and suckers unarmed (Fig. 29.14B). Genital pores unilateral, anterior to middle of segment margin. Testes 3 in number, usually arranged in a transverse row.

LIFE HISTORY. The development of the cysticercoid of this species of tapeworm is rather unique. As observed by Jones and Alicata (1935), the terminal buds arise from the many-branched individual and ultimately develop into infective larvae (Fig. 29.14A). Dung beetles serve as intermediate hosts of this tapeworm. From 2 to 3 weeks are required for the bladderworm to develop into the adult tapeworm in the avian host.

PATHOLOGY. No definite pathological conditions have been associated with this species.

Hymenolepis tenuirostris (Rudolphi 1819) (Slender-beaked tapeworm of poultry)

Cram (1928) reported this parasite to be present in large numbers from the goose in Oregon. Gower (1939) lists this tapeworm as a parasite of the duck in North America.

SYNONYMS. *Taenia tenuirostris* Rudolphi 1819; *Drepanidotaenia tenuirostris* (Rudolphi 1819) Railliet 1893. This species has been placed in the genus *Microsomacanthus* Lopez-Neyra 1942.

DESCRIPTION. Mature worms 10–25 cm long. Rostellum slender, with about 10 hooks, 20–23μ long (Fig. 29.15A). Genital pores unilateral. Testes 3 in number, in a transverse row. Eggs (Fig. 29.15B) not in capsules.

LIFE HISTORY. Unknown.

PATHOLOGY. Cram regarded this species as responsible for heavy losses in geese in Oregon. The affected birds showed symptoms of weakness, emaciation, incoordination, and diarrhea.

Hymenolepis compressa (Linton 1892)

Sprehn (1932) listed this tapeworm as a parasite of ducks and geese from North America.

SYNONYM. *Taenia compressa* Linton 1892. This species has been placed in the genus *Microsomacanthus* Lopez-Neyra 1942.

DESCRIPTION. Mature worms up to 4 cm long. Suckers unarmed (Fig. 29.16A), ros-

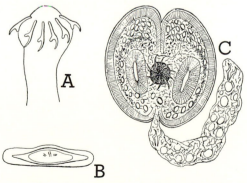

FIG. 29.15—Hymenolepis tenuirostris. *(A) Head with rostellar hooks. (B) Egg. (Krabbe, 1869) (C) Cysticercoid. (Hamann, 1889)*

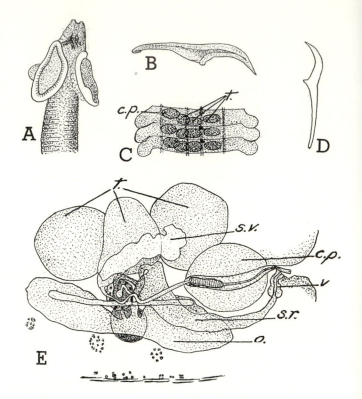

FIG. 29.16—Hymenolepis compressa. (A) Head. (B) Rostellar hook. (Linton, 1892) (C) Mature segments. (D) Rostellar hook. (E) Portion of transverse section through pore of mature segment (c.p., cirrus pouch; o., ovary; s.r., seminal receptacle; s.v., seminal vesicle; t., testis; v., vagina). (Kowalewski, 1907)

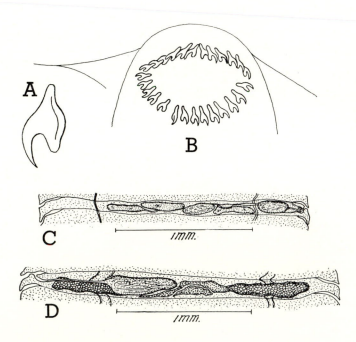

FIG. 29.17—Hymenolepis coronula. (A) Rostellar hook. (B) Hook crown in place. (Krabbe, 1869) (C) Mature segment with male genitalia. (D) Mature segment with female genitalia. (Meggitt, 1920)

tellum with 10 hooks, 50–58μ long (Figs. 29.16B,D). Testes 3 in number, in a more or less straight row across the segment (Fig. 29.16C).

LIFE HISTORY. Unknown.

PATHOLOGY. Unknown.

Hymenolepis coronula (Dujardin 1845)

SYNONYMS. *Taenia coronula* Dujardin 1845; *Weinlandia coronula* (Dujardin 1845) Mayhew 1925. This species has been placed in the genus *Dicranotaenia* Railliet 1892.

DESCRIPTION. Mature worms 1–2 cm long. Suckers unarmed; rostellum armed with a crown of 18–26 hooks, 9–18μ long, with short handle and a strong guard which is almost as long as the blade (Fig. 29.17A,B). Testes 3 in number (Fig. 29.17C). Eggs not contained in capsules.

LIFE HISTORY. Eggs of this tapeworm are ingested by small crustaceans, the embryos hatching and developing to cysticercoids in the body cavity of these animals. When these infected crustaceans are swallowed by waterfowl, the cysticercoids develop to adult tapeworms in the intestines of the birds. Joyeux (1920) demonstrated that snails may carry cysticercoids of this species for a time after having eaten infected crustaceans. Birds may become infected by eating snails infected with cysticercoids.

PATHOLOGY. Pillers (1923) reported a heavy infection with this species and with *H. megalops* and *Aploparaksis furcigera* as "apparently the cause of 'going light' and of deaths" in ducks in England. Kingscote (1932) reported an enzootic in a flock of ducks in Canada caused by this species, the parasites being present in large numbers. Schofield (1932) reported heavy mortality among ducklings in Canada due to *H. coronula*.

Hymenolepis lanceolata (Bloch 1782)
(Lancetlike tapeworm of poultry)

Quortrup and Shillinger (1941) reported *Hymenolepis* sp. (probably *H. lanceolata*) from the Canadian goose in Utah.

SYNONYM. *Taenia lanceolata* Bloch 1782. This species has been placed in the genus *Schistocephalus* Creplin 1829.

DESCRIPTION. Mature worms 3–13 cm long. Segments 20–40 times as wide as long. Suckers unarmed; rostellum with 8 hooks, 31–35μ long, with handle longer than blade, and guard slightly salient (Fig. 29.18C). Genital pore at anterior corner of segment margin, testes 3 in number, in a transverse row (Fig. 29.18D). Eggs not in capsules.

LIFE HISTORY. Ruszkowski (1932) demonstrated that larvae of this species developed to the cysticercoid stage in small crustaceans in about 6 weeks at 9–12° C. The time required for development of the adult worm in the primary host has not been determined.

PATHOLOGY. Emets (1929) described an epizootic, chiefly among young geese but also in some older birds. Muscular incoordination was the chief symptom. Postmortem examination showed a catarrhal inflammation of the intestinal mucosa.

Hymenolepis megalops Nitzsch, in Creplin 1829
(Large-headed tapeworm of poultry)

This tapeworm may be readily distinguished from other species found in poultry by its extraordinarily large head and its preference for the cloaca and bursa of Fabricius. It has been found on a number of occasions in wild ducks.

Green et al. (1937) reported this tapeworm from wild ducks in Minnesota. It has been collected on a number of occasions from wild ducks in Montana by Wehr.

SYNONYMS. *Taenia megalops* Nitzsch, in Creplin 1829; *Weinlandia megalops* (Nitzsch, in Creplin 1829) Mayhew 1925. This species has been placed in the genus *Cloacotaenia* Wolffhügel 1938.

DESCRIPTION. Mature worms 3–6 mm long. Head very large, 1–2 mm wide (Fig. 29.19A). Suckers and rostellum unarmed. Testes 3 in number. Eggs not in capsules.

LIFE HISTORY. Unknown.

PATHOLOGY. Pillers (1923) reported a heavy infection with this worm and with *H. cor-*

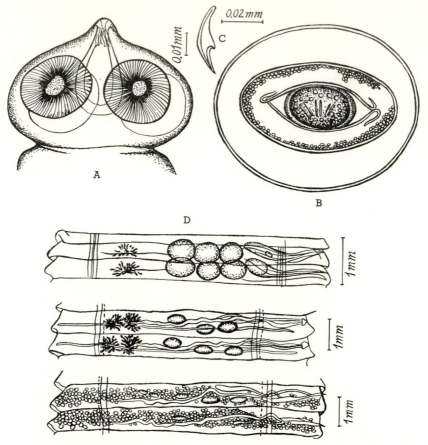

FIG. 29.18—Hymenolepis lanceolata. *(A) Head. (B) Egg. (C) Hook. (D) Proglottids in early and late stages of development. (Potemkinot, 1938)*

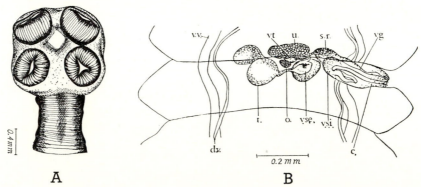

FIG. 29.19—Hymenolepis megalops. *(A) Head. (B) Mature proglottid, dorsal view (c., cirrus; d. v., dorsal excretory vessel; o., ovary; r.s., seminal receptacle; t., testis; u., uterus; vg., vagina; v. s. e., vesicula seminals externa; v. s. i., vesicula seminalis interna; vt., vitelline gland; v. v., ventral excretory vessel). (Yamaguti, 1940)*

onula and *Aploparaksis furcigera* as "apparently the cause of 'going light' and of deaths" in ducks in England.

Hymenolepis tritesticulata Fuhrmann 1906
(Tritesticulated tapeworm of poultry)

This species has been reported by Linton (1927) as occurring in wild ducks of North America.

SYNONYM. *Weinlandia tritesticulata* (Fuhrmann 1906). This species has been placed in the genus *Microsomacanthus* Lopez-Neyra 1954.

DESCRIPTION. Mature worms 25 cm long. Suckers unarmed; rostellum with 10 hooks, 32μ long (Fig. 29.20B). Testes 3 in number. Eggs not in capsules.

LIFE HISTORY. Unknown.

PATHOLOGY. Unknown.

Hymenolepis introversa (Mayhew 1925)

This species has been reported by Mayhew (1925) as occurring in ducks in Illinois. It has been placed in the genus *Dicranotaenia* Railliet 1892.

DESCRIPTION. Mature worms 5–8 cm long. Suckers unarmed (Fig. 29.21A); rostellum

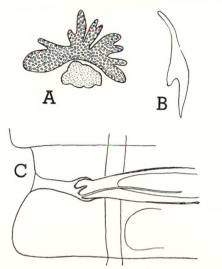

FIG. 29.20—*Hymenolepis tritesticulata.* **(A)** *Ovary and vitelline gland.* **(B)** *Rostellar hook.* **(C)** *Poral region showing part of cirrus pouch with internal sacculus accessorius.* (*Fuhrmann, 1907*)

armed with 20 hooks, $17–20\mu$ long (Fig. 29.21B). Genital pores in anterior region of right segment margins. Testes 3 in number, irregularly lobed.

LIFE HISTORY. Unknown.

PATHOLOGY. Unknown.

Fimbriaria fasciolaris (Pallas 1781)
(Fimbriated Tapeworm)

This tapeworm has been reported by Todd (1946) as occurring in chickens in Tennessee. It has also been recorded as a parasite of wild ducks on several occasions in this country.

SYNONYMS. *Taenia laevis* Bloch 1782; *Diploposthe laevis* (Bloch 1782) Jacobi 1896.

DESCRIPTION. Mature worms 10–50 cm long by 3–9 mm wide. Scolex small, provided with 10 hooks, $16–21\mu$ long, with long handle and very short guard and blade; suckers unarmed. Anterior part of body forms a folded expansion or "pseudoscolex." Genital pores unilateral. Testes 3 in number. Uterus continuous throughout strobila, breaking up posteriorly into tubules, each containing several eggs.

LIFE HISTORY. The water flea *Diaptomus vulgaris* has been reported as harboring the cysticercoid of this tapeworm.

PATHOLOGY. Unknown.

SYMPTOMS

Everything else being equal, the severity of the symptoms resulting from tapeworm infections apparently depends to some extent on the number of worms present, the diet, and the age of the birds. Few if any clinical symptoms are observed in lightly infected birds. Heavily infected birds sometimes show marked retardation in growth rate.

Harwood and Luttermoser (1938) demonstrated experimentally that growth rates of 2–4-week-old chicks fed an adequate diet and having infections at necropsy ranging in numbers from 15 to 155 *Raillietina cesticillus* were definitely retarded. Ackert and Case (1938) reported weight retardation and reduced sugar and hemoglobin content of the blood in 3–4-month-old birds each having at necropsy infections of 4–25 *Raillie-*

*FIG. 29.21—*Hymenolepis introversa. *(A) Head. (B) Hook. (C) Proglottids. (D) Cirrus sac. (E) Reproductive organs. (Mayhew, 1925)*

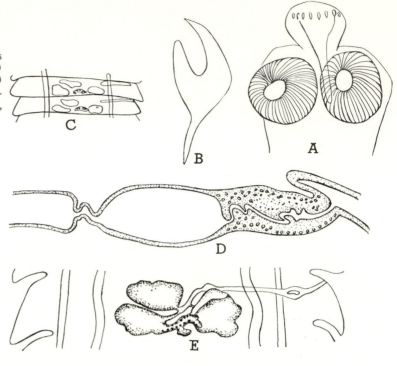

tina cesticillus. Levine (1938) found that the difference between the mean weights of chickens experimentally infected with *Davainea proglottina* when 7 weeks of age and held under observation for 13 weeks was 12% less than the controls. Alicata (1940) experimentally determined that birds receiving animal-protein supplements (fish meal and dry skim milk) had at necropsy an average of 14 tapeworms *(Hymenolepis exigua);* a similar number of birds receiving plant-protein supplements (yeast, sesame meal, peanut oil, and soybean meal) had an average of 66 tapeworms. In contrast to the above observations, Luttermoser (1940) reported that the growth rates of 22 4-week-old Rhode Island Red chickens experimentally fed 1,000 cysticercoids of *Hymenolepis carioca* were practically the same as those of an equal number of controls held under similar conditions.

Birds of all ages harbor tapeworms. However, Ackert and Reid (1937) have demonstrated that concomitant with an increase in age of the bird there is a corresponding increase in resistance to tapeworm infection.

A number of clinical symptoms have been inadvertently ascribed to tapeworm infections. At the present time there is not sufficient experimental evidence to show that such clinical symptoms as cyanosis, lameness, poor feathering, and failure to come into or stay in production are due solely to the presence of these parasites.

GROSS PATHOLOGY

A few tapeworms may produce few or no perceptible gross pathological changes in the intestines. However, in heavy tapeworm infections, a more or less extensive catarrhal enteritis and diarrhea may result. At least one species of tapeworm, *Raillietina echinobothrida,* causes the formation of nodules in the intestinal wall. Inasmuch as this condition closely resembles tuberculosis, it is important that the two conditions be kept in mind in attempting to arrive at a diagnosis. The presence of intestinal nodules— sometimes distinctly visible on the outer surface of the intestinal wall—and the absence of tapeworms are strongly suggestive of tuberculosis. However, a diagnosis of intestinal tuberculosis should not be made without first eliminating tapeworms of this species as a cause of the nodules. Mature specimens of this tapeworm are usually several centimeters long; but observations have shown that, in many cases, infections involved individual tapeworms containing only a very few segments, sometimes only the heads. In such cases the parasites may be easily overlooked if only a casual or hurried examination is made. In doubtful cases the intestine should be scraped with a scalpel or other suitable instrument and a careful examination made of the scrapings under suitable magnification for the presence of small tapeworms or their heads. The presence of tapeworms and the absence of tubercles in the liver and other organs are indicative of tapeworm disease. Another species of tapeworm, *Raillietina tetragona,* which is morphologically very similar to *R. echinobothrida* and often confused with it, has not been definitely associated with tuberculosislike lesions.

Leg weakness and paralysis have frequently been attributable to tapeworm infection. However, the relationship of tapeworms to these diseases is still unknown. Should these conditions be intimately associated with the presence of tapeworms, the mere removal of the parasite should clear up the condition. The fact that birds which had previously shown symptoms of leg weakness and paralysis were free from tapeworms at necropsy seems to disprove the idea that tapeworms are in a large degree responsible for these conditions. Capillary congestion; lymphocyte, polymorphonuclear, and eosinophil infiltration; proliferation of epithelium; and fibrosis are microscopic lesions which have been associated with tapeworm infections.

There is some evidence to show that birds heavily parasitized with tapeworms are not as productive as uninfected ones. Under ordinary conditions birds may tolerate a fairly heavy tapeworm infection, at least for a time. However, young birds and hens in heavy production do not fare so well when heavily infected with these parasites.

DIAGNOSIS

Diagnosis of tapeworm infection by examination of the fresh droppings for the presence of eggs or segments is unreliable. Even in cases of heavy infection, segments or eggs are sometimes absent. It has been shown by Harwood (1938) that segment production in the tapeworm *Raillietina*

cesticillus occurs in cycles, segment production being marked at first by a period of intense segment elimination, alternating with periods in which no segments (or only a relatively few) were eliminated.

The diagnosis of poultry taeniasis is best made at necropsy. The intestine of the supposedly infected bird is slit open with an enterotome, spread out flat on the bottom of a suitable container, and examined carefully for the white ribbonlike worms. If this method of examination reveals no worms, a small amount of water may be added to the container. The water will cause the worms, if present, to float to the surface, or they may be seen swaying back and forth in the water above the opened intestine. In infections involving tapeworms of the smaller species, the individual worms are often so small that they are overlooked. Therefore, examination of the intestinal scrapings under the binocular microscope is frequently necessary to detect such small species as *Davainea proglottina* and *Amoebotaenia sphenoides.*

PREVENTION AND CONTROL

When one considers the number of tapeworms infecting poultry and their various intermediate hosts, the task of prevention of tapeworm infection in birds raised under natural conditions seems impossible. Investigations have shown that many intermediate hosts of varying habits may serve experimentally as intermediate hosts of a single species of tapeworm. To prevent birds from eating the many species of invertebrates (insects, snails, and slugs) is an inconceivable task. However, intermediate hosts of these parasites may be reduced in numbers by application of certain insecticides to the poultry manure (Kartman et al., 1950).

Directions for housefly control are described in Chapter 27. Precautions should be taken to prevent accidental contamination of poultry meat or eggs with insecticides.

A commercially prepared bait containing metaldehyde will control slugs and snails. It is best to apply bait in late afternoon or evening. Ground beetles are difficult to control. These as well as slugs and snails tend to collect under loose boards and other protected places where it is moist. Prompt removal of these mechanical protections and elimination of moist feed wastes from poultry yards will discourage their presence in such places. Grasshoppers are controlled by spraying with the proper insecticides, by poison baits, and to some extent by agricultural practices. The controls for stable flies as well as houseflies are directed toward their breeding places. Moisture is necessary for development of the fly larvae. Therefore, prompt removal of moist feed wastes, weed piles, and other vegetation which has accumulated in piles is essential. Loosely piled strawstacks, if allowed to become wet, are important breeding places of the stable fly. Hence, straw should not be allowed to become wet and decayed before removal. Ants may be controlled by the use of approved ant poisons. Malathion and Sevin may prove useful. The first step in the control of ants is to find the nests. Then an insecticide is applied to the nests and to the surfaces over which the ants crawl. The number of earthworms may be reduced considerably by keeping the yards dry and well drained and by avoiding the accumulation of manure.

Proper disposal of the droppings is unquestionably the most effective preventive measure for control of tapeworm infection if management practices permit. Droppings of infected birds are the source from which the intermediate hosts become infected. Disposal of droppings on pasture lands in such a manner as to prevent the intermediate host from picking up the tapeworm eggs or gravid segments passed in the droppings is of primary importance. Since eggs are short-lived, such a practice must be carried out daily and may be practical in poultry operations involving use of automated cleanout systems.

Body wastes from farm flocks can usually be disposed of by hauling them to the field and spreading thinly over the land. The action of the sun and wind will quickly dry out the droppings and destroy all parasitic material that may be present, since prolonged desiccation is fatal to the infective stages of the parasites. This practice of disposing of poultry droppings not only serves to destroy parasitic material but also adds tremendously to the value of the land for growing crops. Poultry manure, when handled in this way, is said to be an excellent fertilizer for garden and field crops.

Body wastes from backyard flocks usually must necessarily be handled in some other way, as accumulations from such flocks usually exceed the demands of the owner. In communities where large numbers of poultry raisers are within a short distance of each other, the droppings from their birds are sometimes hauled to centrally located storage sheds and retailed to the public at a reasonable price. In order that the fertilizing value of poultry manure may not be lost, it must be stored in a suitable screened-in shed provided with a cement floor and a roof to keep out rain and snow. The screens exclude flying and crawling insects which may serve as intermediate hosts of poultry parasites. This practice naturally raises the question of how safe this manure is if used on land where other poultry are likely to run. Limited experimentation seems to indicate that much destruction of the tapeworm eggs may result from the self-sterilization process which takes place in stored manure.

TREATMENT

Medication has served to reduce appreciably parasitism in many groups of livestock, but its applicability in the control of poultry parasites in general is limited.

A drug, in order to be a satisfactory poultry remedial agent, must be inexpensive, highly effective, nontoxic, and easy to administer. It is highly essential that a drug designed for the purpose of removing parasites from poultry possess the above qualifications, since the unit value of the domestic fowl is usually quite low.

A large number of drugs has been recommended for the removal of tapeworms from poultry. Guthrie and Harwood (1941) reported that mixtures of 0.3–1.0 g of stannous (tin) tartrate and 0.07–0.2 g of synthetic pelletierine hydrochloride removed 86.8% of *Raillietina cesticillus* and 95.0% of *Hymenolepis carioca* from experimentally infected chickens. However, when used by themselves, the tin compounds possessed only slight value for the removal of *R. cesticillus*. By adding small amounts of synthetic pelletierine hydrochloride to any of the various tin compounds, a synergistic action was obtained, thus increasing the effectiveness of the mixture. The above authors (1944) found that a freshly prepared mixture of tin oleate and triethanolamine effectively removed a large percentage of *R. cesticillus* from experimentally infected birds in some tests and only a small percentage in others. Kerr (1948) demonstrated that hexachlorophene (2,2′-dihydroxy-3,3′, 5, 5′, 6, 6′-hexachloro-diphenylmethane) at doses of 25–50 mg per kg body weight possesses a high efficacy in removing *R. cesticillus* from chickens. However, when used at the therapeutic level this drug seriously affects egg production.

Kerr (1952) presented data to show that butynorate was an effective and safe drug for the removal of *R. cesticillus* from chickens. When administered as a single dose by capsule, a dose of 75–150 mg per kg body weight gave efficacies ranging from 86 to 100%. Edgar (1956) reported the above compound to be highly effective in removing six species of tapeworms (*R. cesticillus, R. tetragona, Hymenolepis carioca, Choanotaenia infundibulum, Davainea proglottina,* and *Amoebotaenia sphenoides*) from field-infected chickens when administered in the feed at the rate of 500 mg per kg of feed for 2–6 days, or by capsule at the rate of 125 mg per bird, or in combination with nicotine and phenothiazine. A temporary drop in egg production, which persisted from the 3rd through the 10th day after treatment, resulted from the use of the combination.

Almost complete control of *R. cesticillus* was accomplished using the coccidiostat combination of 0.02% butynorate, 0.03% sulfanitran, 0.02% dinsed, and 0.0025% roxarsone in the feed. However, Botero and Reid (1969) did not recommend use of medication since they found no harmful effects from heavy artificial infection on broilers or layers.

Nugara and Reid (1962) tested Trithiadol in the feed at the rate of 3 lb per ton for 5 days, dibutyltin dilaurate (butynorate) in the feed at a 0.07% level for 5 days, and dibutyltin oxide via capsule at 65-mg and 125-mg doses per bird against the turkey tapeworm *Raillietina georgiensis*. They reported the last to be the most efficacious, removing 100% of the worms at the lower level and 90% at the higher level.

Reid (1940) found that starvation of birds infected with the cestode *Raillietina cesticillus* for 20–48 hours resulted in loss of the strobilae (minus the head) of the worms. The loss of the tapeworm strobilae was apparently directly due to the partial starvation of the parasite, as it was determined that the glycogen store in worms from chickens starved 20 hours was lowered to less than one-twelfth of that found in tapeworms taken from nonstarved birds. However, Reid (1942) demonstrated that the tapeworm head was not affected by the long period of starvation. When normal feeding habits of the fowl were restored, new strobilae or segments were regenerated by the unaffected heads, and gravid segments appeared later in the feces of the birds. Therefore, it is obvious that the practice of starving tapeworm-infected birds has the effect of breaking off the strobilae and leaving the heads attached to the mucosa. Because of its harmful effects on the health and growth of the birds and the rapid regeneration of new segments following the starvation period, such a procedure is not practical.

REFERENCES

Abdou, A. H. 1958. Studies on the development of *Davainea proglottina* in the intermediate host. *J. Parasitol.* 44:484–88.

Ackert, J. E. 1919. On the life cycle of the fowl cestode, *Davainea cesticillus* (Molin). *J. Parasitol.* 5:41–43.

———. 1932. Fowl resistance to parasitism affected by vitamins A and B. *Arch. Zool. Ital. Toreno* 16:1360–79.

Ackert, J. E., and A. A. Case. 1938. Effects of the tapeworm *Raillietina cesticillus* (Molin) on growing chickens. *J. Parasitol.* 24 (Sect. 2): 14.

Ackert, J. E., and W. M. Reid. 1937. Age resistance of chickens to the cestode *Raillietina cesticillus* (Molin). *J. Parasitol.* 23 (Sect. 2): 558.

Adams, F. M., and S. W. Geiser. 1933. Helminth parasites of the chicken, *Gallus domesticus,* in Dallas County, Texas. *Am. Midland Naturalist* 14:251–57.

Alicata, J. E. 1936. The Amphipod, *Orchestia platensis,* an intermediate host for *Hymenolepid exigua,* a tapeworm of chickens in Hawaii. *J. Parasitol.* 22:515–16.

———. 1940. Poultry parasites. *Rept. Hawaii Agr. Expt. Sta.* (1939):65–66.

Alicata, J. E., and M. F. Jones. 1933. The dung beetle, *Atenius cognatus,* as the intermediate host of *Hymenolepis cantaniana. J. Parasitol.* 19:244.

Baer, J. G. 1927. Monographie des cestodes de la famille des Anoplocephalides. *Bull. Biol. France Belg. Suppl.* 10.

Botero, H., and W. M. Reid. 1969. The effects of the tapeworm *Raillietina cesticillus* upon body weight gains of broilers, poults and on egg production. *Poultry Sci.* 48:536–42.

Bushnell, L. E., and C. A. Brandly. 1929. Poultry diseases, their prevention and control. *Kansas Agr. Expt. Sta. Bull.* 247.

Case, A. A., and J. E. Ackert. 1939. Intermediate hosts of chicken tapeworms found in Kansas. *Trans. Kansas Acad. Sci.* 42:437–42.

———. 1940. New intermediate hosts of fowl cestodes. *Trans. Kansas Acad. Sci.* 43:393–96.

Chandler, A. C. 1923. Observations on the life cycle of *Davainea proglottina* in the United States. *Trans. Am. Microscop. Soc.* 42:142–47.

Cram, E. B. 1928. The present status of our knowledge of poultry parasitism. *North Am. Vet.* 9:43–51.

Cram, E. B., and M. F. Jones. 1929. Observations on the life histories of *Raillietina cesticillus* and of *Hymenolepis carioca*, tapeworms of poultry and game birds. *North Am. Vet.* 10:49–51.

Crawley, H. 1922. *Davainea proglottina*, a pathogenic cestode, in American poultry. *J. Am. Vet. Med. Ass.* 61:305–10.

Cuviller, E., and M. F. Jones. 1933. Two new intermediate hosts for the poultry cestode, *Hymenolepis carioca*. *J. Parasitol.* 19:245.

Edgar, S. A. 1956. The removal of chicken tapeworms by di-n-butyl tin dilaurate. *Poultry Sci.* 35:64–73.

Edgar, S. A., and P. A. Teer. 1957. The efficacy of several compounds in causing the elimination of tapeworms from laboratory-infected chickens. *Poultry Sci.* 36:329–34.

Emets, S. 1929. (Cerebellar ataxia in geese as a result of infestation with *Hymenolepis lanceolata*.) (Russian text.) *Vestn. Sovrem. Vet. Mosk.* (94) 5:531–32.

Enigh, K., and E. Stincinsky. 1959a. Zur Biologie und Bekampfung der haufigsten Huhnerbandwuermer. *Arch. Gefluegelk.* 23:247–56.

———. 1959b. Die Zwischenwirte der Huhnerbandwuermer *Raillietina cesticillus, Choanotaenia infundibulum* und *Hymenolepis carioca*. *Z. Parasitenk.* 19:278–308.

Enigh, K., E. Stincinsky, and H. Ergun. 1958. Die Zwischenwirte von *Davainea proglottina* (Cestoidae). *Z. Parasitenk.* 18:230–36.

Ferry, Q. B. 1934. Studies on the cestodes of poultry in and around Douglas County, Kansas. *Am. Midland Naturalist* 15:586–97.

Fuhrmann, O. 1902. Die Anoplocephaliden der Voegel. *Zentr. Bakteriol. 1 Abt. Orig.* 32:122–47.

———. 1907. Bekannte und neue Arten und Genera von Vogeltaenien. *Zentr. Bakteriol. 1 Abt. Orig.* 45:516–36.

———. 1932. Le tenias des oiseaux. *Mem. Universite Neuchatel* 8.

Gage, G. E., and C. L. Opperman. 1909. Nodular taeniasis, or tapeworm disease, of fowls. *Maryland Agr. Expt. Sta. Bull.* 139:73–85.

Gardiner, J. L., and E. E. Wehr. 1949. Some parasites of the wild turkey (*Meleagris gallopavo silvestris*) in Maryland. *Proc. Helminthol. Soc. Wash. D.C.* 16:16–19.

Gower, W. C. 1939. Host-parasite catalogue of the helminths of ducks. *Am. Midland Naturalist* 22:580–628.

Grassi, B., and G. Rovelli. 1889. Embryologische Forschungen an Cestoden. *Zentr. Bakteriol. Parasitenk.* 5:370, 401.

Green, R. G., J. F. Bell, and D. W. Mather. 1937. The occurrence of botulism in waterfowl in western Minnesota. *Rept. of Minn. Wildlife Disease Invest.* 1936–37.

Guberlet, J. E. 1919. On the life history of the chicken cestode, *Hymenolepis carioca* (Magalhaes). *J. Parasitol.* 6:35–38.

Guthrie, J. E., and P. D. Harwood. 1941. Use of tin preparations for the treatment of chickens experimentally infected with tapeworms. *Am. J. Vet. Res.* 2:108–16.

———. 1944. Limited tests of mixtures of tin oleate with ammonium compounds for the removal of experimental tapeworm infections of chickens. *Proc. Helminthol. Soc. Wash. D.C.* 11:45–48.

Hamann, O. 1889. In *Gammarus pulex* lebende Cysticercoides mit Schwanzanhaengen. *Jena Z. Naturw.* 17:1–10.

Hanson, A. J. 1930. The slug as the intermediate host of the microscopic tapeworm of chickens. *Ann. Rept. Western Wash. Expt. Sta. Bull.* 184 (1929–30), N.S.

Harkema, R. 1943. The cestodes of North Carolina poultry with remarks on the life history of *Raillietina tetragona*. *J. Elisha Mitchell Sci. Soc.* 59:127.

Harwood, P. D. 1938. Reproductive cycles of *Raillietina cesticillus* of the fowl. *Livro. Jubilar Lauro Travassos*, Rio de Janeiro, Institute Oswaldo Cruz, pp. 213–20.

Harwood, P. D., and G. E. Guthrie. 1940. Tests with miscellaneous substances for removal of tapeworms from chickens. *J. Am. Vet. Med. Ass.* 97:248–53.

Harwood, P. D., and G. W. Luttermoser. 1938. The influence of infections with the tapeworm, *Raillietina cesticillus*, on the growth of chickens. *Proc. Helminthol. Soc. Wash. D.C.* 5:60–62.

Horsfall, M. W. 1938. Meal beetles as intermediate hosts of poultry tapeworms. *Poultry Sci.* 17:8–11.

Horsfall, M. W., and M. F. Jones. 1937. The life history of *Choanotaenia infundibulum*, a cestode parasitic in chickens. *J. Parasitol.* 23:435–50.

Hudson, J. R. 1934. Notes on some avian cestodes. *Ann. Mag. Nat. Hist.*, Ser. 19(80), 14:314–18.

Jones, M. F. 1929. *Hister (Carcinops) 14-striatus* an intermediate host for *Hymenolepis carioca*. *J. Parasitol.* 15:224.

———. 1930a. A new tapeworm from the guinea fowl, with cysticercoids in a ground beetle. *J. Parasitol.* 16:158.

———. 1930b. Life history of *Metroliasthes lucida*, a tapeworm of the turkey. *J. Parasitol.* 17:53.

———. 1932. Additional notes on intermediate hosts of poultry tapeworms. *J. Parasitol.* 18:307.

———. 1936a. *Metroliasthes lucida,* a cestode of galliform birds, in arthropod and avian hosts. *Proc. Helminthol. Soc. Wash. D.C.* 3:26–30.

———. 1936b. A new species of cestode, *Davainea meleagridis* (Davaineidae), from the turkey, with a key to species of *Davainea* from galliform birds. *Proc. Helminthol. Soc. Wash. D.C.* 3:49–52.

Jones, M. F., and J. E. Alicata. 1935. Development and morphology of the cestode, *Hymenolepis cantaniana* in coleopteran and avian hosts. *J. Wash. Acad. Sci.* 25:237–47.

Jones, M. F., and M. W. Horsfall. 1935. Ants as intermediate hosts for two species of *Raillietina* parasitic in chickens. *J. Parasitol.* 21:442–43.

Joyeux, C. 1920. Cycle evolutif de quelques cestodes. Recherches experimentalis. *Bull. Biol. France Belg. Suppl.* 2:1–219.

Joyeux, C., and J. G. Baer. 1937. Recherches sur l'evolution des cestodes de gallinaces. *Compt. Rend. Acad. Sci.* 205:751–53.

Kartman, L., Y. Tanada, F. G. Holdaway, and J. E. Alicata. 1950. Laboratory tests to determine the efficacy of certain insecticides in the control of arthropods inhabiting poultry manure. *Poultry Sci.* 29:336–46.

Kerr, K. B. 1948. Hexachlorophene as an agent for the removal of *Raillietina cesticillus. Poultry Sci.* 27:781–88.

———. 1952. Butynorate, an effective and safe substance for the removal of *R. cesticillus* from chickens. *Poultry Sci.* 31:328–36.

Kingscote, A. A. 1932. Department of Parasitology. *Rept. Ont. Vet. Coll.* (1931):60–71.

Kowalewski, M. 1907. Studya helmintologiczne czesc X. Przyczynek do blizszej znajamosci dwoch ptasich tasiemcow. *Polska. Akad. Umiejetnosci. Rozprawy Wydzailu. Mat.-Przyro.* 47, s. 3, Vol. 7, Dzial B, pp. 633–43.

Krabbe, H. 1869. Bidrag til Kundskab om Fuglenes Baendelorme K. *Danske Vidensk. Selsk. Skr. Naturw. og Math. Afd.* 5 R., 8: 249–363.

Lang, R. 1929. Vergleichende Untersuchungen an Huehnercestoden der Gattung *Raillietina* Fuhrmann, 1920. *Z. Parasitenk.* 1:562–611.

Levine, P. P. 1938. The effect of infection with *Davainea proglottina* on the weights of growing chickens. *J. Parasitol.* 24:550–51.

Linton, E. 1892. Notes on avian cestodes. *Proc. U.S. Nat. Museum* 15:87–113.

———. 1927. Notes on cestode parasites of birds. *Proc. U.S. Nat. Museum* 70:1–73.

Lopez-Neyra, C. R. 1931. Revision del gebero Davainea. *Mem. Acad. Cienc. Exactas., Fes. Nat. Madrid, a Cienc. Nat.* 1:1–177.

Luttermoser, G. W. 1940. The effects on the growth-rate of young chickens of infections of the tapeworm, *Hymenolepis carioca. Proc. Helminthol. Soc. Wash. D.C.* 7:74–76.

Mayhew, R. L. 1925. Studies on the avian species of the cestode family Hymenolepididae. *Illinois Biol. Monograph* 10:1–125.

Meggitt, F. J. 1914. On the anatomy of a fowl tapeworm *Amoebotaenis sphenoides. Parasitology* 7:262–77.

———. 1916. A contribution to the knowledge of the tapeworms of fowls and sparrows. *Parasitology* 8:390–410.

———. 1920. A contribution to our knowledge of the tapeworms of poultry. *Parasitology* 12:301–9, 313.

———. 1926. The tapeworms of the domestic fowl. *J. Burma Res. Soc.* 15:222–43.

———. 1927. Report on a collection of cestodes mainly from Egypt. 1. Families Anoplocephalidae, Davaineidae. *Parasitology* 19: 314–17.

Mönnig, H. O. 1926. The anatomy and life history of the fowl tapeworm *Amoebotaenia sphenoides. 11th and 12th Rept. Dir. Vet. Educ. Res., Union S. Africa, Dept. Agr.,* Pt. 1, pp. 199–206.

Nugara, D., and W. M. Reid. 1962. Some drug treatments for the turkey tapeworm, *Raillietina georgiensis. Poultry Sci.* 41:674–75.

Pillers, A. W. N. 1923. Notes on parasites during 1922. *Vet. Record* 3:459–60.

Potemkina, V. I. 1938. Biology and diagnosis of *Drepanidotaenia lanceolata* in geese. *Tr. Vses. Inst. Gel'mintol.* 3:97–126.

Quortrup, E. R., and J. E. Shillinger. 1941. 3,000 wild bird autopsies on western lake areas. *J. Am. Vet. Med. Ass.* 99:382–87.

Ransom, B. H. 1899. A new avian cestode—*Metroliasthes lucida. Trans. Am. Microscop. Soc.* 21 (May): 213–16.

———. 1902. On *Hymenolepis carioca* (Magalhaes) and *H. megalops* (Nitzsch) with remarks on the classification of the group. *Trans. Am. Microscop. Soc.* 23 (August): 151–72.

———. 1905. The tapeworms of American chickens and turkeys. *21st Ann. Rept. BAI, USDA.*

Reid, W. M. 1940. Some effects of short starvation periods upon the fowl cestode *Raillietina cesticillus* (Molin). *J. Parasitol.* 26:16.

———. 1942. The removal of the fowl tapeworm *Raillietina cesticillus* by short periods of starvation. *Poultry Sci.* 21:220–29.

———. 1959. Egg characteristics as aids in species identification and control of chicken tapeworms. *Avian Diseases* 3:188–97.

———. 1962. Chicken and turkey tapeworms. Handbook to aid in identification and control of tapeworms found in the United States of America. *Univ. Georgia Coll. Agr.*

Reid, W. M., and D. Nugara. 1961. Description and life cycle of *Raillietina georgiensis* n. sp., a tapeworm from wild and domestic turkeys. *J. Parasitol.* 47:885–89.

Reid, W. M., J. E. Ackert, and A. A. Case. 1938. Studies on the life history and biology of the fowl tapeworm *Raillietina cesticillus* (Molin). *Trans. Am. Microscop. Soc.* 57:65–76.

Rietz, J. H. 1930. Animal parasites of chickens in Ohio and West Virginia. *J. Am. Vet. Med. Ass.* 77:154–56.

Ruszkowski, J. S. 1932. Le cycle evolutif du cestode *Drepanidotaenia lanceolata* (Bloch). *Bull. Int. Acad. Pol. Sci. Lett., Cl. Sci. Math. Nat., s. B.Sc. Nat.* (11) (1–4):1–8.

Sawada, I. 1952a. (Ants as intermediate hosts for chicken tapeworm, *Raillietina tetragona.*) *Nara Gakugei Univ. Bull.* 1:225. (English summary.)

———. 1952b. (On the life history of the chicken cestode, *Raillietina cesticillus.*) *Nara Gakugei Univ. Bull.* 1:235–43. (English summary.)

———. 1953. (Observation on the seasonal variation in infestation rate of cysticercoids of *Raillietina tetragona* and *Raillietina echinobothrida* in the ant, *Tetramorium caespitum jacoti.*) *Dobutsugaku Zasshi* 62:292–96.

———. 1954. Morphological studies on the chicken tapeworm, *Raillietina (Raillietina) echinobothrida.* *Dobutsugaku Zasshi* 63:200–203. (English summary.)

Schofield, F. W. 1932. Heavy mortality among ducklings due to *Hymenolepis coronula.* *Rept. Ont. Vet. Coll.* (1931):49.

Schwartz, B. 1925. The chicken as a host for *Metroliasthes lucida. J. Parasitol.* 12:112.

Southwell, T. 1921. Cestodes from Indian poultry. *Ann. Trop. Med. Parasitol.* 15:161–66.

———. 1930. *Cestodes: The Fauna of British India, Including Ceylon and Burma,* Vol. 2.

Sprehn, C. E. W. 1932. *Lehrbuch der Helminthologie. Eine Naturgeschichte der in deutschen Saugetieren und Vogeln schmarotzenden Wuermer, unter besonderer Beruecksichtigung der Helminthen des Menschen, der Haustiere und wichtigsten Nutztiere.* Gebrueder Borntracger, Berlin.

Stafseth, H. J. 1940. Tapeworm infestation in poultry. Poultry Practice. A collection of discussions on poultry diseases and related subjects. *Vet. Med.* 34:763–65.

Stoddard, H. L. 1931. *The Bobwhite Quail: Its Habits, Preservation, and Increase.* Charles Scribner's Sons, New York.

Todd, A. C. 1946. The nature of helminth infestations in chickens in east Tennessee. *Poultry Sci.* 25:424–32.

Ward, J. W. 1946. A preliminary study of the occurrence of internal parasites of animals in Mississippi. *Proc. Helminthol. Soc. Wash. D.C.* 13:12–14.

Wardle, R. A., and J. A. McLeod. 1952. *The Zoology of Tapeworms.* Univ. Minnesota Press, Minneapolis.

Wehr, E. E., and D. R. Coburn. 1943. Some economically important parasites of the wild turkey and Hungarian partridge of Pennsylvania. *Penn. Game News* 13(11):14, 31.

Wetzel, R. 1932. Zur Kenntnis des weniggliedrigen Huehnerbandwuermes *Davainea proglottina. Arch. Wiss. Prakt. Tierheilk.* 65:595–625.

———. 1933. Zur Kenntnis des Entwicklungskreises des Huehnerbandwuermes *Raillietina cesticillus. Deut. Tieraerztl. Wochschr.* 41:465–67.

Williams, O. L. 1931. Cestodes from the eastern wild turkey. *J. Parasitol.* 18:14–20.

Yamaguti, S. 1940. Studies on the helminth fauna of Japan. Pt. 30. Cestodes of birds. II. *Japan. J. Med. Sci.* Pt. 6. *Bacteriol. Parasitol.* 1:175–211.

———. 1961. The cestodes of vertebrates. In Yamaguti, S., *Systema Helminthum,* Vol. II. Interscience Publ., New York.

Chapter 30

TREMATODES

ELON E. BYRD

Zoology Department
University of Georgia
Athens, Georgia

TREMATODES are parasitic organisms which, as parasites of vertebrates, are devoid of locomotor appendages but possess adhesive organs in the form of suckers or other specialized structures. They belong to the phylum Platyhelminthes (flatworm), a group of multicellular animals conveniently divided into three classes: Turbellaria—ciliated, free-living worms (planarians); Cestoda—segmented, ribbon-like forms (tapeworms); and Trematoda—flat and leaflike (flukes).

The class Trematoda is further divided into Aspidogastrea, Monogenea, and Digenea. The aspidogastrids comprise a small group of species which normally live as parasites of bivalve mollusks but occasionally occur as internal parasites of "shell-eating," cold-blooded vertebrates; very little is known concerning their life history. The monogenetic flukes parasitize cold-blooded aquatic and semiaquatic vertebrates. They have a direct life cycle (egg, embryo, juvenile, and adult) and live on the external surface of the host, although some become embedded in the skin or migrate into cavities (nasal, mouth, cloaca, etc.). The digenetic flukes, on the other hand, are almost exclusively endoparasites, invading practically all cavities and tissues of the body. They have complicated life

cycles, involving an alternation of generations and hosts.

There are thousands of described species of digenetic flukes; this chapter will consider only those which are important or potentially important as parasites of poultry.

GENERAL MORPHOLOGY

In general the body of the adult digenetic fluke is leaflike, occasionally cylindrical, and usually bears one or more recognizable suckers—oral and ventral (acetabulum). The body is covered with a cuticle which may bear fine scalelike spines. Except for the blood flukes (Schistosomatidae) all trematodes of poultry are monoecious; i.e., male and female organ systems are present in a single individual. Usually there are 2 testes, each giving rise to a vas eferens; these unite to form the vas deferens. After entering a saclike cirrus pouch, the vas deferens enlarges to form a sperm reservoir—the seminal vesicle. A muscular, usually eversible, copulatory organ—the cirrus—is present, and this conveys the sperm to the exterior. A single ovary is present. The vitellaria (yolk glands) usually lie lateral to the ceca, in the central third of the body. Fertilization occurs in an oötype. A sperm storage structure—the receptacle—may be present. After fertilization the zygote is enclosed along with some yolk cells in a capsule—the shell—and this is passed into a long, slender, coiling uterine tube, the terminal portion of which may be modified into a metraterm or vagina. The uterus opens alongside the cirrus, and the two organs discharge to the exterior through a common genital pore. In most flukes the genital pore is ventrally located near the ventral sucker. The digestive system consists of the mouth surrounded by the oral sucker, a short prepharyngeal tube, a muscular bulblike pharynx, a slender esophagus, and 2 intestines (ceca). The ceca are lined with a simple epithelium and usually end as blind sacs some distance from the end of the esophagus. In some forms (Cyclocoelidae, Tanaisia) the 2 ceca may become fused posteriorly, or after bifurcating from the esophagus become reunited (Schistosomatidae) into a common cecum which continues to near the posterior end of the body before ending blindly. The nervous system is composed of ganglia located in the pharyngeal region; anteriorly and pos-

Revision and extension of the information contained in this chapter are organized in accord with the data presented originally by the late Emmett W. Price.

teriorly directed nerves originate from the ganglia and pass along the lateral margins of the body as nerve trunks. The excretory system consists of a pore located at or near the body's posterior end, a bladder, and a system of collecting tubules. These tubules branch many times in ramifying the tissues, and each terminates in a flame cell—a tuft of cilia which is associated with a nucleus.

DEVELOPMENT

Customarily the eggs reach the exterior in the excrement of the host. On reaching a favorable external environment, embryonation may be complete within a few hours to many days. In some (e.g., Cyclocoelidae, Schistosomatidae), water provides the favorable environment, and after hatching the miracidium (ciliated first larval stage) swims, actively searching for an appropriate first intermediate host—usually a gastropod snail. In other flukes (e.g., Opisthorchiidae, Dicrocoeliidae) the miracidium does not hatch until after the egg is ingested by the snail host. In either case the liberated miracidium penetrates into the snail's tissues and, on reaching a location of its choice, transforms into or liberates an organism commonly called the mother sporocyst. After a week or two of growth and development the mother sporocyst (e.g., Echinostomatidae, Paramphistomatidae) produces a generation of rediae—organisms provided with a modified digestive system (mouth, sucker, and gut) and locomotor appendages. After a similar period of growth and development each redia produces a number of cercariae—second larval stage. In others (e.g., Schistosomatidae, Strigeidae) the mother sporocyst produces a generation of daughter sporocysts, and these in turn produce the cercariae. Often the number of cercariae resulting from the entrance of a single miracidium into the snail host runs into the thousands or tens of thousands. The cercaria is an immature fluke, usually provided with a tail (for swimming) and other larval structures necessary for survival, penetrating into the next host, and encystment. In some (e.g., Paramphistomatidae, Notocotylidae) the cercariae encyst on objects submerged in water; in others (e.g., Echinostomatidae, Strigeidae) the cercariae penetrate into and encyst within such second intermediate hosts as snails, insects, tadpoles, and fish. At penetration and encystment the purely larval structures are used up or discarded, and the young encysted fluke—the metacercaria—may require a shorter or longer period of encystment before it is infective for the final host, usually a vertebrate. When the infective metacercaria is ingested by the final host the cyst wall is digested away and the young fluke migrates to the site of its selection where it feeds and develops to sexual maturity. In the blood flukes (Schistosomatidae) the metacercarial stage is omitted; the cercariae penetrate the host's skin and the young flukes move along the blood vessels to the sites of their choice.

IMPORTANCE

Compared with roundworms (Nematoda) the trematodes are less important as parasites of poultry. Notwithstanding, there are more than 400 species belonging to about 100 genera and 24 families of digenetic trematodes (Gower, 1939; LaPage, 1961; McDonald, 1965) known to occur in members of the avian orders Anseriformes (ducks and allies), Galliformes (chickens and allies), Columbiformes (pigeons and allies) and Passeriformes (perching birds). Although most of these flukes are rather host specific, some are known from hosts in each of the 4 avian orders listed. This versatility in host selection makes some of the species heretofore unrecorded as poultry parasites potentially dangerous hazards to the industry.

With but few exceptions the fluke species recorded from birds are believed to cause only light to moderate pathology. Some, however, may be a leading cause of pathology among domestic poultry, especially when the parasite burden is heavy. With trematodes as with other parasites, the amount of damage or loss also will depend largely on the organ(s) involved. The fact that domestic birds have parasites in common with wild relatives enhances the possibility that an otherwise "mild-mannered" parasite of a wild natural host could develop into a serious pathogen when introduced into a nonimmune (nonresistant) domestic bird. The poultryman thus should be aware constantly of the possibility that a potentially dangerous parasite can be present in a wild population of the area and that such a parasite could result in reduced profit if introduced into his flock.

TAXONOMY

In recent years taxonomists have divided the subclass Digenea into the superorders Anepitheliocystidia and Epitheliocystidia, basing the separation on whether or not the excretory bladder of the sexual stage is lined with an epithelium. Members of both superorders are present among the fluke parasites of poultry, and these, as indicated above, have representatives in 24 families. Representatives of some of these families do not occur in poultry of North America or are reported as being present under circumstances suggesting accidental parasitism. The more dangerous (or potentially dangerous) trematodes of poultry in the Western Hemisphere have been assigned to 18 families (10 belonging to the Anepitheliocystidia, indicated by a single asterisk, and 8 belonging to the Epitheliocystidia, double asterisk) in the following dichotomous key:

1. Dioecious species (separate sex); parasites in the blood vascular system . . . .
   . . . . . . Schistosomatidae*
   Monoecious species (hermaphroditic); parasites in locations other than blood stream 2

2. Body fleshy, rounded or hemispherical in shape; usually living as pairs in cutaneous cysts . . . . . . Collyriclidae**
   Body elongated, usually flattened; living elsewhere in body 3

3. Monostomate flukes (oral sucker only) . 4
   Distomate flukes (usually prominent oral and ventral suckers present) . . . 6

4. Stout-bodied flukes with intestinal ceca uniting posteriorly; living in respiratory passages . . . . . Cyclocoelidae*
   Smaller flukes; only rarely do ceca unite (Tanaisia) posteriorly; when ventral sucker is present it is small and masked by uterus; not living in respiratory passages 5

5. Pharynx absent; uterus in front of testes; parasites of digestive tube (small intestine and cecum) . . . . Notocotylidae*
   Pharynx present; uterus extends both behind and in front of testes; parasites of the excretory system . . Eucotylidae**

6. Ventral sucker prominent, at extreme posterior end of body . Paramphistomatidae*

Ventral sucker less prominent and elsewhere on ventral surface of body . 7

7. Body divided by constriction into cup or leaflike anterior portion and cylindrical posterior portion; genital pore at extreme posterior end of body . . Strigeidae*
   Body not divided by constriction into 2 parts; genital pore on ventral surface of body 8

8. Testes tandem (one behind the other); vitellaria usually extending from bifurcation of ceca to caudal end of body . . . 9
   Testes not tandemly arranged; vitellaria usually more restricted, extending through about 1/3 of body length . . . 10

9. Oral sucker surrounded by adoral collar or disc bearing relatively large spines . .
   . . . . . . Echinostomatidae*
   Oral sucker not surrounded by armed, adoral collar . . . Psilostomatidae*

10. Gonotyl (genital sucker) present, beside ventral sucker . . . Heterophyidae**
    Gonotyl absent 11

11. Testes in posterior end of body, usually behind other elements of genital system . 12
    Testes more anterior in position, not caudal to other elements of genital system 13

12. Uterine loops overlapping ceca; parasitic in conjunctival sacs of eye . . . . .
    . . . . . . Philophthalmidae*
    Uterine loops confined to area between ceca; parasitic in liver . Opisthorchiidae**

13. Testes in front of ovary; parasitic in liver . . . . . . Dicrocoeliidae**
    Arrangement of testes and ovary otherwise; parasitic elsewhere in body . . . 14

14. Ovary between testes; uterus in front of gonads . . . . . Brachylaimidae*
    Ovary in front of testes; uterus extending into both pre- and post-testicular regions 15

15. Suckers weakly developed; body usually with a conical extension at caudal end; parasitic in kidney . . . Renicolidae*
    Suckers well developed; body without posterior extension; parasitic elsewhere in body 16

16. Ceca short, scarcely reaching level of ventral sucker . . . . Microphallidae**
    Ceca extending beyond level of ventral sucker 17

17. Genital pore close beside oral sucker . .
    . . . . . . Prosthogonimidae**
    Genital pore more caudal in position, usually immediately in front of ventral sucker . . . . Plagiorchiidae**

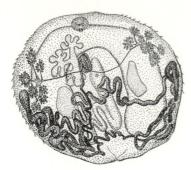

FIG. 30.1—Collyriclum faba, *ventral view.*
(Kossack, 1911)

SKIN

COLLYRICLIDAE

The skin fluke is rather plump of body
and lives as pairs in fibrous, cutaneous
cysts.

Collyriclum faba (Bremser 1831)

SYNONYM. *Collyriclum colei* Ward 1917.

DESCRIPTION. Body hemispherical, 4.2–8.6
mm long by 4.5–5.5 mm wide (Fig. 30.1).
Oral sucker subterminal; acetabulum absent. Testes variable in shape; ovary T-
shaped, with each branch divided into several lobes. Vitellaria in anterior part of
body, somewhat asymmetrical, consisting of
6–9 groups of follicles on each side. Uterus
greatly coiled, in posterior part of body.
Eggs 19–21μ long by 9–11μ wide.

This parasite occurs in cutaneous cysts
in the skin of chickens, turkeys, and a number of passerine birds. The cysts are 4–6
mm in diameter, and each normally contains two flukes, one slightly smaller than
the other. An opening at the summit of
the cyst allows the fluke's eggs to escape.
In the United States the fluke has been reported from poultry in Minnesota where it
was found in young chickens and turkeys
by Riley and Kernkamp (1924). Marotel
(1926) reported it as parasitizing turkey
poults in southeastern France.

LIFE HISTORY. Although the life history of
C. faba is unknown, it, like other flukes,
must require a snail primary host. Because
of its widespread occurrence in passerine
birds, the molluscan host in all probability
is an ordinary garden variety of snail (family Polygyridae), and the second intermediate host an arthropod. Jegen (1917) believed the infection to be direct, since each
egg contained two embryos—young flukes
and not miracidia. Tyzzer (1918), Riley
and Kernkamp (1924), and Riley (1931),
however, observed miracidia (not young
flukes) escaping from the eggs. Riley was
of the opinion that dragonfly larvae may

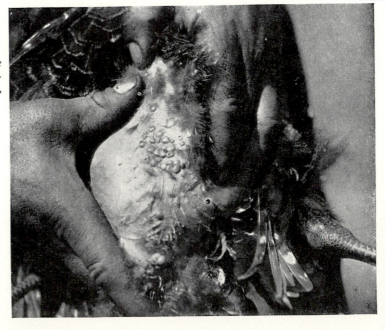

FIG. 30.2—*Abdominal surface
of turkey to show cysts of* Collyriclum faba. *(Kernkamp,
Univ. of Minn.)*

serve as secondary intermediate hosts, because the outbreaks of infection among
chickens and turkeys which he was able to
observe occurred in birds having access to
wet or marshy places at a time in early summer when the dragonfly nymphs were
emerging. Riley also "recovered from these
nymphs metacercariae which suggest closely the characteristics of the adult *Collyriclum*."

PATHOLOGY. The encysted flukes are found
mainly around the vent but may occur elsewhere on the body of the affected bird (Fig.
30.2). In the cases studied in the United
States there were no striking symptoms,
but there is little doubt that extremely
heavy infections in young birds would
prove fatal. In poultry of marketable age
the presence of *Collyriclum* cysts in the
skin greatly decrease the value of the birds.

Farmer and Morgan (1944) summarized
the information available on *C. faba*. They
found it had been recorded from chickens
and turkeys in Minnesota and from turkeys
in France, as well as from wild birds of the
passerine families Corvidae, Motacillidae,
Paridae, Ploceidae, Sittidae, Sturnidae,
Sylviidae, Turdidae and Tyrannidae. In
the United States these infected birds were
taken in Maryland, New Jersey, Massachusetts, Michigan, and Minnesota. The
parasite had been reported from the robin
(family Turdidae) and Byrd (1970) reported it from the brown thrasher in western
Virginia.

EYE

PHILOPHTHALMIDAE

Flukes commonly occurring in the eye
(conjunctival sacs) of birds are relatively
small trematodes with well-developed suckers and a finely spinose cuticle. The gonads
are in the posterior end of the body, with
the ovary in front of the testes. The yolk
glands (vitellaria) lie laterally and usually
are tubular in form. At least 3 genera and
12 species of the family have been reported
from Anseriformes, Galliformes, and Gruiformes and experimentally from mammals.
The family is typified by *P. gralli*.

Philophthalmus gralli
Mathis and Leger 1910

DESCRIPTION. Body lanceolate, 3–6 mm long
by 0.9–1.7 mm wide, yellowish and semi-

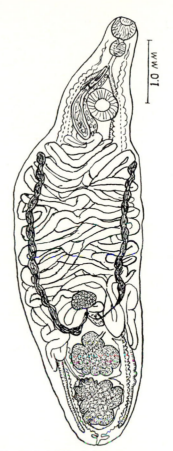

FIG. 30.3—*Philophthalmus gralli, ventral
view. (West, 1961)*

transparent (Fig. 30.3). Oral sucker 285μ
wide; acetabulum about 588μ in diameter
and one-fourth of body length from anteri-
or end. Genital aperture about midway
between the suckers. Cirrus pouch slender,
its base slightly distal to the acetabulum.
Testes oval, tandem, in posterior fourth of
body. Ovary median, pretesticular. Uterus
with numerous transverse loops, filling
greater part of the body from level of anterior margin of testicular zone to base of
cirrus pouch; metraterm slender, as long as
and paralleling cirrus pouch. Vitellaria
tubular, more or less obscured by uterus.
Eggs in uterus $85–120\mu$ long by $39–55\mu$
wide; each contains fully developed miracidium when mature.

LIFE HISTORY. The life cycle has been ascertained by Alicata and Noda (1960) and
Alicata (1962) in Hawaii, and by West
(1961) in Indiana. The freshly oviposited

egg contains a fully developed miracidium in which is found a mother redia. Hatching takes place almost immediately on reaching water. On making contact with a suitable snail (*Tarebia granifera mauiensis* and *Melanoides newcombi* in Hawaii and *Goniobasis* spp. and *Pleurocera acuta* in Indiana), the miracidium penetrates the host's tissues and releases the mother redia. The redia makes its way into the snail's heart where, according to Alicata, two subsequent generations of rediae develop. The final redial generation, giving rise to cercariae, moves from the heart to the digestive gland. The time required for development from mother redia to cercariae is about 3 months. Upon emerging from the snail host, the cercariae encyst on any solid object, including the shells of snails and exoskeletons of crayfish. When eaten by a bird host, the encysted metacercaria excysts in the mouth and crop and the young fluke migrates to the conjunctival sac through the nasolacrimal duct; 1–5 days are required for the young fluke to reach the eye where it matures in about a month.

In a closely related species *Philophthalmus megalurus* (Cort 1914), Khalil and Cable (1969) conclude that there are no less than 5 polymorphic generations in the life cycle. The miracidium contains a well-developed redialike sporocyst in its body cavity on hatching. The sporocyst is released into the tissues of the snail host *Pleurocera acuta* at penetration and makes its way to the snail's heart where it develops a small number of mother rediae. Each mother redia produces many daughter rediae, and these in turn, after leaving the host's heart, produce a few granddaughter rediae and many cercariae. On emerging from the snail the cercariae swim about for a short time before encysting on any solid object, including the surface of the dish in which the host snail is kept. When the water in the dish is replaced with warm (45° C) saline, the metacercariae excysts. When the freed metacercariae are pipetted directly into the eyes of newly hatched Leghorn chickens they develop into mature flukes.

PATHOLOGY. The attachment of the worms by their suckers to the conjunctiva causes congestion and erosion of the membrane. The conjunctival fluid contains blood, fluke eggs, and active miracidia.

Philophthalmus gralli has been reported in natural infections of the chicken, peafowl, turkey, duck, and goose in Indo-China and Formosa, and in experimental infections of chickens in the United States (Hawaii and Indiana). Several other species have been reported from domestic poultry as follows: *P. anatinus* Sugimoto from ducks in China; *P. muraschkinzewi* Tretiakowa from ducks in Russia; and *P. problematicus* Tubangui from chickens and *P. rizalensis* Tubangui from ducks in the Philippines. Recently Penner and Fried (1961) and Fried (1962) reported experimental infections of chicks with an unnamed species of Philophthalmus, later named *P. hegeneri*, obtained from a marine snail *Batillaria minima* from Florida. In spite of successful experimental infections with this species, the fact that a marine snail is involved in the life cycle makes it improbable that domestic poultry would be found infected under natural conditions. Heard (1967) found 3 of 11 clapper rails from Monroe County, Florida, to be infected with *P. hegeneri*.

RESPIRATORY SYSTEM

CYCLOCOELIDAE

Flukes commonly occurring in the respiratory system of domestic fowl are relatively large forms and have flattened oval or lancet-shaped bodies. The oral sucker is weakly developed or absent, and the acetabulum is absent or rudimentary. The branches of the intestine are fused posteriorly, causing the ceca to make one complete circle. The gonads are near the posterior end of the body with the ovary variously arranged with respect to the testes. The family is represented by at least 6 genera and 11 species in birds from around the world, with but 2 genera and 3 species of importance occurring in domestic fowl in North and South America.

Typhlocoelum cymbium (Diesing 1850)

SYNONYM. *Tracheophilus sisowi* Skrjabin 1913.

DESCRIPTION. Body oval, 6–12 mm long by 3–6 mm (Fig. 30.4). Mouth terminal, not surrounded by a muscular sucker; acetabu-

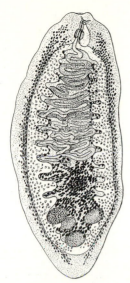

FIG. 30.4—Typhlocoelum cymbium, *ventral view. (Skrjabin, 1913)*

lum absent. Intestinal tract continuous posteriorly and provided with several median diverticula. Ovary and testes in posterior part of body, the latter rounded in shape. Uterus greatly convoluted, in median field. Eggs 154–180μ long by 85–90μ wide.

This species is not uncommon in wild waterfowl in various parts of the world, including the United States, and has been reported from the duck and goose. It occurs in the trachea, bronchi, air sacs, and infraorbital sinus.

LIFE HISTORY. The life history has been ascertained by Szidat (1932) and Stunkard (1934). The eggs, which contain miracidia when deposited, hatch on reaching water. The miracidium swims about and, on coming in contact with suitable snails *(Menetus planorbis, Helisoma trivolvis, Planorbis corneus, Lymnaea palustris,* or *L. ovata),* penetrates the tissues and liberates a redia which is present in the body of the miracidium. The redia increases in size and gives rise to tailless cercariae which escape and become encysted in the vicinity of the redia. Birds become infected by eating the snails harboring the encysted larvae.

PATHOLOGY. The presence of a large number of these flukes in the larynx and tra-

chea may cause death by suffocation. Light infections may cause little or no injury.

Typhlocoelum cucumerinum (Rudolphi 1809)

SYNONYMS. *Typhlocoelum flavum* (Mehlis 1831); *T. obovale* Neumann 1909.

DESCRIPTION. Body oval, 6–15 mm long by 2–7 mm wide, yellowish in color. General features similar to *T. cymbium* except that testes are deeply lobed instead of rounded. Eggs 122–154μ long by 73–81μ wide, each containing a miracidium when oviposited.

This fluke occurs in the trachea of wild waterfowl in North and South America and in Europe; it has been reported from the domestic duck in South America.

LIFE HISTORY. Incompletely known, probably similar to that of *T. cymbium.*

PATHOLOGY. This fluke was reported by Magalhães (1899) in Brazil as the cause of suffocation promptly resulting in death of some domestic ducks; it was present in large numbers in the trachea and bronchi.

Several other cyclocoelids have been reported as parasites of poultry: *Cyclocoelum mutabile* (Zeder) from the goose and turkey in Europe, Asia, and South America; *C. japonicus* Kurisu from the chicken in Japan; and *Hyptiasmus tumidus* Kossack from the goose in Europe.

In addition to flukes of the family Cyclocoelidae, Price (1937) reported *Clinostomum attenuatum* Cort (Clinostomatidae), normally a parasite of bitterns, from the trachea of a chicken in Nebraska. This was apparently a case of accidental parasitism acquired through the ingestion of a tadpole or young frog containing the larvae of the fluke.

DIGESTIVE SYSTEM

The digestive system (liver and digestive tube) is a favorite location for sexually mature trematodes. As many as 290 species belonging to 80 genera and 15 families have been recorded from wild and domestic fowl from this system. Many of these are considered to be accidental parasites (reported but once); others have been experimentally introduced into these hosts.

ECHINOSTOMATIDAE

Flukes of the family Echinostomatidae are generally small in size, have the gonads

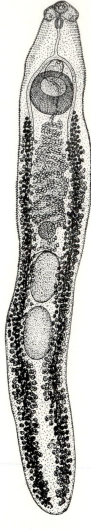

FIG. 30.5—Echinostoma revolutum, *ventral view. (Dietz, 1910)*

by an adoral disc bearing 37 spines—27 marginal and 5 on each ventral lobe. Acetabulum strongly developed, situated a short distance posterior to oral sucker. Testes variable in shape, one behind the other; ovary pretesticular; uterus preovarial. Eggs 94–126μ long by 59–71μ wide.

The fluke occurs in the intestine, ceca, and cloaca of a wide variety of hosts, including members of the avian orders Anseriformes, Podicipediformes, Pelecaniformes, Ciconiiformes, Falconiformes, Galliformes, Gruiformes, Charadriiformes, Columbiformes, Strigiformes, Coraciformes, and Passeriformes and from Marsupialia, Carnivora, Rodentia, Lagomorpha, Artiodactyla, and Primates (man) among mammals. It is cosmopolitan in distribution and has been described under a large variety of names, some of which are indicated above as synonyms. The species has been recorded a total of 93 times in wild and 86 times in domestic ducks.

LIFE HISTORY. The life history of *E. revolutum* is known mostly through the work of Johnson (1920) and Beaver (1937). The egg hatches in 9–14 days on reaching fresh water, and the miracidium penetrates into a snail of the genera *Amerianna, Anisus, Gyraulus, Lymnaea, Helisoma, Physa, Planorbis* or *Semisulcospira*. The cercariae develop in daughter rediae, and on escaping from the snail they enter and encyst in mollusks (members of 18 or more genera), planarians, fish, and amphibians. The final hosts are reached when these second intermediate hosts are ingested.

PATHOLOGY. In most instances and in light infections, this fluke causes little injury. Heavy infections in pigeons have been reported from Europe by Zunker (1925), Krause (1925), Bolle (1925), and Van Heelsbergen (1927b); in these cases losses have resulted. Zunker stated that the small intestine of the affected birds showed hemorrhagic inflammation, and similar findings were reported by Bolle. Krause collected about 5,000 echinostomes, apparently *E. revolutum*, from 8 pigeons at Rostock; the more heavily parasitized birds died, while the more lightly infected ones recovered after sickness lasting several weeks. In the cases studied by Bolle there was hemorrhagic diarrhea; some of the pigeons died in an emaciated condition after being sick for 4 days. Krause reported as early symp-

entirely behind the uterus, and possess an adoral kidney-shaped collar about the anterior end of the body. The collar is armed with stout cuticular spines. No less than 88 species belonging to 15 genera of the family have been reported from fowl. Some of the species are cosmopolitan in distribution; others are rather restricted. Only a few of the more important echinostomes will be considered.

Echinostoma revolutum (Froelich 1802)

SYNONYMS. *Echinostoma echinatum* (Zeder 1803); *E. columbae* Zunker 1925; *E. paraulum* Dietz 1909; *E. miyagawai* Ishii 1932; *E. cinetorchis* Ando and Ozaki 1923.

DESCRIPTION. Body elongated, up to 22 mm long (Fig. 30.5). Oral sucker surrounded

toms the refusal of food, increased thirst, weakness in flight, and pronounced diarrhea; death occurred in 8–10 days following increased weakness. Van Heelsbergen in Holland also reported a severe enteritis in pigeons infected with an echinostome which appears to be *E. revolutum.* The birds showed atrophy of the pectoral muscles, engorged liver, and intestinal congestion; the lumen of the gut was filled with a hemorrhagic catarrhal secretion containing numerous flukes, 1,550 specimens being present in one pigeon. In the United States Beaver (1937) reported a case of experimental infection in a pigeon which developed a bloody diarrhea 10 days after being infected. At necropsy 621 flukes were recovered, the majority being in the lower duodenum and upper ileum. Kitchell et al. (1947) found 40 of 670 turkey poults in Minnesota to harbor *E. revolutum.* A total of 200 parasites was recovered from 4 of the dead poults. Metacercariae of the species were found in *Helisoma trivolvis.*

Echinoparyphium recurvatum (Linstow 1873)

DESCRIPTION. Body 0.7–4.5 mm long, with the anterior part strongly recurved ventrally (Fig. 30.6A). Adoral disc armed with 45 spines in a double row (Fig. 30.6B). General organization similar to that of *Echinostoma revolutum.* Eggs 108–120μ long by 64–84μ wide.

This parasite is widely distributed, being reported from Europe, Asia, Africa, and North America. It has been recorded as many as 45 times in wild fowl and 45 times in domestic birds. The species is known to occur in turkeys in California (Annereaux, 1940), Oklahoma (Self and Bouchard, 1950), Alabama, Arkansas, Florida, Louisiana, and Tennessee (Maxfield et al., 1963). The domestic chicken in both the United States and Mexico harbors the parasite. Among birds generally the species has recorded from Anseriformes, Podicipediformes, Cioniformes, Falconiformes, Galliformes, Gruiformes, Charadriiformes, Columbiformes, Strigiformes, and Passeriformes. Among mammals it is known to occur in Rodentia, Carnivora, and Primates (man). It normally is a parasite of the small intestine.

LIFE HISTORY. Similar to that of *E. revolutum.* The cercariae develop in daughter rediae in several species of freshwater snails (Lymnaea, Physa, Psidium, Bulinus, Gyraulus, Musculinum, Planorbis, Sphaerium, Valvata, Paludina, and Spiralina), and the metacercariae (Fig. 30.6C) encyst in these snail hosts as well as in the tadpoles of Anurans. The fluke matures and begins egg production 8–18 days after reaching the definitive host.

PATHOLOGY. Van Heelsbergen (1927a) reported that in Holland infected chickens showed a severe enteritis. The parasitized birds were emaciated and anemic and developed weakness of the legs. Annereaux (1940) in California observed a "severe inflammation of the intestinal mucosa with cecal involvements consisting of a pasty, cheeselike mass which greatly distended the organs" in a 10-week-old turkey harboring 267 adult flukes in the upper portion of the small intestine. More recently Betz (1941), Soulsby (1955), and Shleikus and Tatarintsevaite (1960) found little or no pathology when the parasite occurs in small or moderate numbers. When present in large numbers, especially in young birds, the infection is accompanied by a severe irritation-inflammation of the mucosa in both the intestine and ceca, a cheeselike exudate in the lumen, droopiness, loss of appetite, and death. Older birds may survive the infection but there may be a loss in weight, a reduction of egg production, and a generalized malaise.

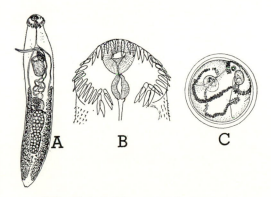

FIG. 30.6—Echinoparyphium recurvatum. (A) Ventral view of entire worm. (B) Anterior end to show head collar. (C) Encysted larva. (After Bittner, 1925)

Hypoderaeum conoideum (Bloch 1782)

SYNONYMS. *Echinostoma oxycephalum* (Rudolphi 1819); *Opisthorchis pianae*

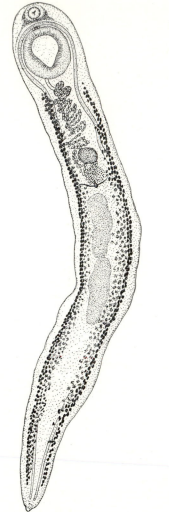

FIG. 30.7—Hypoderaeum conoideum, ventral view. (Dietz, 1910)

Galli-Valerio 1898; *Psilochasmus lecithosus* Otte 1926.

DESCRIPTION. Similar in size and appearance to *Echinostoma revolutum* (Fig. 30.7). Adoral disc poorly developed, bearing 49 short spines in a double row. Eggs 95–108μ long by 61–68μ wide.

The species occurs in the small intestine of numerous wild waterfowl and has been found in the chicken, goose, and pigeon. It was reported from the domestic duck in the United States by Stunkard and Dunihue (1931), and has been recorded at least 52 times in wild and 47 times in domestic fowl. These hosts include Anseriformes, Podocipediformes, Galliformes, and Co-

lumbiformes. It is known from Europe, Africa, and North America.

LIFE HISTORY. Similar to that of *E. revolutum*, with the cercariae developing in daughter rediae in *Lymnaea* and *Planorbis* snails. The metacercariae are in snails of these two genera as well as in other snails, and the young flukes develop to maturity in 8–30 days after being transferred to the definitive host.

PATHOLOGY. The pathology is not well known, but like the other echinostomes its damage to the host depends largely on the number of worms present. Vevers (1923) reported a localized inflammation in the immediate area of the parasite and a progressive weakness leading to death of a bird infected with 40 of the flukes.

A similar species, *Echinoparyphium aconiatum* (Dietz 1910), has been recorded from domestic ducks and chickens and is known to occur in the United States in wild fowl. Its life cycle follows very closely that outlined for the other echinostomes included herein.

PSILOSTOMATIDAE

In general morphology flukes of this family resemble species of the Echinostomatidae but are usually much smaller, often globose, and not provided with the armed adoral disc.

Ribeiroia ondatrae (Price 1931)

SYNONYMS. *Psilostomum ondatrae* Price 1931; *Cercaria marini* Faust and Hoffman 1934.

DESCRIPTION. Elongate oval flukes measuring 1.6–3mm in length (Fig. 30.8) and having a spiny cuticle. Oral sucker and acetabulum well developed. Esophagus with lateral diverticula. Testes in posterior end of body; ovary pretesticular. Vitellaria consisting of relatively large follicles extending from level of esophagus to posterior end of body. Uterus between ovary and acetabulum. Eggs 82–90μ long by 45–48μ wide.

This fluke, originally described from the muskrat in Canada by Price (1931), occurs in the proventriculus of several fish-eating birds including the California gull, green heron, osprey, and Cooper's hawk. It has also been reported in natural infections in the chicken in Colorado (Newsom and

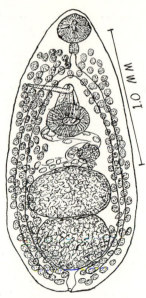

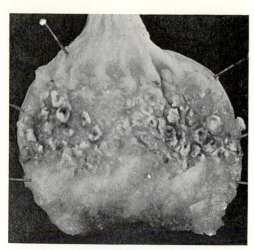

FIG. 30.9—Proventriculus of chicken showing lesions caused by Ribeiroia ondatrae. *(Newsom and Stout, 1933)*

FIG. 30.8–Ribeiroia ondatrae, ventral view. (Price, 1931)

Stout, 1933), in the domestic goose in Canada (Kingscote, 1951), in experimental infections in the chicken, duck, pigeon, and canary (Beaver, 1939), and in the parakeet and pigeon (Riggin, 1956). Yamaguti (1958) erected a new genus Pseudopsilostoma for the reception of this species.

LIFE HISTORY. Similar to that indicated for the echinostomes. Beaver (1939) reported Helisoma to serve as the primary host in the United States, while Riggin (1956) found Australorbis to be the primary host in Puerto Rico. The cercariae develop in daughter rediae and on emerging from the snail enter and encyst mainly in the lateral line organ of fish (perch, rock bass, small mouth black bass, pumpkinseed, blue gill, catfish, guppy, and minnow). The metacercariae are infective in about a week and, after transfer to the final host, reach sexual maturity in 7–10 days. Metacercariae have been found in the nostrils of tadpoles.

PATHOLOGY. Newsom and Stout (1933) reported outbreaks of proventriculitis in two flocks of chickens in Colorado. The birds lost their appetite, stood around with their eyes closed, and gradually wasted away. Gross examination "showed a very noticeable enlargement of the proventriculus. On opening this organ there seemed to be a deep reddening around the orifices of the glands. In the more extreme cases there appeared to be a grayish exudate on the surface, simulating ulceration" (Fig. 30.9). Microscopic examination "showed that the surface of the mucous membrane was covered with a fibrinous exudate, the outer portion of which had become necrotic. Below this necrotic area was a thick zone heavily infiltrated with polymorphonuclear leukocytes. Under this the mucous layer was quite edematous in which were scattered a few polymorphonuclear leukocytes and a few monocytes. In a few places small abscesses had formed in the lower portion of the mucous membrane." Beaver (1939) observed in experimental infections in chickens and canaries that this fluke is fairly pathogenic, each worm forming in the proventriculus a separate lesion which is a deeply eroded pit with a raised orifice surrounded by a conspicuous reddish to purple area. Leibowitz (1962) recorded *R. ondatrae* as the natural cause of death in domestic ducks in the United States.

Sphaeridiotream globulus (Rudolphi 1914)

DESCRIPTION. Body pyriform to globular, 0.5–0.85 mm long (Fig. 30.10). Suckers well developed, acetabulum massive. Genital aperture lateral, at level of posterior margin of oral sucker. Testes in posterior end of body, one dorsal to other. Ovary pretesticular. Vitellaria consisting of large follicles extending from intestinal bifur-

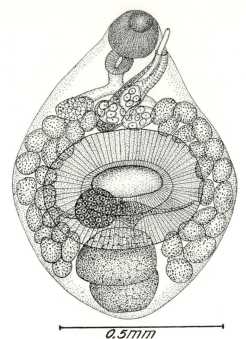

FIG. 30.10—Sphaeridiotrema globulus, *ventral view. (Price, 1934)*

cation to level of anterior margins of testes; uterus relatively short, largely preacetabular. Eggs 90–105μ long by 60–67μ wide.

This fluke occurs in the small intestine of the wild duck in Europe and North America and has been reported from the domestic duck and swan. In the United States it was reported by Price (1934) as causing extensive loss among lesser scaup ducks near Washington, D.C., and it has also been found by Shaw (1947) in the domestic duck in Oregon.

LIFE HISTORY. As determined by Szidat (1937) in Germany, the cercariae develop in rediae in the snail *Bithynia tentaculata*, and the metacercariae encyst between the shell and mantle of the same host. Birds acquire the parasite through ingesting of the infected mollusk; eggs appear in the host's feces 5–6 days later.

PATHOLOGY. This fluke produces in wild fowl a severe ulcerative enteritis. Price (1934) found that on three separate occasions wild ducks evidently had died of a marked congestion, hemorrhaging, and ulceration of the lower third of the small intestine. The lumen of the gut was filled by a cast composed largely of fibrin. Histolog-

ically the layers (serosa, muscular, and mucous) of the gut showed evidence of acute hyperemia; the mucous membrane showed pronounced epithelial desquamation, the villi being entirely denuded in most areas, and the accompanying ulcers extended as deep as the muscularis. These areas contained numerous flukes attached by their powerful suckers. Cornwell and Cowan (1963) and Trainer and Fisher (1963) found similar conditions in ducks and other waterfowl. To date the trematode is known to occur in Anseriformes, Gruiformes, and Charadriiformes from Europe, Asia, and North America.

In a similar species, *Sphaeridiotrema spinoacetabulum* Burns 1961, the individuals inhabit the ceca where they produce pathological changes similar to those described by Price (1934) for *S. globulus*. Since the intestinal ceca of *S. spinoacetabulum* were filled with blood, it was assumed that the flukes live off the host's blood. Evidently the two forms differ mainly in requiring different habitats within the host (ceca for *S. spinoacetabulum* and small intestine for *S. globulus*). Burns (1961) worked out the life cycle for his species and found it to use the snail *Flumincola virens* as the first intermediate host and this snail and *Oxytrema silicula* as the second intermediate hosts. The cercariae developed in rediae and required 16 days for full development as metacercariae. On being ingested, the young flukes developed to sexual maturity in 9 days. In experimental feedings 3 of 7 ducklings 4 weeks old died after being fed 250 metacercariae.

More recently Byrd and Prestwood (1969) reported a new genus and species, *Psilotornus audacirrus*, of the family Psilostomatidae from the cecum of the wild turkey in Alabama. The host was a young bird (previous year's brood) and was collected routinely during the early spring hunt. The cecum of the host bird showed no gross pathological changes even though it contained 87 specimens of the fluke.

STRIGEIDAE

The strigeids are characterized by having the body divided into two parts, an anterior leaf or cup-shaped portion containing the suckers and a peculiar tonguelike adhesive organ—the haptor—and a cylindrical posterior portion containing the reproduc-

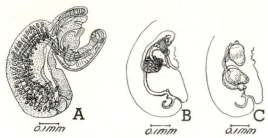

FIG. 30.11—Cotylurus flabelliformis. (A) Lateral view to show digestive and excretory systems. (B) Female genital system. (C) Male genital system. (Van Haitsma, 1931)

tive organs. At least 5 genera and 30 species are known from waterfowl.

Cotylurus flabelliformis (Faust 1917)

DESCRIPTION. Body 0.56–0.85 mm long, anterior cup-shaped portion 0.20–0.28 mm long and posterior cylindrical portion 0.36–0.57 mm long (Fig. 30.11). Genital aperture at posterior end of body. Eggs 100–112μ long by 68–76μ wide.

The fluke occurs in the intestine of a number of wild ducks in the United States and has been reported from the domestic duck; it also has been grown to maturity in chickens. Maxfield et al. (1963) found the species occurring naturally in wild turkeys (17 of 390 birds) from Alabama, Arkansas, Florida, Tennessee, and Virginia.

LIFE HISTORY. The cercarial and precercarial stages occur in snails of the genera Helisoma, Planorbis, Stagnicola, Lymnaea, and Physa. The cercariae, developing in daughter sporocysts in the snail in about 20–30 days, have forked tails. On escaping from the snail host they penetrate into other snails and develop into tetracotylid larvae. When snails containing them are ingested by a definite host, they grow to maturity and begin egg production in 3–4 days. The species normally occurs in birds of the orders Anseriformes and Galliformes in Europe, Asia, and North America.

PATHOLOGY. According to Van Haitsma (1931), C. flabelliformis digests away the epithelium of the intestine of the host and causes a congestion of the subepithelial tissue. The symptoms shown by infected ducks appear to vary greatly; some showed leg weakness, nervous twitchings of the head and wings, dyspnea, diarrhea, and irregular appetite, and others given "heavy doses" of larvae died within a week without showing definite symptoms.

Other strigeid flukes reported from North America as parasites of Anseriformes and Galliformes include Cotylurus cornutus (Rudolphi 1808), Apatemon gracilis (Rudolphi 1819), and A. falconis meleagris Harwood 1931. Although these species can be distinguished from each other and from C. flabelliformis by experts in taxonomy, their general morphology is quite similar, as are their life cycles. Where it is known, the pathology produced by them is similar to that caused by C. flabelliformis (see Feng, 1931). Apatemon falconis meleagris is reported from the domestic turkey in Texas; the other two species are known to occur in Anseriformes in Canada, United States, Cuba, and Venezuela.

BRACHYLAEMIDAE

Flukes of this family are characterized mainly by having the gonads in a linear series in the posterior end of the body, the ovary being situated between the testes. The genital pore is in the zone of the gonads.

Postharmostomum gallinum (Witenberg 1923)

SYNONYMS. Harmostomum (Postharmostomum) horizawai Ozaki 1925; H. annamense Railliet 1925; H. (P.) hawaiiensis Guberlet 1928.

DESCRIPTION. Body linguiform, 3.5–7.4 mm (Fig. 30.12). Oral sucker and acetabulum strongly developed, the latter situated about one-third of body length from anterior end. Intestinal ceca with wide serpentine undulations. Ovary between testes, near posterior end of body. Vitellaria lateral, extending anteriorly as far as posterior margin of acetabulum; uterus in front of gonads, extending anteriorly as far as intestinal bifurcation. Eggs 29–32μ long by 18μ wide.

This trematode occurs in the ceca of the chicken, turkey, guinea fowl, and pigeon in Europe, Asia, and Africa, and in the chicken in Hawaii and Puerto Rico.

LIFE HISTORY. According to Alicata (1940), the egg contains a miracidium when oviposited. When the egg is eaten by the snail

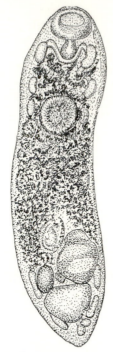

FIG. 30.12—Postharmostomum gallinum, ventral view. (Skrjabin, 1924)

Eulota similaris, hatching occurs, and the miracidium penetrates to the host's liver and develops into a sporocyst. The cercariae, developing in daughter sporocysts, escape and leave the body of the snail; they may reenter the same snail host or enter others of the same or different species where they become encysted in the pericardial cavity. Another land snail, *Subulina octona,* has been shown to harbor the metacercariae. In the Orient *Euhadra peliomphala, Philomycus bilineatus,* and *Eulota sieboldiana minor* have been reported as capable of serving as intermediate hosts.

PATHOLOGY. So far as known, these flukes cause little or no injury to their bird hosts. It is possible that in extreme cases of heavy infection, some irritation or inflammation of the ceca might result.

In addition to *Postharmostomum gallinum* three other members of the family have been found naturally in poultry or have grown experimentally to sexual maturity in these hosts. Two of these belong to the genus *Brachylaemus.* The first, *B. virginiana* (Dickerson, 1930), a species known to occur commonly in the opossum

Didelphis virginiana Kerr was reported by Maxfield et al. (1963) from 17 of 302 wild turkeys *(Meleagris gallopava* subspp.) examined from 6 southeastern states. No infected bird was encountered in Florida, Georgia, Kentucky, and Mississippi. The number of birds searched in these states was 67, 9, 4, and 8 respectively. In Alabama approximately 1 of each 10 birds (total 104) searched harbored the species; in the other states the infection ran as follows: Arkansas, 1 of 76 birds; Louisiana, 2 of 21; Maryland, 1 of 9; Tennessee, 1 of 54; Virginia, 2 of 38.

The life cycle of *B. virginiana* is similar to that of *P. gallinum* except that garden snails and slugs (genera Polygyra, Helix, Helisoma, Deroceras, Succinea, Pseudosuccinea, Agrolimax, and Mesodon) are used as the first intermediate hosts. The sporocyst is branched and the cercariae are tailless. On emerging the cercaria reenters the same snail host or another snail of the same species where it slowly develops to the infective stage. The transfer is made when the final host ingests the snail carrying the infective stage larva. When present in large numbers the sexually mature fluke may cause a marked inflammation of the mucosa of the small intestine.

The second species of the genus Brachylaemus is *B. fuscatus* (Rudolphi 1819). It has been reported from the esophagus, small intestine, and ceca of the duck, pigeon, and chicken as well as from other birds in Europe, Asia, Africa, and North America. The cercariae develop in sporocysts in the kidney of Deroceras, Helicella, Helicopsis, Helix, and Oxychilus, and the metacercariae occur in these same snail hosts; they mature in 7–10 days after being transferred to the final host. In large numbers the fluke can produce considerable inflammation in the mucous membrane of that part of the digestive tract in which they reside.

The third member of the family, *Leucochloridiomorpha constantiae* (Mueller 1935), is a parasite of the bursa of Fabricius of ducks. Allison (1943) found the cercariae to develop in irregularly branching sporocysts in the aquatic snail *Campeloma decisum.* The cercariae have a forked tail and a short tail stem; they are poor swimmers, swimming a very short time before reentering the same snail host where they require a period of about 5 months to develop to the infective stage. The infective larvae (cercariaeum) are capable of reaching sexual maturity in young ducks, young chickens, and raccoons. When infective larvae were fed to fully feathered young chickens, the sexually mature worms did not develop. In bird hosts the fluke moves to the bursa of Fabricius as its location of choice; in mammals it remains in the small intestine.

NOTOCOTYLIDAE

The notocotylids are small to medium-sized monostomes. The ventral surface is usually provided with rows of glands or ridges (absent in Paramonostomum). There is no pharynx, and the tips of the intestinal ceca pass between the testes, which are located in the posterior part of the body. The eggs are small and provided with a long, slender filament at each pole. The family is represented as parasites of waterfowl by at least 6 genera and 42 species. Only the more important and more common species will be included here.

Notocotylus imbricatus (Looss 1893)

SYNONYMS. *Notocotylus gibbus* (Mehlis 1846); *N. seineti* Fuhrmann 1919; *N. urbanensis* Harrah 1922, in part; *N. intestinalis* Tubangui 1932; *N. lucknowensis* (Lal 1935); *N. anatis* Ku 1937; *N. orientalis* Ku 1937.

DESCRIPTION. Body elongate, oval, 2–4 mm long (Fig. 30.13A,B). Ventral surface with 3 linear rows of glands (Fig. 30.13A), 12–16 in median row and 12–17 in each lateral row. Eggs 17–20µ long by 9–12µ wide (Fig. 30.13C).

This species is widely distributed throughout Europe, Asia, Africa, India, and North and South America. It is primarily a parasite of wild waterfowl, although it is known to occur naturally and experimentally in the domestic duck and chicken.

LIFE HISTORY. The cercariae develop in rediae in about 7 weeks. The snail hosts include members of the genera Bithynia, Lymnaea, Paludina, Physa, and Semisulcospira. After emerging the cercariae quickly encyst on vegetation and submerged debris and are infective immediately for the definitive hosts. The metacercariae excyst

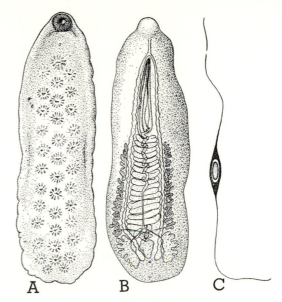

FIG. 30.13—Notocotylus imbricatus. *(A) Ventral view showing distribution of glands. (B) Dorsal view showing internal organization. (C) Egg with filaments. (Fuhrmann, 1919)*

in the small intestine and migrate to the ceca and cloacal region where they reach the egg-laying stage in 10–27 days.

Other species of the genus *Notocotylus*: (1) *N. attenuatus* (Rudolphi 1809) is a species reported more than 60 times from Anseriformes, Galliformes, Gruiformes, and Charadriiformes among birds and from Rodentia (especially the muskrat) among mammals. The species has been recorded over 50 times from domestic ducks and chickens. (2) *N. ephemera* (Nitzsch 1807) occurs in ducks and chickens in Europe. Its cercariae develop in snails of the genus Planorbis. (3) *N. chionis* Baylis 1928 is known from a goose in Europe and from a pigeonlike bird, a sheath-bill, from Patagonia. (4) *N. aegypticus* (Looss 1896) occurs in ducks from Africa.

Catatropis verrucosa (Froelich 1789), a notocotylid having a glandular keel or ridge instead of a median row of glands, occurs in the duck, goose, and chicken in Europe and the chicken in the United States. *Paramonostomum alveatum* (Mehlis 1846) and *P. parvum* Stunkard and Dunihue 1931, species without ventral glands, occur in domestic ducks in Europe and North America respectively. *Paramonostomum philippinensis* Velasquez 1969 has been brought to sexual maturity in chickens and ducks in the Philippine Islands.

PATHOLOGY. Flukes of this family generally cause very little injury to their hosts. It is possible that if present in large numbers they may cause some inflammation to the mucous membrane in that part of the gut in which they reside. Wehrmann (1909) described the type of local reaction ordinarily seen in the mucosa when worms of this variety are present, and Serapin (1957) attributed the death of waterfowl to an unusually heavy infection of *Notocotylus attenuatus* in Poland.

PLAGIORCHIIDAE

Trematodes of this family are rather small forms in which the testes usually are diagonal in position, behind the ovary and posterior to the acetabulum. In descending and ascending the uterus passes between the testes, descending to near the caudal end of the body. The genital pore usually is located in front of the acetabulum. The vitellaria normally extend from the bifurcation of the ceca into the posterior part of the body; they may be entirely lateral to the ceca or spread across the body. When lateral to the ceca the vitellaria are likely to be confined to the central third of the body length. The eggs are small.

Plagiorchis megalorchis Rees 1952

SYNONYMS. *Plagiorchis (Multiglandularis) megalorchis* Rees 1952; *P. laricola* of Foggie 1937.

DESCRIPTION. Body elongated ovoid (Fig. 30.14), 1.70–2.40 mm long by 0.54–0.70 mm wide. Oral sucker subterminal, larger than ventral sucker; ventral sucker in anterior third of body. Ovary to one side of midline, close behind acetabulum. Mehlis' gland median, between ovary and anterior testis. Testes large, slightly diagonal in position, in posterior half of body. Genital pore median or to one side of midline, immediately in front of ventral sucker. Cirrus pouch large, extending from genital pore to beyond ventral sucker. Vitellaria extensive, from oral sucker to caudal extremity. Eggs 30–33μ long by 21–23μ wide.

Although reported as a parasite of turkey poults only from the British Isles, it was associated with a severe enteritis, and the damage done by the parasite makes it

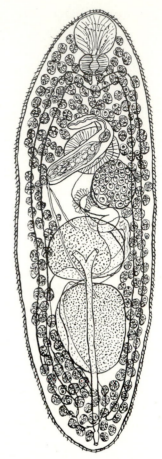

FIG. 30.14–*Plagiorchis megalorchis, dorsal view. (Rees, 1952)*

a potentially dangerous parasite wherever it occurs. Foggie (1937) recorded it as an epidemic-type parasite from the turkey in Northern Ireland; Rees (1952) was able to experimentally infect the turkey; Jordan (1953) found it naturally infecting turkeys in England.

LIFE HISTORY. The eggs hatch after being ingested by Lymnaea and Physa snails. The cercariae develop in daughter sporocysts in about 30 days, and the encysted metacercariae are in Chironomus, Culicoides, and Anatopynia larvae; they require 3–5 days to become infective for the bird host. Sexually mature worms are recovered from the intestine of the final host in 7–10 days.

PATHOLOGY. Foggie (1937), Rees (1952), and Jordan (1953) recorded deaths in young turkey poults as a result of natural and experimental infections with *P. megalorchis*. The worms were associated with a well-developed necrotic enteritis affecting the entire small intestine. The presence of the worms was associated with a droopiness, a failure to put on weight and ultimately death.

Other flukes of the plagiorchid group recorded from poultry include *P. elegans* (Rudolphi 1802), recorded from Anseriformes, Falconiformes, Charadriiformes, Cuculiformes, Strigiformes, Piciformes, and Passeriformes; it has been grown successfully in domestic duck, chicken, and rat in Europe and Asia. Its metacercarial stage is in dragonfly (Odonata) and dipterous larvae. *Plagiorchis maculosus* (Rudolphi 1802) also has been grown experimentally in chickens and turkeys.

MICROPHALLIDAE

Trematodes of this family are small in size and have a moderately long esophagus, short ceca, Y-shaped excretory vesicle, gonads at or behind level of ventral sucker, and variously arranged vitellaria. The ovary usually is anterior to the testes which are symmetrically situated. The cirrus rarely is eversible and sometimes opens into a greatly modified genital atrium. The uterus usually is coiled posterior to the level of the acetabulum, although it may extend well into the anterior portion, especially in freshly harvested specimens in which the excretory bladder is dilated. The vitellaria may be follicular or fused and may be ring-forming in either the posterior or anterior half of the body.

At least 5 genera and 32 species of the family have been recorded as parasites of Anseriformes and Galliformes. Some of the species have been recorded as epizootic in ducks, causing a high mortality when present in appreciable numbers. Only one species is discussed.

Maritrema obstipum (Van Cleave and Mueller 1932)

SYNONYM. *Microphallus obstipus* Van Cleave and Mueller 1932.

DESCRIPTION. Small pyriform to ovate distome with minute cuticular spines and Y-shaped excretory bladder (Fig. 30.15). Body 0.23–0.52 mm long and up to 0.30 mm wide. Oral and ventral suckers present. Ceca short, often diverging laterally

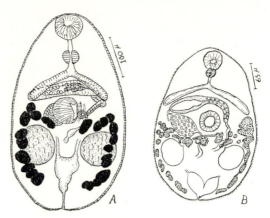

FIG. 30.15—Maritrema obstipum. *(A) Ventral view of young adult. (Van Cleave and Mueller, 1932) (B) Metacercaria. (Etges, 1953)*

from end of esophagus, ending at or in advance of acetabulum. Gonads in or just caudal to zone of acetabulum. Genital pore to one side of ventral sucker. Cirrus pouch long, curving over acetabulum, containing seminal vesicle and small eversible cirrus. Uterus may be confined to posterior half of body or looping into forward portion. Vitellaria often ring-formed. Eggs 19–25μ long and unembryonated when passed in feces of host.

The fluke has been recorded from fish, birds, and mammals, although it appears to be primarily a parasite of birds; it has been recorded in both wild and domestic ducks as well as chickens (Etges, 1953).

LIFE HISTORY. The eggs require several weeks for full development and then must be ingested by the snail host (*Amnicola pilsburyi*) before hatching occurs. The monostomate cercaria bears a stylet and is produced in a sporocyst which when mature has a birth pore. The metacercariae develop to infectivity (5 weeks) in thin-walled cysts adjacent to the main blood vessel in the isopod (*Asellus communis*). On being ingested by ducklings, baby chickens, mice, and hamsters the young flukes develop to sexual maturity in a very few days. In ducks and chickens the mature fluke may live for about a month.

PATHOLOGY. Although as many as 300 mature flukes of the species were removed from the small intestine of a single chicken 48 hours after ingesting several infected isopods, no appreciable change in the appearance of the intestinal mucosa was noted. It is likely the host did not have adequate time to respond to the trematode's presence or the parasite to exert its full influence on the host. In a closely related form *(M. acadiae)*, Swales (1933) found a high mortality rate among young naturally infected ducklings in Canada.

Other than *M. obstipum* and *M. acadiae*, members of the genera Microphallus *(M. pygmaeus* Levinsen 1881) and Levinseniella *(L. brachysoma* Creplin 1846) have been recorded from Anseriformes in North America. Experimentally *M. pygmaeus* has been transferred to cats.

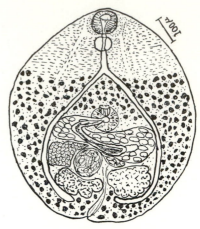

FIG. 30.16—Cryptocotyle concavum, *ventral view. (Wootton, 1957)*

HETEROPHYIDAE

Members of this family are small to very small flukes in which the cuticle is covered by very fine scalelike spines. Ventral sucker is closely associated with the genital sucker (gonotyl). The gonads are posterior to the ventral sucker, and the ovary is usually median to the diagonally or symmetrically placed testes. The vitellaria are diffuse or form groups of follicles behind the gonads. The uterus coils between the gonotyle (near acetabulum) and caudal extremity. Ten genera and 19 species of the family have been recorded from Anseriformes and Galliformes; however, members of a single genus (Cryptocotyle) appear to have significance as a parasite of poultry.

Cryptocotyle concavum (Creplin 1825)

SYNONYMS. *Distoma concairum* Creplin 1825; *Tocotrema concava* (Creplin 1825).

DESCRIPTION. Body usually ovoid in shape, 0.60–0.95 mm long by 0.50–0.80 mm wide, spinose (Fig. 30.16). Oral sucker followed by short prepharynx, muscular pharynx, esophagus (reaching to midpoint between suckers), and slender curving ceca which extend back to near excretory vesicle, behind testes. Ventral sucker small, in anterior wall of spacious muscular genital sinus (gonotyle), located in midline of body. Testes slightly lobed, symmetrical, near caudal extremity. Seminal vesicle well developed, forming long S-shaped organ dorsal to uterus, extending from level of Mehlis' gland to genital sinus. Ovary anterior to right testis, slightly lobed, separated from genital sinus by coils of uterus. Eggs 27–38μ long by 16–20μ wide.

LIFE HISTORY. According to Wootton (1957), the eggs pass undeveloped from host and miracidia require several weeks to complete development. Hatching occurs after the egg is ingested by the snail *Amnicola longinqua*. The mother sporocyst is followed by rediae and these produce the ceracariae. The cercariae penetrate into and encyst in the fins of the fish *Gasterosteus aculeatus*. As the metacercariae mature (3–4 weeks) the cyst accumulates masses of melanophores, often to a point that a heavily infected host may be black in color. When the mature metacercariae are ingested by a suitable host, excystation occurs and the young fluke develops to the egg-producing stage in 24–48 hours. The adults may live about 1 month.

In North America this species has been successfully brought to maturity in both ducks and chickens. In Europe the species has been reported many times in wild ducks, chickens, pigeons, turkeys, and Charadriiformes birds. Experimentally it has been grown in dogs, pigs, and rabbits.

PATHOLOGY. Although the parasite is found in both wild and domestic hosts, it has not been incriminated in severe pathological conditions. The parasite, however, belongs to a family of flukes in which some species are known to cause pathological changes of major proportions. The flukes live deep in the crypts of the intestinal glands, and many of the species are said to burrow into the lamina propria where acute tissue reactions develop. In mammalian hosts many of the heterophyids, normally parasites of birds, wander out of the gut cavity and invade the tissue. From this location their eggs often are caught up in the bloodstream and become filtered into the tissues of other organs where acute pathological changes occur.

Cryptocotyle lingua (Creplin 1825)

This species is known to occur in terns and gulls in North America. Stunkard (1930) obtained development in both the cat and the rat; he was unable to infect ducklings even though he fed them enormous numbers of the metacercariae daily. The species, however, has been recorded from both wild and domestic ducks in Russia.

PARAMPHISTOMATIDAE

This family comprises a large number of flukes from vertebrate hosts around the world. They are characterized by having the ventral sucker situated at the posterior end of the body and in having a well-developed system of lymph tubules. A single species is recorded from poultry (wild and domestic ducks, turkeys, and chickens).

Zygocotyle lunata (Diesing 1836)

SYNONYMS. *Amphistoma lunata* Diesing 1836; *Zygocotyle ceratosa* Stunkard 1916; *Solenorchis travassosi* Hilmy 1949; *Zygocotyle travassosi* (Hilmy 1949).

DESCRIPTION. Body ovate, up to 9 mm long (Fig. 30.17). Oral sucker subventral, provided with two evaginations or pouches. Acetabulum large, at posterior end, its posterior margin provided with a flap which terminates on each side in a conelike projection. Eggs 124–153μ long by 72–94μ wide.

This fluke normally lives in the ceca of wild waterfowl and has been recorded from Russia (Far East), Africa (Rhodesia), North America (United States, Canada, and Mexico), and South America (Brazil). On several occasions it has been found in domestic ducks, turkeys, and chickens and has occurred naturally in cattle and sheep. Experimentally it has been grown in ducks, chickens, and rats. Price (1928) found it in the goose in the United States; Caballero (1941) recorded it from the chicken in Mexico. Recently Byrd and Prestwood (unpublished data) found it in ducks from Argentina.

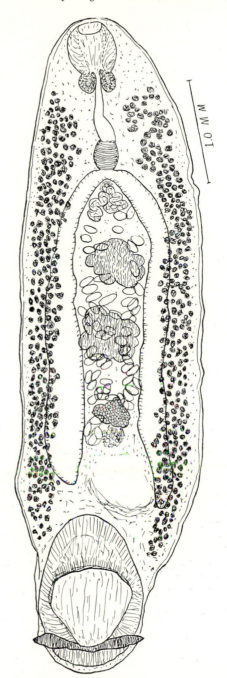

FIG. 30.17—Zygocotyle lunata, *ventral view.*

LIFE HISTORY. The life history of the fluke includes the passage of undeveloped eggs in the feces of the host and the development of cercariae in rediae in snails of the genus Helisoma *(H. antrosum, H. anceps, H. trivolvis).* The metacercariae encyst on debris, aquatic vegetation, and shells of snails (Willey, 1941). These larvae are ingested by the final host with food or drink, and the excysted young flukes migrate down the intestine (usually) to the ceca where they develop to maturity in 3–6 weeks.

PATHOLOGY. Mettrick (1959) recorded a high mortality among ducklings in southern Rhodesia from the parasite. There was widespread inflammation with hemorrhaging, emaciation, and death. Normally the pathology is confined to a simple traumatic injury caused by the powerful ventral sucker.

LIVER

Trematodes occurring in the liver of poultry belong to the families Dicrocoeliidae and Opisthorchiidae. These flukes live in the common bile duct, the gall bladder, and the biliary passages; a few of them may occasionally wander into the pancreas.

DICROCOELIIDAE

Members of this family are small parasites having a flat, oval, elliptical, lanceolate, or subcylindrical body. The ventral sucker is usually larger than the oral sucker and most often lies in the anterior third of the body. The ovary is posterior to the diagonally or symmetrically arranged testes which lie near but caudal to the ventral sucker. The descending and ascending uterus coils between the testes, and the coils extend to near the posterior end of the body. The vitellaria are lateral in position, usually in the central third of the body.

A single representative from each of 5 genera has been reported from poultry and waterfowl. Only one of these is discussed.

Athesmia heterolecithodes (Braun 1899)

SYNONYMS. *Distomum heterolecithodes* Braun 1899; *Athesmia rudecta* Braun 1901; *A. attilae* Travassos 1917; *A. wehri* McIntosh 1937; *A. pricei* McIntosh 1937; *A. butensis* Petri 1942; *A. reelfooti* Denton in Petri 1942; *A. jolliei* Schell 1957.

DESCRIPTION. Body elongated, flattened, suckers close together (Fig. 30.18). Oral sucker larger than acetabulum. Ceca slender, reaching beyond middle of body length. Testes tandem or slightly diagonal, in anterior half of body, in front of ovary.

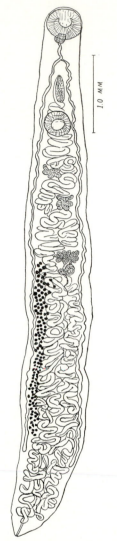

FIG. 30.18—Athesmia heterolecithodes, ventral view.

Uterus voluminous, reaching from ovary to near posterior extremity before turning anteriorly to genital pore, passing between testes. Genital pore immediately in front of ventral sucker. Vitellaria follicular, confined to one side of body, behind level of gonads. Eggs small, 26–38μ long by 17–26μ wide.

The fluke has been reported from both birds and mammals. It was described originally from the gallinule in Europe and Africa, but has been recorded from birds of the orders Charadriiformes (Europe and Africa); Anseriformes, Charadriiformes, Cuculiformes, Falconiformes, Passeriformes, and Strigiformes (South America); and Charadriiformes, Galliformes and Falconiformes (North America) and from mammals (monkeys in South America and bats in Cuba). Recently Lumsden and Zischke (1963) recorded the species from the king rail in Louisiana; Byrd et al. (1967) recorded natural infections in the ruffed grouse and wild turkey in West Virginia, the wild turkey (21 of 43 birds) from Alabama, and from 13 of 74 clapper rails from Alabama, Florida, Georgia, Louisiana, and North Carolina as well as from the two species of tinamou in Argentina.

LIFE HISTORY. Although the life cycle is unknown, it very likely follows the pattern determined for the other dicrocoelids for which some data are known. The snail host probably is a garden variety (family Polygyridae) and there are two generations of sporocysts. The cercariae may or may not have a tail and are passed from the snail in slime balls. The same snail, another snail, or some other invertebrate serves as the host for the metacercaria which, when taken in by the final host, excysts in the intestine and migrates to the liver where it reaches maturity.

The versatility in final host selection by the fluke makes it a potentially important species and suggests the possibility of a wide variety of second intermediate hosts. Further, it is to be suggested that the fluke may be one of those species of trematodes capable of being transferred from one final host to another if the first of these is captured and ingested shortly after the young fluke excysts.

PATHOLOGY. Nothing is known relative to the pathological changes in the host's hepatic areas that can be referred specifically to *A. heterolecithodes*. It is quite likely, however, that severe hepatic disturbances can be produced when the fluke is present in moderate to large numbers (Patten, 1952; Krull and Mapes, 1952–1953).

Other dicrocoeliids from waterfowl include members of the genera Brachylecithum, Lyperosomum, Pancreatrema, and Wetzelitrema.

OPISTHORCHIIDAE

Flukes belonging to this family are small to medium-sized worms in which the body often may be greatly extended. The suckers are weakly developed or absent and the ceca usually reach to the posterior extremity. The testes are more or less tandem, in the posterior third of the body. The ovary is in front of the testes and the uterine coils are preovarian. The genital pore is in front of the weakly developed ventral sucker. The follicular vitellaria usually are lateral to the ceca, in front of the gonads, although sometimes extending to within or just caudal to the zone of the testes. In the latter case the vitelline follicles are grouped into clusters. Eggs small, 18–26μ long.

Twenty-three species representing 5 genera of the family have been recorded from various waterfowl, domestic ducks, and chickens. A single species of the group is discussed.

Amphimerus elongatus Gower 1938

DESCRIPTION. Body narrow, elongated, up to 23 mm long (Fig. 30.19). Greatest width immediately in front of ovary. Oral sucker absent. Ventral sucker small, in anterior third of body. Ceca extending to near caudal extremity. Testes slightly oblique, in posterior eighth of body, separated by excretory bladder. Ovary immediately in front of testes. Uterus extensively coiled in

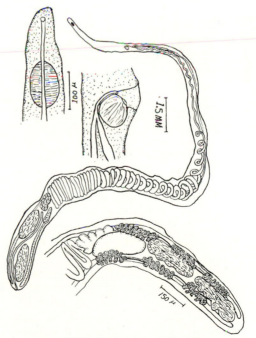

FIG. 30.19–Amphimerus elongatus. *Four sketches showing the several features of the anatomy.* (Gower, 1938)

passing forward between the ceca to the genital pore which lies immediately in front of acetabulum. Vitellaria in clusters, extending from midway between ovary and acetabulum to midregion of caudal testis. Eggs 22μ long by 12μ wide.

LIFE HISTORY. The cercariae develop in rediae in *Amnicola limosa*, the snail host, and after a short swimming period penetrate into several species of fish (Netropis, Pimephalis, Perca, Lepomis, and Micropterus) where they encyst as metacercariae. When ingested by the final host, excystation occurs and the young flukes move quickly up the bile and pancreatic ducts. In chickens the fluke is found entirely in the liver; in ducks and pigeons the majority move into the pancreas (Wallace, 1940). Some metacercariae survive and mature in the liver of mice.

PATHOLOGY. As usual, the number of flukes present will determine the pathological picture. When *Amphimerus elongatus* locates in the pancreas, this organ pales and the walls of the ducts thicken, often to the point that flow of pancreatic juices is blocked. When in the liver typical trematodiasis lesions are produced. Any serious disruption of the flow of juices from the liver and pancreas produces serious consequences in the physiology of the individual—failure to gain weight, cessation of egg production, inflammation of the digestive tube, and death. Gower (1938) reported that of the 15 or more trematodes known to occur in ducks at the W. K. Kellogg Bird Sanctuary (Michigan), *A. elongatus* was the leading cause of mortality from fluke infections. In the turkey (*Amphimerus* sp., North Dakota) there is a marked distention of the bile ducts and extensive pressure atrophy of the liver parenchyma.

Other flukes of this family which have been recorded from the duck, chicken, and allies (and which are potential pathology-producing worms) include *Amphimerus anatis* Yamaguti 1933 from Japan; *Opisthorchis simulans* (Looss 1896) from Europe; *O. longissimus* (Linstow 1883) from Russia; *Metorchis orientalis* Tanabe 1919 from China, Japan, Formosa, and the Far East; and *M. xanthosomus* (Creplin 1846) from Asia and Europe.

URINARY SYSTEM

Trematodes commonly occurring in the kidney of poultry belong to the families Eucotylidae and Renicolidae.

EUCOTYLIDAE

These are small to medium-sized flukes in which the uterus coils posteriorly between the testes in descending and ascending. The genital pore is anteriorly located, a short distance behind the bifurcation of the ceca, and the uterus usually coils in ascending and descending anterior to the pore. The family is divided morphologically into two rather distinct groups, and members of both groups have been reported from Anseriformes and Galliformes hosts.

Tanaisia Group

Small to medium-sized, slender, delicate flukes in which the testes are symmetrical, diagonal, or tandem in respect to each other and are internal to the intestinal ceca. The ceca are joined together near the posterior end of the body, and there is a small but distinct ventral sucker present. Byrd and Denton (1950) are of the opinion that all of the species in this group belong to the genus *Tanaisia* Skrjabin 1924.

Tanaisia bragai (Dos Santos 1934)

SYNONYM. *Tamerlania bragai* Dos Santos 1934.

DESCRIPTION. Body elongated, flat, up to 3 mm long (Fig. 30.20). The oral sucker is subterminal and much larger than the small inconspicuous ventral sucker. Pharynx prominent; esophagus short or absent; ceca uniting posteriorly near caudal extremity of body. Testes more or less symmetrically placed, at or in front of body middle. Ovary pretesticular, in or just posterior to zone of acetabulum. Vitellaria lateral to ceca, extending caudally from near bifurcation of ceca to just anterior to cecal union. Uterus greatly convoluted posterior and anterior to gonads. Genital pore immediately in front of acetabulum. Eggs 30–34μ long by 16–22μ wide.

This fluke is found in the kidney and ureter of pigeons in Brazil, Puerto Rico, and the Philippine Islands and in a large number of Passeriformes in the United States and in the chicken in Brazil.

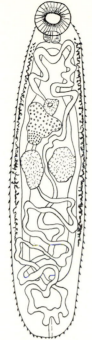

FIG. 30.20—Tanaisia bragai, *ventral view.* (*Dos Santos, 1934*)

LIFE HISTORY. Maldonado (1945) reported that the intermediate host is a land snail *Subulina octona;* the larval cycle is completed in about a month. Birds become infected upon ingestion of infected snails containing encysted metacercariae. Eggs are recoverable in the urine and excreta 23 days after infection.

PATHOLOGY. According to Dos Santos (1934), the presence of flukes in the kidney caused distention of the collecting tubules and thickening of their walls, the lumen of the tubules being filled with amorphous and crystallized detritus. The parenchyma of the kidney showed extensive cellular infiltration, but the cortex was rarely involved. Maldonado and Hoffman (1941) noted similar changes in pigeons in Puerto Rico but were of the opinion that the parasites caused no ill effect; birds that were kept in cages for several months appeared unaffected by the parasites.

Another member of the genus, *T. zarudnyi* (Skrjabin 1924), has been reported from the ruffed grouse (*Bonasa umbellus*) from Ontario and Michigan by Kingston (1965). This author found that *Anguispira alternata* and *Succinea ovalis* served as the mol-luscan host and that cercariae, produced in second-generation sporocysts, were present within 45 days after feeding egg to the snails. The cercariae are brevicercous forms which encyst as metacercariae in the sporocysts giving rise to them. By feeding encysted metacercariae to chickens of various ages, immature and mature ruffed grouse, immature and mature pheasants, and white-throated sparrows, Kingston obtained developing *T. zarudnyi* only in the young ruffed grouse. The older birds did not acquire the infection even when fed large numbers of the metacercariae. Kingston found 13 of 95 ruffed grouse from Algonquin Park, Ontario, infected with the fluke in nature, although none of the 40 grouse taken elsewhere in Ontario carried the fluke. All 5 of the ruffed grouse taken from the southern peninsula of Michigan were infected. Spaulding (1958) recorded the fluke from the ruffed grouse in the northern peninsula of Michigan. Prestwood (1968) found *T. zarudnyi* in young wild turkey poults in Desha County, Arkansas.

Eucotyle Group

Anterior end of body is set off by an annular cervical thickening. The ceca terminate blindly near posterior extremity. The testes are symmetrically situated, usually located extracecally. The ovary is pretesticular and the uterus is intercecal throughout length of the ceca. The acetabulum is absent.

Several species of the genus Eucotyle have been reported from waterfowl, mostly from wild and domestic ducks: *Eucotyle zapharowi* Skrjabin 1920 is recorded at least 14 times in wild ducks and 3 times in domestic ducks from Europe and Asia; *E. cohni* Skrjabin 1924—3 times in wild ducks from similar locations; *E. popowi* Skrjabin and Evranova 1942—4 times in wild and once in domestic ducks; *E. wehri* Price 1930—3 times in wild ducks from North America (U.S.). These species, however, are found infrequently and at widely separated locations. Their life cycles are unknown, and it is believed that they produce very little pathology in their natural hosts.

RENICOLIDAE

Members of this family are small plump flukes with rather globose body; posterior

FIG. 30.21—Renicola hayesan-nieae. *(A) Ventral view of entire worm. (B) Gonads, genital pore, and ends of ceca in relation to ventral sucker.*

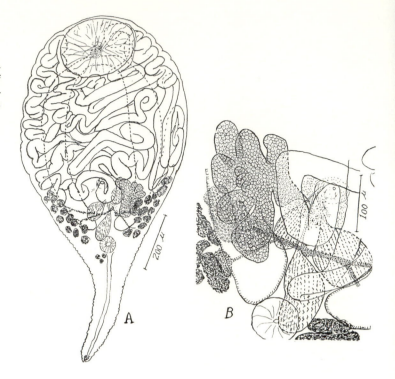

part may taper caudally beyond reproductive organs. The suckers are weakly developed and the oral is the larger. The gonads are close by the ventral sucker, as is the genital pore. The uterus is voluminous, making more than a single passage up and down the length of the body.

Renicola hayesannieae

DESCRIPTION. Medium-sized flukes, 3.15 mm long by 1.56 mm wide, distomate, with teardrop-shaped body and weak musculature (Fig. 30.21). The posterior third of the body is greatly attenuated and contains only the Y-shaped excretory vesicle which opens at the extremity. Oral sucker weak and flat, subterminal in position, much larger than the acetabulum which lies behind the gonads at the base of the attenuated caudal piece. The ovary is large and greatly lobed, mostly in front of the testes and to one side (usually right) of the midline. Testes small, 2 in number, behind the ovary. Vitellaria lateral, in zone and anterior to the gonads. Uterus voluminous, making at least four passes up and down the body (in front of the gonads) before reaching the genital pore which lies medially, left of the ovary. Eggs 28–32μ long.

This is the first member of the genus to be recorded from the wild turkey. The infected birds (7 of 20) were all mature and came from Mississippi (Byrd and Kellogg, 1971).

LIFE HISTORY. Although the life history of *R. hayesannieae* is unknown, its cycle probably is quite similar to that of *R. thaidus*, as worked out by Stunkard (1964), with different molluscan hosts being used. Stunkard found this species to develop its first- and second-generation sporocyst in the oyster drill *Thais lopillus*. On emerging the cercariae entered and encysted in the bivalve mollusks *Mytilus edulis, Pecten irradians,* and *Gemma gemma.* Adult flukes were recovered from the kidneys of the gull *Larus argentatus* 7 weeks after feeding the metacercariae. Stunkard, however, was unable to infect young ducks, chickens, mice, hamsters, and various species of fish by feeding them the metacercariae of *R. thaidus.*

Other members of the genus, recorded from ducks, geese, and allies, include *R. brantae* McIntosh and Farr 1952, from the Canada goose; *R. mediovitellata* Bykhovskaia 1950, recorded 4 times from wild ducks in Western Siberia; *R. mollissima*

Kulachkova 1957, an unusually heavy infection in young ducks (2 weeks old) in Southern Europe (White Sea); and *R. somateriae* Belopol'skaia 1952.

PATHOLOGY. Very little is known concerning the pathology caused by renicolid flukes. The report by Kapitonov (1959) to the effect that *R. somateria* served as an epizootic causing considerable loss in young eider ducklings in Russia is the only case in which definite pathology is indicated. However, the presence of large numbers of these medium-sized flukes in the kidney tubules suggests the possibility of more damage through blockage, cellular infiltration, and erosion of kidney substance than would be desirable to the sound health of the host.

REPRODUCTIVE SYSTEM

PROSTHOGONIMIDAE

These flukes are characterized by having features similar to the Plagiorchiidae but possess symmetrically located testes, more forwardly placed vitellaria, and genital pore well forward, close beside the oral sucker. At least 2 genera and 11 species have been recorded from Anseriformes and Galliformes hosts throughout the world. Many of these species are thought to be synonyms of *Prosthogonimus ovatus* (Rudolphi 1803), a form known to have a wide distribution throughout Europe and Asia. In North America the species most frequently encountered is *P. macrorchis* Macy 1934.

Prosthogonimus macrorchis Macy 1934

DESCRIPTION. Body pyriform in outline, 5.26–7.56 mm long (Fig. 30.22), cuticle spiny. Intestinal ceca simple, extending to near posterior end of body. Genital pore at anterior end of body, slightly to left of oral sucker. Testes oval, opposite each other and about one-third of body length from posterior end. Ovary greatly lobulated, immediately posterior to acetabulum. Vitellaria lateral, extending from acetabulum to testes. Uterus with numerous coils in post-testicular part of the body. Eggs 28μ long by 16μ wide, with spine of variable shape and length at antopercular pole. This fluke occurs in the bursa of Fabricius and oviduct of the duck, chicken, and other birds in the United States; it is

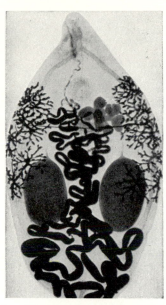

FIG. 30.22—*Prosthogonimus macrorchis* Photomicrograph of ventral view. (Macy, College of St. Thomas)

particularly common in the lake region of Michigan and Minnesota.

LIFE HISTORY. According to Macy (1934), the sporocyst found in the "liver" of *Amnicola limosa porata* produces cercariae directly, without a redia stage. The cercaria swims away from the snail host; if it is drawn into the anal opening of a suitable species of dragonfly naiad by the breathing movements of such a host, the tail of the cercaria is lost and the metacercaria thus formed makes its way to the muscle of the naiad, where it increases to about 5 times its original size. A thick wall with an outer radially striated and an inner homogeneous layer (Fig. 30.23H) now forms about the metacercaria, and the cyst usually settles in the body cavity of the host. If the infected naiad or adult dragonfly is eaten by a suitable avian definitive host, the cyst wall is digested away and the young fluke passes down the digestive tract to the cloaca from whence it enters the bursa of Fabricius or oviduct before developing into the mature trematode. Embryonated eggs produced by the fluke leave the host by way of the cloacal opening; if they reach a lake inhabited by *Amnicola limosa* the latter become infected and sporocysts and cercariae develop (Fig. 30.23). The important dragonfly hosts

FIG. 30.23—Schematic representation of life history of Prosthogonimus macrorchis. Adult fluke (A) in oviduct of bird host (J) produces eggs (B). In water embryonated eggs (C) ingested by snail host (D) in which two generations of sporocysts (E) are produced. Last sporocyst generation produces cercariae (F) which leave snail and enter dragonfly naiads (G) where they encyst as metacercariae (H). Naiads metamorphose into adult dragonflies (I). Infected ones ingested by bird host (J) in whose intestine excystment occurs. Young flukes migrate to oviduct, mature, and produce eggs.

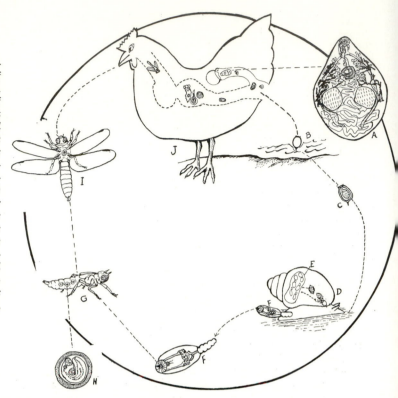

belong to the genera Leucorrhinia, Tetragoneuria, and Epicordulia.

PATHOLOGY. The lesions and symptoms caused by species of Prosthogonimus in Europe have been described by Hieronymi (1921), Reinhardt (1922), De Blieck and Van Heelsbergen (1922), Seifried (1923), and others; in the United States by Kotlan and Chandler (1925) and Macy (1934). The disease in American fowl caused by *P. macrorchis* is essentially the same as that caused by *P. pellucidus* (Linstow, 1873) in Europe. Affected birds lose their normal activity and appetite, and there is a pronounced reduction in egg production. The eggs that are produced frequently have very thin shells or no shells. On necropsy there may be extreme emaciation and anemia and an adhesive peritonitis. The intestines may show pronounced hyperemia and be covered with a fibrinous exudate. The oviduct may show similar changes, be distended, and contain considerable exudate and egg material. In some cases there may be a rupture of the oviduct with the secre-

tions (albumen and yolk material) present in the body cavity. Flukes are present in the oviduct and egg material as well as in the abdominal cavity in the case of oviduct rupture. In some instances the peritonitis may be so pronounced as to be detected in the dead and unopened birds by the bluish red color of the abdominal wall. These lesions and the laying of thin-shelled or shell-less eggs may be due to other causes, but it seems to be an established fact that the flukes may be a contributory cause, if not the actual cause. At any rate, if such conditions are encountered in areas where dragonflies are breeding (lake regions), prosthogonimiasis should be suspected.

Recently Prestwood (1968) reported *Prosthogonimus ovatus* (Rudolphi 1803) from a single wild turkey poult taken in Mississippi; Heard (1967) found a form which he tentatively identified as *P. ovatus* in the bursa of 14 of 158 clapper rails collected from Florida, Georgia, Louisiana, Maryland, New Jersey, North Carolina, South Carolina, and Virginia.

CIRCULATORY SYSTEM

SCHISTOSOMATIDAE

All of the trematodes found in the circulatory system of birds are characterized by having the sexes separate. Several species— *Bilharziella polonica* (Kowalewski), *Pseudobilharziella yokogawai* (Oiso), *Dendritobilharzia pulverulenta* (Braun), *Trichobilharzia ocellata* (La Valette), and *Gigantobilharzia monocotylea* Szidat—occur in domestic waterfowl in Europe and elsewhere; but none of these is known to occur in this country. Several schistosomes are known from wild waterfowl in North America, and some of them probably will be found capable of infecting poultry. In spite of the fact that the blood flukes are serious parasites of man, those infecting poultry do not seem to cause comparable injury to their bird hosts. Szidat (1929) reported that, in infections with *Bilharziella polonica,* the eggs of the fluke in the intestinal wall caused slight connective tissue proliferation and some leukocytic infiltration; in infections with *P. yokogawai,* Oiso (1927) noted pathological changes in the liver and intestine and arrested growth of the bird host.

TREATMENT

Owing to the fact that trematode infections of poultry are rarely diagnosed antemortem, practically nothing is known concerning effective treatment for their removal. Medicinal treatment would appear to be of no value for the removal of the skin fluke *Collyriclum faba,* surgical incision and mechanical removal of the worms seeming to be the rational procedure in such infections.

Flukes occurring in the respiratory system, particularly the nasal passages, trachea, and bronchi, might possibly be removed by inhalations of powdered drugs having vermicidal properties. The most promising of such drugs is barium antimonyl tartrate, which is highly effective against the poultry gapeworm (Wehr, 1941).

For trematodes occurring in the digestive tract, carbon tetrachloride in doses of 1–3 cc, depending on the kind and size of the bird, might be tried. In case the flukes are in the proventriculus or upper part of the intestine, the drug may be introduced directly into the former organ by means of a syringe and rubber catheter. For flukes in the lower part of the intestine or ceca, 2–5 cc of carbon tetrachloride in 3–4 times its volume of a bland oil (mineral or cottonseed), administered by rectal injection, would probably prove effective.

In infections with the oviduct fluke *Prosthogonimus,* carbon tetrachloride is again the most promising treatment. Schmid (1930) reported the administration to a hen of 1.5 cc of this drug in an equal amount of flour paste. On the following day the bird received 1 cc of the drug in 8 cc of paste, and on the third day 1.7 cc of the drug in 8 cc of paste. At this time no more prosthogonimid eggs could be found in the feces. On the day following the last treatment, a mass of egg yolk containing 9 flukes was found in the cage. The bird was then killed, and in the oviduct were found two small egg concretions in which several flukes were lying; other flukes were embedded in collections of mucus. All of the flukes apparently were dead. Other birds in the flock were treated, but the results were inconclusive.

No drug treatment of value is known for the destruction of fluke parasites of the excretory and circulatory systems.

CONTROL

In view of the fact that all of the trematode parasites of poultry require at least one snail intermediate host, measures for the prevention of fluke infections must be directed toward control or eradication of these mollusks or toward keeping poultry away from areas where the parasites may be acquired. The easier and perhaps most certain method of preventing birds from acquiring trematode infections consists of selecting areas for poultry raising that are as far removed as possible from streams or swampy places or of fencing to keep the birds from ranging over such areas.

Control of snail intermediate hosts may be accomplished either by draining the low marshy places or by using chemicals that are toxic to snails. In the case of swampy areas, drainage either by means of open ditches or by the use of agricultural tile will lower the water table to a point where there is insufficient surface moisture to enable the snails to propagate. If drainage should be too expensive or otherwise impractical, the snails may be destroyed by dusting the area with powered copper sulfate or bluestone. The copper sulfate should be mixed with a carrier (fine sand or land plaster) in the proportion of 1:4–8, and spread either by broadcasting by hand or by the use of hand or power dusters. For destroying snails in ponds and small lakes, the powdered copper sulfate may be used as in the case of marshes. The chemical should be spread along the banks and in the water near the shore, as most of the snails will be found in these locations.

For destroying snails in streams, burlap sacks containing large crystals of copper sulfate may be placed in the streams at the uppermost part of the section to be treated, in an amount sufficient to give a concentration of 1 part chemical to about 500,000 parts water. The amount of chemical necessary may be determined by ascertaining the cross-section area of the stream and multiplying by the velocity in order to get the flow in cu ft/sec. This result multiplied by 12 (the amount in pounds of copper sulfate necessary to give a concentration of 1:500,000 for a 24-hour period) equals the amount of copper sulfate needed for the treatment. For example, if a stream is 3 ft wide and 1 ft deep and the velocity is 2 ft/sec, the flow is 6 cu ft/sec; this result times 12 equals 72—the number of pounds of copper sulfate necessary for one treatment. This concentration of the chemical will kill most snails but is not injurious to livestock; it may kill some fish and will destroy algae and moss.

In some instances, especially with Prosthogonimus where the fluke is acquired through the ingestion of dragonflies, keeping poultry away from the shores of ponds or lakes in the mornings when these insects are inactive is recommended.

REFERENCES

Alicata, J. E. 1940. The life cycle of *Postharmostomum gallinum,* the cecal fluke of poultry. *J. Parasitol.* 26:135–43.

——. 1962. Life cycle and developmental stages of *Philophthalmus gralli* in the intermediate and final hosts. *J. Parasitol.* 48: 47–54.

Alicata, J. E., and K. Noda. 1960. Observations on the life history of *Philophthalmus,* a species of eye-fluke of birds in Hawaii. *Libro Homenaje Caballero y Caballero,* pp. 67–73.

Allison, L. N. 1943. *Leucochloridiomorpha constantiae* (Mueller) (Brachylaemidae), its life cycle and taxonomic relationships among digenetic trematodes. *Trans. Am. Microscop. Soc.* 62:127–68.

Annereaux, R. F. 1940. A note on *Echinoparyphium recurvatum* (von Linstow) parasitic in California turkeys. *J. Am. Vet. Med. Ass.* 96:62–64.

Beaver, P. C. 1937. Experimental studies on *Echinostoma revolutum* (Froelich), a fluke from birds and mammals. *Illinois Biol. Monograph* 15:1–96.

——. 1939. The morphology and life history of *Psilostomum ondatrae* Price, 1931 (Trematoda: Psilostomidae). *J. Parasitol.* 25: 383–93.

Betz, W. 1941. Seuchenhafte Trematodenerkrankungen bei Gaensen. *Tieraerztl. Rundschau* 47:526–27.

Bittner, H. 1925. Ein Beitrag zur Uebertragung und zur Morphologie von *Echinoparyphium recurvatum. Berlin. Muench. Tieraerztl. Wochschr.* 41:82–86.

Bolle, W. 1925. Ueber einen Taubentrematoden aus der Gattung *Echinostomum. Deut. Tieraerztl. Wochschr.* 33:529–31.

Burns, W. C. 1961. The life history of *Sphaeridiotrema spinoacetabulum* sp. n. (Trematoda: Psilostomidae) from the ceca of ducks. *J. Parasitol.* 47:933–38.

Byrd, E. E. 1970. Brown thrasher, *Toxostoma rufum* (L.), a new host for *Collyriclum faba* (Bremser). *J. Parasitol.* 56:195–96.

Byrd, E. E., and J. F. Denton. 1950. The helminth parasites of birds. I. A review of the trematode genus *Tanaisia* Skrjabin, 1924. *Am. Midland Naturalist* 43:32–57.

Byrd, E. E., and F. E. Kellogg. 1971. *Renicola hayesannieae,* a new kidney fluke (Digenea: Renicolidae) from the wild turkey, *Meleagris gallopavo silvestris* Vieillot, from Mississippi. *J. Parasitol.* (In press.)

Byrd, E. E., and A. K. Prestwood. 1969. *Psilotornus audacirrus* n. g., n. sp., a new trematode (Digenea: Psilostomatidae) from the wild turkey, *Meleagris gallopavo sylvestris* Vieillot, from Alabama. *Trans. Am. Microscop. Soc.* 88:366–69.

Byrd, E. E., A. K. Prestwood, F. E. Kellogg, and R. W. Heard. 1967. New hosts and locality records for the large liver fluke, *Athesmia heterolecithodes* (Braun, 1899) Looss, 1899 (Dicrocoeliidae) of birds and mammals. *J. Parasitol.* 53:1116–17.

Calballero y. C., Eduardo. 1941. Parasitismo en *Gallus gallus* L. originado por *Zygocotyle lunatum* en la region de Lerma. III. *Ann. Inst. Biol., Univ. Nac. Mexico* 12:123–25.

Cornwell, G. W., and A. B. Cowan. 1963.

Helminth populations of the canvasback (*Aythya valisineria*) and host-parasite-environmental interrelationships. *Trans. 28th N. Am. Wildlife (Nat. Resources) Conf.*, pp. 173–98.

De Blieck, L., and T. van Heelsbergen. 1922. Trematoden als oorzaak van eileider-onsteking en het leggen van windeiren. *Tijdschr. Diergeneesk.* 49:536–39.

Dietz, E. 1910. Die Echinostomiden der Voegel. *Zool. Jahrb.*, Suppl. 12, pp. 265–512.

Dos Santos, V. 1934. Monostomose renal dos aves domesticas. (Portuguese text, French and English summaries.) *Rev. Dept. Nac. Prod. Animal Brasil* 1:203–11.

Etges, F. J. 1953. Studies on the life histories of *Maritrema obstipum* (van Cleave and Mueller, 1932) and *Levinseniella amnicolae* n. sp. (Trematoda: Microphallidae). *J. Parasitol.* 39:643–62.

Farmer, D. S., and B. B. Morgan. 1944. Occurrence and distribution of the trematode *Collyriclum faba* (Bremser) in birds. *Auk* 61:421.

Feng, L. C. 1931. Studies on tissue lesions produced by helminths. *Arch. Schiffs. und Tropen-Hyg.* 35:1–10.

Foggie, A. 1937. An outbreak of parasitic necrosis in turkeys caused by *Plagiorchis laricola* (Skrjabin). *J. Helminthol.* 15:35.

Fried, B. 1962. Growth of *Philophthalmus* sp. (Trematoda) in the eyes of chicks. *J. Parasitol.* 48:395–99.

Fuhrmann, O. 1919. Notes helminthologiques suisse. 2. *Rev. Suisse Zool.* 27:353–76.

Gower, W. C. 1938. Studies on the trematodes of ducks in Michigan with special reference to the Mallard. *Mich. State Coll. Agr. Expt. Sta. Mem.* 3:1–94.

———. 1939. Host-parasite catalogue of the helminths of ducks. *Am. Midland Naturalist* 22:580–628.

Heard, R. W. 1967. Some helminth parasites of the clapper rail, *Rallus longirostris* Boddaert, from the Atlantic and Gulf Coasts of the United States. Master's thesis. Univ. Georgia.

Hieronymi, E. 1921. Ueber eine neue Huehnerenzooetie, bedingt durch *Prosthogonimus intercalandus,* n. sp. I Teil.: Pathologie. *Zentr. Bakteriol. Parasitenk. Abt. I. Orig.* 86:236–40.

Jegen, G. 1917. *Collyriclum faba* (Bremser) Kossack. Ein Parasit der Singvoegel, sein Bau und seine Lebensgeschichte. *Z. Wiss. Zool. Abt. A.* 117:460–553.

Johnson, J. C. 1920. The life cycle of *Echinostoma revolutum* (Froelich). *Univ. Calif. (Berkeley) Publ. Zool.* 19:335–98.

Jordan, F. T. W. 1953. Intestinal infestation in turkey poults with *Plagiorchis* (*Multiglandularis*) *megalorchis* Rees, 1952 and an experimental study of its life cycle. *J. Helminthol.* 27:75–80.

Kapitonov, V. I. 1959. Biology of the eider of the Kandalaksha Gulf. *Tr. Nauchn. Issled. Inst. Sel'skokhoz. Krain. Severs.* 9:216–37 (Russian text.)

Khalil, G. M., and R. M. Cable. 1969. Germinal development in *Philophthalmus megalurus* (Cort. 1914) (Trematoda: Digenea). *Z. Parasitenk.* 31:211–31.

Kingscote, A. A. 1951. A note on *Ribeiroia ondatrae* Price 1931 (Trematoda). *J. Parasitol.* 37:324.

Kingston, N. 1965. On the morphology and life cycle of the trematode *Tanaisia zarudyni* (Skrjabin, 1924) Byrd and Denton, 1950 from the ruffed grouse *Bonasa umbellus* L. *Can. J. Zool.* 43:953–69.

Kitchell, R. L., J. S. Cass, and J. H. Sautter. 1947. An infestation in domestic turkeys with intestinal flukes. *J. Am. Vet. Med. Ass.* 111:379–81.

Kossack, W. F. K. 1911. Ueber Monostomiden. *Zool. Jahrb. Jena Abt. Syst.* 31:491–590.

Kotlan, A., and W. L. Chandler. 1925. A newly recognized fluke disease (prosthogonimiasis) of fowls in the United States. *J. Am. Vet. Med. Ass.* 67:756–63.

Krause, C. 1925. Gehaeuftes Sterben bei Tauben durch Echinostomiden. *Berlin. Muench. Tieraerztl. Wochschr.* 41:262–63.

Krull, W. H., and C. R. Mapes. 1952-1953. Studies on the biology of *Dicrocoelium dendriticum* (Rudolphi, 1819) Looss, 1899 (Trematoda: Dicrocoeliidae) including its relation to the intermediate host, *Cionella lubrica* (Mueller). I-IX. *Cornell Vet.* 41:382–432; 42:253–76, 277–85, 339–51, 464–89, 603; 43:199–202, 389–410.

LaPage, G. 1961. A list of the parasitic protozoa, helminths and arthropoda recorded from species of the family Anatidae (ducks, geese, and swans). *Parasitology* 51:1–109.

Leibowitz, L. 1962. Unusual bird parasite cases and overall parasitic incidence found in a diagnostic laboratory during a five-year period. *Avian Diseases* 6:141–44.

Lumsden, R. D., and J. A. Zischke. 1963. Studies on the trematodes of Louisiana birds. *Z. Parasitenk.* 22:316–66.

McDonald, M. E. 1965. Catalogue of helminths of waterfowl (Anatidae). *Wildlife Dis.* 46:1–392.

Macy, R. W. 1934. Studies on the taxonomy, morphology, and biology of *Prosthogonimus macrorchis* Macy, a common oviduct fluke of domestic fowls in North America. *Minn. Agr. Expt. Sta. Tech. Bull.* 98:1–71.

Magalhães, P. S. 1899. Notes d'helminthologie bresilienne. 9. Monostomose suffocante des canards. *Arch. Parasitol.* 2:258–61.

Maldonado, J. F. 1945. The life cycle of *Tamerlania bragai* Santos 1934 (Eucotylidae), a kidney fluke of domestic pigeons. *J. Parasitol.* 31:306–14.

Maldonado, J. F., and W. A. Hoffman. 1941. *Tamerlania bragai,* a parasite of pigeons in Puerto Rico. *J. Parasitol.* 27:91.

Marotel, G. 1926. Une nouvelle maladie parasitaire: La monostomidose cutanee du dindon. *Rev. Vet. Med.* 78:725–36.

Maxfield, B. G., W. M. Reid, and F. A. Hayes. 1963. Gastrointestinal helminths from turkeys in Southeastern United States. *J. Wildlife Management* 27:261–71.

Mettrick, D. F. 1959. *Zygocotyle lunata.* A redescription of *Zygocotyle lunata* (Diesing, 1836) Stunkard from *Anas platyrhynchos domesticus* in Southern Rhodesia. *Rhodesia Agr. J.* 56:197–98.

Newsom, I. E., and E. N. Stout. 1933. Proventriculitis in chickens due to flukes. *Vet. Med.* 28:462–63.

Oiso, T. 1927. On a new species of avian Schistosoma developing in the portal vein of the duck, and investigations of its life-history. *Taiwan Igakkwai Zasshi, Taihoku* 270:848–65. (Japanese text, English summary.)

Patten, J. A. 1952. The life cycle of *Conspicuum icteridorum* Denton and Byrd 1951 (Trematoda: Dicrocoeliidae). *J. Parasitol.* 38:165–82.

Penner, L. R., and B. Fried. 1961. Studies on ocular trematodiasis. I. Marine acquired Philophthalmiasis. *J. Parasitol.* 47 (Suppl.): 31.

Prestwood, A. K. 1968. Parasitism among wild turkeys *(Meleagris gallopavo silvestris)* of the Mississippi delta. Doctoral dissertation, Univ. Georgia.

Price, E. W. 1928. The host relationship of the trematode genus *Zygocotyle. J. Agr. Res.* 36:911–14.

———. 1931. Four new species of trematode worms from the muskrat, *Ondatra zibethica,* with a key to the trematode parasites of the muskrat. *Proc. U.S. Nat. Mus.* 2870, 79, Art. 4:1–13.

———. 1934. Losses among wild ducks due to infestation with *Sphaeridiotrema globulus* (Rudolphi) (Trematoda: Psilostomidae). *Proc. Helminthol. Soc. Wash. D.C.* 1:31–34.

———. 1937. A note on the occurrence of a trematode of the genus *Clinostomum* in a chicken. *North Am. Vet.* 18:33–36.

Rees, G. 1952. The structure of the adult and larval stages of *Plagiorchis (Multiglandularis) megalorchis* N. Nom. from the turkey and an experimental demonstration of the life history. *Parasitology* 42:92–113.

Reinhardt, R. 1922. Seuchenhaft auftretende Eileiterentzuendungen bei Huehnern durch Invasion von *Prosthogonimus intercalandus. Berlin. Muench. Tieraerztl. Wochschr.* 38: 384.

Riggin, G. T., Jr. 1956. A note on *Ribeiroia ondatrae* (Price, 1931) in Puerto Rico. *Proc. Helminthol. Soc. Wash. D.C.* 23:28–29.

Riley, W. A. 1931. *Collyriclum faba* as a parasite of poultry. *Poultry Sci.* 10:204–7.

Riley, W. A., and H. C. H. Kernkamp. 1924. Flukes of the genus *Collyriclum* as parasites of turkeys and chickens. *J. Am. Vet. Med. Ass.* 64:591–99.

Schmid, F. 1930. Beitrag zur Gefluegelparasiten-Behandlung. *Tieraerztl. Rundschau* 36:313–16.

Seifried, O. 1923. Durch Invasion von Trematoden (Prosthogonimus-Arten) verursachte seuchenhaft auftretende und toedlich verlaufende Eileiter-Erkrankungen bei Huehnern in Mecklenburg. *Deut. Tieraerztl. Wochschr.* 31:541–44.

Self, J. T., and J. L. Bouchard. 1950. Parasites of the wild turkey, *Meleagris gallopavo intermedia* Sinnet, from the Wichita Mountains Wildlife Refuge. *J. Parasitol.* 36: 502–3.

Serapin, C. 1957. W sprawie pojawienia sie przywry *Notocotylus attenuatus* Rudolphi, 1809 u gesi na fermi "C." (On the occurence of the fluke *Notocotylus attenuatus* Rudolphi, 1809 in geese.) *Med. Weterynar.* 13:398–99. (Polish text.)

Shaw, J. N. 1947. Some parasites of Oregon wildlife. *Oregon Agr. Expt. Sta. Tech. Bull.* 11:1-16.

Shleikus, P., and A. Tatarintsevaite. 1960. Ekhinoparifioz-Novyi gelmintoz gusiat v Litouskoi SSR *(Echinoparyphium* infection—a new helminthiasis of geese in the Lithuanian SSR) *Veterinariya* 37:53. (Russian text.)

Skrjabin, K. I. 1913. *Tracheophilus sisowi* n. g., n. sp. Ein Beitrag zur Systematik der Gattung *Typhlocoelum* Stossich und der Verwandten Formen. *Zentr. Bakteriol. Parasitenk. Abt. I. Orig.* 69:90–95.

———. 1924. Nierentrematoden der Voegel Russland. *Zentr. Bakteriol. Parasitenk. Abt. II.* 62:80–90.

Soulsby, E. J. L. 1955. Deaths in swans associated with trematode infection. *Brit. Vet. J.* 111:498–500.

Spaulding, W. M. 1958. A survey of the parasites of ruffed grouse *(Bonasa umbellus)* in the Ottawa National Forest. Unpublished Master's thesis, Univ. Mich.

Stunkard, H. W. 1930. The life cycle of *Cryptocotyle lingua* (Creplin), with notes on the physiology of the metacercariae. *J. Morphol. Physiol.* 50:143–92.

———. 1934. The life history of *Typhlocoelum cymbium* (Diesing, 1850) Kossack, 1911 (Trematoda, Cyclocoelidae). A contribution to the phylogeny of the monostomes. *Bull. Soc. Zool.* 59:447–66.

———. 1964. Studies on the trematode genus

Renicola: Observations on the life-history, specificity, and systematic position. *Biol. Bull.* 126:467–89.

Stunkard, H. W., and F. W. Dunihue. 1931. Notes on the trematodes from a Long Island duck with description of a new species. *Biol. Bull.* 60:179–86.

Swales, W. E. 1933. *Streptovitella acadiae* gen. et. spec. nov. A trematode of the family Heterophyidae from the black duck *Anas rubripes. J. Helminthol.* 11:115–18.

Szidat, L. 1929. Die Parasiten des Hausgefluegels. 3. *Bilharziella polonica* Kow., ein im Blut schmarotzender Trematode unserer Enten, seine Entwicklung und Uebertragung. *Arch. Gefluegelk.* 3:78–87.

———. 1932. Zur Entwicklungsgeschichte der Cyclocoeliden. Der Lebenszyklus von *Tracheophilus sisowi* Skrj. 1923. *Zool. Anz.* 100:205–13.

———. 1937. Ueber die Entwicklungsgeschichte von *Sphaeridiotrema globulus* Rud. 1814 und die Stellung der Psilostomidae Odhner im natuerlichen System. I. Die Entwicklungsgeschichte von *Sphaeridiotrema globulus* Rud. *Z. Parasitenk.* 9:529–42.

Trainer, D. O., and G. W. Fisher. 1963. Fatal trematodiasis of coots. *J. Wildlife Management* 27:483–86.

Tyzzer, E. E. 1918. A monostome of the genus *Collyriclum* occurring in the European sparrow, with observations on the development of the ovum. *J. Med. Res.* 38, N.S. 33:267–92.

Van Cleave, H. J., and J. F. Mueller. 1932. Parasites of the Oneida Lake fishes. Part 1. Description of new genera and new species. *Roosevelt Wild Life Ann.* 3:5–71.

Van Haitsma, J. P. 1931. Studies on the trematode family Strigeidae (Holostomidae). No. XXII. *Cotylurus flabelliformis* (Faust) and its life-history. *Papers Mich. Acad. Sci.* 13:447–82.

Van Heelsbergen, T. 1927a. Echinostomiasis bij kippen door Echinoparyphium. *Tijdschr. Diergeneesk.* 54:413–14.

———. 1927b. Echinostomiasis bij de duif door Echinostoma. *Tijdschr. Diergeneesk.* 54:414–16.

Vevers, G. M. 1923. Observations on the life-histories of *Hypodaerium* (sic) *conoideum* (Bloch) and *Echinostomum revolutum* (Froel.): Trematode parasites of the domestic duck. *Ann. Appl. Biol.* 10:134–36.

Wallace, F. G. 1940. Studies on two species of liver flukes. *J. Parasitol.* 26 (Suppl.):37. (Abstr.)

Wehr, E. E. 1941. Controlling gapeworms in poultry. *USDA Leaflet* no. 207:1–6.

Wehrmann, S. 1909. Sur l'action pathogene des helminthes des oiseaux. *Arch. Parasitol.* 13:204–38.

West, A. Fred. 1961. Studies on the biology of *Philophthalmus gralli* Mathis and Leger, 1910 (Trematoda: Digena). *Am. Midland Naturalist* 66:363–83.

Willey, C. H. 1941. The life history of bionomics of the trematode, *Zygocotyle lunata* (Paramphistomidae). *Zoologica* 26:65–88.

Wooton, D. M. 1957. The life history of *Cryptocotyle concavum* (Creplin, 1825) Fischoeder, 1903 (Trematoda: Heterophyidae). *J. Parasitol.* 43:271–82.

Zunker, M. 1925. *Echinostoma columbae* n. sp. ein neuer Parasit der Haustaube. *Berlin. Muench. Tieraerztl. Wochschr.* 41:483–84.

CHAPTER 31

PROTOZOA

❖

INTRODUCTION

❖

W. MALCOLM REID

Department of Poultry Science
University of Georgia
Athens, Georgia

❖

ALTHOUGH PROTOZOA have usually been defined as unicellular animals, this description is not universally accepted. To emphasize the differences between protozoan organisms, which may contain a complex system of organelles, and the typical cells in multicellular animals (Metazoa), Hyman (1940) defined Protozoa as acellular animals.

Distinctions between Protozoa and Metazoa are not easily drawn since some Protozoa exhibit syncytial stages in their life cycles with no cell membranes being present between the nuclei. Similarly, distinctions between Protozoa and various unicellular plants are difficult to draw. Bacterial and fungal organisms possess a somewhat rigid permeable cell wall while Protozoa have a more flexible pellicle or a plasma membrane. Some of the difficulties in distinguishing protozoan from fungal organisms are dealt with in the section in Sarcosporidia. Following Spindler's observations (1947) showing funguslike structures produced by Sarcosporidia, sarcosporidiosis was moved from the chapter on Protozoa (first edition) to "Diseases Pro-

duced by Fungi" in the second and subsequent editions of this text. The decision to again include Sarcosporidia within the chapter on Protozoa in this edition was made by the Editorial Board for reasons other than the controversial issues covered in Spindler's review.

The role of over 100 species of protozoa in producing avian diseases is reviewed in this chapter by three different authors. Fuller accounts of their role as parasites and classification will be found in other textbooks (Levine, 1961; Soulsby, 1968). At the request of textbook users greater emphasis has been placed on diagnostic procedures for coccidiosis.

The voluminous literature on coccidiostats could be but briefly reviewed through the use of tables. Over 1,000 abstracts dealing with chemotherapy have been listed in recent bibliographies (Merck, 1953, 1961, 1965). Methodology in testing anticoccidial drugs has been reviewed in a symposium involving 25 speakers (Reid, 1970).

Controversial opinions on the etiology of infectious enterohepatitis (blackhead) have been reopened during recent years. Although all recent studies in the United States have generally accepted a role for *Histomonas meleagridis* in etiology of this disease, Schiefer and Mehnert (1963) have revived Enigk's earlier work recognizing *Candida albicans* as a primary etiological agent. His "blastocystis" theory has been briefly reviewed in the first four editions of this text and more extensively by Reid (1967). A restudy using Koch's postulates from case material from the United States (Kemp, 1964; Kemp and Reid, 1966a) and Europe (Reid et al., 1967) would confirm the primary role of *H. meleagridis*. The possibility exists that certain mycoses may produce hepatoenteric lesions superficially resembling those of histomoniasis. Instances include liver involvement in candidiasis, which, however, has rarely been reported in the United States. Lesions in the liver are not as well defined as those illustrated for histomoniasis (see Fig. 31.8). In questionable cases use of the Periodic acid-Schiff differential staining technique has been found useful (Kemp and Reid, 1966b).

Studies using germ-free techniques with turkeys indicate that certain species of bacteria also play a role with *H. meleagridis* in the development of the disease. Using

Grateful acknowledgement is made of the groundwork for this chapter by the late Elery R. Becker and by Marion M. Farr who coauthored this chapter in the 5th edition.

gnotobiotic techniques for introduction of eggs of Heterakis-containing histomonads into bacteriologically sterile poults, a graded series of severity of lesions has been demonstrated (Franker and Doll, 1964a,b; Bradley, 1965; Franker, 1965; Bradley and Reid, 1966; Reid, 1967; Reid et al., 1967; Springer, 1968; Springer et al., 1970), depending upon the species of bacteria established as flora of the digestive tract. In these bacteria-free poults the combination of *H. meleagridis* and either of the organisms *Clostridium perfringens* and *Escherichia* coli alone or together produced the disease syndrome. The lesions were more severe in turkeys (Springer, 1968) when *C. perfringens* was present than when *E. coli* represented the single monoassociated organism with *H. meleagridis*. Mild atypical lesions occurred if *E. intermedia* (Franker and Doll, 1964b) and *Bacillus subtilis* (Bradley, 1965) were introduced before Histomonas was added to germ-free poults. *Proteus mirabilis* (Bradley and Reid, 1966), *B. cereus*, and *Lactobacillus faecalis* (Franker and Doll, 1964b) permitted no disease when introduced as monoassociates.

Fresh cecal contents from normal chickens were required to contaminate germ-free chickens in order to establish blackhead, which then readily developed after introduction of histomonad organisms via heterakid eggs. However, in no instance was the disease produced in chickens when as many as 48 species of bacteria were introduced alone or as single or multiple associates in gnotobiotic chickens, demonstrating a difference between chickens and turkeys in response to causative factors in histomoniasis (Springer, 1968; Springer et al., 1970). The practical significance of these studies is basic to the development of chemotherapeutic agents which may act as antibacterial and antihelminthic as well as antihistomonal agents.

The role of *H. meleagridis* in producing histomoniasis together with new discoveries involving the earthworm is reviewed in the section by Lund. He has also reviewed the role of all other protozoan organisms in producing avian disease.

Demonstration that cats are the natural host of *Toxoplasma gondii* and that the life cycle also involves an oocyst of *Isospora* sp. will change emphasis on control measures as well as on the systematic position of this parasite. It now seems probable that poultry as well as man and other mammals are accidental hosts infected through oocyst infection originating from cats. The announcement of this major discovery made independently from two laboratories (Sheffield and Melton, 1970; Frenkel et al., 1970) was received too close to the press deadline to reorganize classification within the chapter.

REFERENCES

Bradley, R. E. 1965. *Histomonas meleagridis* and several pure bacterial strains in the production of infectious enterohepatitis in gnotobiotic turkeys. Ph.D. dissertation, Univ. Georgia.

Bradley, R. E., and W. M. Reid. 1966. *Histomonas meleagridis* and several bacteria as agents of infectious enterohepatitis in gnotobiotic turkeys. *Exp. Parasitol.* 19:91–101.

Franker, C. K. 1965. Experimental histomoniasis in gnotobiotic turkeys. Ph.D. dissertation, Univ. Notre Dame.

Franker, C. K., and J. P. Doll. 1964a. Effects of some cecal bacteria on Histomonas infection of gnotobiotic turkeys. *Proc. Am. Soc. Microbiol. Bacteriol.*, p. 46. (Abstr.)

——. 1964b. Experimental histomoniasis in gnotobiotic turkeys. II. Effects of some cecal bacteria on pathogenesis. *J. Parasitol.* 50:636–40.

Frenkel, J. H., J. P. Dubey, and N. L. Miller. 1970. *Toxoplasma gondii* in cats: Fecal stages identified as coccidian oocysts. *Science* 167:893–96.

Hyman, Libbie H. 1940. *The Invertebrates: Protozoa Through Ctenophora.* McGraw-Hill, New York.

Kemp, R. L. 1964. The relationship of *Histomonas meleagridis* and *Candida albicans* to infectious enterohepatitis of domestic poultry. Ph.D. dissertation, Univ. Georgia.

Kemp, R. L., and W. M. Reid. 1966a. Studies on the etiology of blackhead disease: The roles of *Histomonas meleagridis* and *Candida albicans* in the United States. *Poultry Sci.* 45:1296–1302.

——. 1966b. Staining techniques for differential diagnosis of histomoniasis and mycosis in domestic poultry. *Avian Diseases* 10:357–63.

Levine, N. D. 1961. *Protozoan Parasites of Domestic Animals and of Man.* Burgess Publ. Co., Minneapolis.

Merck and Co., Inc. 1953. *Coccidiosis.* Annotated Bibliography Pt. I; 1961, Pt. II; 1965, Pt. III.

Reid, W. M. 1967. Etiology and dissemination of the blackhead disease syndrome in turkeys and chickens. *Exp. Parasitol.* 21:249–75.

———. 1970. Anticoccidial drugs. Objectives of symposium on development, selection and testing. *Exp. Parasitol.* 28:1–3.

Reid, W. M., R. L. Kemp, and Joyce Johnson. 1967. Studies on the comparative roles of *Histomonas meleagridis* and *Candida albicans* in the production of blackhead in European poultry. *Zentr. Veterinaermed.* B 14:179–85.

Schiefer, B., and B. Mehnert. 1963. Untersuchungen zur Aetiologie und Pathogenese der Typhlohepatitis der Huehnervoegel. *Zentr. Veterinaermed.* 10 (Reihe B):28–48.

Sheffield, H. G., and Marjorie L. Melton. 1970. *Toxoplasma gondii:* The oocyst, sporozoite, and infection of cultured cells. *Science* 167:892–93.

Soulsby, E. J. L. 1968. *Helminths, Arthropods and Protozoa of Domesticated Animals.* Bailliere, Tindall, and Cassell, London.

Spindler, L. A. 1947. A note on the fungoid nature of certain internal structures of Miescher's sacs (Sarcocystis) from a naturally infected sheep and a naturally infected duck. *Proc. Helminthol. Soc. Wash. D.C.* 14:28–30.

Springer, W. T. 1968. Histomoniasis: Biological aspects of transmission, pathogenesis, and relationships to the indigenous bacterial flora of chickens and turkeys. Ph.D. dissertation, Univ. Georgia.

Springer, W. T., Joyce Johnson, and W. M. Reid. 1970. Histomoniasis in gnotobiotic chickens and turkeys: Biological aspects of the role of bacteria in the etiology. *Exp. Parasitol.* 28:383–92.

❖

COCCIDIOSIS

❖

W. MALCOLM REID

*Department of Poultry Science
University of Georgia
Athens, Georgia*

❖

COCCIDIOSIS is the term applied to the diseased condition caused by infection with one or more of the many species of Coccidia, a subdivision of the great protozoan class Sporozoa. All representatives are parasitic and devoid of specialized organelles of locomotion in the vegetative stages. As emphasized by Tyzzer (1932), whose monumental studies are considered classic descriptions, there are as many kinds of coccidiosis as there are species of coccidia, each with its characteristic signs. Nonpathogenic species or extremely light infections of pathogenic species may produce *coccidiasis*, which indicates an absence of clinical or subclinical coccidiosis. While coccidiosis is cosmopolitan, occurring in practically all kinds of birds, the problem of identification is simplified somewhat by the fact that parasites are host-specific; each species occurs in a single host or in a limited group of closely related hosts. Several bird hosts are known to harbor more than one species of coccidia, which complicates the diagnostic problem. Identification requires recognition of one species and elimination of the other species characteristically present in this host.

As a group, the coccidioses of chickens cause more severe financial losses than is encountered in other domesticated birds. Losses due to mortality following a severe outbreak may be devastating. However, morbidity losses may be even more costly without the producer being aware that his flock has any disease problem. Effects of parasitism may not be apparent until comparative weights are available between parasitized and parasite-free birds. Turkeys, geese, ducks, and guinea fowl suffer less severely from intestinal coccidiosis infection than do chickens; however, economic losses occur under certain conditions of infection in all these birds. Disastrous outbreaks of renal coccidiosis in geese have frequently been recorded. Young pigeons suffer severe mortality from acute at-

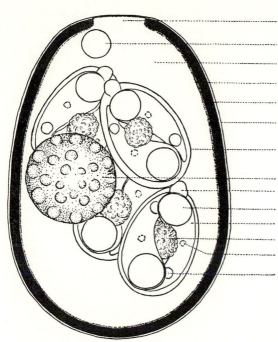

1—Micropyle.

2—Polar inclusion.

3—Oocyst jelly.

4—Endomembrane of cyst wall.

5—Middle or "granular layer" of cyst wall.
6—Exomembrane of cyst wall.

7—Sporocyst or envelope of a spore.

8—Oocystic or extra-residual body.
9—Stieda body of spore.

10—Refractile globule of sporozoite.
11—Sporozoite.

12—Sporocystic or intra-residual body.

13—Nucleus of sporozoite.

14—Small refractile globule at more attenuated end of sporozoite.

FIG. 31.1—*Diagrammatic representation of mature oocyst of genus Eimeria.*
(Becker, 1948)

tacks of diarrhea. Coccidiosis has produced serious losses in pheasants and quail raised in captivity. Coccidiosis of game birds may produce problems, but no satisfactory method of assessing these losses has been developed (Prestwood, 1968).

CLASSIFICATION-TAXONOMIC
RELATIONSHIPS

Of many described genera of Coccidia, the genus Eimeria contains the species of major economic importance in domestic birds. Internal structure of the sporulated oocysts (Fig. 31.1) is the characteristic used to distinguish this genus from several others which may occasionally be encountered. The oocysts of all genera, when freshly passed, consist of a thickened outer wall and a rounded mass of nucleated protoplasm. Not until sporulation has occurred do the distinguishing characteristics become apparent. In the genus Eimeria, four spores or sporocysts develop, each containing two banana-shaped sporozoites.

Isospora, a second genus containing many species from wild birds, may be distinguished from Eimeria by the presence of two sporocysts, each of which contains four sporozoites (Fig. 31.2A). These internal differences are illustrated by *Isospora gallinae* Scholtyseck, 1954. Although described as a new species from a hen, Levine (1961) lists sparrows as a more probable host. Transmission experiments have not been completed with hens.

The genus Wenyonella has four sporocysts, each of which contains four sporozoites (Fig. 31.2B). *Wenyonella gallinae* (Ray, 1945) is the only species reported from the domestic fowl. Although pathogenicity in the form of pinpoint hemorrhages in the posterior portion of the intestine has been described, infection appears to be very rare (Gill, 1955); it has thus far been described only from India.

Eight sporozoites have been described from the genus Tyzzeria by Allen (1936) (Fig. 31.2C). No sporocysts develop in this genus. The type species *T. perniciosa* Allen 1936 parasitizes the duck.

Four free sporozoites with no sporocysts characterize the genus Cryptosporidium. Tyzzer named the parasite *C. parvum*. The specimens used for illustration were considered the same species (Tyzzer, 1912; 1929) from the house mouse (Fig. 31.2D) and the chicken. Those parasitizing chickens were renamed *C. tyzzeria* by Levine

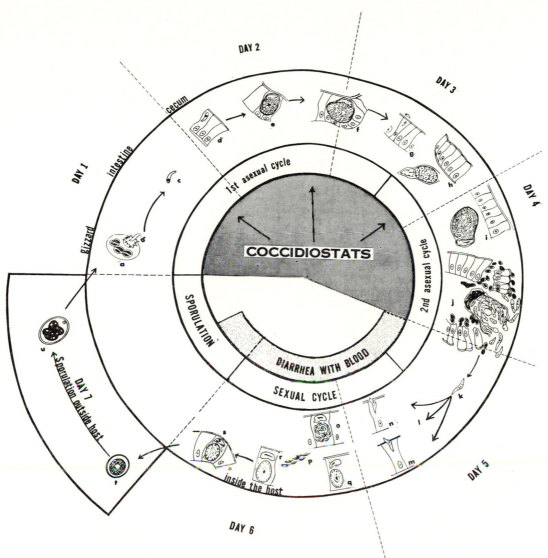

FIG. 31.3—*Life cycle of* Eimeria tenella: *(a) sporulated oocyst; (b) sporozoite being liberated from oocyst and sporozoite; (c) sporozoite; (d) trophozoite parasitizing an epithelial cell; (e) early schizont; (f) mature first-generation schizont; (g) first-generation merozoite parasitizing another epithelial cell; (h) and (i) second-generation schizonts; (j) rupture of second-generation schizont; (k) second-generation merozoite may again parasitize other epithelial cells (l) for a third asexual cycle, or may parasitize an epithelial cell (m) to become a female gametocyte (q); merozoite parasitizing an epithelial cell (n) and becoming a male gametocyte (o); (p) liberated microgametes unite with macrogamete (r) which develops into oocyst (s) and is liberated in the feces by host (t); sporulation (u) of oocyst occurs in outside environment. (After Levine, 1961)*

passed outside the host. Here specific environmental conditions are required to permit sporulation. Nuclear (diploid to haploid) and cellular division occur resulting in the typical 8 sporozoites within 4 sporocysts during a minimum period of 18 hours

(t,u). The entire life cycle may be completed in 6½ days, although the average time is somewhat longer (Edgar, 1955).

Only a small proportion of the millions of oocysts produced by a bird survive and become infective. Essential conditions for survival are: (1) sufficient moisture, (2) oxygen, and (3) suitable temperatures. Sporulation of *E. tenella* is most rapid at 28° C (Ellis, 1938; Edgar, 1954). Oocysts still sporulate at 20° and 32° C but fail to sporulate at 8° C and sporulate slowly at 37° C. If maintained at this higher temperature they soon lose viability. Oocysts are quickly killed by extremes in temperatures. A 10-minute exposure to 55° C kills all oocysts (Fish, 1931). A decrease in refrigerator temperature sufficient to produce a few ice crystals will kill all oocysts (Edgar, 1954). Sporulation is more rapid in the presence of oxygen, although a few may develop under anaerobic conditions (Ellis, 1938). Adequate moisture is also essential for sporulation. This latter need is frequently illustrated in poultry houses by coccidiosis outbreaks following appearance of wet litter. In experimental studies (Ellis, 1938) oocyst survival was extended from 4 to 46 days by increasing humidity from dry (21–34%) to wet conditions (91–93%).

CHICKEN

Coccidiosis remains one of the major disease problems of the poultryman in spite of advances made in prevention and control through chemotherapy. It is one of the most commonly encountered diseases in the diagnostic laboratories. In northeastern United States 16% (Chute et al., 1967) and in southern United States 19% (Murphy et al., 1967) of the consignments submitted to laboratories were diagnosed as coccidiosis. Realistic dollar losses are difficult to determine, but the estimate of $35 million made by the USDA (1965) is far too low. Dollar savings through improved production in broilers by the use of coccidiostats have been estimated at $37 million (Reid, 1969). In all parts of the world where confinement rearing is practiced, coccidiosis represents a major disease problem.

INCIDENCE AND DISTRIBUTION

Unlike many other poultry diseases, coccidia are almost universally found wherever chickens are being raised. The resistant oocysts are readily transported in live birds which sometimes remain carriers for long periods of time. Because most coccidial infections are subclinical, the producer is usually completely unaware of the presence of several species of organisms on his premises until mismanagement permits an explosive development of large numbers of sporulated oocysts. The seriousness of an attack is directly proportional to the number of organisms ingested by a bird at one time. Unlike most viral and bacterial diseases, multiplication within the host is very strictly limited. The greatest number of daughter oocysts produced per oocyst inoculated was 100,000 in experimental trials (Bracket and Bliznick, 1950). This number compares with indefinite multiplication by other classes of organisms.

All species of Eimeria reported from chickens appear to be widely and universally distributed throughout the world. However, this conclusion seems to have been recognized only recently by poultry pathologists who had previously hoped coccidiosis could be contained by quarantine measures. Wherever intensive search has been made, most or all of the recognized species have been identified. This was true in Iowa (Zimmermann, 1957), Alabama (Edgar, 1958a), Maine (Chute et al., 1960), Georgia (Reid et al., 1960, 1965, 1968; Reid, 1963a,b, 1966; Reid and Raja, 1963), Romania (Lungu, 1961), England (Davies, 1963; Long, 1959, 1964, 1967a,b), Greece (Papadopoulas et al., 1963), France (Renault et al., 1965), Germany (Reid et al., 1965; Pohl, 1965a,b), India (Gill, 1955, 1961), and Lebanon (Long and Tanielian, 1965). The worldwide distribution of all species has been confirmed by Roncalli (personal communication, 1967), a veterinarian studying coccidiostat performance in extensive travels in Europe, South America, and Australia. He has indicated that similar coccidiosis problems are encountered by the different species in all areas which he visited. Distribution of the species of coccidia appears to be limited only by distribution of the chicken.

ETIOLOGY

There are 9 recognized species of Eimeria reported from chickens. Identification and recognition of these different species pose a difficult but necessary diagnostic problem. The following characteristics are useful in species identification: (1) zone of intestine parasitized; (2) nature of macroscopic lesions; (3) oocyst size, shape, and color; (4) minimum sporulation time; (5) minimum prepatent period; (6) schizont size and area in which it develops; (7) loca-

TABLE 31.1 ❧ Differential Characteristics for 9 Species of Chicken Coccidia (Reid, 1968)

CHARACTERISTICS	E. acervulina	E. brunetti	E. hagani	E. maxima	E. mivati	E. mitis	E. necatrix	E. praecox	E. tenella
ZONE PARASITIZED									
MACROSCOPIC LESIONS	light infection: transverse, whitish bands of oocysts; heavy infection: paques coalescing thickened wall	coagulation necrosis, mucoid, bloody enteritis	pinhead hemorrhages petechiae	thickened walls, mucoid, blood-tinged exudate, petechiae	light infection: rounded plaques of oocysts; heavy infection: thickened walls coalescing plaques	no lesions, mucoid exudate	ballooning, white spots (schizonts), petechiae, mucoid blood-filled exudate	no lesions, mucoid exudate	onset: hemorrhage into lumen; later: thickening, whitish mucosa, cores clotted blood
MICROSCOPIC CHARACTERISTICS — OOCYSTS REDRAWN FROM ORIGINALS			none available						
LENGTH x WIDTH — LENGTH= WIDTH=	AV = 18.3 x 14.6 (μ) 17.7–20.2 13.7–16.3	24.6 x 18.8 20.7–30.3 18.1–24.2	19.1 x 17.6 15.8–20.9 14.3–19.5	30.5 x 20.7 21.5–42.5 16.5–29.8	15.5 x 13.4 11.1–19.9 10.5–16.2	16.2 x 16.0 14.3–19.6 13.0–17.0	20.4 x 17.2 13.2–22.7 11.3–18.3	21.3 x 17.1 19.8–24.7 15.7–19.8	22.0 x 19.0 19.5–26.0 16.5–22.8
OOCYST SHAPE AND INDEX= LENGTH/WIDTH	ovoid 1.25	ovoid 1.31	broadly ovoid 1.08	ovoid 1.47	ellipsoid to broadly ovoid 1.16	subspherical 1.01	oblong ovoid 1.19	ovoidal 1.24	ovoid 1.16
SPORULATION MINIMUM-HR	17	18	18	30	12	18	18	12	18
SCHIZONT MAX IN MICRONS	10.3	30.0		9.4	17.3	11.3	65.9	20	54.0
PARASITE LOCATION IN TISSUE SECTIONS	epithelial	2nd generation schizonts subepithelial	epithelial	gametocytes subepithelial	epithelial	epithelial	2nd generation schizonts subepithelial	epithelial	2nd generation schizonts subepithelial
PREPATENT PERIOD-HR	97	120	99	123	93	138	99	84	138

tion of the parasite within the epithelial cells; (8) cross-immunization trials. The first six characteristics most commonly used in diagnostic laboratories are summarized in Table 31.1 with the most useful characteristics printed in red. Further explanations are included with the species described in alphabetical order. A presumptive diagnosis is usually possible after a necropsy examination of a recently killed bird and microscopic examination of smear preparations. Confirmation may require cross-immunization experiments. Characteristics listed under (7) and (8) will be of little value in most diagnostic laboratories. Orientation of the parasite with respect to the nucleus of the epithelial cell is described in the final section on histopathology, but such examination will be attempted only in special studies. Cross-immunization trials require pure suspensions of daughter oocysts derived by use of single oocyst isolation techniques for immunization of parasite-free birds. Challenge with the other species likewise requires another pure strain of a single species.

Oocyst size and/or color is useful in identification of some species. It is diagnostic for *E. maxima*. Overlapping sizes of all other species require measurements (see Diagnosis). Oocyst shape differs from species to species. Edgar and Seibold (1964) have classed *E. tenella, E. maxima, E. acervulina,* and *E. brunetti* as being ovoid; *E. necatrix* as oblong; *E. hagani* as broadly ovoid. Since these descriptive terms are subjective, the "shape index" (Becker et al., 1955) may be more useful. It is determined by dividing the mean length by the mean width. The shape index ranked beginning with the most spherical using Edgar and Seibold's measurements (1964) would be: *E. mitis* 1.01, *E. hagani* 1.08, *E. tenella* and *E. mivati* 1.16, *E. necatrix* 1.19, *E. praecox* 1.24, *E. acervulina* 1.25, *E. brunetti* 1.31, and *E. maxima* 1.47.

Eimeria acervulina Tyzzer 1929

Classification and Morphology

In addition to this species, *E. hagani, E. mivati, E. mitis,* and *E. praecox* parasitize the epithelium in the same zone of the digestive tract. *E. acervulina* invades the epithelial cells in the duodenal loop, but infection may extend as far posterior as the

rectum or cecum (Tyzzer, 1929). In light infections whitish lesions may be seen from either the serosal or mucosal surfaces of the digestive tract. These elongated lesions are oriented transversely in "ladderlike" arrangements (Fig. 31.4A,B) and contain colonies of developing oocysts. In heavier infections these colonies become coalesced, whitish yellow or gray, and less distinct.

The oocysts are egg-shaped and frequently show thinning of the shell at the small end and slight elevation of the border of the thinned area. This is called a micropyle by Pellérdy (1965), but Levine (1961) lists the micropyle and residuum as being absent. *E. mivati* is somewhat smaller than *E. acervulina*, as is also *E. mitis*. The latter species and *E. hagani* also differ in being more rounded (shape index 1.01 and 1.08 compared to 1.25). *E. praecox* is somewhat larger than *E. acervulina*. Both the minimum prepatent period of 97 hours and the minimum sporulation time of 17 hours are longer for *E. acervulina* than for *E. mivati* or *E. praecox*.

Pathogenicity

Although older accounts claim but slight pathogenicity for this species (Tyzzer, 1929; Dickinson, 1941; Becker, 1948; Brackett and Bliznick, 1950), it must be regarded as a moderately severe pathogen. Pathogenicity is very directly dependent upon the numbers of oocysts received by the bird. Mortality as high as 75% followed inoculation with 5 million oocysts, a number which might be acquired under natural conditions, according to Morehouse and McGuire (1958). Other investigators have reported light to moderate mortality following heavy inoculations (Edgar, 1958a; Gill and Lall, 1961; Aycardi, 1963; Hegde and Reid, 1969). Moderate to severe reduction in weight gain has followed inoculation of large numbers (500,000–2,000,000) of oocysts (Dickinson, 1941; Moynihan, 1950; Aycardi, 1963; Long, 1968a; Hein, 1968; Reid and Johnson, 1969). Outbreaks in layers cause decrease in egg production (Dickinson, 1941; Peterson, 1949; Edgar, 1958a; Hegde and Reid, 1969). Recovery to the normal rate of lay requires about 3 weeks. Climatic conditions in northwestern United States produce special problems with layers which are associated with changes in moisture levels (Peterson, 1949).

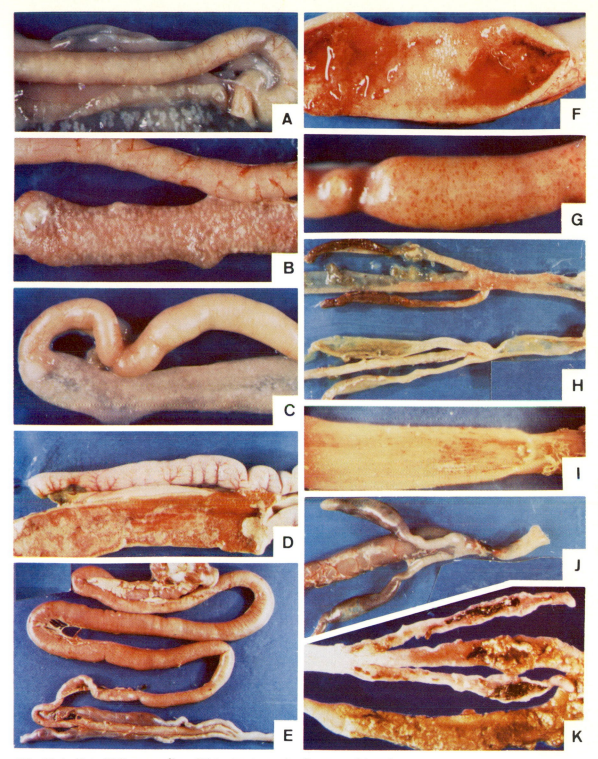

FIG. 31.4—(A to D) E. acervulina. (A) Lesion (scored +2) very mild pathogenicity; (B) lesion (scored +3) moderate pathogenicity; (C and D) severely pathogenic (scored +4). (E to G) E. maxima. (E) Showing ballooning in heavy infection, day 5; (F) mucosal surface 5th day of infection; (G) serosal surface 6th day of infection. (H to K) E. brunetti. (H) Moderate lesions in lower intestine, rectum, and neck of cecum (upper); normal control (lower); (I) moderate infection of rectum; (J) complete blockage (pointer) of the rectum due to E. brunetti infection; (K) field case showing severe coagulation necrosis.

Gross Lesions

The typical ladderlike transverse lesions usually described for *E. acervulina* in the duodenal and upper jejunal area represent light infections. Lesions classified as $+1$ or $+2$ on a visual scoring scale (Fig. 31.4A,B) showed no loss in growth rate (Reid and Johnson, 1969). Heavier inoculations scored as $+3$ or $+4$ produce coalescence in the lesions and thickening of the mucosa. Larger numbers of oocysts cause lesions to be extended further down the intestinal tract (Barber, 1955; Hein, 1968). Color of the intestine may be grayish yellow in light or moderate infections; the bright red congestion described by Morehouse and McGuire (1958) appears in extremely heavy infections and has been seen only in White Rocks in our laboratory.

Histopathology

Histopathological changes associated with *E. acervulina* infection occur in the epithelium resulting in the denuding of the intestinal villi. Parasites may invade every villus in some areas. Thinning out of the epithelial layer occurs as its normal rapid regenerative capacity is taxed by successive swarms of invading organisms. Most of the changes are superficial with little invasion of deeper tissues. Thickening may be severe on the 5th and 6th days in heavily parasitized intestines.

Both schizonts and gametocytes locate above the nucleus of the epithelial cell. First-generation schizonts are smaller ($5-8\mu$) than those of *E. mivati* which measure $9-14\mu$ (Long, 1967c).

Eimeria brunetti Levine 1942

Classification and Morphology

Lesions in the lower small intestine, rectum, and proximal area of the ceca are produced by this species (Fig. 31.4H,I,J,K). None of the other 8 species typically establish themselves in this zone. In severe cases a coagulation necrosis produces a caseous eroded surface over the entire mucosa (Fig. 31.4K). This occurs between the 4th and 7th days of infection. In rare cases the tissue breakdown in the upper rectum may cause a complete blockage of the digestive system (Fig. 31.4J). Although this condition originally described by Levine (1943) was not consistently reproduced in laboratory infections by Boles and Becker (1954),

moderate coagulation necrosis has been demonstrated in bacteria-free birds (Hegde et al., 1969). This investigation proves that moderate necrosis does not require presence of secondary bacterial invaders, although they may be involved in very severe lesions. Sloughing and coagulation of the bloody exudate may sometimes produce soft cores extending into the ceca as well as into the intestine. In light infections hemorrhagic streaks occur in the mucosa; a thick bloody mucoid exudate fills the intestine (Fig. 31.4H,I). At other times feces may be whitish but blood-streaked. Although pathological manifestations are usually noted in the lower half of the digestive tract, initially the parasite establishes itself more anteriorly and moves to posterior zones with the emergence of second-generation merozoites. Lesions are highly variable in character with this species and may appear chiefly as a fibrinous enteritis (Pohl, 1965a). For this reason infections may be entirely overlooked.

The parasite produces moderately large oocysts (av. $23.4 \times 19.7\mu$). Thus it has the second largest oocyst, being surpassed in size only by *E. maxima*. Oocysts resemble those of *E. tenella* in color and shape but are proportionately larger, thicker, and longer. Oocyst size as demonstrated by measurement of a number of oocysts is a reliable differential characteristic. The oocyst has a polar granule but no residuum or micropyle. Schizonts, which are considerably smaller than those of *E. necatrix* and *E. tenella*, are typically found in the lower small intestine, rectum, cloaca, and proximal portions of the ceca.

Pathogenicity

Although less serious than *E. tenella* or *E. necatrix* in producing mortality, *E. brunetti* must be rated as a severe pathogen. The 10% mortality in a pullet flock reported by a local diagnostic laboratory probably represents as severe an outbreak as encountered in the field. In experimental infections relatively few oocysts may sometimes produce mortality in susceptible strains of birds.

Pathogenesis and Epizootiology

Although listed as "uncommon" by Levine (1961), studies in Georgia would indicate that this species is very common

(Reid, 1963a, 1965; Reid and Pitois, 1965). It is reported rather frequently from diagnostic laboratories (Chute et al., 1967; Murphy et al., 1967). For unexplained reasons, clinical flock problems show up at irregular intervals but may affect several flocks in an area. Although undiagnosed until recently in England (Davies et al., 1963; Long, 1964) or in France (Renault et al., 1965), it is now considered fairly common in these areas. Similar observations have been made in Hungary (Pellérdy, 1960). Lesions from milder cases are frequently overlooked if microscopic studies are not made.

Histopathology

Microscopic sections at 3½ days reveal numerous young schizonts, eosinophilia, hyperemia, and some sloughing of the epithelium (Boles and Becker, 1954). Red pinpoint gross lesions may appear in the lower intestine just above the junction of the ceca. The host becomes listless by the 4th day with the intestine appearing whitish and the hemorrhagic areas increasing in size. The epithelium sloughs off, the tips of the villi being more severely invaded than the sides. By the end of the 4th day, large numbers of released merozoites begin to parasitize the epithelium, and sexual stages establish themselves with pinpoint lesions in the lower small intestine and ceca. At this time a caseous core may appear in the cecum and rectum. Few differences are noted on the 5th day, but by the 6th, swelling of the invaded intestine is more intense with the red pinpoint lesions turning brown. The epithelium covering the villi is completely denuded with only the basement membrane remaining. The large multicentric arrangement of developing microgametocytes recently described by Scholtyseck (1959) shows similarities to those of E. maxima. Tyzzer (1929) had previously regarded this as a species characteristic of E. maxima.

First- and second-generation schizonts and most gametocytes occupy the zone above the nucleus in the epithelial cell. Occasionally, however, some gametocytes may develop below the nucleus.

Eimeria hagani Levine 1938

Classification and Morphology

No distinctive characteristics can be included for this upper intestinal species since the endogenous stages of the life cycle have not been described. The original describer (Levine, 1964, personal communication) now regards this species as very rare, and he no longer has oocysts or other stages for study. Edgar (1964, personal communication) has isolated and is describing a strain which he considers identical to the one described by Levine as E. hagani. Until a full description has been published, diagnosis of this species will be considered uncertain.

Levine (1938) listed the following characteristics for differential diagnosis: (1) Entire life cycle takes place in the duodenum and small intestine, unlike E. tenella and E. necatrix which involve the ceca. (2) Prepatent period of 6 days is similar to E. maxima but longer than E. acervulina, E. praecox, and E. mitis. (3) Oocysts are smaller and differently shaped than E. maxima. (4) Cross-immunization studies show differences from 7 other species.

Pathogenicity

The hemorrhagic spots, severe catarrhal inflammation, and fluid contents recorded in the original description (Levine, 1938) would suggest moderate pathogenicity. These lesions could be seen only from the serosal surface. Later Levine (1945) regarded this species as relatively nonpathogenic.

Eimeria maxima Tyzzer 1929

Classification and Morphology

The zone in which epithelial cells are parasitized is localized in the middle intestine, which shows hemorrhagic enteritis associated with thickening of the intestinal wall and some ballooning (Fig. 31.4E). The intestinal contents are brown, orange, pink, or red-brown with a very viscous mucous secretion present.

Recognition of the characteristic oocyst of this species is the most certain method to identify an E. maxima infection. Oocysts differ from the other 8 species in size, appearance, and color. Although the largest oocysts ($42.5 \times 29.8\mu$) offer complete size distinction, smaller E. maxima oocysts may overlap the larger range of other species. The measurement of several oocysts to determine the average length, width, and range may be necessary before species determination is certain. The walls of the oocyst have a characteristic golden brown

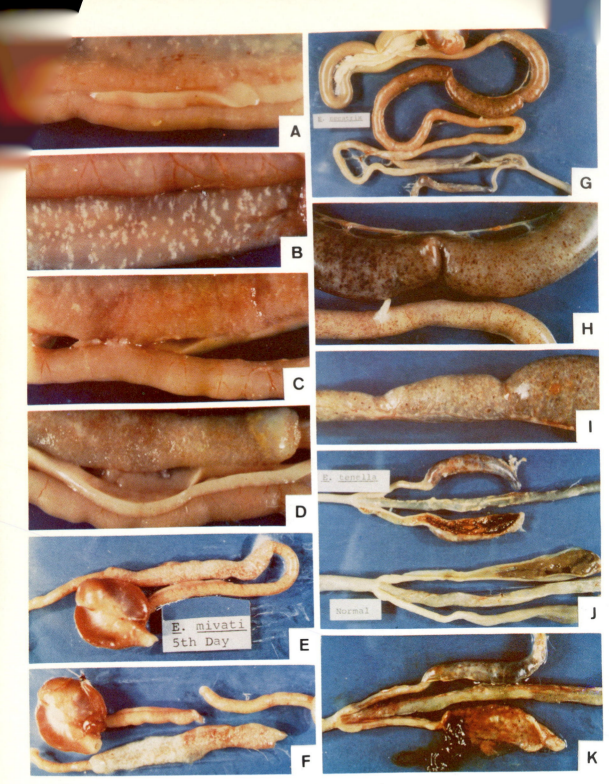

FIG. 31.5—(A to F) Eimeria mivati lesions. **(A)** and **(B)** Light infections (scored +1 and +2); **(C** and **D)** moderate infections (scored +3); **(E)** heavy infection (scored +4); **(F)** shows postmortem changes (see text). **(G to I) E. necatrix. (G)** Ballooning in the midgut region; **(H)** petechiae shown on swollen portion (above) and normal sized intestine (below, 5th day) before yellowish plaques were developed; **(I)** yellowish plaques enclosing islands of schizonts (6th day). **(J and K) E. tenella** with a forming core on the 5th day of infection **(J)** and severe bleeding **(K)**.

color which is distinctive. This characteristic alone may be diagnostic if comparison
is made with other species using similar
light and the same microscope. The walls
of the oocyst occasionally retain a roughened external covering derived from the
parasitized epithelial cell. This characteristic is peculiar to *E. maxima,* and its recognition may assist in species diagnosis.

Pathogenicity

This species should be classed as moderately to severely pathogenic. Mortality has
been reported (Bracket and Bliznick, 1950;
Edgar, 1958a; Pellérdy, 1960; Horton-
Smith, 1960; Supperer, 1961; Reid and
Raja, 1963) following experimental infection. Laying hens in heavy production suffered 50% mortality following artificial
inoculation with 200,000 oocysts each
(Hegde and Reid, 1969). Others have reported less severe pathogenicity (Hunter,
1959; Long, 1959). Morbidity, readily
measured by weight loss in artificial infections, has been demonstrated by all investigators (Scholtyseck, 1959; Park et al.,
1959; Reid and Raja, 1963). In severe cases
there is extreme emaciation; pallor, rough-
ening of feathers, and anorexia occur in
less severe cases. Rapid development of immunity frequently aids in control of *E.
maxima* coccidiosis.

Histopathology

Minimum tissue damage occurs with the
first two asexual cycles which develop superficially in epithelial cells. Not until invasion of deeper tissues on the 5th to 8th
days of the cycle in development of gametocytes does tissue damage become severe. At
this time there is congestion and edema,
marked with subepithelial thickening and
rapid growth in size and number of parasites. Both nucleus and cytoplasm of the
invaded epithelial cells become enormously enlarged and displaced into the subepithelial zone. Microscopic hemorrhages occur near the tips of the villi at this time.
Of the two types of gametocytes, the macrogametocytes are by far the more numerous,
but the microgametocytes are considerably
larger. The latter show a distinctive enlarged nucleus (Scholtyseck, 1956). Few
gross pathological changes are noted from
the serosal surface. Swelling and petechiae
have been noted by Edgar (1959, personal
communication) and confirmed in our lab-

oratory (Fig. 31.4E,G), but they did not
occur in studies by Long (1959). Considerable congestion may occur late in the cycle
(Fig. 31.4F).

The invading gametocyte develops beneath the host cell nucleus. Developing
schizonts usually parasitize the host cell
above the nucleus; rarely are they found
beside the nucleus.

Eimeria mivati Edgar and Seibold 1964

Classification and Morphology

Of the 9 species, *E. mivati* has been the
most recently and most completely described. Undoubtedly the parasite is widely distributed and is new only in name.
Previously it was insufficiently characterized to be recognized as a distinct species.
In earlier studies it has been identified as
"a small strain" of *E. acervulina.* The zone
parasitized may extend from the duodenal
loop to the rectum and ceca. Early lesions
appear in epithelial cells in the anterior
portion of the zone; later the first- and second-generation merozoites infect epithelial
cells in more posterior areas. In light infections individual plaques containing
oocysts appear to be more circular than the
ladder-shaped lesions typical of light *E.
acervulina* infection (Fig. 31.5A to F).
These circular lesions may be seen on either
the serosal or mucosal surface but are rapidly altered by postmortem changes. Thirty
minutes after death, marked congestion
may appear if the gut is exposed to the air
while the unopened portion remains un-
altered (Fig. 31.5F). In heavy infections
petechiae may be either scattered or more
concentrated. The entire surface of the
epithelium may show a coalescing mass of
colonies filled with developing oocysts. Intestinal contents include creamy or white
intestinal materials occasionally streaked
with blood. In the lower intestine the contents may take the form of pellets containing quantities of undigested feed (Cornell
Johnson, 1968, personal communication).

Oocysts are similar to but smaller than
those typical for *E. acervulina,* averaging
2–3μ shorter and 1μ narrower (Table 31.1).
They possess a micropyle, a smooth exterior, a refractile polar granule, and an
oocyst residuum. Peak of oocyst production occurs between the 6th and 7th days
but may continue until the 12th day postinfection. In contrast, peak oocyst produc-

tion of *E. acervulina* is on the 4th and 5th days (Long, 1967c). Minimum sporulation time for *E. mivati* is 12 hours; minimum prepatent period is 93 hours (Edgar and Seibold, 1964). Krassner's (1963) report of a sporulation time of 13 hours for *E. acervulina* probably represented an *E. mivati* infection.

Pathogenicity

Eimeria mivati coccidiosis seldom produces heavy mortality, but occasionally some birds die following heavy artificial inoculations. Experimental infections of 5–10 million oocysts produced only 10% mortality (Edgar and Seibold, 1964). Birds show listlessness, anorexia, ruffled feathers, and watery diarrhea 4 days after infection. Symptoms become more severe on the 5th and 6th days and death occurs on the 6th or 7th day. Signs of recovery with regained appetite begin on the 8th or 9th day but may not be complete until 12–14 days post-infection. Coccidiosis outbreaks occur in both young and adult flocks. Marked reduction in egg production has been reported with poor response to coccidiostat treatment. This species would certainly be rated as pathogenic.

Histopathology

Large numbers of third- and fourth-generation schizonts are the predominant stage present by the 4th day when the first gross lesions are noticed. These schizonts, $9.3 \times 17.3\mu$ in length, are longer than *E. acervulina* (Long, 1967c) but similar in size to those of other intestinal species with the exception of the large schizonts of *E. necatrix*. Eosinophilia, hyperemia, and edema are present in severely affected areas. Most severe lesions occur in the anterior half of the digestive tract where the epithelium sloughs off from the distal half of the villus. Epithelial cells of the posterior small intestine, cecal pouches, and rectum also become invaded. Unlike *E. brunetti* there is no subepithelial invasion of *E. mivati* parasites.

The sporozoites penetrate and develop superficially to the nucleus of the epithelial cell. As many as four generations of schizonts have been recognized.

Eimeria mitis Tyzzer 1929

Classification and Morphology

Although the anterior half of the intestinal tract is the zone parasitized (Table 31.1), gross lesions are not produced by this species (Tyzzer, 1929; Joyner, 1958). The subspherical oocyst is a distinctive characteristic of this species. Except for the presence of a slight tapering at one end, the shape would be called spherical. Several such oocysts should be found before accepting subspherical as characteristic of the infection. The shape index of *E. mitis* (1.01) indicates the almost round (1.0) structure. A polar granule is present but micropyle and oocyst residuum are absent. Minimum sporulation time is 18 hours; minimum prepatent period is 99 hours. Microscopic lesions are seldom found in the posterior intestine or tubular portion of the cecum.

Pathogenicity

Although *E. mitis* was previously regarded as completely nonpathogenic, Joyner (1958) induced some mortality and fairly severe morbidity in young chicks; older birds were resistant. Lack of immunity and repeated reinfection has been reported by Tyzzer (1929). Since no gross lesions are usually detected, coccidiosis is subclinical and pathogenicity would be classed as mild.

Histopathology

Tissue reactions induced by presence of parasites appear to be lacking. Developmental stages have been recognized and drawn (Tyzzer, 1929). By the end of the 4th day, schizonts containing 24–60 merozoites appear scattered among epithelial cells of the villi. Later generations show less regularity in appearance with this than in other species. Uniform distribution of the parasites throughout the epithelium with an absence of colonies is typical of this species. Schizonts, microgametes, and macrogametes may develop superficially or beneath the nuclei of epithelial cells.

Eimeria necatrix Johnson 1930

Classification and Morphology

The midgut near the yolk sac diverticulum is the primary zone parasitized by this species. In severe cases lesions may extend the entire length of the digestive tract. Massive dilation or "ballooning" of the middle intestinal tract suggests the presence of *E. necatrix* coccidiosis (Fig. 31.5G). The intestine may expand to almost twice the normal diameter. However, birds may die due to *E. necatrix* infection in the complete absence of ballooning. Only with *E. maxima* does similar but less extensive swelling occur. Microscopic examination of scrapings from the whitish yellow foci often visible on the serosal surface of the small intestine reveals the distinctive large second-generation schizonts. Scrapings are best secured from the mucosal surface, although they may be so deeply embedded that they will need to be located first on the serosal surface. Presence of pockets of these schizonts (which individually range in size up to 62μ in diameter) is diagnostic for *E. necatrix*. They are easily recognized in smear preparations under low power. Schizonts of other intestinal species do not exceed 31μ in diameter except for those of *E. tenella* which are confined to the cecum. Marked congestion, bleeding, and necrosis occur on the mucosal surface. Intestinal contents may contain much freshly passed or clotted blood and large quantities of mucus, fibrin, and necrotic epithelial tissue. Due to persistent anorexia, little feed is usually present.

Since oocysts of *E. necatrix* develop only in the cecum following the downward movement and establishment of the second-generation merozoites, recovery of oocyst scrapings from the midintestinal wall indicates presence of some other species. *E. necatrix* oocysts develop superficially in scattered areas of the cecal epithelium and show no distinctive characteristics distinguishing them from *E. tenella* oocysts, although they may be slightly smaller and less pointed. They range from 13.2 to 22.7μ in length and 11.3 to 18.3μ in width. They are discharged from the host between the 7th and 18th days. This species produces the fewest oocysts of the 9 species recovered from chickens. Investigators have frequently encountered difficulty in securing sufficient oocysts for experimental studies (Tyzzer et al., 1932; Davies, 1956).

Pathogenesis and Epizootiology

Infected birds show listlessness, drooping wings, humped back, and dehydration; mortality begins on the 5th day, shows greatest severity on the 7th, and extends to the 12th day. *E. necatrix* infection produces higher mortality than any other species except *E. tenella*. In experimental infections, 100% mortality followed inoculation with 100,000 oocysts (Davies, 1956).

Some birds may die before oocysts appear in the feces. Mortality, if present, usually occurs early in the life cycle, but signs of morbidity may continue for a week longer than with most other species. Weight loss becomes apparent on the 6th day and reaches a maximum on the 7th to 9th day. Both young and old birds may suffer attacks which typically occur one or two weeks later than with *E. tenella*.

The term "chronic" has been used to describe *E. necatrix* coccidiosis (Tyzzer et al., 1932). This unfortunate terminology was selected to describe somewhat slower progress of the disease through the flock. Self-limiting immunity requires but little more time to develop with this species than with *E. tenella* infection. The smaller number of oocysts produced contributes to slower spreading in a flock.

The first gross lesions appear 2½–3 days after infection when first-generation merozoites are released. The serosal surface may be bright red and show numerous minute petechiae. Inflammatory cells infiltrate the epithelium and produce an overall thickening of the intestinal wall followed by the pathognomonic appearance of the whitish yellow plaques containing schizonts. Although these schizonts begin to form on the 3rd and 4th days, they are most clearly seen on the 6th day (Fig. 31.5H,I). These colonies formed from second-generation schizonts have developed from released first-generation merozoites.

Histopathology

The numerous parasitized epithelial cells in the second asexual cycle become enormously enlarged, invading and disrupting glandular structures in the subepithelial zone. Necrosis and bleeding occur in the inflammatory congested areas on the 5th and 6th days. These may appear as discrete petechiae or as enlarged coalesced areas. A parasitic granuloma, a focal type reaction, is induced by infection with only this species of coccidia. It appears in the lamina propria and adjacent muscular layers. By the 6th day sloughed epithelium may be replaced by a network of fibrin containing mononuclear cells. If epithelial regeneration is incomplete, scar tissue may invade such areas.

The invasion of the cecal epithelium by second-generation merozoites beginning on the 5th day produces little damage. Most of these parasites produce small third-generation schizonts containing 6–16 merozoites. Both second- and third-generation merozoites may produce gametocytes diffusely scattered in the glands or over the surface of the cecal epithelium.

Parasites produced in the asexual generations are superficial to the nucleus of the epithelial cell; developing gametocytes may occur either above or below the nucleus.

Eimeria praecox Johnson 1930

Classification and Morphology

No gross lesions are produced as the parasite develops in the epithelium of the upper third of the digestive tract. Very mild pathogenicity has been reported (Johnson, 1930; Tyzzer et al., 1932). Intestinal contents sometimes contain mucoid casts. A minimum sporulation time of 12 hours for newly passed oocysts is a characteristic that this species shares with *E. mivati,* according to Edgar and Seibold (1964). The prepatent period of only 84 hours is by far the shortest recorded for any species. Oocyst size is relatively large (av. $21.3 \times 17.1\mu$), being exceeded only by *E. maxima* and *E. brunetti.* Levine (1940) found this species in 13 of 33 examinations of subclinical coccidial infections. Immunity develops promptly after infection.

Pathogenicity

E. praecox has been considered of no economic importance (Tyzzer et al., 1932) since no lesions are found in experimental infections. More recently Edgar (1958, personal communication) has found inclusion of this species necessary in his program of planned immunization to prevent coccidiosis losses. Long (1968a) found no mortality but weight loss and changes in intestinal permeability after heavy artificial infection. *E. praecox* is now regarded as mildly pathogenic, producing subclinical coccidiosis which results in retarded weight gains.

Small pinpoint hemorrhages are seen from the mucosal surface on the 4th and 5th days of infection (Long, 1967b), but no lesions are visible on the serosal surface. Watery intestinal contents appear by the 3rd day; thick mucoid material is evident on the 4th and 5th days.

Histopathology

Although essentially no tissue reaction due to presence of oocysts has been reported (Tyzzer et al., 1932), various parasitic stages of the life cycle continue development and have been described in detail. No wandering cells are found in very heavy infections. The epithelial cells of the sides but not the ends of the villi are most commonly parasitized. Many show multiple infections with two or three parasites per cell. Long (1967b) found three or four asexual generations present. Parasites establish themselves either above or below the nucleus of the epithelial cell.

Eimeria tenella (Railliet and Lucet 1891) Fantham 1909

Classification and Morphology

Cecal or "bloody" coccidiosis is caused by parasitic invasion of the ceca and adjacent areas of the digestive tract of the domestic fowl (Fig. 31.5J,K). Presence of characteristic bleeding from cecal walls on the 5th and 6th days of the cycle or presence of hardened cheesy cores in later stages suggests *E. tenella* infection. Confirmation by demonstration of oocysts or endogenous stages of coccodia is usually required to rule out histomoniasis or presence of blood entering from the small intestine. The most distinctive endogenous stage is the large schizont measuring up to 54μ in diameter. It may be filled with elongated merozoites numbering up to 900 in the first generation and 350 in the second generation. The range of the oocyst (av. $22 \times 19\mu$) overlaps that of other species in both size and shape.

Pathogenicity

Because of the sudden onset of mortality, this species has been most feared by the poultry producer. Flock mortality up to 20% has occurred within a period of 2–3 days. Blood loss from cecal lesions, diarrhea, huddling together of infected birds, and a characteristic odor may be noted shortly before mortality begins. Although birds give the appearance of being chilled, studies by Keener (1963) do not confirm the claim (Herrick, 1950) that a drop in body temperature is typical of early infection. The first sign of morbidity is a refusal to drink and/or eat (Hilbrich, 1963; Reid and Pitois, 1965). Blood loss may be sufficient to cause the bird to bleed to death on the 5th to 7th day (Edgar, 1944). Erythrocyte count and hematocrit values may decrease as much as 50% on the 5th and 6th days of infection and require 8 days to recover to normal ranges (Natt and Herrick, 1955). During the same period, depression in growth rate or weight loss may occur (Joyner and Davies, 1960) with maximum loss on the 7th day postinfection. Weight loss due to dehydration may be rapidly regained during the recovery period, but normal weights are never fully regained during the growing period (S. A. Edgar, 1958, personal communication). Coccidiosis is a self-limiting disease; most birds recover following survival past the 8th day. Birds with gangrenous or ruptured cecal pouches may linger for long periods but never fully recover.

Pathogenesis and Epizootiology

Severity of infection is dependent upon the number of oocysts received at one time. For example, 1–150 oocysts produced no hemorrhage and no mortality; 150–500, slight hemorrhage and no mortality; 1,000–3,000, heavy hemorrhage and light mortality; 3,000–5,000, very heavy hemorrhage and moderate mortality; over 5,000, very heavy hemorrhage and severe mortality (Jankiewicz and Scofield, 1934). Numerous other reports confirm this trend, but the number of oocysts required to produce mortality varies with breed, age, and nutritional status of the chicken and viability of oocysts in the inoculum. Oocysts begin to appear on the 7th day after infection (Reid et al., 1969a), reach a peak of several million per bird on the 8th day, and are reduced in numbers on the 9th and following days. Cessation of oocyst production occurs about the 13th day of infection. Oocysts may be entrapped in the regenerating epithelium or the cecal core, thus delaying their release by weeks or even months.

Histopathology

Pathological changes become progressively more severe (Fig. 31.6) as the parasites proliferate in two or more asexual generations. At the end of the 1st day the only reported histopathological alteration has been the presence of "penetration tubes" in the mucosal layers of the villi as the sporozoites enter and are transported to the epithelial cells lining the gland fundi via macrophages (Patillo, 1959). Small focal areas of denuded epithelium (Bertke, 1955) and focal areas of necrosis in underlying connective tissue are seen after the 2nd day. The first gross changes with some enlargement of the ceca and appearance of small areas of hemorrhage are noted on the 3rd day. Further necrosis of denuded areas occurs separating such areas from the underlying connective tissue. The epithelium may contain sufficient parasitized cells to produce pressure-inducing degeneration of surrounding connective tissues. An evenly distributed increase in eosinophils occurs at this time. Small focal areas of necrosis may appear near blood vessels of the inner circular muscles of the muscularis layer.

By the end of the 4th day the ceca show inflammation over 80% of the distal areas and enlargement to three times normal size (Fig. 31.6d,e). Spotted irregular focal hemorrhagic areas, some large in size, appear on the serosal surface. The lumen is filled with blood and pieces of loosened ulcerated mucosa. Deeper layers contain large areas of congestion while the cecal walls thicken. The connective tissue as well as the muscularis mucosa becomes necrotic; the underlying submucosa is edematous. The submucosa still contains eosinophils while both the mucosa and submucosa show an increase in lymphocytes, monocytes, and plasma cells. Separated bands of muscles become infiltrated with lymphocytes and contain small areas of focal necrosis. By the end of the 5th day most of the mucosa, including the muscularis layer, is destroyed (Fig. 31.6e,f). Edema is present in the submucosa, and large areas of hemorrhage reach the surface through the necrotic mucosa. By the 6th day the lumen contents become hardened and speckled with a grayish core representing clotted blood, mucosal debris, and an increased number of grayish oocysts. At first this core is firmly attached to the mucosa, but later it becomes loosened and is usually expelled by the 8th day. However, it may remain in the cecum for a much longer time.

Regeneration of the epithelium and glands is complete by the 10th day in light infections (Mayhew, 1937). Although the epithelium shows remarkable powers of regeneration, in severe cases surface epithelium between glands may never fully regen-

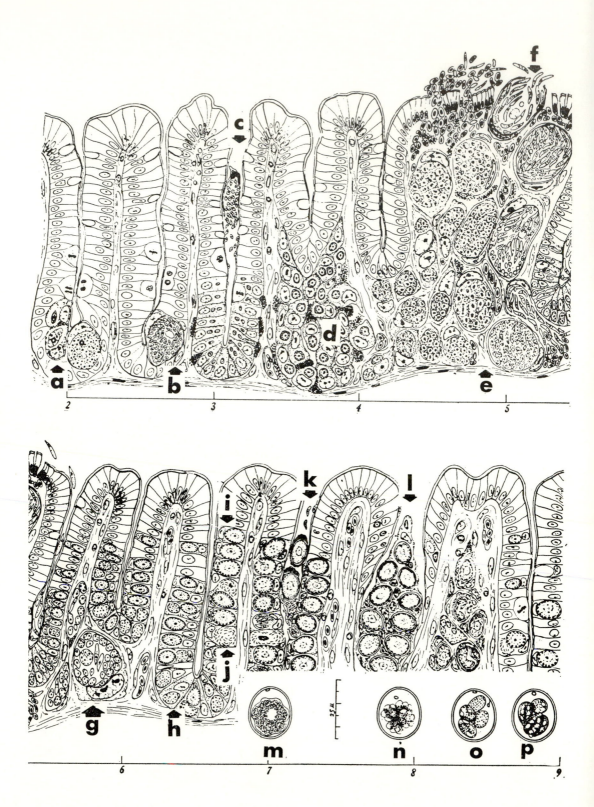

erate. The lost muscularis mucosa is not replaced; the submucosa becomes densely fibrosed. The ceca may remain considerably contracted during this period of recovery. Abnormal renal clearance has been reported (Bertke, 1963). Earlier Bertke (1955) had described necrotic foci on kidneys of infected birds, but he was unable to correlate their appearance with these changes in uric acid clearance.

Both asexual and sexual forms of parasites develop beneath the nuclei of epithelial cells.

EPIZOOTIOLOGY

Natural and Experimental Hosts

The chicken is the only natural host of the 9 described species. Although *E. tenella* has been reported from several species of birds (Levine, 1961; Pellérdy, 1965), these observations must be considered doubtful until confirmed. Following unsuccessful cross-infection trials no other host species is recognized as a carrier of chicken coccidia (Patterson, 1933a; Lund and Farr, 1965).

Day-old chicks are susceptible to coccidiosis (Gordeuk et al., 1951), but outbreaks seldom occur at less than 11 days of age (Edgar and King, 1955; Lund and Farr, 1965). They are more common at 4–6 weeks of age. Partial resistance of newly hatched chicks is due to a carryover of parental immunity (Edgar, 1958a). Increased susceptibility as birds advance in age is most marked with *E. maxima* (Long, 1959) and *E. acervulina* (Krassner, 1963). Nonex-

FIG. 31.6—Developmental stages in cecal epithelium 2–9 days after infection with Eimeria tenella: (a) trophozoite arising from growth of sporozoite; (b) first-generation schizont; (c) first-generation merozoite; (d) second-generation trophozoite; (e) second-generation schizont; (f) second-generation merozoite; (g) retained schizont with failure of merozoites to escape; (h) third-generation schizont; (i) macrogametocyte; (j) microgametocyte; (k) third-generation merozoite; (l) oocysts; (m) oocyst as discharged from intestine; (n) oocyst showing division into 4 sporoblasts; (o) oocyst showing immature spores slightly developed; (p) oocyst with fully developed spores each containing 2 sporozoites. (After Tyzzer, 1929; reproduced with permission of Am. J. Hyg.)

posed adult birds remain highly susceptible to all species (Edgar, 1958a; Hegde and Reid, 1969).

Transmission and Vectors

Ingestion of viable sporulated oocysts is the only natural method of transmission. Artificial methods of transmission using other stages have been demonstrated experimentally (Lund and Farr, 1965; Horton-Smith and Long, 1966). Both diseased and recovered chickens may continue to shed oocysts. It should be recognized, however, that birds stricken with severe coccidiosis may die before oocysts have completed their development.

Man is second only to the chicken as a vector in dissemination of oocysts. Mechanical transmission is commonly accomplished by manure clinging to shoes or by utensils carried about from one pen to another. Hands and clothing may also serve to transmit the single oocyst necessary to start infection cycles. Flies, beetles, cockroaches, rodents, pets, and wild birds have also been incriminated as mechanical vectors (Lund and Farr, 1965).

Oocysts may survive for long periods of time in shaded soil. The maximum period of infectivity was 86 weeks in experimental feeding trials (Farr and Wehr, 1949–1950). Sunlight assists in destruction of oocysts (Patterson, 1933b). Incubator temperatures kill oocysts, so there is no danger of hatchery transmission to baby chicks (Ellis, 1938). Oocysts are so resistant that they survive stringent attempts to kill them. Accidental coccidiosis outbreaks frequently occur following such control measures (Reid and Davis, 1969). Transmission from one pen to another in floor pen trials is to be expected (Reid et al., 1969b). New premises are usually contaminated with all species within the first few weeks of occupancy.

In chickens reared outdoors under range conditions, coccidiosis outbreaks are much more common in the spring and summer months than under cooler fall and winter conditions. Under confinement rearing management, outbreaks may occur at any season of the year. However, there is some evidence of more rapid cycling in spring and summer than in fall and winter (Reid et al., 1968).

That coccidiosis mortality may occur in layers has been known for many years (Johnson, 1932, 1933; Bressler and Gordeuk, 1951; Edgar, 1958a). A decrease in egg production may be expected following coccidiosis from any species of chicken coccidia. Even such mild pathogens as *E. praecox* and *E. mitis* reduce egg production (Johnson, 1932). Edgar (1958b) has reported flocks in 80% production were reduced to a level of 30% following an infection with *E. mitis*. Maximum reduction occurred at the end of the 2nd week following artificial infections with *E. acervulina, E. brunetti, E. maxima, E. mivati,* and *E. tenella* which were severe enough to produce 1–39% mortality (Hegde and Reid, 1969). With *E. necatrix* producing 37% flock mortality, egg production decreased from 80% to zero at the end of the 3rd week. Normal egg production rates were regained in survivors by the end of the 4th week in hens inoculated with all species except *E. necatrix* which required 1–2 weeks longer. Culling rate was not appreciably increased over that shown by unparasitized controls. Prognosis is good for most survivors of uncomplicated coccidiosis outbreaks.

Immunity

Following an outbreak of coccidiosis, birds rapidly develop self-limiting immunity. Resistance may be partial or complete, depending upon the species and number of subsequent reexposures. Graded oral doses of oocysts at weekly intervals (Farr, 1943; Horton-Smith, 1963) induced sufficient immunity to subsequently prevent any infection or oocyst production following challenge. Single severe infections did not confer "solid" immunity but were sufficient to prevent mortality (Waletzky et al., 1949). In many flocks a low level of exposure to all species commonly produces immunity as birds approach maturity (Reid et al., 1968), although the producer may be entirely unaware that any oocysts are present on his premises. This type of protective immunity is relied upon for prevention of coccidiosis in floor-pen managed flocks following coccidiostat withdrawal.

The nature of the immune mechanism which protects against coccidiosis appears to differ from the type demonstrated for viral and bacterial organisms. The major difference is in persistence of localized tissue immunity in the intestine after all evidence of antibodies has disappeared. Serological evidence for the production of a

humoral immune response to coccidiosis has been demonstrated in a number of ways. The classic experiment of Burns and Challey (1959), confirmed by Horton-Smith et al. (1961), has been cited as suggesting a humoral basis for the immunity. One cecum was surgically separated from the digestive tract while the remaining cecum was subjected to an immunizing dose of oocysts. After immunity had been developed from the infection, the isolated cecal epithelium was shown to be resistant following introduction of sporozoites. Serological studies have included agglutination of second-generation schizonts (McDermott and Stauber, 1954), demonstration of precipitins by gel diffusion methods (Rose and Long, 1962; Leathem, 1965), and immobilization of sporozoites and merozoites by use of serum from hyperimmunized birds (Herlich, 1965). However, these antibodies do not appear to be the primary mechanism furnishing protection. In most cases the host showed strong resistance to challenge after evidence of these circulating antibodies had disappeared. Furthermore, all attempts to demonstrate passive transfer of immunity to a normal host have failed (Bachman, 1930; Becker et al., 1932, 1935; Herlich, 1961; Pierce et al., 1963). At the present time no satisfactory answer can be given to the nature of the immune mechanism in coccidiosis.

DURATION. Protective immunity developed under conditions of field-flock management is usually of long duration. Sufficient sporulated oocysts are usually present to permit recycling and reinforcement if immunity levels begin to drop. Furthermore, oocysts may continue to appear in droppings for as long as 7½ months after the initial infection (Herrick et al., 1936). Oocysts from such a source would also make recycling possible.

Investigators have disagreed on the duration of immunity if reinfection is completely prevented. This question takes on practical importance if flocks must be moved to a new location or if temperature extremes (hot or cold) destroy all viable oocysts in the area. Unusual precautions to prevent accidental reinfection are required in experimental tests on duration of immunity. Evidence of decreased immunity 10 weeks after initial immunization with *E. maxima* was reported from studies on a limited number of birds by Long (1962). A similar decrease in immunity level was reported following three graded artificial inoculations with *E. mivati* (Reid and Keener, 1962). Using oocyst counts as well as clinical symptoms following immunization and challenge with *E. tenella,* Leathem and Burns (1968) concluded that symptoms reappeared in birds which had been solidly immune between 42 and 63 days after immunization. They concluded, however, that there was sufficient immunity to protect against mortality for at least 105 days. Immunity was never strong enough to preclude tissue invasion in reinfection experiments. Protection for 6 months against mortality followed three graded inoculations of *E. tenella* (Farr, 1943). Complete resistance to infection for 3 months was reported (Horton-Smith, 1963) under conditions which prevented reinfection.

The most thorough investigation of the duration of immunity has been made by Edgar (1968, personal communication). Using early exposure he found sufficient immunity to protect against economic losses for 6, 12, or 18 months. The planned immunization program (Edgar, 1959) was followed by 12 weeks exposure in floor pens. Afterwards the birds were isolated in cages until time for testing by challenge.

There is experimental evidence that Marek's disease may reduce resistance to coccidiosis by interference with coccidial immunity (Edgar et al., 1968; Biggs et al., 1969). This phenomenon is probably the reason for frequent assertions by poultrymen that there is an interrelationship between coccidiosis and Marek's disease. In an extensive series of experimental trials Brewer et al. (1967, 1968) were unable to demonstrate oocyst transmission of Marek's disease or that coccidiosis induced more severe Marek's disease losses. Similar findings were reported by Long et al. (1968). It seems probable that Marek's disease increases the coccidiosis problems rather than the converse which has usually been the interpretation from field observations.

The flock prognosis with a combination of both coccidiosis and Marek's disease is very poor. The coccidiosis does not respond to either preventive or curative chemotherapy in a normal way. The owner may unsuccessfully shift from one coccidiostat to another without getting a response because normal self-limiting immunity fails to establish itself. Marek's mortality, which may be unusually severe in such cases, may rise to severe proportions. Poultry producers have reported a sharp decrease in this type of flock problem since the turkey herpesvirus vaccine has become widely used by the industry.

Most investigators have accepted the idea that immunity produced by each species is highly specific and that no cross-immunity occurs between species. Each describer of the 9 recognized species (Tyzzer, 1929; Johnson, 1930; Levine, 1938, 1942; Edgar and Seibold, 1964) has demonstrated by appropriate challenge experiments the absence of any cross-immunity as a species characteristic. Rose (1965, 1967), however, has reported evidence of *E. tenella-E. necatrix* and *E. maxima-E. brunetti* cross-immunity. More extensive investigations using single oocyst isolated subcultures will be required to confirm her hypothesis that cross-immunity may interfere with interpreting the geographical studies on species distribution which have been based on the immunity challenge technique (Edgar, 1958a; Reid et al., 1968).

DIAGNOSIS

The poultry diagnostician faces a difficult task in accurate diagnosis of coccidiosis. Four complications increase his difficulties:

1. There are 9 different species producing different types of lesions in different areas. Although 3 species (*E. hagani, E. mitis,* and *E. praecox*) may usually be disregarded, 6 should be diagnosed as to species.

2. The gross lesions change in appearance as infection progresses during the life cycle.

3. The status of different birds in a flock may vary with progress of the disease—some showing acute lesions, some being in a recovery phase, and others remaining unexposed; however, diagnosis and recommendations are required on a total flock basis.

4. Distinction must be made between true clinical coccidiosis requiring treatment and mild subclinical coccidiasis characterized by presence of a few lesions or a few oocysts. Coccidiasis is more common than coccidiosis (Reid and Johnson, 1970). Some diagnosticians record coccidiosis for every accession after finding any parasitic stage. Thus the seriousness of

coccidiosis may be overemphasized in reports from diagnostic laboratories.

Although an experienced diagnostician may attempt a presumptive diagnosis after examining gross lesions in the field, he will want confirmatory microscopic examination of the parasites—a procedure best conducted in the laboratory. Both types of observations are desirable (Edgar, 1959; Reid, 1968). Postmortem changes rapidly obscure lesions useful with some species so that characteristics available on freshly killed specimens may be missing in birds dead for 2–3 hours. Thus transportation of live birds to the laboratory is a necessary procedure.

Examination for Gross Lesions

The entire length of the external surface of the digestive tract from the gizzard to the lower rectum needs to be examined under strong light. This requires freeing the intestine from its mesentery throughout the entire length. Note that *E. acervulina* and *E. mivati* most frequently produce lesions in the duodenal loop (Table 31.1), *E. maxima* and *E. necatrix* in the midgut, and *E. brunetti* in the lower intestine between the ceca and in the rectum. Although *E. tenella* usually appears in the cecum, it may extend into the adjacent intestine or rectum. In examining the serosal surface a search should be made for whitish plaques or petechiae. Whitish streaks or rounded colonies of oocysts in the duodenal area often indicate *E. acervulina* or *E. mivati*. In the midgut area on both sides of the yolk sac diverticulum, whitish plaques may be produced by colonies of *E. necatrix* schizonts.

The intestine needs to be opened in 5 or 6 areas or throughout its entire length with an enterotome. While cutting, examination should be made for thickened areas indicating parasitic invasion of the mucosa or submucosa. Presence of mucus, blood, casts, or cores (which may be either whitish, red, or brown) and presence of cheesy coagulation necrosis should be noted. Examine the appearance of the fecal material as the two ceca are opened, watching for blood, mucus, clots, or cecal cores. Presence of blood in this area suggests a diagnosis of *E. tenella* but may originate from bleeding in more anterior zones of the intestinal tract. Bleeding induced by *E. necatrix* infection in the midintestine produces blood which later appears in the cecum and has led to a misdiagnosis of *E. tenella* infection. Histomoniasis may also produce somewhat similar gross lesions.

Microscopic Examinations

Parasitic stages demonstrated in fresh smear preparations are usually adequate in confirming a diagnosis. Make superficial scrapings of the mucosa using a scalpel. Mount the material on a glass slide and dilute with an equal quantity of saline. Mix with a toothpick and cover with a coverglass. Preparations should be made from several different areas of the intestine, selecting whitish plaques or other lesions for samples. Examine with the 10X and/or 43X objective, looking for oocysts, schizonts, merozoites, macrogametocytes, or microgametocytes. If no suspicious lesions have been noted, select scrapings from (1) the duodenal loop below the entrance of the bile duct, (2) the midgut region near the yolk sac diverticulum, (3) the lower intestinal area just above the union of the cecal pouches, and (4) an area from the middle of the cecum.

Oocysts are the most commonly recognized stage of the life cycle and may be present in large numbers. However, because they develop late in the cycle they may be entirely missing in the presence of severe coccidiosis. Other stages, if found, may be more useful in diagnosis. Presence of distinctive schizonts of *E. necatrix* from the midgut area is pathognomonic for this species. Only *E. tenella* schizonts in the ceca approach those of *E. necatrix* in size, while schizonts of other species do not exceed 30μ in diameter.

Oocyst size and shape are less useful as diagnostic characteristics in chickens than in many other animals. The size ranges overlap and shapes are similar with all species but *E. maxima*. With other species, measurements of a number of oocysts (10 suggested) using an ocular micrometer is required. Full length and width must be determined from a side and not an end view of the oocyst. Thick fecal smears frequently prevent securing the necessary side view of the oocyst. Average length, average width, range in length, and range in width should be determined. Recording length and width measurements in two separate columns hastens calculation of mean and range measurements.

With some species a confirmed diagnosis may be possible after identification of a single distinctive characteristic. More often only a presumptive diagnosis is possible after finding two or more characteristics.

Confirmed Diagnostic Procedures

Studies on the minimum time required for sporulation and the prepatent period may be desirable for confirmed species identification. *E. praecox* may be isolated from a mixed suspension after experimental feeding and recovery of the first oocysts passed, since this species has the shortest prepatent period. The rapid sporulation of *E. mivati* may be useful in separating it from some other species. For such studies oocysts should be aerated in 2.5% potassium dichromate solution at the optimum temperature for sporulation (29° C ± 1) (Edgar, 1955); 2–5 g of fecal material may be satisfactorily sporulated in a petri dish. The material needs to be mixed thoroughly and spread in a thin layer over the surface of the dish. Depth of the suspension should not exceed 1–2 mm, thus permitting adequate oxygen exchange. Aeration of large numbers of oocysts requires a larger volume of fluid. Exposure to bubbling air using a compressed air source or an aquarium aerator produces more uniform sporulation. Use of centrifugation or of strong saline solutions to concentrate oocysts should be avoided to prevent damage to oocysts. Sporulated oocysts, cleaned from fecal debris, may survive for several months if stored in potassium dischromate at 10° C. During transportation, less than half of the bottle should contain liquid.

Critical studies in species identification may require cross-immunity tests using pure suspensions previously derived from single oocyst inoculation (Tyzzer, 1929; Jones, 1932). Stained tissue sections may be useful in demonstrating some of the distinctive endogenous stages of the parasite. In a few cases the location of the parasite in relation to the host cell nucleus may furnish a useful diagnostic characteristic (listed as the final paragraph under the description of each species). Long (1966) has suggested other tissue culture or egg-embryo developmental differences which may prove useful in identification of some species.

TREATMENT

Following discovery of anticoccidial activity of the sulfa drugs (Levine, 1939), attention was directed toward treatment of coccidiosis. The limitations of this approach soon became apparent, as users found that medication was frequently started too late in the life cycle to be effective. Anticoccidial agents (popularly termed coccidiostats) show activity so early in the life cycle that few benefits are derived from treatment after symptoms appear (Fig. 31.3). For this reason the preventive approach for use of drugs has largely superseded the treatment approach. However, producers may find occasional conditions where treatment is beneficial. Treatment with some drugs as late as 96 hours postinfection may sometimes be effective in reducing mortality (Gill et al., 1963; Horton-Smith and Long, 1965).

In evaluating the benefits from treatment, the self-limiting nature of the disease needs to be borne in mind. Many treated flocks would have recovered spontaneously equally as rapidly had no drug been used. Setting aside a group of untreated controls for comparison would offer a much fairer test than placing the entire flock on drug treatment. Such a disease-drug relationship offers real advantages to the unscrupulous drug salesman since his product will look good even if it has no efficacy!

If treatment is to be useful, it must be started promptly. Early recognition of the disease may permit initiation of treatment before all birds have picked up massive doses of oocysts. A few hours delay may be costly, and delay of a full day may render treatment useless. Cautious producers frequently stock a supply of the drug of choice for emergencies. Progress of the disease through the flock needs to be observed and considered. In some situations spreading of oocysts from one end of the house to another may be slow, since individual birds move in very limited areas of a large house.

Many different coccidiostats have been cleared for treatment (Table 31.2). Since numerous precautions and restrictions are required, all directions issued by the manufacturer need to be carefully followed.

TABLE 31.2 ❧ Anticoccidial Drugs Used for Chickens

Coccidiostat (empirical or trade name and manufacturer)	Feed or Water	Active Ingredient: Treatment Duration	First Commerical Use	First Report of Efficacy
Sulfaguanidine American Cyanamid	Feed	1%:2 days on, 4 off, 1 on, 4 off, 1 on; or continuous 3–4 days	1942	Levine, 1941
3-Nitro (sulfanitran) Salsbury Laboratories	Water	0.0076%:up to 10 days; repeat when necessary	1945	Morehouse and Mayfield, 1944
Sulfamethazine American Cyanamid	Water	1%:2 days, 0.5%: 4 days	1947	Horton-Smith and Taylor, 1942
Sulfa Veterinary (4,4'-diaminodiphenyl-sulfone + N' phenyl-sulfanilamide) Salsbury Laboratories	Feed	0.02% diphenylsulfone + 0.1% sulfanilamide:2 days on, 3–4 off; repeat if necessary	1947	Steward, 1947
SQ (sulfaquinoxaline) Merck	Feed	0.1%:2–3 days on, 3 off followed by 0.05%:2 on, 3 off, 2 on	1948	Delaplane et al., 1947
	Water	0.04%:2 days on, 3 off, 2 on		
Sufamerazine American Cyanamid	Feed	0.4–0.5%:2 days 0.2–0.25%:4 days	1948	Swales, 1944
nfz (nitrofurazone) Hess & Clark	Feed	0.11%:5 days	1948	Harwood et al., 1947
nfz soluble (nitrofura-zone) Hess & Clark	Water	0.0082%:5 days	1956	Shumard, 1956
Whitsyn-S (2,4-dia-mino-5-[p-chlorophen-yl]-6-ethyl-pyrimidine + sulfa-quinoxaline) Whitmoyer Laboratories	Water	0.0015%:pyrimidine compound + 0.005% sulfa-quinoxaline: 2–3 days on, 3 off, 2 on	1957	Lux, 1954
Aureomycin (chlortetracycline) American Cyanamid	Feed	0.022% + 0.4–0.55% calcium: not more than 5 days	1960	Seeger et al., 1950
Terramycin (oxytetracycline) Chas Pfizer & Co.	Feed	0.02% + 0.18–0.55% calcium: not more than 5 days	1960	Ball, 1959
Amprol (amprolium) Merck	Water	0.012–0.024%: 3–5 days 0.006%: 1–2 weeks	1960	Cuckler et al., 1960
Esb₃ (sodium sulfa-chloropyrazine mono-hydrate) Gland-O-Lac Co.	Water	0.03%: 3 days	1967	Gabriel et al., 1965
Agribon (sulfadimeth-oxine) Hoffman LaRoche	Water	0.05%: 6 days	1968	Mitrovic and Bauernfeind, 1967

Water vs. Feed Medication

Water has generally been selected as the preferred method of administering coccidiostats for treatment. Medication is more easily dispensed using water barrels or medication proportioners than in feed if mechanical feeders are being used. Water has sometimes been selected as the method of medication because of an often-quoted misstatement: "Ill birds will continue to drink water, but they will not eat in the late stages of the disease" (Jones, 1959). Water consumption is sharply curtailed at the same time that feed consumption is decreased (Hilbrich, 1960). In confirming this finding using 6 different species, it was shown that there is seldom any difference in quantity of drug intake between the two methods (Reid and Pitois, 1965). This fallacious statement needs to be corrected for another reason. A sudden decrease in either water or feed consumption may be the useful first sign of a coccidiosis outbreak.

Preventive Coccidiostats

Before 1936 poultry producers had little assistance from chemotherapy in controlling devastating outbreaks of coccidiosis. Herrick and Holmes (1936) reported that sulfur markedly reduced mortality from *E. tenella* when fed at 1.5% or higher in the diet. Although this product was too toxic for general use, its discovery helped arouse interest in the sulfonamides which were found efficacious against coccidia 3 years later. Levine (1939) described the suppressive action of sulfanilamide against 6 intestinal species but found it ineffective on the more pathogenic *E. tenella* and *E. necatrix*. Subsequently 9 or more different sulfa drugs have been found to show variable activity against pathogenic species. Of the older drugs only sulfaquinoxaline, sulfamethazine (sulfadimidine, sulfamezathine), and sulfanitran are currently being used. The major disadvantage to their use is that high levels for extended periods may result in development of the hemorrhagic syndrome (Davies et al., 1963). Since all commonly used coccidiostats are active in blocking asexual stages of the parasite (Fig. 31.3), it was soon realized that these drugs would be more useful in prevention than in treatment. Such use calls for continuous medication. Inclusion of the coccidiostat in the feed provides the most convenient method of administration, and adoption of this practice brought about a revolution in the feed manufacturing industry. This industry has been forced to assume responsibility for selection, mixing, withdrawal, and investigation of "breaks" on coccidiostats. This program is usually executed by a staff of professional animal health consultants and by service personnel who make regular calls on flock owners.

Some anticoccidials require a 5-day withdrawal before birds are marketed. These regulations should be strictly complied with by poultrymen lest drug levels in excess of tolerance levels occur in meat. Such levels have been established for all anticoccidials.

Problems associated with accidental coccidiostat contamination of layer flock feeds led to requests from feed manufacturers for improvement in coccidiostat manufacturing. Desirable characteristics of potential new coccidiostats presented to the American Feed Manufacturers Association (Edgar, 1958b) are that they: (1) suppress development of the most important species of coccidia, preventing death and morbidity. This should have been demonstrated for at least 3 or 4 chicken coccidia and at least 2 species for control of turkey coccidiosis; (2) be palatable and nontoxic; (3) improve feed conversion of infected birds; (4) not impair growth; (5) be compatible with other common feed additives; (6) not affect feathering; (7) not cause excitability; (8) not harm reproductive organs, production, or hatchability; (9) be readily eliminated by birds and not stored in tissues beyond acceptable limits; (10) not be harmful to other animals or man; (11) be easily mixed with feed; (12) be stable in the processing and storage of feed; (13) not be hydroscopic; (14) not be electrostatic; (15) be subject to accurate and simple analysis in feeds and tissues; (16) possess plus factors (e.g. activity against other infections, possibly bacteria, fungi, and helminths); (17) should have been cleared by the Food and Drug Administration.

To this list other desirable characteristics could be added (Reid, 1961): that they (18) be low in cost ($1/ton of feed suggested); (19) not be toxic to birds of any age; (20) have no flavor or odor; (21) the carrier be registered (thus simplifying governmental approvals); (22) not interfere with development of immunity under field conditions if recommended for replacement flocks. This last point emphasizes the need for immunity after drug withdrawal in replacement flocks where coccidiostats may have decreased oocyst exposure preventing immunity (Reid, et al., 1968).

Intensive screening programs have produced a succession of coccidiostats. Early drugs (Table 31.3) primarily selected for control of *E. tenella* and *E. necatrix* appear to have reduced the incidence of coccidiosis due to these species (Long, 1964; Reid and Murphy, 1966). However, other species such as *E. maxima*, *E. brunetti*, *E. acervulina*, and *E. mivati* have been more frequently reported in recent years. Search for wide-spectrum anticoccidial drugs to

TABLE 31.3 ❧ Preventive Coccidiostats Used in Feed Formulation

Common or Chemical Name and Most Frequently Used Level in Feed	Trade Name	First Commercial Use	First Report of Efficacy
Sulfaquinoxaline (0.0125%)	SQ, Sulquin	1948	Delaplane et al., 1947
Nitrofurazone (0.0056%)	nfz	1948	Harwood et al., 1947
Nitrophenide (0.0125%)	Megasul	1949	Waletzky et al., 1949
Sulfanitran (0.003%) + roxarsone (0.005%)	Nitrosal	1953	Morehouse and Mayfield, 1948
Arsenobenzene (0.002%)	Arzene	1953	
Butynorate (0.02%) + sulfanitran (0.003%) + dinsed (0.02%) and roxarsone (0.005%)	Polystat-3	1954	Zbornik et al., 1955
Nicarbazin (0.0125%)	Nicarb	1955	Barber, 1955
Nitrofurazone (0.0056%) + furazolidone (0.00083%)	Bifuran	1956	Harwood et al., 1956
Bithionol (0.05%) + methiotriazamine (0.01%)	Trithiadol	1957	Coulston and Dennis, 1958
2,4-diamino-5-(p-chlorophenyl)-6-ethyl-pyrimidine + sulfaquinoxaline (0.005%)	Whitsyn-10	1955	Lux, 1954
	Bifuran	1956	Harwood et al., 1956
Furazolidone (0.0055%)	nf-180	1957	Harwood and Stunz, 1954
Glycarbylamide (0.003%)	Glycamide	1958	Cuckler et al., 1958
Nitromide (0.025%) + sulfanitran (0.03%) + roxarsone (0.005%)	Unistat-3	1958	Morehouse and McGuire, 1957
Oxytetracycline (0.02%)	Terramycin	1959	Ball, 1959
Amprolium (0.0125%)	Amprol	1960	Cuckler et al., 1960
Chlortetracycline (0.02%)	Aureomycin	1960	Peterson, 1958
Zoalene (0.0125%)	Zoamix	1960	Hymas and Stevenson, 1960
Amprolium (0.0125%) + ethopabate (0.0004%)	Amprol Plus	1963	Clark, 1964
Nihydrazone (0.011%)	Nidrafur	1963	Morrison et al., 1961
Aklomide (0.025%) + sulfanitran (0.020%)	Novastat, Aclan	1965	Baron et al., 1963
Buquinolate (0.00825%)	Bonaid	1967	Spencer et al., 1966
Clopidol = meticlorpindol (0.0125%)	Coyden	1968	Stock et al., 1967
Decoquinate (0.003%)	Deccox	1970	Ball et al., 1968
Monensin (0.0121%)	Coban	1971	Shumard and Callender, 1967

control other species has lead to use of combinations of two (Bifuran, Trithiadol, Amprol Plus), three (Unistat-3, Novastat), and even four drugs (Polystat) combined as a single coccidiostat. Recently discovered drugs, buquinolate (Spencer et al., 1966), clopidol (clopindol or meticlorpindol) (Stock et al., 1967), and decoquinate (Ball et al., 1968) have shown a wide spectrum of activity against all species of chicken coccidia. These newer drugs have been shown to be more truly coccidiostatic while other drugs such as nicarbazin are coccidiocidal (Reid et al., 1969a).

Drug Resistance

Low levels of coccidiostats used for economic reasons and to permit immunity development provide ideal conditions for development of drug resistance. A field strain of *E. tenella* was isolated in 1954 (Waletzky et al., 1954) which was resistant to sulfaquinoxaline and sulfamethazine.

Two months later Cuckler and Malanga (1955) reported that 17 of 40 field strains were resistant to sulfaquinoxaline, nitrofurazone, or nitrophenide. Although they found no resistance to nicarbazin, Horton-Smith (1958) found this drug to develop partial resistance on the 16th passage under laboratory conditions of exposure with the coccidiostat at use level.

Coccidiostatic drugs vary in the number of generations of exposure to coccidial strains before developing drug resistance (McLoughlin and Gardiner, 1961a, 1962; Gardiner and McLoughlin, 1963a,b). The coccidiostat glycarbylamide developed resistant strains in 9 passages (McLoughlin and Gardiner, 1961b). However, its failure to satisfactorily perform may have been due to resistant strains already present in the field before it was introduced into commercial use. It had shown great promise when tested against several species and laboratory strains (Cuckler et al., 1958; Horton-Smith and Long, 1959). It is generally agreed that anticoccidials, as in the case of antimalarial and trypanocidal compounds, vary greatly as to length of use before resistance is produced (Bishop, 1959). Lack of better criteria for evaluation of drug sensitivity has led to a laboratory exposure program counting the number of generations which have withstood low-level exposure without developing resistance. Some reliance has been placed on 12, 15, or 22 passages. Other methods of predicting field performance would be highly desirable.

Some large-scale producers, becoming overly alarmed at supposed increases in drug resistance, have resorted to frequent "switching" from one coccidiostat to another. In some cases three different coccidiostats have been used within a period of 8 weeks on a single flock of birds. In most cases the disease problem will have run its course before a change in mixed feed can be accomplished. Other flock problems such as those resulting from a change to Unistat in cold weather or nicarbazin in hot weather may be more serious than any improvements resulting from changes. Increases to higher levels than those recommended by manufacturers (Snoeyenbos, 1955) likewise seem unjustified. Cross-resistance between drugs appears to be the exception rather than the rule. Cross-resistance has been reported between gly-carbylamide and nitrofurazone and between zoalene and nitrofurazone (Mc-Loughlin and Gardiner, 1961a, 1962) but was absent with five other coccidiostats. At the time new drugs are discovered little may be known about the metabolic pathways arrested by anticoccidial action, so the chemical nature of drug activity is of little help in prediction of cross-resistance patterns. Physiological studies on individual coccidiostats may eventually assist in interpretation of cross-resistance phenomena.

The intensive screening programs of pharmaceutical companies has continued to make other coccidiostats available to replace ones which have become less effective. Fortunately for the poultry industry, development of a few resistant strains does not immediately nullify usefulness of an otherwise successful product. The new strain is no more dangerous than the original strain for which the drug was de-veloped. The feed manufacturer will find a review of feed efficiency performance a better index of drug usefulness than demonstration of a few lesions or quick forays into the field to make necropsies with competitive sales teams.

Disinfection and Sanitation

Oocysts are extremely resistant to many of the chemical agents used for disinfectant purposes, including 5% formalin, 5% copper sulfate, 10% sulfuric acid (Perard, 1925), 5% potassium hydroxide, 5% potassium iodide (Horton-Smith et al., 1940), and peracetic acid (Doll et al., 1963). Potassium dichromate (2.5%) is the most frequently used solution for preservation. Some phenolic and chlorinated phenolic compounds have anticoccidial activity (Harry, 1967). Formaldehyde fumigation is ineffective, but ammonia gas (Horton-Smith et al., 1940) and methyl bromide (Andrews et al., 1943; Boney, 1948; Clapham, 1950) will kill oocysts under laboratory or poultry house conditions. The problems in application, which include tight sealing of the house and high costs of the gas, have precluded extensive use of these methods.

In experiments where special coccidiosis studies are planned, complete sterilization of the premises from oocyst contamination may be required. Tight closure of the space and heat introduced from a stream jenny may furnish the most practical method. A temperature of 65° C maintained for 15 minutes is usually sufficient to kill viable oocysts. Although a blow-torch will kill oocysts, the time and effort involved makes this method impractical (Horton-Smith and Taylor, 1939).

Under poultry house conditions the benefits to be derived from oocyst elimination using the eradication approach to coccidiosis are highly questionable, since birds reared in complete isolation remain susceptible and may be subjected to severe outbreaks unless permitted to develop immunity by low-level infection (Dorn and Sommerer, 1961). Some of the most severe coccidiosis outbreaks recorded have followed use of extensive sanitary measures taken in control of other disease problems (Reid and Davis, 1969). Coccidiosis frequently occurs in new houses where birds have never been raised before.

The importance of removing droppings

or litter in coccidiosis control seems to have been overemphasized in many poultry health recommendations (Bryant, 1956; Levine, 1961; Pellérdy, 1965; Biester and Schwarte, 1965). Hart et al. (1949) showed some improvement in production records with weekly litter changes but concluded this practice would be impractical in terms of labor and litter costs. In large-scale broiler operations a change of litter while birds are in the house is entirely impractical. Even a change between broods is difficult because of the costs of labor and litter. Litter change to reduce oocyst levels is seldom sufficient reason for recommending such a practice. Although desirable for control of other diseases, changing of boots between farms is not successful in preventing the dissemination of coccidia.

The one recommendation under "sanitation" which requires repeated emphasis with practical poultrymen is the prevention of damp areas in houses. Leaking roofs or waterers frequently precede coccidiosis by 1–2 weeks.

Dietary Control

It has long been known that vitamin K supplementation may drastically reduce mortality due to cecal coccidiosis (Baldwin et al., 1941). More recently the minimum requirements of this vitamin, preferably in the form of menadione sodium bisulfite, have been extensively studied (Harms and Tugwell, 1956; Tugwell et al., 1957; Otto et al., 1958). The marked improvement following supplementation of deficient diets in birds hemorrhaging with coccidiosis has been almost as dramatic as using a coccidiostat. Reduction of blood clotting time prevents serious hemorrhaging. Needs for this vitamin are highest in young chicks or in breeder hens which may produce baby chicks with prolonged clotting time. Although the vitamin is usually present in such feed ingredients as alfalfa and fish meal, increased amounts may be required following sulfa medication. Routine dietary supplementation with menadione sodium bisulfite at the level of 2 g/ton of feed has been recommended (Nelson and Norris, 1957). Other nutritionists recommend twice or half this level of supplementation.

General agreement has not been reached on the effects of high-level (3–7 times NRC recommended levels) vitamin A supplementation on coccidiosis. Successful reports most frequently have been in the presence of hypovitaminosis A (Murphy et al., 1938; Taylor and Russell, 1947; Erasmus et al., 1960; Gerriets, 1961). Supplementation failed to reduce coccidiosis mortality and morbidity in birds fed practical rations containing normal levels of vitamin A (Waldroup et al., 1963; Malik, 1967). There is more general agreement that vitamin A supplementation may hasten recovery following coccidiosis outbreaks.

Protein levels reduced to 5 and 10% of the ration produced less cecal coccidiosis mortality than did the 15% level (Britton et al., 1964). This well-conducted experimental study presents something of an unexplained paradox, since it had previously been assumed that any improvement of the nutritional status of the host increased resistance to parasitism.

Planned Immunization

It has long been known (Johnson, 1927; Tyzzer, 1929; Farr, 1943) that protective flock immunity is readily developed under field conditions. Many producers appear to be unaware of their dependence on this accidentally acquired immunity, which may develop with no evidence of disease but eventually becomes strong enough to forestall coccidiosis losses in the majority of their flocks. Several experimental approaches have been used in attempts to induce flock immunity. Use of oocysts attenuated by heat (Jankiewicz and Scofield, 1934; Uricchio, 1953), freezing, or x-ray (Waxler, 1941; Hein, 1963) has been attempted. All of these investigations appear to lack evidence that the treatment accomplished more than killing a portion of the treated oocysts. Nor did these workers attempt to save less virulent attenuated strains from survivors of the treatment for future immunization trials. Methods thus far described require very large numbers of oocysts, do not preclude use of live oocysts, and appear to provide little promise for practical field applications. A single heavy inoculation followed by prompt treatment (Dickinson et al., 1951; Babcock and Dickinson, 1954) has been used for extensive field trials on the west coast of the United States. Among the practical difficulties of this method are the large number of oocysts required and the problems of providing very strict supervision for administering both inoculum and medication.

The most extensively used program of planned immunization has been developed by Edgar and his colleagues (Edgar and King, 1952, 1955; Edgar, 1958a, 1964). In this method very small numbers of oocysts of 4–8 species are administered in the feed or drinking water during the 1st week of age. Success of the program is dependent on the coccidia becoming established and producing daughter oocysts followed by two or more generations of cycling. Each subsequent release of oocysts reinforces immunity induced by the first exposure. Spot treatment with a coccidiostat was originally recommended on the 13th day following administration. Later, continuous use of a preventive coccidiostat was substituted in the recommended procedure. Failures due to action of the coccidiostat in blocking necessary cycling of the coccidia has resulted in revised recommendations in which no coccidiostat is used (Vezey, 1966). Inspection of the litter is required during the 2nd and 3rd weeks to make certain that moisture conditions are satisfactory to permit oocyst sporulation. Freezing or overheating of suspensions during storage or in shipment has sometimes killed the oocysts and resulted in failures.

Undue fear of this program appears to stem from the following misunderstandings on the nature of this disease problem:

1. It is not generally recognized that the described species of coccidia are universally distributed throughout the world. Absence of documented clinical cases has sometimes led observers to the conclusion that species previously absent are being introduced with the product. However, a growing body of evidence indicates that all important species are uniformly present throughout the world.

2. Coccidiosis differs from viral and bacterial diseases in that multiplication powers of the organisms are definitely limited within a given host. Thus virulence may be controlled by the number of oocysts administered at one time. One oocyst fed to a bird in an experimental feeding produces so few daughter oocysts that the investigator may fail to recover them without an extensive search. Not until reinfection and completion of the second or more fre-

quently the third successive life cycle can the number of oocysts build up to harmful levels. The planned immunization procedure makes maximum use of the natural immunization method using low-level exposure followed by reinfection with increasingly large numbers of oocysts in successive cycles.

The biggest problem with the controlled exposure method has come from failure to secure adequate immunity for all species. Close supervision of every step of the program is required. Use of potent coccidiostats has sometimes prevented either natural or planned immunization from taking place. Even though the coccidiostat does not directly interfere with development of immunity (Cuckler and Malanga, 1956), it may decrease oocyst multiplication and result in reduced opportunities for development of natural immunity under field conditions.

In planning a program for replacement flocks, the producer must choose between use of continuous medication throughout the life of the bird or a program which permits development of immunity. In the latter case reducing the level and discontinuing the use of the coccidiostat as soon as possible is more likely to permit immunity to develop (Reid et al., 1968). Coccidiostats permitting some oocyst production are preferable to others that permit none. Such a program must accept some risk of insufficient coccidiostat protection during the growing period. Recent governmental clearance has made the use of such a program legal in the United States with amprolium (0.0125%), but widespread adoption has not occurred because of costs.

Genetic Resistance

Genetic resistance to coccidiosis has been thoroughly established by a number of investigations (Rosenberg et al., 1948, 1954; Champion, 1954; Millen et al., 1959). Several of these investigators have successfully separated moderately resistant and highly susceptible strains from a singe stock strain. These studies indicate that multiple alleles are probably involved with no simple dominance of hereditary transmission. Sex-linkage, cytoplasmic inheritance, and passive immunity transfer are not involved. This multiple allele hypothesis would account for differences between breeds (Long,

1968b) and differences in susceptibility to different species of coccidia (Rosenberg, 1941; Patterson et al., 1961). Selection for resistance could give poultry producers considerable protection and has been considered in commercial breeding programs (Millen et al., 1959; Hy-Line, 1963). However, economic pressures have given more encouragement for selection of production attributes or for resistance to such diseases as the leukosis complex (Cole, 1967). There appears to be insufficient incentive for primary poultry breeding organizations to select for coccidial resistant strains of poultry at the present time. Selection for genetic resistance still remains a possible means of coccidiosis control.

REFERENCES

Allen, Ena A. 1936. *Tyzzeria perniciosa* gen. et sp. nov., a coccidium from the small intestine of the Pekin duck, *Anas domesticus* L. *Arch. Protistenk.* 87:262–67.

Andrews, J. S., A. L. Taylor, and L. E. Swanson. 1943. Fumigation of soil with methyl bromide as a means of destroying infective stages and intermediate hosts of some internal parasites of mammals. *Proc. Helminthol. Soc. Wash. D.C.* 10:4–6.

Aycardi, J. 1963. Problemes actuels de recherches sur les coccidioses aviaires. *Rec. Med. Vet.* 139:831–46.

Babcock, W. E., and E. M. Dickinson. 1954. Coccidial immunity studies in chickens. 2. The dosage of *Eimeria tenella* and time required for immunity to develop in chickens. *Poultry Sci.* 33:596–601.

Bachman, G. W. 1930. Serological studies in experimental coccidiosis of rabbits. *Am. J. Hyg.* 12:624–40.

Baldwin, F. M., O. B. Wiswell, and H. A. Jankiewicz. 1941. Hemorrhage control in *Eimeria tenella* infected chicks when protected by anti-hemorrhagic factor, vitamin K. *Proc. Soc. Exp. Biol. Med.* 48:278–80.

Ball, S. J. 1959. Antibiotics in chemotherapy of caecal coccidiosis in chickens. *J. Comp. Pathol. Therap.* 69:327–33.

Ball, S. J., M. Davis, J. N. Hodgson, J. M. S. Lucas, E. W. Parnell, B. W. Sharp, and D. Warburton. 1968. A new anti-coccidial drug. *Chem. & Ind. (London)*, pp. 56–7.

Barber, C. W. 1955. Nicarbazin in the prevention of coccidiosis in chickens. *Cornell Vet.* 45:360–66.

Baron, R. R., M. W. Moeller, and N. F. Morehouse. 1963. Further studies on substituted benzamides for the prevention of coccidiosis in chickens. *Poultry Sci.* 42:1255. (Abstr.)

Becker, E. R. 1948. Protozoa, pp. 863–91. In Biester, H. E., and L. H. Schwarte (eds.), *Diseases of Poultry,* 2nd ed. Iowa State Univ. Press, Ames.

Becker, E. R., P. R. Hall, and Anna Hager. 1932. Quantitative, biometric, and host-parasite studies on *Eimeria miyairii* and *Eimeria separata* in rats. *Iowa State Coll. J. Sci.* 6:299–316.

Becker, E. R., P. R. Hall, and R. Madden.

1935. The mechanism of immunity in murine coccidiosis. *Am. J. Hyg.* 21:389–404.

Becker, E. R., W. J. Zimmermann, and W. H. Patillo. 1955. A biometrical study of the oocyst of *Eimeria brunetti,* a parasite of the common fowl. *J. Protozool.* 2:145–50.

Bertke, E. M. 1955. Pathological effects of coccidiosis caused by the protozoan parasite *Eimeria tenella* in chickens. Unpublished thesis, Univ. Wisconsin.

———. 1963. Renal function during the course of *Eimeria tenella* infection. *J. Parasitol.* 49:937–42.

Biester, H. E., and L. H. Schwarte (eds.). 1965. *Diseases of Poultry,* 5th ed. Iowa State Univ. Press, Ames.

Biggs, P. M., P. L. Long, S. G. Kenzy, and D. G. Rootes. 1969. Relationship between Marek's disease and coccidiosis. II. The effect of Marek's disease on the susceptibility of chickens to coccidial infection. *Vet. Record* 83:284–89.

Bishop, Ann. 1959. Drug resistance in protozoa. *Biol. Rev. Cambridge Phil. Soc.* 34:445–500.

Boles, Janet I., and E. R. Becker. 1954. The development of *Eimeria brunetti* Levine in the digestive tract of chickens. *Iowa State Coll. J. Sci.* 29:1–26.

Boney, W. A., Jr. 1948. The efficacy of methyl bromide as a fumigant for the prevention of cecal coccidiosis in chickens. *Am. J. Vet. Res.* 9:210–14.

Brackett, S., and A. Bliznick. 1950. *The Occurrence and Economic Importance of Coccidiosis in Chickens.* American Cyanamid, New York.

Bressler, G. O., and S. Gordeuk. 1951. Effect of cecal coccidiosis on body weight, egg production, and hatchability in chickens. *Poultry Sci.* 30:509–11.

Brewer, R. N., W. M. Reid, and H. Botero. 1967. A study of coccidiosis-leukosis relationships. *Poultry Sci.* 46:1237. (Abstr.)

Brewer, R. N., W. M. Reid, H. Botero, and S. C. Schmittle. 1968. Studies on acute Marek's disease. 2. The role of coccidia in transmission and induction. *Poultry Sci.* 47:2003–12.

Britton, W. M., C. H. Hill, and C. W. Barber.

1964. A mechanism of interaction between dietary protein levels and coccidiosis in chicks. *J. Nutr.* 82:306–10.

Bryant, B. F. 1956. Coccidiosis in poultry. *Central African Pharm. J.* (November):20–24.

Burns, W. C., and J. R. Challey. 1959. Resistance of birds to challenge with *Eimeria tenella. Exp. Parasitol.* 8:515–26.

Challey, J. R., and W. C. Burns. 1959. The invasion of the cecal mucosa by *Eimeria tenella* sporozoites and their transport by macrophages. *J. Protozool.* 6:238–41.

Champion, L. R. 1954. The inheritance of resistance to cecal coccidiosis in the domestic fowl. *Poultry Sci.* 33:670–81.

Chute, H. L., A. Kalavaitis, J. Frazier, D. C. O'Meara, D. D. Payne, and E. F. Waller. 1960. A survey of the species of coccidia in chickens in Maine. *J. Am. Vet. Med. Ass.* 137:261–65.

Chute, H. L., M. S. Cover, G. H. Snoeyenbos, and C. L. Angstron. 1967. Report committee on nomenclature and reporting of disease: Northeastern Conference on Avian Diseases. *Avian Diseases* 11:727–33.

Clapham, Phyllis A. 1950. On sterilizing land against poultry parasites. *J. Helminthol.* 24:137–44

Clarke, M. L. 1964. A mixture of diaveridine and sulphaquinoxaline as a coccidiostat for poultry. II. Efficiency against *Eimeria acervulina, E. brunetti,* and *E. maxima* infections together with a field survey of coccidiosis in S.E. England. *Vet. Record* 76:818–21.

Cole, R. K. 1967. Selection for resistance to Marek's disease by use of the JM virus. *Poultry Sci.* 46:1246. (Abstr.)

Coulston, F., and E. W. Dennis. 1958. Prevention and suppression of coccidiosis in poultry with 2,2′-thiobis (2,4-dichlorophenol). U.S. Pat. 2,844,509.

Cuckler, A. C., and Christine M. Malanga. 1955. Studies on drug resistance in coccidia. *J. Parasitol.* 41:302–11.

———. 1956. The effect of nicarbazin on the development of immunity to avian coccidia. *J. Parasitol.* 42:593–605.

Cuckler, A. C., L. R. Chapin, Christine M. Malanga, E. F. Rogers, H. J. Becker, R. L. Clark, W. J. Leanza, A. A. Pessolano, T. Y. Shen, and L. H. Sarett. 1958. Antiparasitic drugs. II. Anticoccidial activity of 4,5 imidazoledicarboxamide and related compounds. *Proc. Soc. Exp. Biol. Med.* 98:167–70.

Cuckler, A. C., M. Garzillo, Christine Malanga, and E. C. McManus. 1960. Amprolium. 1. Efficacy for coccidia in chickens. *Poultry Sci.* 39:1241. (Abstr.)

Davies, S. F. M. 1956. Intestinal coccidiosis in chickens caused by *Eimeria necatrix. Vet. Record* 68:853–57.

———. 1963. *Eimeria brunetti,* an additional cause of intestinal coccidiosis in the domestic fowl in Britain. *Vet. Record* 75:1–4.

Davies, S. F. M., L. P. Joyner, and S. B. Kendall. 1963. *Coccidiosis.* Oliver and Boyd, Edinburgh.

Delaplane, J. F., R. M. Batchelder, and T. C. Higgins. 1947. Sulfaquinoxaline in the prevention of *Eimeria tenella* infections in chickens. *North Am. Vet.* 28:19–24.

Dickinson, E. M. 1941. The effect of variable dosage of sporulated *Eimeria acervulina* oocysts on chickens. *Poultry Sci.* 20:413–24.

Dickinson, E. M., W. E. Babcock, and J. W. Osebold. 1951. Coccidial immunity studies in chickens. I. *Poultry Sci.* 30:76–80.

Doll, J. P., P. C. Trexler, L. I. Reynolds, and G. R. Bernard. 1963. The use of peracetic acid to obtain germ-free invertebrate eggs for gnotobiotic studies. *Am. Midland Naturalist* 69:231–39.

Doran, D. J. 1966. The migration of *Eimeria acervulina* sporozoites to the duodenal glands of Lieberkuehn. *J. Protozool.* 13:27–33.

Doran, D. J., and Marion M. Farr. 1962. Excystation of the poultry coccidium, *Eimeria acervulina. J. Protozool.* 9:154–61.

Dorn, P., and M. Sommerer. 1961. Treatment of intestinal coccidiosis in fowls. *Monatsh. Tierheilk.* 13:63–69.

Edgar, S. A. 1944. The development of the protozoan parasite *Eimeria tenella* Railliet and Lucet, 1891, in the domestic fowl. Unpublished thesis, Univ. Wisconsin.

———. 1954. Effect of temperature on the sporulation of oocysts of the protozoan, *Eimeria tenella. Trans. Am. Microscop. Soc.* 73:237–42.

———. 1955. Sporulation of oocysts at specific temperatures and notes on the prepatent period of several species of avian coccidia. *J. Parasitol.* 41:214–16.

———. 1958a. Coccidiosis of chickens and turkeys and control by immunization, pp. 415–21, 769. In *Avicultura Moderna.* Mem. XI. Congr. Mondial Avicultura.

———. 1958b. Problems in the control of coccidiosis. *Proc. Semi-Annual Nutr. Council Am. Feed Mfg. Ass.,* pp. 19–26.

———. 1959. Control of cecal coccidiosis by active immunization. *Auburn Vet.* 10:79–81, 116.

———. 1964. Stable coccidiosis immunization. U.S. Pat. 3,147,186.

Edgar, S. A., and D. F. King. 1952. Breeding and immunizing chickens for resistance to coccidiosis. *Ann. Rept. Alabama Polytech. Inst. Agr. Expt. Sta.* 62, 63:36–37.

———. 1955. Coccidiosis vaccine. *J. World Poultry Sci.* 11:29–30.

Edgar, S. A., and C. T. Seibold. 1964. A new coccidium of chickens, *Eimeria mivati* sp.

n. (Protozoa: Eimeriidae) with details of its life history. *J. Parasitol.* 50:193–204.

Edgar, S. A., C. Flanagan, K. F. Tam, and D. Bond. 1968. Factors related to immunity of chickens to coccidiosis. *Poultry Sci.* 47:1668.

Ellis, C. C. 1938. Studies of the viability of the oocysts of *Eimeria tenella* with particular reference to conditions of incubation. *Cornell Vet.* 28:267–74.

Erasmus, J., M. L. Scott, and P. P. Levine. 1960. A relationship between coccidiosis and vitamin A nutrition in chickens. *Poultry Sci.* 39:565–72.

Fantham, H. B. 1909. [The morphology and life history of *Eimeria (coccidium) avium:* Sporozoon causing a fatal disease among young grouse.] *Proc. Zool. Soc. London,* 886–87.

Farr, Marion M. 1943. Resistance of chickens to cecal coccidiosis. *Poultry Sci.* 22:277–86.

Farr, Marion M., and D. J. Doran. 1962. Comparative excystation of four species of poultry coccidia. *J. Protozool.* 9:403–7.

Farr, Marion M., and E. E. Wehr. 1949–50. Survival of *Eimeria acervulina, E. tenella,* and *E. maxima* oocysts on soil under various field conditions. *Ann. N.Y. Acad. Sci.* 52:468–72.

Fish, F. 1931. Quantitative and statistical analyses of infections with *Eimeria tenella* in the chicken. *Am. J. Hyg.* 14:560–76.

Gabriel, K. L., and S. F. Scheidy. 1965. Sulphonamides. *Advan. Vet. Sci.* 10:245–52.

Gardiner, J. L., and D. K. McLoughlin. 1963a. Drug resistance in *Eimeria tenella.* III. Stability of resistance to glycarbylamide. *J. Parasitol.* 49:657–59.

———. 1963b. Drug resistance in *Eimeria tenella.* IV. The experimental development of a nitrofurazone-resistant strain. *J. Parasitol.* 49:947–50.

Gerriets, E. 1961. The prophylactic action of vitamin A in caecal coccidiosis by protection of the epithelium. *Brit. Vet. J.* 117:507–15.

Gill, B. S. 1955. Review on the differential characters of poultry coccidia. *Indian Vet. J.* 32:122–24.

———. 1961. Incidence of *Eimeria necatrix* Johnson infection in Indian poultry. *Indian J. Vet. Sci.* 31:304–9.

Gill, B. S., and N. B. Lall. 1961. A fatal outbreak of *Eimeria acervulina* Tyzzer, 1929, in an experimental flock. *Indian J. Vet. Sci.* 31:315–18.

Gill, B. S., M. N. Malhotra, and N. B. Lall. 1963. Technical note. Studies on the comparative efficacy of sulphamezathine, sulphaquinoxaline and nitrofurazone given in feed, and their soluble salts administered in drinking water in the control of caecal coccidiosis *(Eimeria tenella)* of poultry. *Indian J. Vet. Sci.* 33:56–58.

Gordeuk, S., Jr., G. O. Bressler, and P. J. Glantz. 1951. The effect of age of birds and degree of exposure in the development of immunity to cecal coccidiosis in chicks. *Poultry Sci.* 30:503–8.

Harms, R. H., and R. L. Tugwell. 1956. The effect of experimentally induced prolonged blood clotting time on cecal coccidiosis of chicks. *Poultry Sci.* 35:937–38.

Harry, E. G. 1967. The disinfection and disinfestation of poultry houses. *Vet. Record* 80 (Suppl. 7):3–4.

Hart, C. P., W. H. Wiley, J. P. Delaplane, L. C. Grumbles, and T. C. Higgins. 1949. Medication versus sanitation in the control of coccidiosis. *Poultry Sci.* 28:686–90.

Harwood, P. D., and Dorothy I. Stunz. 1954. Efficacy of furazolidone, a new nitrofuran, against blackhead and coccidiosis. *J. Parasitol.* 40 (Sect. 2):24–25. (Abstr.)

Harwood, P. D., Dorothy I. Stunz, and R. Wolfgang. 1947. An effective new coccidiostat. *J. Parasitol.* 33 (Sect. 2):14–15. (Abstr.)

———. 1956. The efficacy of a nitrofuran mixture as an avian coccidiostat. *J. Protozool.* 3 (Sect. 2):8. (Abstr.)

Hegde, K. S., and W. M. Reid. 1969. Effects of six single species of coccidia on egg production and culling rate of susceptible layers. *Poultry Sci.* 48:928–32.

Hegde, K. S., W. M. Reid, Joyce Johnson, and H. Womack. 1969. Pathogenicity of *Eimeria brunetti* in bacteria-free and conventional chickens. *J. Parasitol.* 55:402–5.

Hein, Helen. 1963. Vaccination against infection with *Eimeria tenella* in broiler chickens. *17th World Vet. Congr.* 2:1443–52.

———. 1968. The pathogenic effects of *Eimeria acervulina* in young chicks. *Exp. Parasitol.* 23:1–11.

Herlich, H. 1961. The serology and immunology of coccidiosis in chickens. *Dissertation Abstr.* 22:1753–54.

———. 1965. Effect of chicken antiserum and tissue extracts on the oocysts, sporozoites, and merozoites of *Eimeria tenella* and *E. acervulina. J. Parasitol.* 51:847–51.

Herrick, C. A. 1950. The effect of coccidia on the metabolism and temperature regulation of chickens. *Poultry Sci.* 29:763. (Abstr.)

Herrick, C. A., and C. E. Holmes. 1936. Effects of sulphur on coccidiosis in chickens. *Vet. Med.* 31:390–92.

Herrick, C. A., G. L. Ott, and C. E. Holmes. 1936. The chicken as a carrier of the oocysts of the coccidia, *Eimeria tenella. Poultry Sci.* 15:322–25.

Hilbrich, P. 1960. Warum prophylaktische Beigabe von Kokzidiostatika zum Gefluegelmischfutter? *Kraftfutter* 43, Jahrgang Heft 10.

———. 1963. *Krankheiten des Gefluegels.*

Hermann Kuhn, Schwenningen am Neckar.

Horton-Smith, C. 1958. Resistance to anticoccidial drugs experimentally induced in a laboratory strain of *Eimeria tenella,* pp. 483–89, 773. In *Avicultura Moderna.* Mem. XI Congr. Mundial Avicultura.

———. 1960. Coccidiosis. *Vet. Record* 72: 967–70.

———. 1963. Immunity to avian coccidiosis. *Brit. Vet. J.* 119:99–109.

Horton-Smith, C., and P. L. Long. 1959. The effects of different anticoccidial agents on the intestinal coccidioses of the fowl. *J. Comp. Pathol. Therap.* 69:192–207.

———. 1965. The development of *Eimeria necatrix* Johnson, 1930, and *Eimeria brunetti* Levine, 1942, in the caeca of the domestic fowl *(Gallus domesticus). Parasitology* 55: 401–5.

———. 1966. The fate of the sporozoites of *Eimeria acervulina, Eimeria maxima* and *Eimeria mivati* in the caeca of the fowl. *Parasitology* 56:569–74.

Horton-Smith, C., and E. L. Taylor. 1939. The efficiency of the blowlamp for the destruction of coccidial oocysts in poultry houses. *Vet. Record* 51:839–42.

———. 1942. Sulphamethazine and sulphadiazine treatment in caecal coccidiosis of chickens. *Vet. Record* 54:516.

Horton-Smith, C., E. L. Taylor, and E. E. Turtle. 1940. Ammonia fumigation for coccidial disinfection. *Vet. Record* 52:829–32.

Horton-Smith, C., J. Beattie, and P. L. Long. 1961. Resistance to *Eimeria tenella* and its transference from one caecum to the other in individual fowls. *Immunology* 4:111–21.

Hunter, J. E. 1959. Considerations for the evaluation of coccidiostats. *Proc. Semi-Ann. Nutr. Council Am. Feed Mfg. Ass.,* pp. 16–19.

Hy-Line Poultry Farms. 1963. Control coccidiosis—And protect egg profits. *Profit Pointers* 2:1–4.

Hymas, T. A., and G. T. Stevenson. 1960. A study of the action of zoalene on *Eimeria tenella* and *Eimeria necatrix* when administered in the diet or the drinking water. *Poultry Sci.* 39:1261–62.

Jankiewicz, H. A., and R. H. Scofield. 1934. The administration of heated oocysts of *Eimeria tenella* as a means of establishing resistance and immunity to cecal coccidiosis. *J. Am. Vet. Med. Ass.* 84:507–26.

Johnson, W. T. 1927. Immunity or resistance of the chicken to coccidial infection. *Oregon Agr. Expt. Sta. Bull.* 230:17.

———. 1930. Coccidiosis investigations. *Oregon Agr. Expt. Sta. Director's Biennial Report (1928–30),* pp. 119–20.

———. 1932. Effect of five species of Eimeria upon egg production of single comb White

Leghorns. *J. Parasitol.* 18 (Sect. 2):122. (Abstr.)

———. 1933. Coccidiosis of the chicken. *Oregon State Coll. Agr. Expt. Sta. Bull.* 314:16.

Jones, E. Elizabeth. 1932. Size as a species characteristic in coccidia: Variation under diverse conditions of infection. *Arch. Protestenk.* 76:130–70.

Jones, L. M. 1959. Avian coccidiosis, pp. 594–602. In *Veterinary Pharmacology and Therapeutics,* 2nd ed. Iowa State Univ. Press, Ames.

Joyner, L. P. 1958. Experimental *Eimeria mitis* infections in chickens. *Parasitology* 48:101–12.

Joyner, L. P., and S. F. M. Davies. 1960. Detection and assessment of sublethal infections of *Eimeria tenella* and *Eimeria necatrix. Exp. Parasitol.* 9:243–49.

Keener, Joyce. 1963. Effects of environmental temperature on birds infected with coccidiosis. Unpublished thesis, Univ. Georgia.

Krassner, S. M. 1963. Factors in host susceptibility and oocyst infectivity in *Eimeria acervulina* infections. *J. Protozool.* 10:327–33.

Leathem, W. D. 1965. Studies on the behavior of the protozoan parasite *Eimeria tenella* in immune chickens. *Dissertation Abstr.* 26:5605.

Leathem, W. D., and W. C. Burns. 1968. Duration of acquired immunity of the chicken to *Eimeria tenella* infection. *J. Parasitol.* 54:227–32.

Levine, N. D. 1961. *Protozoan Parasites of Domestic Animals and of Man.* Burgess Publ. Co., Minneapolis.

Levine, P. P. 1938. *Eimeria hagani* n. sp. (Protozoa: Eimeriidae) a new coccidium of the chicken. *Cornell Vet.* 28:263–66.

———. 1939. The effect of sulfanilamide on the course of experimental avian coccidiosis. *Cornell Vet.* 29:309–20.

———. 1940. Sub-clinical coccidial infection in chickens. *Cornell Vet.* 30:127–32.

———. 1941. The coccidiostatic effect of sulfaguanidine (sulfanilyl guanidine). *Cornell Vet.* 31:107–12.

———. 1942. A new coccidium pathogenic for chickens, *Eimeria brunetti* n. sp. (Protozoa: Eimeriidae). *Cornell Vet.* 32:430–39.

———. 1943. Additional field outbreaks of coccidiosis in chickens due to *Eimeria brunetti. Cornell Vet.* 33:383–85.

———. 1945. Specific diagnosis and chemotherapy of avian coccidiosis. *J. Am. Vet. Med. Ass.* 106:88–90.

Long, P. L. 1959. A study of *Eimeria maxima,* Tyzzer, 1929, a coccidium of the fowl *(Gallus gallus). Ann. Trop. Med. Parasitol.* 53: 325–33.

———. 1962. Observations on the duration of the acquired immunity of chickens to *Ei-*

meria maxima Tyzzer, 1929. *Parasitology* 52:89–93.

———. 1964. Coccidiosis of chickens in Great Britain 1960–1962. Changes in the incidence of different forms of the disease. *Brit. Vet. J.* 120:110–16.

———. 1966. The growth of some species of Eimeria in avian embryos. *Parasitology* 56:575–81.

———. 1967a. Coccidiosis in chickens and turkeys. *Vet. Record* 80:8–12.

———. 1967b. Studies on *Eimeria praecox* Johnson, 1930, in the chicken. *Parasitology* 57:351–61.

———. 1967c. Studies on *Eimeria mivati* in chickens and a comparison with *Eimeria acervulina*. *J. Comp. Pathol.* 77:315–25.

———. 1968a. The pathogenic effects of *Eimeria praecox* and *E. acervulina* in the chicken. *Parasitology* 58:691–700.

———. 1968b. The effect of breed of chickens on resistance to Eimeria infections. *Poultry Sci.* 9:71–78.

Long, P. L., and Z. Tanielian. 1965. The isolation of *Eimeria mivati* in Lebanon during the course of a survey of Eimeria spp. in chickens. *Inst. Rech. Agron. (Liban) Sci. Ser.* 6:1–18.

Long, P. L., S. G. Kenzy, and P. M. Biggs. 1968. Relationship between Marek's disease and coccidiosis. *Vet. Record* 83:260–62.

Lund, E. E., and Marion M. Farr. 1965. Protozoa, pp. 1056–1148. In Biester, H. E., and L. H. Schwarte (eds.), *Diseases of Poultry,* 5th ed. Iowa State Univ. Press, Ames.

Lungu, V. 1961. Observations on the identity and the frequency of types of coccidioses in a center of avian coccidiosis. *Lucrarile Stiint. Inst. Patol. Igiena Animala* 11:425–30.

Lux, R. E. 1954. The chemotherapy of *Eimeria tenella.* 1. Diaminopyrimidines and dihydrotriazenes. *Antibiot. Chemotherapy* 4:971–77.

McDermott, J. J., and L. A. Stauber. 1954. Preparation and agglutination of merozoite suspension of the chicken coccidian, *Eimeria tenella. J. Parasitol.* 40 (Sect. 2):23–24. (Abstr.)

McLoughlin, D. K., and J. L. Gardiner. 1961a. Zoalene tolerance by *Eimeria tenella. J. Parasitol.* 47 (Sect. 2):46. (Abstr.)

———. 1961b. Drug resistance in *Eimeria tenella.* I. The experimental development of a glycarbylamide-resistant strain. *J. Parasitol.* 47:1001–6.

———. 1962. Drug resistance in *Eimeria tenella.* II. The experimental development of a zoalene-resistant strain. *J. Parasitol.* 48:341–46.

Malik, A. Q. 1967. The effect of vitamin A on avian coccidiosis. Unpublished thesis. Texas A & M Univ.

Mayhew, R. L. 1937. Studies on coccidiosis. IX. Histopathology of the caecal type in the chicken. *Trans. Am. Microscop. Soc.* 56:431–46.

Millen, T. W., J. F. Hill, and R. B. Arvidson. 1959. Inheritance of resistance to *Eimeria acervulina. Poultry Sci.* 38:1229. (Abstr.)

Misra, P. L. 1944. On a new coccidian *Wenyonella bahli,* n. sp. from the common grey quail, *Coturnix communis* Bonn. *Proc. Nat. Inst. Sci. India* 10:203–4.

Mitrovic, M., and J. C. Bauernfeind. 1967. Sulfadimethoxine therapy of avian coccidiosis. *Poultry Sci.* 46:402–11.

Morehouse, N. F., and W. C. McGuire. 1957. The effect of 3,5-dinitrobenzamide and its N-substituted derivatives on coccidiosis in chickens. *Poultry Sci.* 36:1143. (Abstr.)

———. 1958. The pathogenicity of *Eimeria acervulina. Poultry Sci.* 37:665–72.

Morehouse, N. F., and O. J. Mayfield. 1944. The effect of some aryl arsonic acids on experimental coccidiosis infection in chickens. *J. Parasitol.* 30 (Sect. 2):6. (Abstr.)

———. 1948. Poultry treatment composition. U.S. Pat. 2,450,866.

Morrison, W. D., A. E. Ferguson, M. C. Connell, and J. K. McGregor. 1961. The efficacy of certain coccidiostats against mixed avian coccidial infections. *Avian Diseases* 5:222–28.

Moynihan, I. W. 1950. The role of the protozoan parasite, *Eimeria acervulina,* in disease of the domestic chicken. *Can. J. Comp. Med.* 14:74–82.

Murphy, C. B., C. F. Hall, and H. W. Yoder, Jr. 1967. Disease reports of the Southern Conference on Avian Diseases. *Avian Diseases* 11:708–26.

Murphy, R. R., J. E. Hunter, and H. C. Knandel. 1938. The effects of rations containing gradient amounts of cod liver oil on the subsequent performance of laying pullets following a natural infection of coccidiosis. *Poultry Sci.* 17:377–80.

Natt, M. P., and C. A. Herrick. 1955. The effect of cecal coccidiosis on the blood cells of the domestic fowl. *Poultry Sci.* 34:1100–1106.

Nelson, T. S., and L. C. Norris. 1957. Cornell studies vitamin K relationship to field hemorrhagic conditions. *Feedstuffs* (February 16):74–75.

Nyberg, P. A., Diana H. Bauer, and S. E. Knapp. 1968. Carbon dioxide as the initial stimulus for excystation of *Eimeria tenella* oocysts. *J. Protozool.* 15:144–48.

Otto, G. F., H. A. Jeske, D. V. Frost, and H. S. Perdue. 1958. Menadione sodium bisulfite complex (Klotogen F) in cecal coccidiosis. *Poultry Sci.* 37:201–5.

Papadopoulos, A., K. Tatsiramos, and A. Tsaglis. 1963. Sur quelques cas de coccidiose a *Eimeria mivati* en Greece. (In Greek, French summary.) *Deltion Ellenikes Kteniatrikes Etaireias* 52:164–70.

Park, S. E., J. E. Porter, F. V. Washko, and D. F. Green. 1959. A study of broiler production with observations on the biology of coccidia in litter. *Conference on Methods of Testing Coccidiostats.* Merck Chem. Div., Rahway, N.J. 1:1–27.

Patillo, W. H. 1959. Invasion of the cecal mucosa of the chicken by sporozoites of *Eimeria tenella. J. Parasitol.* 45:253–58.

Patterson, F. D. 1933a. Cross infection experiments with coccidia of birds. *Cornell Vet.* 23:249–53.

———. 1933b. Studies on the viability of *Eimeria tenella* in soil. *Cornell Vet.* 23:232–49.

Patterson, L. T., L. W. Johnson, and S. A. Edgar. 1961. The comparative resistance of several inbred lines of S. C. White Leghorns to certain infectious diseases. *Poultry Sci.* 40:1442. (Abstr.)

Pellérdy, L. 1960. Investigation into the incidence of *E. brunetti* coccidiosis in Hungary. (In Hungarian, English summary.) *Magy. Allatorv. Lapja* 15:410–13.

———. 1965. Coccidia and coccidiosis. *Akad. Kiado, Budapest,* p. 657.

Pérard, H. C. 1925. Recherches sur les coccidies et les coccidiosis du lapin. *Ann. Inst. Pasteur* 39:505–42.

Peterson, E. H. 1949. Coccidiosis in laying hens due presumably to *Eimeria acervulina. Ann. N.Y. Acad. Sci.* 52:464–67.

———. 1958. Potentiating effect of terephthalic acid upon absorption of chlorotetracycline from the avian alimentary tract. *Univ. Arkansas Agr. Expt. Sta. Rept.* Ser. 74:6.

Pierce, A. E., P. L. Long, and C. Horton-Smith. 1963. Attempts to induce a passive immunity to *Eimeria tenella* in young fowls *(Gallus domesticus). Immunology* 6:37–47.

Pohl, R. 1965a. Ein Beitrag zur Epidemiologie von *Eimeria brunetti. Deut. Tieraerztl. Wochschr.* 71:583–86.

———. 1965b. Ein Beitrag zur Diagnostik der Coccidienarten des Huhnes. *Deut. Tieraerztl. Wochschr.* 72:230–32.

Prestwood, Annie K. 1968. Parasitism among wild turkeys *(Meleagris gallopavo silvestris)* on the Mississippi Delta. Unpublished dissertation, Univ. Georgia.

Railliet, A., and A. Lucet. 1891. Note sur quelques especes de coccidies encore peu etudiees. *Bull. Soc. Zool. France,* pp. 246–51.

Ray, H. N. 1945. On a new coccidium *Wenyonella gallinae* n. sp. from the gut of the domestic fowl, *Gallus gallus domesticus* Linn. *Current Sci.* 14:275.

Reid, W. M. 1961. Coccidiosis control. Symposium on disease, environmental and management factors related to poultry health. USDA ARS 45–2, pp. 48–52.

———. 1963a. *Eimeria brunetti.* Studies on incidence and geographical distribution. *Am. J. Vet. Res.* 25:224–29.

———. 1963b. Control programs and immunity to coccidiosis with broilers and layers. *Proc. 17th World Vet. Congr.* 2:1489–90.

———. 1965. Coccidiosis control in started pullets. *Poultry Tribune* 71:14, 54.

———. 1966. Relationship between layer flock immunity to six species of coccidia and the use of coccidiostats. *Proc. 13th World's Poultry Congr.,* pp. 453–55.

———. 1968 (revised). A diagnostic chart for nine species of fowl coccidia. *Georgia Agr. Expt. Sta. Tech. Bull.* N.S. 39:1–18.

———. 1969. The effects and mechanisms of coccidiostats, histomonostats, and anthelmintics in feed on the performance and health of animals. *Nat. Acad. Sci. Publ.* 1679:87–99.

Reid, W. M., and R. B. Davis. 1969. Severe coccidiosis in a breeder flock following high level medication for mycoplasma and coccidia control. *Avian Diseases* 13:447–52.

Reid, W. M., and Joyce Johnson. 1970. Pathogenicity of *Eimeria acervulina* in light and heavy coccidial infections. *Avian Diseases* 14:166–71.

Reid, W. M., and Joyce Keener. 1962. Laying house coccidiosis. *Proc. 59th Ass. Southern Agr. Workers Meet.,* p. 250 (Abstr.)

Reid, W. M., and C. D. Murphy. 1966. Relationships between coccidiostats and coccidiosis control. *Georgia Vet.* 18:7–10.

Reid, W. M., and M. Pitois. 1965. The influence of coccidiosis on feed and water intake of chickens. *Avian Diseases* 9:343–48.

Reid, W. M., and M. R. Raja. 1963. Incidence in Georgia broilers and pathogenicity studies of the coccidium *Eimeria maxima. J. Vet. Res.* 24:174–78.

Reid, W. M., A. G. Kemler, and M. R. Raja. 1960. Prevalence of various species of coccidia in Georgia. *Poultry Sci.* 39:1287. (Abstr.)

Reid, W. M., K. Friedhoff, P. Hilbrich, Joyce Johnson, and S. A. Edgar. 1965. The occurrence of the coccidium species *Eimeria mivati* in European poultry. *Zentr. Parasitenk.* 25:303–8.

Reid, W. M., H. E. Womack, and Joyce Johnson. 1968. Coccidiosis susceptibility in layer flock replacement programs. *Poultry Sci.* 47:892–99.

Reid, W. M., E. M. Taylor, and Joyce Johnson. 1969a. A technique for demonstration of coccidiostatic activity of anticoccidial agents. *Trans. Am. Microscop. Soc.* 88:148–59.

Reid, W. M., R. N. Brewer, Joyce Johnson, E. M. Taylor, K. S. Hegde, and L. M. Kowalski. 1969b. Evaluation of techniques used in studies on efficacy of anticoccidial drugs in chickens. *Am. J. Vet. Res.* 30:447–59.

Renault, L., W. M. Reid, M. Pitois, and Joyce Johnson. 1965. Identification en France de la coccidiose intestinale aviaire provoquee par *Eimeria brunetti. Rec. Med. Vet.* 5:463–67.

Rose, M. Elaine. 1965. Immunity in the fowl to some species of *Eimeria. Second Int. Conf. Protozool.* Ser. 91:155. (Abstr.)

———. 1967. Immunity to *Eimeria brunetti* and *Eimeria maxima* infections in the fowl. *Parasitology* 57:363–70.

Rose, M. Elaine, and P. L. Long. 1962. Immunity to four species of Eimeria in fowls. *Immunology* 5:79–92.

Rosenberg, M. M. 1941. A study of the inheritance of resistance to *Eimeria tenella* in the domestic fowl. *Poultry Sci.* 20:472. (Abstr.)

Rosenberg, M. M., W. H. McGibbon, and C. A. Herrick. 1948. Selection for hereditary resistance and susceptibility to cecal coccidiosis in the domestic fowl. *Eighth World's Poultry Congr. Offic. Rept.* 1:745–51.

Rosenberg, M. M., J. E. Alicata, and A. L. Palafox. 1954. Further evidence of hereditary resistance and susceptibility to cecal coccidiosis in chickens. *Poultry Sci.* 33:972–80.

Scholtyseck, E. 1954. Untersuchungen ueber die bei Einheimischen Vogelarten vorkommenden Coccidien der Gattung Isospora. *Arch. Protistenk.* 100:91–112.

———. 1956. Cytologische Beobachtungen bei der Entwicklung der Makrogametocyten von *Eimeria maxima. Verhandl. Deut. Zool. Ges. Hamburg* 235–41.

———. 1959. Zur pathologie der *Eimeria maxima*—Coccidiose. *Zentr. Bakteriol.* 175:305–17.

Seeger, K. C., W. C. Lucas, and A. E. Tomhave. 1950. The effect of dried crude Aureomycin on cecal coccidiosis in chickens. *Poultry Sci.* 29:779. (Abstr.)

Shumard, R. F. 1956. The activity of soluble Furacin (nitrofurazone) against the coccidian, *Eimeria necatrix. Proc. 1st Nat. Symp. on Nitrofurans in Agr.,* pp. 36–42.

Shumard. R. F., and M. E. Callender. 1967. Monensin, a new biologically active compound. VI. Anticoccidial activity. *Antimicrobial Agents Chemotherapy* 1967:369–77.

Snoeyenbos, G. H. 1955. Is coccidiosis gaining resistance to drugs? *World's Poultry Sci. J.* 11:223–24.

Spencer, C. F., A. Engle, C. N. Yu, R. C. Finch, E. J. Watson, F. F. Ebetino, and C. A. Johnson. 1966. Anticoccidial activity in a series of alkyl 6, 7-dialkoxy-4-hydroxy-3-quinolinecarboxylates. *J. Med. Chem.* 9:934–36.

Steward, K. S. 1947. The treatment of bovine coccidiosis with 4,4'-diaminodiphenyl-sulfone. *Vet. Record* 59:21–27.

Stock, B. L., G. T. Stevenson, and T. A. Hymas. 1967. Coyden coccidiostat for control of coccidiosis in chickens. *Poultry Sci.* 46:485–92.

Supperer, R. 1961. Beitrag zur Diagnose der Huehner-Kokzidiosen. *Wien. Tieraerztl. Monatschr.* 10:777–83.

Swales, W. E. 1944. On the chemotherapy of caecal coccidiosis *(Eimeria tenella)* of chickens. *Can. J. Res.* 22:131–40.

Taylor, M. W., and W. C. Russell. 1947. The provitamin A requirement of growing chickens. *Poultry Sci.* 26:234–42.

Tugwell, R. L., J. F. Stephens, and R. H. Harms. 1957. The relationship of vitamin K to mortality from cecal coccidiosis. *Poultry Sci.* 36:1245–47.

Tyzzer, E. E. 1912. *Cryptosporidium parvum* (sp. nov.), a coccidium found in the small intestine of the common mouse. *Arch. Protistenk.* 26:394–412.

———. 1929. Coccidiosis in gallinaceous birds. *Am. J. Hyg.* 10:269–383.

———. 1932. Criteria and methods in the investigations of avian coccidiosis. *Science* 75:324–28.

Tyzzer, E. E., H. L. Theiler, and Eliz. E. Jones. 1932. Coccidiosis in gallinaceous birds. II. A comparative study of species of Eimeria of the chicken. *Am. J. Hyg.* 15:319–93.

Uricchio, W. A. 1953. The feeding of artificially altered oocysts of *Eimeria tenella* as a means of establishing immunity to cecal coccidiosis in chickens. *Proc. Helminthol. Soc. Wash. D.C.* 20:77–83.

USDA. 1965. *Losses in Agriculture.* Agr. Handbook 291, pp. 72–84.

Vezey, S. A. 1966. Coccidiosis immunization without the aid of a coccidiostat. *Proc. Poultry Health Conf.,* pp. 37–41.

Waldroup, P. W., C. F. Simpson, D. D. Cox, and R. H. Harms. 1963. The effects of feeding various levels of vitamin A on chicks with cecal coccidiosis. *Poultry Sci.* 42:274–75.

Waletzky, E., C. O. Huges, and M. C. Brandt. 1949. The anticoccidial activity of nitrophenide. *Ann. N.Y. Acad. Sci.* 52:543–57.

Waletzky, E., R. Neal, and I. Hable. 1954. A field strain of *Eimeria tenella* resistant to sulfonamides. *J. Parasitol.* 40 (Sect. 2): 24. (Abstr.)

Waxler, S. H. 1941. Immunization against cecal coccidiosis in chickens by the use of x-ray-attenuated oocysts. *J. Am. Vet. Med. Ass.* 99:481–85.

Zbornik, T. W., N. F. Morehouse, and A. W. Walde. 1955. N, N-(3-nitro-benzenesulfonyl) ethylene-diamine compositions for the treatment of coccidiosis. U.S. Pat. 2,715,600.

Zimmermann, W. J. 1957. Field studies on Eimeria species in Iowa chickens. *Poultry Sci.* 36:184–93.

TURKEY

The coccidioses of turkeys are capable of causing moderate to severe economic losses (Lund and Farr, 1965; Bond, 1966). Mortality losses are variable, ranging from insignificant to as high as 25% or more in untreated outbreaks. Experimental infections may produce 100% mortality following inoculation of as few as 50,000 oocysts per bird (Hawkins, 1952). Since morbidity losses are more difficult to estimate, they have had little consideration but probably are of greater economic importance than mortality (Bond, 1966). Coccidiosis is primarily a disease of young poults, with most of the mortality occurring between 3 and 16 weeks of age (Morehouse, 1949). Drooping wings, listlessness, ruffled feathers, brownish mucoid diarrhea, anorexia, huddling in groups, constant cheeping, and weight loss characterize presence of coccidiosis. Although flecks of blood may appear in the droppings, the copious bloody discharges found in cecal coccidiosis of chickens are not typical of turkey coccidiosis. The character and location of diseased tissues depends upon the severity of infection and the species of coccidia involved.

In a study of the geographical distribution of the different species of turkey coccidia in the United States, Bond (1966) recovered *Eimeria gallopavonis* in 18 of 19 states, *E. adenoides* in 17 states, and *E. meleagridis* in 16 states. Other as yet undescribed species were found in 16 states, while the four relatively nonpathogenic species (Table 31.4) were identified less frequently. These records indicate a very high infection rate considering the very small number of samples available for study. Numerous scattered reports from other parts of the world suggest that the common coccidial species are found wherever turkeys are raised. As pointed out by Davies et al. (1963), distribution of the species of Eimeria is limited only by availability of hosts, since no vector is required and survival requires only moisture and moderate temperatures.

ETIOLOGY

Seven species of Eimeria have been described from the turkey in the United States (Table 31.4); *Isospora haesini* described by Svanbaev (1955) from USSR and *Cryptosporidium meleagridis* by Slavin (1955) from Scotland have not been reported from the United States. The differential characteristics of the 7 species of Eimeria are best compared by use of Table 31.4. Data were compiled from the species descriptions of the original describers, with added observations from other investigators. Bond (1966) demonstrated a shorter minimum sporulation time and prepatent period for *E. dispersa, E. gallopavonis,* and *E. meleagrimitis.* Sporulation was more rapid since optimum temperatures (29° C ± 1) were used.

Descriptions of 7 individual species (arranged alphabetically) are given below. Characteristics used in distinguishing species include: oocyst characteristics, gross and microscopic pathology, minimum time required for sporulation and prepatent period, degree of pathogenicity, morphology of developmental forms, and absence of cross-immunity between species. This final test, requiring purified suspensions of oocysts of 2 or more species and a supply of fully susceptible turkeys, can seldom be accomplished in most diagnostic laboratories. Diagnosis of turkey coccidiosis is attended with the same difficulties found in chicken coccidiosis, plus these added complications: (1) Some species have yet to be fully described (Hawkins, 1952; Bond, 1966; Lin and Edgar, 1970). (2) Since oocyst size is similar with many species, use of this characteristic has strict limitations. (3) At least 3 species (*E. innocua, E. meleagridis,* and *E. subrotunda*) are nonpathogenic. Thus recovery of oocysts (or in some cases finding of lesions) does not always indicate a serious disease problem. Parasites, either oocysts or endogenous stages of coccidia, always should be demonstrated before a diagnosis of coccidiosis is made. Coccidiosis diagnosed on the basis of bloody diarrhea is probably due to some other disease condition (Hinshaw, 1965). Need for a microscopic examination of intestinal scrapings is thus emphasized.

Eimeria adenoides Moore and Brown 1951

Classification

Gross lesions appear in the ceca, lower small intestine, and rectum. Feces contain

TABLE 31.4 ❧ Diagnostic Characteristics of Eimeria in Turkeys*

Species Characteristics	E. adenoides	E. dispersa	E. gallopavonis	E. innocua	E. meleagridis	E. meleagrimitis	E. subrotunda
Zone parasitized							
Macroscopic lesions	liquid feces with mucus and flecks of blood, loose cecal cores	cream-colored serosal surface, dilation of intestine, yellowish mucoid material	edema, ulceration of mucosal ileum, yellow exudate	none	cream-colored ceca, formation of caseous plug, a few petechial hemorrhages	spotty congestion and petechiae from duodenum to ileum, dilation of jejunum, casts	none
Length × Width (in microns) Length = Width =	Av = 25.6 × 16.6 18.9–31.3 12.6–20.9	Av = 26.1 × 21.0 21.8–31.1 17.7–23.9	Av = 27.1 × 17.2 22.7–32.7 15.2–19.4	Av = 22.4 × 20.9 18.57–25.86 17.34–24.54	Av = 24.4 × 18.1 20.3–30.8 15.4–20.6	Av = 19.2 × 16.3 15.8–26.9 13.1–21.9	Av = 21.8 × 19.8 16.48–26.42 14.21–24.44
Oocyst shape and index length/width	ellipsoidal 1.54	broadly ovoid 1.24	ellipsoidal 1.52	*subspherical* *1.07*	*ellipsoidal* *1.34*	ovoid 1.17	*subspherical* *1.10*
Minimum sporulation	24 hr.	35 hr.	15 hr.	under 48 hr.	24 hr.	18 hr.	48 hr.
Prepatent period (minimum)	103 hr.	**120 hr.**	105 hr.	114 hr.	110 hr.	103 hr.	**95 hr.**
Refractile body	yes	no	**yes**	no	yes	yes	no
Pathogenicity	✠✠✠✠	✠	✠✠✠	none	***none***	✠✠✠	none

* Characteristics in italics and solid black portions of drawings = diagnostic.

whitish material composed of oocysts, gametocytes, and cellular debris.

The ellipsoidal oocysts, somewhat narrower at one end, have the highest shape
index (length/width = 1.54) of any of the
7 described species. They contain a refractile body. Sporulation is completed in 24
hours and the minimum prepatent period
is 103 hours (112 hours is more common
[Moore and Brown, 1951] and it may be
as long as 132 hours [Clarkson, 1958]), although with most turkeys the first oocysts
appear somewhat later.

Differentiation is required from *E. gallopavonis* and *E. meleagridis* which often
parasitize the lower small intestine and
cecum. *E. meleagridis* shows less tendency
to localize in the rectum than the other
two species. *E. adenoides* invades more
deeply into the intestinal glands than the
other two species. *E. gallopavonis* is confined to the superficial epithelium covering
the tips of the villi. Both *E. adenoides* and
E. meleagridis produce cecal plugs, but the
latter does not kill or produce weight loss
in the host.

Pathogenesis and Epizootiology

E. adenoides is one of the most pathogenic of the turkey coccidia. Experimental
infections of poults 5 weeks of age have
shown 100% mortality, with death occurring on the 5th to 7th day (Moore and
Brown, 1951). Inoculations of as few as
100,000 oocysts produced similar results
(Clarkson, 1958). These investigators report older birds are less susceptible, but
Edgar (1958) found that turkeys 6 months
of age lost more than 1 lb in weight after
experimental infection and were still highly susceptible. Anorexia, droopiness, and
ruffled feathers are noted beginning on the
4th day after infection. Feces are frequently fluid and blood-tinged and contain mucous casts 2–5 cm in length. Caseous plugs
may be produced in the ceca.

Natural and Experimental Hosts

Only the turkey, wild as well as domestic
(Prestwood, 1968), has been parasitized
with this species. Attempts to infect chickens, guinea fowl, pheasants *(Phasianus colchicus)*, bobwhite quail *(Colinus virginianus)*, and Japanese quail *(Coturnix coturnix)* have been unsuccessful (Moore and
Brown, 1951; Edgar et al., 1964).

Gross Lesions

The mucosal surface of the intestine appears normal on gross examination until
the 4th day after infection when congestion, edema, petechial hemorrhages, and
mucus secretion appear. By the 5th day
orange strands of mucus, streaks of blood,
and solid caseous secretions are seen. During the 6th to 8th day the coloration of the
mucosal surface may become white or
cream-colored due to presence of large numbers of oocysts. The appearance often takes
on a "cottage cheese-like" consistency. The
serosal surface of the lower intestine, ceca,
and rectum are dilated, slightly edematous,
and sometimes whitish in color at the
height of infection.

Histopathology

Invasion of the submucosa by eosinophilic leukocytes is the most marked early host
response (Clarkson, 1958). This reaction is
generalized throughout the intestine early
in the parasitic cycle and becomes concentrated in the lower small intestine, ceca,
and rectum in older infections. Epithelial
cells at the tips of the villi represent the
zone of greatest parasite development.
However, this parasite, unlike *E. gallopavonis* and *E. meleagridis,* invades the deep
glands as well as the villi. Edema is common deep in muscular layers as infection
progresses. After the 5th day cell replacement is rapid. Eighty percent of the first-
generation schizonts locate below the epithelial cell nucleus; the second generation
is found above the nucleus (Clarkson, 1958).

Eimeria dispersa Tyzzer 1929

Classification

The midgut area is the zone most frequently parasitized in turkeys, but some
parasites may invade the epithelium anterior into the duodenum, posterior into the
rectum, or into the neck area of the ceca.
The area parasitized is so extensive that
the zone of parasitism is a less useful characteristic with this species. The large
oocyst size (av. $26.1 \times 21.0\mu$) and the broadly ovoid shape (index 1.24) may assist in
separation from *E. meleagrimitis, E. innocua,* and *E. subrotunda. E. dispersa* lacks a
refractile body, a characteristic shared only
with *E. innocua* and *E. subrotunda.* The
distinction of possessing a single contoured

oocyst wall instead of the double wall described for other species (Hawkins, 1952) has not been fully confirmed. The prepatent period (120 hours) in the turkey is the longest reported for any species. It may be somewhat longer (144 hours) in the bobwhite quail.

Pathogenesis and Epizootiology

Compared to *E. meleagrimitis, E. gallopavonis,* and *E. adenoides,* this species is but mildly pathogenic in turkeys. Infection may cause mild diarrhea and some decrease in rate of weight gains. It is more pathogenic in the bobwhite quail.

Natural and Experimental Hosts

The natural host of this species is the bobwhite quail in which it may produce disease problems (Levine, 1961; Pellérdy, 1965). However, domestic and wild turkeys are frequently infected in nature. Isolations were made from turkeys in 11 states by Hawkins (1952); 12 isolations were found in 6 states by Bond (1966). This coccidium shows less host specificity than any other species found in turkeys. Successful infection attempts have been reported from Hungarian partridge *Perdix perdix* (Hawkins, 1952), ruffed grouse *Bonasa umbellus* and sharp-tailed grouse *Pediocetes phasianellus campestris* (Boughton, 1937), pheasant (Tyzzer, 1929), and Japanese quail *Coturnix coturnix* (Edgar et al., 1964). Tyzzer (1929) reported light infections in chickens, but several other investigators have found this host refractory.

Gross Lesions

Three days after infection the duodenum shows cream-colored changes on the serosal surface. A little later the entire intestine becomes dilated with thickening of the wall. Dilation continues on the 5th and 6th days along with congestion and secretion of a whitish yellow, sticky, mucoid material containing denuded epithelium from the duodenum. Individual villi may become so dilated as to be visible to the naked eye.

Histopathology

The duodenum shows edema and progressively increasing congestion in the capillaries. Separation of the epithelium and basement membranes may result in the lamina propria being exposed to a fibrin network or an open fluid-filled space. The

necrosis, which is common on the distal tips of the villi, is less marked at the base of the villi. Parasites do not invade the glands. In spite of the extensive disruption caused by large numbers of parasites and by lymphocytic infiltration, very few of the epithelial cells are sloughed off. The two forms of developing schizonts generally develop toward the lumen side of the nucleus within the parasitized epithelial cells (Hawkins, 1952).

Eimeria gallopavonis Hawkins 1952

Classification

Lesions are restricted to the area of the intestine posterior to the yolk sac diverticulum and are most severe in the rectum. Milky white exudate consisting mostly of oocysts fills and distends infected areas. *E. adenoides* and *E. meleagridis* localize in the same zone of the intestine and thus require differentiation. Presence of numerous elongate oocysts in the rectum with but limited cecal infection suggests *E. gallopavonis,* as distinguished from *E. meleagridis* and *E. adenoides.* Oocysts average 27.1μ long by 17.2μ in width. The length/width index is 1.52.

Pathogenesis and Epizootiology

Mortality ranging from 10 to 100% was induced in 3–6-week-old poults (Farr et al., 1961) with experimental infections. Mortality appeared 6–12 days postinoculation. No evidence of age resistance was observed by Bond (1966), an observation at variance with findings of Wehr et al. (1962).

Natural and Experimental Hosts

Wild as well as domestic turkeys are the natural hosts (Prestwood, 1968). Experimental infections have been reported in Hungarian partridge *Perdix perdix* by Hawkins (1952). He reported negative transmission experiments for bobwhite quail *Colinus virginianus.* Hawkins (1952) and Edgar et al. (1964) were unsuccessful in infecting chickens, but Gill (1954) reported successful transmission. Further confirmation of this later work is required (Lund and Farr, 1965).

Gross Lesions and Histopathology

Marked inflammatory and edematous changes occur on the 6th day followed by sloughing of soft white caseous necrotic materials containing large numbers of oocysts on the 7th and 8th days. These reactions occur in response to development of gametocyte stages of the parasite. Schizonts always develop below the hypertrophied host cell nucleus (Farr, 1964).

Eimeria innocua Moore and Brown 1952

Classification

This species parasitizes the epithelial cells in the area between the duodenum and the lower ileum. There is a complete absence of any gross lesions. The numerous oocysts are almost spherical, averaging 22.4 $\times$ 20.9μ (shape index 1.07). Oocysts do not differ greatly in shape or size from *E. subrotunda*. This nonpathogenic species tends to localize in more anterior regions of the intestine. The prepatent period of *E. innocua* is 5 days compared to 4 days with *E. subrotunda*.

Pathogenesis and Epizootiology

No macroscopic lesions and no signs of illness were observed by the original describers (Moore and Brown, 1952). The normal well-formed feces showed no blood or mucus. The only suggestion of pathogenicity was a slight retardation in rate of weight gain. Epithelial cells on the tips of the villi in the duodenum (loop area), jejunum, and ileum were parasitized with developmental stages. Fewer parasites were found at the base of the villi. Crypts and deep glands were unparasitized. The patent period during which oocysts were produced was 13 days.

Natural and Experimental Hosts

This species is known to infect only the turkey. Attempts to infect chicks, guinea fowl, and bobwhite quail (*Colinus virginianus*) have proved negative.

Eimeria meleagridis Tyzzer 1929

Classification

Lesions in the ceca sometimes produce cores containing yellow caseous materials. In spite of the presence of visible lesions this species is nonpathogenic. Differentiation from the pathogenic *E. adenoides* and *E. gallopavonis* is required. The latter species shows very limited cecal but common lower intestinal and rectal lesions. Oocysts of these 3 species are of similar length, but

E. meleagridis is wider. Thus the shape index (1.34) for this species is lower than the other 2 species (1.54 *E. adenoides* and 1.52 *E. gallopavonis*).

Pathogenesis and Epizootiology

All recent studies have characterized this species as being almost or entirely nonpathogenic (Moore and Brown, 1951; Hawkins, 1952; Edgar, 1958; Clarkson, 1959b; Lund and Farr, 1965). Two to five million oocysts produced no effect on growth of 4–8-week-old poults (Edgar, 1958). Reports indicating pathogenicity made before the description of *E. adenoides* in 1954 were probably mixed infections. Recovery of this species should be reported as a case of coccidiasis but not of coccidiosis. It is widely distributed throughout the United States.

Natural and Experimental Hosts

Domestic and wild turkeys are the recognized natural hosts of this parasite. Chickens have proved refractory to experimental infection by seven or more thorough investigations. However, two reports of successful transmission have been reported (Steward, 1947; Gill, 1954). Pheasants, bobwhite quail (Tyzzer, 1929; Edgar, 1958), and Coturnix quail (Bond, 1966) have proved refractory.

Gross Lesions

Nonadherent, cream-colored caseous cecal plugs are characteristic of early infections. The plug center may contain normal feces but later becomes solid and may be removed intact. The mucosa is somewhat thickened and may contain petechial hemorrhages in the dilated portions of the ceca. These plugs disappear 5½–6 days after infection, at which time large numbers of oocysts may be found in the cecal contents.

Histopathology

Although indications of some edema and lymphocytic infiltration may be seen on histopathological examination, these are less extensive than with *E. adenoides* or *E. gallopavonis*. First-generation schizonts develop in surface epithelium of the small intestine; later stages occur chiefly in the cecal epithelium (Clarkson, 1959b). Although trophozoites and schizonts usually develop above the epithelial cell nucleus, the sexual stages more often develop below the nucleus.

Eimeria meleagrimitis Tyzzer 1929

Classification

Of the 4 species which locate in the duodenum and upper jejunum, *E. meleagrimitis* is the most pathogenic. All three asexual generations and the sexual cycle are generally completed in this area. Occasional lesions may extend below the yolk sac diverticulum. The small size and subspherical shape of the oocyst (av. 19.2 × 16.3μ) is a useful diagnostic characteristic. Measurement of a number of oocysts is required to establish the mean and the range. Sporulation may be completed in 18 hours (Bond, 1966).

Pathogenesis and Epizootiology

Experimental infections of young poults have shown 100% mortality following inoculation with 50,000 oocysts (Hawkins, 1952). Age resistance began to appear at 4–6 weeks, but older birds continued to show reduced growth rate (Clarkson, 1959a). Age resistance was found most marked at 50 days of age using comparative oocyst output as a criterion (Warren et al., 1963). In an experimental comparison of pathogenicity equal numbers of oocysts killed 1 of 5 poults with *E. meleagrimitis,* 4 of 5 with *E. gallopavonis,* and 1 of 5 with *E. adenoides.*

Natural and Experimental Hosts

Wild as well as domestic turkeys appear to be the natural host (Prestwood, 1968). Bobwhite quail *Colinus virginianus* and pheasants *Phasianus colchicus* were found refractory to infection by Hawkins (1952) and Edgar (1958). Hungarian partridge *Perdix perdix* and Japanese quail *Coturnix coturnix* have also been found refractory (Hawkins, 1952; Edgar et al., 1964). Hawkins (1952) and Edgar (1958) were unable to infect chickens, but Gill (1954) reported successful infection experiments.

Gross Lesions

Infected birds show symptoms of dehydration as indicated by the skin in the breast area adhering to underlying muscle. In the duodenum, enlargement and congestion are most marked on the 5th and 6th days of infection. A reddish brown necrotic core adhering to the mucosa may be present. In other areas petechial hemorrhages may appear on the mucosal surface. Feces may contain occasional flecks of blood and cylindrical casts 3–6 mm in diameter. Death usually occurs on the 5th to 7th day after infection.

Histopathology

The most marked change is the complete denuding of the epithelium from tips of the villi beginning 5 days after infection. Developing gametocytes cause this disruption. Only the intact basement membrane may separate the blood vessels from the lumen, but hemorrhaging of the type seen in chicken coccidiosis is rare. Eosinophilic infiltration similar to that described for *E. adenoides* may begin as early as 2 hours after infection (Clarkson, 1959a).

The first-generation schizont locates below the host cell nucleus. Other stages may develop above or below, with most parasites developing above the nucleus.

Eimeria subrotunda Moore, Brown, and Carter 1954

Classification

This nonpathogenic species is characterized by production of subspherical oocysts (shape index 1.10) which are devoid of a refractile body. *E. innocua* and *E. dispersa* also lack a refractile body. *E. subrotunda* differs from *E. innocua* and *E. dispersa* in localizing in the area of the intestine anterior to the yolk sac diverticulum. It has a shorter prepatent period than these other 2 species (95 hours compared to 114 and 120 respectively). The only confirmatory studies of this description have been made by Bond (1966), who isolated *E. subrotunda* 4 times in submissions of 44 tissues and 55 litter samples from 21 states.

Natural and Experimental Hosts

The turkey is the only reported host for this parasite; chickens, guinea fowl, pheasants, and bobwhite quail *(Colinus virginianus)* were refractory in experimental infections (Moore et al., 1954).

Gross Lesions and Histopathology

No gross or microscopic lesions have been found following heavy infection with large numbers of oocysts. Parasitic stages usually invade the epithelial cells at the tips of the villi, less commonly occur at the base of the villi, but are never found in the crypts and deep glands.

TREATMENT

Turkeys respond favorably to the use of some but not all of the coccidiostats used with chickens. The different species of turkey coccidia may also show variation in drug response. Treatment may be considered in controlling the species *E. adenoides, E. gallopavonis,* and *E. meleagrimitis.* Following a positive diagnosis drug treatment should be instituted as soon as possible. Best response to most drugs occurs if medication is administered at the same time oocyst exposure occurs. Drug effectiveness progressively decreases for the next 5 days, after which little benefit is derived. Although recommendations are still made by Davies et al. (1963) for an intermittent treatment schedule of 3 days on drug, 2 days off, and 3 days on, others find little benefit to be gained by an interrupted schedule. Although such a schedule could provide partial relief for toxic products, nontoxic drugs are now available. Most treatment programs use water as the most convenient method of administering the drug.

Among drugs currently in use in the United States are: 0.025% sulfaquinoxaline, 0.025% amprolium, 0.03% ESB₃, and 0.2% sulfamethazine. Sulfaquinoxaline and sulfamethazine probably interfere with the paraminobenzoic acid-folic acid sequence (Horton-Smith and Long, 1961). Questionable palatability of sulfamethazine for poults (Wilson, 1951) and possible depression in weight gains (Moore, 1949) make this drug less useful. Amprolium probably acts as a substitute for thiamin, blocking the normal metabolism of the coccidia.

PREVENTION AND CONTROL

Many large turkey producers have experienced sufficient problems with coccidiosis outbreaks that they have resorted to use of a preventive coccidiostat for birds 3–8 weeks of age. Preventive coccidiostats provide drug protection earlier in the life cycle of the parasite than does treatment, which frequently comes too late to be very effective. A difficult decision must often be faced as to whether histomoniasis or coccidiosis should be treated. Simultaneous use of two drugs has not been approved by the Food and Drug Administration. Both diseases produce heaviest losses between 1 and 3 months of age. Unfortunately the high cost of obtaining clearance has prevented pharmaceutical companies from developing the data necessary for such approval. Preventive coccidiostat programs are frequently used in eastern, midwestern, and central southern United States. Their use appears to be more limited in southeastern and western areas where use may be restricted to isolated farms or endemic areas showing coccidiosis problems. Coccidiostats are almost universally used in England and western Europe.

Drugs currently approved for use as feed medication include: sulfaquinoxaline (0.0125%), amprolium (0.0125%), Polystat (0.030% sulfanitran, 0.020% butynorate, and 0.020% dinsed), butynorate (0.0375%), 2,4-diamino-5 (para-chlorophenyl)-6-ethyl pyrimidine (0.003–0.006%), 2-sulfanilamidoquinoxaline (0.01–0.02%), and zoalene (0.0125%).

Other methods of prevention are similar to those used in controlling chicken coccidiosis. Immunity usually develops in the course of natural exposure by the time birds are 3 months of age. Control recommendations should include preventing exposure to wet areas on range or in houses.

REFERENCES

Bond, D. S. 1966. The incidence of turkey coccidia in the United States with details on certain species. Ph.D. dissertation, Auburn Univ., Auburn, Ala.

Boughton, R. V. 1937. Endoparasitic infestations in grouse, their pathogenicity and correlation with meteoro-topographical conditions. *Univ. Minn. Agr. Expt. Sta. Tech. Bull.* 121.

Clarkson, M. J. 1958. Life history and pathogenicity of *Eimeria adenoeides* Moore and Brown, 1951, in the turkey poult. *Parasitology* 48: 70–88.

———. 1959a. The life history and pathogenicity of *Eimeria meleagrimitis* Tyzzer, 1929, in the turkey poult. *Parasitology* 49:70–82.

———. 1959b. The life history and pathogenicity of *Eimeria meleagridis* Tyzzer, 1927, in the turkey poult. *Parasitology* 49:519–28.

Davies, S. F. M., L. P. Joyner, and S. B. Kendall. 1963. *Coccidiosis.* Oliver and Boyd, Edinburgh.

Edgar, S. A. 1958. Coccidiosis of chickens and turkeys and control by immunization. *Eleventh World's Poultry Congr. Avicultura* 3:415–21.

Edgar, S. A., R. Waggoner, and C. Flanagan. 1964. Susceptibility of Coturnix quail to certain disease producing agents common to poultry. *Poultry Sci.* 43:1315. (Abstr.)

Farr, Marion M. 1964. Life cycle of *Eimeria gallopavonis* Hawkins in the turkey. *J. Parasitol.* 50 (Sec. 2): 52. (Abstr.)

Farr, Marion M., E. E. Wehr, and W. T. Shalkop. 1961. Pathogenicity of *Eimeria gallopavonis*. *Virginia J. Sci.* 12:150–51.

Gill, B. S. 1954. Transmissibility of turkey coccidia. *(Eimeria meleagridis, E. meleagrimitis* and *E. gallopavonis)* to chickens. *Indian Vet. J.* 31:92–98.

Hawkins, P. A. 1952. Coccidiosis in turkeys. *Mich. State Univ. Agr. Expt. Sta. Tech. Bull.* 226.

Hinshaw, W. R. 1965. Coccidiosis, pp. 1329–31. In Biester, H. E., and L. H. Schwarte, (eds.), *Diseases of Poultry,* 5th ed. Iowa State Univ. Press, Ames,

Horton-Smith, C., and P. L. Long. 1961. Effect of sulfonamide medication on the life cycle of *Eimeria meleagrimitis* in turkeys. *Exp. Parasitol.* 11:93–101.

Levine, N. D. 1961. *Protozoan Parasites of Domestic Animals and of Man.* Burgess Publ. Co., Minneapolis.

Lin, T. C., and S. A. Edgar. 1970. Preliminary report on a coccidium of turkeys, *Eimeria* n. sp. (Protozoa: Eimeriidae). *Poultry Sci.* 49:1406.

Lund, E. E., and Marion M. Farr. 1965. Protozoa, pp. 1056–96. In Biester H. E., and L. H. Schwarte (eds.), *Diseases of Poultry,* 5th ed. Iowa State Univ. Press, Ames.

Moore, E. N. 1949. Sulfaquinoxaline as a treatment for coccidiosis in turkeys. *Cornell Vet.* 39:223–28.

Moore, E. N., and J. A. Brown. 1951. A new coccidium pathogenic for turkeys, *Eimeria adenoeides* n. sp. (Protozoa: Eimeriidae). *Cornell Vet.* 41:124–35.

———. 1952. A new coccidium of turkeys, *Eimeria innocua* n. sp. (Protozoa: Eimeriidae). *Cornell Vet.* 42:395–402.

Moore, E. N., J. A. Brown, and R. D. Carter. 1954. A new coccidium of turkeys, *Eimeria subrotunda* n. sp. (Protozoa: Eimeriidae). *Poultry Sci.* 33:925–29.

Morehouse, N. F. 1949. Coccidiosis as a disease of turkeys. *Ann. N.Y. Acad. Sci.* 52: 501–4.

Pellérdy, L. P. 1965. *Coccidia and Coccidiosis.* Akademiai Kiado, Budapest.

Prestwood, Annie K. 1968. Parasitism among wild turkeys *(Meleagris gallopavo silvestris)* of the Mississippi Delta. Ph.D. dissertation, Univ. Georgia, Athens.

Slavin, D. 1955. *Cryptosporidium meleagridis* (sp. nov.). *J. Comp. Pathol. Therap.* 65: 262–70.

Steward, J. S. 1947. Host-parasite specificity in coccidia: Infection of the chicken with the turkey coccidium, *Eimeria meleagridis*. *Parasitology* 38:157–59.

Svanbaev, S. K. 1955. A new species of coccidia in turkeys. (In Russian.) *Trans. Inst. Zool. Akad. Nauk. Kaz. SSSR.* 3:161–63.

Tyzzer, E. E. 1929. Coccidiosis in gallinaceous birds. *Am. J. Hyg.* 10:269–383.

Warren, E. W., S. J. Ball, and Joan R. Fagg. 1963. Age resistance by turkeys to *Eimeria meleagrimitis,* Tyzzer, 1929. *Nature* 200: 238–40.

Wehr, E. E., Marion M. Farr, and W. T. Shalkop. 1962. Studies on pathogenicity of *Eimeria gallopavonis* to turkeys. *J. Protozool.* 9:8–9.

Wilson, J. E. 1951. Sulphaquinoxaline and sulphamezathine in the treatment of experimentally induced caecal coccidiosis of chickens *(E. tenella)* and in natural outbreaks of coccidiosis in turkeys *(E. meleagridis* and *E. meleagrimitis).* *Vet. Record* 63:373–77.

GOOSE

Renal coccidiosis in geese, a disease producing severe inflammatory reactions confined to the kidneys, has been described frequently in technical reports. The parasitic stages of *Eimeria truncata* localize in the tubules, blocking kidney function, and may produce very high mortality of young goslings in an explosive epizootic. Intestinal coccidiosis is more common than renal coccidiosis (Klimeš, 1963; Pellérdy, 1965) in areas of central Europe, where the goose is a bird of commercial importance. In a review of 10 species from wild geese and swans (Hanson et al., 1957), several species are included from the domestic goose. Wild geese are undoubtedly involved in the introduction and distribution of coccidia to domestic geese.

Eimeria truncata Railliet and Lucet 1891

Flock losses approaching 100% within a period of 2–3 days have occurred in the United States and other parts of the world. In Iowa 87% mortality was found on a farm one year, but the following year mortality was reduced to 12% (McNutt, 1929). Geese affected usually range between 3 and 12 weeks of age. The disease is acute in goslings which show depression, weakness, diarrhea with whitish feces, and anorexia. Eyes become dull and sunken while the wings are drooped. Survivors may show vertigo and torticollis as evidenced by a staggering gait, twisted neck, or lying on the back. Development of flock immunity is generally prompt.

Classification

Oocysts and endogenous stages of *E. truncata* are found only in the kidneys or in the cloaca near the junction of the ureters. The route of infection into the kidneys is unknown, but presence of oocysts and endogenous stages in other parts of the digestive tract is produced by another species. Diagnosis of *E. truncata* is assured by recognition of the distinctive shape and size of the oocyst. The smooth-walled, oval oocyst has a truncated end. A micropyle and polar cap are present and located at the truncated end. Oocysts range from 14–27μ (av. 21.3) in length by 12–22μ (av. 16.7) in width. An oocyst residuum is usually present and a sporocyst residuum is also found. Sporulation time has varied from 1 to 5 days and the prepatent period is 5–6 days.

Pathogenesis and Epizootiology

Some investigators consider the high mortality and explosive nature of outbreaks due to accidental introductions of oocysts into the flock. However, demonstration of oocysts over widespread areas in Hungary and inability to produce severe mortality experimentally suggest that other unknown factors are involved in outbreaks (Pellérdy, 1965). The moist environment near watering places often provides ideal conditions for the accumulating oocysts to sporulate. Gradual development of protective immunity is probably an important factor in preventing disastrous outbreaks.

Natural and Experimental Hosts

Although primarily a parasite of domestic and wild geese (*Anser anser, A. rossi, Branta canadensis*), rare reports of infection in ducks and swans have been described (Pellérdy, 1965). These infections may represent another species. Severe losses attributed to *E. truncata* have been reported in the Canadian goose *Branta canadensis* (Farr, 1954).

Gross Lesions

On necropsy kidneys may appear as enlarged thumb-sized bodies which protrude from the sacral bed. The normal reddish brown color is altered to light grayish yellow or red. Faintly demarcated grayish white foci the size of a pinhead or streaks along with hemorrhagic petechiae may be seen. The grayish white foci contain accumulations of urates and large numbers of oocysts.

Histopathology

Lesions, commonly present in foci, show reaction to mechanical pressure as well as the presence of invading parasites in the epithelium of the kidney tubules. Engorged tubules with discharging parasites, disintegrating host cells, and urates may be 5–10 times normal size. Round-cell aggregations may appear throughout the renal tissue; eosinophilia and signs of necrosis are present in the focal areas. The parasite displaces the host cell nucleus laterally while producing marked hypertrophy of the host cell.

INTESTINAL SPECIES

The 4 species (Klimeš, 1963) or 5 species (Pellérdy, 1965) of coccidia developing in the intestinal tract of the domestic goose vary greatly in pathogenicity. Although each species is somewhat selective in area of digestive tract parasitized, zones of infection are not as clearly demarcated as in the chicken. Severe morbidity problems are caused by infection with *Eimeria anseris*. Most of the goslings dying of infection are parasitized also with *E. nocens*. Although this latter species alone is relatively innocuous, the double infection appears to produce a severe condition. *Tyzzeria parvula* (*E. parvula* or *T. anseris*, according to Klimeš, 1963) does not produce mortality following heavy artificial infection. Extensive destruction of the epithelium covering the tips of the villi suggests that there are morbidity losses from this species. *E. stigmosa* is nonpathogenic and noteworthy chiefly in complicating the problem of diagnosis.

Eimeria anseris Kotlan 1933

Classification

Differences in oocysts are used in recognition of the various species found in the goose. *E. anseris* oocysts are colorless and pear-shaped, average 19.2 × 16.6μ, and have a shape index of 1.16 (Klimeš, 1963).

Differentiation is required from: *E. nocens* Kotlán (1933) which have brown elliptical oocysts averaging $30 \times 23\mu$ and a shape index of 1.28; *E. stigmosa* Klimeš (1963) which have large, brown oval oocysts with a punctate surface, measure $23 \times 16.7\mu$, and have a shape index of 1.38; *E. truncata*, the renal species described above, which have colorless, egg-shaped, truncated oocysts measuring $21.3 \times 16.7\mu$ and a shape index of 1.27; *T. parvula* whose oocysts are colorless, lack a micropyle, are moderately elliptic to spherical, measure $14.8 \times 12.8\mu$, and have an index of 1.16. Oocysts of the last-named species show the usual genus characteristics which include presence of 8 free sporozoites which lack sporocysts.

Differentiation between intestinal coccidiosis and paratyphoid or other bacterial pathogens needs to be considered.

Pathogenesis and Epizootiology

E. anseris may produce hemorrhagic enteritis which terminates fatally in 9-month-old geese (Pellérdy, 1965). Anorexia, tottering gait, debility, and diarrhea are the clinical symptoms. The small intestine becomes enlarged and filled with thin reddish brown fluid. Catarrhal inflammatory lesions are most intense in the middle and lower portions of the small intestine. There may be large whitish nodules or a fibrinous diphtheroid necrotic enteritis. Underneath dry pseudomembranous flakes, the oocysts and endogenous stages of the parasite may be demonstrated in large numbers. Parasitic stages invade the epithelial cells of the posterior half of the intestine in closely packed rows. Developing gametocytes penetrate more deeply into the subepithelial tissues of the villi.

TREATMENT

Various sulfonamide drugs have been used in treatment of both renal and intestinal coccidiosis of geese. Some of these studies have indicated a favorable response, but unfortunately there are no reports of trials in which adequate controls were used. With such a self-limiting disease, inclusion of a group of unmedicated controls is essential before reports can be considered reliable.

PREVENTION AND CONTROL

Control measures have sometimes required removal of flocks from highly contaminated areas (Pellérdy, 1965). Damp areas near watering places containing high concentrations of oocysts should be avoided with young goslings until some protective immunity has developed. Separation of young from older stock has also been suggested. In areas where coccidiosis produces problems, controlled testing of preventive coccidiostats would be worthwhile.

REFERENCES

Farr, Marion M. 1954. Renal coccidiosis of Canada geese. *J. Parasitol.* 40:46.

Hanson, H. C., N. D. Levine, and Virginia Ivens. 1957. Coccidia (Protozoa: Eimeriidae) of North American wild geese and swans. *Can. J. Zool.* 35:715–33.

Klimeš, B. 1963. Coccidia of the domestic goose *(Anser anser dom.).* *Zentr. Veterinaermed.* B 10:427–48.

Kotlán, A. 1933. Zur Kenntnis der Kokzidiose des Wassergefluegels. Die Kokzidiose der Hausgans. *Zentr. Bakteriol. Parasitenk. Abt. I. Orig.* 129:11–21.

McNutt, S. H. 1929. Renal coccidiosis of geese. *J. Am. Vet. Med. Ass.* 75:365–69.

Pellérdy, L. P. 1965. *Coccidia and Coccidiosis.* Akademiai Kiado, Budapest.

Railliet, A., and A. Lucet. 1891. Note sur quelques especes de coccidies encore peu etudiees. *Bull. Soc. Zool. France* 16:246–51.

DUCKS

Coccidiosis outbreaks, although reported sporadically, occur with sufficient frequency to warrant more study than they have thus far received. Cases involving moderate to heavy mortality have been reported on domestic duck farms from New York State (Allen, 1936; Dougherty, 1952) and New Jersey (Leibovitz, 1967, 1968), Hungary (Pellérdy, 1965), and Japan (Inoue, 1967). Wild duck die-offs of the Lesser Scaup *(Aythya affinis)* in north central states (Farr, 1965) and of the Goldeneye *(Bucephala clangula)* in Denmark (Christiansen and Madsen, 1948) have been reported. In samplings from 75% of the duck farms on Long Island, infectious coccidial oocysts in droppings and litter have been recovered from each farm by Leibovitz (1969, personal communication). He concluded that on Long Island (and probably wherever ducks are maintained in large numbers) a continuous cycle of coccidial infection exists, although clinical infection may be undetected. Literature reviews tend to emphasize fatal infections in young susceptible ducklings that appear as explosive, dramatic outbreaks. This feature is probably related to those striking exceptions in normal duck farming where totally susceptible ducklings are placed in heavily contaminated environments.

Use of chemotherapy for preventive medication using sulfaquinoxaline, nicarbazin, glycamide, Trithiadole, and sulfaguanidine were found ineffective (Dougherty, 1952, 1959). The common sulfa drugs (sulfamethazine and sulfaquinoxaline) have been employed successfully in the treatment of clinical coccidiosis (Leibovitz, 1969, personal communication). Avoidance of introducing young stock to areas highly contaminated with oocysts is a very practical recommendation.

CLASSIFICATION

Unfortunately, many of the 15 species of coccidia reported from domestic and wild ducks have been insufficiently described for diagnostic purposes. Until more studies similar to the one conducted by Leibovitz (1968) with *Wenyonella philiplevinei* have been completed, identification of many species will remain in doubt. Species descriptions as outlined by Tyzzer (1932) require establishment of pure strains by single oocyst isolation, adequate description of the endogenous stages, and some description of pathogenicity following artificial infection with a single strain. The common practice of partially describing new species after study of the oocyst alone is a disservice to those interested in the study of poultry diseases. Brief descriptions of sufficiently described species are herein included, while incompletely described species or those known only from wild ducks are mentioned only by name.

Classification to genus by the diagnostician is worthwhile and can readily be accomplished by comparing sporulated oocysts (Figs. 31.1, 31.2). From very incomplete information now available, it may be suggested that the most pathogenic species may belong to the genera Eimeria and Tyzzeria while Wenyonella is of lesser importance. Some species are entirely nonpatho-

genic (Leibovitz, 1969, personal communication). A double infection involving more than one genus is probably more pathogenic than single infections (Davies, 1957; Leibovitz, 1968).

Eimeria saitamae Inoue 1967, described from a disease outbreak in domestic ducks in Japan, has a smooth-surfaced oocyst measuring 18.6μ long $\times$ 13.2μ wide. It has a double wall 0.7–0.8μ thick with a micropyle at the narrower end. Sporulation requires 72 hours; the prepatent period is 4 days. Other described species from the domestic duck include *E. battakhi* Dubey and Pande 1963 from India and *E. danailovi* Grafner, Graubmann and Betke 1965 from Germany. The mallard duck (*Anas platyrhynchos platyrhynchos*) is host for *E. anatis* Scholtyseck 1955 from Germany and *E. boschadis* Walden 1961 from Sweden. The latter description is of doubtful validity since only an unsporulated oocyst is described. *E. aythyae* Farr 1965 has been described from the Lesser Scaup in the United States and *E. bucephalae* Christiansen and Madsen 1948 from the Goldeneye in Denmark.

Tyzzeria perniciosa Allen 1936, found in domestic ducks in the United States, has thin-walled oocysts (0.5μ) which are oval, colorless, and without a micropyle; measure 10–12.3×9–10.8μ; and upon sporulation produce 8 free sporozoites within the oocyst in the absence of sporocysts. Several other species have been described from the oocyst alone from various species of wild ducks.

The oocysts of *Wenyonella philiplevinei* Leibovitz 1968 measure 15.5–21μ (av. 18.7) $\times$ 12.5–16μ (av. 14.4) and contain a micropyle opening 2μ wide, 1–2 polar granules, and no oocyst residuum. The three-layered wall has a yellowish blue middle wall and green striated inner wall. Minimum sporulation time is 33 hours, with sporocysts averaging $9.4 \times 6.1\mu$ and containing a residual mass and 4 sporozoites. But 6–8 merozoites are formed in the first- and second-generation schizonts. The zone of the intestine parasitized extends from the posterior jejunal annular band to the rectum. The prepatent period is 93 hours. *W. pellerdyi* Bhatia and Pande 1966 from the blue-winged teal (*Anas querquedula* L.) and *W. anatis* Pande, Bhatia and Srivastava 1965 from domestic ducks have been described but only from the oocyst. They differ from *W. philiplevinei* in the presence of clear walls.

PATHOGENESIS AND EPIZOOTIOLOGY

Only brief descriptions of symptoms and pathology are available. Anorexia, weight loss, weakness, inability to stand, and continuous distress as indicated by crying were described as symptoms in *T. perniciosa* infection (Allen, 1936). Seven of 10 experimentally infected ducklings died. Hemorrhagic areas were heaviest in the anterior half of the intestine but found throughout its length. Bloody or cheesy exudate was frequent but cores were absent. Sloughing of the epithelial lining occurred in long sheets. Deep invasion of both mucosal and submucosal layers of the intestinal wall penetrated as far as the muscular layers. An outbreak in England showed acute hemorrhagic diarrhea on the 4th day following exposure (Davies, 1957). Peak of mortality occurred on the 5th and 6th days. Both Tyzzeria and Eimeria oocysts were recovered, but species were not recorded.

W. philiplevinei produced pathogenic effects limited to 72–96 hours after inoculation. Occasional petechial hemorrhages were seen in the posterior ileal mucosa. Diffuse congestion was found in the rectal mucosa. One of 120 experimentally infected ducklings died of coccidiosis on the 4th day.

REFERENCES

Allen, Ena A. 1936. *Tyzzeria perniciosa* gen. et sp. nov. a coccidium from the small intestine of the Pekin duck, *Anas domesticus* L. *Arch. Protistenk.* B 87:262–69.

Bhatia, B. B., and B. P. Pande. 1966. On two new species of coccidia from wild anatidae. *Acta Vet. Acad. Sci. Hung.* 16:335–40.

Christiansen, M., and H. Madsen. 1948. *Eimeria bucephalae* n. sp. (coccidia) pathogenic in Goldeneye *(Bucephala clangula* L.) in Denmark. *Danish Rev. Game Biol.* 1:63–73.

Davies, S. F. M. 1957. An outbreak of duck coccidiosis in Britain. *Vet. Record* 69: 1051–52.

Dougherty, E. 1952. Coccidiosis in ducks. *Ann. Rept. N.Y. State Vet. Coll.*, p. 31.

———. 1959. Duck coccidiosis. *Ann. Rept. N. Y. State Vet. Coll.* 89:48.

Dubey, J. P., and B. P. Pande. 1963. A preliminary note on *Eimeria battakhi*, n. sp. (Protozoa: Eimeriidae) from domestic duck *(Anas Platyrhynchos platyrhynchos domesticus)*. *Current Sci.* 32:329–31.

Farr, Marion M. 1965. Coccidiosis of the Lesser Scaup duck *Aythya affinis* (Eyton, 1838) with a description of a new species, *Eimeria aythyae*. *Proc. Helminthol. Soc. Wash. D.C.* 32:236–38.

Gräfner, G., H. D. Graubmann, and P. Betke. 1965. Duenndarmkokzidiose bei Hausenten, verursacht durch eine neue Kokzidiernart, *Eimeria danailovi* n. sp. *Monatsh. Veterinaermed.* 20:141–43.

Inoue, I. 1967. *Eimeria saitamae* n. sp.: A new cause of coccidiosis in domestic ducks *(Anas platyrhyncha* var. *domestica)*. *Japan. J. Vet. Sci.* 29:209–15.

Leibovitz, L. 1967. Anatine coccidiosis. *Ann. Rept. N.Y. State Vet. Coll. 1966–67*, p. 86.

———. 1968. *Wenyonella philiplevinei*, n. sp., a coccidial organism of the White Pekin duck. *Avian Diseases* 12:670–81.

Pande, B. P., B. B. Bhatia, K. M. N. Srivastava. 1965. *Weyonella anatis*, n. sp. (Protozoa: Eimeriidae) from Indian domestic duck. *Sci. Cult. Calcutta* 31:383–84.

Pellérdy, L. P. 1965. *Coccidia and Coccidiosis*. *Akademiai Kiado, Budapest*.

Scholtyseck, E. 1955. *Eimeria anatis* n. sp., ein neues Coccidaus der Stockente *(Anas platyrhynchos)*. *Arch. Protistenk.* B 100:431–35.

Tyzzer, E. E. 1932. Criteria and methods in the investigation of avian coccidiosis. *Science* 75:324–28.

Walden, H. W. 1961. Observations on renal coccidia in Swedish anseriform birds, with notes concerning two new species, *Eimeria boschadis,* and *Eimeria christianseni* (Sporozoa, Telosporidia). *Arkiv. Zool.* 15:97–104.

PIGEONS

Coccidiosis in pigeons is similar but generally less severe than intestinal coccidiosis induced by *E. necatrix* in chickens. Young pigeons suffer greatest losses, but high mortality may occur also in birds as old as 3–4 months. Since pigeons are raised for racing, as carrier pigeons, and in some areas for commercial production of squabs as a food specialty, the avian pathologist may be called upon for advice in diagnosis, treatment, or control of disease.

CLASSIFICATION

Eimeria labbeana (Labbe, 1896) Pinto, 1928, is the species recognized most frequently. Oocysts are spherical to subspherical, averaging 19.1μ (14.5–24.1) in length × 17.4μ (12.1–22.5) in width. The oocysts produced early in the patent period may be considerably smaller than those appearing later (Duncan, 1959). Based on these studies showing size increase with older infections, Levine (1961) has questioned the validity of the species *E. columbarum* Nieschulz, 1935. It had been differentiated from *E. labbeana* chiefly on the basis of greater oocyst size. One other species, *E. columbae* Mitra and Das Gupta 1937, has been incompletely described.

PATHOGENESIS AND EPIZOOTIOLOGY

Mortality is most severe in squabs which have just left the nest. Cases of 60% mortality in the Washington, D.C., area have been reported (Morse, 1908). Of 110 case reports of pigeon disease by Hare (1937) in England, 15% were due to coccidiosis. Problems have been recorded in California and on Long Island (Levi, 1957). In Germany at least 55% of the carrier pigeons and 70% of the racing pigeons were found infected (Hauser, 1959). Older birds rarely show symptoms, but subclinical infection may persist for long periods since little self-limiting immunity is developed. Anorexia, thirst, and greenish diarrhea followed by marked dehydration and emaciation are the typical symptoms. Limited quantities of blood may be passed in severe cases. Inflammation of the entire digestive tract is the principal observation on necropsy. The common condition of "going light" is frequently attributed to coccidiosis (Miller, 1964).

TREATMENT

Favorable response has been reported following administration of sulfonamides (sulfamethazine, sulfaguanidine, or sulfaquinoxaline) or nitrofurazone in drinking water (Hauser, 1959; Miller, 1964). Although Hauser suggests use of the same level of medication used for chickens, Miller advocates half this level. Well-controlled studies on use of medication have not been reported.

PREVENTION AND CONTROL

Control of excess moisture in lofts or cages is the most important management procedure. Oocysts do not remain viable for long periods in a dry environment. Daily cleaning of cages has been suggested for very valuable stock.

REFERENCES

Duncan, S. 1959. The size of the oocysts of *Eimeria labbeana*. *J. Parasitol.* 45:191–92.

Hare, Tom. 1937. A study of 110 consecutive cases of disease in pigeons. *Vet. Record* 49:680–86.

Hauser, K. W. 1959. Erfahrungen bei der Bekaempfung der Kokzidiose der Tauben. *Berlin. Muench. Tieraerztl. Wochschr.* 72:481–83.

Labbe, A. 1896. Recherches zoologiques, cytologiques et biologiques sur les coccidies. *Arch. Zool. Exp. Gen.* 4 (Ser. 3):517–654.

Levi, W. M. 1957. *The Pigeon.* Levi Publ. Co., Sumter, S.C.

Levine, N. D. 1961. *Protozoan Parasites of Domestic Animals and of Man.* Burgess Publ. Co., Minneapolis.

Miller, L. K. 1964. A primer on racing pigeons. *Mod. Vet. Pract.* 45:36–38.

Mitra, A. N., and M. Das Gupta. 1937. On a species of Eimeria (Coccidia: Sporozoa) from the intestine of a pigeon, *Columba intermedia. Proc. Indian Sci. Congr. Ass.* 24:291. (Abstr.)

Morse, G. B. 1908. White diarrhea of chicks. *USDA BAI Circ.* 128:7.

Nieschluz, O. 1935. Ueber Kokzidien der Haustauben. *Zentr. Bakteriol. Parasitenk. Abt. I. Orig.* 134:390–93.

Pinto, C. 1928. Synonymie de quelques especes du genre Eimeria (Eimeriida, Sporozoa). *Soc. Biol.* 1:1564–65.

HISTOMONIASIS

❖

EVERETT E. LUND

Veterinary Sciences Research Division
Agricultural Research Service
United States Department of Agriculture
Beltsville, Maryland

❖

HISTOMONIASIS, also frequently known as enterohepatitis or blackhead, is a protozoan disease of the lower digestive tract (usually the ceca and liver) of turkeys, chickens, and several other gallinaceous birds.

Once a scourge that almost wiped out the turkey industry in the United States, it is presently responsible for the death of only about 0.5% of the birds started each year. From 1962 through 1966, this percentage represented an average annual loss of about $1.7 million. Losses among breeders, although less frequent, were also costly. The average annual mortality loss as a direct result of histomoniasis among turkeys probably exceeded $2 million. Losses sustained as a result of morbidity causing poor feed conversion, delays in marketing, downgrading, and reduced production among breeders have been estimated to exceed those from outright mortality by as much as 1.5 times.

Among chickens the incidence of mortality as a result of histomoniasis is much lower than among turkeys, but the industry is so much larger that the monetary loss sustained by the growers may exceed that of the turkey industry.

Some of our most cherished upland game birds are quite susceptible to histomoniasis. It is not possible to place a monetary value on losses among these species. However, the annual expenditure required to maintain some of them for their esthetic or recreational values is very substantial, and larger because of the annual toll taken by histomoniasis.

HISTORY

Apparently the first published report of the occurrence in the United States of a disease now considered to be histomoniasis was that of Rice (1892). Soon Cushman (1894) gave a brief description of the disease and called it "Black Head."

On the basis of material provided by Cushman, Smith (1895) decided that he was dealing with "a specific infectious disease" and that "the cause of this disease was a protozoan parasite not hitherto recognized." After a more thorough study, Smith gave a detailed description of the disease and of the organism that caused it. He renamed the disease "infectious entero-hepatitis" and named the protozoon that caused it *"Amoeba meleagridis."*

The decade following Smith's work was largely one of recognition of the disease, which actually was already widespread. Chester and Robin (1901) apparently were the first to report it from chickens. However, the most significant progress was made by Curtice (1907a,b), whose major contributions probably were: (1) that chickens are an important source of contamination of soil with blackhead parasites; (2) that adult turkeys may also be important in this respect; (3) that such contamination is more common in heavy moist soils than in light, dry, or barren soils; and (4) that by feeding earthworms from contaminated soils to poults one may sometimes produce enterohepatitis.

The decade following publication of Curtice's works was characterized by the confusion of enterohepatitis with other diseases of poultry, principally coccidiosis and trichomoniasis. Smith (1910, 1915) bitterly protested the confusion that he had cautioned against in his initial report. Ultimately he and an associate, Graybill, discovered that a small parasitic worm, Heterakis, was involved in the transmission of the blackhead parasite (Graybill and Smith, 1920), but they were not clear as to the role played by the parasitic worm. Meanwhile, Dr. Tyzzer discovered that the organism causing blackhead was not an amoeba but a flagellated protozoon capable of amoeboid movement (1920), and he renamed the organism *Histomonas meleagridis.*

During the next 15 years, Tyzzer and his students in more than 20 reports explored almost every phase of histomoniasis that has been studied to this time.

The most important contributions during the first two decades after Tyzzer completed his studies were in the field of drug control. Development of practical measures of chemical control permitted an unprecedented rise in turkey production (see section on Treatment). However, during the past decade there has been a revival of interest in biological control.

More complete historical accounts have been published recently (Reid, 1967; Lund, 1969).

INCIDENCE AND DISTRIBUTION

Histomoniasis has been reported from nearly every region in which susceptible gallinaceous birds exist with the vectors required for transmission of the histomonad. In general, the disease seems to be no problem north of the 60th parallel or south of the 45th parallel. However, such arbitrary boundaries are very deceiving. In much of the temperate zones the disease is absent or almost so, especially where soils are dry and barren or even light and sandy. Also, at higher elevations with long severe winters, histomoniasis seems to be absent among the wild gallinaceous birds that frequent such habitats. The disease is usually not prevalent in areas where earthworms are absent or infrequent.

Before the widespread use of histomonacidal drugs, the incidence of histomoniasis among turkeys bore a conspicuous relationship to soil and climate. Thus in 1952 and 1953 histomoniasis mortality among turkeys in California was only about 0.2% (Lund, 1954). In flocks raised in the dry interior valleys or on the fringe of the desert, the disease was almost absent. About the same time, histomoniasis mortality among turkeys in Virginia and Maryland was about 1.2% (author's unpublished data); it was 1.78% among young birds and 1.85% among breeding turkeys in Minnesota (Bergersen, 1952). Less than a decade later it was only one-third as prevalent in Minnesota. Comparable figures from other areas are not available.

Certainly the incidence of the disease still varies, but, as previously indicated, it is now fairly low. Even in cool climates with soil and rainfall capable of supporting abundant vegetation, mortality in turkeys is probably less than 0.5%.

Histomoniasis may be increasing among chickens (Ohara and Reid, 1961). At least

it has been reported with increasing frequency. As yet, data are meager, but reports from various diagnostic laboratories seem to indicate that the disease now occurs about one-sixth to one-tenth as frequently among chickens as among turkeys reared in the same region.

ETIOLOGY

CLASSIFICATION

Histomonas meleagridis (Smith 1895) Tyzzer 1920 is a flagellated protozoon, long considered to be of the family Mastigamoebidae but recently assigned by Honigberg and Kuldova (1969) to the trichomonad family Monocercomonadidae. *Histomonas meleagridis* is the only known species of the genus Histomonas, the nonpathogenic histomonad formerly known as *H. wenrichi* Lund 1963 becoming *Parahistomonas wenrichi* (Lund 1963) comb. nov.

Tyzzer (1920) established the genus Histomonas for the organism that Smith (1895) had named *Amoeba meleagridis* but later referred to as *Ameba meleagridis* (1915). No other synonyms exist. To the layman the organism is known merely as "the blackhead parasite," a circumstance that has caused much confusion (Reid, 1967).

MORPHOLOGY

In the definitive host, *H. meleagridis* exists in two forms, one that characteristically inhabits the tissues as an intercellular parasite and the other primarily a lumen dweller. Each will be described as it is known from fresh preparations maintained at or near the body temperature of the host and as it is viewed in fixed and stained preparations.

Tissue Form

In fresh preparations resting organisms conform closely with Smith's original description (1895). He observed them as circular or oval, 8–14μ in diameter, and almost structureless except for the nucleus, which had a granular appearance. Actually the diameter of undistorted individuals may vary from about 6 to 20μ. The nucleus is about 3μ in diameter. Several years after Smith had published his original description, he studied the organism again, using a warm chamber. In 1915 he reported as follows: "Some of the freed parasites . . . pushed out small, finger-like pseudopodia, usually one at a time." Tyzzer (1919) depicted organisms showing considerably more motility. We now know that histomonads taken directly from the tissues may possess as many as 6–7 blunt pseudopodia (lobopodia) at one time. Infrequently, tissue-type histomonads may form one or a few filamentous pseudopodia, some of which may be quite long, occasionally branching. The nature of the surroundings probably influences the type of pseudopodia formed. The two types seem not to occur together.

Fixation almost always shrinks Histomonas, a circumstance to which both Smith and Tyzzer called attention. However, stained specimens show more internal structure. Smith (1895) detected an intranuclear "(nucleolar?)" body, and Tyzzer (1919) noted adjacent to the nucleus an "extranuclear body" from which delicate filaments radiated out over the surface of the nuclear membrane. He also noted that division of the extranuclear body resulted in the formation of a paradesmose that persisted until division of the

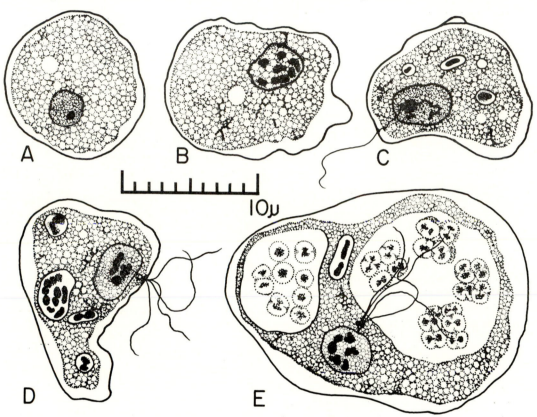

FIG. 31.7—Examples of Histomonas meleagridis (**A**, **B**, and **C**) compared with P. wenrichi (**D** and **E**), showing for each species variations associated with environmental conditions. (**A**) Tissue type H. meleagridis in fresh preparation from liver lesion; viewed with phase contrast. (**B**) H. meleagridis in transitional stage in lumen of the cecum. Pseudopodia have been formed, and the distribution of chromatin suggests that binary fission is approaching. However, the flagellum has not yet appeared. (**C**) An organism in same cecal preparation as **B**, but this one completely adapted as a lumen dweller. (**D**) Small P. wenrichi, structurally distinguishable from H. meleagridis by presence of four flagella. (**E**) P. wenrichi as viewed in stained smear from cecum in which packets of Sarcina were abundant. All figures from camera lucida tracings. Organisms **B**, **C** and **D** from portions of ceca fixed in Zenker's fluid, sectioned at 6 or 8μ, and stained with Heidenhain's (**B** and **C**) or Wiegert's (**D**) iron-hematoxylin. Smear from which **E** was selected was fixed in Schaudinn's fluid with 10% glacial acetic acid. (Lund, original)

nucleus had taken place, after which cell division occurred. Tyzzer had not yet observed a flagellum, probably because it is not often developed by the tissue-dwelling form. Nevertheless, he remarked that "the presence of an extranuclear body resembling the blepharoplast of flagellates and a type of nuclear division characteristic of certain flagellates, sets it apart from all known amoebae." He later concluded that "reclassification of the parasite should not be attempted until additional facts have been obtained concerning its life history." With appropriate stains chromophilic granules may be observed in the nucleus. Often these line the nuclear membrane, but sometimes they are consolidated into discrete bodies suggestive of chromosomes (Fig. 31.7B).

Lumen Form

Scarcely had Tyzzer published his account of an internal structure suggestive of a flagellate before he observed movements so suggestive of flagellar activity that he renamed the organism *Histomonas meleagridis* (Tyzzer, 1920). He had not yet observed an external flagellum. However, he had noted that organisms showing rhythmic rotations through 90–120° that must result from the beat of one or a few flagella did not appear early in the disease. The long-sought flagellum was first observed by Tyzzer and Fabyan (1922) while studying histomonads from the cecal contents of a turkey experimentally infected 28 days earlier. Later, Tyzzer (1924) reported flagellated forms in the ceca of chickens.

In warm, freshly prepared smears, the most conspicuous characteristic of the lumen-dwelling histomonad is unquestionably the brisk turn imparted by the beat of the flagellum. However, at no time do all of the lumen dwellers display such movement. Some move the flagellum only feebly or not at all. Many (sometimes most) of the histomonads form pseudopodia, the positions of which bear no relation to that of the flagellum. With phase microscopy, or with the illumination carefully adjusted, bacteria and other particulate matter can be observed in the endoplasm. Holozoic feeding is as characteristic of the lumen-dwelling histomonad as saprozoic nutrition is of the tissue dweller. Occasionally histomonads in sinusoids of the liver or in areas of liquefaction of tissues develop flagella. They may also feed on cellular debris, so the endoplasm is not homogeneous, but the latter is difficult to observe in unstained preparations.

To study the lumen-dwelling histomonad after fixation and staining, one may start with either histological sections of the cecum or smears of cecal contents. Organisms observed in stained sections show the same characteristic shrinkage noted for tissue dwellers. Organisms observed in smears often appear to have resisted shrinkage because they were distended in the plane of the slide as the liquid in the film spread or evaporated. The endoplasm of the lumen-dwelling histomonad usually stains more deeply than it does in tissue dwellers, and vacuoles and particulate matter give it quite a heterogeneous appearance. Also the blepharoplast is more readily observed, especially if the flagellum can be found, so the area at its base may be studied intently (Fig. 31.7C). Infrequently 2 flagella may be visible before evidence of cell division becomes conspicuous. If more than 2 flagella are observed in either living or preserved organisms, *P. wenrichi* is almost certainly present (see Fig. 31.7D,E).

LIFE CYCLE

The life cycle of *H. meleagridis* varies from extremely simple to rather complex. The parasite is too fragile to endure the hazards of the environment outside the definitive host more than several minutes to a few hours. There is no evidence whatsoever of its transmission through the egg of any gallinaceous bird. Neither is there any evidence of its transmission by biting arthropods that might introduce the organism into the peripheral blood. Consequently, infection by ingestion of *Histomonas* alone or with other organisms is the only plausible means by which a bird may acquire this parasite under natural conditions. Even then the protozoon may require protection before it arrives at a suitable site. Experimentally, histomonads may be introduced in a variety of ways, some of which are quite inapplicable in nature. Not all methods are equally satisfactory. The results of such efforts have been tabulated by Swales (1950).

Direct Infection

After Histomonas is ingested, it must in some way be protected against prolonged exposure to the low pH of the gizzard. Horton-Smith and Long (1955, 1956) accomplished this with chickens by starving them or giving them alkaline solutions. Lund (1956) infected young turkeys by giving large numbers of histomonads suspended in physiologic saline containing a minimum of solids, thus avoiding retention of the material in the gizzard. Obviously, among birds receiving proper care, the conditions required for such transmission should not occur, and this method of transmission is no longer considered important.

Role of Cecal Worm

Reasoning that invasion of the cecal walls was not a normal part of the life cycle of the histomonad, Graybill and Smith (1920) sought some means by which the parasite might readily enter the tissues. Lesions produced by the larvae of the cecal worm *H. gallinarum* might afford the histomonads such an opportunity. By giving embryonated Heterakis eggs to birds also given turkey feces containing histomonads, they produced blackhead, whereas birds given only the turkey feces with histomonads remained well. However, 3 turkeys given only Heterakis eggs developed the disease, creating a dilemma these investigators did not solve (Smith and Graybill, 1920; Graybill, 1921).

Tyzzer's group (Tyzzer et al., 1921) soon confirmed the work of Graybill and Smith and then devised experiments that demonstrated that the histomonad must be carried inside the shell of the cecal worm egg (Tyzzer and Fabyan, 1922). However, Tyzzer (1926) was unable to detect it there microscopically, although he had seen histomonads in the intestinal epithelium of Heterakis larvae 11 days old (Tyzzer, 1927). Later, Swales (1948) showed that larvae separated mechanically from the rest of the egg, washed, treated with H_2O_2, and introduced into the ceca of turkeys could transmit histomonads. However, relatively few eggs harbor larvae that contain the histomonad (Kendall, 1957; Lund and Burtner, 1957), so the search for one in a larva still within the egg would be tedious at best.

Although Niimi (1937) portrayed what may have been histomonads throughout much of the body of some female heterakids, the identity of the minute bodies he represented as histomonads contained within the eggs is questionable. Not so with the bodies that Gibbs (1962) identified as histomonads. Widely distributed in the bodies of some worms of both sexes and also present in some Heterakis eggs, Gibbs's organisms conform in size and appearance with *Histomonas meleagridis* as seen in stained sections of bird tissues.

Just how *H. meleagridis* gets into the Heterakis egg and its developing larva has been a subject of conjecture. Tyzzer (1927) and Gibbs (1962) considered it likely that the protozoon is introduced into the female at copulation. Niimi (1937) believed that the histomonads ingested by the male disappeared rather quickly, whereas those ingested by the female penetrated the gut wall and entered the ovary where they were enveloped by the shells, along with the ova. Niimi gave eggs of Histomonas-free Heterakis to birds that were independently infected with *Histomonas meleagridis* introduced rectally. Some of the worms grown in such birds produced eggs that transmitted the histomonad. Later, Lund (1968) studied the time and frequency of both acquisition and liberation of *Parahistomonas wenrichi* by *Heterakis gallinarum*. Although optimum times for acquisition and liberation of *Parahistomonas wenrichi* differ somewhat from those for *H. meleagridis*, the role played by the cecal worm is very similar. In each generation, some Heterakis larvae must liberate histomonads if the bird is to become infected, and usually some of the female worms must acquire histomonads from the host if the eggs that they produce are to carry the protozoon to another definitive host. Characteristically, it is predominantly the young larvae that effectively liberate the histomonads. Frequently such liberation comes with the death and dissolution of the larva (Lund, 1967a). Presumably the "parasites resembling *Histomonas meleagridis*" observed by Kendall (1959) in a 4-day-old Heterakis larva were in that larva as it entered the bird in which it was found. The histomonads observed by Tyzzer (1927) in an 11-day-old Heterakis larva had almost certainly been acquired by that larva from its surroundings in the cecum of the host in which it was developing. Such histomonads would be involved in transmission only through the subsequent generation of worms.

Role of Earthworm

In 1907 Curtice produced blackhead in poults as a result of feeding earthworms from chicken yards. The role of Heterakis in transmitting this disease had not yet been discovered, and Curtice (1907b) concluded: "The earthworms in this instance were probably carriers of infected soil, and were not necessarily a second host to the parasite." During the next several decades, the earthworm was regarded as merely a mechanical vector of Heterakis (Ackert, 1917; Lund, 1960; Madsen, 1962) and, as such, only of incidental importance in the transmission of Histomonas. In many respects, the sturdy little egg of Heterakis seemed to provide all the protection the delicate histomonad needed to persist from season to season and get from bird to bird. Even the autumn rise in cecal worm counts and incidence of blackhead among birds on soil free of additional contamination could seemingly be explained. Heterakis eggs that had percolated into the soil following thaws and spring rains were brought to the surface by earthworms and other burrowing creatures (Lund, 1960). But this concept did not explain why so many infections with Histomonas and Heterakis apparently had been acquired 1–2 days after a rain. Neither did it explain why so many heterakids were almost the same size or predominantly of two sizes and therefore of two ages (Lund, 1958a).

In 1963 Lund et al. reported experiments that indicated that earthworms were actually transmitting Heterakis larvae and that these larvae were not merely in transit through the digestive tract. Usually the castings alone transmitted nothing and rarely contained either Heterakis eggs or larvae. The results of additional studies were reported later (Lund et al., 1966b), as were reports concerning the significance of earthworm transmission (Lund and Farr, 1965; Lund 1966a, 1967b). Thus, after female heterakids or their ova are voided in the cecal discharges of a bird, 10 days to 3 weeks may be required before the eggs are embryonated and become infective. By this time the discharges have either dried sufficiently to be acceptable to surface-feeding earthworms or have been dispersed by rain to mingle with the uppermost soil lay-

ers where some species of earthworms feed. In either event, once ingested by an earthworm, the embryonated Heterakis eggs hatch, and the larvae burrow into the earthworm's tissues. Here these larvae may remain for many months, some perhaps for the life of the worm. Throughout a summer's feeding, an earthworm may accumulate several hundred such larvae. Many of these do not survive as the earthworm hibernates deep in the soil, below the frost line. But some do, and the following summer additional heterakid larvae may be acquired. However, following rains, earthworms come to the surface, making them ready prey for birds. Thus the tiny larvae, all in approximately the same stage of development, are liberated and carried to the cecum. Here they enter the mucosa, develop for a few days if the host is suitable, and then emerge to the lumen of the cecum and migrate to its quiet distal end. Here the cecal worms develop to maturity and mate, and the cycle nears its completion. Larvae that carry histomonads may liberate them, either as the larvae perish or (perhaps less frequently) as the protozoa escape by other means. In either event histomoniasis could result. Obviously, completion of the life cycle requires acquision of histomonads by some cecal worms that survive to maturity and produce fertile eggs that contain the protozoon and then escape to embryonate on or in the soil.

In a typical agricultural situation in the north central or New England states, for example, earthworms are usually sufficiently abundant to assure the transmission of both Heterakis and Histomonas. However, enough cecal worms must mature in birds that harbor *H. meleagridis* to permit Histomonas-bearing eggs of Heterakis to accumulate in sufficient numbers in earthworms in the summer to compensate for the loss of such larvae (sometimes 75–90%) during the hibernation of the worms. Usually a bird that is highly susceptible to histomoniasis, such as a young poult, cannot assure the survival of enough heterakids to produce the fertile eggs necessary to compensate for the annual loss of embryonated eggs and infective larvae. Although chickens vary considerably in their resistance to histomoniasis (Lund, 1967c), most breeds tolerate the disease well enough to permit sufficient heterakids to mature to spread histomonads if they too are present. Although a simple expression of the life cycle need not involve the earthworm (Lund, 1957), under the field conditions selected for our example the earthworm plays a very important part (Lund, 1967b).

Pathogenicity

The response that *Histomonas meleagridis* invokes in the definitive host (always, so far as is known, a gallinaceous bird) varies considerably. Many factors influence this response. One of the most obvious is the species of host, but the bird's breed, age, and individual tolerance also influence its response. The turkey is one of the most susceptible birds, and especially so from its 4th or 5th week until the end of its first autumn. Obviously, the opportunities for infection are fewer among very young birds and those maturing during the winter. Usually, even among poults, 8–15% either resist infection or escape prolonged or severe involvement.

Populations of histomonads contain individuals that vary from those that are almost harmless to those that invade and spread among the tissues so readily as to provide the bird little opportunity to muster its defenses and repair the damage. At times, probably frequently, these variants are sorted out locally and temporarily (Lund et al., 1966a). Under controlled conditions, as among histomonads grown in culture, a gradual loss of virulence commonly occurs (Tyzzer, 1932, 1934, 1936; Lund et al., 1966a, 1967), to be followed ultimately by a loss of ability to multiply in birds. Such organisms may remain unchanged in many ways and probably emerge as that sector of the initial population that survived prolonged exposure to the restricted environment.

The related parasite *Parahistomonas wenrichi* (Lund, 1963) is not known to multiply appreciably in the tissues of any bird, calls forth no readily detectable host response (Lund, 1959), and is considered nonpathogenic. Otherwise its life cycle appears to be identical with that of *H. meleagridis,* and it is important not to confuse the two organisms.

PATHOGENESIS AND EPIZOOTIOLOGY

NATURAL AND EXPERIMENTAL HOSTS

Gallinaceous birds other than turkeys and chickens that have been reported to develop histomoniasis are ring-necked pheasant *(Phasianus colchicus),* ruffed grouse *(Bonasa umbellus),* greater prairie chicken *(Tympanuchus cupido),* peafowl *(Pavo* sp.), guinea fowl *(Numida meleagris),* chukar partridge *(Alectoris graeca),* bobwhite *(Colinus virginianus)* and Japanese quail *(Coturnix coturnix japonica).* The frequency with which the disease develops in the different species varies greatly. The chukar partridge is at least as susceptible to histomoniasis as is the turkey poult, so it usually thrives best in arid rocky regions where conditions are unfavorable for vectors of the parasites. The ring-necked pheasant is as resistant as some of our breeds of chickens (Lund, unpublished data), and would be an equally dangerous source of contamination of turkey range with heterakids and histomonads if it were abundant there. Bobwhite and Japanese quail are poor hosts for Histomonas and Heterakis. They seldom succumb to histomoniasis, rarely produce heterakids with histomonads, and are therefore unimportant in the spread of the parasites (Lund and Ellis, 1967). Birds of susceptible breeds may develop histomoniasis at any age. However, the disease is most prevalent during the birds' first season of exposure to the vectors of Histomonas and Heterakis. The prevalence of these vectors and their parasite burdens is seasonal and subject to local climatic conditions. Consequently, under some circumstances, more turkeys in a given flock may acquire histomoniasis at 20–25 weeks of age (usually autumn) than did so at 9–10 weeks.

VECTORS

At present we know of no vector that is as effective as Heterakis in protecting the histomonad after it leaves the bird. Several invertebrates may serve as *mechanical* vectors for Heterakis, but hatching of the egg and accumulation of larvae is not known to occur except in earthworms. Invertebrates that can serve as mechanical vectors include certain blowflies (De Volt and Davis, 1936), several species of grasshoppers (Frank, 1953) and under experimental conditions sowbugs (Spindler, 1967) and the field cricket (Spindler, 1968, personal communication). Some outbreaks of histomoniasis among flocks of turkeys grown commercially indicate that unknown vectors may at times be involved.

COURSE OF THE DISEASE

Incubation Period

Probably *Histomonas meleagridis* is most frequently liberated by the Heterakis larvae 1–5 days after the latter have been ingested by the bird. However, liberation may be deferred by several days. Usually 4–5 days of multiplication are required before the histomonads become numerous enough in the cecal discharges to be detected in fresh smears. Caged poults occasionally may show evidences of discomfort as early as the 4th day after infection, but even the practiced eye would hardly notice infected birds in a flock until about the 6th day. Occasionally, histomonads can be detected in cecal discharges at that time.

Signs

By the 7th or 8th day after infection a poult may be obviously ill, walking with a stilted gait and rather inattentive except on provocation. Its interest in food is casual at best. By this time tissue-type histomonads may be found in the cecal droppings should there be any such discharges. Internally, the walls of the ceca are thickened and hyperemic; the entire organ may be distended as the lumen fills with a mucuslike discharge that exudes from the thousands of glands in the swollen cecal mucosa. During the 9th and 10th days, liver lesions may become conspicuous in poults, there may be no cecal discharges, and, instead of the usual semiformed feces, the bird may void fluid, sulfur-colored discharges that frequently stain the perianal feathers. Except when disturbed, the bird, now quite ill, stands or rests with wings drooping, eyes closed, and head drawn closely to the body or tucked under a wing.

At this stage in chickens of most breeds there is no liver involvement. The birds do not void sulfur-colored droppings but may void cecal cores, fragments thereof, or bloody cecal discharges. Such cleansing of the ceca is the prelude to cecal repair, which then proceeds rapidly, leaving few or no macroscopic residual signs of involvement as soon as 18–28 days after infection. However, in chickens of quite susceptible breeds the disease may proceed as in poults. Furthermore, in some individual chickens of any breed, the histomonads may persist and multiply in the lumen of the cecum for many weeks or even several months (Lund, 1967c).

Later Stages of the Disease

Some poults may recover as described above for chickens. However, if liver involvement is extensive, the lesions, usually grayish white or cream colored, continue to increase in size, often with concentric rings surrounding a darker depressed center (Fig. 31.8). Usually not more than 10–15% of the young turkeys involved to this extent

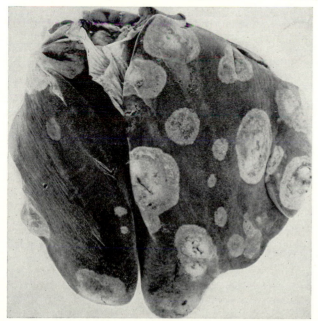

FIG. 31.8—Liver of turkey affected with blackhead. (Graybill, 1925)

survive. Death may come as early as 11–12 days after infection, but it is more common for deaths to start about the 14th day. Mortality usually reaches a peak about the 17th day and then subsides by the end of the 4th week with the deaths of birds that have developed secondary complications, often respiratory. If the cecal walls rupture or are otherwise perforated, peritonitis usually develops. Death may then occur before liver involvement becomes pronounced.

For a detailed account and literature review of the progress of Heterakis-produced histomoniasis in turkeys, consult Clarkson (1962).

Histopathology

Under experimental conditions, the earliest microscopic evidence of cecal involvement is an infiltration of heterophil leukocytes beneath the mucosa 1–3 days after embryonated Heterakis eggs containing histomonads are administered (Clarkson, 1962). This involvement probably is a response to tissue invasion by the larvae. However, histomonads may be detected as early as the 4th or 5th day, sometimes in the vicinity of the remains of Heterakis larvae. Heterophilic infiltration increases, as do the histomonads, until the muscularis is invaded. Meanwhile a core has been building up in the lumen of one or both ceca. It consists of an amorphous matrix containing leukocytes, sloughed mucosal cells, often some erythrocytes, and, especially at its margin, tissue-type histomonads. Sometimes, 12–14 days after infection, large areas of the distal three-fourths of the cecum are almost devoid of mucosa. By this time it is usually difficult to recognize histomonads except perhaps at the interface between the cecal wall and the detached mucosa or the core.

Long before the cecal walls are eroded as described above, histomonads may have escaped into the hepatic portal system in such numbers as to set up foci of infection along the venules of the liver. Again, the first evidence of these foci is an infiltration of leukocytes (Clarkson, 1962), which can occur as early as 6 days postinfection. Presumably, by the 8th day one should find histomonads in sections of such locations. They can be detected in smears of these very early lesions. However, unless histomonads are fairly numerous and fixation

and staining are excellent, the organisms are hard to identify (Tyzzer, 1934). Usually they can be detected more readily in histological sections prepared from birds infected 10–12 days previously (Fig. 31.9). Histomonads should be sought at the margins of the lesions. Once necrosis of the liver cells becomes extensive, as it does near the center of old lesions, histomonads can no longer be found. Descriptions of alterations that occur in the blood of turkeys with histomoniasis were given by Johnson and Lange (1939), McGuire and Cavett (1952), and Malewitz and Calhoun (1957). Clarkson (1961) studied the distribution of blood vessels of the lower digestive tract and the liver of turkeys and suggested an interesting explanation for the occasional involvement of the kidneys in birds with histomoniasis.

IMMUNITY

Active

Curtice (1907a,b) foresaw the possibility of slowly enhancing the natural immunity of turkeys to blackhead by selection, but he apparently had little faith in depending upon acquired immunity as a control measure for this disease.

Higgins et al. (1915) and Tyzzer et al. (1921) were unable to immunize birds by injecting either saline extracts or emulsions of tissues from turkeys with histomoniasis. However, by 1932 Tyzzer reported having immunized chickens with a strain of *Histomonas meleagridis* that had lost its pathogenicity during 2 years of in vitro cultivation. He later (1936) reported comparable results with turkeys, this time using strains of *H. meleagridis* cultivated up to 3 years in vitro to invoke the immunity. In all instances for which details were given, immunizing and challenge doses were administered rectally. Lund et al. (1966a) reported similar results with both chickens and turkeys by employing for immunization a strain of *H. meleagridis* cultivated in vitro more than 6 years. Some tests employed challenge infections of histomonads given rectally, but in some chickens the challenges consisted of Histomonas-bearing Heterakis eggs administered orally. The lower incidence of histomoniasis among the latter birds (20% versus 45% in the controls) suggested that the immunity was to some extent systemic. Birds tested only by rec-

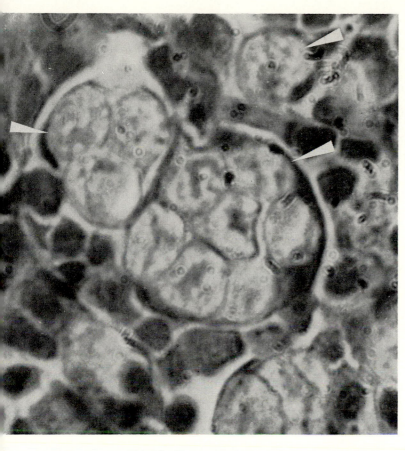

FIG. 31.9—Histomonads in liver of young turkey. In addition to organisms seen in two clusters, at least two appear singly. Tissue fixed in Helly's fluid and sections (6μ thick) stained with Weigert's iron hematoxylin. ×2,000 (Lund, original)

tal challenge infection could have developed only the localized "tissue" immunity such as occurs when *Parahistomonas wenrichi* is used for immunization (Lund, 1959). However, it should be noted that a comparable test, employing Heterakis eggs to transmit virulent histomonads of the challenge dose, has not been reported for turkeys. The results might not be comparable with those for chickens. In any event, with continued in vitro passage the strain of *Histomonas meleagridis* rapidly lost its ability to arouse immune responses in either chickens or turkeys, and eventually these "culture-adapted" histomonads would no longer live in birds (Lund et al., 1967).

With the discovery of drugs effective in controlling blackhead, a new stimulus was given to studies on immunity. Now turkeys could be given initial inoculations with virulent histomonads and still be protected against fatal or extremely severe blackhead, thus assuring the survival of the birds for later challenge doses. However, the results obtained by testing for immunity in drug-treated birds have varied considerably. Sautter et al. (1950) commented that little immunity was obtained from experimental infections if the birds recovered as a result of drug therapy. If any immunity was developed at all, the "turkey must be markedly ill, almost to the point of death, and then recover." DeVolt et al. (1954) obtained essentially the same results. Swales (1950), Kendall (1957), and Clarkson (1963) had some turkeys that resisted Histomonas infections after recovering from blackhead that was kept under control by drugs. Apparently, immunity is absent or negligible if the drug is used in such a way that little tissue invasion occurs as a result of the initial ("immunizing") infection or infections, but it is significant if the drug is not employed until the histomonads are plentiful in the tissues.

Clarkson has demonstrated the presence of serum precipitins as early as 7 days after the antigen could be detected in the cecal content, but by this time there was extensive proliferation of histomonads in the cecal mucosa, and the cecal content contained large numbers of organisms. He made the following pertinent statement: "It is not suggested that the precipitating antibodies demonstrated in turkeys and fowls are a measure of the resistance of the bird to histomoniasis, but, like the protective immune response, serum precipitins are connected with the infection of the cecal mucosa and persist in both turkeys and fowls for a considerable length of time."

Passive

Attempts to obtain passive immunization by injecting whole blood from immunized birds (Sautter et al., 1950) or serum from birds showing precipitating antibodies (Clarkson, 1963) have uniformly failed.

DIAGNOSIS

The early evidences of histomoniasis were described above. The grower should of course become so familiar with his birds that he can detect evidences of distress in time to summon professional assistance before birds begin dying. Should birds be dying before he seeks such assistance, he may wish to see whether their internal appearance suggests a single cause. Or he may choose to submit some dead birds to a professionally trained diagnostician. However, he should certainly submit one or more birds that are still alive but quite ill.

The diagnostician can make a tentative diagnosis of histomoniasis if cores are present, forming, or dissolving in one or both ceca. In turkeys especially, the circular lesions of the liver may be expected (Fig. 31.8). Conclusive diagnosis ordinarily requires demonstrating *Histomonas meleagridis* by microscopic examination. Its appearance has already been discussed.

Smears of cecal material should be prepared from areas where the mucosa is moist, preferably coated with mucus. If these smears are examined at temperatures of 75–80° F, many of the histomonads may be active. This activity greatly simplifies their detection and identification. Some of the histomonads may be forming pseudopodia, whereas others may rotate 60–90° periodically. With phase microscopy the flagellum may be observed on those showing rotary movements.

Smears from the liver should be made with material taken at the margin of a lesion. Rarely are histomonads with flagella found in such preparations. Usually these organisms appear as clear bubblelike spheres, with the nucleus faintly discernible. Amoeboid movement is seldom observed (Fig. 31.7A).

For research purposes or for a permanent record, smears may be fixed and stained, but the study of such preparations is more time-consuming and generally less satisfactory than the study of fresh smears containing living organisms. Each investigator probably has a method of fixation and staining that best meets his own requirements. This author prefers fixation in Schaudinn's fluid with 10% glacial acetic acid and staining with Heidenhain's iron alum hematoxylin.

For some purposes it is desirable to show both the organisms and the host's tissue responses in one permanent preparation. In our laboratory we do not regard this as a *diagnostic* aid, because even with tissues carefully selected from obviously involved organs, faulty fixation or staining can make the identification of Histomonas very uncertain. However, for special purposes, excellent preparations can be made. Kemp and Reid (1966) recommend the Periodic acid-Schiff staining technique for use in differentiating *H. meleagridis* from *Candida albicans* in histologic sections of liver lesions.

TREATMENT

Of the early workers, the few who mentioned treatment of blackhead regarded it as unpromising (Mohler, 1905; Curtice, 1907a). Little reliance can be placed on reports of the efficacy of control measures tested during the decade of confusion of blackhead with coccidiosis (see History).

By the close of World War I, various drugs had been found useful in treating human infections with amoebae, trypanosomes, and spirochetes. Tyzzer tried some of these and some closely related substances for efficacy against Histomonas infections. Certain of these, including tryparsamide (Tyzzer, 1923), had merit but were too expensive for use with birds raised commercially. If the industry was to grow, treatment of birds individually was to be avoided whenever possible. Indeed, even with the use of drugs, prevention was vastly more desirable than attempted cure. Accordingly, the remainder of this section deals almost entirely with the use of drugs at prophylactic levels to control histomoniasis.

By the end of World War II, several drugs had been shown to be effective against coccidiosis in poultry. These successes stimulated the search for drugs comparably effective in combatting Histomonas infections. More reports of such efforts appeared from 1948 to 1952 than had appeared in the preceding 50 years. Two (McGregor, 1949; Waletzky et al., 1949) included results using 2-amino-5-nitrothiazole, a drug that appeared superior to any heretofore tested for controlling histomoniasis. By mid-1950 it became available to turkey growers. The following spring an arsenical, 4-nitro-benzenearsonic acid, was marketed for the prevention of histomoniasis. The turkey industry, already expanding rapidly, responded to the increased security provided by the availability of effective drugs with an unprecedented growth. This growth in turn must have stimulated the quest for additional effective drugs, a search that still goes on.

Some of the reviews on chemical control of histomoniasis have classified the various substances according to their chemical relationships, presented reports of their efficacy under different conditions, and given comprehensive references to original sources (Jerstad, 1957; Wehr et al., 1958; and Joyner et al., 1963, 1966).

Wehr et al. (1958) considered all important contributions to the chemotherapy of blackhead from 1923 to 1957. Among the drugs listed as having therapeutic value were 4-nitro-benzenearsonic acid (previously mentioned), 2-acetylamino-5-nitrothiazole (closely related to 2-amino-5-nitrothiazole mentioned above), N-(5-nitro-2-furylidene)-3-amino-2-oxazolidone (a nitrofuran better known as furazolidone), and 1-ethyl-3-(5-nitro-2-thiazole) urea. Joyner et al. (1963, 1966) dealt with these and with more recently tested drugs: 1,2-dimethyl-5-nitroimidazole (dimetridazole); paramomycin sulfate (an antibiotic); and p-ureidobenzenearsonic acid (an arsenical sometimes used to control certain other protozoan infections).

Peardon and Eoff (1967) tested the efficacy of p-ureidobenzenearsonic acid against blackhead in chickens infected by rectal inoculation with Histomonas. In 1968 Peardon and Ramsay reported the use of the same drug to prevent blackhead in chickens given Histomonas-bearing Heterakis eggs. Whitmore et al. (1968c) tested the efficacy of graded levels of p-ureidobenzenearsonic acid in the control of histomoniasis among turkeys 5 and 13 weeks old. Atkinson et al. (1967) evaluated the effects of this and other antihistomonal drugs on growth and feed efficiency of turkeys. Whitmore et al. (1968a) studied the effects of various levels of vitamin A on the efficacy of several drugs in preventing histomoniasis in turkeys.

Reports of three new antihistomonal drugs have appeared since the latest review was published. The chemical composition of two of these was not disclosed in what appeared to be merely preliminary reports (Peterson, 1967; Vatne et al., 1967). The third drug, given the generic name "ronidazole," is 1-methyl-2-carbamoyloxymethyl-5-nitroimidazole. It was reported as "consistently effective at a level only one-fifth to one-twelfth of the other compounds" (Whitmore et al., 1968b). The compounds with which it was compared were dimetridazole, 4-nitrophenylarsonic acid, and p-ureidobenzenearsonic acid. At this writing these three drugs are not available except perhaps for experimental use by qualified researchers.

One recent report (Morehouse et al., 1968) deals with the use of the drug dimetridazole with "half-grown turkeys exhibiting advanced signs of enterohepatitis."

As the above passages indicate, there is brisk activity in the chemotherapy of histomoniasis. New drugs are being tested and new information is being developed concerning the conditions under which earlier formulations work best. *Histomonas meleagridis* appears to be a relatively immutable parasite (Lund, 1966b), at least in comparison to some of the coccidia such as Eimeria and Isospora. Possibly because of this characteristic and the rather demanding requirements of the life cycle, Histomonas has not quickly developed a tolerance to drugs.

Many circumstances influence the choice of a drug. Among these are local availability, cost, applicability to preferred management practices, and compatibility with other medicants. Each grower should consider what drugs have proved to be effective and feasible in his area and with his mode of operation. Having made a selection, he should always follow the recommendations of the manufacturer. Such recommendations are made on the basis of costly research and in compliance with rigid standards.

The grower must always bear in mind that the use of drugs in no way replaces the need for cleanliness and good management practices. Indeed, it was only *after* the poultry industry had made enormous progress as a result of intelligent, purposeful improvement through good management practices that additional successes were scored through employment of chemotherapy.

PREVENTION AND CONTROL

As was pointed out earlier, poultrymen, and especially turkey growers, had fairly effective means of controlling blackhead before the discovery of satisfactory antihistomonal drugs.

MANAGEMENT PROCEDURES

Curtice (1907a,b) pioneered in the control of blackhead by management. To attain the isolation of poults from chickens and older turkeys, as Curtice advocated, confinement rearing was necessary. When the poults' range could be restricted to well-drained or sandy soil, the results were even better than those achieved with isolation alone. However, the industry was slow in following Curtice's recommendations. To some extent at least, this slowness must be attributed to the confusion of blackhead with coccidiosis and trichomoniasis. Turkey production rose but very slightly in the United States between 1907 and 1920, and both the overall mortality and that resulting from blackhead declined only a little, according to USDA statistics and early reports from experiment stations.

By the time turkey growers and farm advisors became aware of the role of the cecal worm in the transmission of Histomonas, systems for the rotation of range were already being studied and advocated as an adjunct to confinement rearing (Lund, 1969). Growers recognized that they must keep their birds relatively free of parasites if they were to keep their range reasonably free of contamination with these organisms. Conversely, they recognized that on range moderately free of contaminations, some birds (such as poults) could be kept comparably free of parasites. If completion of

the life cycle of the parasite could be kept favorably low by using the same range only every third year, they would do so. If soil and climate permitted using the same range each year, they would do that (Lund, 1954). In each area, experiment stations, farm advisors, and poultry specialists determined the program best suited to local use. Many growers cooperated by keeping good records, reporting accurately, and profiting from each other's experience. It worked, and it still does.

BIOLOGICAL CONTROL

With the widespread use of chemicals to control parasitic infections, it became necessary to designate in some way those practices that relied on other means of preventing excessive parasitism. However, the lines of distinction have by no means always been clear.

As here used, biological control is the employment of any naturally occurring phenomenon of living things to interrupt the life cycle of a parasite, or to reduce the frequency of its appearance or the severity of its effect on the host (Lund, 1966b). Thus, eliminating an organism that serves as a vector for a parasite, regardless of how this is achieved, constitutes biological control of the parasite. Obviously we have long used such means as a part of good management. Draining swamps to rid an area of mosquitoes could be an example of control of malaria by biological means. As yet, no one has attempted the large-scale elimination of earthworms as an aid to the control of Heterakis and Histomonas. At considerable expense it has been tried with small yards or pens used for ornamental pheasants. "Stone yards" discourage earthworms and permit Heterakis eggs to be washed out of the birds' reach.

For more than 2 decades, phenothiazine has been used with chickens and turkeys to remove Heterakis. In some tests it has removed 90–94% of the worms (Wehr and Olivier, 1946; Colglazier et al., 1960). However, it does not attack the worms at a sufficiently early stage of their development to prevent the liberation of Histomonas. Consequently, the incidence of blackhead is not reduced correspondingly (Wehr and Olivier, 1946; Lund, 1958b). The use of phenothiazine substantially reduces contamination of the range with cecal worm eggs. Consequently in 2 or 3 years the worm load of birds using such range should be greatly reduced. Under these conditions the acquisition of Histomonas is reduced proportionately. Phenothiazine does not attack the histomonad, so to this parasite the use of the drug may be considered a form of biological control, even though it is chemical control as far as the vector is concerned.

Other drugs are presently being studied

for the control of cecal worms, and some that are presently marketed principally to remove other helminths have an influence on cecal worms. Formulations vary, so each grower must select according to his needs and use the formulation as directed by the manufacturer.

Immunization is usually considered to be a form of biological control. As yet it has no practical applications in histomoniasis control.

REFERENCES

Ackert, J. E. 1917. A means of transmitting the fowl nematode, *Heterakis papillosa* Bloch. *Science* 46:394.

Atkinson, R. L., J. W. Bradley, J. R. Couch, and J. H. Quisenberry. 1967. Evaluation of blackhead preventive drugs with regard to growth and feed efficiency of turkeys. *Poultry Sci.* 46:1003–8.

Bergersen, R. A. 1952. Minnesota turkeys— Death losses. *Minn. Turkey Growers Ass.*, pp. i–iii, 1–13. (Mimeo.)

Chester, F. D., and A. Robin. 1901. Enterohepatitis or blackhead of fowls, *Twelfth Ann. Rept. Delaware Agr. Expt. Sta.*, pp. 60–66.

Clarkson, M. J. 1961. The blood supply of the liver of the turkey and the anatomy of the biliary tract with reference to infection with *Histomonas meleagridis*. *Res. Vet. Sci.* 2:259–64.

————. 1962. The progressive pathology of Heterakis-produced histomoniasis in turkeys. *Res. Vet. Sci.* 3:443–48.

————. 1963. Immunological responses to *Histomonas meleagridis* in the turkey and fowl. *Immunology* 6:156–68.

Colglazier, M. L., A. O. Foster, F. D. Enzie, and D. E. Thompson. 1960. The anthelmintic action of phenothiazine and piperazine against *Heterakis gallinae* and *Ascaridia galli* in chickens. *J. Parasitol.* 46:267–70.

Curtice, C. 1907a. The rearing and management of turkeys with special reference to the blackhead disease. *Rhode Island Agr. Expt. Sta. Bull.* 123:1–64.

————. 1907b. Further experiments in connection with the blackhead disease in turkeys. *Rhode Island Agr. Expt. Sta. Bull.* 124:65–105.

Cushman, S. 1894. A study of the diseases of turkeys, pp. 286–88. In *6th Ann. Rept. Rhode Island Agr. Expt. Sta., 1893*, Pt. II.

DeVolt, H. M., and C. R. Davis. 1936. Blackhead (infectious enterohepatitis) in turkeys, with notes on other intestinal protozoa. *Maryland Agr. Expt. Sta. Bull.* 392:493–567.

DeVolt, H. M., F. G. Tromba, and A. P. Holst. 1954. An investigation to determine wheth-

er immunity to infectious enterohepatitis (blackhead) of turkeys develops during enheptin treatment. *Poultry Sci.* 33:1256–61.

Frank, J. F. 1953. A note on the experimental transmission of enterohepatitis of turkeys by arthropods. *Can. J. Comp. Med. Vet. Sci.* 17:230–31.

Gibbs, B. J. 1962. The occurrence of the protozoan parasite *Histomonas meleagridis* in the adults and eggs of the cecal worm *Heterakis gallinae*. *J. Protozool.* 9:288–93.

Graybill, H. W. 1921. The incidence of blackhead and occurrence of *Heterakis papillosa* in a flock of artificially reared turkeys. *J. Exp. Med.* 33:667–73.

————. 1925. Blackhead and other causes of loss of turkeys in California. *California Agr. Expt. Sta. Circ.* 291:1–14.

Graybill, H. W., and T. Smith. 1920. Production of fatal blackhead in turkeys by feeding embryonated eggs of *Heterakis papillosa. J. Exp. Med.* 31:647–55.

Higgins, C. H., A. B. Wickware, and N. B. Guiou. 1915. Entero-hepatitis or blackhead in turkeys. Notes and experiments. *Rept. Vet. Director Gen., Dept. Agr. Canada,* pp. 103–10.

Honigberg, B. M., and Jelena Kuldova. 1969. Structure of a nonpathogenic histomonad from the cecum of galliform birds and revision of the trichomonad family Monocercomonadidae Kirby. *J. Protozool.* 16:526–35.

Horton-Smith, C., and P. L. Long. 1955. The infection of chickens *(Gallus gallus)* with suspension of blackhead organism *Histomonas meleagridis*. *Vet. Record* 67:478.

————. 1956. Studies in histomoniasis. I. The infection of chickens *(Gallus gallus)* with histomonad suspensions. *Parasitology* 46:79–90.

Jerstad, A. C. 1957. Furazolidone for infectious enterohepatitis (blackhead) of turkeys. *Am. J. Vet. Res.* 18:174–79.

Johnson, E. P., and C. J. Lange. 1939. Blood alterations in typhlohepatitis of turkeys, with notes on the disease. *J. Parasitol.* 25: 157–67.

Joyner, L. P., S. F. M. Davies, and S. D. Kendall. 1963. Chemotherapy of histomoniasis, pp. 333–49. In Schnitzer, R. J., and F. Hawking (eds.), *Experimental Chemotherapy,* Vol. I. Academic Press, New York.

———. 1966. Chemotherapy of histomoniasis, pp. 425–28. In Schnitzer, R. J., and F. Hawking (eds.), *Experimental Chemotherapy,* Vol. IV. Academic Press, New York.

Kemp, R. L., and W. M. Reid. 1966. Staining techniques for differential diagnosis of histomoniasis and mycosis in domestic poultry. *Avian Diseases* 10:357–63.

Kendall, S. B. 1957. Some factors influencing resistance to histomoniasis in turkeys. *Brit. Vet. J.* 133:435–39.

———. 1959. The occurrence of *Histomonas meleagridis* in *Heterakis gallinae. Parasitology* 49:169–72.

Lund, E. E. 1954. A health report on 376,000 turkeys in southern California. *Turkey World* 29:15, 54–55.

———. 1956. Oral transmission of Histomonas in turkeys. *Poultry Sci.* 35:900–904.

———. 1957. We're learning more about blackhead. *Agr. Res.* 6 (2):12–13.

———. 1958a. Growth and development of *Heterakis gallinae* in turkeys and chickens infected with *Histomonas meleagridis. J. Parasitol.* 44:297–301.

———. 1958b. Studies on "self-cure" and acquired resistance to Heterakis infections in chickens and turkeys. *J. Parasitol.* 44 (4, Sect. 2):27. (Abstr.)

———. 1959. Immunizing action of a nonpathogenic strain of Histomonas against blackhead in turkeys. *J. Protozool.* 6:182–85.

———. 1960. Factors influencing the survival of Heterakis and Histomonas on soil. *J. Parasitol.* 46 (5, Sect. 2):38. (Abstr.)

———. 1961. Acquisition and liberation of nonpathogenic histomonads by *Heterakis gallinarum. J. Protozool.* 8 (Suppl.):6. (Abstr.)

———. 1963. *Histomonas wenrichi* n. sp. (Mastigophora: Mastigamoebidae), a nonpathogenic parasite of gallinaceous birds. *J. Protozool.* 10:401–4.

———. 1966a. The significance of earthworm transmission of Heterakis and Histomonas. *Proc. 1st Int. Congr. Parasitol.,* Vol. I, pp. 371–72. (Abstr.)

———. 1966b. Biological control of animal parasites, pp. 111–16. In *Pest Control by Chemical, Biological, Genetic and Physical Means.* USDA ARS 33–110.

———. 1967a. Acquired resistance to experimental Heterakis infections in chickens and turkeys: Effect on transmission of *Histo-monas meleagridis. J. Helminthol.* 41:55–62.

———. 1967b. USDA makes progress on soil test for blackhead. *Poultry Meat* 4:A40–A42.

———. 1967c. Response of four breeds of chickens and one breed of turkeys to experimental Heterakis and Histomonas infections. *Avian Diseases* 11:491–502.

———. 1968. Acquisition and liberation of *Histomonas wenrichi* by *Heterakis gallinarum. Exp. Parasitol.* 22:62–67.

———. 1969. Histomoniasis. *Advan. Vet. Sci.* 13:355–90.

Lund, E. E., and R. H. Burtner, Jr. 1957. Infectivity of *Heterakis gallinae* eggs with *Histomonas meleagridis. Exp. Parasitol.* 6:189–93.

Lund, E. E., and D. J. Ellis. 1967. The Japanese quail, *Coturnix coturnix japonica,* as a host for Heterakis and Histomonas. *Lab. Animal Care* 17:110–13.

Lund, E. E., and Marion M. Farr. 1965. Protozoa, pp. 1056–1148. In Biester, H. E., and L. H. Schwarte (eds.), *Diseases of Poultry,* 5th ed. Iowa State Univ. Press, Ames.

Lund, E. E., E. E. Wehr, and D. J. Ellis. 1963. Role of earthworms in transmission of Heterakis and Histomonas to turkeys and chickens. *J. Parasitol.* 49 (5, Sect. 2):50. (Abstr.)

Lund, E. E., Patricia C. Augustine, and D. J. Ellis. 1966a. Immunizing action of in vitro-attenuated *Histomonas meleagridis* in chickens and turkeys. *Exp. Parasitol.* 18:403–7.

Lund, E. E., E. E. Wehr, and D. J. Ellis. 1966b. Earthworm transmission of Heterakis and Histomonas to turkeys and chickens. *J. Parasitol.* 52:899–902.

Lund, E. E., Patricia C. Augustine, and Anne M. Chute. 1967. *Histomonas meleagridis* after one thousand in vitro passages. *J. Protozool.* 14:349–51.

McGregor, J. K. 1949. Observations on the prophylactic value of certain drugs for enterohepatitis infection (blackhead) in turkeys. *Can. J. Comp. Med. Vet. Sci.* 13:257–61.

McGuire, W. C., and J. W. Cavett. 1952. Blood studies on histomoniasis in turkeys. *Poultry Sci.* 31:610–17.

Madsen, H. 1962. On the interaction between *Heterakis gallinarum, Ascaridia galli,* "blackhead" and the chicken. *J. Helminthol.* 36:107–42.

Malewitz, T. D., and M. L. Calhoun. 1957. The normal hematological picture of turkey poults and blood alterations caused by entero-hepatitis. *Am. J. Vet. Res.* 18:396–99.

Mohler, J. R. 1905. Blackhead, or infectious

entero-hepatitis, in turkeys. *USDA BAI Circ.* 5 (rev.), pp. 1–8.

Morehouse, N. F., T. A. Rude, and R. D. Vatne. 1968. Liver regeneration in black-head-infected turkeys treated with 1,2-dimethyl-5-nitroimidazole. *Avian Diseases* 12: 85–95.

Niimi, D. 1937. Studies on blackhead. II. Mode of infection. (In Japanese, English summary.) *J. Japan. Soc. Vet. Sci.* 16:23–26, 183–239.

Ohara, T., and W. M. Reid. 1961. Histomoniasis in chickens: Age of greatest susceptibility and pathogenicity studies. *Avian Diseases* 5:355–61.

Peardon, D. L., and H. J. Eoff. 1967. Efficacy of p-ureidobenzenearsonic acid against blackhead in chickens. *Poultry Sci.* 46:1108–12.

Peardon, D. L., and J. R. Ramsay. 1968. Efficacy of p-ureidobenzenearsonic acid against blackhead in chickens exposed orally with *Heterakis gallinae* ova. *Poultry Sci.* 47:312–14.

Peterson, E. H. 1967. Studies on MK–930, a new drug effective against enterohepatitis. *Poultry Sci.* 46:1306. (Abstr.)

Reid, W. M. 1967. Etiology and dissemination of the blackhead disease syndrome in turkeys and chickens. *Exp. Parasitol.* 21:249–75.

Rice, F. E. 1892. Disease among turkeys, p. 96. In *4th Ann. Rept. Rhode Island Agr. Expt. Sta., 1891*, Pt. II.

Sautter, J. H., B. S. Pomeroy, and M. H. Roepke. 1950. Histomoniasis (enterohepatitis) in turkeys. II. Chemotherapy of experimental histomoniasis. *Am. J. Vet. Res.* 11:120–29.

Smith, T. 1895. An infectious disease among turkeys caused by protozoa (infectious entero-hepatitis), pp. 7–38. In *Investigations Concerning Infectious Diseases among Poultry.* USDA BAI Bull. 8.

———. 1910. Amoeba meleagridis. *Science* 32:509–12.

———. 1915. Further investigations into the etiology of the protozoan disease of turkeys known as blackhead, entero-hepatitis, typhlitis, etc. *J. Med. Res.* 33:243–70.

Smith, T., and H. W. Graybill. 1920. Blackhead in chickens and its experimental production by feeding embryonated eggs of *Heterakis papillosa. J. Exp. Med.* 32:143–52.

Spindler, L. A. 1967. Experimental transmission of *Histomonas meleagridis* and *Heterakis gallinarum* by the sow bug, *Porcellio scaber,* and its implications for further research. *Proc. Helminthol. Soc. Wash.* 34:26–29.

Swales, W. E. 1948. Enterohepatitis (blackhead) in turkeys. II. Observations on transmission by the cecal worm *(Heterakis gallinae). Can. J. Comp. Med.* 12:97–100.

———. 1950. Enterohepatitis (blackhead) in turkeys. VII. Experiments on transmission of the disease. *Can. J. Comp. Med.* 14:298–303.

Tyzzer, E. E. 1919. Developmental phases of the protozoon of "blackhead" in turkeys. *J. Med. Res.* 40:1–30.

———. 1920. The flagellate character and reclassification of the parasite producing "blackhead" in turkeys—*Histomonas* (gen. nov.) *meleagridis* (Smith). *J. Parasitol.* 6:124–31.

———. 1923. Arsenical compounds in the treatment of blackhead in turkeys. *J. Exp. Med.* 37:851–73.

———. 1924. The chicken as a carrier of *Histomonas meleagridis* (blackhead): The protozoon in its flagellated stage. *J. Med. Res.* 44:676–77. (Abstr.)

———. 1926. *Heterakis vesicularis* Froelich 1791: A vector of an infectious disease. *Proc. Soc. Exp. Biol. Med.* 23:708–9.

———. 1927. Entero-hepatitis in turkeys and its transmission through the agency of *Heterakis vesicularis. Rep. Proc. Third World's Poultry Congr.,* pp. 286–90.

———. 1932. Problems and observations concerning the transmission of blackhead infection in turkeys. *Proc. Am. Phil. Soc.* 71:407–10.

———. 1934. Studies on histomoniasis, or "blackhead" infection, in the chicken and the turkey. *Proc. Am. Acad. Arts Sci.* 69:189–264.

———. 1936. A study of immunity produced by infection with attenuated culture-strains of *Histomonas meleagridis. J. Comp. Pathol. Therap.* 49:285–303.

Tyzzer, E. E., and M. Fabyan. 1922. A further inquiry into the source of the virus in blackhead of turkeys, together with observations on the administration of ipecac and sulfur. *J. Exp. Med.* 35:791–812.

Tyzzer, E. E., M. Fabyan, and N. C. Foot. 1921. Further observations on "blackhead" in turkeys. *J. Infect. Diseases* 29:268–86.

Vatne, R. D., R. R. Baron, and N. F. Morehouse. 1967. Salfuride, a new antihistomonal compound. *Poultry Sci.* 46:1332. (Abstr.)

Waletzky, E., M. C. Brandt, A. Bliznick, and C. O. Hughes. 1949. Some new chemotherapeutic agents in experimental enterohepatitis (blackhead) of turkeys. *J. Parasitol.* 35 (6, Sect. 2):16. (Abstr.)

Wehr, E. E., and L. S. Olivier. 1946. Limitations of phenothiazine in the control of cecal worms and blackhead disease of turkeys. *Poultry Sci.* 25:199–203.

Wehr, E. E., M. M. Farr, and D. K. McLoughlin. 1958. Chemotherapy of blackhead in poultry. *J. Am. Vet. Med. Ass.* 132:439–45.

Whitmore, J. H., T. W. Sullivan, and O. D. Grace. 1968a. Prophylactic efficacy of vitamin A and certain compounds against histomoniasis in turkeys. *Poultry Sci.* 47:159–64.

———. 1968b. Prophylactic efficacy of 1-methyl-2-carbamoyloxymethyl-5-nitroimidazole against histomoniasis in turkeys. *Poultry Sci.* 47:428–30.

———. 1968c. Efficacy of graded levels of p-ureidobenzenearsonic acid against different levels of exposure to histomoniasis in turkeys 5 and 13 weeks old. *Poultry Sci.* 47: 450–53.

❖

OTHER PROTOZOAN DISEASES

❖

LEUCOCYTOZOONOSIS

THE GENUS Leucocytozoon Danilewsky 1890 is difficult to define but is fundamentally very close to Plasmodium and Haemoproteus. Levine (1961), after examining the life cycles as reported for representatives of each of the three genera, concluded that "there is no point in retaining more than a single family in the suborder" (which he designated as Hemospororina). But Fallis and Bennett (1961), after comparing several stages in the life cycles of members of the three genera, proposed that each genus occupy a separate family, all being in the order Hemosporidiida. Variations in interpretations appear to rest largely on the relative significance ascribed to similarities and differences in the life cycles. The similarities are, of course, impressive.

The gametocytes of Leucocytozoon, supposedly without pigment, appear in the circulating blood inside distorted host cells, presumably leucocytes; multiplication is by schizogony undergone only in the internal organs. As in the malarias, there is a blood-sucking dipterous intermediate host in which fertilization and sporogony take place, very much as in the case of the true malarial parasites. There has been considerable difference of opinion over the nature of the host cell of the gametocytes, but Huff (1942) found evidence that in *Leucocytozoon simondi*, while various types of cells are initially invaded, this stage becomes fully grown only in "monocytes, or more possibly macrophages." Hartman (1929), O'Roke (1934), and others have observed pigment granules in the cytoplasm. Huff (1942), however, pointed out that such granules may not be true hematin such as occurs in malarial parasites that develop in erythrocytes, because it is not visible as pigment in unstained preparations and its optical properties are different from those of malarial pigment. Borg (1953) could remove the pigment from *L. mansoni* with dilute acetic acid and ammonia, but not from Haemoproteus. The nucleus of the male gametocyte is somewhat larger than that of the female, and its cytoplasm stains less deeply. Several stages in the life cycle of Leucocytozoon from turkeys are shown in Fig. 31.10.

Birds seem to be the sole hosts of Leucocytozoon. Coatney (1937) cataloged and host-indexed 68 species up to that year. The card files of the USDA Index-Catalogue of Medical and Veterinary Zoology list almost 100 species of Leucocytozoon, but perhaps a quarter of these are now regarded as synonyms or are otherwise out of use. At least two, and probably three, species occur in domestic birds in North America.

Leucocytozoon simondi Mathis and Ledger 1910

Etiology

L. anatis Wickware (1915), described from tame ducks, appears on morphological grounds to be a synonym of *L.*

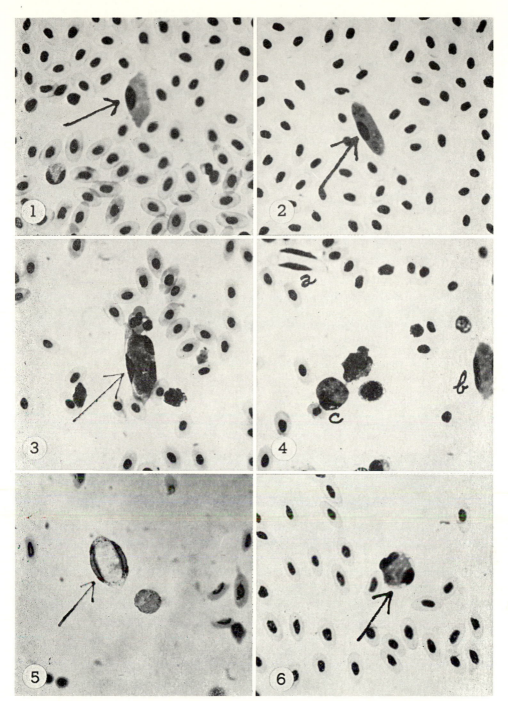

FIG. 31.10—*Photomicrographs of stained turkey blood containing various stages of Leucocytozoon from turkeys. Giemsa, ×750. (1) Microgametocyte with only one lateral bar present. Note light color of parasite. (2) Macrogametocyte with only one lateral bar present. Note dark color of parasite. (3) Macrogametocyte with one bar on one side and two bars on opposite side. (4) Microgametocyte shown at a, and macrogametocyte at b, each with bilateral bars, are most common forms found. At c may be seen a macrogametocyte that has become round to form a macrogamete. Note that one bar is still attached ventrally. (5) Early microgametocyte with distinct difference between density of central body, or what might be the parasite proper, and surrounding cytoplasm connecting the two lateral bars or possible host-cell nucleus. At right and ventrally is a typical granulocyte with eosinophilic rod granules. Note comparative size. (6) Earliest macrogametocyte found. Here again there is well-marked distinction between central body and surrounding cytoplasm including the bilateral bars. (Johnson et al., 1938)*

simondi (Coatney and Roudabush, 1937; Herman, 1938). *L. anseris* Knuth and Magdeburg 1922, described from geese, appears to be another synonym. Fallis et al. (1954) found in cross-infection trials that ducks and geese were suitable hosts for this species, but chickens, turkeys, pheasants, and ruffed grouse were not.

L. simondi, first described from an oriental teal in Tonkin, is found in the blood as gametocytes measuring 14–15μ by 4.5–5.5μ. These usually inhabit elongate spindle-shaped host cells pointed at both ends and about 48μ in length. The parasite lies either beside a conspicuously staining bar or between two such bars representing the nucleus of the host cell. Huff (1942) identifies the latter as a distorted monocyte or macrophage. Fallis et al. (1951) observed round gametocytes in addition to the spindle-shaped, which were mature because of the ability to exflagellate.

Schizogony takes place in such internal organs as the liver, heart, brain, spleen, and lungs. According to Huff (1942), the earliest stages consist of small ovoid bodies inside macrophages, extracellular, or within liver (parenchyma) cells, and showing some degree of separation of their more densely staining material. The "hepatic schizonts" in liver cells, measuring 11–18μ, undergo differentiation into cytomeres which in the final step in schizogony break up into small merozoites. The "megaloschizonts," measuring 60–105μ when mature, usually develop inside cells (possibly lymphoid cells or macrophages) within or outside blood vessels. The earliest stages observed were inside cells and were already multinuclear. Later stages were very large and contained numerous cytomeres (intermediate subdivisions of a schizont) and a large conspicuous "central body" concerning whose true nature Huff is not certain, but he conjectures that it is the hypertrophied nucleus of the host cell. Cowan (1955), however, interprets the "central body" as an integral part of the parasite—a "primordium"—from whose surface bud off the primary cytomeres. In the last step of schizogony the megaloschizont contains many thousands of bipolar merozoites being released into the gametocytes after invading suitable cells. Fallis et al. (1951) noted mature forms in peripheral blood as early as 7 days after exposure to natural infection, and later, 5–6 days af-

ter (Fallis et al., 1956). Parasitemia may terminate in about 30 days after its first appearance (Chernin, 1952c).

Pathogenesis and Epizootiology

L. simondi occurs in domestic ducks and geese and has been reported from many wild anseriform birds. Levine and Hanson (1953) tabulated reports of this parasite from 23 species of wild waterfowl.

O'Roke (1934) first showed a bloodsucking fly, *Simulium venustum,* to be the vector among ducks in Michigan and outlined the development in this insect. Fallis et al. (1951, 1956) have added *S. croxtoni, S. euradminiculum,* and *S. rugglesi* to the list of transmitters, with the suggestion that the latter is the natural vector in Canada. Development in the fly may be completed in a minimal time of 4 days, and a fly may remain infective for as long as 18 days.

There is no doubt about the pathogenicity of *L. simondi* in ducks and geese. O'Roke in Michigan noted 35% mortality in an outbreak among ducks, confirming in general the observations of Wickware (1915) in Canada. Knuth (1922) and Knuth and Magdeburg (1922) reported on a serious and often fatal disease among young geese in Germany apparently caused by the same organism. (See also Stephan, 1922.) About 68% of the fatalities occur 11–19 days after exposure (Chernin, 1952a). Some of the pathological effects of the disease are anemia, leucocytosis, splenomegaly, and liver degeneration and hypertrophy (Fallis et al., 1951). Kocan (1968) reports: "An anti-erythrocyte (A-E) factor was found in the serum of acutely infected ducks which agglutinated and hemolyzed normal untreated duck erythrocytes as well as infected cells." This factor was believed to be a product of the parasite, and its action was intravascular.

Extensive tissue damage was noted by Huff (1942) in the spleens and hearts of ducks carrying megaloschizonts. O'Roke (1930), Chernin and Sadun (1949), and Chernin (1952a) have noted that the greatest number of infections in northern Michigan is coincident with the hottest part of the summer and occurs mostly in July.

O'Roke (1934) and Huff (1942) both observed that the gametocytes decrease in number in the blood until midwinter when they disappear or become scarce and then reappear in the spring. The sporadic occurrence of parasites in the blood during the entire winter, however sparse they may be, indicates that sporogony is proceeding at a low level. After a 3-year investigation of the spring relapse phenomenon, Chernin (1952b) concluded that it was associated with the onset of renewed reproductive activity in both sexes of the avian host. Female ducks subjected to increased hours of artificial light per day in the fall and winter not only commenced egg laying earlier but experienced earlier onset of the relapse parasitemia.

Leucocytozoon smithi Laveran and Lucet 1905

Incidence and Distribution

L. smithi was first seen in turkeys in the eastern United States by Smith (1895), after whom it is named. It has been reported by Volkmar (1929) as occurring in North Dakota and Minnesota, by Skidmore (1932) in Nebraska, by Johnson (1942, 1945) in Virginia, and by Hinshaw and McNeil (1943) in California. Other reports indicate its presence in France, Germany, Crimea, and Canada. The widespread occurrence of the parasite in certain areas is emphasized by the survey of Travis et al. (1939) on adult domesticated turkeys: 289 of 357 were found infected in Georgia, 60 of 67 in Florida, 4 of 12 in Alabama, and 7 of 9 in South Carolina. Mosby and Handley (1943) reported the parasite in 40% of 268 turkeys in Virginia, of which 40 were domestic, 183 were captivity-reared wild turkeys, and 45 were wild. Others who have reported Leucocytozoon in captive wild turkeys are Johnson et al. (1938), Wehr and Coburn (1943), and Travis et al. (1939); Kozicky (1948) found it in all of 5 native wild turkeys taken in the field in Pennsylvania. Byrd (1959), who studied Leucocytozoon in penraised and free-ranging wild turkeys in the Cumberland State Forest of Virginia, reported incidences of almost 100% among mature birds maintained in large open pens in the spring.

Etiology

Positive identification of leucocytozoonosis requires the finding of the organism in the tissues or blood of the turkey at necropsy. Dried blood smears stained with Wright's or Giemsa's stains provide a convenient method of examination. *L. smithi* in general resembles *L. simondi* of Anseriformes, but turkeys are probably not susceptible to the latter (Fallis et al., 1954; Byrd, 1959).

Wehr, studying schizogony in the domestic turkey, found indications that the life cycle of *L. smithi* may differ in some details from that of *L. simondi* in ducks. These observations were in agreement with those of some earlier workers, such as Richey and Ware (1955) and Newberne (1955).

Pathogenesis and Epizootiology

Skidmore (1932) considered *Simulium occidentale* to be the vector concerned in a Nebraska outbreak of leucocytozoonosis in domestic turkeys; Johnson et al. (1938) found *S. nigroparvum* to be the vector in Virginia. Wehr (1962), studying outbreaks of Leucocytozoon infection in domestic turkeys in South Carolina, transmitted the parasite experimentally by intramuscular injections of suspensions of ground black flies, *Simulium slossonae*. He cited communications with others working in the same region who also found this species of black fly to transmit the disease.

Byrd (1959), working with infected mature wild turkeys in Virginia, observed: "Heavy infections, comparable to those reported for *L. simondi* in ducks, do not seem to occur. . . . Few symptoms were observed in wild turkeys that could be attributed to the disease." He attempted to relate this lack of pathogenicity to local factors, such as the time at which suitable vectors were prevalent and the age of the birds at first exposure. With regard to the vector, Byrd observed, "The period of infection for the disease on the Cumberland forest is such that *P.* [*Prosimulium*] *hirtipes* appears to be the only species responsible for its transmission." Byrd considered the possibility, also, that wild turkeys may "have developed some degree of natural resistance to the disease" (leucocytozoonosis).

According to Hinshaw (1965), poults under 12 weeks of age are most affected by outbreaks of leucocytozoonosis in domestic turkeys. The visible signs (loss of appetite, droopiness, and general indisposition) last only 2–3 days, after which the birds either die or recover. Those that recover may harbor parasites in their blood for several months. Some birds develop a chronic form of the disease resulting in a mild indisposition, sometimes expressed in males by a lack of interest in mating. However, terrific losses have been experienced among poults and even adults; Stoddard et al. (1952) reported an outbreak in Georgia wherein a grower suffered a 75% loss in a flock of 1,600 5-month-old turkeys presumably due to Leucocytozoon disease. Flies of the genus Simulium were observed in the vicinity of roosts and feeding troughs.

The pathogenesis of the disease has been described in detail by Newberne (1955).

Leucocytozoon Species from the Chicken

Atchley (1951) described *Leucocytozoon andrewsi*, n. sp., from chickens in South Carolina. It had rounded gametocytes, was present in 15.3% of 400 chickens examined, and represents the only instance in which Leucocytozoon has been reported from chickens in North America. Levine (1961) regards *L. andrewsi* as a synonym of *L. caulleryi,* a species reported by several investigators as present in chickens in southern and eastern Asia, but Atchley considered the regular presence of the nucleus in the host cell sufficient basis for the creation of the new species. He gave no indication of the pathogenicity of this parasite. Levine (1961) concluded, "This species is presumably pathogenic, but accounts of it have been so mixed up with those of *L. sabrazesi* [a species thus far known only from southeast Asia]. . . . that its pathogenicity is uncertain." Wehr (1962) observed, "The status of *L. andrewsi* is in doubt, and cannot be determined until more is known of its development and mode of transmission in the chicken."

L. sabrazesi Mathis and Leger 1910 was frequently found by its describers in chickens in Tonkin. Kuppusamy (1936) considers it a pathogen of economic importance in Malaya. The gametocytes in the blood, like *L. simondi,* are enveloped in elongate spindle-shaped host cells, pointed at both ends. *L. schuffneri* Prowazek 1912, from domestic fowl in Sumatra, may be a synonym. *L. caulleryi* Mathis and Leger 1909 was also observed in the blood of chickens in Tonkin. The gametocytes were enveloped in round host cells which, when the parasites were mature, frequently were without nuclei. In this connection, Pan (1963), studying blood smears from White

Leghorns in Taiwan, proposed a new interpretation of the gametogony of *Leucocytozoon caulleryi.* He believed that the development of the gametocytes differed somewhat, depending on whether a given host cell was parasitized by one or by more than one organism. If by only one, the host cell nucleus was lost. If several organisms entered the same host cell, that cell apparently ruptured. This, he believed, accounted for both the freed stages of gametocytes and the disrupted host cells, both of which he encountered at times.

Leucocytozoon mansoni Sambon 1908

L. mansoni, from the Swedish capercaillie *(Tetrao urogallus),* has been the subject of an intensive investigation by Borg (1953), whose results led him to conclude that this and similar parasites occurring in Swedish forest game birds have no significant role in the widespread mortality in their hosts (capercaillie, black grouse, hazel grouse). Gametocytes were of three types—round, oval, and elongated. The host cells of the latter two types had tails at the two extremities unless they were worn off.

TREATMENT

Drug treatment has been reviewed by O'Roke (1934) and Coatney and West (1937). Pamakin (plasmochin) proved unsatisfactory; quinine showed promise if fed for a time before adult gametocytes showed in the blood but did not affect adult gametocytes. Coatney found that atebrin did attack the adult gametocytes. On the other hand, Fallis (1948) had no success in curing or suppressing infections of *L. simondi* in ducks with paludrine, atebrin, or sulfamerazine. He was inclined to blame the resistance of the tissue stages for the failure.

CONTROL

Control is to be attained only through management. This means principally that duck and turkey culture should not be attempted in regions where there is running water serving as breeding places for an abundance of black flies (Simulium). Otherwise it is necessary to screen the young birds from the flies, which is difficult. Removing parasitized young and adult birds from the flock would also prove helpful in some instances. For ducks, O'Roke (1934) has suggested hatching the ducklings either before or after the main black fly season. For turkeys, Hinshaw (1965) points out that it may be useful to sell adult breeders before young stock is brought in for replacement. If breeders are kept for two laying seasons, the flocks of first- and second-year breeders should be well separated or this system would fail.

Anthony and Richey (1958) attempted to control outbreaks of *L. smithi* in domestic turkeys in South Carolina by spraying the breeding grounds of black flies with

DDT. This was very effective for 2 weeks and moderately so for another 2 weeks. After that, near drought conditions developed, so black fly control actually averaged almost 95% effective over a 10-week period. Nevertheless, poults placed on range 4 weeks after the application of DDT to the black fly breeding grounds started showing Leucocytozoon disease within 2 weeks of release. Within another 4 weeks, 80–100% of the birds were infected. Anthony and Richey suggested that other diptera may have been responsible for the transmission of the disease.

REFERENCES

Anthony, D. W., and D. J. Richey. 1958. Influence of black fly control on the incidence of Leucocytozoon disease in South Carolina turkeys. *J. Econ. Entomol.* 51:845–47.

Atchley, F. O. 1951. *Leucocytozoon andrewsi* n. sp., from chickens observed in a survey of blood parasites in domestic animals in South Carolina. *J. Parasitol.* 37:483–88.

Borg. K. 1953. *On Leucocytozoon in Swedish Capercaillie, Black Grouse and Hazel Grouse.* State Vet. Med. Inst. of Sweden (Stockholm), Lund.

Byrd, M. A. 1959. Observations on Leucocytozoon in pen-raised and free-ranging wild turkeys. *J. Wildlife Management* 23:145–56.

Chernin, E. 1952a. The epizootiology of *Leucocytozoon simondi* infections in domestic ducks in northern Michigan. *Am. J. Hyg.* 56:39–57.

———. 1952b. The relapse phenomenon in the *Leucocytozoon simondi* infection of the domestic duck. *Am. J. Hyg.* 56:101–18.

———. 1952c. Parasitemia in primary *Leucocytozoon simondi* infections. *J. Parasitol.* 38:499–508.

Chernin, E., and E. H. Sadun. 1949. *Leucocytozoon simondi* infections in domestic ducks in northern Michigan with a note on Haemoproteus. *Poultry Sci.* 28:890–93.

Coatney, G. R. 1937. A catalog and host-index of the genus Leucocytozoon. *J. Parasitol.* 23:202–12.

Coatney, G. R., and R. L. Roudabush. 1937. Some blood parasites from Nebraska birds. *Am. Midland Naturalist* 18:1005–30.

Coatney, G. R., and E. West. 1937. Some notes on the effect of atebrine on gametocytes of the genus Leucocytozoon. *J. Parasitol.* 23:227–28.

Cowan, A. B. 1955. The development of megaloschizonts of *Leucocytozoon simondi* Mathis and Leger. *J. Protozool.* 2:158–67.

———. 1957. Reactions against the megaloschizonts of *Leucocytozoon simondi* Mathis

and Leger in ducks. *J. Infect. Diseases* 100:82–87.

Fallis, A. M. 1948. Observations on Leucocytozoon infections in birds receiving paludrine, atebrin, and sulphamerazine. *Can. J. Res.* 26:73–76.

Fallis, A. M., and G. F. Bennett. 1961. Sporogony of Leucocytozoon and Haemoproteus in simuliids and ceratopogonids and a revised classification of the Haemosporidiida. *Can. J. Zool.* 39:215–28.

Fallis, A. M., D. M. Davies, and M. A. Vickers. 1951. Life history of *Leucocytozoon simondi* Mathis and Leger in natural and experimental infections and blood changes produced in the avian host. *Can. J. Zool.* 29:305–28.

Fallis, A. M., J. C. Pearson, and G. F. Bennett. 1954. On the specificity of Leucocytozoon. *Can. J. Zool.* 32:120–24.

Fallis, A. M., R. C. Anderson, and G. F. Bennett. 1956. Further observations on the transmission and development of *Leucocytozoon simondi. Can. J. Zool.* 34:389–404.

Hartman, E. 1929. The asexual cycle in *Leucocytozoon anatis. J. Parasitol.* 15:178–82.

Herman, C. M. 1938. *Leucocytozoon anatis* Wickware, a synonym for *L. simondi* Mathis and Leger. *J. Parasitol.* 24:472–73.

Hinshaw, W. R. 1965. Diseases of the turkey, pp. 1337–40. In Biester, H. E., and L. H. Schwarte (eds.), *Diseases of Poultry,* 5th ed. Iowa State Univ. Press, Ames.

Hinshaw, W. R., and Ethel McNeil. 1943. Leucocytozoon sp. from turkeys in California. *Poultry Sci.* 22:268–69.

Huff, C. G. 1942. Schizogony and gametocyte development in *Leucocytozoon simondi,* and comparisons with Plasmodium and Haemoproteus. *J. Infect. Diseases* 71:18–32.

Johnson, E. P. 1942. Further observations on a blood protozoan of turkeys transmitted by *Simulium nigroparvum* (Twinn). *Am. J. Vet. Res.* 3:214–18.

———. 1945. Blood parasites of turkeys. *Mich.*

State Coll. Vet. 5:144–46, 174.

Johnson, E. P., G. W. Underhill, J. A. Cox, and W. L. Threlkeld. 1938. A blood protozoon of turkeys transmitted by *Simulium nigroparvum* (Twinn). *Am. J. Hyg.* 27:649–65.

Knuth, P. 1922. Demonstration ueber in Deutschland gefundene Leukozytozoen der Hausgaus. *Arch. Schiffs- u. Tropen-Hyg.* 26:315–17.

Knuth, P., and F. Magdeburg. 1922. Ueber ein durch Leukozytozoen verursachtes Sterben junger Gaense. *Berlin. Tieraerztl. Wochschr.* 38:359–61.

Kocan, R. M. 1968. Anemia and mechanism of erythrocyte destruction in ducks with acute Leucocytozoon infections. *J. Protozool.* 15:455–62.

Kozicky, E. L. 1948. Some protozoan parasites of the eastern wild turkey in Pennsylvania. *J. Wildlife Management* 12:263–66.

Kuppusamy, A. R. 1936. *Leucocytozoa sabrazesi* and *Microfilariae seguini* of fowls and *Haemoproteus columbae* of pigeons in province of Wellesley. *Indian Vet. J.* 13:24–35.

Levine, N. D. 1961. *Protozoan Parasites of Domestic Animals and of Man.* Burgess Publ. Co., Minneapolis.

Levine, N. D., and H. C. Hanson. 1953. Blood parasites of the Canada goose, *Branta canadensis interior.* *J. Wildlife Management* 17:185–96.

Mathis, C., and M. Leger. 1910. Leucocytozoon d'une tourterelle *(Turtur humilis)* et d'une sarcelle *(Querquedula crecca)* du Tonkin. *Compt. Rend. Soc. Biol.* 68:118–20.

Mosby, H. S., and C. O. Handley. 1943. *The Wild Turkey in Virginia; Its Status, Life History, and Management.* Commission of Game and Inland Fisheries, Richmond, Va.

Newberne, J. W. 1955. The pathology of Leucocytozoon infection in turkeys with a note on its tissue stages. *Am. J. Vet. Res.* 16:593–97.

O'Roke, E. C. 1930. The incidence, pathogenicity, and transmission of *Leucocytozoon*

anatis of ducks. *J. Parasitol.* 17 (Suppl. 2):112. (Abstr.)

———. 1934. A malaria-like disease of ducks caused by *Leucocytozoon anatis* Wickware. *Univ. Mich. School Forestry and Conserv. Bull.* 4:1–44.

Pan, I.-C. 1963. A new interpretation of the gametogony of *Leucocytozoon caulleryi* in chickens. *Avian Diseases* 7:361–68.

Richey, D. J., and R. E. Ware. 1955. Schizonts of *Leucocytozoon smithi* in artificially infected turkeys. *Cornell Vet.* 45:642–43.

Skidmore, L. V. 1932. *Leucocytozoon smithi* infections in turkeys and its transmission by *Simulium occidentale* Townsend. *Zentr. Bakteriol. Parasitenk. Abt. I. Orig.* 125:329–35.

Smith, T. 1895. An infectious disease among turkeys caused by protozoa (infectious entero-hepatitis). *USDA BAI Bull.* 8:7–38.

Stephan, J. 1922. Ueber eine durch Leukozytozoen verursachte Gaense-und Putenerkrankung. *Deut. Tieraerztl. Wochschr.* 30:589–92.

Stoddard, E. D., J. T. Tumlin, and D. E. Cooperrider. 1952. Recent outbreak of Leukocytozoon infection in adult turkeys in Georgia. *J. Am. Vet. Med. Ass.* 121:190–91.

Travis, B. V., M. H. Goodwin, Jr., and W. E. Gambrell. 1939. Preliminary note on the occurrence of *Leucocytozoon smithi* Laveran and Lucet (1905) in turkeys in the southeastern United States. *J. Parasitol.* 25:278.

Volkmar, F. 1929. Observations on *Leucocytozoon smithi;* with notes on Leukocytozoa in other poultry. *J. Parasitol.* 16:24–28.

Wehr, E. E. 1962. Studies on leucocytozoonosis of turkeys, with notes on schizogony, transmission, and control of *Leucocytozoon smithi.* *Avian Diseases* 6:195–210.

Wehr, E. E., and D. R. Coburn. 1943. Some economically important parasites of the wild turkey and Hungarian partridge of Pennsylvania. *Penn. Game News* 13:14–15.

Wickware, A. B. 1915. Is *Leucocytozoon anatis* the cause of a new disease in ducks? *Parasitology* 8:17–21.

TOXOPLASMOSIS

Toxoplasmosis is an infection of mammals and birds with *Toxoplasma gondii* Nicolle and Manceaux 1909, whose type host is the rodent *Ctenodactylus gundi* of North Africa. Interest in the parasite increased sharply about 1939 when its importance in man became evident. Thereafter interest in toxoplasmosis in all animals burgeoned, partly because of its potentially serious and multifarious effects on human beings and the epidemiological community of interest people share with animals in its dissemination, and partly because of its actual or potential role in causing losses among livestock. Expanding interest reflected in publications on the subject required 2,000 titles by 1956 (Hoare), most of which are listed in two bibliographies (Eyles and Frenkel, 1952, 1954). (See also Markham, 1956). Our interest is primarily in avian toxoplasmosis, dealt with recently by Jacobs and Melton (1966). Their references, together with those given by Siim et al. (1963), will guide the reader to the most significant portions of the vast volume of literature on those phases of the disease that concern us here.

ETIOLOGY

Classification

The taxonomic position of Toxoplasma remains uncertain. Wenyon (1926) placed it among organisms of doubtful nature, perhaps not protozoal at all. Manwell and Drobeck (1953) and Ludvik (1956) have indicated ways in which it resembles Sarcocystis. Goldman et al. (1957) have pointed out structural similarities in *Toxoplasma gondii* and *Besnoitia jellisoni,* although they found these two organisms to be serologically distinct. Lunde and Jacobs (1965) confirm this but note that they "appear to have certain antigens in common." Levine (1961) considered Toxoplasma as belonging to the same order as Sarcocystis, but he separated the two at the family level, placing Toxoplasma in the same family as Besnoitia and Encephalitozoon. Westphal (1954) regarded Toxoplasma as a nonflagellated, kinetoplast-free leishmanial type and suggested that it is a member of the Trypanosomidae, but this view has apparently received little support. Recently Sheffield and Melton (1970) and Frenkel et al. (1970) have presented evidence, both morphological and experimental, that *Toxoplasma gondii* is a coccidium, probably of the genus Isospora. Currently, this conclusion is receiving considerable acceptance. It is still too early to determine the impact of these findings on the concepts already held, and to determine where reappraisals of accepted interpretations are required. Consequently, the terminology previously used has been retained in the remainder of this section.

Morphology

The trophozoite of Toxoplasma is a crescentic body (Fig. 31.11), less rounded at one end than the other, measuring $4–7\mu$ in length and $2–4\mu$ in width. The nucleus is nearest the thicker end. An electron microscope study (Gustafson et al., 1954) has revealed a small hollow cone at the more tapering end and, radiating from the cone's base toward the thicker end, 14–16 homogeneous fibrils. Since that time several workers have used electron microscopy to study the finer structure of Toxoplasma. Sheffield and Melton (1968) not only listed these reports but contributed substantially to the findings of earlier workers and to our knowledge of the changes that occur as the organism reproduces.

Life Cycle

The trophozoite of Toxoplasma is capable of several types of movement of translation (Manwell and Drobeck, 1953). Reproduction is principally by binary fission of this stage inside a vacuole in one of a considerable variety of host cells—macrophages; lymphocytes; parenchymal cells of liver, adrenals, lungs, and brain; microglia; neuroglia; etc. A form of internal budding (endodyogeny) was described by Goldman et al. (1958), and this was in part confirmed by Gangi and Manwell (1961). However, the latter investigators did not see all stages

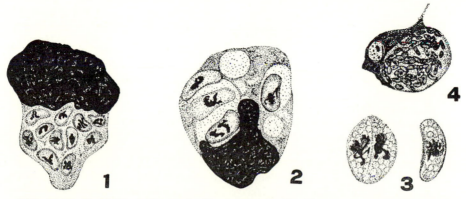

FIG. 31.11—(*1, 2*) *Toxoplasma bodies in lymphoid cells of ground squirrel.* (*3*) *Free Toxoplasma in same host, individual on left in division.* (*4*) *Toxoplasma in cytoplasm of nerve cell of rabbit.* (*1–3, Zasukhin and Gaiskii, 1930; 4, Levaditi and Schoen, 1928*)

characteristic of endodyogeny, and they made the interesting observation that "the inability to demonstrate cytochemically DNA in the parasites stained with silver protein suggests that morphologic structures seen in endodyogeny are not primarily involved with the distribution of gametic material." Repeated binary fissions result in an accumulation of organisms called a terminal colony, occupying the greater part of the host cell. The members of the colony are released by rupture of the cell and invade other cells. In the chronic or latent infection a cystlike stage is characteristic and predominant. It is a round or oval agglomeration of organisms, usually found in the brain, measuring 14.5–37.7μ across and enclosed by a wall of sufficient tenacity to hold the structure together when the surrounding tissue is disintegrated by shaking with glass beads (Rodhain, 1950). Jacobs et al. (1960) reviewed the recent literature dealing with these cystlike bodies and concluded that they may properly be called "cysts" rather than "pseudocysts," as some have suggested. They also demonstrated that the cyst wall was destroyed immediately on contact with a peptic digest solution heated to 37° C, and that the Toxoplasma so liberated remained infective for mice after exposure to the pepsin-HCl solution 1.5–2 hours but not after exposures of 3 hours or more. The cyst wall was digested in 1% trypsin also, and Toxoplasma remained viable in this solution after 6 hours. Proliferative Toxoplasma did not withstand the action of artificial gastric juice for even very brief intervals. For additional details concerning the nature of the cyst wall, its origin, composition, and staining, see Jacobs (1963). One must not confuse these cystlike bodies found in the brain of an infected mouse with the "new cystic form" of Work and Hutchison (1969), which is the oocyst as described and figured by Sheffield and Melton (1970) and Frenkel et al. (1970). The latter body possesses the characteristics of a typical coccidial oocyst (Isospora type) including site of origin, requirements for sporulation, and means of infecting the new host. Some who consider the coccidial nature of Toxoplasma as controversial may be wondering whether all bodies described as stages in the life cycle of Toxoplasma actually belong to the same organism. The postulated life cycle depicted by Frenkel et al. (1970) seems to answer some questions and raise others.

Cultivation

Cook and Jacobs (1958) tabulated the history of in vitro cultivation of Toxoplasma. Kaufman and Maloney (1962) studied the organism's multiplication in tissue culture and suggested that certain relationships may exist between the rate of multiplication of a strain of Toxoplasma and its susceptibility to antimetabolic drugs such as pyrimethamine and the sulfonamides.

PATHOGENESIS AND EPIZOOTIOLOGY

Natural and Experimental Hosts

Spontaneous toxoplasmosis has been reported in at least 27 genera of mammals belonging to 8 orders (Siim et al., 1963), in many species of birds of several orders (Manwell and Drobeck, 1953), and perhaps in certain reptiles also. Some of these hosts (Jacobs, 1956) are moles, gundis, guinea pigs, mice (but laboratory strains do not ordinarily harbor the organism), rats, rabbits and hares, dogs, foxes, cats, swine, sheep, cattle, baboons, chimpanzees, monkeys, man, pigeons, chickens, turkeys, and ducks. Capercaillie, black grouse, hazel grouse (Borg, 1953), crows (Finlay and Manwell, 1956), and barnyard geese (Biering-Sorensen [1957] dye test) may be added to this list.

Transmission, Carriers, Vectors

Considering the uncertainty surrounding the etiology of toxoplasmosis, we can understand why the means of transmission of Toxoplasma are as yet unclear. Congenital transmission has been established in such mammals as human beings (Feldman and Miller, 1956), dogs (Koestner and Cole, 1960), pigs, and cattle. The ingestion of contaminated food or water, including the flesh of an infected animal, surely seems to be another method of transmission. However, the unprotected trophozoites may not always endure the conditions of the digestive tract, which apparently may differ with the age of the animal. Kulasiri (1965), for example, could readily infect chicks 1 day old with an avirulent strain of Toxoplasma by giving the parasites orally. Chicks 3 days old were less readily infected and older chicks were refractory. He cites a report of similar results obtained by using a virulent strain of the parasite.

Transmission by bloodsucking arthropods such as ticks, mites, mosquitoes, fleas, and lice has been suggested and has a certain degree of plausibility because of the occurrence of the parasites in the circulating blood, usually inside monocytes. Wolfson (1941) worked with a strain which she obtained from a worker who had first observed it in a guinea pig which had been "injected with some ticks." A limited number of successful transmissions with certain ticks and a species of louse lends further credence to the hypothesis (Woke et al., 1953).

Course of the Disease

The first report of spontaneous toxoplasmosis in chickens was that by the German veterinarian Hepding (1939), who found the organisms, which he considered secondary invaders, in the retina of a hen with neurolymphomatosis. Other early observers are mentioned by Erichsen and Harboe (1953a). The latter workers studied an outbreak with some fatal illnesses in a small flock of White Leghorns in southern Norway. The outstanding symptoms of the sick birds were anorexia, emaciation, paleness and shrinking of the comb, and in some instances diarrhea and blindness. Nine birds from the flock were necropsied; of these, Toxoplasma was observed in sections of the organs of 5, but not in the eye despite the diffuse chorioiditis. In an important later study by the same authors (1953b), 2 experimentally infected birds and 1 naturally infected bird were found to have developed multiple gliomas in their brains. Intracerebral or intraperitoneal injections of suspensions of tissue from 3 birds resulted in Toxoplasma infection in 3 mice. The most outstanding lesions were focal and diffuse pericarditis, myocarditis, necrotizing encephalitis, necrotic hepatitis, and ulcerative gastroenteritis. The dye tests were either negative or feebly positive.

A rapidly developing outbreak in Brazil, in which the total mortality was 50% and almost the entire flock was affected, was reported by Nobrega et al (1955). Symptoms were similar to those of coccidiosis except that the stools were whitish. Outstanding necropsy findings were enlarged liver and spleen with necrotic foci, heart pale with yellowish white nodules of various sizes, and lungs with extensive areas of congestion and consolidation. Toxoplasma was observed in 10 of 15 chicks examined, both in smears of lungs, liver, and spleen stained with Giemsa and in tissue sections of spleen, heart, and lungs, but with one exception not in the central nervous system. The parasite was demonstrated in mice 4–6 months after intracerebral inoculation with organ suspensions.

Biering-Sorensen (1956) in Denmark diagnosed toxoplasmosis in 35 hens from 21 flocks of 26,000 fowls necropsied. Of these, 11 showed necrosis of the optic chiasm. In an epidemiological study of an area where toxoplasmosis had been found in fowls, the same author (1957) found 15 of 57 hens, all of 6 human beings, 4 of 22 geese, 2 of 6 horses, and 7 of 8 pigs positive to the dye test. Furthermore, mouse inoculation tests showed 8 fowls to be harboring the parasite. Pseudocysts were demonstrated in 8 fowls.

Siim et al. (1963) give a detailed description of toxoplasmosis in the chicken, including observations of results of experimental infections. Their account of the disease in pigeons is equally comprehensive and should be consulted by those who are concerned with this species of bird. They also mention one report of spontaneous toxoplasmosis in turkeys in Germany and one report of the course of the disease in turkeys infected experimentally. Apparently, spontaneous infections are rare among domestic turkeys in the United States, or they are not being sought. Spontaneous infections with *T. gondii* have been detected in ducks in the United States. Siim et al. state that these infections were very mild and suggest that they may occur more frequently than suspected.

DIAGNOSIS

Formerly, the most distinctive characteristic of Toxoplasma was considered to be its capacity to multiply and produce disease in a variety of hosts, including mammals and birds (Sabin, 1939). The organism's morphology, as demonstrated by practical diagnostic methods, could not be trusted as the sole basis for identification (Wolfson, 1940). For these reasons, intracerebral (0.03 ml) and intraperitoneal (0.1 ml) injections of body fluids and suspensions of tissues (brain, liver, lungs, spleen, etc.) of suspect hosts into laboratory mice, hamsters, guinea pigs, or young chicks and subsequent microscopic examinations of both fresh and stained smears of the inoculated hosts are depended upon both for confirmation of positive microscopic diagnosis and for revealing the presence of the etiological agent in cases where the microscopic examination is negative. Of course the actual demonstration of the parasite in the original case is in itself a valuable diagnostic accomplishment. Positive animal transmission adds much to the reliability of the diagnosis. When ascites or other symptoms of illness develop in the experimental host, the peritoneal fluid and smears of brain, liver, lungs, spleen, etc. should be examined for the parasite. If no parasites are found, or if the inoculated animals do not show symptoms in 7–8 days, blind passages should be made from the inoculated animals to another series. With chickens and pigeons a large number of blind subpassages in laboratory mice may be required before the parasite can be observed microscopically, or it may not be demonstrated at all.

Direct impression smears of tissues; smears of peritoneal fluid stained in Giemsa; or tissue sections of brain, lung, liver, spleen, lymph nodes, eye, etc. often serve for the direct microscopic observation of Toxoplasma when the oil-immersion lens is employed. Rarely the parasites are seen in blood smears, inside monocytes or free.

Carver and Goldman (1959) were able to locate organisms, singly or in clusters, in tissues sectioned in paraffin, by the use of fluorescein-labeled antibody.

Siim et al. (1963) list 11 methods that have been reported for laboratory diagnosis of toxoplasmosis. In addition to those methods discussed above, their list includes 7 "quantitative serologic tests," one of which is Sabin and Feldman's (1948) alkaline methylene blue dye test, simply called "the dye test." Recently (1966) Feldman and Lamb developed a modification of this test that requires less material and equipment than the conventional method. Unfortunately, infected chickens often respond weakly to the dye test, but pigeons perform better except in infections of long standing.

TREATMENT

Both sulfonamides (especially sulfadiazine, sulfamethazine, sulfamerazine, and sulfapyrazine) and the 2,4-diamino pyrimidines (especially pyrimethamine = Daraprim) have been shown to be effective in treating mouse and human infection (Eyles, 1956). Eyles and Coleman (1953) discovered that Daraprim and sulfonamides act synergistically, so that it was possible to obtain chemotherapeutic effect with much lower combined dosages than with the two drugs separately.

REFERENCES

Biering-Sorensen, U. 1956. Fjerkraetoxoplasmose. Om forekomsten af endemisk optraedende toxoplasmose (toxoplasmosis gallinarum) i danske honsebesaetninger. (Danish text, English and German summaries.) Nord. Veterinarmed. 8:140–64.

———. 1957. Serological examinations of the occurrence of latent toxoplasmosis in animals and human beings in an environment in which the diagnosis of toxoplasmosis gallinarum was verified. (Danish text, English and German summaries.) Nord. Veterinarmed. 9:129–44.

Borg, K. 1953. On Leucocytozoon in Swedish Capercaillie, Black Grouse and Hazel Grouse. State Vet. Med. Inst. of Sweden (Stockholm), Lund.

Carver, R. K., and M. Goldman. 1959. Staining Toxoplasma gondii with fluorescein-labeled antibody. III. The reaction in frozen and paraffin sections. Am. J. Clin. Pathol. 32:159–64.

Cook, M. Katherine, and L. Jacobs. 1958. Cultivation of Toxoplasma gondii in tissue cultures of various derivations. J. Parasitol. 44:172–82.

Erichsen, S., and A. Harboe. 1953a. Toxoplasmosis in chickens. I. An epidemic outbreak of toxoplasmosis in a chicken flock in southeastern Norway. Acta Pathol. Microbiol. Scand. 33:56–71.

———. 1953b. Toxoplasmosis in chickens. II. So-called gliomas observed in chickens infected with toxoplasms. Acta Pathol. Microbiol. Scand. 33:381–86.

Eyles, D. E. 1956. Newer knowledge of chemotherapy of toxoplasmosis. Ann. N.Y. Acad. Sci. 64:252–67.

Eyles, D. E., and Nell Coleman. 1953. Synergistic effect of sulfadiazine and daraprim against experimental toxoplasmosis in the mouse. Antibiot. Chemotherapy 3:483–90.

Eyles, D. E., and J. K. Frenkel. 1952. A Bibliography of Toxoplasmosis and Toxoplasma gondii. U.S. Public Health Serv. Publ. 247, Washington, D.C.

———. 1954. *A Bibliography of Toxoplasmosis and* Toxoplasma gondii. First Suppl. U.S. Public Health Serv., Washington, D.C. (Mimeo.)

Feldman, H. A., and G. A. Lamb. 1966. A micromodification of the Toxoplasma dye test. *J. Parasitol.* 52:415.

Feldman, H. A., and Louise T. Miller. 1956. Congenital human toxoplasmosis. *Ann. N.Y. Acad. Sci.* 64:180–84.

Finlay, P., and R. D. Manwell. 1956. Toxoplasma from the crow, a new natural host. *Exp. Parasitol.* 5:149–53.

Frenkel, J. K., J. P. Dubey, and N. L. Miller. 1970. *Toxoplasma* gondii in cats: Fecal stages identified as coccidian oocysts. *Science* 167:893–96.

Gangi, D. P., and R. D. Manwell. 1961. Some aspects of the cytochemical anatomy of *Toxoplasma gondii. J. Parasitol.* 47:291–96.

Goldman, M., R. K. Carver, and A. Sulzer. 1957. Similar internal morphology of *Toxoplasma gondii* and *Besnoitia jellisoni* stained with silver protein. *J. Parasitol.* 43:490–91.

———. 1958. Reproduction of *Toxoplasma gondii* by internal budding. *J. Parasitol.* 44:161–71.

Gustafson, P. V., Hilda D. Agar, and Dorothy I. Cramer. 1954. An electron microscope study of Toxoplasma. *Am. J. Trop. Med. Hyg.* 3:1008–21.

Hepding, L. 1939. Ueber Toxoplasmen *(Toxoplasma gallinarum* n. sp.) in der Retina eines Huhnes und ueber deren Beziehung zur Huehnerlaehmung. *Z. Infektionskr. Haustiere* 55:109–16.

Hoare, C. A. 1956. Toxoplasmosis in animals. *Vet. Rev. Annotations* 2:25–34.

Jacobs, L. 1953. The biology of Toxoplasma. *Am. J. Trop. Med. Hyg.* 2:365–89.

———. 1956. Propagation, morphology, and biology of toxoplasmosis. *Ann. N.Y. Acad. Sci.* 64:154–79.

———. 1963. *Toxoplasma* and toxoplasmosis. *Ann. Rev. Microbiol.* 17:429–50.

Jacobs, L., and Marjorie L. Melton. 1966. Toxoplasmosis in chickens. *J. Parasitol.* 52:1158–62.

Jacobs, L., J. S. Remington, and Marjorie L. Melton. 1960. The resistance of the encysted form of *Toxoplasma gondii. J. Parasitol.* 46:11–21.

Kaufman, H. E., and Emily D. Maloney. 1962. Multiplication of three strains of *Toxoplasma gondii* in tissue culture. *J. Parasitol.* 48:358–61.

Koestner, A., and C. R. Cole. 1960. Neuropathology of canine toxoplasmosis. *Am. J. Vet. Res.* 21:831–44.

Kulasiri, C. de S. 1965. Infection of the chicken with avirulent *Toxoplasma gondii. Exp. Parasitol.* 17:65–68.

Levaditi, C., and R. Schoen. 1928. Penetration et pullulation de protozoaires dans la cellule nerveuse (Neuroprotozooses). *Compt. Rend. Acad. Sci.* 186:1584–86.

Levine, N. D. 1961. *Protozoan Parasites of Animals and of Man.* Burgess Publ. Co., Minneapolis.

Ludvik, J. 1956. Vergleichende elektronenoptische Untersuchungen an *Toxoplasma gondii* und *Sarcocystis tenella.* (English summary.) *Zentr. Bakteriol. Parasitenk. Abt. I, Orig.* 166:60–65.

Lunde, M. N., and L. Jacobs. 1965. Antigenic relationship of *Toxoplasma gondii* and *Besnoitia jellisoni. J. Parasitol.* 51:273–76.

Manwell, R. D., and H. P. Drobeck. 1953. The behavior of Toxoplasma with notes on its taxonomic status. *J. Parasitol.* 39:577–84.

Markham, F. S. 1956. Part III. Toxoplasmosis. Introductory remarks. *Ann. N.Y. Acad. Sci.* 64:152–53.

Nobrega, P., E. Trapp, and M. Giovannoni. 1955. Toxoplasmose espontanea de galinha. *Arquiv. Inst. Biol. (Sao Paulo)* 22:43–49.

Rodhain, J. 1950. Formation de pseudokystes au cours d'essais d'immunite croisee entre souches differentes de Toxoplasmes. *Compt. Rend. Soc. Biol.* 144:719–22.

Sabin, A. B. 1939. Biological and immunological identity of Toxoplasma of animal and human origin. *Proc. Soc. Exp. Biol. Med.* 41:75–80.

Sabin, A. B., and H. A. Feldman. 1948. Dyes as microchemical indicators of a new immunity phenomenon affecting a protozoan parasite (Toxoplasma). *Science* 108:660–63.

Sheffield, H. G., and Marjorie L. Melton. 1968. The fine structure of *Toxoplasma gondii. J. Parasitol.* 54:209–26.

———. 1970. *Toxoplasma gondii:* The oocyst, sporozoite, and infection of cultured cells. *Science* 167:892–93.

Siim, J. C., U. Biering-Sorensen, and T. Moller. 1963. Toxoplasmosis in domestic animals. *Advan. Vet. Sci.* 8:335–429.

Wenyon, C. M. 1926. *Protozoology.* Bailliere, Tindall, and Cox, London.

Westphal, A. 1954. Zur Systematik von *Toxoplasma gondii.* Die Toxoplasmen als Trypanosomidae. *Z. Tropenmed. Parasitol.* 5:145–82.

Woke, P. A., L. Jacobs, Frances E. Jones, and Marjorie L. Melton. 1953. Experimental results on possible arthropod transmission of toxoplasmosis. *J. Parasitol.* 39:523–32.

Wolfson, Fruma. 1940. Organisms described as avian Toxoplasma. *Am. J. Hyg.* 32 (3, Sect. C): 88–99.

———. 1941. Mammalian Toxoplasma in

erythrocytes of canaries, ducks, and duck embryos. *Am. J. Trop. Med.* 21:653–58.

Work, K., and W. M. Hutchison. 1969. A new cystic form of *Toxoplasma gondii*. *Acta Pathol. Microbiol. Scand.* 75:191–92.

Zasukhin, D. N., and N. A. Gaiskii. 1930. *Toxoplasma nikanorovi* n. sp.—Parasite de *Citellus pygmaeus*. (Russian text, French summary.) *Vestn. Mikrobiol. Epidemiol. Parazitol.* 9:96–100, 135.

HAEMOPROTEUS INFECTIONS

ETIOLOGY

The genus Haemoproteus belongs to the family Haemoproteidae, which is fundamentally like the family Plasmodiidae (to which the true malaria parasites belong) except that schizogony occurs in endothelial cells of internal organs rather than in circulating blood cells. Ordinarily it is impossible to transfer the infection by inoculation of infected blood, as can be done with the true malarias (cf. Lastra and Coatney, 1950). Haemoproteus differs from Leucocytozoon in two important respects: (1) While in both genera the mature gametocytes are the stages generally occurring in the circulating blood, those of Haemoproteus occupy erythrocytes and those of Leucocytozoon, supposedly, only white cells, such as monocytes or macrophages. (2) True malarial pigment is produced in the gametocytes of Haemoproteus, while the pigmentlike granules of Leucocytozoon, if any, disappear from specimens on stained slides after washing in dilute acetic acid and ammonia.

VECTORS AND HOSTS

The life cycle of Haemoproteus in general parallels that of Plasmodium and Leucocytozoon, but the intermediate hosts of Haemoproteus species are usually hippoboscid flies (louse flies). However, Fallis and Wood (1957) have shown that an orthorrhaphous insect, a biting midge, *Culicoides* sp., is a suitable intermediate host and transmitting agent of *H. nettionis* of ducks. Coatney (1936) published a checklist and host index of the genus Haemoproteus in which appear 45 specific names, most of which are described from birds. The genus occurs widely in passerine birds, owls, flickers, woodpeckers, ducks, and other types of birds, and in certain reptiles as well. Herman (1938a) found 50% of the chipping sparrows on Cape Cod infected.

Haemoproteus lophortyx O'Roke 1929

H. lophortyx is a pathogenic parasite of California valley quail (O'Roke, 1930; Herman and Glading, 1942). It is doubtful if this bird ever completely recovers once it has become infected (Herman and Bischoff, 1949). The vectors are louse flies *Lynchia hirsuta* (cf. O'Roke, 1930) and *Stilbometopa impressa* (cf. Herman and Bischoff, 1949).

Other species of quail have also been found infected as follows: in California— San Quentin, Gambel's, and mountain quail (Wood and Herman, 1943); in New Mexico and Arizona—Gambel's and scaled quail; in District of Columbia and vicinity—the bobwhite (Campbell and Lee, 1953; Hungerford, 1955).

Haemoproteus nettionis Cleland and Johnston 1909

H. nettionis has for its type host the Australian teal, *Anas (= Nettion) castaneum*. Herman (1954), in a critical review, suggests that this is the correct name for the *Haemoproteus* of Anatidae and assigns *H. anatis* Haiba 1946 and *H. hermani* Haiba 1948 to synonymy. The gametocytes do not affect the size of the infected cell but may push the nucleus aside. The following are some of the other known hosts: Indian runner duck, common tame duck (White Pekin) (Chernin and Sadun, 1949), white Chinese goose, Canada goose, whistling swan, mallard, black duck, green-winged teal, blue-winged teal, cotton teal, shoveller, American pintail, wood duck, baldpate, common goldeneye, ring-necked duck, and common merganser (Wetmore, 1941; Wood and Herman, 1943; Herman, 1951, 1954; Levine and Hanson, 1953; Fallis and Wood, 1957). The vector in certain parts of North America is probably a species of Culicoides, since Fallis and Wood have shown that biting midges of this genus occur in areas where the parasite occurs in ducks, will feed on ducks, are suitable hosts for the parasite, and, when infected specimens are ground up and injected into clean ducks, carry the sporozoites capable of producing the infection with an incubation period of 14–21 days. The infection appears to be well tolerated by its hosts.

Haemoproteus danilewskyi Kruse 1890

H. danilewskyi, whose type host is the gray crow and has been found in various

types of birds, was merely recorded as occurring in the Red Jungle Fowl of Malaya
(*Gallus gallus*) by Plimmer (1913). The
bird had been kept in a London zoo.

Haemoproteus canachites Fallis and Bennett 1960

H. canachites occurs in the spruce grouse.
It apparently was this species that Stabler
et al. (1967) found in 54 of 108 spruce
grouse from Alaska's Kenai Peninsula and
in 82 of 110 such birds from the Lake Alek-
nagik area. Of the hematozoa, Haemoproteus was second only to Leucocytozoon in
prevalence. Vectors responsible for transmission have not been established.

Haemoproteus columbae Kruse 1890

Incidence and Distribution

H. columbae occurs in pigeons widely
throughout tropical and subtropical regions and in temperate zones wherever the
insect vector can survive, but only sporadically in a climate such as prevails in Iowa
where the vector ordinarily dies out in winter if introduced by chance during spring
or summer (Drake and Jones, 1930). In
England it occurs in wood pigeons (Baker,
1957). Becker (1959) reported that he frequently found gametocytes of *H. columbae*
in the blood of adult and nestling mourning doves in Iowa but never observed louse
flies on these birds (cf. Hanson et al.,
1957). Stabler found this parasite in all of
51 white-winged doves from Texas examined in June. Stabler and Holt (1963)
found *H. columbae* in 52% of the band-
tailed pigeons and 61% of the western
mourning doves collected in southern Colorado. The times of the collections were not
stated.

Etiology

H. columbae (Fig. 31.12) from the common pigeon and *H. maccallumi* Novy and
MacNeal 1905 from the mourning dove
seem to be morphologically identical. Besides, the parasite from both hosts has been
transferred to the pigeon by means of the
bloodsucking intermediate host *Pseudolynchia canariensis* (= *Lynchia maura* =
P. maura) by Huff (1932). Since it was the
first of the genus to have its life cycle in
the pigeon and louse fly completely outlined, accounts of it appear in standard
works on protozoology such as Wenyon

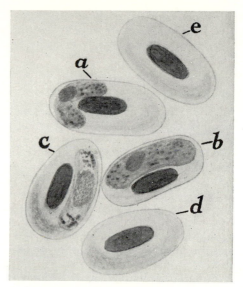

FIG. 31.12—Haemoproteus columbae. *Pigeon blood: (a, b) Macrogametocyte in
erythrocyte. (c) Microgametocyte. (d, e)
Normal erythrocyte. (Drake and Jones,
1930)*

(1926) and Kudo (1966). Although schizogony does not take place in the peripheral
blood, Lastra and Coatney (1950) showed
that it is possible to transfer the infection
by direct injection of considerable quantities of blood or transplantation of tissues
from donor pigeons taken early in the
course of infection.

Pathogenesis and Epizootiology

Levine and Kantor (1959) tabulated reports of Haemoproteus, judged to be *H. columbae*, from 45 species of columbiform
birds. Wood and Herman (1943) recorded
it in the western mourning dove, western
white-winged dove, and band-tailed pigeon.

In addition to *Pseudolynchia canariensis*
two other louse flies, *Microlynchia pusilla*
in South America and *Ornithomyia avicularia* in England, are suspected of being
vectors of *H. columbae* (Baker, 1957).

This parasite is not a severe pathogen,
although Coatney (1933) observed one bird
with a heavy infection whose behavior was
for a while definitely abnormal.

Treatment

Atebrin and pamakin (plasmochin), according to Coatney (1935), affect *Haemoproteus columbae* infection. Atebrin inhibits the development of young gametocytes,

while pamakin (plasmochin) does not. The latter is parasiticidal to adult gametocytes; however, neither seems to affect the schizonts.

Haemoproteus sacharovi Novy and MacNeal 1904

H. sacharovi is one of the numerous species of Haemoproteus described from various wild birds that should be mentioned; while normally a parasite of mourning doves, it occurs at times in the common pigeon (Coatney and West, 1940; Becker et al., 1956). The oval or round gametocytes, unlike those of most other species of Haemoproteus, enlarge their host cells—erythrocytes—about 1.3 times in width and 1.4 times in length and push the nucleus to one side, sometimes surrounding it. The amount of pigment is small. The known bird hosts are the eastern mourning dove, western mourning dove, and western white-winged dove (Wood and Herman, 1943; Herman, 1944; Stabler, 1961; Stabler and Holt, 1963). Huff (1932) transferred this species from the dove to a pigeon, using the louse fly *Pseudolynchia canariensis* for the vector. However, as he points out in a later publication (1963), "demonstration of one means of transmission has often been followed by the dogmatic assumption that this can be the *only* means," and he then cites instances to show how such assumptions may retard research. As Levine (1961) observes, the natural vector of *H. sacharovi* is unknown, but *Culicoides* is a possibility.

Haemoproteus meleagridis Levine 1961

Wetmore (1941) seems to have been the first to record Haemoproteus as a parasite of domestic turkeys (from District of Columbia and vicinity). Morehouse (1945) next observed the gametocytes of Haemoproteus in the blood of a turkey sent from Texas. The infection was a heavy one in an anemic bird from a flock that "seemed to have a good appetite, but just wasted away." The parasite was also observed by Kozicky (1948) in a native wild gobbler and 4 wild turkey hens reared in captivity—a total of 5 of 97 blood smears of wild turkeys collected in 1947. Goldsby (1951) reported the occurrence of Haemoproteus in a flock of turkeys in North Dakota. Three of 10 turkeys examined by Atchley (1951) harbored the parasite. Bierer et al. (1959), also working in South Carolina, found a "Haemoproteuslike" organism in 22 of 52 domestic turkeys; 2 of the birds were heavily parasitized and obviously ill. These workers suggested that wild turkeys might have been the source of infection. Love et al. (1953) found Haemoproteus in 1 of 2 wild turkeys taken in Georgia. Morehouse's figures indicate little or no enlargement of the infected erythrocyte, and the position of the cell nucleus seems to be altered in some but not in others.

REFERENCES

Atchley, F. O. 1951. *Leucocytozoon andrewsi* n. sp., from chickens observed in a survey of blood parasites in domestic animals in South Carolina. *J. Parasitol.* 37:483–88.

Baker, J. R. 1957. A new vector of *Haemoproteus columbae* in England. *J. Protozool.* 4:204–8.

Becker, E. R. 1959. Haemoproteus infections, pp. 888–92. In Biester, H. E., and L. H. Schwarte (eds.), *Diseases of Poultry*, 4th ed. Iowa State Univ. Press, Ames.

Becker, E. R., W. F. Hollander, and W. H. Pattillo. 1956. Naturally occurring Plasmodium and Haemoproteus infection in the common pigeon. *J. Parasitol.* 42:474–78.

Bierer, B. W., C. L. Vickers, and J. B. Thomas. 1959. A parasitism in turkeys due to a Haemoproteus-like blood parasite. *J. Am. Vet. Med. Ass.* 135:181–82.

Campbell, H., and L. Lee. 1953. *Studies on Quail Malaria in New Mexico and Notes on Other Aspects of Quail Populations*. New Mexico Dept. Game and Fish, Santa Fe.

Chernin, E., and E. H. Sadun. 1949. *Leucocytozoon simondi* infections in domestic ducks in northern Michigan with a note on Haemoproteus. *Poultry Sci.* 28:890–93.

Coatney, G. R. 1933. Relapse and associated phenomena in the Haemoproteus infection of the pigeon. *Am. J. Hyg.* 18:133–60.

———. 1935. The effect of atebrin and plasmochin on the Haemoproteus infection of the pigeon. *Am. J. Hyg.* 21:249–59.

———. 1936. A check-list and host-index of the genus Haemoproteus. *J. Parasitol.* 22:88–105.

Coatney, G. R., and E. West. 1940. Studies on *Haemoproteus sacharovi* of mourning doves and pigeons, with notes on *H. maccallumi*. *Am. J. Hyg.* 31(1, Sect. C):9–14.

Drake, C. J., and R. M. Jones. 1930. The pigeon fly and pigeon malaria in Iowa. *Iowa State Coll. J. Sci.* 4:253–61.

Fallis, A. M., and D. M. Wood. 1957. Biting

midges (Diptera: Ceratopogonidae) as intermediate hosts for Haemoproteus of ducks. *Can. J. Zool.* 35:425–35.

Goldsby, A. I. 1951. Poultry parasites new to North Dakota. *Bimonth. N. Dakota Agr. Expt. Sta. Bull.* 13:121–22.

Hanson, H. C., N. D. Levine, C. W. Kossack, S. Kantor, and L. J. Stannard. 1957. Parasites of the mourning dove *(Zenaidura macroura carolinensis)* in Illinois. *J. Parasitol.* 43:186–93.

Herman, C. M. 1938a. The relative incidence of blood protozoa in some birds from Cape Cod. *Trans. Am. Microscop. Soc.* 57:132–41.

———. 1938b. Haemoproteus sp. from the common black duck, *Anas rubripes tristis. J. Parasitol.* 24:53–56.

———. 1944. The blood protozoa of North American birds. *Bird Banding* 15:89–112.

———. 1945. Hippoboscid flies as parasites of game animals in California. *Calif. Fish Game* 31:16–25.

———. 1951. Blood parasites from California ducks and geese. *J. Parasitol.* 37:280–82.

———. 1954. Haemoproteus infections in waterfowl. *Proc. Helminthol. Soc. Wash.* 21:37–42.

Herman, C. M., and A. I. Bischoff. 1949. The duration of Haemoproteus infection in California quail. *Calif. Fish Game* 35:293–99.

Herman, C. M., and B. Glading. 1942. The protozoan blood parasite *Haemoproteus lophortyx* O'Roke in quail at the San Joaquin experimental range, California. *Calif. Fish Game* 28:150–53.

Huff, C. G. 1932. Studies on Haemoproteus of mourning doves. *Am. J. Hyg.* 16:618–23.

———. 1942. Schizogony and gametocyte development in *Leucocytozoon simondi,* and comparisons with Plasmodium and Haemoproteus. *J. Infect. Diseases* 71:18–22.

———. 1963. Experimental research on avian malaria. *Advan. Parasitol.* 1:1–65.

Hungerford, C. R. 1955. A preliminary evaluation of quail malaria in southern Arizona in relation to habitat and quail mortality. *Trans. 20th North Am. Wildlife Conf.,* pp. 209–19.

Kozicky, E. L. 1948. Some protozoan parasites of the eastern wild turkey in Pennsylvania. *J. Wildlife Management* 12:263–66.

Kudo, R. R. 1966. *Protozoology,* 5th ed. Charles C Thomas, Springfield, Ill.

Lastra, I., and G. R. Coatney. 1950. Transmission of *Haemoproteus columbae* by blood inoculation and tissue transplants. *J. Nat. Malaria Soc.* 9:151–52.

Levine, N. D. 1961. *Protozoan Parasites of Domestic Animals and of Man.* Burgess Publ. Co., Minneapolis.

Levine, N. D., and H. C. Hanson. 1953. Blood parasites of the Canada goose, *Branta canadensis interior. J. Wildlife Management* 17:185–96.

Levine, N. D., and S. Kantor. 1959. Checklist of blood parasites of the order Columbiformes. *Wildlife Diseases* 1:1–38. (Microcards.)

Love, G. J., Sara A. Wilkin, and M. H. Goodwin, Jr. 1953. Incidence of blood parasites in birds collected in southwestern Georgia. *J. Parasitol.* 39:52–57.

Morehouse, N. F. 1945. The occurrence of Haemoproteus sp. in the domesticated turkey. *Trans. Am. Microscop. Soc.* 64:109–11.

O'Roke, E. C. 1929. The morphology of *Haemoproteus lophortyx* sp. nov. *Science* 70:432.

———. 1930. The morphology, transmission, and life-history of *Haemoproteus lophortyx* O'Roke, a blood parasite of the California valley quail. *Univ. Calif. Publ. Zool.* 36:1–50.

———. 1932. Parasitism of the California Valley quail by *Haemoproteus lophortyx,* a protozoan blood parasite. *Calif. Fish Game* 18:223–38.

Plimmer, H. G. 1913. Report on the deaths which occurred in the Zoological Gardens during 1912, together with blood-parasites found during the year. *Proc. Zool. Soc. London* (1) Mar., pp. 141–49.

Reis, J., and P. Nobrega. 1936. *Doencas das Aves.* Sao Paulo, Brazil.

Stabler, R. M. 1961. A parasitological survey of fifty-one eastern white-winged doves. *J. Parasitol.* 47:309–11.

Stabler, R. M., and Portia A. Holt. 1963. Haematozoa of Colorado birds. I. Pigeons and doves. *J. Parasitol.* 49:320–22.

Stabler, R. M., Nancy J. Kitzmiller, L. N. Ellison, and Portia A. Holt. 1967. Hematozoa from the Alaskan spruce grouse, *Canachites canadensis. J. Parasitol.* 53:233–34.

Wenyon, C. M. 1926. *Protozoology.* Bailliere, Tindall, and Cox, London.

Wetmore, P. W. 1941. Blood parasites of birds of the District of Columbia and Patuxent Research Refuge vicinity. *J. Parasitol.* 27:379–93.

Wood, S. F., and C. M. Herman. 1943. The occurrence of blood parasites in birds from southwestern United States. *J. Parasitol.* 29:187–96.

AVIAN MALARIA

More than 30 species of Plasmodium have been described from birds of various kinds (Hewitt, 1940), but fewer than half are presently regarded as valid (Bray, 1957; Laird and Lari, 1958; Levine, 1961). The volume of literature on avian malaria is immense, many of the contributions having dealt with drug screening and other studies related to malaricidal properties of various drugs. There are also a great many contributions on other aspects of experimental research, such as studies on immunity, genetics, in vitro cultivation, interrelationship with other infections, and basic physiology and biochemistry. A brief but excellent review of representative contributions to these and other fields of experimental research on avian malaria has been presented by Huff (1963). He was, however, obliged to restrict his coverage largely to the period 1955–62. Still other references to special areas of research will be found in several of the papers presented at the workshop "Research in Malaria" (1966)—articles dealing with the ultrastructure of Plasmodium, its feeding mechanisms, its cultivation, and its cytochemistry. These sum up contemporary views in these special areas of interest and, together with references given in Huff's review, will guide the interested investigator to the literature on almost any aspect of avian malaria.

Most of the avian species of Plasmodium are far less host-specific than are some of the better known mammalian forms. Some occur naturally in a considerable number of species of wild birds, and some have been adapted by experimental passage to develop in birds in which they are not known to occur naturally. Only a few species have been reported as responsible for natural infections in domestic birds, and it is by no means certain that all of these are of veterinary importance.

Naturally occurring Plasmodium infections were found in chickens in the United States for the first time in Wisconsin in 1962 (Krishnamurti et al.). Soon thereafter, several flocks in Wisconsin were found to have birds infected with the same Plasmodium (Krishnamurti et al., 1964). In both reports the authors compare the organism they found with *Plasmodium gallinaceum,* but they do not specifically identify it as such. It produced no mortality, and *P. gallinaceum* characteristically does.

ETIOLOGY

The true malarial organisms belong to the genus Plasmodium, which in turn is closely related to Haemoproteus and Leucocytozoon. The principal significant difference between Plasmodium and the other two genera is that the asexual stages (schizonts) of the former occur in erythrocytes of the circulating blood, while those of the two latter occur in the internal organs (lung, liver, spleen, kidney, etc.). As a result, Plasmodium can be transmitted regularly from one susceptible host to another by injection of infected blood from the vessels or heart. In the case of the other two this procedure will result in infection only at certain times when merozoites are in the blood by chance, because the only stages ordinarily in the blood are gametocytes which continue development in the proper invertebrate host. Like Haemoproteus, Plasmodium contains pigment. The life cycle involves two hosts: an intermediate host, a vertebrate, in which asexual multiplication (schizogony) and the formation of immature sexual forms (gametocytes) occur; and a definitive host, presumably always a mosquito, in which maturation of the gametes, fertilization, and sporogony take place. It is of special interest that mammalian malarias are carried by Anopheles mosquitoes, while those of birds are carried by culicine (Culex, Aedes) mosquitoes, although some of the latter also have anopheline vectors.

The story of the development of Plasmodium in vertebrates from sporozoite (the stage introduced by the mosquito while biting) to the earliest stages observed in erythrocytes was the contribution resulting from the brilliant researches of a number of investigators, among them Huff and Coulston (1944). The sporozoite of *P. gallinaceum* enters a "lymphoid macrophage" cell to develop in about 42 hours into a "cryptozoite," or a schizont undergoing schizogony. The merozoites of this generation enter other similar cells to repeat schizogony in another 40 hours (the "metacryptozoites"). Blood infections then ensue, presumably from the merozoites from the fixed tissue stages. Subsequent development of Plasmodium within the vertebrate host usually follows the general course outlined below.

The parasite (Fig. 31.13) as first seen in the red blood cells in films treated with a Romanowsky stain may have the appearance of a signet ring. The center of the parasite is occupied by a vacuole which does not stain. The surrounding cytoplasm, which stains blue, therefore appears as a ring. The nucleus, also located peripherally,

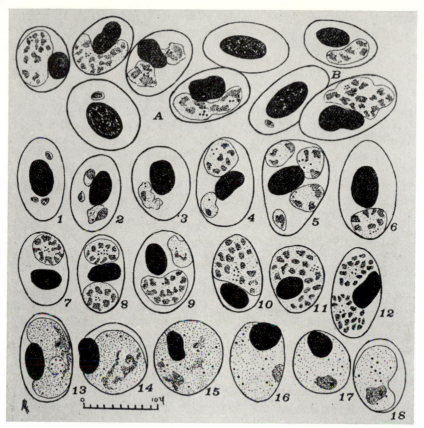

FIG. 31.13—Plasmodium gallinaceum: *(A and B) Group of erythrocytes showing alterations in chromatin of infected cells. (1–12) Simple or multiple infections of erythrocytes by trophozoites and schizonts in different stages of development. 10, 11, and 12 represent formation of merozoites; 13, 14, and 15, male gametocytes; 16, 17, and 18, female gametocytes; 18, female gametocyte in enucleated erythrocyte. Solid black bodies are nuclei of erythrocytes. (Brumpt, 1935)*

stains red. The signet ring effect is observed when this stage, now called a trophozoite, is viewed at right angles to the plane containing the nucleus. The trophozoite grows at the expense of the red cell, actually engulfing hemoglobin which, when digested, leaves a residue of pigment. Eventually the chromatin material divides, followed by the division of the cytoplasm, and the segmenting schizont gives rise to merozoites. The number of merozoites formed depends on the species, as does the time required for their development, at least under fixed conditions. The schizonts of different cells usually mature at about the same time, so large numbers of red blood cells may be destroyed in a short time, resulting in the liberation of toxic products as well as merozoites. The merozoites so liberated now enter other red cells and repeat the asexual cycle until some develop into sexual forms, microgametes and macrogametes, also within red blood cells. These sexual cells undergo no further development until taken up by a mosquito. The gametes and the schizonts, both in the peripheral blood, may be sufficiently characteristic for a given species of Plasmodium to make specific identification possible.

Plasmodium gallinaceum Brumpt 1935

Etiology

The British veterinarian M. Crawford, while stationed in Ceylon, announced in the official 1933 report to his government that cases of bird malaria had developed on that island in chickens recently imported from England, and he described the symptoms and advocated quinine for treatment. He assigned the microorganism to *Plasmodium praecox*. Later, Crawford (1945) carefully narrated the history of the parasite and the manner in which it became available as a satisfactory laboratory war program for obtaining new and better antimalarial drugs. Also, he acknowledged the correct name to be *P. gallinaceum,* described by Brumpt in 1935 from a blood smear presented to him in 1910 by Broussais who had seen the malarial organism in fowls in Indo-China. Brumpt stated that from 1935 to 1948 more than 600 publications on *P. gallinaceum* had enriched practical and theoretical knowledge concerning malaria, and many more papers have appeared since 1948.

The discovery of an exoerythrocytic phase (an asexual developmental cycle in endothelial cells or reticuloendothelial cells of spleen, brain, liver, etc.) by James and Tate (1938) and James (1939) attracted a great deal of attention, because it was formerly believed that the increment of malaria parasites in the vertebrate host occurred entirely within the erythrocytes. For morphological and other details the reader should consult Brumpt's papers. The exoerythrocytic stages preceding the erythrocytic stages described by Huff and Coulston (1944) have been mentioned above. The structural details of stages occurring in the mosquito have been presented by Terzakis et al. (1966), who also called attention to many of the earlier contributions.

Pathogenesis and Epizootiology

As previously indicated, birds acquire Plasmodium from mosquitoes, of which many species belonging to several genera may possibly serve as vectors (Huff, 1954). Experimentally, oral transmission of *P. gallinaceum* was reported by Beltran and Larenas (1941). However, Beckman (1965) was unable to infect 7-day-old chicks of a highly susceptible strain orally by any of several methods.

Crawford (1945) considered jungle fowls to be the natural hosts—*Gallus lafayetti* in Ceylon, *G. bankiva* in India, and *G. sonnerati* in Sumatra. (Brumpt [1935], however, believed the native host to be a still undetected wild bird.) These native fowl (Gallus) are quite resistant to the infection, but when imported breeds are introduced

into areas where the wild fowl are infected, they suffer intense infections which generally lead to death after a brief illness. Birds may at times develop paralysis and die after drug treatment, owing to blocking of brain capillaries with the large non-pigmented exoerythrocytic stages of the parasite discovered by James and Tate (1937, 1938). Because he believed the chicken not susceptible to known avian malarias (see, however, Manwell, 1933), Brumpt felt confident he was dealing with a new species. Ducks, guinea fowl, pigeons, turtle doves, quail, buzzards, canaries, calfats, and finches were later shown by him to be resistant to *P. gallinaceum;* chickens of various breeds, geese, pheasants, partridges, and peacocks were susceptible. The infection assumed a more acute form in young chicks and a more chronic course in the adult birds (Coggeshall, 1938).

Since Crawford's (1945) summary, Haiba (1948) reported the parasite in the blood of a dead chicken in Egypt, but its occurrence in that country has been questioned (Becker, 1959; Levine, 1961). Occurrence of two naturally acquired infections in exotic fowl at the Izatnagar (India) Poultry Farm was first noted by Rao et al. (1951) and later by Das et al. (1952). The symptoms, postmortem lesions, and histopathology observed in fowls infected by direct blood inoculation are described in considerable detail. Kraneveld and Mansjoer (1953) found the parasite in West Java and submitted authority for its occurrence also in Sumatra, Java, and the Celebes.

Beltran (1941a) published a summary of the state of our knowledge concerning this species up to that year, but much information has been added since. Jacobi (1939) studied the pathology of *P. gallinaceum* infection.

Plasmodium juxtanucleare Versiani and Furtado Gomes 1941

P. juxtanucleare occurs chiefly in chickens. Until recently it had been recorded only from Brazil (Versiani and Furtado Gomes, 1941), Mexico (Beltran, 1941b), and Uruguay (Cassamagnaghi, 1946). However, in 1962 Dhanapala reported what he believed to be *P. juxtanucleare* from chickens in Ceylon, and Bennett and Warren (1966a) found what was apparently the same parasite in chickens in the Malay states. The mortality rate among birds parasitized with the Asiatic strain was very low, whereas the American strain was responsible for considerable mortality. Bennett and Warren point out that there are other differences. The American strain commonly has 4 merozoites in a mature schizont; in the strain from the Malay states, 3 or 5 merozoites were usual. Also, the gametocytes of the American strain usually displaced the host cell nucleus, and the parasitized erythrocyte was markedly distorted. Neither of these situations was regularly displayed by the Asiatic strain. Bennett and Warren do not believe that the differences noted to date justify a species separation. Bennett et al. (1966) and Bennett and Warren (1966b) have extended the observation on the biology of this parasite considerably. These reports should be consulted for details on the life history and unique features of the Asiatic strain of *P. juxtanucleare.*

Plasmodium durae Herman 1941

This species was found in a blood smear in 1 of 75 domestic turkeys examined in Kenya Colony, British East Africa. It was capable of afflicting young turkeys fatally.

Plasmodium cathemerium Hartman 1927

P. cathemerium, the type host of which is the English sparrow, resembles *P. relictum* in that it occurs commonly in passerine birds, causes the nucleus of the infected cell to be displaced more or less toward one pole or expelled, and has roundish gametocytes; it differs from that species in that the pigment grains in the gametocytes are relatively coarse and rodlike. An outbreak of *P. cathemerium* in California that cost a canary raiser possibly 165 of 700 birds was reported by Mathey (1955b). The sick birds exhibited swelling in the region of the eyes. The characteristic parasites were found in blood smears. Necropsy disclosed subcutaneous hemorrhage, splenomegaly, and hepatomegaly. Sick birds responded to atebrin. Herman and Vail (1942) reported a fatal case of spontaneous malaria in a canary from Temple City, California. Hewitt (1939) made a special study of splenic enlargement and infarction in infected canaries.

Plasmodium relictum Grassi and Feletti 1891

P. relictum, of which *P. praecox* is a synonym, is a species occurring in many species of wild birds, among them the eastern (Coatney, 1938) and western mourning doves (Herman et al., 1954) and certain wild waterfowl such as the pintail, cinnamon teal (Herman, 1951), wood duck (Mielcarek, 1954), and American coot (Roudabush, 1942). Coatney (1938) observed identical strains from the wild mourning dove and common pigeon. The strain was extremely pathogenic in pigeons, but in doves and canaries the infections were light and transitory. When transferred to chicks, the infections lasted 6–11 days. The first observers of naturally occurring *P. relictum* in pigeons, however, were Sergent and Sergent (1904), working in Algeria. Others were as follows: Pelaez et al. (1951) in Mexico, Mathey (1955a) in California, and Becker et al. (1956) in Iowa. Mathey observed 3 infected pigeons, at least 2 of which succumbed to malaria. He also succeeded in infecting the chick and canary with parasites from the pigeon. This species resembles *P. cathemerium* morphologically, but its pigment grains are roundish instead of elongate. Some strains of it, like *P. cathemerium,* have diurnal periodicity. The infection responds readily to treatment with quinine or atebrin. Wolfson (1938) also obtained infections in ducks with two other strains of *P. relictum.* Hill (1942) has proved rather conclusively that anemia may be regarded as the cause of death of pigeons in *P. relictum* infections.

Plasmodium circumflexum Kikuth 1931

P. circumflexum has for its type host a German thrush *(Turdus pilaris).* Its morphological characteristics are as follows: all stages occur in the circulating blood; elongate gametocytes; 13–30 merozoites produced per schizont; both schizonts and gametocytes tend to encircle the nucleus of the infected cell without displacing it. A Plasmodium morphologically similar in many respects to this one was observed by Fallis (1945, 1946) in ruffed grouse in Ontario, Canada. It developed in canaries but not so readily as in grouse; a canary strain would not develop in grouse. The grouse strain is not pathogenic in grouse, canaries, or ducks and would not develop in chickens or pheasants.

Plasmodium lophurae Coggeshall 1938

This species was isolated by Coggeshall (1938) from a Borneo fireback pheasant,

Lophura igniti igniti, at the New York Zoological Park. It is transmissible to very young chicks but as a rule produces a moderately severe attack that does not terminate fatally. Only mild infections may be produced in adult fowls, and canaries are not susceptible. The original description should be consulted for morphological and other details. Terzian (1941a,b) made an excellent study of the biological characteristics, pathology, and effects of this interesting species in chicks. Laird (1941) showed that *P. lophurae* can be transmitted from duck to duck through the agency of the mosquito *Aedes albopictus,* and he succeeded in infecting also *Culex restuans* and *Aedes atropalpus. Anopheles quadrimaculatus* can also be infected, at least lightly (Coggeshall, 1941; Hurlbut and Hewitt, 1941, 1942). Trager (1952) obtained by selective breeding a strain of *Aedes aegypti* which was more susceptible to *P. lophurae* than the original stock.

Severe infections with high parasitemias are produced in ducks (Wolfson, 1941). Hewitt's (1942) study of host-parasite relationship of *P. lophurae* infection in ducks, with its excellent colored plates of the parasite and types of blood cells affected by the infection, is especially commended to the reader's attention. The course of untreated blood-induced infections in 1,200 young White Pekin ducks was charted by Hewitt et al. (1942). Becker et al. (1949) studied the course of infection in some of the comparatively few ducks that had survived the primary attack and found that in only 1 of 26 did the infection become permanently latent; in all the rest it followed a relapsing course with subpatent periods of varying length alternating with patent periods of varying length and with parasitemias of varying intensity. Ducks exhibit reverse age resistance to this parasite in contrast to chicks, which become more resistant as they grow older (Becker, 1950).

Exoerythrocytic forms (phanerozoites) have never been detected in chickens or ducks, although Becker and Manresa (1950) and Manresa (1953) located them in brain capillaries in turkey infections. As in *P. gallinaceum,* they may cause the death of the host by blocking the capillaries, even though the parasitemia is low. Stauber and Van Dyke (1945) have compared *P. cathemerium* and *P. lophurae* infections in duck embryos. Goslings are highly susceptible (Becker, 1951). This species, like *P. gallinaceum,* has served as an excellent subject for antimalarial investigations. Among the many contributions of this nature is that of Farmer and Breitenbach (1968), who report on the course of *P. lophurae* infections in normal and hormonally bursectomized chicks. These authors cite many reports that, like their own, contribute substantially to our emerging understanding of the development of immunity to malaria.

For information on domesticated birds as experimental hosts of avian plasmodia, the reader is referred to Wolfson (1941), Manwell (1933, 1943, 1952), and Huff (1963).

REFERENCES

Becker, E. R. 1950. Mortality in relation to age in young white pekin ducks with blood-induced *Plasmodium lophurae* infection. *Proc. Iowa Acad. Sci.* 57:435–38.

———. 1951. The course of blood-induced *P. lophurae* malaria in young goslings and guinea fowl chicks. *J. Parasitol.* 37 (5, Sect. 2):12. (Abstr.)

———. 1959. Protozoa, pp. 828–916. In Biester, H. E., and L. H. Schwarte (eds.), *Diseases of Poultry,* 4th ed. Iowa State Univ. Press, Ames.

Becker, E. R., and M. Manresa, Jr. 1950. Phanerozoites in turkeys succumbing with blood-induced *Plasmodium lophurae* infection. *Iowa State Coll. J. Sci.* 24:353–54.

Becker, E. R., C. E. Brodine, and Bonnie L. Clappison. 1949. The post-crisis in blood-induced *Plasmodium lophurae* infections in white pekin ducks. *Iowa State Coll. J. Sci.* 23:237–47.

Becker, E. R., W. F. Hollander, and W. H. Pattillo. 1956. Naturally occurring Plasmodium and Haemoproteus infection in the common pigeon. *J. Parasitol.* 42:474–78.

Beckman, H. 1965. Attempted oral infection of chicks with *Plasmodium gallinaceum. J. Parasitol.* 51:845–46.

Beltran, E. 1941a. Estado actual de nuestros conocimientos acerca del *Plasmodium gallinaceum* Brumpt, 1935. *Rev. Inst. Salubridad Enfermedades Trop., Mex.* 2:95–113.

———. 1941b. Hallazgo de *Plasmodium juxtanucleare* Versiani y Furtado en gallinas de Chiapas. *Rev. Inst. Salubridad Enfermedades Trop., Mex.* 2:353–54.

Beltran, E., and M. R. Larenas. 1941. Production de malaria aviar con *Plasmodium gallinaceum* por via oral. *Rev. Inst. Salubridad Enfermedades Trop., Mex.* 2:87–94.

Bennett, G. F., and McW. Warren. 1966a. Biology of the Malaysian strain of *Plasmo-*

dium juxtanucleare Versiani and Gomes, 1941. I. Description of the stages in the vertebrate host. *J. Parasitol.* 52:565–69.

———. 1966b. Biology of the Malaysian strain of *Plasmodium juxtanucleare* Versiani and Gomes, 1941. III. Life cycle of the erythrocytic parasite in the avian host. *J. Parasitol.* 52:653–59.

Bennett, G. F., McW. Warren, and W. H. Cheong. 1966. Biology of the Malaysian strain of *Plasmodium juxtanucleare* Versiani and Gomes, 1941. II. The sporogonic stages in *Culex (Culex) sitiens* Wiedmann. *J. Parasitol.* 52:647–52.

Bray, R. S. 1957. Studies on the exo-erythrocytic cycle in the genus Plasmodium. *London School Hyg. Trop. Med., Mem. Ser.* 12:1–192.

Brumpt, E. 1935. Paludisme aviaire: *Plasmodium gallinaceum* n. sp. de la poule domestique. *Compt. Rend. Acad. Sci.* 200: 783–85.

Cassamagnaghi, A., Jr. 1946. Plasmodiosis (malaria o paludismo) en las aves del Uruguay. *Ann. 3rd Congr. Brasil. Vet.* 13:625–38.

Coatney, G. R. 1938. A strain of *Plasmodium relictum* from doves and pigeons infective to canaries and the common fowl. *Am. J. Hyg.* 27:380–89.

Coggeshall, L. T. 1938. *Plasmodium lophurae,* a new species of malaria parasite pathogenic for the domestic fowl. *Am. J. Hyg.* 27:615–18.

———. 1941. Infection of *Anopheles quadrimaculatus* with *Plasmodium cynomolgi,* a monkey malaria parasite, and with *Plasmodium lophurae,* an avian malaria parasite. *Am. J. Trop. Med.* 21:525–30.

Crawford, M. 1945. *Plasmodium gallinaceum,* a malarial parasite of the domestic fowl. *Vet. Record* 57:395–96.

Das, J., S. B. V. Rao, and D. R. Ramnani. 1952. Studies on *Plasmodium gallinaceum.* *Indian Vet. J.* 29:14–26.

Dhanapala, S. B. 1962. The occurrence of *Plasmodium juxtanucleare* Versiani and Gomes, 1941 in domestic fowls in Ceylon. *Rev. Malariol.* 41:39–46.

Fallis, A. M. 1945. Population trends and blood parasites of ruffed grouse in Ontario. *J. Wildlife Management* 9:203–6.

———. 1946. *Plasmodium circumflexum* (Kikuth) in ruffed grouse in Ontario. *J. Parasitol.* 32:345–53.

Farmer, J. N., and R. P. Breitenbach. 1968. *Plasmodium lophurae* infections and related serum protein changes in 2-week-old normal and hormonally bursectomized chickens. *J. Parasitol.* 54:137–49.

Haiba, M. H. 1948. Plasmodia of common Egyptian birds. *J. Comp. Pathol. Therap.* 58:81–93.

Herman, C. M. 1951. Blood parasites from California ducks and geese. *J. Parasitol.* 37:280–82.

Herman, C. M., and E. L. Vail. 1942. A fatal case of spontaneous malaria in a canary. *J. Am. Vet. Med. Ass.* 101:502.

Herman, C. M., W. C. Reeves, H. E. McClure, E. M. French, and W. McD. Hammon. 1954. Studies on avian malaria in vectors and hosts of encephalitis in Kern County, California. *Am. J. Trop. Med. Hyg.* 3:676–95.

Hewitt, R. I. 1939. Splenic enlargement and infarction in canaries infected with a virulent strain of *Plasmodium cathemerium.* *Am. J. Hyg.* 30 (Sect. C):49–63.

———. 1940. Bird malaria. *Am. J. Hyg., Monograph Ser.* 15:1–228.

———. 1942. Studies on the host-parasite relationships of untreated infections with *Plasmodium lophurae* in ducks. *Am. J. Hyg.* 36:6–42.

Hewitt, R. I., A. P. Richardson, and L. D. Seager. 1942. Observations on untreated infections with *Plasmodium lophurae* in twelve hundred young white pekin ducks. *Am. J. Hyg.* 36:362–73.

Hill, C. McD. 1942. Anemia as a cause of death in bird malaria. *Am. J. Hyg.* 36:143–46.

Huff, C. G. 1954. A review of the literature on susceptibility of mosquitoes to avian malaria, with some unpublished data on the subject. *Res. Rept. Naval Med. Res. Inst.* 12:619–44.

———. 1963. Experimental research on avian malaria. *Advan. Parasitol.* 1:1–65.

Huff, C. G., and F. Coulston. 1944. The development of *Plasmodium gallinaceum* from sporozoite to erythrocytic trophozoite. *J. Infect. Diseases* 75:231–49.

Hurlbut, H. S., and R. I. Hewitt. 1941. Sporozoites of *Plasmodium lophurae,* an avian malaria parasite, in *Anopheles quadrimaculatus.* *Public Health Rept.* 56:1336–37.

———. 1942. The transmission of *Plasmodium lophurae,* an avian malaria parasite, by *Anopheles quadrimaculatus.* *Public Health Rept.* 57:1891–92.

Jacobi, L. 1939. Beitraege zur Pathologie der Infektion des Huhnes mit *Plasmodium gallinaceum* (Brumpt). *Arch. Exp. Pathol. Pharmakol.* 191:482–91.

James, S. P. 1939. The incidence of exo-erythrocytic schizogony in *Plasmodium gallinaceum* in relation to the mode of infection. *Trans. Roy. Soc. Trop. Med. Hyg.* 32:763–69.

James, S. P., and P. Tate. 1937. New knowledge of the life-cycle of malaria parasites. *Nature* 139:545.

———. 1938. Exo-erythrocytic schizogony in

Plasmodium gallinaceum Brumpt, 1935. *Parasitology* 30:128–39.

Kraneveld, F. C., and M. Mansjoer. 1953. Onderzoekingen over bloedparasieten voorkomen. VII. Het van *Plasmodium gallinaceum* (Brumpt, 1935) in Indonesia. *Indonesie Zoa* 60:234–48.

Krishnamurti, P. V., D. L. Peardon, A. C. Todd, and W. H. McGibbon. 1962. A Plasmodium from chickens in Wisconsin. *Poultry Sci.* 41:685–90.

Krishnamurti, P. V., A. C. Todd, and W. H. McGibbon. 1964. Prevalence of a Plasmodium in Wisconsin chickens. *J. Parasitol.* 50:98.

Laird, R. L. 1941. Observations on mosquito transmission of *Plasmodium lophurae*. *Am. J. Hyg.* 34 (Sect. C):163–67.

Laird, R. L., and F. A. Lari. 1958. Observations on *Plasmodium circumflexum* Kikuth and *P. vaughani* Novy and MacNeal from East Pakistan. *J. Parasitol.* 44:136–52.

Levine, N. D. 1961. *Protozoan Parasites of Domestic Animals and of Man.* Burgess Publ. Co., Minneapolis.

Manresa, M., Jr. 1953. The occurrence of phanerozoites of *Plasmodium lophurae* in blood-inoculated turkeys. *J. Parasitol.* 39:452–55.

Manwell, R. D. 1933. The behavior of the avian malarias in the common fowl, an abnormal host. *Am. J. Trop. Med.* 13:97–112.

———. 1943. Malaria infections by four species of Plasmodium in the duck and chicken, and resulting parasite modifications. *Am. J. Hyg.* 38:211–19.

———. 1952. Turkeys and ducks as experimental hosts for *Plasmodium hexamerium* and *P. vaughani*. *Exp. Parasitol.* 1:274–82.

Mathey, W. J., Jr. 1955a. Two cases of *Plasmodium relictum* infection in domestic pigeons in the Sacramento area. *Vet. Med.* 50:318.

———. 1955b. Malaria in canaries. *Vet. Med.* 50:369–70.

Mielcarek, J. E. 1954. The occurrence of

Plasmodium relictum in the wood duck (*Aix sponsa*). *J. Parasitol.* 40:232.

Pelaez, D., A. Barrera, F. de la Jara, and R. Perez Reyes. 1951. Estudios sobre hematozoarios. II. Interes de las investigaciones sobre el paludismo en los animales. *Rev. Palud. Med. Trop.* 3:59–76.

Rao, S. B. V., J. Das, and D. R. Ramnani. 1951. Fowl malaria. *Indian Vet. J.* 28:99–101.

Research in Malaria. 1966. An International Panel Workshop. *Military Med.* (Suppl.), 131:847–1272.

Roudabush, R. L. 1942. Parasites of the American coot (*Fulica americana*) in central Iowa. *Iowa State Coll. J. Sci.* 16:437–41.

Sergent, Ed., and Et. Sergent. 1904. Sur les hematozoaires des oiseaux d'Algerie. *Compt. Rend. Soc. Biol.* 56:132–33.

Stauber, L. A., and H. B. Van Dyke. 1945. Malarial infections in the duck embryo. *Proc. Soc. Exp. Biol. Med.* 58:125–26.

Terzakis, J. A., H. Sprinz, and R. A. Ward. 1966. Sporoblast and sporozoite formation in *Plasmodium gallinaceum* infection of *Aedes aegypti*. Research in Malaria. *Military Med.* (Suppl.), 131:984–92.

Terzian, L. A. 1941a. Studies on *Plasmodium lophurae*, a malarial parasite in fowls. I. Biological characteristics. *Am. J. Hyg.* 33 (Sect. C):1–22.

———. 1941b. Studies on *Plasmodium lophurae*, a malarial parasite in fowls. II. Pathology and the effects of experimental conditions. *Am. J. Hyg.* 33 (Sect. C):33–53.

Trager, W. 1942. A strain of the mosquito *Aedes aegypti* selected for susceptibility to the avian malaria parasite *Plasmodium lophurae*. *J. Parasitol.* 28:457–65.

Versiani, W., and B. Furtado Gomes. 1941. Sobre um novo hematozoario da galinha, *Plasmodium juxtanucleare* n. sp. (Nota previa). *Rev. Brasil. Biol.* 1:231–33. (English summary.)

Wolfson, Fruma. 1938. The common duck as a convenient experimental host for avian Plasmodium. *Am. J. Hyg.* 28:317–20.

———. 1941. Avian hosts for malaria research. *Quart. Rev. Biol.* 16:462–73.

AVIAN PIROPLASMOSIS

The protozoon involved was seen by Balfour (1907, 1914) in Sudanese fowl. His first interpretation of the organism was that it represented intracellular developmental phases of the fowl spirochete *Treponema anserinum* which accompanied the infection. Hindle (1912) and Wenyon (1926) suggested that the intracellular granular bodies represented portions of nuclei extruded into the cytoplasm of the red cell as a result of concomitant spirochete infection.

Balfour (1914) and Carpano (1929) believed that the spirochete infection and the infection with the granular bodies in the blood cells were distinct, for either could occur in the absence of the other; Carpano found that subinoculations with the pure protozoon infection at no time produced spirochetes. He found the protozoon in both ducks and geese in Egypt, named it *Aegyptianella pullorum,* and considered it a piroplasm (Fig. 31.14). It appears to be

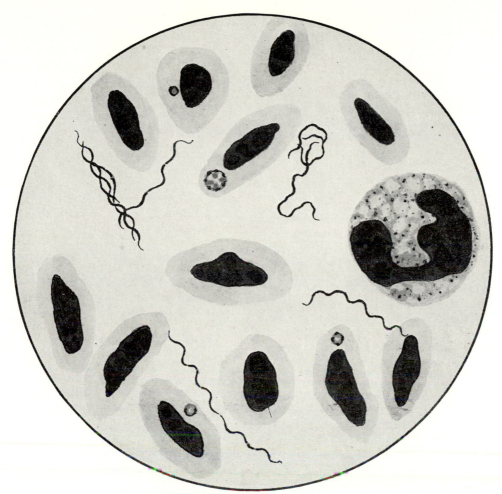

FIG. *31.14*—Aegyptianella pullorum *and* Spirochaeta gallinarum. *(Carpano, 1929)*

predominantly distributed in Africa and Mediterranean countries, having been reported from Egypt, the British and French Sudan, Tunis, South Africa, Transcaucasia, Greece, Yugoslavia, and Albania.

ETIOLOGY

Classification

Organisms resembling *A. pullorum* have been described by several investigators under a variety of names. Laird and Lari (1957), who found one of these forms in the heart blood of an Indian house crow, have reviewed the literature on the avian babesiids, compared the findings of the several investigators, and suggest that all of these organisms should be included in the genus Babesia. They liken the organisms found by Shchurenkova (1938), Henry (1939),

Toumanoff (1940), and Mohamed (1952) in the eagle, chicken, heron, and Egyptian kestrel, respectively, to that found in the crow and suggest that all be considered as belonging to "a single polymorphic species," *Babesia moshkovskii* (Shchurenkova 1938). Levine (1961), for convenience and pending further details on life cycles, prefers to retain *Aegyptianella pullorum* as the name of the organism described above and considers the rest under the name *A. moshkovskii* (Shchurenkova 1938) Poisson 1953. In doing so, he includes as organisms of uncertain relationships those of Coles (1937), McNeil and Hinshaw (1944), Abdussalam (1945), and Rousselot (1947). These last were found in chickens, turkeys, and pheasants and presumably could be found to be of veterinary importance. The accounts of

Laird and Lari (1957) and Levine (1961) should be consulted by those interested in studying the avian babesiids in detail.

Morphology

Carpano's (1929) definition of the genus Aegyptianella is as follows: Protozoa of red cells; of small size; in shape, rounded, oval or pyriform; not producing pigment; producing no change in size or shape of infected cell; multiplying in circulating blood by schizogony, producing up to 25 minute merozoites.

A. pullorum can vary in size from 0.5 to 4.0μ, depending on the stage of development. The parasites are infrequently found in the circulating blood (and when found are present for only a day or two) but may be encountered in the lungs, heart, liver, spleen, and bone marrow. In life the parasites may show slow movements of translation. Since the organisms stain with difficulty and the size is small, morphological study is difficult.

PATHOGENESIS AND EPIZOOTIOLOGY

A. pullorum is found naturally in ducks, geese, chickens, and turkeys and has been transmitted experimentally to various other birds (see Levine, 1961).

Carpano (1929) believed that the frequent presence of Treponema and Aegyptianella in the same bird indicated that *Argas persicus,* the tick transmitter of *T. anserinum,* is also the vector of *A. pullorum.* According to Reis and Nobrega (1936),

Coles and Bedford demonstrated carriage by *A. persicus,* although Chaillot and Saunie in 1932 could not confirm it. Coles (1939) stated that only adults of this species act as transmitters.

The protozoan infection may appear in the acute, subacute, or chronic form. Native fowl usually show the chronic form. However, Ahmed and Soliman (1966) report the loss of 3 of 31 native chickens 8–10 weeks old as the disease was noted. Among imported birds the acute form of the disease is not uncommon. Fowl crossed with foreign strains show the subacute or chronic form.

The symptoms are ruffing of the feathers, anorexia, hyperthermia, immobility, drooping, paralysis of the joints, and often diarrhea. Necropsy shows anemia, swollen spleen, enlarged liver, yellowish green kidneys, punctiform hemorrhage in the serosa, and sometimes an infiltration of gelatinous hemorrhage in the coronary sulcus.

Ahmed and Soliman (1966), comparing aegyptianellosis and spirochetosis, state: "A common finding in both infections was anemia associated with a significant decrease in hemoglobin content and packed cell volume. However, Aegyptianellosis lacked the marked changes which characterized the differential leucocytic picture in spirochete infection."

Brumpt (1930) reported that splenectomy of fowl recovered from heavy infections caused a reappearance of the parasites in the blood. The fowl recovered from this artificially induced relapse.

REFERENCES

Abdussalam, M. 1945. Piroplasmosis of the domestic fowl in Northern India. *Indian J. Vet. Sci.* 15:17–21.

Ahmed, A. A. S., and M. K. Soliman. 1966. Observations made during a natural outbreak of aegyptianellosis in chickens. *Avian Diseases* 10:390–93.

Balfour, A. 1907. A peculiar blood condition, probably parasitic, in Sudanese fowls. *J. Trop. Med. Hyg.* 10:153–57.

———. 1914. Notes on the life-cycle of the Sudan fowl spirochaete. *Trans. 17th Int. Congr. Med.,* Sect. 21, Pt. 2:275–78.

Brumpt, E. 1930. Rechutes parasitaires intenses, dues a la splenectomie, au course d'infections latentes a Aegyptianella, chez la poule. *Compt. Rend. Acad. Sci.* 191: 1028–30.

Carpano, M. 1929. Su di un Piroplasma osservati nei polli in Egitto (*"Aegiptianella pullorum"*). Nota preventiva. *Clin. Vet.* 52:339–51.

Coles, J. D. W. A. 1937. A new blood parasite of the fowl. *Onderstepoort J. Vet. Sci. Animal Ind.* 9:301–7.

———. 1939. Aegyptianellosis of poultry. *Proc. 7th World's Poultry Congr.,* pp. 261–65.

Henry, C. 1939. Presence dans les hematies de poulets d'elements rappelant les corps de Balfour. *Bull. Soc. Pathol. Exotique* 32: 145–49.

Hindle, E. 1912. The inheritance of spirochaetal infection in *Argas persicus. Proc. Cambridge Phil. Soc.* 16:457–59.

Laird, M., and F. A. Lari. 1957. The avian blood parasite *Babesia moshkovskii* (Shchurenkova, 1938), with a record from *Corvus splendens* Vieillot in Pakistan. *Can. J. Zool.* 35:783–95.

Levine, N. D. 1961. *Protozoan Parasites of Domestic Animals and of Man.* Burgess Publ. Co., Minneapolis.

McNeil, Ethel, and W. R. Hinshaw. 1944. A blood parasite of the turkey. *J. Parasitol.* 30 (Suppl.):9. (Abstr.)

Mohamed, A. H. H. 1952. Protozoan blood parasites of Egyptian birds. *Trans. Roy. Soc. Trop. Med. Hyg.* 46:1. (Abstr.)

Reis, J., and P. Nobrega. 1936. *Doencas das Aves.* Sao Paulo.

Rousselot, R. 1947. Parasites du sang de divers animaux de la region de Tehran. *Arch. Inst. Hessarek* 5:62–72.

Shchurenkova, A. I. 1938. *Sogdianella moshkovskii* gen. nov. sp. nov.—A parasite belonging to the Piroplasmidae in a raptorial bird: *Gypaetus barbatus* L. *Med. Parazitol. i Parazitarn. Bolezni* 7:932–37.

Toumanoff, C. 1940. Le parasite sanguin endoglobulaire du heron cendre de l'Indochine (*Ardea cinerea* var. *rectirostris* Gould), *Babesia (Nicollia) ardeae* nov. sp. *Rev. Med. Franc. Extreme-Orient* 18:491–96.

Wenyon, C. M. 1926. *Protozoology.* Bailliere, Tindall, and Cox, London.

SPIROCHETOSIS

Although spirochetes were discussed in this chapter in earlier editions, they are not protozoa and are now dealt with in Chapter 12 of this book.

TRYPANOSOMIASIS

Trypanosomes have been reported as occurring naturally in a large number of wild birds and in the chicken, pigeon, and guinea fowl. In most instances the organism was known only from the vertebrate host, and frequently it was designated as a new species if its morphology differed from that of trypanosomes previously reported from birds. Sometimes the organism observed was named as a new species merely because a similar trypanosome had not previously been reported from that particular host. It is now known that most of the trypanosomes of birds can vary considerably morphologically, and that some, at least, are not specific as to the vertebrate host. They may indeed show considerably more specificity for the invertebrate host (Bennett, 1961). Pending additional studies, it may be well to regard them as Levine (1961) has: "They all look very much alike and probably belong to a relatively few species. However, extensive cross-transmission studies are needed to establish their relationships, and, until these are carried out, it is probably best to refer to them by the names under which they were first described."

Trypanosoma avium Danilewsky 1885

Etiology

Baker (1965a) gave a good description of the strain of *T. avium* used in his studies and included references to all pertinent literature. The morphological characteristics of the trypanosome varied somewhat according to the vertebrate host, as well as showing the usual variation within a given host, but in summary Baker described his flagellate as follows:

"The trypanosome in question is a large spindle-shaped form, measuring an average of 48.2μ in length (excluding flagellum) and 5.5μ in width. There is a tapering aflagellar region extending 14.1μ (on the average) beyond the kinetoplast. This trypanosome is assigned to the species *T. avium* Danilevsky, 1885."

Bennett (1961), who also reviewed the literature, including the work of Baker, tabulated measurements for the trypanosomes he found in several species of birds and came to similar conclusions regarding the morphology and identity of the organism, but he recognized that "many physiologically distinct strains or species may exist" in what he termed the "*avium* complex."

Baker (1956c) has given for *Trypanosoma avium* the most complete description of the life cycle in both the vertebrate and invertebrate hosts that has thus far been presented for an avian trypanosome.

Pathogenesis and Epizootiology

T. avium was first reported from owls and roller birds in Europe. Since then, trypanosomes regarded as being of this species have been reported by numerous workers. Among these are Diamond and Herman (1954), who found it in Canada geese; Baker (1956a), who obtained it from rooks (*Corvus frugilegus* L.) and jackdaws (*C. monedula spermologous* Vieill.); Bennett (1961), who observed it in more than 30 species of birds belonging to more than a dozen orders; and Stabler et al. (1966), who found it in 100 species of birds in Colorado.

T. avium is not known to occur in chickens. However, in view of the intricate relationships between it (or its "complex") and the many vertebrate and invertebrate hosts from which it has been reported, natural infection of domestic birds can hardly be ruled out. Like infections with other avian trypanosomes, it would probably be of little or no economic importance. *T. avium* is considered at length here because it is the only avian trypanosome to have received much attention in recent years.

The natural methods of transmission of the trypanosomes presently considered to be members of this "complex" are by no means clear. Baker (1956b) described experimental transmission by the hippoboscid *Ornithomyia avicularia* L. He concluded: "The metacyclic trypanosomes develop in the insect's hind-gut, and infect birds by penetrating the membranes of buccal cavity and/or esophagus and crop." Transmission did not occur by the bite of infected louse flies, and he had only very limited success with efforts to produce infections in canaries by rubbing fecal matter from infected flies into scarifications in the skin. Bennett (1961) obtained quite different results using infected mosquitoes (*Aedes aegypti*) and ornithophilic simulids. Infections could be produced by ingestion of macerated insects but not by feeding the insects intact. Emulsions of material from the hind-gut or feces of infected insects readily produced infections after having been rubbed into scarifications in the skin. The flagellates apparently were unable to penetrate unbroken membranes. However, trypanosomes from some species of birds were quite unable to develop in some insects that successfully transmitted the flagellates acquired from birds of other species. Bennett summed up the situation as follows: "New criteria for the identification of avian trypanosomes must be developed. It is suggested that the ability of the trypanosome to develop in and produce infective flagellates in a variety of bloodsucking Diptera, whether or not such Diptera are true vectors, be used as criteria. Other criteria, such as serological evidence, or perhaps, the ability to develop on cultures lacking certain chemicals, may yet be needed to definitely separate the species."

Diagnosis

Diamond and Herman (1954) described a technique "for the cultural isolation of trypanosomes from avian bone marrow obtained from living birds or at autopsy." They found the method to be vastly superior to those of merely examining stained smears or of culturing heart blood as a means of detecting trypanosome infections. By examining, but not culturing, the bone marrow from the femur of freshly killed birds, Stabler (1961) detected *T. avium* in 81% of the birds, whereas a study of blood films revealed the organism in only 6% of the specimens. For a Colorado study (Stabler et al., 1966) both methods were again used. This time *T. avium* was detected in bone marrow from 334 birds, whereas only 33 were found to have trypanosome parasitemia. Consequently, reports of the incidence of infection with avian trypanosomes probably have little meaning unless the methods of detection are comparable or can be brought to comparable bases.

Trypanosoma hannai Pittaluga 1905

Hanna in 1903 observed a trypanosome in scanty numbers in the blood of domesticated pigeons in India (Fig. 31.15). It was named *Trypanosoma hannai* by Pittaluga (1905). The parasite was also observed by

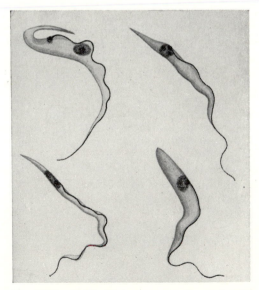

FIG. 31.15—Trypanosoma hannai. (De Beaurepaire Aragao, 1927)

De Beaurepaire Aragao (1927) in the blood of a pigeon in Brazil.

The mode of transmission is still unknown, although De Beaurepaire Aragão noted numerous flagellates of the crithidia type in the alimentary tracts of hippoboscid flies, *Lynchia maura,* which had fed upon a pigeon infected with trypanosomes, but none in flies that had fed upon uninfected birds. Two types of crithidias were noted, the respective dimensions being $40.0 \times 3.0\mu$ and $49.0 \times 1.5\mu$. Attempts to transmit the infection to clean pigeons by the bite of the fly, by injection of the emulsified intestines of infected flies, or even by blood inoculation were unsuccessful.

Trypanosoma gallinarum Bruce, Hamerton, Bateman, Mackie, and Bruce 1911

This trypanosome, and another described about the same time by Mathis and Leger (1911) under the name *Trichomonas calmelli,* were both found in chickens. The flagellate described by Bruce et al. (1911) was about 1.5 times as long and slightly broader than that of Mathis and Leger, but many years ago Wenyon (1926) suggested that they were possibly the same trypanosome. Bennett (1961) went even further, suggesting that both *T. gallinarum* and *T. calmelli* could be considered as belonging to the complex presently regarded as *T. avium.*

REFERENCES

Baker, J. R. 1956a. Studies on *Trypanosoma avium* Danilewsky, 1885. I. Incidence in some birds of Hertfordshire. *Parasitology* 46:308–20.

———. 1956b. Studies on *Trypanosoma avium* Danilewsky, 1885. II. Transmission by *Ornithomyia avicularia* L. *Parasitology* 46:321–34.

———. 1956c. Studies on *Trypanosoma avium* Danilewsky, 1885. III. Life cycle in vertebrate and invertebrate hosts. *Parasitology* 46:335–52.

Bennett, G. F. 1961. On the specificity and transmission of some avian trypanosomes. *Can. J. Zool.* 39:17–33.

Bruce, D., A. E. Hamerton, H. R. Bateman, F. P. Mackie, and Mary Bruce. 1911. *Trypanosoma gallinarum* n. sp. *Rept. Sleeping Sickness Committee Roy. Soc.* 11:170–74.

De Beaurepaire Aragão, H. 1927. Evolution de l'*Haemoproteus columbae* et du *Trypanosoma hannai* dans la *Lynchia maura* Bigot. *Compt. Rend. Soc. Biol.* 97:827–29.

Diamond, L. S., and C. M. Herman. 1954. Incidence of trypanosomes in the Canada goose as revealed by bone marrow culture. *J. Parasitol.* 40:195–202.

Hanna, W. 1903. Trypanosoma in birds in India. *Quart. J. Microscop. Sci.* 47:433–38.

Levine, N. D. 1961. *Protozoan Parasites of Domestic Animals and of Man.* Burgess Publ. Co., Minneapolis.

Mathis, C., and M. Leger. 1911. *Recherches de Parasitologie et de Pathologie Humaines et Animales au Tonkin.* Masson et Cie., Paris.

Pittaluga, G. 1905. Estudios acerca de los Dipteros y de los parasitos que transmiten al hombre y a los animales domesticos. *Rev. R. Acad. Cienc. Exact. Fis. y Natur. Madrid* 3:292–362, 402–504.

Stabler, R. M. 1961. Comparison of trypanosome incidence in blood and bone marrow from 79 Colorado birds. *J. Protozool.* 8:122–23.

Stabler, R. M., Portia A. Holt, and Nancy J. Kitzmiller. 1966. *Trypanosoma avium* in the blood and bone marrow from 677 Colorado birds. *J. Parasitol.* 52:1141–44.

Wenyon, C. M. 1926. *Protozoology.* Bailliere, Tindall, and Cox, London.

INTESTINAL FLAGELLATES

TRICHOMONIASIS

Trichomonads are flagellated protozoa that are characterized by the possession of a longitudinal axial rod—the axostyle, an undulating membrane bordered by a posteriorly directed flagellum, and 3–5 "free" flagella that arise (as does the marginal flagellum) from basal granules near the front end of the body. Some students of this group of protozoa have attempted to classify the trichomonads on the basis of the number of "free" flagella characteristic of the genus; others have regarded the nature of the axostyle, the undulating membrane, and other organelles as better criteria for grouping the trichomonads. For our purposes we may consider all species that are likely to be found in domestic poultry as of the genus Trichomonas ex-

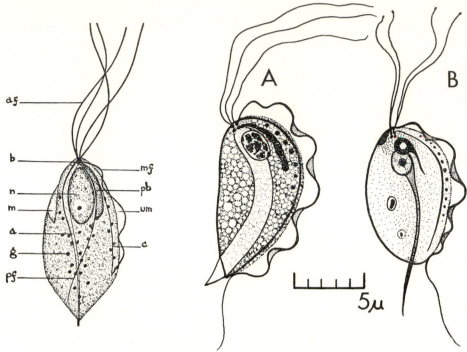

FIG. 31.16—(Left) Trichomonas gallinae, semidiagrammatic: **a.** axostyle; **af.** anterior flagellum; **b.** blepharoplast; **c.** costa; **g.** cytoplasmic granules; **m.** mouth; **mf.** marginal filament; **n.** nucleus; **pb.** parabasal body; **p.f.** parabasal fibril; **um.** undulating membrane. (Stabler, 1941a) **(Right)** Diagrammatic representations of two common trichomonads of lower digestive tract of domestic birds, as favorable specimens fixed in Schaudinn's fluid and stained with Heidenhain's haematoxylin may appear. **(A)** Tritrichomonas eberthi. **(B)** Trichomonas gallinarum. (Lund, in Lund and Farr, 1965)

cept for one cecal form for which the name *Tritrichomonas eberthi* has been generally accepted. The reader who has a special interest in presumed evolutionary relationships and the systematics of the trichomonads and related protozoa should consult Honigberg (1963) and Honigberg and Kuldova (1969) and some of the papers in the extensive list of references therein.

The principal structural components of Trichomonas are designated in Figure 31.16A which depicts *T. gallinae* semidiagrammatically. Figure 31.16B shows semidiagrammatically how two other trichomonads of poultry differ in details from each other and from *T. gallinae*. These are *Trichomonas gallinarum* and *Tritrichomonas eberthi,* mentioned above.

Inasmuch as trichomonads do not form cysts, infection by the ingestion of trophozoites in contaminated food or water must be assumed. However, the intervention of

insects, such as flies, as mechanical carriers has long been postulated.

The vast body of literature on the physiology of the trichomonads has been reviewed by Shorb (1964).

Trichomonas gallinarum Martin and Robertson 1911

Etiology

T. gallinarum varies considerably in both shape and size. Usually it is pyriform, but sometimes many or most of the individuals may be spherical or slightly elongate. Living organisms viewed in wet smears or hanging drops commonly range in length from 7 to 15μ and in breadth from 4 to 10μ. The axostyle extends well beyond the body and is slender and pointed. The undulating membrane is prominent, traversing the entire length of the body and ending near the point at which the axostyle emerges. The marginal flagellum often extends well beyond the axostyle. Characteristically there are 4 anterior flagella, which in living specimens are best seen by the use of a dark-field or phase-contrast microscope. For a detailed description of structures visible in stained preparations, see McDowell (1953). Fixation usually shrinks the organisms (Theodorides and Olson, 1965), but smears fixed in vapors of osmium tetraoxide retain their form and dimensions quite faithfully.

Although the usual habitat of *T. gallinarum* is the cecum, organisms may often be found in the adjacent small intestine. Several observers have reported finding this trichomonad in the liver of turkeys, and Wichmann and Bankowski (1956) found it in the liver of chukar partridges that were dead upon arrival at the laboratory. Indeed, most if not all reports of the finding of *T. gallinarum* in the livers of gallinaceous birds have been based on studies of birds dead long enough to permit postmortem invasion or on studies of birds heavily parasitized by *Histomonas meleagridis*. The livers of birds so parasitized were probably only secondarily invaded by the trichomonad. Rarely, trichomonads may escape into the coelomic cavity and multiply profusely on the serous membranes. Such was the origin of strain TG79 (Soc. Protozool. Comm. on Cultures, 1958). In that instance, apparently, ulceration of the cecum attributable to histomoniasis provided the trichomonads access to the peritoneal and pleural cavities (Lund and Farr, 1965). It is questionable that *T. gallinarum* unaided may invade sites other than the ceca and adjacent intestine.

Pathogenesis and Epizootiology

T. gallinarum was said by Martin and Robertson (1911) to be one of the most common of the flagellates of fowls. McDowell (1953) found it in more than 60% of "several hundred fowl of varying ages and from many sources." Chickens and turkeys are the hosts from which *T. gallinarum* is most frequently reported, but it has been found in guinea fowl by several observers and in chukar partridges by Wichmann and Bankowski (1956). Diamond (1957) found "a *T. gallinarum*-like form" in the Canada goose, and Lund (Lund and Farr, 1965) observed trichomonads resembling this species in the ceca of pheasants raised in captivity.

McDowell's guarded statement (1953) concerning the possible ill effects of heavy cecal infections may approximate the impressions of many workers who have studied farm flocks of either chickens or turkeys. He comments as follows: "The present study discloses that there is a definite association of a yellowish foamy discharge from the caeca and the presence of many *T. gallinarum* in both young fowl and adults, but this diarrhea is most common on range in June and July when every two- to three-month-old fowl will show bedraggled feathers and general unthriftiness as indications of this disease. Severe emaciation may ensue followed occasionally by death." There does indeed appear to be a "definite association," but even if a specific parasitic disorder such as hexamitiasis is ruled out, the presence of harmful bacteria or viruses must be considered.

Kemp and Reid (1965) tested 3 strains of *T. gallinarum* for influence on weight gains in young chickens and on egg production in laying hens. All 3 strains were recovered from flocks "with a history of low egg production reportedly induced by this organism." The authors concluded that the more common strains of *T. gallinarum* are probably harmless.

Tritrichomonas eberthi (Martin and Robertson 1911) Kofoid 1920

This trichomonad inhabits the cecum of chickens and turkeys and has once been reported from ducks (Kotlan, 1923). According to McDowell (1953), who found it in 35% of the several hundred chickens he examined, it occurs principally in older birds, and usually in association with *Trichomonas gallinarum* and *Chilomastix*.

The body of *Tritrichomonas eberthi* was described by McDowell as "carrot-shaped," with an average length in fixed specimens of 13μ and a width of 6.5μ. There is considerable variation in size, however, and spherical forms sometimes occur. The undulating membrane is prominent and traverses virtually the entire length of the body. The marginal flagellum trails well behind. In these respects *T. eberthi* resembles *Trichomonas gallinarum*. However, it is frequently rather larger, and the cytoplasm is more heavily vacuolated than that of *T. gallinarum*. Also, the axostyle of *Tritrichomonas eberthi* is more massive and tends to taper more abruptly at its posterior end than does that of *Trichomonas gallinarum*. Usually only 3 anterior flagella can be demonstrated, and, according to McDowell, it is their beating in unison that imparts to the organism its jerky movement. McDowell also gives in considerable detail the distinctive internal features visible in stained preparations.

Tritrichomonas eberthi is nonpathogenic, and the modes of transmission are assumed to be similar to those for *Trichomonas gallinarum*. Diamond (1957) cultivated *Tritrichomonas eberthi* axenically for the first time.

Trichomonas gallinae (Rivolta 1878) Stabler 1938

Etiology

SYNONYMS. *T. columbae* auct.; *T. hepaticum* (Rivolta 1878); *T. diversa* Volkmar 1930; *T. halli* Yakimoff 1934. According to Stabler (1938a), the turkey and pigeon trichomonad of the upper digestive tract are identical species, and the correct name is *T. gallinae* (Stabler, 1938b) (Fig. 31.16A).

Among the better accounts of the morphology of *T. gallinae* are those of Levine and Brandly (1939), Stabler (1941a, 1954), and Abraham and Honigberg (1964). The organism is roughly pear-shaped but may be rounded under adverse conditions. It ranges in length from 6 to 19μ and in width from 2.5 to 9μ, averaging 10.5 by 5.2μ. As in *T. gallinarum*, there are 4 free anterior flagella, but the body is more elongate, the undulating membrane and costa are shorter, and the marginal flagellum terminates at the end of the undulating membrane as shown in Figure 31.16A. Mattern et al. (1967) gave a detailed account of the ultrastructure of *T. gallinae;* their electron micrographs are excellent.

Various strains of *T. gallinae* differ considerably in virulence (Stabler, 1948a,b, 1951b). That of one strain ("Jones' Barn") was so great that 5 of 10 clean pigeons that received a single trichomonad became infected and died in 8–13 days (Stabler and Kihara, 1954). On one occasion Stabler (1953) passed organisms of this strain successively through 119 Trichomonas-free pigeons, of which 114 died. Continued in vitro passage was accompanied by a gradual loss in pathogenicity, but this was sub-sequently restored by successive passages in pigeons. Pathogenicity was not reduced by holding the organisms at −19° C or −72° C for as long as a year (Stabler et al., 1964). Honigberg and Goldman (1968) cultivated *T. gallinae,* Jones' Barn strain, in vitro longer than 3 years and confirmed that the pathogenicity declined. However, the antigenic nature of organisms cultured 1 year and more than 3 years remained similar to that of highly virulent trichomonads maintained in pigeons, as determined by quantitative fluorescent antibody studies.

Pathogenesis and Epizootiology

T. gallinae occurs almost universally in pigeons, and this bird is probably the primary host (Stabler, 1951a). Its occurrence in the pigeon in America was first reported by Waller (1934), who compiled a brief historical account. Its natural host range includes several varieties of domestic pigeons, the band-tailed pigeon, eastern mourning dove, western mourning dove, and ring-necked dove; various hawks, falcons, and owls; and turkeys and chickens (Stabler, 1941b; Stabler and Herman, 1951; Locke and James, 1962). It can easily be transferred from one of these hosts to another, as from doves to clean pigeons (Stabler, 1951b) or from pigeons to hawks or falcons (Stabler and Shelanski, 1936). Levine et al. (1941) transmitted *T. gallinae* from chickens to the turkey, quail, canary, and English sparrow with lesions and to a duckling without lesions. Additional accounts of transfer experiments with *T. gallinae* are given in Stabler's excellent 1954 review of virtually all of the important literature on this organism.

T. gallinae of pigeons occurs in the mouth, pharynx, esophagus, and crop of apparently healthy carriers. The squabs become infected through the ingestion of their natural food, "pigeon milk." The infection can probably be spread also through contamination of feed or water. The incidence in pigeons and doves may be very high. Stabler (1951a) in Colorado found infection in 19.3% of trapped band-tailed pigeons, 23% of western mourning doves, and 60% of captured common pigeons. Pigeon fanciers call the disease "canker." Falconers refer to it as "frounce."

Obviously the course of the disease in pigeons varies with the strain of *T. galli-*

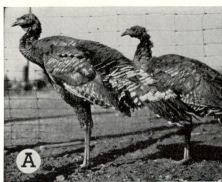 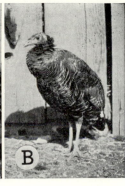

FIG. 31.17—*Posture typical in trichomoniasis of crop. Note especially sunken appearance of crop area. (Hinshaw, in Hinshaw and Rosenwald, 1951)*

nae (Stabler, 1947; Stabler and Herman, 1951). In chronic infections there are no lesions, but in mild cases the apparently healthy bird may show "small, yellowish, adherent masses in the oral or upper oesophageal regions of the digestive tract," which may disappear later. More severe cases frequently end in death, even certain cases where the lesions appear to be slight and confined to the mouth and pharynx. First, yellowish lesions appear on the oral mucosa. These grow into large caseous lumps which may prevent swallowing food or drink. The bird wastes away and may die on about the 8th day of infection. Involvement of internal organs may be noted at necropsy, particularly the liver, which may show only a few yellowish necrotic spots or more extensive caseation. Perez Mesa et al. (1961) described in detail and illustrated the histopathological changes in pigeons experimentally infected with the virulent Jones' Barn strain of *T. gallinae.*

Wild mourning doves are frequently victims of this form of trichomoniasis. The 1950 Alabama outbreak killed many thousands of these birds (Haugen, 1952). Most of the deaths occurred after the spring migration or during the nesting season. The dead birds were emaciated and showed throat swellings that probably had made it impossible for them to swallow food or drink. Herman (1953) prepared a brief paper on recognition of the disease in doves.

T. gallinae infections were once fairly common in turkeys on range frequented by pigeons. Hinshaw (1965) described the epizootiology of one such outbreak that was typical of many that he had observed in California over a period of several years. In this instance the turkeys were on rice stubble and had access to irrigation ditches

and stagnant pools. However, pigeons were abundant in the area and undoubtedly fed on fallen rice, as did the turkeys. Most of the outbreaks that Hinshaw observed were among birds 16–30 weeks old, thus occurring from midsummer through the usual market time for the holiday trade.

The outward signs of the disease are not particularly distinctive. Heads are darkened, sinuses shrunken, and feathers unkempt. Most distinctive perhaps is the sunken chest, occasioned partly by the empty crop and partly by the posture assumed (Fig. 31.17). Such birds lack appetite, drool, and emit a foul odor but seldom have diarrhea. Except in very acute cases, obvious emaciation precedes death. At necropsy, ulceration of the crop is the most common finding. Hinshaw (1965) described other necropsy findings as follows:

The lower esophagus and, less often, the proventriculus and upper esophagus may be involved. The lower digestive tract and the other organs are, as a rule, normal. Aspergillosis of the lungs may be secondary to the necrotic ulceration of the upper digestive tract.

The lesions involve the glandular tissue and vary in size from a few to 15 mm in diameter at the base (Figs. 31.18A, B, 31.19). They taper to a point in concentric rings of piled-up necrotic tissue to as much as 5 mm above the surface. They may extend into the tissue 3 or 4 mm. The surface protruding into the lumen of the organ is rough, irregular, and surrounded at the base by a circular hemorrhagic ring. The lesions in the esophagus are usually smaller than those in the crop but are similar in shape and structure. When the proventriculus is involved, the esophageal portion is most affected. The lesions in the proventriculus are, as a rule, coalesced and may appear as a solid ring of necrotic material causing a marked thickening of the tissues and resulting in partial to com-

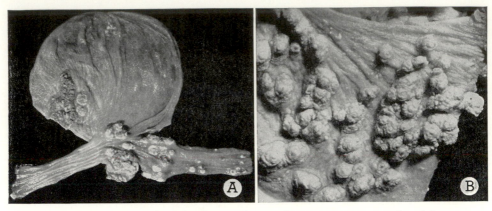

FIG. 31.18—(A) Necrotic ulceration of the esophagus and crop seen in trichomoniasis. (B) Close-up of typical pyramidlike necrotic ulcers characteristic of trichomoniasis of upper digestive tract. (Hinshaw, in Hinshaw and Rosenwald, 1951)

plete occlusion of the lumen. Impactions of the lower esophagus have been noted in such cases.

Prevention and Control

Prevention of trichomoniasis of the upper digestive tract of turkeys is achieved primarily through sanitation. It is particularly important that no contact with pigeons be permitted. Should any turkeys be found to have the disease, they should be isolated and cared for last, using the usual precautions to prevent the organisms being carried to healthy birds.

Treatment

Drugs have been used for the treatment of *T. gallinae* infections in pigeons. Stabler et al. (1958) found that sol-uble Enheptin (2-amino-5-nitrothiazole) used in a concentration of 6.3 g/gal of water was satisfactory. Bussieras et al. (1961) successfully used metronidazole (1-beta-hydroxyethyl-2-methyl-5-nitroimidazole) at a level of 60 mg/kg body weight over a 5-day period. A more convenient means of administering the drug was used by McLoughlin (1966), who found that *T. gallinae* infections were suppressed by giving 0.05% dimetridazole (1,2-dimethyl-5-nitroimidazole) in the drinking water for 3–6 days. It appears likely that any of these drugs could be used for treating *T. gallinae* infections in other birds. Stabler and Kitzmiller (1967) give suggestions for certain hawks, but doses are based on a single administration of the drug Enheptin or dimetridazole in tablet form in this report.

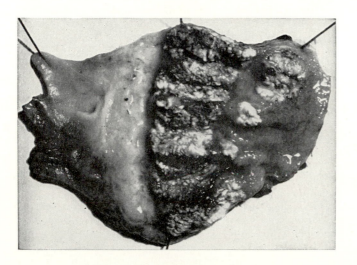

FIG. 31.19—Necrotic ulceration of the proventriculus often seen in trichomoniasis of this organ. (Hinshaw, in Hinshaw and Rosenwald, 1951)

Trichomonas anatis (Kotlan 1923)

SYNONYM. *Tetratrichomonas anatis,* Kotlán, 1923.

Kotlán (1923) made a study of the intestinal flagellates of ducks. His work, except for some random observations, is the only information on this subject available. *T. anatis* has a broadly beet-shaped body which measures 13–27μ in length and 8–18μ in breadth. There are 4 free anterior flagella of about the same length as the body. The well-developed undulating membrane has a sturdy marginal flagellum along its border.

The habitat is the posterior region of the intestine of *Anas boschas dom.* Kotlán states that massive infections are established only when the mucosa is in a catarrhal condition.

Trichomonas anseri Hegner 1929

Hegner (1929) inoculated 3-day-old chicks with cecal material from a goose containing a very few trichomonads. Some of the chicks became heavily infected. The description of the species is based upon the forms which appeared in the chicks. Hegner finds that *T. anseri* has peculiarities which distinguish it from other trichomonads. The body is oval in shape; size, 6–9μ × 3.5–6.5μ with a mean of 7.9μ × 4.7μ. There are 4 free anterior flagella which arise from 2 blepharoplasts, and a fifth one which forms the border of the undulating membrane and becomes a free lash near the posterior end. The chromatic basal rod is distinct; the axostyle is broad and hyaline and protrudes considerably; the nucleus contains an eccentric karyosome and is otherwise filled with minute chromatin granules. Bacteria are ingested into the cytoplasm through a prominent cytostome.

CHILOMASTIX INFECTIONS

Chilomastix gallinarum Martin and Robertson 1911

Etiology

This flagellate and its cysts were first reported from fowls by Martin and Robertson (1911). The best account is that of Boeck and Tanabe (1926), who also described the process of binary fission in detail (Fig. 31.20) (McDowell, 1953).

The trophozoites of Chilomastix are pyriform, somewhat asymmetrical, and plastic. They vary considerably in size, the

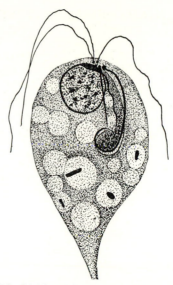

FIG. 31.20—Chilomastix gallinarum, *semi-diagrammatic, illustrating details of morphology.* ×5,000. *(Boeck and Tanabe, 1926)*

length ranging commonly from 11 to 18μ and the width from 5 to 12μ. Occasionally a considerable number of individuals reach a length of 20μ or slightly more. After fixation with Schaudinn's fluid the dimensions are 10–20% less. A large cytostomal groove originates near the anterior end and terminates as a pouch just short of the center of the body. It contributes to the asymmetry of the trophozoite, and because it spirals slightly, the organism sometimes seems to be somewhat twisted. The margin of the cytostome appears to be supported by fibrils, but their exact nature, number, extent, and function have been interpreted in various ways. As shown in Figure 31.20, Chilomastix has 3 free anterior flagella and a fourth flagellum that undulates in the cytostome and aids in the ingestion of bacteria and other food particles. The blepharoplasts which give rise to the flagella, supporting fibrils, and peristomal flagella are difficult to count, but there seem to be 4 of them with the relationships to the other organelles shown in the figure. The nucleus is rounded and of the vesicular type.

Cysts are infrequently observed in fresh cecal material, but McDowell (1953) asserts that they are common in cultures. They measure 7–8.5μ in length and 4.5–5.5μ in width. The internal structures are similar to those in the motile form except that the nucleus has moved to a more central position.

For additional details concerning the structure of either the trophozoites or the cysts, as well as for information on a simple method of culturing the organism, the reader is referred to McDowell (1953).

Pathogenesis and Epizootiology

Chilomastix gallinarum is a common and usually harmless inhabitant of the ceca of chickens and turkeys. McDowell reported having found it in 40% of the "several hundred fowl of varying ages" used in his studies. Lund (Lund and Farr, 1965) stated that there is considerable variation in the incidence in both chickens and turkeys from season to season and year to year. The factors responsible for these variations have not been determined. Only rarely is Chilomastix present alone, so some of the circumstances favoring infections with trichomonads, amebas, and coccidia are probably operative.

Lund (Lund and Farr, 1965) pointed out that Chilomastix has been observed at various times in ring-necked pheasants reared in close confinement and that it has also appeared in pen-raised chukar partridges. Kimura (1934) reported having found it in ducks, and May (1963) and Davis et al. (1964) described outbreaks in quail.

HEXAMITIASIS

The USDA (1954) estimated the annual losses attributable to hexamitiasis of turkeys to have averaged about $667,000 for the period 1942–51. During the decade following that period, the number of turkeys raised in the United States doubled (USDA, 1963), but there were no indications that losses attributable to this disease increased proportionately. However, the organism is easily missed, and other indications of the disease are not highly distinctive.

Etiology

Hexamitiasis, a disease usually of importance only in young poults, is caused by a small flagellate *Hexamita meleagridis*. Although the disease had been observed for many years, particularly in California, trichomonads were assumed to be responsible. Hinshaw et al. (1938a,b) were the first to associate the disorder with a species of Hexamita, and in 1941 McNeil et al.

named the causal agent *Hexamita meleagridis*. They described the parasite as follows:

This organism (minus flagella) varies in length from 6 to 12.4μ (average 9μ) and in width from 2 to 5μ (average 3μ). The nuclear membrane is distinct, and the karyosomes are round and fairly large (two-thirds diameter of the nucleus). Anterior to the nuclei are 2 large blepharoplasts (or groups of blepharoplasts) from which arise the 4 anterior and 2 antero-lateral flagella. The flagella are all of about the same length, measured from the point of emergence from the body. The 4 anterior flagella are usually curved back along the body. Just posterior to these 2 large blepharoplasts are 2 others from which arise the 2 caudal flagella. These flagella pass posteriorly in a granular line of cytoplasm to their pockets of emergence near the posterior end of the body (Fig. 31.21).

As McNeil (1958) pointed out, the symptoms of hexamitiasis and blue comb are very similar, and there may have been some confusion of the two diseases. Furthermore, they undoubtedly occur together at times, and it would be of interest to know whether the relationship is more than one of mere coincidence.

Pathogenesis and Epizootiology

Hexamita meleagridis has been found in quail, pheasants, chukar partridges, and peafowl (Hinshaw and McNeil, 1941; Levine et al., 1952; McNeil, 1958) as well as in turkeys. It can be transmitted to chickens and ducks, but natural infections do not seem to occur in these species. This parasite has been reported from several regions of the United States, including California, Connecticut, Illinois, Indiana, and Virginia. It has also been observed in Alberta (Vance and Bigland, 1956), in Scotland (Campbell, 1945), and in England (Slavin and Wilson, 1953; Wilson and Slavin, 1955).

Lund (1956) described the course of a typical outbreak as follows:

Light cases usually show no symptoms, and outbreaks commonly start this way because only a few parasites were introduced. These infected birds soon shed many parasites, however; contamination increases, and other poults pick up enough organisms to be affected seriously. They soon have a ragged appearance, are nervous, keep on the move, and chirp incessantly, but

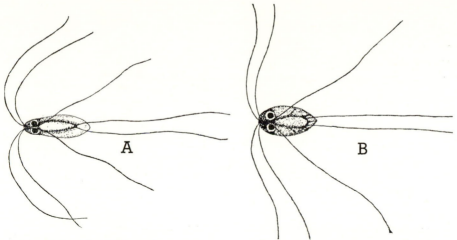

FIG. 31.21—(*A, B*) Hexamita meleagridis *from intestine of turkey, showing indi-vidual variation in size and shape.* ×1,875. *(McNeil et al., 1941)*

do not gain. Small poults especially tend to crowd close to the hover.

As the infections become more severe, the droppings become fluid and foamy and often are yellow. Water is voided faster than it is replaced, and the poults lose weight rapidly.

In the later stages of the disease, the birds stand with heads drawn in, feathers ruffled, and wings drooping, as they do with several other disorders, particularly those of the lower digestive tract. Chirping is less frequent and more muffled than before.

In the final stages, the birds go into a coma, struggle convulsively, and die.

The greatest changes internally are in the upper intestine, just below the gizzard. The intestinal wall is inflamed, and the cavity contains mucus, which may be thin and watery or heavy and like phlegm. The flesh of birds dying with hexamitiasis is usually dark and dry.

The diagnosis of hexamitiasis depends on finding the organism, which is very small, even as parasites go, and hard to identify. If hexamitiasis is suspected, several sick birds should be taken to the nearest diagnostic laboratory, State agricultural experiment station, or a veterinarian who includes poultry in his practice.

A comprehensive paper by Wilson and Slavin (1955) on symptomatology, pathology, and diagnosis of hexamitiasis of turkeys in Great Britain and a previous paper by Slavin and Wilson (1953) describe a complicated life cycle for *Hexamita meleagridis* involving schizogony and cysts. According to Hoare (1955), this unusual life cycle cannot be accepted without more plausible evidence.

Mature turkeys often harbor Hexamita without showing any signs of disease. Outbreaks among poults still in the brooder house probably occur as a result of the grower having introduced the fragile parasite from nearby yards occupied by older birds. Mud and droppings on boots, tires, buckets, and other utensils or equipment may permit the parasite to live for several hours. Outbreaks that appear after the poults are on range could have originated in the brooder house, or contamination of the surroundings may have occurred shortly after the birds were out. Often several stress factors operate more or less simultaneously as the birds are moved to the less sheltered environment. Occasionally, wild birds may introduce the parasite among turkeys on range. The usual hygienic precautions go far in protecting the younger birds from parasites that are better tolerated by older birds, especially breeders.

Treatment and Control

Several drugs are available that may be used at appropriate levels in the feed or water as a preventive measure, or even to control the disorder among birds already somewhat involved. Among these are chlortetracycline, oxytetracycline, and nithiazide. Inasmuch as the preparations available commercially are compounded in various ways, each should be used according to the directions given for the product. In any instance, such a control program must have the support of good management practices.

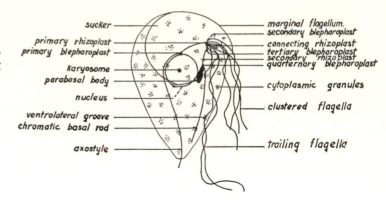

FIG. 31.22—*Cochlosoma. Diagrammatic drawing naming structures. (Travis, 1938)*

Labels (left side): sucker, primary rhizoplast, primary blepharoplast, karyosome, parabasal body, nucleus, ventrolateral groove, chromatic basal rod, axostyle

Labels (right side): marginal flagellum, secondary blepharoplast, connecting rhizoplast, tertiary blepharoplast, secondary rhizoplast, quarternary blepharoplast, cytoplasmic granules, clustered flagella, trailing flagella

MISCELLANEOUS FLAGELLATES

Cochlosoma anatis Kotlan 1923

This curious flagellate has a sharply outlined depression at the anterior end of one side. This concavity, similar to the sucking disc of Giardia, marks the ventral surface. The dorsal surface shows a convexity at the anterior end. The body measures 10–12μ by 6–7μ. From a blepharoplast on the anterior border of the body there arises a tuft of about 6 flagella, all of which are directed posteriad adjacent to the surface of the body. Two axial fibrils (axostyle?) arise from a granule near the blepharoplast and traverse the body to beyond the caudal tip. A vesicular nucleus lies in about the center of the body. Ovoid cysts with 4 or more nuclei are formed. Reproduction is either by binary fission of the trophozoite or by multiplication within the cysts (Fig. 31.22).

This organism was found in the feces and intestinal mucus of a duckling which was suffering with coccidiosis of the intestine, and in the ceca of a growing duck. Travis located them also in the cloaca and large intestine of ducks. Kotlán found the same flagellate in *Nyroca ferruginea* and *Fulica atra*. Pathogenicity of the flagellate has not been proved. Travis (1938) observed it in the wild mallard, shoveler, pintail, lesser scaup, and domesticated mallard. Other species were observed in the magpie and eastern robin.

A severe outbreak of cochlosomiasis, attributed to *C. anatis,* in poults of 2–10 weeks on a turkey farm in Scotland was recorded by Campbell (1945). The birds were affected with a condition clinically indistinguishable from infectious catarrhal enteritis due to Hexamita. The symptoms were as follows: intense thirst, frothy diarrhea, depression, ruffled plumage, drooping head, closed eyes, loss of appetite, weakness, coma, and death. Only 2 or 3 days intervened between the first appearance of symptoms and death. Among the findings at necropsy was the atonic intestine with dilations or bullae filled with yellow fluid swarming with the jerkily swimming flagellates. The flagellate was revealed in every case. Trichomonas and Hexamita were also usually present, but Cochlosoma predominated.

Cochlosoma rostratum Kimura 1934

This species was found by Kimura (1934) in Muscovy and White Pekin ducks in California. It measured 6–10μ by 3.9–6.7μ. McNeil and Hinshaw (1942) have found it throughout the intestinal tract of turkey poults and in the region of the cecal tonsil in adults. It occurred in turkeys associated with Hexamita or in combinations of Hexamita and Salmonella. The true significance of this parasite in turkey poults or ducklings has not been determined.

Protrichomonas anatis Kotlan 1923

This species, observed by Kotlán in the duck, has a more or less pear-shaped body measuring 10–13μ × 4–6μ. There are 3 active flagella which arise from an anterior blepharoplast. It appears as if the axostyle is formed of 2 fibrils which arise from the blepharoplast, pass posteriad, and meet at a point a considerable distance from the caudal tip of the body. The nucleus appears to lie between the fibrils at about the middle of the body.

REFERENCES

Abraham, R., and B. M. Honigberg. 1964. Structure of *Trichomonas gallinae* (Rivolta). *J. Parasitol.* 50:608–18.

Boeck, W. C., and M. Tanabe. 1926. *Chilomastix gallinarum,* morphology, division and cultivation. *Am. J. Hyg.* 6:319–36.

Bussieras, J., R. Dams, and J. Euzeby. 1961. Prophylaxie de la trichomonose du pigeon par le metronidazole. *Bull. Soc. Sci. Vet. Lyon* 63:307–12.

Campbell, J. G. 1945. An infectious enteritis of young turkeys associated with Cochlosoma sp. *Vet. J.* 101:255–59.

Davis, D. E., L. D. Schwartz, and Helen E. Jordan. 1964. A case report: Chilomastix sp. infection in pen-raised quail. *Avian Diseases* 8:465–70.

Diamond, L. S. 1957. The establishment of various trichomonads of animals and man in axenic cultures. *J. Parasitol.* 43:488–90.

Haugen, A. O. 1952. Trichomoniasis in Alabama mourning doves. *J. Wildlife Management* 16:164–69.

Hegner, R. W. 1929. Transmission of intestinal protozoa from man and other animals to parasite-free fowls. *Am. J. Hyg.* 9:529–43.

Herman, C. M. 1953. Recognition of trichomoniasis in doves. *Bird-Banding* 24:11–12.

Hinshaw, W. R. 1965. Diseases of the turkey, pp. 1253–63. In Biester, H. E., and L. H. Schwarte (eds.), *Diseases of Poultry,* 5th ed. Iowa State Univ. Press, Ames.

Hinshaw, W. R., and Ethel McNeil. 1941. Carriers of *Hexamita meleagridis. Am. J. Vet. Res.* 2:453–58.

Hinshaw, W. R., and A. S. Rosenwald. 1951. Trichomoniasis of the upper digestive tract. *Calif. Agr. Exp. Sta. Man.* 3 (Sect. 5):1–2.

Hinshaw, W. R., Ethel McNeil, and C. A. Kofoid. 1938a. The presence and distribution of Hexamita sp. in turkeys in California. *J. Am. Vet. Med. Ass.* 93:160.

———. 1938b. The relationship of Hexamita sp. to an enteritis of turkey poults. *Cornell Vet.* 28:281–93.

Hoare, C. A. 1955. Life cycle of *Hexamita meleagridis. Vet. Record* 67:324.

Honigberg, B. M., and M. Goldman. 1968. Immunologic analysis by quantitative fluorescent antibody methods of the effects of prolonged cultivation on *Trichomonas gallinae. J. Protozool.* 15:176–84.

Honigberg, B. M., and Jelena Kuldova. 1969. Structure of a nonpathogenic histomonad from the cecum of galliform birds and a revision of the trichomonad family Monocercomonadidae Kirby. *J. Protozool.* 16:526–35.

Hughes, W. F., and D. V. Zander. 1954. Isolation and culture of Hexamita free of bacteria. *Poultry Sci.* 33:810–15.

Kemp, R. L., and W. M. Reid. 1965. Pathogenicity studies on *Trichomonas gallinarum* in domestic poultry. *Poultry Sci.* 44:215–21.

Kimura, G. G. 1934. *Cochlosoma rostratum* sp. nov., an intestinal flagellate of domesticated ducks. *Trans. Am. Microscop. Soc.* 53:102–15.

Kotlán, A. 1923. Zur Kenntnis der Darmflagellaten aus der Hausente und anderen Wasservoegeln. Vorlaeufige Mitteilung. *Zentr. Bakteriol. Parasitenk. Abt. I. Orig.* 90:24–28.

Levine, N. D., and C. A. Brandly. 1939. A pathogenic trichomonas from the upper digestive tract of chickens. *J. Am. Vet. Med. Ass.* 95:77–78.

Levine, N. D., L. E. Boley, and H. R. Hester. 1941. Experimental transmission of *Trichomonas gallinae* from the chicken to other birds. *Am. J. Hyg.* 33:23–32.

Levine, N. D., P. D. Beamer, and Ethel McNeil. 1952. Hexamita (Protozoa: Mastigophora) from the golden pheasant. *J. Parasitol.* 38:90.

Locke, L. N., and Pauline James. 1962. Trichomonad canker in the Inca dove, *Scardafella inca* (Lesson). *J. Parasitol.* 48:497.

Lund, E. E. 1956. *Hexamitiasis of Turkeys.* USDA Agr. Yearbook, pp. 444–46.

Lund, E. E., and Marion M. Farr. 1965. Protozoa, pp. 1056–1148. In Biester, H. E., and L. H. Schwarte (eds.), *Diseases of Poultry,* 5th ed. Iowa State Univ. Press, Ames.

McDowell, S., Jr. 1953. A morphological and taxonomic study of the caecal protozoa of the common fowl, *Gallus gallus* L. *J. Morphol.* 92:337–99.

McLoughlin, D. K. 1966. Observations on the treatment of *Trichomonas gallinae* in pigeons. *Avian Diseases* 10:288–90.

McNeil, Ethel. 1958. Hexamitiasis. *Merck Agr. Memo.* 3:5.

McNeil, Ethel, and W. R. Hinshaw. 1942. *Cochlosoma rostratum* from the turkey. *J. Parasitol.* 28:349–50.

McNeil, Ethel, W. R. Hinshaw, and C. A. Kofoid. 1941. *Hexamita meleagridis* sp. nov. from the turkey. *Am. J. Hyg.* 34 (Sect. C):71–82.

Martin, C. H., and Muriel Robertson. 1911. Further observations on the caecal parasites of fowls, with some reference to the rectal fauna of other vertebrates. Part I. *Quart. J. Microscop. Sci.* 57:53–81.

Mattern, C. F. T., B. M. Honigberg, and W. A. Daniel. 1967. The mastigont system of *Trichomonas gallinae* Rivolta as revealed by electron microscopy. *J. Protozool.* 14:320–39.

May, W. O. 1963. Chilomastix infection in quail. *Southeastern Vet.* 14:100–102.

Perez Mesa, C., R. M. Stabler, and M. Berthrong. 1961. Histopathological changes in the domestic pigeon infected with *Trichomonas gallinae* (Jones' Barn strain). *Avian Diseases* 5:48–60.

Shorb, Mary S. 1964. The physiology of trichomonads, pp. 383–457. In Hunter, S. F. (ed.), *Biochemistry and Physiology of Protozoa*. Vol. III. Academic Press, New York.

Slavin, D., and J. E. Wilson. 1953. *Hexamita meleagridis. Nature* 172:1179–81.

Society of Protozoologists, The Committee on Cultures. 1958. A catalogue of laboratory of strains of free-living and parasitic protozoa. *J. Protozool.* 5:1–38.

Stabler, R. M. 1938a. The similarity between the flagellate of turkey trichomoniasis and *T. columbae* in the pigeon. *J. Am. Vet. Med. Ass.* 93:33–34.

———. 1938b. *Trichomonas gallinae* (Rivolta, 1878), the correct name for the flagellate in the mouth, crop, and liver of the pigeon. *J. Parasitol.* 24:553–54.

———. 1941a. The morphology of *Trichomonas gallinae* (= *columbae*). *J. Morphol. Physiol.* 69:501–15.

———. 1941b. Further studies on trichomoniasis in birds. *Auk* 58:558–62.

———. 1947. *Trichomonas gallinae*, pathogenic trichomonad of birds. *J. Parasitol.* 33:207–13.

———. 1948a. Variations in virulence of strains of *Trichomonas gallinae* in pigeons. *J. Parasitol.* 34:147–49.

———. 1948b. Protection in pigeons against virulent *Trichomonas gallinae* acquired by infection with milder strains. *J. Parasitol.* 34:150–57.

———. 1951a. A survey of Colorado band-tailed pigeons, mourning doves, and wild common pigeons for *Trichomonas gallinae*. *J. Parasitol.* 37:471–72.

———. 1951b. Effect of *Trichomonas gallinae* from diseased mourning doves on clean domestic pigeons. *J. Parasitol.* 37:473–78.

———. 1953. Observations on the passage of virulent *Trichomonas gallinae* through 119 successive domestic pigeons. *J. Parasitol.* 39 (4, Sect. 2): 12. (Abstr.)

———. 1954. *Trichomonas gallinae*: A review. *Exp. Parasitol.* 3:368–402.

Stabler, R. M., and C. M. Herman. 1951. Upper digestive tract trichomoniasis in mourning doves and other birds. *Trans. North Am. Wildlife Conf.* 16:145–62.

Stabler, R. M., and J. T. Kihara. 1954. Infection and death in the pigeon resulting from the oral implantation of single individuals of *Trichomonas gallinae*. *J. Parasitol.* 40: 706.

Stabler, R. M., and Nancy J. Kitzmiller. 1967. Emtryl in the treatment of trichomoniasis in pigeons and hawks. *Am. Falconers' Ass.* 6:47–49.

Stabler, R. M., and H. A. Shelanski. 1936. *Trichomonas columbae* as a cause of death in the hawk. *J. Parasitol.* 22:539–40. (Abstr.)

Stabler, R. M., Stella M. Schmittner, and W. M. Harmon. 1958. Success of soluble 2-amino-5-nitrothiazole in the treatment of trichomoniasis in the domestic pigeon. *Poultry Sci.* 37:352–55.

Stabler, R. M., B. M. Honigberg, and Vera M. King. 1964. Effect of certain laboratory procedures on virulence of the Jones' Barn strain of *Trichomonas gallinae* for pigeons. *J. Parasitol.* 50:36–41.

Theodorides, V. J., and W. A. Olson. 1965. Observations on the size of *Tetratrichomonas gallinarum. Avian Diseases* 9:232–36.

Travis, B. V. 1938. A synopsis of the flagellate genus Cochlosoma Kotlan, with the description of two new species. *J. Parasitol.* 24: 343–51.

USDA. 1954. *Losses in Agriculture. A Preliminary Review.* USDA ARS 20–1.

———. 1963. *Agricultural Statistics, 1962.* U.S. Govt. Printing Office, Washington, D.C.

Vance, H. N., and C. H. Bigland. 1956. Hexamitiasis: A report of cases in Alberta turkey flocks. *Can. J. Comp. Med. Vet. Sci.* 20:337–42.

Waller, E. F. 1934. A preliminary report on trichomoniasis of pigeons. *J. Am. Vet. Med. Ass.* 84:596–602.

Wichmann, R. W., and R. A. Bankowski. 1956. A report of *Trichomonas gallinarum* infection in chukar partridges (*Alectoris graeca*). *Cornell Vet.* 46:367–69.

Wilson. J. E., and D. Slavin. 1955. Hexamitiasis of turkeys. *Vet. Record* 67:236–42.

PARASITIC AMEBAS

Entamoeba gallinarum Tyzzer 1920

This ameba was described by Tyzzer (1920) from the cecal excrement of both young turkeys and the common fowl. The trophozoites measure 9–25μ in diameter; average size, 16–18μ. They are continuously and actively motile at room temperature. Pseudopod formation is said by Tyzzer to be gradual rather than eruptive in charac-

ter, but Hegner (1929b) finds that it is almost as explosive as in *E. histolytica*. The ectoplasm is differentiated from the endoplasm. The latter stains intensely and usually contains a variety of inclusions such as cell fragments, flagellates, amebas of the genus Endolimax, and other material from the cecal contents. Tyzzer stated that bacteria are not utilized as food, but McDowell (1953) disagrees. The nucleus is spherical and measures 3–5μ across. A dense layer of chromatin is closely applied to the nuclear membrane. Tyzzer states that the endosome is centrally located, but in his figures he shows it in an eccentric position (McDowell, 1953).

The cysts contain 8 nuclei when mature, but immature quadrinucleate forms occur. The cysts are spheroidal and have an average size of 12 × 15μ.

This ameba is not known to affect the host adversely in life, but within a short time after death the organisms migrate through the tissue and can be found in large numbers throughout the cecal mucosa and submucosa. Under these conditions the parasite may also ingest epithelial cells. Several workers have found this ameba in blackhead lesions in livers of turkeys along with other microorganisms.

If it should eventually be determined that this Entamoeba is identical with that found in the red grouse, the correct name would be *E. lagopodis* Fantham 1910. Although only four-nucleate cysts of the latter species were noted by Fantham, it is not unlikely that the mature cysts possess 8 nuclei. What seems to be *E. gallinarum* was reported from guinea fowls by Hegner (1929b).

Endolimax gregariniformis (Tyzzer 1920)

SYNONYMS. *Pygolimax gregariniformis* Tyzzer 1920; *Endolimax janisae* Hegner 1926.

This small ameba, found by Tyzzer (1920) in the ceca of diseased and normal turkeys, is ovoid in shape with a posterior protuberance. It measures, according to Tyzzer, 3.9–13.3μ; average size, 8.75 × 5.3μ. The movement is quite sluggish at room temperature. The ectoplasm is not noticeably differentiated from the endoplasm. The cytoplasm shows a variable number of food vacuoles in which bacteria or other bodies may be enclosed. The nucleus usually shows a large, deeply staining, centrally situated karyosome separated from an achromatic membrane by a clear space. The diameter of the nucleus is 1.5–2.0μ; that of the karyosome 0.8–1.3μ. The cysts, which rarely occur, measure 9.7 × 6.6μ on the average, are oval and provided with a thin wall, and when mature contain 4 nuclei (McDowell, 1953).

A similar ameba was described from the chicken by Hegner (1926) under the name *Endolimax janisae*. Levine (1961) regards this as a synonym for *Endolimax gregariniformis*.

Tyzzer was able to transmit this species readily to young chicks by feeding small amounts of the feces of infected adult birds. Myriads of the small amebas were present in the cecal discharges of the chicks 4 days after the inoculation. Hegner (1929b) found what seems to be the same ameba in guinea fowls. He also inoculated chicks per os and per rectum with the cecal contents of a goose. There appeared in the ceca of the chicks large numbers of an Endolimax ameba. They measured 4.5–11 × 4.5–8μ; average size 7.8 × 6.2μ. Cysts were observed, but no measurements were given. Hegner is uncertain whether this form is cospecific with *E. gregariniformis* of chickens or represents a new species. In addition, the same investigator noted an Endolimax in cecal material of a duck and succeeded in cultivating it in chicks.

Endolimax numidae Hegner 1929

This small species described from guinea fowls in the United States differs from *Endolimax gregariniformis* in its smaller average size, which is given as 4.2 × 3.4μ. The mature cyst is tetranucleate. Levine (1961) considers Hegner's *Endolimax numidae* to be a "small race" of *E. gregariniformis*.

Entamoeba anatis Fantham 1924

Fantham (1924) in Africa found this histolyticalike Entamoeba in the feces of a duck which had died of an acute enteritis. The appearance, structure, and size of the trophozoites and the presence of erythrocytes in the endoplasm all indicated a similarity to *E. histolytica* of man. In addition the cysts were spherical or subspherical, uninucleate and tetranucleate, thin-walled, possessed of thin needlelike chromatoid bars, and measured 13 × 14μ. A further study should be made of this unusual organism.

Entamoeba sp.

Hegner found in chicks previously inoculated with cecal material from the duck an Entamoeba resembling that from the guinea fowl. The nucleus, however, was spherical in shape and not irregular, and the chromatin was massed in conspicuous clumps on the membrane. The motile forms ranged from 14 to 22.5μ in diameter; average, 17.78μ. No cysts were observed.

OTHER AMEBAS

Hegner (1929a) was unsuccessful in transmitting per rectum or per os the human amebas *Entamoeba coli, Endolimax nana,* and *Iodamoeba williamsi* to chicks 3–18 days of age. *Entamoeba histolytica, E. muris,* and *E. caviae,* however, persisted in the cecum up to 2 days, 5 days, and 20 hours respectively. Later (1929b) he found that an Endolimax from the stomach of sheep could establish itself in the ceca of chicks for as long as 21 days. The cecal discharges contained both trophozoites and cysts.

Hegner (1929b) also succeeded in infecting chicks with the following entozoic amebas of birds: *Entamoeba* sp. and *Endolimax numidae* of guinea fowls, *Entamoeba anatis* (?) of the duck, *Endolimax* sp. from the goose, and *Endolimax* sp. supposedly from the feces of the screech owl.

REFERENCES

Fantham, H. B. 1924. Some parasitic protozoa found in South Africa. VII. *S. African J. Sci.* 21:435–44.

Hegner, R. W. 1926. *Endolimax caviae* n. sp. from the guinea-pig and *Endolimax janisae* n. sp. from the domestic fowl. *J. Parasitol.* 12:146–47.

———. 1929a. Transmission of intestinal protozoa from man and other animals to parasite-free fowls. *Am. J. Hyg.* 9:529–43.

———. 1929b. The infection of parasite-free chicks with intestinal protozoa from birds and other animals. *Am. J. Hyg.* 10:33–62.

Levine, N. D. 1961. *Protozoan Parasites of Domestic Animals and of Man.* Burgess Publ. Co., Minneapolis.

McDowell, S., Jr. 1953. A morphological and taxonomic study of the caecal protozoa of the common fowl, *Gallus gallus* L. *J. Morphol.* 92:337–99.

Tyzzer, E. E. 1920. Amoebae of the caeca of the common fowl and of the turkey. *Entamoeba gallinarum,* sp. n., and *Pygolimax gregariniformis* gen. et spec. nov. *J. Med. Res.* 41:199–209.

❖

SARCOSPORIDIOSIS

❖

LLOYD A. SPINDLER

Beltsville Parasitological Laboratory
Animal Disease and Parasite
Research Division
Agricultural Research Service
U.S. Department of Agriculture
Beltsville, Maryland

❖

SARCOSPORIDIOSIS ("sarco") is an infection with organisms of the genus Sarcocystis. The disease name was derived from that of the protozoan order Sarcosporidia, where the genus was originally classified. The infections might now be called toxoplasmoridiosis, since Levine (1961b) reclassified the genus in order Toxoplasmorida.

The striated muscles of mammals are involved principally; a few reptiles and a variety of birds may be affected. Among mammals sarco is most prevalent in range cattle and sheep and in swine. Several cases in man have been reported. Sarco appears neither widespread nor economically important in domestic fowl. Cornwell (1963) stated that in wild ducks it "warrants consideration from economic and esthetic standpoints since hunters commonly discard infected birds." The literature is extensive, refers mostly to mammals, and establishes little. Information on sarcosporidiosis in birds must be based largely on available knowledge of the infection in mammals. Scott's (1930, 1943a,b) reports (which include extensive literature reviews), Babudieri (1932), Eisenstein and Innes (1956), and Levine (1961a,b) should be consulted.

HISTORY

Sarcosporidiosis was first observed by Miescher (1843) in the mouse and was soon found in a variety of animals and some wild birds. The first report for chickens was by Kühn (1865) in Europe. In United States Stiles (1893) found *Sarcocystis* in a wild mallard, and in 1894 reported the infection in a chicken. Since these initial findings, numerous reports of the parasite in wild birds have appeared.

INCIDENCE AND DISTRIBUTION

Although avian sarcosporidiosis apparently is worldwide, information on incidence and distribution is imperfect, because most reports constitute incidental findings in postmortem examinations. Five records for domestic fowl were published before 1943. Hawkins (1943) found the infection in a chicken in Michigan. Apparently there are no reports for turkeys. An incidence of about 20% was reported in limited numbers of ducks collected in specific localities in the United States (Erickson, 1940; Cornwell, 1963).

ETIOLOGY

CLASSIFICATION

Parasites of the genus *Sarcocystis* (= *Miescheria* Blanchard, 1885; *Balbiania* Blanchard, 1885) have commonly been called sarcocysts, sarcocystis, Miescher's sacs, and Miescher's tubes. Historically the genus has been included in phylum Protozoa, class Sporozoa, order Sarcosporidia. Levine (1961b) reclassified the genus in class Toxoplasmasida, order Toxoplasmorida. However, the biological nature of the parasite is undetermined, and therefore its systematic position is uncertain. Wenyon (1926) discussed the organism under the heading, "Parasites of Undetermined Position." Opinions on classification by Crawley (1916), Wenyon (1926), Babudieri (1932), Scott (1943a), Eisenstein and Innes (1956), and Levine (1961a,b) should be consulted. *Sarcocystis rileyi* (Stiles, 1893) is the name generally applied to the parasite in ducks. Other names are *Balbiania rileyi* and *S. anatina;* Hawkins (1943) concluded that these names are synonymous with *S. rileyi.* Levine (1961a) called the *Sarcocystis* of birds *S. rileyi* and listed the other names as synonyms. The literature contains about 50 species names, designated primarily with

respect to the host. Sarcocysts from some birds have been called *Sarcocystis* sp. Opinions that there may be only one species in animals and birds were expressed by Aléxeieff (1913), Wenyon (1926), and others. If there is one species, the parasites would be known as *S. miescheriana* (Kühn, 1865); otherwise, this term would apply only to the infections in swine.

There have been discussions on whether *Sarcocystis* is a protozoon or a fungus. Opinions favoring the protozoal nature of the organism are based on its morphology, its serological resemblance to Toxoplasma (a protozoon) (Levine, 1961a), statements that the internal sporelike bodies become active when removed from the sarcocyst, and reports of direct transmission by feeding infected flesh. Contrary to the last opinion is the rarity of natural infections in Carnivora and their prevalence in Herbivora. Siebold (1853) believed that the organisms are funguslike Entophytes, because he failed to see animal-like movement of the Miescher's sacs or of the sporelike bodies, and the nuclear arrangement appeared like that of plants. Wenyon (1926) stated that it is doubtful if *Sarcocystis* is a "Protozoa." Craig and Faust (1940) believed that there is no good reason for considering *Sarcocystis* a protozoon, especially since *Rhinosporidium seeberi,* a related parasite, is a fungus, one of the Aspergillus species. Observations on *Sarcocystis* by several investigators indicate that this organism may also be a fungus or closely related to the fungi. The evidence, however, is incomplete, considered controversial, and lacks verification. A summarization follows.

Spindler and Zimmerman (1945) published in part, an investigation in which an Aspergillus was recovered by aseptically rupturing sarcocysts from swine into sterilized dextrose solution. Growth was completed on semisolid dextrose or prune agar; an early growth stage in dextrose is shown in Figure 31.23B. Pigs were inoculated with or fed conidia from the cultures. At 6 months, half of the pigs harbored typical sarcocysts. Mature ones were cultured; a fungus resembling the one administered was recovered.

The following observations are unpublished. Signs like mycotoxicosis developed in some other exposed pigs, most of which died or were killed in extremis within a week; the others were killed within a

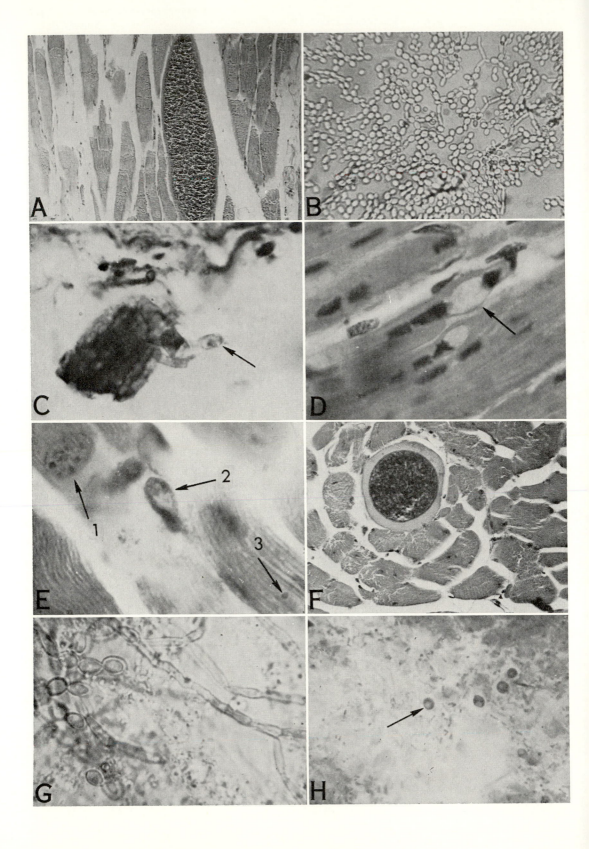

month because of their poor physical condition. Typical sarcocysts were not found, but in histological sections of muscles, varying numbers of fibers contained inclusion bodies (Figs. 31.23C,D,E1,2); some were thought to be young sarcocysts, but the identification was uncertain. Typical sarcocysts (Fig. 31.23F) were found at necropsy in the muscles of another pig continuously exposed to straw moistened daily with urine voided by a worker during 3 months after accidental inhalation of fungus spores from a sarcocyst culture. Straw cultures yielded Aspergillus and other fungi. A litter mate similarly exposed to urine of unexposed volunteers was negative. Cultures of mature sarcocysts from a wild bird (Maryland yellowthroat) and from a sheep (natural infections) yielded a fungus that resembled the one in cultures of swine sarcocysts. Pigs were exposed to conidia from the former cultures, and rabbits were exposed to those from the latter; some animals of each group harbored immature Miescher's sacs at 8 weeks. Rats were fed sarcocysts from a naturally infected hog. At 15 days an almost microscopic, sacculate, funguslike growth was found attached to the mucosa of the ileum of some rats. Yeastlike bodies resembling those shown in Figure 31.23H were seen in sacculate portions of the growth and in the animals' intestinal contents and droppings. Cultures yielded a fungus resembling that in cultures of swine sarcocysts. Ciesla (1951) cultured sarcocysts from bovines, and Holz

(1954) cultured sacs from sheep; both workers reported a funguslike growth in the cultures. Akün and Holz (1955) reported that histochemical studies on sarcocysts from sheep indicated a relationship with the fungi. Spindler (1947) made histological sections of sheep and duck sarcocysts, after draining off most of the internal banana-shaped bodies, and stained the sections with a fungus stain. Portions of the internal network appeared jointed, somewhat like hyphae. In duck sarcocysts, parts of the network appeared tubular with transverse septalike divisions. Delicate jointed branching structures receptive to a fungus stain were seen in residues of sarcocysts from cattle, sheep, ducks, and swine (Fig. 31.23G) after heating with 30% KOH solution.

Observations summarized here, unverified and divergent from the generally accepted idea that Sarcocystis is a protozoon, remain unexplained. Possibly an unidentified organism morphologically similar to Sarcocystis or an unrecognized type of sarcocyst may have been used. The parasite may be capable of behaving either as a protozoon or as a fungus. Or sarcocysts at some stage may contain either funguslike or protozoal elements or both simultaneously; in culturing sarcocysts from swine, growth was most likely to be obtained from the fully mature ones. The sporelike bodies in sarcocysts are said to be motile when removed to isotonic solutions; this is considered indicative of their protozoal nature. However, ripe seeds of some plants are said to be capable of movement, and zoospores of certain freshwater algae move by terminal cilialike organelles. Sarcocyst "spores" with terminal cilialike organelles have been pictured. However, Spindler and Zimmerman (1945), Ciesla (1951), and Holz (1954) failed to show that the growths reported as occurring in cultures of sarcocysts actually originated from the sarcocyst materials placed in culture. Moreover, Spindler and Zimmerman (1945) were unable to eliminate fortuitous infection as a possibility in their successful transmission trials with sarcocysts. However, if the infections were fortuitous, the occurrence was selective for the exposed animals. The result is that the biological nature of Sarcocystis still is undetermined, and the concept that the organism is a protozoon remains based on morphological affinities.

FIG. 31.23—*(A)* Sarcocystis rileyi *in breast muscle of chicken. Longitudinal section.* ×*125.* **(B)** *Early stage of fungus in sarcocyst culture, dextrose solution.* ×*500.* **(C, D, E1** *and* **2)** *Inclusion bodies, presumably young sarcocysts, in muscle fibers of pigs exposed to Aspergillus from sarcocyst cultures.* **(E3)** *Coccoid body in muscle fiber in* **C.** *The body has been displaced from a broken fiber.* **(F)** *Sarcocyst in muscle of pig exposed to urine voided by worker after inhalation of fungus spores from sarcocyst culture.* ×*250.* **(G)** *Contents of Miescher's sac from pig, showing branching divided structure.* ×*1,800.* **(H)** *Yeastlike bodies presumed to be a transmitting stage of Sarcocystis, in intestinal contents of pig 15 days after consuming flesh containing sarcocysts.* ×*980.*

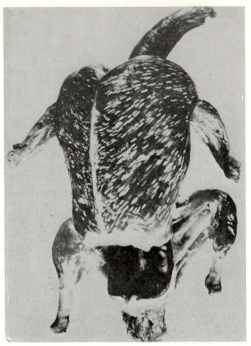

FIG. 31.24—Severe sarcosporidiosis in a wild mallard, natural infection. (Bureau of Sport, Fisheries and Wildlife. Fish and Wildlife Service, U.S. Department of the Interior)

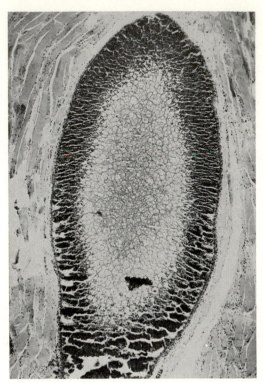

FIG. 31.25—Sarcocystis rileyi in breast muscle of wild duck. Longitudinal section showing internal reticulum (septa).

MORPHOLOGY

Sarcocystis rileyi was described by Stiles (1893), Crawley (1911), and Levine (1961a). Sarcocysts often escape detection except by microscopic examination. When larger and present in considerable numbers, as in some ducks, the musculature has a streaked or wormy appearance (Fig. 31.24). The large cysts have been called *Balbiania*. Stiles (1893) stated that sarcocysts of *S. rileyi* are 1.0–6.0 mm long by 0.48 mm broad. Crawley (1911) gave the size as 6–6.5 mm long by 0.6–1 mm broad. Cysts 5 cm long have been reported from some mammals. Sarcocysts are usually elongate with the long axes parallel to the muscle fiber. When removed they are whitish and cylindroid or spindle-shaped with somewhat pointed ends; the surface may appear lobulated. According to Levine (1961a), *S. rileyi* sarcocysts microscopically have double-layered smooth walls; in some other species the walls appear striated with one layer. Sarcocysts are divided internally into compartments by a reticulum (Fig. 31.25) historically called septa. The arrangement resembles that of the coenobium of certain freshwater algae. When mature, interspaces in the reticulum contain banana-shaped bodies called Rainey's corpuscles—naked trophozoites, according to Levine (1961b). If Sarcocystis is a fungus, the corpuscles might be called zoospores. Spindler (1947) reported that Rainey's corpuscles in sarcocysts appeared to be in chains like some conidia, originating from strands of the reticulum and best seen by microdissection. The trophozoite size varies with the species. Crawley (1911) gave the size for *S. rileyi* as 14–15μ long by 2–3μ broad. Levine (1961a) gave the size as about 8μ long by 2μ wide. In some *S. rileyi* sarcocysts the central compartments are empty. It is not known if these sarcocysts are degenerating or developing. Sarcocysts start development within muscle fibers, but as they enlarge, the fibers may become so compressed that the cysts appear extracellular (Figs. 31.23A,F; 31.25).

LIFE CYCLE

The Sarcocystis life cycle is incompletely known. Smith (1901, 1905) and others reported transmission, particularly in mice, by feeding flesh containing sarcocysts. Possibly this would not have been accomplished had coprophagy been prevented; Minchin (1903) believed that carnivores may discharge infective stages in their feces after consuming infected flesh, without themselves becoming parasitized. Négre's (1907, 1918) transmission trials with mice (reviewed by Scott, 1943b) and those with swine reported by Spindler et al. (1946) appear confirmatory. The latter failed to infect pigs by feeding swine flesh containing sarcocysts and preventing coprophagy. When coprophagy was permitted, infections occurred. Infections occurred in other pigs fed feces (often contaminated with the urine) of pigs, dogs, rats, and chickens (donors) fed infected swine flesh. As reported by Négre for mice, transmission was obtained at about 15 days when minute yeastlike bodies (Fig. 31.23H), thought to be a transmitting stage, occurred in fecal and some urine samples from the donors. The feces were mixed with clean straw on soil. Six months later, pigs maintained thereon acquired overwhelming Sarcocystis infections; some pigs died. The magnitude of the infections seemed disproportionate to the numbers of yeastlike bodies in the feces originally demonstrated (unpublished). Possibly an aging or multiplicative process had occurred. Observations on transmission indicate that hosts in nature may acquire Sarcocystis directly or indirectly from feces of predator or scavenger animals and birds, and that a stage of the parasite may (like Histoplasma and Coccidioides) grow saprophytically on soil, in feces, or even in shallow water. If saprophytic growth occurs, that might throw light on the widespread occurrence of sarcosporidiosis in hosts that are not known to be primarily carnivorous or coprophagous.

In all reported transmission trials, an unexplained latent period elapsed before sarcocysts were detected. Spindler (unpublished) studied blood films from pigs moribund after exposure to fungus spores from sarcocyst cultures and from pigs moribund after consuming feces from animals that had been fed flesh containing sarcocysts. The blood contained numerous minute, somewhat wedge-shaped bodies and some coccoid forms. Many of the former were extracellular, some positioned with the blunt end against erythrocytes, platelets, and phagocytes. Others were inside these cells, usually one per erythrocyte or platelet; many phagocytes were packed with them. The coccoid bodies, about 0.1μ in diameter, were intracellular in erythrocytes and platelets, usually one per cell; occasionally one was in the nucleus of a phagocyte. In histological sections of muscles, coccoid bodies were within erythrocytes in blood vesels, in endothelium of the vessels, and in muscle fibers (Fig. 31.23E3). The relationship of the two types of bodies to each other and to Sarcocystis was not determined.

RESISTANCE TO PHYSICAL & CHEMICAL AGENTS

The resistance of sarcocysts and their stages to physical and chemical agents has not been established. According to Scott (1943a), Négre reported that the "spores" could withstand drying or heating for 5 minutes to 65° C but were killed by heating for 5 minutes at 85–90° C.

PATHOGENICITY

The pathogenicity of sarco in birds is undetermined. Apparently sarcocysts are not noticeably injurious to them. Most reports, however, are on birds considered normal when killed. Very heavy infections may possibly cause disease signs. Infected ducks are said to fly low and slowly. Unthriftiness, emaciation, skin irritation, lameness, incoordination, partial to complete paralysis, and death have occurred in experimentally infected swine, naturally infected sheep and horses, pigs exposed to fungus spores from sarcocyst cultures, and pigs that consumed feces deposited by animals and chickens after eating flesh containing sarcocysts. These signs, if observed in wild birds in nature, might not be attributed to Sarcocystis. Sarcocysts contain "endotoxin" called sarcocystin, said to be an enzyme, injurious to the central nervous system, heart, adrenal glands, and intestines of inoculated rabbits and sparrows. Some species of Aspergillus contain endotoxins. In mammals exfoliation of the intestinal epithelium may follow ingestion of sarcocysts. Exfoliation was observed in chickens experimentally fed swine flesh containing sarcocysts, in rats and mice fed sarcocystin, and in pigs and rats given intraperitoneal injections of fungus spores from sarcocyst cultures of swine origin.

PATHOGENESIS AND EPIZOOTIOLOGY

NATURAL AND EXPERIMENTAL HOSTS

Naturally occurring sarcosporidiosis has been found in a variety of birds (Erickson, 1940; Cornwell, 1963; Vande Vusse, 1966). Older birds seem most likely to be infected. Erickson (1940) compiled the then existing host records which included birds of 20 species in 19 genera, 13 families, and 8 orders. Cornwell (1963) listed the reports that appeared after Erickson's compilation and recorded for the first time infections in redhead, canvasback, and goldeneye ducks. In 1966 Vande Vusse stated that sarcosporidiosis had up to that time been reported from 53 species of birds representing 10 orders and 19 families; he listed, as new host records, infections in the great horned owl, eastern kingbird, and brown thrasher. Better-known wild bird hosts include mallard, black duck, gadwell, American pintail, blue-winged teal, spoonbill, snipe, great blue heron, turkey vulture, English sparrow, slate-colored junco, blackbird, common grackle, sage grouse, and red-legged partridge. Ducks of the puddling or dabbling varieties are likely to be infected.

TRANSMISSION, CARRIERS, VECTORS

Transmission through feces has been reported for some mammals but apparently has not been demonstrated for birds. Sarcosporidiosis is most prevalent in hosts that frequent or drink from shallow, quiet, and even stagnant water (puddling ducks, cattle and sheep on ranges, and swine). Quiet shallow water may be an important ecological factor in natural transmission. *Rhinosporidium seeberi* is said to occur most often in persons with frequent exposure to water of streams and pools. As hosts without disease signs may fit the definition of carriers, most infected birds might be called carriers.

Whether a vector is involved in Sarcocystitis is unknown. Stable flies have been said to transmit the Sarcocystic-like Besnoitia. Therefore, the possibility that a vector may be involved in Sarcocystis transmission should not be disregarded, although attempts have failed to find one. Possibilities are coprophagous beetles, other terrestrial and aquatic invertebrates, and parasitic invertebrates, both external and internal.

HISTOPATHOLOGY

The only histopathology described for birds is fatty degeneration of muscles, enlargement and occasional rupture of parasitized fibers, and inflammatory reactions around some fibers with sarcocysts, especially in older infections. In cattle, sheep, and swine there is generally proliferation of sarcolemmal nuclei and often massive infiltrations of eosinophilic leukocytes with focal tissue degenerations around some sarcocysts. Glomerular and tubular nephritis, intralobular necrosis (liver), and proliferation of sarcolemmal nuclei were prominent in swine fed feces containing the presumed infective stage of the parasite and in others exposed to fungus spores from sarcocyst cultures. It is not known if these disorders occur in birds with sarcosporidiosis.

IMMUNITY

Neither active nor passive immunity has been demonstrated in avian sarcosporidiosis. Repeated natural infections of sheep in successive seasons were reported by Scott (1943a). According to Levine (1961a), animals can be immunized against sarcocystin by repeated injections of untreated or formalin-treated toxin; blood serum of immunized animals protects other animals against the toxin. Whether injections of sarcocystin will protect against infections of the parasite has not been established.

DIAGNOSIS

ISOLATION AND IDENTIFICATION OF CAUSATIVE AGENT

To find sarcocysts by histological examination, muscle tissue is fixed in Bouin's or other standard fixatives, sectioned at 10μ, and stained with hematoxylin-eosin, using standard procedures. The parasites stain blue, as shown in Figure 31.23A,F. Direct examinations are more rapid and utilize more muscle than sectioning. Small pieces of tissue are finely minced, flattened by compression between glass plates, and examined with high magnifications of the dissecting microscope without staining. Sarcocysts appear as elongate saclike bodies within the fiber; they can be easily removed. The more active muscles, such as the masseter and heart, are favorable sites for sampling. For presarcocyst stages, tissues should be sectioned 10μ or thinner and some stained with hematoxylin-eosin and others with fungus stains for comparison. Tissues indicated for sampling include ileum, liver, spleen, kidney, and muscles from the sites mentioned.

SEROLOGY

Serologic reactions have not been used to any extent in diagnosis of Sarcocystis infections in birds. Differential diagnosis is not indicated since the parasites in birds are considered to be of one species. Sera of laboratory animals fed sarcocysts from sheep react positively to the dye test with Toxoplasma trophozoites; sera of naturally infected sheep also react positively. Sarcocystis serology was summarized by Levine (1961a); it is similar to that for Toxoplasma, a protozoon. Both parasites react with cytoplasm-modifying antibody in the Sabin-Feldman dye test; cross-reactions are common.

TREATMENT

Treatments are unknown and may be unwise, because sarcocysts contain sarcocystin which may be damaging to the host. If many sarcocysts were destroyed at one time, sarcocystin might leave the sacs, come into contact with the tissues, stimulate cellular reactions and focal tissue degenera-

tions, and damage the host in other ways. However, according to Scott (1943b), administrations of potassium iodide have been beneficial in sarcosporidiosis.

PREVENTION AND CONTROL

MANAGEMENT PROCEDURES

Management procedures have not been determined. Potentially helpful measures are garbage cooking, disposing of infected flesh and carcasses, provisions for clean water, sanitation to prevent coprophagy, and predator control.

IMMUNIZATION

It is not known if infections can be prevented by inoculations of vaccines prepared from sarcocysts or their stages.

Progress in prevention and control of sarcosporidiosis awaits determination of the biological nature of the parasite, recognition of the transmitting stage, determination of its location in the environment of hosts and the natural modes of transmission, identification of the migrating and developmental stages in the host, identification of the organs and tissues involved in presarcocyst development, and elucidation of other aspects of the infection and of the parasite's life cycle.

REFERENCES

Akün, R. S., and J. Holz. 1955. Histochemische Untersuchungen an Sarkozysten. *Monatsh. Tierheilk.* 7:49–52.

Aléxeieff, A. G. 1913. Recherches sur les Sarcosporidies. I. Etude morphologique. *Arch. Zool. Exp. Gen.* 51:521–69.

Babudieri, B. 1932. I sarcosporidi e le Sarcosporidiosi (Studio monografico). *Arch. Protistenk.* 76:421–580.

Ciesla, E. 1951. Studia nad sarkosporidioza swierzat rzeznych (Sarcosporidiosis of slauterous animals). (In Polish, English summary.) *Ann. Univ. Mariae Curie-Skodowska, Lublin-Polonia Sec. DD* 6:193–215.

Cornwell, G. 1963. New waterfowl host records for *Sarcocystis rileyi* and a review of sarcosporidiosis in birds. *Avian Diseases* 7:212–16.

Craig, C. F., and E. C. Faust. 1940. Parasites of undetermined nature, pp. 220–21. In Craig, C. F., and E. C. Faust, *Clinic Parasitology.* Lea & Febiger, Philadelphia.

Crawley, H. 1911. Observations on *Sarcocystis rileyi* (Stiles). *Proc. Acad. Nat. Sci., Phila.* 63:457–68.

———. 1916. The zoological position of the sarcosporidia. *Proc. Acad. Nat. Sci., Phila.* 68:379–88.

Eisenstein, R., and J. M. R. Innes. 1956. Sarcosporidiosis in man and animals. *Vet. Rev. Annotations* 2:61–78.

Erickson, A. B. 1940. Sarcocystis in birds. *Auk* 57:514–19.

Hawkins, P. A. 1943. *Sarcocystis rileyi* (Stiles, 1893) in the domestic fowl, *Gallus gallus. Parasitology* 29:300.

Holz, J. 1954. Ueber die Morphologie der Sarkocystes tenella. *Monatsh. Tierheilk.* 6:166–72.

Kühn, J. 1865. Untersuchungen ueber die Trichinenkrankheit der Schweine. *Mitt. Landwirtsch. Inst. Univ. Halle,* pp. 1–84.

Levine, N. D. 1961a. Genus Sarcocystis Lankester, 1882, pp. 318–25. In Levine, N. D., *Protozoan Diseases of Domestic Animals and Man.* Burgess Publ. Co., Minneapolis.

———. 1961b. Problems in the systematics of the "Sporozoa." *Protozoology* 8:442–51.

Miescher, F. 1843. Ueber eigenthuemliche Schlaeuche in den Muskelen einer Hausmaus. *Ber. Verhandl. Naturforsch. Ges. Basel (1840–42).* 5:198–202.

Minchin, E. A. 1903. Protozoa. The sporozoa, pp. 150–360. In Lankester, E. Ray (ed.), *A Treatise on Zoology,* Pt. 1, fasc. 2. A. and C. Black, London.

Négre, L. 1907. Sarcosporidiose experimentale. *Compt. Rend. Soc. Biol.* 68:374–75.

———. 1918. Recherches experimentales sur l'evolution de la sarcosporidie de la souris. These-doctorat esciences naturelles. Laval Univ., Quebec.

Scott, J. W. 1930. The sarcosporidia. A critical review. *J. Parasitol.* 16:111–30.

———. 1943a. Life history of sarcosporidia, with particular reference to *Sarcocystis tenella. Wyoming Agr. Exp. Sta. Bull.* 259: 1–63.

———. 1943b. Economic importance of sarcosporidia, with especial reference to *Sarcocystis tenella. Wyoming Agr. Expt. Sta. Bull.* 262:1–53.

Siebold, C. T. 1853. Zusatz to v. Hessling, Theodor, 1853. *Z. Wiss. Zool. Abt. A.* 5: 199–200.

Smith, T. 1901. The production of sarcosporidiosis in the mouse by feeding infected muscular tissue. *J. Exp. Med.* 6:1–21.

———. 1905. Further observations on the trans-mission of *Sarcocystis muris* by feeding. *J. Med. Res.* 13:429–30.

Spindler, L. A. 1947. A note on the fungoid nature of certain internal structures of Miescher's sacs (Sarcocystis) from a naturally infected sheep and a naturally infected duck. *Proc. Helminthol. Soc. Wash. D.C.* 14:28–30.

Spindler, L. A., and Harry E. Zimmerman, Jr. 1945. The biological nature of Sarcocystis. *J. Parasitol.* 31 (December suppl.):13.

Spindler, L. A., Harry E. Zimmerman, Jr., and D. S. Jaquette. 1946. Transmission of Sarcocystis to swine. *Proc. Helminthol. Soc. Wash. D.C.* 13:1–11.

Stiles, C. W. 1893. Notes on parasites-18: On the presence of sarcosporidia in birds. *USDA BAI Bull.* 3:70–88.

———. 1894. Notes on parasites-28: New American finds of sarcosporidia. *Vet. Mag.* 1:727–28.

Vande Vusse, F. J. 1966. Sarcocystis (Protozoa: Sarcocystidae) from three new avian hosts. *J. Parasitol.* 52:22.

Wenyon, C. M. 1926. Parasites of undetermined position, pp. 760–89. In Wenyon, C. M., *Protozoology,* Vol. 1, Bailliere, Tindall, and Cox, London.

CHAPTER 32

VICES AND MISCELLANEOUS DISEASES

❖

M. C. PECKHAM

Department of Avian Diseases
New York State Veterinary College
Cornell University
Ithaca, New York

❖

VICES of poultry are undesirable behavior patterns manifested by one or many birds in the flock which result in injury, death, or financial loss.

CANNIBALISM

Many forms of cannibalism occur in domestic fowl and game birds reared in captivity. Weaver and Bird (1934) indicated that the light breeds of the Mediterranean class are much more prone to these vices than the heavier breeds of the American and Asiatic classes.

ETIOLOGY

Many causes of cannibalism have been suggested, but often outbreaks of cannibalism occur in one pen whereas similar environmental conditions or feeding practices in other pens on the same farm do not cause any difficulty. Conditions reported as predisposing to cannibalism are: feeding only pellets or compressed feed, cafeteria system of feeding, excess corn in the ration, insufficient feeder or drinker space, being without feed too long, insufficient nests, nests too light, excessively light pens, high-density rearing systems, too much heat, nutritional and mineral deficiencies, and irritation by external parasites (Huston et al., 1956; Ostrander, 1957).

Grateful acknowledgement is made to Dr. L. H. Schwarte, original author of this chapter, for much of the material in this section pertaining to chickens, and to Dr. W. R. Hinshaw for the material pertaining to turkeys.

TYPES

Vent Picking

Picking of the vent or the region of the abdomen several inches below the vent is the severest form of cannibalism. This type is generally seen in pullet flocks in high production. Predisposing factors are prolapsus or tearing of the tissues by passage of an abnormally large egg. After birds have tasted blood they will continue their cannibalistic habits without provocation. Many poultrymen will pick up dead birds day after day without observing that they have been picked about the vent and in some instances eviscerated.

Feather Pulling

This is most frequently seen in flocks kept in close confinement with lack of sufficient exercise. Nutritional and mineral deficiencies may be contributing factors. Irritation caused by lice and mites may induce feather pulling (see Chap. 27).

Toe Picking

This is most commonly seen in domestic chicks or young game birds. Hunger often initiates this vice. Chicks may not find the feed because the feed hoppers are too high or too far from the heat source. Feeder space may be inadequate, and the smaller or more timid chicks may be kept from eating by aggressive birds. It is a common practice to start chicks on paper for the first few days to keep them from eating litter. If the chick cannot find feed he will pick at his own or his neighbor's toes. It is a good practice to put mash on newspapers or chick box covers and place them under the hover the first few days of brooding.

Head Picking

This usually follows injuries to the comb or wattles caused by freezing or by fighting among males. A different form of cannibalism is now being observed in debeaked birds kept in cages. In this type the area about the eyes is black and blue with subcutaneous hemorrhage, the wattles are dark and swollen with extravasated blood, and the ear lobes are black and necrotic (Fig. 32.1). Even though the birds are debeaked and kept in separate cages, they will reach through the wire and peck at the neighboring bird or grasp the ear lobes or wattles of the bird and shake their heads in much

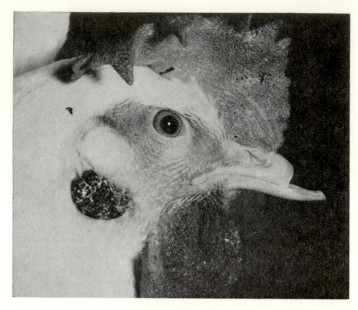

FIG. 32.1—Cannibalism. This bird was a victim of its pen mates even though they were debeaked. Note black and necrotic ear lobe and blackening around eye and wattles due to subcutaneous hemorrhage.

the same fashion as a terrier shaking a rat (C. I. Angstrom, 1962, personal communication).

Wing and Tail Picking

These frequently follow feather pulling or external injuries. Pin feathers are highly vascular, and bleeding follows their removal or breakage. Birds will exsanguinate themselves by continual picking at a feather follicle that oozes blood or by pecking at a small lesion on the foot or other part of the body.

Nose Picking in Quail

Bass (1939) reported an unusual form of cannibalism in quail. It was termed "nose picking" as the birds peck at the top of the nose where the fleshy portion merges with the beak. The condition is generally seen in birds 2–7 weeks of age kept under crowded conditions. The bird may die as the result of blood loss. If the bird survives, the beak will be permanently deformed and the males will be unsatisfactory for breeding stock. This vice occurs only when birds are brooded under artificial conditions. It seldom develops in large pens on the ground in which there is opportunity to pick and scratch. Bass also observed that the addition of raw meat to the ration was very effective in preventing and controlling outbreaks. It may be necessary to withhold the grain ration for a few days until the birds become accustomed to the meat.

Blueback and Cannibalism in Turkeys

Blueback, as the name indicates, is a condition in which the backs of the affected turkeys are discolored blue or black. It is caused by an injury to the quills of the feathers at the point of entrance into the skin which allows the pigment to escape and tattoo the surrounding skin (Fig. 32.2). Feather picking is the immediate cause. Exposure to sunlight after picking is necessary to produce the pigmented condition. Some of the other causes are overcrowding in the brooder, keeping the poults too long on the sun porch, and lack of sufficient fiber in the ration. After picking becomes a habit, the vice is difficult to control; the financial loss due to lowering of the market grade of the carcass may be considerable. Another form of cannibalism which often results in evisceration may also be started by feather picking.

PREVENTION

Cannibalism can best be prevented by providing adequate feed and water space and by not permitting the birds to go without feed for extended periods of time. Overcrowding should be avoided; in cages where high-density rearing is practiced it may be necessary to debeak before housing. Careful attention to ventilation and light intensity may preclude an outbreak of cannibalism.

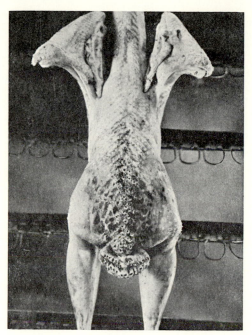

FIG. 32.2–"Blueback" of turkeys. (Ralston Purina Co.)

Chickens

In the past, many remedies have been used to stop cannibalism: hanging cabbages or sugar beets in the pen, putting pine boughs on the floor, painting the windows red, using a red light bulb, darkening the pen and nests, applying pine tar to picked birds, using no-pick salves, using repellent sprays, adding salt to the feed or water, and feeding oats. Miller and Bearse (1937) reported that an increase in fiber content of the ration reduced the incidence of cannibalism. Kennard and Chamberlin (1936) reported that feather pulling and other vices in confined birds largely disappeared when the ration was supplemented with oats. Kull (1948) found that cannibalism and feather picking were stopped by the addition of manganese sulfate and horn meal to the mash. Nelson (1952) reported effective results in 24–48 hours in many instances by the addition of several vitamin preparations to the feed. Willimon and Morgan (1953) reported that the addition of minor nutrient mineral elements to the ration did not show any consistent effect on feather pulling and cannibalism under experimental conditions. Neal (1956) reported that DL-methionine was effective in controlling cannibalism in laying hens, but Creek and Dendy (1957) claimed their investigations did not indicate that methionine counteracted cannibalistic tendencies.

DEBEAKING. When cannibalism becomes established in a flock, the most positive control measures are application of mechanical devices (specs or pickguards) or debeaking. The mechanical devices have several disadvantages as they can be put only on birds of pullet size or larger, they are relatively expensive, and it takes considerable time to put them on. These devices cannot be used on birds kept in cages because they interfere with eating and drinking. They do have an advantage as the operation needs to be done only once, whereas it may be necessary to debeak several times.

Today the most widely accepted means of preventing and stopping cannibalism is by debeaking with an electric cautery. Debeaking can be done on birds of any age from 1 day to maturity. Ostrander (1957) described and illustrated in detail the various debeaking techniques. Many broiler growers and some egg producers have their chicks debeaked at 1 day of age (Lonsdale et al., 1957; Morgan, 1957). Care must be used in debeaking chicks to prevent adverse effects. If the beak is not cut squarely across, the chick may develop crossed beaks. About one-third of the upper beak and just the tip of the lower beak are removed. Care should be observed in cauterizing the beaks of chicks. Too little cauterization results in excessive bleeding, and too much causes necrosis of the tissues. The incidence of "starve-outs" (failure to eat) is much higher in debeaked chicks. Therefore, every effort should be made to have the feed and water readily available for the first few days.

Many poultrymen debeak their laying stock before housing time, particularly where they are kept under close confinement in colony cages. The upper beak is cut and cauterized with the electric debeaker midway between the point of the beak and the nostrils. Some also advocate cutting the lower beak. If debeaking is done on a flock in production because of an emergency, it is best to debeak only to the "quick." This will usually stop cannibalism but will not upset production. If an electric debeaker is not available, a temporary form of debeaking can be done by using a sharp jackknife. A nick is made in the beak about ¼ inch from the tip; with the thumb holding the cut portion of

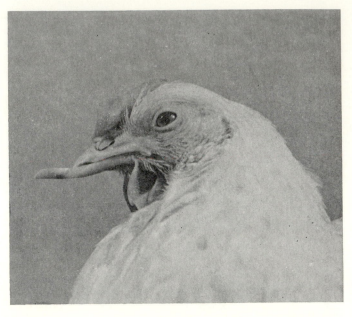

FIG. 32.3—*Debeaking. Note how lower beak has become excessively long following debeaking of upper beak. This interferes with eating and drinking.*

the beak against the blade, the knife is rolled around the tip of the beak tearing off the horny portion and exposing the "quick." If properly done there is little bleeding following debeaking. If birds are debeaked severely, the lower beak may grow very long in time and interfere with eating and drinking (Fig. 32.3). If this occurs it may be necessary to cut off the lower beak to permit the bird to eat and drink properly.

Turkeys

A mechancial device similar to a small hog ring can be used to prevent cannibalism in turkeys. The ring is passed through the nasal septum and between the upper and lower beaks to prevent them from closing tightly. Debeaking can be done with a sharp jackknife or an electrically heated cauterizing knife. Figure 32.4 shows an electric cauterizing knife and a turkey that has been properly debeaked.

EGG EATING

This costly vice of chickens is similar in some respects to cannibalism, for once a few individuals acquire the habit it quickly spreads throughout the flock. Predisposing factors to egg eating are conditions which favor egg breakage—inadequate nesting facilities, insufficient nesting ma-

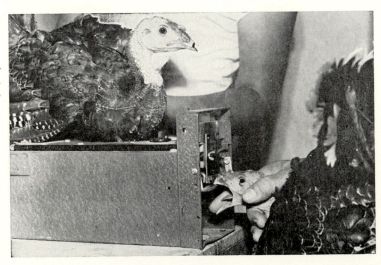

FIG. 32.4—*Electric debeaker in use. Upper beak is removed halfway between tip and nostril. (Payne, 1956)*

terial, failure to collect eggs frequently, and soft-shelled or thin-shelled eggs. If many soft-shelled or thin-shelled eggs are being laid, conditions that may be responsible for these abnormal eggs should be investigated (see section on abnormal eggs).

The prevention of this vice is best accomplished by eliminating those conditions which favor egg breakage. Stopping the egg-eating habit is very difficult. If the birds have not been debeaked, this should be done immediately. When birds have developed a liking for eggs they will not only eat broken eggs but will deliberately eat any egg whether or not it has an intact shell. Debeaking will make the end of the beak sensitive for a few days and the birds will be reluctant to peck against a hard shell. Darkening the nests by putting bags over the front or end of the nests will aid in stopping the habit. The frequent collection of eggs is mandatory if the egg-eating habit is to be checked.

PICA

This condition is the abnormal consumption of material not generally used as food. The cause is not always readily apparent, but lack of feed, boredom, nutritional and mineral deficiencies, parasitic diseases, and sudden exposure to new types of litter may be predisposing factors. It may take the form of litter eating, feather eating, or even the ingestion of fecal material or hot ashes taken from a brooder stove. The incidence of this condition has decreased with improvements in management and feeding practices. Control is based upon detection of the cause and adoption of corrective measures.

MISCELLANEOUS DISEASES

The diseases discussed in this section are those which cannot be classified as to etiology. They vary considerably in their economic importance and frequency of occurrence. Many diseases can be diagnosed from the appearance of the gross lesions, by demonstration of the causative agent, by serological tests, or by histological changes. Some diseases and conditions do not produce pathognomonic signs or lesions; in these cases the ultimate diagnosis depends upon the acumen and experience of the observer. For some diseases and conditions the etiology is unknown or controversial and control measures are lacking at the present time. However, it is no less impor-

tant to recognize a disease of unknown etiology or one without a satisfactory treatment than it is to diagnose a disease of specific etiology or one that has positive control measures.

INJURY

THERMAL

Frostbite

Freezing of the comb and wattles may occur in the northern climate. Male birds are more susceptible to freezing because of the large comb and wattles. The increase in the started pullet business has necessitated the trucking of pullets during the winter months. Unless the crates are properly covered, exposure to wind and cold will rapidly cause freezing of the unfeathered parts. The frosted appendage first becomes red and swollen followed by gangrene, necrosis, and sloughing. After the frozen appendage thaws, the bird experiences intense pain and remains inactive and does not eat. This results in decreased egg production from the layers and diminished activity by the males. In addition other birds will peck at the injured part, leading to further discomfort and possibly death. Affected individuals can be segregated and the injured part can be removed surgically. If the frostbite is detected early and the value of the bird warrants, it can be given individual treatment. The construction of the house should be such as to prevent subfreezing temperatures. If this is not possible, surgical removal of the comb (dubbing) and wattles (cropping) should be done at an early age.

Heat Prostration

CHICKENS. Birds in production are particularly susceptible to high temperatures accompanied by high humidity. As birds lack sweat glands, their only means of cooling off is by rapid respiration with mouths open and wings relaxed and hanging loosely at their sides. Closed nests and community-type nests predispose to heat prostration when temperature and humidity are high. An attempt to cool the birds can be made by dipping or by spraying them with water. Every effort should be made to increase the circulation of air by opening doors and windows and using fans. Cooling the air can be accomplished by using a hose to wet down the floor, walls, ceiling, and outside roof. Additional drinkers should be added to provide readily available water. Preventive measures consist of installation of fans, proper construction of ventilating ducts, insulation of the building, and using white or aluminum paint on the outside to reflect the heat. In southern climates where low production and mortality from heat are constant problems, the installation of foggers and sprinklers may be necessary.

TURKEYS. Heat prostration is usually associated with high humidity or very low humidity on excessively hot days. Stiles (1943) reported a case of heat exhaustion in a flock of 3-week-old turkey poults which were abruptly transferred from cool battery brooders to quarters where the heat inside the building and on the sun porches was extreme. Wilson and Woodard (1955) found that air temperatures above 90° F cause hyperthermy in turkeys and that the body temperature is definitely influenced by the amount of shade at such temperatures.

The symptoms are labored breathing, weakness, excessive thirst, and high temperature followed by complete prostration. Losses can be prevented by furnishing ample shade facilities, especially for poults just transferred from the brooder house to an open yard or range. If a house is available on the range, young poults may well be sheltered in it during the hottest part of the day, but with all the windows open for ample circulation of air. As soon as the poults become accustomed to the new quarters, they will stay inside during the excessive heat; water and feed should be left both inside and outside the house for the first few weeks. Out of doors, trees make the best shade, but an abundance of cheap artificial shade can be made from old lumber and posts. Thatched roofs may be used advantageously if material for covering the shelter can be secured. Pure fresh water must be available at all times. It should be kept in a shady place and in enough containers to enable the birds to find it readily. If, in spite of all precautions, turkeys are overcome by the heat, they should be put in a shady well-protected place and sprayed with cold water. Used in time, this procedure will save a large number. Filling the crop with cold water by means of rubber tubing and a funnel is also advisable. Dipping the birds in cold water may be effective, but care must be taken to prevent drowning. As the birds may be weak for several days, they should be kept in the shade with food and water easily accessible.

PHYSICAL

Mechanical Feeder Trauma

In chicks an unusual injury of the toes is caused by mechanical feeder trauma. This has been observed in flocks where there is no wire guard over the metal thrust rod that pushes against the chain link in the trough. The motor operating the movement of the chain runs intermittently, and chicks develop a conditioned response to the sound of the motor as they know fresh feed will enter the beginning of the trough when the motor starts. As a consequence, chicks crowd around the beginning of the feeder, and some of them have their toes crushed between the thrust bar and chain link. There is little or no bleeding associated with the injury, and scab formation is followed by gangrene, necrosis, and sloughing of the toe (Fig. 32.5).

Emphysema

Subcutaneous emphysema is caused by an injury or defect in the respiratory tract that permits the accumulation of air beneath the skin (Fig. 32.6). This condition

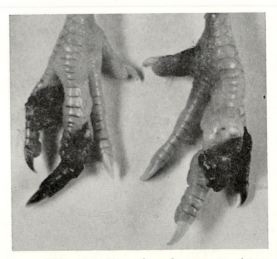

FIG. 32.5—*Necrosis and gangrene of toes in chick as the result of crushing in a mechanical feeder. (Courtesy P. P. Levine, Cornell Univ.)*

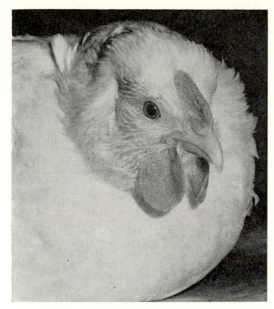

FIG. 32.6—*Subcutaneous emphysema. Note ballooning of skin over crop, neck, and head region.*

has been observed following rough handling and caponizing. After the caponizing operation the skin incision may heal before the opening in the body wall, with a subsequent accumulation of air beneath the skin. This condition, commonly called a "windpuff," can be alleviated by puncturing the skin with a sharp instrument. In aquatic or flying birds some of the pneumatic bones such as the humerus, coracoid, and sternum may fracture, allowing air to accumulate beneath the skin.

Keel Bursitis

This occurs most commonly in heavy, rapidly growing birds. Pressure of the keel on the roost causes irritation and inflammation followed by callus formation or infection of the bursa. The accumulation of cheesy exudate caused by the infection produces a blemish resulting in downgrading of the carcass. Van Ness (1946) reported the isolation of *Staphylococcus citreus* from the livers, joints, and sternal bursae of birds with keel bursitis. In this case the birds were injuring the skin on sharp pieces of wire protruding from the floor of the porch. Infection developed at the site of injury and metastasized to various parts of the body. Losses ceased after the sharp ends of the wire were covered. Cur-

vature or deformity of the sternum is also associated with certain strains and breeds. Nutrition and management may play a role in the development of this condition.

Improper Sexing Technique

Levine (1952) reported finding ascites, nephritis, and mortality in chicks resulting from physical injury during sexing. Affected chicks were inactive, the skin on the medial aspect of the shanks was wrinkled, and the beaks were bluish in color. These chicks died within 24–48 hours. The abdomen was distended with a cloudy but odorless fluid. Marked nephritis was present. Nearly all the chicks had ruptured yolk sacs. In addition there was an ecchymotic, hemorrhagic area in the inner musculature of the pelvis adjacent to the cloaca. It was found that the output of one Japanese sexer suffered a 15% mortality. Losses did not occur in chicks sexed by other workers or in unsexed chicks.

Cranial Injury

Injury to the skull and brain is most commonly seen in quail, pheasants, and pet birds such as canaries and parakeets. Quail and pheasant take off from the ground with great thrust and will fly directly into objects under the stress of fear. The force of the impact will cause hemorrhage in the cancellous bone of the skull and intracranial hemorrhage. Sudden death in a quail or pheasant in excellent physical condition with no evidence of internal lesions or infectious disease should prompt one to examine the skull for injury. Pet birds that escape from their cages or are released for exercise in the house will frequently fly against windows or walls and sustain cerebral injury. The bird does not die immediately but generally succumbs within a period of hours following the accident. The bird may act sleepy or manifest nervous symptoms prior to death. A history of acute death in a well-nourished pet bird with no obvious sign of disease should lead one to investigate the possibility of cranial injury.

Smothering

This condition is generally caused by birds crowding or piling up in a corner. It may occur when birds are moved to new quarters, when they are frightened, or in young birds when they are chilled. The

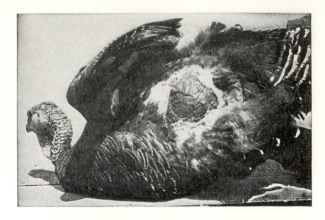

FIG. 32.7—Turkey hen with severe laceration caused by male during mating process. (Hinshaw, Univ. of Calif.)

history of the case indicates that mortality occurs only at night and the flock in general looks healthy. Smothering of baby chicks can occur in chick boxes that are piled too high without an air space between each box, in boxes that do not have sufficient ventilation holes, or in boxes that are placed in a closed compartment such as the trunk of a car. Postmortem examination of chicks that have smothered usually does not reveal enough gross pathology to make a positive diagnosis, but a thorough examination will eliminate other possible causes of death. In broilers and older birds that have smothered there is congestion of the trachea and lungs, and the feathers will be worn off the birds where they have been trampled. Smothering of chicks in the brooder house can be controlled by putting a circle of corrugated cardboard around the hover for the first week and gradually widening its diameter as the chicks get older. This will prevent the chicks from piling up in a corner during the night. When birds are moved to new quarters, the use of a dim light or lantern the first few nights will decrease the possibility of smothering. Birds transferred to new quarters should be checked late in the evening for signs of piling. Frequent observation of the flock is very important the first few days after acquiring a group of new chicks or grown birds.

Mating Turkeys

Severe losses occur in many breeding flocks because of the females' backs being badly torn by the male during the mating process (Fig. 32.7). Badly torn females seldom recover sufficiently to produce fertile eggs during the remainder of the season; if the wound does heal, the area is tender and easily torn when the bird is trodden again.

Some males are much more vigorous and rough in the mating than others, and many of the losses can be traced to one or two individuals in a flock. These males

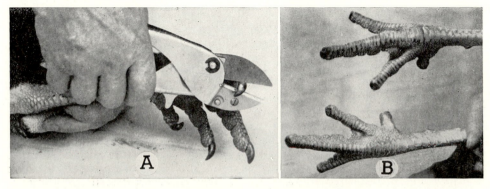

FIG. 32.8—(A) Method of trimming toenails of male turkey to prevent injuries during mating. (B) Feet of male turkey after trimming toenails. (Hinshaw, Univ. of Calif.)

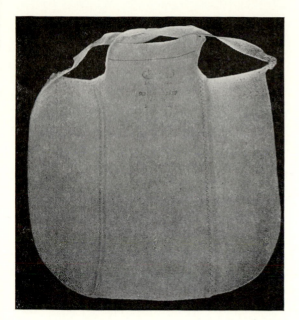

FIG. 32.9—A type of "apron" or "saddle" in common use for prevention of injuries to females during mating. (Hinshaw, Univ. of Calif.)

should immediately be replaced by reserves. One method of prevention is removal of the toenails from the males about a week before the breeding pens are put into the breeding pens (Fig. 32.8). A convenient instrument for removing the toenails is a pair of pruning shears of the roll-cut type shown in Figure 32.8A. An electric soldering iron or some other form of searing iron can be used for searing the cut surface to stop hemorrhage.

Another method of preventing breeding females from being torn is to fit a canvas saddle over the back (Figs. 32.9, 32.10). These saddles, which can be purchased at a reasonable price, are recommended for general use. Care should be taken to purchase saddles which fit correctly in order to prevent strangulation or injury to the body or wings.

If an injured hen is discovered immediately, the torn edges of skin should be sutured. The bird should then be placed in a pen where there are no males and left for about 2 weeks. An antiseptic dusting powder will induce healing and prevent attacks by flies. As soon as the wound begins to heal normally, the hen can be fitted with the canvas saddle described above and returned to the breeding pen.

She should be watched carefully, however, and if again injured by the males, should be returned to the isolation pen.

Where several males are in one pen, the transfer of one male to a pen of injured females may be a better procedure than putting the injured hens back in the regular pen. The time required for complete recovery depends on the extent of the injury and the efficiency of the treatment. Whether or not treatment is worthwhile depends on the value of the individual and the time available.

Vertebrae, Turkeys

Injury to the vertebrae usually occurs in the cervical or thoracic region. With cervical injuries the bird is found with its head and neck extended close to the ground, and it cannot change this position. The neck muscles are swollen and hot to the touch. There may be feathers missing from the side of the neck and evidence of a bruise. Correction of the dislocation by massage and tension gives relief and complete recovery in 2–6 weeks. The bird should be isolated until recovered to protect it from other birds.

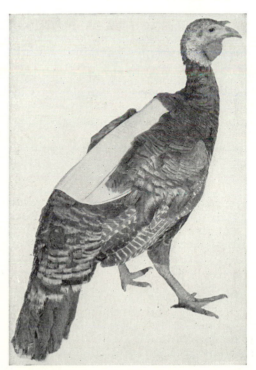

FIG. 32.10—Turkey hen with "saddle" in place. (Hinshaw, Univ. of Calif.)

Sudden inability to stand or walk in a previously healthy turkey is characteristic of a broken back. The injury usually occurs between the 5th and 6th thoracic vertebrae and can readily be seen upon postmortem examination (Moore, 1954).

Moorhead and Mohamed (1968) reported a crooked neck syndrome in 10% of 8,000 18-week-old turkeys. The principal lesion was an osteodystrophy of the cervical vertebrae; investigation of the flock suggested an inherited defect.

Fighting

Males are more likely to be injured from fighting than are females, and a valuable male should be separated from its pen mates if it not able to defend itself successfully. A male which has been away from the flock for any length of time or has just been purchased must be protected when placed with other males, because they will invariably fight it.

Minor injuries seldom require treatment and will heal readily if the bird is unmolested. Severe lacerations about the head usually respond to an antiseptic dusting powder.

Rupture of Gastrocnemius Tendon

An unusual lameness of chickens described as rupture of the gastrocnemius tendon was first reported in the United States by Bullis and Van Roekel (1944). Subsequent reports were made in Scotland by Harriss (1947), in Canada by Chute (1950a,b), in England by Jordon (1955) and Carnaghan and Hanson (1958), and in Belgium by Devos (1963). Harris (1963) reported rupture of the gastrocnemius tendon in a 6-week-old and a 7-month-old turkey.

ETIOLOGY. The etiology of ruptured tendons is unknown. Bullis and Van Roekel (1944) observed the condition in the spring in birds hatched out of season. They suggested that the tendons may lack strength and are predisposed to rupture under the strain of jumping from roosts, nests, or feeders. Chute (1950a,b) failed to find any bacterial agent using aerobic and anaerobic techniques. He discussed three theories as to the possible etiology—nutrition and management, genetics, and predation—but drew no conclusions. The results of Carnaghan's experiment (1958) suggest that a susceptibility to the condition may be inherited.

Jordan (1955) was of the belief that genetic factors were concerned in the etiology, although he believed that out-of-season hatching, environmental conditions, and early maturity were contributing factors. Devos (1963) stated that the condition appeared to be the result of genetic selection for fast growth, increased weight, and broad-breastedness, coinciding with accidental stress factors. He observed no correlation between ruptured tendons and nutrition, seasonal incidence, or sexual maturity.

INCIDENCE. Harriss (1947) reported a flock incidence of 3.8%, but Bullis and Van Roekel (1944) and Devos (1963) reported an incidence of 10%, and Chute (1950a, b) reported 15% affected in one flock. In one experiment where the offspring were derived from previously affected parents, Carnaghan (1958) observed 20% of the flock affected.

SIGNS. The condition is characterized by an acute lameness of one or both legs. If both legs are affected, the bird will rest on its hocks with the toes flexed. At the onset affected birds are in good condition, are alert, and may even be in production. Harriss (1947) indicated that birds 3–9 months of age were affected. Bullis and Van Roekel (1944 and Chute (1950a,b) observed that the disease occurred most frequently in birds 4–7 months of age which were just starting to lay. The same investigators noted that fall-hatched chicks had a higher incidence than chicks hatched in the spring.

Bullis and Van Roekel (1944) observed the condition only in females, whereas Harriss (1947) and Chute (1950a,b) reported that males, capons, and pullets were affected. It was noted by Carnaghan (1958) that females were affected at an earlier age than males, and this tended to coincide with sexual maturity. Ruptured tendons have been reported in light breeds, heavy breeds, and crosses among heavy breeds.

GROSS LESIONS. Externally the lesion is manifested by a bluish green discoloration of the skin above the hock. It is often possible to palpate a break in the gastrocnemius tendon in the live bird. Fibrosis and thickening occur around the tendon in old lesions, and indurated areas can be palpated through the skin. The gastrocnemius

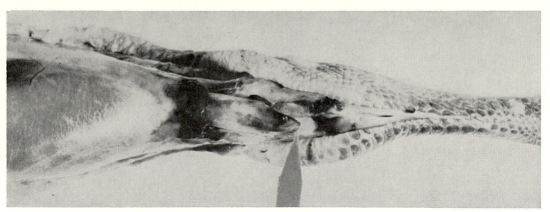

FIG. 32.11—Ruptured tendon. Skin reflected from hock joint revealing ruptured and hemorrhagic end of gastrocnemius tendon.

tendon may have a complete transverse break (Fig. 32.11), or the tendon may have a gray water-soaked appearance. Hemorrhage into the affected area may be slight or extensive.

HISTOPATHOLOGY. On histological examination, Harriss (1947) noted round cell infiltration in the grossly thickened tendons but none where complete rupture without fibrosis had occurred. Chute (1950a,b) found that muscle fibers were degenerated and some had disappeared adjacent to its tendinous attachment. There was hyaline degeneration of the tendon. Adjacent to this area was a network of collagen which surrounded lacunae containing individual, variously shaped, darkly blue staining cells. Proliferating fibroblasts were present which constituted the thickening about the tendon. Upon examination of blood from affected birds, Chute (1950a,b) did not find any abnormalities in the hemoglobin content, red cell count, white cell count, and differential count.

Dehydration

Dehydration can occur in birds of any age. It is generally caused by failure of birds to find water, inability to reach the water, and in some cases by a deterring factor in the water. Baby chicks can survive several days without water but will start to die by the 4th or 5th day if they have not had any. Mortality will reach its peak during the fifth and sixth days and terminate abruptly thereafter if water is provided. The chicks that are not drinking will have succumbed by this period, and the survivors are those that have found the water and are drinking. Dehydration can be detected in a chick as it is unable to "peep" during the later stages. The chick lacks sufficient weight for its size and age, and the skin on the medial aspect of the shanks is dehydrated and wrinkled. Other changes in a dehydrated chick are blue discoloration of the beak, dry and dark breast musculature, dark kidneys, an accumulation of urates in the ureters, and darkening of the blood. Symptoms and lesions in older birds are similar to those in chicks, and the loss in weight is much more noticeable. To prevent dehydration in chicks the water fountains should be placed at the edge of the hover directly upon the litter without any platform. When a change is made from a small drinker to a larger type or to automatic drinkers, the old type of drinker should be kept for a few days and moved toward the new source of water supply to gradually accustom the birds to the change. When birds are moved from range shelters to laying houses, drinking pans should be placed on the floor for the first few days until the birds become adjusted to their new environment.

On occasion an electrical charge may be present in the water caused by faulty electrical heating devices used to prevent water from freezing. The drinkers will be full of water and the owner will be unaware that dehydration is occurring if the system is automatic. Even if the problem of dehydration is made known to the owner, he may be unaware of the reason the birds are not drinking unless he puts his hand in the water. On one occasion a short circuit was occurring in the laying house and the same water pipes also supplied the drinkers on range. The owner put temporary drinkers in the laying house because the birds had become conditioned to the electric shock and refused to drink from the old drinkers. However, he was unaware that the same situation had occurred on the range; only after more mortality had occurred and the situation was reevaluated at the laboratory did he realize that the birds on range had also been conditioned by the electric shock and would not drink from the usual pans.

Laying birds need a constant water supply or production will drop. Frozen pipelines or frozen water pans are followed by dips in the production charts. Cold weather followed by a drop in production should lead to an investigation of the possibility of a frozen water supply.

CHEMICAL

Fuel Oil Burns

Bullis and Van Roekel (1944) reported exfoliation of the cranial skin in chicks caused by contact with kerosene or fuel oil. This problem occurred where a kerosene brooder stove had a small leak in the fuel line which dampened the bottom of the pipe. The chicks became exposed by brushing their heads against the pipe. Kerosene causes irritation and necrosis, and an eschar is formed which eventually drops off, leaving the surface smooth and devoid of down. The shrinkage of the skin on top of the head produces tension on the eyelids causing distortion and angulation (Fig. 32.12). This combination of bald head and angular eyelids has led to a description of the condition as "china boy" disease. The chicks rapidly recover once the source of irritation is removed.

Dickinson and Clark (1946) reported brooder stove residue burns in turkey poults. The poults came in contact with the tarlike residue that leaked from the pipes of brooder stoves burning gas briquettes, causing severe coagulation necrosis of the skin over the skull and on the back of the neck. It was discovered that exposure to sunlight was necessary for irritation and subsequent lesions to occur. Birds exposed to sunlight would rub the base of the skull and neck over the wings and back. Some birds would shake their heads so violently as to fall over. The intense irritation would cause the birds to scratch almost continually, and scratches or lacerations would be produced on the head and eyelids. Birds with severe irritation would quickly get relief when removed from the sunlight. In one experiment, four 6-week-old poults were rubbed with residue on the head and neck. The birds were exposed to sunlight for 2 hours on 4 successive days. Three of the birds died on the 4th day. Four other poults treated with the same material but not exposed to sunlight developed a mild dermatitis but showed no visible signs of discomfort. The condition was readily corrected by confin-

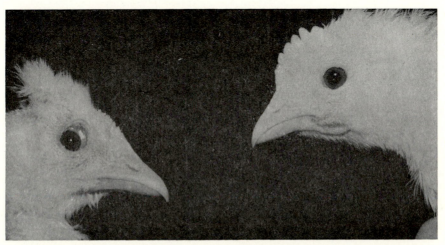

FIG. 32.12—Angular eyelids and loss of down on top of head in chick on left caused by kerosene burn. Normal chick on right.

ing affected birds for 10–14 days until the lesions healed.

Ammonia Burns

Barber (1947) first described a kerato-conjunctivitis in chickens caused by exposure to ammonia fumes produced from unsanitary conditions. Bullis et al. (1950) thoroughly investigated the circumstances under which the condition appeared and concluded that it was caused by exposure to ammonia fumes. Experimental reproduction of the syndrome was carried out by Faddoul and Ringrose (1950). Wright and Frank (1957) recorded the condition in Canada, and Saunders (1958) and Carnaghan (1958) described affected broiler flocks in England. Dorn et al. (1964) described keratoconjunctivitis in chickens associated with intranuclear inclusion bodies in the palpebral conjunctiva suggesting a viral etiology. However, they were not successful in isolating an etiological agent and could not effect transmission. The clinical signs and gross pathology were identical to those cases caused by ammonia burn.

The condition is usually seen in young birds during the winter and spring months. The first symptoms manifested are a rubbing of the head and eyes against the wing. The bird remains quietly in one spot with the eyelids closed as there is a marked photophobia (Fig. 32.13). Upon close examination of the conjunctiva, edema and inflammation are evident and the surface of the cornea may be roughened or opaque (Fig. 32.14). The center of the cornea may

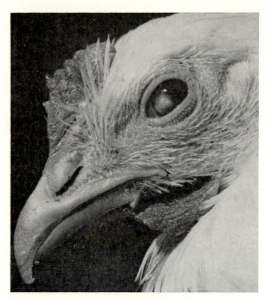

FIG. 32.14—Corneal opacity caused by ammonia burn.

have a shallow ulceration with irregular edges; the remaining area of the cornea is normal in appearance. Generally the condition is bilateral but may be unilateral. In chronic cases the outline of the eyelids is irregular. Affected birds do not eat and rapidly become emaciated.

The condition is apparently caused by continued exposure to ammonia fumes generated by decomposition processes occurring in the droppings (Bullis et al., 1950; Wright and Frank, 1957; Saunders, 1958).

Experimental exposure of birds to ammonia fumes by Faddoul and Ringrose (1950), Wright and Frank (1957), and Saunders (1958) resulted in the production of lesions similar to those occurring in field cases. Prevention of this condition is based on sound management practices with particular attention to ventilation, clean litter, and adequate floor space. Affected birds may take a month or longer to recover even though removed to well-ventilated quarters. Under commercial conditions disposal of severely affected birds is indicated.

Blepharoconjunctivitis, Turkeys

Bierer (1956, 1958) and Sanger et al. (1960) described a disease of breeder turkeys characterized by inflammation of the eyelids, lacrimation, and in severe cases destruction of the eyeball. This disease usu-

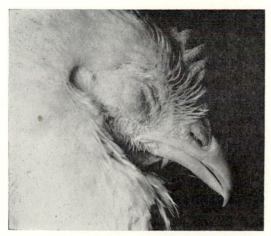

FIG. 32.13—Photophobia in chicken with keratoconjunctivitis caused by ammonia burn.

ally appears during the fall and winter months. When warm weather appears, new cases do not develop and mildly affected birds recover. Mortality is low but morbidity may reach 15–40%. Economic losses result from lowered egg production, decreased fertility, and poor finish when dressed. Mature hens and toms are usually affected, but younger birds may be afflicted.

ETIOLOGY. The etiology has not been established. Bierer (1958) presents evidence that suboptimal vitamin A levels predispose birds to this syndrome. However, Sanger et al. (1960) stated that vitamin A deficiency is not considered to be a factor as the disease occurred in flocks receiving adequate vitamin A, and supplementation of rations fed to affected flocks did not produce discernible improvement. The disease has not been reproduced experimentally. Sanger et al. (1960) were unable to effect contact transmission by placing mature turkeys in a small pen with affected birds. There was no evidence of egg transmission when fertile eggs from affected hens were hatched and the poults reared to maturity. All attempts to isolate significant bacteria or viruses were negative.

SIGNS. The first sign of the disease is a white frothy foam at the anterior canthus of one or both eyes. (Fig. 32.15). As the bird exhales, air passes up the nasolacrimal duct producing the frothing of the ocular secretions. Holding a small feather at the anterior canthus will demonstrate quite conclusively that air is being expelled via the nasolacrimal duct; holding the feather at the nares on the same side as the affected eye will show that air is not being

expelled through this orifice. It may be that the primary problem is swollen turbinates which interferes with normal respiration. The accumulation of fluid in the eye irritates the birds, and they scratch the affected eye and rub their heads on the wings.

LESIONS. Frothing of the eye is followed by ulceration of the eyelid at the mucocutaneous junction. The eyelids become swollen, caseous exudate accumulates, and the lids may become encrusted and closed. Ulceration of the cornea is followed by infection and panophthalmitis. Destruction of the eyeball results in atrophy of the globe, the lids become thickened and distorted by scar tissue, and the palpebral fissure is reduced to a small opening (Fig. 32.16).

DIFFERENTIAL DIAGNOSIS. A number of reports on eye involvements in turkeys must be differentiated from this disease. Included are Manson's eyeworm disease (Schwabe, 1950), *Plasmodium lophurae* infection (Becker et al., 1949), aspergillosis (Moore, 1953), salmonellosis (Evans et al., 1955), paracolon infections (Hinshaw and McNeil, 1946), and granulomatous chorioretinitis (Saunders and Moore, 1957). Similar signs and lesions are sometimes seen in turkeys that have been vaccinated against fowl pox at an early age and exposed several months later after the initial immunity has been reduced or lost. These cases usually develop in old breeders following fighting. In such cases the causative virus can be easily isolated.

TREATMENT. Injection with 250 mg streptomycin for 4 days gives immediate improvement (Sanger et al., 1960). When affected birds are placed in clean warm quarters, spontaneous recovery occurs. Bierer (1958) suggests treating the affected birds with ophthalmic antibiotic ointment and high levels of vitamin A in addition to supplementing the ration with vitamin A. Affected birds should be isolated to prevent cannibalism.

DISEASES OF THE DIGESTIVE SYSTEM

STOMATITIS

Mathey (1956) reported the occurrence of diphtheritic patches in the oral cavity of chickens caused by *Spirillum pulli* sp. *nova* (Fig. 32.17). The organism could be demonstrated in fresh scrapings taken from salivary glands or diphtheritic lesions and ex-

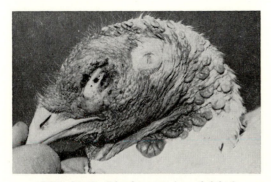

FIG. 32.15—*Blepharoconjunctivitis in turkey with frothy exudate at anterior canthus of eye.*

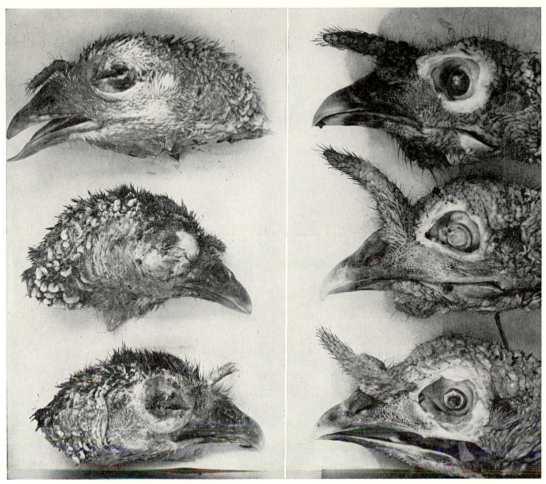

FIG. 32.16—Keratoconjunctivitis. **Left:** *(upper) severe conjunctivitis; (middle) thickened eyelids and conjunctival sac filled with cheesy matter; (lower) eyelids removed to show cheesy matter.* **Right:** *(upper) ulceration of cornea, eyelids removed; (middle) severe keratitis with extensive destruction of corneal tissue; (lower) eyelids removed. (Bierer, 1956)*

amined by dark-field illumination or in Giemsa-stained preparations. The organism was not grown in pure culture, but transmission was accomplished by experimental inoculation of tissue suspensions and by contact.

STRING EATING

Respiratory distress caused by string looped around the base of the tongue and passing down the esophagus has been observed in chickens and turkey poults. Poults are commonly reared in batteries with crinoline cloth covering the floor. Strands of thread protrude from the cut edges and the poults ingest these fibers, some of which become looped around the tongue. Con-

tinual swallowing movements draw the string tighter until it cuts into the tissue, causing edema of the glottis. Although the condition could easily be alleviated, it is usually detected only at necropsy. Chickens frequently pick up the long white strings used to stitch together the tops of feed sacks. The string becomes looped around the base of the tongue (Fig. 32.18), and the bird will keep extending its head and neck in much the same manner as a bird with laryngotracheitis.

Occasionally pieces of grain or pellets become lodged in the larynx or trachea. Frequently they may be retracted through the oral cavity with a suitable instrument. Foreign bodies which cannot be reached

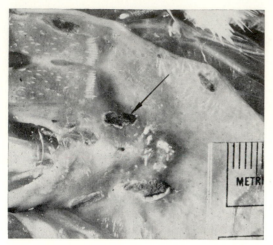

FIG. 32.17—Diphtheritic patches in mouth of chicken caused by Spirillum pulli *infection.*

in this manner can be removed by tracheotomy. Procaine is suitable for local anesthesia.

BEAK NECROSIS

Beak necrosis is now a condition of the past because of modern feeding practices. It is caused by a gradual accumulation of feed inside the mouth along the edge of the lower beak.

Infection and necrosis gradually occur followed by sloughing of the beak. Barr (1965) gives a recent account in which 80% of 300 cockerels were affected; 15% of the birds had lost the lower beak. Virtually none of the 3,000 females had lesions. It

was observed that the maxilla was more convex in the males than in the females; this prevented proper closure of the beaks, allowing fine particles of feed to accumulate. Substituting pellets for the mash alleviated the condition in a few days. Peckham (1961) saw a severe case of beak necrosis and sloughing of the mandible in a pigeon.

Beak necrosis is more common where finely ground feed is used or when feeds contain a high gluten content. Supplying grain, crumbles, or pellets will correct the condition.

CURLED TONGUE CONDITION

The first report of this condition was made by Hudson (1939), who reported on a curled tongue condition in turkey poults a few days old (Fig. 32.19); 25% of a flock of 200 poults were affected. The outcome or cause was not discussed.

Grau and Almquist (1945) first noted that chicks fed a diet deficient in any one of three amino acids (leucine, isoleucine, and phenylalanine) developed a folded condition of the tip of the tongue (Fig. 32.20). They could cure the condition in a few days by adding the deficient amino acid to the diet. In the same chicks the condition reappeared when one of the amino acids was withheld from the diet.

Sanger et al. (1953) described a curled tongue condition occurring in Broad Breasted Bronze and Beltsville White turkeys over a period of several years. In one case the birds received a commercial feed; in another case a home-mixed ration was

FIG. 32.18—String looped around base of tongue and larynx of chicken.

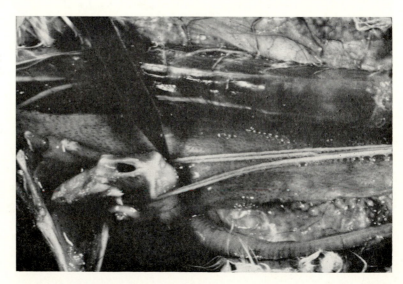

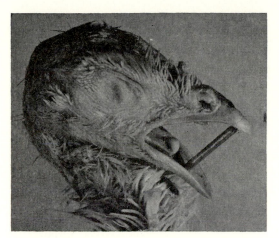

FIG. 32.19–Curled tongue condition in turkey poult.

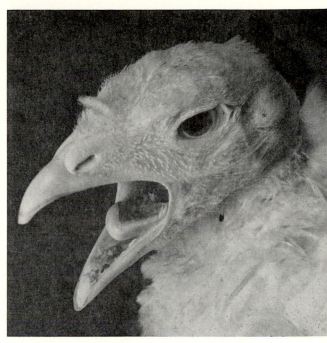

FIG. 32.21–Curled tongue condition in Beltsville White turkey. (Courtesy V. L. Sanger, Ohio State Univ.)

fed. The condition was first noticed at 10 days of age, and by 6 weeks of age 200 in a flock of 4,000 were affected (Fig. 32.31). In addition to its folded state the tongue rested in a submandibular pocket that protruded between the rami of the mandible (Fig. 32.22). Feed adhered to the floor of the mouth in the anterior portion of the intermandibular space. Surgical removal of the curled portion of the tongue did not improve the ventral displacement. Histological examination of the tongue revealed nothing unusual.

The defect in the tongue had interfered with feed intake, and affected birds were below normal weight. Although the ration was changed to commercial crumbles at 6 weeks of age, the condition was not improved in affected birds, but no new cases developed. It is possible that the pathological change had reached an irreversible

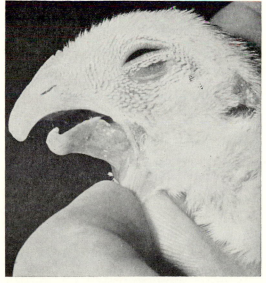

FIG. 32.20–Curled tongue condition in young chick.

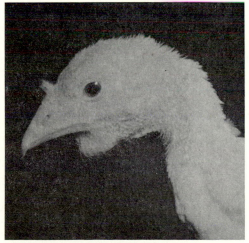

FIG. 32.22–Submandibular pocket caused by ventral displacement of tongue in turkey with curled tongue condition. (Courtesy V. L. Sanger, Ohio State Univ.)

state even though the causative factor or factors had been removed.

Scott, in 1951, quoted by Bragg (1953), found a high incidence of curled tongue condition among poults used in an experiment testing various high-energy ingredients from carbohydrate sources. The leucine, isoleucine, and phenylalanine were calculated to be 1.3 times the known chick requirement. He concluded that the condition was not caused by an amino acid deficiency in this case but was probably due to a high amount of red dog flour in the ration which caused pasting in the beaks of the poults and caused the tongue to curl back mechanically. He further stated that when the level of red dog flour was reduced or replaced by cornmeal, pulverized oats, or standard middlings, no cases of curled tongue condition occurred.

Bragg (1953) conducted extensive experiments in studying the curled tongue condition in poults and made several observations: (1) Some cases of curled tongue occur at hatching time. He stated, "This may be explained by a fairly rare recessive genetic factor or a genetic difference in the nutritional requirements of the breeding hen, or the differential depletion of nutrients in a few breeder hens in the flock supplying the hatching eggs." (2) A greater incidence of the condition occurs among poults fed fine mash than among those fed a coarser type ration. (3) Under normal growing conditions it appears that the deformity is not caused by a deficiency of the amino acids (leucine, isoleucine, or phenylalanine) in the poult's diet.

Wright and Temperton (1955) in Great Britain reported that poults of four different breeds and one cross-breed group developed typical symptoms of curled tongue when fed a home-mixed dry mash. The condition also occurred when commercial mash was fed in the dry state; 5–26% of the poults became affected. When the rations were fed in a moistened condition from the time of hatching, only an isolated case of curled tongue was observed. A large proportion of affected poults recovered when a change was made from dry to wet mash feeding. These authors concluded that the primary cause of curled tongue condition in turkey poults is the feeding of

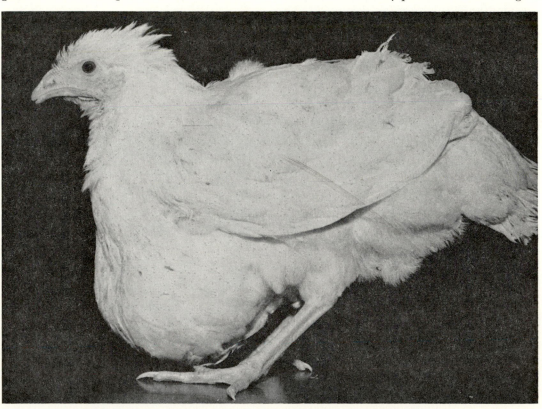

FIG.32.23—Marked distension of crop caused by impaction with straw.

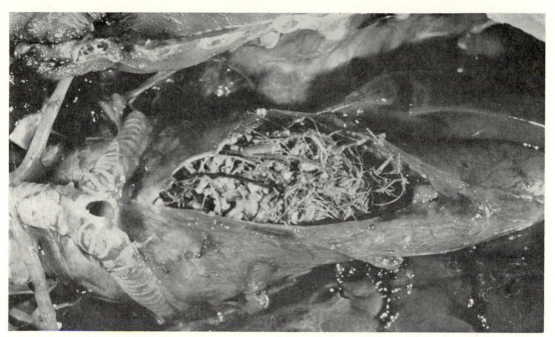

FIG. 32.24—*Large fibrous mass lodged in lower end of esophagus. Note how pressure of mass has flattened primary bronchi.*

a dry mash of fine physical consistency during the first few weeks of life.

IMPACTION

Crop impaction occurs when large amounts of fibrous material are ingested (Fig. 32.23). This is apt to occur when birds are first put on range that has long tough grass. If birds are allowed to go without feed for any length of time and there is straw or grass available, they will eat this material. In some cases where straw is used for litter, birds will eat this material even though feed is available. The fibrous material will form a ball in the crop, and if not too large it will begin to pass through the remainder of the digestive tract. It may become lodged at any point along the digestive tract (Fig. 32.24). Birds with impaction may survive for days, but gradually they become emaciated and die of inanition. Early detection of crop impaction can be corrected by surgery. If the condition is allowed to remain too long, atony of the muscles may occur.

PENDULOUS CROP, TURKEYS

Etiology

Serious losses from pendulous crop (Fig. 32.25A) in some flocks are, according to Hinshaw and Asmundson (1936) and Asmundson and Hinshaw (1938), the result of a hereditary predisposition toward the condition. Turkeys with the inherent weakness develop pendulous crops after increased liquid intake during the first wave of excessively hot weather. The crop, once expanded, seldom returns to normal size, especially if the hot dry weather continues. It may contract for a few days if the weather becomes cool and then expand again during the next hot spell. Although a few birds recover, the majority continue to have pendulous crops. In this condition the crop does not empty normally; stagnant, sour liquid contents are retained in the bulbous portion. As time goes on, the mucous membrane thickens and may become ulcerated (Fig. 32.25B) due to secondary microbial infections.

Studies by Rigdon et al. (1958) and Manfre et al. (1958) indicate that the normal diets fed turkeys do not greatly influence the incidence of pendulous crops in a flock. However, they experimentally produced pendulous crops in turkeys by feeding a ration containing cerelose as a substitute for starch. When such birds were returned to a starch ration, the pendulous crops regressed. No mention is made as to whether the turkeys used were from parent

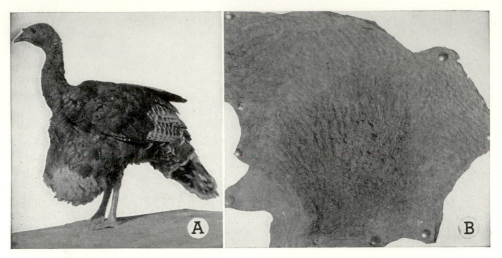

FIG. 32.25—(A) An 8-month-old female turkey with pendulous crop of about 5 months' duration. (B) Section of pendulous crop showing thickening and ulceration of mucous membrane. (Hinshaw, Univ. of Calif.)

stock having a hereditary tendency to this condition. These workers also found that *Saccharomyces tellustris* grows and multiplies rapidly in crops of turkeys fed cerelose. This yeast produces a large amount of gas which is thought to be the cause of the expansion of the crops of cerelose-fed birds. *Candida albicans* was also found to be a common inhabitant of the crops of the turkeys used in the cerelose experiments, but it did not multiply when cerelose was fed, and no frank cases of candidiasis developed.

Signs

The appetite is not greatly affected, but digestion is hindered. The feed and water remaining in the crop may increase until the crop and its contents equal one-fourth of the total live weight of the bird. The bird may continue to grow but will remain unthrifty and may become emaciated.

The course of the disease is chronic; as mentioned above, very few birds recover even with treatment. Some live for as long as 2 years, but the mortality of the affected birds in a flock may exceed 50%.

The causes of death are (1) rupture of the crop by the bird's toes in its attempt to walk or run, (2) mechanical pneumonia from the seepage of crop contents into the bronchi during mechanical efforts to drain the crop or as a result of a backflow when the bird lowers its head, and (3) starvation due to insufficient intake of food or to improper digestion.

Pendulous crops caused by an inherent weakness must be distinguished from similar conditions that sporadically result from impactions, mycosis, trichomoniasis, and other crop infections. These conditions, however, may be exaggerated in flocks having a hereditary tendency towards pendulous crops.

Lesions

Necrotic ulcers, varying in nature according to type of contents and severity of the case, frequently occur. Scraping the necrotic membrane from the surface leaves a denuded bleeding area. This type of necrosis is distinguished from that seen in trichomoniasis by the tendency of the latter to form individual pyramidal ulcers as compared with the diffuse, spreading nature of the former. Demonstration of trichomonads furnishes a further means of differentiation. In a few cases, lesions typical of moniliasis (thrush) have also been observed. In these cases fungi are readily demonstrated. The contents of the crops have varied from a watery, sour-smelling mass to a solid bolus of mud, feces, and grain. Semiliquid contents have been most common. The contents usually suggest a depraved appetite.

Few or no changes in any organ except the crop and possibly the lower esophagus are seen on necropsy. The mucous membrane of the bulbous portion of the crop is thickened and in folds. Areas of diseased lung tissue varying in size are easily seen in those cases where the cause of death has been inhalation pneumonia caused by the entrance of crop contents into the lung. In such cases, food particles are found in the bronchi when the latter are carefully dissected. The air sacs are sometimes involved, and foreign matter can be seen when scrapings from them are examined microscopically.

Treatment and Control

Many methods for "curing" pendulous crops have been described by turkey growers. These have included various operations, the use of cloth vests or supporters, and methods of portioning out the water supply to the affected birds. Most of the methods have produced few actual recoveries.

Removing a portion of the crop surgically results in a high percentage of recoveries, but the time consumed probably does not warrant the procedure as a routine practice. Washing out the crop with warm water containing a weak antiseptic and then tying off a portion of the skin over the enlarged crop will yield temporary relief until market time. If only a few cases appear, it is more economical to kill the affected birds.

Since pendulous crops are usually associated with a hereditary weakness, the best preventive measure is to avoid mating any birds that have a family history of this weakness. Although this is a difficult procedure in a flock that is not trapnested, much can be done to prevent the condition from becoming established. Poults with affected crops should be caught and toe-marked or banded so they can be eliminated at the time turkeys are selected for breeding.

Sufficient shade during the hot months will reduce the numbers of pendulous crops in a flock. It is doubtful, however, whether any procedure other than eliminating the inherent tendency will remove the possibility of having a few cases.

PROVENTRICULAR HYPERTROPHY

A peculiar hypertrophy of the proventriculus in 4-week-old chicks fed a purified diet was reported by Newberne et al. (1956). Approximately 15% of the chicks which originated from 3 different sources were affected. It was suggested that the condition may have been dietary in origin. The author has also noted unusual enlargement of the proventriculus in chicks fed a commercial ration.

TRAUMATIC VENTRICULITIS AND ENTERITIS

Traumatic ventriculitis is generally caused by a sharp object such as a nail, wire, or stick perforating the wall of the gizzard. Contraction of the powerful gizzard muscle forces the object through the wall (Fig. 32.26). Birds with this condition become emaciated and die. On postmortem examination adhesions and inflammatory

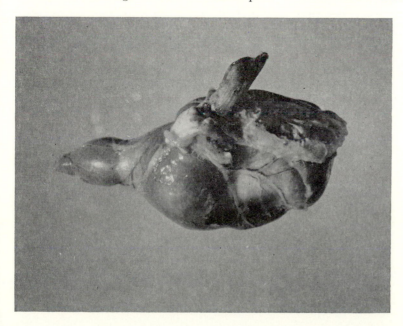

FIG. 32.26—Traumatic ventriculitis in pheasant. A sharp pointed stick has been forced through gizzard muscle.

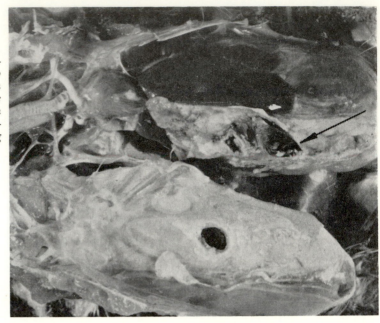

FIG. 32.27—Traumatic ventriculitis in pheasant. A sharp pointed stick (**arrow**) has been forced through gizzard muscle and has eroded a hole through sternal muscles. Note inflammatory exudate surrounding injured area.

exudate mark the site of the injury (Fig. 32.27). A high incidence of traumatic ventriculitis was observed in a cage-reared flock by Angstrom (1961, personal communication). Each bird had a slender piece of wire an inch long piercing the gizzard. He discovered that the owner was using a wire brush to clean the drinking trough. Switching to a fiber brush stopped the losses.

Wickware (1945) reported that grasshoppers may cause death of turkeys by mechanically injuring the walls of the crop and intestine. In some cases the walls of these organs were punctured by grasshopper legs. He suggests that such losses can be prevented by feeding plenty of mash to turkeys that have access to ranges where grasshoppers are abundant.

HERNIA

Hernias seldom occur in fowl. They are most frequently seen following caponizing where the incision has failed to heal properly. Rough handling and overfeeding should be avoided for several days after caponizing. Carlson (1962) reported abdominal hernia of undetermined etiology in 25% of a flock of 500 Broad Breasted Bronze female poults 1 month of age. The hernia was lateral to the median line and about 1 cm anterior to the vent on the left side of the abdomen. Peckham (1964) observed abdominal hernia in 3% of 1,000

White Leghorns 9 months of age kept in cages (Fig. 32.28). The lesions did not appear to cause any discomfort to the birds and did not inhibit production. Cause was unknown.

INTUSSUSCEPTION

Intussusception rarely occurs in the fowl. The invagination of the upper portion of the intestine into the lower portion with subsequent circulatory arrest and adhesions of the involved parts make the diagnosis obvious. The cause is not always apparent,

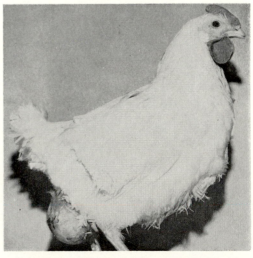

FIG. 32.28—Herniation of abdominal wall.

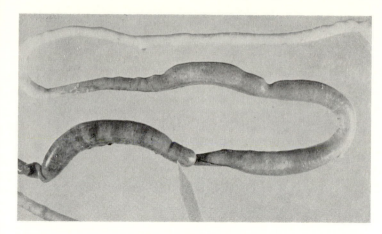

FIG. 32.29—Intussusception. Note congestion caused by circulatory arrest at origin of invagination.

but cases have been observed where the birds were affected with ulcerative enteritis and coccidiosis (Fig. 32.29). Birds may show signs of illness for several days before death. If an early diagnosis were made, resection of the affected intestine could be performed in a valuable bird.

TYPHYLITIS

Mathey and Zander (1955) described a typhylitis of chickens, turkeys, and pheasants characterized by caseous granulomas (Figs. 32.30, 32.31). A spirochete which they believed was *Spironema ceci-gallorum* was isolated from the lesions (Fig. 32.32). The organism could not be grown in artificial media but was grown in embryonating eggs. The feeding of cecal tissues containing spirochetes to 1-week-old chicks produced cecal nodules 30 days postinoculation. Spirochetes were demonstrated in the lesions of the inoculated chicks. Lesions were not produced with pure cultures.

ANOMALY

Occasionally an anomaly of the cecum is encountered in which only one cecum is present with a bifurcation forming two cul-de-sacs at its blind end (Fig. 32.33).

DISEASES OF THE SKIN AND INTEGUMENT

STUNTED CHICK DISEASE

During the decade between 1943 and 1953 a condition in chicks characterized by stunting and mortality during the first weeks of life was of common occurrence. In subsequent years the number of cases has declined, according to diagnostic laboratory reports. Typical symptoms reported by Robertson et al. (1949) are rough feathering, with brittle and broken primary and secondary wing feathers producing a characteristic ragged appearance. Some chicks have encrustations at the commissures of the mouth and granulations on the eyelids

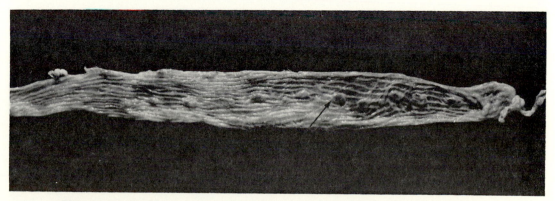

FIG. 32.30—Turkey cecum with small nodules on mucosal surface in typhylitis. (Courtesy W. J. Mathey, Jr., Washington State Univ.)

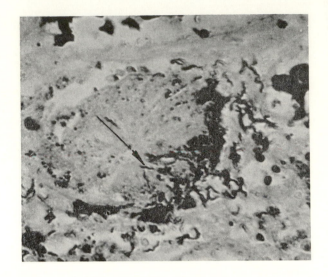

FIG. 32.31—Histological section of nodule in turkey cecum containing many spirochetes. Levaditi stain, ×800. (Courtesy W. J. Mathey, Jr., Washington State Univ.)

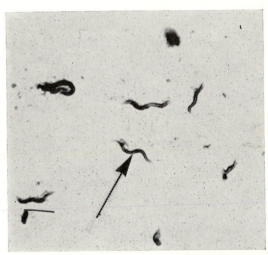

FIG. 32.32—Spirochetes in smear taken from cecal nodule. ×1,350. (Courtesy W. J. Mathey, Jr., Washington State Univ.)

FIG. 32.33—Cecal anomaly in chicken. Only one cecum present with bifurcation of its tip.

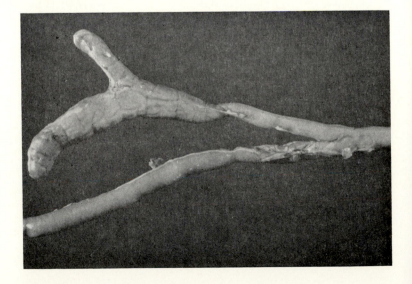

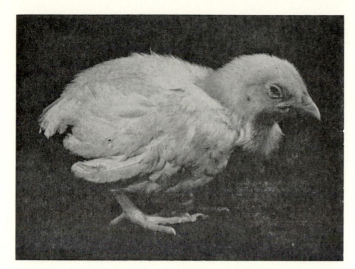

FIG. 32.34—Stunted chick disease. Ragged feathering, granulations on eyelids, and encrustations at commissures of mouth in 19-day-old chick. (Courtesy P. P. Levine, Cornell Univ.)

causing them to adhere. Growth is severely depressed (Fig. 32.34). Mortality progressively increases to a peak, ranging from 25 to 75% at about the 4th week. Survivors at 5–6 weeks of age recover and grow normally and at maturity show no ill effects from their earlier condition. Field trials were conducted by Robertson et al. (1949) in an effort to find the cause of this condition.

The addition of 5% liver meal or 5% dried brewer's yeast to the ration improved weight gains but did not prevent the condition. Once the condition became established, the injection of 100 μg of pantothenic acid or riboflavin had little effect although growth was slightly improved. It was concluded from their field trials that neither feed nor source of chicks appeared to be predisposing factors in the production of stunted chick disease. The problem may have been the result of several factors, primarily mismanagement, rather than a single etiological factor (Angstrom, 1962, personal communication). Wide fluctuations in brooding temperatures were noted, and overheating frequently occurred. The feed hoppers contained large amounts of litter and feed was spilled into the litter.

VESICULAR DERMATITIS AND PHOTOSENSITIZATION

Vesicular dermatitis in chickens was reported by Newson and Feldman (1920), who designated the condition "sod disease" because outbreaks occurred on unbroken prairie sod in eastern Colorado during the months of May, June, and July. It was characterized by vesicle and scab formation on the feet and toes and occasionally on the unfeathered portions of the head. Involvement of the joints was followed by necrosis and sloughing of the toes. Some birds recovered in 2–3 weeks, but the feet and toes were severely distorted.

Hoffman (1939) reported an outbreak of vesicular dermatitis in a flock of adult White Leghorns. He observed vesicles on the comb, wattles, face, feet, and shanks. Rupture of the vesicles was followed by scab formation (Fig. 32.35). Egg production was reduced and mortality was 10%. Hoffman isolated a staphylococcus from the vesicles which, when inoculated into scarified areas, reproduced the clinical symptoms. However, he could not transmit the disease by contact. Perek (1958) and Trenchi (1960) isolated staphylococcus from lesions of vesicular dermatitis but were unable to reproduce the disease with these cultures.

Thomas et al. (1952) described a vesicular dermatitis in Light Sussex cockerels in England. There was a reddening of the skin and swelling of the feet and metatarsal region, accompanied by lameness. Affected birds walked in a "goose-stepping" fashion. Erythema was followed by vesicle formation and scab formation. A few birds had small lesions on the head. Cultures of the vesicle fluid were sterile. The condition could not be transmitted by inoculation or contact trials. There was no mortality, and affected birds recovered in 2 weeks. The etiology was undetermined, but it was suggested that it might be an allergic reaction.

Faddoul and Fellows (1958) reported a

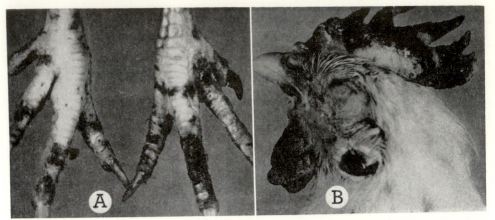

FIG. 32.35—(A) Scabs on feet and shanks resulting from vesicle formations in skin. (B) Scabs on comb as a result of second attack approximately 5 weeks following first attack. (Hoffman, J. Am. Vet. Med. Ass.)

vesicular dermatitis due to photosensitization in a flock of 800 10-week-old White Holland turkeys. Affected birds exhibited restlessness, shaking of the head, and rubbing of eyes on the wings. Vesicle formation involved the face and head. An edematous swelling was present in the throat region. Morbidity was 20% and mortality was 1%. The condition became apparent within 48 hours following the ingestion of blossoming buckwheat plants which were growing on new range. The photodynamic effect was confined to those areas exposed to direct sunlight and lacking the protection of pigment and feathers.

Perek (1958) studied outbreaks of vesicular dermatitis in Israel and reproduced lesions in chickens by feeding *Lolium temulentum* seeds contaminated with *Cladosporium herborum*. The early lesions were small vesicles on the comb and wattles which tended to coalesce forming larger ones containing a milky fluid. The ruptured vesicles were covered by a light green crust. Vesicles which developed between the toes and on the lower portion of the shanks became ulcerated. Facial involvement was accompanied by adhesion of the eyelids. Recovery took place in 3–5 weeks but the comb and wattles remained shrunken. In young chickens growth was retarded and 25% mortality occurred. Laying flocks decreased their feed consumption, egg production dropped 30–50%, and up to 10% mortality occurred. Necropsy did not reveal any internal lesions. Experimental feeding of the fungus-contaminated *Lolium*

temulentum produced vesicles in 7–14 days. The lesions were not the result of photodynamic action as the experimental birds were confined and not exposed to direct sunlight (Perek, 1968, personal communication). The feeding of fungus-free *Lolium temulentum* seeds caused no ill effects.

Cassamagnaghi and Cassamagnaghi (1946) and Trenchi (1960) reported that ingestion of *Ammi visnaga* seeds caused photosensitization in chickens and ducks and subsequent exposure to sunlight caused vesicular dermatitis. The lesions and course of the disease were similar to those described by Hoffman (1939) and Perek (1958).

Trenchi (1962) reported on comparative experimental studies of the lesions produced by ergot poisoning and vesicular dermatitis produced by photosensitization after the ingestion of *Ammi visnaga* seeds. He stated that vesicles were not produced by ergot poisoning and that it took 2 weeks for lesions to appear, whereas lesions appeared in 4–7 days following ingestion of *Ammi visnaga* seeds.

Williams and Binns (1968) reported experimental photosensitization in chicks by feeding spring parsley, *Cymopterus watsonii*. The chicks had marked erythema and swelling of scales on legs and feet, with acute erythema around the eyes, beak, and comb. In severely affected chicks the combs, eyelids, and feet cracked and bled.

Clapham (1950) reported photosensitization in pheasants following the continuous feeding of phenothiazine. There was increased secretion from the lachrymal glands

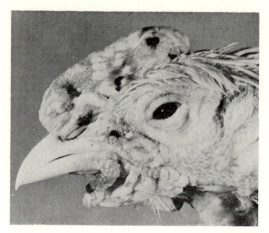

FIG. 32.36—*Vesicular dermatitis. Vesicles and scabs on comb and wattles of White Leghorn.*

and edema of the circumorbital tissues. The cornea became cloudy and rapidly thickened until it became opaque. In severe cases ulceration and secondary bacterial infection rendered the eye useless.

Peckham (1968, unpublished data) observed vesicular dermatitis in highly inbred White Leghorn cockerels for 4 consecutive years. One thousand 4-month-old males were moved from the growing quarters to range shelters on old sod in April for the first three outbreaks. Within 3 weeks, 5% of the flock had yellow blisters on the comb, wattles, eyelids, and toes (Fig. 32.36). Vesicle rupture led to scab formation. Affected birds kept inside made an uneventful recovery. The condition persisted in the flock for about 3 weeks. Attempts to transmit the condition by contact or inoculation were unsuccessful. The fourth annual outbreak occurred when the males were moved to colony brooder houses. The birds were confined and did not have access to grass and were not fed green forage. Only 3 of 30 houses became affected, with an overall incidence of 2%. The affected houses had the most exposure to direct sunlight and were of close genetic origin. All houses had been heavily painted with carbolineum several months before use. Although the character of the lesion and its subsequent appearance within a few weeks after exposure to direct bright sunlight would suggest photosensitization, the dietary or toxic product responsible for the photosensitization was not determined.

XANTHOMATOSIS

Reports of this unusual skin condition have originated from the United States and from Belgium (Thoonen et al., 1959). Hudson (1953, personal communication) observed three flocks of White Leghorns with swollen wattles and cutaneous swellings. Clinical cases and investigational studies were reported by Peckham (1955), Corner et al. (1959), Greve and Moses (1961), Meinecke et al. (1962), Johnson and Sanger (1963), and Sanger and Lagace (1966).

The condition has been observed primarily in White Leghorns of different genetic origin. Lesions usually became evident at 6–7 months of age. Meinecke et al. (1962) reported that birds may range from 5 weeks to 18 months of age when the signs of xanthomatosis appear. Lesions in the 5-week-old chicks were confirmed by histological examination. The percentage of birds affected in a flock may vary from 1 to 60. The condition develops slowly in a flock, and new cases may appear over a period of several months. In general, egg production and feed consumption are unimpaired. Even severely affected birds may be bright, active, and in production. The lesions are permanent and do not regress, notwithstanding changes in feed or environment. Johnson and Sanger (1963) reported the disease in males and females of the same flock. Pistor, quoted by Greve and Moses (1961), reported that the condition may occur in caged birds as well as in those on litter, slats, or range.

Etiology

The etiology of this condition remains uncertain. Johnson and Sanger (1963) determined that xanthomatous tissue contained 40 times as much hydrocarbon as did normal tissues. In a continuation of these studies, Sanger and Lagace (1966) noted that alimentary toxemia (edema disease) and xanthomatosis appeared almost simultaneously throughout the United States. The toxic principle causing alimentary toxemia was a hydrocarbon present in waste animal fat being incorporated in the feed. They postulated that the toxic principle accumulated under the skin and acted as an irritant leading to the development of xanthomas. Support for this theory was not offered by experimental repro-

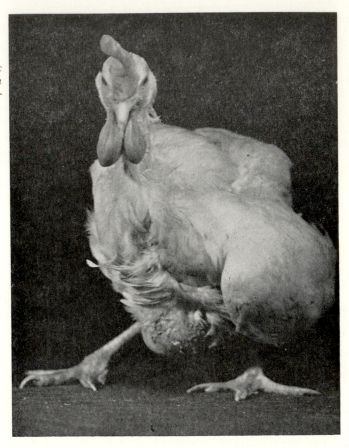

FIG. 32.37—Swollen wattles and cystic swelling on breast of bird with xanthomatosis. (Courtesy P. P. Levine, Cornell Univ.)

duction of the field syndrome. Control measures are lacking until more is learned regarding the etiology of the condition.

Gross Lesions

Early lesions are a unilateral or bilateral swelling of the wattles (Fig. 32.37). In some cases the wattles are unaffected and the intermandibular tissue is edematous. These soft, fluctuating swellings contain a honey-colored transudate. Early lesions on the breast and abdomen are thick and doughy and contain yellow transudate similar to that in the wattles. The character of the skin lesion gradually changes from soft to firm, and thickened or nodular areas may be found on the breast, abdomen, or feathered portion of the legs (Fig. 32.38). The epidermis becomes orange-yellow and the thick layer of tissue beneath the epidermis is taffy colored (Fig. 32.39). Chalky-white areas of cholesterol deposits may be interspersed throughout the abnormal subcutaneous tissue. Some of the swellings on the legs become spherical in shape, and there may be a dimpled

effect where the feather follicles are indented (Fig. 32.40). Cystic swellings containing a yellow watery fluid may develop on the ventral portions of the body.

Histopathology

Greve and Moses (1961) reported on the histopathologic changes occurring in xanthomatosis. The microscopic lesions vary, but all have similarities depending upon the stage of the lesion. Early lesions are infiltrated with vacuolated lipoid-laden macrophages commonly called "foam cells" (Fig. 32.41). Lymphocytes, occurring singly or in clumps, are characteristic and often numerous. A striking feature is the presence of lenticular spaces or clefts produced by cholesterol deposits in the tissue (Fig. 32.42). Multinucleated giant cells may surround the cholesterol crystals. Frozen sections when viewed with polarized light reveal birefringent, rhombic crystals (Fig. 32.43) and the typical "maltese cross" effect of cholesterol esters (Fig. 32.44). Schultze's histochemical test for cholesterol and related substances is positive on frozen skin

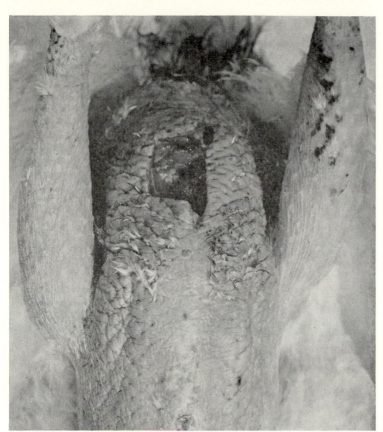

FIG. 32.38—Markedly thickened skin over breast and abdomen of chicken with xanthomatosis. (Courtesy P. P. Levine, Cornell Univ.)

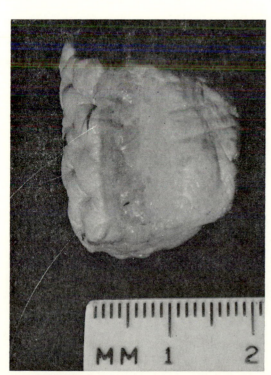

FIG. 32.39—Xanthomatosis. Cross-section of thickened abdominal skin from bird in Fig. 32.38. (Courtesy P. P. Levine, Cornell Univ.)

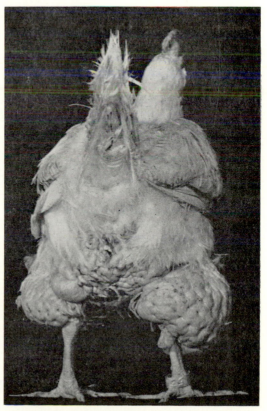

FIG. 32.40—Nodular swellings on abdomen and thighs of chicken with xanthomatosis.

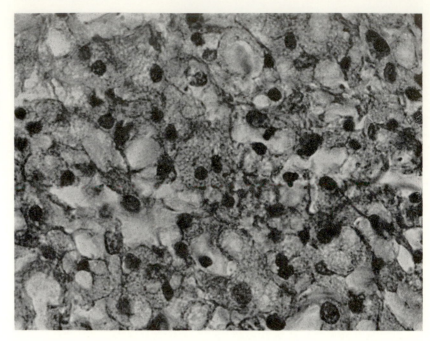

FIG. 32.41—Histological section of xanthomatous lesion illustrating vacuolated structure of cytoplasm in foam cells. ×470. (AFIP 54–7256.)

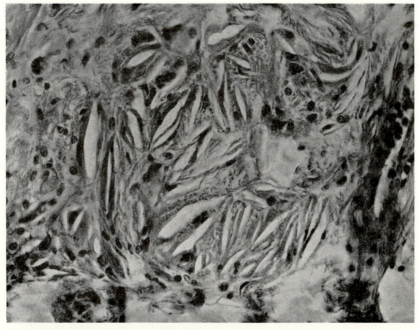

FIG. 32.42—Histological section of xanthomatous skin showing lenticular spaces produced by deposits of cholesterol crystals. ×470. (AFIP 54–5394.)

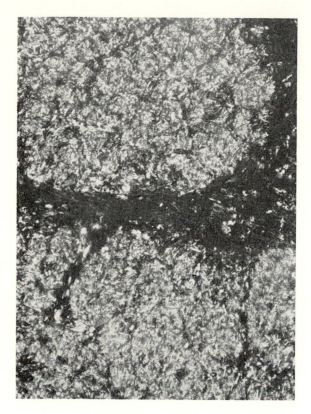

FIG. 32.43—Frozen, unstained, histological section of xanthomatous lesion as seen by polarized light. Birefringent property of cholesterol crystals (white areas) is contrasted against black background of tissue. ×100. (Courtesy J. H. Greve and H. E. Moses, Purdue Univ.)

FIG. 32.44—Frozen, unstained, histological section of xanthoma viewed by polarized light. Birefringent "maltese cross" effect of cholesterol esters is visible against black background. ×400. (Courtesy J. H. Greve and H. E. Moses, Purdue Univ.)

sections. Cholesterol determinations on the affected skin show a marked increase over normal. Blood cholesterol determinations are normal. The skin lesions are permanent and affected birds are unfit for meat consumption.

BUMBLEFOOT, CHICKENS

This term is used to designate a localized infection in the foot causing bulbous swelling of the foot pad and surrounding tissues. The condition may be unilateral or bilateral. Generally only a few individuals in the flock are affected, but in some cases it is widespread throughout the flock. Infection is believed to occur by means of an injury to the ball of the foot. As infection progresses, the lesion enlarges and the ball of the foot and the tissue between the toes become distended (Fig. 32.45). Eventually the swelling will ulcerate through the plantar surface (Fig. 32.46). The birds become lame, have a diminished appetite, and stop laying. Staphylococci may be isolated from the lesion, and where ulceration has occurred, mixed infections will be encountered. If treated early, surgery and antibiotic therapy may alleviate the condition. In commercial flocks, disposal of the affected bird is generally indicated.

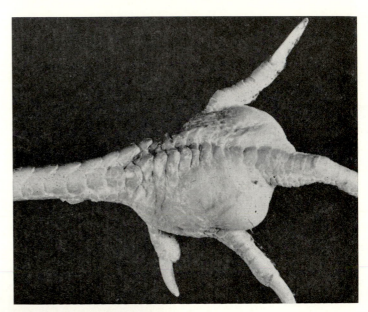

FIG. 32.45—Bumblefoot. Marked swelling of foot pad and surrounding tissues in chicken.

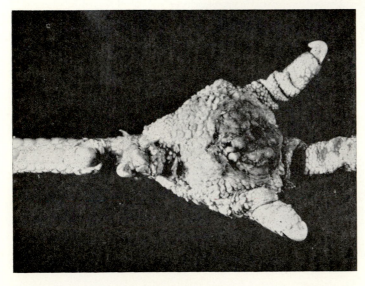

FIG. 32.46—Bumblefoot in turkey with ulceration of plantar surface.

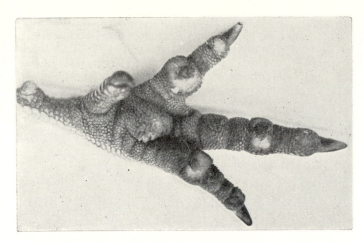

FIG. 32.47—*Abscesses of foot pads (bumblefoot). (Hinshaw, Univ. of Calif.)*

ABSCESSED FOOT PADS, TURKEYS

Turkeys sometimes suffer from abscesses of the foot pads. (Fig. 32.47). These may resemble corns and are similar to the condition commonly called bumblefoot in chickens. The cause is not known, but the abscess probably starts from an infection following an injury to the foot pad. Some of the cases observed have resembled foot rot as seen in other animals. In these instances the affected turkeys have been in yards that were in constant use and were covered with several months' collection of feces; cases usually appeared after the fall rains when the yards became very muddy. No doubt many cases of abscesses of the foot pads are also identical with staphylococcal arthritis.

Putting the birds in clean dry quarters and treating the diseased pad will cure many cases. If pus is present, it should be removed and the area cleaned and treated with an antiseptic healing ointment or tincture of iodine.

Rotating the runs and removing the birds to a clean well-drained yard just before the breeding season are recommended as preventive measures.

PLANTAR NECROSIS

Angstrom (1961, personal communication) observed a condition in adult chickens characterized by necrosis and exfoliation of the skin on the plantar surface of the feet (Fig. 32.48). The litter in the pens was wet and filthy, and masses of fecal material were caked on the feet. The hardened masses of material on the feet did not allow for normal exfoliation of the epithelial cells, and the accumulation of dead tissue and moisture provided a favorable site for growth of organisms of the necrophorus type. When litter conditions were improved, the problem stopped.

ABSCESS OF THE UROPYGIAL GLAND

The uropygial gland is a sebaceous gland located on the back of the bird at the base of the tail. Infection of the gland or obstruction of the excretory duct may cause an accumulation of cheesy exudate. When this happens, the area surrounding the gland becomes inflamed and swollen. Incising the area, removing the exudate, and applying an antibiotic will generally cure the condition.

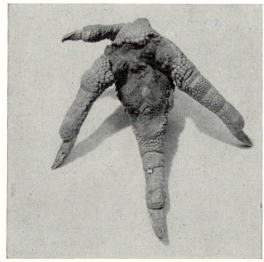

FIG. 32.48—*Plantar necrosis. Necrosis and exfoliation of skin on foot pad and toes of chicken.*

DISEASES OF THE CARDIOVASCULAR SYSTEM

ROUND HEART DISEASE

This is an acute cardiac arrest causing sudden death in pullets, cockerels, and hens. Many descriptive terms have been given to the disease, usually reflecting the striking changes manifested in the heart. Eber and Pallaske-Eber (1934) and Matzke (1942) in Germany described the syndrome as "Eierherzen" (egg heart). Fischel (1946) reported on cases of "enzootic fatal syncope" (toxic heart degeneration) which he observed in New Zealand as early as 1941. In Ireland Luke (1947) coined the term "round heart disease" which has found popular usage. Adsersen (1948) indicated the disease was prevalent in Denmark since 1936 where it was described by the term "yellow heart degeneration."

Incidence and Distribution

The incidence of round heart disease is very low in the United States, and only two reports describing six outbreaks have been published (Levine, 1958; Kilian et al., 1964). Europe, England, Ireland, and Scotland experience significant losses from this disease every year. Adsersen (1948) reported an incidence of 1–4.5% in accessions submitted for diagnosis during the period 1936–47. Schröter (1952) in Germany reported that 3% of all cases submitted for diagnosis had round heart disease. Wilson (1957) recorded 277 outbreaks in Scotland during the period 1950–56. The disease is worldwide in distribution, having been reported in Germany (Matzke, 1942; Rasch and Matzke, 1949; Schröter, 1952), New Zealand (Fischel, 1946), Ireland (Luke, 1947), England (Blaxland and Markson, 1947), Scotland (Wilson, 1948), Belgium (Geurden and Thoonen, 1950), British Columbia (Bankier, 1954), Czechoslovakia (Kóna and Belobrad, 1956), United States (Levine, 1958), India (Iyer et al., 1959), and Bulgaria (Natscheff, 1965).

Etiology

The etiology of round heart disease is unknown. Extensive investigations into possible causes and predisposing factors have been conducted by many investigators. All attempts to isolate or demonstrate an infectious agent have been unsuccessful, and transmission attempts with tissues from affected birds have been unsuccessful (Luke, 1947; Adsersen, 1948; Gerriets, 1955; Wilson, 1957; Kilian et al., 1964; Shishkov et al., 1968). Fischel (1946) was of the opinion that the clinical and pathological features suggested a toxic etiology with a tropism for cardiac muscle. Rasch and Matzke (1949) supported the toxin theory in conjunction with an "inherited disposition." Shishkov et al. (1968) reported the pathology of the heart and kidney suggested damage by a toxin. The litter or toxic agents in the litter as possible etiologies have been proposed by several investigators with considerable circumstantial evidence offered to support these theories. Siegmann and Woernle (1954) reported success in producing round heart in chickens by placing them on litter in a pen where the disease had occurred in another flock. Wilson (1957) also expressed the view that there is an association between round heart disease and the built-up litter system of poultry management. In two experiments he produced the disease in pullets by placing them on litter previously used by affected birds. Of 216 affected flocks, 174 were on built-up litter, 31 on range, and 11 were kept semi-intensively. No outbreaks occurred in laying batteries. Shishkov et al. (1968) stated that the use of old litter in poultry houses contributed to the appearance of the disease but was not the sole etiologic factor.

Gerriets (1955) expressed the opinion that round heart disease was caused by zinc poisoning from feeding potatoes stored in zinc containers. However, he was unable to reproduce the syndrome by feeding potatoes kept in zinc containers or by oral administration of zinc oxide or zinc acetate (Gerriets, 1957).

Natscheff (1965) reported the successful treatment of round heart disease with sodium selenite administered in the drinking water, thus implying that the disease was related to the vitamin E and selenium deficiency complex. These observations are not supported by the investigations of Wilson (1957), who kept 36 birds on a vitamin E free diet for over 2 years without any deaths from round heart disease. Shishkov et al. (1968) reported that treatment of affected flocks with selenium dioxide was ineffective. The author has seen numerous flocks affected with encephalomalacia and transudative diathesis but has failed to see a single bird from these flocks affected with round heart disease either during the growing period or at maturity.

Geurden and Thoonen (1950) were of the opinion that the condition was an expression of an allergic reaction caused by bacterial emboli. Stonebrink (1949) investigated 8 outbreaks and could not find any etiologic relationship between the feed, strain of birds, or management conditions.

Pathogenesis and Epizootiology

CHICKENS. Most breeds of chickens are susceptible, but when an outbreak occurs on a farm where there are several breeds the mortality rate is often much higher in one breed. Wilson (1957) states that the disease occurs most often in Leghorns, viz. Black, Brown, White, and Exchequer. Chickens of any age are susceptible to round heart disease, but the highest mortality occurs between 6 and 12 months of age. Luke (1947) and Adsersen (1948) reported ages ranging from 3 to 18 months, Rasch and Matzke (1949) observed the disease in birds 2–14 months old, and Iyer et al. (1959) reported the disease in birds ranging in age from 1 week to 19 months. Wilson (1957) reported a range in ages of 4 days to 6 years.

GEESE. A condition similar to round heart disease in chickens was reported in a 6-week-old gosling by Kurtze (1948). Two outbreaks in 6-week-old goslings with a loss of 14 birds of 102 in one flock and 30 birds of 900 in another was reported by Franze (1961). He further stated that by changing the feed the losses stopped. It has been observed in many outbreaks of round heart disease in chickens that the losses may stop as abruptly as they begin; therefore any conclusions drawn from a change in regimen would require carefully controlled studies.

TURKEYS. Magwood and Bray (1962) described two grossly different pathological changes in two flocks of young turkeys. The two conditions appeared independently, affecting birds 1–3 weeks of age and birds 6–10 weeks of age. The pathology in the younger group differed from the classical description of round heart disease in chickens. The right ventricle always showed the greatest distortion and the wall was flaccid. The color of the muscle was unchanged and the coronary veins were engorged. The lungs were frequently edematous and the kidneys and liver enlarged. Excess pericardial and peritoneal fluid was noted. The condition affected primarily the males, and in one flock only males suffered mortality. Premonitory signs were absent and the flocks appeared healthy.

A different cardiac pathology was observed in four 6–10-week-old males and one adult female from previously affected flocks. The lesions in these birds resembled typical round heart disease of chickens. The etiology was undetermined, but as the strains and management conditions were different for the two flocks these factors did not appear to be implicated. Sautter et al. (1968) gave a detailed report on the pathogenesis of round heart syndrome in turkeys. They noted that the condition was often associated with stress. Young poults had ruffled feathers, drooping wings, and an unthrifty appearance. Mortality was highest at the end of the 2nd week and stopped after the 3rd week. Myocardial lesions were congestion, myocardial degeneration, foci of macrophages, infiltration of heterophils, and fibroplasia in the coronary groove.

TRANSMISSION. All attempts to transmit the disease by inoculation of tissue suspensions from affected birds into experimental chickens have failed (Fischel, 1946; Blaxland and Markson, 1947; Adsersen, 1948; Luke, 1948).

Wilson (1957) reported on extensive transmission trials. Intestinal contents from affected birds were cultured in broth and filtered through glass wool and instilled into the crops of birds for periods varying from 3 to 96 days. Fowls were injected with emulsions of heart and liver tissue from affected cases. All of the inoculated birds remained healthy. Two investigators reported they were able to reproduce the disease in pullets by placing them on litter where the disease had previously occurred (Siegmann and Woernle, 1954; Wilson, 1957). Six weeks elapsed before the first deaths occurred. It is not uncommon for the disease to recur on the same farm in succeeding years (Levine, 1958; Kilian et al., 1964; Shishkov et al., 1968).

SIGNS. The majority of birds that die with round heart disease do not manifest any premonitory signs. Death usually occurs during sudden exertion and often mani-

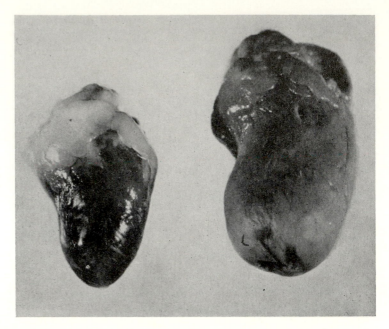

FIG. 32.49—"Round heart" (right) with enlarged and dimpled apex. Normal heart on left.

fests itself at feeding time. Occasionally birds will topple off the roosts.

Wilson and Siller (1954) indicated that in some outbreaks, individual birds may have slight cyanosis of the combs and be lethargic for several days before death. Levine (1958) and Kilian et al. (1964) noted a drop in egg production during the course of an outbreak.

MORBIDITY AND MORTALITY. All reports of round heart disease have indicated that morbidity is very low and may be absent. The mortality rate is variable but may exceed 50%. Luke (1947) reported a range of 2–54% with an average of 15%; Fischel (1946) reported 15–50% mortality; Kilian et al. (1964) observed 1–15% mortality in 3 flocks in Oregon.

GROSS LESIONS. The most striking and consistent lesion found at necropsy is enlargement, distortion, and discoloration of the heart. The cardiac musculature is pale and presents a parboiled appearance. The coronary vessels are markedly distended. The normal tapered appearance of the heart is lost and the apex presents a blunt or rounded appearance. The musculature may be whorled at the apex with an invagination causing a dimpled effect (Fig. 32.49). The left ventricle is markedly thickened although some pathology may occur in the right ventricle. The pericardial sac may

be distended with amber-colored transudate in a fluid or gelatinous state. Ascitic fluid may be present and a gelatinous layer may adhere to the liver. The lungs are often edematous. The liver may be enlarged and show chronic passive congestion. The spleen and kidneys occasionally show evidence of congestion but often appear unchanged. The ovary is usually inactive as invariably birds stop laying before dying from round heart disease.

HISTOPATHOLOGY. Fischel (1946) stated that the main microscopic lesions occurred in the heart muscle. Loss of cross-striations, granular degeneration, and cloudy swelling were evident. The cytoplasm of the myofibrils had lost its eosinophilic properties. Shishkov et al. (1968) described two types of myocardial lesions. Early lesions were fatty degeneration leading to the accumulation of fatty droplets in the individual muscle fibers which were swollen and devoid of cross-striations. In more advanced lesions, the muscle fibers had disappeared and were replaced by fat. In severe cases the sarcolemma of the muscle fibers was destroyed and replaced by confluent fatty accumulations. In 40% of the cases the degenerative changes were accompanied by interstitial lymphocytic infiltration or perivascular infiltration. Most of the cases had degeneration of the epithelial cells of the renal tubules. The livers were congested and occasionally had periportal lympho-cytic infiltration. Kilian et al. (1946) re-ported muscular degeneration, fatty degen-eration, and infiltration by eosinophils. Wilson and Siller (1954) and Iyer et al. (1959) described intranuclear inclusion bodies in the cardiac muscle.

Diagnosis

The diagnosis of round heart disease is based primarily on a history of sudden death and the finding of an enlarged heart with a round or dimpled apex. Routine bacteriological culture will eliminate pul-lorum and listerella infections that may cause enlargement and necrosis of the car-diac muscle. These bacterial infections usually produce changes in other organs that will aid in making a differential diag-nosis.

Treatment

Until the etiology of round heart disease is known, treatment for affected flocks will be empirical. Sassenhoff (1947) reported favorable results by treating birds with vitamin A and vitamin B complex. Nats-cheff (1965) reported the administration of sodium selenite in a daily dosage of 0.1–0.25 mg per bird in the drinking water was followed by cessation of all mortality due to round heart disease within 3 weeks. Shishkov et al. (1968) did not see any flock improvement following administration of sodium selenite. Kilian et al. (1964) re-ported that the addition of high levels of trace minerals to the feed appeared to have a beneficial effect. Levine (1958) reported that changing the feed and water produced a statistically significant drop in mortality. Chemotherapy was used by many investi-gators without the slightest evidence of improvement. As birds have come down with round heart disease when placed on litter previously used by an affected flock (Siegmann and Woernle, 1954; Wilson, 1957) and have stopped dying when re-moved from affected pens (Levine, 1958), it would appear that removal of the litter was indicated during an outbreak.

Prevention and Control

Preventive and control measures that can be assured of success are lacking. However, in view of the many outbreaks on old or built-up litter and apparent cessation of losses when birds are moved to clean quar-ters, it would appear advisable to use fresh litter with each flock and to clean out the litter in the event of an outbreak. Medica-tion is not deemed advisable until con-trolled studies have proved its efficacy.

AORTIC RUPTURE (DISSECTING ANEURYSM)

This disease is characterized by sudden death in young, rapidly growing turkeys caused by internal hemorrhage through a rupture in the abdominal aorta. The con-dition was first reported by Durrell et al. (1952) in Vermont, Minnesota, Indiana, and Washington. The disease is of con-siderable economic significance as it may cause up to 20% mortality (Krista et al., 1967).

Incidence and Distribution

The relatively high incidence of the dis-ease is indicated by the 62 cases reported from northeastern United States and On-tario, Canada, in 1966 (Angstrom et al., 1967). In addition to its wide occurrence in the United States it was reported in England (Carnaghan, 1955).

Etiology

The etiology of this disease has been the subject of several investigators; all are in accord that an infectious agent is not involved.

RATION. It is generally observed that the ruptured aorta condition occurs in the heaviest and fastest-growing birds. These observations have led to investigations con-cerning the influence of the dietary regi-men on the disease.

McSherry et al. (1954) reported that the diet of an affected turkey flock contained 28% protein the first 6 weeks, 24% protein the next 6 weeks, and 20% protein to market age. Grain was fed at 15 weeks of age. They further stated that this feeding program was not generally recommended and that turkeys were much heavier than birds of a comparable age in flocks not being force-fed. Ruptured aorta did not occur in the next flock when the feeding program was changed to 28% protein for 10 days, 24% protein to 6 weeks of age, and 20% protein to finish. Grain was given at 7 weeks of age. Pritchard et al. (1958) con-ducted dietary studies and found that high levels of protein and fat increased the inci-dence of dissecting aneurysm. Turkeys fed low-protein, high-fat rations did not de-velop aneurysm. Krista et al. (1965) reported that although blood cholesterol levels were increased by the addition of 1% cholesterol and 10% fat it did not increase the incidence of ruptured aortas.

HORMONES AND BLOOD PRESSURE. The male turkey displays a much higher incidence of dissecting aneurysm and has a higher blood pressure than the female. The inference has been drawn that high blood pressure is causative in the production of the aneurysm (Speckmann and Ringer, 1962). Krista et al. (1965) found that the mortality rate due to ruptured aorta was 50% less in hypotensive poults than in hypertensive poults. However, it has been established by Krista et al. (1963, 1965) that the administration of diethylstilbestrol decreased blood pressure and paradoxically caused a significant increase in dissecting aneurysms. Krista et al. (1967) did find, however, that two-thirds of the birds which died of ruptured aortas after estrogen administration had blood pressure higher than the mean within their respective groups. The apparent increase in the rate of dissecting aneurysms following the implantation of stilbestrol is of considerable interest, since it is a recorded fact that stilbestrol produces atheromata in chickens (Chaikoff et al., 1948). In several field outbreaks of ruptured aorta it was observed that the males had been implanted with diethylstilbestrol pellets (Pritchard et al., 1958). Krista et al. (1965) found that testosterone injections which did not affect blood pressure almost completely abolished all deaths due to aortic rupture.

BETA-AMINOPROPIONITRILE. Beta-aminopropionitrile (BAPN) is a toxic product that occurs under natural conditions in the sweet pea (Lathyrus odoratus). BAPN was used by several investigators to produce aortic rupture (Barnett et al., 1957; Pritchard et al., 1958; Waibel and Pomeroy, 1958). Barnett et al. (1957) investigated the effect of BAPN on turkey poults. Administration of BAPN-HCl at the rate of 0.03–0.125% caused pericardial hemorrhages, pulmonary hemorrhages, and ruptured aortas. They further stated that the ruptured aortas showed degenerative changes quite similar to those produced in the natural disease. However, Krista et al. (1965) stated that their studies showed many morphological and etiological differences between the field sydnrome and that pro-

duced by BAPN. They further stated that this disparity emphasized the need for study of the condition as it occurred under natural conditions. Sweet peas are not used in turkey rations and have not been incriminated as an etiologic agent in any field cases of ruptured aorta. No other natural source of BAPN has been reported.

Pathogenesis and Epizootiology

NATURAL HOST. Naturally occuring dissecting aneurysm of the abdominal aorta has been reported only in the turkey. Siller (1962) reported two cases of a ruptured ascending aorta in chickens, but these would seem to be quite different from the condition found in turkeys. Primarily Broad Breasted Bronze and Broad Breasted White turkeys are affected, although Pritchard et al. (1958) reported seeing the condition in Beltsville White turkeys. The condition occurs in birds at 7–24 weeks of age with a peak mortality between 12 and 16 weeks.

SIGNS. Affected birds do not show any premonitory signs, and the first indication of the condition is the sudden death of large, rapidly growing, healthy looking birds. The general appearance of the flock is one of excellent health and good growth.

MORBIDITY AND MORTALITY. The morbidity rate is difficult to assess as there are no indications of sick or listless birds in the flock. Mortality rates up to 50% have been reported, but the majority of flocks experience a 1–2% loss.

GROSS LESIONS. Excellent descriptions of the gross and microscopic lesions are given by McSherry et al. (1954) and Pritchard et al. (1958). At necropsy the head, skin, and musculature are anemic. Occasionally blood will run out the mouth or the oral cavity will be bloodstained. Upon internal examination large clots of blood will be found in the abdominal cavity and beneath the capsule of the kidney. Clotted blood may be present in the pericardial sac, lungs, and leg muscle. Invariably a longitudinal slit will be present in the aorta between the external iliac artery and the sciatic artery. In this region the aorta is dilated; the wall is thin and has lost its elasticity. The tunica intima and media are thrown into deep folds and partially separated from the tunica adventitia.

HISTOPATHOLOGY. The fibers of the tunica media may show mild to severe degenerative changes and infiltration with heterophils, and macrophages may be present. Degenerative changes and areas of erosion and cellular infiltration are present in the adventitia (McSherry et al., 1954).

Pritchard et al. (1958) reported that examination of field cases revealed either a marked intimal thickening or a large fibrous intimal plaque in the region of the rupture. Sudan II stains revealed lipid accumulations in the affected intima. Dissolution or disappearance of the elastic laminae of the media occurred at the site of the rupture. Thickening of the media was caused by fibroblastic proliferation and an increase in ground substance.

Diagnosis

The diagnosis of ruptured aorta will be apparent by the presence of large blood clots in the body cavity at necropsy, and careful dissection of the abdominal aorta between the kidneys will reveal the rupture.

Treatment

Uncontrolled field studies suggest favorable results in the treatment of ruptured aorta with reserpine. Speckmann and Ringer (1962) thought the action of reserpine was related to its depressing effect on the turkey's unusually high blood pressure. They also found that reserpine administration at levels of 0.1 and 0.2 ppm in the feed did not offer any protection against the increase in plasma cholesterol or the severity of arteriosclerosis with advancing age. Mean systolic blood pressures were not reduced. Waibel et al. (1962) found that the feeding of reserpine at 1 ppm to turkeys 7–28 days of age, depressed weight gains significantly. The loss in weight gains could be counteracted by feeding 220 ppm of chlortetracycline or 110 ppm of procaine penicillin.

In a study of the influence of reserpine on late growth in 6-month-old turkeys, Craig et al. (1962) found that the reserpine-treated group had poorer feed efficiency and retarded growth compared to the controls. A tranquilizing effect was not noted in the reserpine-treated birds.

Prevention and Control

The role of nutrition, particularly high-protein and high-fat levels in the diet, should be carefully investigated. If the condition continues to recur on the same feeding regimen, the advice of a qualified nutritionist should be sought. Selective breeding for lines with low blood pressure as a means of diminishing losses has been suggested by Krista et al. (1967). The efficacy of reserpine should be investigated further.

HEMORRHAGIC SYNDROME

This condition is a blood dyscrasia of chickens characterized by hemorrhages in the muscles, internal organs, and aplastic bone marrow.

Gordon (1951) in England reported a disease in 5–6-month-old cockerels and pullets characterized by anemia and hemorrhages. Cosgrove (1953) and Baker and Jaquette (1953) reported on the hemorrhagic syndrome. Later investigations concerning the etiology, hematology, and pathology of hemorrhagic syndrome were reported by Gray et al. (1954), Sadek et al. (1955), Cover et al. (1955), and Hanley (1962).

Incidence and Distribution

In some areas the disease has reached an incidence of alarming proportions. Cover et al. (1955) reported that the malady was the third most prevalent disease in the Delmarva area. In Florida Hanley (1962) reported that 74 cases were diagnosed in one year in flocks totaling nearly a quarter of a million birds.

The disease is found throughout the United States and has been reported from Israel (Bornstein and Samberg, 1954), England (Gordon, 1951), and Denmark (Marthedal and Velling, 1961).

Etiology

The etiology of hemorrhagic syndrome has not been elucidated to the extent that there is widespread agreement on one etiologic factor. However, several possible causes have been investigated, and these are discussed.

TRICHLOROETHYLENE. When hemorrhagic syndrome first appeared, it was noted that the pathological and hematological changes were similar to those of aplastic anemia in cattle caused by feeding trichloroethylene-extracted soybean oil meal; this prompted investigation into the role of trichloroethylene-extracted soybean oil meal in the hemorrhagic syndrome. Pritchard et al. (1952) and Sautter et al. (1952) reported that chickens were unaffected by eating soybean oil meal that was toxic for cattle. Eveleth and Goldsby (1953) reported mortality, retarded growth, pliable bones, and lowered resistance to disease in chicks fed experimentally a ration containing trichloroethylene-extracted soybean oil meal. Gray et al. (1954) indicated the hematology of birds fed trichloroethylene-extracted soybean oil meal did not indicate the marked depression in numbers of blood cells found in birds severely affected with the hemorrhagic syndrome. Baker and Jaquette (1953), Gray et al. (1954), and Washko and Mushett (1955) reported hemorrhagic syndromes occurring in flocks that had not been fed trichloroethylene-extracted soybean oil meal. Present evidence indicates that it is unlikely that trichloroethylene-extracted soybean oil meal plays a role in the hemorrhagic syndrome of chickens.

INFECTIOUS AGENTS. All attempts to isolate or demonstrate an infectious agent from cases of hemorrhagic syndrome have failed. Baker and Jaquette (1953) indicated that culture and embryo inoculation trials were negative. Cover et al. (1955) failed to transmit the disease by parenteral inoculation of chicks with blood, liver, spleen, and kidney from affected chickens. Embryo inoculations with tissue suspensions were negative. Washko and Mushett (1955) reported that cultural examination of blood and tissues failed to yield an etiologic agent. Hanley (1962) reported that aerobic and anaerobic culture attempts and bird inoculation trials were negative.

VITAMIN K. The significance of vitamin K in the role of hemorrhagic syndrome is not fully understood. Baker and Jaquette (1953) reported that the addition of alfalfa leaf meal to the ration did not alleviate the hemorrhagic syndrome. Gray et al. (1954) stated that they could not correlate some of their findings to those of vitamin K deficiency. Cover et al. (1955) made a detailed comparison of hemorrhagic syndrome and experimentally produced vitamin K deficiency. They noted that birds affected with hemorrhagic syndrome did not have the increased prothrombin time and extensive hemorrhages that are characteristic of vitamin K deficiency. They concluded that a comparison of the two syndromes showed

them to be definitely distinct and dissimilar. Washko and Mushett (1955) found that prothrombin times and whole blood clotting times were within normal limits in most cases. Hence they did not consider it likely that vitamin K deficiency per se could be responsible for the hemorrhagic syndrome seen in the field.

FUNGI. The role of toxic fungi in the hemorrhagic syndrome was investigated by Forgacs and Carll (1955) and Forgacs et al. (1958, 1962). They stated that one of the paramount features of the hemorrhagic syndrome is the variability, both within and between affected flocks, in epizootiology, clinical symptoms, hematologic findings, course of mortality, and pathologic changes. They noted that these variations are strikingly similar to those observed among the hosts afflicted with known mycotoxicoses. Forgacs and Carll (1955) isolated various fungi from feed spilled in the litter of broiler houses where the hemorrhagic syndrome was enzootic. Some of these fungi, when cultured on a mixture of grains and subsequently dried, ground, and fed to day-old chicks, caused morbidity and mortality. At necropsy hemorrhages were found in the subcutaneous tissue, skeletal muscles, heart, gastrointestinal tract, liver, and kidneys. Forgacs et al. (1958) reported attempts to produce the hemorrhagic syndrome in chickens under simulated field conditions. The chicks were placed on wood shavings and fed a broiler mash inoculated with a 0.5% mixture of dry fungal substrate. The birds manifested depression and diarrhea, and on necropsy at the end of 8 weeks, lesions similar to those of the hemorrhagic syndrome were found. Although experimental studies have indicated that fungi may produce toxins capable of causing hemorrhages, further evidence is needed that the feed or litter in field outbreaks contains sufficient toxin to produce the field syndrome. The role of fungi in the hemorrhagic syndrome needs further investigation.

COCCIDIOSTATS. The widespread use of coccidiostats and the appearance of hemorrhagic syndrome occurred almost simultaneously. The observation prompted investigation into the role of coccidiostats in the hemorrhagic syndrome. Gray et al. (1954) and Marthedal and Velling (1961) indicated that in their cases of hemorrhagic syndrome the flocks had been treated with sulfaquinoxaline or other coccidiostats. In the author's examination of cases of hemorrhagic syndrome submitted to the diagnostic laboratory for the past 10 years, most of the cases (particularly the severest) have been associated with sulfonamide medication. That the condition is not a simple case of sulfonamide intoxication per se is indicated by the many flocks not showing hemorrhagic syndrome yet receiving the same amount of medication as affected birds. However, there have been reports of the hemorrhagic syndrome in flocks which were not receiving coccidiostats or sulfonamides (Baker and Jaquette, 1953; Goldhaft and Wernicoff, 1954; Cover et al., 1955). Sanger et al. (1956) reported that in their observation where certain drugs had been used, especially sulfonamides, the hemorrhagic syndrome suggested a manifestation of drug allergy. (See Chapter 33 for further information relative to sulfonamide intoxication.)

All cases of hemorrhagic syndrome have not been ascribed as being due to a single etiology. It may be that similar clinical and pathological syndromes may be produced by different causes acting independently or simultaneously.

Pathogenesis and Epizootiology

NATURAL HOST. The disease has been reported primarily in chickens ranging in age from 3 to 15 weeks, with most cases occurring between 5 and 9 weeks of age.

SIGNS. Affected birds show a paleness or icteric discoloration of the tissues about the head. Hemorrhage may be present in the anterior chamber of the eye (Fig. 32.50). The feathers are ruffled, the birds act droopy and have a tendency to huddle. A diarrhea has been noted in some cases (Gray et al., 1954; Cover et al., 1955). Washko and Mushett (1955) indicated that the course of the disease was usually about 3 weeks, and in many flocks the prime causes of economic loss were decreased feed consumption and poor feed conversion with a resultant delay in marketing.

MORBIDITY AND MORTALITY. Outbreaks of hemorrhagic syndrome may vary in severity ranging from only a few affected individuals to signs in the entire flock. Mortality

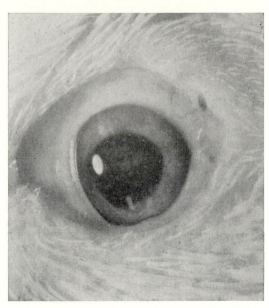

FIG. 32.50—*Hemorrhage in anterior chamber of eye in chicken with hemorrhagic disease.*

is variable, ranging from 1 to 40%, with an average of 5–10% (Baker and Jaquette, 1953; Gray et al., 1954; Goldhaft and Wernicoff, 1954).

GROSS LESIONS. At necropsy hemorrhages may be found in the skin, musculature, and viscera. The blood may be cherry red and have a watery consistency. An occasional bird may have hydropericardium (Fig. 32.51). The most consistent lesion and of great aid in making a diagnosis, if extensive hemorrhagic changes have not occurred, is a pale and fatty bone marrow (Fig. 32.52E). This change in the appearance of the bone marrow is due to a decrease in hematopoietic elements which are replaced by fatty tissue (Gray et al., 1954). Irregular scattered hemorrhages may be present in the breast and thigh muscles (Fig. 32.52B,C). Punctate hemorrhages may be present in the mucosa of the proventriculus at its junction with the gizzard, and hemorrhage may occur beneath the gizzard lining causing blackening and sloughing (Fig. 32.52F). Focal hemorrhages may be found on the external surface of the crop, and "paintbrush" splotches may occur in the myocardium. The intestine may have punctate hemorrhages in the mucosal and serosal surfaces (Fig. 32.52D),

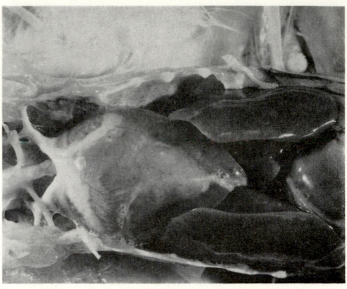

FIG. 32.51—Hydropericardium associated with hemorrhagic disease.

and occasionally a bloody core is present in the cecum. Gray et al. (1954) reported that subcutaneous hemorrhage of the shanks and feet frequently resulted in the formation of ulcers. Hemorrhages may be present in the liver, spleen, and kidney. The liver may be ocher colored and studded with small hemorrhages, or it may present a reticulated network particularly along the edges (Marthedal and Velling, 1961) (Fig. 32.52A). Occasionally a yellow gelatinous transudate may be noted in the subcutis of the neck, breast, and thighs (Hanley, 1962). The kidneys may show evidence of nephritis. Marthedal and Velling (1961) noted hemorrhages and fungal granulomas in the lungs which they regarded as a manifestation of reduced resistance. This observation has been confirmed by others, and it behooves the diagnostician to make a differentiation between primary and secondary lesions. Gray et al. (1954) noted liver necrosis and intestinal ulcers associated secondarily with hemorrhagic syndrome during the terminal course of the disease. These liver and intestinal lesions are the hallmark of ulcerative enteritis which is an opportunist that follows in the wake of debilitating diseases.

HEMATOLOGY. Gray et al. (1954) found leukopenia and anemia associated with depressed bone marrow activity. The anemia was the normocytic, normochromic type. Abnormal thrombocytes were consistently observed on blood smears. These cells were enlarged, more circular than normal, and highly vacuolated. Cover et al. (1955) observed similar blood changes and noted that the prothrombin time was never prolonged. Hanley (1962) confirmed the results of earlier investigators and noted that the hemogram indicated a reduction in red blood cells, granulocytes, and thrombocytes.

HISTOPATHOLOGY. Gray et al. (1954) reported that the marrow of affected birds was devoid of hematopoietic elements and replaced by fatty tissue. Most of the sinusoids were collapsed. Hypoplastic bone marrow showed conspicuous reduction of myelocytic elements. In extreme cases only sinusoidal endothelial cells, interstitial reticular cells, and fat cells were present. A few lymphocytic foci were seen. Cover et al. (1955) noted varying degrees of hemorrhage and necrosis in the liver. The parenchyma adjacent to the surface was most frequently involved. Vessels in the affected area were congested and bile stasis was evident. The lymphoid nodules of the spleen had indistinct borders and appeared hypoplastic. Irregular areas of hemorrhage were seen in the red pulp. Hyalinized material was common in the adenoid sheaths and lymphoid nodules. The kidney showed evidence of coagulation necrosis in the tubular epithelium and infiltration of lymphocytes.

Diagnosis

The diagnosis of hemorrhagic syndrome is based primarily on signs and lesions rather than demonstrating a specific etio-

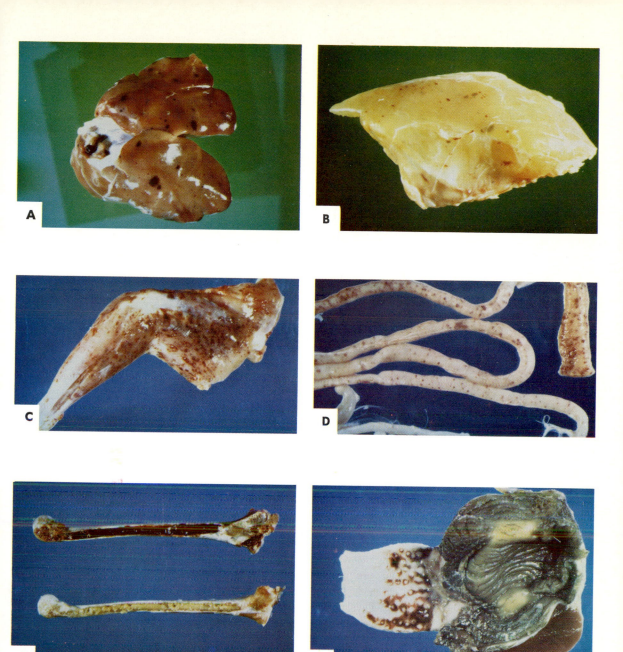

FIG. 32.52—Lesions of hemorrhagic disease. (A) Punctate hemorrhages in pale liver. (B) Hemorrhages in breast muscle of chicken. (C) Hemorrhages in thigh and leg muscles of chicken. (D) Punctate hemorrhages in mucosal surface of duodenum. (E) Pale aplastic marrow in tibia from chicken with hemorrhagic disease (bottom) contrasted with the dark red marrow in tibia from normal bird (top). (F) Hemorrhages in proventriculus.

logic agent. The consideration and elimination of diseases having similar signs and lesions but caused by a specific etiology is mandatory.

DIFFERENTIAL DIAGNOSIS. The consideration of the "bloody triumvirate" is of prime importance in making a differential diagnosis between cecal coccidiosis, ulcerative enteritis, and hemorrhagic syndrome. Blood in the intestinal tract and ceca necessitates making a microscopic examination for the presence of coccidia. The indiscriminate use of sulfonamides when hemorrhages are found in the intestinal tract can result in disaster if the lesions are caused by hemorrhagic syndrome. Ulcerative enteritis may cause punctate hemorrhages in the intestine, cecal ulcerations, and blood in the lumen. However, if an adequate number of specimens are examined, the diagnosis of ulcerative enteritis can be established by finding focal yellow areas of necrosis in the liver. A stained smear of these liver lesions will reveal the etiologic agent, a gram-positive spore-forming rod.

Not infrequently two diseases may dovetail each other in the same flock. Coccidiosis is usually the first disease to appear in these dual infections and sets the stage for hemorrhagic syndrome or ulcerative enteritis. Only by a careful review of the history and proper evaluation of the postmortem findings can the diagnostician make appropriate recommendations.

Treatment

Until the etiology of hemorrhagic syndrome has been elucidated, a specific treatment cannot be recommended. Where coccidiostats or other medications are being given, careful attention should be paid to dosage and duration of treatment. Management and environmental factors should be carefully investigated for detection of conditions that could cause mycotoxicosis. Although supplementary feeding of vitamin K in the form of alfalfa leaf meal or menadione bisulfate has been used in cases of hemorrhagic disease, there is no controlled evidence that this treatment has been uniformly successful.

Prevention and Control

The observance of good husbandry and management practices is suggested as a means of minimizing the possibility of an outbreak of hemorrhagic syndrome. Poor litter conditions and spillage of feed should be carefully avoided to prevent the growth of fungi and the ultimate possibility of mycotoxicosis. The use of coccidiostats, particularly sulfonamides, should be attended with utmost caution and vigilant observation for unfavorable response. Stress factors such as reducing the heat and vaccinations should be avoided during the period when hemorrhagic syndrome is likely to occur.

ENDOCARDITIS

Vegetative endocarditis is rarely reported in the records of diagnostic laboratories. It probably would be found more frequently if the hearts of all birds were carefully examined at necropsy.

Etiology

Kernkamp (1927) and Peckham (1966) found vegetative endocarditis in outbreaks of streptococcosis. Dauber and Katz (1943) reported vegetative endocarditis on the aortic and mitral valves associated with extensive pericarditis. The etiology of the pericarditis was undetermined, but on histological examination the valvular vegetations were found to contain masses of bacteria and fibrin. Povar and Brownstein (1947) described many cases of valvular endocarditis observed during routine postmortem examination of birds dying from miscellaneous conditions on a large breeding farm. Approximately 15% of 551 females over 40 weeks of age had some degree of valvular endocarditis. Only 3% of the birds between 10 weeks and 40 weeks of age were affected. It was noted that birds affected with chronic infections had a significantly greater incidence of valvular endocarditis than did birds dying of all other causes. Birds with salpingitis had the highest frequency of lesions, followed by birds with hepatitis and those with bumblefoot. Cultures from the heart valves yielded staphylococci and streptococci. Gross and Domermuth (1962) reported the experimental production of endocarditis in chickens and turkeys by intravenous inoculation of cultures of *Streptococcus fecalis, Staphylococcus aureus,* and *Pasteurella multocida* isolated from the livers of naturally infected birds. Bacteremia was followed by valvular lesions, and later infarcts were produced in the liver, spleen, and myocardium. The peak of mortality in

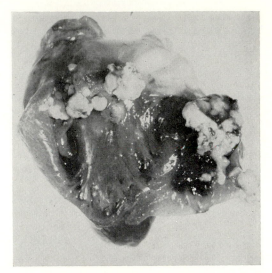

FIG. 32.53—*Vegetative endocarditis. Nodular vegetations on heart valve caused by* Streptococcus zooepidemicus.

birds with endocarditis occurred between the 5th and 16th day postinoculation.

Lesions

Povar and Brownstein (1947) described the lesions as variable in size from small, punctiform, edematous nodules to yellowish, friable masses 0.75 cm in diameter. The smaller lesions lined the edge of the valves in a glistening row. The larger lesions were caseous and extremely friable (Fig. 32.53). The semilunar valves of the pulmonary artery were most often affected, followed by the right atrioventricular valves and the semilunar valves of the aorta. The left atrioventricular valves were

affected with the lowest frequency but had the largest lesions.

DISEASES OF THE URINARY SYSTEM

CYSTS AND AGENESIA

The kidneys occasionally have small cysts 5 mm in diameter that contain a clear amber-colored fluid. The cysts are distributed throughout the parenchyma. It is possible that they represent anatomical defects as they do not appear to be associated with infectious disease processes. Rarely a single large cyst may involve the kidney. It is not unusual to find agenesia of one kidney in a healthy bird. The single kidney apparently compensates for the added load and the bird is not unduly handicapped. The kidneys are frequently the site of tumors and inflammatory conditions associated with specific diseases.

GOUT

Although not of common occurrence, gout has been observed in both young and mature turkeys and chickens (Schlotthauer and Bollman, 1934a; Jungherr, 1935). The predisposing factors are not always known, but some cases have been associated with conditions that impose a stress on the kidneys such as a high-protein diet, sodium bicarbonate intoxication, vitamin A deficiency, and bluecomb disease. The articular or visceral form may occur singly or in combination. Schlotthauer and Bollman (1934b) produced articular gout in turkeys by increasing the protein level of the feed to 40% with the addition of horse meat and 5% urea. Gout tophi appeared on the

FIG. 32.54—*Gout in mature chicken causing enlargement and deformity of toes and feet.*

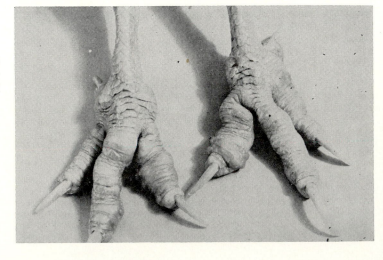

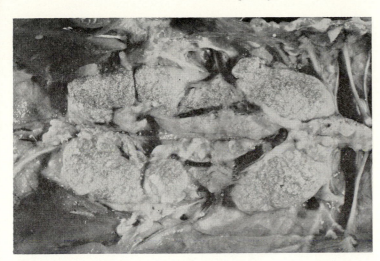

FIG. 32.55—Visceral gout. Urate deposits in kidney of chicken.

feet of those birds in which the blood values for uric acid were 15 mg/100 ml for at least 2 weeks. In articular gout, urate deposits may occur on the articular surfaces and in the periarticular tissues (Fig. 32.54). Bullis and Van Roekel (1944) observed visceral gout in chicks less than 3–4 days of age. The losses were usually less than 5% and the cause was unknown. In the visceral form the kidney tubules are distended with urates, and white deposits of uric acid crystals may be found on the surface of the viscera (Figs. 32.55, 32.56). Lloyd et al. (1949) reported experimental production of articular gout involving the feet of young poults fed a 38% protein ration. The birds gradually recovered after the protein level was reduced to 20%. The condition did not occur in groups fed a lower level of protein.

Snoeyenbos et al. (1962) reported naturally occurring gout in a flock of 400 11-month-old Broad Breasted White turkeys. About 20% of the group were affected including both males and females. The flock was provided with adequate feed and water. The birds had been eating a 20% protein feed for 6 weeks. At necropsy numerous tophi were observed in the periarticular tissues of the feet, and uric acid crystals were present in the tendon sheaths and joints of the wings, hocks, and feet. Urate crystals and erosions were present on some of the articular surfaces. Serum uric acid levels were about 15 mg/100 ml. Colchicine was fed to affected birds at a level of 0.4 mg per lb of body weight per day for a week, but this treatment failed to lower serum uric acid levels or alter the course of the disease. This dose was about 8 times the maximum dose necessary to control the disease in man. The flock was

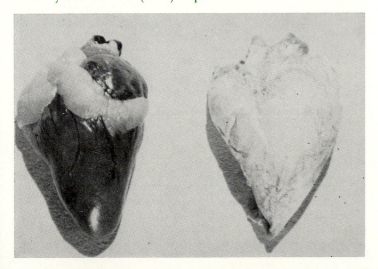

FIG. 32.56—Visceral gout. Heart covered with layer of urates.

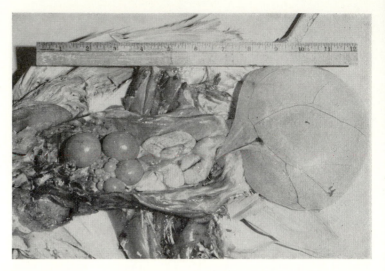

FIG. 32.57—Cystic right oviduct in chicken.

placed on a 15% protein ration for 11 days and then returned to the original ration. One month after the first signs were noted, the flock appeared to have recovered except for 6 severely affected birds. Egg production and hatchability were normal.

DISEASES OF THE REPRODUCTIVE SYSTEM

CYSTIC RIGHT OVIDUCT

In the developing female chick two ovaries and two oviducts are present. As the bird matures the left ovary and oviduct become functional and the right ovary and oviduct remain immature. However, there have been reports of finding two functional oviducts in fowl. Of common occurrence is a cystic right oviduct. This structure may vary in size from a small 1-inch elongated cyst to a ballooned sac containing a pint of clear watery fluid (Fig. 32.57). The small cysts are of little consequence but large cysts compress the vital organs. Ascites, the accumulation of fluid in the abdominal cavity, is colloquially termed "water-belly" by poultrymen. In addition to a cystic oviduct, ascites may be produced by pathological conditions involving the heart, kidneys, liver, and mesentery.

CYSTIC LEFT OVIDUCT

Goldhaft (1956) reported the occurrence of massive cysts in the left oviduct and the dorsal ligament of the oviduct in a flock of White Leghorn pullets. Where cysts occurred in the oviduct, the anterior and posterior portions of the oviduct were nor-mal but the middle of the oviduct was a blind sac distended with over a pint of clear fluid in some cases. It was estimated that 5% of a flock of 2,800 7-month-old birds were affected with these cysts during the previous 30-day period. The cause of the high percentage of cysts in this flock was not determined. Hutt et al. (1956) also observed discontinuous cysts in the oviduct similar to those described by Goldhaft (1956). They postulated that discontinuity of the oviduct probably resulted from accidental degeneration of part or parts of the Mullerian duct during development of the embryo. They also described another defect in which the anterior end of the oviduct was closed by cohesion of the lips of the infundibulum causing a cystic oviduct.

Atresia of the Oviduct

Finne and Vike (1951) described hereditary atresia of the oviduct in the region of the isthmus. The layers looked normal, but the egg yolks were discharged into the body cavity. Peritonitis developed and the birds usually died at 5–6 months of age shortly after coming into production.

OVIDUCT DYSFUNCTION

False Layer

The term "false layer" has been used to describe the bird which has the characteristics of a bird in production and acts like a normal layer but in reality does not lay eggs. Hutt et al. (1956) described the ovulating nonlayer hen as a bird that has the external characteristics of a layer, visits the nest regularly, yet does not lay eggs, as verified by trap nest records. This bird has a normal appearing ovary and oviduct, but the infundibulum fails to engulf the ovum after it has been ovulated. At necropsy these birds show excessive amounts of orange-colored fat and have liquid yolk or coagulated yolk in the body cavity.

SEQUEL TO INFECTIOUS BRONCHITIS. Broadfoot et al. (1954) reported that natural infection of chicks with infectious bronchitis during the first week of age may interfere with later egg production. Flocks 7 months of age that had bronchitis as chicks were laying only 50% whereas birds of the same breeding that did not have bronchitis as chicks laid at a normal rate. Birds in the poor laying flock looked healthy and had the appearance of good layers. Trap-nesting records of the flock for 14 days showed that 43% of the birds visited the nests on 3–5 successive days without laying. Some of these birds visited the nest as many as 3 times in a single day. Postmortem examination of 26 of these birds revealed that the viscera were surrounded by a heavy layer of mottled oily fat. Cheesy yolks with roughened and pitted surfaces were found in the body cavity. The oviducts were not full size and many were less than 20% normal size. The striking fact about these birds was that the ovaries were found to be fully active. In a subsequent report Broadfoot et al. (1956) experimentally infected chicks of different ages with virulent bronchitis virus and vaccine strains of bronchitis. The results of these experiments confirmed their field observations that exposure to virulent bronchitis virus during the 1st week of age produced an increasing number of false layers at maturity; chicks exposed to a mild vaccine strain of bronchitis virus did not experience an adverse effect on egg production at maturity.

Internal Layer

In some birds soft-shelled eggs or fully formed eggs may be found in the peritoneal cavity. This indicates that the yolk progressed normally through the oviduct to a certain point and then reverse peristalsis discharged the egg into the body cavity. A bird with a large accumulation of eggs in the peritoneal cavity may assume a penguinlike posture.

Impaction

Occasionally an impacted oviduct is observed in which the oviduct is occluded by masses of yolk, coagulated albumen, shell membranes, and in some instances fully formed eggs. Large masses of yolklike material may be found in the oviduct, and upon transection these masses have the appearance of concentric rings.

EGG BOUND

"Egg bound" is the term used to describe the condition where an egg is lodged in the cloaca but cannot be laid. It may result from inflammation of the oviduct, partial paralysis of the muscles of the oviduct, or the production of an egg so large that it is physically impossible for it to be laid. Young pullets laying an unusually large egg are more prone to the problem. This condition may be relieved by inserting a lubricated finger into the cloaca and exerting pressure on the abdomen with the other hand. If expulsion of the egg is not possible in this way, the egg may be held in position at the vent opening, the shell broken with a sharp object, and the contents and pieces of the shell removed. If the chicken has been egg bound for a considerable period of time before the condition is detected, there is apt to be an eversion of the cloacal tissues after the egg is removed. The bloodstained tissues invite cannibalism, and the bird should be placed in separate quarters until fully recovered.

OVARIAN DYSFUNCTION

The ovary reflects the general health of the mature bird. Many infectious diseases and physiological disturbances immediately produce retrogressive changes in the ovary. The normal, yellow, turgid ovum may become wrinkled and the contents almost black with hemorrhage. At other times the yolk is coagulated or "cooked" in appearance. Discolored, pedunculated, and inspissated ova are the hallmark of pullorum disease. Cauliflowerlike growths from the ovary are indicative of lymphomatosis. Multiple cystic ova filled with clear fluid may occur occasionally.

ABNORMAL EGGS AND DEPRESSED PRODUCTION

Eggs differing in size and shape may be laid in any flock, but in the average healthy flock there is remarkable uniformity of eggs. There are many conditions which affect egg size, shape, shell texture, internal quality, and rate of lay. Wilson (1949) found that environmental temperatures had a marked effect on the strength and thickness of the shell. As the temperature rises above 70° F, the blood calcium drops progressively; at 100° F the shell averages about two-thirds the normal thickness. This would explain why the eggshell is thicker and stronger in the winter months. Increased humidity also has an unfavorable effect on shell thickness but not as marked as increased temperature. Jull (1930) indicated that the production of soft-shelled eggs is more prevalent in the spring when production is at its peak. Respiratory diseases such as infectious bronchitis and Newcastle disease may affect the size, shape, shell texture, and internal quality of eggs (Gordeuk and Bressler, 1950; Biswall and Morrill, 1954).

Mann and Keilin (1940) reported sulfanilamide to be a very powerful inhibitor of the enzyme carbonic anhydrase. Since then several reports have appeared describing the inhibitory effects of certain sulfonamides on the formation of eggshells. Hinshaw and McNeil (1943) found that a single dose of sulfanilamide, 0.5 grain per pound of live weight, caused turkeys to lay eggs with very thin shells or without shells the next day. When 1.5 grains of sulfanilamide per pound of live weight was fed to leghorn hens, the same result was produced. This inhibitory action of small dosages of sulfanilamide on the secretion of shell material was confirmed by Benesch et al. (1944), Gutowska and Mitchell (1945), and Tyler (1950). Scott et al. (1944) observed that in addition to thin shells, sulfanilamide also caused a bleaching of the pigment in brown eggs. Bankowski (1948) reported a decrease in egg production following sulfamerazine and sulfamethazine medication. Mehring et al. (1955) reported that two unsubstituted sulfonamides, Diamox and benzenesulfonamide, caused pullets to lay eggs with very thin shells or with no shells, beginning with the first egg laid after the initial dose. Nicarbazin, a coccidiostat, may cause mottled yolks, loss of shell pigment, decreased egg size, and low egg production (Weiss, 1957; Baker et al., 1957). Arasan, a fungicide used in the treatment of seed corn, has been reported to cause misshapen and soft-shelled eggs,

retarded production, and finally complete cessation of production (Waibel et al., 1955; Johnson et al., 1955). Trematodes and ascarids sometimes enter the cloaca and pass up the oviduct where they are swept along with the yolk and albumen and become encased by the shell.

CLOACITIS

Cloacitis, or vent gleet as it is commonly known, is a chronic inflammatory process of the cloaca with a very offensive odor. A yellow diphtheritic membrane may form on the mucosal surface of the vent, and urates and inflammatory exudate contaminate the skin and feathers beneath the vent. The disease is more common in laying hens than in males. A very small percentage of birds in a flock are affected at one time, and the disease does not appear to be very contagious. The specific cause of this disease is unknown. Transmission experiments carried out by Gwatkin (1925) and Scherago (1925) were unsuccessful. Removal of affected birds is advised in commercial flocks. Valuable birds can be treated by cleansing the affected area and applying a broad-spectrum antibiotic in dust or ointment form.

CAGE LAYER FATIGUE

The marked increase in the number of birds kept in cages during the past decade has given rise to a new problem. The condition, called cage layer fatigue, is characterized by inability of the birds to stand and marked fragility of the bones. The long bones are not soft but exceedingly thin and break or splinter at the slightest pressure. There may be beading of the ribs at the costochondral junction and the rib cage may be sunken along this line. In addition to losses from paralysis the rearing of birds in cages has resulted in dressing plant downgrading. The marked fragility of the bones results in fractures when the birds are removed from the cages, and more injury occurs when the birds are subjected to the pounding of the picking machines in the dressing plants. The bone splinters become lodged in the meat, creating a hazard when the meat is used for human consumption.

It has been observed that birds will recover in 4–7 days if removed from the cages and placed on the floor. Francis

(1957) noted significant differences in the incidence of cage layer fatigue between various strains. During a 10-week observation period 0.65% of one strain was affected compared to a high of 3.95% in another strain; 80% of the birds recovered when removed from the cages. According to Grumbles (1959), this condition occurs more often during the summer months in young pullets that are producing at a high rate and have a good feed efficiency ratio. The percentage affected will vary from 1 to 20. Fisher, quoted by Grumbles (1959), stated that in his experience, cage fatigue has not occurred when the calcium level of the diet was maintained at 2.5%. Harms et al. (1961) reported leg weakness in caged hens fed diets containing 0.34% phosphorus. The lameness resembled cage layer fatigue, and addition of phosphorus to the diet caused a reduction in mortality and leg weakness. In an extension of these studies Simpson et al. (1964) studied the effect of low-calcium and low-phosphorus diets on cage layers. The control diet contained 3% calcium and 0.7% phosphorus; the low-calcium diet contained 2% calcium and 0.7% phosphorus; the low phosphorus diet contained 3% calcium (the same amount as the control diet) and 0.34% phosphorus. The birds on the low-phosphorus diet developed leg weakness after 96 days. No leg weakness was observed in the groups fed the low-calcium or control diets. In bone-breaking tests for fragility ratings, bones from birds on the low-phosphorus diet were more fragile than those from birds fed the other two diets. On histological examination the diaphysis of the tibia of birds fed the low-phosphorus diet contained large broad trabeculae that often coalesced. The spicules contained a small amount of centrally located calcified matrix and a prominent peripheral layer of osteoid, or were composed entirely of osteoid. This constituted a histological picture of osteomalacia.

FATTY LIVER SYNDROME

The shift from floor-reared layers to cage confinement was not without the creation of new problems, some of which have yet to be satisfactorily explained or controlled. Among these is the fatty liver syndrome which is characterized by fat deposits, fatty livers, and a drop in egg production.

Etiology

The precise mechanism or chain of events which leads to the development of this disease has not been clearly elucidated. The disease is seen in different strains and breeds of chickens, and all major feed companies have faced the problem. Various theories have been advanced to explain the development of the disease, but controlled studies whereby the field syndrome is reproduced have yet to be published. One theory is that the syndrome is the result of excessive caloric intake and/or decreased energy utilization (Tudor, 1967). The explanation is that birds on the floor can consume the same amount of feed but because of increased movement more of the caloric intake is transformed into heat and energy instead of fat. Although this explanation may have theoretical validity, it does not explain the sporadic appearance of the disease in replicate flocks on the same feed.

Couch (1964) stated that from the results of his experiments, the fatty liver syndrome was not necessarily caused by high-energy feed formulas. He further stated that it was impossible to predict the time or conditions under which the disease might occur. He added that the stress of high egg production, improved breeding for egg production, and the use of high-energy feeds might possibly be contributing factors. The actual precipitation of overt signs was caused by a "low level disease of some type." These observations were based on field information.

Signs

The rate of lay decreases from the normal of 75–85% to 45–55%. The birds appear healthy and in good physical condition. There is usually a 25–30% increase in body weight. Birds in excellent condition may suddenly die without premonitory signs.

Lesions

Birds that die acutely from ruptured livers have pale combs, wattles, and musculature. The capsule of the liver is torn, and large blood clots are present on the surface of the liver and in the body cavity (Fig. 32.58). Small hemorrhagic areas may be seen beneath the liver capsule. The liver is

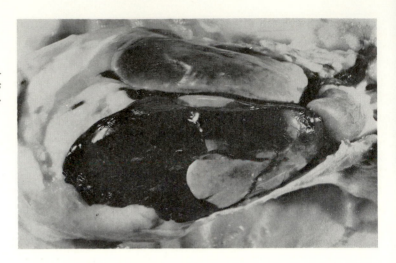

FIG. 32.58—Fatty liver syndrome. A large blood clot is molded over one lobe of liver. Note excess abdominal fat.

yellow, greasy, and of mushlike consistency. Large deposits of fat may line the abdomen and cover the intestines.

Control

Until the etiology of fatty liver syndrome is established, it will be difficult to recommend rearing and feeding programs that will prevent the appearance of this syndrome.

Couch (1968) has suggested the following treatment of field cases. Add to each ton of mash, in addition to the amounts normally recommended: 1,000 g choline chloride, 10,000 I.U. vitamin E, 12 mg vitamin B$_{12}$, and 2 lb inositol.

CONGENITAL AND INHERITED CONDITIONS

CONGENITAL LOCO

Durant (1926, 1927) first noted this nervous disorder in newly hatched White Leghorn chicks. Subsequently Knowlton (1929) conducted breeding trials and concluded that the defect was inherited as a simple Mendelian recessive. Peckham (1967) observed a high percentage of loco in White Leghorn chicks in one pedigree hatch of a breeder from highly inbred matings (Fig. 32.59). An apparently identical syndrome was reported in turkey poults by Cole (1957). After a thorough investigation of the genetic factors involved, he concluded that the condition was an obligate postnatal lethal syndrome caused by the homozygous state of the recessive gene lo. Hatchability is not affected and the poults are in excellent physical condition. Symptoms manifested are opisthotonus or sagging of the head and neck until the beak touches the floor. The birds can stand normally for only a few seconds at a time and then involuntarily or in response to external stimuli thrust themselves vigorously into a backward somersault. They lie on their backs or sides kicking aimlessly (Fig. 32.60). The anatomical defect responsible for this syndrome is unknown. The brain appears normal upon gross and microscopic examination. Affected birds die since they are unable to eat or drink.

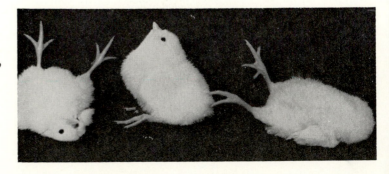

FIG. 32.59—Congenital loco in day-old chicks.

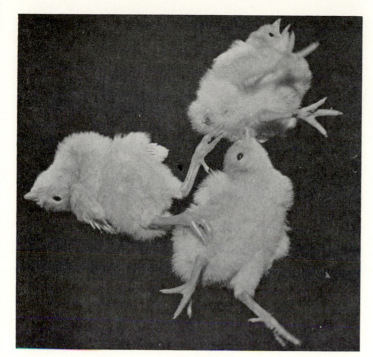

FIG. 32.60—Congenital loco in turkey poults. Affected birds manifest opisthotonus and thrust themselves over backward.

CONGENITAL ALOPECIA

Congenital alopecia is occasionally encountered in newly hatched chicks. Certain avian hybrids develop a partial alopecia which is characteristic of the cross-breeding.

CONGENITAL OPISTHOTONUS

Caskey et al. (1944) described congenital opisthotonus occurring in chicks at hatching due to manganese deficiency in the maternal diet. The symptoms persisted at maturity even though adaquate manganese was given. The progeny resulting from the mating of affected males and females did not manifest opisthotonus, thus indicating it was not of genetic origin.

CEREBELLAR HYPOPLASIA

Avian cerebellar hypoplasia and degeneration, according to Winterfield (1953), is probably an inherited defect. The condition was first observed in 12-week-old pullets in 15 different flocks with 3–10% becoming affected. Affected birds did not die and came into production at 6 months of age. Symptoms were weaving and bobbing of the head; when the birds were excited they became ataxic. Gross pathology was confined to the cerebellum which was about one-fourth normal size. Neuronal degeneration was present in the cerebellar cortex, and there was degeneration and disappearance of the Purkinje cells. In England Markson et al. (1959) described a similar condition affecting Light Sussex pullets.

CROOKED TOE DISEASE

Crooked toes may occur in young or adult birds. This condition should not be confused with "curly toe paralysis" which is caused by riboflavin deficiency. In the crooked toe condition the toes have a lateral curvature but the bird still walks on the plantar surface of the foot (Fig. 32.61). However, in "curly toe paralysis" the toes curl under and the bird walks on the dorsal surface of the toes. Birds with riboflavin deficiency have difficulty in walking and rest on their hocks when not trying to walk. In "curly toe paralysis" a histological section of the sciatic nerve will enable a positive diagnosis to be made.

The tendency for crooked toes is inherited, and any birds so affected should not be used for breeding. Black et al. (1952) reported strain differences in the manifestation of crooked toe condition in chicks when brooded under the bright emitter type of infrared lamp. Chicks from one strain manifested none of the abnormality, whereas 100% of the offspring from

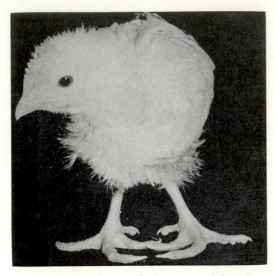

FIG. 32.61—Crooked toe condition in a 3-week-old chick.

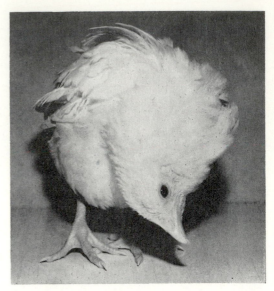

FIG. 32.62—Wry-neck condition in young chicken.

crooked-toed parents of another strain had crooked toes when brooded under infrared lamps. However, when the two stocks were reared under ordinary electrical heating, crooked toes did not develop in either strain. This is an example of the interactions which frequently occur between inheritance and environment. Norris et al. (1940) found that the development of the crooked toe condition was influenced by the type of floor covering on which the birds were reared. Smooth surfaces such as newspaper greatly increased the percentage of affected birds if the birds carried a genetic susceptibility. Crooked toes are under the influence of genetic factors; however, these genes express themselves differently in various environments.

SCOLIOSIS

This condition is commonly spoken of as wry neck and is characterized by torsion and lateral curvature of the neck (Fig. 32.62). Jull and Quinn (1931) reported that the defect appeared in half-grown chicks and became worse with advancing age. Males and females heterozygous for the condition were mated; 27 crooked-neck chicks and 129 normal chicks were produced. An autosomal recessive gene was considered responsible for the condition. Conner and Shaffner (1953) reported an arched-neck defect in New Hampshire chickens that resembled the nervous signs of Newcastle disease. They considered re-cessive genes as a probable cause. Although birds with this condition manage to eat and drink, it is generally best to remove them as they never recover.

COLOBOMA OF THE IRIS

This condition is manifested as a unilateral or bilateral teardrop shape of the pupil or as a circular pupil with a defect in the iris. Wilcox (1958) presented evidence that the condition was inherited in White Leghorns by finding coloboma in 22% of the offspring obtained from mating affected birds. Because of the dark pigmentation of the iris in chicks the defect was not readily discernible until 6 weeks of age. The defect was much more obvious when observed in bright light in which the iris was maximally constricted. In some of the offspring without coloboma, a pronounced bulging of the cornea occurred, presumably from increased intraocular pressure in the anterior chamber of the eye. In one case bulging developed in an eye previously classified as coloboma. Another abnormality observed occasionally in this stock was a sunken eye, which was reduced considerably in size. Recognition of the existence of coloboma in chickens is important in making a differential diagnosis of ocular lymphomatosis. A histological examination of the eye would enable one to differentiate between these two conditions.

REFERENCES

Adsersen, J. 1948. On the occurrence of the so-called round heart disease in Denmark. *Proc. 8th World's Poultry Congr.*, p. 702.

Angstrom, C. I., H. L. Chute, M. S. Cover, and G. Snoeyenbos. 1967. Report-committee on nomenclature and reporting of disease, Northeastern Conference on Avian Diseases. *Avian Diseases* 1:727–33.

Asmundson, V. S., and W. R. Hinshaw. 1938. On the inheritance of pendulous crop in turkeys *(Meleagris gallopavo)*. *Poultry Sci.* 17:276–85.

Baker, H. R., and D. S. Jaquette. 1953. Observation concerning the "hemorrhagic syndrome" in poultry. *Proc. 25th Ann. Conf. Lab. Workers in Pullorum Disease Control.*

Baker, R. C., F. W. Hill, A. Van Tienhoven, and J. H. Bruckner. 1957. The effect of Nicarbazin on egg production and egg quality. *Poultry Sci.* 36:718–26.

Bankier, J. C. 1954. Poultry disease problems in British Columbia. *Proc. Am. Vet. Med. Ass. 91st Ann. Meet.* 350–54.

Bankowski, R. A. 1948. A decrease in egg production following sulfamerazine and sulfamethazine medication. *J. Am. Vet. Med. Ass.* 113:49–50.

Barber, C. W. 1947. Studies on the avian leukosis complex. *Cornell Vet.* 37:349–67.

Barnett, B. D., H. R. Bird, J. J. Lalich, and F. M. Strong. 1957. Toxicity of beta-amino-propionitrile for turkey poults. *Proc. Soc. Exp. Biol. Med.* 94:67–70.

Barr, M. 1965. Mandibular disease in stock cockerels. *Vet. Record* 77:677–79.

Bass, C. C. 1939. Control of "nose-picking" form of cannibalism in young closely confined quail. *Proc. Soc. Exp. Biol. Med.* 40:488–89.

Becker, E. R., C. E. Brodine, and A. A. Marousek. 1949. Eyelid lesion of chicks in acute dietary deficiency resulting from blood induced *Plasmodium lophurae* infection. *J. Infect. Diseases* 85:230–38.

Benesch, R., N. S. Barron, and C. A. Mawson. 1944. Carbonic anhydrase, sulfonamides, and shell formation in the domestic fowl. *Nature* 153:138.

Bierer, B. W. 1956. Keratoconjunctivitis in turkeys: A preliminary report. *Vet. Med.* 51:363–66.

———. 1958. Keratoconjunctivitis in turkeys. II. The relationship of vitamin A, infectious agents and environmental factors to the disease. *Vet. Med.* 53:477–83.

Bierer, B. W., and C. L. Vickers. 1959. The effect on egg size and production of fungicide-treated and fumigated grains fed to hens. *J. Am. Vet. Med. Ass.* 134:452–53.

Biswall, G., and C. C. Morrill. 1954. The pathology of the reproductive tract of laying pullets affected with Newcastle disease. *Poultry Sci.* 33:880–97.

Black, D. J. G., J. Getty, and T. R. Morris. 1952. Infra-red brooding and the crooked toe problem in chicks. *Nature* 170:167.

Blaxland, J. D., and L. M. Markson. 1947. Toxic heart degeneration, or "round heart disease" of poultry. *Brit. Vet. J.* 103:401–5.

Bornstein, S., and Y. Samberg. 1954. Field cases of vitamin K deficiency in Israel. *Poultry Sci.* 33:831–36.

Bragg, D. D. 1953. An attempt to determine the cause of curled or deformed tongues in young Beltsville White turkeys. *Poultry Sci.* 32:294–303.

Brion, A. J., and M. Fontaine. 1958. A hemorrhagic and rachiticlike syndrome in chickens due to nitrofural medicated feed. *Poultry Sci.* 37:1071–74.

Broadfoot, D. I., B. S. Pomeroy, and W. M. Smith, Jr. 1954. Effects of infectious bronchitis on egg production. *J. Am. Vet. Med. Ass.* 124:128–30.

———. 1956. Effects of infectious bronchitis in baby chicks. *Poultry Sci.* 35:757–62.

Bullis, K. L., and H. Van Roekel. 1944. Uncommon pathological conditions in chickens and turkeys. *Cornell Vet.* 34:313–20.

Bullis, K. L., G. H. Snoyenbos, and H. Van Roekel. 1950. A keratoconjunctivitis in chickens. *Poultry Sci.* 29:386–89.

Carlson, H. C. 1962. Abdominal hernia in turkey poults. *Can. Vet. J.* 3:263–64.

Carnaghan, R. B. A. 1955. Atheroma of the aorta associated with dissecting aneurysm in turkeys. *Vet. Record* 67:568–69.

———. 1958. Keratoconjunctivitis in broiler chicks. *Vet. Record* 70:35–37.

Carnaghan, R. B. A., and B. S. Hanson. 1958. Rupture of the gastrocnemius tendon in fowls. *Brit. Vet. J.* 114:360–66.

Caskey, C. D., L. C. Norris, and G. F. Heuser. 1944. A chronic congenital ataxia in chicks due to manganese deficiency in the maternal diet. *Poultry Sci.* 23:516–20.

Cassamagnaghi, A., and A. Cassamagnaghi, Jr. 1946. Accidentes de fotosensibilizacion de origen alimenticio en los animales domesticos. *Bul. Min. Gan. Agr. Montevideo*, pp. 541–49.

Chaikoff, I. L., S. Lindsay, F. W. Lorenz, and C. Entenman. 1948. Production of atheromatosis in the aorta of the bird by the administration of diethylstilbestrol. *J. Exp. Med.* 88:373–87.

Chute, H. L. 1950a. Rupture of the gastrocnemius tendon in chickens. *Can. J. Comp. Med. Vet. Sci.* 14:218–21.

———. 1950b. Ruptured gastrocnemius tendons. *Proc. 22nd Ann. Conf. Lab. Workers in Pullorum Disease Control.*

Clapham, Phyllis A. 1950. Keratitis in pheasants following treatment with phenothiazine. *J. Helminthol.* 24:61–62.

Cole, R. K. 1957. Congenital loco in turkeys. *J. Heredity* 48:173–75.

Conner, M. H., and C. S. Shaffner. 1953. An arched-neck character in chickens. *J. Heredity* 44:223–24.

Corner, A. H., J. M. Isa, and G. L. Bannister. 1959. Xanthomatosis in White Leghorns in Canada. *Can. J. Comp. Med. Vet. Sci.* 23: 199–202.

Cosgrove, A. S. 1953. Hemorrhagic disease in chickens. *Delaware Poultry Handbook* 8: 86.

Couch, J. R. 1964. The fatty liver syndrome in laying hens. *Res. Digest* 2:1–2.

———. 1968. Fatty liver syndrome. *Feedstuffs* December 7:48–51.

Cover, M. S., W. J. Mellen, and E. Gill. 1955. Studies of hemorrhagic syndrome in chickens. *Cornell Vet.* 45:366–86.

Craig, F. R., W. L. Blow, R. J. Monroe, and C. W. Barber. 1962. The influence of reserpine on late growth of turkeys. *Poultry Sci.* 41:711–13.

Creek, R. D., and M. Y. Dendy. 1957. The relationship of cannibalism and methionine. *Poultry Sci.* 36:1093–94.

Cuckler, A. C., and W. H. Ott. 1955. Tolerance studies on sulfaquinoxaline in poultry. *Poultry Sci.* 34:867–79.

Dauber, D. V., and L. N. Katz. 1943. Experimental atherosclerosis in the chick. *Arch. Pathol.* 36:473–92.

Devos, A. 1962. Xanthomatose bij grasparkieten. *Vlaams Diergeneesk. Tijdschr.* 31:211.

———. 1963. Rupture of the gastrocnemius tendon in chickens. *Avian Diseases* 7:451–56.

Dickinson, E. M., and W. G. Clark. 1946. Brooder stove residue burns on turkey poults. *Cornell Vet.* 36:314–17.

Dorn, P., M. F. el-Etreby, and R. Weber. 1964. Keratoconjunctivitis mit intranukleaeren Einschlusskoerperchen beim Huhn. *Berlin. Muench. Tieraerztl. Wochschr.* 77:262–66.

Durant, A. J. 1926. Inherited incoordination of muscles in newly hatched chicks. *Missouri Agr. Expt. Sta. Bull.* 244:60–61.

———. 1927. Inherited incoordination of muscles in newly hatched chicks. *Missouri Agr. Expt. Sta. Bull.* 256:102.

Durrell, W. B., B. S. Pomeroy, W. S. Carr, and A. C. Jerstad. 1952. Discussion. *Proc. Ann. Meet. Am. Vet. Med. Ass.* 1952:280.

Eber, A., and Ruth Pallaske-Eber. 1934. *Die durch Obduktion Feststellbaren Gefluegelkrankheiten.* M. & H. Schaper, Hanover.

Evans, W. M., D. W. Bruner, and M. C. Peckham. 1955. Blindness in chicks associated with salmonellosis. *Cornell Vet.* 45:239–47.

Eveleth, D. F., and A. I. Goldsby. 1953. Toxicosis of chickens caused by trichloroethylene-extracted soybean meal. *J. Am. Vet. Med. Ass.* 123:38–39.

Faddoul, G. P., and G. W. Fellows. 1958. *Eighth Ann. Rept. Vet. Pathol.*, Poultry Diagnostic Lab., Waltham Field Station, Univ. Mass.

Faddoul, G. P., and R. C. Ringrose. 1950. Avian keratoconjunctivitis. *Vet. Med.* 45: 492–93.

Finne, I., and N. Vike. 1951. A new sub-lethal factor in hens. *Poultry Sci.* 30:455–65.

Fischel, W. G. 1946. Enzootic fatal syncope (toxic heart degeneration) of fowls. *Australian Vet. J.* 22:144–49.

Forgacs, J., and W. T. Carll. 1955. Preliminary mycotoxic studies on hemorrhagic disease in poultry. *Vet. Med.* 50:172.

Forgacs, J., H. Koch, W. T. Carll, and R. H. White-Stevens. 1958. Additional studies on the relationship of mycotoxicoses to the poultry hemorrhagic syndrome. *Am. J. Vet. Res.* 19:744–53.

———. 1962. Mycotoxicoses. I. Relationship of toxic fungi to moldy feed toxicosis in poultry. *Avian Diseases* 6:363–80.

Francis, D. W. 1957. Strain differences in the incidence of cage layer fatigue. *Poultry Sci.* 36:181–83.

Franze, F. 1961. Beobachtungen ueber herztodahnliche Erkrankungen bei Jungenten. *Monatsh. Veterinaermed.* 16:109–10.

Fritzche, K., and E. Gerriets. 1959. *Gefluegelkrankheiten.* Verlag Paul Parey, Berlin, Hamburg.

Gerriets, E. 1955. Zur Aetiologie des enzootischen Herztodes der Huehner. *Monatsh. Veterinaermed.* 10:416–18.

———. 1957. Experimentelle Untersuchung beim enzootischen Herztod des Huhnes. *Berlin. Muench. Tieraerztl. Wochschr.* 70: 238–40.

Gerry, R. W., and J. F. Witter. 1952. Sulfaquinoxaline toxicity in growing chickens. *Proc. 24th Ann. Conf. Lab. Workers in Pullorum Disease Control.*

Geurden, L. M. G., and J. Thoonen. 1950. Onderzoekingen over round heart disease. *Vlaams Diergeneesk. Tijdschr.* 19:29–39.

Gibson, E. A., and P. H. DeGruchy. 1955. Aortic rupture in turkeys subsequent to dissecting aneurism. *Vet. Record* 67:650–54.

Gill, E. 1956. Clinical and pathological observations in a hemorrhagic syndrome of chickens. M.S. thesis, Univ. Delaware.

Goldhaft, T. M. 1956. Massive cysts in the dorsal ligament of the oviduct in White Leghorn pullets. *Cornell Vet.* 46:223–27.

Goldhaft, T. M., and N. Wernicoff. 1954. A report on a hemorrhagic condition occurring in poultry in the United States. *Proc. Tenth World's Poultry Congr.*, pp. 278–82.

Gordeuk, S., Jr., and G. O. Bressler. 1950. Infectious bronchitis; its effect on rate of egg production and egg quality. *Penn. State Coll. Agr. Progr. Rept.* 36.

Gordon, R. F. 1951. Observations on an outbreak of disease in fowls possibly associated with sulfaquinoxaline poisoning. *Proc. Ninth World's Poultry Congr.* 3:95–101.

Grau, C. R., and H. J. Almquist. 1945. Deformity of the tongue associated with amino acid deficiencies in the chick. *Proc. Soc. Exp. Biol. Med.* 59:177–78.

Gray, J. E., G. H. Snoeyenbos, and I. M. Reynolds. 1954. Hemorrhagic syndrome of chickens. *J. Am. Vet. Med. Ass.* 125:144–51.

Greve, J. H., and H. E. Moses. 1961. Histopathologic changes in xanthomatosis in chickens. *J. Am. Vet. Med. Ass.* 139:1106–10.

Gross, W. B., and C. H. Domermuth. 1962. Bacterial endocarditis of poultry. *Am. J. Vet. Res.* 23:320–29.

Grumbles, L. C. 1956. Some current poultry disease problems in Texas. *Southwestern Vet.* 9:256–58.

———. 1959. Cage layer fatigue (cage paralysis). *Avian Diseases* 3:122–25.

Gutowska, Marie S., and C. A. Mitchell. 1945. Carbonic anhydrase in the calcification of the egg shell. *Poultry Sci.* 24:159–67.

Gwatkin, R. 1925. Vent gleet (cloacitis). *Ann. Rept. Ont. Vet. Coll.* 1924, pp. 65–66.

Hanley, J. E. 1962. Observations on avian aplastic anemia in Florida. *Avian Diseases* 6:251–57.

Harms, R. H., C. R. Douglas, and P. W. Waldroup. 1961. The effect of feeding various levels and sources of phosphorus to laying hens. *Florida Agr. Expt. Sta. Bull.* 644.

Harris, A. H. 1963. Rupture of the gastrocnemius tendon in the turkey. *Vet. Record* 75:969–70.

Harriss, S. T. 1947. Rupture of the tendon achilles in chickens. *Vet. J.* 103:356–57.

Henderson, W., W. R. Pritchard, and Doris B. Taylor. 1957. Observations on aplastic anemia in chickens. *Poultry Sci.* 36:1125. (Abstr.)

Hinshaw, W. R., and V. S. Asmundson. 1936. Observations on pendulous crops in turkeys. *J. Am. Vet. Med. Ass.* 88:154–65.

Hinshaw, W. R., and Ethel McNeil. 1943. Experiments with sulfanilamide for turkeys. *Poultry Sci.* 22:291–94.

———. 1946. The occurrence of type 10 paracolon in turkeys. *J. Bacteriol.* 51:281–86.

Hoffman, H. A. 1939. Vesicular dermatitis in chickens. *J. Am. Vet. Med. Ass.* 95:329–32.

Hudson, C. B. 1939. Curled tongue in young poults. *J. Am. Vet. Med. Ass.* 94:662.

Huston, T. M., H. L. Fuller, and C. K. Laurent. 1956. A comparison of various methods of debeaking broilers. *Poultry Sci.* 35:806–10.

Hutt, F. B., K. Goodwin, and W. D. Urban.

1956. Investigations of nonlaying hens. *Cornell Vet.* 46:257–73.

Iyer, P. K. R., R. C. Pathak, and A. Singh. 1959. Observations on round heart disease in fowls. *Indian Vet. J.* 36:1–5.

Johnson, E. L., P. E. Waibel, and B. S. Pomeroy. 1955. The toxicity of Arasan-treated corn to hens and chicks. *Proc. Am. Vet. Med. Ass., 92nd Ann. Meet.*, pp. 322–23.

Johnson, R. M., and V. L. Sanger. 1963. Lipids in avian xanthomatous lesions. *Am. J. Vet. Res.* 24:1280–82.

Jordan, F. T. W. 1955. Rupture of the gastrocnemius in the fowl. *Vet. Record* 67:548–51.

Jull, M. A. 1930. *Poultry Husbandry.* McGraw-Hill, New York.

Jull, M. A., and J. P. Quinn. 1931. Inheritance in poultry. *J. Heredity* 22:147–54.

Jungherr, E. 1935. Disease of brooder chicks. *Storrs Agr. Expt. Sta. Bull.* 202.

Kennard, D. C. 1937. Chicken vices. *Ohio Agr. Expt. Sta. Bimonthly Bull.* 184, 22:33.

Kennard, D. C., and V. D. Chamberlin. 1936. Oats for chickens. *Ohio Agr. Expt. Sta. Bimonthly Bull.* 181, 21:95.

Kernkamp, H. C. H. 1927. Idiopathic streptococcic peritonitis in poultry. *J. Am. Vet. Med. Ass.* 70:585–96.

Kilian, J. G., W. E. Babcock, and E. M. Dickinson. 1964. A report on round heart disease in Oregon chickens. *Avian Diseases* 8:56–61.

Knezevic, N., and L. Kozic. 1962. Keratoconjunctivitis (ammoniacal blindness) in poultry. *Vet. Glasn.* 16:943–47.

Knowlton, F. L. 1929. Congenital loco in chicks. *Oregon Agr. Expt. Sta. Bull.* 253: 1–15.

Kóna, E., and G. Belobrad. 1956. (Round heart disease in chickens.) *Vet. Casopis* 5:390–94.

Krista, L. M., R. E. Burger, and P. E. Waibel. 1963. The influence of various drugs on the growth and beta-aminopropionitrile-induced dissecting aneurysm of turkeys. *Poultry Sci.* 42:522–26.

Krista, L. M., P. E. Waibel, and R. E. Burger. 1965. The influence of dietary alterations, hormones, and blood pressure on the incidence of dissecting aneurysms in the turkey. *Poultry Sci.* 46:15–22.

Krista, L. M., P. E. Waibel, R. N. Shoffner, and J. A. Sautter. 1967. Natural dissecting aneurysm (aortic rupture) and blood pressure in turkeys. *Nature* 214:1162–63.

Kull, K. E. 1948. Prevention and treatment of cannibalism and feather eating fowls. *Proc. Eighth World's Poultry Congr.* 1:124.

Kurtze, H. 1948. Ein Fall von ploetzlichem Herztod bei einer Ente. *Deut. Tieraerztl. Wochschr.* 55:201.

Levine, P. P. 1952. Ascites and nephritis of traumatic origin in day old chicks. *Proc.*

24th Ann. Conf. Lab. Workers in Pullorum Disease Control.

———. 1958. Case report—Round heart disease in the United States. *Avian Diseases* 2:530–36.

Lloyd, M. D., C. A. Reed, and J. C. Fritz. 1949. Experiences with high protein diets for chicks and poults. *Poultry Sci.* 28:69–74.

Lonsdale, M. B., R. M. Vondell, and R. C. Ringrose. 1957. Debeaking at one day of age and the feeding of pellets to broiler chickens. *Poultry Sci.* 36:565–71.

Luke, D. 1947. Round heart disease in poultry. *Vet. J.* 103:17–20.

———. 1948. Round heart disease in poultry. *Proc. Eighth World's Poultry Congr.* 1:692–96.

McSherry, B. J., A. E. Ferguson, and J. Ballantyne. 1954. A dissecting aneurysm in internal hemorrhage in turkeys. *J. Am. Vet. Med. Ass.* 124:279–83.

Magwood, S. E., and D. F. Bray. 1962. Disease condition of turkey poults characterized by enlarged and rounded hearts. *Can. J. Comp. Med. Vet. Sci.* 26:268–72.

Manfre, A. S., H. O. Wheeler, G. L. Feldman, R. H. Rigdon, T. M. Ferguson, and J. R. Couch. 1958. Fungi in the crop of turkeys. *Am. J. Vet. Res.* 19:689–95.

Mann, T., and D. Keilin. 1940. Sulfanilamide as a specific inhibitor of carbonic anhydrase. *Nature* 146:164.

Markson, L. M., R. B. A. Carnaghan, and G. B. Young. 1959. Familial cerebellar degeneration and atrophy—A sex-linked disease affecting Light Sussex pullets. *J. Comp. Pathol. Therap.* 69:223–30.

Marthedal, H. E., and Grethe Velling. 1961. Hemorrhagic syndrome in poultry. *Brit. Vet. J.* 117:357–65.

Mathey, W. J. 1956. A diphtheroid stomatitis of chickens apparently due to *Spirillum pulli,* species nova. *Am. J. Vet. Res.* 17:742–46.

Mathey, W. J., and D. V. Zander. 1955. Spirochetes and cecal nodules in poultry. *J. Am. Vet. Med. Ass.* 126:475–77.

Matzke, M. 1942. Ein Beitrag zum sogenannten, "Eierherzen" bei Huehnern. *Berlin. Muench. Tieraerztl. Wochschr.* 37/38:283–89.

Mehring, A. L., Jr., H. W. Titus, and J. H. Brumbaugh. 1955. Effects of two sulfonamides on the formation of egg shells. *Poultry Sci.* 34:1385–88.

Meinecke, C. F., A. I. Flowers, and J. N. Beasley. 1962. Observations of xanthomatosis in chickens. *Poultry Sci.* 41:1207–10.

Miller, W. M., and G. E. Bearse. 1937. The cannibalism-preventing properties of oats. *Poultry Sci.* 16:314–21.

Moore, E. N. 1953. *Aspergillus fumigatus* as a cause of ophthalmitis in turkeys. *Poultry Sci.* 32:796–99.

———. 1954. Diseases of turkeys. *Vet. Med.* 49:314–17.

Moorhead, P. D., and Y. S. Mohamed. 1968. Case report: Pathologic and microbiologic studies of crooked-neck in a turkey flock. *Avian Diseases* 12:476–82.

Morgan, W. 1957. Effect of day-old debeaking on the performance of pullets. *Poultry Sci.* 36:208–10.

Natscheff, B. 1965. Beitrag zur Behandlung des enzootischen Herztodes beim Huhn. *Berlin. Muench. Tieraerztl. Wochschr.* 78:334–35.

Neal, W. M. 1956. Cannibalism, pick-outs and methionine. *Poultry Sci.* 35:10–13.

Nelson, C. L. 1952. Cannibalism. *Iowa Vet.* 23:28.

Newberne, P. M., M. E. Muhrer, R. Craghead, and B. L. O'Dell. 1956. An abnormality of the proventriculus of the chick. *J. Am. Vet. Med. Ass.* 128:553–55.

Newsom, I. E., and W. H. Feldman. 1920. Sod disease of chickens (Vesicular dermatitis). *Colo. Agr. Expt. Sta. Bull.* 262.

Norris, L. C., C. D. Caskey, and J. C. Bauernfeind. 1940. Malformation of the tarsometatarsal and phalangeal bones of chicks. *Poultry Sci.* 19:219–23.

Ostrander, C. E. 1957. Control cannibalism in your poultry flock. *Cornell Ext. Bull.* 992.

Payne, L. F. 1956. Growing turkeys in Kansas. *Kansas Agr. Expt. Sta. Bull.* 376:38.

Peckham, M. C. 1955. Xanthomatosis in chickens. *Am. J. Vet. Res.* 16:580–83.

———. 1961. Poultry diagnostic laboratory accessions. *Ann. Rept. N.Y. State Vet. Coll. 1961–62,* p. 165.

———. 1964. Poultry diagnostic laboratory accessions. *Ann. Rept. N.Y. State Vet. Coll. 1964–65,* p. 202.

———. 1966. An outbreak of streptococcosis (apoplectiform septicemia) in White Rock chickens. *Avian Diseases* 10:413–21.

———. 1967. Poultry diagnostic laboratory accessions. *Ann. Rept. N.Y. State Vet. Coll. 1967–68,* p. 223.

Perek, M. 1958. Ergot and ergot-like fungi as the cause of vesicular dermatitis (sod disease) in chickens. *J. Am. Vet. Med. Ass.* 132:529–33.

Povar, M. L., and B. Brownstein. 1947. Valvular endocarditis in the fowl. *Cornell Vet.* 37:49–54.

Pritchard, W. R., C. E. Rehfeld, and J. H. Sautter. 1952. Aplastic anemia of cattle associated with ingestion of trichloroethylene-extracted soybean oil meal. *J. Am. Vet. Med. Ass.* 121:1–8.

Pritchard, W. R., W. Henderson, and C. W. Beall. 1958. Experimental production of dissecting aneurysms in turkeys. *Am. J. Vet. Res.* 19:696–705.

Rasch, K., and M. Matzke. 1949. Enzootischer Herztod und regressive Leberverfettung der Huhner. *Deut. Tieraerztl. Wochschr.* 43/44:357–59.

Rigdon, R. H., T. M. Ferguson, G. L. Feldman, H. O. Wheeler, and J. R. Couch. 1958. A study of the mechanism of the experimentally induced pendulous crop in the turkey. *Am. J. Vet. Res.* 19:681.

Ringer, R. K. 1961. The effect of beta-aminopropionitrile on the blood pressure of turkeys. *Poultry Sci.* 40:1001–4.

Robertson, E. I., C. I. Angstrom, H. C. Clark, and M. Shimm. 1949. Field research on "stunted chick" disease. *Poultry Sci.* 28:14–18.

Sadek, S. E., L. E. Hanson, and J. O. Alberts. 1955. Suspected drug-induced anemias in the chicken. *J. Am. Vet. Med. Ass.* 127:201–3.

Sanger, V. L., and A. Lagace. 1966. Avian xanthomatosis. Etiology and pathogenesis. *Avian Diseases* 10:103–11.

Sanger, V. L., D. M. Chamberlain, C. R. Cole, F. L. Docton, and R. L. Farrell. 1953. A disease of turkeys characterized by deformity of the tongue. *J. Am. Vet. Med. Ass.* 122:207–10.

Sanger, V. L., H. Yacowitz, and E. N. Moore. 1956. Micropathological changes in an experimental hemorrhagic syndrome in chickens fed sulfaquinoxaline and suggested cause of the disease. *Am. J. Vet. Res.* 17:766–70.

Sanger, V. L., E. N. Moore, and Norma A. Frank. 1960. Blepharoconjunctivitis in turkeys. *Poultry Sci.* 39:482–87.

Sassenhoff, Irmgard. 1947. Enzootischen Herztod bei Huhnern. *Tieraerztl. Umschau* 15/16:181–83.

Saunders, C. N. 1958. Keratoconjunctivitis in broiler birds. *Vet. Record* 70:117–19.

Saunders, L. Z., and E. N. Moore. 1957. Blindness in turkeys due to granulomatous chorioretinitis. *Avian Diseases* 1:27–36.

Sautter, J. H., C. E. Rehfeld, and W. R. Pritchard. 1952. Aplastic anemia of cattle associated with ingestion of trichloroethylene-extracted soybean oil meal. II. Necropsy findings in field cases. *J. Am. Vet. Med. Ass.* 121:73–79.

Sautter, J. H., J. A. Newman, S. H. Kleven, and C. T. Larsen. 1968. Pathogenesis of the round heart syndrome in turkeys. *Avian Diseases* 12:614–28.

Scherago, M. 1925. Ulcerative cloacitis in chickens. *J. Am. Vet. Med. Ass.* 67:232–38.

Schlotthauer, C. F., and J. L. Bollman. 1934a. Spontaneous gout in turkeys. *J. Am. Vet. Med. Ass.* 85:98–103.

———. 1934b. Experimental gout in turkeys. *Proc. Staff Meet. Mayo Clinic* 9:560.

Schröter, A. 1952. Ueber den enzootischen Herztod bei huehnern. *Monatsh. Veterinaermed.* 7:271–73.

Schwabe, C. W. 1950. The tropical eyeworm of poultry. *Am. J. Vet. Res.* 11:286–90.

Scott, H. M., E. L. Jungherr, and L. D. Matterson. 1944. The effect of feeding sulfanilamide to the laying fowl. *Poultry Sci.* 23:446–53.

Shishkov, N., C. Obreshkov, and St. Enchev. 1968. Round heart disease of the domestic fowl *(Gallus gallus)* in Bulgaria. *Pathol. Vet.* 5:41–50.

Siegmann, O., and H. Woernle. 1954. Beitrag zum enzootischen Herztod der Huhner. *Arch. Exp. Veterinaermed.* 8:465–77.

Siller, W. G. 1962. Two cases of aortic rupture in fowls. *Pathol. Bacteriol.* 83:527–33.

Simpson, C. F., P. W. Waldroup, C. B. Ammerman, and R. H. Harms. 1964. Relationship of dietary calcium and phosphorus levels to the cage layer fatigue syndrome. *Avian Diseases* 8:92–100.

Snoeyenbos, G. H., I. M. Reynolds, and T. Tzianabos. 1962. Articular gout in turkeys. *Avian Diseases* 6:32–36.

Speckmann, E. W., and R. K. Ringer. 1962. The influence of reserpine on plasma cholesterol, hemodynamics and arteriosclerotic lesions in the broad breasted bronze turkey. *Poultry Sci.* 41:40–45.

Stafseth, H. J. 1934. Diseases of adult poultry. *Mich. State Coll. Ext. Bull.* 54. (Revised.)

Stiles, G. W. 1943. Heat exhaustion in young turkeys. *Poultry Sci.* 22:242–47.

Stonebrink, B. 1949. Round heart disease bij kippen. *Tijdschr. Diergeneesk.* 74:337–41.

Thomas, R. J., F. T. W. Jordan, and J. D. Blaxland. 1952. A vesicular dermatitis in poultry resembling sod disease. *Vet. Record* 64:223–24.

Thoonen, J., J. Hoorens, and E. Van Meirhaeghe. 1959. Xanthomatose beim Huhn. *Arch. Gefluegelk.* 23:314–18.

Trenchi, H. 1960. Ingestion of *Ammi visnaga* seeds and photosensitization—The cause of vesicular dermatitis in fowls. *Avian Diseases* 4:275–80.

———. 1962. A comparative study of the lesions produced by ergot and photosensitization induced by *Ammi visnaga*. *Proc. Fourth Pan. Am. Congr. Vet. Med. and Zootechnics*, pp. 187–89.

Tudor, D. C. 1967. The fatty liver syndrome in chickens. *Merck Agr. Memo.* 39:1–4.

Tyler, C. 1950. The effect of sulphanilamide on the metabolism of calcium carbonate, phosphorus chloride, and nitrogen in the laying hen. *Brit. J. Nutr.* 4:112.

Van Ness, G. 1946. Staphylococcus citreus in the fowl. *Poultry Sci.* 25:647–48.

Waibel, P. E., and B. S. Pomeroy. 1958. Studies on the production of aortic hemorrhage in growing turkeys with beta-aminopropionitrile. *Poultry Sci.* 37:934–38.

Waibel, P. E., B. S. Pomeroy, and E. L. Johnson. 1955. Effect of Arasan treated corn on laying hens. *Science* 121:401.

Wannop, C. C. 1957. Some observations on the hemorrhagic syndrome in chicks. *World's Poultry Sci. J.* 13:310.

Washko, F. V., and C. W. Mushett. 1955. Some observations on the pathology of the hemorrhagic condition of chickens. *Proc. Ann. Meet. Am. Vet. Med. Ass.* 360–63.

Weaver, C. H., and S. Bird. 1934. The nature of cannibalism occurring among adult domestic fowls. *J. Am. Vet. Med. Ass.* 85:623–37.

Weiss, H. S. 1957. Further comments on the effect of nicarbazin on the egg. *Poultry Sci.* 36:589–91.

Wickware, A. B. 1945. Grasshoppers, a potential danger to turkeys. *Can. J. Comp. Med. Vet. Sci.* 9:80–81.

Wilcox, F. H. 1958. Studies on the inheritance of coloboma of the iris in the domestic fowl. *J. Heredity* 49:107–10.

Williams, M. C., and W. Binns. 1968. Experimental photosensitization by spring parsley *(Cymopterus watsonii)* in chicks. *Am. J. Vet. Res.* 29:111–15.

Willimon, C. P., and C. L. Morgan. 1953. The effect of minor nutrient mineral elements in the diet of chickens on feather pulling and cannibalism. *Poultry Sci.* 32:309–13.

Wilson, J. E. 1948. Round heart disease in poultry in Scotland. *Proc. 8th World's Poultry Congress,* pp. 697–702.

———. 1957. Round heart disease in poultry. *J. Comp. Pathol. Therap.* 67:239–50.

Wilson, J. E., and W. G. Siller. 1954. Round heart disease in the fowl. *J. Comp. Pathol. Therap.* 64:41–51.

Wilson, W. O. 1949. High environmental temperatures as affecting the reaction of laying hens to iodized casein. *Poultry Sci.* 28:581–92.

Wilson, W. O., and A. Woodward. 1955. Some factors affecting body temperatures of turkeys. *Poultry Sci.* 34:369–71.

Winterfield, R. W. 1953. Avian cerebellar hypoplasia and degeneration. *J. Am. Vet. Med. Ass.* 123:136–38.

Wright, G. W., and J. F. Frank. 1957. Ocular lesions in chickens caused by ammonia fumes. *Can. J. Comp. Med. Vet. Sci.* 21:225–27.

Wright, M. M., and H. Temperton. 1955. Curled tongue in turkey poults. *Vet. Record* 67:510–13.

Yacowitz, H., E. Ross, V. L. Sanger, E. N. Moore, and R. D. Carter. 1955. Hemorrhagic syndrome in chicks fed normal rations supplemented with sulfaquinoxaline. *Proc. Soc. Exp. Biol. Med.* 89:1–7.

CHAPTER 33

POISONS AND TOXINS

❖

M. C. PECKHAM

Department of Avian Diseases
New York State Veterinary College
Cornell University
Ithaca, New York

❖

THE LITERATURE CONTAINS many reports of acute and chronic poisoning of birds due to the ingestion of toxic substances, but numerical and monetary losses are insignificant compared with losses caused by infectious, parasitic, and nutritional diseases. Despite the infrequency of poisoning the pathologist should be cognizant of the signs and lesions caused by noxious agents and by toxic levels of coccidiostats, growth stimulants, and other chemotherapeutic agents euphemistically regarded as harmless.

Today our poisons are occult and insidious and masquerade under the guise of chemotherapeutic agents, fungicides, and insecticides. Drugs and chemicals used for the control of infectious and parasitic diseases may have therapeutic levels that impinge on toxic levels, and errors in computation or improper mixing can easily result in toxic levels in the feed. It is a widely known but little publicized fact that, "what is on the tag is not necessarily in the bag." Disinfectants properly used play an important role in the first line of defense against the invasion of diseases, but careless or indiscriminate use can lead to disaster. The treatment of seed grains with fungicides is a universal practice, and

Grateful acknowledgement is made of the groundwork for this chapter by Dr. L. H. Schwarte, Veterinary Medical Research Institute, Iowa State University, Ames.

treated grain has been used in laying mash with tragic results. Insecticides can be deadly for avian species, and indiscriminate repeated saturation of large areas may lead to the accumulation of toxic levels in different species of the biologic food chain as we ascend the phylogenetic scale. It is now recognized that the time required for complete chemical disintegration of some chlorinated hydrocarbons can only be measured in millennia.

Phytointoxication may occur when birds eat poisonous plants because of their succulent nature or attractive appearance. Birds confined to small yards or ranges devoid of grasses may eat toxic plants if forced to go without feed. Poisonous seed such as *Crotalaria spectabilis* may accidentally be incorporated in the feed.

The treatment of individual birds for poisoning is seldom practical in commercial flocks. However, if the source of poisoning can be determined in large flocks, appropriate remedial measures can be instituted.

The metabolic pathways which detoxify poisons vary considerably in different animals. There is also a variation in the tolerance of different species for toxic agents. Sherwin and Crowdle (1922) found that the detoxification process in chickens was similar to that in dogs.

AUTOINTOXICATION

Autointoxication, endogenous in origin, is caused by the absorption of waste products of metabolism or products of decomposition within the intestine. In young chicks autointoxication may be the result of injudicious feeding practices. The use of feed high in fiber content may cause obstruction of the digestive tract with subsequent absorption of the products of decomposition. Hay chaff used for litter may result in the ingestion of sufficient quantities to cause impaction of the digestive tract. Chicks raised in confinement and fed chopped green feed may consume enough fibrous material to cause intestinal obstruction. This material frequently kills young poults which are supplied with green feed containing short pieces of fibrous stems.

The chilling of chicks may cause pasting and occlusion of the vent. The resulting stasis of the intestinal contents leads to autointoxication.

The signs observed in birds suffering

from autointoxication are anorexia, increased water consumption, and depression, followed by weakness and prostration. Nervous signs typical of a generalized toxemia may appear shortly before death.

COCCIDIOSTATS

The advent of coccidiostats was the beginning of modern chemotherapy and mass medication. The uncontrolled, unsupervised, and unwise use of coccidiostats soon led to the realization that even "wonder drugs" had their limitations when it came to toxicity. If a given percentage of drug was added to the feed mix, it was assumed that this percentage of drug was evenly distributed throughout the feed. The electrostatic properties of some chemicals caused them to adhere to the interior of the mixer and prevented proper mixing. This situation created a compound felony. First, the poultrymen expecting a prophylactic or therapeutic level of coccidiostat in his feed was short-changed and could experience heavy losses from coccidiosis because of inadequate coccidiostat in the feed. If the flock did not experience losses from coccidiosis, the poultryman blithely assumed it was because of the "protection" he had purchased. On the other hand, if the flock did break out with coccidiosis, the drug companies suggested that a resistant strain of coccidium had developed on the farm or that the exposure had been too heavy for adequate control.

The second aspect of the felony was the anomalous situation in which a feed buyer was getting more than he paid for. The next batch of feed prepared in the mixer following coccidiostat mix often picked up significant concentrations of the residual coccidiostat. If the contaminated feed was a laying mash, the mistake was reflected in a drop in egg production, off-color shells, thin shells, reduced egg size, and inferior internal quality or mottled yolks. In one instance a dog food prepared in a mixer used for poultry feed became contaminated with sufficient coccidiostat to cause poisoning and mortality in dogs that ate it (Elsasser et al., 1950).

SULFONAMIDES

Sulfonamides were among the first of the so-called "wonder drugs" to be used for poultry medication following World War II. Their effectiveness in the treatment of war injuries led to extensive use in veterinary medicine. The most significant and enduring use of sulfonamides for poultry was in their treatment of coccidiosis. Gradually it became evident that although sulfonamides exerted inhibitory action against invading pathogens, they also effected pronounced physiologic and metabolic changes in the host. The pathologic effect induced by toxicity was one of blood dyscrasia, kidney dysfunction, disrupted liver function, and superinfection. The therapeutic level of a sulfonamide may impinge on the toxic level, and caution is the watchword in respect to dosage, age of birds, duration of treatment, previous medication, and concomitant feeding of several drugs.

Levine (1939), in a study of the efficacy of sulfanilamide against coccidiosis, found that concentrations of 0.2, 0.3, and 0.4% in the mash fed for a period of 2 weeks was decidedly toxic for chickens. Hinshaw and McNeil (1943) reported sulfanilamide was toxic for 4-week-old turkeys at a level of 3 grains per pound of body weight. Farr and Wehr (1945) reported that a level of 0.25% sulfamerazine in the feed of chickens caused retarded growth and necrosis of the liver and spleen. These studies were extended and confirmed; it was noted that 6-week-old chickens were more sensitive to high levels of sulfamerazine than younger chickens (Farr and Jaquette, 1947). Levine and Barber (1947) found hemorrhagic infarcts, necrosis, and swelling of the spleens in chickens following the feeding of 0.5% sulfamethazine, 0.5% sulfamerazine, and 1% sulfaguanidine in the mash for 8 days. Sulfamethazine was most toxic and sulfaguanidine least toxic. Delaplane and Milliff (1948) reported that laying pullets which were fed sulfaquinoxaline in the mash at a level of 0.25% for a period of 8–10 days rapidly declined in egg production; became droopy, weak, and anemic; and eventually died. Davies and Kendall (1953) and Davies (1954) found that sulfaquinoxaline added to the drinking water in a concentration of 0.0645% was toxic for chickens after 5 days of treatment.

Yacowitz et al. (1955) reported that the feeding of 0.1% sulfaquinoxaline in the presence of 3–5% alfalfa and 5 mg menadione per pound of feed resulted in the occurrence of a hemorrhagic syndrome in chicks similar to spontaneous cases. The feeding of iodinated casein and penicillin appeared to increase the toxicity of sulfaquinoxaline. The whole blood clotting time was increased but the prothrombin time was normal. Joyner and Davies (1956) also observed an increase in whole blood clotting times in chickens given sulfaquinoxaline at a level of 0.06% in the water. The incidence of lesions and mortality was highest in birds 4–8 weeks of age. These investigators made the observation that the administration of vitamin K or synthetic analogues of vitamin K reduced the blood clotting time of birds receiving sulfaquinoxaline but did not reduce the incidence of hemorrhages or splenic lesions. The results of this study suggest that it is most unlikely that the toxicity of sulfaquinoxaline is due solely to a deficiency of vitamin K caused by inhibition of the intestinal bacterial flora or by a shortage of the vitamin in the ration.

Marthedal and Velling (1961) indicated that macroscopic changes were produced in 5–8-week-old chickens in 4 days following administration of 0.05% sulfaquinoxaline in the drinking water.

Faddoul et al. (1967) conducted toxicity studies on sulfaquinoxaline and observed a mitigating effect on the toxicity of sulfaquinoxaline by previous low level continuous medication. They postulated that this reduction in toxicity indicated an adaptive phenomenon possibly involving detoxifying processes in the liver. One group of previously unmedicated 19-week-old chickens experienced 11% mortality when fed 0.05% sulfaquinoxaline for 4 weeks, whereas another group of birds that had been continuously fed 0.0125% sulfaquinoxaline since 1 day of age experienced no mortality when fed 0.05% of the drug for 4 weeks.

Cuckler and Ott (1955) reported that continuous administration of 0.05% sulfaquinoxaline in the feed or of 0.025% in water for as long as 12 weeks had no adverse effects on chickens. Similarly there was no evidence that the intermittent administration of 0.05% in the feed or of 0.025% in the water for 2–5 weeks had any deleterious effects. The continuous administration of 0.025% sulfaquinoxaline solu-

tion to turkeys retarded growth slightly, but there was no mortality or other adverse effect. Ducks tolerated up to 0.1% sulfaquinoxaline in the feed for 9 weeks without growth retardation or mortality. Cuckler and Ott (1955) found that the feeding of 0.1% and 0.2% sulfaquinoxaline in the ration for 2–3 weeks or 0.015% for 11 weeks had no detectable effect on blood clotting times. Prothrombin times of chicken blood were not prolonged by feeding 0.1% and 0.2% sulfaquinoxaline in the feed. An excessive dosage of 0.4% sulfaquinoxaline in the feed was required to produce a prolongation in whole blood clotting time, but this dosage produced only a slight increase in prothrombin time.

Therefore, it appears that given levels of sulfonamide medication may at times exert no ill effect, whereas on other occasions toxic manifestations are evident.

Signs

Sulfonamide toxicity is manifested in growing birds by ruffled feathers, depression, paleness and icteric discoloration of the tissues about the head, poor weight gains, and an increase in blood clotting time (Farr and Jaquette, 1947; Delaplane and Milliff, 1948; Joyner and Davies, 1956).

Hinshaw and McNeil (1943) and Scott et al. (1944) reported on the adverse effect of feeding sulfanilamide to chickens and turkeys in production. Sulfanilamide in the diet caused a marked decrease in production, soft-shelled eggs, thin shells, rough shells, and depigmentation of brown eggs. According to Scott et al. (1944), the thinness of the shell (or lack of it) could not be attributed to premature expulsion of the egg as it remained in the shell gland for the normal length of time. The adverse effect of sulfamethazine on egg production was noted by Asplin and Boyland (1947); Delaplane and Milliff (1948) observed that sulfaquinoxaline caused a marked drop in egg production. Asplin and Boyland (1947) noted precocious sexual development in young cockerels after 10 days of treatment with sulfamethazine. Growth of the comb and wattles was accelerated and the testes were enlarged. On microscopic examination hyperplasia of the seminiferous tubules was evident.

Faddoul et al. (1967) reported that drug fever was a common manifestation of sulfaquinoxaline toxicity; rectal temperatures were 1–4° F above normal. Asplin and Boyland (1947) reported body temperatures up to 110° F in pullets suffering from sulfamethazine toxicity.

Gross Lesions

Excellent descriptions of the gross and microscopic pathology are given by Delaplane and Milliff (1948) and Faddoul et al. (1967).

Hemorrhage in the skin, muscles, and internal organs is the most consistent and extensive lesion of sulfonamide intoxication. Hemorrhage may be present in the comb, eyelids, face, wattles, anterior chamber of the eye, and musculature of the breast and thighs. The dark red color of normal bone marrow in growing birds changes to pink in mild cases and yellow in severe cases. The entire length of the intestinal tract may be spotted with petechial and ecchymotic hemorrhages, and the cecal lumen may contain blood. Hemorrhage may be present in the proventriculus and beneath the lining of the gizzard. The liver is swollen and ocher or icteric in color and may be studded with petechiae or focal necrosis. The spleen is commonly affected and is enlarged, has hemorrhagic infarcts, and contains gray nodular areas (Farr and Wehr, 1945). Hemorrhages of the paintbrush type occur in the myocardium. Delaplane and Milliff (1948) noted gray nodular areas in the myocardium similar to lesions they found in the spleen, liver, kidneys, and lungs of chickens poisoned by sulfaquinoxaline.

Histopathology

Comprehensive descriptions of the histopathology of sulfaquinoxaline toxicity were given by Delaplane and Milliff (1948) and Faddoul et al. (1967). Areas of caseation necrosis surrounded by a mantle of giant cells occurred in the liver, spleen, lungs, and kidneys. The giant cells ranged from 30 to 200μ in size. Lymphocytic and heterophilic infiltration was present at the periphery of the necrotic foci. Lymphoid hypoplasia around the splenic adenoid sheaths, edema and fibroplasia of the capsule, and macrophages containing hemosiderin were common. Early changes in the liver were periportal mononuclear infil-

tration associated with bile duct hyperplasia. Hemosiderin deposits were present in the necrotic areas, and thrombosis of the portal vessels was present. An early change in the kidneys was interstitial lymphocytic infiltration. Degeneration and necrosis of the tubular epithelium were associated with albuminous casts. The glomeruli were hyperplastic and Bowman's capsule was dilated with albuminous casts.

The lungs were congested with interlobular and interstitial edema. The interstitial tissues contained mononuclear foci.

In the femoral bone marrow there was a decrease in intrasinusoidal erythropoiesis and a focal increase in extrasinusoidal lymphopoiesis, and in some instances myelopoiesis. There was a decrease in hemopoiesis and cellular degeneration in advanced lesions. There were also focal areas of hyalinization, necrosis, and fibroplasia. Hemosiderin deposits and extrasinusoidal edema were present.

NITROFURAZONE

Nitrofurazone (5-nitro-2-furaldehyde-semicarbozone) was introduced in 1949 for treatment and prevention of coccidiosis. Harwood and Stunz (1949a) found that a single dose of 150–200 mg of nitrofurazone per kg of body weight given to 10–14-week-old chickens caused toxic signs. These authors subsequently found that when nitrofurazone was fed continuously for 14 days at a level of 0.022% in the mash it retarded growth. A similar effect on growth was reported by Gardiner and Farr (1954) when the drug was fed at this level for 7 days, and by Peterson and Hymas (1950) who noted that 0.04 and 0.05% of the drug in the diet of 4-week-old chicks caused retarded growth and mortality when fed for 9 days.

Blount (1955) described a case of nitrofurazone poisoning in 3–6-week-old chicks in which the feed contained 10 times the recommended level of 0.01% nitrofurazone in the feed. Mortality started 10 days after feeding the poisoned feed, and 60% of the birds died.

Jordan (1955) reported accidental nitrofurazone poisoning in day-old chicks that received 0.04–0.07% of the drug in the feed for 3 days; 30% of the chicks died and growth was retarded in the survivors.

Klimes and Kruza (1962) reported that

the feeding of 0.022% nitrofurazone for 2 weeks caused 50% mortality in 14-day-old White Pekin ducklings. Clinical signs did not appear and death occurred suddenly.

Signs

The signs manifested by nitrofurazone toxicity depend on dosage and duration of administration. At levels of 0.011% in the feed for 28 days or 0.222% for 7–14 days it caused retarded growth (Harwood and Stunz, 1949b; Horton-Smith and Long, 1952; Gardiner and Farr, 1954). Harwood and Stunz (1949a) described the signs of acute toxicity as depression in some chicks and hyperexcitability in others. The latter signs were manifested by rapid movements, loud squawking, extended rigid legs and wings, opisthotonus, and aimless flying about. Birds thus affected usually died in 2–3 days. In addition to depression Jordan (1955) also noted hyperexcitability in 2-day-old chicks. The chicks cheeped in a high-pitched shrill note, dashed wildly about, whirled in circles, flopped and jumped about like decapitated birds, and finally succumbed. Blount (1955) reported that chicks poisoned by nitrofurazone were very quiet, stood motionless, had rough feathers, and lacked interest in feed or water.

Moore and Brown (1950) observed that the MLD of nitrofurazone in turkeys was 75 mg/kg of body weight; signs of intoxication were ruffled feathers, incoordinated movements, spasmodic head and body movements, and finally exhaustion and death.

Gross Lesions

Harwood and Stunz (1949a) reported catarrhal enteritis and marked congestion of the kidneys, meninges, and cranial bones. Edema of the body and venous congestion, especially of the lungs, were noticed by Jordan (1955). Blount (1955) noted enteritis and cardiac degeneration.

Histopathology

Lesions were not present in the brain or meninges of chicks examined by Jordan (1955). Klimes and Kruza (1962) reported that livers of ducklings showed degeneration of the trabecular structure, edema of the interstitial tissue, and dilatation of the capillaries. Nephrosis was also noted.

NICARBAZIN

Nicarbazin, an equimolecular complex of 4,4'-dinitrocarbanilide and 2-hydroxy-4, 6-dimethylpyrimidine, was introduced as a coccidiostat in 1955. Berg et al. (1956) reported that a level of 0.0125% in the feed depressed feed efficiency significantly, and a level of 0.02% depressed the rate of growth and impaired feed efficiency. Contrary to the previous report, Ott et al. (1956) reported that continuous feeding of 0.01–0.02% nicarbazin to young chickens did not interfere with growth, feed efficiency, or sexual maturity. Baker et al. (1957) reported that egg production was markedly reduced by feeding levels of 0.0125% nicarbazin to White Leghorns and as little as 0.009% to heavy breeds. Egg size was reduced by 0.006% nicarbazin in the feed. Depigmented eggs were produced by heavy breed hens fed 0.009% nicarbazin. Perhaps the most widely known adverse effect of nicarbazin and most damaging to the image of the poultry industry in the eyes of the consumer is the production of mottled yolks. Baker et al. (1957) found that as little as 0.006% nicarbazin in the feed caused large numbers of severely mottled yolks. The mottling was accentuated if the eggs were kept several days. Ott et al. (1956) found that nicarbazin caused disastrous effects when fed to New Hampshire breeders. At levels of 0.04% in the feed the eggshells became chalk white within 2 days after medication was started and returned to normal just as rapidly after withdrawal of the drug. Shape, texture, and thickness of the eggshell were normal. Hatchability was severely affected; at a level of 0.02% nicarbazin in the diet less than 10% of the eggs hatched.

Signs

Newberne and Buck (1957) described the signs produced by toxic levels of nicarbazin fed to day-old chicks. After feeding 0.025% nicarbazin for 1–2 weeks the chicks were dull, listless, and weak and showed signs of ataxia, jerky incoordination, and a stilted gait. The birds appeared to develop some tolerance to the effects of high levels of the drug as signs and mortality decreased after consuming the drug for 3–4 weeks. It is interesting to note that this "adaptive phenomenon" to prolonged ingestion of toxic drugs was also noted by Faddoul et al. (1967) in birds consuming sulfaquinoxaline.

Histopathology

A good description of the histopathologic lesions caused by nicarbazin toxicity is given by Newberne and Buck (1957).

The first microscopic changes were fatty metamorphosis in the liver followed by cellular degeneration, pyknotic nuclei, reticulation of the cytoplasm, and degeneration of the renal tubular epithelium. A marked hyperplasia of the lymphoid follicles of the lung was evident about the primary and secondary bronchi, and ossified nodules occurred in the lung. In the spleen there was an increase of the white pulp and Malpighian bodies during the early stages of medication; later the white pulp decreased and the Malpighian bodies were reduced in number and size.

Hemopoietic dysfunction was reflected in a reduction in heterophils and an increase in thrombocytes.

ZOALENE

The toxicity of Zoalene (3, 5-dinitro-o-toluamide) for chickens has been reported by Morrison et al. (1961), Bigland et al. (1963), and Henk and Hromalka (1967). When Zoalene was fed at 2 and 4 times the recommended level (0.025 and 0.05%), growth and feed efficiency were depressed (Morrison et al., 1961). Bigland et al. (1963) reported that concentrations of 0.083 and 0.086% accidentally incorporated in two lots of broiler feed caused nervous signs and depressed growth and feed efficiency. They also noted that it was apparently necessary for the drug to accumulate 4–7 days in the tissues before signs were noted and that birds showing nervous signs in the evening might look normal in the morning due to decreased intake of the drug. This rapid remission of signs has also been noted in nitrophenide intoxication (Blount, 1955).

Signs

Bigland et al. (1963) reported that signs included an extended "stiff" neck with eyes cast downward, staggering, vertigo, and tumbling over when excited. In addition to ataxia and opisthotonus, Henk and Hromalka (1967) noted increased mortality.

Lesions

Gross lesions are not produced by Zoalene toxicity, and microscopically only slight edema is present in the white matter of the cerebellum (Bigland et al., 1963).

NITROPHENIDE

Nitrophenide (m, m'-dinitro-diphenyl-disulfide) was first introduced as a coccidiostat in 1949 by Lederle Laboratories as a 25% premix under the name of Megasul. Blount (1955) recalls an interesting account of poisoning where a feed company miscalculated and added 4 times the recommended amount to the feed. Peckham (1950) saw several cases of nitrophenide intoxication. The diagnosis of nitrophenide intoxication in a research flock was received with disbelief and consternation on the part of the nutritionist who had personally supervised the mixing and swept out the inside of the mixing drum after completion of the operation. In fact, he confided that the portion he swept out of the mixer was the feed currently in use. Unwittingly the nutritionist had given the answer to how the overdosage occurred. Nitrophenide possessed marked electrostatic properties and the greater portion of the drug adhered to the wall of the mixer. The sweepings he had carefully husbanded were subsequently found by his own admission to contain 4 times the recommended amount of 0.025%.

Signs

Waletzky et al. (1949) stated that toxic levels of nitrophenide produce marked signs in chickens: disturbances of posture and locomotion, retardation of growth, and mortality. Postural disturbances include a tilted position of the head, tremor of the neck, and difficulty in "righting" reactions when the bird is placed on its back.

Blount (1955) described the signs in 14-week-old chickens fed 0.4%. Four days after the onset of feeding nearly all the birds were showing nervous signs, and feed consumption dropped by half. Some birds were ataxic or off their legs. Others would run about and leap up into the air. No mortality occurred and the flock returned to normal within 48 hours after changing feed. Peckham (1950) observed that many birds showing nervous signs would act completely normal the next day when held in the laboratory overnight.

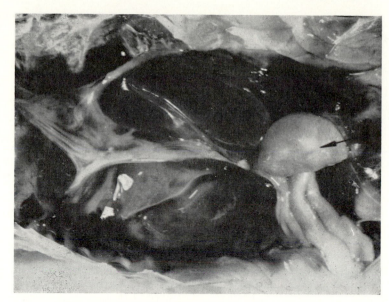

*FIG. 33.1—Cresol poisoning. Liver is gray and shrunken with rounded edges. Ascitic fluid and coagula (**arrow**) in body cavity.*

DISINFECTANTS

CRESOL

Bullis and Van Roekel (1944) first reported the injurious effects of carbolineum and creosote products for young chicks. West (1957) confirmed these observations, and Bierer et al. (1963) studied the effect of feeding 1% coal tar and other disinfectants to chicks for a 2-week period.

Bressler et al. (1951) reported on the effect of salt and carbolineum in the experimental production of ascites in turkey poults.

Signs

Detailed descriptions of the signs and lesions were given by Bullis and Van Roekel (1944) and West (1957). Cresol poisoning usually occurs at 3–6 weeks of age. Affected chicks are depressed, weak, and have a tendency to huddle. The flock is generally uneven in size and has ragged feathering. Respiratory signs are rales, gasping, wheezing, and extension of the head and neck. Chicks with anasarca may waddle or walk stiff-legged.

Lesions

The lesions depend upon the severity and duration of exposure. The ventral subcutis is infiltrated with a yellow transudate. The breast muscles are pale. A clear amber-colored fluid may cause ascites. Yellow fibrinous coagula form a mantle on the surface of the liver. Early liver lesions are enlargement and mottling, whereas chronic lesions are atrophy and cirrhosis (Fig. 33.1). The spleen is pale and atrophied. The kidneys are usually swollen and pale. The myocardium is pale and hypertrophied with hydropericardium. The lungs may be edematous and have areas of hepatization. Mucus may be present in the trachea; Bullis and Van Roekel (1944) observed blood in the mouth and trachea of some chicks. West (1957) observed pale and hydropic bone marrow and detected the odor of coal tar in the internal tissues of three cases. He reported mortality of 2–56% and indicated that morbidity and mortality depend upon several factors: concentration of the toxic agent, chick density, composition of the floor, weather conditions, and ventilation.

Control

As medicinal treatment is lacking, further injury may be prevented by moving the chicks to new quarters. If this is not possible, the pen should be thoroughly ventilated and old litter removed. Prevention of complications of creosote derivative disinfectants requires caution. After application of the disinfectant the building should be heated to volatilize residual disinfectant and kept well ventilated for several days before putting in the litter and chicks.

Differential Diagnosis

In arriving at a diagnosis of cresol poisoning, the syndromes of salt poisoning, "toxic fat" poisoning, crotalaria poisoning, and transudative diathesis must be considered. These syndromes occur in birds of the same age group and resemble each other in their clinical manifestations, making it exceedingly difficult for the diagnostician to establish a positive diagnosis.

POTASSIUM PERMANGANATE

This chemical is frequently used in the drinking water for poultry and can be decidedly toxic if used to excess. Gallagher (1919) conducted toxicity studies and reported the toxic dose for mature chickens was 30 grains, with death ensuing within 24 hours after administration. A 1:500 solution in the drinking water for several weeks caused no ill effects. After administration of the toxic dose clinical signs were not observed prior to death. Lesions consisted of a severe cauterization of the crop wall with blackening of the submucosa and skin on the lower surface of the crop. Extensive hemorrhages were found in the crop where the crystals of potassium permanganate came in contact with the mucosa, the caustic action of the chemical being localized in the tissues which it contacted. All other organs appeared normal.

QUATERNARY AMMONIUM COMPOUNDS

The great increase in the number of birds being raised in cages with automatic watering systems has led to increased usage of sanitizers and disinfectants in the drinking water. The sanitizers are metered into the water system by an automatic measuring device which could get out of adjustment. Mayeda (1968) described the toxic effects of a quaternary ammonium compound for turkey poults and demonstrated that the recommended level and toxic level were perilously close. The approved dosage for the product he tested was 100 ppm; when 150 ppm were given, 50% mortality occurred in 12 days and growth was depressed in the survivors. Dam and Norris (1962) reported that a 1:2,000 dilution of Zephiran in the drinking water of layers caused reduced feed and water consumption and depressed egg production.

Signs

Mayeda (1968) indicated that the toxicosis caused by a quaternary ammonium compound produced signs and lesions which constituted a distinctive pathognomonic syndrome. He described the clinical signs as follows: reluctance to drink, cry of discontent, restlessness, persistent swallowing, continual spitting, foamy ocular discharge, sniffling and discharge from the nostrils, facial swelling, gasping, occasional violent head shaking, scratching of eyes and mouth with toes, adhesion of eyelids, distinct lump visible in throat region, incessant coughing and chirping, ataxia, convulsions, and death.

Lesions

Mayeda (1968) described an early lesion as a diphtheritic caseous ulcer at the base of the tongue. Later similar pseudomembranous lesions were observed elsewhere in the mouth. The mucosa of the esophagus, crop, and proventriculus appeared thickened and manifested small pseudomembranous lesions. The gizzard lining characteristically manifested a circumscribed erosion at the proventricular orifice.

Histopathology

Oral lesions in poults were characterized by focal necrosis of the stratified squamous epithelium and heterophilic infiltration with minor extension to the underlying muscle and glands.

DRUGS

AMMONIUM CHLORIDE

This drug was formerly administered to poultry for prevention and treatment of ascites. Gallagher (1919) reported the nontoxic dose was 15–45 grains and the lethal dose 60 grains.

Clinical signs of toxicity are anorexia, depression, weakness, coma, and death. Gross lesions are absent.

BORIC ACID

Boric acid was formerly used for the preservation of home-canned foods. Leftover canned food was frequently fed to chickens with fatal results. Gallagher (1924) reported that canned string beans with 9 g boric acid/qt were toxic to chickens.

Clinical signs are anorexia, diarrhea, depression, coma, and death. Lesions are severe gastroenteritis with the mucosa of the crop becoming thickened and necrotic.

COPPER SULFATE

Copper sulfate, commonly known as blue vitriol, has occasionally been used as water-soluble medication. If birds drink a concentrated solution or ingest undissolved crystals, intoxication may occur. Gallagher (1919) found 20 grains of the crystalline salt or 15 grains in solution was a lethal dose for fowl.

Pullar (1940) reported the MLD in g/kg body weight to be 0.9 copper sulfate crystals, 0.3–0.5 copper sulfate when mixed with twice its weight in sodium chloride, and 0.9 copper carbonate. Copper sulfate and copper carbonate in doses of 1.0–1.5 g/kg body weight were MLD for pigeons; for ducks the range was 0.4–0.9 g. Pullar (1940) considered the maximum daily intake of copper carbonate to be 0.06 g/kg body weight for chickens and 0.029 for mallard ducks. Toxic effects were not observed from administration of 1:4,000 dilution of copper sulfate in the drinking water.

Lander (1926) reported that salts of copper form soluble albuminates in the stomach which are rapidly absorbed. The albuminates are deposited in the liver, lungs, and kidneys. These products are slowly eliminated in the bile and urates.

Hinshaw and Lloyd (1931) reported that turkeys were poisoned by concentrations greater than 0.2% in the drinking water. Turkeys do not like copper sulfate solutions in any dilution and will reduce their water intake.

Signs

In mild cases of poisoning there may be temporary depression followed by uneventful recovery. Toxic doses cause a primary stimulation and activity followed by severe depression and weakness. Convulsions, paralysis, and coma precede death.

Gross Lesions

There is a greenish catarrhal gastroenteritis. Coagulation necrosis may occur in the mucosa of the lower esophagus and crop. Severe degenerative changes may occur in the liver and kidneys.

KAMALA

Kamala is a strong intestinal irritant formerly used as an anthelmintic. Egg production is reduced following its use. Hall and Shillinger (1926) considered 15 grains an effective dose for chickens. Cram (1928) cautioned against the use of kamala in chickens with complicating diseases. Beach (1930) reported that turkeys were less tolerant than chickens, and Hawn (1933) found that kamala was neither safe nor efficient for turkeys.

MERCURY COMPOUNDS

The oxides and chlorides of mercury are extremely toxic whereas the insoluble sulfides are relatively nontoxic. The chlorides are commonly used as disinfectants and medicinal agents; the oxides are used in paint. Glover (1932) reported toxic effects in chickens caused by application of excessive amounts of mercurial ointment for the control of lice.

Gallagher (1919) reported the lethal dose of bichloride of mercury to be 4 grains whereas 3 grains were nontoxic. According to Nunn (1907), mercury compounds are not quickly eliminated but are deposited in the liver and kidneys.

Signs

Progressive incoordination and leg weakness is followed by complete prostration. The birds may be depressed.

Lesions

Gastroenteritis accompanied by hemorrhages may be observed throughout the digestive tract, accompanied by greenish gelatinous exudate. Necrosis and sloughing of the mucosa may occur. The kidneys are pale and often studded with minute white foci. Fatty degeneration is evident in the liver. A green viscid fluid is present in the abdominal cavity.

A single dose of 2 grains of calomel is lethal for geese. The signs and lesions are similar to those seen in chickens but the degenerative changes are more severe. Figure 33.2 shows the formation of crystals in a necrotic focus of the kidney.

McNeil and Hinshaw (1945) reported that a 1:4,000 dilution of mercuric chloride in the drinking water was toxic for turkeys. Lesions on necropsy were thickening and necrosis of the gizzard lining, escharotic thickening of the crop, and sloughing of the mucous membrane of the proventriculus.

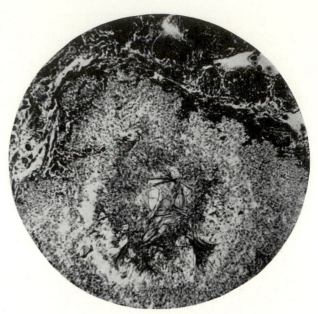

FIG. 33.2—Calomel poisoning in goose showing crystals in necrotic focus of kidney. ×320.

NITRATES

The nitrates of potassium and sodium may be poisonous for poultry. Sodium nitrate is commonly used in the form of saltpeter as fertilizer and may be mistaken for magnesium sulfate. Guberlet (1922) reported 60–70 grains were lethal for fowl and smaller doses caused diarrhea.

Signs

These are excessive thirst, anorexia, vomition, diarrhea, subnormal temperature and cyanosis of the comb, wattles, and skin. Terminal convulsions may occur.

Lesions

Varying degrees of gastroenteritis are present. Degenerative changes may be present in the heart, liver, and kidneys.

SODIUM BICARBONATE

It used to be common practice for poultrymen to "flush" their flocks with various chemicals in the drinking water, one of which was sodium bicarbonate. Pathologists observed that chicks with visceral gout often had a history of receiving sodium bicarbonate as a flush. Subsequent investigation revealed that overdosing with sodium bicarbonate caused nephritis and visceral gout (Delaplane, 1934). Jungherr (1935) reported that single doses or repeated small doses of sodium bicarbonate may cause visceral gout. He also observed gout in 2-day-old chicks that were not medicated. Bullis and Van Roekel (1944) stated that excess sodium bicarbonate would produce visceral gout. They also observed gout in chicks 3–4 days of age that had not received sodium bicarbonate.

Witter (1936) reported toxic reactions but no mortality in 2-week-old chicks which were given a 0.6% solution of sodium bicarbonate. Doubling the dosage caused toxic reactions in 2 days and death in 4 days. A 2% solution given to chicks 6–8 weeks of age caused morbidity in 2 days and mortality by the 3rd day. A 2.4% solution given to yearlings caused toxic signs and mortality in 5 days.

Signs

Clinical signs include depression, weakness, increased water consumption, and watery droppings.

Lesions

The primary lesion occurs in the kidneys which become pale and swollen, followed by marked distension of the tubules and ureters with urates. Urate deposits are found on the epicardium and the surface of the liver and lungs (Fig. 33.3).

Scrivner (1946) reported that 0.1% sodium bicarbonate in the drinking water for 18 days was nontoxic for day-old poults. Concentrations of 0.3, 0.5, and 0.6% caused heavy mortality in 2–3 weeks. Lesions in

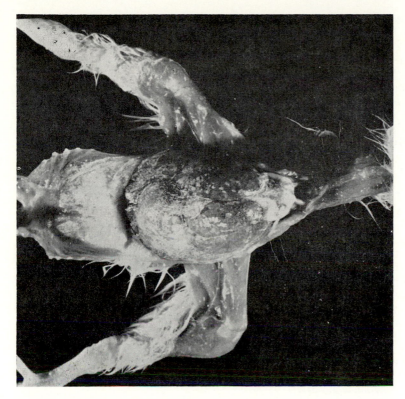

FIG. 33.3—Sodium bicarbonate poisoning. Five-day-old chick with urate deposits over viscera and muscles.

the dead poults were subcutaneous edema and ascites; there were no lesions of visceral gout.

Scrivner (1946) investigated the toxic effect of sodium citrate, sodium iodide, sodium sulfate, and sodium hydroxide for poults. At toxic levels in the drinking water these compounds produced ascites and edema.

SODIUM CHLORIDE

Chickens, turkeys, ducks, and pigeons are susceptible to salt poisoning. Young birds are more frequently affected than adults because of increased feed intake in relation to body weight. Salt poisoning can be acute or chronic. The acute form occurs when birds are accidently exposed to large amounts of salt such as rock salt used in chilling brine, fish brine, salt boxes for livestock, or mixed with sand for highways. Chronic salt poisoning is more common and often occurs where well or pond water is being used. Excess salt in the feed is another common cause of chronic poisoning.

Gallagher (1919) concluded the MLD for chickens was 4 g/kg of body weight. Paver et al. (1953) found levels of 0.98–3.25% in

the mash nontoxic for chicks. Concentrations above 3.5% were toxic. They found that a gradual increase in the salt content of the diet from 2 to 50% when fed to chickens over 1 month of age severely depressed growth but was not necessarily fatal. It was postulated that this was due to the lower feed requirements of older birds in relation to liveweight and possibly increased renal efficiency in older birds. Doll et al. (1946) reported 0.25% sodium chloride in drinking water was not toxic when given to chicks for 4 weeks. Sodium chloride at a level of 0.5% and above in drinking water was toxic. Blaxland (1946) observed that 5–10% salt in the mash caused heavy mortality in baby chicks. He also reported that 0.9% sodium chloride in the drinking water caused 100% mortality in baby chicks within 5 days. Kare and Biely (1948) reported that chicks receiving over 4% salt in the mash had ascites and hydropericardium.

Gordon et al. (1959) reported the production of a condition resembling "toxic fat" disease in 4-week-old chickens fed purified diets containing 20% blood meal, 2% corn oil, and 0.88% sodium chloride. A similar diet containing 30% blood meal and 22%

corn oil caused no ill effects. When ether-extracted blood meal was fed with the high level of sodium chloride, edema did not result. Supplementation of isolated soybean protein diets with high levels of sodium chloride resulted in edema only in chickens fed diets low in fat. It was concluded that there is an ether-soluble factor present in blood meal which disturbs salt regulation of the young chicken. In addition, high levels of fat can counteract the edematous effects of a high dietary sodium chloride level.

Bigland (1950) reported on field cases of salt poisoning in turkey poults and found that in some instances the feed contained an excess of 1% salt over the recommended amount. In addition to the excess salt in the feed some sources of drinking water contained salt. He also found that the salt content of the mash in the feed hoppers was higher than that in the bags. The salt by virtue of its specific gravity and physical characteristics gravitated to the bottom of the feed hopper. Mortality of 10–20% started at 8 days of age with daily losses of 1–3% for 10 days.

Bressler et al. (1951) reported mortality in young poults when 0.9% salt was added to the ration. Scrivner (1946) fed 2.5% salt in the mash to day-old poults and caused 40% mortality in 7 days. The administration of 2% sodium chloride in the water and 0.5% in the feed to day-old poults caused listlessness in 2 days and 100% mortality in 4 days. Lowering the salt content in the water to 0.5% in addition to feeding 0.5% salt in the mash caused 80% mortality in 10 days with lesions of subcutaneous edema and ascites. Gibson (1957) reported 2% salt in a turkey mash caused 5–11% mortality in poults. Turkeys 8–31 weeks of age can tolerate salt levels up to 6% in the ration without adverse effect on weight gains and development (Roberts, 1957).

Shaw (1929) reported that less than 5 g of salt was nontoxic for ducks weighing 600 g, while larger doses were fatal. Torrey and Graham (1935) reported 4 doses of 5 g of salt were fatal to half-grown Pekin ducks. The ducks tolerated 1–2 g of salt daily for 29 days. Clinical signs of toxicity were anorexia, incoordination, progressive weakness, and death. Lesions varied from mild to severe enteritis and nephritis.

Edwards (1918) reported that 3.3 g sodium chloride/kg body weight was fatal for pigeons.

Signs

Signs include loss of appetite, somnolence, thirst, dyspnea, opisthotonus, convulsions, and inability to stand. Krakower and Goettsch (1945) noted that increasing the salt content of the diet caused a marked increase in water consumption.

Lesions

Lesions in poults are anasarca, ascites, hydropericardium, cardiac hypertrophy, edema of the lungs, and enteritis with edema of the intestinal wall (Bigland, 1950). Lesions in chicks are nephritis, myocardial hemorrhage, ascites, and subcutaneous edema (Doll et al., 1946; Barlow et al., 1948).

Treatment

According to Buckley et al. (1939), there is no antidote for sodium chloride poisoning. However, every effort should be made to provide the birds with fresh water and a salt-free diet.

FUMIGANTS AND GASES

CARBON MONOXIDE

Carbon monoxide poisoning is due primarily to poorly ventilated brooders or defective coal or oil heating units.

Signs

Signs of acute carbon monoxide poisoning include restlessness, drowsiness, stupor, labored breathing, and incoordination. The birds gasp, lie on their sides, and exhibit opisthotonus. Spasms and convulsions commonly occur prior to death. In subacute cases the feathers may appear rough, the appetite is diminished, and the birds do not develop normally. Stiles (1940) found 0.04–0.05% carbon monoxide was sufficient to produce toxicity.

Lesions

The principal lesion observed in acute carbon monoxide poisoning is a bright cherry-red color of the lungs and blood. The lesions may be somewhat confusing in subacute cases and are insufficient for accurate clinical diagnosis. Such cases necessitate laboratory tests.

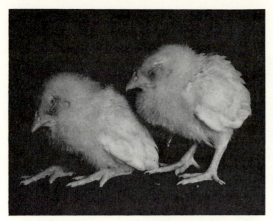

FIG. 33.4—*Photophobia in young chicks caused by prolonged exposure to formaldehyde fumes.*

FORMALDEHYDE

Formalin has been highly recommended and widely used as a disinfectant in controlling hatchery-borne infections. However, some poultrymen use a higher concentration of formaldehyde than recommended and follow the dangerous practice of disinfecting while the chicks are hatching.

Lesions

Prolonged exposure to formaldehyde causes irritation of the respiratory tract with subsequent gasping and distress; also conjunctivitis and photophobia (Fig. 33.4). To determine if White Leghorn chicks have been exposed to formaldehyde after hatching, the down can be moistened with water which will turn a telltale bright yellow.

Bierer (1958) noted lesions in newly hatched poults similar to those in chicks after exposure to double the recommended amount of disinfectant. Lesions were subcutaneous edema and inflammation of the mouth, pharynx, and larynx. He did not observe air sac lesions or ascites.

Scrivner (1946) reported on the results of exposing newly hatched poults for 1 hour to formaldehyde at a concentration of 2 oz formalin and 30 g potassium permanganate per 268 cu ft air space. By the 16th day after exposure 8 poults had died with lesions of ascites or edema.

NAPHTHALENE

Naphthalene was formerly added to the nest in the form of moth balls to protect chickens against lice and mites. The naphthalene is volatile and the moth balls gradually decrease in size and may be ingested by the birds. Hudson (1936) reported the loss of 40 chickens in a flock of 400 caused by naphthalene poisoning. Clinical signs were congestion of comb and wattles, abnormally bright eyes, greenish black diarrhea, progressive paralysis, and death. Death occurred within 3 days following the first signs.

NICOTINE SULFATE

Nicotine, the toxic alkaloid of tobacco, is used for the control of insects. According to Carpenter (1931) the development of the commercial Black Leaf 40, a standardized 40% solution of nicotine sulfate, made it possible to standardize the dosage and obtain more efficient results in the treatment of internal parasites of poultry. Mature fowls apparently tolerate greater doses of nicotine sulfate than do mammals. Bleecker and Smith (1933b) reported toxic reactions in birds treated for internal parasites with Black Leaf 40; the toxic dose was 0.5–1.0 ml (Bleecker and Smith, 1933a). Some birds became depressed and prostrate and died in a short time.

Parker (1929) found that baby chicks were quite susceptible to poisoning with nicotine sulfate. Doses of 0.2 ml in various concentrations were given with the following results: 8% solution killed all treated chicks; 6% solution was fatal to 70%; 3% solution, though producing a toxic reaction and coma for about 15 minutes, resulted in very few deaths.

The application of nicotine sulfate to the roosts shortly before fowls go to roost has been effective in controlling lice and mites. According to Carpenter (1931), nicotine is highly volatile at 100–105° F and is volatilized by the body temperature of the fowl. Severe intoxication has been reported from improper use of the product. Proper ventilation of the poultry house will prevent accumulation of toxic quantities of the vapor.

Signs

Signs observed in nicotine poisoning are severe depression, retarded respiration, cyanosis, and coma followed by death.

Lesions

The lesions usually observed are congestion of lungs and liver, ecchymoses of lungs

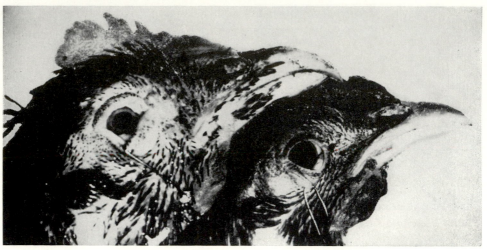

FIG. 33.5—Nicotine sulfate poisoning in chickens showing dilatation of pupil.

and heart, congestion of nictitating membranes, dilatation of the pupil (Fig. 33.5), and cyanosis.

FUNGICIDES

Organic seed protectants are applied to nearly all commercially produced seed corn. In practice it usually happens that the demand for seed is overestimated. This leaves substantial dealer stocks which are often salvaged by incorporating in livestock feed after washing to remove the fungicide. Treated corn looks like untreated corn. Detreatment methods are available but some of these are not efficient. Some states now require that all treated seeds used for grain be colored with a dye.

ARASAN

The toxic effect of Arasan (tetramethylthiuram disulfide—TMTD) for laying hens and young chicks was reported by Johnson et al. (1955), Waibel et al. (1955), and Heuser and Schumacher (1956). Seed corn treated with Arasan-SFX (containing 75% TMTD) may have levels of TMTD as high as 750–1,000 ppm. Swanson et al. (1956) found that levels of Arasan as low as 10 ppm caused production of soft-shelled eggs. From a comparison of the TMTD content of treated corn and the small amount necessary to cause toxic signs, it is obvious that the inclusion of only a small fraction of treated corn in commercial laying mash could have a deleterious effect. The contamination of commercial feed with Arasan was discussed by Waibel et al. (1955) after investigation of several flocks that began to lay misshapen and soft-shelled eggs.

The toxicity of TMTD for chicks was studied by Ackerson and Mussehl (1955) and Waibel et al. (1957). The severity of signs was dependent upon the concentration of TMTD in the ration and duration of exposure to the toxic feed. It is interesting to note that chicks receiving 20 ppm of TMTD made faster weight gains than the controls. Waibel et al. (1957) stated that this indicated a slight stimulation in growth is often produced by small amounts of toxic substances, the use of arsenicals in broiler feed being a case in point. However, increasing the level of TMTD above 20 ppm caused depressed growth, and at levels above 125 ppm growth rate was less than half that of the controls. Affected chicks walk with a stilted gait and continually rest on their hocks. The toes are crooked or curled under in much the same manner as with riboflavin deficiency. The hock joint is enlarged and the gastrocnemius tendon may slip medially. Some chicks become spraddle-legged whereby both legs extend laterally in an extreme splay-footed manner because of joint deformity. Some birds have an abnormal bending of the femur and tibiotarsus.

The presence of Arasan in the mash of layers has an almost immediate effect on production and egg quality (Swanson et al., 1956). With levels as low as 10 ppm nearly 4% of all eggs had little or no shell deposition. At 200 ppm only soft-shelled eggs were laid after 36 hours on the experimental diet. The laying of the shell-less eggs occurred almost exclusively during the night. Another manifestation of TMTD toxicity is the production of a characteristically misshapen egg. The small end of the egg is enlarged and irregular in outline. Frequently the irregular area is covered with a network of blind cracks. Interior egg quality as measured by Haugh units declines with increasing levels of TMTD; at 50 ppm of Arasan it averaged 14 Haugh units. On withdrawal of TMTD from the diet the egg quality returns to normal within 7 days.

Waibel et al. (1957) found that turkey poults were more resistant than chicks to TMTD and tolerated 200 ppm in the diet. At levels of 400 ppm and above in the ration they had leg deformities, reduced growth rate, an unsteady gait, enlarged hocks, and the gastrocnemius tendon slipped medially.

Goslings have the same relative sensitivity as chicks and display similar signs. Affected goslings are unable to walk normally and exhibit a splay-footed condition whereby the legs are extended laterally (Waibel et al., 1957).

CAPTAN

Captan is an organic seed protectant (N-trichloromethylthiotetrahydrophthalimide) applied to seed corn in the commercial form of orthocide. This seed protectant is considerably less toxic for chicks than Arasan (Ackerson and Mussehl, 1955; Link et al., 1956). Orthocide at the rate of 0.043% in the diet of chicks retarded growth the first 3 weeks, but by the 4th week the weight of the treated group equalled controls. Link et al. (1956) did not observe any retardation in chicks fed orthocide. Its effect on egg production or egg quality was not studied.

PESTICIDES—CHLORINATED HYDROCARBONS AND ORGANOPHOSPHORUS COMPOUNDS

CHLORDANE

Rosenberg and Adler (1950) and Rosenberg and Tanaka (1950) reported on the toxicity of the chlorinated hydrocarbon chlordane for chicks. When a 0.25% chlordane was fed in the diet to week-old chicks, mortality started within 30 hours; by 30 days the majority of the chicks were dead.

Chlordane at a level of 0.05% in the feed killed 66% of week-old chicks within 14 days. It was noted that the older the birds were when chlordane was given, the longer it took for the group to die off. However, the percentage of mortality was the same in all age groups.

The toxicity of chlordane for laying pullets was investigated by Rosenberg et al. (1950). A level of 0.05% in the feed did not affect livability, hatchability, or egg production during the 4-week trial. At a level of 0.15%, production dropped to 7% in 4 weeks. Chlordane levels of 0.25 and 0.5% caused complete cessation of lay in 14 days; 1 of 4 treated birds died in each group with lesions of chlordane toxicity. The effect on egg quality was not mentioned. Molting occurred in all treated groups.

Signs

Chicks chirp nervously, rest on their hocks, and lie on their sides. In the terminal stages hyperexcitability is evident. Mucous exudate is present in the nasal passages.

Chlordane toxicity in layers causes reduced feed consumption, decreased body weight, molting, and severely depressed egg production. The comb and wattles atrophy and become cyanotic.

Lesions

The pericardial sac is distended with amber-colored transudate. The heart is enlarged and distorted and the coronary vessels are prominent.

Post (1951) compared the toxic effect of chlordane and toxaphene in pheasants and chukar partridges. The minimum toxic dose of chlordane was 200 mg/kg of body weight for both species. Pheasants survived for 56 days when given the minimum toxic dose but lived for only 10 days when given 5,000 mg/kg of body weight. Partridges died much sooner than pheasants, the shortest survival time being 2 hours and the maximum 72 hours.

The minimum lethal dose of toxaphene was 200 mg/kg of body weight for pheasants. Death occurred within 20 days when the minimum toxic level was fed and within 4 hours when 5,000 mg/kg were fed. The minimum lethal dose for partridges was 50 mg/kg of body weight.

Moore and Carter (1954) reported heavy mortality in 6-week-old poults 3–6 days after spraying the room and cages with 2% chlordane and 0.4% lindane. The chlordane residues on the cages were toxic for poults at least 7 days after spraying.

DIELDRIN

Dieldrin is a chlorinated cyclic hydrocarbon used as a seed protectant. Carnaghan and Blaxland (1957) investigated the toxicity of this product for pigeons and pheasants after circumstantial evidence indicated that these species were being poisoned in the wild. During their investigations these workers found that seed protectants containing organo-mercurials and gamma benzene hexachloride were nontoxic to pigeons and pheasants. However, dieldrin-treated wheat killed pigeons and pheasants. The administration of washings from 45 g of dieldrin-treated grain killed adult pigeons within 4–10 days.

Signs

The birds are listless and have a "hunched-up" attitude. In flight they are ungainly and tend to lose balance when lighting. Nervous signs become pronounced before death and are characterized by rapid lateral movements of the head with slight tremor of the head and neck. There is constant blinking of the eyelids, and death ensues during a violent convulsion. At necropsy the liver and kidneys are congested. The gizzard lining is degenerated and the underlying muscle contains ecchymotic hemorrhages.

DDT (DICHLORO-DIPHENYL-TRICHLOROETHANE)

Rubin et al. (1947) investigated the toxicity of DDT for laying hens. A level of 0.031% DDT in the diet caused a 20% drop in production within a month, and 0.25% caused a 70% drop in 30 days and almost 100% within 60 days. Hatchability was not lowered by 0.031% DDT in the diet but was reduced to zero by 0.125%. Woodward et al. (1944) reported 0.05% DDT in the feed caused 100% mortality in 4–16 days when fed to young chicks.

Signs

Manifestations of DDT toxicity in layers are initial loss of weight, molting, cessation of lay, marked tremors, ataxia, downward bending of the neck, and a marked tendency to rest on the hocks or lie on its side. Chicks manifest nervous signs, hyperexcitability, and fine tremors (Rosenberg and Adler, 1950).

Lesions

Gross and microscopic lesions are absent in DDT poisoning (Rosenberg and Adler, 1950).

Marsden and Bird (1947) investigated the effect of DDT on 19-week-old turkeys. At levels in the diet up to 0.038%, DDT had no adverse effect on males or females for an 8-week period. A level of 0.075% depressed growth rate and caused mortality, whereas doubling this amount caused a severe depression in growth and almost 100% mortality within 30 days. In analyzing the DDT content of the body tissues, it was found that the concentration of DDT in the body fat was 4–8 times the concentration in the diet. The accumulation of DDT in body tissues has serious implications in the biological food chain. By means of extrapolation with the figures obtained from experimental studies, Marsden and Bird (1947) determined that it would be virtually impossible to poison turkeys by using 1 gal of 5% DDT spray for 100 turkeys. Kingscote and Jarvis (1946) stated the dry form or water-dispersible preparations of DDT are less hazardous than oil preparations.

Signs

Toxicity is manifested by moderate to violent continual muscular tremors resembling shivering.

LINDANE

Bootes (1962) reported immediate signs of poisoning in day-old turkey poults after 300 g of an insecticide containing 10% lindane was dusted on 81 sq ft of floor space. Losses continued for a week even though the poults were removed from the litter. Godfrey et al. (1953) found that a 0.5% lindane spray when used on laying chickens did not affect egg production or livability.

Signs

Bootes (1962) reported that the poisoned poults stopped eating and began to squeak noticeably. Shortly thereafter they manifested opisthotonus, flapping of the wings, clonic muscle spasms, backward somersaults, and coma shortly before death.

CHLORINATED BIPHENYL

McCune et al. (1962) reported that chicks reared in a battery freshly painted with an epoxy-resin paint developed ascites and hydropericardium similar to the lesions found in the "toxic fat" syndrome. Various fractions of the paint were mixed with the mash; the most toxic fraction was chlorinated biphenyl which was added to the paint as a plasticizer. A level of 0.04% biphenyl in the mash caused signs and mortality within 3 weeks.

Signs

The chicks made poor weight gains and had dyspnea and rales.

Lesions

At necropsy the most striking lesion was hydropericardium. Some crops contained bloody fluid. Yellow gelatinous transudate was present beneath the skin. Yellow ascitic fluid and coagula were in the abdominal cavity. The liver was enlarged and mottled. The kidneys were pale, swollen, and sometimes hemorrhagic.

Histological lesions were a severe renal tubular dilatation with numerous basophilic casts. Small vessels of the liver had lymphocytic cuffing.

ORGANOPHOSPHORUS INSECTICIDES AND RELATED COMPOUNDS

Dimethoate

Sherman et al. (1963, 1964) reported that the administration to poultry of insecticide-treated feed or water was successful in preventing the development of various species of diptera in the droppings. This method of insect control has a great advantage in the simplicity of administration, particularly in warmer climates where insect control is a continual problem. Technical and emulsifiable dimethoate was given in the drinking water at the rate of 30 ppm to laying hens for 59 weeks. The results were as follows: feed consumption and weight gains were reduced; egg production declined initially but returned to normal; there was no detrimental effect on egg size, shell quality, internal quality, or shell color. In another study Sherman et al. (1964) reported on the acute and subacute

toxicity of 14 organophosphorus insecticides for White Leghorn cockerels.

Diazinon

A commercial thiophosphate insecticide ordinarily used for chicken premises proved highly toxic when used in a pen housing White Pekin ducklings (Dougherty, 1957). Diazinon was mixed at a level of 32 lb Diazinon 25W per 100 gal of spray according to the manufacturer's recommendations; 100% of the 1–2-week-old ducklings died 1 hour after exposure, and ducks 3–5 weeks of age suffered 75% mortality in 24 hours. In comparative toxicity studies on White Pekin ducks, the lethal oral dosage of Malathion was 1,100 mg/kg of body weight compared to 14 mg/kg of body weight for Diazinon. This points out the extreme toxicity of Diazinon; insecticides considered safe for chickens may be highly toxic for other species of birds.

SIGNS. Affected ducklings were unable to stand and manifested tremors of the head and neck. Microscopic pathology was limited to acute congestion of the lungs.

Malathion

Gaafar and Turk (1957) determined the LD_{50} of an organophosphorus insecticide (Malathion) for 3-week-old chickens to be 200–400 mg/kg of body weight and 150–200 mg for yearlings. If birds survived for 16 hours after dosing, they usually recovered. It was found that 4% Malathion was not toxic when chickens were dusted 4 times at weekly intervals. Golz and Shaffer (1955) reported that feeding 100–1,000 ppm Malathion in the mash for 10 weeks was nontoxic to chickens. Malathion at a level of 5,000 ppm or an average daily consumption of 450 mg/kg was decidedly toxic.

SIGNS. Chickens become sleepy, ataxic, and reluctant to move, resting on their hocks; and finally paralysis and death ensue. Stringy mucus hangs from the beak, cyanosis is evident, and a blood-tinged diarrhea may be seen. At no time do the birds show evidence of hyperexcitability, which may aid in making a differential diagnosis.

LESIONS. The heart is congested and darker than normal. The subcutaneous vessels are injected.

Parathion

One of the most toxic organophosphorus insecticides is parathion, and it should be used with utmost caution to avoid human or livestock poisoning. Dougherty (1962) relates two cases of poisoning in White Pekin ducks that were bedded on straw contaminated with parathion. Mortality started immediately and 126 ducks died within 30 minutes. McFarland and Lacy (1968) studied the pharmacological effect of parathion toxicity in mallard ducks (*Anas platyrhynchos*), pintail ducks (*Anas acuta*), and Japanese quail (*Coturnix coturnix japonica*). Intravenous toxic doses for the mallards were 0.61–1.70 mg parathion/kg body weight, for pintails 1.57–2.02 mg parathion, and for the quail 3.59–5.7 mg parathion. The birds died within 30 minutes to 2 hours postinjection.

SIGNS. Acute parathion poisoning caused these signs in the order of their appearance: increased salivation and lacrimation as indicated by varying amounts of foam and fluid dripping from the mouth and eyes; miosis; intermittent swallowing and gasping; clonic muscular convulsions associated with dyspnea; muscle tremors; ataxia; a tonic convulsion at time of death.

Tri-Ortho-Cresyl Phosphate (TOCP)

Although not used as an insecticide, tri-ortho-cresyl phosphate compounds have caused accidental poisoning in chickens. Hartwigk (1950) relates a fascinating account of an unexplainable lameness appearing in many flocks from the region of Saxony. After careful consideration of the histories, it was learned that most of the affected birds belonged to shoemakers. The causal relationship between the sick birds and the shoemakers became apparent when it was discovered that the shoemakers were using synthetic soles which contained Igelit, a plastic softened with TOCP. Scraps that were discarded by the cobblers were being eaten with fatal results by the chickens. In one instance all members of the family had synthetic soles, and large chunks were breaking off and being consumed by the birds.

SIGNS. Toxic signs were manifested after feeding 5 g Igelit (Hartwigk, 1950) or 1 ml TOCP/kg of body weight (Cavanagh,

1954). There is a latent period of 10–14 days after which the birds become ataxic, are reluctant to walk, rest on their keels or hocks, and finally become prostrate with legs outstretched similar to Marek's disease. During the initial stages the birds eat normally and may survive for several weeks.

LESIONS. Gross changes are absent; the primary microscopic lesions are in the peripheral nerves leading from the brachial and sciatic plexus and in the long tracts of the spinal cord. Cavanagh (1954) reported degeneration of axis cylinders and myelin sheaths.

METALS

LEAD

Commercial preparations of lead which may cause lead poisoning include the oxides and carbonates of lead, lead acetate, lead arsenate, and metallic lead. The oxides and carbonates are found in paints; lead acetate is used in industrial and medicinal products; lead arsenate is incorporated in orchard and garden sprays; metallic lead, especially in the form of spent shot, causes alarming losses in waterfowl. In an effort to decrease the losses in waterfowl, munitions manufacturers have attempted to manufacture shot from metals other than lead or to make lead alloys that would be less toxic. Irby et al. (1967) described the relative toxicity of lead and selected substitute shot for mallards. Plastic-coated lead shot were as toxic as commercial lead shot. The average mortality in mallards fed lead-magnesium alloy shot was about 50% less than the group fed plain lead. Mortality in mallards fed iron, copper, or zinc-coated iron or molybdenum-coated iron shot was not significantly greater than the controls.

Toxic Levels

Wetmore (1922) reported that the usual number of shot found in dead waterfowl was 15–40. Hanzlik and Presho (1923) observed clinical signs in pigeons 8–10 days after the introduction of lead shot directly into the crop. They estimated the minimum lethal dose of metallic lead to be 0.16 g/kg body weight. Coburn et al. (1951) determined the critical daily dosage of lead to be 6–8 mg/kg body weight when lead was given as an aqueous solution of lead nitrate. Birds survived about 4 weeks after dosing. McIntosh and Staples, quoted by Salisbury et al. (1958), failed to produce any signs or gross lesions of lead poisoning by feeding single massive doses of red lead and white lead in amounts up to 1,000 mg/kg body weight. Trainer and Hunt (1965a), in a survey of lead poisoning in whistling swans *(Olor columbianus)*, recovered 0–201 lead shot from the gizzards, with an average of 50 pellets per bird. Bagley et al. (1967) found 0–8 lead shot in Canada geese *(Branta canadensis)* dying from lead poisoning. The amount of lead in the liver ranged from 6 to 20 ppm wet weight. These levels were high enough to reflect lead intoxication on the basis of evidence given by Adler (1944) and Cook and Trainer (1966). Salisbury et al. (1958) reported lead poisoning in chicks caused by feeding a grit composed of "frit," an ingredient used in the manufacture of enamelware. Analysis of the "frit" revealed 32% lead oxide content. Levels of lead in the liver were above 10 ppm in the wet tissue. Rac and Crisp (1954) reported lead poisoning in domestic ducks; analysis of the liver revealed 60 ppm lead.

Natural Host

Most of the losses from lead poisoning occur in waterfowl, which may be a reflection of their eating habits rather than inherent susceptibility. Reports of lead poisoning in species other than waterfowl are as follows: guinea fowl (Costigan, 1940), White Leghorns (Salisbury et al., 1958), pigeons (Hanzlik and Presho, 1923), mourning doves *(Zenaidura macroura)* (Locke and Bagley, 1967), scaled quail *(Callipepla squamata)* (Campbell, 1950), and bobwhite quail *(Colinus virginianus)* (Westemeier, 1966).

Signs

Salisbury et al. (1958) reported 70% mortality in a flock of 600 2-week-old chicks. Apparently the chicks did not manifest any striking signs as none were reported. They conducted feeding trials with the toxic grit in adult White Leghorn hens and observed loss of weight, drop in egg production, and green diarrhea in the later stages. Costigan (1940) observed leg weakness and paralysis in poisoned guinea fowl.

Trainer and Hunt (1965a,b) observed green diarrhea, general weakness, prostration, and emaciation in whistling swans. Bagley et al. (1967) observed that Canada geese became emaciated, could barely fly, and emitted a striking high-pitched call. Cook and Trainer (1966) reported that lead poisoning signs in Canada geese were similar to those described for the mallard and included anorexia, weight loss, listlessness, weakness, and green diarrhea.

Gross Lesions

Salisbury et al. (1958) found severe necrosis of the gizzard lining and submucosal hemorrhage and edema in chickens. The birds had severe anemia, but there was no evidence of basophilic stippling.

Excellent descriptions of lead poisoning in Canada geese *(Branta canadensis)* were given by Cook and Trainer (1966) and Bagley et al. (1967). Necropsy findings included impaction of the proventriculus, roughened and greenish stained gizzard lining, edema of the head, discharge from the eyes and nares, severe enteritis, distended gall bladder, discolored liver, and flaccid heart (Fig. 33.6).

Histopathology and Clinical Findings

Key (1924) studied the blood changes in rabbits with lead poisoning and observed basophilic stippling of the red blood cells. Although this is an interesting phenomenon, its specificity and frequency are greatly overemphasized. Hass et al. (1964) state that man and rabbit are two species in which basophilic stippling of the red blood cells occurs. However, they further state that stippled cells in man rarely exceeds 1%. They also indicate that stippling in both species is not restricted to lead poisoning. This diminishes its diagnostic value.

Johns (1934) reported the stippling of red blood cells in ducks with lead poisoning. This pathological finding has not been described for other avian species. Coburn et al. (1951) indicated they were unable to find evidence of stippling in red blood cells in any avian species. They did find abnormally shaped erythrocytes which included dumbbell, bottle, oat, sickle, and teardrop forms. Enucleated erythrocytes may be found in blood smears from chickens with lead poisoning (Fig. 33.7). Punctate stippling of erythrocytes was not found in Canada geese or whistling swans

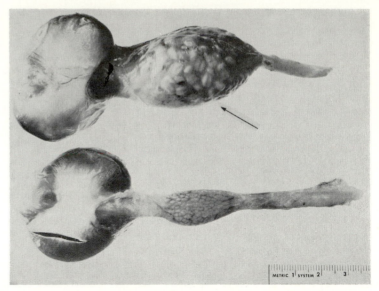

FIG. 33.6—Lead poisoning. Distended proventriculus in duck that had 15 lead shot in its gizzard.

(Trainer and Hunt, 1965b; Cook and Trainer, 1966).

Locke et al. (1966) made the highly significant observation that lead poisoning may produce acid-fast intranuclear inclusion bodies in the cells of the kidney tubules. Mallards *(Anas platyrhynchos)* given 1–8 #6 lead shot and fed grain developed intranuclear inclusion bodies, whereas no acid-fast inclusion bodies developed if a duck pellet ration was fed. The inclusion bodies were pale yellowish pink when stained with hematoxylin and eosin and exhibited a metallic sheen. When stained with the Ziehl-Neelsen technique the intranuclear inclusion bodies were reddish violet to scarlet in color and varied in size and shape, ranging from small discrete spheres 1–3μ in size to irregular bands 6 $\times$ 10μ in dimension (Fig. 33.8). In general, the size and number of inclusion bodies were dependent upon dosage and survival time after ingestion of lead. Locke and Bagley (1967) found acid-fast inclusion bodies in the kidney cells of a mourning dove *(Zenaidura macroura)*. The liver and tibia contained 72 ppm and 187 ppm lead respectively. The inclusion bodies were similar in

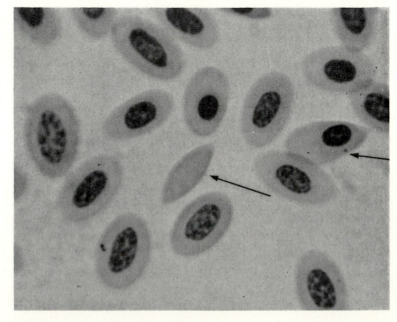

FIG. 33.7—Lead poisoning. Blood smear from chicken. Note enucleated, spindle-shaped erythrocyte and teardrop-shaped erythrocyte.

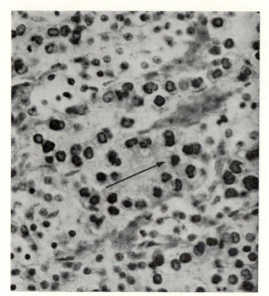

FIG. 33.8—*Lead poisoning. Acid-fast intranuclear inclusion bodies in kidney of mallard duck. ×480. (Courtesy L. N. Locke, Patuxent Wildlife Research Center, Laurel, Md.)*

staining reactions to those in mallards but differed in morphological characteristics. The inclusion bodies appeared as individual granules, flakes, or clumps of granules ranging in size from 0.5 to 3.5μ. Bagley et al. (1967) found acid-fast inclusion bodies in the kidneys of a Canada goose (*Branta canadensis*) afflicted with lead poisoning.

Cook and Trainer (1966) gave a detailed description of the histopathology of lead poisoning in Canada geese. Large quantities of brownish pigment were present in the hepatic cells and Kupffer cells. Kidney nephrosis consisted of degeneration, necrosis, and sloughing of tubular epithelium, with large amounts of brownish pigment in tubular epithelium cells. The heart had patchy myocardial necrosis associated with hyaline or fibrinoid necrosis of the blood vessels. Hyperemia and hemorrhages were regularly seen in the lungs. The pancreas had necroses of both acinar and islet tissues.

Diagnosis

Diagnosis of lead poisoning cannot be made upon finding lead particles in the gizzard contents. Neither can lead poisoning be eliminated as the cause of death by failure to find lead in the digestive tract. In arriving at a diagnosis the history, signs, and macroscopic lesions must be carefully considered. The lead content of the brain, liver, and tibia should be determined by the dithizone method (A.O.A.C. with the modifications by Snyder, 1947). High concentrations of lead in the liver usually indicate recent ingestion of lead, whereas high concentrations in the bone indicate chronic exposure. Histopathological studies should be conducted and the kidneys examined for the presence of acid-fast inclusion bodies. Positive findings have far greater significance than negative observations. Rosen and Bankowski (1960) described a diagnostic technique and treatment for lead poisoning in swans. They injected swans showing flaccid neck paralysis with 1.5 ml calcium versenate intravenously; within 24 hours the birds appeared normal. Calcium versenate is a chelating agent, and the lead replaces the calcium to form a soluble compound that is excreted. However, as the calcium versenate becomes depleted in the blood stream, more lead is resorbed into the vascular system and the paralysis reappears within 24 hours. This remission of signs was considered as additional evidence for a diagnosis of lead poisoning. These authors reported that the daily administration of 1.5 ml calcium versenate in the median wing vein eventually cured some swans of lead poisoning.

SELENIUM

Franke et al. (1934) reported that grains grown in certain areas of South Dakota were toxic for livestock. The so-called alkali disease was caused by toxic levels of selenium in the feed. Losses of livestock from selenium poisoning were reported by Moxon (1937). Studies at the South Dakota Experiment Station revealed that toxic grain fed at levels containing 15 ppm of selenium caused loss of body weight, marked reduction in egg size, and hatchability reduced to practically zero. Poley et al. (1937) found that 5 ppm of selenium in the diet did not significantly affect hatchability although some evidence of selenium poisoning was apparent.

PHOSPHORUS

The two most common forms of phosphorus are the yellow and red. The former is very active, oxidizing readily, being highly inflammable and extremely toxic. It is incorporated in suitable vehicles as poison baits for mice, rats, and other rodents. It is also used in the manufacture of matches and fireworks. Red phosphorus, an amorphous form, is relatively nontoxic. Occasionally birds will accidentally consume sufficient amounts of poison bait to produce a fatal toxemia. Turkeys on range may be poisoned by consuming fragments of firecrackers and fireworks which remain following holiday celebrations and pyrotechnic displays. Dissolved or finely divided phosphorus may be absorbed as such, absorption being facilitated by the emulsifying action of the bile. The absorbed phosphorus is eliminated principally through the lungs and kidneys. The toxic dose for fowls is 0.3 grain (Lander, 1926).

Signs

Signs include depression, anorexia, increased water consumption, diarrhea, ataxia, paralysis, coma, and death. Acute toxicity may cause sudden death without premonitory signs.

Lesions

In peracute cases there may not be any lesions, but fragments of the toxic material may be found in the digestive tract. Beaudette et al. (1933) reported that the characteristic odor of phosphorus, which smells like burnt matches, can be detected in the crop or gizzard contents. The author has detected phosphorus poisoning in chickens that ate rat poison by taking the crop contents into a totally black room where a characteristic luminescence was observed. In less acute cases gastroenteritis may be seen. Areas of necrosis may occur on the mucosa of the crop, proventriculus, and intestines. The liver is enlarged, congested, and friable. The kidneys show evidence of degeneration. Petechiae may be present in the serous surfaces and parenchymatous organs.

MYCOTOXINS

ERGOT

Ergot is the sclerotium of the fungus *Claviceps purpurea* which infects the seed-bearing heads of maturing rye and other grains (Fig. 33.9). In European countries where rye is commonly used as poultry feed, ergotism is frequently encountered. Ergot is unpalatable and will not be eaten if other feed is available. Trenchi (1962) reported a comparative study of the pathogenesis of *Ammi visnaga* and ergot.

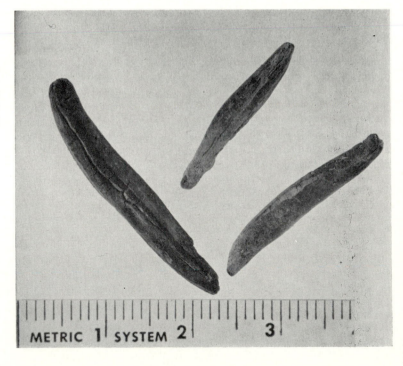

FIG. 33.9—Ergot. Black, hard, spindle-shaped masses are sclerotia fungus Claviceps purpurea *which infects seed of maturing rye.*

Signs

In acute ergot poisoning the comb is cold, wilted, and cyanotic. The birds are listless and do not eat but have an abnormal thirst accompanied by diarrhea. General debilitation is followed by convulsions, paralysis, and death.

Lesions

In chronic poisoning the comb, wattles, and toes may become black and necrotic followed by sloughing. Enteritis may be present in conjunction with degenerative changes in the heart, liver, and kidneys.

Treatment

Chickens will make a prompt recovery when placed on an ergot-free diet.

ASPERGILLUS FLAVUS
(BRAZILIAN GROUNDNUT POISONING)

In Great Britain during the spring and summer of 1960 over 500 cases of turkey "X" disease were diagnosed with an estimated loss of 100,000 turkeys (Blount, 1961). Most of the cases occurred within a radius of 100 miles of London. At first only turkeys were affected, but later sporadic cases were seen in ducklings and pheasants. At that time there were no reports of the disease in chickens. All efforts to isolate a causative agent or transmit the disease failed, and this led to the suspicion that the disease was caused by a toxin. Feed from affected farms was fed to experimental turkeys which succumbed with the same signs and lesions as the field cases. This observation by Blount (1961) pinpointed the source of the trouble as it was the first positive indication that proprietary feeds might be the cause. An intensive study was then conducted to determine the nature of the toxic substance in the feed. Examinations for many of the known poisons and toxins were negative. A careful summary of the first 50 outbreaks revealed that all the feed was manufactured at only one of two mills in London. Both mills were owned by the same company, and this raised the question as to why feed from one mill was toxic and not the other. Suddenly outbreaks of turkey "X" disease appeared in the Cheshire area, and the feed for this area was manufactured at Selby. It was quickly discovered that the common ingredient used between the Selby mill and the one

in London producing toxic feed was Brazilian groundnut meal. The feed company having the problem had purchased 5,000 tons of groundnut meal from Brazil for the first time shortly before turkey "X" disease began to appear.

During the period that losses were occurring in turkeys, Asplin and Carnaghan (1961) described a new syndrome in ducks. It was found that the protein source for these ducks was Brazilian groundnut, and feeding trials confirmed that this contained the toxic agent. Reports were received from Kenya and Uganda of severe losses in ducklings, and the signs and lesions were similar to those of ducks dying in Great Britain (Carnaghan and Sargeant, 1961). Extracts were prepared from samples of East Africa groundnut meal, and these proved to be highly toxic for ducklings. The toxicity of Brazilian groundnut meal for chickens was discovered when a group of experimental chicks were found to be stunted at 2 weeks of age. The feed contained 6.25% groundnut meal, and feeding trials substantiated that this ingredient was toxic.

Allcroft et al. (1961) demonstrated toxic activity in a two-step solvent extract from a peanut cake meal sample. Sargeant et al. (1961a) extracted the toxic factor in Brazilian nut meal and found it 250 times more concentrated than the original meal. By dosing young ducklings, they determined that this was a rapid and sensitive method for testing the toxicity of groundnut meals. In a continuation of the studies by Sargeant et al. (1961b), it was suspected that the toxic substance might be a fungal metabolite, as a highly toxic sample of nuts from Uganda which had been associated with the death of ducklings in Kenya was seen to be heavily contaminated with fungi.

Pure cultures of 8 fungal species in this sample were produced on Czapek's agar and extracted with chloroform. The extract from one of these was shown to contain a fluorescent material, Rf 0.7 in *n*-butanol 5% acetic acid. These extracts were given to groups of day-old ducklings, and those receiving the fluorescent extract died and had histologic lesions in the liver typical of toxic groundnut poisoning. The single toxin-producing fungus was grown on heat sterilized, nontoxic groundnuts. Extracts from the grossly moldy nuts were shown to contain the blue fluorescent material and to be lethal for day-old ducklings with the production of lesions typical for groundnut poisoning. The toxin-producing fungus was identified as *Aspergillus flavus* Link ex Fries.

De Iongh et al. (1964) indicated that toxin-containing extracts of either groundnut meals or *Aspergillus flavus* cultures can be resolved by thin layer chromatography into several zones which are fluorescent when viewed under ultraviolet light. Administration to ducklings of extracts of the fluorescent spots showed that at least two substances were toxic to ducklings and that although the toxin is more concentrated in a fraction B_1, the combined fractions B_1 and B_2 apparently exert greater toxicity. Another report by Nesbitt et al. (1962) confirmed that extracts of groundnut meal or cultures of *A. flavus* contained at least two toxic components, viz. B(C17 H12 06) and G(C17 H12 07), the former being approximately 3 times more toxic than the latter.

In addition to the identification of aflatoxin in peanut oil cake meal from 13 producing countries, it has been demonstrated in maize meal and in cottonseed oil cake meal. Richmond et al. (1962) isolated toxin-producing strains of *Aspergillus flavus* from the litter and dust of poultry houses. Extracts from the substrate on which these fungi were grown produced toxicosis when fed to ducklings. This points out the possibility that aflatoxicosis may occur not only from imported products but by indigenous strains of *Aspergillus flavus* growing on toxigenic substrates. Not all strains of an *Aspergillus* species are toxigenic, and under various environmental conditions the toxigenic potential may not be expressed. Aspergilli are predominantly storage fungi, and only rarely can plant products be infected prior to harvest. Peanuts can be infected and toxin demonstrated within 48 hours of reaping. Moisture or high humidity will exacerbate *Aspergillus* infection and resultant toxicity. Blount (1961) records that the outbreak attributed to the Brazilian peanut oil cake meal was associated with the wet season crop.

Economic and Public Health Significance

An area requiring more detailed examination is that of the possibility of toxicity in man following consumption of meat or products derived from animals fed diets containing aflatoxin. Allcroft and Carnaghan (1963) reported that cows fed toxic groundnut meal excreted in the milk a toxic factor having a biological effect in ducklings similar to that caused by aflatoxin. The toxic factor was not found in the cow's liver or in eggs from hens fed toxic groundnut meal. In support of this finding Van der Linde et al. (1964) demonstrated excretion of aflatoxin in milk from cows receiving 8 mg of aflatoxin B_1 daily. However, Brown and Abrams (1965) were unable to produce aflatoxicosis in ducklings fed diets containing milk and eggs obtained from cows and hens fed highly toxic rations. Lancaster et al. (1961) noted the development of hepatomas in rats fed Brazilian groundnut meal. Newberne (1964) reported a high incidence of hepatocellular carcinomas induced in rats fed aflatoxin-contaminated peanut meal grown and processed in the United States. Ubiquitous toxigenic *Aspergillus* species capable of growing under a variety of environmental conditions represent a serious threat to animals and public health and to the economic stability of many tropical agricultural areas.

Natural Hosts

Young turkey poults, ducklings, and pheasants have succumbed in field outbreaks (Blount, 1961). Archibald et al. (1962) described Brazilian groundnut toxicosis in broiler chickens reared in Canada. Losses in poults usually occur at 2–4 weeks of age but may persist up to 16 weeks of age.

Signs

In turkeys there is a gradual loss of appetite, and the birds have a tendency to eat litter. The birds are lethargic, the wings droop, and the feathers are ruffled and broken. Occasionally nervous signs are present, and the birds may exhibit opisthotonus and die with the legs rigidly extended backwards. Losses of 50–90% are not uncommon (Blount, 1961).

Ducklings are more susceptible to aflatoxin than turkeys, pheasants, or chickens, and this sensitivity makes them the bird of choice when testing feed for toxicity. Blount et al. (1963) in feeding trials determined that Khaki Campbell ducklings were more sensitive to aflatoxin than Penines. In field outbreaks there may be an interval of 2 weeks between the feeding of toxic groundnut meal and the onset of mortality. At first there is decreased feed intake and poor growth. A conspicuous change sometimes observed in young white-skinned ducklings is lameness and purple discoloration of feet and legs caused by subcutaneous hemorrhage. Young ducklings develop ataxia followed by convulsions shortly before death and die in opisthotonus. Ducklings are most susceptible to aflatoxin at approximately 0.75 ppm in the ration (Brown and Abrams, 1965).

A striking feature of the outbreaks in chickens in South Africa was the susceptibility of the New Hampshire breed, whereas White Rocks, White Leghorns, and Rhode Island Reds consuming the same feed grew normally (Brown and Abrams, 1965). Chickens have depressed weight gains when fed toxic peanut meal but experience little or no mortality.

Lesions

Siller and Ostler (1961) described the gross and microscopic lesions in turkeys. The carcasses were congested and there was general slight edema. Livers were congested, enlarged, and very firm. The gall bladder was distended. The kidneys were swollen and congested. The myocardium was congested, and amber-colored fluid distended the pericardial sac. Catarrhal enteritis was present in the duodenum. Blount (1961) reported hemorrhages and pale necrotic lesions in the liver.

Asplin and Carnaghan (1961) described the gross and microscopic lesions in ducklings and chickens. The lesions in ducklings vary according to survival time and age of the birds. In newly hatched ducklings dying within a week from aflatoxicosis, the liver is gray and enlarged. The kidneys are pale, swollen, and have a few petechiae. Petechiae are present in the pancreas. In ducklings surviving to 3 weeks of age the liver changes become more pronounced. A pale reticulated network is seen throughout the liver substance, and this is associated with atrophy and cirrhosis. Hydropericardium and ascites may be present although never severe. Petechiae are present in the kidneys and pancreas.

In older ducklings which generally survive for longer periods, the cirrhosis is more marked and eventually progresses to the stage of nodular hyperplasia. Hydro-

pericardium and ascites may be pronounced. Petechiae may occur in the pancreas, and more diffuse hemorrhages may be in the kidneys. The kidneys may be swollen, but this feature is not as prominent as in turkeys. A gelatinous subcutaneous transudate may be present in older ducklings which have survived for a long period. A distinctive and almost pathognomonic lesion in older birds is severe subcutaneous hemorrhage in the shank and web of the foot causing a purplish discoloration in white-skinned birds.

Asplin and Carnaghan (1961) and Carnaghan et al. (1966) have described the biochemical and pathological aspects of groundnut poisoning in chickens. After 3 weeks on an experimental diet containing an aflatoxin B_1 content of 1.5 ppm, the livers were enlarged and gray with a reticulated network. The consistency was soft and petechial hemorrhages were present. Thereafter, there was a reduction in size of the liver with increasing firmness of texture until the 7th week when well-defined, raised nodular lesions were seen on the surface. Diffuse white pinhead-sized foci were visible from the 6th week. Archibald et al. (1962) noted that kidneys were enlarged and pale and had a fine network of urate deposits.

Histopathology

The histopathology of turkey "X" disease was described in detail by Siller and Ostler (1961) and Wannop (1961). With hematoxylin and eosin stain the parenchymal cells were swollen and had a homogeneous eosinophilic appearance and were occasionally vacuolated. The large vesicular nuclei with marginated chromatin had prominent spherical nucleoli. There was diffuse necrosis of nearly all the perisinusoidal regions. These areas were characterized by cell debris, karyorrhexis, and karyolysis. Early lesions were degenerative, and these were replaced by groups of regenerating liver cells in advanced cases. The groups of regenerating cells were basophilic, often containing large vacuoles, sometimes multinucleated and arranged as distinct tubules. The bile ducts were hyperplastic. At this stage small groups of lymphocytes, blast cells, and occasional plasma cells and fibroblasts could be seen.

In the kidneys only the glomeruli and proximal convoluted tubules were signifi-

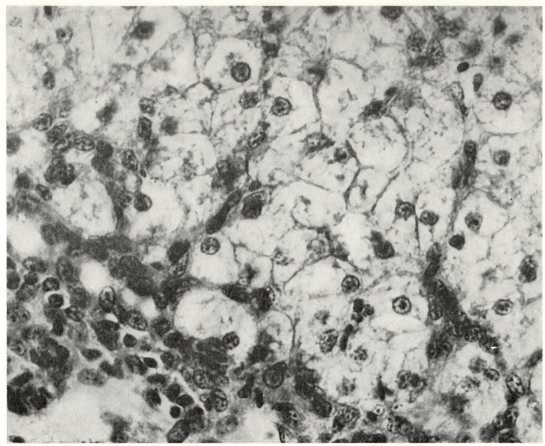

FIG. 33.10—Aflatoxicosis. Early liver lesion from duck fed toxic peanut meal. Degenerative changes in liver parenchyma and bile duct hyperplasia. H & E, ×1,000. (Courtesy P. N. Newberne, Mass. Inst. Technol.)

cantly changed. In the glomeruli a pronounced thickening of the capillary basement membrane was seen. The membranes were dense and stained deeply with P.A.S. (Periodic-Acid-Schiff). Ischemia was evident in the most severely affected glomeruli, and P.A.S.-positive spherical granules were seen in Bowman's capsule. In sections stained with P.A.S. tubular lesions when present were striking but sparsely distributed. The epithelium of the proximal convoluted tubules was swollen and the cytoplasm was completely filled by P.A.S.-positive hyaline droplets.

Newberne et al. (1964) reported on the histopathology of ducklings fed toxic peanut meal and aflatoxin. After 1 week the liver and parenchymal cells were swollen and the cytoplasm was granular and eosinophilic. The more degenerate cells were shrunken and deeply eosinophilic, and the cytoplasm was homogeneous. The nuclei of the liver cells were enlarged, the nucleolus was prominent, and mitosis was evident. Birds killed after 10 days had marked cytoplasmic vacuolization of hepatic cells and proliferation of bile duct epithelium in the periportal zone (Fig. 33.10). A concomitant alteration was the formation of hepatic cells into cylindrical ductlike structures with a centrally placed lumen. After 17 days on experiment, bile duct hyperplasia was more pronounced and widespread with the ductular epithelium radiating from the periportal zone toward the centrolobular area. After 4 weeks on the diet, widespread nodular hyperplasia of the parenchyma was present and regenerative areas were separated by numerous bands of proliferating bile duct epithelium arranged in

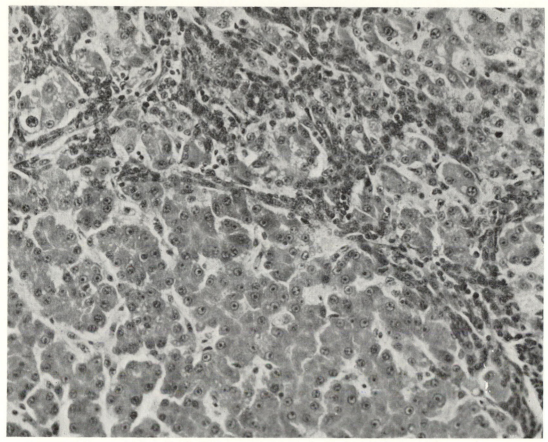

FIG. 33.11—*Aflatoxicosis. Liver from duck fed toxic peanut meal. Nodular hyperplasia of liver parenchyma and bile duct hyperplasia are present. H & E, ×398. (Courtesy P. N. Newberne, Mass. Inst. Technol.)*

parallel rows, single cell groups, or cylindrical ductules (Fig. 33.11). Asplin and Carnaghan (1961) reported that multiple and diffuse hemorrhages in the interstitial tissue of the kidneys are a constant feature but the glomerular changes which were described in turkeys (Siller and Osler, 1961) are not seen in ducklings. Newberne et al. (1964) reported the most striking change was the presence of large bizarre nuclei in the tubular epithelium (Fig. 33.12). In the pancreas diffuse areas of acinar degeneration are invariably present.

In chickens retrogressive and regenerative parenchymal changes in the liver occur similar to those in turkeys (Asplin and Carnaghan, 1961). The cells are not as basophilic as those in ducklings. Between 3 and 4 months of age lymphoid hyperplasia occurs in those areas where regenerative cells are still active. Polymorphonuclear leuko-

cytes and lymphocytes are present around the portal tracts.

Acinar degeneration of the pancreas occurs, and the renal changes are similar to those in ducklings.

Diagnosis

A presumptive diagnosis of aflatoxin poisoning in turkeys and ducklings could be made on the basis of a typical history and characteristic gross and histological lesions. Confirmation by biological testing of the suspect feed should be performed by feeding it to day-old ducklings. In addition, samples of the feed should be analyzed by chromatography for the detection of aflatoxin. Feed and feed ingredients should be sampled at the feed mill, as *Aspergillus flavus* is a common contaminant and production of toxin in the feed could occur in the storage bins on the poultry farm.

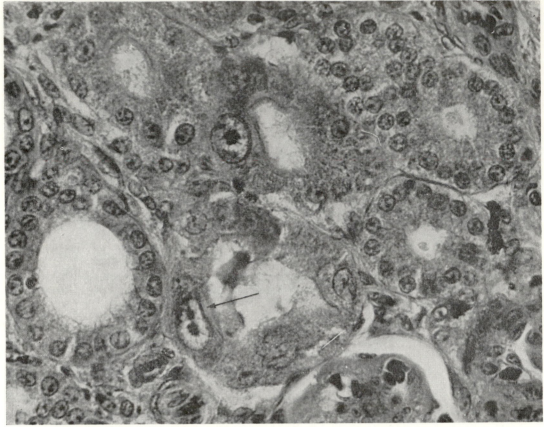

FIG. 33.12—Aflatoxicosis. Kidney from duck fed toxic peanut meal. Proximal tubules are dilated, epithelium is undergoing necrosis, and some nuclei have enlarged bizarre form with prominent nucleoli. H & E, ×1,000. (Courtesy P. N. Newberne, Mass. Inst. Technol.)

Treatment

It has been observed that poultry make a rapid recovery if the source of aflatoxin is removed from the diet. Medication is not deemed necessary.

PHYTOTOXINS

Phytotoxins may be considered as any toxic substance derived from plants, including the roots, stems, leaves, flowers, and seeds. The seeds and foliage are the plant structures most often consumed by birds. Some plants are toxic throughout the entire growing season; others are toxic only during certain stages of development. Most toxic plants are unpalatable and ordinarily not eaten by birds.

BLACK LOCUST

Barnes (1921) reported the leaves of the black locust *(Robinia pseudoacacia)* were toxic during July and early August and caused mortality in fowls after being eaten. Signs in toxic birds are depression and paralysis, with death ensuing in 12–24 hours. The principal lesion is a severe hemorrhagic enteritis.

CORN COCKLE

The corn cockle *(Argostemma githago)* is a weed commonly found in wheat fields throughout the world. The seeds of this plant are highly toxic but very unpalatable and rarely eaten by birds in their original state. The seeds are harvested accidentally with the wheat and become incorporated in poultry feeds. Quigley and Waite (1931) found the toxic dose to be about 0.2% of the body weight and the lethal dose 0.25%. Heuser and Schumacher (1942) reported that 5% of the ration or 0.3% of the body weight was toxic for 8-week-old chickens.

The birds developed a tolerance to the toxin, and 0.5% of the body weight could be consumed without affecting growth. Ten percent corn cockle in the ration was lethal to some of the fowls. Bierer and Rhodes (1960) fed a ration containing 5% corn cockle to 7-week-old chickens for 6 weeks without ill effect. They concluded that under routine methods of preparing poultry rations there appeared to be little danger of poisoning from corn cockle.

Signs

There is a marked decrease in respiration and heart rate. Diarrhea is present.

Lesions

Caseous exudate adheres to the mucosa of the pharynx and crop. Hydropericardium and edema of the intestine is present. Petechiae are present in the myocardium. Congestion and degeneration are common liver lesions.

COTTONSEED MEAL

Gossypol, a phenolic compound present in cottonseed meal, is toxic for birds and mammals. Cottonseed meal is used as a protein supplement and if properly used in a mixed grain ration is a valuable and economical protein supplement. Kaupp (1933) observed that toxic signs were readily produced in birds consuming 1 oz cottonseed meal daily or its equivalent in gossypol. Clinical signs were cyanosis, loss of appetite, and emaciation. Death ensued within a few days after the onset of signs. Lesions included enteritis and degeneration of the liver and kidneys.

COYOTILLO

Losses in poultry from the consumption of the fruit and seed of the coyotillo plant (*Karwinskia humboldtiana*) were reported by Marsh et al. (1928). The plant is indigenous to Texas and Mexico. The onset of clinical signs may occur from several days to 3 weeks after ingestion of the seed. The toxic dose for chickens was 0.3% or more of the bird's weight, fed as dried fruit or seed. Signs of generalized toxemia are followed by paralysis and death.

CACAO

Black and Barron (1943) reported the effect of feeding cacao waste from the cacao bean (*Theobroma cacao*) to poultry. The product consisted primarily of the cacao shell, and the theobromine content was 1.7%. Incorporation of 7% of the cacao product in the ration did not cause any adverse effect, but levels of 15% or higher were toxic. Signs of toxicity were depressed appetite, decreased egg production, diarrhea, and mortality after several months.

CROTALARIA SEED

Although crotalaria seed was shown to be toxic for chickens, quail, and doves by Thomas (1934), livestock poisoning did not become a serious problem until the introduction of mechanical harvesters for corn and soybeans coupled with increased use of crotalaria in the Southeast to supplement the humus and nitrogen content of the soil (Kelley et al., 1961).

Toxic Species

Smith and Osborne (1962) reported that of the many species of crotalaria, only a few are toxic for poultry. *Crotalaria spectabilis* is one of the most toxic species; *C. giant striata* is also toxic (Kelley et al., 1961); and Emmel (1937b) found *C. retusa* toxic for chickens. The small seeds are black or greenish brown with a smooth glossy surface and a characteristic mitten shape (Fig. 33.13). Extracts prepared from seeds, leaves, and stems of *C. spectabilis* contained a principal toxic for chickens and other species

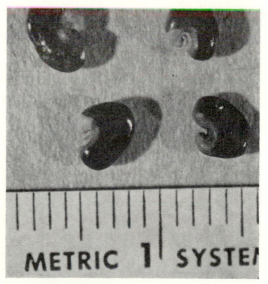

FIG. 33.13—Crotalaria spectabilis *seeds. Note smooth glossy seed coat and mitten-shaped appearance.* ×4.

(Thomas et al., 1935). An alkaloid, designated monocrotaline, was isolated from the extracts (Neal et al., 1935). The molecular formula of monocrotaline was reported by Adams and Rogers (1939).

Toxic Levels

Bierer et al. (1960) reported 0.2 lb *Crotalaria spectabilis* seeds per ton of feed (0.01%) was toxic for chickens. A 1% level of the seeds in the ration of day-old chicks caused 100% mortality in 4 weeks (Kelley et al., 1961). Caylor and Laurent (1961) reported a level of 0.05% *C. spectabilis* fed to laying birds for 4 weeks depressed production and had a pronounced effect after 6 weeks. At a 0.1% level, production practically ceased after 6 weeks. Harms et al. (1963) confirmed the adverse effect of *Crotalaria sp.* on egg production but reported the inclusion of 64 *C. spectabilis* seeds in each pound of feed did not cause mortality when fed to pullets for 9 weeks. Allen (1963) fed 1% *C. spectabilis* to 4-week-old turkey poults; 100% died during the 3rd and 4th weeks. A level of 0.5% crotalaria caused 40% mortality.

Signs

Poisoning may occur in acute or chronic form, terminating fatally in 1 day or several months. Chicks are droopy and inactive with ruffled feathers. The birds tend to huddle, and feed consumption decreases. Growth is retarded and the birds are stunted and inactive (Fig. 33.14). Ascites cause the chicks to manifest a ducklike attitude when walking. In layers the comb and wattles are pale and egg production declines with a corresponding increase in mortality. One of the first signs in turkey poults is a change in the color of the urates from a cream color to a bright greenish yellow (Allen, 1963).

Lesions

In chickens the type and severity of the lesions depend on duration of exposure to the toxin and age of the birds. Young birds have subcutaneous edema and ascites. Hydropericardium may be present but is not a consistent lesion. In the acute form the liver is swollen and mahogany colored. In chronic cases the liver is atrophied and cirrhotic (Fig. 33.15). Mature birds die suddenly from a ruptured liver (Allen et al., 1960). Nephritis and mottling of the liver is evident. Emmel (1937a) reported petechiae in the serous membranes and visceral fat (Fig. 33.16). Simpson et al. (1963) found thickening of the pericardium and air sacs in pullets fed crotalaria-contaminated diets for 9 weeks. The lungs were edematous and the proventriculus was thickened. The livers were either dark and swollen or atrophied, knobby, and grayish tan. The spleens were swollen and pulpy.

Simpson et al. (1963) reported the most prominent lesions in turkey poults were focal or diffuse hemorrhages on the surface of the liver and extending into the parenchyma. There were hemorrhages on the epicardium and in the pectoral muscles. Rupture of the capsule of the liver with subsequent acumulation of blood in the abdominal cavity was noted by Allen (1963). He also noted hydropericardium, hydrothorax, pulmonary edema, and ascites

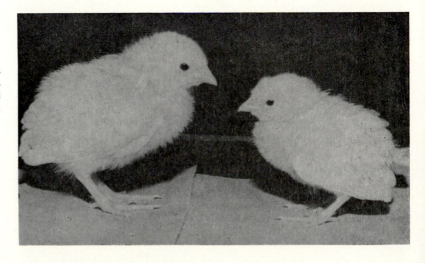

FIG. 33.14—Crotalaria spectabilis poisoning. Note stunting of chick on right compared with normal chick on left.

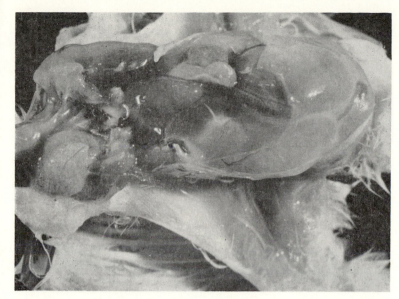

FIG. 33.15—Crotalaria spectabilis *poisoning in 2-week-old chick. Visible lobe of liver is yellow and atrophied; other lobe is covered by ascitic fluid.*

in poults surviving longer than 35 days on the toxic diet. Blood clotting time was markedly increased, averaging 25 minutes for the group fed 1% crotalaria compared to 5 minutes for the controls.

Histopathology

Crotalaria spectabilis causes extensive liver lesions. Details were given by Kelley et al. (1961) and Simpson et al. (1963).

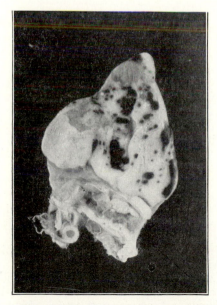

FIG. 33.16—*Hemorrhages of epicardium and myocardium in acute* Crotalaria spectabilis *seed poisoning in chicken. (Emmel, 1937a)*

There is a fibrous thickening of the liver capsule and vacuolation or granular degeneration of the hepatic cells. Productive tissue changes are present in the region of the portal triad associated with the bile duct hyperplasia and increased connective tissue. Swollen endothelial cells and subendothelial edema cause occlusion of the small branches of the portal veins. Allen et al. (1963) reported that a 0.25% level of *C. spectabilis* in the diet caused hydropic degeneration, necrosis, and eventual cirrhosis in the livers of growing turkeys. The kidneys may have interstitial edema, dilatation of Bowman's space, and hyaline casts in some tubules. In the spleen there is a depletion of the splenic corpuscles and necrosis of persistent germinal centers. Occasionally there is a lymphocytic interstitial myocarditis and separation of myocardial fibers by edema. Hypoplasia of the bone marrow is found in chicks.

Diagnosis

The gross and microscopic lesions of crotalaria poisoning in young birds are not sufficiently pathognomonic for a positive diagnosis. Tissues from affected birds and the suspected feed sample can be analyzed for the presence of monocrotaline, the toxic alkaloid in *Crotalaria spectabilis* seed. In acute cases of poisoning the presence of the characteristic mitten-shaped seeds in the crop or gizzard will aid in diagnosis.

The lesions produced by crotalaria poisoning in young birds are similar to those produced by "toxic fat," salt poisoning, cresol poisoning, and transudative diathesis caused by selenium and vitamin E deficiency. The diagnosis of these diseases is discussed under their respective headings.

DAUBENTONIA SEEDS

The Daubentonia *(Daubentonia longifolia)*, also called the Sesbania, is native to Mexico but was introduced to the southern states as an ornamental shrub. The seeds of this plant are readily eaten by poultry and are extremely toxic. According to Shealy and Thomas (1928), the ingestion of as few as 9 seeds will cause death in birds. The first clinical sign observed is a staggering gait, accompanied by drooping of the wings. Depression, general debility, and unthriftiness soon become apparent. The comb becomes cyanotic, and the head may hang to one side. Muscular twitching, diarrhea, emaciation, and extreme weakness are followed by death in 24–72 hours after appearance of the first symptoms. The lesions include severe gastroenteritis with ulceration of the proventriculus and gizzard, together with degenerative changes of the liver.

DEATH CAMAS

The death camas belongs to the genus *Zygadenus*. Members of this genus generally conceded to be poisonous are *Z. glaberrimus, Z. intermedius, Z. mexicanus, Z. nuttallii, Z. paniculatus,* and *Z. venenosus* (Marsh et al., 1915). Niemann (1928) reported a case of poisoning in the domestic fowl due to *Z. nuttallii*. The plant is not palatable and is only eaten by birds on the range in early spring and late fall when other green feed is scarce. When 5–10 g were fed to chickens, clinical signs were apparent in 12 hours. Salivation, incoordination, muscular weakness, and diarrhea were followed by prostration and death. Specific lesions were not reported.

GLOTTIDIUM SEED

Glottidium vesicarium (Jacq.) Harper is quite common along the coastal plain from North Carolina to Florida and Texas, having been introduced from the West Indies. The seeds of this plant are toxic for poultry. Under ordinary conditions fowl do not select these seeds as food, but if underfed they may consume sufficient quantities to be toxic. Emmel (1935) produced toxic effects by experimental feeding of *G. vesicarium* seeds to fowl. The clinical signs in acute poisoning are prostration and cyanotic appearance of comb and wattles accompanied by diarrhea. In chronic cases the feathers become ruffled, copious yellow diarrhea persists, and the birds may become emaciated. The combs appear light in color and become scaly. The most characteristic lesions include necrotic enteritis, necrotic areas in the lining of the gizzard, and degenerative changes in the liver and kidneys.

GELSEMIUM SEMPERVIRENS

Williamson et al. (1964) reported on the effect of feeding *Gelsemium sempervirens* (yellow jassamine) to young chickens and turkeys. The toxicity of *G. sempervirens* is caused by alkaloids that affect motor nerve endings. Ten percent *G. sempervirens* in the ration caused a marked depression of growth rate during the 1st week, but the rate returned to normal by the 4th week. Histopathologic examinations of selected tissues were negative, and the birds did not show signs of paralysis. Under the conditions of the experiment, *G. sempervirens* was not very toxic for chicks or poults, but because of depressed weight gain it is not advisable to range turkeys on areas where *G. sempervirens* is growing.

VETCH

The common vetch *Vicia satvia*, L. var. *Willamette* and hairy vetch *Vicia villosa*, var. *glabrescens* Koch are grown extensively in Oregon and other states as seed crops and may contaminate other cereal grain crops unless destroyed by chemical sprays. Vetches belong to the family Leguminosae and are related to the legumes Lathyrus, Pisum, and Ervum. Lathyrism refers to the degenerative process of the spinal cord which occurs in animals and humans fed one of the related legumes, and odoratism is used to describe the skeletal and vascular lesions induced in animals by *Lathyrus odoratus*. Stockman (1931) regarded early reports of lathyrism in birds showing nervous signs following the use of Lathyrus peas as controversial. Anderson et al. (1925) indicated that the seed of *Lathyrus sativus* is not toxic. Horvath (1945) reported that the vetchling *Lathyrus cicera* when comprising the entire ration seemed to exert a toxic effect on hens causing a loss of weight. Harper and Arscott (1962) reported that the seed of common vetch *Vicia sativa* was toxic and lethal for poults and chicks when it comprised 20–40% of the ration; 30% of the vetch in the feed caused 70% mortality in poults and 100% in chicks within 1–4 weeks after administration. Affected poults and chicks exhibited excitability, muscular incoordination, respiratory distress, and violent convulsions terminating in death. Autoclaving the ground vetch seed at 15 psi for 8 hours reduced its toxicity. The seed of hairy vetch *Vicia villosa* was less toxic for poults and chicks. Ressler (1962) isolated β-cyano-L-alanine from seeds of *Vicia angustifolia* and *Vicia sativa* and determined its identity by a comparison of its physical, chemical, and biological properties with the synthetic product, a neuroactive amino acid.

MILKWEED

Two of our common species of milkweed, *Asclepias tuberosa* and *A. incarnata,* contain the bitter glucoside asclepidin, which apparently is toxic to animals and birds. Pammel (1911) includes *A. vestita* and *A. mexicana* in the list of toxic species of the milkweed family. Campbell (1931) reported serious losses in poultry caused by consumption of the narrow-leaved, whorled milkweed *A. mexicana*. Experimental investigations indicated that all parts of the plant are toxic. Pammel (1917) reported milkweed poisoning in chickens resulting in the loss of approximately 500 birds. Stiles (1942) reported extensive losses in turkey poults resulting from consumption of whorled milkweed *Asclepias galioides*. Poultry as well as other species of livestock are not likely to eat milkweed except when it is the only succulent feed available.

Clinical signs may vary considerably, depending on the quantity of the toxic material eaten. The first sign observed was lameness which developed rapidly into complete loss of muscular control. The neck became twisted and the head drawn back. The affected birds often lay on their sternums or sat on their hocks, alternately extending and retracting their heads at frequent intervals. This condition did not seem to be a true paralysis but appeared to be an overstimulation of the motor nerve centers with complete loss of coordination. At times the birds would fall over and struggle, with violent convulsive movements of the legs. In some instances the signs gradually subsided, followed by recovery. In fatal cases the signs became progressively worse, followed by prostration, coma, and death. No characteristic lesions were found upon necropsy.

NIGHTSHADE

The black nightshade *(Solanum nigrum)* is a common weed in yards and poor pasture land. The immature fruit of this plant contains the alkaloids solanin and solanidin which are toxic to man and animals. The toxicity of the plants is believed to be influenced by the soil, climate, and degree of plant maturity. Hansen (1925) reported fatal poisoning in chickens and ducks attributed to black nightshade. The clinical signs include incoordination, prostration, paralysis, and death. The pupils of the eyes may be dilated. No characteristic lesions are reported except evidence of severe toxemia.

POTATOES

Under certain conditions the potato *(Solanum tuberosum)* is poisonous to domesticated animals and poultry. Greened tubers (produced by exposure to light) and young potato sprouts contain considerable amounts of the alkaloid solanin which is highly toxic. Analyses have shown that the solanin content of the sprouts and peelings is higher than that of the interior of the tuber. Hansen (1927) reported several outbreaks of poisoning in poultry resulting from ingestion of potato sprouts. Losses ocurred within a few hours after consumption of the toxic sprouts. Temperton (1944) reported losses in ducks as the result of eating either cooked or uncooked sprouted potatoes. This type of poisoning is similar to that of poisoning by other plants of the nightshade family. However, where large amounts of potatoes are fed to poultry, it is advisable as a safety measure to cook green or sprouted potatoes and to discard the residual water. From the standpoint of nutrition, raw potato starch is poorly digested by poultry, and cooking will result in a more efficient utilization of this type of feed.

LILY OF THE VALLEY AND OLEANDER

The flowers, leaves, and stems of the lily of the valley *(Convallaria majalis)* and the leaves of the oleander (*Nerium oleander*) were reported by Bardosi (1939) to be poisonous for geese, ducks, and hens. The lily of the valley flowers were found to be lethal to geese in doses of 13 g and to ducks in doses of 12 g. Doses of 30 g produced only a mild enteritis in mature chickens.

The dried leaves of the oleander plant of the previous season's growth proved fatal to geese in 24 hours after the ingestion of 6 g. The lethal dose for ducks was found to be 3 g. The young leaves of this plant proved fatal to hens in doses of 15 g.

McNeil and Denny (1939), quoted by Hinshaw (1965), were able to kill 4-week-old poults by inserting leaves of oleander sprouts into the crop. The poults died in 24 hours and had a severe hemorrhagic enteritis at necropsy. Three adult turkeys were fed succulent oleander shoots mixed with grain for 2 weeks but the birds refused to eat them.

The clinical signs of oleander poisoning include general depression, weakness, diarrhea, accelerated heart rate, impaired vision, muscular incoordination, and in some instances paralysis of the wings. Various degrees of gastroenteritis and liver degeneration occur in fatal cases.

TOBACCO

The tobacco plant (*Nicotiana tobacum* L.) contains the toxic alkaloid nicotine. Hunter and Haley (1931) and Hunter et al. (1934) reported chicks over 3 weeks of age can tolerate as much as 0.06% nicotine in the ration without any toxic reaction. The feeding of the same nicotine levels in the form of ground cigar clippings having only 0.86% nicotine content retarded the growth and development of chicks, causing some losses. Toxic doses of tobacco produce similar reactions to those of nicotine sulfate poisoning.

ALGAE

Certain types of algae, including *Microcystis aeruginosa* which grows abundantly in lakes under certain conditions, may become concentrated in localized areas by the action of strong winds blowing the surface of the water in one direction for a number of days. Great quantities of algae are deposited on the banks and in shallow waters along the shore line. The disintegration of this material produces toxins which are responsible for the loss of various species of wildlife as well as domesticated animals and birds. This condition has frequently been called "water bloom." Fitch et al. (1934) reported losses of livestock from this cause in Minnesota. Brandenburg and Shigley (1947) reported this condition in North Dakota. It has also been reported in northern Iowa and in parts of Canada. It usually occurs in the latter part of July, August, and September. The exact nature of the toxin is not known at the present time. Apparently the toxin is an intermediate product of disintegration, as these toxic properties disappear during later stages of decomposition.

The toxicity of this material is directly proportional to the concentration. Some waters taken from the shores of lakes are extremely toxic to birds and animals. Under experimental conditions oral dosages of 10–30 cc will produce death in mature ducks and chickens in 10–45 minutes. The toxin is thermostable and is affected little if any by boiling. The signs include restlessness, twitching of muscles, nervous manifestations, spasms, convulsions, paralysis, and death. These clinical manifestations resemble strychnine poisoning in many respects. The postmortem lesions include generalized cyanosis; dark, tar-colored blood; liver congested and dark in color; heart dilated and distended; muscles also congested and dark in color. No characteristic hemorrhages are observed. Ashworth and Mason (1946) described in detail the signs and lesions associated with algae poisoning in laboratory animals.

Because of the highly toxic nature of this material and the rapidity with which it acts, there are no therapeutic measures effective. Poultry should be restricted to areas free from toxic material.

Nontoxic algae may be responsible for considerable losses in young chickens. Mature birds are seldom affected, but young chicks which wade out along the shore line and feed on insects alighting on the floating scum or masses of algae invariably swallow various amounts of this material. This scum becomes lodged in the nostrils and digestive and respiratory passages, causing strangulation and suffocation. Postmortem examination reveals obstruction of the nostrils and respiratory passages as well as those of the digestive tract.

Losses of poultry associated with the ingestion of algae should be investigated at once. The toxicity of algae can be determined readily by injecting 2 ml or more of a sample filtered through gauze intraperitoneally into laboratory animals or chickens. Toxic material will produce typical symptoms in a short time and death within an hour or so. A prompt determination of toxicity may prevent serious losses to all species of livestock.

RODENTICIDES

ALPHA NAPHTHYL THIOUREA

This rodenticide, commonly known as ANTU, is highly toxic for domestic animals and poultry. Anderson and Richter (1946) reported that 3–5-week-old chicks showed toxic signs and mortality within 24 hours after being fed 3% ANTU in the mash. Those surviving after 24 hours recovered if given untreated feed.

Signs

These include depression, anorexia, listlessness, incoordination, weakness, prostration, and death.

Lesions

Pulmonary edema and hydropericardium are the most common lesions. Fatty degeneration of the liver and myocardial degeneration may be present.

SODIUM MONOFLUORACETATE

Commonly designated as "Compound 1080," this product is highly toxic for animals and birds. Cottral et al. (1947) conducted tolerance studies in White Leghorns and determined the LD_{50} was approximately 6 mg/kg of body weight for laying hens. The birds died within 48 hours after treatment. By extrapolation it was estimated a pullet would not ingest a lethal dose of poison if it ate a mouse that died of poisoning.

Signs

These include depression, weakness, reluctance to move, edema of the wattles, cyanosis of the comb and wattles, and distension of the crop with fluid. Diarrhea is present in some birds. Several hours before death dyspnea and rales are present.

Lesions

The blood is dark red and remains unclotted in the heart and major blood vessels. The lungs are hemorrhagic and edematous. Clotted blood may be present in the thoracic air sacs and trachea. Hematomas may be present in the comb. Petechiae are present in the pericardial and mesenteric fat. Severe enteritis is present. The liver, spleen, and kidneys are often congested.

Diagnosis

There is no chemical test for "1080" and only a presumptive diagnosis could be given on the basis of history, signs, and lesions.

ARSENIC

Arsenical compounds are commonly used in the control of rodents and insects. Van Zyl (1929) states that birds are more resistant to arsenic poisoning than domestic animals. Gallagher (1919) and Barber and Hubster (1933) reported the lethal dose of arsenous acid to be 4–5 grains for chickens. Cooley et al. (1923), Whitehead (1934), and Wilson and Holmes (1936) claimed that birds will not be poisoned by picking up well-scattered poisoned bran used to kill grasshoppers. Furthermore, grasshoppers killed by feeding on the poisoned bran and fed to poultry produced no ill effect. Weber et al. (1932) reported arsenic trioxide poisoning in adult chickens. DeLay (1940) reported losses in 10-week-old poults from eating grasshopper bait containing sodium arsenate and bran. The bait was spread unevenly and the birds had access to clumps of moistened bran. In feeding trials, poults consuming an equivalent of 0.25 g of arsenic trioxide died in 1–3 days, and a level of 0.5 g killed poults in 2–12 hours.

Signs

These include dropping of the wings, ruffled feathers, ataxia, and a spasmodic jerking of the head which finally becomes twisted to one side. The comb and wattles become cyanotic and watery fluid is regurgitated.

Lesions

Inflammatory changes in the crop, gizzard, and intestine are accompanied by catarrhal exudate. Fluid may accumulate in the gizzard, and the lining is easily detached. Hemorrhage and gelatinous exudate are present beneath the gizzard lining. The liver is friable and yellowish brown.

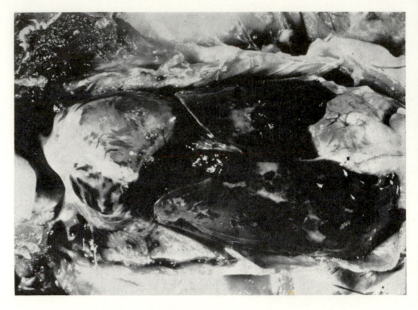

FIG. 33.17—Arsenic poisoning in duck. Hemorrhages in myocardium and yellow-green necrotic areas in liver.

In ducks yellow-green irregular necrotic areas may occur in the liver, and there are myocardial hemorrhages (Fig. 33.17). The kidneys are swollen and degenerated. The fat is soft, edematous, and orange colored. In chronic cases the heart is enlarged and flabby. The blood is scarlet and watery, having little tendency to clot.

ZINC PHOSPHIDE

Five percent of this compound in the ration is toxic for birds, domestic animals, and rodents. The lethal dose for birds is 7–15 mg/kg of body weight. Hare and Orr (1945) reported cases of accidental poisoning in geese and chickens.

Signs

Clinical signs may appear within an hour after ingestion of a lethal dose. The birds are depressed and the feathers are ruffled. Diarrhea is manifest and the birds become progressively weaker. In the terminal stages the birds lie on their sides with head retracted over the back and legs extended. Convulsions may develop shortly before death. Large doses may kill the birds without premonitory signs. Sublethal doses are followed by depression and green diarrhea.

Lesions

Hydropericardium and ascites are present. Enteritis is seen in the duodenum. A characteristic pungent odor of phosphorus can be detected in the content of the crop and gizzard in birds which have ingested large quantities.

STRYCHNINE

Accidental strychnine poisoning may occur in animals and birds consuming poisoned baits. Heinekamp (1925) stated that the toxic dose in fowls depends on the quantity and nature of the crop contents. If the crop contents are fluid in nature, the strychnine is more readily absorbed. Gallagher (1919) stated that lethal dose for chickens was 0.08 g/kg of body weight given per os. Turkeys dislike grain coated with strychnine and after the first taste will not eat the poisoned bait. Toxic doses cause tonic spasms, paralysis, respiratory failure, and death.

MISCELLANEOUS

COAL TAR

Carlton (1966) reported on experimental coal tar poisoning in White Pekin ducks by feeding clay pigeons used in trap-shooting. Clay pigeons at levels of 0.5, 0.75, and 10% of a 21% protein duck starter diet were acutely toxic to ducklings and resulted in depressed growth and reduced packed-cell volume. Lesions were subcutaneous edema, hydropericardium, ascites, and fibrin deposits on the viscera. Histologic liver lesions were focal necrosis, increase in lymphoid follicles, and, most significantly, bile duct cell hyperplasia. Hepatocyte alterations were cellular enlargement, nuclear hypertrophy, a prominent nucleolus, and margination of chromatin. Other compounds which provoke bile duct cell hyperplasia in ducks are aflatoxins, dimethylnitrosamine, cycasin, and lithocholic acid. Edema and ascites are not prominent features of aflatoxin poisoning, which aids in the differentiation between these two conditions.

ETHYLENE GLYCOL

Riddell et al. (1967) reported a field case of ethylene glycol poisoning in geese and the results of experimental intoxication in 6-week-old chickens. They determined the lethal dose of ethylene glycol was 6.7 ml/kg of body weight. Wescott and McDougle (1967) described ethylene glycol toxicosis in chickens following administration of a suspension of oocysts that was exposed to ethylene oxide gas. The gas was hydrated to ethylene glycol during exposure of the oocysts.

Signs

Chickens have ruffled feathers and watery droppings and become listless and ataxic. In the terminal stages the birds assume a characteristic recumbent posture, the wings droop, the eyes are closed, and the head rests on the floor with the beak used as a prop. When the birds are handled, they offer little resistance, and fluid runs out of the mouth.

Lesions

The primary gross lesion is pale and swollen kidneys. Histopathologic lesions are characteristic and of great aid in establishing a diagnosis. Ethylene glycol forms calcium oxalate crystals in the tissues, particularly the kidneys and sometimes other organs such as the lumen of the duodenum (Riddell et al., 1967). These crystals vary in shape from fans to rosettes or elongated prisms. They are found in the proximal tubules, loops of Henle, and collecting tubules. The crystals are more numerous and easier to detect in unstained frozen sections viewed under polarized light. Urates may also appear birefringent with polarized light but appear amorphous and lack the sharp angular edges of a crystal. Crystals may be seen in hematoxylin and eosin stained slides but with considerable difficulty. Foci of heterophils may be present in the collecting renal tubules and inter-

stitial tissue. The composition of the suspect crystals can be determined by histochemical means. The crystals are insoluble in 2 M acetic acid, give off carbon dioxide with sulfuric acid after microincineration, and react positively with alizarin red S stain.

TOXIC FAT

During the spring and fall of 1957 severe outbreaks of a new disease syndrome characterized by ascites, hydropericardium, and subcutaneous edema occurred in broilers in central and southeastern United States. Schmittle et al. (1958) and Sanger et al. (1958) conducted investigations on this disease and determined that certain samples of fat or feed containing this fat would cause this syndrome. A similar syndrome was reported in Great Britain by Wannop and Chubb (1961), who stated that fat had been added to the suspect feed.

Etiology

After it was determined by Schmittle et al. (1958) that the toxic factor was in the fat added to the ration, investigations were undertaken to determine the precise identity of the toxic substance. It appears that still residues, fatty acid distillates and their derivatives, and some vegetable fat sources may contain the chick edema factor (Friedman, 1962). Large quantities of fatty acids are used industrially, and low grades of fat are split into fatty acids and glycerol. The fatty acids are triple-distilled; the first distillate is a high-grade mixture of fatty acids, the second distillate yields low-grade fatty acids used for rubber on highways, and the third distillate yields a low-grade product. It was the third distillate that had been blended with feed grade fat for use in feeds. Close study of the various stages of fatty acid production soon revealed that the toxic factor was distillable and present to some extent in the first distillates which were used in the manufacture of foods. It was demonstrated that the toxic factor was entirely in the unsaponified portion of the fat. Ott et al. (1961) described a chick assay procedure for detecting the toxic factor in fat or feed. Detectable hydropericardium was produced by feeding 7 parts of pure edema-producing factor per billion parts of diet in a 20-day feeding period. Mortality was produced when the diet contained 64 parts per billion of the toxic factor. From comparative assay results it was concluded that the concentration of the pure factor in the toxic fat standard was approximately 0.5 ppm. After storage for 21 months the toxic fat retained 72% of its toxicity. This comparatively small loss in the activity of the chick edema factor demonstrates its stability. Schmittle et al. (1958) found that the toxic factor was still active after heating for 20 minutes at 121° C.

Wootton et al. (1962) reported the isolation of three hydropericardium-producing factors from a toxic fat. Two of the compounds were isolated in pure form, and it was determined that they had a high melting point and high molecular weight. They were found to be crystalline compounds containing six chlorine atoms per mole and having an aromatic nucleus. It was estimated that 5 μg of one fraction designated alpha 3.02 is enough to kill one chick.

Hosts

The chicken appears to be the most susceptible host, although Simpson et al. (1959) indicated that clinical cases occurred in turkeys as well. Ducks and turkeys did not appear highly susceptible, as Edgar et al. (1958) fed 4% toxic fat to ducks and turkeys for 6 and 11 weeks respectively but failed to produce any pronounced signs or lesions of the disease. The disease usually appears in birds 3 weeks of age, and losses may continue up to 10 weeks of age.

Signs

Signs may appear at 3 weeks of age and include dyspnea, ruffled feathers, listlessness, paleness, stunting, and sudden death. Some chicks may waddle like a duck, have an unsteady gait, or assume a penguinlike posture. Feed consumption was never noticed to drop more than 10% (Sanger et al., 1958). Pullets and laying birds do not show pronounced clinical signs but have lowered weight gains, poor production, and poor hatchability. Dunahoo et al. (1959) reported that pullets receiving 5% toxic fat in the diet between 12 and 14 weeks of age came into production 2 weeks later than the controls. Production was 20% below normal and hatchability was decreased. Pullets receiving 5% toxic fat in the ration for 61 days did not come into production and had a depressed growth rate; 67% mortality was experienced in the group receiving toxic fat for the full growing period. When layers were fed 5% toxic

fat, production practically ceased in 2 weeks time. Hatchability was markedly decreased and production was only slightly improved 6 weeks after the feeding of toxic fat was discontinued.

Allen and Lalich (1962) fed 4-week-old cockerels toxic fat at levels of 0.25, 0.5, and 1.0% in the feed for 5 months. At all levels the birds had testicular hypoplasia, and at the two higher levels ascites and hydropericardium were produced. Despite the testicular hypoplasia the secondary sex characteristics such as enlarged comb and body conformation were not inhibited. It would appear that in immature chickens testicular hypoplasia is a more sensitive indicator of toxic fat in the diet than is hydropericardium or ascites. Flick et al. (1967) conducted chronicity studies; although the outward appearance of the birds was normal, ascites and edema were present on necropsy.

Morbidity and Mortality

The morbidity initially is low, but as the disease progresses it reaches serious proportions with correspondingly high mortality. Mortality rates of 50–90% were reported.

Gross Lesions

Birds in advanced stages of the disease have large, fluctuating, distended abdomens containing clear straw-colored fluid with large fibrinous clots (Fig. 33.18). Sub-

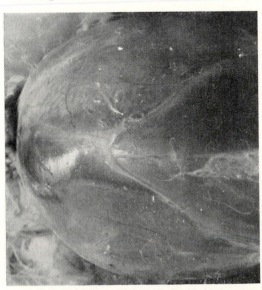

FIG. 33.18—Toxic fat syndrome. Abdomen distended by ascitic fluid in 7-week-old chicken.

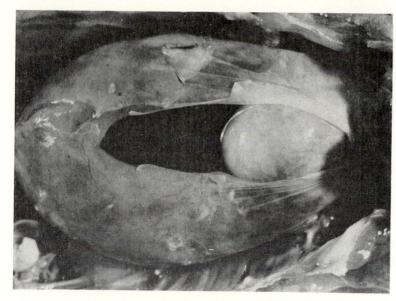

FIG. 33.19—*Toxic fat syndrome. Marked distension of pericardial sac with fluid.*

cutaneous edema may occur in the region of the breast, abdomen, and thighs. The most consistent lesion is a greatly distended pericardial sac filled with amber-colored fluid (Fig. 33.19). The myocardium is pale and the heart may be slightly or greatly enlarged. Allen (1964) noted dilatation and hypertrophy of the right ventricle. Petechiae may be present in the myocardium. Hemorrhages may occur in the skeletal muscles but are not a consistent feature of the disease. The crop contents may be bloody and the buccal cavity, beak, and head region may be bloodstained. The lesions in the liver are variable depending upon the duration of the disease. A layer of coagulated serum may cover the surface (Fig. 33.20). In acute cases the liver is enlarged and mottled with irregular, diffuse, light-colored areas resembling fatty change interspersed with red streaks or patches. In chronic cases the liver is shrunken, nodular, firm, and has a nutmeg or bronze color. The kidneys are pale and enlarged. Pulmonary edema may be present.

Hematology

Simpson et al. (1959) reported a marked anemia with erythrocyte counts as low as 800,000 per cu mm. In blood smears there were many immature erythrocytes. There was an increased proportion of heterophils and a decreased proportion of lymphocytes.

Alexander et al. (1962) reported serum

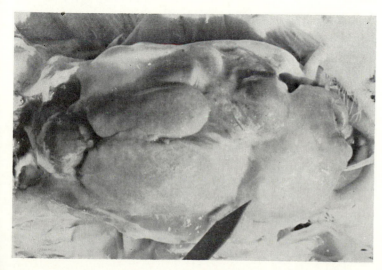

FIG. 33.20—*Toxic fat syndrome. Liver is gray with rounded edges. Coagulated ascitic fluid in body cavity.*

albumin levels below normal in affected birds. These workers noted that severity of hydropericardium was directly related to the sodium chloride content of the feed and hydropericardium was not produced when sodium chloride was omitted from the diet.

Histopathology

Simpson et al. (1959) and Sanger et al. (1958) described in detail the histological changes. In the liver, bile duct hyperplasia with severe degeneration of epithelium including desquamation, hydropic degeneration, and necrosis is observed. Patent bile ducts often contain inspissated bile and crystallized bile salts in the form of rosettes. Centrolobular and peripheral necrosis is common. Occasionally fatty degeneration and thickening of the liver capsule are present. Hemorrhages are present in the liver in early lesions. Aggregates of lymphocytes and heterophils are distributed throughout the liver and around the portal triad.

The kidneys have enlarged glomeruli that are bloodless due to the proliferation and swelling of the endothelial cells of the capillaries. The epithelial cells of Bowman's capsule may be proliferated. Interstitial lymphocytic infiltration and edema are present in some cases. Proteinaceous debris may accumulate in the space between the layers of Bowman's capsule. Hyaline droplets or urate crystals are frequently seen in the lumen of the tubules.

Heart lesions consist of swollen degenerated muscle fibers separated by edema. Some hydropic degeneration of muscle fibers and lymphocytic and granulocytic infiltration may be present. The pericardium is thickened due to the accumulation of fibrinonecrotic debris. Focal subepicardial hemorrhages may be present.

Vascular changes consisting of proliferation and swelling of the endothelial cells of arterioles and small arteries occur most frequently in the vessels of the spleen, lung, kidney, and liver.

Marked degenerative changes may be seen in the pectoral muscles of birds with ascites. Muscle fibers are swollen, fragmented, globular, necrotic, and widely separated by edematous fluid.

Diagnosis

Uncomplicated and inexpensive laboratory tests have not been developed for establishing a positive diagnosis of toxic fat poisoning. It would involve lengthy and expensive feeding trials to establish the fact that it was the fat in the ration causing the disease in question. The precise identity of the toxic compound(s) has yet to be determined. Only by a process of elimination and careful evaluation of the history, clinical signs, and lesions could a presumptive diagnosis be made.

Diseases that would come under consideration in making a differential diagnosis would be cresol poisoning, salt poisoning, crotalaria poisoning, and transudative diathesis.

Cresol poisoning occurs only sporadically whereas in the toxic fat syndrome there are likely to be reports of several flocks having the same problem. In addition, in a given area the toxic fat syndrome is likely to show up in flocks receiving the same brand of feed. A careful history would reveal that a cresol disinfectant had been used in cases of cresol poisoning.

Salt poisoning caused by excessive amounts of sodium chloride in the feed or water could be detected by analysis of these dietary components for their salt content. Sanger et al. (1958) indicated that the extreme liver necrosis found in the toxic fat syndrome was not found upon histological examination in cases of salt poisoning.

Crotalaria poisoning would be more

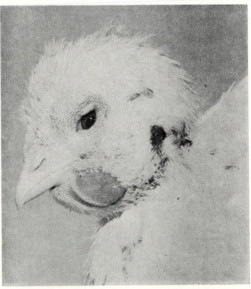

FIG. 33.21—Transudative diathesis. Edema of head and wattles, necrosis of skin on neck.

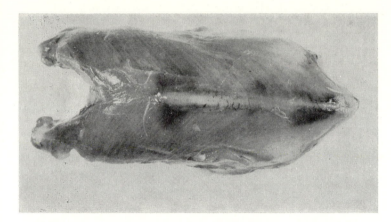

FIG. 33.22—*Transudative diathesis. Hemorrhage and degenerative streaks in breast muscle.*

likely to occur in those regions where this crop is grown and therefore would tend to be regional in occurrence. Feed suspected of containing *Crotalaria spectabilis* could be analyzed for the toxic alkaloid monocrotalin.

Transudative diathesis may superficially resemble toxic fat syndrome, but an experienced diagnostician having representative specimens could distinguish between the two diseases. Transudative diathesis is characterized by subcutaneous edema of the head region, breast, and abdomen (Fig. 33.21). The edematous fluid has a blue-green cast that can be seen beneath the abdominal skin. The subcutaneous fat contains hemorrhages, and white streaks of degeneration are present in the breast muscle (Fig. 33.22). The legs are red and swollen in the early stages, and later the skin of the feet and shanks becomes green. Necrosis and scab formation appear on the head and neck, beneath the wing tips, and above the hocks (Fig. 33.23). The internal fat is white, hard, and lumpy and has been described as having an "oatmeal" appearance. The consistent and pronounced hydropericardium seen in toxic fat syndrome is not a prominent feature of transudative diathesis. If transudative diathesis is suspected, a portion of the flock could be injected with a commercial preparation of *alpha*-tocopherol and selenium.

INSECTS

Rose Chafer

Rose chafers *(Macrodactylus subspinosus)* are abundant during the latter part of May, June, and early July in Canada and eastern United States, extending as far west as Colorado. Toxic properties of the insect for chickens have been reported by Bates (1916), Gallagher (1920), and Lamson (1916, 1922). Young chickens are fatally poisoned by eating rose chafers but mature birds are seldom killed. Chickens will feed ravenously upon these insects; 15–20 rose chafers will kill a week-old chicken; 3-week-old birds show a toxic reaction after eating 25 or more of these insects. The birds usually die within 24 hours or gradually recover. Water extracts of crushed rose chafers are toxic for chickens. The nature of the toxin or its mode of action have not been determined.

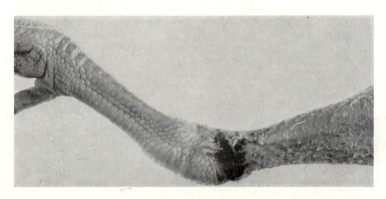

FIG. 33.23—*Transudative diathesis. Necrosis of skin above hock.*

Clinical signs include drowsiness, incoordination, weakness, prostration, convulsions, and opisthotonos. Death usually ensues within 1 hour after the onset of signs. On necropsy the coronary vessels are injected.

REFERENCES

Ackerson, C. W., and F. E. Mussehl. 1955. Toxicity of treated seed corn in rations for chicks. *Poultry Sci.* 34:728–29.

Adams, R., and E. F. Rogers. 1939. The structure of monocrotaline, the alkaloid in *Crotalaria spectabilis* and *Crotalaria retusa*. I. *J. Am. Chem. Soc.* 61:2815–19.

Adler, F. E. W. 1944. Chemical analyses of organs from lead poisoned Canada geese. *J. Wildlife Management* 8:83–85.

Alexander, J. C., R. J. Young, C. M. Burnett, and H. D. Hathaway. 1962. Hydropericardium assay and safety of fats and fatty acid products. *Poultry Sci.* 41:22–32.

Allcroft, Ruth, and R. B. A. Carnaghan. 1963. Groundnut toxicity: An examination for toxin in human food products from animals fed toxic groundnut meal. *Vet. Record* 75:259–63.

Allcroft, Ruth, R. B. A. Carnaghan, K. Sargeant, and J. O'Kelley. 1961. A toxic factor in Brazilian groundnut meal. *Vet. Record* 73:428.

Allen, J. R. 1963. *Crotalaria spectabilis* toxicity studies in turkeys. *Avian Diseases* 7:318–24.

———. 1964. The role of "toxic fat" in the production of hydropericardium and ascites in chickens. *Am. J. Vet. Res.* 25:1210–19.

Allen, J. R., and J. J. Lalich. 1962. Response of chickens to prolonged feeding of crude "toxic fat." *Proc. Soc. Exp. Biol. Med.* 109:48–51.

Allen, J. R., G. R. Childs, and W. W. Cravens. 1960. *Crotalaria spectabilis* toxicity in chickens. *Proc. Soc. Exp. Biol. Med.* 104:434–36.

Allen, J. R., J. J. Lalich, and S. C. Schmittle. 1963. *Crotalaria spectabilis* induced cirrhosis in turkeys. *Lab. Invest.* 12:512–17.

Anderson, L. A. P., A. Howard, and J. L. Simonsen. 1925. Studies on lathyrism. *Indian J. Med. Res.* 12:613.

Anderson, W. A., and C. P. Richter. 1946. Toxicity of alpha napthyl thiourea. *Vet. Med.* 41:302–3.

Archibald, R. McG., H. J. Smith, and J. D. Smith. 1962. Brazilian groundnut toxicosis in Canadian broiler chickens. *Can. Vet. J.* 3:322–25.

Ashworth, C. T., and M. F. Mason. 1946. Observations on the pathological changes produced by a toxic substance present in bluegreen algae *(Microcystis aeruginosa)*. *Am. J. Pathol.* 22:369–83.

Asplin, F. D., and E. Boyland. 1947. The effects of pyrimidine sulfonamide derivatives upon the blood-clotting system and testes of chicks and the breeding capacity of adult fowls. *Brit. J. Pharmacol.* 2:79–92.

Asplin, F. D., and R. B. A. Carnaghan. 1961. The toxicity of certain groundnut meals for poultry with special reference to their effect on ducklings and chickens. *Vet. Record* 73:1215–19.

Bagley, G. E., L. N. Locke, and G. T. Nightingale. 1967. Lead poisoning in Canada geese in Delaware. *Avian Diseases* 11:601–8.

Baker, R. C., F. W. Hill, A. Van Tienhoven, and J. H. Bruckner. 1957. The effect of nicarbazin on egg production and egg quality. *Poultry Sci.* 36:718–26.

Barber, P. G., and E. B. Hubster. 1933. Arsenic poisoning in poultry. *Vet. Med.* 28:500–502.

Bardosi, Z. 1939. Toxicity of lily of the valley and oleander leaves for fowls. Thesis, Budapest; *Abstr. Vet. Bull.* (1940) 10:624. (Trans. title.)

Barlow, J. S., S. J. Slinger, and R. P. Simmer. 1948. The reaction of growing chicks to diets varying in sodium chloride content. *Poultry Sci.* 27:542–52.

Barnes, M. F. 1921. Black locust poisoning of chickens. *J. Am. Vet. Med. Ass.* 59:370–72.

Bates, J. M. 1916. The poisonous character of rose chafers. *Science* 43:209.

Beach, J. R. 1930. Intestinal worms of poultry. *North Am. Vet.* 11 (November):45–48.

Beaudette, F. R., C. B. Hudson, and A. L. Weber. 1933. Phosphorous poisoning in poultry. *North Am. Vet.* 14 (July):39–42.

Berg, L. R., C. M. Hamilton, and G. E. Bearse. 1956. Nitrofurazone and nicarbazin as growth stimulants and coccidiostatic agents for young chicks. *Poultry Sci.* 35:1394–96.

Bierer, B. W. 1958. The ill effects of excessive formaldehyde fumigation on turkey poults. *J. Am. Vet. Med. Ass.* 132:174–76.

Bierer, B. W., and W. H. Rhodes. 1960. Poultry ration contaminants. *J. Am. Vet. Med. Ass.* 137:352–53.

Bierer, B. W., C. L. Vickers, W. H. Rhodes, and J. B. Thomas. 1960. Comparison of the toxic effects of *Crotalaria spectabilis* and *Crotalaria giant striata* as complete feed contaminants. *J. Am. Vet. Med. Ass.* 136:318–22.

Bierer, B. W., C. F. Risher, and D. E. Roebuck. 1963. Effect of ingested disinfectants on chicks. *J. Am. Vet. Med. Ass.* 142:512–13.

Bigland, C. H. 1950. Ascites and edema of brooded turkey poults in Alberta, Canada. *Can. J. Comp. Med. Vet. Sci.* 14:144–56.

Bigland, C. H., J. Howell, and A. J. Da Massa. 1963. Zoalene toxicity in broiler chickens. *Avian Diseases* 7:471–80.

Black, D. J. G., and N. S. Barron. 1943. Observations on the feeding of a cacao waste product to poultry. *Vet. Record* 55:166–67.

Blaxland, J. D. 1946. The toxicity of sodium chloride for fowls. *Vet. J.* 102:157–73.

Bleecker, W. L., and R. M. Smith. 1933a. Further studies on the relative efficiency of vermifuges for poultry. *J. Am. Vet. Med. Ass.* 83:76–81.

———. 1933b. Nicotine sulfate as a vermifuge for the removal of ascarids from poultry. *J. Am. Vet. Med. Ass.* 83:645–55.

Blount, W. P. 1955. Recent advances in poultry therapeutics. *Vet. Rec.* 67:1087–97.

———. 1961. Turkey "X" disease. *J. Brit. Turkey Fed.* 9:52.

Blount, W. P., D. M. Fraser, D. Knight, and W. M. Dowling. 1963. The use of ducklings for the detection of aflatoxin. *Vet. Record* 75:35.

Bootes, B. W. 1962. Poisoning of turkey poults with lindane. *Australian Vet. J.* 38:67–68.

Brandenburg, T. O., and F. M. Shigley. 1947. "Water Bloom" as a cause of poisoning in livestock in North Dakota. *J. Am. Vet. Med. Ass.* 110:384–85.

Bressler, G. O., S. Gordeuk, Jr., and G. H. Pritham. 1951. The effect of salt and carbolineum in producing ascites in turkey poults. *Poultry Sci.* 30:738–44.

Brown, J. M. M., and L. Abrams. 1965. Biochemical studies on aflatoxicosis. *Onderstepoort J. Vet. Res.* 32:119–46.

Buckley, J. S., H. Bunyea, and Eloise B. Cram. 1939. Diseases and parasites of poultry. *USDA Farmers' Bull.* 1652.

Bullis, K. L., and H. Van Roekel. 1944. Uncommon pathological conditions in chickens and turkeys. *Cornell Vet.* 34:313–20.

Campbell, H. 1950. Quail picking up lead shot. *J. Wildlife Management* 14:243–44.

Campbell, H. W. 1931. Poisoning in chickens with whorled milkweed. *J. Am. Vet. Med. Ass.* 79:102–4.

Carlton, W. W. 1966. Experimental coal tar poisoning in the White Pekin duck. *Avian Diseases* 10:484–502.

Carnaghan, R. B. A., and J. D. Blaxland. 1957. The toxic effect of certain seed dressings on wild and game birds. *Vet. Record* 69:324–25.

Carnaghan, R. B. A., and K. Sargeant. 1961. The toxicity of certain groundnut meals to poultry. *Vet. Record* 73:726–27.

Carnaghan, R. B. A., G. Lewis, D. S. P. Patterson, and Ruth Allcroft. 1966. Biochemical and pathological aspects of groundnut poisoning in chickens. *Pathol. Vet.* 3:601–15.

Carpenter, C. D. 1931. The use of nicotine and its compounds for the control of poultry parasites. *J. Am. Vet. Med. Ass.* 78:651–57.

Cavanagh, J. B. 1954. The toxic effects of tri-ortho-cresyl phosphate on the nervous system. *J. Neurol. Neurosurg. Psychiat.* 17:163–72.

Caylor, J. F., and C. K. Laurent. 1961. Effect of level of *Crotalaria spectabilis* on egg production of White Leghorn hens. *Poultry Sci.* 40:818.

Coburn, D. R., D. W. Metzler, and R. Triechleer. 1951. A study of absorption and retention of lead in wild waterfowl in relation to clinical evidence of lead poisoning. *J. Wildlife Management* 15:186–92.

Cook, R. S., and D. O. Trainer. 1966. Experimental lead poisoning of Canada geese. *J. Wildlife Management* 30:1–8.

Cooley, R. A., J. R. Parker, and A. L. Strand. 1923. Improved methods of controlling grasshoppers. *Montana Agr. Expt. Sta. Circ.* 112.

Costigan, S. M. 1940. Lead poisoning in guinea fowl. *J. Am. Vet. Med. Ass.* 97:451.

Cottral, G. E., G. D. Dibble, and B. Winton. 1947. The effect of sodium fluoroacetate ("1080" rodenticide) on White Leghorn chickens. *Poultry Sci.* 26:610–13.

Cram, E. B. 1928. The present status of our knowledge of poultry parasitism. *North Am. Vet.* 9:43–50.

Cuckler, A. C., and W. H. Ott. 1955. Tolerance studies on sulfaquinoxaline in poultry. *Poultry Sci.* 34:867–74.

Dam, R., and L. C. Norris. 1962. Studies of the effect of some antibacterial and antifungal agents on growth and egg production of chickens. *Poultry Sci.* 41:78–87.

Davies, S. F. M. 1954. Sulfonamide poisoning in chickens treated for coccidiosis. *Proc. Tenth World's Poultry Congress,* pp. 275–78.

Davies, S. F. M., and S. B. Kendall. 1953. Toxicity of sulfaquinoxaline for chickens. *Vet. Record* 65:85–88.

Delaplane, J. P. 1934. Some of the tissue changes in poultry resulting from the ingestion of sodium bicarbonate. *Ohio State Univ. Vet. Alumni Quart.* 21:149.

Delaplane, J. P., and J. H. Milliff. 1948. The gross and micropathology of sulfaquinoxaline poisoning in chickens. *Am. J. Vet. Res.* 9:92–96.

De Lay, P. D. 1940. Grasshopper poison bait and turkey poult mortality. *J. Am. Vet. Med. Ass.* 97:149.

Doll, E. R., F. E. Hull, and W. M. Insko. 1946. Toxicity of sodium chloride for baby chicks. *Vet. Med.* 41:361–63.

Dougherty, E., III. 1957. Thiophosphate poisoning in White Pekin ducks. *Avian Diseases* 1:127–30.

Dougherty, E., III. 1962. Fly sprays can poison ducks. *Farm Research,* March, p. 14.

Dunahoo, W. S., H. M. Edwards, Jr., S. C. Schmittle, and H. L. Fuller. 1959. Studies on toxic fat in the rations of laying hens and pullets. *Poultry Sci.* 38:663–67.

Edgar, S. A., D. S. Bond, P. Melius, and C. R. Ingram. 1958. The effect of a toxic substance in fat on poultry. *Poultry Sci.* 37: 1200.

Edwards, J. T. 1918. Salt poisoning in pigs and poultry. *J. Comp. Pathol. Therap.* 31: 40.

Elsasser, D. S., R. W. Grundish, and J. W. Ralston. 1950. An unusual type of food poisoning in dogs. *North Am. Vet.* 32: 839–40.

Emmel, M. W. 1935. The toxicity of *Glottidium vesicarium* (Jacq.) Harper seeds for the fowl. *J. Am. Vet. Med. Ass.* 87:13–21.

———. 1937a. The pathology of *Crotalaria spectabilis* Roth seed poisoning in the domestic fowl. *J. Am. Vet. Med. Ass.* 90:627–34.

———. 1937b. The toxicity of *Crotalaria retusa* L. seeds for the domestic fowl. *J. Am. Vet. Med. Ass.* 91:205–6.

Faddoul, G. P., S. V. Amato, M. Sevoian, and G. W. Fellows. 1967. Studies on intolerance to sulfaquinoxaline in chickens. *Avian Diseases* 11:226–40.

Farr, Marion M., and D. S. Jaquette. 1947. The toxicity of sulfamerazine to chickens. *Am. J. Vet. Res.* 8:216–20.

Farr, Marion M., and E. E. Wehr. 1945. Sulfamerazine therapy in experimental cecal coccidiosis of chickens. *J. Parasitol.* 31:353–58.

Fitch, C. P., L. Bishop, and W. L. Boyd. 1934. "Water Bloom" as a cause of poisoning in domestic animals. *Cornell Vet.* 24:30–39.

Flick, D. F., R. G. O'Dell, and U. C. Ross. 1967. Studies of the chick edema disease. *Poultry Sci.* 46:186–91.

Franke, K. W., T. D. Rice, A. G. Johnson, and H. W. Schoening. 1934. Report on a preliminary field survey of the so-called "alkali disease" of livestock. *USDA Circ.* 320.

Friedman, L. 1962. Progress in the chick edema problem. *Feedstuffs* 34:18.

Gaafar, S. M., and R. D. Turk. 1957. The toxicity of malathion in chickens. *Am. J. Vet. Res.* 18:180–82.

Gallagher, B. A. 1919. Experiments in avian toxicology. *J. Am. Vet. Med. Ass.* 54:337–56.

———. 1920. Rose-chafer poisoning in chickens. *J. Am. Vet. Med. Ass.* 57:692–95.

———. 1924. Canned goods preserved with boric acid poisonous to chickens. *North Am. Vet.* 5:125–30.

Gardiner, J. L., and Marion M. Farr. 1954. Nitrofurazone for the prevention of experi-

mentally induced *Eimeria tenella* infections in chickens. *J. Parasitol.* 40:42–49.

Gibson, E. A. 1957. An outbreak of sodium chloride poisoning in turkey poults. *Vet. Record* 69:1115–17.

Glover, J. S. 1932. Mercurial poisoning in fowl. *Rept. Ont. Vet. Coll.* 1931:56.

Godfrey, G. F., D. E. Howell, and E. Graybill. 1953. Effect of lindane on egg production. *Poultry Sci.* 32:183–84.

Golz, H. H., and C. B. Shaffer. 1955. Malathion, summary of pharmacology and toxicology. *Am. Cyanamid Co. Tech. Bull.,* pp. 1–14.

Gordon, R. S., R. A. Mulholland, L. J. Machlin, and K. H. Maddy. 1959. Hydropericardium and ascites caused by excess salt and a factor in blood meal. *Poultry Sci.* 38: 1209.

Guberlet, J. E. 1922. Potassium nitrate poisoning in chickens with a note on its toxicity. *J. Am. Vet. Med. Ass.* 62:362.

Hall, M. C., and J. E. Shillinger. 1926. Kamala, a satisfactory anthelmintic for tapeworms in poultry. *North Am. Vet.* 7 (March):52–56.

Hansen, A. A. 1925. Nightshade poisoning in chickens and ducks. *J. Am. Vet. Med. Ass.* 66:502–3.

———. 1927. Stock poisoning by plants in the nightshade family. *J. Am. Vet. Med. Ass.* 71:221–24.

Hanzlik, P. J., and E. Presho. 1923. Comparative toxicity of inorganic lead compounds and metallic lead for pigeons. *J. Pharmocol. Exp. Therap.* 21:123.

Hare, T., and A. B. Orr. 1945. Poultry poisoned by zinc phosphide. *Vet. Record* 57:17.

Harms, R. H., P. W. Waldroup, and C. F. Simpson. 1963. Effect of feeding various levels of *Crotalaria spectabilis* seeds on the performance of chicks, turkeys, and pullets. *J. Am. Vet. Med. Ass.* 142:260–63.

Harper, J. A., and G. H. Arscott. 1962. Toxicity of common and hairy vetch seed for poults and chicks. *Poultry Sci.* 41:1968–74.

Hartwigk, H. 1950. Laehmungen bei Huehnern durch Weichigelit. *Monatsh. Veterinaermed.* 5:53–55.

Harwood, P. D., and Dorothy Stunz. 1949a. Nitrofurazone in the medication of avian coccidiosis. *J. Parasitol.* 35:175–82.

———. 1949b. Nitrofurazone and coccidiosis. *Ann. N.Y. Acad. Sci.* 52:538–42.

Hass, C. M., D. V. L. Brown, R. Eisenstein, and Ann Hemmens. 1964. Relations between lead poisoning in rabbit and man. *Am. J. Pathol.* 45:691–727.

Hawn, M. C. 1933. The value of kamala as a tenicide for young turkeys. *J. Am. Vet. Med. Ass.* 83:400–404.

Heinekamp, W. J. R. 1925. The resistance of

fowl to strychnine. *J. Lab. Clin. Med.* 11: 209–14.

Henk, F., and L. Hromalka. 1967. Experimentelle Dot-vergiftung beim Gefluegel. *Wien. Tieraerztl. Monatschr.* 5:23–24.

Heuser, G. F., and A. E. Schumacher. 1942. The feeding of corn cockle to chickens. *Poultry Sci.* 2:86–93.

———. 1956. Feeding chemically treated seed grains to hens. *Poultry Sci.* 35:160–63.

Hinshaw, W. R. 1965. In Biester, H. E., and L. H. Schwarte (eds.), *Diseases of Poultry.* Iowa State Univ. Press, Ames.

Hinshaw, W. R., and W. E. Lloyd. 1931. Studies on the use of copper sulfate for turkeys. *Poultry Sci.* 10:392–93.

Hinshaw, W. R., and Ethel McNeil. 1943. Experiments with sulfanilamide for turkeys. *Poultry Sci.* 22:291–94.

Horton-Smith, C., and P. L. Long. 1952. Nitrofurazone in the treatment of cecal coccidiosis in chickens. *Brit. Vet. J.* 108:47–57.

Horvath, A. A. 1945. Toxicity of vetch seed for chickens. *Poultry Sci.* 24:291–95.

Hudson, C. B. 1936. Napthalene poisoning in poultry. *J. Am. Vet. Med. Ass.* 89:219.

Hunter, J. E., and D. E. Haley. 1931. The effect of various concentrations of nicotine in tobacco on the growth and development of fowls. I. A study of the nicotine tolerance of growing chicks. *Poultry Sci.* 10:61–67.

Hunter, J. E., D. E. Haley, and H. C. Knandel. 1934. Effect of concentrations of nicotine on growth and development. II. Growth and development of chicks as influenced by the addition of ground tobacco to the ration. *Poultry Sci.* 13:91–94.

Iongh, H. de, R. O. Vles, and P. de Vogel. 1964. The occurrence and detection of aflatoxin in food. *Proc. Int. Symp. Mycotoxins in Foodstuffs.* M.I.T. Press, Cambridge, Mass.

Irby, H. D., L. N. Locke, and G. E. Bagley. 1967. Relative toxicity of lead and selected substitute shot types to game farm mallards. *J. Wildlife Management* 31:253–57.

Johns, F. M. 1934. A study of punctate stippling as found in the lead poisoning of wild ducks. *J. Lab. Clin. Med.* 19:514–17.

Johnson, E. L., P. E. Waibel, and B. S. Pomeroy. 1955. The toxicity of Arasan-treated corn to hens and chicks. *Proc. Am. Vet. Med. Ass. 92nd Ann. Meet.,* pp. 322–23.

Jordan, F. T. W. 1955. Accidental nitrofurazone poisoning in baby chicks. *Vet. Record* 67:514–16.

Joyner, L. P., and S. F. M. Davies. 1956. Sulfaquinoxaline poisoning in chickens. *J. Comp. Pathol. Therap.* 66:39–48.

Jull, M. A. 1930. *Poultry Husbandry.* McGraw-Hill, New York.

Jungherr, E. 1935. Diseases of brooder chicks. *Storrs Agr. Expt. Sta. Bull.* 202.

Kare, M. R., and J. Biely. 1948. The toxicity of sodium chloride and its relation to water intake in baby chicks. *Poultry Sci.* 27:751–58.

Kaupp, B. F. 1933. *Poultry Diseases,* 6th ed. Alexander Eger, Chicago.

Kelley, J. W., C. W. Barber, D. D. Pate, and C. H. Hill. 1961. Effect of feeding crotalaria seed to young chickens. *J. Am. Vet. Med. Ass.* 139:1215–17.

Key, J. A. 1924. Lead studies. IV. Blood changes in lead poisoning in rabbits with especial reference to stippled cells. *Am. J. Physiol.* 70:86–99.

Kingscote, A. A., and C. H. Jarvis. 1946. Report on experiments conducted to establish the tolerance of turkeys to DDT. *Can. J. Comp. Med. Vet. Sci.* 10:211–18.

Klimes, B., and B. Kruza. 1962. Toxicity of nitrofurazone for young ducklings. *Vet. Record* 74:167–68.

Krakower, C. A., and Marianne Goettsch. 1945. Effect of excessive ingestion of sodium chloride on the chick, with particular reference to renal changes. *Arch. Pathol.* 40: 209–19.

Lamson, G. H., Jr. 1916. The poisonous effects of the rose chafer upon chickens. *Science* 43:138.

———. 1922. The rose chafer as a cause of death of chickens. *Storrs Agr. Expt. Sta. Bull.* 110:115.

Lancaster, M. C., F. P. Jenkins, and J. McL. Philp. 1961. Toxicity associated with certain samples of groundnuts. *Nature* 192: 1095–96.

Lander, C. D. 1926. *Veterinary Toxicology.* Alexander Eger, Chicago.

Levine, P. P. 1939. The effect of sulfanilamide on the course of experimental avian coccidiosis. *Cornell Vet.* 29:409–20.

Levine, P. P., and C. W. Barber. 1947. The comparative efficiency of some coccidiostatic agents against experimental infection with *Eimeria tenella. Cornell Vet.* 37:155–59.

Link, R. P., Jean C. Smith, and C. C. Morrill. 1956. Toxicity studies on captan-treated corn in pigs and chickens. *J. Am. Vet. Med. Ass.* 128:614–16.

Locke, L. N., and G. E. Bagley. 1967. Lead poisoning in a sample of Maryland mourning doves. *J. Wildlife Management* 31:515–18.

Locke, L. N., G. E. Bagley, and H. D. Irby. 1966. Acid-fast intranuclear inclusion bodies in the kidneys of mallards fed lead shot. *Bull. Wildlife Disease Ass.* 2:127–31.

McCune, E. L., J. E. Savage, and B. L. O'Dell.

1962. Hydropericardium and ascites in chicks fed a chlorinated hydrocarbon. *Poultry Sci.* 41:295.

McFarland, L. Z., and Paula B. Lacy. 1968. Acute anticholinesterase toxicity in ducks and Japanese quail. *Toxicol. Appl. Pharmacol.* 12:105–14.

McNeil, Ethel, and W. R. Hinshaw. 1945. Effects of mercuric chloride on turkeys and on *Hexamita meleagridis*. *Poultry Sci.* 24:516–21.

Marsden, S. J., and H. R. Bird. 1947. Effects of DDT on growing turkeys. *Poultry Sci.* 25:3–6.

Marsh, C. D., A. B. Clawson, and H. Marsh. 1915. Zygadenus or death camas. *USDA Bull.* 125.

Marsh, C. D., A. B. Clawson, and G. C. Roe. 1928. Coyotillo *(Karwinskia humboldtiana)* as a poisonous plant. *USDA Tech. Bull.* 29.

Marthedal, H. E., and Grethe Velling. 1961. Hemorrhagic syndrome in poultry. *Brit. Vet. J.* 177:357–65.

Mayeda, B. 1968. The toxic effects in turkey poults of a quaternary ammonium compound in drinking water at 150 and 200 ppm. *Avian Diseases* 12:67–74.

Moore, E. N., and J. A. Brown. 1950. The effect of nitrofurazone on normal and coccidiosis infected poults. *J. Parasitol.* 36:43. (Suppl.)

Moore, E. N., and R. D. Carter. 1954. Toxicity of chlordane to turkey poults. *Poultry Sci.* 33:654–55.

Morrison, W. D., A. E. Ferguson, M. C. Connell, and J. K. McGregor. 1961. The efficacy of certain coccidiostats against mixed avian coccidial infections. *Avian Diseases* 5:222–28.

Moxon, A. L. 1937. Alkali disease or selenium poisoning. *S. Dakota Agr. Expt. Sta. Bull.* 311.

Neal, W. M., L. L. Rusoff, and C. F. Ahmann. 1935. The isolation and some properties of an alkaloid from *Crotalaria spectabilis* Roth. *J. Am. Chem. Soc.* 57:2560–61.

Nesbitt, Brenda F., J. O'Kelly, K. Sargeant, and Ann Sheridan. 1962. Toxic metabolites of *Aspergillus flavus*. *Nature* 195:1062–63.

Newberne, P. M. 1964. Carcinogenicity of aflatoxin-contaminated peanut meals. *Proc. Int. Symp. Mycotoxins in Foodstuffs.* M.I.T. Press, Cambridge, Mass.

Newberne, P. M., and W. B. Buck. 1957. Studies on drug toxicity in chicks. *Poultry Sci.* 36:304–12.

Newberne, P. M., W. W. Carlton, and G. N. Wogan. 1964. Hepatomas in rats and hepatorenal injury in ducklings fed peanut meal or *Aspergillus flavus* extract. *Pathol. Vet.* 1:105–32.

Niemann, K. W. 1928. Report of an outbreak of poisoning in the domesticated fowl, due to death camas. *J. Am. Vet. Med. Ass.* 73:627–30.

Nunn, J. A. 1907. *Veterinary Toxicology*. Bailliere, Tindall, and Cox, London.

Ott, W. H., S. Kuna, C. C. Porter, and A. C. Cuckler. 1956. Biological studies on Nicarbazin, a new anticoccidial agent. *Poultry Sci.* 35:1357–67.

Ott, W. H., A. M. Dickinson, and A. Van Iderstine. 1961. A chick assay procedure for the edema-producing factor in toxic fat. *Poultry Sci.* 40:1016–22.

Pammel, L. H. 1911. *A Manual of Poisonous Plants*. Torch Press, Cedar Rapids, Iowa.

———. 1917. Milkweed poisonous to chickens. *Am. J. Vet. Med.* 12:236–37.

Parker, S. L. 1929. Effects of early handicaps on chickens as measured by yolk absorption and body weight to twenty weeks of age. *Hilgardia* 4:1.

Paver, H., A. Robertson, and J. E. Wilson. 1953. Observations on the toxicity of salt for young chickens. *J. Comp. Pathol. Therap.* 63:31–47.

Peckham, M. C. 1950. Diagnostic accession. *Ann. Rept. N.Y. State Vet. Coll.* 1950–51.

Peterson, E. H., and T. A. Hymas. 1950. Sulfaquinoxaline, nitrofurazone and nitrophenide in the prophylaxis of experimental *Eimeria necatrix* infection. *Am. J. Vet. Res.* 11:278–83.

Poley, W. E., A. L. Moxon, and K. W. Franke. 1937. Further studies of the effects of selenium poisoning on hatchability. *Poultry Sci.* 16:219–25.

Post, G. 1951. Effects of toxaphene and chlordane on certain game birds. *J. Wildlife Management* 15:381.

Pullar, E. M. 1940. The toxicity of various copper compounds and mixtures for domesticated birds. *Australian Vet. J.* 16:147–62, 203–13.

Quigley, G. D., and R. H. Waite. 1931. Miscellaneous feeding trials with poultry. *Maryland Agr. Expt. Sta. Bull.* 325:343.

———. 1932. Salt tolerance of baby chicks. *Maryland Agr. Expt. Sta. Bull.* 340:345.

Rac, R., and C. S. Crisp. 1954. Lead poisoning in domestic ducks. *Australian Vet. J.* 30:145–46.

Ressler, Charlotte. 1962. Isolation and identification from common vetch of the neurotoxin B-cyano-L-alanine, a possible factor in neurolathyrism. *J. Biol. Chem.* 237:733–35.

Richmond, J. W., N. H. Sutcliffe, N. W. R. Daniels, P. W. Russell Eggitt, and J. B. M. Coppock. 1962. Factors other than groundnut relating to "turkey X disease." *Vet. Record* 74:544–45.

Riddell, C., S. W. Nielsen, and E. J. Kersting. 1967. Ethylene glycol poisoning in poultry. *J. Am. Vet. Med. Ass.* 150:1531–35.

Roberts, R. E. 1957. Salt tolerance of turkeys. *Poultry Sci.* 36:672–73.

Rosen, M. H., and R. A. Bankowski. 1960. A diagnostic technique and treatment for lead poisoning in swans. *Calif. Fish Game* 46: 81–90.

Rosenberg, M. M., and H. E. Adler. 1950. Comparative toxicity of DDT and chlordane to young chicks. *Am. J. Vet. Res.* 11: 142–44.

Rosenberg, M. M., and T. Tanaka. 1950. Toxicity of chlordane to growing chickens. *Am. J. Vet. Res.* 11:233–35.

Rosenberg, M. M., T. Tanaka, and H. E. Adler. 1950. Toxicity of chlordane to laying pullets. *Am. J. Vet. Res.* 11:236–39.

Rubin, M., H. R. Bird, N. Green, and R. H. Carter. 1947. Toxicity of DDT to laying hens. *Poultry Sci.* 26:410–13.

Salisbury, R. M., E. L. J. Staples, and M. Sutton. 1958. Lead poisoning of chickens. *New Zealand Vet. J.* 6:2–7.

Sanger, V. L., L. Scott, A. Hamdy, C. Gale, and W. D. Pounden. 1958. Alimentary toxemia in chickens. *J. Am. Vet. Med. Ass.* 33:172–76.

Sargeant, K., J. O'Kelley, R. B. A. Carnaghan, and Ruth Allcroft. 1961a. The assay of a toxic principle in certain groundnut meals. *Vet. Record* 73:1219–23.

Sargeant, K., Ann Sheridan, J. O'Kelley, and R. B. A. Carnaghan. 1961b. Toxicity associated with certain samples of groundnuts. *Nature* 199:1096–97.

Schmittle, S. C., H. M. Edwards, and D. Morris. 1958. A disorder of chickens probably due to toxic feed—preliminary report. *J. Am. Vet. Med. Ass.* 132:216–19.

Scott, H. M., E. L. Jungherr, and L. D. Matterson. 1944. The effect of feeding sulfanilamide to the laying fowl. *Poultry Sci.* 23: 446–53.

Scrivner, L. H. 1946. Experimental edema and ascites in poults. *J. Am. Vet. Med. Ass.* 108:27–32.

Shaw, P. A. 1929. Duck disease studies. II. Feeding of single and mixed salts. *Proc. Soc. Exp. Biol. Med.* 27:120–22.

Shealy, A. L., and E. F. Thomas. 1928. Daubentonia seed poisoning of poultry. *Univ. Fla. Agr. Expt. Sta. Bull.* 196.

Sherman, M., Ernest Ross, F. F. Sanchez, and M. T. Y. Chang. 1963. Chronic toxicity of dimethoate to hens. *J. Econ. Entomol.* 56: 10–15.

Sherman, M., Ernest Ross, and M. T. Y. Chang. 1964. Acute and subacute toxicity of several organophosphorus insecticides to chicks. *Toxicol. Appl. Pharmacol.* 6:147–53.

Sherwin, C. P., and J. H. Crowdle. 1922. Detoxication in the organism of the fowl. *Proc. Soc. Exp. Biol. Med.* 19:318–20.

Siller, W. G., and D. C. Ostler. 1961. The histopathology of an enterohepatic syndrome of turkey poults. *Vet. Record* 73: 134–38.

Simpson, C. F., W. R. Pritchard, and R. H. Harms. 1959. An endotheliosis in chickens and turkeys caused by an unidentified dietary factor. *J. Am. Vet. Med. Ass.* 134:410–16.

Simpson, C. F., P. W. Waldroup, and R. H. Harms. 1963. Pathologic changes associated with feeding various levels of *Crotalaria spectabilis* seeds to poultry. *J. Am. Vet. Med. Ass.* 142:264–71

Smith, F. H., and C. J. Osborne. 1962. Toxic effects of crotalaria seed. *Vet. Med.* 57:234–37.

Snyder, L. J. 1947. Improved dithizone method for determination of lead. *Ind. Eng. Chem.* 19(9):684–87.

Stiles, G. W. 1940. Carbon monoxide poisoning of chicks and poults in poorly ventilated brooders. *Poultry Sci.* 19:111–15.

———. 1942. Poisoning of turkey poults from whorled milkweed *(Asclepias galioides)*. *Poultry Sci.* 21:263–70.

Stockman, R. 1931. The poisonous principle of Lathyrus and some other leguminous seeds. *J. Hyg.* 31:550–62.

Swanson, M. H., P. E. Waibel, N. V. Helbacka, and E. L. Johnson. 1956. Egg shell quality as affected by Arasan in the diet. *Poultry Sci.* 35:92–95.

Temperton, H. 1944. Effect of green and sprouted potatoes on laying pullets. *Vet. Med.* 39:13–14.

Thomas, E. F. 1934. The toxicity of certain species of crotalaria seed for the chicken, quail, turkey, and dove. *J. Am. Vet. Med. Ass.* 85:617–22.

Thomas, E. W., W. M. Neal, and C. F. Ahmann. 1935. Toxicity of *Crotalaria spectabilis* Roth to livestock and poultry. *J. Am. Soc. Agron.* 27:499–500.

Torrey, J. P., and R. Graham. 1935. A note on experimental salt poisoning in ducks. *Cornell Vet.* 25:50–53.

Trainer, D. O., and R. A. Hunt. 1965a. Lead poisoning of waterfowl in Wisconsin. *J. Wildlife Management* 29:95–103.

———. 1965b. Lead poisoning of whistling swans in Wisconsin. *Avian Diseases* 9:252–64.

Trenchi, H. 1962. A comparative study of the lesions produced by ergot and photosensitization induced by *Ammi visnaga*. *Fourth Pan. Am. Congr. Vet. Med. Zootechnics.*

Van der Linde, J. A., A. M. Frens, and G. J. Van Esch. 1964. Experiments with cows fed groundnut meal containing aflatoxin, in mycotoxins in foodstuffs. *Proc. Int. Symp. Mycotoxins in Foodstuffs.* M.I.T. Press, Cambridge, Mass.

Van Zyl, J. P. 1929. *Ann. Rept. Dir. Vet. Serv. Union S. Africa* 15:1189.

Waibel, P. E., B. S. Pomeroy, and E. L. Johnson. 1955. Effect of Arasan-treated corn on laying hens. *Science* 121:401–2.

Waibel, P. E., E. L. Johnson, B. S. Pomeroy, and L. B. Howard. 1957. Toxicity of tetramethylthiuram disulfide for chicks, poults and goslings. *Poultry Sci.* 36:697–703.

Waletzky, E., C. O. Hughes, and M. C. Brandt. 1949. The anticoccidial activity of nitrophenide. *Ann. N.Y. Acad. Sci.* 52:541–57.

Wannop, C. C. 1961. The histopathology of turkey "X" disease in Great Britain. *Avian Diseases* 5:371–81.

Wannop, C. C., and L. G. Chubb. 1961. Possible fat intoxication in chickens. *Vet. Record* 73:586.

Weber, A. L., F. R. Beaudette, and C. B. Hudson. 1932. Arsenic poisoning in poultry. *North Am. Vet.* 13:46–47.

Westcott, R. B., and H. C. McDougle. 1967. Ethylene oxide toxicosis in chickens. *J. Am. Vet. Med. Ass.* 151:935–38.

West, J. L. 1957. Disinfectant poisoning in chicks. *Vet. Med.* 52:40–42.

Westemeier, R. L. 1966. Apparent lead poisoning in a wild bobwhite. *Wilson Bull.* 78(4):471–72.

Wetmore, A. 1922. Lead poisoning in waterfowl. *USDA Bull.* 793.

Whitehead, F. E. 1934. The effect of arsenic, as used in poisoning grasshoppers, upon birds. *Oklahoma Agr. Expt. Sta. Bull.* 218.

Wickware, A. B. 1940. Lead poisoning in ducks following ingestion of shot. *Can. J. Comp. Med. Vet. Sci.* 4:201–3.

———. 1945. Grasshoppers: A potential danger to turkeys. *Can. J. Comp. Med. Vet. Sci.* 9:80–81.

Williamson, J. H., F. R. Craig, C. W. Barber, and F. W. Cook. 1964. Some effects of feeding *Gelsemium sempervirens* (yellow jassamine) to young chickens and turkeys. *Avian Diseases* 8:183–90.

Wilson, H. F., and C. E. Holmes. 1936. Effect on chickens of arsenic in grasshopper bait. *J. Econ. Entomol.* 29:1008.

Witter, J. F. 1936. A preliminary report on the injurious effect of sodium bicarbonate in chicks. *Poultry Sci.* 15:256–59.

Woodward, G., A. A. Nelson, and H. O. Calvery. 1944. Acute and subacute toxicity of DDT (2,2–bis (p–chlorophenyl) –1, 1, 1–Trichloroethane) to laboratory animals. *J. Pharmacol. Expt. Therap.* 82:152–58.

Wootton, J. C., N. R. Artman, and J. C. Alexander. 1962. Isolation of three hydropericardium-producing factors from a toxic fat. *J. Ass. Offic. Agr. Chemists* 45:739–46.

Yacowitz, H., E. Ross, V. L. Sanger, E. N. Moore, and R. D. Carter. 1955. Hemorrhagic syndrome in chicks fed normal rations supplemented with sulfaquinoxaline. *Proc. Soc. Exp. Biol. Med.* 89:1–7.

INDEX

❖

❖